LATEST APPROVED METHODS OF TREATMENT
FOR THE PRACTICING PHYSICIAN

Edited by
ROBERT E. RAKEL, M.D.

Professor and Chairman, Department of Family Medicine
Associate Dean for Academic and Clinical Affairs
Baylor College of Medicine, Houston, Texas

W.B. SAUNDERS COMPANY
A Division of Harcourt Brace & Company
Philadelphia
London   Toronto   Montreal   Sydney   Tokyo

Conn's **Current Therapy**

W.B. SAUNDERS COMPANY
A Division of
Harcourt Brace & Company

The Curtis Center
Independence Square West
Philadelphia, Pennsylvania 19106

Library of Congress Cataloging-in-Publication Data

Current therapy; latest approved methods of treatment for the practicing physician. 1949–

v. 28 cm. annual.

Editors: 1949–   H. F. Conn and others.

1. Therapeutics.   Therapeutics, Surgical.   3. Medicine—
   Practice.   I. Conn, Howard Franklin, 1908–1982 ed.

RM101.C87   616.058   49–8328 rev*

ISBN 0–7216–3804–X

Conn's Current Therapy 1994   ISBN 0–7216–3804–X

Printed in the United States of America.

Last digit is the print number: 9   8   7   6   5   4   3   2   1

Contributors

JAMES L. ACHORD, M.D.

Professor and Director, Division of Digestive Diseases, University of Mississippi; Staff Physician, University Medical Center, Jackson, Mississippi
Peptic Ulcer Disease

DAVID B. ADAMS, M.D.

Associate Professor of Surgery and Head, Section of General and Gastrointestinal Surgery, Medical University of South Carolina, Charleston, South Carolina
Acute Pancreatitis

MYOUNG OCK AHN, M.D., Ph.D., M.P.H.

Director, Maternal Fetal Medicine, Cha Women's Hospital of Seoul; Clinical Assistant Professor, Yon Sei University College of Medicine, Seoul, Korea; Staff Physician, Cedars Sinai Medical Center, Beverly Hills, California
Antepartum Care

ABDULKARIM AL-ASKA, M.D.

Professor of Medicine, College of Medicine, King Saud University; Consultant and Head, Infectious Diseases Division, Department of Medicine, King Khalid University Hospital, Riyadh, Saudi Arabia
Brucellosis

CHARLES G. ALEX, M.D.

Assistant Professor of Medicine, Loyola University of Chicago, Stritch School of Medicine, Chicago; Staff Physician, Edward Hines, Jr., Department of Veterans Affairs Hospital, Hines; Attending Physician, Foster G. McGaw Hospital and Loyola University Medical Center, Chicago, Illinois
Chronic Obstructive Pulmonary Disease

CHARLES C. ALLING III, D.D.S., M.S., D.Sc.(Hon.)

Adjunct Professor, University of Iowa School of Dentistry, Iowa City, Iowa; Staff, Brookwood Medical Center, Birmingham, Alabama
Temporomandibular Disorders

ALEX F. ALTHAUSEN, M.D.

Associate Professor of Surgery, Harvard Medical School; Senior Urologist, Massachusetts General Hospital, Boston, Massachusetts
Epididymitis

ROY D. ALTMAN, M.D.

Professor of Medicine, University of Miami School of Medicine; Chief, Arthritis Section, Miami Department of Veterans Affairs Medical Center, Miami, Florida
Paget's Disease of Bone

JAMES W. ANDERSON, M.D.

Professor of Medicine and Clinical Nutrition, University of Kentucky; Chief, Metabolic Endocrine Section, Veterans Affairs Medical Center and University of Kentucky Hospital, Lexington, Kentucky
Diabetes Mellitus in Adults

ROBERT J. ANDERSON, M.D.

Associate Professor of Medicine and Biomedical Sciences, Creighton University School of Medicine, and Chief, Section of Endocrinology and Metabolism, Veterans Affairs Medical Center, Omaha, Nebraska
Hypopituitarism

ROBERT J. ANDERSON, M.D.

Professor of Medicine, University of Colorado Health Sciences Center, and Chief, Medical Service, Denver Veterans Affairs Medical Center, Denver, Colorado
Acute Renal Failure

RODNEY U. ANDERSON, M.D.

Professor of Urology, Stanford University School of Medicine, Stanford; Chief of Urology, Santa Clara Valley Medical Center, San Jose, California
Prostatitis

LOWELL B. ANTHONY, M.D.

Assistant Professor of Medicine, Vanderbilt University; Active Staff, Vanderbilt University Hospital and Veterans Affairs Medical Center; Courtesy Staff, St. Thomas Hospital, Nashville, Tennessee
Nausea and Vomiting

JOSEPH J. APUZZIO, M.D.

Professor of Obstetrics, Gynecology, and Radiology, and Director, Prenatal Diagnosis and Infectious Diseases, New Jersey Medical School; Attending Physician, University Hospital, Newark, New Jersey
Chlamydia Trachomatis Infection

MOSHE ARDITI, M.D.

Assistant Professor of Pediatrics, University of Southern California; Assistant Professor of Pediatrics, Children's Hospital, Los Angeles, California
Measles (Rubeola)

EDWARD L. ARSURA, M.D., F.A.C.P.

Associate Clinical Professor of Medicine, UCLA School of Medicine, Los Angeles; Chairman, Department of Medicine, Kern Medical Center, Bakersfield, California
Myasthenia Gravis

LARS ASMIS, M.D.

Resident, Clinic of Internal Medicine, Inselspital, University of Bern, Bern, Switzerland
Goiter

BARBARA L. ASSELIN, M.D.

Assistant Professor of Pediatrics, University of Rochester School of Medicine; Assistant Professor and Attending Pedia-

trician in Hematology/Oncology, Strong Memorial Hospital, Rochester, New York
Nonimmune Hemolytic Anemia

BALU H. ATHREYA, M.D.

Professor of Pediatrics, University of Pennsylvania School of Medicine; Director, Pediatric Rheumatology Center, Children's Seashore House and Children's Hospital of Philadelphia, Philadelphia, Pennsylvania
Juvenile Rheumatoid Arthritis

PAUL S. AUERBACH, M.D., M.S.

Professor and Chief, Division of Emergency Medicine, Stanford University Medical Center; Attending Physician, Stanford University Hospital, Stanford, California
Spider Bites and Scorpion Stings; Injury Received From Hazardous Marine Animals

MILES AUSLANDER, M.D.

Assistant Clinical Professor of Medicine, University of California, Los Angeles; Staff Physician, Division of Gastroenterology, Valley Presbyterian Hospital, Van Nuys, California
Gaseousness and Indigestion

SAMI T. AZAR, M.D.

Assistant Professor of Medicine, Department of Endocrinology and Metabolism, American University of Beirut, Beirut, Lebanon
Primary Aldosteronism

JASON BACHARACH, M.D.

Glaucoma Fellow, Jules Stein Eye Institute, University of California, Los Angeles, Los Angeles, California
Glaucoma

JOHN W. BACHMAN, M.D.

Consultant, Department of Family Medicine, Mayo Clinic and Mayo Foundation, and Associate Professor of Medicine, Mayo Medical School, Rochester, Minnesota
Cardiac Arrest: Sudden Cardiac Death

ROBERT L. BAEHNER, M.D.

Professor of Pediatrics, University of Southern California School of Medicine; Vice President, Pediatrics, Children's Hospital of Los Angeles, Los Angeles, California
Neutropenia

JOHN G. BANWELL, M.D.

Professor of Medicine, Case Western Reserve University School of Medicine; Attending Physician, University Hospital of Cleveland, Cleveland, Ohio
Malabsorption Syndromes

JAMIE S. BARKIN, M.D.

Professor of Medicine, University of Miami, School of Medicine; Chief, Division of Gastroenterology, Mt. Sinai Medical Center, Miami Beach, Florida
Diverticula of the Alimentary Tract

LARRY BARMAT, M.D.

Senior Resident, Department of Obstetrics and Gynecology; Albert Einstein Hospital, Philadelphia, Pennsylvania
Dysmenorrhea

URIEL S. BARZEL, M.D.

Professor of Medicine, Albert Einstein College of Medicine; Attending Physician, Division of Endocrinology and Metabolism, Montefiore Medical Center, Bronx, New York
Osteoporosis

JAMES W. BASS, M.D., M.P.H.

Professor of Pediatrics, Uniformed Services University of the Health Sciences (Tripler Army Medical Center Affiliate); Clinical Professor of Pediatrics, University of Hawaii John A. Burns School of Medicine; Chairman, Department of Pediatrics, Tripler Army Medical Center, Honolulu, Hawaii
Streptococcal Pharyngitis

ROBERT W. BAUMHEFNER, M.D.

Associate Professor of Neurology, UCLA School of Medicine; Staff Neurologist, Veterans Affairs Medical Center–West Los Angeles, Los Angeles, California
Multiple Sclerosis

J. ERIC BAUWENS, M.D.

Clinical Instructor, University of Washington and Harborview Medical Center, Seattle; Clinical Consultant, Fred Hutchinson Cancer Research Center, Seattle; Private Practice, Infectious Diseases, Providence Hospital, Everett; General Hospital Medical Center, Everett; Cascade Valley Hospital, Arlington, Washington
Granuloma Inguinale (Donovanosis); Lymphogranuloma Venereum (LGV)

GREGORY P. BECKS, M.D., F.R.C.P.C.

Assistant Professor, Department of Medicine, Division of Endocrinology and Metabolism, University of Western Ontario; Staff Physician, Department of Medicine, St. Joseph's Health Centre, London, Ontario, Canada
Thyroiditis

IRIS R. BELL, M.D., PH.D.

Assistant Professor of Psychiatry, University of Arizona College of Medicine; Attending Psychiatrist, University Medical Center; Attending Psychiatrist, Tucson Veterans Affairs Medical Center, Tucson, Arizona
Mood Disorders

WILLIAM R. BELL, JR., M.D.

Professor of Medicine-Radiology-Nuclear Medicine; Edythe Harris Lucas Chair and Clara Lucas Lynn Professor of Hematology; Co-Director, Division of Hematology, Department of Medicine; and Director, Special Coagulation Laboratory, The Johns Hopkins University Hospital, Baltimore, Maryland
Disseminated Intravascular Coagulation; Thrombotic Thrombocytopenic Purpura–Hemolytic Uremic Syndrome

BARBARA BENNETT, M.D.

Assistant Professor, Department of Obstetrics and Gynecology, University of Florida; Staff Physician, Shands Teaching Hospital, Gainesville, Florida
Thrombophlebitis in Obstetrics and Gynecology

ROBERT M. BENNETT, M.D.

Professor of Medicine and Chairman, Division of Arthritis and Rheumatic Diseases, Oregon Health Sciences University, Portland, Oregon
Bursitis, Tendinitis, Myofascial Pain, and Fibromyalgia

JOEL E. BERNSTEIN, M.D.

Private Practice, Lincolnshire, Illinois
Pigmentary Disorders of the Skin

G. MICHAEL BESSER, M.D., D.SC.

Professor of Medicine, St. Bartholomew's Hospital, West Smithfield, London, United Kingdom
Cushing's Syndrome

HENRY R. BLACK, M.D.

Charles J. & Margaret Roberts Professor and Chairman, Department of Preventive Medicine, Professor, Internal Medicine, Senior Attending Physician, Preventive Medicine and Internal Medicine, Rush-Presbyterian-St. Luke's Medical Center; Professor of Health Resources Management, School of Public Health, The University of Illinois at Chicago, Chicago, Illinois
Hypertension

MICHAEL S. BLAISS, M.D.

Associate Professor of Pediatrics and Assistant Professor of Medicine, University of Tennessee, Memphis; Consultant, Allergy, LeBonheur Children's Medical Center, Memphis, Tennessee
Anaphylaxis and Serum Sickness

JOHN F. BOHNSACK, M.D.

Associate Professor of Pediatrics, University of Utah School of Medicine; Attending Physician, University of Utah Hospital, Salt Lake City, Utah
Rheumatic Fever

WILLIAM Z. BORER, M.D.

Associate Professor, Department of Pathology, Thomas Jefferson University; Director, Clinical Chemistry, Thomas Jefferson University Hospital, Philadelphia, Pennsylvania
Reference Values for the Interpretation of Laboratory Tests

DENISE BRATCHER, D.O.

Assistant Professor of Pediatrics, University of Louisville School of Medicine, Kosair Children's Hospital, Louisville, Kentucky
Conjunctivitis

J. DOUGLAS BREMNER, M.D.

Assistant Professor of Psychiatry, Yale University School of Medicine, New Haven; Attending Physician, Psychiatry Service, West Haven Veterans Affairs Medical Center, West Haven, Connecticut
Anxiety Disorders

DOREEN B. BRETTLER, M.D.

Associate Professor of Medicine, University of Massachusetts Medical School; Director, New England Hemophilia Center, Medical Center of Central Massachusetts, Worcester, Massachusetts
Platelet-Mediated Bleeding Disorders

GREGORY A. BRODERICK, M.D.

Assistant Professor of Surgery of Urology, Director, Center for the Study of Male Sexual Dysfunction, and Co-Director, Neurourology Program, Hospital of the University of Pennsylvania, Philadelphia, Pennsylvania
Genitourinary Trauma

LYNN BROOKS, M.D.

Staff, Clear Lake Regional Medical Center, St. John Hospital—Nassau Bay, Houston, Texas
Vulvovaginitis

ROBERT A. BROUGHTON, M.D.

Associate Professor of Pediatrics, University of Kentucky Medical Center, Lexington, Kentucky
Mumps

RICHARD B. BROWN, M.D.

Associate Professor of Medicine, Tufts University School of Medicine, Boston; Chief, Infectious Disease Division, Baystate Medical Center, Springfield, Massachusetts
Acute Bronchitis

JOHN R. BURNS, M.D.

Professor of Urology, University of Alabama at Birmingham, Birmingham, Alabama
Renal Calculi

JASON H. CALHOUN, M.D., M.Eng.

Associate Professor, University of Texas Medical Branch; Chief of Orthopaedic Surgery, University of Texas Medical Branch; Orthopaedic Surgeon, St. Mary's Hospital; Orthopaedic Surgeon, Shriners Burn Institute, Galveston, Texas
Osteomyelitis

JEFFREY P. CALLEN, M.D.

Professor of Medicine (Dermatology) and Chief, Division of Dermatology, University of Louisville School of Medicine, Louisville, Kentucky
Cutaneous Vasculitis

THOMAS R. CARACCIO, Pharm.D., A.B.A.T.

Assistant Professor of Emergency Medicine, State University of New York at Stony Brook, Stony Brook; Assistant Professor of Pharmacology/Toxicology, New York College of Osteopathy, Old Westbury; Assistant Professor of Clinical Pharmacy, St. John's University College of Pharmacy, Jamaica; Assistant Director of Long Island Regional Poison Control Center, Winthrop University Hospital, Mineola, New York
Acute Poisonings

ANTONINO CATANZARO, M.D.

Associate Professor of Medicine, University of California, San Diego (UCSD), School of Medicine; Attending Physician, UCSD Medical Center, San Diego, California
Coccidioidomycosis

D. C. CATTRAN, M.D., F.R.C.P., F.A.C.P.

Professor of Medicine, University of Toronto; Consultant Nephrologist, The Toronto Hospital, Toronto, Ontario, Canada
Primary Glomerular Diseases

AMITABH CHAK, M.D.

Assistant Professor, Case Western Reserve University School of Medicine; Attending Physician, University Hospitals of Cleveland, Cleveland, Ohio
Malabsorption Syndromes

BRUCE P. CHANDLER, M.D., M.P.H.

Staff Pediatrician, Providence Hospital, Anchorage, and Alaska Regional Hospital, Anchorage, Alaska
The Typhus Fevers

DENNIS S. CHARNEY, M.D.

Professor of Psychiatry and Associate Chairman for Research, Yale University School of Medicine, New Haven; Chief of the Psychiatry Service, West Haven Veterans Administration Medical Center, West Haven, Connecticut
Anxiety Disorders

ELLIOT CHESLER, M.D.

Professor of Medicine, University of Minnesota; Chief, Cardiovascular Division, Veterans Administration Hospital, Minneapolis, Minnesota
Mitral Valve Prolapse

H. JANE CHIHAL, M.D., Ph.D.

President of the Medical Staff, Trinity Medical Center, Carrollton, Texas
Premenstrual Syndrome

PAUL M. CHOI, M.D.

Assistant Professor of Medicine, UCLA School of Medicine; Director of Clinical Research, Inflammatory Bowel Disease Center, Cedars-Sinai Medical Center, Los Angeles, California
Ulcerative Colitis

ANTHONY W. CHOW, M.D., F.R.C.P.C., F.A.C.P.

Professor of Medicine and Head, Division of Infectious Diseases, Department of Medicine, University of British Columbia; Head, Division of Infectious Diseases, Department of Medicine, Vancouver General Hospital, Vancouver, British Columbia, Canada
Toxic Shock Syndrome

ROBERT E. CLARK, M.D., Ph.D.

Director, Dermatologic Surgery and Cutaneous Oncology Unit, Duke University Medical Center, Durham, North Carolina
Cancer of the Skin

WILLIAM R. CLARK, Jr., M.D.

Professor of Surgery and Active Staff, University Hospital, State University of New York Health Science Center at Syracuse, Syracuse, New York
Burns

WILLIAM L. CLARKE, M.D.

Professor of Pediatrics, University of Virginia Health Sciences Center, Charlottesville, Virginia
Diabetes Mellitus in Children and Adolescents

JACK C. CLEMIS, M.D.

Chief of Otolaryngology, Mercy Hospital and Medical Center, Chicago, Illinois
Tinnitus

JOSE A. COBOS, M.D.

Resident, Orthopaedic Surgery, University of Texas Medical Branch, Galveston, Texas
Osteomyelitis

MARY B. CONNOLLY, M.B., B.Ch.

Neurology Fellow, Department of Pediatrics, University of British Columbia, Vancouver, British Columbia, Canada
Epilepsy in Infants and Children

JOSEPH M. CONNORS, M.D.

Clinical Associate Professor, British Columbia Cancer Agency, University of British Columbia, Vancouver, British Columbia, Canada
Non-Hodgkin's Lymphoma

CATHY CONRY-CANTILENA, M.D.

Senior Staff Fellow, Department of Transfusion Medicine Clinical Center, National Institutes of Health, Bethesda, Maryland
Therapeutic Use of Blood Components

DAVID S. COOPER, M.D.

Associate Professor of Medicine, The Johns Hopkins University School of Medicine; Director, Division of Endocrinology, Sinai Hospital of Baltimore, Baltimore, Maryland
Hyperthyroidism

RONALD H. COOPER, M.D.

Staff, Madigan Army Medical Center, Tacoma, Washington
Gonorrhea

JOSHUA A. COPEL, M.D.

Professor, Obstetrics and Gynecology, Yale University School of Medicine; Director, Obstetrics, Yale-New Haven Hospital, New Haven, Connecticut
Hemolytic Disease of the Newborn (Fetal Isoimmunization)

JOHN D. CORSON, M.B., Ch.B., F.R.C.S. (Eng), F.A.C.S.

Professor of Surgery, The University of Iowa School of Medicine; Director, Vascular Surgery Section, Department of Surgery, The University of Iowa Hospitals and Clinics, Iowa City, Iowa
Deep Venous Thrombosis of the Lower Extremities

NILDE COSTANTE, M.D.

Immunodermatology Fellow, Section of Dermatology, University of Chicago, Chicago, Illinois
Parasitic Diseases of the Skin

EDWARD C. COVINGTON, M.D.

Head, Section of Pain Management, Department of Psychiatry, Cleveland Clinic Foundation, Cleveland, Ohio
Alcoholism

GEOFFREY S. COX, M.D., F.R.A.C.S.

Vascular Surgeon, The Royal Melbourne Hospital, Melbourne, Australia
Acquired Diseases of the Aorta

DEREK J. CRIPPS, M.D. (London), M.Sc., F.A.C.P.

Professor and Head of Dermatology, University of Wisconsin, Madison, Wisconsin
Pruritus (Itching)

BARBARA A. CROSSE, B.Sc., M.B.Ch.B.

Senior Registrar in Infectious Diseases, Seacroft Hospital, Leeds, United Kingdom
Psittacosis (Ornithosis)

JAMES P. CROWLEY, M.D.

Professor of Medicine, Brown University School of Medicine; Director, Clinical Hematology, Rhode Island Hospital, Providence, Rhode Island
Autoimmune Hemolytic Anemia

GARY V. DAHL, M.D.

Professor of Pediatrics (Hematology/Oncology), Stanford University School of Medicine; Co-Director of Section of Oncology, Lucile Salter Packard Children's Hospital at Stanford, Palo Alto, California
Acute Leukemia in Childhood

ADNAN S. DAJANI, M.D.

Professor of Pediatrics, Wayne State University School of Medicine; Chief, Division of Infectious Diseases, Children's Hospital of Michigan; Attending Physician, Children's Hospital of Michigan, Detroit, Michigan
Infective Endocarditis

LAWRENCE J. D'ANGELO, M.D., M.P.H.

Professor of Pediatrics, Medicine, and Health Care Science, George Washington University Medical School; Senior At-

tending Physician, Children's National Medical Center, Washington, D.C.
Infectious Mononucleosis

STEVEN K. DAUGHERTY, M.D.

Post-Doctoral Fellow of Infectious Diseases, University of Wisconsin Medical School; Clinical and Research Fellow, Infectious Diseases, University of Wisconsin Hospitals and Clinics, Madison, Wisconsin
Bacteremia and Septicemia

TERENCE M. DAVIDSON, M.D.

Professor of Surgery and Associate Dean, Continuing Medical Education, University of California at San Diego; UCSD Medical Center, Veterans Administration Hospital, San Diego, California
Snake Venom Poisoning

GEORGE S. DEEPE, JR., M.D.

Associate Professor, University of Cincinnati College of Medicine; Staff Physician, University of Cincinnati Hospital, Cincinnati, Ohio
Histoplasmosis

PAUL DICK, M.D., C.M.

Assistant Professor, Department of Paediatrics, Division of General Paediatrics, University of Toronto; Staff Physician, The Hospital for Sick Children, Toronto, Ontario, Canada
Childhood Enuresis

JERRY F. DONIN, M.D.

Clinical Professor of Ophthalmology and Neurology, University of Southern California School of Medicine, Los Angeles; Attending Physician (Emeritus), Pomona Valley Hospital Medical Center, Pomona, and Los Angeles County–University of Southern California Medical Center, Los Angeles, California
Optic Neuritis

PETER DRESCHER, M.D.

Research Fellow in Urology, Veterans Administration Hospital and University Hospital, University of Wisconsin School of Medicine, Madison, Wisconsin
Benign Prostatic Hyperplasia

EDWARD J. DROPCHO, M.D.

Associate Professor of Neurology, University of Alabama at Birmingham School of Medicine; Director, Neuro-Oncology Program, University of Alabama Comprehensive Cancer Center, Birmingham, Alabama
Brain Tumors

PATRICK DUFF, M.D.

Professor, Department of Obstetrics & Gynecology and Division of Maternal-Fetal Medicine, University of Florida College of Medicine; Staff Physician, Shands Teaching Hospital, Gainesville, Florida
Thrombophlebitis in Obstetrics and Gynecology

N. FRED EAGLSTEIN, D.O.

Courtesy Clinical Assistant Professor, Department of Community Health and Family Medicine, University of Florida College of Medicine, Jacksonville; Staff Physician, Orange Park Medical Center, Orange Park, and St. Vincent's Hospital, Baptist Hospital, and University Hospital, Jacksonville, Florida
Bullous Disorders

PAUL H. EDELSTEIN, M.D.

Associate Professor of Pathology and Laboratory Medicine and Associate Professor of Medicine, University of Pennsylvania School of Medicine; Director of Clinical Microbiology and Attending Physician, Hospital of the University of Pennsylvania, Philadelphia, Pennsylvania
Legionnaires' Disease and Pontiac Fever

MARLA S. EGLOWSTEIN, M.D.

Assistant Professor, Department of Obstetrics and Gynecology, Albany Medical College; Attending Physician, Department of Obstetrics and Gynecology, Division of Maternal-Fetal Medicine, Albany Medical Center Hospital, Albany, New York
Vaginal Bleeding in Late Pregnancy

DRORE EISEN, M.D., D.D.S.

Private Practice, Cincinnati, Ohio
Diseases of the Mouth

GEORGE H. ELDER, M.D.

Professor of Medical Biochemistry, University of Wales College of Medicine; Honorary Consultant in Medical Biochemistry; University Hospital of Wales, Cardiff, Wales, United Kingdom
The Porphyrias

KENNETH A. ELLENBOGEN, M.D.

Associate Professor of Medicine, Assistant Professor of Surgery, and Director, Clinical Electrophysiology and Pacing Laboratory, Medical College of Virginia and McGuire Veterans Administration Medical Center, Richmond, Virginia
Tachycardia

JERRY J. ELLER, M.D.

Clinical Professor of Pediatrics and Community Medicine, University of Alabama School of Medicine, Birmingham; Staff Physician, Hill Hospital, York; Adjunct Staff Physician, The Children's Hospital of Alabama, Birmingham; Rush Medical Group, Livingston, Alabama
Diphtheria

CRAIG A. ELMETS, M.D.

Associate Professor of Dermatology and General Medical Sciences (Oncology), Case Western Reserve University; Attending Dermatologist, University Hospitals of Cleveland; Attending Dermatologist, Cleveland Veterans Administration Hospital, Cleveland, Ohio
Papulosquamous Diseases

JANET ENGLUND, M.D.

Assistant Professor, Department of Microbiology and Immunology, and Pediatrics, Baylor College of Medicine; Staff Physician, Ben Taub Hospital, Texas Children's Hospital, Houston, Texas
Viral Respiratory Infections

CHARLES D. ERICSSON, M.D.

Professor of Medicine, University of Texas Medical School; Staff, Hermann Hospital and LBJ General Hospital, Houston, Texas
Acute Infectious Diarrhea

DAVID S. ETTINGER, M.D.

Professor of Oncology and Medicine, The Johns Hopkins University School of Medicine; Associate Director for Clinical Affairs, The Johns Hopkins Oncology Center, Baltimore, Maryland
Primary Lung Cancer

JOSEPH EVERS, M.D.

Instructor in Medicine and Fellow in Hematology-Oncology, Georgetown University Medical Center, Washington, D.C.
Pernicious Anemia and Other Megaloblastic Anemias

MEHDI FARHANGI, M.D.

Associate Professor of Medicine, University of Missouri-Columbia School of Medicine; Staff Physician, Ellis Fischel Cancer Center, and University of Missouri Hospital and Clinics, Columbia, Missouri
Multiple Myeloma

KEVIN FARRELL, M.B., Ch.B.

Associate Professor, Department of Pediatrics, University of British Columbia; Director of Epilepsy Service, British Columbia's Children's Hospital, Vancouver, British Columbia, Canada
Epilepsy in Infants and Children

WILLIAM FELDMAN, M.D.

Professor of Pediatrics and of Preventive Medicine and Biostatistics, University of Toronto; Head, Division of General Pediatrics and Medical Director, General Pediatrics Program, Hospital for Sick Children, Toronto, Ontario, Canada
Fever; Childhood Enuresis

NEIL A. FENSKE, M.D.

Professor of Medicine and Pathology and Director, Division of Dermatology and Cutaneous Surgery, University of South Florida College of Medicine; Chief, Dermatology Section, James A. Haley Veterans Administration Hospital and Chief, Dermatology Section, H. Lee Moffitt Cancer Center and Research Institute, Tampa, Florida
Warts (Verruca Vulgaris)

ENRIQUE S. FERNANDEZ, M.D., M.S.Ed.

HIV Clinical Consultant, Infectious Disease Service, Walter Reed Army Medical Center, Washington D.C.; Chief, HIV and Substance Abuse Services Branch, Bureau of Primary Health Care, Health Resources and Services Administration, United States Public Health Service, Rockville, Maryland
Management of the Patient with HIV Disease

LAURENCE FINBERG, M.D.

Professor and Chairman of Pediatrics, SUNY/Children's Medical Center of Brooklyn; Staff Physician, University Hospital of Brooklyn and Kings County Hospital Center, Brooklyn, New York
Normal Infant Feeding

JORDAN N. FINK, M.D.

Professor of Medicine and Chief, Allergy-Immunology Division, Medical College of Wisconsin; Attending Physician, Milwaukee County Medical Complex and Veterans Administration Medical Center; Consultant, Columbia Hospital, Milwaukee, Wisconsin
Hypersensitivity Pneumonitis

ROGER S. FOSTER, Jr., M.D.

Professor of Surgery, Emory University; Chief of Surgery, Crawford Long Hospital of Emory University, Atlanta, Georgia
Diseases of the Breast

JEFFREY M. FOWLER, M.D.

Assistant Professor, Division of Gynecologic Oncology, Department of Obstetrics and Gynecology, University of Minnesota; Staff Physician, University of Minnesota Hospital and Clinics, Minneapolis, Minnesota
Endometrial Cancer

SANDRA L. FOWLER, M.D.

Assistant Professor of Pediatrics, Division of Infectious Diseases and Clinical Immunology, Medical University of South Carolina, Charleston, South Carolina
Varicella (Chickenpox)

MARTIN J. FRANK, M.D.

Professor of Medicine and Radiology, Medical College of Georgia, Augusta, Georgia
Congestive Heart Failure

ANDREW G. FRANTZ, M.D.

Professor of Medicine, Columbia University College of Physicians and Surgeons; Attending Physician, Presbyterian Hospital, New York, New York
Hyperprolactinemia

CHAD I. FRIEDMAN, M.D.

Associate Professor, Department of Obstetrics and Gynecology, Ohio State University; Director, Division of Reproductive Endocrinology, Ohio State University Hospital, Columbus, Ohio
Dysfunctional Uterine Bleeding

ANTHONY J. FURLAN, M.D.

Head, Section of Adult Neurology and Director, Cerebrovascular Program, Cleveland Clinic Foundation, Cleveland, Ohio
Focal Ischemic Cerebrovascular Disease

PAUL E. GARFINKEL, M.D., M.Sc., F.R.C.P.(C)

Professor and Chair, Department of Psychiatry, University of Toronto; Director and Psychiatrist-in-Chief, Clarke Institute of Psychiatry, Toronto, Ontario, Canada
Bulimia Nervosa

ALAN J. GELENBERG, M.D.

Professor and Head, Department of Psychiatry, University of Arizona College of Medicine; Chief of Service, Department of Psychiatry, University Medical Center; Consultant, Tucson Veterans Affairs Medical Center, Tucson, Arizona
Mood Disorders

STEPHEN P. GLASSER, M.D.

Professor of Medicine (Cardiology) and Director, Division of Clinical Pharmacology, the Cardiovascular Unit for Research and Education and the Lipid Disorders Clinic, University of South Florida, Health Sciences Center, Tampa, Florida
Angina Pectoris

A. DAVID GOLDBERG, M.D.

Assistant Professor of Medicine, University of Michigan, Ann Arbor; Director of Holter Laboratory and Director of Clinical Trials, Division of Cardiovascular Medicine, Henry Ford Hospital, Detroit, Michigan
Premature Beats

FRANZ GOLDSTEIN, M.D.

Professor of Medicine, Jefferson Medical College of Thomas Jefferson University, Philadelphia; Attending Physician, Gastroenterology, Lankenau Hospital, Wynnewood, Pennsylvania
Gastritis

JOHN L. GOLLAN, M.D., Ph.D.

Associate Professor of Medicine, Harvard Medical School; Director, Gastroenterology Division and Senior Physician, Brigham and Women's Hospital, Boston, Massachusetts
Cirrhosis; Bleeding Esophageal Varices

YVONNE GOLLIN, M.D.

Instructor, Yale-New Haven Hospital, New Haven, Connecticut
Hemolytic Disease of the Newborn (Fetal Isoimmunization)

DAVID F. GRAFT, M.D.

Clinical Associate Professor, University of Minnesota School of Medicine; Chairman, Allergy Department, Park Nicollet Medical Center, and Attending Staff, Methodist Hospital, Minneapolis, Minnesota
Allergic Reactions to Insect Stings

THEODOR B. GRAGE, M.D., Ph.D.

Professor of Surgery, University of Minnesota Medical School; Director, Surgical Oncology, University of Minnesota Hospitals, Minneapolis, Minnesota
Tumors of the Stomach

LESLIE C. GRAMMER, M.D.

Professor of Medicine, Northwestern University Medical School; Attending Physician, Northwestern Memorial Hospital, Chicago, Illinois
Allergic Reactions to Drugs

GREGORY A. GRANT, M.D., F.R.C.P.C.

Senior Fellow, Division of Infectious Diseases, Department of Medicine, University of British Columbia and Vancouver General Hospital, Vancouver, British Columbia, Canada
Toxic Shock Syndrome

CLIVE E. H. GRATTAN, F.R.C.P.

Consultant Dermatologist, Norfolk and Norwich Hospital, Norwich, Norfolk, United Kingdom
Urticaria and Angioedema

ARTHUR GREENBERG, M.D.

Associate Professor of Medicine, Renal-Electrolyte Division, University of Pittsburgh School of Medicine; Staff Physician, Presbyterian University Hospital, Montefiore University Hospital, and Department of Veterans Affairs Medical Center, Pittsburgh, Pennsylvania
Diabetes Insipidus

STEPHEN B. GREENBERG, M.D.

Professor of Medicine, Baylor College of Medicine; Chief, Medicine Service, Ben Taub General Hospital, Houston, Texas
Bacterial Pneumonia

JOSEPH GREENSHER, M.D.

Professor of Pediatrics, State University of New York at Stony Brook, Stony Brook; Medical Director and Associate Chairman, Department of Pediatrics, Winthrop University Hospital; Associate Director, Long Island Regional Poison Control Center, Winthrop University Hospital, Mineola, New York
Acute Poisonings

HANS W. GRÜNWALD, M.D., F.A.C.P.

Chief, Division of Hematology-Oncology, Queens Hospital Center, Jamaica, New York
Acute Leukemia in Adults

GREG GUTIERREZ, M.D.

Director, Division of Sports Medicine, Family Practice Department, St. Joseph Hospital; Clinical Faculty, University of Colorado Health Science Center, Denver, Colorado
Common Sports Injuries

LISA A. HAGLUND, M.D.

Assistant Professor of Clinical Medicine, The University of Cincinnati, College of Medicine; Staff Physician, University Hospital and Good Samaritan Hospital, Cincinnati, Ohio
Histoplasmosis

ECKART HANEKE, M.D.

Head, Department of Dermatology, Ferdinand-Sauerbruch Hospital, Teaching Hospital of the University of Düsseldorf; Professor and Chairman, Department of Dermatology, Ferdinand-Sauerbruch Hospital, Wuppertal, Germany
Diseases of the Nails

JOSEPH P. HANNA, M.D.

Clinical Associate, Department of Neurology, Cleveland Clinic Foundation, Cleveland, Ohio
Focal Ischemic Cerebrovascular Disease

PETER HANSON, M.S., M.D.

Professor of Medicine (Cardiology), University of Wisconsin Medical School; Co-director, Preventive Cardiology, University Hospital and Clinics, Madison, Wisconsin
Disturbances Due to Heat

M. SCOTT HARRIS, M.D.

Clinical Associate Professor of Medicine, Gastrointestinal Section, University of Wisconsin Medical School; Section Head, Gastroenterology, Sinai Samaritan Medical Center, Milwaukee, Wisconsin
Constipation

CHRISTOPHER J. HARRISON, M.D.

Associate Professor of Pediatrics, Creighton University School of Medicine and University of Nebraska School of Medicine; Staff Physician, AMI-St. Joseph Hospital, Children's Memorial Hospital, and University of Nebraska Medical Center, Omaha, Nebraska
Conjunctivitis

DON C. HARTING, M.D.

Private Practice, Cleveland, Tennessee
Contact Dermatitis

JACK HARVEY, M.D.

Director, Sports Medicine, Orthopaedic Center of the Rockies, Fort Collins, Colorado
Common Sports Injuries

VICTOR W. HENDERSON, M.D.

Professor of Neurology, Gerontology, and Psychology, University of Southern California; Chief of Neurology Service, Los Angeles County—University of Southern California Medical Center, Los Angeles, California
Alzheimer's Disease

HARRY R. HILL, M.D.

Professor of Pathology and and Pediatrics, University of Utah School of Medicine; Attending Staff, University of Utah Hospital Primary Childrens Medical Center, Salt Lake City, Utah
Rheumatic Fever

CHESLEY HINES, Jr., M.D.

Clinical Associate Professor of Medicine, Tulane University School of Medicine; Clinical Associate Professor of Medicine, Louisiana State University; Active Staff, Southern Baptist

Hospital; Visiting Staff, Charity Hospital and Veterans Administration Hospital, New Orleans, Louisiana
Crohn's Disease

DONALD W. HOSKINS, M.D.

Clinical Associate Professor of Medicine, Cornell University Medical College; Vice-President, Medical Affairs, Associate Medical Director, and Attending Physician, Beth Israel Medical Center; Associate Attending Physician, New York Hospital–Cornell University Medical Center, New York, New York
Trichinellosis

GORDON B. HUGHES, M.D.

Clinical Staff, Department of Otolaryngology and Communicative Disorders, Cleveland Clinic Foundation, Cleveland, Ohio
Acute Peripheral Facial Paralysis (Bell's Palsy)

ROBIN P. HUMPHREYS, M.D., F.R.C.S.C., F.A.C.S., F.A.A.P.

Professor, Department of Surgery, Faculty of Medicine, University of Toronto; Associate Surgeon-in-Chief and Senior Neurosurgeon, Hospital for Sick Children, Toronto, Ontario, Canada
Acute Head Injuries in Children

CHRISTOPHER W. IVES, M.D.

Gastroenterology Fellow, Louisiana State University School of Medicine, New Orleans, Louisiana
Crohn's Disease

A. J. JENKINS, M.D., F.R.C.S. (GLASGOW)

Senior Lecturer and Honorary Consultant Neurosurgeon, Department of Surgery (Neurosurgery), The Medical School, University of Newcastle upon Tyne, Newcastle upon Tyne, United Kingdom
Acute Head Injury in Adults

MARK D. JOHNSON, M.D.

Associate Professor, Department of Anesthesia, University of Texas Southwestern; Director, Division of Obstetric Anesthesia, Parkland Hospital, Dallas, Texas
Obstetric Anesthesia

BRIAN T. JONES, M.D.

Instructor, Department of Surgery, University of Virginia, and University of Virginia Health Sciences Center, Charlottesville, Virginia
Cholecystitis and Cholelithiasis

R. SCOTT JONES, M.D., F.A.C.S.

Stephen H. Watts Professor of Surgery and Chairman, Department of Surgery, University of Virginia, Charlottesville, Virginia
Cholecystitis and Cholelithiasis

DAVID B. JOSEPH, M.D.

Associate Professor of Surgery, University of Alabama at Birmingham; Chief of Pediatric Urology, The Children's Hospital of Alabama, Birmingham, Alabama
Bacterial Infections of the Urinary Tract in Girls

NORMAN J. KACHUCK, M.D.

Assistant Profesor of Clinical Neurology, University of Southern California (USC) School of Medicine; Director, USC Multiple Sclerosis and Immunologic Disorders Clinic, Los Angeles, California
Viral Meningitis and Encephalitis

RUTH DITZIAN KADANOFF, M.D., PH.D.

Assistant Professor-Adjunct, Chicago Medical School; Chief of Rheumatology, Mount Sinai Hospital, Chicago, Illinois
Rheumatoid Arthritis

PHILLIP H. KALEIDA, M.D.

Associate Professor of Pediatrics, University of Pittsburgh School of Medicine; Staff Pediatrician, Children's Hospital of Pittsburgh, Pittsburgh, Pennsylvania
Otitis Media

DEBRA CHESTER KALTER, M.D.

Assistant Professor of Dermatology, Uniformed Services University of Health Sciences, Bethesda, Maryland, and George Washington University, Washington, D.C.; Consultant, Washington Hospital Center, Washington, D.C.; National Institutes of Health, Bethesda, Maryland; and Walter Reed Army Medical Center, Washington, D.C.
Leishmaniasis

J. E. KASIK, M.D., PH.D.

Professor of Internal Medicine, University of Iowa College of Medicine and Veterans Administration Medical Center; State University of Iowa Hospitals and Clinics, Department of Veterans Affairs Hospital, Iowa City, Iowa
Tuberculosis and Other Mycobacterial Diseases

LOUIS KATTINE, M.D.

Staff Physician, St. Patrick Hospital and Community Medical Center, Missoula, Montana
Pleural Effusion and Empyema Thoracis

SOL KATZ, M.D.

Professor of Medicine, Georgetown University; Professorial Lecturer, George Washington University, Washington, D.C.
Primary Lung Abscess

CAROL A. KAUFFMAN, M.D.

Professor of Internal Medicine, University of Michigan Medical School; Chief, Infectious Diseases Section, Ann Arbor Veterans Affairs Medical Center, Ann Arbor, Michigan
Blastomycosis

RUSSEL E. KAUFMAN, M.D.

Associate Professor of Medicine, Assistant Professor of Biochemistry, and Director, Division of Hematology/Oncology, Duke University Medical Center, Durham, North Carolina
Thalassemia

J. WILLIAM KELLY, M.D.

Clinical Assistant Professor of Medicine, University of Texas Health Science Center, San Antonio; Infectious Disease Service, Brooke Army Medical Center, Fort Sam Houston, Texas
Acute Bacterial Meningitis

ELAINE KEOHANE, M.S.

Associate Professor of Clinical Laboratory Sciences, Department of Clinical Laboratory Sciences, University of Medicine and Dentistry of New Jersey School of Health Related Professions, Newark, New Jersey
Rat-Bite Fever

JACOB KERBESHIAN, M.D.

Clinical Professor of Neuroscience, University of North Dakota School of Medicine; Medical Programs Director, Behavioral Health Division, United Hospital, Grand Forks, North Dakota
Gilles de la Tourette Syndrome

JOHN H. KERR, D.M.

Clinical Lecturer in Anaesthetics, University of Oxford; Consultant Anaesthetist, Nuffield Department of Anaesthetics, Radcliffe Infirmary, Oxford, England
Tetanus

JAY S. KEYSTONE, M.D., M.Sc. (C.T.M.)

Associate Professor of Medicine and Microbiology, University of Toronto; Director, Tropical Disease Unit, The Toronto Hospital, Toronto, Ontario, Canada
Malaria

DAVID A. KHAN, M.D.

Fellow, Division of Allergic Diseases and Internal Medicine, Mayo Clinic and Foundation, Rochester, Minnesota
Asthma in Adolescents and Adults

MUHAMMAD ASIM KHAN, M.D., F.R.C.P.

Professor of Medicine, Case Western Reserve University School of Medicine; Director, Division of Rheumatology, Metro Health Medical Center, Cleveland, Ohio
Ankylosing Spondylitis

BARBARA K. KINDER, M.D.

Professor of Surgery, Yale University School of Medicine; Chief, Surgical Service, West Haven Veterans Administration Medical Center; Attending Physician, Yale New Haven Hospital, New Haven, Connecticut
Thyroid Cancer

BRIAN KIRSHON, M.D.

Associate Professor, Obstetrics & Gynecology, Baylor College of Medicine; Staff Physician, St. Luke's Episcopal Hospital, Methodist Hospital, and Ben Taub General Hospital, Houston, Texas
Hypertensive Disorders of Pregnancy

CRAIG S. KITCHENS, M.D.

Professor and Vice-Chairman, Department of Medicine, University of Florida; Chief, Medical Service, Gainesville Veterans Administration Medical Center, Gainesville, Florida
Iron Deficiency Anemia

HARVEY G. KLEIN, M.D.

Chief, Department of Transfusion Medicine, Warren G. Magnuson Clinical Center, National Institutes of Health, Bethesda, Maryland
Therapeutic Use of Blood Components

VERNON KNIGHT, M.D.

Professor of Biotechnology, Baylor College of Medicine; Senior Attending Physician, Methodist Hospital, Houston, Texas
Viral Respiratory Infections

HERB KOFFLER, M.D.

Professor of Pediatrics, Obstetrics, and Gynecology, University of New Mexico School of Medicine, Albuquerque, New Mexico
Care of the High-Risk Neonate

GERALD B. KOLSKI, M.D., Ph.D.

Associate Professor of Clinical Pediatrics, Columbia University College of Physicians and Surgeons, New York; Pediatrician-in-Chief, Mary Imogene Bassett Hospital, Cooperstown, New York
Asthma in Children

PETER KOPP, M.D.

Senior Resident, Clinic of Internal Medicine, Inselspital, University of Bern, Switzerland
Goiter

MARK J. KORUDA, M.D.

Assistant Professor, University of North Carolina School of Medicine, Chapel Hill, North Carolina
Parenteral Nutrition in Adults

LYNN Y. KOSOWICZ, M.D.

Assistant Professor of Medicine, University of Connecticut School of Medicine; Attending Physician, John Dempsey Hospital, University of Connecticut Health Center, Farmington, Connecticut
Cough

FREDERICK T. KOSTER, M.D.

Professor of Medicine, University of New Mexico School of Medicine; Staff Physician, University of New Mexico Hospital, Albuquerque, New Mexico
Q Fever

MARGARET KOTZ, D.O.

Staff Psychiatrist, The Cleveland Clinic Foundation, Cleveland, Ohio
Alcoholism

WAYNE KRAMER, M.D.

Fellow, Department of Maternal-Fetal Medicine, Baylor College of Medicine, Houston, Texas
Hypertensive Disorders of Pregnancy

DANIEL F. KRIPKE, M.D.

Professor of Psychiatry in Residence, University of California, San Diego, School of Medicine, La Jolla; Staff Psychiatrist, Veterans Affairs Medical Center, San Diego, and Scripps Clinic and Research Foundation, La Jolla, California
Insomnia

NORMAN J. LACAYO, M.D.

Fellow in Pediatric Hematology-Oncology, Stanford University School of Medicine; Fellow in Pediatric Hematology-Oncology, Department of Pediatrics, Division of Hematology-Oncology, Lucile Salter Packard Children's Hospital at Stanford, Palo Alto, California
Acute Leukemia in Childhood

STANFORD I. LAMBERG, M.D.

Associate Professor of Dermatology, Johns Hopkins University School of Medicine; Staff Physician, Johns Hopkins Hospital and Sinai Hospital of Baltimore, Baltimore, Maryland
Cutaneous T Cell Lymphoma

R. ALLEN LAWHEAD, Jr., M.D.

Associate Clinical Professor, Department of Obstetrics and Gynecology, Medical College of Georgia, Augusta; Director of Gynecologic Oncology, Cancer Center of Georgia at Georgia Baptist Medical Center, Atlanta, Georgia
Neoplasms of the Vulva

JOSEPH L. LEACH, M.D.

Assistant Professor of Otolaryngology, University of Texas Southwestern Medical School; Staff Physician, Zale-Lipshy University Hospital, Parkland Hospital, Veterans Administration Medical Center, John Peter Smith Hospital, Childrens Medical Center, and St. Paul Hospital, Dallas, Texas
Sinusitis

JACQUES R. LECLERC, M.D.

Associate Professor of Medicine, McGill University; Director, Hematology Division, Montreal General Hospital, Montreal, Quebec, Canada
Pulmonary Embolism

J. DOUGLAS LEE, M.D.

Associate Clinical Professor, Department of Medicine, University of Wisconsin, Madison; Staff Physician, St. Joseph's Hospital, Marshfield, Wisconsin
Relapsing Fever

ANN M. LEES, M.D.

Assistant Professor of Medicine, Harvard Medical School; Associate Director, Boston Heart Foundation; Research Staff Physician, Deaconess Hospital, Boston, Massachusetts
Hyperlipoproteinemia

ROBERT S. LEES, M.D.

Professor of Health Sciences and Technology, Harvard University and Massachusetts Institute of Technology, Cambridge; President, Boston Heart Foundation; Physician, Deaconess Hospital; Member, Cardiac Unit, Massachusetts General Hospital, Boston, Massachusetts
Hyperlipoproteinemia

STEPHEN S. LEFRAK, M.D.

Professor of Medicine, Washington University School of Medicine; Director, Medical Intensive Care Unit, The Jewish Hospital of St. Louis at Washington University Medical Center; Director, Internal Medicine House Staff Training Program, The Jewish Hospital of St. Louis at Washington University Medical Center, St. Louis, Missouri
Acute Respiratory Failure

LINDA BAKER LESTER, M.D.

Fellow in Endocrinology, Diabetes, and Clinical Nutrition, Oregon Health Sciences University and Providence Medical Center, Portland, Oregon
Hyperparathyroidism and Hypoparathyroidism

ROBERT S. LESTER, B.A., M.D., F.R.C.P.C.

Associate Professor of Medicine (Dermatology), University of Toronto; Consultant, Dermatology, and Vice-President, Medical, Sunnybrook Health Sciences Centre, Toronto, Ontario, Canada
Atopic Dermatitis

PETER A. LeWITT, M.D.

Professor of Neurology, Wayne State University School of Medicine; Director, Clinical Neuroscience Program, Sinai Hospital, Detroit, Michigan
Parkinson's Disease

JAMES T. C. LI, M.D., PH.D.

Consultant in Allergy and Internal Medicine, Mayo Clinic, Rochester, Minnesota
Asthma in Adolescents and Adults

R. B. LIBMAN, M.D.

Assistant Professor of Neurology, Albert Einstein College of Medicine, Bronx; Attending Neurologist and Head, Section of Cerebrovascular Disease, Long Island Jewish Medical Center, New Hyde Park, New York
Parenchymatous Brain Hemorrhage

MICHAEL B. LIPPMANN, M.D.

Assistant Clinical Professor, Washington University School of Medicine; Pulmonary Attending Physician, The Jewish Hospital of St. Louis at Washington University Medical Center; Director, Medical Intensive Care Unit, John Cochran Veterans Administration Medical Center, St. Louis, Missouri
Acute Respiratory Failure

GERALD L. LOGUE, M.D.

Professor of Medicine and Head, Division of Hematology, State University of New York at Buffalo School of Medicine and Biomedical Sciences; Chief of Staff, Department of Veterans Affairs Medical Center, Buffalo, New York
Polycythemia Vera

DONALD P. LOOKINGBILL, M.D.

Professor of Medicine (Dermatology) and Chief, Division of Dermatology, The Pennsylvania State University College of Medicine, Hershey, Pennsylvania
Acne Vulgaris and Rosacea

RODNEY A. LORENZ, M.D.

Director, Pediatric Endocrinology and Associate Professor of Pediatrics, Vanderbilt University School of Medicine, Nashville, Tennessee
Diabetic Ketoacidosis

MARK O. LOVELESS, M.D.

Assistant Professor of Medicine, Oregon Health Sciences University, Portland, Oregon
Rabies

ANTHONY A. LUCIANO, M.D.

Professor, Obstetrics and Gynecology, University of Connecticut School of Medicine, Farmington; Director, Center for Reproductive Endocrinology and Infertility, New Britain General Hospital, New Britain, Connecticut
Endometriosis

STEVEN W. LUGER, M.D.

Assistant Clinical Professor, Department of Medicine, Tufts New England Medical Center, Boston, Massachusetts; Attending Physician, Kaiser Permanente, Rocky Hill, and Hartford Hospital, West Hartford, Connecticut
Lyme Disease

JEANNE M. LUSHER, M.D.

Professor of Pediatrics and Marion Barnhart Hemostasis Research Professor, Wayne State University School of Medicine; Co-Director, Division of Hematology-Oncology and Director, Regional Comprehensive Hemophilia Center, Children's Hospital of Michigan, Detroit, Michigan
Hemophilia and Related Conditions

SHERWOOD C. LYNN, JR., M.D.

Associate Professor, Department of Obstetrics and Gynecology, University of South Alabama College of Medicine; Staff Physician, University of South Alabama Medical Center, Mobile, Alabama
Pelvic Inflammatory Disease

SCOTT A. MacDIARMID, M.D.

Fellow in Reconstructive Urology and Urodynamics, Division of Urologic Surgery, Duke University Medical Center, Durham, North Carolina
Urethral Stricture

ABE M. MACHER, M.D.

Medical Consultant to the National AIDS Education and Training Centers Program, HIV Health Professions Education Branch, Health Resources and Services Administration, United States Public Health Service, Rockville, Maryland
Management of the Patient with HIV Disease

JON T. MADER, M.D.

Professor, Department of Internal Medicine; Acting Chief, Division of Infectious Diseases; and Chief, Division of Hyperbaric Medicine, University of Texas Medical Branch, Galveston, Texas
Osteomyelitis

PAUL O. MADSEN, M.D., Ph.D.

Professor Emeritus of Urology, University of Wisconsin School of Medicine, Madison, Wisconsin
Benign Prostatic Hyperplasia

JAMES A. MAGNER, M.D.

Associate Professor of Medicine, Section of Endocrinology, East Carolina University School of Medicine, Greenville, North Carolina
Hypothyroidism

DILIP MAHALANABIS, M.B., B.S.

Associate Director, Clinical Sciences Division and Senior Consultant, Clinical Research and Service Centre, International Centre for Diarrhoeal Disease Research; B Dhaka, Bangladesh
Cholera

STEPHEN R. MARDER, M.D.

Professor of Psychiatry, University of California, Los Angeles, School of Medicine; Chief, Psychiatry Service, West Los Angeles Veterans Affairs Medical Center, Los Angeles, California
Schizophrenia

DAVID H. MARTIN, M.D.

Harry E. Dascomb, M.D. Professor of Medicine and Chief, Section of Infectious Diseases, Louisiana State University Medical Center; Medical Staff Member, Medical Center of Louisiana at New Orleans, and Tulane University Hospital, New Orleans, Louisiana
Chancroid

JOHN A. MATA, M.D.

Associate Professor, Department of Urology, Louisiana State University Medical Center; Staff Physician, Louisiana State University Hospital, Shriners Hospital, and Schumpart Medical Center, Shreveport, Louisiana
Bacterial Infections of the Urinary Tract in Females; Nongonococcal Urethritis in Men

NINAN T. MATHEW, M.D.

Clinical Professor, Restorative Neurology and Human Neurobiology, Baylor College of Medicine; Staff Physician, Methodist Hospital, St. Luke's Hospital, Hermann Hospital, and Park Plaza Hospital, Houston, Texas
Headache

ALEXANDER MAUSKOP, M.D.

Assistant Professor of Neurology, State University of New York Health Science Center at Brooklyn, Brooklyn; Director, New York Headache Center, New York, and Associate Attending Neurologist, Long Island College Hospital, Brooklyn, New York
Pain

JOHN H. McANULTY, M.D.

Professor of Medicine, Oregon Health Sciences University; Staff Physician, University Hospital, Oregon Health Sciences University, Portland, Oregon
Atrial Fibrillation

ANNE E. McCARTHY, M.D., F.A.C.P., F.R.C.P.(C.), D.T.M.&H.

Infectious Disease Fellow, University of Ottawa, Ottawa, Ontario, Canada
Malaria

MICHAEL R. McCLUNG, M.D.

Associate Professor of Medicine, Oregon Health Sciences University; Director, Center for Metabolic Bone Disorders, Providence Medical Center, Portland, Oregon
Hyperparathyroidism and Hypoparathyroidism

SALLY McDONALD, M.D.

Clinical Faculty, Northwestern Medical School; Volunteer Attending Staff, Mercy Hospital and Medical Center, Chicago, Illinois
Tinnitus

MARILYNNE McKAY, M.D.

Associate Professor of Dermatology and Gynecology, Emory University School of Medicine; Chief, Dermatology Service, Grady Memorial Hospital, Atlanta, Georgia
Skin Diseases of Pregnancy

JAMES C. MELBY, M.D.

Professor of Medicine and Director, Division of Endocrinology and Metabolism, Boston University School of Medicine, Boston, Massachusetts
Adrenocortical Insufficiency; Primary Aldosteronism

A. D. MENDELOW, M.D., Ph.D., F.R.C.S. (Edinburgh) (Surgical Neurology), Ph.D.

Reader and Honorary Consultant Neurosurgeon, Department of Surgery (Neurosurgery), The Medical School, University of Newcastle upon Tyne, Newcastle upon Tyne, United Kingdom
Acute Head Injury in Adults

COL. RODNEY A. MICHAEL, M.D.

Associate Professor, Uniformed Services University of Health Sciences, Bethesda, Maryland; Chief, Department of Retrovirology, United States Army Medical Component, Armed Forces Research Institute of Medical Science, Bangkok, Thailand
Gonorrhea

JOHN M. MILLER, M.D.

Associate Professor of Medicine, Temple University School of Medicine; Director of Electrophysiology Services, Temple University Hospital, Philadelphia, Pennsylvania
Heart Block

LESTER D. MILLER, M.D.

Rheumatologist, Active Staff, Department of Internal Medicine, Dominican Santa Cruz Hospital, Santa Cruz, California
Connective Tissue Diseases

PAUL F. MILNER, M.D.

Professor, Pathology and Medicine, Medical College of Georgia; Medical College of Georgia Hospital and Clinics, Augusta, Georgia
Sickle Cell Disease

HOWARD C. MOFENSON, M.D.

Professor, Pediatrics and Emergency Medicine, State University of New York at Stony Brook, Stony Brook; Professor, Pharmacology and Toxicology, New York School of Osteopathy, Old Westbury, and St. John's University College of Pharmacy, Jamaica; Director, Long Island Regional Poison Control Center, Mineola; Staff, Winthrop University Hospital, Nassau County Medical Center, Mineola, New York
Acute Poisonings

J. P. MOHR, M.D.

Sciarra Professor of Clinical Neurology, College of Physicians and Surgeons, Columbia University; Director, Neurovascular Unit, The New York Neurological Institute, New York, New York
Parenchymatous Brain Hemorrhage

ALISON MOLITERNO, M.D.

Assistant Professor of Medicine, Department of Medicine/Division of Hematology, The Johns Hopkins University School of Medicine; Staff Physician, The Johns Hopkins University Hospital, Baltimore, Maryland
Disseminated Intravascular Coagulation

GARY D. MONHEIT, M.D.

Assistant Professor, University of Alabama Medical Center; Staff, Eye Foundation Hospital, Health South Medical Center, Baptist Montclair, Brookwood Medical Center, St. Vincents Hospital, and Veterans Administration Hospital Staff, Birmingham, Alabama
Premalignant Lesions of the Skin

PETER MORGAN-CAPNER, F.R.C.PATH.

Consultant Virologist, Royal Preston Hospital, Preston, United Kingdom
Rubella and Congenital Rubella

MICHAEL J. MOSKAL, D.O.

Broadlawns Medical Center, Iowa Methodist Medical Center, Des Moines, Iowa
Mycoplasmal and Viral Pneumonias

JOSEPH A. MUCCINI, M.D.

Resident, Department of Dermatology, Harvard Medical School; Massachusetts General Hospital, Boston, Massachusetts
Erythema Multiforme and Other Erythematous Disorders

DAVID G. MUTCH, M.D.

Assistant Professor and Director, Division of Gynecologic Oncology, Washington University School of Medicine, St. Louis, Missouri
Carcinoma of the Uterine Cervix

STEVEN R. NEISH, M.D.

Assistant Professor of Pediatrics, University of Colorado School of Medicine, Denver; Pediatric Cardiologist, Fitzsimons Army Medical Center, Aurora, and The Children's Hospital, Denver, Colorado
Congenital Heart Disease

RICHARD NEWMAN, M.D.

Associate Clinical Professor of Pathology, University of California, Irvine, School of Medicine; Associate Director, Blood Bank Director, HLA and Coagulation Laboratories at UCI Medical Center, Orange, California
Adverse Reactions to Blood Transfusion

S. K. NOORDEEN, M.D.

Chief Medical Officer, Leprosy Unit, Division of Control of Tropical Disease, World Health Organization, Geneva, Switzerland
Leprosy

RICHARD B. NORTH, M.D.

Associate Professor, Department of Neurosurgery, The Johns Hopkins University School of Medicine, Baltimore, Maryland
Trigeminal Neuralgia

MIRIAM OLIVEROS DE ANGULO, M.D.

Professor, School of Medicine, University of Caraboro, Valencia, Venezuela; Visiting Professor, University of Kentucky, Lexington, Kentucky
Diabetes Mellitus in Adults

JOSEPH F. O'NEILL, M.D., M.S., M.P.H.

Assistant Professor of Medicine, The Johns Hopkins University School of Medicine; Clinical Assistant Professor of Medicine, University of Maryland School of Medicine, Baltimore, Maryland
Management of the Patient with HIV Disease

NICHOLAS A. ORFAN, M.D.

Assistant Professor of Clinical Medicine, Columbia University College of Physicians and Surgeons, New York; Staff Physican, Mary Imogene Bassett Hospital, Cooperstown, New York
Asthma in Children

BERNHARD ORTEL, M.D.

Universitätsdozent (Associate Professor), Department of Dermatology, University of Vienna School of Medicine, Vienna; Staff, Division of Special and Environmental Dermatology, Vienna, Austria
Sunburn and Photosensitivity

FRED D. OWENS, M.D.

President, Dallas Foundation of Otology; Assistant Chief, Otolaryngology, Baylor University Medical Center, Dallas, Texas
Meniere's Disease

SANTIAGO L. PADILLA, M.D.

Staff Physician, Fertility Center of Maryland, Department of Gynecology, Greater Baltimore Medical Center, Baltimore, Maryland
Ectopic Pregnancy

BIFF F. PALMER, M.D.

Assistant Professor of Internal Medicine, University of Texas Southwestern Medical School; Associate Medical Director of Renal Transplantation, Parkland Memorial Hospital, Dallas, Texas
Chronic Renal Failure

CLAIRE B. PANOSIAN, M.D., D.T.M.&H.

Associate Clinical Professor of Medicine, Division of Infectious Diseases, and Director, Travel and Tropical Medicine, University of California, Los Angeles, School of Medicine; Director, Travel and Tropical Medicine, UCLA Medical Center, Los Angeles, California
Tularemia

JOHN E. PARKER, M.D.

Adjunct Associate Professor, Section of Pulmonary and Critical Care Medicine, Department of Medicine, West Virginia University Health Sciences Center; Attending Physician,

Ruby Memorial Hospital, West Virginia University Medical Center, and Mountainview Regional Rehabilitation Hospital; National Institute for Occupational Safety and Health, Morgantown, West Virginia
Silicosis

JOHN C. PARTIN, M.D.

Professor of Pediatrics, Department of Pediatrics, School of Medicine, State University of New York at Stony Brook, Stony Brook, New York
Reye's Syndrome

JOSÉ F. PATIÑO, M.D., F.A.C.S. (HON.)

Special Professor of Surgery, Universidad Nacional de Colombia, Bogotá; Visiting Professor of Surgery, Yale University School of Medicine, New Haven, Connecticut; Chairman, Department of Surgery, Fundación Santa Fe de Bogotá, Bogotá, Colombia
Necrotizing Skin and Soft Tissue Infections

ROBERT L. PENN, M.D.

Professor of Medicine, Louisiana State University School of Medicine in Shreveport; Chief, Infectious Diseases Section, Louisiana State University Medical Center, Shreveport, Louisiana
Toxoplasmosis

JEFFREY P. PHELAN, M.D., J.D.

Co-Director, Maternal-Fetal Medicine, Pomona Valley Hospital Medical Center, Pomona; Attending Physician, San Antonio Community Hospital, Upland, California
Antepartum Care

GEORGE PHILLIPS, JR., M.D.

Assistant Professor of Medicine, Hematology/Oncology, Duke University Medical Center; Assistant Professor of Medicine and Director of Adult Hemoglobinopathy and Thalassemia Clinic, Duke University Medical Center, Durham, North Carolina
Thalassemia

F. XAVIER PI-SUNYER, M.D.

Professor of Medicine, Columbia University College of Physicians and Surgeons; Director, Division of Endocrinology, Diabetes, and Nutrition, St. Luke's-Roosevelt Hospital Center New York, New York
Obesity

MARK H. POLLACK M.D.

Assistant Professor of Psychiatry, Harvard Medical School; Director, Anxiety Disorders Program, Massachusetts General Hospital, Boston, Massachusetts
Panic Disorder and Agoraphobia

LAWRIE W. POWELL, M.D., PH.D.

Professor of Medicine, University of Queensland; Director, Queensland Institute of Medical Research; Consultant Physician (Internist) and Hepatologist, Royal Brisbane Hospital, Herston, Brisbane, Queensland, Australia
Hemochromatosis

RICHARD A. PROCTOR, M.D.

Professor of Medicine and Medical Microbiology/Immunology, University of Wisconsin Medical School; Staff Physician, University of Wisconsin Hospital, Madison, Wisconsin
Bacteremia and Septicemia

SIMON S. RABINOWITZ, PH.D, M.D.

Assistant Professor of Pediatrics and Chief, Pediatric Gastroenterologist and Nutrition, Children's Medical Center of Brooklyn, Brooklyn, New York
Normal Infant Feeding

PETER V. RABINS, M.D., M.P.H.

Professor of Psychiatry, The Johns Hopkins University School of Medicine; Full-Time Staff, The Johns Hopkins University Hospital, Baltimore, Maryland
Delirium

REBECCA B. RABY, M.D.

Fellow, Division of Clinical Immunology, Department of Pediatrics, University of Tennessee; Staff Physician, LeBonheur Children's Medical Center, Memphis, Tennessee
Anaphylaxis and Serum Sickness

JUSTIN D. RADOLF, M.D.

Associate Professor of Internal Medicine and Microbiology, University of Texas Southwestern Medical Center; Attending Physician, Parkland Memorial Hospital and Zale-Lipshy University Hospital, Dallas, Texas
Syphilis

JOEL M. RAPPEPORT, M.D.

Professor of Medicine and Pediatrics, Yale University School of Medicine; Director, Bone Marrow Transplant Program, Yale-New Haven Hospital, New Haven, Connecticut
Aplastic Anemia

JONATHAN I. RAVDIN, M.D.

Professor and Vice-Chairman of Medicine, Case Western Reserve University; Chief of Medical Service, Veterans Affairs Medical Center, Cleveland, Ohio
Amebiasis

MARCIA L. REEDER, M.D.

Resident in Dermatology, University of Wisconsin, Madison, Wisconsin
Pruritus (Itching)

ALEXANDER REITER, M.D.

Assistant Professor, Baylor College of Medicine, Houston, Texas
Postpartum Care

WILLIAM O. RICHARDS, M.D.

Assistant Professor of Surgery, Vanderbilt University School of Medicine; Staff Surgeon and Physician, Nashville Veterans Administration Medical Center; Staff Physician, Vanderbilt University Hospital, Nashville, Tennessee
Chronic Pancreatitis

HARRIS D. RILEY, JR., M.D.

Professor of Pediatrics, Vanderbilt University School of Medicine; Staff Physician, Vanderbilt Children's Hospital, Vanderbilt University Medical Center, Nashville, Tennessee
Whooping Cough (Pertussis)

PETER B. RINTELS, M.D.

Instructor, Brown University School of Medicine; Associate Director, Clinical Hematology, Rhode Island Hospital, Providence, Rhode Island
Autoimmune Hemolytic Anemia

RICHARD S. RIVLIN, M.D.

Professor of Medicine, Cornell University Medical College; Program Director, Clinical Nutrition Research Unit, Memorial Sloan-Kettering Cancer Center, New York; Attending Physician, GI-Nutrition Service, MSKCC; Chief, Nutrition Division, New York Hospital-Cornell Medical Center, New York, New York
Vitamin Deficiency

DAVID J. ROBERTS, M.D.

Clinical Associate Professor, University of Minnesota, Minneapolis, Medical School; Staff Emergency Physician and Consultant, Toxicology, North Memorial Medical Center, Minneapolis, Minnesota
Drug Abuse

JAMES A. ROBERTS, M.D.

Professor and Associate Chairman, Tulane University School of Medicine; Active Staff, Tulane University Hospital and St. Tammany Parish Hospital; Attending Staff, Charity Hospital, New Orleans, Louisiana
Pyelonephritis

HENRY H. ROENIGK, Jr., M.D.

Professor of Dermatology, Northwestern University Medical School and Northwestern Memorial Hospital, Chicago, Illinois
Venous (Stasis) Ulcers

WARD B. ROGERS, M.D.

Assistant Professor of Medicine and Radiology, Medical College of Georgia, Augusta, Georgia
Congestive Heart Failure

DONALD A. ROMIG, M.D.

Associate Clinical Professor of Medicine, University of New Mexico School of Medicine; Staff Physician, St. Vincent Hospital, Santa Fe, New Mexico
Plague

JERROLD F. ROSENBAUM, M.D.

Associate Professor of Psychiatry, Harvard Medical School; Chief, Clinical Psychopharmacology and Behavioral Therapy Unit, and Director, Outpatient Psychiatry Division, Massachusetts General Hospital, Boston, Massachusetts
Panic Disorder and Agoraphobia

ALLAN M. ROSS, M.D.

Professor of Medicine, George Washington University; Staff Physician, George Washington University Medical Center, Washington, D.C.
Acute Myocardial Infarction

FREDERICK L. RUBEN, M.D.

Professor of Medicine, University of Pittsburgh School of Medicine; Head, Infectious Disease Division, Montefiore University Hospital; Director, Infection Control, University of Pittsburgh Medical Center, Pittsburgh, Pennsylvania
Influenza

RONALD A. SACHER, M.D., F.R.C.P.(C)

Professor of Medicine and Pathology, Georgetown University Medical Center, Washington, D.C.
Pernicious Anemia and Other Megaloblastic Anemias

KENNETH E. SACK, M.D.

Clinical Professor of Medicine and Director of Clinical Programs in Rheumatology, University of California, San Francisco, San Francisco, California
Osteoarthritis

THEODORE J. SACLARIDES, M.D.

Assistant Professor of Surgery, Rush Medical College; Head, Section of Colon and Rectal Surgery, Rush-Presbyterian-St. Luke's Medical Center, Chicago, Illinois
Tumors of the Colon and Rectum

JOHN L. SAWYERS, M.D.

John Clinton Foshee Distinguished Professor of Surgery, and Chairman, Department of Surgery, Vanderbilt University School of Medicine; Surgeon-in-Chief, Vanderbilt University Hospital, Nashville, Tennessee
Chronic Pancreatitis

STEVEN D. SCHAEFER, M.D., F.A.C.S.

Professor and Chairman, Department of Otolaryngology, New York Eye and Ear Infirmary, New York Medical College, New York; Attending Physician, Lincoln Medical and Mental Health Center, New York Eye and Ear Infirmary, St. Vincent's Hospital and Medical Center of New York, New York; and Westchester County Medical Center, Valhalla, New York
Sinusitis

ISAAC SCHIFF, M.D.

Joe Vincent Meigs Professor of Gynecology, Harvard Medical School; Chief, Vincent Memorial Gynecology Service, Women's Care Division, Massachusetts General Hospital, Boston, Massachusetts
Menopause

JAY S. SCHINFELD, M.D.

Clinical Associate Professor, Department of Obstetrics and Gynecology, Thomas Jefferson Medical College and University, Philadelphia; Chief, Reproductive Endocrinology, Abington Memorial Hospital, Abington, Pennsylvania
Dysmenorrhea

GEORGE B. SEGEL, M.D.

Professor of Pediatrics, Medicine, and Genetics and Associate Chair, Department of Pediatrics, University of Rochester School of Medicine; Pediatrician and Physician, Strong Memorial Hospital, Rochester, New York
Nonimmune Hemolytic Anemia

PAULO SERAFINI, M.D.

Director, Reproductive Endocrinology and Infertility, Huntington Memorial Hospital, Pasadena, California
Amenorrhea

WILLIAM R. SEXSON, M.D.

Associate Professor of Pediatrics, Emory University; Director of Nurseries, Grady Memorial Hospital, Atlanta, Georgia
Neonatal Resuscitation

GAIL G. SHAPIRO, M.D.

Clinical Professor of Pediatrics, University of Washington School of Medicine; Staff Physician, Children's Hospital and Medical Center, Seattle, Washington
Allergic Rhinitis Due to Inhalant Factors

OM P. SHARMA, M.D.

Professor of Medicine, University of Southern California School of Medicine; Physician Specialist, USC University Hospital and Los Angeles County–University of Southern California Medical Center, Los Angeles, California
Sarcoidosis

KAUSHIK A. SHASTRI, M.D.

Research Assistant Professor of Medicine, Division of Hematology, State University of New York at Buffalo School of

Medicine and Biomedical Sciences; Staff Physician, Department of Veterans Affairs Medical Center, Buffalo, New York
Polycythemia Vera

THOMAS W. SHEEHY, M.D.

Distinguished Professor Emeritus, University of Alabama at Birmingham (UAB); Staff Physician, UAB Hospitals, Birmingham, Alabama
Disturbances Due to Cold

PHILIP D. SHENEFELT, M.D.

Assistant Professor of Medicine, University of South Florida; Staff Physician, Tampa General Hospital, James A. Haley Veterans Hospital, and H. Lee Moffitt Cancer Center and Research Institute, Tampa, Florida
Malignant Melanoma

ELIZABETH F. SHERERTZ, M.D.

Professor and Vice-Chairman of Dermatology, Bowman Gray School of Medicine of Wake Forest University, Winston-Salem, North Carolina
Occupational Dermatitis

GLENN K. SHOPPER, M.D.

Associate Professor, University of Missouri, Kansas City, School of Medicine; Director of Obstetric Anesthesia, Truman Medical Center, Kansas City, Missouri
Obstetric Anesthesia

WILLIAM SIEVERT, M.D.

Senior Lecturer in Medicine, Monash University Department of Medicine, Melbourne; Consultant Gastroenterologist, Fairfield Hospital, Melbourne, Victoria, Australia
Acute and Chronic Hepatitis

RICHARD T. SILVER, M.D.

Clinical Professor of Medicine, Cornell University Medical College; Director, Section of Clinical Oncology Chemotherapy Research; Attending Physician, New York Hospital-Cornell Medical Center, New York, New York
Chronic Myeloid Leukemia

GARY L. SIMON, M.D., PH.D.

Professor of Medicine, George Washington University School of Medicine; Associate Chairman, Department of Medicine, George Washington University Medical Center, Washington, D.C.
Food-Borne Illness

BARRY SKIKNE, M.D.

Professor of Medicine and Staff Physician, University of Kansas Medical Center, Kansas City, Kansas
Vitamin K Deficiency

DAVID L. SMITH, M.D.

Clinical Associate Professor, University of Kansas Medical Center, Kansas City, Kansas
Rocky Mountain Spotted Fever

L. KENT SMITH, M.D., M.P.H.

Arizona State University and Baylor University; Director, Cardiac Rehabilitation and Director, Ambulatory Drug Research, Arizona Heart Institute and Foundation; Staff Physician, Healthwest Regional Medical Center, Phoenix, Arizona
Coronary Rehabilitation

GARWIN B. SOE, M.D.

Staff Physician, Kaiser Foundation Hospital, Walnut Creek; Kaiser Foundation Hospital, Martinez; and Kaiser Permanente Medical Center, Antioch, California
Nontyphoidal Salmonellosis

KEYOUMARS SOLTANI, M.D.

Professor and Chief, Section of Dermatology, University of Chicago, Chicago, Illinois
Parasitic Diseases of the Skin

KATHY R. SONENTHAL, M.D.

Adult Allergist, Cook County Hospital, Chicago, Illinois
Allergic Reactions to Drugs

CHRISTOPH SPARWASSER, M.D.

Research Fellow in Urology, Veterans Administration Hospital and University Hospital, University of Wisconsin School of Medicine, Madison, Wisconsin
Benign Prostatic Hyperplasia

ROBERT E. SPERRY, M.D.

Instructor, Department of Medicine, Medical College of Virginia, Richmond, Virginia
Tachycardia

GARY SPIEGELMAN, M.D.

Staff Physician, Fort Sanders Park West Medical Center, Knoxville, Tennessee
Diverticula of the Alimentary Tract

HEATHER T. SPONSEL, M.D.

Clinical Fellow, Renal Division, University of Colorado Health Sciences Center, Denver, Colorado
Acute Renal Failure

JAMES C. STANLEY, M.D.

Professor of Surgery, University of Michigan Medical School; Head, Section of Vascular Surgery, University of Michigan Hospital, Ann Arbor, Michigan
Peripheral Arterial Disease

PERRY STARER, M.D.

Assistant Professor, Department of Geriatrics and Adult Development, Mount Sinai School of Medicine; Attending Physician, The Jewish Home and Hospital for the Aged; Chief, Geriatrics Section, Elmhurst Hospital Center, New York, New York
Urinary Incontinence

FREDERIC W. STEARNS, M.D.

Instructor, School of Aerospace Medicine, San Antonio, Texas; Clinical Assistant Professor, Oklahoma School of Medicine, Tulsa; Active Staff, St. Francis Hospital, Tulsa, Oklahoma
Superficial Fungal Infections of the Skin

WILLARD D. STECK, M.D., F.A.C.P.

Senior Physician, Department of Dermatology, The Cleveland Clinic Foundation, Cleveland, Ohio
Decubitus Ulcer

ROBERT S. STERN, M.D.

Associate Professor, Department of Dermatology, Harvard Medical School; Staff Physician, Beth Israel Hospital, Boston, Massachusetts
Erythema Multiforme and Other Erythematous Disorders

J. C. STEVENSON, M.B., F.R.C.S.(ENG.)

Clinical Research Associate, Department of Neurosurgery, University of Newcastle upon Tyne Medical School; Registrar, Newcastle General Hospital, Newcastle upon Tyne, England
Acute Head Injury in Adults

STEPHEN P. STONE, M.D.

Clinical Associate Professor (Medicine), Southern Illinois University School of Medicine; Staff Physician, The Dermatology Center, Memorial Medical Center, and St. John's Hospital, Springfield, Illinois
Pruritis Ani and Vulvae

DAVID J. STRAUS, M.D

Associate Professor of Clinical Medicine, Cornell University Medical College; Associate Attending Physician, Memorial Sloan-Kettering Cancer Center, New York, New York
Hodgkin's Disease: Chemotherapy

MICHAEL STREIFF, M.D.

Fellow in Hematology, The Johns Hopkins University School of Medicine and The Johns Hopkins University Hospital, Baltimore, Maryland
Thrombotic Thrombocytopenic Purpura–Hemolytic Uremic Syndrome

JAMES D. STROUD, M.D.

Clinical Associate Professor, Department of Dermatology, Wayne State University; Active Staff, Providence Hospital and Beaumont Hospital, Detroit, Michigan
Hair Disorders

HUGO STUDER, M.D.

Professor of Medicine and Chief, Clinic of Internal Medicine, Inselspital, University of Bern, Bern, Switzerland
Goiter

S. H. SUBRAMONY, M.D.

Professor of Neurology, University of Mississippi Medical Center; Attending Physician, University Hospital; Consultant, Veterans Administration Hospital, Jackson, Mississippi
Peripheral Neuropathies

MATTHEW O. SWARTZ, M.D.

Consultant in Rheumatology, Prince William Hospital, Manassas; Fauquier Hospital, Warrenton; and Fairfax Hospital, Falls Church, Virginia
Polymyalgia Rheumatica and Giant Cell Arteritis

MORTON N. SWARTZ, M.D.

Professor of Medicine, Harvard Medical School; Chief, James Jackson Firm Department of Medicine, Massachusetts General Hospital, Boston, Massachusetts
Bacterial Diseases of the Skin

ROBERT A. SWERLICK, M.D.

Assistant Professor, Department of Dermatology, Emory University School of Medicine; Staff Physician, Emory University Hospital, Atlanta, Georgia
Skin Diseases of Pregnancy

NICHOLAS J. TALLEY, M.D., PH.D.

Associate Professor of Medicine, Mayo Medical School; Consultant, Division of Gastroenterology and Internal Medicine and Department of Health Sciences Research, Mayo Clinic and Mayo Foundation, Rochester, Minnesota
Irritable Bowel Syndrome

STEPHAN R. TARGAN, M.D.

Professor of Medicine, UCLA School of Medicine; Director, Inflammatory Bowel Disease Center and Cedars-Sinai Medical Center, Los Angeles, California
Ulcerative Colitis

UDELE V. TAYLOR, M.D.

Staff Physician, Jamaica Hospital, Jamaica, New York
Chlamydia Trachomatis Infection

W. SCOTT TAYLOR, M.D.

Clinical Assistant Professor, Department of Obstetrics and Gynecology, George Washington University Medical School; Associate Chairman, Department of Obstetrics and Gynecology, Washington Hospital Center; Director, Department of Obstetric-Gynecologic Ultrasonography, Washington Hospital Center, Washington, D.C.
Leiomyomas of the Uterus

JULIUS L. TEAGUE, M.D.

Chief, Pediatric Urology, Brooke Army Medical Center, San Antonio, Texas
Genitourinary Tumors

IAN M. THOMPSON, M.D.

Chief, Urology Service, Brooke Army Medical Center, San Antonio, Texas
Genitourinary Tumors

MARK A. THOMPSON, M.D.

Assistant Clinical Professor of Medicine, Consulting Cardiologist, and Attending Cardiologist, George Washington University Medical Center, Washington, D.C.
Acute Myocardial Infarction

STEPHEN E. THURSTON, M.D.

Clinical Assistant Professor of Neurology, Jefferson Medical College, Philadelphia, Pennsylvania
Episodic Vertigo

MARTIN J. TOBIN, M.D.

Professor of Medicine, Loyola University of Chicago Stritch School of Medicine, Chicago; Staff Physician, Department of Veterans Affairs Edward Hines, Jr. Hospital, Hines; Attending Physician, Foster G. McGaw Hospital and Loyola University Medical Center, Chicago, Illinois
Chronic Obstructive Pulmonary Disease

N. V. TODD, M.D., F.R.C.S. (ENG.)

Consultant Neurosurgeon, Department of Surgery (Neurosurgery), The Medical School, University of Newcastle upon Tyne, Newcastle upon Tyne, United Kingdom
Acute Head Injury in Adults

PRENTICE A. TOM, M.D.

Clinical Assistant Professor of Surgery and Attending Physician, Emergency Medicine, Stanford University Hospital, Stanford; Attending Physician, South Valley Hospital, Gilroy, California
Spider Bites and Scorpion Stings

WALLACE W. TOURTELLOTTE, M.D., PH.D.

Professor and Vice-Chairman, Department of Neurology, UCLA School of Medicine; Chief, Neurology Service, Veterans Affairs Medical Center–West Los Angeles; Staff Physician, UCLA Medical Center, Los Angeles, California
Multiple Sclerosis

HOWARD TRACHTMAN, M.D.

Associate Professor of Pediatrics, Albert Einstein College of Medicine of Yeshiva University, Bronx; Staff Nephrologist, Schneider Children's Hospital, New Hyde Park, New York
Parenteral Fluid Therapy for Infants and Children

PETER J. TRAINER, M.B.

Lecturer, St. Bartholomew's Hospital, West Smithfield, London, United Kingdom
Cushing's Syndrome

MORRIS TRAUBE, M.D.

Associate Professor of Medicine, Yale University School of Medicine; Director, Gastrointestinal Procedure Center, and Attending Physician, Yale-New Haven Hospital, New Haven, Connecticut
Dysphagia and Esophageal Obstruction

JUAN ANTONIO TREJO Y PÉREZ, M.D.

Professor of Pediatrics, Universidad Nacional Autónoma de México; Staff Physician, Division of Pediatrics, Children's Hospital, National Medical Center, Mexican Institute of Social Security, Mexico, D.F., Mexico
Typhoid Fever

ALLAN R. TUNKEL, M.D., PH.D.

Assistant Professor of Medicine, Medical College of Pennsylvania; Attending Physician, Medical College Hospitals/Main Clinical Campus, Philadelphia, Pennsylvania
Brain Abscess

PETER A. TUXEN, M.D.

Staff Physician, St. Joseph's Medical Center, San Joaquin General Hospital, Stockton, California
Hemorrhoids, Anal Fissure, and Anorectal Abscess and Fistula

LEO B. TWIGGS, M.D.

Professor and Head, Department of Obstetrics and Gynecology, University of Minnesota Medical School, Minneapolis, Minnesota
Endometrial Cancer

LOUISE B. TYRER, M.D.

Medical Director, Association of Reproductive Health Professionals, Washington, D.C.
Contraception

STEPHEN K. TYRING, M.D., PH.D.

Professor of Dermatology, Microbiology and Internal Medicine, University of Texas Medical Branch, Galveston, Texas
Viral Diseases of the Skin

JOUNI UITTO, M.D., PH.D.

Professor of Dermatology, Biochemistry, and Molecular Biology, Jefferson Medical College; Chairman, Department of Dermatology, Thomas Jefferson University Hospital, Philadelphia, Pennsylvania
Keloids

BASIM M. UTHMAN, M.D.

Assistant Professor, Department of Neurology, College of Medicine, University of Florida; Acting Chief, Neurology Service, Department of Veterans Affairs Medical Center, Gainesville, Florida
Epilepsy in Adolescents and Adults

RAMON VALLARINO, M.D.

Assistant Clinical Professor, Physical Medicine and Rehabilitation, State University of New York Health Sciences Center at Brooklyn; Director of Physical Medicine and Rehabilitation, Victory Memorial Hospital, Brooklyn; Attending Physician, Physical Medicine and Rehabilitation, The Methodist Hospital, Brooklyn, New York
Rehabilitation of Persons with Stroke

KEITH N. VAN ARSDALEN, M.D.

Associate Professor, University of Pennsylvania School of Medicine; Chief of Urology, Hospital of the University of Pennsylvania, Veterans Administration Medical Center, Philadelphia, Pennsylvania
Bacterial Infections of the Urinary Tract in Males

MARY LEE VANCE, M.D.

Associate Professor of Medicine, University of Virginia Health Sciences Center, Charlottesville, Virginia
Acromegaly

L. GEORGE VEASY, M.D.

Professor of Pediatrics, University of Utah School of Medicine; Attending Physician, Primary Children's Medical Center, University of Utah Hospital, Salt Lake City, Utah
Rheumatic Fever

SATISH R. C. VELAGAPUDI, M.D.

Assistant Professor of Urology, State University of New York, Buffalo; Associate Chief, Department of Urologic Oncology, Roswell Park Cancer Institute, Buffalo, New York
Genitourinary Trauma

JOSEPH G. VERBALIS, M.D.

Professor of Medicine, Division of Endocrinology and Metabolism, University of Pittsburgh School of Medicine; Attending Physician, University of Pittsburgh Medical Center and Department of Veterans Affairs Medical Center, Pittsburgh, Pennsylvania
Diabetes Insipidus

JENNIFER L. VESPER, M.D.

Dermatology Resident, University of South Florida College of Medicine, Tampa, Florida
Warts (Verruca Vulgaris)

GEORGE J. WALKER, M.D.

Fellow, University of Wisconsin Medical School, Milwaukee Clinical Campus, Milwaukee, Wisconsin
Constipation

BRIAN W. WALSH, M.D.

Assistant Professor of Obstetrics, Gynecology, and Reproductive Biology, Harvard Medical School; Director, Menopause Clinic, Brigham and Women's Hospital, Boston, Massachusetts
Menopause

INDIRA WARRIER, M.D.

Associate Professor of Pediatrics, Wayne State University School of Medicine; Associate Hematologist and Associate Director, Regional Comprehensive Hemophilia Center, Children's Hospital of Michigan, Detroit, Michigan
Hemophilia and Related Conditions

WATTS R. WEBB, M.D.

Professor of Surgery, Tulane University School of Medicine; Staff Physician, Tulane University Medical Center, Medical

Center of Louisiana, Veterans Administration Medical Center, New Orleans, Louisiana
Atelectasis

GEORGE D. WEBSTER, M.B., F.R.C.S.

Professor of Urologic Surgery, Duke University Medical Center, Durham, North Carolina
Urethral Stricture

LESLIE P. WEINER, M.D.

Professor, School of Medicine, University of Southern California, Los Angeles, California
Viral Meningitis and Encephalitis

ERIC L. WEISS, M.D., D.T.M.&H.

Assistant Professor of Surgery, Emergency Medicine, Stanford University; Director, Stanford Travel Medicine Service; Staff Physician, Stanford University Hospital, Stanford, California
Injury Received From Hazardous Marine Animals

LOUIS M. WEISS, M.D., M.P.H.

Assistant Professor of Medicine, Division of Infectious Diseases, and Assistant Professor of Pathology, Division of Parasitology and Tropical Medicine, Albert Einstein College of Medicine of Yeshiva University; Attending Physician, Bronx Municipal Hospital, Jack D. Weiler Hospital of the Albert Einstein College of Medicine of Yeshiva University, and Montefiore Medical Center, Bronx, New York
Rat-Bite Fever

WILLIAM B. WHITE, M.D.

Professor of Medicine, University of Connecticut School of Medicine; Chief, Section of Hypertension and Vascular Diseases; Attending Physician, John Dempsey Hospital, University of Connecticut Health Center, Farmington, Connecticut
Cough

B. J. WILDER, M.D.

Chief, Neurology Service, Department of Veterans Affairs Medical Center; Professor of Neurology and Neuroscience, University of Florida College of Medicine, Gainesville, Florida
Epilepsy in Adolescents and Adults

M. ROY WILSON, M.D., M.S.

Associate Professor, Jules Stein Eye Institute, UCLA, and Charles R. Drew University of Medicine and Science, Los Angeles, California
Glaucoma

RANDALL K. WOLF, M.D.

Attending Thoracic Surgeon, The Christ Hospital and The Jewish Hospital of Cincinnati, Cincinnati, Ohio
Pleural Effusion and Empyema Thoracis

MARTIN S. WOLFE, M.D.

Clinical Professor of Medicine, George Washington University Medical School; Clinical Associate Professor of Medicine, Georgetown University Medical School, Washington, D.C.
Intestinal Parasites

GAYLE E. WOODSON, M.D.

Professor of Otolaryngology, University of Tennessee, Memphis, College of Medicine; Staff Physician, Methodist Hospital, LeBonheur Children's Medical Center, Baptist Memorial Hospital, University of Tennessee Bowld Hospital Regional Medical Center, Memphis, Tennessee
Hoarseness and Laryngitis

CREIGHTON B. WRIGHT, M.D.

Clinical Professor of Surgery, Uniformed Services University; Director, Department of Surgery, Jewish Hospital of Cincinnati, Cincinnati, Ohio
Pleural Effusion and Empyema Thoracis

JOACHIM YAHALOM, M.D.

Associate Professor, Cornell University Medical College; Associate Member, Memorial Sloan-Kettering Cancer Center, New York, New York
Hodgkin's Disease: Radiation Therapy

ROBERT A. YOOD, M.D.

Assistant Professor of Medicine, University of Massachusetts Medical School; Director of Rheumatology, Saint Vincent Hospital, Worcester, Massachusetts
Hyperuricemia and Gout

EDWARD M. YOUNG, JR., M.D.

Private Practice, Sidell Erikson, McLeary, and Young Dermatology Surgical and Medical Group, Sherman Oaks, California
Nevi

JAMES B. YOUNG, M.D.

Professor of Medicine, Baylor College of Medicine; Staff Physician, The Methodist Hospital, Houston, Texas
Pericarditis

WILLIAM F. YOUNG, JR., M.D.

Associate Professor of Medicine, Mayo Medical School; Consultant, Division of Hypertension and Division of Endocrinology, Metabolism and Internal Medicine, Mayo Clinic and Mayo Foundation, Rochester, Minnesota
Pheochromocytoma

SETH M. ZEIDMAN, M.D.

Senior Resident, Department of Neurosurgery, The Johns Hopkins University School of Medicine, Baltimore; Clinical Associate, Surgical Neurology Branch, National Institute for Neurological Disorders and Strokes, National Institutes of Health, Bethesda, Maryland
Trigeminal Neuralgia

JAIME ZIGHELBOIM, M.D.

Senior Gastroenterology Fellow, Mayo Clinic, Rochester, Minnesota
Irritable Bowel Syndrome

MARJORIE L. ZUCKER, M.D.

Clinical Associate Professor, University of Kansas Medical Center, Kansas City, Kansas; Clinical Pathologist, St. Luke's Hospital, Kansas City, Missouri
Vitamin K Deficiency

STEPHEN D. ZUCKER, M.D.

Instructor in Medicine, Harvard Medical School; Associate Physician, Brigham and Women's Hospital, Boston, Massachusetts
Cirrhosis; Bleeding Esophageal Varices

Preface

This is the 46th year that *Current Therapy* has been published since the first edition in 1949. As always, this is a completely new book when compared with the 1993 edition. More than 80% of the authors are new, and the continuing authors have thoroughly revised and updated their material. This extensive annual updating is necessary to remain current with the rapidly changing technical and therapeutic advances in medicine.

Practitioners who have extensive experience treating each problem and who are at the leading edge of new developments share their favorite methods and medications, some of which may not yet have the approval of the U.S. Food and Drug Administration. In addition, this year's author may have a different approach to the problem from that of previous authors, giving the reader a variety of options. Our goal is to speed the transfer of knowledge acquired in the research laboratory to the field, where it can be put to practical use.

Our primary mission remains unchanged: to provide the practicing physician with a concise, practical reference containing the most recent advances in therapy in a format that is easily accessible and reasonably priced. The editorial staff at W. B. Saunders has done an excellent job of keeping the text concise and easy to read. With the renewed attention to the need for primary care, physicians trained in subspecialties who are being called on to provide an increasing amount of this care will find the up-to-date management of common problems presented in this text particularly helpful.

The treatment of injuries caused by hazardous marine animals is a new addition this year and seems appropriate with the increasing popularity of snorkeling and scuba diving. As in previous editions, there is extensive coverage of acute poisonings and a thorough index.

My special thanks to Ray Kersey and the excellent staff at W. B. Saunders; Jeanne Ullian, my editorial assistant who organizes and manages deadlines and communication with authors; and my wife, Peggy, who assists Jeanne and me in so many ways. I also want to thank the many physicians who rely on these annual editions to remain current with advances in medicine and who send me their comments and suggestions.

ROBERT E. RAKEL, M.D.

NOTICE

Medicine is an ever-changing field. Standard safety precautions must be followed, but as new research and clinical experience broaden our knowledge, changes in treatment and drug therapy become necessary or appropriate. The editors of this work have carefully checked the generic and trade drug names and verified drug dosages to ensure that the dosage information in this work is accurate and in accord with the standards accepted at the time of publication. Readers are advised, however, to check the product information currently provided by the manufacturer of each drug to be administered to be certain that changes have not been made in the recommended dose or in the contraindications for administration. This is of particular importance in regard to new or infrequently used drugs. It is the responsibility of the treating physician, relying on experience and knowledge of the patient, to determine dosages and the best treatment for the patient. The editors cannot be responsible for misuse or misapplication of the material in this work.

THE PUBLISHER

Contents

SECTION 1. SYMPTOMATIC CARE PENDING DIAGNOSIS

SECTION 2. THE INFECTIOUS DISEASES

SECTION 3. THE RESPIRATORY SYSTEM

SECTION 4. THE CARDIOVASCULAR SYSTEM

SECTION 5. THE BLOOD AND SPLEEN

SECTION 6. THE DIGESTIVE SYSTEM

SECTION 7. METABOLIC DISORDERS

SECTION 8. THE ENDOCRINE SYSTEM

SECTION 9. THE UROGENITAL TRACT

SECTION 10. THE SEXUALLY TRANSMITTED DISEASES

SECTION 11. DISEASES OF ALLERGY

SECTION 12. DISEASES OF THE SKIN

SECTION 13. THE NERVOUS SYSTEM

SECTION 14. THE LOCOMOTOR SYSTEM

SECTION 15. OBSTETRICS AND GYNECOLOGY

SECTION 16. PSYCHIATRIC DISORDERS

SECTION 17. PHYSICAL AND CHEMICAL INJURIES

SECTION 18. APPENDICES AND INDEX

Symptomatic Care Pending Diagnosis

PAIN

method of
ALEXANDER MAUSKOP, M.D.
New York Headache Center
New York, New York

PHARMACOTHERAPY

Pharmacologic management has been the mainstay of treatment for many pain syndromes; however, nonpharmacologic therapies can at times be more effective and should not be used as methods of last resort. Examples include biofeedback for patients with headaches and physical therapy for patients with many forms of chronic low back pain.

The three major groups of drugs used in pain management are nonsteroidal anti-inflammatory drugs (NSAIDs), opiates, and adjuvant medications.

Nonsteroidal Anti-Inflammatory Drugs

Aspirin and ibuprofen (Advil, Motrin) are sold over the counter, and many patients try them before seeking medical care. It is necessary for the physician to establish that the dosage and the frequency of self-administration were sufficient before giving up on this group of medications. Failure of one NSAID to relieve pain does not mean that another one is not effective. Side effects can also be idiosyncratic. For example, naproxen (Naprosyn) and indomethacin (Indocin) can produce gastrointestinal side effects in a particular patient, whereas naproxen sodium (Anaprox) and diclofenac sodium (Voltaren) do not.

NSAIDs can be surprisingly effective in the relief of pain from metastatic bone disease. Opiates and NSAIDs have different mechanisms of action and together can have a synergistic effect. This combination may reduce the dose requirement of an opiate and consequently reduce its side effects. Longer acting NSAIDs, such as piroxicam (Feldene) given at 20 mg once a day, diflunisal (Do-lobid) given at 500 mg twice a day, choline or magnesium salicylate (Trilisate) given at 1500 mg twice a day, nabumetone (Relafen) given at 1000 mg once a day, and sustained-release indomethacin (Indocin SR) given at 75 mg once a day, are preferred in patients who have continuous pain. Short-acting NSAIDs include ibuprofen (Motrin, Advil) given at 400 to 600 mg every 4 hours, aspirin given at 650 to 1000 mg every 3 to 4 hours, and ketoprofen (Orudis) given at 50 mg four times a day. Ketorolac tromethamine (Toradol) is the first NSAID to be available in a parenteral form; the efficacy of a 30-mg intramuscular injection is comparable with that of an injection of 10 mg of morphine. Ketorolac (60 mg IM) has replaced dihydroergotamine (DHE-45) as the author's drug of first choice for office management of a patient with an acute migraine attack. Sometimes the author injects ketorolac in the office to relieve acute low back or neck pain.

Opiates

Important characteristics of opiate drugs and their relative potencies are shown in Table 1. Unlike NSAIDs, opiate drugs do not have a ceiling effect. This means that with the development of tolerance in order to regain pain relief, the dose of an opiate can be escalated indefinitely. Usually, the development of side effects limits such escalation, although some patients can tolerate an equivalent of up to several grams of morphine a day, given parenterally. These patients remain functional because gradual escalation of the dose leads to the development of tolerance not only to pain relief but also to side effects. The development of tolerance to an opiate is usually manifested by a shorter duration of action. Because cross-tolerance between different opiates is incomplete, switching to a different opiate may forestall escalation of the dose. Combinations of NSAIDs and adjuvant analgesics with opiates constitute another useful approach. Development of tolerance and physical dependence is often

TABLE 1. **Dosing Data for Opioid Analgesics**

Drug	Approximate Equianalgesic Oral Dose	Approximate Equianalgesic Parenteral Dose
Opioid Agonist		
Morphine	30 mg q 3–4 h (around-the-clock dosing)	10 mg q 3–4 h
	60 mg q 3–4 h (single dose or intermittent dosing)	
Codeine	130 mg q 3–4 h	75 mg q 3–4 h
Hydromorphone (Dilaudid)	7.5 mg q 3–4 h	1.5 mg q 3–4 h
Hydrocodone (in Lorcet, Lortab, Vicodin, others)	30 mg q 3–4 h	Not available
Levorphanol (Levo-Dromoran)	4 mg q 6–8 h	2 mg q 6–8 h
Meperidine (Demerol)	300 mg q 2–3 h	100 mg q 3 h
Methadone (Dolophine, others)	20 mg q 6–8 h	10 mg q 6–8 h
Oxycodone (Roxicodone, also in Percocet, Percodan, Tylox, others)	30 mg q 3–4 h	Not available
Oxymorphone (Numorphan)	Not available	1 mg q 3–4 h
Opioid Agonist-Antagonist and Partial Agonist		
Buprenorphine (Buprenex)	Not available	0.3–0.4 mg q 6–8 h
Butorphanol (Stadol)	Not available	2 mg q 3–4 h
Nalbuphine (Nubain)	Not available	10 mg q 3–4 h
Pentazocine (Talwin, others)	150 mg q 3–4 h	60 mg q 3–4 h

Adapted from Agency for Health Care Policy and Research: Acute Pain Management in Adults: Operative Procedures (Pub. No. 92-0032). Washington, DC, Public Health Service, U.S. Department of Health and Human Services, 1992.

mistakenly equated with addiction. In a tolerant patient receiving a high dose of an opiate drug, symptoms of withdrawal can appear within 6 hours of the last dose. Addiction, in contrast, is characterized by craving for the drug, efforts to secure a supply of the drug, and not following a physician's directions regarding usage.

Both physicians and patients have an instinctive fear of opiates because of the potential for addiction. Sometimes the use of an opiate in a cancer patient is equated with imminent death. A large amount of data indicates that the risk of iatrogenic opiate addiction is extremely small and can be predicted in the majority of cases by a patient's history of prior addictions. The author always brings up this topic because many patients do not verbalize their fears and, if not reassured, are reluctant to take sufficient amounts, if any, of the drug. Another obstacle to the proper use of opiates is an exaggerated concern about respiratory and central nervous system (CNS) depression. Tolerance to these side effects of opiates develops quickly. Patients do not become oversedated or stop breathing while in pain. When a patient receiving a steady dose of an opiate suddenly becomes drowsy or demonstrates respiratory depression, the most likely cause is a new systemic problem, such as an infection or liver or kidney failure. When pain can be controlled only with some degree of sedation, a stimulant, such as dextroamphetamine (Dexedrine) given at 5 mg twice a day, may not only improve the alertness but provide analgesia as well. Dextroamphetamine has mild analgesic properties synergistic with opioid analgesics.

The major side effect of opiates that must be anticipated is constipation. Senna concentrate (Senokot) is an anecdotal favorite used to combat this problem. Transdermal fentanyl (Duragesic) tends to produce less constipation than do oral opiates.

Meperidine (Demerol) is a popular drug, but it is the only opiate that should not be used continuously for more than a few days. Meperidine is metabolized into normeperidine, which is a CNS stimulant. With chronic administration, meperidine can cause irritability, tremor, and generalized seizures.

Until recently, the preferred route of administration of medications has been oral. With the introduction of transdermal fentanyl (Duragesic), the author has found that many patients do better with a fentanyl patch. This product provides a steady level of an opiate drug with practical and psychologic benefits. The patches last for about 3 days and come in four strengths. Because of the long half-life of the drug, the process of determining the optimal dose of the patch may take up to a few weeks. While this adjustment is being made, patients should be given a short-acting opiate such as oxycodone (Percocet, Percodan), morphine sulfate (Roxanol), or hydromorphone (Dilaudid) for breakthrough pain. This also applies to the titration phase of other long-acting oral opiates, including sustained-release morphine (MS Contin, Oramorph SR), methadone (Dolophine), and levorphanol (Levo-Dromoran). Methadone is an excellent analgesic with good absorption and, in the author's experience, fewer side effects than other opiates. It is also one of the most inexpensive opiates, although it can be difficult to obtain from some pharmacies.

Rectal suppositories of morphine, hydromorphone, and oxymorphone (Numorphan) are useful for patients who cannot take oral preparations. The rectal route is not practical for long-term management and when high doses are needed.

Intranasal administration of butorphanol (Stadol NS) produces a rapid onset of action. The limitation of this drug in current formulation is that the dose contained in each spray is excessive for many patients. This results in a high incidence of CNS side effects. Reformulation at a low dose may improve the utility of this drug. Butorphanol is not a controlled substance because it is a partial agonist-antagonist drug with a lower potential for addiction. It should not be given to patients who are maintained on opiates that are pure agonists (see Table 1) because the antagonist properties can lead to a withdrawal reaction when the drug is discontinued. Patients on chronic opiate maintenance become very sensitive to all opiate antagonists. Should a need arise to reverse the effect of an opiate in such a patient, naloxone (Narcan) must be diluted with saline and infused very gradually.

When a patient with continuous pain cannot take oral medications, subcutaneous (SC) infusion of opiates is an alternative to the transdermal route and has many advantages over intravenous infusion. The patch should be tried first, but when it is ineffective at a high dose (e.g., two Duragesic-100 patches) or causes side effects, SC infusion is the method of choice. SC infusion is administered with the use of a programmable, portable pump that can be filled with a solution of any opiate, including morphine, hydromorphone, methadone, and levorphanol. The pump is connected to a 25-gauge butterfly needle that can be inserted subcutaneously by the patient or a family member. An intravenous infusion of an opiate may be necessary only if a patient requires a very large volume of an opiate or if other routes are not tolerated.

The use of opiate analgesics has been limited mostly to cancer patients. Their prolonged use in non–cancer patients with pain remains controversial. Many anecdotal reports and the author's personal experience suggest that under strict supervision, selected non-cancer patients with pain can derive great benefits from chronic opiate therapy. Such patients are usually those who do not develop significant tolerance and can remain on a steady dose for long periods of time with few side effects. The author obtains an informed consent from such patients, sees them at least once a month, and tries to make opiates only a part of the pain management program.

Adjuvant Analgesics

This is a diverse group of medications that were not known to have analgesic properties when they were first introduced. The most useful drugs for chronic pain and headache management are tricyclic antidepressants (TCAs). Among the TCAs, amitriptyline (Elavil) has been studied most extensively but nortriptyline (Pamelor), imipramine (Tofranil), and desipramine (Norpramin) are also effective and may produce fewer anticholinergic side effects. If one TCA is ineffective or produces unacceptable side effects, another TCA should be tried.

The starting doses for any TCA are 25 mg in young or middle-aged patients and 10 mg in elderly persons. The average effective dose is 50 to 75 mg taken once a day in the evening. Some patients may require and tolerate antidepressant doses of up to 300 mg or more a day in order to achieve pain or headache relief. Patients must be told that these medications are antidepressants but that they are also used for chronic painful conditions, even if there is no associated depression. If patients discover from other sources that TCAs are antidepressant drugs, they may become angry and noncompliant; they may think that their complaints were interpreted as depressive symptoms and not real pain. Warning patients about possible side effects such as dryness of the mouth, drowsiness, and constipation also improves compliance. Some of the contraindications for the use of TCAs include concomitant use of monoamine oxidase inhibitors, recent myocardial infarction, cardiac arrhythmias, glaucoma, and urinary retention. An electrocardiogram should be obtained before the initiation of treatment in all elderly patients.

Other antidepressants including fluoxetine (Prozac), bupropion (Wellbutrin), sertraline (Zoloft), and phenelzine (Nardil) may have some utility in pain management. No large trials of these drugs have been conducted in pain patients to show any benefits beyond their antidepressant effect.

Anticonvulsants that are commonly used for pain relief are carbamazepine (Tegretol) and phenytoin (Dilantin). It has been suggested that anticonvulsants are more effective for sharp, lancinating pain, whereas TCAs are better for burning, dysesthetic pain.

Hydroxyzine (Vistaril, Atarax) has mild analgesic properties, but what makes it a useful adjuvant analgesic is its reduction of anxiety and nausea.

Caffeine has been shown to enhance the effect of other analgesics and to have mild analgesic properties of its own. It is useful in a variety of pain syndromes, but it is most commonly used for headaches. Overuse of caffeine in drinks (coffee, tea, colas) and medications (Excedrin, Anacin, Fiorinal, Esgic, Norgesic) can lead to severe withdrawal headaches and other symptoms when use of the drug is stopped. As little as three cups of coffee a day can lead to a withdrawal syndrome.

Corticosteroids can be effective in relieving pain from various causes. Long-term side effects and loss of efficacy limits their use to treatment of acute pain syndromes, such as those involving the spinal cord, a plexus, or nerve compression.

PSYCHOLOGICAL METHODS

These methods are indispensable in the management of patients with chronic pain. Pain affects all aspects of chronic pain patients' lives and the lives of people who live and work with them. For this reason, the psychologist is a crucial member of the pain management team. Chronic pain of long duration is very unlikely to respond to a single treatment modality. Patients should not be allowed to pick and choose their treatment. The author explains to such patients that pain control can be achieved only by attacking the problem with several methods at the same time. Psychological methods may include behavior modification, cognitive psychotherapy, biofeedback, and relaxation training. On occasion, in an anxious patient with acute or cancer pain, simple reassurance may reduce the need for opiate analgesics. In some patients, music therapy can have beneficial effects. Benzodiazepines usually have little utility in pain management, except for acute pain of muscle spasm. However, in an anxious patient with cancer pain, a short course of diazepam (Valium) or clonazepam (Klonopin) may help.

ANESTHETIC APPROACHES

Muscle spasm is a common primary cause of pain, and it often accompanies pain of other types. Trigger point injections are very effective in the management of acute pain caused by muscle spasm. They usually involve the use of a long-acting local anesthetic, bupivacaine (Marcaine).

Nerve blocks can provide temporary relief of pain in patients with local pain. Some physicians use them to predict possible efficacy of a nerve ablation. The author much more commonly injects a corticosteroid such as betamethasone (Celestone Soluspan) or methylprednisolone (Depo-Medrol) into an area surrounding the nerve. Although such an injection cannot be considered a nerve block, a similar technique is used. Examples of conditions that benefit from corticosteroid injections include carpal tunnel syndrome, meralgia paresthetica, and occipital neuralgia.

Sympathetic block is the most effective procedure for the treatment of reflex sympathetic dystrophy, especially when blocks are combined with vigorous physical therapy and, if necessary, pharmacotherapy and psychological methods. This combined treatment works best if it is started early in the course of the disease.

Epidural and spinal infusions of opiates and local anesthetics are useful in some cancer patients and in a few selected patients with a "failed back syndrome."

NEUROSURGICAL METHODS

In attempting to stop transmission of pain signals along the nervous system, neurosurgeons have tried placing lesions anywhere from the peripheral nerves all the way up to the frontal cortex. Nerve section can be effective in patients with meralgia paresthetica, occipital neuralgia, and some other focal neuropathic pains. It is not effective, however, in patients with postherpetic neuralgia. Some patients with trigeminal neuralgia find temporary relief when the nerve leading to the trigger area is sectioned. A lesion in the dorsal root entry zone can sometimes relieve pain caused by brachial plexus avulsion and anesthesia dolorosa. Section of half of the spinal cord (cordotomy) is effective in patients with cancer who have unilateral pain below the waist. Bilateral cordotomy usually leads to loss of sphincter control and should be reserved for cancer patients who have already lost such control. Hypophysectomy should be considered in women whose pain is resistant to other modalities and who have hormonal (breast or ovarian) cancers.

PHYSICAL METHODS

Physical therapy is the main treatment modality for most patients with low back and neck pain. It is also essential in the management of reflex sympathetic dystrophy. Patients with almost any pain syndrome benefit from regular exercise. Improved cardiovascular and pulmonary function from aerobic exercise is of significant benefit in itself, but it also provides important psychological benefits. Patients feel that they are regaining some control over their bodies and feel less helpless and hopeless. Regular exercise helps to alleviate stress, which is a major contributing factor in chronic headaches, back pain, and other pain syndromes.

Other physical methods include transcutaneous electrical nerve stimulation and acupuncture. Neither method has been scientifically proved to be effective; however, a large body of anecdotal evidence indicates that they can be very helpful in some patients. Results of experiments detailing opiate and nonopiate mechanisms of acupuncture analgesia in animals, as well as the successful use of acupuncture in veterinary medicine, suggest that the effect of acupuncture is superior to placebo. The author usually uses acupuncture in elderly patients, patients who do not tolerate any medications, and patients who have tried a variety of treatments without relief. In patients with chronic pain, acupuncture should be used as a part of multidisciplinary approach.

NAUSEA AND VOMITING

method of
LOWELL B. ANTHONY, M.D.
Vanderbilt University
Nashville, Tennessee

Nausea and vomiting are protective reflexes activated by a wide range of gastrointestinal and nongastrointestinal causes. Even though nausea is usually an accompanying symptom, vomiting can occur with little or no warning. The general approach to the management of nausea and vomiting is to narrow the differential diagnosis by first using subjective and objective data and then treating the most probable underlying cause. For the control of cancer chemotherapy induced emesis, an effective antiemetic scheduled regimen should be administered before and after the emetogenic stimuli.

Nausea and emesis result from efferent stimuli from the medullary vomiting center to striated muscles of the chest and abdomen and the smooth muscles of the gastrointestinal system. This final coordinating center in the medulla receives input not only from other areas within the brain (the medullary chemoreceptor trigger zone, the cerebrum, and the limbic and vestibular systems) but also from visceral stimuli (cardiac and gastrointestinal neuroreceptors). Central and peripheral neurotransmitters that play an important role in nausea and vomiting include dopamine, acetylcholine, serotonin, histamine, and endorphins.

INITIAL ASSESSMENT AND DIFFERENTIAL DIAGNOSIS

Gastrointestinal, central nervous system, iatrogenic, and systemic disorders may produce nausea and vomiting as an initial or a late manifestation of an underlying disorder (Table 1). Iatrogenic causes may also be an unexpected warning of drug toxicity or are anticipated side effects from treatment. The patient's history provides crucial information regarding any relationship to meals and the onset, character, frequency,

and intensity of nausea and emesis. Pertinent historical data also include the presence of fever, pain (abdominal or cephalic), changes in bowel habits, gallstones, kidney stones, jaundice, weight loss, medications, concomitant illnesses, previous operations, and personal habits.

Objective evaluation includes the physical, laboratory, and radiologic examinations. The physical examination allows for not only observing signs accompanying the illness but also assessing hydration and the cardiovascular status in order to initiate supportive measures before the final diagnosis is made. Screening laboratory tests include serum chemistries documenting acid-base electrolyte status, glucose, calcium, urinary abnormalities, human chorionic gonadotropin–beta (hCG-β) (if pregnancy is suspected), amylase, gastrointestinal bleeding, drug levels (including urinary toxicologic screening if drug overdose is being evaluated), and peritoneal aspirate along with evaluating renal, cardiac, and hepatic functions. Radiologic tests, including chest x-ray and

TABLE 1. **Some Causes of Nausea and Vomiting**

Gastrointestinal Disorders
Peptic ulcer disease/gastritis
Intestinal obstruction/ileus/perforation
Cholelithiasis/cholecystitis
Constipation/fecal impaction
Adhesions
Gastric cancer
Pancreatitis/pancreatic tumors
Motility disorders
Autonomic neuropathy
Central Nervous System Disorders
Migraine
Motion sickness
Vestibular dysfunction/Ménière's disease
Brain tumor/carcinomatous meningitis
Brain abscess
Hydrocephalus
Iatrogenic Causes
Medications:
Antineoplastic agents
Morphine/analgesics
Theophylline
Digitalis/digoxin
Anesthetic agents
L-Dopa/bromocriptine
Radiation therapy
Postoperative factors
Systemic Causes
Pregnancy
Infectious causes/food poisoning
Diabetic ketoacidosis
Uremia
Chronic hepatic disease
Adrenal insufficiency
Paraneoplastic syndromes
Hypercalcemia
Drug overdose
Heavy metal poisoning
Psychogenic Causes

flat and upright abdominal films, and abdominal ultrasonography complete the initial evaluation and usually result in narrowing the diagnostic focus to one major organ system.

Assessment of Causes of Nausea and Vomiting in Cancer Patients

Special consideration is required in order to determine whether nausea and vomiting are iatrogenic or indications of disease-related effects. Mechanical or nonmechanical bowel obstruction should be carefully ruled out. Not only may adhesions from prior operations develop, but inactivity, metabolic effects, and drugs can decrease bowel motility. Constipation and fecal impaction, accompanying the use of moderate to strong analgesics, must be considered as causes of nausea and vomiting in cancer patients. Central nervous system metastases can manifest with nausea and emesis as the initial indications of disease spread.

Cancer chemotherapy–induced nausea and emesis are usually temporally related to drug administration. The severity of nausea and vomiting is dependent on which drug or drugs are administered (Table 2). Nausea and emesis in cancer patients can also result from conditioning that occurs when antiemetic protection is not complete. These anticipatory symptoms develop in about 25% of patients and can affect compliance with the treatment regimen.

Delayed nausea and vomiting occur more with

TABLE 2. **Emetic Potency of Chemotherapeutic Agents**

Severe
Cisplatin
Dacarbazine
Nitrogen mustard
Streptozocin
Moderately Severe
Cyclophosphamide
Ifosfamide
Doxorubicin
Nitrosoureas
Actinomycin D
Moderate
Cytarabine
Procarbazine
Mitomycin C
High-dose methotrexate
Mild
Etoposide
5-Fluorouracil
Hydroxyurea
Bleomycin
Vinblastine
Vincristine
Chlorambucil
Low-dose methotrexate

cisplatin-based regimens and usually resolve within 4 to 14 days after the treatment ends. Patients in whom pain, protracted nausea and emesis, fever, and metabolic effects develop and do not respond to effective antiemetic measures should be evaluated for other causes of emesis.

TREATMENT

General Considerations

Successful control of nausea and vomiting is dependent on identifying the most likely cause of the symptoms. Because antiemetics are routinely used empirically in many instances (except pregnancy and drug overdose), initiating treatment with these agents alone or with intravenous fluids allows the patient to be comfortable while evaluation is underway. If abdominal pain accompanies nausea and vomiting, surgical opinion may preclude early pharmacologic intervention.

Treatment of nausea and vomiting can be divided into pharmacologic and nonpharmacologic interventions. The latter encompasses dietary restrictions during pregnancy, behavioral techniques for conditioned behavior developing during cancer therapy, Alcoholics Anonymous for alcoholism, dialysis for uremia or drug overdose, radiation therapy or craniotomy or both for central nervous system tumors, nasogastric tube for possible diagnostic and therapeutic intervention, lithotripsy for kidney stones, abdominal surgery for intestinal obstruction and refractory peptic ulcer disease, and cholecystectomy for cholelithiasis and cholecystitis.

Pharmacologic approaches include antiemetic and nonantiemetic agents, depending on the underlying cause. Treatment of the underlying disease with antibiotics, insulin, nitrates, calcium channel blockers, steroids, anticonvulsants, and H_2 antagonists, among other agents indicated for specific diseases, may be accompanied by the empiric use of antiemetics for symptom control.

Antiemetics can be divided into eight major categories (Table 3). Classifying these drugs according to mechanisms of action enables the selection of drugs from different classes when the emetic stimuli is strong and combination drug therapy is warranted. Avoiding combinations of two drugs within the same class decreases the likelihood of an adverse drug reaction, such as acute dystonic reactions with the dopamine antagonists.

A patient's sensitivity, existing diseases, and severity of symptoms determine which specific antiemetic or antiemetic regimen is used. An effective combination regimen (Table 4) for preventing cisplatin-induced emesis includes a serotonin antagonist such as ondansetron (Zofran), a

TABLE 3. **Antiemetic Classification and Recommended Dosages/Schedules**

Drug	Trade Name	Dosage/Administration
Serotonin Antagonists		
Ondansetron	Zofran	0.15–0.36 mg/kg q 4- 8 h IV or a single 32-mg IV dose
		8 mg q 8 h PO
		4 mg q 8 h PO (ages 4–12 years)
Dopamine Antagonists		
PHENOTHIAZINES		
Prochlorperazine	Compazine	5–20 mg q 4–6 h PO or IM
		10–40 mg q 3 h IV
		25 mg q 4–6 h rectally
Thiethylperazine	Torecan	10 mg q 6–8 h PO or IM, rectally
Promethazine	Phenergan	25 mg q 4–6 h PO or IM, rectally
		12.5 mg q 4–6 h IV
Perphenazine	Trilafon	8–16 mg q 4–6 h PO
Chlorpromazine	Thorazine	10–25 mg q 3–6 h PO or IV
		50–100 mg q 6–8 h rectally
BUTYROPHENONES		
Droperidol	Inapsine	1–2 mg q 6–8 h PO or IM
		0.5–10 mg q 2–4 h IV
Haloperidol	Haldol	1–3 mg/kg q 2 h IV
SUBSTITUTED BENZAMIDES		
Metoclopramide	Reglan	1–3 mg/kg q 2 h IV
		10 mg 30 min a.c. PO
Steroids		
Dexamethasone	Decadron	10–20 mg once PO or IV
Methylprednisolone	Solu-Medrol	250–500 mg q 4–6 h IV
Antihistamines		
Diphenhydramine	Benadryl	25–100 mg q 6–8 h PO, IM, or IV
Hydroxyzine	Vistaril	25–100 mg q 6–8 h PO or IV
Meclizine	Antivert	20–50 mg q 24 h PO
Dimenhydrinate	Dramamine	50 mg q 4–8 h PO or IV
Benzodiazepines		
Lorazepam	Ativan	1.0–1.5 mg/m^2 IV or IM
Diazepam	Valium	5–10 mg q 6–8 h PO or IV
Cannabinoids		
Dronabinol	Marinol	5–10 mg/m^2 q 4–6 h PO
Nabilone*	Cesamet	1–2 mg q 12 h PO
Anticholinergics		
Scopolamine	Transderm Scōp	1 patch q 3 days behind ear
Miscellaneous		
Trimethobenzamide	Tigan	100 mg q 4–6 h PO or IM
Benzquinamide	Emete-con	50 mg q 3–4 h IM
		25 mg IV (1 mg/min)

Abbreviations: IV = intravenous; PO = orally; IM = intramuscularly; a.c. = before meals.
*Not available in the United States.

steroid such as dexamethasone (Decadron), and a benzodiazepine such as lorazepam (Ativan). If cost is a primary consideration, a dopamine antagonist such as metoclopramide (Reglan) can be substituted for ondansetron in this regimen. However, ondansetron is the antiemetic of choice if the patient is less than 30 years old, has a history of motion sickness, or has had a previous dystonic reaction to dopamine antagonists.

Antiemetic Drugs

Serotonin Antagonists

The most recent development in antiemetic pharmacology has been the introduction of ondansetron (Zofran), a selective 5-HT$_3$ (serotonin) receptor antagonist. Ondansetron is highly effective in controlling cisplatin-induced emesis and produces few side effects. Headache, which is mild and usually controlled with non-narcotic an-

TABLE 4. **Combination Antiemetic Regimens**

Regimen 1	
Ondansetron	0.15–0.36 mg/kg q 4 h × 3 IV
Dexamethasone	10 mg IV
Lorazepam	1.0–1.5 mg/m^2 IV
Regimen 2	
Metoclopramide	2 mg/kg q 2–4 h × 3 IV
Dexamethasone	10 mg IV
Lorazepam	1.0–1.5 mg/m^2 IV
Diphenhydramine	25–50 mg q 6–8 h IV

Abbreviation: IV = intravenous.

algesics, occurs in about 15% of patients. Some patients also report lightheadedness, and serum transaminase elevations can occur transiently. Extrapyramidal symptoms occurring with dopamine antagonists are rarely seen with serotonin inhibitory drugs. The usual dose is 0.15 mg per kg. A single 32-mg intravenous dose has been shown to be equivalent to 32 mg in divided doses.

Dopamine Antagonists

Phenothiazines. These agents have been the most widely used in controlling non–cisplatin-based cancer chemotherapy–induced emesis. Prochlorperazine (Compazine) is usually given in doses ranging from 5 to 20 mg orally, rectally, or intramuscularly every 4 to 6 hours on an as-needed basis. Thiethylperazine (Torecan), chlorpromazine (Thorazine), perphenazine (Trilafon), and promethazine (Phenergan) are alternative drugs in this class. Unfortunately, the activity of this class of drugs is modest at best, and dose escalation is associated with increased toxicity, including hypotension, extrapyramidal effects, sedation, orthostasis, and anticholinergic effects, which restrict their use in controlling a strong emetic stimulus.

Butyrophenones. The limitations to these agents are similar to those of the phenothiazines. Droperidol (Inapsine), 0.5 to 10 mg every 2 hours, can effectively control cisplatin-induced emesis. Sedation as well as diarrhea can occur at these doses. Adverse effects are similar to the phenothiazines.

Substituted Benzamides. The most widely used agent in controlling cisplatin-induced emesis is metoclopramide (Reglan). Successful dose escalation to 2 mg/kg every 2 hours for five doses, starting one half hour before cisplatin, controls nausea and emesis effectively. Its action in these larger doses most likely involves nonselective serotonin blockade in addition to its dopamine antagonism.

A limitation to the use of metoclopramide is a relatively high incidence of extrapyramidal side effects, including acute dystonic reactions, which can be lessened somewhat with antihistamines or cogentin. Even though these side effects can be anticipated and controlled, they can be alarming to the patient, the patient's family, and sometimes the hospital staff. Somnolence, anxiety, and diarrhea may also be observed.

Another disadvantage to the use of metoclopramide is the lack of a high-dose oral tablet. Even though it has been shown that high-dose oral and intravenous metoclopramide have bioequivalence, the U.S. Food and Drug Administration has approached the high-dose oral formulation as a new drug requiring dose-response efficacy trials. In the outpatient setting, patients take 5 to 15 of the 10-mg tablets every 2 hours if metoclopramide is to be used.

Steroids

Dexamethasone (Decadron) and other steroids have moderate antiemetic activity when used as single agents (10 to 20 mg) with little, if any, toxicity. This class of drugs is generally used in combination with dopamine or serotonin antagonists. The mechanism by which steroids act as antiemetics is unknown. Lower doses of steroids have shown activity when used as single agents in low-dose cisplatin regimens. Because of transient rectal pain that sometimes occurs with rapid dexamethasone infusion, slow infusion is recommended.

Antihistamines

Diphenhydramine (Benadryl) among others, has modest antiemetic activity and is generally used alone for weak emetic stimuli or in combination with metoclopramide for cisplatin-based chemotherapy. This class of drugs can potentially lessen the impact of extrapyramidal symptoms induced by dopamine antagonists. Antihistamines may be administered orally, intramuscularly, or intravenously; the major side effects are sedation and anticholinergic symptoms.

Benzodiazepines

The antiemetic action of benzodiazepines is their effect on cortical pathways and possibly on the medullary vomiting center. Amnesia accompanies the use of benzodiazepines, and this pharmacodynamic effect may be desired because it lessens the conditioning of behavior resulting from emetogenic therapy. This class of antiemetics may also assist in controlling the extrapyramidal side effects of the dopamine antagonists. Lorazepam (Ativan), commonly used because of its short half-life, is given in 1.0- to 1.5-mg/m² doses. Even though benzodiazepines have a wide therapeutic index, respiratory depression can occur.

Cannabinoids

In younger patients (less than 40 years of age), particularly those with a history of marijuana use, cannabinoids may be an effective antiemetic. The antiemetic efficacy of this class of drugs is improved when used in combination with prochlorperazine. Current guidelines require that synthetic cannabinoids be used before a request to the government for legal marijuana use is submitted. Dronabinol (Marinol) is representative of this class and is given in oral doses of 5 to 10 mg/m² every 4 to 6 hours, starting an hour before chemotherapy. The high incidence of central nervous system side effects (including hallucinations, nightmares, anxiety) severely limits their broader use, particularly in older patients (over 60 years of age).

Anticholinergics

This class of antiemetics is used mostly for motion sickness and is represented by scopolamine (Transderm Scōp) formulated as a patch placed behind the ear and changed every third day. Patients should be warned about the proper method of handling the scopolamine patch. After placing the patch, wearers should wash their hands so as to prevent getting the drug in their eyes should they inadvertently rub their eyes. Not washing hands could result in the sudden onset of anisocoria. Even though the antiemetic activity of some of the other drug classes may be explained in part by anticholinergic mechanisms, drugs in this class are not generally used as single agents in suppressing cancer chemotherapy–induced emesis.

Miscellaneous

Other drugs are used more often with less serious emetic stimuli. They are well tolerated and produce few side effects. Representative agents include trimethobenzamide (Tigan) and benzquinamide (Emete-con).

Special Circumstances in Controlling Nausea and Vomiting

Cancer Chemotherapy–Induced Nausea and Vomiting

Preventing nausea and vomiting from emetogenic therapy is dependent on giving antiemetics prophylactically and in combination (see Table 4). Antiemetics used as rescuing agents are not as effective but are generally offered anyway. Avoiding rescue drugs in the same class as those given previously may lessen the likelihood of an adverse reaction.

Drug Overdose

Nausea and vomiting accompanying drug overdose may be a contraindication to antiemetic therapy until the risk for central nervous system or cardiac complications is lessened.

Parkinson's Disease and Pheochromocytoma

Parkinson's disease and pheochromocytoma are two situations in which dopamine antagonists used to treat nausea and vomiting can exacerbate the underlying disease. Carbidopa (Sinemet) has fewer gastrointestinal effects than L-dopa. In approximately 15% of patients treated with bromo-

criptine (Parlodel), significant nausea and vomiting develop. The use of serotonin antagonists is an additional treatment option.

Diabetes Mellitus

Promotility agents such as metoclopramide in low doses may be the antiemetics of choice for nausea and vomiting resulting from diabetic gastroparesis. Ten milligrams of metoclopramide taken 30 minutes before meals may ameliorate these symptoms.

Carcinoid Tumor/Syndrome

Nausea and vomiting accompanying carcinoid syndrome, a hyperserotonergic state, is usually secondary to the effects of the tumor and not to serotonin stimulation of the chemoreceptor trigger zone or vomiting center. Octreotide (Sandostatin), a somatostatin analogue, should be considered in the management of nausea and vomiting in patients with hormonally active neoplasms.

Delayed Emesis After Cancer Chemotherapy

Prolonged nausea associated with anorexia and vomiting beginning 24 hours or more after cisplatin-based chemotherapy are referred to as delayed emesis. Cytotoxic damage to the gastrointestinal mucosa may account for nausea and emesis that occur when the noxious stimulus is no longer present. Continuing effective antiemetics, such as oral ondansetron, metoclopramide, or a phenothiazine for at least 4 days after chemotherapy treatment may be indicated. Because sustained use beyond 4 to 7 days may cause adverse effects, the administration of antiemetics on an as-needed basis is preferred should nausea persist for longer than a week after cisplatin therapy.

Anticipatory Emesis

The development of nausea and vomiting after an aversive experience occurs in 25 to 40% of patients receiving cancer chemotherapy. Effectively controlling emesis is the best method of preventing the occurrence of this conditioned response. The amnestic effect of the benzodiazepines may also help reduce the incidence of anticipatory emesis if the antiemetic regimen is only partially effective. Behavioral methods employing relaxation and imagery, guided by an experienced clinician, is an additional treatment option if conditioning interferes with compliance.

Nausea and Vomiting Accompanying Pregnancy

Morning or evening sickness is common during the first trimester of pregnancy. These symptoms usually abate during the second trimester. More severe symptoms may be associated with multiple pregnancy or with a hydatidiform mole.

Pharmacologic intervention is usually unnecessary. Reassurance, rest, frequent small meals, and dietary restrictions may be all that is required. For some patients, 50 to 100 mg of pyridoxine (vitamin B_6) a day is beneficial. If symptoms are more persistent and protracted, as in hyperemesis gravidarum, hospitalization and intravenous fluids may be required. No antiemetic drugs have been approved for use during pregnancy. The selection of any pharmacologic agent should be based on the severity of symptoms and the potential risk to the fetus. Metoclopramide and the phenothiazines are effective in controlling pregnancy-related nausea and vomiting.

Postanesthesia Nausea and Vomiting

About 80% of patients have nausea and vomiting during the peri- or postoperative period. Use of ondansetron may avoid the sedation, hypotension, and extrapyramidal reactions associated with the phenothiazines and substituted benzamides.

Motion Sickness

Anticholinergics and antihistamines are commonly used in the management of motion sickness. Small, bland meals may be another effective measure. Scopolamine placed behind the ear may be convenient for patients exposed to motion for long periods.

GASEOUSNESS AND INDIGESTION

method of
MILES AUSLANDER, M.D.
Encino, California

Gaseousness and indigestion are among the most common of gastrointestinal symptoms. Although they often coexist, they may have very different etiologies and significances.

GASEOUSNESS

The nonspecific complaints of eructation, flatus, bloating, and distention may be evidence of serious bowel obstruction or simple dietary indiscretion. Increased abdominal gas may be caused by excessive air swallowing, such as occurs in patients with chronic obstructive pulmonary disease or in anxious patients with aerophagia. In other patients, the excessive gas is hydrogen, methane, and carbon dioxide produced by the fer-

mentation of nondigestible carbohydrates. High-fiber foods, especially vegetables such as broccoli and cauliflower, tend to produce gas. Many people maldigest the lactose of milk, ice cream, and soft cheeses. Blacks and Asians are particularly prone to lactase deficiency and experience gaseousness (as well as diarrhea) with excessive intake of dairy products. Other carbohydrates such as fructose and sorbitol that are found in certain fruits, apple juice, and dietetic sweeteners produce similar symptoms. Excessive gas from these mechanisms is also increased in patients with prolonged intestinal transit times. The spastic colon with chronic constipation causes gas retention and increased fermentation time within the colon.

Many patients with the irritable bowel syndrome feel gassy and bloated but do not actually have more gas than do normal people. Part of the functional disease of the gut is a heightened sensitivity to distention with resultant discomfort. Obstruction of the intestinal tract also causes gaseous distention. Gastric outlet obstruction distends the stomach, and adhesions may block the small bowel. Tumor, ischemia, inflammation, and ileus can all result in intestinal distention.

The evaluation of patients with gas should include a careful history and physical examination with special attention to diet and bowel movement patterns. The need for diagnostic tests is increased if the patient reports rectal bleeding, weight loss, localized pain, nausea, or vomiting. Physical findings of a mass, localized tenderness, and occult gastrointestinal blood loss also mandate evaluation.

For patients with acute symptoms or in whom the degree of gaseousness is in question, abdominal flat and upright radiographs can diagnose gastric outlet or bowel obstruction. The finding of a normal gas pattern but considerable retained fecal matter suggests constipation with a functional bowel. If dietary carbohydrate maldigestion is suspected on the basis of the history, breath tests for hydrogen and intestinal gas analysis can be performed. A simple elimination diet, however, is effective for diagnosis as well as for therapy. When more significant disease is suspected, the intestinal tract should be evaluated by means of barium contrast radiographs or endoscopic examination.

The therapy of gaseousness depends on the etiology. Aerophagia can be reduced by teaching the patient to recognize and avoid air swallowing and to limit the use of chewing gum and drinking straws. Because irritable bowel is a common cause of gaseousness, the restriction of gas-forming foods, antispasmodic medications such as dicyclomine (Bentyl) (20 mg before meals and bedtime), and stool softening and laxative combinations such as docusate sodium with cas-anthranol (Peri-Colace) (one at bedtime) are effective. Bulk-acting laxatives such as psyllium (Metamucil) and methylcellulose (Citrucel) may actually produce gas or a feeling of fullness, in which case they should be avoided. Dietary gaseousness resulting from lactose maldigestion can be improved by using lactase-pretreated milk (LactAid milk) or supplemental lactase enzyme (LactAid Tablets). The maldigested carbohydrates of beans and certain vegetables can be reduced by pretreatment with alpha-d-galactosidase (Beano liquid). Various antigas agents such as simethicone (Mylicon) and charcoal have limited use only for stomach gas resulting from swallowed air.

INDIGESTION

The sense of upper abdominal discomfort ranging from burning to mild nausea to a full, dull aching sensation may be termed "indigestion." In patients with the acute onset of symptoms, often with related fever and diarrhea, an infectious or toxic etiology may be suspected, and the illness is often self-limited. If the symptoms are recent but persistent, with burning pain in the epigastrium or lower chest and related to food, peptic disease is likely. The current recommendations for suspected, uncomplicated peptic disease is to treat the patient with one of the following H_2 blocking agents: cimetidine (Tagamet), 800 mg at bedtime; ranitidine (Zantac) or nizatidine (Axid), 150 mg twice per day; or famotidine (Pepcid), 20 mg twice per day. If the patient responds to the therapy within 10 days, the diagnosis is considered confirmed, and therapy is continued for 6 to 8 weeks. If symptoms persist, diagnostic evaluation, preferably by upper gastrointestinal endoscopy, is suggested. For resistant peptic disease, especially symptomatic esophageal reflux, omeprazole (Prilosec), 20 mg each morning for 6 to 8 weeks, is more effective.

Indigestion can be caused by gallbladder or biliary disease, suspected on the basis of the pattern of illness (occurring during the night, sometimes after a heavy or fatty meal, and associated with nausea and sometimes fever). Diagnostic ultrasonography can confirm gallstones, whereas nuclear biliary imaging can demonstrate the cystic duct obstruction of acute cholecystitis. Although gallbladder disease may be treated expectantly or by stone-dissolving medication, most confirmed cases are best managed by laparoscopic cholecystectomy. Early pancreatitis, bowel obstruction, hepatitis, or any abdominal catastrophe may manifest as indigestion, but the clinical picture soon points toward the correct diagnosis and therapy.

An increasingly recognized cause of indigestion is nonulcer dyspepsia. This functional disease of the upper intestinal tract causes upper abdominal discomfort, nausea, a feeling of fullness, early satiety, and general malaise, but it does not cause systemic features such as fever, weight loss, or gastrointestinal bleeding. Many patients also complain of fatigue, insomnia, and general anxiety. The diagnosis of nonulcer dyspepsia is made by exclusion. Upper gastrointestinal endoscopy is negative. *Helicobactor pylori* gastritis is sometimes detected; however, therapy does not improve symptoms. Solid-phase nuclear medicine gastric emptying is sometimes prolonged, and as in diabetics with gastric paresis, metoclopramide (Reglan), 10 mg before meals and bedtime, may help. For many patients with indigestion, emotional support, low-fat diets, and nonspecific measures, including acid reduction, antispasmodics, and tranquilizers, may control symptoms while newer diagnostic and therapeutic options are awaited.

ACUTE INFECTIOUS DIARRHEA

method of
CHARLES D. ERICSSON, M.D.
University of Texas Medical School, Houston
Houston, Texas

Acute infectious diarrhea is common worldwide and is a cause of serious morbidity and mortality in developing countries, especially in infants and small children. The usual life-threatening event is dehydration and electrolyte imbalance, which are special concerns in malnourished persons, infants, and the elderly. Because of differences in the mix of infective enteropathogens, the approach to laboratory evaluation and empiric therapy is different for adults and infants residing long-term in developed and developing countries, for travelers from industrialized to developing countries, and for homosexual men and persons with AIDS.

The definition of acute infectious diarrhea is variable and differs by age. Many clinical studies have defined diarrhea in adults as the passage of three or more unformed stools in a 24-hour period whether the patient has additional symptoms or not. Less frequent stooling has been defined as diarrhea only when it is accompanied by enteric symptoms such as nausea, vomiting, abdominal pain or cramps, tenesmus, or temperature elevation. Definitions involving passage of increased volumes of unformed stool are important for the physiologist but are not as clinically helpful. The presence of fever and passage of grossly bloody stool even in very small volumes is usually indicative of infection with an invasive enteropathogen such as *Shigella*. As a general rule, clinical symptoms are poorly predictive of the causal agent of diarrhea. A careful history should help to distinguish acute infectious diarrhea from food poisoning; malabsorption syndromes; and diarrhea caused by laxatives, alcohol, antacids, ulcerative colitis, Crohn's disease, and certain malignant tumors. A history of prior antimicrobial use suggests the possibility of *Clostridium difficile* cytotoxin–mediated diarrhea (pseudomembranous enterocolitis).

LABORATORY TESTS

As outlined in Table 1, the use of expensive laboratory tests can sometimes be circumvented in favor of empiric therapy. When laboratory evaluation of diarrhea is indicated, the useful tests include assessment of fecal blood and leukocytes, stains for ova and parasites, and cultures for bacterial enteropathogens. When indicated, stools can be assessed for the presence of *Clostridium difficile* cytotoxin. Tests for rotavirus are available and can be useful in the evaluation of children. Other tests to identify toxin-producing bacteria or genes for invasiveness are research tools at present.

TREATMENT (Table 2)

Symptomatic Relief

The cornerstone of therapy is oral rehydration, which can be lifesaving in the very young and old and in patients with voluminous losses caused by cholera or cholera-like illness. One liter of a typical oral rehydration solution contains the following in grams: NaCl, 3.5; trisodium citrate, 2.9 (or NaHCO$_3$, 2.5); KCl, 1.5; and glucose, 20. This hypertonic solution is used to begin rehydration, and free water is added ad libitum. After rehydration, maintenance solutions containing less sodium (40 to 50 mEq per liter) are administered. Examples include Pedialyte, Lytren, Infalyte, and Resol. Although such oral rehydration solutions may save lives, use of the solution may actually increase diarrheic output. Newer oral rehydration solutions that are cereal based, but require cooking, actually treat the diarrhea while rehydrating the patient. Most travelers or residents in developing countries do not develop dehydrating diarrhea. Any number of beverages taken ad libitum with saltine crackers usually suffice to sustain hydration in these patients. Also, many countries sell flavored (glucose-containing) mineral waters that have an electrolyte content that is sufficient for hydration in non–cholera-like disease.

Bismuth subsalicylate (Pepto-Bismol) has been found to be effective in a number of causes of diarrhea; however, it is not as effective as loperamide (Imodium), which is preferred for moderate to severe diarrhea. Antimotility agents can potentiate disease caused by invasive enteropathogens, and so, alone, they are not used empirically when the patient has fever or is passing bloody stools. Opiates or products containing diphenoxylate (e.g., Lomotil) are not preferred over

TABLE 1. **Approaches to Empiric Therapy and Laboratory Evaluation of Acute Infectious Diarrhea**

Host factor	A	A	A$_T$	I	I	A$_{HM}$	A$_{AIDS}$	E
Location diarrhea acquired	D	U	U	D	U	D, U	D, U	D, U
Common causes of diarrhea	V>>B>>P	V>B, P	B>>V>P	V>>B>>P	B>V>P	B>V>P	B, P, V	B, P, V*
Empiric Approach								
Fever or bloody stools present	1	1 or 2	2	1	1 or 2	2 or 1	1	1
Moderate to severe diarrhea	3	3	4	3	3	2 or 1	1	2 or 3
Mild diarrhea	5	5	4 or 6	5	5	3	3	5

Hosts
A, adult
A$_T$, traveler from developed country
I, infant
A$_{HM}$, homosexual male
A$_{AIDS}$, person with acquired immunodeficiency syndrome (AIDS)
E, elderly
Locations
D, developed country
U, developing country
Causes (>, more common than; >>, much more common than)
V, viral
B, bacterial
P, parasitic
*, causes in the elderly are similar to causes in other adults by location, except that the elderly are more prone to bacteremic salmonellosis
Empiric Approaches (all patients should be rehydrated as necessary)
1. Antimicrobial plus stool evaluation
2. Antimicrobial, stool evaluation if treatment failure
3. Symptomatic therapy plus stool evaluation
4. Combination antimicrobial plus loperamide; stool evaluation if treatment failure
5. Symptomatic therapy; stool evaluation if treatment failure
6. Symptomatic therapy; add antimicrobial if symptoms persist; stool evaluation if symptoms still persist

TABLE 2. **Empiric Therapy for Acute Infectious Diarrhea**

Therapy Type	Dosages		Comments
	Adult	*Pediatric*	
Symptomatic Therapy			
Bismuth subsalicylate (Pepto-Bismol)	30 mL q 30 min for eight doses	3–8 yr: 5 mL 6–9 yr: 10 mL 9–12 yr: 15 mL (q 30 min for eight doses)	If needed, repeat on day 2; black tongue and stools
Loperamide (Imodium)	4 mg, then 2 mg after each loose stool—do not exceed 16 mg/day	2–5 yr: 1 mg tid	OTC preparations: do not exceed 8 mg/day; usually not necessary after first 1–2 days of treatment
Antimicrobials			
Trimethoprim-sulfamethoxazole (Bactrim, Septra); DS tablets (160/800 mg) or suspension (40/200 mg/5 mL)	1 DS tablet bid for 3 days 2 DS tablets, stat	0.5 mL/kg bid for 3 days (do not exceed adult dosage)	Rash <5%, resistance reported; not active against *Campylobacter*
Ciprofloxacin (Cipro) 500-mg tablets 750-mg tablet	1 tablet bid for 3 days 1 tablet stat	— —	Contraindicated in children; rash 1–5%
Furazolidone (Furoxone), 100-mg tablets or 50 mg/15 mL	1 tablet qid for 5 days	8 mg/kg/day in three divided doses for 7 days	Has activity against *Giardia*; not as effective as trimethoprim-sulfamethoxazole or ciprofloxacin

Abbreviation: OTC = over the counter.

loperamide, because they are habit forming and have a less satisfactory safety profile.

A number of other drugs or approaches, such as anticholinergic agents, absorbents (kaolin, charcoal), and aciduric bacteria (*Lactobacillus, Bifidobacterium, Streptococcus faecium*), have shown disappointing results in clinical trials.

Antimicrobial Agents

Most cases of traveler's diarrhea are caused by bacteria (or their toxins), and empiric use of antimicrobial agents has proved useful. Trimethoprim-sulfamethoxazole (Bactrim, Septra) is still effective in central Mexico. However, resistance to trimethoprim-sulfamethoxazole limits its usefulness in most other places in the world. Also, *Campylobacter* is inherently resistant to trimethoprim-sulfamethoxazole. For these reasons, the use of quinolones such as ciprofloxacin (Cipro) has become popular as empiric therapy of bacterial diarrhea. Likewise, *Campylobacter* is an occasional cause of diarrhea among homosexual men or persons with AIDS, so that ciprofloxacin is a logical choice for empiric therapy in these conditions as well.

A single large dose of trimethoprim-sulfamethoxazole or a quinolone has been effective in shigellosis and traveler's diarrhea. The combination of trimethoprim-sulfamethoxazole with loperamide was very effective in traveler's diarrhea

when the predominant organism was enterotoxigenic *Escherichia coli*. A quinolone with loperamide was somewhat more effective than either agent alone when enterotoxigenic *E. coli* was common; however, when *Campylobacter* was common, the combination was only minimally more effective than either drug alone.

Certain antimicrobials are indicated for a specific organism. When cholera is suspected, tetracycline (Sumycin, 500 mg four times daily for 3 to 5 days) is the drug of choice. Erythromycin (E.E.S., E-Mycin, ERYC, 500 mg four times daily for 3 to 5 days) can be used for *Campylobacter*. Metronidazole (Flagyl) is indicated for the treatment of giardiasis (2 grams daily for 3 days) or amebiasis (750 mg three times a day for 5 days). *Clostridium difficile* cytotoxin–mediated colitis can be treated with oral vancomycin (Vancocin), 125 mg four times a day for 7 to 10 days, or metronidazole (Flagyl), 250 mg three times a day for 7 to 10 days.

PREVENTION OF DIARRHEA

Both bismuth subsalicylate and antimicrobial agents have been studied and are effective in the prevention of traveler's diarrhea. The latter are generally not recommended. Bismuth subsalicylate, taken as two tablets chewed four times a day beginning on the first day of travel, confers 65% protection. Travelers need to be warned about the probability of developing black tongues and stools, and this approach should not be used longer than 3 weeks or in persons who cannot otherwise take salicylates.

CONSTIPATION

method of
GEORGE J. WALKER, M.D., and
M. SCOTT HARRIS, M.D.

University of Wisconsin Medical School,
Milwaukee Clinical Campus
Milwaukee, Wisconsin

Constipation is one of the most common gastrointestinal complaints in the United States. It accounts for approximately 2.5 million visits to physicians each year. More than $3.5 million is spent annually on over-the-counter laxatives. At least 120 laxative products are currently available. Although constipation affects people of all ages, both males and females, and people of all educational and socioeconomic levels, it is more common in the elderly, and women are affected two to three times more often than are men.

Although constipation is a common problem, it is one that is poorly understood. Constipation represents an abnormality of bowel function. The term "abnormality" implies a deviation from normal, but there is no agreement as to what constitutes normal bowel habits. Physicians know what constipation is but have trouble accurately defining it. Patients may complain of bowel movements that are too infrequent or stools that are too hard, or they may be referring to defecation that feels incomplete. These symptoms may or may not imply specific abnormalities in bowel function. Because stool frequency is the easiest factor to measure, it is often used as a definition. Three stools per week is the most commonly accepted definition of normal bowel function, but great variation in bowel frequency exists in the general population.

ASSESSMENT

A variety of diseases and conditions cause or are associated with constipation (Table 1). Medications should always be considered as a cause of constipation. Chronic stimulant laxative abuse can result in cathartic colon from damage to neural elements. Depressed patients are more likely to become constipated, but many of the drugs used to treat depression are themselves constipating. In many patients, no immediate cause is identified.

Evaluation of patients with constipation requires understanding of normal function of the colon and anorectal area. In normal persons, approximately 1500 to 2000 mL of water is delivered from the small intestine each day. The colon is able to reduce the water content of the stool to

about 100 to 200 mL. A phase change from liquid to semisolid occurs in the right and transverse colon. This is accomplished partly as a result of the to-and-fro action of colonic motility. Derangements in neural or muscular tone may disturb this function. When colonic transit time is prolonged (colonic inertia), excess fecal water reabsorption and retention may occur. The rectosigmoid acts as a reservoir that retains stool before defecation. Additional water and electrolytes are recovered before elimination, and the stool becomes harder. Motility in the rectosigmoid is

TABLE 1. **Conditions Associated with Constipation**

Systemic
Metabolic-Endocrine Abnormalities
Hypothyroidism
Hyperthyroidism
Hyperparathyroidism
Addison's disease
Cushing's syndrome
Diabetes mellitus
Hypercalcemia
Hypokalemia
Uremia
Pregnancy
Drug Effects
Antacids (with aluminum or calcium)
Iron sulfate supplements
Opiates (codeine, diphenoxylate, hydrocodone)
Anticholinergics (antidepressants, neuroleptics, antihistamines)
Antihypertensives (calcium channel antagonists, clonidine, disopyramide)
Antiparkinsonian drugs
Barium sulfate
Diuretics
Sympathomimetics (isoproterenol, phenylephrine, phenylpropanolamine, pseudoephedrine)

Gastrointestinal
Colonic Disorders
Tumors
Intussusception
Inflammatory strictures
Systemic sclerosis
Diverticular disease
Irritable bowel syndrome
Anorectal Disorders
Hirschsprung's disease
Rectocele
Anal stenosis
Anterior mucosal prolapse
Anal fissure
Perianal abscess
Ulcerative proctitis

Neurologic
Intestinal pseudo-obstruction
Multiple sclerosis
Parkinson's disease
Spinal cord disease
Paraplegia
Cauda equina tumor
Autonomic neuropathy

stimulated by eating (gastrocolic reflex). In the rectum, the pelvic floor muscles (levator ani, puborectalis) and anal sphincters (internal and external) regulate fecal retention and defecation. The puborectalis suspends the rectosigmoid and imposes an acute angle, which facilitates continence. The urge to defecate is signaled by the propulsion of feces from the sigmoid colon to rectum. Distention of the rectum causes transient relaxation of the internal anal sphincter. Defecation proceeds as the external anal sphincter and puborectalis voluntarily relax and the perineum descends, permitting straightening of the anorectal angle. Defecation is facilitated by squatting or sitting and by increasing intra-abdominal pressure. Abnormalities in muscular relaxation, either congenital (Hirschsprung's disease) or acquired (anismus), may result in functional outlet obstruction.

Evaluation of constipated patients should begin with a history and a physical examination. Patients should be asked what they mean by "constipation" and what their normal bowel habits are. The duration of symptoms, frequency of bowel movements, consistency of stools, straining or pain, sense of complete evacuation, and presence of blood should be documented. Rectosigmoid neoplasm should be suspected in any patient over 40 with a change in bowel habit of short duration, with gross or occult blood, or with a family history of colorectal carcinoma. Medications, including the use of over-the-counter laxatives, should be reviewed, and dietary fiber intake should be quantified by a careful diet history. A digital rectal examination should be performed to evaluate anal sphincter tone, perineal descent, and puborectalis relaxation and to detect signs of tenderness, obstructing masses, rectocele, or occult blood. Screening laboratory studies should include a complete blood count, a chemistry profile, and a thyroid panel. An abdominal x-ray is useful for ruling out megacolon and fecal impaction.

If an underlying pathologic process is suspected, structural evaluation of the colon by either radiography (barium enema) or endoscopy (flexible sigmoidoscopy or colonoscopy) is indicated. In selected patients, specialized studies may be employed. Colonic transit can be evaluated by retention of radiopaque markers (Sitzmarks) on abdominal plain film 5 days after ingestion. Significant marker retention in the right colon implies diffuse colonic inertia; accumulation in the rectosigmoid suggests pelvic outlet obstruction. Anorectal manometry can be used to measure resting and squeezing anal sphincter pressures, rectal sensation, compliance, and sphincter response. It is important to rule out Hirschsprung's disease in patients with constipa-

tion dating back to birth. This entity stems from congenital denervation of anorectal smooth muscle and may manifest in adults as well as children. Anorectal manometry demonstrates incomplete relaxation of the internal anal sphincter in response to rectal distention. To rule out Hirschsprung's disease in adults, a full-thickness biopsy of the anal smooth muscle may be indicated. Defecography evaluates completeness of rectal expulsion, identifies anatomic abnormalities, and evaluates puborectalis muscle relaxation by radiographic techniques.

MANAGEMENT

The management of constipation includes education of patients about bowel function and diet, behavior modification, drug therapy, and, infrequently, surgery. Patients should be encouraged to exercise regularly, to maintain a diet high in fiber, and to respond to the urge to defecate. Reassurance is sufficient in many patients. Time should be allowed for a bowel movement each day, and patients should be encouraged to attempt bowel movements after eating in order to make use of the gastrocolic reflex. Constipating medications should be changed if possible. Laxatives should be discontinued so that response to treatment can be accurately assessed. Patients should also be educated about laxatives and their side effects.

Fiber additives are the safest, most effective way to prevent or treat constipation. Fiber absorbs many times its weight in water, swelling within the colon and producing larger, softer stools that can pass quickly and easily through the digestive tract. The diet of many Americans contains only 10 to 15 gm of fiber per day. Typically, an additional 15 to 20 grams is recommended for therapeutic benefit. Foods high in fiber include beans and legumes, whole grains, and certain fruits and vegetables. Most patients find dietary manipulation unacceptable because of impalatability and inconvenience. Therefore, the authors generally start with commercially available fiber supplements. These supplements, often referred to as the bulk-forming agents, include products containing psyllium seed (Metamucil, Konsyl) or carboxymethyl cellulose (Citrucel, Fibercon) derivatives. Bulk-forming agents agents are available in a variety of formulations (e.g., granular, powder, cookie, or tablet) and flavors that improve compliance. The dose should be increased gradually because patients may initially experience abdominal cramping, bloating, and flatulence as a result of gas production by colonic bacteria.

Laxatives act by stimulating colonic water and

electrolyte secretion. So-called surface-acting agents or stool softeners, which include docusate salts (Colace, Surfak), are surfactant fatty acids that may also provide some lubricating function. They are poorly named inasmuch as they work primarily by stimulating colonic secretion and may cause frank diarrhea. These products may be useful for short-term therapy (1 to 2 weeks) when straining at defecation is to be avoided, as in acute perianal disease, after rectal surgery, during pregnancy, or after myocardial infarction. In the authors' experience, they have little value in treating chronic constipation. Osmotic agents include magnesium salts (milk of magnesia, magnesium citrate, Maalox, Mylanta), phosphate salts (Fleet Phospho-Soda), lactulose (Chronulac, Cephulac), and glycerin. These agents are fast-acting and are available for both oral and rectal administration. Glycerin suppositories, which are useful in children and elderly patients, promote defecation by stimulating evacuation through a hyperosmotic action on the rectal mucosa. Glycerin also lubricates the stool and eases passage. Osmotic agents are generally reserved for patients who are bedridden and those whose disease is refractory to bulk-forming agents. Caution is advised against use of osmotic agents in patients prone to volume depletion (elderly patients, patients with cardiac failure) or with potential for phosphate or magnesium toxicity (i.e., renal failure).

Colonic lavage solutions (Colyte, GoLYTELY) containing polyethylene glycol may be administered when rapid catharsis is desired. These solutions are best suited for purging the bowel before colonoscopy or barium enema examinations. They have the theoretical benefit of maintaining water and electrolyte balance but should be used with caution when impaction or obstruction is suspected.

Contact agents, also known as stimulant laxatives, stimulate both water and electrolyte secretion and a vigorous pattern of intestinal motility. These laxatives consist of the anthraquinone derivatives (cascara, sennosides, and casanthranol), the diphenylmethane derivatives (bisacodyl and phenolphthalein), and castor oil. Chronic use of stimulant laxatives may damage the myenteric plexus, leading to cathartic colon syndrome with chronic dilatation and motility abnormalities. Melanosis coli is a reversible brown-black pigmentation of the intestinal mucosa that results from deposition of lipofuscin in the histiocytes of the mucosa. This condition is common in patients who are chronically dependent on anthraquinone derivatives. Phenolphthalein (Ex-Lax, Feen-A-Mint) is partially absorbed and may cause skin eruptions and prolonged discoloration. The effect of phenolphthalein may last for several days be-cause it undergoes enterohepatic circulation and is repeatedly re-excreted into the bowel lumen via bile. Castor oil, which is metabolized to ricinoleic acid (a surfactant), is sometimes included in the list of stimulant laxatives, but its use has declined in recent years. Stimulant laxatives should normally be reserved for severe episodes of constipation or failure of other regimens and, in the authors' opinion, are contraindicated for long-term use. They should be given only under supervised conditions because of their potential for dependency. Patients with a long-standing history of laxative abuse should be encouraged to discontinue the laxatives on a gradual basis.

The value of enemas and manual disimpaction should not be ignored. If there is significant stool in the rectosigmoid, forceful catharsis by any of the aforementioned agents, especially lavage, may result in significant proximal fluid retention and abdominal distention. Disimpaction via enema or digital manipulation should be considered the first step in the treatment of chronically constipated or institutionalized patients. Tap water and Fleet Phospho-Soda (Fleets) enemas appear to have equal efficacy. Soapsuds enemas should not be used because they have been shown to cause a chemical colitis.

Lubricating agents (mineral oil) are a simple, inexpensive, and yet effective alternative to many laxative regimens, particularly when pelvic outlet obstruction is suspected. One tablespoon administered four times per day evokes a bowel movement even in the most severely constipated patients. Subsequently, only 1 to 2 tbsp per day is required. Because of the potential danger of aspiration, caution must be exercised in giving mineral oil to bedridden patients or to patients with swallowing difficulties secondary to neurologic impairment. Chronic use of mineral oil has been reported to cause malabsorption of fat-soluble vitamins, but this has been seen only in children ingesting mineral oil with meals. We therefore recommend that mineral oil be given between meals when used over a long term.

A new class of drugs that may be useful in treating constipation is the prokinetic agents. Domperidone and cisapride are investigational drugs currently being tested. Cisapride is a substituted benzamide that acts indirectly by stimulating release of acetylcholine from neurons in the gastrointestinal tract. In preliminary trials, cisapride has increased the number of bowel movements and decreased laxative use in chronically constipated patients. It has also been shown to accelerate colonic transit in patients with idiopathic constipation.

Biofeedback is becoming a popular treatment modality for constipation associated with functional pelvic floor dysfunction. The biofeedback sessions can include the monitoring of relaxation of the puborectalis muscle and external anal sphincter. Patients are instructed to practice decreasing pressures during expulsion efforts and then use this technique while attempting to defecate.

The role for surgery in chronic idiopathic constipation is controversial. Surgery is an infrequent option in selected patients and should be advised with caution. Total abdominal colectomy with ileorectal anastomosis is a possible option in a small subset of patients who have failed conservative management for documented colonic inertia, but a comprehensive anorectal physiologic investigation is mandatory before any surgical intervention. Surgery for pelvic floor dyssynergia involving division of the puborectalis muscle has not been promising because patients fail to improve and are often left with significant side effects. Abnormalities associated with constipation that are successfully corrected by surgical means include classic Hirschsprung's disease and rectoceles.

FEVER

method of
WILLIAM FELDMAN, M.D.
Hospital for Sick Children
Toronto, Ontario, Canada

In all parts of the world, fever and the subjective and objective changes in persons with fever constitute a major (in the case of children, *the* major) reason for a medical visit. Some of the anxiety caused by fever is related to the alarming (to parents) febrile seizure, which is almost always quite benign and occurs in about 3% of children under 6 years of age. Another concern is that a small percentage of febrile episodes are caused by serious bacterial infections.

DEFINITIONS OF FEVER

By consensus, fever is defined as an oral temperature above 99° F (37.2° C), rectal temperature above 100.4° F (38° C), and axillary temperature above 99° F (37.2° C). In some healthy persons, normal temperatures may be slightly higher.

RISKS AND BENEFITS OF TREATING FEVER

The risks of treating fever can be divided into practical and theoretical risks. Practical risks include toxic or idiosyncratic reactions to pharmacologically active agents, the discomfort associated with physical means of lowering body temperature, and the possibility that treatment of fever will mask an underlying serious disease.

Toxic or idiosyncratic reactions to pharmacologic agents include hepatotoxicity with massive acetaminophen overdose, salicylate poisoning with overdose, the rare association of salicylate and Reye's syndrome, allergic reactions to salicylate, and the rare poisoning caused by isopropyl alcohol absorbed via the skin after sponging.

The discomfort caused by sponging with tepid or cool water is universal and is attributable to the fact that if the hypothalamic regulatory center is not affected by centrally acting medication, the body attempts to conserve heat and shivering is increased.

Concern about antipyretic measures masking serious underlying disease should be lessened in view of a recent study showing that no cases of bacterial meningitis were missed even after fever was lowered in infants in whom high fever had no obvious focus.

A theoretical risk associated with fever-lowering measures is that important host defense mechanisms associated with fever may be impaired, thereby causing the underlying condition to last longer or to worsen clinically. Although elevating the temperature in the laboratory has been shown to enhance in vitro host defense mechanisms, there is little evidence that antipyretic measures cause patients' illnesses to last longer or to worsen. In a randomized controlled trial of 225 children between the ages of 6 months and 6 years with fever caused presumably by viral illness, those given acetaminophen did not have longer or more severe illnesses than did those given placebo. In another randomized controlled trial in which acetaminophen was used for chickenpox, time to complete healing was no different between the placebo and the treatment groups. This study is commonly quoted by authors who believe that the study provides evidence that antipyresis impairs healing; time to total scabbing was 1 day less in the placebo group, but, as mentioned, there was no difference in healing.

The benefits of treating fever are based on many observers' years of clinical experience, as well as on at least one excellent randomized double-blind controlled trial. In that study, mentioned earlier, children with fever who were given acetaminophen were rated by their parents as more active and alert than were those given placebo. In addition, there was a trend for treated children to be in a better mood and to be eating better. The authors of that study point out that many parents refused entry of their children into the study because they were convinced about the benefits of antipyresis for their children.

METHODS OF FEVER CONTROL

There are two main approaches to fever control: physical and chemical. Physical approaches include sponging in an attempt to lower body temperature, using either water alone or water in which there is a dilute mixture of isopropyl alcohol. Because of the reports of coma caused by skin absorption of isopropyl alcohol, this approach is rarely used now. There are two reasons why sponging even with water alone is being used less and less. First, it does not work. In one controlled trial of sponging, there was no significant difference in lowering of body temperature between children who were sponged and those who were not. Second, it is very unpleasant to the patient, whose feeling of being cold is made worse.

Chemical or pharmacologic means of lowering body temperature are effective. Acetaminophen or aspirin in doses of 10 to 15 mg per kilogram of body weight every 4 to 6 hours for children and 300 to 600 mg every 4 to 6 hours for adults may be used. Acetaminophen is a potent antipyretic and analgesic agent, and although it has few, if any, anti-inflammatory properties in comparison with aspirin or other nonsteroidal anti-inflammatory drugs, its safety and efficacy have made it the drug of first choice in children and a widely used alternative to aspirin in adults.

The benefits of controlling fever outweigh the risks when an antipyretic such as acetaminophen is used carefully. Physicians should attempt to lower the anxiety that many patients feel about fever: it is a symptom, not a disease, but appropriate treatment of the symptom helps to make those affected feel better.

COUGH

method of
LYNN Y. KOSOWICZ, M.D., and
WILLIAM B. WHITE, M.D.

University of Connecticut School of Medicine
Farmington, Connecticut

Cough normally serves to clear the tracheobronchial tree of secretions and foreign substances. Cough and expectoration become important when the mucociliary apparatus is overloaded by inhaled particles or mucus. Cough is produced after deep inhalation when there is an increase in pleural pressure against a closed glottis, which is then suddenly opened to release this pressure, resulting in high flow rates and clearing of secretions and foreign substances.

Afferent cough receptors are located in the larynx and respiratory tract, including the nasopharynx, trachea, bronchi, and bronchioles. Cough can also result from stimulation of the pleura, acoustic duct, stomach, and diaphragm. Mechanical, inflammatory, chemical, or thermal stimuli trigger afferent signals, which are carried via trigeminal, glossopharyngeal, superior laryngeal, and vagus nerves to the medullary cough center. Efferent responses travel via the recurrent laryngeal and spinal motor nerves to produce the cough response.

DIAGNOSTIC EVALUATION

Cough is one of the most common reasons why patients seek medical treatment. It should be considered a symptom and not a diagnosis. Several well-designed prospective studies have shown that a specific cause can be identified in almost all patients with cough, and in up to 25% of patients, more than one cause may be identified.

Initial evaluation should begin with a careful history, including distinguishing acute cough from chronic cough. Acute cough is usually secondary to an acute inflammatory disease such as tracheitis or bronchitis and improves as the illness resolves. Chronic cough is usually defined when symptoms have been present for more than 3 weeks. The most common causes of chronic cough are postnasal congestion, bronchial asthma, gastroesophageal reflux (GER), smoking, chronic bronchitis, and bronchiectasis. Chronic cough may also be associated with angiotensin-converting enzyme (ACE) inhibitor therapy, congestive heart failure, sarcoidosis, and pulmonary tumors (Table 1).

Diagnostic evaluation of chronic cough includes a careful history, physical examination, and in most cases a chest x-ray. Further evaluation might include sinus films, upper endoscopy, barium swallow, 24-hour esophageal pH monitoring, spirometry with inhalation challenge, sputum culture, and cytologic studies. Bronchoscopy has been shown to be most helpful only if specifically indicated, as in the example of an abnormal chest x-ray (Table 2).

TABLE 1. **Common Causes of Chronic Cough (>3 Weeks' Duration)**

Postnasal congestion
Asthma
Gastroesophageal reflux
Smoking
Chronic bronchitis/bronchiectasis
Miscellaneous: ACE inhibitor therapy, CHF, sarcoidosis, tuberculosis and other chronic infections, pulmonary tumor, pneumonia, tracheal compression, foreign body, toxic exposures, cystic fibrosis, psychogenic causes

Abbreviations: ACE, angiotensin-converting enzyme; CHF, congestive heart failure.

TABLE 2. **Diagnostic Evaluation of Chronic Cough**

History
Physical examination
Pulmonary function testing
Methacholine inhalational challenge
Upper endoscopy/upper gastrointestinal images/24-hour
  esophageal pH monitoring
Sinus films
Chest X-ray
Bronchoscopy

THERAPY

Specific Therapy

Principles of therapy are similar for acute and chronic cough. Specific therapy aimed at the underlying cause of the cough is nearly always effective.

Acute Upper Respiratory Infection (URI). Cough associated with an acute viral URI has been shown to decrease in frequency and severity during treatment of postnasal drip with antihistamine/decongestant combinations (e.g., 6 mg of dexbrompheniramine and 120 mg of pseudoephedrine sulfate twice a day).

Postnasal Congestion. Chronic cough secondary to postnasal congestion can be further categorized as secondary to sinusitis, allergic rhinitis, perennial non–allergic rhinitis, post–infectious rhinitis, and vasomotor rhinitis. Effective therapy includes antihistamines, decongestants, nasal steroids or cromolyn sodium, and antibiotics.

Asthma. Cough may be the single presenting symptom of asthma, and diagnosis can be difficult. A high index of suspicion must be maintained, and spirometry with inhalation challenge may be necessary for revealing the diagnosis. Specific therapy for the asthma (e.g., bronchodilators or steroids) is usually effective in eliminating the cough.

Gastroesophageal Reflux. GER may be the cause of chronic cough in up to 20% of patients with cough. In up to 40% of these patients, cough is the sole manifestation of underlying GER, and barium swallow, endoscopy, and 24-hour esophageal pH monitoring may be needed in order to establish the diagnosis. Appropriate therapy (e.g., H_2 blockers) may be quite successful in eliminating the cough, although it may take several months for complete resolution.

Chronic Bronchitis. Chronic bronchitis can usually be identified from the patient's history and sputum production. The most effective treatment is cessation of cigarette smoking. Ipratropium bromide (Atrovent), postural drainage, and iodinated glycerol have been shown to be useful in many cases.

Angiotensin-Converting Enzyme Inhibitor–Induced Cough. ACE inhibitors induce bronchospasm and cough by increasing circulating levels of bradykinin. The incidence of cough in patients taking ACE inhibitors ranges from 4 to 15%. The nonsteroidal anti-inflammatory drug sulindac may be helpful in treating ACE inhibitor–induced cough in patients in whom ACE inhibitor therapy cannot be discontinued.

Nonspecific Therapy

Because of the success of specific therapy in treating cough, every effort should be made to identify the underlying cause. Nonspecific therapy is indicated if the cause of cough is unknown, if definitive therapy is unsuccessful, and if the cough interferes with sleep or is potentially hazardous to the patient. Complications of cough include muscle strain, fatigue, rib fracture, syncope, pneumothorax or pneumomediastinum, nausea and vomiting, and epistaxis.

It has been difficult to scientifically study the efficacy of various nonspecific therapies for cough. Most studies have involved the use of artificially induced cough in healthy volunteers or have been conducted in patients with bronchitis; these results may not apply to general populations of patients. It has also been difficult to objectively measure cough severity and efficacy.

Supportive therapy comprises two major categories: expectorant/mucolytic and antitussive agents.

Expectorants/Mucolytics

The goal in the use of expectorants and mucolytics (Table 3) is to improve the efficacy of the cough. Expectorants are thought to act by stimulating cough or increasing the volume of secretions, whereas mucolytics change the consistency of the mucus. Although some of these agents have been shown to produce these effects in vitro, ac-

TABLE 3. **Treatment of Cough: Expectorants/Mucolytics**

Drug	Adult Dose	Side Effects
Guaifenesin (Robitussin)	200–400 mg every 4 hr	Nausea, vomiting
Iodinated glycerol (Organidin)	60 mg qid with additional liquids	Gastrointestinal irritation, hypersensitivity, rash, goiter
Acetylcysteine (Mucomyst)	3–5 mL of 20% solution or 6–10 mL of 10% solution three to four times daily via nebulizer	Stomatitis, nausea and vomiting, drowsiness, bronchoconstriction

tual clinical benefit has not been demonstrated. These agents are widely used despite lack of evidence of efficacy.

1. Guaifenesin acts by thinning bronchial secretions, theoretically promoting respiratory tract drainage, and making dry, nonproductive coughs more productive and less frequent. Adverse reactions include nausea, vomiting, dizziness, headache, and rash.

2. Iodinated glycerol increases the output of thin respiratory fluid and helps liquify thick mucus in the bronchial tree. It has been shown to be effective in patients with chronic bronchitis, but its role in other types of cough is unclear. Adverse reactions include gastrointestinal irritation, rash, hypersensitivity, and thyroid gland enlargement.

3. Potassium iodide acts in a manner similar to that of iodinated glycerol but with more numerous side effects and has generally been replaced by iodinated glycerol.

4. N-acetylcysteine is a mucolytic agent that reduces the viscosity of pulmonary secretions through reduction of mucoprotein disulfide linkages. It has not consistently been shown to be more efficacious than adequate humidification alone.

5. Aerosolized hypertonic saline has been shown to improve cough clearance in patients with chronic bronchitis but has not been studied as a nonspecific expectorant and may trigger bronchospasm.

6. Oral or intravenous hydrations and humidified air are often recommended but have not been evaluated in appropriately designed clinical trials.

7. Ammonium chloride, syrup of ipecac, and guaiacol sulfonate are occasionally used in combination preparations without objective evidence of benefit.

8. Terpin hydrate has been studied and found to have no measurable effect on cough.

Antitussive Agents

Antitussive agents (Table 4) are used to suppress or eliminate cough. In general, they should not be given to patients with productive cough. Antitussive agents are often categorized by site of effect as peripheral- or central-acting, but many agents have effects at both sites. Another method of classification is by abuse potential (i.e., narcotic or non-narcotic).

NON-NARCOTIC AGENTS

Aromatic chest rubs and cough drops or lozenges (which may contain agents such as menthol, camphor, and eucalyptus oil) and other demulcents (often containing sugars) are thought to act by soothing irritated mucosa. Several of these agents have been shown to decrease cough frequency in artificially induced cough in healthy volunteers but have not been demonstrated to offer clinical benefit in patients with cough.

1. Intravenous lidocaine is quite effective in suppressing cough during, for example, intraophthalmologic surgery, bronchoscopy, and intubation.

2. Benzonatate (Tessalon) is an anesthetic agent similar to tetracaine that acts by increasing the threshold or latency, or both, of the afferent limb of the cough reflex and probably has

TABLE 4. **Treatment of Cough: Antitussive Agents**

Drug	Adult Dose	Side Effects
Non-Narcotic		
Benzonatate (Tessalon Perles)	100 mg q 8 h (up to q 4 h if necessary)	Dizziness, vertigo, nausea, oral anesthesia if chewed
Dextromethorphan (Robitussin)		
Regular preparations	10–20 mg q 4 h; 30 mg q 6–8 h	Minimal side effects, mild nausea, dizziness, CNS depression
Extended-release preparations	60 mg bid	Same as for regular preparations
Narcotic		
Codeine	10–20 mg q 4–6 h	Constipation, sedation, nausea, CNS and respiratory depression at high doses
Hydrocodone		
Regular preparations	5–10 mg q 4–6 h	Lightheadedness, gastrointestinal upset, sedation, constipation, increased CNS and respiratory depression at high doses
Extended-release preparations	10 mg q 12 h	Same as for regular preparations
Commercially available only in combination products (e.g., Hycodan, Hycomine, Hycomine Compound, Hycotuss Expectorant, Ru-Tuss with Hydrocodone liquid, Tussend, Tussionex)		

Abbreviations: CNS, central nervous system.

both peripheral and central sites of action. Side effects may include dizziness, vertigo, or nausea. If chewed, it may cause an unpleasant taste or oral anesthesia.

3. Caramiphen has local anesthetic and anticholinergic effects and is available only in combination products.

4. Dextromethorphan is chemically derived from opiates, but at prescribed doses, it has no sedative or analgesic effects and little potential for abuse. Therefore, it is usually classified as non-narcotic. The antitussive efficacy of dextromethorphan is similar to that of codeine. It acts centrally with side effects of nausea and dizziness, and overdose can lead to depression of the central nervous system.

5. Diphenhydramine, an antihistamine, is an effective antitussive agent with both central and peripheral effects. It may cause drowsiness, gastrointestinal irritation, and anticholinergic side effects.

6. Bronchodilators, cromolyn sodium, and steroids have not been shown to be helpful for cough in the absence of bronchospasm.

NARCOTIC AGENTS

The phenanthrene alkaloid narcotics (e.g., morphine and codeine) are very effective antitussive agents that act by increasing the threshold or latency, or both, of the cough receptor. They are effective in doses that are lower than analgesic doses; this may be because of separate opiate cough receptors in the central nervous system. There is some evidence that narcotic antitussive agents may also act on the afferent sensory nerve endings that initiate cough. Because these agents are effective at low doses, tolerance and addiction are not as common as often feared if they are prescribed appropriately.

1. Codeine is the most commonly prescribed narcotic antitussive. Its primary effect is thought to be at the cough center in the medulla. It is very effective at doses associated with little respiratory depression. Codeine also causes drying of respiratory tract mucosa and increases mucus viscosity. A 10- to 20-mg oral dose of codeine is effective in suppressing cough; increased cough-suppressing effects are observed at higher doses.

2. Hydrocodone also suppresses the cough center in the medulla and causes drying of the respiratory tract mucosa. Its antitussive effect may be slightly greater than that of codeine, but it is more sedating. It is commercially available only in combination products (e.g., with phenylpropanolamine, chlorpheniramine, guaifenesin, or pseudoephedrine hydrochloride).

3. Other opiates, such as morphine and hydromorphone, have antitussive activity but with more adverse reactions and dependence potential. They are generally used only if cough is associated with another disorder such as severe pain or anxiety.

CONCLUSION

In treating patients with cough, a thorough evaluation is indicated so as to identify an underlying cause. Specific therapy is successful in alleviating or eliminating cough. If no cause is found or if specific therapy is not effective *and* there is sufficient reason to treat the cough, a non-narcotic antitussive agent (e.g., dextromethorphan) is reasonable initial nonspecific therapy. Expectorants/mucolytics have not been demonstrated to be efficacious as a primary therapy of cough. They may be useful in treating irritative cough associated with scant, thick sputum production, but they generally have a limited therapeutic role. Combined suppressant and expectorant therapy is illogical and should be avoided. If necessary, narcotic antitussives (e.g., codeine) are very effective in suppressing cough. Initial dosages should be low and titrated for effect.

HOARSENESS AND LARYNGITIS

method of
GAYLE E. WOODSON, M.D.
University of Tennessee, Memphis
Memphis, Tennessee

Hoarseness, a change in the voice, is a symptom commonly encountered in medical practice. The precise nature of the complaint varies greatly. Patients may describe a change in the quality of the voice as roughness, pitch change, or breathiness. They may notice volume loss, increased effort in speaking, easy fatigue, or a total loss of the voice. The specific characteristics of the vocal change serve as clues to the mechanism of the problem. In the majority of cases of acute hoarseness, the voice is recovered within 2 weeks with expectant conservative management.

PATHOPHYSIOLOGY

Voice is produced by passive vibration of the vocal folds (commonly known as the vocal cords),

TABLE 1. **Requirements for Normal Voice**

1. Breath support
2. Appropriate laryngeal closure
3. Normal vocal fold mucosa
4. Control of length and tension
5. Normal resonance

induced by exhaled air (Table 1). Hence the voice is exquisitely sensitive to minor alterations in the larynx. Mass lesions, edema, or even alterations in mucus can result in irregular vibration, which produces a rough quality. Patients with edematous vocal folds use more effort in speaking because more energy is required to induce vibration. A gap between the vocal folds allows excess air escape during phonation, which is perceived as breathiness. If the gap is too large, no periodic sound is produced (aphonia). In contrast, if the vocal folds are closed too tightly, the voice requires more driving pressure and sounds strained or strangled. Such tight closure is usually caused by a neurologic abnormality, but it may also have a psychogenic basis. Pulmonary insufficiency can impair the driving pressure for phonation, resulting in a weak voice. Neurologic motor abnormalities can induce tremor or spasms, resulting in a wavering or jerky voice or in sudden pitch changes. Inflammation or tumors in the nose can change the resonance of the vocal tract and thereby significantly alter vocal quality, giving it a hyponasal sound. Similar processes in the mouth or pharynx can produce a muffled, or "hot potato," voice, a characteristic sign of acute epiglottitis.

A sudden loss or drastic change of voice that occurs during Valsalva's maneuver or extreme vocal effort may indicate vocal fold hematoma. This most commonly occurs in premenstrual females but can also occur in males. Anticoagulant medications and aspirin are other risk factors. Vocal fold hematoma can sometimes result in a persisting vocal handicap, caused by scarring or formation of a polyp. This risk is greater if bleeding recurs. Whenever a vocal fold hematoma is suspected, strict voice rest is prescribed, and the patient should be referred for a laryngeal examination as soon as possible.

Vocal breathiness indicates that the vocal folds are not achieving sufficient closure during vibration. A tumor or another mass lesion of the vocal fold itself can manifest with breathiness if the mass precludes complete approximation. However, such lesions develop over time, and the onset of voice change is gradual rather than acute. Most often, acute breathiness is caused by laryngeal paralysis, which in turn is commonly the presenting sign of a serious underlying medical problem. For example, the most common cause of laryngeal paralysis is metastatic lung cancer. In any event, patients with a very breathy voice are unlikely to recover quickly with conservative therapy and may have a serious underlying problem.

Hoarseness that occurs immediately after external trauma may indicate a laryngeal fracture or hematoma. This can result from blunt or penetrating trauma or from strangulation. In such a case, the patient is at risk for airway obstruction. This can develop suddenly, even if breathing seems unimpaired initially or for several hours after the injury. Immediate examination of the larynx is indicated, preferably with a flexible laryngoscope, and a tracheotomy may be urgently required. Endotracheal intubation in such a patient could be disastrous.

Hoarseness after intubation is a common occurrence and is in general much less ominous, usually resolving in a day or two. However, if after extubation a patient not only is hoarse but also has pain on swallowing, arytenoid dislocation must be suspected. This injury is uncommon but, if present, requires immediate endoscopic reduction.

COMMON CAUSES OF ACUTE HOARSENESS

Most patients with acute onset of vocal roughness or limitation of pitch range have inflammation and swelling of the larynx. The laryngeal mucosa is delicate, and there are many potential causes of its irritation, including mechanical trauma, infection, and gastroesophageal reflux (GER). A given case may be multifactorial.

Trauma

Mechanical trauma caused by excessive glottic closure is a frequent cause of laryngeal irritation. Vocal abuse, coughing, and throat-clearing all generate high pressure on the delicate mucosa, resulting in edema or even abrasion or hematoma. Vocal abuse includes shouting, excessive singing, and prolonged speaking over noise or under stress. When hoarseness develops after a patient attends a sports event and can recall giving vigorous oral support, vocal abuse is clearly the cause. Frequent and vigorous coughing often result from an upper respiratory infection, with resultant hoarseness. Less commonly, the larynx is irritated by purulent mucus drainage or is directly involved by an infection. Similarly, allergic inflammation most often affects the vocal folds indirectly, by causing sneezing and coughing. In addition, any factor that causes nasal obstruction leads to drying of the mouth and larynx. This deprives the larynx of protective lubrication, so that even normal phonation results in irritation.

Chemical Irritation

GER is another common cause of acute onset of hoarseness. Some patients with reflux laryngitis have a history of heartburn, belching, or ulcer disease, but many have acid reflux that is otherwise asymptomatic, commonly occurring only at night. Asymptomatic GER is common in the general population and usually does not result in laryngeal involvement. However, reflux laryngitis may occur in the presence of cofactors, such as trauma or infection, or if the severity of the reflux increases. Even as minor a trauma as a misguided potato chip can abrade the larynx, producing a wound that is vulnerable to acid. Coughing, throat-clearing, and voice abuse are other cofactors. Even intact mucosa may become inflamed if the pH of the reflux diminishes or if the volume or frequency increases.

A typical patient with reflux laryngitis notices hoarseness on awakening in the morning and may recall having ingested a late heavy or spicy meal the night before. Another suggestive sign is a foul taste in the mouth on awakening. Some patients are awakened at night by severe coughing or bronchospasm. Acidic gastric contents induce a chemical burn of the larynx, which may require several days or weeks to completely heal.

Smoking is another cause of laryngeal irritation. It induces gradual changes in the laryngeal mucosa but may also be responsible for acute hoarseness. Smokers may experience a sudden deterioration of vocal function as a result of a heavy binge of smoking. Chemicals in the smoke are direct irritants. Also, nicotine relaxes the gastroesophageal sphincter and stimulates acid production, and so smoking may also exacerbate GER.

Psychogenic Hoarseness

The voice is a major means of expression of emotion, and therefore it is not surprising that a vocal problem may be a result of emotional or psychiatric problems. For example, sudden total aphonia, in the absence of any signs of organic disease, is likely to represent a conversion disorder.

TREATMENT OF ACUTE HOARSENESS

Most patients with acute laryngitis eventually recover spontaneously, but appropriate management (Table 2) can hasten the healing process and reduce the chance of permanent sequelae. The key therapeutic goals are to put the larynx at rest and to eliminate or diminish the factors that caused or contribute to the problem.

Voice Rest

Voice rest is the most important component of treatment for acute laryngitis. The normal vocal

TABLE 2. **Treatment of Acute Hoarseness**

1. Voice rest
2. Management of contributing factors
   Cough suppression
   Acid suppression
   Antibiotics
   Hydration
   Relief of nasal obstruction
3. Sympathomimetics
4. Steroids *not* generally recommended, but useful in selected cases
5. Allow time for resolution

fold is uniquely constructed to withstand repetitive high collision pressures during phonation, but when the integrity of this structure is compromised, even a little talking can be traumatic and delay healing. Thus laryngitis becomes a self-perpetuating cycle. Nevertheless, total voice rest can be very frustrating for a patient, who may resort to loud whispering or frequent throat clearing in attempts to communicate. Both actions can further traumatize the larynx and are to be discouraged. Furthermore, total voice rest greatly restricts use of laryngeal muscles and may thereby contribute to persisting vocal dysfunction long after the inflammation has resolved. The optimal program of voice rest conserves but does not prohibit voice use.

Patients with hoarseness need to be counseled in order to convince them of the need for voice rest and to instruct them in how to accomplish it. An analogy is frequently helpful; for example, talking with laryngitis is like hiking with blisters on the feet: although healing may eventually occur if the activity persists, there may be scarring or callus formation. Optimal healing requires elimination of continued trauma. Voice rest consists of using as few words as possible to communicate and using a comfortable pitch and a comfortable loudness. Whispering is *not* acceptable because it is quite stressful on the larynx. The patient should not shout or attempt to talk over loud noises, and long telephone conversations should be avoided. If the patient's occupation involves talking, the routine should be altered to decrease or eliminate voice use. If this is not possible, the patient should consider staying home. Professional voice users, such as singers and actors, in whom laryngitis develops are advised not to utter a word for which they are not paid. It is very helpful to request cooperation from family and co-workers, who should not call to the patient from a distance, expecting an answer, and should avoid asking open-ended questions, requesting simple "yes" and "no" responses whenever possible.

Elimination of Throat Clearing

Patients with laryngitis frequently perceive laryngeal swelling as "something in the throat" or "postnasal drip." This misconception results in frequent throat-clearing, which perpetuates the problem. It is difficult for patients to resist the impulse to clear the throat. They are almost always able to expectorate some mucus with the maneuver, inasmuch as the average person produces about one quart of mucus every day. Patients also notice a transient feeling of improvement after throat-clearing. However, throat-clearing is extremely detrimental to the larynx and should be strongly discouraged.

Cough Suppression

Repetitive or vigorous coughing is traumatic to the larynx. If the cough is productive, as in pneumonia or bronchitis, cough suppression is not recommended. However, if a cough is irritative, as in asthma, allergy, or a viral upper respiratory infection, cough suppression can be very beneficial for protecting the larynx or hastening resolution of laryngitis. Two to four teaspoons of an over-the-counter preparation of guaifenesin and dextromethorphan is frequently sufficient, but some patients may require codeine. Cough syrups containing atropine or antihistamine should be avoided because they tend to dry the nose and throat. The resultant thicker mucus is more difficult to expectorate, and this leads to more laryngeal trauma.

Management of Laryngitis Caused by Gastroesophageal Reflux

Medical management of GER in general involves suppression or neutralization of gastric acid secretion, modification of diet, and mechanical maneuvers to decrease the incidence of reflux. Management of reflux laryngitis includes, in addition to the preceding components, voice rest and often requires more stringent acid control than that used in treatment of heartburn or peptic ulcer. Controlled studies have demonstrated that resolution of reflux esophagitis necessitates a higher dose of H_2 blockers than is used for treatment of peptic ulcer disease. This is presumably because normal esophageal mucosa is more sensitive to acid than is gastric mucosa. In the author's clinical experience, effective treatment of reflux laryngitis also requires at least high doses of H_2 blockers, such as ranitidine (Zantac), 300 mg twice daily, and frequently even this is not sufficient. The best response is obtained with omeprazole (Prilosec), 20 mg daily. Also, suppression of acid secretion does not eliminate the reflux of gastric contents, which, even when not acidic, could be irritating. For this reason, metoclopramide (Reglan) is recommended for facilitating gastric emptying, 10 to 15 mg four times a day, before meals and at bedtime.

Reflux laryngitis is essentially a burn and requires time to heal. Reduction or elimination of acidity does not directly promote mucosal healing, but it does remove a cause of the injury, so that repair can take place. Therefore, improvement should not be expected overnight, and complete resolution may take 6 to 8 weeks. However, if no response at all is seen in 2 to 3 weeks, it is best to refer patient for a laryngeal examination so that in cases of tumor or granuloma the diagnosis is not delayed.

Like other burns, acid-induced laryngitis may become superinfected. This is particularly true if an infectious process is a cofactor in development. Therefore, in patients with reflux laryngitis who also have pain or productive, purulent sputum, a short course of antibiotics is indicated. In view of the usual flora of the upper respiratory tract, penicillin is usually adequate. In the presence of sinusitis, amoxicillin, with or without clavulanate (Augmentin), is preferable. In case of penicillin allergy, appropriate alternate drugs should of course be used.

Hydration

If the mucus blanket over the vocal folds does not provide adequate lubrication, even minimal phonation can be traumatic. Mucus can become thick and sticky as a result of even mild degrees of dehydration, such as that incurred by a long airplane flight. Adequate liquid intake (at least eight glasses of water a day) should be maintained. The late laryngologist to a well-known opera company used to advise his patients to drink sufficient liquids to keep the urine dilute, specifically using the words "Pee pale."

Decongestants

Nasal congestion can also affect mucus, inasmuch as the resultant mouth breathing bypasses the normal humidification function of the nose. In the management of acute hoarseness, relief of nasal obstruction is important and should be accomplished by topical or oral sympathomimetic medication, such as pseudoephedrine (Sudafed). Oral sympathomimetic medication may also reduce laryngeal swelling. Most antihistamines should be avoided because they are drying and result in thicker mucus. If an antihistamine is indicated for treatment of an allergic manifestation, the use of one with little drying effect, such as terfenadine (Seldane), is recommended.

When the Show Must Go On

Although vocal rest is the best recommendation for patients with hoarseness, there is sometimes a pressing need for continued speech. A patient may have an important speaking engagement or vocal performance. In such a situation, if laryngeal examination rules out vocal fold hemorrhage or abrasion, the voice can sometimes be temporarily improved by administration of steroids, orally or parenterally, to reduce vocal fold edema. Prednisone, 40 mg about 4 hours before the event, is usually effective and may be repeated once if necessary. A long-acting topical vasoconstrictor, such as oxymetazoline (Afrin), may also be applied directly to the laryngeal mucosa so as to further reduce edema.

These measures should be used only to permit limited periods of vocal use, not to enable the patient to return to full voice use. Although steroids and vasoconstrictors diminish the swelling, they do not promote healing, nor do they protect the vocal folds from sustaining further damage with use. Such temporary measures should be resorted to only if there is no evidence of vocal fold hemorrhage or laceration.

The use of cocaine and topical steroids in this situation is not recommended. Cocaine can achieve impressive decongestion of the vocal folds, but the accompanying anesthesia may result in severe vocal injury, because pain feedback is eliminated. Topical administration of steroids is no more effective than systemic administration, and the inhalant preparations can damage the larynx.

PREVENTION

Patients who have repeated bouts of laryngitis can benefit from education in vocal hygiene or vocal retraining. A major objective is to avoid vocal abuse: do not shout, do not whisper, and avoid talking over loud background noise, particularly during an upper respiratory infection. Patients should strive to speak with adequate breath support and to relax the face and throat. Hydration is also important. In addition, the patient should be screened for signs of contributing conditions, such as allergy, sinusitis, or GER.

CHRONIC LARYNGITIS

Organic Causes. If hoarseness lasts more than a couple of weeks, history taking and a physical examination, including a laryngeal ex-

TABLE 3. Etiology of Chronic Hoarseness

Chronic Laryngitis
Vocal abuse or misuse
Allergy
Chronic sinusitis
Gastroesophageal reflux
Benign Vocal Cord Lesions
Nodules
Polyp
Contact ulcer or granuloma
Papilloma
Cancer
Vocal Cord Paralysis
Systemic Illness
Aging
Psychogenic Causes

amination, are indicated, to identify the mechanism of hoarseness (Table 3). Chronic hoarseness is the cardinal presenting sign of laryngeal cancer. Even if the laryngeal examination is negative, the neck should be carefully palpated in order to detect metastatic nodes. Laryngeal cancer is primarily a disease of men in the sixth or seventh decade of life who have smoked tobacco and ingested alcohol regularly over many years. However, it also occurs, although less frequently, in women and in younger people. Other mass lesions of the vocal fold are common, usually resulting from either vocal abuse or chronic inflammation. Laryngeal papilloma, seen most often in young children, is caused by a virus. Untreated, it can lead to severe airway obstruction. Systemic diseases, such as rheumatoid arthritis, and mucosal disorders, such as pemphigus, may involve the larynx. Hormonal changes caused by menopause or hypothyroidism may also adversely affect the voice. Vocal fold mobility must be assessed. Finally, chronic laryngeal irritation, caused by chronic sinusitis or GER, must be considered.

Aging. The voice changes profoundly with age. This is a natural process, and the age of an individual is frequently reflected in the sound of the voice. Calcification of thyroid cartilage and increasing stiffness of vocal fold tissues tend to elevate the vocal pitch, and this accounts for the characteristic high-pitched voice in elderly men. In women, the same changes take place, but at menopause, a second process begins: the accumulation of mucoid edema in the submucosal space. This change results in a lower pitch, which outweighs the trend to a higher pitch. In women who smoke, the edema can become very pronounced, even resulting in large sessile polyps (Reinke's edema). Vocal muscle atrophy is also common with increasing age, frequently resulting in impaired vocal fold closure and a weak or breathy voice.

Functional Dysphonia

Hoarseness that cannot be attributed to organic causes but occurs in a patient who does not have psychiatric problems is most likely caused by poor vocal habits and is termed "functional dysphonia." A common form is postviral dysphonia, or persisting hoarseness after resolution of laryngitis. It is analogous to limping after a leg injury. It may be caused by habitual misuse or by weakness of specific muscles. Some young men have a persisting high voice after puberty, termed "mutational dysphonia." There are many other types of dysphonias, and in general, they respond quite well to voice therapy.

INSOMNIA

method of
DANIEL F. KRIPKE, M.D.
University of California, San Diego
La Jolla, California

There are few areas of medicine in which actual practice differs so widely from scientific indications as in the current treatment of insomnia.

The most widespread practice is prescription of hypnotic agents. About half of all hypnotic agents dispensed are refills. Most hypnotic agents are being prescribed for chronic insomnia, but the expert consensus is that hypnotic agents are neither safe nor effective for the treatment of chronic insomnia.

CHRONIC INSOMNIA

Prevalence

Approximately one-third of American adults report insomnia from time to time. Among a smaller proportion, symptoms persist for months or years. Insomnia complaints increase with aging. There is an abrupt increase in insomnia complaints among women at menopause, past which women receive hypnotic agents about twice as often as men. Most insomnia complaints brought to the attention of physicians signify chronic disorders, for which hypnotic agents are not effective treatment.

Whenever an insomnia complaint suggests a chronic disorder, the physician should obtain a detailed history sufficient for exploring the etiology of the disorder and then select specific treatments. Chronic insomnia commonly has complex causes that necessitate multimodal, specific treatments.

Depression

Depressive disorders are probably the most common cause of insomnia seen in primary practice. Major depressive disorders, minor depressive disorders, dysthymia, depressive adjustment reactions, and bereavement are usually accompanied by complaints of insomnia, which are often the outstanding presenting symptom. When insomnia is a sign of depression, treatment should be focused on the underlying depressive disorder.

Antidepressant drugs are the first-line treatment for depressive disorders with symptomatic insomnia. In general, a sedative antidepressant such as nortriptyline (10 to 100 mg), doxepin (25 to 300 mg), or trazodone (25 to 300 mg) is administered; the entire daily dosage is given shortly before bedtime. The sedative effects of these antidepressants aid sleep immediately, although the full antidepressant effects may require several weeks to develop. When the entire daily dosage is taken before the patient goes to bed, sedative and other side effects are minimized, efficacy of the drug is at least as good, and compliance with the regimen may be better. Less sedative antidepressants such as fluoxetine (Prozac), bupropion (Wellbutrin), and desipramine (Norpramin), may have fewer anticholinergic and cardiac side effects and are at least as effective for primary depression, but they are much less likely to improve sleep rapidly, and they are unlikely to be tolerated well in single bedtime dosages. Although often effective as antidepressants, monoamine oxidase inhibitors such as tranylcypromine (Parnate) are more likely to disturb sleep than to lead to improvement.

Cognitive and interpersonal psychotherapies are effective in treating depression, but the benefits for insomnia appear more slowly than with medication.

There is no evidence that hypnotic agents provide additional benefit, if an adequate dosage of a sedative antidepressant is given at bedtime. There is virtually no evidence that hypnotic agents are themselves antidepressant, but the risk of hypnotic overdose is particularly high when depression is recognized. Barbiturate hypnotic agents and glutethimide should never be used in the presence of depression because barbiturates commonly make depressive symptoms worse. The risk of lethal barbiturate overdosage is excessive.

Menopause

When insomnia complaints begin shortly before or after the onset of menopause, a hormonal factor may be suspected. Among women beyond age 45, hot flashes may not be sufficiently recognized as a source of frequent sleep awakenings. When insomnia complaints are present, potential benefits of estrogen replacement in alleviating insomnia should be balanced with the other benefits and risks of estrogen replacement.

Habit Disorders

Bedtime behavioral disorders are important causes of chronic insomnia. Physicians can often correct these disorders with simple counseling. Even when other problems such as depression, alcohol abuse, or body clock disturbances are present, concomitant correction of maladaptive habits is often essential for resolving chronic insomnia.

When worries are brought to bed, they bring insomnia with them. Good sleep requires relaxing bedtime habits of mind. Although some patients believe that reading or watching television in bed is relaxing, other patients find that these activities disrupt the habit of going to bed to quiet the mind. Patients with a chronic habit of worrying in bed may actually benefit if they train themselves to worry in a different part of the home and to get out of bed whenever they do not feel sleepy. Hot baths, a glass of low-fat milk, prayers, and relaxation exercises may ready the mind for sleep.

Paradoxically, one of most common causes of lying in bed awake is spending too long in bed. The more that some patients lie in bed desperately trying to sleep, the more they associate their beds with frustrating hours of insomnia. Controlled studies show that for many insomniacs, restricting time in bed to 7, 6, or even 5 hours a night produces a remarkable increase in objective sleep time. Patients should be reassured that the increased sleepiness that results from restricting time in bed is part of the cure. Once a patient has learned to sleep solidly for all of a restricted sleep time, the time in bed can sometimes be judiciously extended. Restricted time in bed should be combined with a regular time for arising.

Sleep Apnea

Beyond age 40, most adults experience some apneas (cessations of respiration) during sleep. These apneas are terminated by very brief arousals, which in some patients lead to complaints of insomnia and midsleep awakenings, in others lead to complaints of excessive daytime sleepiness, and in still others lead to both insomnia and sleepiness. Apnea is so common that no treatment other than weight control is advisable in mild cases, but apneas are sometimes made worse by alcohol and sedatives.

Periodic Limb Movements in Sleep

A remarkable concomitant of aging is the development of brief Babinski-like withdrawal movements in the legs, which may appear rhythmically during sleep in association with dozens or even hundreds of brief arousals. Such periodic limb movements are apparently a minor factor in chronic aging-related insomnia; unfortunately, no long-term treatment has demonstrated benefits superior to risks.

Slow and Fast Body Clocks

Increasing evidence implicates the circadian (about 24-hour) body clock in insomnia. Among young adults, the body clock commonly runs a bit late, so that patients have trouble falling asleep at night and trouble getting up in the morning. People with this difficulty—called "delayed sleep phase syndrome"—may be chronic night owls who have difficulty getting to work on time. Increasing the bright light exposures of such patients early in the morning often helps control their symptoms. Such patients should make it a habit to spend an hour or two in daylight soon after awakening or else increase the artificial lighting wherever they spend their mornings. A regular time of arising and, especially, not sleeping late on weekends are important.

Aging patients, especially women, may find that their body clocks run too fast, so that they fall asleep too early in the evening and then awaken too early, before dawn. This pattern, called "advanced sleep phase syndrome," is sometimes indistinguishable from mild forms of depression. Bright evening light helps such patients remain awake in the evening, which in turn helps them sleep past dawn. Simply adding a few hundred watts of fluorescent or incandescent lighting to the area near the television sometimes produces appreciable benefit. Figure 1 explains the principles of adjusting body clocks with bright light.

Alcohol

Alcohol is a hypnotic compound with a very short blood half-life. Because alcohol produces vigorous withdrawal rebound, some patients experience sleep-onset insomnia after drinking at dinner time, whereas other patients may suffer early awakening related to imbibing in the evening or at bedtime. Although drinking up to 1 ounce of alcohol per day may have no adverse effect on survival or sleep, heavier drinking almost always causes insomnia when the patient is sober. Drinking to avoid insomnia, which alcohol produces, often becomes a part of the vicious circle

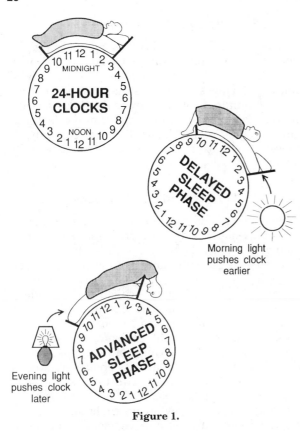

Figure 1.

of alcoholism. Abstinence is the primary long-term treatment.

Hypnotic Habituation

Hypnotic agents such as triazolam (Halcion) and temazepam (Restoril) with relatively short half-lives cause withdrawal insomnia. After just a few doses, sleep is objectively worse whenever the patient skips taking the drug than if the patient had been taking placebo. It is common to find patients whose chronic insomnia can be largely resolved merely by encouraging them to accept a few nights of abstinence-related insomnia.

Hypnotic agents produce little or no benefit for patients with chronic insomnia. Specifically, continuous use of hypnotics for months or years does not produce significantly more subjective or objective sleep than does similar use of placebos, according to available evidence. Chronic use of hypnotic agents may impair daytime alertness, memory, performance, and judgment; may create weakness and increase the risk of falls in the elderly; and possibly may even increase mortality. Pharmaceutical manufacturers have been unable to prove that chronic use of hypnotic agents produces any benefits that counterbalance these

risks. Accordingly, no prescription drug is approved or marketed in the United States for chronic hypnotic use.

Physicians often prescribe hypnotic agents for their patients to express caring, without any diagnostic rationale.

TRANSIENT INSOMNIA

Transient insomnia is a temporary symptom that may arise for a few days (not more than 4 weeks). Stresses, worries, shift work, and jet lag can cause transient insomnia. Transient insomnia can produce difficulty in falling asleep, mid-sleep awakenings, early awakening, nonrestorative sleep, or any combination of these. In many cases, the wisest treatment focuses on relieving the causes of transient insomnia, which are usually apparent.

Flurazepam (Dalmane), quazepam (Doral), temazepam (Restoril), estazolam (ProSom), and triazolam (Halcion) are licensed in the United States for symptomatic relief of transient insomnia. In general, these hypnotic agents transiently increase a patient's sleep by 15 to 45 minutes, and this increase is accompanied by subjective relief and decreased worry. In most circumstances, this minor increase in sleep is not sufficient to improve the insomniac's alertness or performance on the following day. Quite the contrary, alertness and performance are usually impaired, especially if the patient drinks any alcohol.

Both quazepam and flurazepam are metabolized rapidly to intermediates and ultimately in part to desalkylflurazepam, which has a plasma half-life of several days. Because of these long half-lives, desalkylflurazepam accumulates with nightly use. Thus hangover increases, especially when more than 15 mg is taken nightly. Because quazepam and flurazepam are self-tapering, the risk of withdrawal insomnia is minimal. Receptor specificity may render the benefit/risk ratio of quazepam somewhat superior to that of flurazepam, but adequate proof is not available.

Temazepam (Restoril) and estazolam (ProSom) have a somewhat shorter duration of action than do quazepam and flurazepam. Consequently, temazepam and estazolam may produce somewhat less hangover at the price of increased likelihood of withdrawal insomnia.

Triazolam (Halcion) has such a short half-life that hangover effects are often negligible; in fact, after taking triazolam, some patients experience withdrawal anxiety the following morning. After a patient discontinues triazolam, withdrawal insomnia is prompt and impressive. Some evidence suggests that triazolam produces more memory disturbances (especially within a few hours after administration) and more frequent idiosyncratic personality disturbances than do the other hypnotic agents. Anecdotal reports of idiosyncratic triazolam risks are not supported by sound epidemiologic studies.

Lorazepam and oxazepam are frequently used as hypnotics, although they are not marketed for that purpose. These drugs are too slowly absorbed to be efficient for promoting sleep onset, but their duration of action is roughly equivalent to that of temazepam. Diazepam is also frequently used as a hypnotic agent. Rapid distribution into lipid stores makes diazepam effectively short-acting in the first dose, although with nightly dosing, its metabolites accumulate much like desalkylflurazepam. Some physicians prescribe diphenhydramine at bedtime because this antihistamine may produce less physical dependence than do benzodiazepines; however, diphenhydramine produces typical hangover and more anticholinergic side effects than do benzodiazepines.

PRURITUS
(Itching)

method of
MARCIA L. REEDER, M.D., and
DEREK J. CRIPPS, M.D.
University of Wisconsin
Madison, Wisconsin

Pruritus, or itching, consists of an uncomfortable sensation that provokes scratching. It is the most common symptom of skin disease but occasionally indicates an internal disorder.

Evaluation of itching in a patient should include a complete history and physical examination. Pertinent questions should focus on location and duration of the pruritus, provoking and relieving factors, severity, and past or present treatment. Physical examination should include identification of both primary and secondary changes. A primary skin lesion is usually characteristic of a particular group of skin disorders, whereas secondary changes are less specific but may indicate where the patient has manipulated the skin. Table 1 lists some of the most common primary pruritic dermatologic conditions and their associated physical findings. Secondary skin changes often seen in pruritic disorders include excoriations (scratch marks), lichenification (papular change caused by rubbing), burnished fingernails, and impetiginization (secondary infection). Additional tests that may facilitate diagnosis include skin scrapings for scabies mites, potassium hydroxide examination for fungal hyphae, and skin biopsy.

Generalized pruritus in the absence of diagnostic primary skin lesions, as well as pruritus that awakens the patient from sleep, are two features that may indicate an underlying systemic disorder. Table 2 lists some systemic causes of such pruritus. Affected patients have persistent pruritus that does not respond to initial work-up and management. Subsequent history and selective use of laboratory tests help identify the underlying disorder.

TREATMENT

Ideally, treatment of the pruritus involves pinpointing and treating the underlying cause. However, symptomatic care while the process of diagnosis is in progress provides the patient with much relief.

Patients first should be instructed to reduce the dryness of their skin. Dryness exacerbates pruritus, regardless of the cause. Bathing in lukewarm water for 10 minutes daily, avoidance of harsh soaps and irritating fabrics such as wool, and increasing environmental humidity are important factors. Air conditioning and heating of surroundings tend to reduce the ambient humidity and therefore contribute to dryness. Applying a cool, wet washcloth to a particular pruritic area and keeping nails trimmed short may help break the itch-scratch cycle.

Topical care should first include discontinuance of any agent that may be causing an irritant or allergic dermatitis. Patients often resort to home remedies as well as over-the-counter topical me-

TABLE 1. **Common Pruritic Skin Disorders and Accompanying Skin Changes**

Scabies	Burrows and excoriations in web spaces, periumbilical and periareolar areas, elbows, and body folds
Insect Bites	Urticarial papules, especially on the extremities
Atopic Dermatitis	Papules and patches with excoriations in antecubital fossae, neck, and eyelids
Seborrheic Dermatitis	Erythema and white scales on scalp, eyebrows, ears, and nasolabial folds
Contact Dermatitis	Sharply demarcated or linear patches located at site of contact; also, eczematous changes of eyelids
Dermatophytosis (Ringworm)	Single patch with central clearing and red scaling border
Psoriasis	Erythematous plaques with silvery scale, especially on scalp, elbows, knees, and buttocks
Dermatitis Herpetiformis	Grouped vesicles or crusts on elbows, knees, buttocks, and scalp
Xerosis of the Elderly	Fine white scale on a dull background with exaggerated skin lines
Pruritus Ani	Erythema, maceration, and lichenification of funnel-shaped anus

TABLE 2. **Systemic Disorders Causing Generalized Pruritus**

Hematologic
Polycythemia vera
Iron deficiency
Hepatobiliary
Obstructive biliary disease
Hepatic cholestasis
Infections and Infestations
Pruritus of HIV
Hookworm
Trichinosis
Ingestants
Opiates
Aspirin
Quinidine
Drugs causing cholestasis (e.g., phenothiazines and
    contraceptives)
Malignancy
Lymphoma
Leukemia
Multiple myeloma
Metabolic
Diabetes mellitus
Hyperthyroidism
Neurologic/Psychogenic
Multiple sclerosis
CNS tumor
Delusions of parasitosis
Renal
Chronic renal failure with uremia

Abbreviations: HIV, human immunodeficiency virus; CNS, central nervous system.

dicaments before presenting for medical evaluation. Persistent questioning by the examiner is sometimes required in order to elicit this history of use of topical agents containing neomycin, vitamin E, or other potential sensitizers. The patient should be encouraged to bring in all systemic and topical medications for evaluation.

Additional topical treatment consists of moisturizers, topical agents that impart a cooling sensation, and topical corticosteroids. Moisturizers may be in lotion, cream, ointment, or oil form. Lotions are the least effective but most cosmetically acceptable to patients. Ointments retain more moisture but feel greasy; therefore, heavier creams and ointments are best used at night. Moisturizers have two effective components: emollients and humectants. Emollients increase hydration of the stratum corneum by occlusion; petrolatum, mineral oil, and lanolin derivatives are emollients that are frequently found in moisturizers. Humectants increase hydration of the stratum corneum by drawing moisture into the skin; common examples are lactic acid, glycerin, and propylene glycol. The patient should apply the moisturizer to damp skin after bathing and reapply once or twice more daily.

Topical agents that impart a cooling sensation contain camphor in a 1 to 3% concentration or menthol in a 0.25 to 2% concentration. These may be found in various preformulated products such as Sarna Lotion or Prame Gel or may be compounded with a moisturizer by the pharmacist.

Topical corticosteroids are effective if a specific steroid-responsive problem, such as atopic or seborrheic dermatitis, is present. The prescribing physician should be familiar with the potency of the specific corticosteroid preparation in order to avoid untoward side effects such as cutaneous atrophy.

Systemic therapy of itching begins with oral antihistamines. H_1 receptor blockers such as diphenhydramine (Benadryl), 25 to 50 mg, or hydroxyzine (Atarax), 10 to 25 mg, may be taken once at bedtime or every 6 hours. Patients should be warned about sedation and should not operate a motor vehicle or drink alcohol while taking these drugs. Less sedating options include terfenadine (Seldane), 60 mg twice daily, or astemizole (Hismanal), 10 mg daily. Elevated plasma levels of both drugs have been associated with life-threatening cardiac arrhythmias; therefore, patients should be cautioned not to take more than the recommended dose. In addition, patients with significant liver dysfunction should not use either medicine; terfenadine is contraindicated in patients taking ketoconazole (Nizoral) or erythromycin. Selected patients may respond to psychotropic medications such as doxepin (Sinequan), 25 to 75 mg at bedtime. Sedation and anticholinergic side effects can occur.

Systemic corticosteroids and anxiolytics generally should not be used in the patient with pruritus of unknown etiology.

More disease-directed systemic therapies may be implemented if a specific condition is diagnosed. Several examples are as follows:

1. Cholestyramine (Questran), 4 gm twice daily, may relieve pruritus in obstructive biliary disease by binding pruritogenic substances in the gut.

2. Ultraviolet B and psoralen plus ultraviolet A (PUVA) therapies are useful in treating psoriasis, pruritus of human immunodeficiency virus (HIV), and pruritus associated with uremia.

3. Dapsone, 25 to 150 mg daily, is effective in controlling dermatitis herpetiformis.

These therapies should be administered by clinicians familiar with the side effects and appropriate monitoring techniques.

TINNITUS

method of
JACK C. CLEMIS, M.D., and
SALLY McDONALD, M.D.

Mercy Hospital and Medical Center
Chicago, Illinois

Tinnitus, the perception of noise in the head or ears, is a common and sometimes debilitating problem. Although in a soundproof room nearly 95% of a normal population would hear some form of tinnitus, 37 million Americans actually complain of tinnitus. Of these, 20% describe the problem as severe enough to interfere with their quality of life: diminishing mental concentration, creating anxiety, and impairing sleep.

Although the majority of patients with tinnitus are over the age of 40, it can occur at any age, and males and females are equally affected. Fifty percent of patients perceive unilateral tinnitus; the others complain of bilateral tinnitus or noise in their heads.

Although not all patients with tinnitus are aware of it, a majority are found to have a measurable hearing loss when tested.

The differential diagnosis of tinnitus is vast and includes all causes of conductive and sensorineural hearing loss, including common problems such as cerumen impaction, serous otitis, and perforation of the tympanic membrane; less common causes such as retrocochlear lesions (acoustic neuroma, meningioma, vascular malformations), myoclonus of tensor palatini or tensor tympani muscles, patulous eustachian tube, temporomandibular joint syndrome, head trauma, and drug toxicity must be included in the differential diagnosis.

As with any medical problem, the cornerstone of diagnosis is a thorough history and physical examination. Pertinent historical points in a patient with tinnitus include the age of the patient at the onset of symptoms, the progression of the problem, and other audiovestibular symptoms. An attempt to elicit a family history of audiologic problems should be made. The exact location of the sound and the quality (buzzing, ringing, pulsatile, and so forth) may help define the problem. A history of infection or trauma is pertinent, as is a survey of the patient's other medical problems and the medications taken.

The physical examination should be complete and include a record of the vital signs. Special attention should be focused on the examination of the head and neck, particularly the ears. The auricle, external canal, and tympanic membrane should be examined for evidence of infection, foreign body, cerumen, or trauma; an attempt to auscultate the tinnitus with a stethoscope or Toynbee ear speculum can be made, and if successful, an effort should be made to change the tinnitus with venous compression.

Additional evaluation should include a baseline complete audiogram, including tympanograms and assessments of acoustic delay, stapedial reflexes, speech reception thresholds, and speech discrimination. If symptoms and audiologic results suggest unilateral disease or a retrocochlear lesion, a magnetic resonance image (MRI) with gadolinium infusion is obtained. If symptoms are suggestive of underlying medical causes, helpful laboratory tests can include microhemagglutination assay—*Treponema pallidum* (MHA-TP), to evaluate for neurosyphilis; thyroid function tests; and a serum glucose test. In selected patients with pulsatile tinnitus, an angiogram may be useful.

TREATMENT

Obviously, it would be ideal to identify a cause for the tinnitus and treat it. Treatable causes include most conductive hearing losses: causes treatable by cerumen removal, treatable serous otitis, and stapedectomy in otosclerosis. The majority of affected patients report improvement or complete resolution of symptoms after treatment. Similarly, a majority of patients who undergo removal of an acoustic neuroma report less tinnitus postoperatively.

The majority of tinnitus is associated with sensorineural hearing loss, which is somewhat more difficult to treat successfully. For approximately 75 to 80% of patients with tinnitus, reassurance that it is not a sign of serious pathologic processes is all the treatment that is necessary, along with simple suggestions such as blocking or masking the noise with a competitive sound such as that from a fan or radio station static. In the remaining patients, tinnitus can be quite difficult to manage, necessitating much more time and attention.

Patients who desire intervention and who do not have a surgically correctable problem can be given a trial of masking therapy. Masking is an attempt to block tinnitus awareness by amplifying environmental noise or introducing broadband noise into the affected ear with either a hearing aid or a tinnitus masker. Some patients do not experience control of tinnitus for 2 to 3 months, and so an adequate trial must be used. After masking, approximately 10% of patients experience complete or partial resolution of the tinnitus.

Because severe tinnitus can cause anxiety and depression, these problems should be identified and treated. Appropriate measures include biofeedback stress management and, at times, referral to a mental health professional.

Pharmacotherapy can play an important role in the treatment of tinnitus. The simplest pharmacotherapy, often overlooked, is the cessation of drugs known to cause tinnitus: aspirin, quinine, quinidine, oral contraceptives, and many psychoactive drugs. It may take as long as 1 month for the tinnitus to lessen after cessation of an offending drug.

First-line drug therapy for many practitioners includes carbamazepine (Tegretol), phenytoin (Dilantin), and valproic acid (Depakene). Carbamazepine is generally the drug of choice, starting with 100 mg each night and increasing 100 mg per day each week until the dose is 200 mg three times per day. White blood cell counts and serum levels must be checked. If carbamazepine is ineffective or cannot be used because of an allergic reaction, phenytoin can be tried, starting at 30 mg three times per day and increasing to a daily dose of 400 mg. Valproic acid is generally reserved for use in patients with allergies to carbamazepine or phenytoin.

Antidepressants and tranquilizers can be used in patients suffering from depression and anxiety as a result of tinnitus, but any significant problem of this nature is better left to a qualified psychiatrist.

The authors' choice for pharmacotherapy is histamine. In a study awaiting publication, nearly 70% of patients treated with histamine achieved complete or partial resolution of their symptoms.

Section 2

The Infectious Diseases

MANAGEMENT OF THE PATIENT WITH HIV DISEASE

method of
ENRIQUE S. FERNANDEZ, M.D., M.S.Ed.

Health Resources and Services Administration,
  United States Public Health Service
Rockville, Maryland,

ABE M. MACHER, M.D., and
JOSEPH F. O'NEILL, M.D., M.S., M.P.H.

Chase-Brexton Clinic and the Baltimore
  Community Research Initiative
Baltimore, Maryland

The World Health Organization estimates that 1.2 million children and up to 14 million men and women have been infected with human immunodeficiency virus (HIV). By the year 2000, 30 to 40 million people will have contracted HIV infection. Current projections indicate that by 1996, over 7 million persons worldwide will have succumbed to the acquired immunodeficiency syndrome (AIDS).

In the United States, the number of individuals with HIV infection is estimated to be between 1 and 1.5 million. As of March 1993, 4470 cases of AIDS in children less than 13 years old and 289,320 cases of AIDS in adolescents and adults had been reported to the U.S. government's Centers for Disease Control and Prevention (CDC). Although the majority of reported cases in the United States are found in gay and bisexual men, other demographic groups are composing an ever larger proportion of AIDS cases and in some communities are the majority incidence group.

In the United States, the highest rates of new transmission of HIV is expected to be found among heterosexuals. With effective means of protecting the blood supply in place since 1985, the incidence of new HIV-1 infection via transfusion of blood products is near zero in developed countries. HIV infection and AIDS associated with injection drug use (IDU) continue to account for a significant proportion of HIV disease in the United States (currently about 22% of adult AIDS cases).

Of particular note is the fact that HIV/AIDS disproportionately affects African Americans and Hispanics in the United States. For example, over 50% of women

The views represented in this article are those of the authors and do not necessarily represent the policy of the Health Resources and Services Administration.

and children with AIDS are African Americans, whereas African Americans compose only 12% of the U.S. population. Likewise, although the number of new diagnoses of AIDS in gay men generally appears to be leveling off, there remains a marked upward trend among ethnic minority and IDU gay men.

It is important for the primary care provider to be aware of these trends because of the crucial role that he or she must play in the prevention of new cases of HIV transmission. It is incumbent upon the provider to assess every patient's risk behaviors by careful interview; the provider should offer or facilitate HIV testing when appropriate.

NATURAL HISTORY OF HIV INFECTION

Patients infected with HIV proceed through a spectrum of disease stages that range from (1) an acute symptomatic viral illness to (2) an asymptomatic "latent" state characterized only by laboratory evidence of HIV infection to (3) an early symptomatic lymphadenopathic syndrome characterized by persistent generalized lymphadenopathy to (4) an advanced symptomatic syndrome (chronic constitutional symptoms, oral candidiasis or hairy leukoplakia, etc.) to, finally, (5) a syndrome resulting from a serious opportunistic complication associated with severe immunoincompetence (pneumocystosis, etc.).

HIV infection may be initiated when an individual is inoculated with the virus (either directly into the bloodstream; or by exposure of broken skin, an open wound, or mucous membranes to HIV-contaminated fluids; or by perinatal transmission from infected mother to infant). After inoculation, HIV infects and begins to replicate in one or more types of susceptible cells, including lymph node tissue. Circulating CD4 lymphocytes and macrophages are most commonly affected, although epithelial cells of the gastrointestinal tract, uterine cervical cells, glial cells of the central nervous system, and other cells may also be targets. In most cases, HIV then proceeds to sufficiently replicate to produce detectable levels of viral antigens and elicit host antibody production within a few weeks to months. It is during this period that the patient often experiences a few days of clinical symptoms suggestive of a viral (mononucleosis-like) illness that may include aseptic meningitis.

As the host's immune system mounts its initial antibody response to HIV, viral antigen is neutralized and disappears or is detectable only at low levels. The patient usually becomes asymptomatic and remains so for a period that may range from weeks to many years; HIV antibodies, but usually not HIV antigens, are detectable in the serum, and viral nucleic acid is detectable in infected cells. The majority of infected individuals exist in this clinical latent state and can be identified by screening of serum for HIV antibody. In most if not all cases, viral replication progresses or accelerates. The subsequent rate of progression of disease and the specific clinical syndromes that appear vary from person to person.

As viral replication proceeds, CD4 lymphocytes are destroyed by HIV infection and cell fusion, and monocyte-macrophages are rendered dysfunctional. Damage to these key cells leads to abnormal activation of other immune mechanisms and accounts for the observed dysfunction of B cell (hypergammaglobulinemia, thrombocytopenia) and cytotoxic T cell response. The clinical syndromes observed at any time depend partly on the degree of immunosuppression and partly on direct effects of HIV. AIDS is diagnosed when CD4 levels fall below 200 cells per mm^3 or when a disease indicative of *severe* immunoincompetence appears (*Pneumocystis carinii* pneumonia, *Candida* esophagitis, pulmonary/extrapulmonary tuberculosis, recurrent pneumonia, invasive cervical cancer, cytomegalovirus retinitis, HIV wasting syndrome or encephalopathy, etc.). Syndromes of *less* severity are placed under the category of "symptomatic" HIV disease and represent HIV infection that has not yet progressed to AIDS (persistent generalized lymphadenopathy, unexplained weight loss with fever or diarrhea, oral candidiasis, oral hairy leukoplakia, dermatomal herpes zoster, psoriasis, seborrheic dermatitis). As the immune system progressively deteriorates, the host not only becomes increasingly vulnerable to opportunistic complications, but also is less able to slow the process of HIV replication. Antibodies to HIV p24 antigen decrease in titer and may become undetectable, and viral core antigens reappear. Eventually, an untreatable opportunistic complication can occur, which will result in death.

The CD4 lymphocyte count is used to make important clinical management decisions regarding the implementation of antiretrovirals and prophylaxis for *P. carinii* infection. Although the average count in healthy persons is 1100 per mm^3, there is substantial intralaboratory variation and even greater interlaboratory variation. Large fluctuations may reflect the technology of the test rather than the biology of the disease; for this reason, trends are more important than a single test result, and the test should be repeated when the results determine important therapeutic decisions. In HIV-infected individuals, the average decline in CD4 lymphocyte counts is 85 to 100 per mm^3 per year. Studies have indicated that use of zidovudine (AZT, Retrovir) in patients with CD4 levels below 500 cells per mm^3 or with early onset of symptoms prolongs the AIDS-free state. This benefit, however, is CD4 dependent and is time limited. The clinical benefits of AZT therapy may be lost in as little as 1.5 years if the therapy is started when CD4 counts are less than 300 cells per mm^3. Also, AZT has generally not been shown to improve survival in patients with early HIV disease who are asymptomatic.

As the CD4 lymphocyte count continues to diminish and approaches 200 cells per mm^3, patients become increasingly susceptible to develop severe opportunistic complications, including *P. carinii* infections. *P. car-*

inii prophylaxis has proved to be of considerable value for HIV-infected patients; prophylactic regimens for the prevention of mycotic, toxoplasmal, and other life-threatening opportunistic infections are also being investigated.

Surrogate HIV Markers

Neopterin appears during the metabolism of folic acid and has been found in increased amounts in the serum and urine of patients with viral infections and malignancies, including patients with HIV disease. Beta$_2$-microglobulin occurs on the surface of all nucleated cells and is released into serum during cell turnover, it is considered a marker of infectious, inflammatory, or malignant, and autoimmune disease activity, and elevated levels are observed in patients with HIV disease. The precise use of neopterin and beta$_2$-microglobulin levels in clinical management is yet to be determined.

The p24 antigen is the major HIV core protein, and serum levels increase shortly after HIV infection and decline when p24 antibody appears. Both a low level antibody or a subsequent decrease in anti-p24 antibody and a high level antigen or an increase in p24 antigen correlate with disease progression and a poor prognosis. Levels of p24 antigen are used in studies to monitor efficacy of drug treatments; p24 antigen levels have been shown to decrease during successful therapy with zidovudine. Nevertheless, details of how to use p24 antigen levels for clinical management are not yet defined.

MANAGEMENT OF THE ASYMPTOMATIC HIV-SEROPOSITIVE PATIENT

Initial Baseline Laboratory Studies

The baseline laboratory evaluation of the asymptomatic HIV-infected patient should include the following: (1) complete blood count (CBC) with differential (a platelet count is suggested if platelets are decreased on the peripheral smear or if there is evidence by history or physical examination of thrombocytopenia); (2) chemistry panel (SMA 12, 14, or 20); (3) CD4 cell count and percentage; (4) purified protein derivative (PPD) skin test with anergy panel; (5) Venereal Disease Research Laboratory (VDRL) or rapid plasma reagin (RPR) test; and (6) hepatitis B serologic testing for surface antibody (HBsAb), advocated for any patient who is being considered for hepatitis B vaccination (see later discussion). Some clinicians also obtain a baseline chest x-ray and toxoplasmosis titers.

A follow-up visit is recommended 1 to 2 weeks after the initial evaluation in order to review laboratory results and to provide additional counseling. The CD4 cell count will be available and should be used in establishing the care plan. Decisions regarding the initiation of anti-retroviral therapy and *P. carinii* pneumonia prophylaxis for asymptomatic patients are based on the CD4 cell count. Recommendations for monitoring are based on the observation that the CD4 test shows considerable variation and that major therapeutic decisions based on values that are near the decision point need to be confirmed.

In general, CD4 lymphocyte counts should be evaluated every 6 months. If a significant drop (e.g., greater than 10% annual fall) has occurred since the last evaluation or if the CD4 count is at a point where therapeutic decisions are being made, the frequency of monitoring should be increased. Significant changes in CD4 cell counts seldom occur within a period of 3 months. A given result can normally vary by as much as 50 cells per mm^3 from the prior CD4 count. Profound changes in CD4 absolute counts should be correlated with the percentage of CD4 cells, and confirmation testing may be required within 1 to 2 weeks.

Use of Anti-Retroviral Medications

Currently, three medications possessing antiretroviral properties are licensed by the U.S. Food and Drug Administration (FDA) for use in HIV infection (AZT, ddI, and ddC). Although the optimal use (i.e., single vs. combination therapy, early vs. late use, etc.) of these and other antiretroviral medications under development remains controversial, most physicians in the United States have made them an important part of their approach to HIV/AIDS treatment. The decision regarding timing of anti-retroviral therapy initiation, selection of anti-retroviral therapy regimens, changing regimens, or stopping therapy altogether must be made with the fully informed participation of the patient. Because the current state of the art in antiretroviral therapy is in flux, individualized therapy becomes important, pending the identification of a superior regimen. Many factors, including preferences of the patient, are essential considerations

For most clinicians, AZT remains the first-line treatment for HIV-infected patients with CD4 cell counts below 500 cells per mm^3. Some clinicians, however, will not treat at this level and prefer to wait until there is clinical evidence of advancing disease (signs, symptoms, or an increase in the rate of decline of CD4 counts). Clearly, however, the role of AZT is limited by toxicities, viral resistance, and the drug's inability to do more than slow viral replication. Discouraging evidence that long-term AZT monotherapy has little or no impact on survival can be seen as less an argument for abandonment of the drug than as support for

continuing the search for ways of using it that are better than long-term single-agent therapy. Many providers use AZT in combination with ddI or with ddC, and others alternate AZT therapy with ddI therapy (e.g., monthly alternating use of AZT and ddI as single agents). The potential benefits of preventing the development of viral resistance by combining or alternating therapies are theoretical and await the results of clinical trials.

It is common practice in many centers, therefore, to offer treatment with AZT (100 mg orally five times daily and spaced apart every 4 hours, or 200 mg orally three times daily) when CD4 levels fall below 500 cells per mm^3 or when advancing disease is suspected. Regardless of lack of symptomatic disease, many clinicians encourage a patient who has not yet initiated anti-retroviral therapy to consider doing so when CD4 counts fall below the 200- to 300-cell-per-mm^3 range.

In general, after 12 to 24 months of AZT monotherapy, there is evidence of more rapid disease progression, which is often thought to be related to the emergence of viral resistance. The clinician attempts, by careful evaluation, physical examination, and CD4 measurement, to identify this point and then to add a second drug, to switch to ddI, or to alternate therapies. Determining that a particular drug has failed may prove difficult. General guidelines to follow include the development of a new or recurrent opportunistic infection or malignancy, the onset or persistence of debilitating clinical symptoms (weight loss, diarrhea, unexplained fevers, progressive oral thrush, etc.), or when the CD4 count falls by 50% or more within a 1- to 2-year period.

Because ddC is licensed only for use in combination with AZT, the authors generally prefer to add ddC (AZT, 200 mg orally three times daily with ddC, 0.375 mg orally three times daily) (the higher dose of ddC 0.75 mg orally three times daily is less often needed) and hold ddI in reserve. This is because as HIV disease progresses, patients often become less able to tolerate AZT either alone or in combination. Should this occur, the patient will still be ddI naive, and consequently this third option remains available. Moreover, some data support the change to therapy with ddI (200 mg orally twice daily for patients weighing more than 60 kg, 125 mg orally twice daily for those weighing less than 60 kg) in patients whose CD4 counts are below 300 cells per mm^3 and have been on AZT for 4 months or longer.

Other clinicians prefer to begin immediately with a combination of drugs and avoid monotherapy whenever possible. However, because of the similar side effect profile, ddI and ddC should not be used in combination with each other.

Anti-Retroviral Toxicity

Common side effects early in treatment with AZT include nausea, headache, insomnia, myalgias, and vomiting; these usually resolve while the drug is continued. However, if symptoms become intolerable, the dose may be lowered temporarily (100 mg three times daily) and later increased to full dosage as tolerated. AZT also causes a macrocytosis that does not respond to vitamin B$_{12}$ or folic acid. Macrocytosis alone is not an indication for cessation of therapy. The major side effect with long-term use of AZT is bone marrow suppression with anemia or granulocytopenia. Options for medical management of granulocytopenia and anemia ascribed to AZT are as follows: If the hemoglobin decreases to 7.5 grams per dL or less, the drug should be discontinued; options at this juncture are to (1) await bone marrow recovery and then reinitiate AZT at a lower dosage (e.g., 100 mg three times a day); (2) consider periodic transfusions and continue AZT in full dose or reduced dose; (3) administer recombinant human erythropoietin (EPO) (Epogen, Procrit) in a dosage of 24,000 units per week if the baseline EPO is less than 500 milliunits per mm^3, or (4) combinations of these tactics. Similarly, if the absolute neutrophil count is less than 750 per mm^3, the drug should be discontinued, the dosage should be reduced, or AZT should be given concurrently with granulocyte colony-stimulating factor (G-CSF) or granulocyte-macrophage colony-stimulating factor (GM-CSF). Therapies involving other marrow-suppressive drugs should be re-evaluated. Other side effects occasionally encountered with AZT include rash, fever, agitation, confusion, and myopathy; the last-named complication is usually seen after at least 1 year of treatment and tends to resolve when AZT is discontinued.

With continued use of AZT, in vitro resistance is believed to be common in patients with AIDS and is sometimes associated with clinical deterioration; whether drug resistance is the cause of the clinical deterioration is unclear. In vitro resistance emerges more slowly in patients with less advanced disease. Renewed susceptibility to AZT has been reported after treatment with the drug was stopped. Strains of HIV resistant in vitro to AZT may be susceptible to dideoxyinosine (ddI) (Videx) or dideoxycytidine (ddC; zalcitabine [HIVID]).

Dideoxyinosine, which has in vitro activity similar to that of AZT, has been approved by the U.S. Food and Drug Administration (FDA) for use in patients who are intolerant of AZT or who have demonstrated significant clinical or immunologic deterioration during AZT therapy.

Data suggest that the use of ddI can transiently increase CD4 lymphocyte counts, decrease serum p24 antigen levels, and lead to weight gain in patients with AIDS or symptomatic HIV disease. The most frequent adverse effects of ddI have been abdominal cramps and diarrhea resulting from the osmotic effects of the drug vehicle. Major treatment limiting toxicities have been peripheral neuropathy and acute pancreatitis; hepatic failure has also occurred; patients with a history of pancreatitis or alcoholism should not take ddI. Dideoxycytidine, another inhibitor of HIV reverse transcriptase, is now available as an adjunct to AZT therapy to treat patients with AIDS and symptomatic HIV disease. Adverse effects include rash, stomatitis, fever, peripheral neuropathy, and, rarely, pancreatitis. Studies are under way to determine whether concurrent or sequential use of AZT with either ddI or ddC could delay emergence of resistance and clinical deterioration.

Detection and Prophylaxis of Tuberculosis

There is an increased incidence of active tuberculosis in patients with AIDS because progressive immunoincompetence is associated with reactivation of latent tuberculous infections. This has led to the general recommendation for a PPD skin test for all persons with HIV infection and for HIV serologic testing for all persons with active tuberculosis. The following applies for all HIV-infected patients: (1) Standard screening test should be the Mantoux method with the intradermal injection of 5 TU of PPD; (2) induration of 5 mm or greater is considered positive; (3) anergy in the later stages of HIV infection is likely to account for high rates of false-negative tests in persons with low CD4 lymphocyte counts, and some clinicians consider *any* amount of induration in a patient with advanced HIV disease to be a positive test result; (4) patients with positive skin tests should have a chest x-ray and examination for extrapulmonary tuberculosis; (5) patients who are anergic should have a routine chest x-ray; (6) persons with inactive disease should receive isoniazid in a dosage of 300 mg per day for a period of 12 months.

There have been reports of the nosocomial transmission of multidrug-resistant tuberculosis, primarily among HIV-infected persons. It is not known whether "standard" prophylactic therapy (isoniazid) can effectively prevent the development of active tuberculosis in persons who are infected with multidrug-resistant strains of tuberculosis. Immunocompromised persons likely to have been infected with multidrug-resistant tuberculosis may require prophylaxis with isoniazid and an additional agent (e.g., rifampin), on the basis of knowledge of the TB-strain sensitivities in the local setting.

Treatment of active multi-drug-resistant tuberculosis should be undertaken in consultation with infectious disease specialists and appropriate public health institutions.

Vaccinations

The influenza and pneumococcal vaccines should be routinely administered to HIV-infected patients; other vaccines to consider include those for hepatitis B and *Haemophilus influenzae*. All single-dose vaccines should be given as early as possible in the course of HIV infection to obtain an optimal immune response.

Influenza Vaccine

There is no evidence that influenza is more frequent or more severe in persons with HIV infection. Nevertheless, these possibilities have not been excluded, and influenza may pose a diagnostic dilemma when other conditions such as *P. carinii* pneumonia are considered. Patients with HIV infection should receive the annual influenza vaccine, preferably in November or earlier. The importance of influenza vaccine is even greater for persons with HIV infection in chronic care facilities, those over 65 years of age, and those with chronic disorders of the cardiovascular or pulmonary systems.

Pneumococcal Vaccine

The frequency of pneumococcal pneumonia and bacteremia is clearly increased in persons with HIV infection. The efficacy of pneumococcal vaccine is debated, but this vaccine is recommended for all persons with HIV infection, according to current CDC guidelines. Re-vaccination should be considered in those who received the vaccine 6 or more years previously.

Hepatitis B Vaccine

Hepatitis B vaccine is advocated for persons who lack serologic evidence of hepatitis B virus markers and are in any of the following risk groups: active intravenous drug abusers, sexually active homosexual men, and household or sexual contacts of hepatitis B virus surface antigen carriers. The usual serologic test to screen vaccine candidates is surface antibody (HBsAb). The usual regimen involves three serial vaccinations of 1-mL doses of Recombivax HB or Engerix-B, given at 0, 1, and 6 months.

Haemophilus influenzae Vaccine

There appears to be an increased frequency of *H. influenzae* pulmonary infections in persons with HIV infection. However, the efficacy of this vaccine in any adult population has not been demonstrated, and it is also not clear that the predominant infecting strains are Type B, which are the *only* strains against which this vaccine provides protection. No clear recommendation for adults can be made, although some providers may wish to give this vaccine, particularly to HIV-infected persons with chronic lung disease.

Poliovirus, DTP, Measles, Mumps, and Rubella Vaccines

Live attenuated virus vaccines routinely administered to children are polioviruses, measles, mumps, and rubella. Persons with compromised humoral immunity, particularly those who lack IgG-bearing B cells, are at risk for severe central nervous system infection with enteroviruses; chronic enterovirus meningoencephalitis and paralytic poliomyelitis associated with attenuated vaccine polioviruses have been reported in children with congenital agammaglobulinemia. However, *neither* of these illnesses has been reported in children with HIV infection. Nevertheless, administration of *inactivated* polio vaccine (IPV) and avoiding direct exposure to live oral polio vaccine (OPV) with resulting diminished possibility of vaccine-associated paralytic disease are prudent in the United States, where the alternative of inactivated poliovirus vaccine is available. Administration of IPV also reduces the inadvertent exposure of other household members (who may be HIV infected) to vaccine virus (OPV) excreted in the stool by the vaccinee. The administration of diphtheria, tetanus, and pertussis (DTP) and measles, mumps, and rubella (MMR) vaccines is recommended for HIV-infected children, and these vaccines can be safely administered to adolescents and adults according to standard practice.

MANAGEMENT OF HIV ENCEPHALOPATHY

The AIDS dementia complex is a common disorder characterized by cognitive, motor, and behavioral dysfunction. The disorder represents a continuum from a mild cognitive defect, noted only on sophisticated testing, to a severe and fatal illness. The early manifestation includes mild forgetfulness and reduced ability to concentrate, slowed verbal and motor responses and decreased coordination, and a wide range of behavioral abnormalities varying from apathy to depression to agitation. Patients who present with depression should be evaluated for early AIDS dementia complex. Likewise, any patient exhibiting signs of dementia should be evaluated for depression. The late manifestation of AIDS dementia complex includes obvious dementia, focal motor and cerebellar findings, urinary and fecal incontinence, and ultimately a nearly vegetative state.

Management of AIDS dementia complex includes a combination of empiric therapies and antiretroviral treatment. AZT improved neurologic function in adults in the first placebo-controlled trial of the drug. However, all of the trials in adults have used oral doses of at least 200 mg every 4 hours; it is not known if the currently recommended lower doses (100 mg every 4 hours) achieve adequate levels in the CNS to be useful in treating AIDS dementia complex. While dose comparison studies are underway, patients with *adequate* hematopoietic reserve should be treated with the higher doses. The neurologic efficacy of alternative antiretroviral agents (ddI, ddC) remains to be determined.

Psychoactive medications have a role in the management of both the cognitive and the behavioral manifestations of AIDS dementia complex. All psychoactive drugs must be used cautiously, because patients with organic brain disease are prone to exaggerated and adverse responses. Methylphenidate has been used in patients with slow responses or decreased attention. Antidepressants in modest and gradually titrated doses can be useful when clinically evident depression causes or contributes to the cognitive impairment and apathy. Minor and major tranquilizers can be useful in persons with agitation or frank psychosis complicating AIDS dementia complex; these patients may have a higher incidence of extrapyramidal reactions to the tranquilizers.

MANAGEMENT OF OPPORTUNISTIC INFECTIONS (Table 1)

Protozoa

Pneumocystis carinii

Pneumonia caused by *Pneumocystis carinii* is the most common life-threatening opportunistic infection in patients with AIDS. As an extracellular protozoan, *P. carinii* exists within the pulmonary alveoli of humans. In the immunocompromised host, proliferation of organisms results in consolidation of pulmonary parenchyma and progressive hypoxemia manifested by chills, fever, diaphoresis, nonproductive cough, dyspnea on exertion, and fatigue. Physical examination of the chest is often unremarkable, or findings are minimal despite advanced signs and symptoms.

Prominent adventitious sounds suggest an etiology other than *P. carinii* pneumonia. In some patients with AIDS, hematogenous dissemination of *P. carinii* may result in extrapulmonary clinical disease characterized by hepatosplenomegaly, lymphadenopathy, mucocutaneous lesions, choroiditis, etc. With the more widespread use of aerosolized pentamidine for prophylaxis and treatment, there has been a rise in the number of extrapulmonary infections caused by *P. carinii*.

Radiographically, a diffuse or perihilar infiltrative pattern, occasionally with peripheral sparing, is the most common presentation of *P. carinii* pneumonia; however, some patients present with local patchy interstitial infiltrates (including unilateral disease), lobar consolidation, nodular lesions, cystic or cavitating lesions, or unilateral or bilateral pneumothoraces. Radiographic presentation with patchy upper lobe consolidation mimicking tuberculosis also occurs; although relapses were observed before the use of aerosolized pentamidine, they have been increasingly reported as upper lobe infiltrates in patients on prophylactic aerosolized pentamidine (NebuPent). Pleural effusions are very uncommon in patients with *P. carinii* pneumonia; when present, particularly if they are large, they should raise suspicions of pleuropulmonary Kaposi's sarcoma, tuberculosis, lymphoma, and bacterial or fungal infections. Finally, 5 to 10% of patients with *P. carinii* pneumonia may present with normal chest radiographs. Therefore, chest x-ray alone is unreliable as an indicator of active *P. carinii* pneumonia. Clinical features such as cough, fever, shortness of breath, and headache along with laboratory findings of hypoxemia in a patient with low CD4 lymphocyte counts should imply active *P. carinii* pneumonia until otherwise ruled out. Evaluation of the lung using gallium 67 scanning at 48 and 72 hours is very sensitive (90 to 100%) for *P. carinii* pneumonia, but the specificity is as low as 20%.

Arterial blood gas measurements (with the patient breathing room air) generally show a moderate hypoxemia, although oxygen tension values vary widely, depending on the severity of the pneumonia; up to 25% of patients have arterial oxygen tensions of 80 mmHg or above; the blood gas pattern usually shows an uncompensated respiratory alkalosis with an increased alveolar-arterial oxygen tension difference. With regard to pulmonary function testing, the most consistent finding is a marked decrease in the single-breath diffusing capacity for carbon monoxide (DL_{CO}). After therapy for *P. carinii* pneumonia, pulmonary function can be expected to return toward normal; many patients return to baseline, but some may have a mild restrictive pattern with or without a reduced DL_{CO}.

TABLE 1. **Treatment of Opportunistic Infections**

Pneumocystis carinii	Trimethoprim (15 mg/kg/day) + sulfamethoxazole (75–100 mg/kg/day) PO or IV × 21 days in three to four daily doses Pentamidine (4 mg/kg/day) IV or IM × 21 days Dapsone (100 mg/day) PO + trimethoprim (5 mg/kg) PO or IV q 8 hr × 21 days Clindamycin (600–900 mg) IV q 6 hr × 10 days, then 450 mg PO q 6 hr × 11 days + primaquine (15 mg base) PO qd Atovaquone (Mepron), 750 mg PO tid with food Maintenance therapy: Trimethoprim-sulfamethoxazole, one double-strength tablet PO qd for 7 days/wk or 2 double-strength tabs PO three times/wk (Monday, Wednesday, Friday) Dapsone 100 mg PO three times/wk Aerosol pentamidine, 300 mg monthly via nebulizer Pyrimethamine + sulfadoxine (25 mg/500 mg, Fansidar) PO each week
Toxoplasma gondii	Pyrimethamine, 50–100 mg PO qd, + sulfadiazine, 1–2 gm PO q 6 hr + folinic acid, 5–20 mg PO qd hr Clindamycin, 450–600 mg PO q 6 hr, or 600 mg IV q 6 hr, + sulfadiazine, 1–2 gm PO q 6 hr Maintenance therapy: Pyrimethamine, 25–50 mg PO qd, + sulfadiazine, 500–1000 mg PO q 6 hr Pyrimethamine, 25–50 mg qd, + clindamycin, 300 mg PO q 6 hr
Cryptosporidium	Paromomycin, 500 mg PO q 6 hr
Isospora belli	Trimethoprim-sulfamethoxazole, one double-strength tablet q 6 hr × 10 days Maintenance therapy: Trimethoprim-sulfamethoxazole, one double-strength tablet three times weekly
Enterocytozoon bieneusi	Metronidazole, 500 mg PO q 6 hr

Candida species
  Oral thrush
 	
  Esophagitis
	Nystatin solution or tablets, 500,000–1,000,000 U PO three to five times/day
	Clotrimazole troches, 10 mg PO five times/day
	Ketoconazole, 200 mg PO qd
	Fluconazole, 50–100 mg PO qd
	Ketoconazole, 200–400 mg qd
	Fluconazole, 100–400 mg PO or IV qd
	Amphotericin B, 0.3 mg/kg IV qd
	
	Maintenance therapy:
	Ketoconazole, 200 mg qd
	Fluconazole, 50 mg qd

Cryptococcus neoformans	Amphotericin B, 0.6 mg/kg/day IV Amphotericin B, 0.3 mg/kg/day IV + flucytosine 100–150 mg/kg/day PO in four divided doses Fluconazole, 400 mg PO qd Maintenance therapy: Amphotericin B, 1.0 mg/kg IV weekly Fluconazole, 200 mg PO qd

Table continued on following page

P. carinii cannot be readily cultured; hence diagnosis is dependent upon direct visualization of the protozoan. The diagnosis is usually established with specimens of induced sputa (this procedure involves inhalation of a hypertonic saline mist generated by an ultrasonic nebulizer and collection of the subsequent expectorated sputum) or bronchoalveolar lavage; alternative methods involve specimens obtained by transbronchial or open lung biopsies.

Treatment of Acute Infection. The preferred treatment of *P. carinii* pneumonia includes trimethoprim (15 mg per kg per day) plus sulfamethoxazole (75 to 100 mg per kg per day) orally or intravenously for up to 21 days in three to four daily doses. Alternative therapy involves pentamidine (4 mg per kg every 24 hours) intravenously or intramuscularly for up to 21 days. Alternative treatments for patients unable to tolerate a full course of these agents include (1) dapsone (100 mg orally every 24 hours) plus trimethoprim (5 mg per kg orally or intravenously every 8 hours) and (2) clindamycin (600 to 900 mg intravenously every 6 hours for 10 days, then 450 mg orally

TABLE 1. **Treatment of Opportunistic Infections** *Continued*

Histoplasma capsulatum	Amphotericin B, 0.6 mg/kg IV qd Itraconazole, 200 mg PO bid Maintenance therapy: Itraconazole, 100 mg PO bid
Coccidioides immitis	Amphotericin B, 0.6 mg/kg IV qd Maintenance therapy: Amphotericin B, 1.0 mg/kg/wk
Mycobacterium tuberculosis	See text
Mycobacterium avium	Clarithromycin (Biaxin), 1 gm PO bid, plus rifampin, 600 mg PO qd, or rifabutin, 300–450 mg PO qd, + ethambutol, 15–25 mg/kg PO qd, + Clofazimime, 100–300 mg PO qd, + ciprofloxacin, 750 mg PO bid, +/− amikacin, 7.5 mg/kg IV or IM qd
Treponema pallidum	See text
Salmonella species	Ampicillin, 8–12 gm/day IV × 2 wk, followed by amoxicillin, 500 mg PO tid × 2 wk Ciprofloxacin, 750 mg PO bid × 2–4 wk Trimethoprim (5–10 mg/kg/day) + sulfamethoxazole IV or PO × 4 wk Maintenance therapy: Amoxicillin, 250 mg PO bid Ciprofloxacin, 500 mg PO qd or bid Trimethoprim (2.5 mg/kg) + sulfamethoxazole PO bid

Herpes simplex virus
  Mild mucocutaneous
  Severe mucocutaneous
 	
  Visceral
	Acyclovir, 200 mg PO five times/day for at least 10 days
	Acyclovir (15 mg/kg/day) IV
	Vidarabine (15 mg/kg/day) IV
	Foscarnet (90 mg/kg/day) IV
	
	Maintenance therapy:
	Acyclovir, 200 mg PO tid
	Acyclovir, (30 mg/kg/day) IV for at least 10 days
	Vidarabine (15 mg/kg/day) IV for 10 days

Herpes zoster / varicella
  Dermatomal
 	
  Ophthalmic, visceral,
    disseminated
	Acyclovir, 800 mg PO five times/day
	Acyclovir (30 mg/kg/day) IV
	Acyclovir (30 mg/kg/day) IV

Cytomegalovirus Retinitis	Foscarnet, 60 mg/kg IV q 8 hr Ganciclovir, 5 mg/kg IV q 12 hr Maintenance therapy: Foscarnet, 90 mg/kg/day IV infusion Ganciclovir, 5 mg/kg/day IV, or 6 mg/kg IV 6 days/wk

Abbreviations: PO = orally; IV = intravenously; IM = intramuscularly.

every 6 hours) plus primaquine (15 mg base orally per day). A new oral agent, atovaquone (Mepron), is also showing promising results in patients who have failed standard therapy. It appears to be effective and generally well tolerated.

It is not uncommon for the radiographic appearance of *P. carinii* pneumonia to worsen early in the course of therapy. In the more severe cases, there may be progression to air-space consolidation; however, if the deterioration continues beyond 7 to 10 days, failure of therapy should be considered. When patients are switched to an alternate regimen because of therapeutic failure, a minimum of 2 to 3 weeks of effective therapy is desirable. Patients presenting with moderately severe or severe pneumonia (arterial oxygen tension of less than 70 mmHg) should receive corticosteroids (prednisone, 40 mg orally twice a day for 5 days, then 40 mg every day for 5 days, then 20 mg per day to completion of treatment).

Prophylaxis. *P. carinii* pneumonia prophylaxis is advocated for all patients with HIV infection with a CD4 lymphocyte count less than 200 per mm³ (less than 20% CD4 lymphocytes), for those who have recovered from an episode of *P. carinii* pneumonia, and for those with constitutional symptoms such as thrush or unexplained fever higher than 100°F for 2 weeks or more (regardless of their CD4 lymphocyte count).

The preferred prophylactic regimen is trimethoprim-sulfamethoxazole, one double-strength tablet by mouth once or twice daily for 3 to 7 days per week. This regimen is inexpensive, is convenient, and is likely to prevent common infections by pathogens other than *P. carinii,* including *Streptococcus pneumoniae, H. influenzae,* and *Legionella, Nocardia, Salmonella,* and possibly *Toxoplasma* spp.; furthermore, there is clinical evidence that trimethoprim-sulfamethoxazole has superior efficacy with regard to preventing or delaying recurrent *P. carinii* pneumonia (secondary prophylaxis). Therefore, the major reason for an alternative prophylactic regimen is an adverse drug reaction to trimethoprim-sulfamethoxazole. Adverse drug reactions to trimethoprim-sulfamethoxazole have been noted in up to 50% of HIV-infected patients and include leukopenia, thrombocytopenia, anemia, hepatitis, rash, fever, nausea, and azotemia; these symptomatic side effects are usually transient and should not hasten a decision to discontinue the drug. However, if the symptoms do become intolerable, an option is to use a lower dosing regimen of trimethoprim-sulfamethoxazole, because most adverse drug reactions are dose related; an alternative consideration is one single-strength tablet daily, or three times a week. Other alternative treatments include (1) dapsone, 100 mg three times per week orally; or (2) aerosol pentamidine, 300 mg monthly via Respigard II nebulizer (generally well tolerated, especially if given with a bronchodilator); or (3) pyrimethamine plus sulfadoxine (Fansidar), one tablet (25 mg/500 mg) orally each week.

Toxoplasma gondii

Toxoplasma encephalitis is the most common cause of intracerebral lesions among patients with AIDS. The onset of cerebral toxoplasmosis is subacute, manifesting with headache, focal neurologic deficits, altered mental status, or seizures, alone or in combination. Fever is often present. Suspicion of toxoplasmosis should prompt imaging of the brain. Magnetic resonance imaging (MRI) is more sensitive than computed tomography but is less readily available. Although *Toxoplasma* lesions have a radiologic appearance similar to brain abscess, pathologically the lesions are nonencapsulated areas of coagulation necrosis. Lesions of toxoplasmal encephalitis are usually round with either solid (diffuse) enhancement or ring enhancement. *Toxoplasma* encephalitis is a multifocal disease, and single lesions are the exception. Most of the other entities causing focal brain disease in patients with AIDS (lymphoma, tuberculoma, cryptococcoma, Kaposi's sarcoma) can have an identical appearance. *Toxoplasma* lesions characteristically occur in the cerebral cortex at the gray-white junction and in the basal ganglia; however, lesions can occur in other locations, including the cerebellum and brain stem. Typically, the degree of neurologic impairment is less than what would be expected from the number and size of the lesions and associated edema. This contrasts with progressive multifocal leukoencephalopathy (PML), in which the degree of impairment is disproportionately greater than the abnormalities on scanning.

Because toxoplasmal encephalitis is usually a reactivation disease, the great majority of patients have detectable levels of anti-*toxoplasma* (IgG) antibody. Changes in antibody titer over time do not necessarily occur in AIDS-associated reactivation toxoplasmosis and need not be looked for. The definitive diagnosis is made by brain biopsy. However, the prompt clinical and radiologic response of *toxoplasma* encephalitis in AIDS patients allows a presumptive diagnosis to be made on a characteristic presentation and a documented response to empiric therapy (obviating the need for biopsy of the brain in many cases). The antifolate agent pyrimethamine (Daraprim) given with sulfadiazine is the treatment of choice for *Toxoplasma* encephalitis. Standard therapy includes pyrimethamine, 50 to 100 mg per day orally, with sulfadiazine, 1 to 2 grams orally every 6 hours; folinic acid or leucovorin, 5 to 20 mg orally daily, offers some protection to mammalian cells without interfering with the anti-*Toxoplasma* activity. Patients generally receive treatment for at least 6 weeks. Patients who cannot tolerate sulfa drugs or who have severe pre-existing hematologic abnormalities can be treated with clindamycin. Clindamycin is taken in doses of 450 to 600 mg every 6 hours orally, or 600 mg intravenously every 6 hours, during acute therapy. For patients with severe cerebral edema, dexamethasone can be used; a loading dose of 10 mg is followed by 4 to 6 mg orally or intravenously every 6 hours.

A clinical and radiologic response is usually evident within 10 to 14 days. If unambiguous improvement is not seen on imaging, brain biopsy should be performed (unless neurosurgically contraindicated). The clinical improvement is usually dramatic, with return of mental status and motor and sensory abnormalities to normal or near normal. Without maintenance therapy, up to 80% of patients experience relapse within 1 month. Chronic suppression regimens include pyrimethamine, 25 to 50 mg per day orally, plus sulfadiazine, 500 to 1000 mg orally every 6 hours;

or pyrimethamine, 25 to 50 mg per day, plus clindamycin, 300 mg orally every 6 hours.

Cryptosporidium

Cryptosporidia cause self-limited diarrhea in immunocompetent persons. However, in patients with severely depressed cell-mediated immunity, cryptosporidia can cause chronic disabling diarrhea with malabsorption, as well as biliary tract disease, including acalculous cholecystitis and sclerosing cholangitis. In specimens of stool, the organism is readily identified with a modified acid-fast stain. In fixed tissue specimens of intestine, liver, and gallbladder, the organism is readily identified on routine hematoxylin and eosin staining.

Clinical responses have been reported in controlled trials of treatment with either bovine colostrum or bovine transfer factor; however, these agents are not generally available. One uncontrolled study reported decreased diarrhea and weight gain in 30 of 31 episodes of cryptosporidiosis with oral paromomycin, 500 mg every 6 hours. Standard treatment is based on symptoms, with attention to fluid balance and nutritional needs. Somatostatin has been utilized with variable success in relieving intractable diarrhea.

Isospora belli

Isospora belli causes a diarrheal disease similar to cryptosporidiosis. However, the disease responds to treatment with oral trimethoprim-sulfamethoxazole, one double-strength tablet every 6 hours for 10 days. Recurrences occur in 50% of treated patients within 2 months but can be prevented by maintenance therapy with trimethoprim-sulfamethoxazole, one double-strength tablet three times weekly. In patients who are intolerant to sulfa, pyrimethamine, 25 to 50 mg orally daily, with 5 to 10 mg of folinic acid daily may be tried, but there are no published data to support this regimen.

Enterocytozoon bieneusi (Microsporidiosis)

Microspora have been found on electron microscopic examination of small bowel biopsy samples in AIDS patients with diarrhea, fever, wasting, and abnormalities of small intestinal mucosa. Some researchers have been able to identify the microsporidia on light microscopic examination of small bowel biopsy samples and in special studies of stool.

Clinical responses have been described among some patients treated with metronidazole (Flagyl), 500 mg orally every 6 hours, in uncontrolled series; among a few patients treated with alben-

dazole*; and in one of two patients treated with octreotide (Sandostatin).

Mycoses

Candidiasis

Approximately 80% of AIDS patients experience candidiasis at some time during their illness, and it is the most frequent cause of esophagitis in this population. The most common presentation of oral candidiasis is the pseudomembranous form, which appears as creamy white or yellowish plaques on red or normal-appearing plaques that can be easily removed, leaving a bleeding surface. These plaques can occur anywhere in the oral cavity but are seen most often on the tongue (dorsal and lateral surfaces), palate, and buccal and gingival mucosa. Diagnosis is by clinical examination and detection of budding yeast and branching pseudohyphae on smears treated by potassium hydroxide. Treatment regimens for oral candidiasis include nystatin solution or tablets, 500,000 to 1,000,000 U orally three to five times per day; or clotrimazole troches, 10 mg orally five times per day. Alternative regimens include ketoconazole, 200 mg per day orally, and fluconazole, 50 to 100 mg orally per day.

Candida esophagitis is the most common cause of odynophagia (pain with swallowing) in patients with AIDS. However, in AIDS patients, *Candida* rarely invades the mucosa of the gastrointestinal tract distal to the esophagus and rarely causes disseminated disease. In patients with *Candida* esophagitis, endoscopic examination reveals diffuse mucosal ulcerations associated with a white discharge. Biopsy specimens reveal the budding yeast and pseudohyphae of *Candida*. Treatment is usually initiated with orally absorbed systemic antifungals, because there is a substantial failure rate with topical therapy. Only in rare circumstances is systemic therapy with amphotericin B required.

Ketoconazole (Nizoral), 200 to 400 mg once daily, is the least expensive oral antifungal for this purpose. Gastric acid is necessary for absorption; therefore, concomitant use of antacids and H$_2$ blockers should be avoided. Ketoconazole should be administered 12 hours after rifampin administration to avoid an interaction that causes low serum levels of both agents. Occasional hepatic toxicity occurs. Fluconazole (Diflucan), 100 mg daily, is also effective. Although it is more costly than ketoconazole, fluconazole does *not* depend on gastric acid for absorption. Fluconazole is available as an intravenous preparation

---

*Not available in the United States.

as well, which can be used in the rare patient who cannot tolerate oral therapy initially. A treatment course of either drug usually lasts 2 to 3 weeks. An alternative regimen utilizes amphotericin B, 0.3 mg per kg intravenously every day for 7 days.

Because relapses of *Candida* esophagitis are common, continuous suppressive therapy with oral antifungals (ketoconazole, 200 mg daily, or fluconazole, 50 mg daily) is indicated. It is possible that early prophylactic use of fluconazole can prevent first episodes of both *Candida* esophagitis and cryptococcosis; prospective placebo-controlled trials, in which fluconazole (200 mg daily) is used in the treatment arm, are under way to define the risks, costs, and benefits of this approach among persons with fewer than 200 CD4 cells.

Cryptococcus neoformans

Meningoencephalitis caused by *Cryptococcus neoformans* occurs in 5 to 15% of persons with AIDS. Extrapulmonary cryptococcosis typically occurs in persons with fewer than 200 CD4 cells per mm^3. The portal of entry for *C. neoformans* is the lung, followed by lymphohematogenous dissemination; AIDS patients may present with cryptococcal fungemia.

Patients with cryptococcal meningitis often present with fever, headache, and stiff neck of several days to several weeks' duration. In some patients with relatively minimal cerebrospinal fluid pleocytosis, the meningismus is subtle and the disease manifests as unexplained fever. In other patients, depressed mental status and cranial nerve abnormalities are present. Focal enhancing intracerebral mass lesions occur and are termed "cryptococcomas."

Cryptococcosis can manifest as pneumonia or pleural effusion; lymphadenopathy; infiltrative hepatic disease; and/or multifocal cutaneous disease with umbilicated lesions that mimic molluscum contagiosum. Patients with AIDS and systemic cryptococcosis may have a clinically inapparent meningitis and therefore require a spinal tap before initiating antifungal treatment. The diagnosis of cryptococcal meningitis is readily accomplished by examination and culture of cerebrospinal fluid. There are a lymphocytic pleocytosis, elevated protein levels, and hypoglycorrhachia. Encapsulated budding yeasts are visualized on the Gram stain or India ink preparation of centrifuged cerebrospinal fluid in the majority of cases. Cryptococcal antigen is detected in the cerebrospinal fluid in 90% of cases and in the serum in 95% of cases.

Treatment regimens include amphotericin B with or without flucytosine; fluconazole; and the investigational drug itraconazole (200 mg orally twice a day). The administration of intravenous amphotericin B begins with a 1-mg test dose, then 0.3 mg per kg per day for 2 days, followed by daily doses of 0.6 mg per kg; after 2 weeks, alternate-day or three-times-weekly amphotericin can be administered to provide the equivalent weekly dose as with daily therapy.

The test dose is administered in 50 mL of D5W over 20 minutes, in order to evaluate the severity of the patient's reaction to amphotericin. Therapeutic doses are administered in 500 mL of D5W (never in saline) and can be infused over 2 to 4 hours. Most patients experience acute symptoms such as fever, chills, nausea, and vomiting during amphotericin B infusion. These symptoms can be minimized by administering acetaminophen, 650 mg orally, and diphenhydramine, 25 to 50 mg orally, before the therapeutic infusion. If shaking chills recur, they can be prevented by pretreatment with oral or parenteral meperidine, 50 to 100 mg. Pretreatment with 25 to 50 mg of hydrocortisone orally or intravenously reduces the severity of these symptoms. Patients usually become tolerant to the immediate effects of amphotericin, and the steroids can usually be discontinued after 1 or several weeks. Additional side effects of amphotericin include anemia, renal potassium and bicarbonate wasting, and renal insufficiency. Aggressive hydration and sodium replacement minimize the azotemia. Replacement of red blood cells, potassium, and bicarbonate are often necessary during the course of therapy.

Amphotericin B (with or without flucytosine; see later discussion) is continued until the cerebrospinal fluid is sterile. Examination of the cerebrospinal fluid is repeated every 2 weeks. When the fungal culture has remained sterile for 7 days, therapy may be continued with amphotericin B, or changed to oral fluconazole (400 mg daily) to complete at least 10 weeks of induction therapy. Examination of the cerebrospinal fluid is repeated after 10 total weeks of therapy. If the cerebrospinal fluid is sterile, chronic suppressive therapy may be initiated with either intravenous amphotericin B at 1.0 mg per kg weekly or oral fluconazole at 200 mg daily. Lifelong maintenance therapy should be provided to all AIDS patients after initial treatment of cryptococcosis.

If tolerated, 5-flucytosine (Ancobon) can be added to the initial amphotericin regimen. The drug causes leukopenia, especially when serum levels are elevated as a result of renal insufficiency. The usual dose of flucytosine in patients with normal renal function is 100 to 150 mg per kg per day in four divided doses. The drug causes gastrointestinal distress, and 500-mg tablets may have to be taken several minutes apart. In the ideal case, serum flucytosine levels should be monitored to minimize systemic toxicity.

Fluconazole (Diflucan), 400 mg orally daily, is also licensed by the FDA for use as initial therapy. Associated side effects include elevated transaminases; gastrointestinal distress; and rash, including a small number of cases of Stevens-Johnson syndrome. Fluconazole, unlike ketoconazole, appears to be well absorbed even in the absence of gastric acid and in patients taking antacids or H_2 blockers. Fluconazole probably has the same interactions with rifampin and other drugs as does ketoconazole. Therefore, fluconazole should be given 12 hours apart from rifampin. AZT therapy is more likely to be tolerated by patients taking fluconazole rather than amphotericin, because the former has no hematologic toxicity.

Histoplasma capsulatum

AIDS patients with histoplasmosis usually present with disseminated disease manifested by fever, weight loss, respiratory complaints, hepatomegaly, lymphadenopathy, splenomegaly, anemia, leukopenia, thrombocytopenia, mucocutaneous lesions, renal insufficiency, chorioretinitis, meningitis, and/or encephalitis. Although tests for anti–Histoplasma capsulatum antibodies may be positive, the definitive diagnosis depends on the identification and/or culture of the organism from specimens of blood, bone marrow, bronchoalveolar lavage fluid, lymph node, liver, or other tissues or body fluids suspected to be infected on clinical grounds. Examination of peripheral blood smear or buffy coat may reveal intracellular and/or extracellular yeast, providing a rapid means of diagnosis; cultures of blood and urine are frequently positive. Skin testing with histoplasmin has no role in the diagnosis of histoplasmosis.

Initial (induction) treatment with intravenous amphotericin B is highly effective, reversing the clinical manifestations of infection in approximately 80% of cases. However, nearly all patients experience relapse within 1 year after completing courses of amphotericin B of 35 mg per kg or more, supporting the use of maintenance treatment to prevent recurrence. Wheat and colleagues at Indiana University administer an induction phase of 15 mg per kg of amphotericin B given over 4 to 6 weeks, followed by lifelong maintenance therapy with 50 to 100 mg of amphotericin B given once or twice weekly, or biweekly. An alternative regimen involves a 12-week induction phase with the investigational agent itraconazole at 200 mg orally twice a day, followed by lifelong suppressive maintenance therapy of 100 mg orally twice a day.

Coccidioides immitis

AIDS patients with coccidioidomycosis most often present with focal or diffuse pulmonary disease, meningitis, extrathoracic lymphadenopathy, hepatic disease, and/or cutaneous lesions. Although the majority of cases have presented in areas endemic for coccidioidomycosis, some have presented outside of the endemic areas; hence all practitioners, regardless of geographic location, should consider coccidioidomycosis in the differential diagnosis of opportunistic infections among those infected with HIV. Furthermore, in a study of 77 HIV patients who developed coccidioidomycosis, sera from 39% of the patients were positive for tube precipitin antibodies, whereas 74% had complement-fixing antibodies (11 of the seronegative patients had focal or diffuse pulmonary coccidioidomycosis); therefore, histopathologic studies and culture remain the most reliable methods for the diagnosis of disseminated coccidioidomycosis in the HIV-infected host.

Intravenous amphotericin B, 0.6 mg per kg per day, is the standard treatment; the length of treatment is determined by clinical response, usually at least 8 weeks; this is followed by lifelong chronic suppressive therapy with intravenous amphotericin B, 1.0 mg per kg per week. Alternative suppressive regimens include fluconazole, 200 to 400 mg orally per day; or oral ketoconazole, 400 mg per day.

Bacteria

Mycobacterium tuberculosis

Pulmonary and extrapulmonary lymphohematogenously disseminated tuberculosis is on the increase in the United States because of HIV-associated immunosuppression. In patients with HIV disease, active tuberculosis usually represents reactivation of latent disease but can also occur as a primary infection. Although HIV-infected patients with pulmonary tuberculosis may present with typical upper lobe infiltrates or cavitary disease, many with advanced HIV disease present with atypical lower lobe infiltrates or a miliary pattern (suggesting disseminated disease). Because decreased cell-mediated immunity makes skin reactivity less sensitive, up to 50% of patients with AIDS and active tuberculosis have a negative PPD test result. Other diagnostic measures such as chest x-ray and blood cultures are important in this group of patients.

Persons with pulmonary tuberculosis may be infectious to others before the initiation of therapy. Infectiousness is greatest in patients with both a productive cough and positive sputum smears for acid-fast bacilli. Local health departments usually attempt to reach contacts of the index patient and provide PPD testing and referrals for treatment. The risk of person-to-person spread falls rapidly as soon as treatment is initiated. Patients hospitalized with suspected or proven pulmonary tuberculosis require respiratory isolation. Patients are usually no longer infectious after 10 to 14 days of therapy.

Disseminated tuberculosis most commonly manifests as pulmonary, lymphadenopathic, hepatic, splenic, and/or bone marrow involvement, often with mycobacteremia; patients may also present with meningitis or intracerebral tuberculomas.

The initial course of treatment for tuberculous disease should include a four-drug regimen (isoniazid, rifampin, pyrazinamide, and either ethambutol or streptomycin) until drug susceptibility results are available; the regimen can be adjusted accordingly.

The authors also recommend directly observed therapy to ensure compliance and to decrease the likelihood that drug resistance will develop.

Mycobacterium avium

Several clinical syndromes are associated with *M. avium* infection in patients with AIDS. Unexplained persistent fever and night sweats are a common manifestation and may be accompanied by wasting. Infiltrative disease of the liver manifests with mild hepatic tenderness and enlargement. Typically, the serum alkaline phosphatase level is elevated and is associated with modest elevations of aminotransferase (transaminase) levels and normal bilirubin levels. Hepatocyte function is relatively intact, reflected by normal coagulation studies. Infiltrative disease of mesenteric and para-aortic lymph nodes also occurs and can cause persistent (sometimes severe) abdominal pain. Infiltrative disease of the bone marrow can manifest as anemia, leukopenia, and/or thrombocytopenia; aspirates and biopsies of bone marrow reveal intrahistiocytic mycobacteria. Chronic diarrhea also occurs because these patients have acid-fast bacilli in specimens of stool as well as mycobacteremia. Pulmonary disease is most often characterized by enlarged mediastinal and hilar lymph nodes; nonspecific patchy pulmonary infiltrates may also occur.

Clinically apparent *M. avium* infection is almost always disseminated and manifested by sustained mycobacteremia. A single blood culture for mycobacteria is a simple, noninvasive, and reasonably sensitive technique to use when the diagnosis is suspected. Bone marrow aspiration and biopsy is another excellent technique for diagnosing disseminated *M. avium* infection. Treatment regimens for disseminated *M. avium*

disease remain controversial. Nevertheless, symptomatic improvement and suppression of mycobacteremia have been achieved in many patients.

Prophylaxis for *Mycobacterium avium* Complex

Patients with HIV infection and fewer than 100 $CD4^+$ lymphocytes should receive rifabutin prophylaxis, 300 mg orally daily, against *Mycobacterium avium* complex. Before the administration of rifabutin prophylaxis, patients should be assessed to ensure that they do not have active disease due to *Mycobacterium avium* complex. Rifabutin monotherapy for active *Mycobacterium avium* complex disease is inadequate, and thus the presence of active disease must be identified so that appropriate multiple-drug therapy can be initiated. The concern regarding tuberculosis is due to the likelihood that the administration of rifabutin monotherapy to patients with active disease could lead to the proliferation of rifabutin/rifampin-resistant organisms. Such organisms can present major clinical and public health consequences.

Adverse effects of rifabutin may include neutropenia, thrombocytopenia, rash, and gastrointestinal disturbances. Rifabutin, like rifampin, increases the hepatic metabolism of certain drugs, such as zidovudine, thus lowering their serum concentrations, as reflected by area under the concentration time curve. Whether this is clinically significant is unknown, but clinicians must be cognizant of the potential for such interactions.

Therapy for Disseminated *Mycobacterium avium* Complex

Studies have not yet identified an optimal regimen. Although no drugs are currently approved by the FDA for the therapy of *Mycobacterium avium* complex disease, every regimen should contain either azithromycin or clarithromycin; many experts would chose ethambutol as a second drug. Many clinicians frequently add one or more of the following as second, third, or fourth agents: clofazimine, rifabutin, rifampin, ciprofloxacin, and, in some situations, amikacin. Isoniazid and pyrazinamide have no role in the therapy of *Mycobacterium avium* complex disease. Adverse effects of these regimens have included nausea, anorexia, and hepatitis.

Treponema pallidum (Syphilis)

Both HIV and *Treponema pallidum* are sexually transmitted pathogens, and therefore persons at risk for infection with one are at risk for infection with both. Furthermore, ulcerative genital disease (including primary syphilis, herpes simplex virus, and chancroid) increases the likelihood of sexual transmission of HIV. The natural history of syphilis may be altered in patients with coexistent HIV infection; syphilis may manifest with an accelerated clinical course, prominent neurologic involvement, and relapse despite standard treatment regimens; there have been several case reports of retinal syphilis and severe neurosyphilis, especially meningovascular syphilis manifesting as strokes, occurring within a few months or years of early syphilis (in non–HIV-infected persons, meningovascular syphilis typically occurred later in the course, 7 to 12 years after primary infection).

Nearly all patients with HIV infection and primary or secondary syphilis have positive serum RPR or VDRL tests. Because of biologic false-positive results in HIV-infected patients, a confirmatory serum test for specific antibody against *T. pallidum* (FTA-ABS) must be performed to verify that the result is a true positive. A positive cerebrospinal fluid VDRL is unequivocal evidence of central nervous system infection with *T. pallidum*; however, a negative cerebrospinal fluid VDRL does not rule out neurosyphilis.

Although the CDC continues to recommend a single dose of benzathine penicillin (2.4 million units intramuscularly) as treatment for primary and secondary syphilis and latent syphilis of less than 1 year's duration (early latent), some clinicians suggest that these patients should be treated with three weekly doses of 2.4 million units of benzathine penicillin; others, suggesting that all HIV-associated syphilis should be treated with a reliable regimen against neurosyphilis, recommend 10 days of intramuscular procaine penicillin (2.4 million units per dose) with 500 mg of probenecid four times a day for 10 days. Patients with penicillin allergy can be treated with ceftriaxone (Rocephin), 250 mg intramuscularly daily for 10 days; or 1 gram intramuscularly on alternate days for five doses. Another alternative regimen includes oral amoxicillin, 3 grams twice a day for 14 days, with probenecid, 500 mg orally twice a day for 14 days. Serologic follow-up should be performed; treatment is considered a failure if the RPR or VDRL does not fall fourfold after 3 months (primary and secondary syphilis) or 6 months (early latent syphilis).

The CDC recommends that patients with late latent syphilis (more than 1 year's duration, without neurosyphilis) receive 2.4 million units of intramuscular benzathine penicillin weekly for three doses; however, some clinicians suggest more aggressive therapy utilizing 10 days of intramuscular procaine penicillin (2.4 million units daily) with oral probenecid, 500 mg four times a day for 10 days, followed by 2.4 million units of intramuscular benzathine penicillin weekly for two or three doses.

Patients with neurosyphilis may be treated with (1) 10 to 20 million units of intravenous aqueous penicillin G daily for 10 to 14 days, followed by three weekly doses of 2.4 million units of intramuscular benzathine penicillin, or (2) 2.4 million units of intramuscular procaine penicillin daily for 10 to 14 days, with oral probenecid, 500 mg four times a day, followed by three weekly doses of 2.4 million units of intramuscular benzathine penicillin. Patients with a positive cerebrospinal fluid VDRL or a cerebrospinal fluid pleocytosis should have repeated cerebrospinal fluid examinations every 6 months for 2 years, or until the VDRL is consistently negative or the cell counts are normal; failure to normalize the cerebrospinal fluid is reason to re-treat.

Salmonellosis

Recurrent bacteremia with non-typhi *Salmonella* (most often typhimurium) occurs with increased frequency in patients with AIDS. After oral acquisition from undercooked poultry or eggs, the salmonella can cause a self-limited enteritis or can disseminate and cause bacteremia. After successful treatment of the bacteremia, repeated septicemic episodes with the same organism are common.

Regimens for acute therapy include (1) intravenous ampicillin (8 to 12 grams per day) for 2 weeks, followed by oral amoxicillin, 500 mg three times a day, for an additional 2 weeks; (2) oral ciprofloxacin, 750 mg twice a day for 2 to 4 weeks; and (3) trimethoprim (5 to 10 mg per kg per day) plus sulfamethoxazole intravenously or orally for 4 weeks. Chronic suppressive maintenance regimens include (1) amoxicillin, 250 mg orally twice a day; (2) ciprofloxacin, 500 mg orally once or twice a day; and (3) trimethoprim (2.5 mg per kg) plus sulfamethoxazole orally twice a day. Although it is common practice to continue oral antibiotics indefinitely to prevent recurrences of *Salmonella* bacteremia, breakthrough septicemias can occur despite such treatment. Nevertheless, in patients who can tolerate sulfa drugs, the use of trimethoprim-sulfamethoxazole for *Salmonella* suppression also provides effective prophylaxis against *P. carinii* infections.

Viruses

Herpes Simplex Virus

The initial manifestation of HIV infection may be severe recurrent episodes of painful ulcerative mucocutaneous lesions caused by herpes simplex virus (HSV). Initial treatment of mild mucocutaneous disease is acyclovir (Zovirax), 200 mg by mouth five times per day for at least 10 days (until lesions are crusted); treatment of severe mucocutaneous disease is with intravenous acyclovir (15 mg per kg per day); alternative regimens include intravenous vidarabine (Vira-A), (15 mg per kg per day) or foscarnet (90 mg per kg per day) intravenously; chronic suppressive maintenance therapy utilizes oral acyclovir, 200 mg three times a day. Visceral disease is treated with intravenous acyclovir (30 mg per kg per day) for at least 10 days; an alternative regimen involves vidarabine (15 mg per kg per day) intravenously for 10 days.

Herpes Zoster/Varicella Virus

Polydermatomal, disseminated, and visceral infections do not necessitate maintenance antiviral therapy. Dermatomal infections are treated with acyclovir intravenously (30 mg per kg per day) or orally (800 mg) five times per day for at least 7 days (until the lesions crust). Ophthalmic, disseminated, or visceral disease is treated with intravenous acyclovir (30 mg per kg per day) for at least 7 days.

Oral Hairy Leukoplakia

A unique oral complication associated with HIV infection is hairy leukoplakia, believed to be caused by the Epstein-Barr virus. Clinically, the lesion often appears as a corrugated white plaque on one or both lateral borders of the tongue; the plaque does not scrape off, as in lingual lesions of oral candidiasis. The majority of patients have asymptomatic lesions that do not necessitate therapy.

Cytomegalovirus

Many patients with AIDS have persistent cytomegaloviremia, and cytomegalovirus is a major cause of dysfunction in a variety of organs. Patients may present with retinitis (subclinical or symptomatic), pneumonia, esophagitis, colitis with extensive ulcerations and perforation, meningoencephalitis, radiculitis with polyneuropathies, and hepatitis. Cytomegalovirus induces cellular gigantism (cytomegaly) with characteristic intranuclear and intracytoplasmic viral inclusions.

Cytomegalovirus retinitis is the most common sight-threatening disease in patients with AIDS. Patients often present with decreased visual acuity without pain, and concurrent involvement of other organs by cytomegalovirus may not be clinically apparent; however, postmortem examinations have revealed the presence of disseminated cytomegalovirus infection.

Retinal findings include perivascular exudates and hemorrhages that are often bilateral; progressive disease leads to retinal necrosis and detachment. Cytomegalovirus retinitis, colitis, and esophagitis often respond to antiviral treatment with foscarnet (Foscavir) or ganciclovir (Cytovene). Foscarnet is the drug of choice for cytomegalovirus retinitis. Foscarnet does not have the hematologic toxicity of ganciclovir (neutropenia is a frequent dose-limiting adverse effect of ganciclovir; if concomitant AZT ganciclovir treatment is administered, more than 80% of patients have dose-limiting hematologic toxicity). Ganciclovir-resistant cytomegalovirus isolates have emerged in patients receiving chronic ganciclovir therapy. Furthermore, in a prospective trial comparing induction and maintenance therapy, although foscarnet and ganciclovir were equivalent in preventing progression of cytomegalovirus retinitis, survival was longer among patients receiving foscarnet. Finally, foscarnet itself has anti-retroviral (anti-HIV) activity.

Foscarnet induction therapy involves infusions of 60 mg per kg every 8 hours for 14 days (each infusion is over 2 hours). Patients with serum creatinine concentrations above 2.0 mg per dL probably will not tolerate foscarnet; patients with a calculated creatinine clearance below 1.2 mL per kg per minute may have better survival if they take ganciclovir rather than foscarnet; if the serum creatinine level rises to above 2.9 mg per dL on therapy, foscarnet should be withheld until the creatinine falls below 2.0 mg per dL. Creatinine, calcium, magnesium, potassium, and hemoglobin levels should be determined three times weekly during induction. A repeat ophthalmologic examination should be performed at the end of 2 weeks to verify that there has been a response before the regimen converts to maintenance therapy. In addition to renal dysfunction, adverse effects of foscarnet include fever, nausea, anemia, diarrhea, vomiting, headache, hypocalcemia, hypokalemia, seizures, and granulocytopenia.

After a successful response to induction, maintenance therapy with foscarnet is administered at 90 mg per kg per day through a central line with an infusion pump. Creatinine, calcium, magnesium, potassium, and hemoglobin concentrations should be determined weekly during maintenance therapy. Foscarnet has also successfully been used to treat patients with cytomegalovirus esophagitis and colitis, as well as patients with acyclovir-resistant herpes simplex and varicella zoster infections.

Ganciclovir induction therapy involves 5 mg per kg intravenously every 12 hours for 14 days with monitoring of the complete blood count and ophthalmologic follow-up. With effective therapy, progression of the retinitis is aborted; although there is no recovery within the foci of retinal necrosis, vision may improve as edema and inflammation subside. Granulocytopenia is the most frequent adverse effect, and ganciclovir therapy is discontinued as the total granulocyte count falls below 750 cells per mm³. Granulocytopenia often occurs among patients receiving both ganciclovir and AZT, and the combination is to be avoided. Patients requiring ganciclovir (renal insufficiency) may be eligible for antiretroviral therapy with dideoxyinosine or dideoxycytidine.

After a successful response to induction, maintenance therapy is administered as single intravenous daily doses of 5 mg per kg or 6 mg per kg six days a week. The white blood cell count should continue to be monitored.

Progressive Multifocal Leukoencephalopathy

Progressive multifocal leukoencephalopathy (PML) is a central nervous system demyelinating disorder caused by polyomaviruses of the papova family. Patients may present with a wide variety of deficits, including limb weakness, cognitive dysfunction, visual loss, and incoordination or ataxia.

Computed tomographic (CT) scans of the brain may demonstrate focal hypodense white matter lesions without contrast enhancement or mass effect; however, CT scanning is relatively insensitive, and a severely ill patient may have an unremarkable study; MRI is more sensitive. HIV encephalopathy can also cause progressive neurologic deterioration and white matter abnormalities on MRI; therefore, it may be difficult to distinguish these two disorders on clinical and radiologic criteria alone. Histopathologic sections of brain biopsy specimens stained with hematoxylin and eosin demonstrate patchy areas of demyelination, necrosis, and gliosis; within these areas are large, bizarre astrocytes as well as oligodendroglia whose nuclei are filled with eosinophilic to amphophilic viral inclusions; these polyomavirus inclusions can be further demonstrated by immunohistochemical staining.

Although the neurologic findings may wax and wane, PML usually progresses to death in a matter of months. There is no known effective treatment.

MANAGEMENT OF OPPORTUNISTIC TUMORS

Kaposi's Sarcoma

Kaposi's sarcoma (the most common tumor in patients with AIDS) manifests as mucocutaneous, lymphadenopathic, and/or visceral disease. Characteristic mucocutaneous lesions may appear as erythematous to violaceous macules, infiltrative plaques, and/or nodules. Treatment of Kaposi's sarcoma is not appropriate for every patient. Subgroups of patients for whom treatment will be most beneficial have been defined; the primary goals of therapy for Kaposi's sarcoma are palliation of symptoms and cosmesis. Cosmesis is perhaps the most common indication for therapy and often the most important. Achievement of good cosmetic results not only may improve appearance but also may significantly improve the patient's overall outlook. Several situations have been identified in which palliative therapy may be indicated: (1) painful or uncomfortable intraoral lesions may interfere with eating or swallowing and may even result in airway compromise; (2) severe lymphedema involving the face or lower extremities; (3) painful or bulky lesions that may occur at any site (including intestinal obstruction); lesions involving the plantar surfaces of the feet may be particularly uncomfortable during ambulation; and (4) pulmonary involvement that may be associated with severe respiratory compromise and failure.

Radiotherapy involving a single dose of 800 rad or the equivalent fractionated dose can be effective in achieving local palliation. Radiotherapy is not appropriate for the patient with widespread disease but is best suited for the patient with a single or a few locally symptomatic areas, as well as areas of lymphedema (although radiation of cutaneous lesions is well tolerated, radiation of intraoral lesions is often complicated by mucositis). Intralesional chemotherapy may be utilized for cosmetic purposes in small cutaneous lesions; this may be accomplished by intralesional injection of 0.01 mg of vinblastine in 0.1 ml of sterile water through a tuberculin syringe; a hyperpigmented area frequently remains after treatment. Cryotherapy with liquid nitrogen has also been used for the treatment of isolated small lesions.

For patients with more rapidly progressive disease or with advanced widespread symptomatic disease, systemic therapy may be most appropriate. The combination of bleomycin (10 units per M² every 14 days) and vincristine (2 mg every 14 days) has significant antitumor activity and may be especially useful for patients with granulocytopenia who are likely to be intolerant of more myelosuppressive regimens (doxorubicin, etoposide, vinblastine). Interferon-alpha (5 to 15 million units subcutaneously or intramuscularly daily) used as a single agent has significant antitumor activity; however, it appears to be most effective in patients with CD4 lymphocyte counts higher than 400 per mm³.

Central Nervous System (CNS)/ Extranodal Lymphoma

Non-Hodgkin's lymphoma confined to the CNS is the second most common cause of enhancing

CNS mass lesions in AIDS patients. Although systemic non-Hodgkin's lymphoma can metastasize to the brain, it usually causes a carcinomatous meningitis rather than discrete intracerebral mass lesions. In patients with AIDS, single or multiple discrete lesions are the most common findings on computed tomography or MRI of the brain; frontal lesions are most common supratentorially, and cerebellar lesions predominate infratentorially. The most common presenting symptoms have been confusion, lethargy, memory loss, hemiparesis, aphasia, seizures, cranial nerve palsies, and headache. Therefore, *Toxoplasma* encephalitis and CNS lymphoma can mimic each other in clinical manifestation and on imaging studies. Cytologic examination of the cerebrospinal fluid provides a diagnosis of lymphoma in up to 25% of cases; more often, the diagnosis is established by biopsy of the brain. Histopathologically, sections of brain most often demonstrate large-cell perivascular pathology of B cell origin with varying degrees of mitosis and necrosis (the majority of B cell lymphomas in patients with AIDS are classified as diffuse large-cell tumors of either intermediate-grade type or the high-grade immunoblastic type, or high-grade small non–cleaved-cell variety).

Standard therapy consists of whole-brain irradiation with 4000 to 5000 rad delivered over 3 to 4 weeks; some patients may also be able to tolerate surgical resection (for circumscribed tumors) and/or chemotherapy. The median length of survival for AIDS patients with CNS lymphoma and a history of opportunistic infection has been 2 months (range, 0 to 11 months), and the median length of survival for those with no history of opportunistic infection has been 12 months (range, 2 to 28 months); therefore, patients with AIDS-related CNS lymphoma with *no* history of opportunistic infection appear to have improved survival. Nevertheless, AIDS patients are often too ill to tolerate aggressive surgery or systemic treatment, and in such cases radiotherapy alone may be an acceptable alternative.

Patients with AIDS may also present with extranodal non-Hodgkin's lymphoma beyond the central nervous system. Involved sites have included the gastrointestinal tract, bone marrow, liver, subcutaneous and soft tissue, lung, pleura, heart, pericardium, kidney, spleen, common bile duct, gingiva, parotid gland, and paranasal sinus. Treatment regimens have included cyclophosphamide, doxorubicin, vincristine, and dexamethasone.

WOMEN AND HIV INFECTION

HIV transmission among heterosexuals continues to increase at an alarming rate; women in particular are facing the fastest rate of increase. It is projected that by the year 2000, the number of women in the United States with HIV infection will equal the number of HIV-infected men. Currently, the majority of AIDS diagnoses occur in women of childbearing age (15 to 44 years), and a significant proportion are diagnosed between the ages of 20 and 29, indicating that many of these women were infected as teenagers and young adults. Factors associated with male-to-female transmission of HIV include failure to use condoms; anal intercourse; advanced disease state of the infected partner; and the presence of genital sores, infections, and inflammation. The risk of transmission appears to be reduced if the infected partner is receiving antiretroviral therapy. Sexual intercourse during menses may increase the risk of female-to-male transmission.

In general, the manifestations of AIDS and HIV-related illnesses in women fall within the same spectrum as those in men. However, certain AIDS-defining conditions are more commonly found in women, including esophageal candidiasis, wasting syndrome, cytomegalovirus disease, tuberculosis, disseminated *M. avium* infection, HIV encephalopathy, and chronic herpes simplex virus ulcerative disease. Although *P. carinii* pneumonia remains the most common AIDS-defining condition in women on a national basis, Kaposi's sarcoma occurs rarely. Because women are inappropriately not considered at increased risk for HIV, they remain undiagnosed for longer periods of time, present with more advanced immune impairment, and consequently have shortened life expectancies. However, survival rates for women with HIV are similar to those of men when a timely diagnosis of infection is made and treatment is initiated.

There are particular gynecologic and other medical conditions that should be addressed in the evaluation of any female patient. The medical history includes questions about abnormal cervical cytologies, pelvic inflammatory disease (occurs more frequently and is often more severe, necessitating prolonged hospitalization and more frequent surgery for treatment of abscesses), genital warts, genital ulcers (herpes simplex virus, chancroid, syphilis), and vaginal yeast infections. Any history of abnormal menstrual cycles, specifically amenorrhea and intermenstrual bleeding, is also important to elicit. Recognizing these gynecologic signs that may accompany HIV infection is critical to the early diagnosis and treatment of women. Similarly, changes or progression of certain gynecologic conditions may be indicators of advancing immunoincompetence.

Recurrent and refractory vaginal candidiasis occurs in early stages of HIV infection and may be associated with only a mild degree of immune impairment. Although vaginal candidiasis may respond readily to standard topical agents, a need for systemic antifungal therapy with ketoconazole or fluconazole may arise, particularly in advanced stages of immunoincompetence. With regard to the relationship of HIV disease and human papillomavirus infection, many clinicians believe that progression of dysplasia and cervical intraepithelial neoplasia occurs more frequently and is more severe and aggressive in coinfected women.

HIV-infected women have a significant increase in abnormal Pap smears and in the development of cervical intraepithelial neoplasia (CIN). According to current CDC recommendations, all HIV-infected women are advised to have an initial pelvic examination and a Pap smear. A normal Pap smear should be followed by a repeat smear in 6 months to rule out false-negative results. If both Pap smear results are normal, testing can be repeated annually. If a Pap smear shows severe inflammation or reactive squamous cell changes, the smear should be repeated in 3 months. Any diagnosis of a squamous intraepithelial lesion (SIL) or atypical squamous cells of undetermined significance should be followed by a colposcopic examination. Current recommendations for colposcopic evaluation and treatment of dysplasia found on screening Pap smears in HIV-positive women are the same as for women who are HIV-negative. Colposcopic characteristics and response to treatment appear to be different in HIV-infected women because they have a tendency to manifest high-grade lesions and more extensive cervical disease. Standard therapies tend to yield fewer cures, and recurrences are more common than in seronegative women. Preliminary studies suggest that the rate of progression from cervical intraepithelial neoplasia to cervical cancer is more rapid in immunocompromised HIV-infected patients. Invasive cervical carcinoma has been added to the list of AIDS-defining conditions.

The recommendations for the initiation of antiretroviral therapies, prophylaxis, and treatment of *P. carinii* infections and other opportunistic infections in HIV-positive women do not differ from those of HIV-positive men. Some treatment decisions may be altered during various stages of pregnancy, while consideration is still given to the overall status and needs of the mother. A discussion of treatment options during pregnancy is beyond the scope of this article. The authors believe that any treatment considerations that are made during pregnancy should involve the informed advice and full consent of the mother before being instituted or withheld.

CONCLUSION

The treatment of HIV disease and AIDS will continue to evolve during the coming years. With the potential availability of newer anti-retrovirals that attack HIV replication, assembly, and release or that inhibit entry into target cells, the potential benefits of combination or alternating chemotherapy become apparent. Not only can toxicity to any one agent be reduced, but also susceptibility of the virus can theoretically be increased, resulting, it is hoped, in the dramatic slowing of disease progression. Similarly, more efficacious and less toxic agents are likely to be developed for prophylaxis and treatment of opportunistic infections and malignancies. Research studies under way to find effective drugs that bolster the immune system, along with the development of vaccines to prevent HIV infection, hold promise but remain elusive.

Nevertheless, the basic tenets of care for the HIV-infected patients will remain unchanged. A well-grounded understanding of the natural history of the disease and points of intervention will stand the practitioner in good stead with regard to management of patients; the monitoring of CD4 lymphocyte counts and percentages will remain the mainstay for evaluation of the degree of immune impairment. Knowing the stage of the patient's illness can assist the practitioner in formulating the appropriate differential diagnosis and in avoiding undue concern and evaluation for conditions that are uncommon at mild to moderate degrees of altered immunity. The practitioner may be further assisted by the availability of other surrogate markers that herald significant HIV activity, drug resistance, or rapid disease progression. In the future, there may be clinical utility in monitoring CD4 lymphocyte counts below 200 per mm^3 (institution of new prophylactic antifungal, antiprotozoal, antiviral, and antibacterial regimens; altering anti-retroviral regimens).

By virtue of the breadth of medical knowledge as well as understanding of psychological and social issues, the primary care practitioner is well suited to care for the HIV-infected patient. Despite the tendency to feel overwhelmed by the daunting task of caring for patients with HIV infection, the practitioner should be reassured by the relatively straightforward nature of disease progression and by standard approaches to patient care. Total care of the HIV-infected patient includes an awareness of existing clinical trials and evaluating patients with regard to their meeting of enrollment criteria. Information about all HIV-related clinical trials, both federally and non–federally sponsored, is available by calling the AIDS Clinical Trials Information Service at 1-800-TRIALS-A, Monday through Friday, 9:00 A.M. to 7:00 P.M. Eastern Time. The practitioner can keep updated on developments in HIV and AIDS care and can enhance clinical HIV care skills by participating in programs sponsored by federally funded Regional AIDS Education and Training Centers; this national program was established to complement and enhance local resources and to provide didactic and clinical training activities for the health care provider; further information about local programs can be obtained by writing the authors.

AMEBIASIS

method of
JONATHAN I. RAVDIN, M.D.
Case Western Reserve University
Cleveland, Ohio

Entamoeba histolytica is an enteric protozoan that infects approximately 10% of the world's population. The cyst is the infective form; following excystation in the small bowel, trophozoites colonize the large bowel. Excystation with excretion of up to 45 million cysts per day results in transmission of disease. Current evidence indicates that there are genotypically distinct pathogenic and nonpathogenic strains. Nonpathogenic *E. histolytica* has never been associated with invasive colitis or liver abscess; intestinal infection spontaneously clears without treatment in 8 to 12 months. Apparently, all individuals with pathogenic infection mount a serum antibody response, only 1 in 10 go on to develop systemic invasive amebiasis. It is unknown whether clearance of pathogenic infection, spontaneously or by chemotherapy, results in any degree of host immunity to subsequent invasive amebiasis.

EPIDEMIOLOGY

It is important for clinicians to identify individuals at greater risk for infection and patients who when infected are more likely to suffer severe invasive disease. The infective dose can be as little as a single cyst, although a higher inoculum results in a shorter incubation period (1 to 3 days). High-risk groups for acquisition of infection include travelers to or immigrants from highly endemic areas (such as Mexico, India, Bangladesh, South Africa, and South America), sexually promiscuous individuals who engage in oral-anal or anal-genital-oral sex, chronically institutionalized populations (especially the mentally retarded), and Mexican-Americans in the Southwest United States. Individuals at risk for fulminant amebiasis include pregnant women, the malnourished, the very young (less than 1 year of age), and patients on corticosteroid therapy. Whether infection with human immunodeficiency virus (HIV) results in increased frequency or severity of invasive amebiasis remains unclear.

CLINICAL SYNDROMES

The main clinical syndromes that result from *E. histolytica* infection include asymptomatic intestinal infection, acute amebic rectocolitis, chronic intestinal amebiasis, and amebic liver abscess. Infections of the peritoneum, lung, and pericardium are unusual manifestations resulting from extension of an amebic liver abscess or colonic perforation. Lung or brain abscesses are rare presentations resulting from hematogenous dissemination. In general, 60 to 90% of individuals with asymptomatic intestinal infection harbor nonpathogenic strains. Such patients are detected by routine or incidental stool examination. Nonpathogenic *E. histolytica* infection does not elicit a serum antibody response. In a nonendemic area, a positive serologic test result for anti-amebic antibodies suggests infection with pathogenic amebae.

Acute amebic rectocolitis is characterized by bloody mucus in stools, tenesmus, and abdominal pain, with the onset of symptoms occurring over 7 to 10 days rather than more acutely. Only one-third of patients are febrile; virtually all will have stools positive for occult blood. Fulminant colitis is characterized by colonic dilatation, toxemia, and peritonitis (often with associated perforation). Chronic intestinal amebiasis is clinically identical to idiopathic inflammatory bowel disease. The disease can last for years, is intermittent in nature, and is characterized by abdominal pain with bloody diarrhea. The mistaken treatment of such patients with corticosteroids can result in fulminant disease. Ameboma, another form of chronic intestinal amebiasis, presents as a focal colonic mass, usually in the right colon, which is often mistaken clinically for colonic carcinoma. Amebic liver abscess, which presents acutely with right upper quadrant pain and fever, is indistinguishable from infection of the biliary tract. Patients with a more chronic infection have abdominal pain and weight loss. A minority are febrile and many are initially misdiagnosed as having primary or metastatic liver cancer. Amebic liver abscess can be differentiated from pyogenic infection by its occurrence at any age, its association with specific epidemiologic risk factors, the finding of *E. histolytica* in the stool (20 to 60%), and the presence of serum antiamebic antibodies.

DIAGNOSIS

Diagnosis of intestinal infection still rests upon expert microscopy of fecal samples. However, errors are frequent, and multiple stool samples are required. Although antigen detection tests have been successful to date only as research tools, they should soon be available commercially. Serologic testing is extremely helpful in the diagnosis of invasive amebiasis or asymptomatic pathogenic infection. Ninety percent of infected patients will be seropositive by the seventh day of illness. Asymptomatic patients harboring a pathogenic infection will also be seropositive. In nonendemic areas, serologic testing is a cost-effective way to differentiate inflammatory bowel disease from chronic intestinal amebiasis. After the treatment of pathogenic infection by most serologic methods, patients remain seropositive for years, which is why in endemic areas up to 25% of noninfected controls have serum anti-amebic antibodies. However, a negative test does reduce the likelihood of invasive amebiasis. Colonoscopy with scrapings or biopsy of the ulcer edge is the gold standard for diagnosis and is especially helpful in acute colitis or to rule out amebiasis before treatment of presumed inflammatory bowel disease with corticosteroids. A periodic acid-Schiff stain (PAS), which highlights trophozoites in tissues, should always be requested. Not only are barium studies not useful in diagnosis, but they also prevent any yield in stool examinations for ova and parasites for 1 to 2 weeks. Because it differentiates biliary tract disease from a primary liver process, abdominal ultrasonography is the most important study in evaluation of patients with right upper quadrant pain and fever. Amebic liver abscesses commonly appear as multiple nonhomogeneous defects by modern imaging techniques, especially in acute disease of less than 10 days' duration. Computed tomography (CT) and magnetic resonance imaging add little in evaluation at increased cost and radiation exposure. Amebic liver abscess cannot be differentiated from necrotic hepatoma or pyogenic abscess by imaging alone. The serologic results and the presence of epidemiologic risk factors are usually sufficient to establish the diagnosis. Well over 90% of patients will be seropositive after 7 days of symptomatic illness. If necessary, fine-needle aspiration under CT guidance can be used to rule out pyogenic disease, but this approach is rarely required for making an accurate diagnosis. Amebic liver abscesses contain proteinaceous fluid (not pus), and trophozoites are usually not found, as they are in the tissues at the periphery of the lesion.

TREATMENT

Treatment of amebiasis is complicated by the need to use multiple agents and the lack of physician familiarity with an appropriate therapeutic response.

Pharmacology of Antiamebic Agents

The drugs recommended for use in treatment of amebiasis are listed in Table 1. Luminal agents include diloxanide furoate, paromomycin, and diiodohydroxyquin. Diloxanide furoate is highly efficacious (95% clearance of patients), relatively nontoxic, and clearly the drug of choice to eradicate *E. histolytica* from the intestinal lumin. However, it is not widely available except through the Drug Service at the Centers for Disease Control in Atlanta, Georgia (telephone, 1–404–639–3670 during the daytime and 1–404–639–2888 in off-hours). Paromomycin, an oral aminoglycoside, is effective in clearing asymptomatic infection and in the setting of little or no inflammation is not absorbed. Therefore, this drug is especially helpful if one elects to treat asymptomatic infection in pregnant women. Paromomycin may cause mild gastrointestinal irri-

TABLE 1. Drugs Recommended for Treatment of Amebiasis by Site of Action

Drug	Advantages/ Disadvantages
Luminal amebicides	
Diloxanide furoate (Furamide)	Low toxicity; high efficacy; available only from CDC
Paromomycin (Humatin)	Nonabsorbable; useful in pregnancy
Diiodohydroxyquin (Diiodoquin, Yodoxin)	20-day course required; potential optic toxicity
Useful in intestinal disease only	
Tetracyclines Erythromycin	Must combine with luminal agent; not effective against liver abscess
Active in all tissues	
Metronidazole (Flagyl) Tinidazole (Simplotan)	Very effective; in vitro resistance not described; frequent nausea and vomiting; Antabuse effect with ethanol

Abbreviation: CDC = Centers for Disease Control.

tation or fungal overgrowth. Diiodohydroxyquin has been used extensively but requires high compliance to complete a 20-day course. This drug can cause optic atrophy, and the author prefers to avoid its use for this reason. The tetracyclines and erythromycins have a long history of successful treatment of invasive intestinal disease; however, they are not nearly as active in vitro against trophozoites as metronidazole and are ineffective in liver abscess. Therefore, these agents are usually used as second-line drugs in combination with a luminal agent to treat mild symptomatic amebic colitis. Given the risks of recurrent or chronic infection, the author would reserve them for patients who experience neurotoxicity or otherwise cannot tolerate metronidazole.

The nitroimidazoles are the mainstays of therapy for invasive amebiasis. They are directly amebicidal in vitro, penetrate well into all tissues, and have shown no parasite resistance to their amebicidal activity. However, gastrointestinal intolerance is common, and individuals must be cautioned to avoid ethanol due to an Antabuse effect. These agents are metabolized in the liver, and high serum levels are associated with neurotoxicity, including seizures. However, most patients tolerate these drugs and they have long been used in the treatment of trichomoniasis. Carcinogenic risks suggested by in vitro mutagenesis studies have not been borne out by long-term follow-up (10–20 years); nevertheless, caution in use of metronidazoles should be exercised. Teratogenesis is a concern; however, uncontrolled studies suggested reasonable safety during the third trimester. Tinidazole is better tolerated and highly efficacious but is not currently available in the United States.

Historically utilized to treat invasive amebiasis, the emetines, although directly amebicidal, are no longer recommended because of significant cardiovascular toxicity (hypotension, precordial chest pain, tachycardia). In addition, parenteral therapy with hospitalization is necessary and neuromuscular toxicity is common. There are no studies that demonstrate that the addition of emetines to metronidazole improves the outcome in invasive amebiasis.

Asymptomatic Infection

This is an area of ongoing controversy. There is no evidence that infection with nonpathogenic *E. histolytica* represents a health risk to the index case or close contacts. However, long-term follow-up studies to assess symptoms and general health status have not been performed. The possibility of asymptomatic pathogenic infection can be addressed by testing for serum anti-amebic antibodies. A positive amebic serology is an indication for presumptive therapy, even in an endemic area. Treatment of asymptomatic infected patients who have negative results on hemoccult and serologic testing should be individualized. In an endemic area, there are no indications for treating such individuals, but treatment is recommended when there is adequate sanitation and the risk of reinfection is low. This recommendation is based on the lack of follow-up studies and complete agreement that nonpathogenic infection is entirely innocuous. For seronegative individuals, treatment with a luminal agent (see Table 2 for regimens) is adequate. In seropositive individuals, a tissue active agent should be added. This may be the only circumstance in which use of a tetracycline with a luminal agent seems a reasonable alternative to metronidazole.

TABLE 2. **Therapeutic Regimens for Adults with Amebiasis**

Asymptomatic Infection (Seronegative)
(1) Diloxanide furoate, 500 mg PO tid for 10 days
(2) Paromomycin, 10 mg/kg PO tid for 10 days
(3) Diiodohydroxyquin, 650 mg PO tid for 20 days
Asymptomatic Infection (Seropositive)
(4) Metronidazole, 750 mg PO tid for 7 days followed by (1), (2), or (3)
(5) Doxycycline, 250 mg PO bid for 14 days followed by (1), (2), or (3)
Invasive Colitis or Liver Abscess
(6) Metronidazole, 750 mg PO tid for 10 days, followed by (1), (2), or (3)
(7) Metronidazole, 2.4 grams PO once daily for 2 days, followed by (1), (2), or (3)

Acute or Chronic Amebic Colitis

Metronidazole (Table 2) is recommended for all invasive *E. histolytica* infections. Treatment with a luminal agent must follow, especially if shorter courses of metronidazole are utilized. It is unwise to use both agents simultaneously due to gastrointestinal intolerance, but there is no direct contraindication if compliance is a major issue. Patients respond promptly to metronidazole therapy; there is no benefit from adding additional tissue amebicides. In patients with fulminant amebiasis, intestinal leakage and bacterial peritonitis may necessitate broader antibacterial therapy. Surgery is usually not indicated as it is difficult to handle colonic tissues and conservative management is more likely to be successful. The only (rare) exception is toxic megacolon, often a result of inadvertent corticosteroid therapy, which may require a total colectomy. Localized chronic amebiasis (ameboma) responds well to therapy with metronidazole.

It is imperative that successful clearance of infection be documented, as relapses can occur. At least two separate stool examinations should be performed after therapy to assess outcome. As mentioned, serum anti-amebic antibody titers remain elevated for years and are not helpful in assessing the resolution of disease. In patients with persistent nonspecific abdominal complaints or underlying inflammatory bowel disease, post-treatment colonoscopy with biopsy is necessary to rule out relapse. In addition, occasional patients may experience onset of an idiopathic colitis after treatment in which amebae cannot be demonstrated in biopsies of tissue, there is no response to metronidazole, and standard therapy for inflammatory bowel disease is also not helpful. These patients are difficult to manage; however, their symptoms usually resolve within a year after cure of the amebic infection. This syndrome is presumably an autoimmune phenomenon: circulating amebic antigen-antibody complexes have been identified during colonic amebiasis.

Amebic Liver Abscess

The overwhelming majority of patients with amebic liver abscess respond to therapy with metronidazole (Table 2) with gradual defervescence, decreased pain, and improved appetite over a 3- to 5-day period. There is no need to add potentially toxic agents such as chloroquine or dehydroemetine. A lack of response to metronidazole indicates a need to reconsider the diagnosis and perform a fine-needle aspiration of the abscess under CT guidance. Patients with amebic liver abscess who respond promptly to aspiration should receive a complete course of metronidazole therapy, and all patients should be treated with a luminal agent after completion of metronidazole therapy. Recent studies suggest that intestinal colonization, leading to a recurrence of amebic liver abscess, is more frequent than previously recognized. Regardless of whether the stool examination was initially positive, a complete course of diloxanide furoate or paromomycin is essential.

Whether fine-needle aspiration of the liver abscess should be done immediately upon presentation depends on the experience and skill of the physician and the resources of the local medical center. Although such aspiration is unnecessary in 90% of individuals, occasionally it is recommended. Examples include very large abscesses with only a thin capsule of liver preventing rupture, a patient in extreme distress requiring rapid relief, and lastly, a high likelihood that primary or secondary bacterial infection is present. Complications of amebic liver abscess such as peritonitis or lung involvement are best treated conservatively. However, an empyema or pericardial effusion must be drained. Amebic pericarditis is a fulminant disease that is often misdiagnosed; ultrasonography revealing a left lobe liver abscess suggests the diagnosis and immediate action is necessary.

Once the patient responds, there is no need to follow the hepatic lesion by expensive imaging studies. This creates undue anxiety and expense, as the lesion usually takes months to resolve. If the patient remains asymptomatic, there is no indication for therapy for a persistent defect, even 6 months after treatment. Only a recurrence of symptoms merits investigation.

BACTEREMIA AND SEPTICEMIA

method of
STEVEN K. DAUGHERTY, M.D., and
RICHARD A. PROCTOR, M.D.

University of Wisconsin
Madison, Wisconsin

Although the terms "bacteremia," "viremia," "fungemia," and "parasitemia" are commonly used to indicate states in which associated microbial pathogens are found in the blood, these terms fail to differentiate between those conditions in which the microorganism is only transiently present and those that are accompanied by fever, acidosis, and multiple organ dysfunction (i.e., the sepsis syndrome). The terms "septicemic" and "bacteremic" are often used interchangeably; however, it seems preferable to reserve the terms "sepsis," "septic," and "septicemia" for those patients showing clinical evidence of the pathophysiologic process, which

is more easily recognized than defined (Table 1). A positive blood culture may be found in the septic patient, but it should not be considered essential to the diagnosis of sepsis.

The circulatory sentinels—antibodies, polymorphonuclear cells, complement, and sinusoidal macrophages—are called upon daily to clear the blood of low levels of bacteria. Positive blood cultures have been obtained from up to one-fourth of study subjects after such innocuous tasks as brushing the teeth. This transient low-level bacteremia rarely has any untoward effects; the bloodstream usually becomes sterile within 30 minutes of onset of bacteremia. For a clinically significant infection to develop, one or more of the following factors must exist: (1) the inoculum is sufficient to overwhelm the host's normal defenses; (2) the organism possesses virulence factors that evade the host's defenses; or (3) the host's defenses have been impaired by concomitant infection, trauma, congenital defect, ischemia, or other factors that weaken normal barriers, such as indwelling infusion or monitoring devices.

Bacteremia is classified as either primary or secondary on the basis of the presence or absence of an

TABLE 1. **Clinical Signs and Symptoms of Sepsis**

Pathologic Event	Clinical and Laboratory Findings
Bacteremia	Fever, chills, nausea, lethargy, clouded sensorium
	Tachycardia
	Leukocytosis (with a leftward shift, toxic granulations); occasionally leukopenia
	Positive blood cultures
Circulatory instability	Cool, clammy skin, diaphoresis
	Tachycardia, "thready" pulse (occasionally bounding pulse, early)
	Hypotension and/or organ hypoperfusion
Organ dysfunction	Listlessness, delirium, or obtundation
	Dyspnea with tachypnea
	Hypoxemia (hypocarbia early)
	Elevated liver enzymes
	Decreased urinary output with rising serum urea nitrogen and creatinine
Disseminated intravascular coagulation (DIC)	Petechiae, purpura, mucosal hemorrhage
	Ecchymosis, persistent oozing from venipuncture sites
	Thrombocytopenia
	Fragmented erythrocytes
	Prolonged prothrombin time
	Decreased fibrinogen levels
	Increased fibrinogen degradation products
Multiorgan failure	Azotemia progressing to anuria and frank renal failure
	Encephalopathy
	Metabolic acidosis with increased lactic acid levels
	Acute respiratory failure
	Cardiac failure

identifiable anatomic source of infection. In *primary bacteremia* there is no identifiable anatomic focus; *secondary bacteremia* occurs in the presence of a local infectious process. Some common diseases giving rise to secondary bacteremia are genitourinary, cardiovascular, or respiratory infections; ascending cholangitis; intra-abdominal abscesses; and cellulitis. Secondary bacteremia is further classified as continuous, intermittent, or transient. Examples of continuous, often referred to as "high-grade" bacteremia, include early-stage infection with *Salmonella typhi*, acute brucellosis, infective endocarditis, and other intravascular infections. Intermittent recovery of bacteria from blood culture is seen in association with abscesses, osteomyelitis, pneumonias, and urinary tract infections. Breakthrough bacteremia can also occur during the early treatment period or with inadequate therapy. Transient bacteremia with an identifiable source is usually due to contaminated infusion devices or manipulation of colonized or infected tissues and is typically without clinical significance in the immunocompetent host unless there is resultant seeding of the cardiac valves or development of osteomyelitis. Of course, this is true only if the proper measures are taken to prevent it from becoming continuous bacteremia.

"Septic shock" denotes the advanced and frequently rapid clinical decline that can accompany sepsis. The spectrum of signs and symptoms range from alterations in thermoregulation and difficulty in maintaining an adequate mean arterial blood pressure to multiorgan dysfunction and death. The authors refer to this as "immunotoxicity" caused by a host immune response that becomes deleterious. Septic shock may follow infection with either gram-positive or gram-negative organisms as well as fungi. In a review of almost 700 cases of sepsis in one center, the proportions due to either gram-positive (45.5%) or gram-negative (43.5%) organisms were nearly equivalent. In this series, 7.8% of the cases were attributed to a mixed infection and 3.2% were fungal in origin.

Whereas the presentation of frank sepsis is overt, the manifestations of bacteremia may be subtle. The earliest symptoms of bacterial invasion of the bloodstream are nonspecific and include general lassitude, lethargy, malaise or occasionally agitation (clostridial bacteremia), myalgias, nausea with or without emesis, fever, chills (occasionally with rigors), and diaphoresis. In the elderly or infirm, heart failure may precede the development of hypotension, and a decline in the normal level of consciousness may be one of the earliest signs.

On clinical examination, the vital signs may also exhibit nonspecific alterations. The heart and respiratory rates are commonly increased. Although fever is typical, normal or even subnormal body temperature may be present, especially in the elderly. Early in the course of sepsis, the blood pressure may be normal with a bounding arterial pulse. Alternatively, the ominous finding of hypotension may herald impending shock.

Although the clues to be uncovered on physical examination may be myriad, a few features deserve attention for empiric purposes. Pallor may be evidence of diminished effective circulatory support leading to a shift of volume away from the periphery. Rash, petechiae, purpura, Janeway lesions, Osler nodes, or splinter hemorrhages of the nailbeds suggest endovascular infection. A diffuse petechial rash may be seen with infections due to *Neisseria meningitidis, Rickettsia, Listeria monocytogenes,* or even staphylococci. Ecthyma gangrenosum suggests gram-negative sepsis, especially in the presence of *Pseudomonas aeruginosa.* Embolic phenomena suggest a cardiovascular origin and may hasten initiation of specific empiric therapies for infective endocarditis. Examination of the fundi may provide further evidence of emboli, such as conjunctival hemorrhages as well as the cotton-like lesions of candidemia. Nuchal rigidity should arouse suspicion of meningitis as the cause of the septic presentation.

Particular attention should be paid to the chest examination. Moist rales and rhonchi are suggestive of pneumonia, and rubs may occur with pneumococcal, staphylococcal, and gram-negative pneumonias. Deliberate evaluation of the heart tones with directed maneuvers to isolate and accentuate each portion of the cardiac cycle may identify valvar leakages due to vegetations and valve destruction.

Intra-abdominal abscesses, hepatobiliary disease, and even gastrointestinal malignancies can give rise to bacteremia. Their presence may be readily recognized; more often, specific evaluation will be required to identify them as the cause of bacterial invasion. Anaerobic and mixed bacteremias are a hallmark of intra-abdominal infections. The isolation of organisms resident in the gastrointestinal tract, such as *Escherichia coli, lactobacilli,* or *Bacteroides fragilis,* should lead the clinician to redouble efforts to identify intra-abdominal pathology. Close attention should also be given to the genitourinary system, including evaluation of the prostate, which can harbor a wide variety of organisms that can enter the bloodstream.

Therapeutic delay can be avoided by implementing empiric therapy when the definitive diagnosis may not be forthcoming for several days or at best several hours. Knowing the likely pathogens associated with a given clinical picture can suggest appropriate empiric therapy (Table 2).

The microbiology laboratory is invaluable in identifying the etiologic organism and its source. The optimal time for blood sampling for culture is not clearly established. If the clinical situation allows, it is probably best to collect two sets of cultures 30 minutes apart. However, in more critical situations, two sets of cultures from two different sites before or at the inception of therapy will suffice. In a review of 292 confirmed cases of bacteremia and fungemia in adults in which three consecutive cultures were obtained, 91.5% were found to be positive after only one set. A second sampling identified an additional 7.8% as positive. Therefore, 99.3% of bacteremic or fungemic episodes were identified with two separately obtained blood cultures. A third set of cultures in this series identified only one additional case.

When properly collected through the use of aseptic techniques, less than 3% of all cultures should be contaminated. Whether an isolate is a contaminate is a clinical decision. In the review of bacteremias and fungemias just mentioned, gram-positive, gram-negative, and anaerobic organisms were isolated but determined to be contaminants. The most frequently identified contaminants were *Staphylococcus epidermidis* (94% con-

TABLE 2. **Bloodstream**

Source	Predisposing Factors	Common Organisms
Sources and Underlying Factors		
Primary bacteremia	Contaminated phlebotomy device	*Serratia*
	Intravascular catheters	*S. aureus, S. epidermidis, Enterobacter, Klebsiella, Candida*
	Parenteral hyperalimentation	*Candida*
	Contaminated IV fluids	*Klebsiella, Enterobacter*
	Contaminated blood products	*Enterobacter, Salmonella*
Skin and soft tissue	Trauma	*S. aureus*, group A streptococci, anaerobes, gram-negative bacilli
	Burns	*Enterobacter cloacae, S. aureus, P. aeruginosa, Candida,* "mixed"
	Surgery	Anaerobes
	Pressure ulcers	*P. aeruginosa, S. aureus*, enterics
	Diabetes, neutropenia	*S. aureus*, group A streptococci, anaerobes
Respiratory tract	Viral infection	Meningococci, *Haemophilus*
	Post influenza	*S. aureus, H. influenzae*
	Pneumonia—community-acquired	*S. pneumoniae, H. influenzae, Legionella, Mycoplasma, Chlamydia*
	Pneumonia—nosocomial	*Pseudomonas*, other gram-negative bacilli, *S. aureus, Legionella*
	Pneumonia—hypogammaglobulinemia	*Pneumococcus, K. pneumoniae*
	Pneumonia—aspiration (seizure disorder, drug use)	Oral anaerobes, *Enterobacter*
	Pneumonia—alcoholic	Gram-negative bacilli (*Klebsiella*)
Gastrointestinal tract	Achlorhydria	Salmonella, *M. tuberculosis*
	Trauma, perforation, or abscess	*B. fragilis*, enterococci, *E. coli, Enterobacter, Clostridia*
	Hepatobiliary obstruction or surgery	Gram-negative bacilli, enterococci, anaerobes
	Diverticulitis	Enterobacteriaceae, Bacteroides, enterococci
	Peritonitis—nephrotic or cirrhotic	*E. coli, S. pneumoniae, K. pneumoniae, S. aureus*
	Peritonitis—chronic ambulatory dialysis	*S. epidermidis, S. aureus*, streptococci, Enterobacteriaceae, *Candida*
	Colonic carcinoma	*Clostridium septicum*
	Neutropenia	Gram-negative bacilli, enterococci, anaerobes
Gynecologic tract	Postpartum or postsurgical	Group B streptococci
	Pelvic inflammatory disease	*N. gonorrhoeae, Chlamydia, Bacteroides,* Enterobacteriaceae
Urinary tract	Intercourse	*E. coli*
	Obstruction, catheterization	Enterobacteriaceae, *Pseudomonas, Enterococcus, S. saprophyticus*
Cardiovascular system	Endocarditis—native valve	Viridans group streptococci, enterococci, *S. aureus*
	Endocarditis—IV drug abuse	*S. aureus, Pseudomonas*, group D streptococci
	Endocarditis—culture-negative	HACEK organisms,† nutritionally-deficient streptococci
	Endocarditis—prosthetic valve	All of the above plus aerobic gram-negative organisms and coagulase-negative staphylococci
	Infected vascular grafts	*S. epidermidis, S. aureus, E. coli, Klebsiella, Serratia*
Central nervous system	Meningitis—normal host	*S. pneumoniae, N. meningitidis,* (*H. influenzae* in children) *Listeria monocytogenes*
	Meningitis—immunosuppressed or elderly	*L. monocytogenes*
	Meningitis—postsurgical	*S. aureus, Pseudomonas*, coagulase-negative staphylococci, gram-negative bacilli
	Primary brain abscess	Polymicrobial: viridans group streptococci, anaerobic streptococci, *Bacteroides,* Enterobacteriaceae
Miscellaneous	Postsplenectomy or functional asplenism	*S. pneumoniae, N. meningitidis, H. influenzae, Salmonella*
	Neutropenia	*P. aeruginosa, S. aureus*, gram-negative bacilli, *Candida*
	Rheumatoid arthritis, diabetes	*S. aureus*

Invasion

Empiric Therapy*	
Treatment of Choice	**Alternative**
Identify and remove source Cephalosporin (III)	Vancomycin + TMP/SMX
Same as above plus consider amphotericin Identify and remove source	Same as above plus consider amphotericin
Identify and remove source Imipenem or ampicillin/sulbactam	Nafcillin or vancomycin + clindamycin + gentamicin
Vancomycin + tobramycin + ticarcillin	Vancomycin + ceftazidime or imipenem/cilastatin
Ampicillin/sulbactam or ticarcillin/clavulanate	Imipenem or clindamycin
Ampicillin/sulbactam	Ciprofloxacin + clindamycin
Nafcillin or clindamycin or cefoxitin	Vancomycin
Cephalosporin (III) or cefuroxime	Ampicillin/sulbactam or TMP/SMX
Nafcillin or cefuroxime	TMP/SMX
Cefuroxime + erythromycin	TMP/SMX + erythromycin
Ticarcillin + tobramycin	Imipenem/cilastatin
Ampicillin or cephalosporin (II or III) + IV gamma globulin	TMP/SMX + IV gamma globulin
Ampicillin/sulbactam	Clindamycin
Tobramycin + cefazolin	Ticarcillin/clavulanate
Ciprofloxacin or ceftriaxone; anti-TB drugs	TMP/SMX (resistance has been reported)
Ampicillin/sulbactam + gentamicin	Imipenem/cilastatin
	Ciprofloxacin + metronidazole
Ampicillin/sulbactam	Cefperazone + metronidazole
Clindamycin + gentamicin + ampicillin	TMP/SMX + metronidazole
Imipenem	Cefoxitin + gentamicin
Vancomycin + tobramycin (intraperitoneal)	IV vancomycin
Penicillin G	Clindamycin
Imipenem or ceftazidime	Tobramycin + ticarcillin
Ampicillin/sulbactam + doxycycline	Cephalosporin (III) + clindamycin
Cefoxitin + doxycycline	Clindamycin + gentamicin
Ampicillin + gentamicin	Cephalosporin (I) or TMP/SMX + gentamicin
Ticarcillin + tobramycin	Cephalosporin (III) + gentamicin ± ampicillin
Nafcillin + ampicillin + gentamicin	Vancomycin + gentamicin
Nafcillin + ticarcillin + tobramycin	Vancomycin + ceftazidime + tobramycin
Ampicillin or penicillin + gentamicin	Vancomycin + gentamicin
Vancomycin + gentamicin + rifampin	Nafcillin + gentamicin + rifampin or cefuroxime + gentamicin
Nafcillin + tobramycin + ticarcillin	Vancomycin + tobramycin + ticarcillin
Cephalosporin (III)	Penicillin or ampicillin/sulbactam
Ampicillin + cephalosporin (III) + gentamicin	TMP/SMX
Vancomycin or nafcillin + ticarcillin + tobramycin + IV ciprofloxacin	Vancomycin + ceftazidime
Penicillin G + metronidazole + cephalosporin (III, but not cefoperazone)	Chloramphenicol + cephalosporin (III) or aztreonam Imipenem
Ampicillin/sulbactam	TMP/SMX
Imipenem or ceftazidime; or ticarcillin + tobramycin	Amphotericin B
Nafcillin	Cefazolin

Abbreviations: I = first-generation; II = second-generation; III = third-generation; TMP/SMX = trimethoprim-sulfamethoxazole; IV = intravenous.

*These are general guidelines for empiric therapy; however, specific decisions should be made on the basis of clinical situations, drug allergies, renal and hepatic function, and local susceptibility patterns.

†*Haemophilus, Actinobacillus, Cardiobacterium, Eikenella, Kingella.*

sidered contaminant), *Staphylococcus aureus* (25%), *Propionibacterium acnes* (99%), *Corynebacterium* species (79%), *Bacillus* species (94%), and *Clostridium perfringens* (50%). In contrast, *Streptococcus pneumoniae,* group B streptococci, and *Listeria monocytogenes* were never considered to be contaminants. In general, the isolation of gram-negative bacteria, either aerobic or anaerobic, or fungi should be considered representative of true bacteremia or fungemia due to their low rate of contamination.

TREATMENT

Deciding on appropriate therapy in the septic patient requires attention to numerous interrelated circumstances. Certainly, the clinical presentation of the patient is the most important. Local microbial pathogens with their antimicrobial susceptibility patterns, host immune status, and drug allergies and interactions should also be weighed in the decision-making process. Most prescribing errors are due to reflexive ordering of antibiotics rather than reasoned decision-making based on clinical and laboratory data. Failure to consider the correct diagnosis in the differential diagnosis leads to the most serious errors.

Empiric Therapy

Treatment undertaken before the offending pathogen is known is considered to be empiric. Although therapeutic decisions must often be made with incomplete or inadequate data, they should not be considered as blind or random. Empiric therapy is most successful when there is an identifiable focus of infection. This information allows prediction of the most likely organisms and thereby narrows the choice of initial therapy (see Table 2). A Gram's stain alone permits the selection of the correct antibiotics in 85% of cases. Once the pathogen or pathogens have been identified, therapy can be definitive, which usually results in a change in or narrowing of the coverage.

The following guidelines are valuable in implementing empiric therapy:

1. The most reliable cultures are obtained before or early in the course of antibiotic therapy.
2. Empiric therapy generally requires the use of broad-spectrum antimicrobial agents (Table 3) but overly long use may in fact increase morbidity and mortality by fostering the development of resistant organisms, superinfections, and alterations in normal flora, an important component of host defenses. The emergence of antibiotic-resistant *Enterococcus* and *Neisseria gonorrhoeae,* oxacillin-resistant *S. aureus,* and penicillin-resistant *Streptococcus pneumoniae* testifies to the need for therapeutic moderation.

3. Empiric therapy should be re-evaluated frequently, but certainly after 48 to 72 hours. The need for continuation of antibiotic therapy should then be addressed, because the large majority of cultures become positive by this time.
4. Definitive therapy should be implemented as soon as specific pathogens are identified.
5. Further modifications should be made once the susceptibility patterns are known. Of note, prospective studies have shown that physicians change to appropriate therapy less than 50% of the time after susceptibility patterns are reported!

Intravascular Device–Associated Infections

The use of intravascular infusion devices and intravascular monitoring devices has done much to improve patient treatment; however, these developments have also brought an increase in bacteremia and sepsis. Because many patients requiring both short- and long-term intravascular access are already quite ill, the added stress of an intravascular infection can significantly increase morbidity and mortality.

Both the type of catheter and the type of infusate influence the risk of infusion-associated infection. The risk of infection is ten times higher with short-term central venous catheters than with temporary peripheral intravascular catheters. The surgically placed long-term cuffed central venous catheter has a much lower rate of infection and is a low-risk option for patients requiring long-term intravenous access.

Identifying a central access catheter as the source of infection can be difficult. The access site should be examined carefully. If there is purulence or if a peripheral or central line is suspected of being the source of infection (positive blood culture, no other site to explain sepsis), it should be removed promptly, a warm compress applied, and the affected part elevated if possible. A Gram's stain of purulent material should be done to aid in directing therapy while cultures are in process. Any abscess requires surgical drainage. The extensively thrombosed, infected peripheral vein is best managed by surgical resection of the infected segment of the vein in addition to administration of intravenous antibiotics. Semiquantitative cultures of the catheter tip have been shown to correlate with catheter-associated sepsis. Therefore, all suspected catheter tips should be cultured by rolling the resected catheter tip across an agar plate. The growth of 15 colonies or more on a culture plate is diagnostic of line sepsis.

Central vein thrombosis deserves specific men-

TABLE 3. **Parenteral Antibiotics for Major Infections**

Drug	Normal Daily Dosage*	Dose for 70-kg adult†
Penicillins		
Penicillin G	2–300,000 U/kg	2–4 million U q 4 h
Ampicillin	150–200 mg/kg	1–2 gm q 4–6 h
β-*Lactamase–resistant penicillins*		
Nafcillin, oxacillin	100–200 mg/kg	1–2 gm q 4–6 h
Antipseudomonal penicillins		
Ticarcillin	250–300 mg/kg	3 gm q 4–6 h
Piperacillin	250–300 mg/kg	3–4 gm q 4–6 h
Penicillins combined with β-*lactamase inhibitors*		
Ampicillin/sulbactam		3 g q 6 h
Ticarcillin/clavulanate		3.1 gm q 4–6 h
First-generation cephalosporin		
Cefazolin		1–2 gm q 8 h
Second-generation cephalosporins		
Cefuroxime		0.75–1.5 gm q 8 h
Cefoxitin		1–2 gm q 4–8 h
Cefotetan		1–3 gm q 12 h
Third-generation cephalosporins		
Cefotaxime, Ceftizoxime	100 mg/kg	2 gm q 6–8 h
Ceftriaxone	50–75 mg/kg	1–2 gm q 24 h‡
Ceftazidime	50–100 mg/kg	2 gm q 8 h
Cefoperazone		2 gm q 12 h (4 gm q 6 h for *Pseudomonas aeruginosa*)
Carbapenem		
Imipenem/cilastatin	30–50 mg/kg	0.5–1.0 gm q 6 h
Monobactam		
Aztreonam	50–100 mg/kg	1–2 gm q 8 h
Aminoglycosides		
Tobramycin, gentamicin	5–7 mg/kg§	180–240 mg q 12 h
Amikacin	15–20 mg/kg§	600–750 mg q 12 h
Miscellaneous		
Ciprofloxacin	15 mg/kg	400 mg (IV) q 12 h
Trimethoprim/sulfamethoxazole	10–20/mg TMP/kg‖	240 mg TMP q 6 h
Vancomycin	30 mg/kg	500 mg q 6 h¶
Rifampin	10 mg/kg	600 mg q 24 h
Erythromycin	15–40 mg/kg	0.5–1.0 gm q 6 h
Doxycycline		100 mg q 12 h
Chloramphenicol	30–50 mg/kg	1 gm q 6 h
Metronidazole	30 mg/kg	500 mg q 6–8 h
Clindamycin	20–30/mg/kg	600–900 mg q 8 h
Amphotericin B	0.25–1.0 mg/kg	15–70 mg q 24 h

*Assumes normal hepatic and renal function.
†Dose range given as a general guideline; actual dose will depend on clinical situation.
‡Two grams every 12 hours for meningitis.
§Dose calculation based on lean body weight.
‖Dose calculation based on trimethoprim component.
¶May also use 1 gram every 12 hours.

tion. As vein resection is not an option, definitive therapy for the infected, thrombosed central vein requires prolonged antibiotic therapy (4 to 6 weeks of intravenous bactericidal antibiotics) and full anticoagulant therapy for at least 3 months.

Infective Endocarditis

Definitive treatment of infective endocarditis is organism specific (Table 4). Because host defenses are minimally effective at killing organisms in a vegetation, the antibiotics must be bactericidal. To be sure that the susceptibility pattern of an organism is known and that proper levels of antibiotics are used, minimal inhibitory and bactericidal concentrations (MICs and MBCs, respectively) are obtained, and doses are given to achieve peaks of 8 to 64 times and troughs of 4 times the MIC. The toxicity of the drugs (aminoglycosides) used to treat gram-negative endocarditis may not permit such levels to be achieved, however.

In general, most patients who develop infective endocarditis have underlying cardiac abnormalities leading to changes in jet flow of the bloodstream. These patients should be identified, and

TABLE 4. **Recommended Therapy for Gram-Positive Organism Endocarditis**

Setting/Organism	Treatment	Alternative	Comments
Native-valve endocarditis			
Penicillin-susceptible streptococci (MIC less than 0.1 μg/ml)	Penicillin G 10–20 million U/day (continuous infusion or q 4 h for 4 weeks) or 2 week course: Penicillin G 10–20 million U per day plus gentamicin 1 mg/kg q 12 h	Vancomycin 30 mg/kg/day (may divide into 2 or 4 daily doses) or Cefazolin 1 gm q 8 h or Ceftriaxone 1–2 gm q 24 h (continue therapy for 4 weeks)	Prevents relapse in 99% of all cases
Nutritionally deficient streptococci or viridans group streptococci with relative penicillin resistance (MIC between 0.1 and 0.5 μg/ml)	Penicillin G 20 million U/day for 4 weeks plus gentamicin 1 mg/kg q 12 h during the initial 2 weeks	As above	
Enterococci or penicillin-resistant streptococci	Penicillin G 20–30 million U/day plus gentamicin 1 mg/kg q 8 h for 4–6 weeks	Vancomycin 30 mg/kg/day (in 4 divided doses) plus gentamicin 1 mg/kg q 8 h for 4–6 weeks	Laboratory evidence of synergism should be demonstrated
Staphylococcus aureus or *S. epidermidis*	Nafcillin 2 gm q 4–6 h for 4–6 weeks plus gentamicin 1 mg/kg every 8 h during the initial 3–5 days	Vancomycin 30 mg/kg/day in 4 divided doses for 4–6 weeks	In methicillin-resistant strains use vancomycin regimen
Prosthetic valve endocarditis			
Streptococci	Penicillin G 10–20 million U/day for 6–8 weeks plus gentamicin 1 mg/kg q 12 h during the initial 2 weeks	Vancomycin 30 mg/kg/day in 4 divided doses for 6–8 weeks plus gentamicin 1 mg/kg q 8 h during the initial 2 weeks	If MIC is less than 0.1 μg/ml, then 2–4 week regimen is satisfactory
S. aureus or *S. epidermidis*	Nafcillin 2 gm q 4 h plus rifampin 300 mg (PO) q 8 h for 6–8 weeks plus gentamicin 1 mg/kg q 8 h during the initial 2 weeks	Vancomycin 30 mg/kg/day in 4 divided doses for 6–8 weeks plus gentamicin 1 mg/kg q 8 h during the initial 2 weeks	In methicillin-resistant strains, use the vancomycin plus gentamicin regimen

Abbreviations: MIC = minimal inhibitory concentration; PO = orally administered.

recommendations for prophylaxis for high-risk procedures should be emphasized (Table 5). Native valve endocarditis is caused by viridans group streptococci in nearly two-thirds of the cases. *S. aureus* is the second most likely agent with an attributable rate of 20%. Enterococci are identified in up to 10% of all cases; gram-negative organisms and fungi account for the rest.

Prosthetic valve endocarditis exhibits different epidemiologic features. Those episodes occurring less than 2 months after implantation are commonly caused by coagulase-negative or coagulase-positive staphylococci, and gram-negative organisms account for a larger proportion of cases, as do fungi. Cases occurring more than 2 months after surgery reflect a microbiologic spectrum similar to that for native valve endocarditis except for a larger number of cases due to coagulase-negative staphylococci.

Pre-existing valvular abnormalities are not a prerequisite for endocarditis in intravenous drug abusers, in whom *S. aureus* is causative in over 50% of cases, the right-sided valves being involved in nearly 90%. The remainder of cases are attributable to streptococci and enterococci. Gram-negative organisms or fungi are occasional etiologic agents.

Neutropenia

The commonly encountered problem of the neutropenic patient who presents with early signs and symptoms suggestive of bacteremia warrants special mention. The septic neutropenic patient must be evaluated rapidly but thoroughly. Particular care should be taken to exclude common foci of infection, such as an indwelling venous catheter, periodontal abscess, thrush or candidal esophagitis, endophthalmitis, infection of the central nervous system, skin or soft tissue infection or abscess, pneumonia, intra-abdominal perforation or abscess, and perianal infections. If a

TABLE 5. **Prophylaxis Against Bacterial Endocarditis in Susceptible Patients***

	Standard Regimen†		Alternative Regimen(s)
Dental, Oral, or Upper Respiratory Tract Procedures			
NO PENICILLIN ALLERGY		UNABLE TO TAKE ORAL MEDICATIONS	
Amoxicillin	3.0 gm PO 1 h prior to the procedure; then 1.5 gm 6 h after the first dose	Ampicillin	2.0 gm IV or IM 30 min prior to the procedure; then 1.0 gm IV or IM 6 h later (alternative second dose: amoxicillin 1.5 gm PO given 6 h after first dose)
PENICILLIN-ALLERGIC PATIENT			
Erythromycin	Ethylsuccinate 800 mg PO 2 h prior to the procedure; then 400 mg 6 h after the first dose	Clindamycin	300 mg IV 30 min prior to the procedure; then 150 mg PO or IV 6 h later
Erythromycin	Stearate 1.0 gm PO 2 h prior to the procedure; then 500 mg 6 h after the first dose	"High-Risk" patients with penicillin allergy Vancomycin	1.0 gm IV given over 1 h prior to the procedure; no subsequent dose necessary
Clindamycin	300 mg PO 1 h prior to the procedure; then 150 mg 6 h after the first dose		
Genitourinary or Gastrointestinal Procedures			
NO PENICILLIN ALLERGY		LOW-RISK PATIENTS:	
Ampicillin	2.0 gm IV	Amoxicillin	3.0 gm PO 1 h prior to the procedure; then 1.5 gm 6 h later
Plus gentamicin	1.5 mg/kg IV (not to exceed 80 mg) given 30 min prior to the procedure		
Then amoxicillin or repeat the initial regimen 8 h later	1.5 gm PO 6 h later		
PENICILLIN-ALLERGIC PATIENTS			
Vancomycin	1.0 gm given IV over 1 h prior to the procedure		
Plus gentamicin	1.5 mg/kg IV or IM (not to exceed 80 mg) given 1 h prior to the procedure		
Then repeat the initial regimen 8 h later			

*These regimens are based on the revised recommendations of the American Heart Association: Prophylaxis against bacterial endocarditis in susceptible patients. JAMA 264:2919, 1990. Copyright 1990, American Medical Association.
†Adult dose.
Abbreviations: PO = by mouth; IV = intravenously; IM = intramuscularly.

focus for infection is identified, empiric therapy should be directed toward normal flora found at that site. However, in the patient who appears septic but has no identifiable source of infection after thorough evaluation, empiric therapy is still indicated. The authors have recommended using single drug therapy such as imipenem or ceftazidime in patients who have not received a course of antibiotic therapy within the last 6 months.

Neutropenic patients who do not qualify for single-drug therapy should receive empiric treatment with an extended-spectrum penicillin plus an aminoglycoside. Tobramycin plus ticarcillin is a satisfactory combination, with the addition of vancomycin if there is reasonable suspicion of line sepsis, methicillin-resistant *S. aureus,* or multiply resistant enterococci. Antibiotic therapy should be continued for 7 to 10 days if the fever and signs of sepsis resolve; however, if there is no response by 72 hours, therapy should be re-evaluated. While clinical studies to define the next course of action are being done, broad-spectrum antibiotics can be stopped in patients whose cardiovascular status is stable, and further work-up can proceed. It has been the authors' practice to start amphotericin B after 3 to 5 days if the patient continues to be febrile. Other alternatives include initiating empiric therapy for infection with *Legionella pneumophila, Pneumocystis carinii,* and herpes viruses.

TABLE 6. **Prevention of Sepsis**

Conditions	Recommendations
Indwelling intravenous catheters	1. Good handwashing plus routine use of gloves when handling or manipulating any part of the system 2. Limited manipulation of the infusion system (e.g., blood draws, medications administration) 3. Peripheral venous catheters (and infusions sets) should be removed after 72 h 4. Central venous catheters should be removed after 4 days if the patient is in the intensive care unit (central venous catheters in patients outside of the intensive care unit may remain in place indefinitely) 5. Central venous access catheters with the least number of ports necessary should be used 6. Coumadin 1 mg PO per day in patients requiring long-term central venous catheters may decrease risk of thrombosis and subsequent infection without increasing risk of hemorrhage
Indwelling arterial lines	1. Replace continuous flow devices and chamber domes after 48 h 2. Replace arterial lines after 7 days
Indwelling urinary catheters	1. Good handwashing plus routine use of gloves when handling or manipulating any part of the system 2. Limit manipulation or accessing of the closed system as much as possible
Postsplenectomy or functional asplenism	1. Vaccinate (before splenectomy if possible): polyvalent pneumococcal—repeat every 6 y, *H. influenzae,* type B meningococcal A and C 2. Benzathine penicillin G 1.2 million U every month for 2–3 y following splenectomy
Prosthetic heart valve, prior episode of infective endocarditis, congenital heart defects, mitral valve prolapse with regurgitant heart murmur, hypertrophic cardiomyopathy, rheumatic or other acquired valvular heart disease	1. These patients considered "at risk" and should receive prophylaxis prior to dental, oral, respiratory, genitourinary, or gastrointestinal procedures (see Table 5 for recommendations)
History of rheumatic fever or chronic lymphedema	1. Benzathine penicillin G 1.2 million U IM every month *or* penicillin V or G 200,000 U PO per day, *or* sulfadiazine 1.0 gm PO per day until the patient is 40–50 years old (or continue as long as lymphedema persists)
AIDS (children and adults), multiple myeloma, chronic lymphocytic leukemia, congenital agammaglobulinemias, common variable immunodeficiency, Wiskott-Aldrich Syndrome	1. Monthly infusions of IV immune globulin 100 mg/kg as replacement therapy (400 mg/kg for patients with CLL, AIDS, or hypogammaglobulinemia)

Abbreviations: PO = by mouth; IM = intramuscularly; IV = intravenously; CLL = chronic lymphocytic leukemia.

Septic Shock

This systemic process is initiated by the host's inflammatory response to the presence of either a cell surface component (lipopolysaccharide) or an exotoxin. The signs and symptoms of septic shock appear on the continuum of "sepsis" as outlined in Table 1. Septic shock can be described as hemodynamic instability due to increased vascular permeability, hypoxia, or both. As tissue perfusion fails to keep up with tissue demand for metabolic needs, metabolic acidosis develops, and rapid intervention is necessary to prevent multiorgan failure.

Current therapies for septic shock carry an unacceptably high failure rate, making prevention all the more important (Table 6). Initiating appropriate antibiotic therapy is critical, but this alone is insufficient to stave off the cascade of events set in motion by hyperstimulation of the inflammatory response in 30 to 50% of patients. Adjunctive therapies are also important. The first priority is to maintain adequate tissue perfusion through fluid infusion as assessed by urine output, mental status, cardiac and liver perfusion, and reduction of acidosis. When volume replacement alone is not sufficient to maintain adequate tissue perfusion, vasopressors such as dopamine are added. Caution should be taken in using dopamine at rates higher than 15 to 20 µg per kg per minute because renal perfusion may be impaired.

Recent reports have shown that immunotherapy with monoclonal antibody against endotoxin may decrease mortality rates by 10%, but these studies are controversial, and at best, improved survival rates were observed only in subgroups of patients. At present, methods to identify subgroups prospectively are not available, making monoclonal antibody therapy unwarranted. A better understanding of the immune response at the molecular level should bring new options for intervention.

BRUCELLOSIS

method of
ABDULKARIM AL-ASKA, M.D.
College of Medicine
King Saud University and King Khalid
University Hospital
Riyadh, Saudi Arabia

Brucellosis is a zoonotic disease caused by any one of several species of *Brucella*. The three members known to infect humans are *B. melitensis, B. abortus,* and *B. suis.* Domestic animals are the reservoir of these small, gram-negative, aerobic, nonmotile coccobacilli, and abortion may be the only sign of a herd infection.

Brucellosis is endemic in many developing countries and remains a health problem in some developed countries. Humans become infected by a variety of routes, including ingestion of contaminated raw dairy or animal products, particularly milk, and contact with infected animal tissues. Therefore, shepherds and farm, dairy, and abattoir workers are at high risk. Inhalation of infected aerosols occasionally leads to the development of the disease.

When *Brucella* invades the intact mucous membranes, it is ingested by phagocytes. Either it may be eradicated without consequences or it may replicate, infecting other cells and disseminating throughout the body. Although a variety of pathologic lesions have been reported, brucellosis is usually associated with granuloma formation in various organ systems. Suppuration and periodic release of the microorganism to the bloodstream (relapse) is not uncommon. Clinically, brucellosis in humans is characterized by nonspecific manifestations, including prolonged fever (sometimes relapsing in nature), myalgia, arthralgia, low back pain, and hepatosplenomegaly. Occasionally, localized infection (sometimes referred to as a complication) is the only manifestation of the disease. Brucellosis is best diagnosed by isolating the microorganism from body fluids or biopsy tissues. In clinical practice, however, serologic methods, such as the standard tube agglutination test, are commonly used. A titer of 1:160 and above in a symptomatic patient is considered indicative of active brucellosis.

TREATMENT

Because of the organism's intracellular localization and survival within the phagocytic system, the ideal antimicrobial drug should have good tissue penetration and intracellular activity. The best regimen for the treatment of acute brucellosis has not yet been established, but the most common regimen is a combination of oral tetracycline, 2 gm in four divided doses, and intramuscular streptomycin, 14 to 20 mg per kg body weight, for 14 to 21 days followed by tetracycline alone for a total duration of 42 days. Of similar effectiveness is the combination of tetracycline and rifampin (15 mg per kg body weight). Although this regimen is more convenient to the patient in terms of compliance and cost, caution should be exercised in areas where tuberculosis is also common, as this therapy can accelerate the emergence of rifampin-resistant mycobacteria. Doxycycline, 200 mg in two divided doses, is an alternative to tetracycline and may increase patient compliance.

Initial response to trimethoprim-sulfamethoxazole (Bactrim, Septra), 8 mg per kg trimethoprim and 40 mg per kg sulfamethoxazole per day in two divided doses, for the treatment of acute brucellosis is good, but the relapse rate is high, indicating that combined drug therapy is desirable. When combined with tetracycline, trimethoprim-sulfamethoxazole has a satisfactory cure rate, and it can also be combined with streptomycin or rifampin to improve long-term results.

Recently developed antibiotics such as cephalosporins and fluorinated quinolones have been used in the treatment of brucellosis. Quinolones are known to have very low minimum inhibitory concentration (MIC) and good tissue penetration. However, there is evidence that relapses are common when these drugs are used alone.

Osteoarticular Brucellosis

Osteoarticular involvement is reported in 20 to 40% of patients with brucellosis. The same drug combinations used in acute brucellosis are employed for the treatment of osteoarticular brucellosis. Although 6 weeks of chemotherapy is adequate in most infections, the relapse rate is high (17%). Therefore, prolonged therapy for 8 to 12 weeks is recommended. In addition, drainage of paraspinal abscesses, either surgically or under imaging control, may be required.

Neurobrucellosis

Doxycycline, 100 mg every 12 hours, and rifampin, 10 to 15 mg per kg, are the drugs of choice for neurobrucellosis because, in addition to their in vitro activity, they easily cross the blood-brain barrier. These drugs are given for 3 to 6 months. High levels of drug concentration are also achieved in the cerebrospinal fluid with trimethoprim–sulfamethoxazole, and some authors recommend adding it to the aforementioned regimen. Others favor the addition of aminoglycosides for the first 3 weeks despite the fact that only small amounts cross the blood-brain barrier. Corticosteroids can be considered if cerebral edema develops.

Brucella Endocarditis

Brucella endocarditis is the most serious complication of brucellosis. A combination of tetracycline, streptomycin, and rifampin (or trimethoprim-sulfamethoxazole) is recommended. Optimal duration of therapy, with conventional doses, is not yet established but should not be less than 2 months. Most patients require surgical intervention and valve replacement. Antimicrobial chemotherapy should be continued for several weeks after surgery.

Brucellosis in Pregnancy

Untreated pregnant women are at risk of abortion, particularly in the first and second trimesters. Combination therapy with doxycycline, 100 mg orally every 12 hours, and rifampin, 15 mg per kg for 6 weeks, is recommended during the first trimester. In the second and third trimesters, rifampin alone in the same dose is relatively safe. We do not advise the use of tetracyclines in late pregnancy because of their effect on developing bones and teeth. Although trimethoprim-sulfamethoxazole (in combination with rifampin) is frequently used in this period, it is potentially teratogenic (at least in animals) and may increase the incidence of kernicterus during late pregnancy. Streptomycin is contraindicated in late pregnancy because of its ototoxicity.

Childhood Brucellosis

Doxycycline, 3 mg per kg orally for 6 weeks, and streptomycin, 14 to 20 mg per kg for 2 weeks, are recommended for children over 8 years of age. An alternative regimen is either doxycycline and trimethoprim-sulfamethoxazole, 30–60 mg per kg for 6 weeks, or doxycycline and rifampin, 15 mg per kg for 6 weeks. Younger children are treated with a combination of trimethoprim-sulfamethoxazole and either rifampin or streptomycin in the same doses and for the same duration as for older children.

CONJUNCTIVITIS

method of
DENISE BRATCHER, D.O.
Children's Hospital Medical Center
Cincinnati, Ohio

and

CHRISTOPHER J. HARRISON, M.D.
Creighton University Medical Center
Omaha, Nebraska

Conjunctivitis may result from allergies, bacterial or viral infections, or an inflammatory response to chemicals or parasites, or may be part of a systemic illness. Patients typically present with diffuse hyperemia or infection of the conjunctiva and drainage that varies from watery to frankly purulent. The patient may describe a foreign body sensation or gritty feeling. There may be edema of the lid and conjunctiva (chemosis). No truly pathognomonic clinical features exist; however, purulent drainage suggests a bacterial cause, whereas nonpurulent drainage suggests viral, allergic, or chemical/toxic causes (Table 1). Lesions, such as a chalazion, hordeolum, or skin break/pustule, generally are associated with *Staphylococcus aureus*. Common infectious causes of "pink eye," or acute conjunctivitis, are nontypable *Haemophilus influenzae, Streptococcus pneumoniae,* adenovirus, and enterovirus. Three pathogens that always require more than empiric topical treatment are *Neisseria gonorrhoeae, Chlamydia,* and herpes simplex virus (HSV). *S. aureus* conjunctivitis may necessitate systemic therapy. Conjunctival inflammation without drainage may be one sign of rickettsial infections, rubeola, Stevens-Johnson syndrome, or Kawasaki's disease. Conjunctivitis may also occur in collagen vascular diseases. The oculoglandular syndrome, Parinaud's syndrome, may be caused by cat-scratch disease or tularemia.

LABORATORY EVALUATION

Although treatment of conjunctivitis is usually empiric, laboratory evaluation is important for conditions for which empiric topical agents alone are inadequate. These include ophthalmia neonatorum or disease caused by HSV, *Chlamydia,* and *N. gonorrhoeae,* when stains (Gram's or Giemsa) of eye drainage and, at times, cultures for specific agents are invaluable. Clues that an evaluation is necessary include extreme pain (foreign body, HSV), suspected corneal involvement (HSV, foreign body, trauma), vesicles near the eye or elsewhere on the body (HSV), and refractory or recurrent conjunctivitis (*Chlamydia, N. gonorrhoeae,* or HSV infection; allergy; or hypersensitivity). Conjunctivitis in newborns nearly always necessitates culture, Gram's stain, or fluorescein dye application to rule out HSV, *Chlamydia,* and *N. gonorrhoeae.*

TREATMENT
Supportive Care

Treatment of all forms of conjunctivitis includes cool, moist compresses after removal of

TABLE 1. **Presumed Causes of Conjunctivitis by Patient Age Group***

	Purulent Conjunctivitis	Nonpurulent Conjunctivitis
Neonate	Chemical (silver nitrate)	Chemical
	Gonococcal†	Herpes simplex†
	Chlamydia†	*Chlamydia*†
	Pneumococcal	Allergic
	H. influenzae	
	Mixed flora (tear duct obstruction)	
Older child, adolescent, or adult	*H. influenzae*	Allergic
	Pneumococcal	Adenovirus
	Group A streptococcus†	Enterovirus
	Gonococcal†	Chemical
	Chlamydia†	Herpes simplex/varicella†
	S. aureus	Systemic illness
	Hordeolum	Rubeola
	Chalazion	Kawasaki's disease
	Pustule	Stevens-Johnson syndrome
		Rocky Mountain spotted fever
		Collagen vascular disease

*Conjunctivitis in the neonate has a higher risk of requiring specific therapy involving more than empiric topical antibacterials. Strong consideration should be given to use of a laboratory evaluation of the drainage.
†Requires specific systemic treatment; see text.

matted exudate from the eyelashes with warm soaks. Patching is not recommended. Irrigation may decrease the gritty sensation and is especially important in gonococcal disease. Caretakers must wash their hands frequently to avoid acquiring or transmitting infection.

Empiric Antibacterial Treatment of Simple Purulent Conjunctivitis

Gram's stain of purulent eye drainage usually reveals more than 20 polymorphonuclear white blood cells per high-power field. This microscopic finding almost always indicates bacterial infection, the most common causes outside the neonatal period being *S. pneumoniae* or nontypable *H. influenzae*. Although bacterial conjunctivitis caused by agents other than *Chlamydia* or *N. gonorrhoeae* is self-limiting, recovery is hastened by topical antimicrobial therapy. Many topical preparations are available for empiric therapy of uncomplicated purulent conjunctivitis. The authors recommend sodium sulfacetamide ointment (Sulamyd) applied twice daily for 5 to 7 days. If sulfa allergy or infection from group A streptococci or *S. aureus* is suspected, bacitracin/polymyxin (Polysporin) applied twice daily is a better choice. Ten days of oral penicillin (250 mg four times daily) should also be provided to patients with group A streptococcal conjunctivitis. The authors avoid neomycin because it may cause hypersensitivity conjunctivitis. Although ointments transiently distort vision, they allow precise and twice-daily administration.

Obstructed Tear Duct

This unilateral chronic condition arises in infants less than 6 months of age. Cultures yield mixed flora, often including *S. aureus*. Treatment consists of topical bacitracin/polymyxin ointment (Polysporin) applied twice a day for 2 to 3 weeks. Massage of the duct may be helpful. Some obstructed ducts require probing by an ophthalmologist.

Otitis-Conjunctivitis Syndrome and Otitis-Prone Children

Conjunctivitis plus otitis media has been designated the otitis-conjunctivitis syndrome. Topical therapy in addition to the customary 10 days of oral antibiotics for otitis media is not necessary, but because the pathogen is nearly always nontypable *H. influenzae* (20 to 70% produce betalactamase), drugs minimally affected by betalactamases are recommended (e.g., trimethoprim-sulfamethoxazole [Septra], based on 8 mg per kg per day of trimethoprim divided every 12 hours; amoxicillin-clavulanate [Augmentin], 10 mg per kg every 8 hours; or cefixime [Suprax], 8 mg per kg every 24 hours). In otitis-prone children, treatment of purulent conjunctivitis should include an oral beta-lactamase-resistant drug even when otitis media is absent in order to reduce the nearly 50% risk of acute otitis media in the subsequent 2 to 4 weeks.

Staphylococcus Aureus

Hallmarks of *S. aureus*-associated conjunctivitis are lesions such as a chalazion, hordeolum, or periocular skin pustule. Treatment consists of supportive care plus topical bacitracin applied twice daily to the inner aspect of the lower eyelid for 2 to 3 weeks. Occasionally, oral cefadroxil (Duricef), 30 mg per kg per day divided in two doses daily, or incision and drainage are necessary to resolve recalcitrant chalazia. *S. aureus* blepharitis can be associated with lice infestation of the lashes.

Neisseria Gonorrhoeae

Ceftriaxone (Rocephin), 50 mg per kg every 24 hours intravenously for 7 days, should be used empirically for neonatal gonococcal conjunctivitis unless susceptibility to penicillin is established, in which case aqueous penicillin G, 100,000 U per kg per day intravenously divided every 6 hours, can be used. The mother and her sexual partner should be treated. In infected children beyond the neonatal period, sexual abuse should be strongly suspected. Older children and adults may be adequately treated with intramuscular ceftriaxone (250 mg) if no evidence of dissemination exists. A search for other sexually transmitted diseases (STDs), such as chlamydial infection and syphilis, is required, as is consideration of potential human immunodeficiency virus (HIV) infection.

Chlamydia

Culture of conjunctival scrapings obtained with a dry calcium alginate swab is the standard for diagnosis of chlamydial infection. Giemsa stains may demonstrate basophilic chlamydial intracytoplasmic inclusion bodies in epithelial cells. Chlamydial infections necessitate oral therapy. In neonates, this may prevent development of pneumonia. Treatment of the infant's parents or the sexual partners of older patients is also necessary. Treatment for children less than 8 years old consists of erythromycin (Ilosone), 40 to 50 mg per kg per day divided in four doses for 3 weeks; and in older patients doxycycline (Vibramycin), 100 mg twice daily. Topical erythromycin (Ilotycin) can be added to oral treatment. Investigation for other STDs is warranted.

Nonherpes Viral Conjunctivitis

Treatment of conjunctival infection caused by viral agents, excluding HSV, is supportive. Because it may be difficult to distinguish clinically between acute viral and bacterial causes, empiric topical antimicrobial agents are often used.

Herpes Simplex Virus

This condition may be missed without careful examination of the cornea. The minimal examination should include application of fluorescein dye to seek dendritic erosions or pits in the corneal surface. Slit-lamp examination may be needed for diagnosis. Culture remains the most sensitive confirmatory method. HSV infections in neonates necessitate intravenous acyclovir (Zovirax), 30 mg per kg per day divided every 8 hours for 2 to 3 weeks, to prevent dissemination to deep organs or the CNS. Topical trifluorothymidine (Viroptic), one drop every 2 hours, is recommended regardless of age because the cornea is avascular and even intravenous acyclovir may not be effective. Topical steroids can also lead to enucleation of the eye if administered during active HSV keratitis. Ophthalmologic consultation is advised in all cases of primary HSV conjunctivitis. Recurrent HSV keratitis should also be confirmed, if need be, by an ophthalmologist and treated topically with Viroptic to limit visual loss. Topical ocular steroid treatment is contraindicated for patients with a history of HSV ocular disease unless done in consultation with an ophthalmologist.

Varicella-Zoster Virus

Conjunctivitis during varicella can lead to corneal varicella-zoster virus (VZV) involvement. Topical Viroptic, one drop every 2 hours, is used to limit ocular involvement when vesicles occur on or near the conjunctiva.

Allergies

The hallmark of allergic conjunctivitis is itching. Profuse tearing may occur. The conjunctivae may have "cobblestoning" from hyperplasia of the papillae. Nasal symptoms may be noted. Allergic conjunctivitis can be seasonal (e.g., ragweed), specific (e.g., animals), or chronic (e.g., dusts or molds). Allergic conjunctivitis is usually a clinical diagnosis. Treatment varies with the severity of symptoms. Oral or topical antihistamines plus vasoconstrictors may be effective for mild cases, whereas more severe symptoms may require topical steroids (Decadron ophthalmic ointment) four times daily for 5 to 7 days. Topical steroids should not be prescribed if HSV or other infectious causes are suspected, and should be tapered over a 5- to 7-day period to prevent potential sequelae of long-term use (glaucoma or cataracts).

Chemical Conjunctivitis

Chemical conjunctivitis occurs in the neonate owing to silver nitrate prophylaxis and may be purulent or nonpurulent. Children and adults exposed to environmental fumes or to heavily chlorinated water from swimming pools or hot tubs also may present with nonpurulent conjunctivitis. Treatment involves avoidance of the irritant and supportive care.

VARICELLA
(Chickenpox)

method of
SANDRA L. FOWLER, M.D.
Medical University of South Carolina
Charleston, South Carolina

Varicella (chickenpox) is a ubiquitous viral infection affecting over 3 million persons per year in the United States, the majority of whom are children. Although generally a benign infection, 100 varicella-associated deaths are reported each year, primarily in the very young (less than 1 year old) and in adults. Adolescents and secondary household cases may also experience more severe clinical disease. Varicella is highly contagious with an attack rate of 85 to 95% in susceptible household contacts. Transmission is believed to occur via respiratory droplets and through direct contact. The incubation period ranges from 8 to 21 days; most cases occur 10 to 14 days after exposure. After infection, lifelong immunity is established, although latent virus may reactivate to produce zoster (shingles), especially with advancing age.

VARICELLA IN NORMAL CHILDREN

The characteristic exanthem of varicella virus infection may be preceded by nonspecific symptoms such as fever and malaise. These are soon followed by a pruritic vesicular eruption that begins on the face and trunk and spreads centrifugally to all areas of the skin, including palms and soles, and may involve mucous membranes. Lesions first appear as erythematous papules and then evolve into vesicles filled with clear fluid, which subsequently appear pustular. Central umbilication is followed by crusting. New crops of lesions continue to appear up to 5 days after the initial eruption, and all stages of lesion development may be present at one time. Crusting is usually complete by 7 to 9 days.

Complications occur in 10% of normal children with chickenpox, the most common of which are skin and soft tissue infections due to group A streptococcus and *Staphylococcus aureus*. These infections typically present as superficial impetiginous lesions consisting of large pustules surrounded by erythema, although more invasive infections such as fasciitis and myositis may also develop. Bacteremia may occur and result in osteomyelitis, septic arthritis, or bacterial pneumonia.

Cerebellitis, the most commonly recognized neurologic complication, begins in the later part of the illness and is characterized by ataxia, nystagmus, vomiting, and slurred speech. Fever is not usually present, and mental status is normal. Recovery is complete but may be prolonged for weeks or months. Varicella-associated encephalitis is described, but an accurate characterization is complicated by the inclusion of cases of Reye's syndrome in earlier reports of varicella-associated neurologic illnesses. Varicella encephalitis is likely to be associated with fever, mental status changes, and cerebrospinal fluid (CSF) pleocytosis. Reye's syndrome, which has been linked with aspirin use during varicella, is associated with a rapid decline in mental status, but patients are likely to be afebrile and do not have CSF pleocytosis. Severe liver dysfunction with marked elevations of aspartate aminotransferase (AST) and alanine aminotransferase (ALT), hyperammonemia, and hypoglycemia are hallmarks of Reye's syndrome. Other rare neurologic complications include transverse myelitis, aseptic meningitis, and cranial nerve palsies. Treatment of neurologic complications is generally supportive. It is unclear whether neurologic complications result from ongoing viral replication or from as yet undefined immunologic responses. Use of specific antiviral therapy is of unknown benefit.

Pneumonia is the third most common complication of varicella and may be due to varicella itself or to secondary bacterial infection with the pneumococcus, *Haemophilus influenzae*, or group A beta-hemolytic streptococci. Subclinical hepatitis with mild elevations in AST and ALT occurs in one-third of normal children. Hemorrhagic complications such as thrombocytopenia and purpura fulminans are uncommon.

Diagnosis

Varicella infections are usually diagnosed clinically by the appearance of the rash, although the characteristic vesicular lesions may fail to develop in immunocompromised patients or it may be difficult to distinguish the vesicular lesions of varicella zoster virus (VZV) infections from other vesicular rashes. In these circumstances, viral cultures may be useful, especially to identify infections due to herpes simplex virus (HSV). VZV is generally more difficult to isolate and requires a longer incubation in tissue culture. In laboratories with the personnel and equipment to perform fluorescence microscopy, scrapings from the lesion base can be stained with fluorescent antibodies specific for VZV or HSV. Serologic tests are generally not useful in identifying acute disease but may be helpful in confirming prior infection. The enzyme-linked immunosorbent assay (ELISA) for varicella is widely available but is less sensitive than the fluorescent antibody to membrane antigen (FAMA) test, whose use is limited primarily to research laboratories.

Control of Transmission of Varicella Zoster Virus

Varicella infections are highly transmissible via the airborne route and by direct contact with lesions. The degree of exposure influences the likelihood of transmission; secondary cases occur more frequently after household than after classroom contact. The period of communicability begins 1 to 2 days before the onset of the rash and continues until all lesions have crusted.

The highly communicable nature of this virus poses a special problem in hospitals. The admission screening should include questions regarding possible exposure to varicella. Elective hospitalizations should be delayed beyond the incubation period, if possible. Susceptible individuals who require hospital admission should be placed in respiratory isolation from day 8 to day 21 after exposure because the period of communicability begins before onset of the rash. Persons admitted with active chickenpox require strict isolation. Zoster is less likely to result in nosocomial transmission if the lesions can be covered, but because of the risk that varicella may pose to other hospitalized patients, drainage/secretion precautions should be followed until all lesions have crusted. Immunocompromised patients with zoster should be placed in isolation.

TREATMENT

Until recently, treatment of varicella has been limited to symptomatic therapy. In 1992, the U.S. Food and Drug Administration (FDA) approved the use of oral acyclovir (Zovirax), 20 mg per kg per dose four times daily (maximum of 800 mg per dose), for the specific antiviral therapy of chickenpox in normal children. This recommendation was based on data showing a decrease in the total number of lesions, more rapid cessation of new lesion formation, and accelerated resolution of pruritus and fever in normal children receiving acyclovir in comparison with placebo controls. Whether these statistically significant improvements are of sufficient clinical significance to warrant the routine use of acyclovir is controversial. These studies did not demonstrate a shortened disease course or a more rapid progression to complete crusting, which is the criterion used for return to school. There are no data to suggest that antiviral treatment reduces complications from varicella in normal children.

Although universal treatment of otherwise normal children is not recommended at this time, therapy may be useful for patients at increased risk for the development of severe varicella such as adolescents and secondary household cases. Adults, who also develop severe disease and in whom the incidence of varicella pneumonitis is higher, should be considered for routine antiviral therapy with oral acyclovir, 800 mg five times per day. Therapy should begin within 24 hours of onset of rash in order to be effective.

Children who are immunocompromised by virtue of an underlying disease or antineoplastic or anti-inflammatory therapy are at risk for severe chickenpox and continued new lesion formation beyond the first week of illness. They are also much more likely to develop pneumonitis or disseminated varicella, both of which are associated with a high mortality rate in this population. Bone marrow transplant recipients with varicella have a 45% risk of experiencing cutaneous or visceral dissemination. Immunocompromised patients who develop zoster (shingles) are also at risk for disseminated disease and should be treated as if they have primary varicella infection. Patients with hematologic or solid malignancies, transplant recipients, patients with human immunodeficiency virus infection or other cellular immune deficiencies, and patients on steroid therapy who experience varicella zoster virus infections (chickenpox or shingles) should receive antiviral therapy, preferably with parenteral acyclovir initially (1500 mg per m^2 per day divided every 8 hours), followed by oral acyclovir as the clinical condition warrants. Therapy is usually continued until symptoms improve and lesions are crusted.

Symptomatic treatment of varicella may include the use of antipyretics such as acetaminophen (Tylenol) or ibuprofen and antipruritics such as diphenhydramine (Benadryl). Calamine lotions or cool compresses can also be used to relieve itching. Although it is important to keep the lesions clean by washing with soap and water, warm baths may increase pruritus. Excessive scratching may predispose to bacterial superinfection and scarring. *Aspirin should not be used in children with chickenpox.*

Varicella in Adults

Most adults who have no history of chickenpox have serologic evidence of prior infection with VZV. Varicella in adults is likely to be accompanied by fever, malaise, and exanthem that are more severe than those that occur in children. The incidence of pneumonitis increases to approximately 15% and is associated with a mortality rate of up to 17%. The overall case-to-fatality ratio for varicella occurring in adults is 17:100,000 in comparison with 0.7:100,000 in normal children. Acyclovir therapy should be considered for any adult who develops varicella. Adults with symptoms or signs of pneumonitis, such as cough, dyspnea, or radiographic abnormalities, should receive prompt antiviral therapy.

Varicella in Pregnancy

It has been estimated that each year, 7000 pregnancies are complicated by varicella. Varicella may be even more severe in pregnant women than in other adults. It is unclear whether pregnancy predisposes to pneumonitis, but among pregnant women who develop this complication, the mortality rate is 40%, in comparison to 17% among all adults. Exposed, susceptible pregnant women thus should be considered for passive immunoprophylaxis with varicella zoster immune globulin (VZIG). Consideration should also be given to specific antiviral therapy with acyclovir when chickenpox complicates pregnancy, especially if there is evidence of pneumonitis. (Use of acyclovir for this indication is not approved or suggested by the manufacturer.)

Gestational varicella during the first half of pregnancy may uncommonly result in the fetal varicella syndrome, characterized by cicatricial skin lesions, limb hypoplasia, microcephaly, eye malformations, and mental retardation. There is no reliable method for determining whether the fetus is affected by maternal varicella infection, although limb hypoplasia may be evident on prenatal ultrasonograms. Fortunately, the syndrome is rare and termination of pregnancy is rarely warranted. Whether VZIG administered to the mother prevents infection of the fetus is unknown.

Onset of maternal varicella between 5 days before and 2 days after delivery places the newborn at risk for disseminated varicella, characterized by rash, pneumonitis, and visceral involvement. Administration of VZIG to these infants may not prevent the development of varicella but does reduce the risk of disseminated disease and its associated mortality. Use of VZIG should also be considered for infants exposed to chickenpox within the first 2 weeks of life if their mothers have no history of previous varicella. Infants born before 28 weeks' gestation should receive VZIG for exposure during the first month of life regardless of the maternal history. Newborns who develop varicella within the first 2 weeks of life should be observed closely and considered for antiviral therapy with acyclovir.

Varicella Zoster Immune Globulin

Chickenpox may be prevented or its course modified by the use of postexposure prophylaxis with VZIG. The preparation should be given at a dose of one vial per 10 kg (one vial for newborns up to a maximal dose of five vials for adults) intramuscularly within 96 hours of exposure. Postexposure prophylaxis is recommended for persons at high risk for severe chickenpox or its complications. This population includes the immunocompromised, infants born to mothers who developed varicella between 5 days before and 2 days after delivery, infants born at less than 28 weeks' gestation who are exposed during the first month of life, and full-term infants who are exposed to chickenpox in the first 2 weeks of life and whose mothers have no history of varicella. Drawbacks to its use include its cost ($450 for an adult dose), the necessity that it be given soon after exposure, and the observation that it may prolong the incubation period from 21 to 35 days. VZIG has no role in the treatment of varicella or zoster.

Varicella Vaccine

A live, attenuated varicella vaccine prepared from the Oka strain of VZV was developed in Japan and has been used in that country since the 1970s. The vaccine is highly immunogenic, eliciting both humoral and cell-mediated responses in normal children. Its efficacy in normal children has ranged from 86 to 100% and is about 85% in leukemic children. For those in whom vaccine failures occurred, disease tended to be very mild. There is accumulating evidence that the vaccine does not result in an increased incidence of zoster.

Despite these observations, the vaccine is not without controversy. There are concerns that vaccine-induced immunity may not be long-lived, resulting in a population of adults who are susceptible to varicella and the complications attendant in this age group. The vaccine is awaiting licensure in the United States and is more likely to be approved for use in immunocompromised children than in the general population.

CHOLERA

method of
DILIP MAHALANABIS, M.B., B.S.
International Centre for Diarrhoeal Disease Research
Dhaka, Bangladesh

Although cholera carries a case fatality rate of 50% or more when untreated, almost all patients recover fully and rapidly when treated adequately. With rapid rehydration, a seriously ill patient in profound shock with no detectable pulse or blood pressure is able to sit, talk, and eat within a few hours and can return to work or school within 2 to 3 days. This lifesaving and dramatic treatment can be rendered at a very low cost; this is important because cholera affects mainly poor people in the least developed countries.

Cholera is caused by the bacteria *Vibrio cholerae*, which colonizes the mucosal lining of the small intestinal lumen. The toxin released is an 84-kilodalton protein consisting of an active A subunit (with A_1 and A_2 peptides) and a cluster of five B subunits. The B subunits bind the toxin molecule to the mucosal receptor GM_1 ganglioside; the active A subunit enters the cell and stimulates the secretion of water and electrolytes, resulting in secretory diarrhea.

TREATMENT

On examination, a typical cholera patient is extremely weak and thirsty, has a hoarse voice, and often complains of muscle cramps. Signs of dehydration include decreased skin turgor, sunken eyes, dry mucous membranes, and a weak or undetectable radial pulse. Patients often have severe metabolic acidosis. A remarkable aspect of the disease is how a healthy person can become so sick after only a few hours of diarrhea and vomiting. However, much less severe episodes of cholera are common, and mild cases cannot be distinguished clinically from other acute watery diarrheal diseases. Such an acute dehydrating diarrhea syndrome is sometimes caused by other etiologic agents, most notably the enterotoxigenic *Escherichia coli*.

Patients are assessed for signs of dehydration to estimate severity and fluid requirements. Rapid assessment is important because a severely dehydrated patient may literally be within minutes of death unless fluid therapy is started immediately. Clinical assessment is adequate for formulating a treatment plan for individual patients; laboratory tests (e.g., hematocrit, plasma specific gravity, total serum proteins) are used in research studies to compare groups of patients but are superfluous for clinical management. Clinical manifestations of severe cholera are mostly due to the loss of salts and water in the stool and vomitus. Complications arise only when

appropriate rehydration is not accomplished rapidly.

Objectives of treatment are (1) rapid replacement of water and salts already lost; (2) maintenance of normal hydration until diarrhea stops, by replacing fluid losses as they occur; (3) reduction of the magnitude and duration of diarrhea with suitable antimicrobials; and (4) introduction of a normal diet as soon as the patient is able to eat without waiting for diarrhea to stop.

Until the early 1970s, fluid losses in cholera could be replaced only by intravenous therapy. Treatment has been revolutionized by the introduction of oral rehydration therapy (ORT), in which a solution containing glucose and three salts is used (Table 1). It has made cholera therapy practical, simple, inexpensive, and highly effective, particularly under field conditions. ORT is based on the fact that glucose-linked enhanced absorption of sodium and water from the small intestine remains largely intact during the massive secretory state of cholera. ORT is optimally employed by starting administration of the solution at the first sign of diarrhea in an amount equal to the losses that occur and continuing it until diarrhea stops. This may reduce the number of severe cases requiring intravenous therapy, conserving scarce medical resources. Research in the 1980s has shown that replacing 20 grams of glucose with 50 grams of rice flour (which requires cooking; see Table 1) for 1 liter of oral rehydration salt solution increases absorption and reduces fluid stool losses by 35 to 40% in

TABLE 1. **Oral Rehydration Salt Solution***

Amount of Oral Rehydration Salts Needed to Prepare 1 Liter of Solution

Sodium chloride	3.5 gm
Trisodium citrate dihydrate	2.9 gm
OR	
Sodium hydrogen carbonate (sodium bicarbonate)	2.5 gm
Potassium chloride	1.5 gm
Glucose anhydrous†	20.0 gm

Molar Concentration of Solution (mmol/L)

	Citrate Solution	Bicarbonate Solution
Sodium	90	90
Potassium	20	20
Chloride	80	80
Citrate	10	—
Bicarbonate	—	30
Glucose	111	111

*Formula recommended by the World Health Organization was first used in 1971.

†50 gm rice powder can replace 20 gm glucose. To prepare a rice-ORS solution, put 50 gm rice flour in 1100 mL water and bring to a boil. Continue boiling for about 7–10 min. When the mixture is opalescent, cool, add the three salts. Serve warm and discard after 8 h. Rice-ORS can reduce purging by 30–40% in comparison with glucose-ORS.

comparison with glucose oral rehydration salt (ORS) solution.

Intravenous rehydration still plays a critical role in the treatment of cholera: in patients who present with severe dehydration and shock, infusion of appropriate intravenous fluids can be lifesaving. Intravenous fluids should replace the electrolyte losses via cholera stool, which in the severely affected patient range from 100 to 140 mmol per liter of sodium, 30 to 50 mmol per liter of bicarbonate, and 15 to 30 mmol per liter of potassium with an osmolality close to that of plasma (Table 2). Lactated Ringer's (Hartmann's) solution is commercially available and has a suitable composition (see Table 2). In cholera-endemic areas, special polyelectrolyte fluids can be prepared especially for diarrhea treatment (e.g., Dhaka solution). Normal saline with or without glucose should be used only if a more suitable polyelectrolyte solution is not available. In such a situation, a complete ORS solution should be given as early as possible to provide the base and potassium.

Patients with severe dehydration and signs of hypovolemia should be rehydrated intravenously to achieve complete rehydration in 2 to 4 hours. After initial complete rehydration, most patients can be maintained with ORT, although about 10 to 15% of hospitalized patients may need an additional short course of intravenous therapy because of high purging rates and recurrence of signs of dehydration. A single solution is adequate for all age groups in cholera.

Rehydration and Maintenance Therapy

The severity of dehydration must be assessed and the fluid requirement estimated quickly. A severely dehydrated patient with a deficit of about 10% of body weight is very weak with very poor skin turgor, sunken eyes, and a barely perceptible or absent radial pulse. As an example, the estimated deficit in a 50-kg adult with severe dehydration is 5 liters. A moderately dehydrated patient whose deficit is estimated at about 7.5% has obvious signs of dehydration with dry mucous membranes, sunken eyes, and poor skin turgor; the radial pulse is palpable but soft and rapid. In severely dehydrated patients, intravenous fluids are infused rapidly to quickly restore circulating volume. As a guide, half of the estimated volume of fluid required in a severely dehydrated patient should be given over the first hour, initially as fast as possible until the radial pulse is palpable. The patient should be fully hydrated in 2 to 4 hours, at which time intravenous therapy may be discontinued and oral rehydration therapy started and continued until diarrhea stops.

For most patients with mild and moderate dehydration, ORT can be given both for initial rehydration and for replacement of ongoing fecal losses (see Table 2). ORT can continue in spite of some vomiting, which is common; with persistence and with small frequent feedings, most patients retain enough fluid to become rehydrated.

Adequate replacement is signaled by the return of the radial pulse to normal strength and rate (the pulse rates in an adult are usually below 90 beats per minute), return of skin turgor to normal, and a feeling of well-being. Children who are drowsy or stuporous may not become fully alert for 12 to 18 hours despite adequate rehydration. In addition, weight gain of about 8 to 10% in a severely dehydrated patient is observed. Return of urine output usually occurs within 12 to 20 hours of initial rehydration.

Patients are most conveniently treated with a cholera cot, which allows efficient collection and measurement of stool. In its simplest configuration, a cholera cot consists of a foldable canvas camp cot covered by a plastic sheet with a suitable hole in the center. A sleeve fits into the hole and guides the diarrheal stool into a plastic bucket underneath the cot so that it can be measured periodically. A vomit basin should also be available. A simple input-output chart at bedside

TABLE 2. **Electrolyte Composition of Cholera Stool and Some Intravenous Solutions***

Concentration (mmol/L)	Cholera Stool		Ringer's Lactate†	Dhaka Solution‡	Normal Saline§
	Adults	*Children*			
Na+	135	105	131	133	154
K+	15	25	4	13	0
Cl−	100	90	111	98	154
HCO3−	45	30	26	48	0

*Do not use 5% dextrose in water to treat dehydrating diarrheal diseases.

†The best commercially available solution. Lactate yields bicarbonate; low potassium concentration is made up by optimum use of oral rehydration therapy.

‡In use for many years to treat cholera at the International Centre for Diarrhoeal Disease Research, Bangladesh. It is not commercially available but serves as a good example of a polyelectrolyte solution for cholera.

§Sodium concentration is high for children and solution does not contain a base or potassium. Prompt introduction of oral rehydration therapy may prevent potential problems.

shows the amounts of intravenous and ORS solutions and the volume of stool. A few hospitalized cholera patients may show signs of dehydration while on ORT. If dehydration occurs, additional intravenous fluids are given rapidly as for initial rehydration, after which oral maintenance should be resumed.

Antimicrobial Therapy

The goal of antimicrobial therapy is to drastically reduce or eliminate *V. cholerae* from the intestinal lumen so that no more cholera toxin is produced and only the residual toxin already bound to the gut mucosa remains. The use of a suitable antibiotic such as tetracycline reduces the duration of diarrhea by about 50%, to an average of 2 days, reduces the volume of diarrhea after start of treatment by about 50%, and reduces the duration of *Vibrio* excretion to an average of 1 to 2 days. Therefore, the use of an appropriate antibiotic has a profound effect on the cost and convenience of treatment.

Antibiotics are usually given after completion of initial rehydration, i.e., about 4 to 6 hours after starting treatment. Tetracycline, the antibiotic of choice, is given to adults at 500 mg every 6 hours for 48 to 72 hours and to children at 50 mg per kg per day in four divided doses for 48 to 72 hours (tetracycline should be avoided in children under 8 years of age). Doxycycline can also be used in a single dose of 300 mg in adults and 6 mg per kg body weight for children under 15 years of age; doxycycline may cause nausea and should be given after the patient eats some food. Alternative antibiotics are furazolidone, 100 mg every 6 hours (for children, 5 mg per kg per day in four divided doses) for 72 hours; erythromycin, 250 mg every 6 hours (for children, 30 mg per kg per day in three divided doses) for 72 hours; or trimethoprim-sulfamethoxazole (8 mg of trimethoprim and 40 mg of sulfamethoxazole per kg per day in two divided doses for 72 hours). Chloramphenicol is also effective in the same dosage as tetracycline but is usually not used because of potential serious side effects. Prophylactic antibiotics are not recommended because of the risk of the emergence of antibiotic-resistant strains.

Diet

Patients should be offered normal food as soon as the dehydration and acidosis are corrected and they feel able to eat.

COMPLICATIONS

Complications of cholera are rare if correct treatment is provided quickly since most result from delay in therapy or provision of inappropriate fluid therapy. Risks of pyrogen reaction, excessive hydration, or too rapid correction of hyper- or hyponatremia or acidosis are minimized by optimal use of ORT and early resumption of a normal diet. Pneumonia, a not uncommon problem, may be due to aspiration of vomitus or altered tissue resistance secondary to shock and acidosis.

PREVENTION

The only effective means of preventing cholera is to ensure that healthy individuals are not infected with *V. cholerae* through food and drink. Therefore, washing hands with soap and water, using clean water for drinking and washing utensils and other activities, and appropriate excreta disposal are useful preventive measures. The injectable killed bacterial vaccines are not recommended because protection is inadequate, short-lived, and ineffective in children. Oral killed whole-cell vaccines with or without added B subunit are more effective and their usefulness in the public health field is being evaluated.

DIPHTHERIA

method of
JERRY J. ELLER, M.D.
Rush Medical Group
Livingston, Alabama

Diphtheria is an acute infectious disease caused by a pleomorphic gram-positive bacillus, *Corynebacterium diphtheriae*. The organism usually colonizes mucous membranes of the upper respiratory tract and less commonly the skin, and it produces a powerful exotoxin. Diphtheria toxin (DT) production is under control of a phage gene. Virulence of strains is under control of bacterial genes and is a result of the capacity to establish infection, multiply rapidly, and quickly produce toxin. One domain of DT is responsible for interference with protein synthesis by inactivating the elongation factor EF 2. DT binds to a specific receptor on the surface of cells identified as heparin-binding epidermal growth factor (EGF)–like precursor. The bound toxin is reabsorbed by endocytosis into the cytosol. DT causes local cellular necrosis and then diffuses into the circulation, which can result in serious damage to the heart or to nerves (myocarditis or polyneuritis). Death may occur early from respiratory obstruction or from overwhelming toxemia and circulatory collapse, or somewhat later from cardiac damage. Patients usually survive neurotoxic injury if they are medically attended and given supportive care. The hallmark of the disease is the presence of a diphtheritic pseudomembrane that is produced by exotoxin. It is composed of necrotic epithelium plus an exudate of fibrin, red and white blood cells, and colonizing bacteria. The clinical course of diphtheria depends on (1) the location and extent of the membrane, (2) the amount of toxin produced and absorbed, (3) early institution of treatment with antitoxin, and (4) the patient's age and immune status.

Three biotypes of *C. diphtheriae—gravis, intermedius,* and *mitis—*may be identified. All toxigenic strains can produce the same exotoxin. *Mitis* strains produce less severe clinical disease than do the other strains.

Transmission of *C. diphtheriae* is by intimate contact with infected droplets, nasopharyngeal secretions, or skin exudates. A carrier state develops when a person with toxigenic immunity harbors the organism in the nasopharynx or on the skin but remains free of symptoms. Such a carrier must be identified by appropriate cultures. A convalescent carrier state after clinical disease also develops. These carriers constitute the reservoir of infection from which susceptible persons contract the disease. The incubation period is 1 to 6 days.

Although now rare, respiratory diphtheria must be considered if clinical findings are suggestive. Currently in the United States and other industrialized countries, "herd immunity" remains high among persons 5 to 25 years of age. Importation of the organism from developing countries where diphtheria remains endemic poses a constant threat to (1) inadequately immunized infants and children, (2) adult drug and alcohol abusers who lack protective antitoxin levels, (3) elderly persons with lapsed immunity, and (4) the increasing proportion of immunocompromised individuals. The case fatality rate has continued to be in the range of 5 to 10% but may be higher in more vulnerable persons.

PREVENTION

Diphtheria is a preventable disease; everyone should be immunized. The following recommended schedules for active immunization, found in the 1991 report of the Committee of Infectious Diseases of the American Academy of Pediatrics, are endorsed: A normal infant should receive 0.5 mL of diphtheria and tetanus toxoid combined with pertussis vaccine (DPT) at 2, 4, and 6 months, with a booster at 1½ years of age. A booster is also given at age 4 to 6 years. At age 14 to 16 years, an adult-type combined tetanus and diphtheria toxoid (Td) injection is given; thereafter it is given every 10 years. For a child younger than 7 years of age, a DPT injection is given at the first visit and then boosters are given 2 and 4 months later. A repeat injection is given 6 to 12 months later or in school. For children 7 years of age and older and for adults, a Td injection is given on the first visit, and a repeat injection is given 2 months later, which is followed by a booster 6 to 12 months later. A Td injection should be given every 10 years. A serum antitoxin level of 0.01 IU per mL or higher is protective. Primary care physicians should maintain protective levels by giving Td boosters to adult patients.

DIAGNOSIS

Diagnosis is a clinical judgment (Table 1). In general, direct smears are unreliable; methylene blue staining of a throat smear is only suggestive of the diagnosis. Although this procedure can be done quickly, its usefulness is limited because diphtheroids normally found in the throat are indistinguishable from *C. diphtheriae.* The organisms responsible for Vincent's angina also resemble *C. diphtheriae,* and some patients have Vincent's angina in association with diphtheria. Albert's stain of a smear is more reliable if it is carried out and interpreted by an experienced technologist. Identification by the fluorescent antibody technique is reliable only when done by experienced personnel.

The first step is to obtain material from the nose and throat and from skin lesions, if present, for culture. It is best to carry the material by hand to the laboratory and tell the technologist that the patient is suspected of having diphtheria. Swabs are usually streaked on Loeffler's blood agar, tellurite, or fresh Pai's or Tinsdale's media. From 16 to 48 hours of incubation are required before *C. diphtheriae* colonies can be identified. A toxigenicity test must then be carried out, preferably by using the modified Elek's diffusion technique. A positive reaction consists of a white streak, which usually appears at 16 to 24 hours.

TREATMENT

Specific Management

Antitoxin

Every effort must be made to administer diphtheria antitoxin as soon as possible after the disease is suspected (Table 2). Delay beyond 48 hours must be avoided because the administration of even very large doses of antitoxin after

TABLE 1. **Clinical Diagnosis of Diphtheria**

Findings	Characteristics
Clinical	Yellow to gray-green membrane on tonsils that (1) bleeds if dislodged with swab (2) crosses anatomic barriers
Laboratory	Smears usually unreliable Culture of nose, throat, or skin that grows on Loeffler's and other media in 16–48 h; then positive toxigenicity test (Elek's diffusion technique) in 16–24 h

TABLE 2. **Treatment of Diphtheria**

1. Preliminary sensitivity testing to horse serum—skin test and eye test
   If either test result is positive, use rapid desensitization before IV antitoxin; if both results are negative, then give
2. IV antitoxin, then start
3. Antibiotics
   If patient is not allergic to penicillin and
   (a) can swallow: penicillin V, 250 mg PO tid × 10 days
   (b) cannot swallow: procaine penicillin G, 600,000 U IM q 12 h × 10 days*
   If patient is allergic to penicillin and
   (a) can swallow: erythromycin, 25–50 mg/kg/day PO qid × 10 days
   (b) cannot swallow: clindamycin, 25–40 mg/kg/day IV q 6 h × 10 days*

Abbreviations: IM = intramuscularly; PO = orally; IV = intravenously.
*Or until able to swallow.

TABLE 3. **Desensitization of Persons Allergic to Horse Serum**

Serial doses given every 15 min provided no reaction occurs

1. SC, 0.05 mL of 1:30 dilution of antitoxin
2. SC, 0.05 mL of 1:10 dilution of antitoxin
3. SC, 0.1 mL of undiluted antitoxin
4. SC, 0.2 mL of undiluted antitoxin
5. IM, 0.5 mL of undiluted antitoxin
6. IV, 0.1 mL of undiluted antitoxin
7. Then a therapeutic dose, given slowly IV, in 200 mL isotonic saline over 30 min

Abbreviations: SC = subcutaneous; IM = intramuscular; IV = intravenous.

this time may have little effect on the incidence or severity of complications. A syringe containing 1 mL of epinephrine chloride (1:1000) solution should always be available when antitoxin is being injected. The dose is 0.01 mL per kg of a 1:1000 aqueous solution, with a maximal dose of 0.5 mL.

Preliminary sensitivity testing (including both a skin test and an eye test) to horse serum should always be done before antitoxin is administered. For the skin test, 0.1 mL of a 1:1000 dilution in isotonic saline of antitoxin should be injected intradermally. A positive skin test result consists of the appearance of a significant wheal and flare at the injection site 15 to 20 minutes after instillation. If either of these test results is positive, the patient is considered to be sensitive to horse serum, and desensitization should be accomplished. Before desensitization, diphenhydramine hydrochloride (Benadryl) should be given as indicated: in children 2 to 5 years of age, 25 mg intramuscularly; in adults, 50 to 100 mg intramuscularly. Serial injections of diluted antitoxin as indicated in Table 3 may be given at intervals of 15 minutes if no reaction occurs. If a reaction occurs after an injection, the physician should wait 1 hour and then repeat the last dose that failed to cause a reaction.

The intravenous route is preferable in all cases. A single dose should suffice; retreatment should never be necessary because of the serious risk of increasing sensitization to horse serum. Diphtheria antitoxin (available from the Centers for Disease Control) is administered on the basis of the following schedule (Table 4): for mild pharyngeal diphtheria or when careful examination indicates that the membrane is small or confined to the anterior nares or tonsils, 40,000 units; for moderate pharyngeal diphtheria, 80,000 units; for severe pharyngeal or laryngeal diphtheria, combined types, or late cases, 120,000 units. Diphtheria antitoxin in 200 mL of isotonic saline is infused during a 30-minute period.

Immediate allergic reactions to antitoxin occur with an overall incidence of about 15%. However, such early reactions bear no relation to subsequent development of serum sickness. In children older than 10 years of age and in adults, the incidence of serum sickness is 20 to 30%. Clinical manifestations occur between the seventh and sixteenth days after antitoxin administration and last 2 to 6 days. The prophylactic use of antagonists of vasoactive amines seems to be worthwhile for the prevention of serum sickness when the agents are orally administered during the period of significant risk after the infusion of horse serum products. Both cyproheptadine and hydroxyzine are effective.

Antibiotics

Antibiotics eliminate the organism from the respiratory tract and skin, terminate the carrier state, stop exotoxin production, and eliminate secondary bacterial infections, particularly those caused by beta-hemolytic streptococci.

Penicillin is the drug of choice. If the patient can swallow, 250 mg of phenoxymethyl penicillin is given by mouth three times a day. Patients unable to swallow may receive intramuscular procaine penicillin G, 600,000 units twice daily for 10 to 14 days. For patients who are allergic to penicillin, erythromycin is given, 25 to 50 mg per

TABLE 4. **Dosage of Diphtheria Antitoxin**

Type of Disease	Dosage (U)
Nasal, tonsillar, mild pharyngeal diphtheria	40,000
Moderate pharyngeal diphtheria	80,000
Severe pharyngeal or laryngeal diphtheria, combined types, late cases	120,000

In 200 mL isotonic saline, infused over 30 min

kg per day, preferably by the oral route, for 10 to 14 days. In vitro sensitivity testing must confirm that the strain is sensitive to erythromycin, because resistant strains are increasing. Clindamycin (Cleocin), 150 mg by mouth every 6 hours for 10 days, has also been used successfully. For patients who are allergic to penicillin and unable to swallow, intravenous erythromycin produces an unacceptable incidence of thrombophlebitis. Instead, clindamycin, 25 to 40 mg per kg per day intravenously, divided into four doses every 6 hours, is efficacious until the patient can take oral medications.

Myocarditis

Patients who develop electrocardiographic changes during the course of diphtheria should have continuous cardiac monitoring for serious arrhythmias and heart block. Monitoring is usually done in special intensive care or cardiac care units. Strict bed rest is enforced. Pharmacologic agents such as lidocaine and procainamide are used to suppress or control specific arrhythmias when indicated. Ventricular tachycardia or fibrillation is treated according to published recommendations by the American Heart Association for Advanced Cardiac Life Support. Transvenous or transthoracic pacing electrodes may need to be inserted for emergency treatment of heart block. Congestive heart failure is usually treated by careful monitoring of fluids and restriction of salt intake. Use of digitalis with congestive heart failure related to diphtheritic myocarditis has been controversial. However, short-acting digitalis preparations are recommended for severe congestive heart failure. Circulatory collapse and shock are managed according to guidelines for treatment of gram-negative sepsis and shock. The value of adrenocorticosteroid therapy is difficult to assess. However, prednisone in the usual doses may be given for approximately 2 weeks to lessen the severity of myocarditis. Bed rest is continued for at least 1 month; activity is gradually increased as tolerated.

Laryngeal and Bronchial Diphtheria

Bronchoscopy may be used to remove dislodged membrane from larger bronchi, where it may cause death by asphyxia. Tracheostomy may be required early for severely ill patients. Secondary bronchopneumonia caused by hospital-acquired gram-negative bacilli should be watched for. Corticosteroids may be of use in acute laryngeal diphtheria. Hydrocortisone sodium succinate (Solu-Cortef), 5 mg per kg per day intramuscularly or intravenously, is given in three divided doses for 1 or 2 days or longer. An equivalent dose of prednisone is then given orally when possible and gradually reduced over 5 to 8 days.

Neurologic Complications

Palatal paralysis, the most common and often the only form of paralysis, usually appears early during the course of diphtheria. Intravenous therapy or nasogastric feeding may be required. Paralysis of respiratory muscles usually appears from 6 to 8 weeks after the onset of pharyngitis. Assisted or controlled mechanical ventilation is indicated until the patient can resume spontaneous respiration with satisfactory alveolar ventilation.

General Management

Bed rest in the hospital for 10 to 14 days is usually required. No special food restrictions or additions are needed. Food that can be swallowed comfortably and a nutritionally adequate diet are sufficient. Parenteral therapy is indicated only for patients who cannot swallow, generally because of dysphagia, palatal paralysis, or airway obstruction. Patients may have considerable pharyngeal discomfort during the first few days of illness, and irrigation of the pharynx with warm isotonic saline solution may be helpful. Occasionally, codeine phosphate, 3 mg per kg per day divided into six doses, may be helpful; it is given either orally or subcutaneously.

Isolation

All patients must be isolated from other people until antibiotic treatment has rendered the respiratory secretions noninfectious. A private room is preferable. Because antibiotic administration is effective in eliminating the carrier state, many patients may be free of organisms early in the course of the disease (1 to 7 days). Isolation can usually be discontinued after 5 days of specific antibiotics. The staff should wear gowns and masks and wash their hands thoroughly after attending patients with diphtheria. Patients should be actively immunized during convalescence.

Contact Prophylaxis

Any patient with a clinical diagnosis of diphtheria should be reported to the local health department. Specimens from household members and close contacts of the patient are cultured. This is followed by observation at home for at least 7 days for clinical diphtheria, administration of antimicrobial prophylaxis, and appropriate immunization with toxoid. A single dose of intramuscular benzathine penicillin G (600,000 units for persons less than 6 years of age and 1.2 million units for persons older than 6 years of age) or a 7- to 10-day course of oral erythromycin

(40 mg per kg per day for children and 1 gram per day for adults) is recommended for prophylaxis. Repeat cultures should be obtained from identified carriers a minimum of 2 weeks after completion of the antimicrobial course to ensure eradication of the organism. Persistent carriers should be retreated with a 10-day course of oral erythromycin.

FOOD-BORNE ILLNESS

method of
GARY L. SIMON, M.D., PH.D.
The George Washington University
Washington, D.C.

A variety of chemicals, microorganisms, and microbial toxins have been implicated as etiologic agents in food-borne illness. The clinical manifestations of such illnesses are predominantly gastrointestinal, although neurologic symptoms are frequently noted in patients who have ingested toxins.

The onset of disease is usually heralded by nausea, vomiting, abdominal cramps, and diarrhea. Fever and other systemic symptoms are variable accompaniments, depending on the causative agent. Paresthesias, weakness, and even paralysis may be present in patients who have ingested neurologic toxins.

Identification of the specific microbial agent is important from both a therapeutic and a public health standpoint. A number of criteria can be used to help establish the etiologic diagnosis: (1) An epidemiologic and dietary history, including the type and preparation of the suspected food, recent travel, season of the year, and the presence of similar symptoms in companions or family members, should be obtained. It may be necessary to contact the local health department in some cases. (2) The clinical features of the illness, including incubation period, type and severity of gastrointestinal symptoms, and the presence of extraintestinal manifestations, should be defined. (3) Appropriate specimens of blood, feces, and gastric aspirate and samples of the food should be sent for laboratory confirmation of the diagnosis.

TREATMENT

The mainstay of therapy for patients with food-borne illness is supportive care. This includes adequate hydration, monitoring of vital signs and other parameters, removal of unabsorbed toxin when appropriate, and symptomatic therapy.

The state of hydration should be determined by assessment of skin turgor and mucous membranes and by measuring heart rate and blood pressure in several positions in order to demonstrate orthostatic changes. The volume of stool output as reported by the patient is rarely accurate, whereas reports of decreased urine output can be very helpful. Prompt repletion of fluid and electrolytes is indicated in dehydrated patients to restore intravascular volume. In many, this may be adequate therapy without specific antimicrobial treatment. Pulse, blood pressure, urine output, and respiratory status should be monitored to ensure the adequacy of fluid replacement and to avoid overhydration.

Rehydration may be accomplished either orally or parenterally, depending on the severity of illness, available facilities, and the patient's ability to tolerate an oral preparation. A standard oral preparation containing 3.5 grams of NaCl, 1.5 grams of KCl, 2.5 grams of $NaHCO_3$, and 20 grams of glucose in 1 liter of boiled water may be used. Sucrose (table sugar) can be substituted for glucose, and a home-made oral replacement solution can be prepared by mixing 4 level tablespoons of sugar, ¾ tablespoon of salt, 1 teaspoon of sodium bicarbonate, and 1 cup of orange juice in 1 liter of water. Infants who are not severely ill can be treated with Pedialyte, a commercially available oral rehydration solution.

Hospitalization is necessary for individuals who are severely dehydrated and for many infants, young children, and elderly patients, who can rapidly become dehydrated. These patients often require rehydration with intravenous solutions. Children with severe hypernatremia must be closely monitored because a rapid decrease in serum sodium can lead to cerebral edema.

In some patients with toxigenic food poisoning, unabsorbed toxin may be present in the gastrointestinal tract. Syrup of ipecac, 15 to 30 mL orally, is an effective emetic. Emetics should be avoided in any patient who is neurologically impaired to prevent aspiration of gastric contents. Gastric lavage and activated charcoal may be administered to aid in removal of toxin. Cathartics such as magnesium citrate and sodium sulfate are effective at speeding transit through the gut.

Persistent nausea and vomiting can be controlled with antiemetics. Prochlorperazine (Compazine), 5 to 10 mL orally, 25 mg by rectal suppository, or 10 mg intramuscularly, may be given to adults. Trimethobenzamide hydrochloride (Tigan), 250 mg orally or 200 mg rectally, can be used as an alternative agent in children. These drugs should be avoided in children less than 2 years of age.

The use of antidiarrheal agents is controversial. In many patients with food-borne illness, diarrhea is relatively brief and may actually aid in removing toxin. Antidiarrheal agents such as loperamide hydrochloride (Imodium), 4 mg followed by 2 mg after each stool to a maximal daily dose of 16 mg; diphenoxylate hydrochloride with atropine (Lomotil), 5 mg every 6 hours; or Paregoric, 4 mL every 2 hours, can be used in selected patients with moderate or severe persistent diarrhea. However, these agents reduce peristalsis and are contraindicated in patients with fever, fecal leukocytes, or other features that suggest the presence of an invasive pathogen such as *Campylobacter, Salmonella, Shigella,* or *Entamoeba histolytica.* Bismuth subsalicylate (Pepto-Bismol) has been used in patients with traveler's diarrhea. The dose is 2 tablespoons or 2 tablets every 30 to 60 minutes for eight doses. This drug should not be used by patients with aspirin sensitivity, renal failure, or gout or by individuals receiving warfarin (Coumadin) or oral hypoglycemic agents.

Diarrhea Caused by Microbial Agents or Their Toxins

Enterotoxigenic strains of *Staphylococcus aureus* and *Bacillus cereus* are associated with the acute onset of nausea, vomiting, and diarrhea, usually within 1 to 6 hours of ingestion of the preformed toxin. Nearly three-fourths of the patients with staphylococcal disease experience vomiting, and a similar percentage develop diarrhea. Fever and other systemic symptoms are not common. Staphylococcal infection is often caused by contamination of food by an infected or colonized food handler, followed by improper storage at room temperature, which allows the bacteria to multiply and produce toxin. Ham, poultry, egg salad, and cream-filled pastries are frequently implicated.

Illness attributable to *Bacillus cereus* is usually associated with eating reheated fried rice. With this organism, food poisoning may present with either of two syndromes. A short-acting emetic form of the illness caused by ingestion of preformed toxin is characterized primarily by nausea and vomiting with onset within 1 to 6 hours. Some patients may also have diarrhea. In a second long–incubation period form of the illness, diarrhea is the prominent clinical feature, and the illness usually occurs 8 to 16 hours after ingestion. In the long-acting syndrome, illness occurs as a result of toxin formation in vivo.

Another enterotoxin-mediated illness follows ingestion of food contaminated by *Clostridium perfringens.* This syndrome is characterized by onset of symptoms 8 to 16 hours after ingestion. This longer incubation time is due to production of toxin in vivo. The predominant symptoms are abdominal cramps and diarrhea; fever and vomiting are infrequent.

These illnesses are self-limited and usually resolve within 24 hours. Therapy is aimed at maintaining adequate intravascular volume with fluid replacement and providing symptomatic relief with antiemetic or antiperistaltic agents if necessary. Antibiotics have no role in the treatment of these intoxications.

Vibrio cholerae is the prototypic diarrheal illness. Cholera may occur in individuals who have recently traveled to an endemic area. The organism has been isolated from the bayous of Louisiana, and infection can be transmitted via contaminated shellfish. Massive fluid loss results from the effects of the cholera enterotoxin, and rehydration is of paramount importance in the treatment of this illness. Intravenous therapy is usually required with either lactated Ringer's or Dhaka solution (0.5% NaCl, 0.4% NaHCO$_3$, 0.1% KCl). Oral replacement therapy can be used in patients with mild disease (when the volume of stool is less than 100 mL per kg per 24 hours). Antibiotics are of benefit in ameliorating symptoms, reducing stool volume, and shortening the duration of excretion of the organism. Tetracycline, 250 mg every 6 hours or 2 grams once daily for 2 days, is the drug of choice for adults; children should receive ampicillin, 50 mg per kg per day in divided doses. Trimethoprim-sulfamethoxazole and quinolones are alternative agents. (Cholera is discussed in greater detail on page 70.)

Another vibrio species, *Vibrio parahaemolyticus,* has enterotoxic as well as invasive properties. This organism is halophilic and is frequently found in coastal waters. Infection occurs when contaminated seafood, especially crab or shrimp, is eaten raw or is inadequately cooked and then stored at room temperature for several hours before being eaten. Clinical illness usually occurs within 48 hours of ingestion of contaminated seafood and is characterized by abdominal cramps and watery, explosive diarrhea. The disease is self-limited, and no treatment other than supportive measures is necessary. Antimicrobial agents have little impact on the severity or duration of symptoms.

Disease caused by organisms that produce their effects by tissue invasion, such as *Campylobacter jejuni, Salmonella,* and *Shigella,* is characterized by fever, abdominal cramps, and diarrhea. Vomiting may occur, but less frequently than with staphylococcal or bacillus intoxications. In general, these invasive forms of enteric disease tend to have a longer incubation period, usually more than 16 hours and occasionally several days. The diagnosis is made by isolation of the pathogen from stool cultures. In most patients, symptoms resolve within 1 week. Antibiotics (specific agents are covered elsewhere) should be included in the treatment regimen for patients with shigellosis and campylobacteriosis. Uncomplicated salmonella gastroenteritis does not require antibiotic therapy.

Escherichia coli has been implicated in a variety of diarrheal syndromes, and it is the most commonly identified agent in traveler's diarrhea (see next section). Most strains of *E. coli* isolated from travelers produce an enterotoxin, although disease has also been reported with enteroadherent isolates that do not produce enterotoxin but, rather, adhere closely to the enterocyte surface and cause destruction of the microvilli.

Disease caused by enterohemorrhagic *E. coli* has been recognized since 1982, when hemorrhagic colitis associated with eating undercooked hamburgers from a fast food restaurant was reported. This outbreak resulted from contamination of the meat with verotoxin containing *E. coli* serotype 0157:H7. Numerous additional cases have been reported, including an outbreak associated with an unchlorinated water supply in a small urban area. An association with hemolytic-uremic syndrome has been described.

Finally, enteroinvasive *E. coli* strains penetrate intestinal cells and produce a clinical illness similar to that seen with *Shigella* infection. Outbreaks related to food contaminated with this organism have also been described.

In general, all of these *E. coli*–related syndromes should be treated with antibiotics. Trimethoprim-sulfamethoxazole, ampicillin, tetracycline, or one of the quinolones can be used.

Traveler's Diarrhea

A major health problem of international travel is the development of diarrhea. Up to 60% of travelers to developing countries develop acute, watery diarrhea in their first month of travel. Enterotoxigenic *E. coli* (ETEC) is the most frequently identified etiologic agent, but other bacterial pathogens may also be encountered, as well as viruses such as rotavirus and parasites such as *Entamoeba histolytica* and *Giardia lamblia*. The incubation period for traveler's diarrhea due to ETEC is usually less than 48 hours. If left untreated, infection may last 5 to 7 days.

Careful attention to diet is the best way to prevent traveler's diarrhea. Boiled or bottled water and especially carbonated beverages are safer than untreated tap water. Raw fruits and vegetables, inadequately cooked or cold meats, and dairy products should be avoided.

Most cases are self-limited, and dehydration is usually not a significant problem. Oral rehydra-tion is sufficient for most adults, but treatment with antibiotics may shorten the duration of illness. Doxycycline, 100 mg twice daily, trimethoprim-sulfamethoxazole, one double-strength tablet twice daily, or a quinolone such as ciprofloxacin, 500 mg twice daily, is a useful agent for travelers with this syndrome.

Many clinicians advocate the use of prophylactic agents. Bismuth subsalicylate (Pepto-Bismol) is effective, but the dose is rather large, 60 ml four times a day. Chewable tablets may be better tolerated. Doxycycline has also been shown to be an effective prophylactic agent, but many strains are resistant and the side effect of sun sensitivity makes this a poor choice for many vacationers. Other possible agents include trimethoprim-sulfamethoxazole and quinolones such as ciprofloxacin (Cipro), or ofloxacin (Floxin). Although these drugs are effective, prophylactic use may hasten the development of resistance. A better approach is to provide travelers with these agents so that they can begin treatment as soon as symptoms develop.

Botulism

Nausea and vomiting followed by symptoms of neurologic dysfunction (weakness, dry mouth, diplopia, and dysphagia) may indicate infection with *Clostridium botulinum*. Diarrhea is an early symptom, although constipation is more common once the clinical syndrome is established. In some patients, the illness may progress very rapidly, with respiratory compromise that requires ventilatory support. Clinical suspicion of botulism mandates hospitalization and intensive monitoring; the fatality rate is 25%. The duration of illness is weeks to months.

Botulism occurs most commonly as a result of eating contaminated home-processed fruits, vegetables, or meat. The incubation period is quite variable and ranges from 6 hours to 8 days, depending on the quantity of toxin ingested.

Infant botulism is caused by ingestion of *C. botulinum* spores with production of toxin in vivo. Some pediatricians suggest that infants not be given honey because it may contain *C. botulinum*.

The mainstay of therapy is respiratory support. Removal of excess toxin by cathartics and emetics may be useful. A trivalent A,B,E antiserum is available from the Centers for Disease Control. If botulism is suspected, the Centers can be contacted at any time (1–404–329–3753 days and 1–404–329–3644 nights) for advice about this rare disorder. Penicillin has been advocated for food-borne botulism, but there are few data to support its use. In another experimental therapy, guanidine hydrochloride has been used to enhance the release of acetylcholine from terminal nerve fibers.

Fish and Shellfish Poisoning

Ciguatera Fish Poisoning

Ingestion of contaminated fish or shellfish can cause illnesses that have both gastrointestinal and neurologic manifestations. Ciguatera fish poisoning is the result of consuming marine fish that have been contaminated through the food chain with ciguatoxin, a product of the dinoflagellate *Gambierdiscus toxicus*. More than 400 species of fish found between latitudes 35°N and 35°S have been noted to contain ciguatoxin. Most cases in the United States occur in Hawaii and Florida, but travelers to the Caribbean are also at risk. The fish species most frequently associated with ciguatera fish poisoning are grouper, red snapper, and barracuda; the last has been a problem among North Carolina surf fisherman who catch and consume this fish. Ciguatoxin is not affected by heating or cooling, may persist for weeks, and is difficult to detect because it does not alter the taste, color, or odor of the contaminated fish.

The incubation period is 1 to 6 hours, after which the initial symptoms are gastrointestinal and include nausea, vomiting, abdominal cramps, and diarrhea. These symptoms are followed by pruritus; paresthesias of the extremities, mouth, tongue, and throat; shooting pains in the legs; and a sensation of looseness and pain in the teeth. Dry mouth, headache, myalgias, blurred vision, and photophobia have been reported. In severe cases there may be transient blindness, other cranial nerve palsies, reversal of hot and cold temperature sensation, bradycardia, hypotension, and respiratory paralysis requiring ventilatory support. Presumed sexual transmission of the toxin has been reported.

The duration of illness is quite variable. Some patients have complete resolution within a few days, whereas symptoms may persist for more than 6 months in a substantial number of infected individuals. It appears that longer incubation periods are associated with prolonged duration of symptoms.

A variety of therapeutic agents have been used with little proven benefit. In severe cases, pralidoxime chloride (Protopam), 1 to 2 grams in 100 mL of saline, is given intravenously over 15 to 30 minutes to patients with life-threatening weakness and low blood cholinesterase concentrations. Cathartics and enemas may help to remove unabsorbed toxin. Chronic symptoms have been treated with amitriptyline, tocainide, and a variety of other drugs, but further experience is needed in order to define potential benefit.

Scombroid Poisoning

Marine bacteria that catalyze the decarboxylation of histidine, producing scombrotoxin, or "saurine," may infect the flesh of tuna, mackerel, bonito, skipjack, and mahimahi. Eating fish contaminated with scombrotoxin results in a histamine-like reaction. Within 30 minutes of ingestion, there is headache, flushing, nausea, vomiting, pruritus, urticaria, and, in severe cases, bronchospasm. Symptoms generally resolve within 4 hours, but in the interim antihistamines and bronchodilators may provide symptomatic relief.

Puffer Fish Poisoning

Tetrodotoxin is a neurotoxin found in the tissues of the puffer fish. Ingestion of improperly cleaned fish may result in paralysis of nerve transmission with subsequent respiratory failure, necessitating mechanical ventilation.

Paralytic Shellfish Poisoning

Paralytic shellfish poisoning is caused by ingestion of clams, oysters, mollusks, or scallops that have ingested dinoflagellates, most commonly *Gonyaulax catenella* and *G. tamarensis*. These dinoflagellates produce neurotoxins, notably saxitoxin, that cause a clinical syndrome characterized by paresthesias of the face and extremities, nausea, vomiting, and diarrhea. Dysphonia, dysphagia, paralysis, and respiratory compromise may occur in severe cases. The incubation period varies inversely with the amount of toxin ingested and can range from 1 to 10 hours. Treatment is primarily supportive. Cathartics and enemas should be used to reduce the concentration of the toxin in the gastrointestinal tract provided that no ileus is present. The duration of symptoms is a few hours to a few days.

Paralytic shellfish poisoning is often associated with "red tides," which may signal high concentrations of dinoflagellates. However, not all such tides are contaminated, and paralytic shellfish poisoning has been seen in the absence of red tides. The toxin is heat-stable and not affected by cooking.

Neurotoxic Shellfish Poisoning

Neurotoxic shellfish poisoning is caused by a toxin produced by another dinoflagellate, *Gymnodinium breve*. Shellfish contaminated by this organism are usually harvested from the Atlantic Ocean or the Gulf of Mexico during the spring and fall. Symptoms usually appear within 3 hours of ingestion and are similar to those of paralytic shellfish poisoning except that paralysis does not occur. The illness is self-limited and requires only symptomatic therapy.

Fungal Poisoning

Mushroom Poisoning

There are seven established groups of toxic mushrooms, each elaborating different toxins and producing different clinical syndromes. Many different genera of mushrooms can cause a gastrointestinal syndrome with nausea, vomiting, abdominal cramping, and diarrhea. This syndrome is self-limited, and only supportive therapy is necessary.

Mushrooms of the *Clitocybe* and *Inocybe* groups elaborate muscarinic compounds that produce an anticholinergic syndrome of sweating, salivation, lacrimation, bradycardia, abdominal cramping, vomiting, retching, and other signs of parasympathetic dysfunction 30 minutes to 2 hours after ingestion. Symptoms usually resolve within 24 hours. Severe cases may be lethal and should be treated with atropine sulfate, 1 to 2 mg every 2 to 6 hours, titrated to symptoms.

Amanita species contain ibotenic acid and isoxazole derivatives, which cause a syndrome resembling acute alcoholic intoxication with confusion, restlessness, and visual disturbances. In more severe cases, ataxia, dizziness, stupor, and convulsions may be seen. Specific therapy is usually not necessary except for the most severely affected patients; they may be treated with physostigmine. Barbiturates and benzodiazepines should be avoided because they may exacerbate the symptoms.

Mood elevation, hallucinations, hyperkinetic activity, and muscle weakness are seen in patients who have ingested *Psilocybe* or *Panaleus* mushrooms containing psilocybin, psilocin, and related indoles. Onset is rapid, usually occurring within 30 minutes of ingestion. Treatment is symptomatic; benzodiazepines such as diazepam (Valium) can be administered to relieve agitation.

Another short-incubation syndrome is caused by *Coprinus* species, which produce coprine. This mycotoxin causes a disulfiram-like reaction after alcohol ingestion. Patients develop headache, nausea, vomiting, and flushing up to 5 days after eating the mushrooms. Therapy is simply to avoid alcohol.

Amanita phalloides as well as several other species of mushrooms produce amatoxins and phallotoxins, which are associated with most cases of fatal mushroom poisoning. These toxins cause a biphasic illness: abdominal pain, vomiting, and diarrhea begin 6 to 12 hours after ingestion and usually resolve within 24 hours, after which the patient appears well. However, several days later, renal and hepatic failure ensue. Intensive support is necessary, including careful monitoring of fluid and electrolytes, opiates for pain relief, and glucose for hypoglycemia. Hemoperfusion may be helpful in removing circulating toxin. The mortality rate is 30 to 50%.

Mushrooms of the genus *Gyromitra* contain gyromitrin, which is converted in vivo to methylhydrazine, a competitive inhibitor of pyridoxal phosphate. Initial symptoms of nausea and vomiting are followed by hemolysis with methemoglobinemia and hepatic failure. Pyridoxine hydrochloride, 25 mg per kg, may be administered intravenously for treatment of neurologic symptoms such as convulsions or coma.

Other Fungal Poisoning

Claviceps purpurea, a fungus that contaminates wheat and rye, produces ergot, a smooth-muscle vasoconstrictor that acts by stimulating alpha-adrenergic receptors. Symptoms of ergotism include headache, severe muscle and abdominal pain, paresthesias, and convulsions. Ischemic necrosis and gangrene can occur. Treatment of severe cases includes anticoagulation to prevent vascular thrombosis and vasodilatation with intravenous sodium nitroprusside, 50 µg or more per minute, titrated against the blood pressure.

Another fungal toxin is aflatoxin, which has been found in commercial peanut butter in the United States; it can also contaminate corn and other grains in warmer climates. Ingestion of aflatoxin has been associated with gastrointestinal bleeding, hepatocellular injury, and hepatoma.

Tricothecenes are heat-stable mycotoxins that occasionally contaminate grains in colder climates. Ingestion of these toxins in contaminated flour may result in nausea, vomiting, bloody diarrhea, and anemia. Treatment is supportive.

Plant Poisoning

The Italian broad (fava) bean has been associated with acute hemolytic crisis in individuals with glucose-6-phosphate dehydrogenase deficiency. Massive hemolysis necessitating transfusions can occur, especially in patients of Mediterranean descent. Rare fatalities have been reported.

Lathyrism is a slowly progressive spastic paraplegia that can follow chronic ingestion of *Lathyrus sativus* (sweet peas). These peas are often eaten during times of famine in Africa and Asia. Early symptoms of lathyrism include muscle spasm, cramps, and leg weakness, which are followed by signs of degeneration of the posterolateral tracts of the thoracolumbar spinal cord with paralysis and incontinence. Subcutaneous neostigmine methylsulfate (Prostigmine), 0.5 mg daily, may be beneficial, especially in patients whose symptoms are of short duration.

Ingestion of leaves from rhubarb, beets, spinach, or the houseplants philodendron and dieffenbachia can result in oxalic acid poisoning. Calcium oxalate formation can lead to hypocalcemic tetany. Treatment includes intravenous fluids and diuretics to prevent renal tubular cell damage and calcium gluconate, 10 mL of a 10% solution, if tetany develops. Oral calcium is given in order to reduce oxalate concentration by precipitation of calcium oxalate in the gastrointestinal tract.

Tubers, vines, leaves, and new sprouts of potatoes, the leaves and fruit of the Jerusalem cherry, and the leaves and stems of tomato plants contain solanine. This toxin is also present in jimson weed and may be ingested by humans who drink milk from cattle that eat jimson weed. Intoxication is characterized by headache, abdominal pain, diarrhea, and confusion. The toxin is heat-labile and destroyed by bottling. Treatment is supportive.

Foxglove and oleander, sometimes used to prepare home-brewed teas, can cause digitalis intoxication. Such patients should be admitted to the hospital and require electrocardiographic monitoring. Potassium supplementation, antiarrhythmics, and temporary pacemaker insertion may be necessary. Digoxin-immune Fab (Digibind) is a preparation of antidigoxin antibody used to treat life-threatening digoxin overdose. The specificity of this preparation for the products that may result from ingestion of these home-brewed teas is unknown. Nevertheless, there is little toxicity associated with Digoxin-immune Fab, and it may be administered to patients with severe intoxication. Advice should be sought from the manufacturer (Burroughs-Wellcome) before the drug is administered in this situation.

Cyanide poisoning is a very rare complication of ingesting large numbers of seeds from fruits and vegetables that contain cyanoglycosides or free hydrocyanic acid; these foods include apples, cherries, pears, peaches, plums, apricots, and cassava and lima beans. Symptoms occur within 5 minutes of ingestion and include headache, faintness, anxiety, dyspnea, tachycardia, and a burning sensation in the throat. Cyanosis, bradycardia, hypotension, opisthotonos, convulsions, coma, and death can occur in severe cases. Removal of cyanide from intracellular sites is accomplished by binding of the anion to ferric ions. Amyl nitrite converts hemoglobin to methemoglobin, which contains the ferric ion. The patient inhales amyl nitrite for 30 seconds every minute, and a new capsule is used every 3 minutes. Alternatively, intravenous sodium nitrite* may be cautiously given in order to achieve a methemoglobin concentration of 26%. Excessive concentrations of methemoglobin result in chocolate-brown cyanosis, acidosis, coma, convulsions, and death. Sodium thiosulfate can be given to promote excretion of cyanide ions.

---

*Not available in the United States.

Miscellaneous Intoxications

Ingestion of metals such as copper, zinc, tin, and cadmium may be followed by the acute onset of nausea, vomiting, and abdominal pain within 5 to 15 minutes. This syndrome most commonly occurs when acidic citric juices come into prolonged contact with these metals. Symptoms are self limited and resolve with removal of the metal from the gastrointestinal tract.

Monosodium L-glutamate (MSG) is the presumed etiologic agent of the "Chinese restaurant syndrome." Symptoms include headache, flushing, diaphoresis, and a burning sensation of the skin within 10 to 15 minutes of ingestion. There is no specific therapy, and symptoms resolve within several hours.

NECROTIZING SKIN AND SOFT TISSUE INFECTIONS

method of
JOSÉ F. PATIÑO, M.D.
Fundación Santa Fe de Bogotá
Bogotá, Colombia

The necrotizing lesions of the skin and soft tissues are very severe, progressive, often lethal, usually mixed synergistic gangrenous infections not infrequently seen in daily clinical practice. The favored encompassing label for these lesions is "necrotizing fasciitis," a term that some authors consider inadequate, as the majority of such cases do not affect the deep muscular fasciae; actually it refers to the subcutaneous fasciae: that is, the superficial fatty layer known as fascia of Camper and the deeper fibrous layer known as fascia of Scarpa, the anatomic structures that become gangrenous as a result of the necrotizing infections. Well over 1000 cases are reported annually in the United States and are associated with severe disability and high mortality rates.

The necrotizing infection may be caused by a single organism, classically a group A beta-hemolytic streptococcus (*Streptococcus pyogenes*) causing only *cellulitis* (superficial infection confined to the skin). However, more frequently the infection is caused by a mixed and rich variety of organisms, aerobic and anaerobic, in synergistic-type associations that inflict massive tissue damage, causing *necrotizing fasciitis* (destruction of the subcutaneous tissues) or *myonecrosis* (destruction of muscle mass) and inducing profound systemic toxicity. Mycotic infections of the zymomycetic type, known as mucormycosis, can also produce fulminating and highly lethal gangrene of the skin and soft tissues.

The necrotizing infections tend to occur in compromised elderly and debilitated hosts, but younger persons who sustain wounds or are subjected to surgical procedures on the gastrointestinal tract, women in the postpartum state, and intravenous drug abusers are at increased risk. The lesions may also occur in previously healthy persons after minor trauma and lacerations, after clean operations, and after blunt nonpenetrating trauma. Moreover, they can also develop spontaneously, usually in obese, alcoholic, and diabetic individuals.

ETIOLOGY

Sixty years ago, Meleney described the "acute hemolytic streptococcal gangrene" and the gangrene caused by the synergistic association of hemolytic streptococcus and staphylococcus, and many authors still refer to the necrotizing infections as "Meleney's gangrene."

Although necrotizing cellulitis, affecting the skin only, is generally the result of infection by a single organism—ordinarily, but not exclusively, a staphylococcus or a streptococcus—it is now well known that most necrotizing lesions are the result of polymicrobial infections by a variety of microorganisms, including both anaerobic gram-positive cocci and gram-negative bacilli. Streptococci and staphylococci are frequently identified, and gram-negative bacteria (Enterobacteriaceae) and *Bacteroides* predominate; marine vibrios have also been recognized as causative agents.

Patients can be categorized according to bacteriology into two distinct groups, although their respective lesions are indistinguishable on clinical or microscopic appearance: in *Type I,* the infection is by anaerobic and facultative anaerobic bacteria, such as Enterobacteriaceae and streptococci (other than group A) in combination, and no anaerobic bacteria are isolated alone; in *Type II,* the infection is by group A streptococci, which can be isolated alone or in combination with *Staphylococcus aureus* or *S. epidermidis.*

Zygomycetes can cause gangrenous cellulitis and fasciitis, and the mucormycotic infection must be considered in the differential diagnosis of the progressive necrotizing lesions of the soft tissues inasmuch as mucormycosis (synonyms: phycomycosis, zygomycosis) is recognized today as a major cause of massive and extremely aggressive gangrenous lesions.

DIAGNOSIS, PATHOLOGY, AND CLINICAL COURSE

Undermining and dissection of the subcutaneous tissue (fascial planes of Camper and Scarpa) as a result of destruction and liquefaction of the fat, with initial preservation of the skin and sparing of the muscular fasciae and masses, is the pathognomonic pathology; gas is generally present in the tissues, produced mainly by the anaerobes *(Peptococcus, Bacteroides)* but also by aerobic gram-negative bacilli (*E. coli, Klebsiella,* enterobacter, pseudomonas) and, in cases of true gas gangrene, by clostridia. Gas per se, therefore, is not a diagnostic sign of clostridial gangrene.

The rapid performance of frozen-section biopsy establishes the diagnosis on the basis of the typical histologic changes: subcutaneous necrosis, polymorphonuclear (PMN) infiltration, fibrinous vascular thrombosis and necrosis, microorganisms within the destroyed fascia and dermis, and sparing of muscle. Early tissue biopsy also permits the identification of zygomycetes in the tissues, with characteristic invasion and occlusion of vessels, for prompt institution of antifungal therapy.

The clinical course of the necrotizing infections is characterized by moderate pain, moderate fever, and marked edema of the skin, which is initially spared from necrosis—a feature that often causes errors and delays in the diagnosis. The destruction of the fat under the edematous skin, which typically exhibits minimal pain or tenderness, permits the easy and painless diagnostic introduction of an instrument into the dissected subcutaneous space. Progression of the occlusive vascular process brings about delayed (meaning not immediate) frank cutaneous gangrene. There is marked systemic toxicity, and if prompt and radical treatment is not established, the condition advances rapidly into severe systemic sepsis and fatal multiple organ failure.

Overall mortality rates range from 9% to over 60%. In the author's experience with the numerous victims of the 1985 Colombian volcanic disaster, the global mortality rate was 47.4%, but it was 75% for the patients who developed mucormycosis.

CLASSIFICATION

Classification of the necrotizing lesions is necessary in order to institute rational treatment. Although many complex and often confusing classification schemes have appeared in the literature, investigators have recently tended to group these syndromes into a unified category of progressive necrotizing infections, recognizing that although the etiology is varied, there is much overlap in symptoms, presentation, and clinical course. The classification into three major categories that appears in Table 1 has shown to be of prac-

TABLE 1. **Classification of the Necrotizing Lesions of the Skin and Soft Tissues**

Necrotizing Cellulitis
A monomicrobial infection in which only the skin is affected, usually by a group A beta-hemolytic streptococcus, but also by staphylococci, aerobic coliforms, clostridia, *Haemophilus influenzae,* and other organisms. The subcutaneous tissue is spared, and débridement does not have to be carried out beyond the limits of the affected necrotic skin.

Necrotizing Fasciitis
The most frequent and typical mixed aerobic-anaerobic gas-producing bacterial infection and/or zygomycetic (mucormycotic) infection that affects primarily and extensively the subcutaneous tissues, associated with marked systemic toxicity. Extensive radical débridement is mandatory.

Myonecrosis
The entity known as gas gangrene, or clostridial myonecrosis, caused primarily by *C. perfringens,* is characterized by profound systemic toxicity, necrosis of the muscle with the presence of gram-positive rods but absence of polymorphonuclear cells in the wound discharge, and gas formation as a rather late manifestation. A fierce, rapidly progressing, and highly lethal entity that extensively destroys the deep muscle, clostridial myonecrosis mandates radical muscle resection and/or amputation.

tical use: (1) necrotizing cellulitis; (2) necrotizing fasciitis; and (3) clostridial myonecrosis (gas gangrene).

In many instances of necrotizing cellulitis, and also of fasciitis, clostridial organisms can be isolated from the wound. Clostridia can be found in three main clinical settings: (1) clostridial contamination; (2) clostridial cellulitis (no systemic toxicity); and (3) clostridial myonecrosis or gas gangrene (extreme systemic toxicity).

Gas gangrene (clostridial myonecrosis) is the most feared of the soft tissue infections; however, necrotizing fasciitis of the polybacterial aerobic-anaerobic and/or mycotic variety, also a gas-forming lesion, is more common and potentially just as lethal.

A form of myositis, the anaerobic streptococcal myositis, produced by anaerobic streptococci, S. pyogenes, and other group B streptococci, is characterized by less toxicity than gas gangrene, no myonecrosis (muscle appears inflamed but is viable and capable of contracting), abundant gas and crepitation, blebs, and many PMNs in the discharge from the wound. The treatment implies removal of surrounding necrotic tissues, but not of the inflamed muscle.

TREATMENT

There is a clear, direct relationship between promptness in diagnosis, initiation of surgical therapy, and survival; the mortality rate is almost doubled among patients for whom more than 24 hours occurs before operation. The physician must keep a high index of suspicion, viewing any area of spreading cellulitis with extreme caution under close monitoring, performing immediate needle aspiration for bacterial examination and culture, and performing biopsies of the affected tissues and the advancing edge. The cornerstone for the successful management of necrotizing infections is *early diagnosis and emergency radical resection* of all necrotic tissue, until healthy and unaffected tissue is reached, accompanied by *wide-spectrum antibiotic coverage* and full hemodynamic and physiologic monitoring for vigorous *organ and metabolic support.*

At the outset, under the preliminary guidance of gram-stained smears while aerobic and anaerobic tissue and blood cultures—and possible biopsies—are under way, a triple regimen of antibiotic coverage is favored to cover the diverse and varied causative flora:

Penicillin for clostridia, the enterococci, and peptostreptococci.

Clindamycin (or metronidazole or chloramphenicol) for the anaerobes, B. fragilis, and peptostreptococci.

Gentamicin (or another aminoglycoside) for the enterobacteriacea and the variety of gram-negative organisms.

In the author's experience, metronidazole and chloramphenicol are adequate substitutes for clindamycin for the control of the anaerobes. Imipenem, by virtue of its very high beta-lactamase resistance and ample wide-spectrum efficacy, may be the agent of choice if only one antibiotic is to be used.

The antibiotic coverage is subsequently tailored according to the results of the meticulous microbiology monitoring that is mandatory in these patients.

Patients with mucormycosis and progressive necrotizing lesions are at high risk of death. Once invasive mucormycosis has been demonstrated, treatment with amphotericin B, currently the agent of choice, must be promptly started. However, not all cases of mucormycosis respond to amphotericin B. The newer antimycotic preparations should demonstrate more reliable protection. Fluconazole (Diflucan) has been utilized in cases of pulmonary mucormycosis.

Antitoxin has no place in the treatment of gas gangrene.

Tetanus prophylaxis with adsorbed tetanus toxoid and passive immune coverage with tetanus hyperimmune globulin are indicated in the management of all high-risk wounds because tetanus is a frequent complication of severe lesions of this nature.

Aggressive débridement is undertaken as soon as initial resuscitation has ensured hemodynamic stability. The management of these entities constitutes a major surgical emergency. Minor drainages and débridements are attended by prohibitive mortality rates, and the experienced surgeon must undertake a radical resection of all affected tissues, regardless of tissue loss and aesthetic considerations, for this is a matter of life and death!

Amputation is rarely needed in cases of necrotizing fasciitis (unless the viability of limb has been impaired by an encircling fasciitis), but it is often necessary in cases of clostridial gas gangrene of the extremities.

A mandatory second look is performed within 24 hours after initial radical resection of the affected tissues and overlying skin. Its purpose is for the careful exploration of the wound and the identification of residual foci and any advancing edge of the necrotizing infection. Similar radical resection is correspondingly performed, with the pertinent cultures and biopsies. A daily regimen of exploration and dressings under general anesthesia in the operating room is instituted, until the patient's condition allows the dressings to be performed in the intensive care unit or the ward without anesthesia. The wound is best covered with saline-soaked dressings; the author does not advocate the use of topical antibiotic or antiseptic agents or of biologic dressings. In patients with loss of the abdominal wall, he prefers the use of a plastic sheath (an open parenteral fluid bag is quite adequate) rather than a mesh, which can become adherent to the bowel wall and may cause enterocutaneous fistula.

Hyperbaric oxygen has not demonstrated consistent value in the treatment of the necrotizing lesions; its true value remains controversial, even in the case of gas gangrene, and the decision to use it, which ordinarily implies transferring the patient to a distant facility, may result in undesirable and potentially fatal delays in the initiation of adequate surgical management.

INFLUENZA

method of
FREDERICK L. RUBEN, M.D.
Montefiore University Hospital
Pittsburgh, Pennsylvania

Influenza is a seasonal viral respiratory illness with outbreaks occurring virtually every winter. The changing surface antigens (the hemagglutinin and neuraminidase designated H and N) and the decline of antibodies, both naturally acquired and vaccine induced, ensure that most individuals are susceptible to infection each year. In most recent years, two different types of influenza A, H1N1 and H3N2, as well as influenza B have been present in outbreaks. Influenza A strains usually predominate in adults, whereas the influenza B strains tend to infect children and, on occasion, the elderly.

The severe impact of influenza on the population has gone unchecked as a result of the poor efforts toward prevention with vaccines and the underuse of amantadine hydrochloride (Symmetrel), an effective agent against influenza A.

PREVENTION

The cornerstone of prevention of influenza is the annual use of influenza vaccines. These killed vaccines are updated each year to contain the virus strains anticipated that year. Current vaccines have three different strains. Both whole-virus and split-virus killed vaccines induce protective antibodies against the H and N antigens. Vaccines generally afford about 70% protection against clinical illness and even greater protection against death from influenza. The outbreak of Guillain-Barré syndrome that accompanied mass immunization with swine influenza vaccines in 1976 has not recurred with subsequent influenza vaccines. Sore arm, redness at the in-

jection site, and low-grade fever are the most frequent side effects. A history of anaphylactic hypersensitivity to eggs or egg products is a contraindication to receiving influenza vaccines.

The updated vaccine should be given each fall. If this is not accomplished, vaccine can be effectively given up to the time of and even during an outbreak of influenza, if the patient is given a concomitant 14-day course of amantadine to provide protection while antibodies rise to protective levels.

Patients who cannot take vaccine can be protected by using amantadine prophylactically during the local outbreak. The drug should be started as soon as possible after the outbreak is recognized and continued until it ends, usually in about 6 weeks. The dosage should be based on renal function as indicated further on.

Priorities have been set for targeting influenza vaccines. The highest priority groups for vaccine are the following: persons of any age with cardiovascular or pulmonary conditions that necessitate regular medical follow-up; residents of nursing homes and other chronic care facilities, regardless of age; and medical personnel who have contact with and can therefore transmit influenza to high-risk patients. At slightly lower risk, but for whom immunization is still important, are otherwise healthy persons over 65 years of age and adults and children with other chronic diseases (diabetes mellitus, renal dysfunction, anemia, immunosuppression, or asthma). Split-virus vaccine should be used in children; the dose is 0.5 mL for children 3 to 8 years of age and 0.25 mL for those 6 to 35 months old. A second dose 4 weeks or more after the first is needed if the child has never received influenza vaccine. Children 9 to 12 years of age should receive one 0.5-mL dose of split-virus vaccine. Adults can be given either whole- or split-virus vaccine as a 0.5-mL dose. All vaccines should be given intramuscularly.

TREATMENT

The availability of an effective agent against influenza A virus, the major cause of influenza, is widely unappreciated. If one waits for diagnostic viral culture results or for serologic studies, treatment will not be as useful. The antiviral drug

TABLE 1. **Recommended Amantadine (Symmetrel) Dosage by Age**

Age (Years)	Dosage
1–9	5 mg/kg/day once daily or divided twice daily (total dosage not to exceed 150 mg/day)
10–64	200 mg once daily or divided twice daily
≥65	100 mg once daily

TABLE 2. **Recommended Amantadine Dosage* in Patients with Renal Disease**

Creatinine Clearance (mL/min/1.73 m²)	Dosage
≥80	100 mg twice daily
60–79	200 mg alternated with 100 mg daily
40–59	100 mg once daily
30–39	200 mg twice weekly
20–29	100 mg three times weekly
10–19	200 mg alternated with 100 mg every 7 days

*Source: Centers for Disease Control. (Adapted from Morbidity and Mortality Weekly Report 35:317–331, 1986.)

amantadine has been licensed for use in treating all types of influenza A for two decades, and numerous controlled studies demonstrate 70% or greater efficacy in reducing symptoms. The drug also decreases viral shedding and can thus prevent the spread of influenza. It is not effective against influenza B.

A person with a febrile respiratory illness during a documented influenza outbreak is an ideal candidate for amantadine. The likelihood that the illness is due to another virus in this setting is small. Amantadine should be started as early in the course of illness as possible (preferably within 24 hours to 48 hours after onset). Thus individuals suspected of having influenza can be treated empirically with amantadine. The drug should be continued for 48 hours after symptoms subside but not more than a total of 5 to 7 days. Most patients can be treated with 200 mg per day. The dosage must be adjusted for diminished renal function. Central nervous system side effects such as insomnia, lightheadedness, irritability, and difficulty concentrating occur in up to 10% of persons. These are usually mild and cease shortly after the drug is stopped. Tables 1 and 2 list dosages of amantadine by age and level of renal function.

Patients with type A influenza being treated with amantadine may shed influenza virus resistant to the drug. For this reason, amantadine should not be used for both prophylaxis and treatment in the same household, unless the ill patient can be isolated from the persons receiving prophylaxis. In the setting of a nursing home, concurrent amantadine treatment and prophylaxis should incorporate adequate case isolation (i.e., ill patients receiving amantadine should be confined to their room for 7 days).

Bacterial superinfections should be treated with antibiotics chosen on the basis of appropriate Gram's stains and cultures of specimens from the respiratory tract. Supportive therapy with hydration and antipyretics is beneficial; however, aspirin should not be used in persons under 16 years of age suspected of having influenza (or any other viral illness) because of the risk of Reye's syndrome. Acetaminophen (Tylenol) rather than aspirin should be used to reduce fever.

LEISHMANIASIS

method of
DEBRA CHESTER KALTER, M.D.
Uniformed Services University of Health Sciences
Bethesda, Maryland

"Leishmaniasis" refers to a pleomorphic collection of clinical diseases resulting from infection with the protozoan *Leishmania*. In most regions, leishmaniasis is a zoonosis, but humans may serve as the reservoir. Infection is transmitted by the bite of an infected female phlebotomus sandfly (typically *Phlebotomus* species, Old World, or *Lutzomyia* species, New World). Blood meals are required for oviposition. Infectious promastigotes are regurgitated into the animal or human host in the act of feeding. Host macrophages phagocytize the flagellates, which quickly convert to amastigotes intracellularly. Paradoxically, they survive and proliferate within the macrophage phagolysosome. Once internalized, the species of *Leishmania* largely determines the clinical outcome, whether visceral or cutaneous, whether lesions are few or multiple, and whether mucocutaneous or diffuse dissemination is likely. Genetic predisposition to resistance or susceptibility to infection has been shown to be of great importance prognostically in murine models and may play some as yet undetermined role in human infection. The immune system of the host certainly influences the degree of disease manifestation. As parasite speciation has become more readily available, it is obvious that almost any species is capable of producing almost any clinical syndrome, although there are typical patterns of expression.

CLINICAL SYNDROMES

The two main clinical syndromes are visceral leishmaniasis (VL) and cutaneous leishmaniasis (CL). VL has been documented in India, Pakistan, southern Russia, China, Africa, the countries bordering the Mediterranean, and South and Central America. Systemic infection results from parasitization of cells of the reticuloendothelial system with *Lutzomyia donovani*. VL is manifest gradually during the course of infection by increasing hepatosplenomegaly and lymphadenopathy. Within 2 to 6 months of parasite introduction by sandfly bite, disease is marked by intermittent fevers, malaise, weight loss, abdominal discomfort, diarrhea, skin darkening, ecchymoses, and epistaxis. Laboratory findings include pancytopenia, hypergammaglobulinemia, mildly elevated levels of liver enzymes, and antigen-specific anergy. Serologic screening of endemic populations indicates that subclinical infection occurs.

In symptomatic infection, however, therapeutic intervention is necessary because the mortality rate is high. Secondary bacterial infection is common and adds to the morbidity.

More cases of VL, and to a lesser extent CL, have been reported within the growing number of immunosuppressed individuals, whether iatrogenically produced or caused by infection with the human immunodeficiency virus. In severe cases, VL may disseminate to involve the skin. Leishmaniasis in this scenario has been considered an opportunistic infection and may be difficult to eradicate.

A new visceral syndrome has recently been described in American soldiers who traveled to the Persian Gulf area in 1990–1991. Systemic infection was documented in the majority to be caused by *Lutzomyia tropica*, an etiologic agent of CL in the Middle East. The manifestations include an acute to subacute febrile illness with fatigue, resembling mononucleosis or gastroenteritis. Some soldiers spontaneously recovered without therapy, whereas others progressed to a more chronic condition, associated with adenopathy or splenomegaly. The symptomatic individuals were treated with standard parenteral pentavalent antimony therapy with apparent resolution. *L. tropica* has been rarely reported previously as the etiologic agent in kala azar.

Cutaneous leishmaniasis (CL) most often is manifest by one or more nodulo-ulcerative lesions at the site of parasite inoculation. Lesions may be singular and sharply localized or may be multiple with satellite or metastatic nodules or lymphangitic spread. The most typical configuration of CL is of a centrally ulcerated nodule, with a volcano-like shape. Papular, verrucous, acneiform, keloidal, lupoid, sporotrichoid, and psoriasiform patterns are also seen. *L. tropica, L. major,* and *L. aethiopica* are etiologic in Old World CL (Middle East, Mediterranean basin, Russia, India, Africa). *L. tropica* has been associated with the dry or urban Oriental sore, in which lesions are few in number and slowly heal over a 10- to 15-month period. Wet or rural Oriental sore is attributed to *L. major,* in which many lesions may be present simultaneously, but healing is quicker (over 6 to 8 months). New World CL is ascribed primarily to *L. mexicana* and *L. brasiliensis,* each with multiple subspecies (South and Central America, Caribbean, Texas). Eventual involvement of mucosal membranes of the nasopharynx occurs in a minority of individuals in South or Central America infected with *L. brasiliensis.* Mucocutaneous leishmaniasis (MCL) is uncommon in the Old World, but has been reported to be caused by *L. aethiopica,* and occurs in the Sudan in areas endemic for VL, where the etiologic agent is uncertain. Other persistent forms of cutaneous disease are referred to as diffuse cutaneous leishmaniasis (DCL) and leishmaniasis recidivans (LR). In DCL, the individual's immune recognition of *Leishmania* is singularly diminished, and the parasite proliferates extensively throughout the dermis, indolently progressing to involve large tracts of skin. These patients respond poorly to therapy. LR is a chronic nonhealing or relapsing cutaneous infection. In contrast to patients with DCL, these individuals are hypersensitive to parasite antigens, and organisms are few.

Patients with VL may have cutaneous manifestations. After apparently successful therapy of kala azar, hypopigmented patches, nonulcerative papulonodules, and plaques may develop on the face and body, at times simulating leprosy. This syndrome of post–kala azar dermal leishmaniasis (PKDL) is most common in India, but it occurs in Africa as well. Despite a history of adequate therapy, infectious organisms are found within the dermis and serve as a continuing reservoir of *Leishmania.* Another nonulcerative cutaneous eruption has been described in relation to infection with *L. donovani chagasi* in Honduras, in an area endemic for kala azar. Twenty-five cases were reported of small, flattened papular lesions resembling sarcoid or leprosy in children aged 4 to 15 years, with no systemic complaints and no history of VL or of antileishmanial therapy. Leishmania was encountered in skin scrapings and biopsies. CL of more typical appearance caused by *L. donovani infantum* has been described in France, Italy, and Algeria.

DIAGNOSIS

Definitive diagnosis is made upon demonstration of the infecting parasite. If VL is suspected, splenic or bone marrow aspirate is performed. In CL or MCL, the border of an active lesion may be scraped (slit skin smear), or a needle aspirate can be made after injection of 0.1 mL of sterile saline. Aspirates are utilized for direct examination and for leishmanial culture. In addition, punch or wedge biopsy of the lesion margin provides tissue for histopathologic study, touch preparations (tissue impression slides), and culture. The base of the ulcer or secondarily infected lesions are avoided because parasite yield is low. For direct examination, aspirated material can be dropped or cytospun onto microscope slides. Smears, touch preparations, and aspirates are handled identically. They can be fixed and stained with Giemsa or with monoclonal antibodies directed against *Leishmania,* if available. The latter technique is far more sensitive and specific when performed by experienced clinicians. Histopathologic sections of tissue are stained routinely with hematoxylin and eosin, and Giemsa should be requested.

Amastigotes or Leishman-Donovan (LD) bodies are 2- to 5-micron oval cytoplasmic inclusions that can be seen within tissue macrophages, whether from smears, aspirates, or skin sections. Ideally, the kinetoplast is visible as a smaller, dense inclusion close by the larger nuclear mass, both enclosed within a limiting plasma membrane. It can be difficult, however, to differentiate LD bodies from other intracytoplasmic organisms, such as those causing histoplasmosis, rhinoscleroma, and granuloma inguinale.

Both aspirate and tissue may be cultured for *Leishmania.* Best results have been obtained by using Nicolle's modification of Novy and McNeal's medium (NNN) or Schneider's drosophila medium overlaid with 23% fetal bovine serum. Cultures are maintained for 3 weeks. Amastigotes grown in culture rapidly convert to the flagellated promastigote form. The promastigotes from one species cannot be morphologically distinguished from those of another. Therefore, cultured organisms must be harvested when sufficient in number, to speciate the *Leishmania.* This information is not of academic interest alone, inasmuch as therapy and prognosis may vary with different species. In vitro cultures require some degree of finesse and experience. Alternatively, cultures can be performed in vivo by inoculating infected material into hamster footpads or nose. This method is slow and does not allow speciation but can be useful.

Isoenzyme analysis is the most commonly utilized method for speciation. New techniques are being developed for practical application and are used in some laboratories; these techniques include species-specific monoclonal antibodies, DNA hybridization with restriction enzymes and specific kinetoplast DNA probes, polymerase chain reaction, and pulse field electrophoresis.

It is not always possible to identify the parasite directly. Serologic studies can be helpful in these cases. In endemic areas, because positive serologic results may relate to previous subclinical infection, they must be interpreted with caution. Direct agglutination test (DAT), indirect hemagglutination assay (IHA), immunofluorescent antibody test (IFA), and enzyme-linked immunosorbent assay (ELISA) have all been utilized in serologic assessment. Sensitivity and specificity may vary among different laboratories. Delayed type hypersensitivity testing (Montenegro test), an intradermal injection similar to the purified protein derivative (PPD), is positive in all forms of leishmaniasis except for active kala azar and in cases of DCL and other forms of immunosuppression. Serologic assays may also be negative in severe immunosuppression.

TREATMENT

In the United States, virtually all diagnosed cases of leishmaniasis are treated with parenteral sodium stibogluconate (Pentostam). This pentavalent antimony (Sb) is available only through the Centers for Disease Control in Atlanta, Georgia (telephone: 1-404-639-3670). In many other parts of the world, meglumine antimonate (Glucantime) is the available pentavalent antimony. They are roughly equivalent. The most accepted regimen for the treatment of CL is 20 mg Sb per kg per day (with no maximal dose) as a single intravenous (in 50 mL of dextrose 5% in water over 10 to 45 minutes) or intramuscular dose for 20 days, or until clinical response. The treatments for VL, PKDL, and MCL are identical but are extended for a minimum of 28 days. Therapy of 4 months' duration has been shown to be necessary to cure some patients. In a study of Indian kala azar, patients were treated with the aforementioned regimen, with the modification of a maximal dose of 850 mg per day, for 20, 30, or 40 days. Cure rates were 71%, 83%, and 94%, respectively, indicating that the longer course of therapy is significantly superior. The World Health Organization has recommended the maximal total daily dose of 850 mg. This would limit the dose in a 70-kg adult to 12 mg per kg per day, which is inadequate in many cases. Toxicity was

shown to be equivalent and reversible at doses of Pentostam at 10 mg per kg per day and at 20 mg per kg per day for 20 days in a study of CL, whereas efficacy was significantly improved at the higher dose (76% vs. 100% cure, respectively). Toxicity and subjective complaints tend to increase thereafter with higher doses and longer duration of therapy and may limit drug administration in some individuals. Multiple courses of Sb of 20 to 30 days' duration may be given, separated by 10- to 14-day drug holidays.

"Clinical response" is an unfortunately vague term, generally implying an absence of amastigotes by bone marrow, splenic aspirate, or lesional smear, aspirate, or biopsy. In VL, clinical response also includes a reversal of clinical stigmata of disease, such as anemia, neutropenia, fever, and hepatosplenomegaly. In MCL, clinical response is determined by a loss of erythema and induration of involved tissue, in association with re-epithelialization of ulcerated areas. It is well documented, however, that in cutaneous lesions, persistent parasites may be encountered at the end of therapy, yet the lesion may proceed to complete cure by 3- or 6-month follow-up.

Relapse in all forms of leishmaniasis is unfortunately common and may not be obvious for months to years. Certainly MCL is less responsive to therapy and is more inclined to relapse than is CL. In a study of 16 Panamanians with mild to moderate MCL (caused by *L. braziliensis panamensis*) treated with Pentostam 20 mg per kg per day intravenously for 28 days, 3 of 16 patients failed to complete the full course of therapy because of toxicity. None of these patients were cured of their disease. Of the 13 who completed therapy, 3 suffered relapse within 12 months. The cure rates were 77% of those completing therapy and 63% of all patients treated. The identical treatment plan was administered to 29 Peruvian patients with mild MCL (8 cases, disease confined to the nose) and severe MCL (21 cases, involvement of the oropharynx). Although 62% responded to therapy, only 8 of 29 (30%) were cured by the time of the 12-month follow-up examination. Of the 8 patients cured, 6 were from among the mild MCL group. A more encouraging response to therapy was recorded in a 4-year follow-up of the study group from Tres Bracos, Brazil. After apparent cure from initial Sb treatment, 6 (10%) of 62 CL patients experienced a cutaneous relapse, 2 (3%) of 62 CL patients developed new mucosal lesions, and 2 (17%) of 17 MCL patients suffered a relapse of mucosal disease.

There are numerous drawbacks to therapy with pentavalent antimonials. Parenteral administration by experienced medical personnel in a closely monitored environment is necessary for a prolonged period, although hospitalization is not absolutely required. This is expensive and inconvenient and often impossible in rural settings. Toxicity with these drugs is tolerable and completely reversible but not trivial. Muscle pain results from repeated intramuscular administration. Systemic toxicity includes electrocardiogram changes (10 to 30%); elevation of liver function test results (26 to 36%); arthralgia and myalgia (90%); thrombocytopenia (11%); anorexia (30%); and thrombophlebitis. Patients may also complain of lethargy, headache, nausea, vomiting, metallic taste, or pruritus. The most common electrocardiogram changes are nonspecific ST and T wave changes or T wave inversion and prolongation of the QT interval (corrected QT interval greater than 0.50 seconds) at higher doses. Only the latter change is an indication to stop therapy, inasmuch as sudden death from arrhythmia has occurred after prolonged, high-dose intravenous Sb. Acute renal failure has been reported in a few cases as well. Symptomatic relief of some side effects may be provided by nonsteroidal anti-inflammatory agents. Before initiating therapy, patients should be thoroughly evaluated by history and physical examination, and baseline laboratory evaluations should be obtained, including serum chemistry profile, complete blood cell count with differential and platelet count, urinalysis, and electrocardiogram. If no significant cardiac, renal, or hepatic contraindications exist, therapy can begin, with twice-weekly electrocardiograms and weekly laboratory examinations throughout the treatment period. Patients should be re-examined at 3, 6, 9, and 12 months after therapy.

Not all VL or MCL patients respond to therapy with pentavalent antimony, which may become evident during primary treatment or with subsequent relapse. The second-line drug used in the Western hemisphere is amphotericin B (AmB), whereas pentamidine isethionate may be more commonly utilized elsewhere. Like the antimonials, both require parenteral administration under supervision and have significant toxicities. AmB therapy is begun with a test dose of 1 mg intravenously. Steroids and antihistamines for intravenous administration should be immediately available at all times during therapy, in case of severe hypersensitivity reaction. The daily dose is administered slowly in 500 mL of dextrose 5% in water, and is increased incrementally by 5 mg daily up to a maximum of 1 mg per kg per day. Thereafter, AmB is administered every other day until cure or a total dose of 1.5 to 2.0 grams has been administered. Renal function must be monitored closely. Liposomal amphotericin B* is now commercially available (AmBisome, Vestar, San Dimas, CA) and has been used in a small number of patients with success. Because liposomes are preferentially taken up by macrophages (the parasitized reservoir of *Leishmania* within the host), active drug is theoretically delivered in higher local concentrations precisely where it is most needed. Toxicity and total necessary dose may be minimized by this targeted approach. Pentamidine is administered intravenously or intramuscularly at a dose of 4 mg per kg three times weekly for several months. Recombinant human gamma interferon (IFNg) has been studied extensively in vitro and has been shown to greatly enhance microbicidal activity of human macrophages. In eight patients with VL unresponsive to multiple courses of Glucantime, six responded to combination therapy of 20 mg Sb per kg per day with IFNg 100 to 400 µg per M² body surface area per day for 10 to 40 days. Eight of nine patients with untreated VL, and one patient with refractory CL caused by *L. tropica,* responded quickly to the foregoing combination therapy, with no recurrences after 8 months. The main side effects are fever and flu-like symptoms. Oral agents have also been used in combination with Sb in refractory VL, such as allopurinol ribonucleoside (20 mg per kg per day in three divided doses) or rifampin (600 to 1200 mg daily).

Therapy in CL is far less regimented than the foregoing description would imply. Outside of the United States, CL is as likely to be treated by alternative medications as by parenteral antimony, determined by regional practices and secondary to the prevalent species of *Leishmania.* Curative therapy must be the goal in any locale where *L. brasiliensis* may be etiologic, inasmuch as MCL is a serious sequela to inadequately treated CL. In areas such as the Middle East, where CL is a self-limited disease with eventual spontaneous resolution, a number of therapeutic approaches have been applied with reasonable success. The most exciting recently introduced agent is topical paromomycin sulfate 15% plus methylbenzethonium chloride 12% in white soft paraffin (P-ointment, UK Patent GB117237A; Teva Pharmaceutical Industry, Jerusalem, Israel*). In a study of 67 patients treated in Israel, 87% of those with CL were cured after twice-daily application locally for 10 to 30 days. Although an irritant reaction is common with the use of this ointment, scarring was less than typically found after spontaneous resolution. Untreated distant cutaneous lesions were also reported to resolve within 2 months of the treated lesions. P-ointment has been curative in CL caused by *L. major,*

---

*Investigational drug in the United States.

*Not available in the United States.

L. tropica, L. aethiopica, and L. mexicana mexicana.

Many oral agents have been used with good results in CL, although the literature is full of conflicting reports of efficacy. Ketoconazole* (Nizoral), 600 mg per day, was administered orally for 28 days to 21 patients with CL caused by L. braziliensis panamensis with a cure rate of 76% by 3 months. No placebo-treated individuals healed during this time. Liver enzyme levels were transiently elevated in 27%, whereas all males had an asymptomatic and reversible 70% depression of testosterone levels. Itraconazole at doses of 200 to 400 mg orally per day may prove to be of equal or greater efficacy in some forms of leishmaniasis, with less hepatic toxicity. Dapsone has also been reported to be an effective oral agent in Indian CL, with a cure rate of 82% of 60 patients treated with 100 mg every 12 hours for 6 weeks. Rifampin has also been advocated at doses of 600 to 1200 mg daily for 28 days. These oral medications have been used in combination with other modalities, although combined agents have not been adequately compared with standard regimens.

Intralesional Sb (0.5 to 5 mL three times a week to once a week for 4 to 8 weeks) with or without adjunctive therapy has been used successfully for localized CL. Adjunctive and alternative agents include cryotherapy, heat (40° to 50° C repeatedly), CO_2 laser, parenteral paromomycin sulfate† (aminosidine), intralesional IFNg, topical antimony potassium tartrate 5% cream† (cream of tartar), and topical chlorpromazine ointment.† In Venezuela, promising results have come from the use of immunotherapy for the treatment, and potentially the prevention, of CL. Viable bacille Calmette-Guerin (BCG) plus heat-killed Leishmania promastigotes were injected intradermally into CL patients for three doses at 6- to 8-week intervals. The cure rate was greater than 90%, equivalent to that in the standard Sb therapy control group. Although this method is unlikely to become first-line therapy in the United States, it may be of great utility in areas of endemic disease.

---

*This use of ketoconazole is not listed in the manufacturer's official directive.
†Not available in the United States.

LEPROSY

method of
S. K. NOORDEEN, M.D.
World Health Organization
Geneva, Switzerland

Leprosy is an age-old disease affecting large populations in developing countries and a few isolated pockets in developed countries. It is estimated that there are about 5.5 million patients in the world. There are pockets of infection in the southern United States, mainly in Louisiana and Texas, in California, and in Hawaii; however, the large majority of leprosy patients diagnosed in the United States are immigrants. The major concern in leprosy is the physical deformity it causes in about one-third of the patients and the consequent social stigma.

Leprosy as a chronic disease affects mainly the skin, mucous membranes, and peripheral nerves, although in very advanced states it can affect most body systems. The disease is caused by *Mycobacterium leprae,* an intracellular acid-fast organism not cultivable in vitro even though it was identified by Armauer Hansen as early as 1873. Recently, however, it has become possible to reproduce the disease to a limited extent in the footpads of mice and extensively in the nine-banded armadillo. The human being is the only significant reservoir of infection, although natural leprosy is known to occur in the nine-banded armadillo, found particularly in Louisiana. The disease is transmitted through inhalation of organisms released in nasal discharges of multibacillary leprosy patients and also through skin-to-skin contact. Leprosy has a long incubation period (sometimes as long as 20 years) and it affects all ages and both sexes.

CLINICAL MANIFESTATIONS

The clinical manifestations of leprosy vary widely, depending on the cellular immunity of the individual. The spectrum of disease encompasses lepromatous leprosy, in which the immune response is low; borderline leprosy, in which the immune response is moderate; and tuberculoid leprosy, in which the immune response is high. Further subclassifications according to the Ridley-Jopling classification include polar lepromatous (LL) leprosy, borderline lepromatous (BL) leprosy, mid-borderline (BB) leprosy, borderline tuberculoid (BT) leprosy, and polar tuberculoid (TT) leprosy. In addition, a very early form of leprosy called indeterminate (I) leprosy is also recognized. For the purposes of chemotherapy, the disease in recent years has been broadly classified into multibacillary (MB) leprosy, consisting of LL, BL, BB, and a proportion of BT leprosy, in which the skin smears show acid-fast bacilli; and paucibacillary (PB) leprosy, consisting of I, TT, and a proportion of BT leprosy, in which the skin smears do not show any acid-fast bacilli. In general, in MB leprosy, the skin lesions, which consist of macules, papules, and nodules as well as diffuse infiltration, are numerous with varying degrees of sensory loss. The lepromin test result is usually negative. In PB leprosy, the skin lesions consist mostly of well-defined macules and papules and are limited in number. The skin patches show definite sensory loss, and the lepromin test result is positive. In both MB and PB leprosy, peripheral nerves (e.g., ulnar, lateral popliteal, and facial) are affected, leading to sensory loss over the limbs and paralysis of the small muscles of the hands and feet; this results in the classic deformities of leprosy, such as claw hand. Involvement of the facial nerve may lead to lagophtholmos, exposure keratitis, and, if unattended, ultimately blindness. Extensive sensory loss over the limbs may cause such problems as trophic ulcers of the feet and loss of digits.

DIAGNOSIS

The diagnosis of leprosy is relatively easy in most cases. Examination includes inspection of the skin lesions, palpation of the nerve trunks, and testing for sensory loss for light touch, pain, and temperature. Skin smears are examined for evidence of acid-fast bacilli (AFB). Leprosy is diagnosed on the basis of characteristic skin lesions, sensory loss, nerve thickening, and presence of AFB in the skin smears. Histopathologic examination of lesions is often useful. Serologic tests such as enzyme-linked immunosorbent assay (ELISA) for antibodies to *M. leprae*–specific phenolic glycolipid I are of little diagnostic value as their sensitivity is quite low.

COMPLICATIONS

The most important complications are lepra reactions, which consist of two distinct entities. The first, which is referred to as reversal reaction (RR), or Type I reaction, seen mostly in BT leprosy, is mainly due to a rapid increase in cellular hypersensitivity and is characterized by erythematous lesions with edema, either fresh or over the existing skin lesions, often accompanied by severe neuritis. The second, referred to as erythema nodosum leprosum (ENL), or Type II reaction, seen mostly in LL and BL leprosy, is due to humoral hypersensitivity involving an immune complex mechanism. This form is characterized by evanescent tender and erythematous skin nodules, often accompanied by systemic features such as fever, malaise, and nerve pain. A third type of reaction, called the Lucio phenomenon, occurs mainly in Central America. It is due to vasculitis and is characterized by punched-out skin ulcers resulting from hemorrhagic infarcts. If not properly treated, lepra reactions can result in deformities. Other complications in MB leprosy include neuritis, iridocyclitis, arthritis, and rhinitis. The major complication in PB leprosy, apart from RR, is neuritis leading to deformities.

TREATMENT

The treatment of leprosy itself is primarily through multidrug chemotherapy. The treatment of leprosy patients, however, should encompass all the problems faced by the patients, including complications and deformities as well as the psychological and social effects. Although the duration of chemotherapy for leprosy itself is relatively short, many leprosy patients require long-term care for the sequelae of the disease such as residual sensory loss, deformities, and trophic ulcers.

Until the 1940s, the treatment of leprosy was a frustrating experience because no effective drugs were available. The advent of sulfone drugs, of which dapsone is the most important, finally brought effective treatment, although therapy had to last for several years and often life-long. The subsequent discovery of highly effective antileprosy drugs such as rifampin and clofazimine changed the situation further. The widespread employment of monotherapy with dapsone through the 1970s, however, resulted in the emergence of sulphone-resistant *M. leprae*, making treatment increasingly ineffective. This challenge has since been met through multidrug therapy (MDT). A major development in this direction came through the recommendations of a Study Group on Chemotherapy of Leprosy for control programs set up by the World Health Organization (WHO) in 1981. The Study Group recommended standard drug regimens for MB and PB leprosy with finite durations of treatment. Since 1982, the WHO/MDT regimen has been widely implemented in disease-control programs, and over 3 million patients were cured between 1982 and 1992. This has also contributed to a reduction of over 50% of the registered cases in the world. The objective of MDT is to prevent drug resistance and make treatment more effective and practical.

Drugs and dosages for MB leprosy are shown in Table 1. Treatment should continue for at least 2 years and, wherever possible, up to smear neg-

TABLE 1. World Health Organization Multidrug Therapy for Multibacillary Leprosy

Rifampin (Rifadine, Rimactane)	600 mg once a month, supervised
Dapsone	100 mg/day, self-administered
Clofazimine (Lamprene)	300 mg once a month, supervised; 50 mg/day, self-administered

From World Health Organization: Chemotherapy of leprosy for control programmes—Report of a WHO Study Group. Technical Report Series 675. Geneva, World Health Organization, 1982.

ativity. If it is not possible to administer clofazimine because of toxicity or total nonacceptance by the patient, ethionamide-protionamide,* 375 mg a day, is an alternative. However, in view of the risk of serious hepatotoxicity, particularly when combined with rifampin, ethionamide-protionamide should be administered under strict medical supervision, with periodic evaluation for hepatotoxicity.

The standard WHO/MDT regimen for PB leprosy consists of rifampin, 600 mg once a month (supervised) for 6 months, plus dapsone, 100 mg daily (unsupervised) for 6 months.

As mentioned earlier, the WHO/MDT regimens are quite effective and, in general, there is no need to try other variations. If new regimens are required for some reason, however, it is important to ensure that patients receive a three-drug combination for MB leprosy and a two-drug combination for PB leprosy, in order to prevent drug resistance. The individual drugs employed in the treatment of leprosy or others that have potential to be employed in the future are discussed in the following sections.

Dapsone

Although dapsone was synthesized in 1908, it was first used in leprosy in 1946, initially as a parenteral preparation and later as tablets. The drug is a synthetase inhibitor in the folate synthesis of *M. leprae*. The dose is 1 to 2 mg per kg of body weight, and a general adult dose is 100 mg per day; in this dose, it acts essentially as a bacteriostatic substance, although with weak bactericidal properties. The drug is extremely well absorbed and has an average half-life of 28 hours. An advantage of dapsone is that after ingestion of a single dose of 100 mg, the peak blood level attained is 500 times the minimal inhibitory concentration, and measurable amounts can be found in the blood even 10 days later.

The drug is generally well tolerated with relatively few side effects and can be administered during pregnancy. Side effects include hemolytic

*Not available in the United States.

anemia, leukopenia, methemoglobinemia, fixed drug eruptions, peripheral neuropathy, exfoliative dermatitis, nephritis, hepatitis, and psychosis. The hemolytic anemia is a particular problem in patients with complete glucose-6-phosphate dehydrogenase (G6PD) deficiency. The dapsone syndrome reported by some to occur around the fifth week of treatment is quite rare and consists of exfoliative dermatitis, lymphadenopathy, and hepatitis with potentially fatal consequences. In such instances dapsone should be immediately stopped and patients treated with steroids.

As mentioned previously, in spite of the drug's effectiveness, dapsone resistance became a major problem mainly because of its use as monotherapy, which facilitated selection of drug-resistant mutants, particularly with the very large bacillary populations found in lepromatous leprosy. It took several years of monotherapy with dapsone before resistance came to be identified as a significant problem. This is because resistance of *M. leprae* to dapsone occurs in a stepwise fashion and because it takes a long time to identify treatment failures in leprosy. However, because of several other advantages, including its low cost, dapsone continues to be used as part of MDT.

Clofazimine

Clofazimine (Lamprene) is a bright red dye and an imino-phenazine derivative that was discovered in 1954 and found to be effective against leprosy in 1962. It is reasonably well absorbed when formulated in a microcrystalline oilwax base and is deposited predominantly in the adipose tissue, skin, and reticuloendothelial cells. Even though the exact mechanism of action is not clear, clofazimine is believed to intercalate within the DNA helix of *M. leprae*. In addition, clofazimine has anti-inflammatory properties and is therefore a useful drug for the treatment of Type II (ENL) reactions. The adult dose of clofazimine is 50 to 100 mg per day for treatment of leprosy itself and up to 300 mg per day for Type II reactions. In WHO/MDT, the dose is 50 mg daily together with a loading dose of 300 mg once a month. The drug is essentially bacteriostatic with weak bactericidal properties. The antileprosy effect is almost the same as that of dapsone. Only rare cases of resistance of *M. leprae* to clofazimine have been reported so far. Among the side effects of clofazimine, the most important is the reddish-black pigmentation produced by deposition of the drug in the skin, which occurs within 4 to 8 weeks of starting therapy. After stopping therapy, the discoloration disappears over a period of 6 to 12 months. Red coloration can also be seen in the mucous membranes, sweat, feces, and urine. Other side effects of clofazimine include xerosis, ichthyosis, abdominal pain, and diarrhea. The drug can be administered during pregnancy. Clofazimine is of value mainly in MB leprosy and should be administered in combination with rifampin and dapsone as in WHO/MDT. Even with a dose of 50 mg per day (WHO/MDT), clofazimine appears to reduce the frequency and intensity of Type II reactions.

Rifampin

Rifampin (Rifadin, Rimactane) is the most potent antileprosy drug. A semisynthetic derivative of a fermentation product of *Streptomyces mediterranei*, it acts by inhibiting the DNA-dependent RNA polymerase of the organisms, thereby interfering with bacterial RNA synthesis. The drug is rapidly absorbed from the gastrointestinal tract and has a half-life of only 3 to 4 hours after a single dose of 600 mg. Rifampin has a much higher bactericidal activity against *M. leprae* than against *Mycobacterium tuberculosis:* a single dose of 600 to 1200 mg of rifampin is capable of killing 99.9% of the organisms. It is because of this extremely high bactericidal activity that the WHO/MDT regimen specifies using the drug only once a month at a dose of 600 mg for adults. At this dose and interval, the drug is extremely well tolerated; the rare side effects include skin rashes, drowsiness, thrombocytopenia, and hepatitis. Hepatotoxicity is increased when the drug is administered with ethionamide-protionamide. Rifampin also causes red discoloration of the urine. The "flu syndrome" often reported in the treatment of tuberculosis is quite rare in the treatment of leprosy. Rifampin can be safely administered during pregnancy. Although rifampin is highly bactericidal, it should not be employed as monotherapy because bacterial resistance to the drug can emerge very rapidly. It is therefore extremely important to use rifampin only as part of MDT.

Ethionamide-Protionamide

These two drugs are closely related, and cross-resistance between them has been well established. They have significant bactericidal activity and are used mainly as a substitute in WHO/MDT for patients who cannot take clofazimine. The dose of is 250 to 375 mg per day. The drugs have significant side effects, including gastrointestinal disturbances, allergic reactions, dermatitis, peripheral neuropathy, and rheumatic pain, apart from hepatotoxicity. The latter complication is particularly enhanced when these drugs are combined with rifampin. Ethionamide-protionamide is therefore recommended for treatment of leprosy only under exceptional circumstances and with close medical supervision, including periodic assessment of serum transaminase levels.

Ofloxacin

Ofloxacin (Floxin) is an orally administered antibacterial drug belonging to the group of fluorinated quinolones. It acts by inhibiting the enzyme DNA gyrase, which controls supercoiling of DNA in bacteria. Among the fluoroquinolones, ofloxacin* is the most promising in the treatment of leprosy; animal experiments and short-term clinical trials suggest that its bactericidal activity is second only to that of rifampin. As with other antileprosy drugs, it should not be given as monotherapy. A large-scale, WHO-supported, multicenter trial is currently under way to find out whether a combination of rifampin and ofloxacin can reduce the treatment period of MB leprosy to just 1 month. The side effects attributed to ofloxacin include gastrointestinal pain, diarrhea, hypersensitivity reactions, and vertigo.

Minocycline

Minocycline (Minocin)† is a semisynthetic tetracycline that has recently been found to have bacterial activity against *M. leprae* similar to that of ofloxacin. It has a fairly long half-life of 13 hours and is effective at a dose of 100 mg per day. Clinical trials are under way to identify the best way to employ the drug in the treatment of leprosy.

Clarithromycin

Clarithromycin (Biaxin)‡ is a macrolide recently identified to have both in vitro and in vivo bactericidal activity against *M. leprae,* probably at the same level as ofloxacin and minocycline. Clinical trials are in progress.

Treatment of Complications

Complications of leprosy, most of which lead to deformities if unattended, necessitate prompt and effective treatment. Educating patients to identify problems early and seek treatment is crucial to the prevention of sequelae. Apart from specific complications such as Type I and Type II reactions, neuritis, and arthritis, which can cause permanent incapacitation, the loss of peripheral sensation over the extremities has lifelong consequences in terms of risk of injury, ulceration, and loss of digits.

---

*This use of ofloxacin is not listed in the manufacturer's official directions.

†This use of minocycline is not listed in the manufacturer's official directions.

‡This use of clarithromycin is not listed in the manufacturer's official directions.

Type I Reactions

The most important goals in the treatment of Type I, or reversal, reactions are to prevent nerve damage through treatment of the acute neuritis that is part of most reactions and to control inflammation of the skin lesions. There is no need to interrupt antileprosy treatment during the reaction. In mild reactions, analgesics are sufficient, particularly when there is no evidence of neuritis. However, the patient should be closely observed for any exacerbation. In severe reactions, particularly when there is evidence of acute neuritis with pain, tenderness, and loss of nerve function, the patient should be hospitalized whenever possible, and treatment with steroids should be initiated together with analgesics. The painful nerves should be rested and the affected limb splinted. Treatment with steroids should preferably start with 40 mg of prednisone daily which should be maintained for at least 2 weeks, and depending on the response, the dose can be reduced every 1 to 2 weeks by 5 to 10 mg. Most patients with severe reactions require at least 12 weeks of treatment with steroids.

Type II Reactions

Although Type II (ENL) reactions are less important from the point of view of nerve damage, the consequences of repeated and severe reactions can be quite grave due to the associated systemic effects. Mild reactions can be easily managed on an ambulatory basis with analgesics and drugs such as chloroquine* (150 mg three times a day) or antimonials (e.g., stibophen,† containing 8.5 mg of antimony per mL given in a dose of 2 to 3 mL intramuscularly on alternate days for a maximal total dose of 30 mL). Thalidomide in a dose of 400 mg daily is very effective in controlling ENL reactions. The drug should never be given to women of child-bearing age, in view of its teratogenic effects.

Patients with severe ENL reactions require hospitalization. The treatment of choice for such patients is thalidomide, which can be administered for prolonged periods. The alternative is treatment with either steroids or clofazimine, the latter in doses of 300 mg per day.‡ Both carry significant risks for patients who are treated for long periods. Patients can become steroid-dependent, which makes withdrawal of the drug difficult. Long-term use of clofazimine in high doses can cause severe gastrointestinal side effects due to crystal deposition in the intestinal tract. Often a judicious combination of any two of the drugs thalidomide, prednisolone, or clofazimine can help in achieving dose reduction and ultimately drug withdrawal.

Neuritis

Inflammation of the peripheral nerve trunk with enlargement, pain, and tenderness can occur by itself in the course of either MB or PB leprosy or accompany either Type I or Type II reactions. The treatment of choice is prednisolone. In addition, the nerve trunk should be rested through splinting and appropriate analgesics. If pain is intractable and persistent, surgical intervention through nerve decompression is of value. Leprosy patients should be closely monitored for sensory and motor changes as these can occur insidiously without acute neuritis. This phenomenon, referred to as "quiet nerve paralysis," also requires management with steroids.

Iridocyclitis

Apart from exposure keratitis and other complications arising from lagophthalmos, iridocyclitis is the most important cause of blindness in leprosy and therefore should be treated promptly and vigorously. Acute iridocyclitis should be treated with mydriatics, such as 1% atropine or 0.25% scopolamine, and anti-inflammatory drugs such as 1% hydrocortisone. Chronic iridocyclitis should be treated on similar lines but for longer periods, and periodic assessment of ocular pressure should be done.

Deformities in Leprosy

Common paralytic deformities in leprosy include claw hand, foot drop, lagophthalmos, and wrist drop; common disabilities due to sensory loss over the extremities include trophic ulcers and absorption of digits. The disease process can also cause problems such as depressed nose, loss of eyebrows, gynecomastia, and blindness resulting from lagophthalmos and iridocyclitis.

Once deformities and disabilities set in, their management poses major problems; therefore, every effort should be made to prevent their development through early treatment. Care of anesthetic hands and feet calls for intensive patient education and use of appropriate footwear. Physiotherapy and splinting are important in preventing and controlling deformities. A number of effective surgical procedures have enabled correction of deformities of hands, feet, nose, and eyes. Patient re-education, physiotherapy, and occupational therapy are important adjuncts to surgical reconstruction.

LEPROSY CONTROL

The strategy of leprosy control today involves essentially secondary prevention through early

---

*This use of chloroquine is not listed in the manufacturer's official directions.

†Not available in the United States.

‡Exceeds dosage recommended by the manufacturer.

detection of cases and effective drug therapy so that the reservoirs of infection can be eliminated and transmission of infection interrupted. So far, there is no primary preventive strategy available for leprosy, although bacilli Calmette-Guérin (BCG) is known to have a protective effect against the disease, particularly in certain parts of the world. The widespread application of WHO-recommended MDT over the last 10 years has had a significant impact in reducing the disease burden in the world, raising hopes of eliminating the disease as a public health problem in the not-too-distant future.

MALARIA

method of
ANNE E. McCARTHY, M.D.
University of Ottawa
Ottawa, Ontario, Canada

and

JAY S. KEYSTONE, M.D., M.Sc.
The Toronto Hospital
Toronto, Canada

Malaria is one of the most prevalent and important diseases in the world. Annually, it affects more than 250 million people and results in 5 million deaths. The majority of infections occur in the developing world, where malaria is a leading cause of morbidity and mortality. The disease is severe in nonimmune individuals, including children, pregnant women, travelers, and immigrants. The epidemiology of malaria has changed in recent years, partly because of the marked spread of drug resistance.

In the United States, about 1000 cases of malaria per year are reported to the Centers for Disease Control (CDC). This is probably a significant underestimate, even though malaria remains a reportable disease. The vast majority of infections seen in North America occur in travelers or immigrants arriving from Africa and Asia. Other sources of infection in patients without a travel history include blood transfusion, use of contaminated needles, and local malaria transmission. The last mentioned has occasionally been reported in California and more recently in New Jersey.

ETIOLOGY

Malaria is caused by the blood protozoan *Plasmodium,* of which there are four human species: *P. falciparum, P. vivax, P. ovale,* and *P. malariae.* The disease is transmitted from the bite of an infected female anopheline mosquito, during which sporozoites from its salivary gland are inoculated into the human bloodstream during feeding. Within 30 minutes, sporozoites are cleared from the bloodstream and enter hepato-

cytes, where they undergo division and development (primary exoerythrocytic phase). Within 7 to 10 days, new forms called merozoites develop and enter the bloodstream, where they infect red blood cells, in which they undergo further division and development (erythrocytic phase). Newly formed merozoites are released from erythrocytes, reinvade and multiply in red blood cells, or mature to sexual forms (gametes), which are picked up by a feeding anopheline mosquito to complete the cycle.

Although all species of human malaria initially infect hepatocytes, only *P. vivax* and *P. ovale* leave behind latent forms called hypnozoites that are capable of causing relapses of infection up to 3 years later. Because *P. malariae* has the potential for lifelong persistence in red blood cells, recrudescences can occur many years after the primary infection.

P. falciparum is the species responsible for severe disease and death. High levels of parasitemia occur because *P. falciparum* has the ability to infect red blood cells of all ages (other species infect only young or old erythrocytes) and to release large numbers of merozoites from the liver because of rapid asexual reproduction. These high levels of parasitemia occur in association with cytoadherence of infected erythrocytes to postcapillary venules. Consequently, sludging of red cells causes blood vessel obstruction, particularly in the central nervous system. Other *Plasmodium* species are very rarely associated with severe disease or death. In the United States, the case fatality rate of *P. falciparum* infections is estimated to be between 2 and 4%.

TRANSMISSION AND RESISTANCE

Malaria transmission occurs in sub-Saharan Africa, the Indian subcontinent, Southeast Asia, the Middle East, Oceania, limited areas of the Caribbean, and large areas of Central and South America. The risk of acquiring malaria varies within these geographic regions, depending on the season, altitude, degree of rural travel, and use of personal protection measures to prevent mosquito bites. In North America, approximately 80% of cases of imported *P. falciparum* malaria were acquired in Africa.

The development of resistance to antimalarial drugs has complicated malaria therapy and prophylaxis. Chloroquine-resistant strains of *P. falciparum* have spread throughout most malarious areas of the world, leaving only Central America, Haiti, the Dominican Republic, Egypt, and parts of the Middle East unaffected (Fig. 1). Resistance to the combination of pyrimethamine and sulfadoxine (Fansidar) is prevalent in some areas of Southeast Asia, the Amazon basin of South America, and parts of Africa. In areas of Southeast Asia, *P. falciparum* malaria has shown a reduced susceptibility to the standard 7-day course of quinine and must be treated with two drugs. Mefloquine and halofantrine resistance are clinically important along the Thai-Cambodian and Myanmar (Burmese) borders. The results of in vitro studies from several countries in West Africa and South America, where mefloquine had

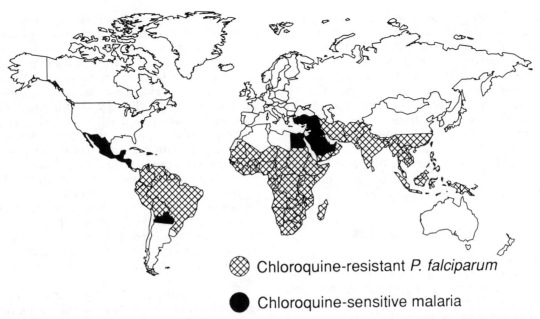

Figure 1. Distribution of malaria and chloroquine-resistant *Plasmodium falciparum*, 1991. From Centers for Disease Control: Health Information for International Travel 1992. Atlanta, U.S. Department of Health and Human Services, 1992, p 99.

not yet been used, suggest that some strains of *P. falciparum* may have an inherently decreased sensitivity to mefloquine.

Recently, chloroquine-resistant *P. vivax* malaria has been reported from Papua New Guinea and Indonesia. Although the extent and frequency of this problem is unclear, recent studies suggest that *P. vivax* malaria from these geographic areas should be assumed to be chloroquine-resistant and treated with quinine. In contrast, primaquine resistance is well-established in Southeast Asia and Oceania, where up to one-third of patients with *P. vivax* infections suffer relapse after a standard 14-day course of therapy. Resistance to primaquine is uncommon in other *P. vivax*–endemic areas of the world.

CLINICAL MANIFESTATIONS

Depending on the species involved, the incubation period for malaria usually ranges from 9 to 30 days but may be as long as 9 months. It may be prolonged in patients taking chemoprophylaxis and in those who have developed partial immunity (known as semi-immune status) from repeated malaria infections. Clinical symptoms of malaria are produced when newly formed merozoites are released from red blood cells at the completion of a development cycle. Hepatic and sexual forms are not associated with symptoms. When the majority of parasites within red blood cells undergo maturation (schizogony) at the same time, episodes of symptoms recur at 48-hour intervals, except for *P. malariae* infections, which have a 72-hour erythrocytic cycle. In most patients with *P. falciparum,* development is asynchronous, and consequently fever occurs at varying intervals.

Typical symptoms of malaria include fever, chills, myalgia, arthralgia, and headache. Abdominal pain, cough, and diarrhea may also occur. Frequent clinical

and laboratory findings include hepatosplenomegaly, anemia, and thrombocytopenia. Pulmonary or renal dysfunction (in the absence of dehydration) and changes in mental status occur in complicated *P. falciparum* malaria. The initial symptoms of infection may be modified by immunity acquired from previous infections or by antimalarial drugs. In such cases, illness may intensify more slowly or appear milder than expected.

DIAGNOSIS

Malaria should be considered in any febrile patient with a history of travel to or residence in a malarious area, even if the patient gives a history of chemoprophylaxis. A detailed travel history should be obtained in order to ascertain the risk of exposure to drug-resistant strains of *P. falciparum* and *P. vivax* malaria.

Thick and thin blood films should be prepared for any patient suspected of having malaria. A low level of parasitemia may be detected only on a thick blood film. Initial blood films may be negative in a patient who ultimately develops significant parasitemia. Therefore, a diagnosis of malaria cannot be excluded on the basis of a single negative blood smear. Films should be repeated every 12 hours in any patient in whom malaria is suspected until the diagnosis is either confirmed or excluded. Most patients with clinical symptoms due to malaria have detectable parasites on repeated, well-stained, thick blood films within 48 hours.

The optimal time to examine blood for malaria is at or soon after a fever spike. However, the first blood film should be done as soon as the diagnosis is considered. The Giemsa stain is optimal for thick and thin malaria blood films; Wright's stain can be used for thin smears. In addition to species identification, the degree of parasitemia should be estimated, because it has prognostic value for severe *P. falciparum* infections. Parasite density can be quickly estimated from a thin blood film by counting parasitized cells in an area in which the red blood cells are evenly spaced. It is assumed that there are between 300 and 500 red blood cells per high-powered (40×) field and 100 to 150 cells per oil immersion (100×) field.

ANTIMALARIAL DRUGS

Chloroquine phosphate (Aralen) and chloroquine sulfate* (Nivaquine) are 4-aminoquinolines that act on the erythrocytic stage of all species of *Plasmodium*. Chloroquine is the drug of choice for sensitive strains of malaria. This therapy is usually well tolerated. Side effects, which affect approximately 25% of users, include gastrointestinal upset, visual disturbances, headache, and nonallergic pruritus in African North Americans. With intravenous therapy, hypotension and heart block may occur, especially if the drug is administered too rapidly.

Mefloquine (Lariam, Mephaquin*) is an effective schizontocidal antimalarial for all four species of human *Plasmodium*. In North America, mefloquine is generally recommended only as prophylaxis for drug-resistant *P. falciparum* malaria; it is not as well tolerated in the higher doses required for treatment. Mefloquine therapy and prophylaxis have been associated with neuropsychiatric side effects, such as severe vertigo, convulsions, and psychosis. Present data suggest that these severe neuropsychiatric reactions can occur in up to 1% of those who are treated with mefloquine, in comparison with 1 in 13,000 of those who use the drug for prophylaxis. Mefloquine is contraindicated in children weighing less than 15 kg, pregnant women, and patients with a history of epilepsy or psychiatric disorders. It should also be avoided in patients who are known to have cardiac conduction disturbances. In theory, quinine or quinidine may exacerbate the cardiodepressant effects of mefloquine.

Quinine sulfate is the oral form and quinine dihydrochloride* the intravenous form of this cinchona alkaloid, which has been used for centuries. Parenteral quinidine gluconate or sulfate may be substituted for quinine when the latter is not immediately available. Quinine and quini-

---

*Not available in the United States.

dine are active against asexual erythrocytic stages of all four malaria species and are also active against gametocytes other than those of *P. falciparum*. Quinine is the first-line drug for the oral treatment of chloroquine-resistant malaria; quinidine is reserved for critically ill patients requiring parenteral therapy. Quinine has a bitter taste and is associated with the well-recognized syndrome of cinchonism: headache, nausea, abdominal pain, tinnitus, and transient loss of hearing. These symptoms usually begin after 48 hours of therapy and subside quickly when the drug is stopped. Both quinine and quinidine cause insulin release from the pancreas and have been associated with hypoglycemia when parenteral forms have been used. Because of potential toxicity, parenteral quinidine should be administered only with constant electrocardiographic monitoring.

Pyrimethamine-sulfadoxine (Fansidar) is used primarily by travelers as a standby drug for self-treatment of suspected malaria when fever develops and medical care is not readily available. Weekly Fansidar prophylaxis is no longer recommended because of the occurrence of severe cutaneous adverse reactions with the long-acting sulfa component (1 case per 5000 to 8000 users). Because drug failures after therapy for chloroquine-resistant falciparum malaria have been reported, medical attention should be obtained as soon as possible after self-treatment. Fansidar should not be used by patients with a history of sulfa allergy. It can cause hemolytic anemia in patients with glucose-6-phosphate dehydrogenase (G6PD) deficiency.

Halofantrine (Halfan), currently available as an oral preparation in France and a number of African countries and recently licensed in the United States, is effective for the treatment of drug-resistant *P. falciparum* except in multidrug-resistant areas of Thailand. The current preparation of halofantrine has variable absorption by the oral route and therefore cannot be relied upon for prophylaxis or for the treatment of severe infections. Side effects include cough, pruritus, hemolytic anemia, and QTc prolongation. Electrocardiographic changes are more severe when mefloquine is in the circulation. Although the drug is generally well tolerated, it should be avoided in persons with cardiac conduction defects.

Ginghaosu derivatives from the Chinese herb *Artemisia annua* have potent antimalarial properties. Recent treatment trials in severe *P. falciparum* malaria have shown that ginghaosu derivatives, including artesunate, a new oral form, produce a more rapid clearing of parasitemia and symptoms than does quinine. Although further trials are needed, these compounds appear to be promising additions to the therapeutic armamentarium for severe *P. falciparum* infections.

Primaquine is used to prevent relapses of *P. vivax* and *P. ovale* malaria. Because primaquine can cause hemolysis in G6PD deficiency, a G6PD level should be estimated before this drug is prescribed, particularly to African North Americans, Asians, and patients from the Mediterranean area. Primaquine is contraindicated during pregnancy because the G6PD status of the fetus cannot be easily ascertained.

TREATMENT

During the initial evaluation of a patient suspected of having malaria, certain factors must be considered. These include the presence of *Plasmodium* species, parasite density, geographic area of potential acquisition of infection, coexisting medical complications, and the patient's ability to take oral medication. The geographic area of acquisition must be considered when the possibility of drug-resistant *P. falciparum* malaria is assessed. Although therapeutic decisions are best determined by epidemiologic considerations and by the clinical and laboratory findings, a precise diagnosis is not always possible. In most malarious areas, different species causing malaria and both chloroquine-sensitive and -resistant strains of *P. falciparum* coexist. Treatment decisions should always include the worst-case scenario. Therefore, when speciation is not possible, treatment should be initiated for *P. falciparum* malaria. Also, when there is a possibility that the malaria was acquired in a chloroquine-resistant area, treatment should be directed against resistant strains (Table 1). Chemotherapy should be initiated as soon as possible, especially in patients with severe *P. falciparum* malaria, in whom there is a significant association between delayed chemotherapy and increased mortality rates. Clinical experience has shown that even patients with apparently stable *P. falciparum* malaria may deteriorate rapidly before or during appropriate therapy.

COMPLICATIONS

Complications of severe malaria are generally limited to infection with *Plasmodium falciparum* and develop as the parasite density increases. Multiple organ system involvement occurs frequently with parasitemias greater than 5%. Exchange transfusion should be considered for patients with parasitemia of 10% or greater.

Cerebral malaria is a life-threatening complication of *P. falciparum* malaria. Coma or impairment in mental status resulting from malaria should be distinguished from other causes of neurologic symptoms such as hyperpyrexia, hypoglycemia, and concurrent infection. Signs of cerebral malaria range from disorientation to focal neurologic signs to unarousable coma with posturing. Seizures are common in earlier stages and are frequently associated with hyperpyrexia. In pediatric patients, cerebral malaria should be differentiated from febrile seizures. Coma lasting longer than 30 minutes after a generalized seizure is suggestive of an underlying infectious etiology rather than a postictal phenomenon. Because cerebral edema is not a factor in the pathogenesis of cerebral malaria, corticosteroid therapy is not recommended. Dexamethasone prolongs coma and increases the rate of complications such as pneumonia and gastrointestinal bleeding. Antipyretics, antiemetics, and anticonvulsants may be indicated as adjunct therapy. Fluid intake and output should be monitored closely to avoid fluid overload and subsequent pulmonary edema.

Hypoglycemia is a frequent complication of severe *P. falciparum* malaria, especially in children and pregnant women. Hypoglycemia results from increased glucose consumption by both parasite and febrile patient, impaired gluconeogenesis, and glycogen depletion. Also, quinine and quinidine cause insulin to be released from the pancreas. Symptoms of hypoglycemia range from sweating, tachycardia, pallor, and nervousness to more severe symptoms, such as convulsions, extensor posturing, and coma.

Pulmonary edema, resembling the adult respiratory distress syndrome (ARDS), is a serious and often fatal complication of severe *P. falciparum* infection. Although often associated with fluid overload, it can occur with normal fluid balance and a normal pulmonary artery wedge pressure. Pulmonary edema can occur unexpectedly after several days of therapy even when the patient seems to be recovering. ARDS is more common in pregnant women than in other adults.

Renal impairment is often caused by dehydration; normal renal function usually returns with correction of fluid balance. Patients with high parasite density can develop renal failure that is unresponsive to rehydration. Diuretics, vasopressors, and dialysis may be required.

Thrombocytopenia is a frequent finding in *P. falciparum* and *P. vivax* malaria at all levels of parasitemia. Although the platelet count may drop as low as 10×10^9 per liter, thrombocytopenia is rarely accompanied by significant bleeding. The platelet count typically increases rapidly with appropriate antimalarial therapy. Disseminated intravascular coagulation is an infrequent complication of *P. falciparum* malaria and occurs

TABLE 1. **Drugs Used to Treat Malaria**

Drugs	Adult Dosage	Pediatric Dosage
All Plasmodium Except Chloroquine-Resistant P. falciparum		
ORAL DRUG OF CHOICE		
Chloroquine phosphate	600 mg base (1 gm), then 300 mg base (500 mg) 6 h later, then 300 mg (500 mg) base at 24 and 48 h	10 mg base/kg (max 600 mg base), then 5 mg base/kg 6 h later, then 5 mg base/kg at 24 and 48 h
PARENTERAL DRUG OF CHOICE		
Quinidine gluconate	10 mg/kg loading dose (max 600 mg) in normal saline slowly over 1 h, followed by continuous infusion of 0.02 mg/kg/min for 3 days maximum	Same as adult dose
or		
Quinine dihydrochloride	20 mg salt/kg loading dose in 10 mL/kg 5% dextrose over 4 h, followed by 10 mg salt/kg over 2–4 h q 8 h (max 1800 mg/day) until oral therapy started	Same as adult dose
Chloroquine-Resistant P. falciparum		
ORAL DRUGS OF CHOICE		
Quinine sulfate + pyrimethamine-sulfadoxine	650 mg tid × 3 days 3 tabs at once on last day of quinine	25 mg/kg/day in 3 doses × 3 days <1 year old: ¼ tablet 1–3 years old: ½ tablet 4–8 years old: 1 tablet 9–14 years old: 2 tablets
or + tetracycline	250 mg qid × 7 days	20 mg/kg/day in 4 doses × 7 days (<8 years old)
or + clindamycin	900 mg tid × 3 days	20–40 mg/kg/day in 3 doses × 3 days
ALTERNATIVES		
Mefloquine	1250 mg once	25 mg/kg once (weight <45 kg)*
or		
Halofantrine†	500 mg q 6 h × 3 doses; repeat in 1 week	8 mg/kg q 6 h × 3 doses (weight <40 kg); repeat in 1 week
PARENTERAL DRUG OF CHOICE		
Quinidine gluconate	Same as above	Same as above
or		
Quinine dihydrochloride	Same as above	Same as above
>10% PARASITEMIA		
Exchange transfusion + parenteral therapy	Same as above	Same as above
Prevention of Relapses: *P. vivax and P. ovale only*		
Primaquine phosphate	15 mg base (26.3 mg)/day × 14 days or 45 mg base (79 mg)/week × 8 weeks	0.3 mg base/kg/day × 14 days or 0.9 mg base/kg/week × 8 weeks

*Contraindicated in children weighing less than 15 kg.
†3 days of therapy without a repeat should be used along the Thai-Cambodian and Burmese borders.

most often in patients who are terminally ill with hyperparasitemia and multiple organ failure.

Anemia occurs frequently with malaria and may be severe when parasite density is high.

Pregnancy complicated by *P. falciparum* malaria carries a high risk for both mother and fetus. Malaria may cause maternal or fetal death, prematurity, or low birth weight. Chloroquine can be used safely during pregnancy. Quinine and quinidine have been shown to have oxytocic effects when given at term. However, they have been used successfully and safely in severe malaria during pregnancy. The risks of malaria to mother and child far outweigh any concerns about the use of these drugs. Although there is a theoretical risk of inducing hyperbilirubinemia and subsequent kernicterus with the use of sulfonamides in late pregnancy, this has not occurred with the doses of Fansidar used for malaria treatment. Tetracycline and primaquine are contraindicated in pregnancy. To avoid relapses of *P. vivax* or *P. ovale* malaria during pregnancy, chloroquine treatment should be followed by chloroquine prophylaxis for the duration of the pregnancy. Primaquine should be administered after delivery.

Congenital malaria was thought to be rare but has recently been shown to be common in neonates born to women living in endemic areas. It is diagnosed by detecting parasitemia in the neo-

TABLE 2. **Drugs Used to Prevent Malaria**

Drugs	Adult Dosage	Pediatric Dosage
Chloroquine-Sensitive Areas DRUG OF CHOICE* Chloroquine phosphate	300 mg base (500 mg salt) PO once per week	5 mg/kg base (8.3 mg/kg salt) once per week, up to adult dose of 300 mg base
Chloroquine-Resistant Areas DRUG OF CHOICE* Mefloquine alone	250 mg PO once per week	Weight 15–19 kg: ¼ tab Weight 20–30 kg: ½ tab Weight 31–45 kg: ¾ tab Weight >45 kg: 1 tab
or Doxycycline alone†	100 mg daily	Age >8 years: 2 mg/kg/day (max 100 mg/day)
or Chloroquine phosphate + proguanil‡ (in Africa south of Sahara)	Same as above 200 mg daily	Same as above Age <2 years: 50 mg/day Age 2–6 years: 100 mg/day Age 7–10 years: 150 mg/day Age >10 years: 200 mg/day
+ pyrimethamine-sulfadoxine (as presumptive treatment)	Carry a single dose (3 tabs) for self-treatment of febrile illness when medical care is not immediately available	Age <1 year: ¼ tab Age 1–3 years: ½ tab Age 4–8 years: 1 tab Age 9–14 years: 2 tabs Age >14 years: 3 tabs

Abbreviation: PO = orally.
*Begin all drugs 1 week before (except doxycycline, for which start 1 to 2 days before) and continue until 4 weeks after last exposure.
†Drug of choice for the Thai-Cambodian and Burmese borders; start 1 to 2 days before departure.
‡Not available in the United States.

nate within the first few weeks of life, assuming that there is no possibility of postpartum mosquito-borne infection.

PREVENTION

At present, the solution to the malaria problem is prevention. Control of malaria has been unsuccessful in many areas of the world because of mosquito resistance to insecticides, parasite resistance to antimalarial drugs, and the breakdown of malaria control programs. Because vaccine development has met some significant obstacles, a vaccine is not likely to be available in the near future.

Personal protection measures against mosquito bites are important for minimizing the risk of malaria. Because the anopheline mosquito bites from dusk to dawn, individuals should wear clothing that minimizes the amount of exposed skin and remain in well-screened areas during this time. Insect repellents containing diethyltoluamide (DEET) should be applied before outdoor activities during hours of malarial transmission. However, DEET can be dangerous to young children; in rare instances, seizures and nervous system damage have been reported with prolonged use and high concentrations of this repellent. Therefore, high concentrations of DEET should be used sparingly on young children. Newer formulations of DEET allow for prolonged protection at lower concentrations. The use of permethrin-impregnated bed nets has been shown to significantly reduce the incidence of malaria among children living in endemic areas. Insect sprays containing pyrethrum should be used in sleeping quarters before people retire, and if practical, bed nets should be used by travelers.

The choice of an appropriate prophylactic regimen is determined by the exact itinerary of the traveler, the length of stay in the malarious area, the estimated intensity of exposure, and pre-existing conditions such as age, pregnancy, allergies, and concurrent medications (Table 2). No chemoprophylactic regimen guarantees protection against malaria. Because most antimalarials act in the bloodstream, beyond the initial liver phase, infection is not prevented; rather, clinical symptoms are suppressed by inhibition of parasite replication in red blood cells. When counseling a patient about malaria chemoprophylaxis, one should check an up-to-date source of information on the location and extent of drug-resistant *Plasmodium* species. Detailed recommendations for the prevention of malaria can be obtained on a 24-hour basis by calling the CDC Malaria Hotline at 1-404-332-4555.

Antimalarial drugs should be taken by those

who travel to endemic areas, regardless of the length of stay. Prophylactic drugs (except doxycycline) should be started 1 to 2 weeks before departure to optimize blood levels and ensure tolerance. As noted previously, antimalarials do not prevent the initial liver phase of the malaria cycle in the human host. Consequently, these drugs must be continued for 4 weeks after a person leaves an endemic area to ensure the eradication of any parasites that are released from the liver after the traveler has departed from a malarious area.

Some travelers carry presumptive therapy for self-treatment of malaria. These regimens are recommended only for the few travelers who are not likely to have access to immediate medical care or who are unable to tolerate or take the optimal regimen for a particular geographic area. Once self-therapy has been administered, the traveler is advised to seek medical attention to confirm the response to therapy. Regardless of the antimalarial regimen employed, travelers should seek medical attention for any flu-like illness occurring within the first year after visiting a malarious area and should remind their health care providers of their travel history. As a rule, more than 90% of individuals with imported *P. falciparum* malaria present with symptoms within the first 2 months of their departure from an endemic area.

With the increasing prevalence of infection and the problem of drug resistance, malaria remains an important cause of morbidity and mortality worldwide. The ease and speed of international travel make it likely that many more physicians will be required to care for patients with malaria. The most important step in the evaluation and management of malaria is consideration of the diagnosis itself in any patient with a history of fever who has recently returned from a malarious area. Treatment, particularly of *P. falciparum* malaria, should be initiated as soon as possible. Because drug-resistant strains of malaria are becoming more prevalent in many areas of the world, an up-to-date source of information on this subject should be consulted. If there is any question about the possibility of drug resistance, treatment for the worst-case scenario should be undertaken. However, in spite of its potential to cause severe disease and death, malaria is very much a preventable infection. Regular use of antimalarials and rigorous adherence to personal protection measures against mosquito bites are simple and effective ways to reduce the risk of infection in travelers to malarious areas.

ACUTE BACTERIAL MENINGITIS

method of
J. WILLIAM KELLY, M.D.*
Brooke Army Medical Center
Ft. Sam Houston, Texas

Acute bacterial meningitis is a medical emergency requiring rapid and decisive action to prevent death or permanent neurologic sequelae. Since the introduction of antibiotics, the mortality rate has remained between 5 and 40%; of the survivors, 30% suffer significant residual neurologic deficits. The prognosis is largely related to the time between the onset of symptoms and the start of effective therapy; therefore, presumptive diagnosis and empiric therapy are necessary. This article focuses on these aspects of initial management.

DIAGNOSIS

Acute bacterial meningitis must be considered in the differential diagnosis of any patient presenting with fever, headache, and signs of meningeal irritation. The presentation may be quite subtle, particularly in the very young and very old and in patients who have received antibiotics; therefore, particular care is required in order to avoid overlooking patients whose only symptoms are changes in mental status. Once suspicion has been raised, the diagnosis of bacterial meningitis rests on the cerebrospinal fluid (CSF) examination. If there are no signs of papilledema or focal neurologic deficits, lumbar puncture should be performed immediately. If there are signs suggestive of an intracranial mass, blood cultures should be obtained and empiric antibiotics administered while one awaits the results of computed tomography (CT) of the head. The classic CSF findings in bacterial meningitis include a cell count of over 1000 per mm^3 with a predominance of neutrophils, a protein concentration over 150 mg per dL, and a glucose concentration below 40 mg per dL. These values are not absolute, and any single parameter may be normal in 10 to 30% of patients with proven bacterial meningitis.

The most valuable study is a careful examination of a Gram-stained sediment of centrifuged CSF. In patients who have not received antibiotics, the CSF Gram's stain is positive in 80 to 90% of culture-confirmed cases. In patients who have been previously treated, Gram's stain is positive in 60 to 70%. In patients who have negative CSF Gram's stains, especially those whose stains may have been rendered negative by prior antibiotics, latex agglutination methods to detect bacterial antigens may increase the sensitivity over that of

---

*The views expressed in this article are those of the author and not of the United States Army.

TABLE 1. **Cerebrospinal Fluid Gram's Stain Morphology and Antibiotic Recommendations**

Morphology	Common Pathogens	Treatment of Choice	Alternative Therapy
Gram-positive cocci in short chains and pairs	*Streptococcus pneumoniae* Group B streptococci	Penicillin G	Cefotaxime* or chloramphenicol
Gram-positive cocci in clusters	*Staphylococcus aureus*	Nafcillin	Vancomycin†
Gram-positive bacilli	*Listeria monocytogenes*	Ampicillin ± aminoglycosides‡	Trimethoprim-sulfamethoxazole
Gram-negative cocci	*Neisseria meningitidis*	Penicillin G	Cefotaxime* or chloramphenicol
Gram-negative coccobacilli	*Haemophilus influenzae*	Cefotaxime*	Ampicillin + chloramphenicol
Gram-negative bacilli	*Escherichia coli* *Klebsiella* *Pseudomonas aeruginosa*	Cefotaxime* Ceftazidime + aminoglycoside	Trimethoprim-sulfamethoxazole —§
No definitive Gram's stain		Ampicillin + cefotaxime*	

*Ceftriaxone may be subtituted for cefotaxime.
†Vancomycin penetration in CSF may be variable.
‡Gentamicin, tobramycin, and amikacin may all be used based on local susceptibilities.
§No alternative therapy has been clinically proven reliable. Infectious diseases consultation is recommended in these difficult cases.

the Gram's stain alone. Clinical judgment is required, and no single test should be the basis for withholding antibiotics.

ANTIBIOTIC SELECTION

Because the timeliness of therapy is a prime predictor of outcome in bacterial meningitis, antibiotics usually must be chosen before the results of CSF cultures are known. If organisms are seen on Gram's stain, therapy may be directed by the morphology. Table 1 lists likely CSF pathogens and treatments of choice based on Gram's stain morphology. When Gram's stain fails to show any organisms, antibiotics must be chosen empirically on the basis of age of the patient (Table 2) and other epidemiologic clues (Table 3). Once culture results are known, these empiric

choices can be modified according to the culture and sensitivity data.

It is important that the antibiotics used be rapidly bactericidal and have adequate penetration into the CSF. It is also important that antibiotics be given in maximal doses (Table 4), because bactericidal activity of antibiotics in the CSF is dose dependent, and CSF penetration under the best of conditions is only a fraction of the serum level. Finally, care should be taken not to use combinations of bacteriostatic and bactericidal drugs, in order to avoid antagonizing the bactericidal activity of the therapy.

SPECIAL CONSIDERATIONS

Over the past 10 years, first in Europe and then in the United States, there has been a slow

TABLE 2. **Antibiotic Recommendations, by Age Group**

Age Group	Common Pathogens	Empiric Drug of Choice	Alternative Drug
Neonates (<1 month)	Group B streptococcus *Escherichia coli* *Listeria monocytogenes*	Ampicillin + aminoglycoside†	Cefotaxime* + aminoglycoside†
Infants (1–3 months)	*Haemophilus influenzae* *Neisseria meningitidis* *Streptococcus pneumoniae* Group B streptococci *Listeria monocytogenes*	Ampicillin + cefotaxime*	Ampicillin + aminoglycoside†
Young Children (3 months–7 years)	*H. influenzae* *S. pneumoniae* *N. meningitidis*	Cefotaxime*	Ampicillin + chloramphenicol
Older Children and Adults (>7 years)	*N. meningitidis* *S. pneumoniae*	Penicillin G	Cefotaxime*

*Ceftriaxone can be substituted.
†Gentamicin, tobramycin, and amikacin can all be used on the basis of local susceptibilities.

TABLE 3. **Antibiotic Recommendations for Special Hosts**

Condition	Common Pathogens	Empiric Choice
Transplant patients	*Listeria monocytogenes*	Ampicillin + aminoglycoside
Closed head trauma	*Streptococcus pneumoniae*	Penicillin G
Asplenia	*Neisseria meningitidis*	Cefotaxime*
	S. pneumoniae	
	Haemophilus influenzae	
Terminal complement deficiency	*Neisseria meningitidis*	Penicillin G
Post neurosurgical procedure	Gram-negative bacilli	Nafcillin + ceftazidime
	Pseudomonas aeruginosa	
	Staphylococcus aureus	
	S. epidermidis	
CSF shunts	*S. epidermidis*	Vancomycin† + ceftazidime
	S. aureus	
	Gram-negative bacilli	
Elderly patients	*S. pneumoniae*	Penicillin G
Recurrent meningitis	*S. pneumoniae*	Penicillin G
Alcoholic patients	*S. pneumoniae*	Penicillin G + cefotaxime*
	Gram-negative bacilli	

Abbreviation: CSF = cerebrospinal fluid.
*Ceftriaxone can be substituted for cefotaxime.
†May also consider shunt removal and intraventricular vancomycin.

but steady increase in the percentage of strains of *Streptococcus pneumoniae* that demonstrate relative resistance to penicillin. At present these account for approximately 5 to 15% of blood and CSF isolates in the United States. There have been a number of treatment failures when penicillin was used alone to treat meningitis due to these strains. All pneumococcal isolates should be screened with an oxacillin disc, and if found to be resistant to oxacillin, the treatment of choice is cefotaxime (Claforan) or ceftriaxone (Rhocephin).

Meningitis due to *Pseudomonas aeruginosa* should be treated with ceftazidime (Fortaz) and an aminoglycoside. Data regarding the effectiveness of intrathecal aminoglycosides are insufficient to warrant their routine use. Patients with organisms resistant to ceftazidime or who fail to respond to conventional therapy might benefit from intraventricular aminoglycosides. Infectious disease consultation should be obtained to assist in this decision.

Patients with ventriculoatrial or ventriculoperitoneal shunt–associated meningitis are most reliably treated by shunt removal in addition to antibiotics. Certain patients may be treated with the shunt in place; however, infectious disease consultation should be obtained before this is attempted.

Traditionally, the duration of therapy for meningococcal, pneumococcal, and *Haemophilus influenzae* meningitides has been 2 weeks; 3 weeks are recommended for gram-negative bacillary meningitis. However, more recent research has shown that 7 to 10 days of therapy are probably sufficient for *Neisseria meningitidis* and *H. influenzae* infections. Patients must be monitored carefully, and treatment should be prolonged in those who are slow to respond.

TABLE 4. **Antibiotic Doses in Bacterial Meningitis**

Antibiotic	Daily Adult Dose	Daily Pediatric Dose	Dose Interval
Amikacin (Amikin)	15 mg/kg	20 mg/kg	8 h
Ampicillin (Polycillin)	12 gm	200 mg/kg	4 h
Cefotaxime (Claforan)	12 gm	200 mg/kg	4 h
Ceftazidime (Fortaz)	6 gm	150 mg/kg	8 h
Ceftriaxone (Rocephin)	2 gm	100 mg/kg*	12 h
Chloramphenicol (Chloromycetin)	4 gm	75 mg/kg†	6 h
Gentamicin (Garamycin)	5 mg/kg	7.5 mg/kg	8 h
Nafcillin (Unipen)	12 gm	200 mg/kg	4 h
Penicillin G	24 million U	250,000 U/kg	4 h
Tobramycin (Nebcin)	5 mg/kg	6 mg/kg	8 h
Trimethoprim-sulfamethoxazole (Bactrim)	10 mg/kg‡	10 mg/kg	8 h

*Ceftriaxone is not recommended for neonates (<28 d) because it may displace bilirubin from albumin-binding sites.
†Ideally serum levels should be monitored in pediatric patients.
‡Dosing based on trimethoprim component.

Repeated lumbar punctures are not necessary in patients who respond well to therapy and may serve only to confuse the issue. Follow-up cultures to document sterilization of the CSF are indicated in patients who have an inadequate clinical response or who deteriorate on therapy and in those in whom the diagnosis is unclear or the meningitis is due to unusual organisms (e.g., *Listeria*).

ADJUNCTIVE THERAPY

A great deal of attention has recently been given to the use of corticosteroids in bacterial meningitis. Several studies have shown that neurologic sequelae, particularly hearing loss, are significantly decreased in pediatric patients given corticosteroids. The recommended steroid dose in infants and children is 0.15 mg of dexamethasone per kg every 6 hours for 4 days beginning at the time of the first dose of antibiotics. Although some data support the use of corticosteroids in adults with bacterial meningitis, it is not possible to make a firm recommendation for their general use at this time.

Infants and children with meningitis should have fluids restricted to 800 to 1000 ml per mm^2 per day to prevent cerebral edema. Mannitol may be employed if hypotension or dehydration require use of additional intravenous fluids. The head of the bed should be elevated to approximately 30 degrees. Intracranial pressure monitoring should be considered for children with alteration of consciousness.

Hearing impairment has been reported in 3 to 30% of children with bacterial meningitis. Evoked response audiometry is the most sensitive technique to detect subtle hearing loss and should be performed before the patient's hospital discharge. If the initial results are abnormal, audiometry should be repeated in 6 to 8 weeks, as hearing loss noted early may improve or disappear during a period of weeks to months.

PREVENTION

Prophylactic antibiotics are employed in documented cases of meningitis due to *N. meningitidis* and *H. influenzae* in order to eliminate nasopharyngeal carriage of the organisms among contacts and prevent invasive disease. In meningococcal meningitis, prophylaxis is indicated only for household or intimate contacts of an index case and is not necessary for casual contacts or medical personnel except those who have performed mouth-to-mouth resuscitation. The preferred agent for prophylaxis is rifampin at a dose of 10 mg per kg (or 600 mg in adults) twice a day for 2 days.

Chemoprophylaxis for *H. influenzae* meningitis is recommended for all household contacts of an index case if one of the contacts is less than 4 years old. It is also necessary for the index case in *H. influenzae* because *Haemophilus* organisms are not reliably eradicated from the nasopharynx by intravenous antibiotics. The preferred regimen for prophylaxis against *H. influenzae* is rifampin, 20 mg per kg (or 600 mg in adults) for 4 days.

INFECTIOUS MONONUCLEOSIS

method of
LAWRENCE J. D'ANGELO, M.D., M.P.H.
Children's National Medical Center
Washington, D.C.

Infectious mononucleosis is characterized by fever, malaise, pharyngitis, and diffuse lymphadenopathy. Laboratory findings of atypical lymphocytosis, mild hepatitis, and the presence of heterophile antibodies help to confirm the diagnosis.

Most cases of infectious mononucleosis are caused by the Epstein-Barr virus. Illnesses indistinguishable clinically from that caused by this virus include acute infections with cytomegalovirus, *Toxoplasma gondii*, herpesvirus 6, adenovirus, Coxsackie B virus, and the human immunodeficiency virus. However, taken together these agents account for only a little more than 10% of all cases of infectious mononucleosis. For this reason, this discussion is limited to illness caused by the Epstein-Barr virus.

While individuals of any age can be infected by this member of the herpesvirus family, overt illness is most common in adolescents and young adults. Acute infection in children usually results in a brief febrile illness, with or without other symptoms. In contrast, those between the ages of 13 and 29 are usually ill for at least 2 to 3 weeks, with particularly persistent fatigue seen in approximately 10% of those affected. The usual incubation period varies from 21 to 49 days. After acute symptoms subside, infected individuals may shed virus in their saliva intermittently for years.

TREATMENT

In immunocompetent hosts, Epstein-Barr virus infections will spontaneously improve and ultimately remit without specific treatment. The most common symptoms of pharyngitis, fever, and lymphadenopathy deserve attention, however.

Symptomatic treatment of pharyngitis with warm salt water gargles followed by anesthetic gargles (lidocaine, 2%, or phenol, 1.4%) speeds the resolution of throat symptoms. All patients with infectious mononucleosis should have routine throat cultures since 8 to 33% will have concomitant infection with beta-hemolytic *Strepto-*

coccus pyogenes. Those with positive cultures should be treated with phenoxymethyl penicillin (Pen VK), 500 mg twice daily. This regimen is as effective as the more common 250 mg four times a day and greatly improves compliance, particularly in adolescents.

Fever usually lasts from 5 to 14 days. Acetaminophen, 650 to 1000 mg every 4 to 6 hours, is preferred over aspirin and other nonsteroidal anti-inflammatory agents because of their potential to exacerbate the splenic or antibody-induced thrombocytopenia that can occur.

Lymphadenopathy is rarely problematic unless manifested by tonsillar hypertrophy that threatens to compromise the airway or by massive splenomegaly with concomitant pain, thrombocytopenia, and anemia. Prednisolone, in tapering dosage from 60 to 5 mg over a 2-week course, can reverse the lymphoid hyperplasia that produces these symptoms. While the administration of glucocorticoids to patients with acute infection seems intuitively questionable, most objections are theoretical or based solely on anecdotal evidence.

More important than specific drug therapy for splenomegaly is the avoidance of all contact sports for at least 4 weeks after the diagnosis of infectious mononucleosis, regardless of the examiner's ability to demonstrate splenomegaly. Persistence of splenomegaly beyond this period requires avoidance of risky activities until 2 weeks after a palpable spleen can no longer be demonstrated.

COMPLICATIONS

Acute airway compromise resulting from tonsillar hypertrophy necessitates an aggressive approach, with 60 mg of intravenous methylprednisolone given every 6 hours. Tracheal intubation may be difficult, so appropriate preparations for tracheostomy should be made. After intravenous therapy is discontinued, oral glucocorticoids should be tapered as suggested previously.

Patients who develop left upper quadrant pain should be evaluated for either traumatic or spontaneous splenic rupture. While this complication occurs in fewer than 0.2% of patients with infectious mononucleosis, virtually all affected patients should undergo splenectomy.

Patients who develop hemolytic anemia, severe granulocytopenia, or immune thrombocytopenic purpura will usually need corticosteroid therapy. While the regimen discussed in the previous section is appropriate, a longer course of therapy may be necessary.

Neurologic complications include Bell's palsy, aseptic meningitis, encephalitis, Guillain-Barré syndrome, and transverse myelitis. The first two conditions usually require no special therapy. While support for its use in encephalitis is not universal, acyclovir (Zovirax), 5 to 10 mg per kg intravenously every 8 hours, may help. Early plasmapheresis is important in patients with Guillain-Barré syndrome. Given its usual poor outcome, transverse myelitis may warrant a combination of prednisolone and acyclovir.

Pulmonary and cardiac manifestations are rare. Glucocorticoids probably will help in more protracted cases.

When Epstein-Barr infection occurs in an individual with X-linked immunodeficiency (Duncan's syndrome), an overwhelming progressive and potentially fatal infection may result. Some combination of acyclovir, glucocorticoids, and intravenous gamma globulin may ultimately prove to be lifesaving. Unfortunately, no such regimen has been tested.

Finally, despite much controversy, there is little factual information to suggest that the small subset of patients with persistent or recurrent symptoms ("chronic mononucleosis") require specific therapy.

MUMPS

method of
ROBERT A. BROUGHTON, M.D.
University of Kentucky Medical Center
Lexington, Kentucky

Mumps is a moderately debilitating communicable disease of children and young adults that is caused by the paramyxovirus mumps virus.

After the introduction of the live mumps virus vaccine in 1967 and recommendation of its routine use in 1977, the incidence of mumps decreased steadily in the United States through 1985. However, a relative resurgence of mumps occurred beginning in 1986 and extending at least through 1989. Accompanying this increase in incidence was a change in the age distribution of reported cases, with the most dramatic increases occurring among 10 to 19 year olds, a cohort of individuals not vaccinated in infancy. Increases in incidence occurred primarily in states lacking comprehensive mumps immunization laws; this suggests that much of the increase in incidence was due to a failure to vaccinate, rather than vaccine failure. Recently, however, mumps outbreaks have been reported in highly vaccinated populations, suggesting that mumps vaccine failure has played a role in continued mumps virus activity in the United States. The relative contribution of primary vaccine failure and of secondary vaccine failure (waning immunity) to continuing mumps activity remains an unresolved issue.

Mumps virus is transmitted via the respiratory route; the disease is considered only slightly less contagious than measles and varicella. Most cases occur in late winter and early spring. Subclinical infection is seen in 30%. Infection usually provides lifelong immunity, although re-infection has been described in 1 to 2%.

The incubation period is usually 16 to 18 days, with a range of 12 to 25 days. The period of communicability is usually 1 to 2 days but occasionally as long as 7 days before onset of parotid swelling and usually extends 5 days, but occasionally as long as 9 days, after onset.

Mumps is a systemic disease that can involve multiple organs. Like many other viral infections, mumps is more severe in older children and adults. Parotid swelling is the most commonly recognized manifestation, although other salivary glands may be involved. Glandular pain when salivation is stimulated is a variable sign. Parotitis may be preceded or accompanied by a variety of nonspecific symptoms.

Epididymo-orchitis is the most common nonsalivary manifestation, occurring primarily in postpubertal males (incidence 30 to 38%). Testicular involvement is usually unilateral, but in 17 to 38% of cases is bilateral. Atrophy of the involved testis may occur, but sterility is a rare complication.

Meningoencephalitis is relatively common in mumps. Meningeal signs are reported in as many as 15% of patients and may be accompanied by cerebrospinal fluid mononuclear pleocytosis, elevated protein, and normal or low glucose concentrations. Encephalitis complicates 0.5% of cases and has an average case fatality rate of 1.4%. Nerve deafness can occur in the absence of meningoencephalitis.

Other complications of mumps include arthritis, renal dysfunction, mastitis, oophoritis, thyroiditis, myocarditis, and pancreatitis. Women who acquire mumps in the first trimester of pregnancy have an increased rate of spontaneous abortion, but there is no evidence that mumps infection produces congenital malformations.

Diagnosis of mumps infection can be established by culture or serology. The virus has been isolated from throat swabs, urine, and spinal fluid. Production of antibody can be assayed by complement fixation, hemagglutination inhibition, enzyme immunoassay, and neutralization tests; the latter two techniques are the most reliable, but they are not as readily available.

THERAPY

In the absence of specific therapy for mumps, which is a self-limited infection, supportive measures are employed. Analgesics may be necessary for discomfort due to parotitis or orchitis as well as headache. Acetaminophen is usually effective, although some patients with orchitis require narcotics such as codeine or meperidine. Either warm or cool compress applications may help individual patients; topical ointments are not beneficial. Particular attention should be paid to maintenance of adequate hydration and nutrition. Some patients may have exacerbation of parotid pain with acid foods, such as orange juice.

Rarely, parenteral administration of fluids may be necessary for patients with persistent vomiting associated with meningoencephalitis or pancreatitis.

No antiviral agent is indicated for the treatment of mumps. Administration of antibody in the form of gamma globulin is not appropriate; mumps immune globulin is no longer available.

PREVENTION

The principal strategy to prevent mumps is to achieve and maintain high immunization levels, particularly in infants and young children.

Live mumps vaccine is prepared in chick embryo cell culture from the Jeryl Lynn strain of mumps virus. Mumps vaccine is available both in monovalent form and in combination with rubella or measles and rubella.

In controlled trials with up to 20 months of follow-up, mumps vaccine was 95% effective in preventing disease. In outbreak-based studies, however, vaccine efficacy has been lower, ranging from 75 to 91%.

All susceptible children, adolescents, and adults should be vaccinated against mumps, in the absence of contraindications (discussed later). According to the Immunization Practices Advisory Committee, persons should be considered as susceptible to mumps unless they have documentation of (1) physician-diagnosed mumps, (2) adequate immunization with live mumps vaccine on or after their first birthday, or (3) laboratory evidence of immunity to mumps. Most persons born before 1957 are likely to have been infected naturally between 1957 and 1977 and generally may be considered to be immune, even if they did not have clinically recognized mumps. However, this does not preclude vaccination of possibly susceptible persons born before 1957 who may be exposed in outbreak situations. Persons who are unsure of their mumps disease history or vaccination history should be vaccinated; testing for susceptibility before vaccination is not necessary, since the vaccine is not harmful when inadvertently given to immune individuals.

Mumps vaccine should be given routinely to children after the first birthday. It is usually given in combination with measles and rubella vaccines (MMR) at 15 months of age. A second dose of MMR is now recommended at entry to middle school (sixth grade) or elementary school (kindergarten); mumps revaccination is especially advisable since infection can occur in highly vaccinated populations. Mumps vaccination is of particular value for children approaching puberty and for adolescents and adults who have not had mumps. It may be given simultaneously with other vaccines.

When given after exposure to mumps, mumps vaccine may not provide protection; however, immunization will provide protection against subsequent exposures.

Adverse reactions attributable to mumps vaccine are uncommon. Mild parotitis, fever, and rash have been reported; orchitis is very rare. The frequency of central nervous system complications after mumps vaccination is no greater than the observed background rate of CNS dysfunction in the general population.

In regard to precautions and contraindications, it is prudent to avoid immunization of pregnant women or women who anticipate becoming pregnant within 3 months, even though there is no evidence that mumps vaccine causes congenital malformations. Mumps vaccine is produced in chick embryo cell culture and contains trace amounts of neomycin. Patients with a history of anaphylactic reactions to egg should be given vaccine only with extreme caution using established protocols. Patients with nonanaphylactic reactions to egg as well as those with allergies to chickens or feathers can be vaccinated in the usual manner. Persons who have experienced anaphylactic reactions (not contact dermatitis) to neomycin should not be vaccinated. Since passively acquired antibody can interfere with the response to live, attenuated virus vaccines, mumps vaccine should be given at least 2 weeks before or 3 months after administration of immune globulin or blood transfusion. Mumps vaccine, being a live vaccine, should be avoided in patients with primary or secondary immunodeficiency states, such as those with immunodeficiency diseases and those receiving immunosuppressive drug or radiation therapy. The exception is children with human immunodeficiency virus infection, who should receive MMR vaccine at the usual age. The risk of mumps exposure for immunosuppressed patients may be reduced by vaccinating their close contacts; vaccinated persons do not transmit mumps vaccine virus. Vaccine administration need not be postponed in children with minor illnesses, with or without fever; those with more serious illnesses should generally not be vaccinated until they have recovered.

For controlling mumps outbreaks in closed populations such as schools, exclusion of susceptible individuals from affected institutions and those judged by local health authorities to be at risk for transmission should be considered. Excluded individuals can be readmitted immediately following vaccination; those who have been exempted from mumps vaccination should be excluded until at least 26 days after the onset of parotitis in the last person with mumps in the affected institution.

PLAGUE

method of
DONALD A. ROMIG, M.D.
University of New Mexico School of Medicine
Santa Fe, New Mexico

Plague is an ancient infection caused by *Yersinia pestis,* an encapsulated gram-negative bacterium. The disease is acquired incidentally by humans entering the flea-animal-flea cycle. The disease exists worldwide, but it is uncommon in the United States. Most recent cases in the United States have been reported in New Mexico; scattered cases have occurred in several other states, including California, Nevada, Arizona, Idaho, Colorado, and Utah.

Epidemics of plague periodically swept through Europe, most notably in the fifteenth century, fueled by the abundant rat population in both urban and rural communities. In the United States, the disease is transmitted by fleas that infect wild rodents and other animals such as coyotes, prairie dogs, domesticated animals, and rabbits. The pressure of population growth has caused deeper invasion of the territory of wild animals, allowing greater exposure of humans and their domestic animals to the natural reservoir of wild animals and their infected fleas.

Most cases of plague are acquired by humans whose occupational or avocational activities make contact with flea-carrying animals likely. Domestic pets that hunt represent an increasing reservoir for transmission to humans as witnessed by the plethora of infected domestic cats in New Mexico in 1992. An urban epidemic is still possible, since some urban rat populations have been found to be infected with *Y. pestis.*

Plague is generally recognized early in its course in endemic areas and treated promptly and appropriately. However, in this time of rapid travel, persons who leave endemic areas with incubating plague may not be diagnosed and treated promptly or appropriately when symptoms develop.

CLINICAL MANIFESTATIONS

Plague must be considered in the differential diagnosis of fever and painful lymphadenopathy. Factors of historical significance include exposure in an endemic area, exposure to hunting domestic pets, an exposure time 2 to 7 days before onset of symptoms, fever, malaise, diarrhea, and a history of flea bites, although the latter is often unknown or absent. The physical examination may reveal in addition to fever an exquisitely tender bubo—a lymph node with marked surrounding edema and often erythema. Most cases of plague (85 to 90%) present with a bubo, i.e., bubonic plague. The disease presents classically in two other forms: septicemic (10 to 15%) and primary pneumonic (less than 1%).

Most buboes occur in the inguinal or femoral nodes, but other lymph nodes may be involved, depending upon the site of the initial flea bite. In septicemic plague, no buboes are detected and systemic symptoms predominate, such as fever, diarrhea, nausea, vomiting, and malaise. Shock may follow with skin changes that gave rise to the term "black death." Approximately 5 to 10% of septicemic plague cases have concomitant pneumonia infiltrates, hilar or mediastinal adenopathy, or both. Cough, shortness of breath, tachypnea, and cyanosis may or may not be present. These patients pose a hazard to family members, health personnel, and others having close contact because coughing can aerosolize the plague organisms. Primary pneumonic plague, which is acquired by inhaling these aerosolized organisms, is rare but rapidly fatal in 2 to 3 days.

DIAGNOSIS

The major obstacle to correct diagnosis of plague is failure to include it in the differential diagnosis. The nature of this infectious process is primarily revealed through a detailed history, including information about travel, wild and domestic animal exposure, and occupational and avocational activities. The physical examination and laboratory values are used in a confirmatory way in the differential diagnostic process.

When a bubo is obvious, a rapid diagnosis can be obtained by aspiration of the node, under strict precautions to guard against aerosolization, followed by stains, cultures, and fluorescence studies. The Gram stain and preferably the Wayson stain can be done immediately; the Wayson stain more commonly shows the characteristic bipolar rods resembling a safety pin. Smears from blood cultures can be stained similarly. However the fluorescent antibody test specific for Y. pestis is the most sensitive and specific staining technique; it is available upon request from state health laboratories and can be obtained on an emergent basis. When no bubo is observed, yet the epidemiology and the constitutional symptoms suggest plague, blood cultures are the most productive diagnostic technique. At least two blood cultures are recommended.

Patients with a suggestive epidemiologic history should be treated as if septicemic plague were present, before bacteriologic confirmation and shortly after blood cultures are obtained. Reexamination of a patient suspected to have septicemic plague may yield a previously undiscovered bubo, which can still be aspirated for a more rapid diagnosis by fluorescent staining techniques if blood cultures have not yet demonstrated the organism. The organisms in the bubo will retain their specific fluorescent staining pattern even after appropriate therapy has begun.

Blood cultures may require 2 or 3 days of incubation before becoming positive. Informing the bacteriologic laboratory that plague is suspected will yield dividends because processing, staining, and transportation to state laboratories are facilitated and the diagnosis expedited. In some instances Y. pestis can be demonstrated on ordinary blood smears when the level of bacteremia is very high.

Certain other hematologic studies are extremely helpful. Although septicemia from organisms other than Y. pestis may present with similar features, special attention should be directed to the total white blood cell count (WBC) and the differential. The WBC is characteristically elevated, with numerous banded polymorphonuclear leukocytes. In addition, and characteristically, the platelet count is low (below 150,000/mL). Fibrin split products may be elevated. Other nonspecific chemical abnormalities may be present, but these are less helpful.

Serologic studies to diagnose plague are quite sensitive. Since these tests do not become positive until 10 days to 2 weeks after infection, they are relatively useless for planning initial therapy. If all cultures are negative then serologic studies are used to confirm the diagnosis of plague, especially if initial therapy has been appropriate.

Differential diagnosis of plague includes diseases that mimic sepsis or systemic toxicity with painful localized lymphadenitis: streptococcal or staphylococcal disease, cat scratch fever, tularemia, unidentified sepsis, and incarcerated inguinal hernia. Rarely is plague considered in the differential diagnosis of lymphadenopathy with a more indolent presentation, such as granuloma inguinale, genital herpetic infections, adenopathy associated with human immunodeficiency virus, and low-grade fungus infection of the groin with some secondary bacterial involvement.

Plague meningitis occurs in approximately 6% of persons with septicemic plague. It usually does not appear until 7 to 10 days after treatment has been started, and often the cerebrospinal fluid is sterile by culture with no organisms seen by staining techniques. Meningeal involvement should be suspected in every patient with septicemic plague who has continued fever, persistent headache, or signs of meningeal irritation on examination.

TREATMENT

Treatment must begin as soon as possible, even before definitive diagnosis. The mortality rate of untreated plague is high: 50% in bubonic plague and much higher—up to 100% in some reports—in septicemic and pneumonic plague. Suspected plague should be promptly reported to state public health officials to facilitate contact tracing and epidemiologic investigations.

If on initial evaluation no respiratory symptoms are present and chest x-rays, including a lateral film, are negative, therapy can proceed without isolation. If symptoms or x-ray findings indicate pulmonary involvement, strict respiratory isolation should be maintained for 72 to 96 hours after the start of therapy.

Streptomycin is the drug of choice for all types of plague. Clinical experience with intravenous gentamicin shows it to be equally effective, but no in vivo studies are available to confirm this impression. If shock is present or absorption of intramuscular medication (streptomycin) is problematic, intravenous gentamicin is preferable. Gentamicin may be the drug of choice in suspected plague when the presenting signs are those of septicemia.

The dose of streptomycin is 30 mg per kg per day in two divided doses intramuscularly for 10 days. The dose of gentamicin is 3 to 5 mg per kg per day in three divided doses. Usually a loading dose of 2 mg per kg is given initially. The course of streptomycin may be shortened in milder cases: streptomycin is given for 3 to 5 days, then the 10-day course is completed with oral tetracycline at a dose of 15 mg per kg per day in four divided doses. Streptomycin toxicity is rarely seen except in pregnant women and in the elderly with pre-existing vestibular or auditory disease. Tetracycline should not be used in children, to avoid staining of immature teeth. Trimethoprim-sulfamethoxazole has been reported to be effective in the treatment of plague. Plague meningitis or plague involving unusual locations, (e.g., tonsils or localized abscesses) is best treated with chloramphenicol, 25 to 40 mg per kg per day in four divided doses intravenously or by mouth. Chloramphenicol penetrates tissue sites and easily crosses the blood-brain barrier.

In light of the large number of organisms in buboes and several reported cases of recurrent plague meningitis, treatment for longer than 10 days may occasionally be warranted. Treatment for longer than 10 days is indicated if *Y. pestis* is demonstrated by staining techniques or culture from draining buboes. On rare occasions, persistent painful buboes may need either excision or drainage to facilitate healing. If reculture of these incised or excised buboes shows organisms other than *Y. pestis,* another antibiotic may be needed. In vitro sensitivities of plague organisms may be misleading, so time-honored antibiotics are indicated.

PREVENTION

Avoidance of plague is obviously desirable, but exposure can occur by indirect contact. Handling of flea-bearing wild animals or their carcasses is to be avoided. Rodent habitats and food sources around homes in endemic areas should be destroyed. Domestic pets with potential contact with rodents and carcasses should undergo regular flea control procedures at 2- to 3-week intervals during the summer months.

Vaccination against plague is available and may be beneficial for occupationally high-risk individuals. Although not a preventative, the vaccine does reduce the severity of plague.

Prevention of plague in household contacts, laboratory workers, hospital personnel, and other inadvertently exposed persons can be accomplished with one of two oral antibiotics. Tetracycline (15 mg/kg/day) or trimethoprim-sulfamethoxazole (40 mg/kg/day of sulfa) is administered by mouth. Antibiotic prophylaxis is indicated when exposure to aerosolized organisms is suspected or proved.

PSITTACOSIS
(Ornithosis)

method of
BARBARA A. CROSSE, B.Sc., MB.ChB.
Leeds, United Kingdom

Psittacosis is a worldwide human disease caused by *Chlamydia psittaci* of avian origin. The organism is an obligate intracellular bacterium. Approximately 300 cases are reported in the United States annually. Atypical pneumonia in a young or middle-aged adult is the usual presentation; infection is rare in children. Antibiotics have reduced the mortality rate from 20% to 1%. Recognized sources include parrots, budgerigars, pigeons, ducks, and poultry, hence the term "ornithosis." Infected birds, often asymptomatic, shed the organism in feces, especially when stressed. Humans become infected by inhaling aerosolized feces or from infected secretions. Sporadic cases arise from pets, pet shops, aviaries, and pigeon lofts. Outbreaks have occurred on poultry farms and processing factories. Human-to-human transmission is rare.

Chlamydia pneumoniae, recently recognized, also causes respiratory disease. It is transmitted between humans, and there is no known animal reservoir. Infection is common and affects all ages.

The ovine strain of *C. psittaci* causes enzootic abortion in sheep. Pregnant women are particularly susceptible to this potentially lethal infection.

CLINICAL MANIFESTATIONS

The incubation period is 1 to 2 weeks, and the onset is variable. Typical symptoms are fever, a dry or minimally productive cough, chills, myalgia, and prominent headache. Gastrointestinal symptoms and altered mentation are relatively frequent. Inspiratory crackles are often the only respiratory sign. Splenomegaly and relative bradycardia may be present. The leukocyte count is usually low or normal. X-ray changes often exceed clinical findings. Consolidation is common in the lower lobes and frequently multilobar. Rare manifestations include a typhoid-like presentation, meningitis, encephalitis, erythema nodosum, hepatitis, and endocarditis.

Chlamydia pneumoniae usually causes mild pneumonia, with sore throat or hoarseness and a single subsegmental lesion on x-ray. It also causes sinusitis, otitis media, and acute bronchitis.

Ovine psittacosis can present as pneumonia but more frequently manifests as overwhelming sepsis.

DIAGNOSIS

Diagnosis requires a high degree of suspicion, and the physician should enquire about contact with birds. The major differential diagnoses are influenza and infection with *Mycoplasma pneumoniae*, *Legionella* species, and *Coxiella burnetii*. Typhoid and brucellosis should also be considered.

The diagnosis is confirmed serologically by the complement fixation test. Antibodies usually rise within 2 weeks and a fourfold rise or fall confirms infection. A titer of greater than 1:32 with a compatible clinical illness is suggestive. The microimmunofluorescence test distinguishes between *Chlamydia* species. Diagnostic criteria for *C. pneumoniae* infection are a fourfold change in antibody levels, a titer greater than 1:512, and the presence of IgM. Antibodies may not rise for 4 weeks.

TREATMENT

Tetracyclines are the treatment of choice for *C. psittaci* infection. Two grams daily, orally, for 10 to 14 days should be prescribed. Erythromycin, 500 mg orally every 6 hours, can be used as an alternative in pregnant women and children. Therapy should continue for at least 1 week after defervescence to avoid relapse. Repeat treatment should be with tetracycline when possible. These recommendations also apply to *C. pneumoniae* infection.

Experience with other drugs is limited. Potential advantages of clarithromycin (Biaxin) and azithromycin (Zithromax), are lower doses and fewer side effects. Ofloxacin (Floxin), may yet prove useful, but quinolones are not generally recommended for the treatment of community-acquired pneumonia.

Isolation is unnecessary. Case reporting is obligatory in the United States.

PREVENTION

Infected avian sources should be identified and either treated or destroyed. Premises should be quarantined and other infected birds identified. Imported exotic birds are quarantined for 35 days, during which tetracycline may be given. Prolonged treatment is required to eradicate infection and is often not completed. All persons exposed to a known source of infection should be monitored for signs of disease. No vaccine is available.

Pregnant women should avoid handling lambing or aborting ewes.

Q FEVER

method of
FREDERICK T. KOSTER, M.D.
University of New Mexico Hospital
Albuquerque, New Mexico

Q fever is a worldwide zoonotic disease caused by the rickettsia *Coxiella burnetii*. Humans become infected primarily by inhaling aerosols emanating from infected placenta, excrement, or hides or by ingestion of infected animal meat or milk. *C. burnetii* in these contaminated products, usually from cattle, sheep, goats, or cats, may survive for months in the inanimate environment.

PRESENTATION AND DIAGNOSIS

The acute phase has an incubation of 4 to 40 days and may be without clinical signs or marked by symptoms of fever, headache, myalgias, arthralgias, and malaise. An atypical pneumonitis may develop, accompanied by cough and dyspnea. A subacute hepatitis may occur, with elevated serum transaminase levels and right upper quadrant tenderness. Myocarditis and endometritis are rare. The chronic phase follows months after the acute phase, consists of hepatitis with or without culture-negative endocarditis, and is often fatal if untreated. Diagnosis of acute Q fever is made by specific serologic tests in which complement fixation or indirect immunofluorescence (IFA) antibody assays are used. Diagnosis of Q fever endocarditis is aided by high titers of anti–Phase I antibody, particularly in the IgA subclass.

TREATMENT

Although most cases of acute Q fever are self-limiting, diagnostic work-up and treatment should be pursued when pneumonitis or hepatitis is present because in these cases, endocarditis may be more likely to develop, especially if there is pre-existing valvular heart disease. On the basis of clinical experience, the drug of choice remains doxycycline (Vibramycin), 100 mg twice daily for 14 days; this treatment may reduce the duration of fever if begun within 3 days of the onset of the illness. Doxycycline is available generically. Alternative antibiotics are tetracycline, 500 mg four times daily; ofloxacin (Floxin), 400 mg twice daily; ciprofloxacin (Cipro), 500 mg twice daily; and norfloxacin (Noroxin), 400 mg twice daily. In vitro studies show that most isolates of *C. burnetii* are more sensitive to ofloxacin than to the other antibiotics just listed. Children may be treated with trimethoprim or chloramphenicol.

The optimal treatment of chronic Q fever is unclear because the use of tetracyclines is associated with relapses and clinical failures, and isolates from such cases are resistant in vitro to tetracyclines. Ciprofloxacin, 750 mg twice daily, or ofloxacin, 400 mg twice daily, may be the best choice, and synergy studies suggest that the addition of rifampin (Rifadin), 600 mg daily, may enhance the effect of the fluoroquinolones. Because cardiac valve replacements have been followed by repeated relapses, lifelong treatment may be necessary. It is unclear whether decreasing antibody titers provide a reliable index of therapeutic success.

PREVENTION

Prevention should be directed at individuals in high-risk occupations, such as abattoir workers, veterinarians, and people engaged in research on animals, particularly pregnant ungulates. In these groups, serosurveys should be conducted to detect recent *C. burnetii* infection, research ungulates should be vaccinated and infected animals handled in such a way that aerosols are avoided and contained. No human vaccine against *C. burnetii* is yet available.

RABIES

method of
MARK O. LOVELESS, M.D.
Oregon Health Sciences University
Portland, Oregon

Hieroglyphic writings of Egypt described rabies nearly 4500 years ago, and the Eshnunna Code of ancient Mesopotamia outlined animal control measures 2000 years ago. Time and technology have not blunted the terror that people feel at the threat of rabies. Many developed countries have successfully controlled most animal rabies, but it remains a major health risk for people in many of the world's poorer communities. There is no effective treatment for clinical rabies, and the case fatality rate is essentially 100%. In contrast, early identification and prophylaxis of rabies exposure completely prevents disease.

The exact number of human rabies cases is unknown. Approximately 100,000 cases of human rabies occur worldwide each year. This is 5 to 10 times the number of reported cases. Under-reporting is due to inadequate resources for public health and epidemiology, social stigma against persons with rabies, and the lack of any effective medical therapy, which results in reluctance to seek medical care. Fewer than 1% of all the reported cases of human rabies occur outside the tropics. In the developed world, the economic and emotional impact of evaluating animal bites for rabies prophylaxis exacts a much greater toll than the disease itself.

Infection of the peripheral nerve tissue at the site of infection initiates a sequence of events that inexorably leads to the death of the patient. If neutralization of the virus does not occur, the virus binds to specific receptors on the surface of peripheral nerves. The virus then ascends the nerve by retrograde axoplasmic flow to the ganglia and then into the central nuclei in the brain. Infection of the brain parenchyma is progressive; the virus spreads to most parts of the brain. There is a predilection for the limbic system, the reticular formation, the pontine tegmentum, and the nuclei of the cranial nerves at the floor of the fourth ventricle. Intracytoplasmic inclusion bodies (Negri bodies) are identifiable in nerve cells at this stage of infection and are pathognomonic of rabies. Histologic specimens demonstrate spongiform encephalopathy; however, there is very little inflammatory response and minimal necrosis. The relative lack of inflammation and neuronal damage in contrast to the profound encephalitic manifestations raises the possibility of interference with neurotransmission as a pathogenic mechanism.

At the height of cerebral infection, the virus moves back to the peripheral nerves and invades highly innervated areas such as the cornea, the skin of the head and neck, and the buccal mucous membranes. There is heavy secretion of the virus into saliva at a time when agitation and aggressive biting behavior are present, increasing the risk of transmission.

CLINICAL HUMAN RABIES

The differential diagnosis of any rapidly progressive encephalitis must include rabies. The disease progresses through a nonspecific prodrome to encephalopathy and death within 10 to 30 days. The prodromal period of rabies usually follows the bite by 2 to 8 weeks; however, incubation periods of more than 1 year are well documented. Bites to the head and neck and bites to highly innervated areas may result in a shorter incubation period. Local cutaneous symptoms include paresthesias, pain, and itching at the site of the inoculation, probably caused by viral excitation of the sensory ganglia. Constitutional symptoms include fatigue, sore throat, anorexia, headaches, fevers, cough, nausea, vomiting, and diarrhea. The patients who developed rabies after corneal transplant from an infected person reported retro-ocular pain.

The acute neurogenic period (furious or agitated rabies) follows the prodrome by 2 to 10 days. A generalized increase in neurologic activity is observed in association with agitation and aggressive behavior. The most profound and characteristic clinical manifestation is hydrophobia, an exaggerated respiratory protective reflex that results in violent but painless contractions of the diaphragm and inspiratory accessory muscle, triggered by attempts to swallow. Other cranial nerve manifestations include choking, drooling, and diplopia. Along with hydrophobia, there is central nervous system excitation with anxiety, disorientation, photophobia, and seizures. Autonomic excitation results in labile hypertension, hyperventilation, priapism, panic attacks, palpitations, hypothermia, and hyperthermia.

The paralytic phase (dumb rabies) may follow the agitated phase, or the disease may progress directly to the paralytic phase from the prodrome. Ascending symmetrical or asymmetrical paralysis leads to respiratory arrest and the need for mechanical ventilatory support. Hypothalamic and hypophyseal dysfunction may contribute to wasting, and myocardiopathy has been described. Ultimately, rabies culminates in coma and generalized multiorgan failure that inevitably leads to death.

LABORATORY DIAGNOSIS

Routine laboratory tests are nonspecific. Computed tomography and magnetic resonance scans are not diagnostic because of the lack of inflammation and edema. Electroencephalographic patterns reveal diffuse encephalitic and encephalopathic changes, but these findings are also nonspecific, not diagnostic of rabies.

Direct histologic and immunohistologic examination of infected tissue produces a definitive diagnosis of rabies. Biopsy specimens of brain, the skin from the head and neck area, the buccal mucous membranes, or touch imprints of the cornea should be submitted for immunofluorescent rabies antigen detection. A positive result on a test for rabies antigen in the cornea, buccal mucosa, or saliva has a high predictive value for rabies and may be positive before the serum antibody is present. The presence of Negri bodies in brain biopsy specimens is pathognomonic. Serum neutralizing antibodies, detected by any one of several methods, develop within 1 to 2 weeks of the onset of the prodrome. Positive antibodies are diagnostic in patients who have not received rabies immune globulin. Spinal fluid antirabies antibody at any titer is also highly predictive of rabies.

CLINICAL MANAGEMENT

Pre-exposure rabies prophylaxis is appropriate for veterinarians, animal handlers, and laboratory workers. In addition, any person who is likely to come into contact with wild or domestic animals that might be infected with rabies should consider vaccination. For example, this includes anyone who frequently explores caves where there are bat colonies and persons spending extended periods studying animals in India, Africa, or South America. Pre-exposure prophylaxis consists of 1.0 mL of human diploid cell vaccine (HDCV) (Imovax), given intramuscularly on days 0 (day of exposure), 7, and 21 or 28. Boosters are recommended every year.

Animal bites raise the issue of postexposure rabies immunotherapy (prophylaxis). When a patient has been bitten by an animal, the first step in the medical management is to define whether the exposure is rabies-prone. If the animal is one that is essentially rabies-free in the wild (rodents, birds, rabbits, opossums, reptiles), the patient should have appropriate local wound care with reassurance that no rabies prophylaxis is required.

If the bite or injury was caused by a rabies-prone animal that is captured, the postexposure protocol is initiated if (1) the animal has been observed and demonstrates signs of infection or (2) the animal has been euthanized and the brain specimen is positive for rabies infection. If the bite occurred during an unprovoked attack by a wild animal that escapes capture and evaluation, the postexposure immunotherapy protocol should be initiated.

Postexposure immunotherapy (prophylaxis), when performed according to the following protocol, is remarkably successful in preventing human rabies:

1. Wearing gloves, wash the wound thoroughly to remove any residual saliva that might contain rabies virus and to remove devitalized tissue.

2. Administer rabies immune globulin (RIG), 20 IU per kg: 50% around the wound itself and 50% in the buttock.

3. Administer HDCV (Imovax) in the deltoid muscle. The dose is 1.0 mL on days 0, 3, 7, 14, and 28 after the exposure.

4. Start empiric antibiotics, inasmuch as bacterial infections are common after animal bites.

5. Test serum rabies neutralizing antibody titers at 2 to 3 weeks and after the last dose; a titer of 1:5 or higher is associated with protection.

Some experts have suggested the use of local interferon injections; however, studies have not documented the efficacy of this approach. Several newer vaccine strategies with nonhuman cell culture systems (e.g., purified chick embryo cell [PCEC] and purified Vero cell rabies vaccine [PVRV]) are more economical for developing countries. The Semple vaccine, prepared from nerve tissue, should not be used unless absolutely necessary because of the risk of neuroparalytic complications.

Without postexposure prophylaxis, there is a 10 to 15% chance that rabies will develop after the bite of a rabid animal. Only three people have survived documented rabies. Each of these patients required prolonged supportive therapy, including mechanical ventilation, and suffered significant neurologic residua. There is no effective antiviral therapy for rabies once the neurologic infection has been established. Limited trials with alpha-interferon have been unsuccessful. There are no antiviral medications with significant activity, and the intraneuron site of the infection is a profound barrier to the penetration of any therapeutic agent. Corticosteroid therapy should be avoided because inflammation plays very little role in the pathogenesis of rabies and there is a risk of more rapid progression of infection and higher viral titers in the saliva. Supportive and symptomatic therapy may include antiseizure medications, sedatives, analgesics, and neuroleptics.

INFECTION CONTROL

The rabies virus may enter through breaks in the skin or intact mucous membrane, may be inhaled as an aerosol, or may be acquired in an infected corneal graft. Blood products do not transmit rabies. Four cases of corneal transplant–associated rabies are the only known examples of human-to-human rabies transmission. Human rabies has never occurred after the bite of an infected person. There has never been a case of rabies transmission from a patient to a health care worker. In a recent human case diagnosed in Oregon, the strict adherence to universal body substance precautions minimized the fear of infection on the part of health care providers and markedly reduced the need for postexposure rabies prophylaxis.

The control and prevention of animal and human rabies is a great public health challenge for many areas of the world. Cost-effective prophylaxis must be made available for those who have suffered animal bites. Strict animal control measures must be implemented, and oral rabies vaccines, if successful in ongoing trials, may provide another tool in the quest for worldwide rabies eradication.

RAT-BITE FEVER

method of
LOUIS M. WEISS, M.D., M.P.H.
Albert Einstein College of Medicine
Bronx, New York

and

ELAINE KEOHANE, M.S.
New Jersey School of Health Related Professions
Newark, New Jersey

Rat-bite fever is a single designation for two similar systemic febrile illnesses caused by two different bacterial species transmitted by the bite of rodents. Clinical manifestations depend upon the etiologic agent producing the disease and include rash, arthritis, adenitis, and a local lesion at the site of the bite. The responsible pathogens are *Spirillum minus,* which is common in Asia, and *Streptobacillus moniliformis,* which is implicated in most cases in the United States. These diseases are worldwide in distribution and most commonly affect individuals exposed to rodents, especially rats.

Illness due to rat bite has been known since antiquity in India and in Japan, where the disease was known as *sodoku* (so: rat, doku: poison). The characteristic syndrome of rat-bite fever was first reported in the United States in 1839. In 1926 it was recognized that one of the types of rat-bite fever could be transmitted in an epidemic form through food (Haverhill fever or erythema arthriticum epidemicum), and the responsible organism (*S. moniliformis*) was isolated.

Both organisms are part of the normal oropharyngeal flora of various rodents, especially rats, and can be excreted in urine. *S. moniliformis* is found in the nasopharynx of 50 to 100% of rats worldwide, and *S. minus* was demonstrated in the oropharynx, conjunctivae, and blood of 25% of wild rats. Infection is acquired through contact (usually bites or scratches) with rodents or occasionally from contact with carnivores, such as cats, that feed on rodents. Transmission to humans from rodents kept as pets or used in laboratories has been reported. *S. moniliformis* infection has also been associated with food- or water-borne spread, presumably due to contamination with rodent excreta. Infection with *S. minus* has not been demonstrated by this route.

BACTERIOLOGY

Streptobacillus moniliformis is a microaerophilic, pleomorphic, nonmotile, unencapsulated gram-negative rod that forms branching filaments and bead-like chains. It requires 8 to 10% CO_2 and 10 to 20% serum or 2.5% Panmede supplementation of media (Trypicase soy agar) for optimal growth. In broth media typical "puff ball" colonies appear within 3 days. The organism can be recovered from routine blood culture media; however, sodium polyanethol sulfonate (Liquoid, which is added routinely to anaerobic broths) at concentrations of 0.0125% inhibits growth. A lysis centrifugation system* or the addition of resin to liquid media may improve the yield from blood culture if this organism is suspected. L forms resistant to penicillin have been found in culture.

Spirillum minus is a gram-negative spiral rod that demonstrates darting motility on dark-field microscopy. *S. minus* has traditionally been considered a spirochete but recently it has been suggested that this organism belongs to the *Campylobacter* genus. This organism has not been cultured on artificial media, and animal inoculation is required for isolation and definitive diagnosis. *S. minus* can be identified directly in blood or material obtained from skin lesions or lymph nodes by dark-field examination or Giemsa stain to establish a presumptive diagnosis.

CLINICAL MANIFESTATIONS

After inoculation of the pathogen from the rodent bite, two similar but distinct diseases may develop. Both illnesses are associated with fever, chills, headache, and other constitutional symptoms. Both may be relapsing, and if untreated the disease may recur for several months. Complications of both pathogens, though rare, include amnionitis, anemia, fever of unknown origin, chronic arthritis, myocarditis, endocarditis, meningitis, hepatitis, and localized abscesses. The features that distinguish these illnesses are summarized in Table 1.

In infection caused by *S. moniliformis* an incubation period of generally less than 3 days is followed by fever, chills, headache, vomiting, and severe migratory arthralgias and myalgias. At the time of clinical presentation, the original rat

---

*Dupont Isolator.

TABLE 1. **Distinguishing Features of Rat-Bite Fever Syndromes**

	Streptobacillus moniliformis	Spirillum minor
Incubation period	<10 days	≥7 days
Reaction at site of inoculation	Rare	Ulceration or eschar
Lymphadenopathy	Rare	Frequent in nodes adjacent to area of ulceration
Rash	Morbilliform, petechial	Maculopapular with red-brown coloration
Joints	Arthralgia, arthritis common	Rarely arthralgia
False positive test for syphilis	<25%	≥50%

bite is often healed or otherwise inapparent. By the second to fourth day of fever, a macular rash over the palms, soles, and extremities appears, often associated with asymmetrical polyarthritis or septic arthritis. Symptoms gradually resolve over 2 weeks, but febrile relapses can occur for weeks to months. Pharyngitis is common in food- or water-borne disease (Haverhill fever). Fatalities are rare, but a rapidly fatal case of disseminated *S. moniliformis* infection was reported in an infant who received several rat bites.

S. minus infection is characterized by a longer incubation time of 1 to 4 weeks before presentation with fever. The site of the rodent bite is characteristically swollen and purple, often with an ulcer or eschar and associated regional adenopathy. A generalized macular rash may been seen in the first week of fever. Untreated, the illness resolves in 1 to 2 months, but febrile relapses have been reported to occur for several years following infection.

DIAGNOSIS

The diagnosis of rat-bite fever should be considered in individuals with fever, a history of animal exposure (especially to rodents), and leukocytosis. Supporting evidence includes arthritis, a false-positive test result for syphilis, and a rash. Confirmation of the diagnosis requires either isolation of the organism for *S. moniliformis* or, in the case of *S. minor* infection, direct visualization of characteristic spirochetes in blood, exudate, or lymph node tissue by Giemsa or Wright's stain or dark-field microscopy. Gas-liquid chromatographic analysis of fatty acids has also been used for the rapid diagnosis of *S. moniliformis* infection. In this form of rat-bite fever, infection-specific agglutinins appear within 10 days of the onset of illness, and a titer greater than 1:80 or a fourfold rise in titer is considered diagnostic. No specific serologic test exists for *S. minus*.

Streptobacillary disease accounts for most of rat-bite fever cases in the United States, while *S. minus* infection has been reported mainly in Asia. The differential diagnosis is broad and includes disseminated neisserial infections, secondary syphilis, rickettsial diseases, leptospirosis, borreliosis, endocarditis, viral exanthems, drug eruptions, and collagen vascular diseases.

TREATMENT

The drug of choice for rat-bite fever caused by either organism is penicillin. Patients should receive 400,000 to 600,000 units intravenously every 4 to 6 hours or 600,000 units of procaine penicillin intramuscularly every 12 hours. Individuals who do not require hospitalization can be treated orally with penicillin V, 500 mg every 6 hours. Response to therapy is often dramatic. A 10- to 14-day course of therapy is recommended. Treatment of *S. minus* infection is often associated with a Jarisch-Herxheimer reaction. In patients allergic to penicillin, tetracycline, 500 mg every 6 hours, or doxycycline, 100 mg every 12 hours, can be used. Streptomycin, 15 mg per kg per day, given intramuscularly in two divided doses has also been effective.

In cases of endocarditis, therapy with 12 to 24 million units of penicillin per day should be given for at least 4 weeks. Streptomycin, 15 mg per kg per day in two divided doses, is often added to enhance activity against L forms, which are penicillin-resistant. Ciprofloxacin, ampicillin, cefuroxime, and cefotaxime have in vitro activity against *S. moniliformis*; however, there is limited clinical experience with these drugs in these infections.

PREVENTION

Prevention of rat-bite fever involves careful pest control and the wearing of gloves when handling rodents. All rodent bites should be thoroughly cleansed with an antiseptic solution and the need for tetanus vaccination evaluated. A three-day course of penicillin V, 500 mg every 6 hours, or tetracycline, 500 mg every 6 hours, would be reasonable as antibiotic prophylaxis. Although no data exist on the efficacy of this regimen, given the ability of these organisms to cause endocarditis it seems justifiable, particularly in patients with known valvular heart disease.

RELAPSING FEVER

method of
J. DOUGLAS LEE, M.D.
Marshfield Clinic
Marshfield, Wisconsin

Relapsing fever is an acute febrile infectious disease caused by the genus *Borrelia* that occurs in worldwide distribution in epidemic (louse-borne) and endemic

TABLE 1. **Features of Relapsing Fever**

Feature	Endemic	Epidemic
Organism	*Borrelia* spp.	*Borrelia recurrentis*
Vector	Tick	Louse
Reservoir	Rodents	Humans
Distribution	Worldwide	Third world
Severity	Less severe	More severe
Jarisch-Herxheimer reaction	35%	90%

(tick-borne) forms. The major differences between the forms are outlined in Table 1.

The relapsing nature of the illness is due to sequential alterations in the antigenic makeup of the organism, which allow cyclic re-emergence of the spirochete into the vascular space, causing fever. Diagnosis, suspected by the clinical history of relapsing febrile illness in an individual with tick or louse exposure, is proved by demonstration of spirochetes in the peripheral blood smear during the febrile interval by examination by dark-field microscopy or by Wright's or Giemsa stains. Epidemic disease may coexist with other louse-borne diseases, such as scrub typhus, and with infections associated with contaminated water sources, crowding, and lack of sanitation.

TREATMENT

Since this is a bacteremic disease, all organ systems can be affected, and the spectrum of disease ranges from mild illness to hypotensive shock and even coma. Complications include encephalopathy, myocarditis, vascular collapse, renal failure, disseminated intravascular coagulation, and liver failure. Management consists of (1) supportive therapy, (2) antibiotic therapy to eradicate the spirochete, (3) management of the Jarisch-Herxheimer reaction, and (4) disease prevention by louse eradication or tick avoidance.

Supportive Care

Initial management should include rapid fluid replacement with a physiologic electrolyte solution, the volume dictated by the initial state of dehydration. The Jarisch-Herxheimer reaction begins about 1 to 2 hours after antibiotics are started, causing a decrease in peripheral vascular resistance and blood pressure, so fluid replacement should be generous and intravascular volume high at this stage. If available, oncotic agents, such as plasma or albumin, can be given if congestive heart failure is absent and blood pressure is low after hydration with electrolyte solutions. These agents, in a dose of 0.5 to 1.5 grams of protein per kg of body weight, will allow significant intravascular volume expansion.

Fever should be managed with tepid water baths, alcohol sponging, or cooling blankets if hyperpyrexia (temperature greater than 105° F) occurs. Pain can be controlled with meperidine, 25 to 100 mg intramuscularly or 10 to 25 mg intravenously. Codeine, 30 to 60 mg orally, or other nonantipyretic analgesics may be given.

Antibiotic Therapy

The recommendations for treatment of relapsing fever are different for endemic and epidemic disease. Epidemic disease can be treated with a single dose of any of the drugs listed in Table 2 to

TABLE 2. **Louse-Borne Relapsing Fever:
Antibiotics**

Drug	Dose	Route	Number of Doses
PAM*	1,200,000 U	IM	1
Tetracycline	500 mg	PO	1
Tetracycline	250 mg	IV	1
Doxycycline	100 mg	IV or PO	1
Erythromycin	500 mg	IV or PO	1

Abbreviations: IM = intramuscular; PO = oral; IV = intravenous.
*Penicillin aluminum monostearate.

achieve a relapse rate of less than 1%. Single-dose regimens of procaine penicillin or ampicillin have unacceptable failure rates, but penicillin aluminum monostearate* in a single dose is effective. Tetracycline is considered the drug of choice since it causes most rapid clearing of the spirochetemia. The penicillins or erythromycin can be used in children and pregnant women.

No large series of patients has been studied to determine drug efficacy or minimal therapy for tick-borne, or endemic, relapsing fever. Five- to ten-day courses as described in Table 3 are effective.

Jarisch-Herxheimer Reaction

Most patients with epidemic relapsing fever and approximately one-third of patients with endemic relapsing fever experience a rise in temperature and a fall in blood pressure, white cell count, and peripheral vascular resistance within 2 hours of the initial dose of antibiotics. This Jarisch-Herxheimer reaction correlates with the clearing of the spirochetemia and is not modified by the use of steroids, antipyretics, or narcotics. This reaction is less intense but more prolonged with penicillins, the significance of which is not clear in terms of choosing therapy. Intensification of the initial support measures, particularly optimizing intravascular volume, is paramount. All patients should be monitored for evidence of congestive heart failure, shock, disseminated intravascular coagulation, and renal failure. Main-

*Not available in the United States.

TABLE 3. **Tick-Borne Relapsing Fever: Antibiotics**

Drug*	Dose	Frequency	Route
Penicillin	500 mg	qid	IV or PO
Ampicillin	500 mg	qid	IV or PO
Doxycycline	100 mg	bid	IV or PO
Tetracycline	500 mg	qid	IV or PO
Erythromycin	500 mg	qid	IV or PO

Abbreviations: IV = intravenous; PO = oral.
*All 5- to 10-day courses orally if patients are able.

tenance of adequate intravascular volume and avoidance of hyperpyrexia should be routine. Pressor and oncotic agents may be needed, used as they would be for gram-negative sepsis.

PREVENTION

Relapsing fever is prevented by avoiding vector exposure. Patients with louse-borne relapsing fever should be deloused by applying lindane (Kwell) shampoo to the entire skin surface, with particular attention to hair-bearing areas. This should be rinsed off thoroughly and the application repeated in 7 days. Clothing and bedclothes should be laundered or dry cleaned and ironed to avoid reinfection. The complete removal of lindane from the skin by adequate rinsing and limiting of skin exposure to 4 to 5 minutes are important, particularly in children and infants, as the drug is absorbed through the skin and is potentially toxic. Other agents, such as pyrethrins, piperonyl butoxide (RID), or malathion (Prioderm Lotion) may be used. The use of insecticides in lice-infested dwellings should be considered. Close contacts should be examined and deloused if infested.

RHEUMATIC FEVER

method of
JOHN F. BOHNSACK, M.D.,
L. GEORGE VEASY, M.D., and
HARRY R. HILL, M.D.
*University of Utah School of Medicine
Salt Lake City, Utah*

Acute rheumatic fever is a nonsuppurative sequela of group A streptococcal pharyngitis that can affect the heart, joints, integument, and central nervous system. The most important affected site is the heart; long-term damage to valvular structures can result from the initial attack and, even more so, from recurrent rheumatic fever. Although the number of cases of acute rheumatic fever has declined in the United States and other developed countries, the incidence remains high in developing countries. Furthermore, recent outbreaks in several areas of the United States demonstrate that rheumatic fever is not a relic of the past, even in developed countries.

Acute rheumatic fever occurs from early childhood through adult life but has its peak incidence in children 5 to 15 years of age. Diagnosis of the initial attack of rheumatic fever relies on the use of the revised Jones criteria (Table 1). The presence of two major or one major and two minor

TABLE 1. **Jones Criteria (Revised) for the Diagnosis of the Initial Attack of Rheumatic Fever**

Major	Minor
Carditis	Fever
Polyarthritis	Arthralgia
Chorea	Elevated erythrocyte
Erythema marginatum	sedimentation rate or
Subcutaneous nodules	C-reactive protein
	Prolonged PR interval

plus

Supporting evidence of preceding streptococcal infection: positive throat culture for group A *Streptococcus* or elevated or rising anti-streptococcal antibody serum titer

From Special Writing Group of the Committee on Rheumatic Fever, Endocarditis, and Kawasaki Disease of the Council on Cardiovascular Disease in the Young of the American Heart Assn: Guidelines for the diagnosis of rheumatic fever: Jones criteria, 1992 update. JAMA 268:2069–2073, 1992. Copyright 1992, American Medical Association.

manifestations indicates a high probability of acute rheumatic fever, *if* supported by evidence of a recent streptococcal infection.

Particular attention should be paid to establishing or ruling out the presence of *carditis,* since it is the only life-threatening manifestation of acute rheumatic fever and because damage to the heart is the only significant cause of residual morbidity. In children and young adults, carditis is predominantly manifested by mitral regurgitation, although pancarditis can involve all portions of the heart. Aortic regurgitation may also be present, but it is usually associated with mitral valve involvement. Thus confirmation of carditis in children depends upon hearing a new murmur of mitral regurgitation, which is a high-frequency systolic murmur heard at the apex with transmission to the left axilla.

If one is unsure of the physical findings, regurgitant flow can be confirmed by echocardiography (see next section). In the young patient with moderate to marked mitral regurgitation, echocardiography will often demonstrate prolapse of the anterior leaflet due to chordal elongation. In the older (>30 years) individual, the predominant hemodynamic alterations and clinical manifestations are due to mitral stenosis. The differing clinical picture of rheumatic heart disease in the older patient is best explained by repeated attacks of rheumatic fever or by a continued low-grade inflammatory reaction that results in the contraction and fusion of the chordae and deformity and fusion of the mitral leaflets. Therefore, a change in the murmur, or the appearance of a new murmur, is necessary to establish the diagnosis of acute rheumatic carditis in the adult. These changes can be subtle and may only be recognized by a skilled cardiologist. Thus when

carditis is suspected or confirmed at any age, it is advisable to refer the patient to an experienced cardiologist.

Arthritis has always been considered the "Achilles heel" of the Jones criteria. Because there is virtually an unending list of diseases that can present with arthritic symptoms, there must be strong evidence of a preceding streptococcal infection to support the diagnosis of rheumatic fever. Recent experience suggests that pulsed Doppler ultrasonography can demonstrate mitral regurgitation when it cannot be heard, and thus help establish the diagnosis in patients with polyarthritis. If Doppler ultrasonography is used, strict criteria must be employed to avoid overdiagnosis. Specifically, echocardiography using pulsed Doppler ultrasound should confirm regurgitant flow to be holosystolic and detected back to the left atrial wall. In addition, with color flow Doppler ultrasonography, mosaic color changes (aliasing) should be present, indicating high-velocity turbulence. Strict adherence to these criteria will distinguish the trivial or nonpathologic mitral regurgitation seen occasionally in individuals without heart disease.

The American Heart Association currently recommends that auscultatory confirmation of valve involvement be accepted as the sole criterion for valvulitis. However, the authors believe it is appropriate to use Doppler evidence of silent mitral regurgitation as a minor manifestation in the same way that electrocardiographic evidence of prolonged atrioventricular conduction is used. In this way the diagnosis of acute rheumatic fever can never be made without the presence of major criteria and those who need more stringent follow-up are identified.

The latent period for presentation of *Sydenham's chorea* is 6 weeks to several months after the preceding streptococcal infection, making it difficult to establish a preceding streptococcal infection. Doppler echocardiography may be useful in "pure" chorea as in isolated arthritis.

In the authors' experience, the skin manifestations of acute rheumatic fever, while strongly diagnostic, are characteristically seen only with another manifestation, for example, *erythema marginatum* with arthritis or carditis and *subcutaneous nodules* only with carditis.

Much evidence indicates that rheumatic fever is a sequela of streptococcal pharyngitis. Thus, it is imperative to establish the diagnosis of a recent streptococcal infection in an individual suspected of having acute rheumatic fever. A throat culture for beta-hemolytic streptococci should be obtained, and evidence sought for a serologic response to group A streptococci. Throat cultures are frequently negative at the time of the initial presentation and should not be used as the sole test to determine streptococcal infection. Several serologic tests (e.g., the antistreptolysin O, anti-hyaluronidase, and antideoxyribonuclease B titers) enhance the sensitivity of serologic diagnosis. Repeated determinations over 2 to 4 weeks can document a rise in serologic titer and establish the diagnosis of preceding streptococcal infection. The anti-DNase B test is useful in cases of isolated chorea.

TREATMENT

Acute rheumatic fever varies in its presentation and severity. The following treatment recommendations are offered as guidelines to be adapted to the individual patient's particular manifestations. Eradication of residual streptococci and prophylaxis of recurrent attacks, however, are an indispensable part of every patient's management, since further cardiac damage results from recurrences of acute rheumatic fever.

Bed Rest

In the past, patients with rheumatic fever were placed on prolonged bed rest, but the value of this therapy was probably overestimated. On the other hand, no one denies that the patient with acute rheumatic fever improves both symptomatically and objectively when placed on bed rest. The physician should severely restrict activity and carefully observe the patient during the first 2 weeks of illness, since carditis will usually appear during that time. If the patient improves and there is no evidence of carditis, the return to full activity can be rapid. If the patient has moderate to severe carditis, activity should be resumed slowly and cautiously with frequent and thorough clinical assessment. Return to full activity is permitted after signs and symptoms have resolved and the acute phase reactants have returned to normal.

Eradication of Streptococci

Antibiotic therapy to eradicate residual streptococci is instituted as soon as the diagnosis of acute rheumatic fever is established, even when the throat culture is negative. A single intramuscular injection of benzathine penicillin G (600,000 units intramuscularly for children under 30 kg, and 1.2 million units for heavier patients) is recommended. Alternatively, oral penicillin V (125 to 250 mg four times a day for 10 days) can be used. In the penicillin-allergic patient, erythromycin, 30 to 50 mg per kg per day in three divided doses may be substituted if erythromycin-resistant group A streptococci are not prevalent

in the geographic area. Clindamycin is another alternative for the penicillin-allergic patient, but sulfa drugs should not be used to eradicate streptococci. Prophylaxis of recurrent infection should begin immediately following the eradicating regimen (see later discussion).

Anti-Inflammatory Agents

Aspirin

Aspirin is extremely effective in the control of arthritis and is used to suppress carditis when there is no associated cardiomegaly and no evidence of congestive heart failure. Aspirin is generally started at an oral dose of 100 mg per kg per day given in four equally divided doses. The dose is usually decreased to 70 mg per kg per day after 2 to 3 days. This lower dose is usually adequate to maintain a therapeutic serum level of 20 to 25 mg per dL. Because absorption can be quite variable, the serum salicylate level should be measured 3 to 5 days after the start of treatment. The salicylate level should also be determined if the patient continues to complain of pain since aspirin consistently provides relief at therapeutic levels. Aspirin should be given until the sedimentation rate returns to normal. Because of the risk of Reye's syndrome, aspirin should be discontinued if the patient develops influenza or varicella.

Corticosteroids

Corticosteroids are recommended for moderate or severe carditis. Although symptomatic relief is often dramatic, there is no clear consensus that corticosteroids reduce the amount of residual cardiac disease. Prednisone, 2 mg per kg per day, is given orally in four divided doses and continued at this level until all clinical evidence of inflammatory activity has disappeared and the sedimentation rate has returned to normal. At this dosage, all patients will experience undesirable side effects, including moon facies, acne, and hirsutism. The patient should be monitored for the development of hypertension. Oral antacids may be given to prevent peptic ulcer. All side effects should disappear gradually after the medication is discontinued. Prednisone should not be discontinued abruptly but rather tapered over a 2- to 3-week period. To avoid rebound inflammation, aspirin should be started during the initiation of the taper and continued for 2 to 3 weeks after steroids have been totally discontinued.

Therapy to suppress inflammation should not be instituted before the diagnosis of rheumatic fever is clearly established since the symptoms may dramatically improve or disappear in response to salicyclates or steroids.

Congestive Heart Failure

Congestive heart failure should be managed in a conventional manner with oxygen, diuretics, and digoxin. Rapid digitalization should probably be avoided because of possible sensitivity in the presence of myocarditis. It is also important that the patient rest comfortably to reduce cardiac demand. Death from refractory congestive heart failure during acute rheumatic fever is rare. When congestive heart failure fails to respond to vigorous medical management, surgical restoration of valvular competence can be lifesaving.

Sydenham's Chorea

Sydenham's chorea generally resolves after several months but can last for over a year. Management of chorea varies with its severity. When chorea is mild, the patient requires only mild sedation and a more tranquil environment; this usually means removal from school for a limited period. Hospitalization may be required for chorea so severe that the patient is unable to feed or dress him or herself. Recently, the anticonvulsants sodium valproate and carbamazepine have been used with some success. Prednisone in the same dosage used for carditis has been employed by the authors with encouraging results. Haloperidol has also been used successfully, but toxicity can be a problem, and it should be used only in hospitalized patients under careful observation.

PREVENTION

Prevention of Primary and Recurrent Rheumatic Fever

As the incidence of rheumatic fever has declined, sentiment has grown among physicians that vigorous diagnosis and treatment of streptococcal pharyngitis in the United States may be unwarranted. However, the recent outbreaks of rheumatic fever in the United States demonstrate that such complacency is dangerous, particularly in areas where rheumatic fever is endemic. (The treatment of streptococcal pharyngitis is discussed elsewhere in this text.)

Estimates of the incidence of recurrent rheumatic fever after an episode of streptococcal pharyngitis range from 5 to 50% per infection. Evidence exists that treatment of streptococcal pharyngitis with antibiotics prevents recurrent rheumatic fever.

All patients diagnosed as having rheumatic fever, including those without apparent carditis, should receive antibiotic prophylaxis. The best regimen is benzathine penicillin, 1.2 million units intramuscularly every 4 weeks. In developing countries, many physicians prefer to give the same dose every 3 weeks. Oral penicillin G or V, 250 mg twice a day, is an alternative, but compliance is easier with intramuscular injections. The penicillin-allergic patient can be treated with sulfadiazine (0.5 to 1.0 grams daily) or erythromycin (250 mg twice a day). The physician should consider the possibility of local erythromycin-resistant streptococci before using this antibiotic.

Although the incidence of recurrent rheumatic fever decreases as the interval from the primary attack increases, it is prudent to administer lifelong antibiotic prophylaxis. Compliance with regimens may require considerable effort and education on the part of the patient. Special emphasis should be placed on high-risk patients: children and adolescents; those in crowded living situations, such as military camps, prisons, or schools; teachers and others whose occupations bring them into contact with children; persons living in or visiting endemic areas or areas experiencing rheumatic fever outbreaks; and most importantly, patients with residual rheumatic heart disease.

Prophylaxis Against Bacterial Endocarditis

Patients with cardiac valvular abnormalities secondary to rheumatic fever are at increased risk for developing infective endocarditis during episodes of transient bacteremia, as can occur during dental work or genitourinary or gastrointestinal surgery or instrumentation. A careful search for evidence of valvular disease in patients with suspected rheumatic fever (by echocardiography if necessary) is mandatory. Recommendations for antibiotic prophylaxis for bacterial endocarditis during procedures likely to cause transient bacteremia are discussed elsewhere (see Table 5, page 61). One should stress the value of good dental hygiene in preventing endocarditis in patients with rheumatic heart disease.

Routine follow-up of patients with acute rheumatic fever should include at least yearly examinations to document the presence and extent of residual or developing cardiac disease. In addition to monitoring disease activity, such examinations give the physician the opportunity to re-emphasize and re-educate the patient about prevention of recurrent rheumatic fever and prophylaxis against bacterial endocarditis.

LYME DISEASE

method of
STEVEN W. LUGER, M.D.
Kaiser Permanente
Rocky Hill, Connecticut

Lyme disease, a tick-transmitted spirochetal infection, is the most common arthropod-transmitted illness in the United States. Although probably present in Europe since the late 1890s and in the United States since the 1940s, it went unrecognized as a clinical entity until described by Steere in 1976. *Borrelia burgdorferi,* a flagellated spirochete, lives primarily in rodents, which act as a reservoir. The vector for Lyme disease, *Ixodes dammini* in the northeast and north central United States and related ticks elsewhere, acquires the spirochete from infected rodents and can then transmit it to humans or other hosts. The various clinical manifestations most commonly involve the skin, heart, joints, and nervous system. Some patients may never manifest clinical symptoms but may seroconvert after exposure. Although cases have been diagnosed in 46 states, the majority of patients reside in the northeastern states, Minnesota, and Wisconsin. In 1992, 9677 cases were reported to the Centers for Disease Control.

CLINICAL MANIFESTATIONS

Early Lyme Disease

Localized (Stage 1)

Erythema migrans is the most common manifestation of Lyme disease, seen in about 80% of patients with early disease. It begins at the site of the tick bite as a small papule and expands in a centrifugal pattern over a period of days to weeks. It can occur as early as 3 days or as late as 30 days after the bite. The rash is usually a flat circle or oval 2 to 15 inches in diameter, which may have a slightly raised border, is red or violaceous in color, and is warm to the touch. Erythema migrans is generally painless (although dysesthesias may be present), nonscaly, and usually nonpruritic. Many patients with erythema migrans have no systemic symptoms; however, a febrile illness with generalized systemic symptoms may precede, accompany, or follow the rash. This usually consists of fever, arthralgias, myalgias, headache, and neck stiffness. Though a "flu-like illness" is frequently mentioned in reference to early Lyme disease, coryza, coughing, exudative pharyngitis, and frequent vomiting and diarrhea are usually absent. When these symptoms predominate, other diagnoses should be strongly considered. More than 50% of patients with early Lyme disease will develop later manifestations if left untreated. Lyme serologic results are negative in as many as 50% of patients at this stage.

Disseminated (Stage 2)

Multiple erythema migrans lesions occur in 20 to 30% of patients with Lyme disease. This indicates hematogenous spread of the spirochete, and therefore other organ involvement should be considered.

Cardiac manifestations, primarily atrioventricular block, occur in about 8% of untreated patients, usually within 2 to 3 months of exposure. Whereas the most common finding is a prolonged PR interval on electrocardiography, complete heart block and myopericarditis can occur. Although some patients may be asymptomatic, others may present with bradycardia or syncope.

Acute neurologic involvement occurs in 15% of untreated patients, usually within 2 to 3 months of exposure. Cranial neuropathies, most often Bell's palsy (either unilateral or bilateral), lymphocytic meningitis, encephalitis, and radiculopathies, are common findings in early neurologic Lyme disease.

Arthritis occurs in about 50% of untreated Lyme disease patients, usually within the first 6 months following exposure. It is characteristically a large-joint asymmetric mono- or oligoarthritis with the knee being the most commonly involved joint. Joint swelling and warmth are the most common manifestations, with severe pain being unusual. The joint fluid is inflammatory.

Late Lyme Disease (Stage 3)

If Lyme disease goes untreated or if antibiotic therapy has been unsuccessful, arthritis can recur or persist for months to years. It can even progress to erosive synovitis, particularly in patients who are HLA DR 2 or DR 4 positive.

Neurologic manifestations, including chronic polyneuropathies, spastic paraparesis, chronic encephalopathy, and peripheral neuropathies, can occur from months to years after initial infection.

DIAGNOSIS AND LABORATORY TESTING

Lyme disease is diagnosed on the basis of the clinical features supported by laboratory confirmation. It is important for the clinician to remember that Lyme disease serology tests only for the presence of antibodies and not for the presence of clinical disease. Just as a positive rubella titer does not mean that a patient has active German measles, neither does a positive Lyme titer mean that a patient has Lyme disease (in the absence of appropriate symptoms). Also, positive serology cannot distinguish patients with active Lyme disease from patients who have been cured,

TABLE 1. **Duration of Symptoms After Adequate Treatment**

Manifestation	Time from Treatment Initiation to Symptom Resolution
Erythema migrans	3–21 days, median 8 days
Facial palsy	3–270 days, median 26 days
Carditis	3–150 days, median 10 days
Arthritis	7–90 days
Chronic neurologic involvement	1–12 months

as titers can remain positive for years after cure. Too frequently, patients with nonspecific complaints who have weakly reactive Lyme titers are incorrectly diagnosed as having Lyme disease. Physicians should interpret weakly reactive Lyme titers with the same degree of caution that they use in interpreting weakly reactive antinuclear antibody tests or rheumatoid factors.

There is marked interlaboratory variability in Lyme disease serology, with up to 20% false positivity in some laboratories as well as problems with false negatives. When in doubt, a university laboratory doing active Lyme disease research should be consulted. The Western blot for Lyme disease has not been standardized and should be interpreted with caution. False-positive Lyme disease serology can occur in many illnesses, including rheumatoid arthritis, lupus erythematosus, infectious mononucleosis, chickenpox, and periodontal disease. Serology may be negative in 50% of Lyme disease patients with erythema migrans; however, serology is almost always positive in individuals with manifestations of disseminated or chronic Lyme disease.

TREATMENT

No standard treatment is universally successful in all patients; however, a lack of response to proper therapy should bring the diagnosis into question. Treatment of patients with early Lyme disease should not be withheld in suspected cases as serology is frequently negative for the first few weeks of illness. Antibiotic therapy does not need to be continued until all of the patient's symptoms have resolved; the goal of antimicrobial therapy is the eradication of the spirochetosis. In patients with central nervous system involvement, fatigue and mild encephalopathic symptoms may take as long as 6 to 12 months to resolve. In addition, a lack of understanding of the normal course of symptom resolution (Table 1) in successfully treated patients has lead to experimental, expensive, dangerous, and unnecessary treatment.

A Jarisch-Herxheimer reaction (an intensification of symptoms including fever, headache, myalgia, and arthralgia) can occur in up to one-third of patients treated for early Lyme disease. It is thought to be the result of the release of

TABLE 2. **Treatment of Lyme Disease**

Manifestation	Complications and Additional Information	Duration of Treatment	Antibiotic and Dose
Erythema migrans	No (or minimal) symptoms	14–21 days	Doxycycline‡ 100 mg PO bid or
	Constitutional symptoms	21–28 days	Amoxicillin 500 mg PO tid or
	Multiple lesions	21–28 days	Cefuroxime axetil (Ceftin), 500 mg PO bid
Facial palsy	Normal CSF	21–28 days	Doxycycline 100 mg PO bid–tid or Amoxicillin 500 mg PO tid–qid
Facial palsy	Pleocytosis or elevated CSF protein	21–28 days	Ceftriaxone (Rocephin) 2 gm IV q d or
Lymphocytic meningitis		21–28 days	Cefotaxime (Claforan) 2 gm IV q 8 h or
Radiculopathy		21–28 days	Penicillin 5 million U IV q 6 h
Carditis	PR < 0.28	21–28 days	Doxycycline 100 mg PO bid–tid or Amoxicillin 500 mg PO tid–qid
	PR > 0.28 Myopericarditis Complete block*	21–28 days	Ceftriaxone 2 gm IV q d or Cefotaxime 2 gm IV q 8 h or Penicillin 5 million U IV q 6 h
Arthritis	Acute, first episode	28 days	Doxycycline 100 mg PO bid–tid or Amoxicillin 500 mg PO tid–qid
Arthritis	Recurrent or persistent†	21–28 days	Ceftriaxone 2 gm IV q d or Cefotaxime 2 gm IV q 8 h or Penicillin 5 million U IV q 6 h
Chronic neurologic or late neurologic	Central or peripheral	21–28 days	Ceftriaxone 2 gm IV q d or Cefotaxime 2 gm IV q 8 h or Penicillin 5 million U IV q 6 h

*Temporary pacing may be necessary in patients with high-degree block.
†Arthroscopic synovectomy may be necessary in patients whose synovitis does not resolve.
‡Tetracyclines should not be used in pregnant or lactating women or children less than 8 years old.

TABLE 3. **Second-Line Antibiotics**

Antibiotic	Comment
Penicillin	May be less effective than amoxicillin
Erythromycin	Less effective in erythema migrans than doxycycline
Azithromycin (Zithromax)	Less effective than amoxicillin when short course used for erythema migrans
Chloramphenicol	May be effective in some patients with late neurologic disease

breakdown products of killed spirochetes and should resolve within 24 to 48 hours.

Treatment recommendations for Lyme disease are given in Table 2. Alternative antibiotics are listed in Table 3, and ineffective antibiotics are shown in Table 4.

Special Circumstances

Asymptomatic Tick Bites

The risk of acquiring Lyme disease after a tick bite depends on many factors, including the percentage of infected ticks in the area, the duration of tick attachment, and host factors. It is rare for ticks attached for less than 24 hours to transmit Lyme disease. Even in endemic areas, the risk of getting Lyme disease after a single *Ixodid* tick bite is probably 1% or less. Therefore, it is generally thought that antibiotic prophylaxis is not necessary. Exceptions may be made for very anxious patients, pregnant women, and patients living high-risk areas who find attached, fully engorged ticks.

Pregnancy

The effect of Lyme disease during pregnancy on the well-being of the fetus is unclear. Reports of transplacental transmission of *Borrelia burgdorferi,* although rare, raise concern. Although there has been no direct proof of fetal damage from perinatal Lyme disease, because Bb has been found in multiple fetal organs it has been the author's policy to treat all pregnant women with active Lyme disease with parenteral antibiotic therapy. Exceptions may be made for patients with only erythema migrans and no systemic symptoms; they can be treated with oral antibiotics. Pregnant patients who are asymptomatic and merely have positive titers do not need treatment

TABLE 4. **Antibiotics Ineffective in Lyme Disease**

First-generation cephalosporins (e.g., cephalexin)
Quinolones (e.g., ciprofloxacin)
Trimethoprim-sulfamethoxazole (Septra, Bactrim)
Aminoglycosides

as there is no increased risk of adverse fetal outcome.

Treatment Failure

The most common cause of treatment failure is incorrect diagnosis. Prior to embarking on longer and more costly therapy, the physician should re-examine the clinical and laboratory findings and consider other possibilities. Even if treatment has been effective, some symptoms may persist (see Table 1). Post–Lyme disease fibrositis is relatively common and does not respond to further antibiotic therapy. It is not a treatment failure; rather, it is a result of the disease. If the patient truly has recurrence of objective signs of Lyme disease, then repeat therapy with parenteral antibiotics should be undertaken or referral made to an appropriate specialist.

Steroids

Although there are no convincing data that corticosteroids are effective in Lyme disease, they may play a limited role. In patients with complete heart block or facial paralysis, a short course of steroids (prednisone, 60 mg daily tapered over 7 to 14 days) along with appropriate antibiotics may be helpful. Intra-articular steroids may be of value in patients with refractory synovitis.

ROCKY MOUNTAIN SPOTTED FEVER

method of
DAVID L. SMITH, M.D.
University of Kansas Medical Center
Kansas City, Kansas

Rocky Mountain spotted fever (RMSF) is an acute febrile infectious vasculitis caused by the rickettsial organism *Rickettsia rickettsii.* The disease was first described by Dr. Howard Ricketts in the late 1800s. His observations were made in the Bitter Root and Snake River Valleys of Montana and Idaho.

The term "Rocky Mountain spotted fever" refers both to the geographic region in which the disease was first observed and its characteristic clinical feature, a rash. At present, this illness is rarely seen in the Rocky Mountain region and the rash itself may be absent in approximately 10% of cases. RMSF occurs most commonly in the south and Oklahoma.

From 1985 to 1990, approximately 650 cases per year were reported to the Centers for Disease Control (CDC) in Atlanta, Georgia. Of these, approximately 50% were serologically confirmed. In 1990, the four states reporting the most cases were North Carolina (178), Oklahoma (70), Tennessee (58), and South Carolina (43). Colorado and Montana report fewer than five cases per year. Almost all cases of RMSF occur between April 1 and September 30. The disease is twice as common in males, and 50% of patients are less than 20 years of age. There is no racial predilection. Ninety percent of patients report visiting brushy, wooded areas, and 60 to 70% have a history of tick bite. Many also report exposure to dogs and cats.

CLINICAL MANIFESTATIONS

The pathophysiologic lesion of RMSF is an acute vasculitis; thus, all organs can be affected. The onset of the illness may be either gradual or abrupt. The characteristic disease triad is that of fever, headache, and rash.

The illness often begins in a nondescript manner with fever and headache. A rash appears on day two through five of the illness. Characteristically, the rash is first seen on the ankles and wrists and spreads centripetally. At some point the palms and soles usually become involved. The rash is initially blanching but may become petechial, purpuric, or in some cases gangrenous.

The central nervous system is commonly involved. This manifests as headache, often very severe, with encephalopathic changes.

Other systems that are involved include (1) musculoskeletal (myalgias); (2) gastrointestinal (nausea, vomiting, abdominal pain, abnormal liver function, and hepatomegaly); (3) hematologic (thrombocytopenia and splenomegaly); (4) metabolic (hyponatremia); (5) respiratory (cough, rales, abnormal chest x-ray, and abnormal gas exchange); and (6) renal (increase in creatinine).

Left untreated the disease may progress to multiorgan failure and death in 20 to 30% of cases.

DIAGNOSIS

The diagnosis of RMSF must be made on epidemiologic and clinical grounds. It may be supported indirectly by nonspecific laboratory tests (Table 1).

The epidemiologic features mentioned earlier may suggest the possibility of RMSF in the acutely febrile patient. The problem early in the evolution of the disease is that prior to the appearance of the characteristic rash the symptoms

TABLE 1. **Common Laboratory Abnormalities in Rocky Mountain Spotted Fever**

Laboratory Value	Patients Affected
Serum sodium < 130 mEq/L	95%
SGOT increased above normal	78%
Creatine phosphokinase increased above normal	54%
Platelet Count < 150,000/mm³	32%

Abbreviation: SGOT = serum glutamic-oxaloacetic transaminase.

are so nonspecific that the physician is likely to diagnose the illness as a self-limited viral process. The severity of the headache and subtle mental status alterations are early clues that may suggest RMSF.

With the appearance of the rash, the characteristic triad is present and the disease should be strongly considered. However, the rash may be difficult to detect or completely absent, and is easily missed in the dark-skinned patient. Even when the rash is present, the differential diagnosis is still wide. Some of the more common illnesses that can present in like manner include enteroviral infections, typical and atypical measles, infectious mononucleosis, rubella, secondary syphilis, and *Neisseria meningitidis* infection. Drug fever with a cutaneous eruption can also confuse the picture.

Confirmatory tests for Rocky Mountain spotted fever include the commonly available nonspecific Weil-Felix test. A variety of more specific and more sensitive tests, including the indirect hemagglutination and complement fixation tests, are available from reference laboratories. Antibodies develop in the second to third week of illness; thus, none of the confirmatory tests can exclude RMSF in the acute phase; they can, however, provide late serologic confirmation of the illness. The major confirmatory test, which is useful in the acute phase, is the rapid response to specific antimicrobial therapy.

TREATMENT

Tetracyclines are the drugs of choice for Rocky Mountain spotted fever for nonpregnant individuals over 8 years of age. Doxycycline (Vibramycin) is the recommended tetracycline. For adults and children weighing more than 45 kg, the loading dose is 200 mg followed by 100 mg every 12 hours. In children over 8 years of age but weighing less than 45 kg the dose is 2.2 mg per kg every 12 hours for 1 day and then 2.2 mg per kg per day (safety has not been established in children less than 8 years of age). Intravenous and oral doses are identical. Chloramphenicol (Chloromycetin) is used in children younger than 8, pregnant women, and situations in which meningococcal disease is a strong consideration. The dosage for adults is 50 mg per kg per day intravenously or orally divided into 4 doses at intervals of every 6 hours, and for children, 50 to 75 mg per kg per day (intravenously initially) every 6 hours, then 50 mg per kg per day (orally) every 6 hours. The duration of antibiotic therapy is usually 10 to 14 days or until the patient has been afebrile for 72 to 96 hours.

Tetracyclines are favored because clinicians are

generally much more willing to give empiric courses of these drugs than they are to give chloramphenicol. This is probably because of the better safety profile of tetracyclines in most age groups. Another reason to favor tetracyclines has been the emergence of human ehrlichiosis caused by the rickettsial organism *Ehrlichia chaffeensis.* Thirty-eight cases of this disease were reported to the CDC in 1989, but the true number is probably much greater. This infective agent is not susceptible to chloramphenicol but is susceptible to tetracyclines and rifampin. Ehrlichiosis closely resembles rashless RMSF. Therapy with tetracycline thus covers both rickettsial possibilities.

Appropriate supportive therapy to replace lost intravascular volume and to treat end-organ damage is mandatory. Patients usually recover without sequelae. The mortality in treated patients is around 2%.

PREVENTION

Tick repellents, protective clothing, and total body search and removal of ticks after exposure are the bedrocks of prevention. Ticks should be removed carefully with steady, gentle pressure with forceps, tweezers, or impermeable tissue. Postexposure prophylaxis is not generally recommended because fewer than 5% of ticks are infected with RMSF. No protective vaccine is available.

RUBELLA AND CONGENITAL RUBELLA

method of
PETER MORGAN-CAPNER, F.R.C.Path.
Royal Preston Hospital
Preston, United Kingdom

Rubella (German measles) is now an uncommon infection in countries that have achieved a high uptake of measles, mumps, and rubella (MMR) vaccine in infants. It must still be considered, however, on all occasions when rashes or contact with rubelliform illness occur during pregnancy as recent clusters of congenital rubella in the United States demonstrate.

CLINICAL MANIFESTATIONS

Up to 50% of cases of rubella in children are subclinical, but with increasing age the proportion of subclinical infection falls, and in a majority of adults infection is symptomatic. Rubella usually presents as a maculopapular, pinkish-red rash with an incubation period of 14 to 21 days

(usually 15 to 17 days). The rash starts on the face and neck but rapidly spreads to involve the body and limbs. The individual spots may coalesce, but the rash usually clears within 3 to 4 days. Itching is uncommon. The rash is often preceded by a few days of nonspecific illness with fever and upper respiratory tract symptoms. Conjunctivitis can occur but is seldom as severe as that seen in measles. Lymphadenopathy is common, with the suboccipital nodes most often involved. It frequently precedes the rash and may persist for some days. Fever is usually mild and, particularly in children, may be absent. Children usually have only mild disease with little or no systemic upset and only a fleeting rash.

COMPLICATIONS

The major complication of rubella is the potential for adverse effects on the fetus when infection occurs early in pregnancy (see further on). Although arthralgia is rare in children, it occurs in up to 30% of adults. The small joints are most frequently involved, particularly the hands and wrists. Although the joint symptoms usually resolve within a month they can persist for much longer. Thrombocytopenia and postinfectious encephalitis are rare complications, the latter occurring in about 1 in 10,000 cases. Infection in the immunocompromised patient is not unduly severe nor does it have an unusual presentation.

DIFFERENTIAL DIAGNOSIS

The clinical diagnosis of rubella is notoriously unreliable, even during epidemics. Infection with other viruses, such as enteroviruses, particularly echoviruses, parvovirus B19, and even measles, can be easily confused with rubella. Differentiating the rash of parvovirus B19 infection from rubella is particularly problematic in adults, with arthralgia of small joints a common complication of both, and the characteristic malar erythema of parvovirus B19 infection in children a rare manifestation in adults. Nonspecific pinkish-red macular rashes are not uncommon, particularly in children and may also be due to noninfective causes such as allergy. As rubella becomes increasingly rare, further difficulties arise since the infection may not even be considered in the differential diagnosis by medical practitioners unfamiliar with its manifestations.

CONGENITAL RUBELLA

Primary rubella in the first 16 weeks of pregnancy presents a major risk to the fetus. Although transplacental infection can occur throughout pregnancy, the risk of fetal damage varies with gestation. Infection in the first 8 weeks will cause intrauterine death or major malformations in up to 85% of fetuses. The risk falls progressively with gestational age, so that at 12 to 16 weeks the risk is 20% and the only damage likely is sensorineural deafness. Beyond 16 weeks, although occasional cases of deafness may be attributable to intrauterine infection, the risk to the fetus is very remote and is probably close to zero for infections past 24 weeks' gestation. Rubella prior to conception carries minimal, if any, risk to the fetus.

Infection in the first 12 weeks is associated with a wide range of congenital abnormalities. The classic triad of the congenital rubella syndrome consists of deformities of the eye (cataract, micro-ophthalmia, chorioretinitis), heart (patent ductus arteriosus, pulmonary artery stenosis), and ear (sensorineural deafness). Neurologic complications such as microencephaly and mental retardation also occur, and a wide range of other manifestations may be present (intrauterine growth retardation, purpura, hepatosplenomegaly). Further problems may develop after birth and include immune-mediated pneumonitis, progressive rubella panencephalitis, and diabetes mellitus.

EPIDEMIOLOGY

Patients are infectious for 7 days prior to and after onset of rash. Transmission is by direct nasopharyngeal droplet spread with no evidence for survival of infectious virus in the environment or spread by fomite. There is no animal reservoir. Infants with congenital rubella can remain infected for many years, although infectivity for susceptible contacts is negligible after 1 year of age, and failure to isolate virus may be demonstrated in even younger patients. Before widespread infant immunization, epidemics of rubella were seen every 7 to 10 years, but the current pattern is one of low-level endemic infection with localized outbreaks, infection being most common in the spring.

DIAGNOSIS

Primary Rubella

Since clinical diagnosis is so unreliable, laboratory investigation must be performed to make the specific diagnosis. As has been demonstrated in recent clusters, a history of past vaccination or positive antibody screening, even if documented, does not necessarily exclude recent rubella. Hence, it is essential to investigate all rubelliform rashes in pregnancy. As subclinical primary rubella can occur and damage the fetus, it is wise to also investigate all pregnant contacts of patients with rubelliform illness. If possible, the source patient should also be tested to ascertain the validity of the diagnosis of rubella.

Virus isolation has no place in the diagnosis of postnatal primary rubella as it is unreliable and may take some weeks. Diagnosis is serologic and serum should be obtained as soon as possible after contact or onset of illness. Procedures and tests vary by laboratory, but it is essential for correct testing and interpretation of results that full clinical details are given, including any past testing and immunization. Most laboratories will test either for total antibody by hemagglutination inhibition (HI) or for specific IgG by a wide variety of tests, and if the titer is high enough, for specific IgM. The detection of specific IgM is usually considered indicative of recent primary rubella, but all specific IgM assays may occasionally give false-positive results, and care is needed in their interpretation. False-positive specific IgM results can occur in infectious mononucleosis and parvovirus B19 infection, both of which may be clinically confused with rubella. Depending on the results obtained with the first serum, it will often be necessary to repeat tests 1 to 4 weeks later. The final interpretation will depend on the serologic results taken in conjunction with the clinical details and history of antibody testing and vaccination.

Reinfection

Reinfection is usually diagnosed in the laboratory by demonstrating a rise in antibody titer after recent contact with rubella by someone who has had natural rubella or successful immunization. The risk to the fetus posed by reinfection in early pregnancy is ill defined but likely to be less than 10%, substantially less than the risk with primary rubella. Reinfection is rarely symptomatic, but the differentiation of primary rubella from reinfection in the asymptomatic patient is critical to determining proper treatment. Routine rubella antibody tests may not be able to distinguish these conditions, however, since rubella-specific IgM can often be detected in reinfections, albeit usually at a lower concentration than in primary rubella.

If primary rubella or reinfection is diagnosed in pregnancy, further management will depend on patient counseling, including assessment of the degree and type of risk to the fetus and the possible prognosis for the baby.

Congenital Rubella

Isolation of virus from urine, throat swab, or tissue is of value in diagnosing congenital rubella, but sufficient virologic expertise for reliable isolation and identification is often not readily available. The detection of specific IgM in neonatal or infant serum is highly reliable, as almost all babies with congenital rubella are seropositive for the first 3 months of life, and most remain so for 6 months. At older ages, but before administration of MMR, persistence of specific IgG or total antibody is diagnostic, as maternal antibody will decline to negativity during the first year of life.

Rubella Antibody Screening

To determine whether a patient is susceptible to rubella, and hence should be immunized, testing for rubella-specific IgG or total antibody is required. There are many reliable assays, including HI, latex agglutination, radial hemolysis, and enzyme-linked immunosorbent assay (ELISA). Sensitivity of the assays varies, and debate continues about the protective efficacy of low concentrations of antibody. Although immunization may be advised for those with low concentrations of antibody (less than 15 IU), it may not boost their antibody levels. Protection against primary rubella can be assumed if two or more doses of vaccine have been given, even if the antibody concentration does not increase.

TREATMENT

There is no justification for the routine administration of gamma globulin to susceptible women after contact with rubella. Although there may be some attenuation of illness, no prophylactic effect or reduced transmission to the fetus has been demonstrated.

Antiviral drugs have not been used for the treatment of postnatal or congenital rubella.

RUBELLA VACCINE

Rubella vaccine (RA 27/3 strain) is available either as a component of MMR or as a single vaccine. It induces protection in more than 95% of recipients. Widespread administration of MMR vaccine to infants at age 15 months has had a major impact on the incidence of rubella. To ensure a continued low incidence, it is necessary to maintain high immunization levels by enforcing school entry laws and targeting socioeconomically deprived groups. Continued efforts must also be made to identify susceptible adolescent and adult women who would benefit from immunization. Screening in occupational health departments, prenatal clinics, family planning services, and college health services should continue.

Rubella vaccine is a live attenuated virus, and rarely a mild rubelliform illness will be seen 2 to 3 weeks after immunization. Arthralgia may occur, but an association with long-term arthritis is disputed and seems unlikely. Administration during pregnancy should be avoided, and an immunized female should not become pregnant for 3 months afterward. If inadvertent immunization in pregnancy does occur, the risk to the fetus is remote; no congenital abnormalities have been found in term infants (maximum risk is 2%, similar to that for nonexposed babies), although in occasional cases the fetus may have been infected.

Vaccination in immunocompromised individuals, including those infected with human immunodeficiency virus, has not been associated with significant side effects, but further guidance should be sought if immunization of such individuals is considered.

Immunization should be postponed for 3 months after administration of intramuscular gamma globulin or blood transfusion. Anti-D antibody does not interfere with development of immunity, although follow-up serologic testing is advisable. Vaccine virus cannot be transmitted between the immunized individual and susceptible contacts.

MEASLES
(Rubeola)

method of
MOSHE ARDITI, M.D.
*University of Southern California
and Children's Hospital, Los Angeles*
Los Angeles, California

Worldwide, measles continues to be a major killer among vaccine-preventable diseases. In developing countries, an estimated 2 million children die from measles each year. Prior to the introduction of measles vaccine in 1963, 400,000 to 700,000 cases were reported annually in the United States. During the next 20 years cases declined significantly. However, since 1989, there has been a serious resurgence of measles in this country, mostly involving preschool, inner-city, indigent, unimmunized children and infants, predominantly African-American and Hispanic. Recent measles outbreaks in the United States have clearly demonstrated deficiencies in compliance with vaccine recommendations. The failure has not been that of vaccine efficacy but of access to health care for infants and children living in poverty.

EPIDEMIOLOGY

The measles virus, classified as a paramyxovirus, has an outer envelope composed of lipoglycoproteins and an internal core of RNA. Only one antigenic type is known. The virus is found in nasopharyngeal secretions, blood, and urine during the prodromal period and for a short time after the rash appears. It remains active for at least 24 hours at room temperature. Measles is one of the most contagious childhood diseases and is transmitted during the prodromal period (catarrhal stage). Transmission to susceptible contacts often occurs before the diagnosis of the index case. The attack rate in household contacts is almost 90%, while less intimate contact (e.g., in school) leads to attack rates of 25 to 40%. Clinical severity, the case fatality rate, or both may be higher among secondary cases exposed to two or more index cases than among those exposed to only one index case. An infected person becomes contagious before the onset of symptoms (the catarrhal phase), which is usually 3 to 5 days before the onset of rash. The patient continues to be contagious until the fifth day after the rash appears. The virus is transmitted by direct contact with infectious respiratory droplets.

The epidemiology of measles in the United States has changed dramatically in the postvaccine era. In the 1960s before routine childhood immunization, more than 400,000 cases were reported annually, compared with fewer than 4000 cases reported annually in the early 1980s. From 1988 to 1990, the incidence of measles increased eightfold. In 1989, 18,913 cases were reported with 41 deaths; in 1990, 27,672 cases with 89 deaths. Nearly 50% of the cases in 1990 occurred in preschool children, 81% of whom were unvaccinated. More than 60% of the cases were reported in California (12,479) and Texas (4,403). These shifts in the age-prevalence of measles have led to a rise in hospitalization rates, with 21% of the 1990 patients requiring hospital care. Together with the preschool predominance, a surprising rise in cases has been reported in individuals over 20 years of age (17% of the total cases in 1989, including 10 deaths; 23% of the total in 1990, including 27 deaths). These findings suggest that the resurgence of measles in infants and young children may be due in part to lower levels of protective antibody against measles in women entering their child-bearing years.

Outbreaks continued in 1991 with new areas of activity. It is important to stress that the majority of cases reported in the past 2 years have never received a single dose of vaccine at a time when two doses of measles vaccine have been recommended.

Measles is endemic over most of the world. Prior to the introduction of the vaccine and currently in developing countries, epidemics usually occur during winter and spring, in urban areas, and every 2 to 3 years.

CLINICAL MANIFESTATIONS

The incubation period of acute measles is 8 to 12 days; however, the rash usually appears an average of 14 days after exposure (range 7–8 days). Measles is characterized by three stages: (1) During the incubation period, there are few if any signs or symptoms. (2) In the prodromal stage, the initial symptoms of coryza, conjunctivitis, and cough are seen. Measles coryza is indistinguishable from that of the common cold. The cough is nonproductive at first and increases in frequency, then slowly subsides over a period of 1 to 2 weeks. Fever usually appears with catarrhal symptoms and increases in intensity until the peak of the rash. Shortly after the start of this catarrhal stage (before the appearance of the rash), Koplik's spots develop on the buccal mucosa. These spots coalesce to form an erythematous base with multiple pinpoint whitish elevations. Considered to be pathognomonic for measles, Koplik's spots usually disappear by the second day of the rash and evolve into stomatitis. (3) In the final stage, a maculopapular rash appears (usually on the third or fourth day of disease), erupting successively over the neck and face, body, arms, and legs. The rash begins to subside in the same manner (from head down) by the third day. Thus, the total duration of illness in uncomplicated cases is 7 to 10 days. If fever persists beyond the third day of the rash, a complication should be suspected.

Acute measles is associated with immunologic abnormalities, including suppression of delayed hypersensitivity (depressed skin test responses), depressed total T-cell population, and in particular significantly depressed T4 helper/inducer subsets. A return to normal T4 and T4/T8 levels usually occurs 4 weeks later. Activation of the immune system is followed by production of measles-specific antibodies.

COMPLICATIONS

Death occurs in 1 of every 3000 reported measles cases in the United States, presumably as a result of respiratory and neurologic complications. However, in developing countries, mortality rates vary from 5% to 50%.

Complications are most common in infants and adults. Otitis media and pneumonia are relatively frequent complications. Pneumonia may be due to direct measles virus invasion or superimposed viral or bacterial infections. Among viral pathogens, adenovirus, herpesvirus, parainfluenza virus, and coxsackievirus play a major role. Among bacteria causing superinfection of the lungs are *Staphylococcus, Streptococcus, Pseudomonas,* and *Klebsiella.* Development of respiratory distress should alert the physician to the possibility of superimposed pneumonia.

During a recent epidemic of measles in southern California, 440 cases were seen between January and June of 1990 at a single children's hospital in Los Angeles. Ninety percent of the children were less than 5 years old and 50% were less than 15 months old. Forty-four percent required hospitalization for measles complications. The most frequent indications for admission were respiratory complications (pneumonia, croup) and dehydration; 7% required intensive care and 5% required assisted ventilation. Diarrhea, vomiting, or both were observed in almost half the patients admitted to the hospital. Clinical or radiographic evidence of pneumonia was seen in 36% of patients, and laryngotracheobronchitis (croup) was observed in slightly more than one-third of the children with pneumonia. Laryngotracheobronchitis (LTB) was diagnosed in 18% (82/440) of children with measles, corresponding to previously reported high rates of this complication in underdeveloped countries. Children with LTB were significantly younger (1.2 $\pm$ 0.7 years) than the group as a whole (2.1 $\pm$ 2.5 years). Physicians caring for young children with measles need to be alert to this potential complication because intensive care and assisted ventilation may be needed.

Subacute sclerosing panencephalitis (SSPE) is a late complication of measles. The incidence of SSPE is 1 in 100,000 cases of measles. In SSPE, the persistence of infection in the central nervous system without production of mature infectious virus may cause a degenerative disease, characterized by progressive behavioral and intellectual deterioration and followed by involuntary myoclonic seizures and death. The mean incubation period for SSPE is 7 years.

Acute measles encephalitis develops in approximately 1 of every 2000 cases. Although the virus generally cannot be isolated from brain tissue, immune system abnormalities persist for long periods with evidence of immune reactivity against myelin basic protein. The usual presentation of acute encephalitis is drowsiness, (which may progress to coma), seizures, vomiting, and headaches. Neck stiffness, and abnormal Kernig's and Brudzinski's signs may be found on physical examination. Mortality may be as high as 10%, and 25% of patients may develop neurologic sequelae. Results of cerebrospinal fluid examination range from normal to an aseptic picture (lymphocytosis with mildly elevated protein and normal glucose).

Less common complications of measles include severe keratoconjunctivitis with corneal ulceration, appendicitis, myocarditis, reactivation of tuberculosis, hepatitis, and premature labor or spontaneous abortion in pregnant women.

MODIFIED MEASLES

A modified form of measles is observed in individuals given gamma globulin during the incubation period and in infants less than 1 year of age who possess maternal antibody. In these patients, the catarrhal phase may be limited after a prolonged incubation period of up to 3 weeks and the rash may be less pronounced. The infection may be entirely subclinical.

ATYPICAL MEASLES

In individuals previously immunized with the killed virus vaccine, the diagnosis of measles may be difficult because of the unusual presentation. Atypical measles is seen in children or young adults exposed to natural measles months to years after primary immunization with killed, but rarely with attenuated, measles vaccine. Clinical presentation consists of a 2- to 3-day prodromal stage with high fever and headache and a rash that appears 1 to 5 days later. The rash usually takes the form of symmetrical eruptions on the extremities that can vary from macular-papular to purpuric lesions to vesicles. Pneumonia is a frequent feature of this syndrome. Elevated liver enzymes, disseminated intravascular coagulation, and myalgias may be seen. This atypical presentation may be a manifestation of delayed hypersensitivity and Arthur's reactions as demonstrated by skin biopsies.

MEASLES IN IMMUNOCOMPROMISED HOSTS

The number of immunocompromised children has increased as a result of cytotoxic chemotherapy to treat malignancies and the increasing prevalence of human immunodeficiency virus (HIV) infection. In the immunocompromised host, measles may have an atypical clinical presentation and is associated with serious complications in 80% of cases. Pneumonitis is present in 60%, compared with 1 to 5% in the general patient population, encephalitis occurs in 20% of these patients, compared with 0.1% in immunologically normal measles patients. Mortality rate from measles in patients with immunosuppression is 55% compared with only 0.1% in immunologically normal patients. In HIV-infected patients, pneumonitis is also the principal complication (70%) and is the cause of all measles deaths. In both groups, the clinical presentation is frequently atypical, with 27 to 40% of patients having no rash.

TREATMENT

Uncomplicated measles is a self-limited disease, and only symptomatic treatment is generally recommended. This includes acetaminophen for headache and fever, fluids to prevent dehydration, and bed rest in a dark room because of photophobia. The complications of otitis media and pneumonia require appropriate antimicrobial therapy.

Oral ribavirin* (10 mg per kg per day every 6 hours for 5 to 7 days) has been used in children with intact immunity. This compound has anti-measles activity in vitro, and in clinical trials in healthy children it appears to shorten the duration of illness, especially if given before the appearance of the rash. However, because measles is usually a mild disease in the normal host, ribavirin therapy is not recommended routinely. In one study, ribavirin, primarily in its aerosolized form, was given to 11 immunocompromised patients with measles pneumonitis, 5 of whom died. A significant improvement in survival could not be demonstrated in this small number of patients. While ribavirin therapy may appear logical in this situation, its effectiveness requires further study.

Other treatments for measles pneumonitis include immunoglobulin, interferon, and vitamin A. The efficacies of intravenous immunoglobulin and interferon have not been rigorously evaluated. However, treatment with oral vitamin A (200,000 IU) for 2 consecutive days reduces morbidity and mortality in poorly nourished children with severe measles in the developing world. Measles keratitis, often resulting from xerosis in children with hypovitaminosis A, is the third most frequent cause of blindness in children in Western Africa. The World Health Organization recommends vitamin A supplementation for children with measles in areas where vitamin A deficiency is a recognized problem and the measles-related mortality rate is 1% or more. The recommended dose is 200,000 IU by mouth at the diagnosis of measles (100,000 IU for children <1 year of age), repeated 24 hours later and again in 4 weeks if clinical signs of vitamin A deficiency are still present. A pilot study from Long Beach California of 20 children with measles found that more than 28% had vitamin A deficiency. Further studies to ascertain whether routine vitamin A supplementation would be beneficial in this group of children in the United States appear warranted. Pediatricians in practice should assess vitamin A status in young children with severe measles or associated complications and offer supplementation as appropriate.

---

*Investigational drug in the United States as an oral preparation.

PREVENTION

Postexposure Passive Immunization

To prevent measles, susceptible individuals who have been exposed can benefit from immunoglobulin (IG) given within 6 days of exposure. The usual dose is 0.25 ml per kg of IG given intramuscularly. The benefit of IG in preventing severe measles complications and death in immunocompromised children is less clear. The usual dose of IG for immunocompromised patients (including HIV-infected persons), regardless of their measles vaccination status, is doubled (0.5 ml per kg, not to exceed 15 ml). The only exception to this rule is HIV-infected children routinely receiving intravenous gamma globulin (IVIG) whose last IVIG dose was given 2 to 3 weeks before the exposure; these patients do not require further IG.

Postexposure Active Immunization

If exposure occurred within 72 hours, vaccination with live attenuated measles vaccine will protect the normal host. Vaccination of immunodeficient individuals with live vaccine is usually contraindicated; however, in HIV-infected children, measles immunization with live virus is recommended 3 months after IG administration if the child is older than 15 months. No adverse effects of live measles vaccine have been demonstrated among more than 100 HIV-infected children. Seroconversion following the vaccination of HIV-infected children occurred in 12% to 25% as demonstrated by ELISA.

Prevention of measles in immunocompromised individuals could be enhanced by vaccination of close contacts, especially siblings. Recent data also suggest that live measles vaccine may, under certain circumstances, be given safely to immunocompromised children with cancer. The American Academy of Pediatrics and the Immunization Practices Advisory Committee (ACIP) state that patients with leukemia in remission can be vaccinated against measles if they have not received chemotherapy in the previous 3 months.

Active Immunization

Vaccination produces a mild or inapparent noncommunicable infection that induces active immunization in more than 95% of recipients. Vaccine-induced protection persists for many years, and although reinfection with measles has occasionally been observed in apparently successfully immunized children, it does not appear that waning immunity is of epidemiologic significance.

The vaccine of choice is the measles-mumps-rubella (MMR) vaccine, which should be given at 15 months of age for maximal seroconversion rate. Measles vaccine is also available as a monovalent (measles alone) vaccine or combined with rubella vaccine (MR). Presently, a two-dose schedule is recommended for live measles vaccination. This is because of the clustering of cases among high school and college students considered to be due to the normal 3 to 5% primary vaccine failure rate. The ACIP and the American Academy of Pediatrics recommend different ages for the second dose; at school entry (ages 5 to 6) or before entrance to middle school (ages 9 to 12), respectively. However, these differences may not be important as long as all vaccinees receive two doses.

Vaccine administration schedules should be adjusted to meet local needs: in endemic or epidemic areas, all children 6 to 9 months of age and older should receive their first dose of measles (monovalent) vaccine; in high-risk areas, first doses of MMR should be given at 12 months of age. In children who were initially vaccinated before 12 months of age, a second vaccination should be administered at 15 months of age. One reason why children fail to receive measles vaccination is the presence of a minor illness such as an upper respiratory tract infection. However, it is a misconception that such children cannot receive live-virus vaccines.

Side Effects

The vaccine is quite safe, and serious complications are exceedingly rare. About 15% of vaccinees develop fever above 39° C (102.5° F), usually 5 to 10 days after the immunization. About 5% of vaccinees develop a transient rash. Serious neurologic disease (Reye's syndrome, encephalitis, cerebellar ataxia, or Guillain-Barré syndrome) following immunization occurs at a rate of about one case per million doses of vaccine.

Contraindications

Fever is not a contraindication for vaccination unless it represents a serious illness. Because the vaccine is prepared in chicken embryo tissue culture, it is widely believed that allergy to eggs is a contraindication for immunization. This assumption is incorrect; only those having had anaphylactic reactions are at increased risk. Live measles vaccine should not be administered to pregnant women or to severely immunocompromised (impaired cell-mediated immunity) individuals. This includes patients with leukemia or lymphoma, and those receiving high-dose steroid, radiation, or antimetabolite therapy. In all instances, the relative risk of measles in the patient should be considered in relation to the risk of immunization.

TETANUS

method of
JOHN H. KERR, D.M.
Nuffield Department of Anaesthetics
Radcliffe Infirmary, Oxford, England

The spores of *Clostridium tetani* are widespread in dust and soil, particularly in warmer climates and in intensively cultivated areas. If they enter the body through a wound and find an anaerobic environment (e.g., in dead tissue or by a foreign body), they may germinate and multiply. A potent neurotoxin, tetanospasmin, is synthesized within the cell and is released into the extracellular fluid when autolysis occurs. The toxin diffuses away from the wound and is taken up by nerve fibers both close to the wound and, if the toxin reaches the bloodstream, throughout the body.

Once within nerve fibers, the toxin migrates toward the spinal cord, where it exerts its effects after passing in a retrograde manner from the motor neurons in the anterior horn to the presynaptic terminals of the spinal interneurones. Here it interferes with the release of the inhibitory transmitters, leading to an increase in muscle tone (e.g., lockjaw), simultaneous contraction of agonist and antagonist muscle groups (e.g., muscle spasms), and impaired muscular coordination. The tetanospasmin that is taken up by autonomic fibers eventually reaches the lateral horns of the spinal cord and has an analogous disinhibitory effect on the sympathetic nervous system. Once inside the nerve fiber or central nervous system (CNS), tetanospasmin cannot be neutralized by tetanus antitoxin in the bloodstream.

Depending on the distribution of the toxin, symptoms may be restricted to the muscles of the wounded limb (*local tetanus*) or to those of the head (*cephalic tetanus*); if the toxin has been spread around the body in the bloodstream, *generalized tetanus* occurs. In such cases, symptoms usually manifest in muscles served by short axons (e.g., masseteric, pharyngeal, and back muscles) and appear several hours later in muscles with longer axons (e.g., abdominal or limb muscles). When symptoms of increased tone first appear at the end of the incubation period, they indicate only that some toxin has reached the spinal interneurons but give little information about the amount still in transit to the CNS within nerve fibers. It is difficult, therefore, to predict the ultimate severity of an individual case with much certainty, and so all patients should be managed as if potentially severely affected.

ESTABLISHED TETANUS

Diagnosis

In the early stages of tetanus, the trismus of a dental abscess may be confused with lockjaw, but sensitivity to phenothiazines is the most common differential diagnosis. A single dose of a phenothiazine such as perphenazine (Trilafon), or other antiemetic agents such as metoclopramide (Reglan), can produce abnormal but variable muscular activity such as stiffness, tremors, and unwillingness to open the mouth in a sensitive patient, but these symptoms are more often seen in patients receiving large doses of the drugs. The symptoms respond rapidly to anticholinergic drugs such as benztropine (Cogentin). Although strychnine poisoning may be mistaken for fully developed tetanus, its rapid lethality makes the distinction academic.

TREATMENT

All patients with established tetanus require basic measures regardless of severity. To these, specific additional measures should be added as appropriate (Table 1).

Basic Measures

Any patient who is suspected of having tetanus should be moved immediately to an intensive care unit that is equipped and staffed to provide 24-hour nursing and artificial ventilation. All patients should receive a 5-day course of penicillin (1 million units every 6 hours intramuscularly)

TABLE 1. **Management of Established Tetanus**

General Measures for All Patients
Observe carefully in intensive care unit
Antibiotics—penicillin or erythromycin or cefuroxime plus metronidazole
Tetanus immune globulin (human)
Thorough débridement of any wound
Active immunization with toxoid

Symptomatic Measures As Required
Diazepam or chlorpromazine *for muscular hypertonicity*
Careful mouth toilet *for trismus*
Oral intubation followed by formal tracheostomy *for dysphagia*
Therapeutic paralysis and intermittent positive pressure ventilation *for muscle spasms*
Mild sedation and analgesia plus reassurance *for anxiety*
Adequate nutrition preferably via nasogastric tube but by parenteral route if absorption impaired by ileus
Adequate fluid intake *to replace large insensible losses*
Anticoagulation *to protect against deep venous thrombosis*
Adrenergic blockade *for sympathetic overactivity*
Atrial pacing *for refractory bradycardia*
Rapid infusion of colloid *if patient "shocked"* (hypotensive, tachycardiac, pyretic, sweating profusely, and sudden onset of ileus)

If Intensive Care Is Not Available
Diazepam or chlorpromazine in very large doses *for muscular symptoms*
Tracheostomy *to protect against laryngeal spasms and aspiration pneumonia*
Nasogastric feeding and fluid administration
Consider intrathecal antitoxin (immediately after diagnosis) *to reduce severity*

or cefuroxime (Zinacef) (750 mg every 8 hours intramuscularly) plus metronidazole (500 mg every 8 hours intravenously).

Human tetanus immune globulin (TIG[H]) (Hyper-Tet) should be given both intravenously (1000 units) and intramuscularly (2000 units). If visible (check the ear and nose carefully), any wound should be explored thoroughly and excised widely *after* the intravenous TIG(H) so that the large amounts of tetanospasmin present in the tissues surrounding the lesion will be neutralized. If TIG(H) is not available, it is doubtful whether the benefits of antitoxin of animal (usually equine) origin outweigh their allergenic risks.

The value of antitoxin given by the intrathecal route is still uncertain after 20 years of use, although there are strong theoretical reasons for its efficacy. If used, a single injection of a special preparation of TIG(H) (*lacking the usual preservatives*) should be given in combination with prednisolone as soon as possible after the diagnosis has been made. In adults, 1000 units of TIG(H) plus 25 mg of prednisolone should be given, and in neonates, 250 units of TIG(H) plus 12.5 mg of prednisolone.

Because having had tetanus does not confer immunity to the disease, active immunization should be commenced with adsorbed toxoid (10 Lf units by deep intramuscular injection into a limb other than the one into which the intramuscular TIG[H] has been given). Further doses should be given 6 weeks and 6 months later.

Symptomatic Measures

Muscular stiffness, which usually manifests in the masseters or injured limb, should be treated with diazepam (Valium), 10 to 20 mg every 3 to 4 hours. The patient's inevitable anxiety should be alleviated by a careful and reassuring explanation of the symptoms and their management. If the hypertonicity extends to involve the pharyngeal muscles, dysphagia develops and there is an immediate risk of laryngeal spasm and inhalation pneumonia. The airway must be protected without delay (and *before* the patient is moved within or between hospitals) by orotracheal intubation under general anesthesia. Tetanus patients respond normally to induction agents (e.g., thiopental) and succinylcholine (1 mg per kg of body weight intravenously). Formal tracheostomy under general anesthesia should follow when convenient. Tracheostomy under local anesthesia is contraindicated in tetanus because laryngeal spasm may be provoked before cannulation is established.

A nasogastric tube should be inserted while the

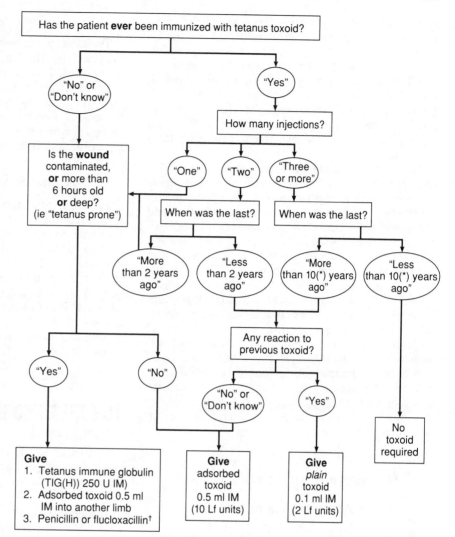

Figure 1. Tetanus prophylaxis for the injured patient. (*) Five years if the wound is "tetanus prone" or if the patient is over 60 years old. ‡Not available in the United States.

patient is anesthetized, and further doses of diazepam should be given by this route. If hypertonicity becomes generalized and if muscle spasms develop, the drug may have to be given intravenously and in large doses in order to keep the patient comfortable. The patient may then fluctuate between poorly controlled spasms and a semicomatose state in which hypoventilation and hypostatic pneumonia occur. In this state, and if the muscle spasms themselves interfere with ventilation, therapeutic paralysis should be instituted with the use of a curariform drug (d-tubocurarine, 15 to 30 mg; alcuronium,* 10 to 20 mg; or pancuronium [Pavulon], 4 to 8 mg up to half hourly intravenously) and artificial ventilation commenced with a volume-preset ventilator. Meticulous ventilatory care is required for 2 to 5 weeks, during which time mild hypnosis should

be induced with diazepam, midazolam, or a barbiturate. The need for heavy sedation and analgesia can be reduced by repeated reassurance and adequate relaxation.

The maintenance of fluid balance in the tetanus patient is complicated by the fact that because trismus is the most common presenting symptom, patients are usually dehydrated by the time that the diagnosis is established. Subsequently, excessive insensible fluid losses in the form of profuse sweating at night and unswallowed saliva tend to prolong this state, which, if allowed to persist, may lead to deep venous thrombosis and fatal pulmonary embolism. Fluid intake, preferably via the nasogastric tube, should be sufficient to allow the production of 1.5 to 2 liters of urine each day with a specific gravity of 1.015 or less. Anticoagulation with warfarin or subcutaneous heparin is indicated to reduce further the risk of pulmonary embolism, which has

---

*Not available in the United States

been a common and often fatal complication in patients with severe tetanus from limb wounds.

If gastrointestinal stasis occurs in conjunction with severe sweating in a sympathetic storm, hypovolemia (shown by tachycardia, hypotension, and diminished urine flow) may develop suddenly. The rapid restoration of the circulating fluid volume with infusion of both colloids and crystalloids is required in order to prevent a fatal outcome.

The involvement of the autonomic nervous system in patients with severe tetanus is analogous to the muscular disturbances. Both hypertonicity (in the form of hypertension and tachycardia) and spasms (as the simultaneous constriction of both arterioles and veins) occur and, if they persist, probably contribute to the high mortality rate in paralyzed and ventilated patients. These symptoms usually appear a day or so after the muscle spasms but may persist after the muscular symptoms have abated. They should be controlled by adrenergic blocking agents such as labetalol (Trandate), 100 mg every 2 to 4 hours intravenously or via nasogastric tube, but pure beta-adrenergic blocking agents should be avoided. An infusion of magnesium sulfate sufficient to maintain a blood magnesium level of 2.5 to 4 mmol per liter has been recommended to control the cardiovascular overactivity.

PREVENTION AND PROPHYLAXIS

Active Immunization

Almost everyone can be protected completely against tetanus by active immunization with tetanus toxoid. After the age of 3 months, unimmunized subjects should be given three injections of adsorbed toxoid (10 Lf units intramuscularly) at intervals of 4 to 6 weeks and 4 to 6 months. To maintain immunity, booster doses of adsorbed toxoid (10 Lf units intramuscularly) are required at about 10-year intervals until the age of 60 years, when the interval should be reduced to 5 years. In patients who suffer disabling swelling and pain after the injection of adsorbed toxoid, a lower dose (1 to 2 Lf units) of plain toxoid should be given by *deep* intramuscular injection. This appears to be equally effective in maintaining immunity by stimulating antitoxin production in such sensitive individuals.

In countries where death from neonatal tetanus remains common, the problem may be reduced markedly if mothers are immunized by at least two injections of toxoid during pregnancy. Antibodies cross the placenta and protect the child for the first 6 months of life.

Passive Immunization

Temporary protection against tetanus can be provided by the parenteral injection of tetanus antibodies. TIG(H) is now used exclusively in the developed world, rather than the equine variety with its high incidence of serious allergic reactions. A protective antibody level is usually maintained for about 4 weeks after an intramuscular injection of 250 units of TIG(H).

Tetanus Prophylaxis After Injury

Figure 1 indicates the need for passive or active immunization after injury, because the treatment required depends on both the immunologic status of the patient and the characteristics of the wound. The other components of tetanus prophylaxis after injury include prompt and aggressive wound surgery and antibiotics. Patients who have not been immunized previously against tetanus and who have been given their initial dose of toxoid should receive further doses at 4 to 6 weeks and 4 to 6 months.

TOXOPLASMOSIS

method of
ROBERT L. PENN, M.D.
Louisiana State University School of Medicine
Shreveport, Louisiana

Toxoplasmosis is caused by infection with the obligate intracellular parasite *Toxoplasma gondii*. Not all *Toxoplasma* infections result in clinical illness and not all require therapy. In fact, asymptomatic infection is much more common than active, symptomatic toxoplasmosis. Seroprevalence studies have found antibody evidence of asymptomatic infection in up to 70% of adults in the United States and 95% of adults in France. The rate of seropositivity generally increases with age through childhood into adult years and may vary widely among different groups within the same country. Factors that increase the risk of exposure to *T. gondii* include the presence of cats, a warm and moist climate, eating raw or undercooked meats, and abattoir work.

T. gondii is capable of infecting most mammals and many birds, but completes its life cycle only in members of the cat family. Oocysts, produced only within cat intestines, are excreted in feces. After several days in the appropriate environmental conditions, sporulation of freshly passed oocysts yields infectious oocysts. The other two forms of *T. gondii* are the trophozoite, the form that invades and grows within host cells, and the tissue cyst, which contains viable trophozoites. Cysts can form in any tissue, persist for life, and be responsible for later reactivation of toxoplasmosis. An effective host immune response is required to control the infection and contain the cysts; this involves antibody, sensitized T cells, and cytokines such as interleukin-2 and interferon-gamma. Immunosuppression can result in reactivation of infection by permitting breakdown of tissue cysts and release of trophozoites, causing local abscess formation, disseminated illness, or both.

Humans most commonly become infected with *T. gondii* by ingestion of infectious oocysts or cysts or by transplacental transmission to the fetus from a mother with active toxoplasmosis. Oocysts can be ingested during childhood play or while gardening, changing cat litter, or eating contaminated food or drink. Cysts can be ingested in raw or poorly cooked meats. Both oocysts and cysts are capable of releasing viable parasites that invade the intestinal wall and subsequently spread hematogenously to any organ in the body, where they can form tissue cysts containing numerous viable trophozoites. Common sites of involvement are the retina, brain, muscle, and heart. If *T. gondii* circulate during pregnancy, they can infect the placenta, causing congenital toxoplasmosis. Less common means of transmitting *T. gondii* are transfusion of whole blood, platelets, or leukocytes, transplantation of organs obtained from a seropositive donor into a seronegative recipient, and percutaneous infection as a result of laboratory accidents.

TREATMENT

The decision to treat *T. gondii* infection is made by considering the immunocompetency of the patient, the route of infection, and the clinical manifestations (Table 1).

Normal Adults

Hosts with normal immune systems usually remain asymptomatic, are diagnosed with latent infection only on the basis of a positive serology, and do not require treatment. Lymphadenopathy is the most common manifestation of acute toxoplasmosis in otherwise healthy people; it is usually self-limited, resolving within 1 to 3 weeks. Treatment for acute lymphadenopathic toxoplasmosis is given only if systemic symptoms are severe or prolonged. Rarely, immunologically normal patients with acute infection will present with dissemination and vital organ involvement (myocarditis, pneumonia, encephalitis), and they require treatment. Acute infections resulting from laboratory accidents or from transfusions should be treated because they are potentially severe.

The treatment of choice is a combination of pyrimethamine (Daraprim) and sulfadiazine or trisulfapyrimidine, given for 4 to 6 weeks or longer if symptoms persist. Pyrimethamine is given orally as a loading dose of 1 mg per kg twice daily for 2 days, up to a maximum of 50 to 100 mg per day in older children and adults. This is followed by daily or every other day therapy with 1 mg per kg pyrimethamine, up to a maximum of 25 to 50 mg per dose in older children and adults. Sulfadiazine or trisulfapyrimidine is given orally as a single loading dose of 75 mg per kg (maximum of 4 grams), followed by 100 mg per kg per day (maximum of 6 to 8 grams per day) in two divided doses. Oral folinic acid (leucovorin) is given to prevent pyrimethamine-induced hematologic toxicity; a dose of 5 to 10 mg per day three times a week is suggested to start and is increased to daily dosing (up to 20 mg per day) based on the results of weekly or twice-weekly complete blood cell and platelet counts.

Ocular Toxoplasmosis

Chorioretinitis almost always represents reactivation of latent congenital *T. gondii* infection and characteristically is bilateral; chorioretinitis

TABLE 1. **Therapy for Toxoplasmosis**

Host Status	Initial Treatment of Choice*
Normal Immunity	
Asymptomatic	None
Lymphadenopathy	Rarely needed (pyrimethamine† + sulfadiazine)
Dissemination	Pyrimethamine + sulfadiazine
Laboratory or transfusion acquired	Pyrimethamine + sulfadiazine
Chorioretinitis	Pyrimethamine + sulfadiazine‡
Congenital infection	Pyrimethamine + sulfadiazine‡
Pregnancy	
Acute infection	Spiramycin ± pyrimethamine + sulfadiazine
Chronic infection	None
Immunosuppression	
Encephalitis	Pyrimethamine + sulfadiazine
Chorioretinitis	Pyrimethamine + sulfadiazine‡
Dissemination	Pyrimethamine + sulfadiazine

*See text for indications, dosages, and alternatives.
†Folinic acid is given to patients receiving pyrimethamine.
‡Corticosteroids may be added if there is significant inflammation (see text).

from reactivation of acquired infection occurs much less often and usually is unilateral. In immunocompromised patients, eye involvement also may be part of disseminated toxoplasmosis, caused by either acute or reactivated infection. Diagnosis of ocular toxoplasmosis is made on the basis of the characteristic funduscopic appearance, together with the appropriate serologic studies.

All forms of *Toxoplasma* chorioretinitis need treatment because of their propensity to relapse with risk of visual loss. The drugs of choice are pyrimethamine and sulfadiazine or trisulfapyrimidine with folinic acid in the dosages described in the previous section. Clindamycin is often used as an alternative to the sulfonamides because it concentrates in the retina; the dose in adults is 300 mg every 6 hours. However, the efficacy of clindamycin when used alone for ocular toxoplasmosis has been questioned. Recently, co-trimoxazole (Bactrim, Septra), (160 mg trimethoprim and 800 mg sulfamethoxazole twice a day for 4 to 6 weeks) has been reported to be another effective oral agent, although clinical experience is limited. Treatment should be given for at least 1 month and should lead to a response within the first 10 days. Corticosteroids can be added if inflammation of the macula, optic nerve head, or papillomacular bundle threatens vision. Photocoagulation and vitrectomy may be required in individual cases. Treatment of ocular toxoplasmosis should always be undertaken in collaboration with an ophthalmologist.

Congenital Infection

Congenital toxoplasmosis can take a variety of forms, from no obvious changes present at birth to the classic syndrome of fever, hydrocephalus or microcephalus, hepatosplenomegaly, jaundice, retinitis, intracerebral calcifications, and abnormal spinal fluid. However, most asymptomatic newborns will eventually develop clinical evidence of active infection. Thus, all infants suspected of having congenital toxoplasmosis should be treated until the diagnosis is established, and all infants proven to have been infected in utero with *T. gondii* should be treated whether or not they are symptomatic. Experience to date suggests that treatment of active disease ameliorates clinical symptoms and can improve the functional prognosis in all but the most severely affected.

The optimal treatment is not known. A national collaborative trial is still accepting patients with congenital toxoplasmosis to compare several empiric regimens. (Patients may be considered for enrollment by contacting Dr. Rima McLeod in Chicago, Illinois, at 1-312-791-4152.) All children receive 1 year of therapy. Loading doses of pyrimethamine (2 mg per kg for 2 days) and sulfadiazine or trisulfapyrimidine (100 mg per kg once) are given, followed by daily therapy for 2 months with pyrimethamine (1 mg per kg) and sulfadiazine or trisulfapyrimidine (100 mg per kg in two divided doses). Over the next 4 months, pyrimethamine is given on Monday, Wednesday, and Friday with daily sulfadiazine or trisulfapyrimidine. The final 6 months of treatment for less severely affected and asymptomatic infants may be either Monday/Wednesday/Friday pyrimethamine plus daily sulfonamide or Monday/Wednesday/Friday pyrimethamine plus daily sulfonamide in months 8, 10, and 12 alternated with spiramycin alone (50 mg per kg twice daily) in months 7, 9, and 11.

Patients with more significant neurologic involvement or severe systemic illness are managed in the same way for the first 2 months. They may then be given either Monday/Wednesday/Friday pyrimethamine plus daily sulfonamide for the next 10 months or daily pyrimethamine plus daily sulfonamide for the first 6 months before changing to Monday/Wednesday/Friday pyrimethamine plus daily sulfonamide for the last 6 months.

Folinic acid should be given whenever pyrimethamine is being used; the dose is 5 to 10 mg three times a week or more frequently, adjusted to prevent the hematologic side effects of pyrimethamine. Prednisone, 1 mg per kg per day in divided doses, should be added when retinal inflammation threatens vision or when the cerebrospinal fluid protein is 1000 mg per dL or higher; steroids are tapered and discontinued once these problems are controlled. Outcome also may be improved by the early detection of and management of hydrocephalus.

Pregnancy

Latent toxoplasmosis acquired before pregnancy is not a threat to the fetus in the immunologically normal mother. Maternal acquisition of *T. gondii* in the last trimester carries the greatest risk for congenital fetal infection, but most of these infants are asymptomatic. Congenital infections are less frequent when *T. gondii* is acquired earlier in pregnancy, but these infants are more likely to have severe clinical involvement. Immunosuppression increases the risk of reactivation of latent *T. gondii* infection; if this should occur during pregnancy, the fetus may become infected. Thus, it is recommended that spiramycin be given throughout pregnancy to immunosuppressed women with previously acquired latent toxoplasmosis (seropositivity acquired before pregnancy).

Treatment of mothers with toxoplasmosis

newly acquired during pregnancy significantly reduces the risk of fetal infection. However, if the fetus already has been infected, subsequent maternal treatment will not arrest the fetal disease. Thus, infants born with congenital toxoplasmosis should be treated even if the mother was treated during pregnancy.

Prenatal diagnosis should be performed in all pregnant women with newly acquired toxoplasmosis. Readily available and useful techniques include ultrasonography, amniocentesis, and fetal blood sampling. If fetal infection is not documented, then oral spiramycin, 1.5 grams twice daily, is given throughout pregnancy. If fetal infection is documented and the pregnancy is not terminated, then 3 weeks of spiramycin is alternated with 3 weeks of sulfadiazine or trisulfapyrimidine (3 to 4 grams per day) plus pyrimethamine (25 to 50 mg per day) and folinic acid (5 to 15 mg per day). The complete blood count and platelet count should be monitored once or twice a week. Pyrimethamine is potentially teratogenic and should not be used in the first 16 weeks of pregnancy; spiramycin is usually used during this time.

AIDS Patients

Patients infected with human immunodeficiency virus (HIV) are at unusually high risk for clinical toxoplasmosis, and this correlates with their degree of immunosuppression. In the United States, most infections present as encephalitis from reactivation disease when the CD4 lymphocyte count is less than 100 per mm³. *Toxoplasma* pneumonia is less frequently diagnosed and is likewise felt to represent reactivation illness. Acute infections also occur and can take a variety of clinical forms.

The combination of pyrimethamine and sulfadiazine or trisulfapyrimidine has had the most extensive use in treating *Toxoplasma* encephalitis in patients with acquired immunodeficiency syndrome (AIDS). Because serum levels of pyrimethamine are unpredictable in these patients, 50 to 100 mg are usually given per day, after a loading dose of 100 mg every 12 hours for two doses. The sulfonamide is given as a 75-mg per kg loading dose (maximum of 4 grams), followed by 100 mg per kg per day in two divided doses (maximum of 6 to 8 grams a day). This initial treatment, which is given for 6 weeks, should also include folinic acid, 10 to 20 mg per day. Successful control of encephalitis is marked by improvement shown clinically within 7 to 10 days and demonstrated on computed tomography or magnetic resonance imaging by 3 weeks. Lifetime suppressive therapy, needed in part because this regimen does not kill cysts, should immediately

follow the initial treatment. The suppressive regimen of choice is 25 to 50 mg per day of pyrimethamine with 2 to 4 grams per day of sulfadiazine; folinic acid, 5 to 10 mg per day, also is given to prevent pyrimethamine's hematologic toxicities. There is a very high incidence of side effects with this regimen, including rash, cytopenias, crystalluria, renal stones, and renal failure. Zidovudine may contribute to hematologic toxicity and in vitro is a pyrimethamine antagonist; the clinical importance of the latter observation is unknown.

The sulfonamide alternative that has received the most attention is clindamycin. Given either intravenously or orally, clindamycin, 2400 to 4800 mg per day in four divided doses plus pyrimethamine is as effective as sulfadiazine plus pyrimethamine (in the doses described earlier) for initial therapy. The lower dose of clindamycin is preferred because of its many side effects, including diarrhea, rash, *Clostridium difficile* enterocolitis, neutropenia, and myopathy. A small number of patients have been successfully treated acutely for *Toxoplasma* encephalitis with pyrimethamine, 75 mg per day, plus clarithromycin (Biaxin),* 1 gram orally twice daily. Atovaquone (Mepron) 750 mg four times daily, was successful in 6 of 10 AIDS patients with *Toxoplasma* encephalitis who had either failed to respond to or were unable to take pyrimethamine plus sulfadiazine.

Many patients who experience rash during the initial phase of treatment can be successfully continued on sulfadiazine for chronic suppression. Patients who are truly sulfonamide intolerant must either be desensitized or given another drug. Maintenance therapy with clindamycin is less well studied; one regimen is 450 mg every 8 hours plus pyrimethamine, 25 mg daily, along with folinic acid. A recent report involving small numbers of patients suggests that twice-weekly pyrimethamine with either sulfadiazine or clindamycin may also be effective. Pyrimethamine alone in a dose of 75 mg per day, with 10 mg per day of folinic acid, may be used for chronic suppression if sulfadiazine or clindamycin cannot be given.

Failures have been reported with doxycycline, co-trimoxazole, spiramycin, and trimetrexate when used for either acute treatment or suppression.

Among the promising drugs currently under study are dapsone, roxithromycin,† clarithromycin, azithromycin (Zithromax), aprinocid,† atovaquone, and recombinant interferon-gamma. Azithromycin, aprinocid, and atovaquone are of

---

*This use of clarithromycin is not listed in the manufacturer's official directive.

†Investigational drug in the United States.

particular interest because they are active against *T. gondii* cysts.

Other Immunosuppressed Patients

Toxoplasmosis poses similar problems in patients immunosuppressed by drugs or diseases other than AIDS. Patients undergoing bone marrow transplantation are at particular risk for reactivation illness during the initial 6 months after transplant. In contrast, recipients of solid organs are at highest risk for new infection acquired from seropositive donors. Pyrimethamine, sulfadiazine or trisulfapyrimidine, and folinic acid in the doses given previously are the drugs of choice. Treatment should be given for 4 to 6 weeks after clinical resolution of illness. If possible, immunosuppressive drugs should be eliminated or dosages minimized.

PREVENTION

Toxoplasmosis can be prevented by educating seronegative patients at risk about how to avoid exposure to *T. gondii* (Table 2). This is particularly important for pregnant women and for those with HIV infection or other immunosuppressive disorders.

Primary chemoprophylaxis is useful in heart transplantation. Acute toxoplasmosis can be prevented by pyrimethamine, 25 mg per day for the initial 6 weeks following transplantation of a heart from a seropositive donor into a seronegative recipient. Whether this regimen also is of benefit to seronegative patients receiving other solid organs from seropositive donors is not known. Recommendations about the chemoprevention of toxoplasmosis in other high-risk seronegative patients, such as those with HIV infection, must await future studies.

Small and often retrospective studies have evaluated the primary chemoprophylaxis of reactivation toxoplasmosis in seropositive HIV-infected patients. When used for *Pneumocystis* pneumonia prophylaxis, co-trimoxazole and pyrimethamine-sulfadoxine (Fansidar) have been associated with reduced rates of presumed *T. gondii* encephalitis. Spiramycin, trimetrexate, and clar-

TABLE 2. **Prevention of Toxoplasmosis**

Do not handle cat feces or cat litter
Do not drink raw milk
Do not eat raw or undercooked eggs or meats
Do not touch the mouth or eyes when handling raw meats
Wash hands and tabletops after handling raw foods
Keep insects and cockroaches away from foods
Wash or peel all fruits and vegetables
Wear gloves while gardening or working in outdoor
    sandboxes

ithromycin used alone are not effective. One prospective study comparing clindamycin with pyrimethamine for this purpose was reportedly terminated after preliminary analysis found excessive toxicity from clindamycin and no demonstrable benefit from pyrimethamine. Thus, at present no single-drug regimen is of proven efficacy for primary prophylaxis of toxoplasmosis in seropositive HIV-infected individuals. The results of prospective controlled trials are needed before co-trimoxazole, the newer agents with anticyst activity (azithromycin, aprinocid, and atovaquone), or combination regimens can be recommended.

Drugs

Pyrimethamine is available only in oral form. Blood levels are unpredictable in individual patients, but measurements of the serum pyrimethamine concentration are not readily available as a routine test in most laboratories. Pyrimethamine's half-life ranges from 1.5 to 5 days, so daily therapy may not be needed in all cases. It is lipid soluble, concentrates in the brain, and yields cerebrospinal fluid levels that are about 10 to 25% of serum levels. The major toxicities of pyrimethamine stem from its antifolate activity and include thrombocytopenia, anemia, and leukopenia. Thus, it is important to monitor blood cell counts once or twice weekly. Folinic acid can minimize bone marrow suppression by pyrimethamine without affecting its activity against *T. gondii* and should be given to all persons receiving daily pyrimethamine and to any child receiving pyrimethamine. Less common side effects of pyrimethamine include headache, gastrointestinal distress, and an unusual taste.

Sulfonamides exert a synergistic effect with pyrimethamine against *T. gondii*. Sulfadiazine and trisulfapyrimidine are the most active, with sulfamethoxazole and other sulfonamides clearly less active. The half-life of these agents is about 12 hours, so twice daily dosing may be used. Tablet and liquid oral forms and an intravenous preparation are available. Hypersensitivity reactions including rash and fever are frequent in HIV-infected patients. A potentially more serious complication of sulfonamide therapy is crystalluria, which can be asymptomatic, associated with hematuria, or result in oliguric acute renal failure. For this reason, patients should be urged to drink at least 2 liters of fluids daily and to report decreased urine output. Some investigators recommend routine urinalysis for sulfonamide crystals, and if present, adding oral sodium bicarbonate (6 to 12 grams per day) to alkalinize the urine. Other side effects from sulfonamides include gastrointestinal reactions and leukopenia.

The macrolide spiramycin is widely used outside the United States for the treatment of pregnant patients and the newborn. It is best absorbed when taken on an empty stomach. It is usually well tolerated and does not suppress the bone marrow but can cause gastrointestinal reactions. Permission to use spiramycin in the United States must be obtained from the Antivirals Division of the Food and Drug Administration prior to obtaining it from the manufacturer (Rhone-Poulenc Rorer, Collegeville, PA).

Clindamycin is available in both oral and intravenous forms. Despite poor penetration into the cerebrospinal fluid, it has been shown to be effective in the treatment of *Toxoplasma* encephalitis in AIDS patients. Unfortunately, its side effects commonly lead to its discontinuation: these include diarrhea, rash, *C. difficile* enterocolitis, neutropenia, and myopathy.

Atovaquone was recently released as an oral agent for the acute therapy of mild to moderate *Pneumocystis carinii* pneumonia. It also is active against *T. gondii,* including cysts, and may prove to be effective alone for the suppression or prevention of toxoplasmosis. The optimal dosages and schedules for toxoplasmosis are currently being evaluated. Atovaquone is best absorbed when taken with food, and its half-life is between 2 and 3 days. Side effects include cutaneous reactions and mild abnormalities in the levels of neutrophils, platelets, and serum transaminases.

TRICHINELLOSIS

method of
DONALD W. HOSKINS, M.D.
Cornell University Medical College
New York, New York

Muscle pain and tenderness, fever, and periorbital edema together with striking eosinophilia are the hallmarks of trichinellosis. Beginning 10 to 21 days after infection, symptoms are caused by the wide dissemination of larvae in skeletal muscle. Although larvae enter most organs and produce, in a few patients, myocarditis, pneumonitis, or meningoencephalitis, the infection is transient with encystment only in skeletal muscle. The greater the number of larvae ingested, the larger the worm burden. In turn, the larger the worm burden, the more larvae are produced, the earlier the onset of symptoms is, and the more seriously ill the patient is.

The disease is acquired by the ingestion of larva-infected raw or poorly cooked meat, primarily pork and pork products, especially sausage. Commercially prepared pork products account for fewer cases now than decades ago, as a result of lower swine infection rates (less than 1%) by required cooking of nongrain hog feeds. There are, however, increasing reports of outbreaks of trichinellosis after ingestion of bear meat, wild pig meat, walrus meat, and even cougar meat.

INTESTINAL PHASE

Few symptoms are reported days 1 to 5 after ingestion of infected meat. A brief self-limited gastroenteritis occasionally results. The ingested larvae mature rapidly into adult *Trichinella spiralis.* After fertilization, gravid females burrow into the mucosa of the proximal small bowel, discharging up to 1500 larvae per female into the bloodstream and lymphatic vessels. Larval production, which begins as early as 5 days after ingestion, continues for 2 to 5 weeks, in some patients for several months.

DIAGNOSIS

Muscle biopsy specimens demonstrating larvae prove the diagnosis. Characteristic symptoms and findings together with marked eosinophilia, especially in the setting of an outbreak with an identifiable meal from a common source, are acceptable criteria without biopsy. Serologic tests are usually confirmatory but are rarely positive less than 30 days after ingestion of infected meat or 1 to 2 weeks after onset of symptoms.

TREATMENT

Several broad-spectrum anthelminthics—including pyrantel pamoate (Antiminth), 10 mg per kg orally once daily for 4 days; mebendazole (Vermox), 7.5 mg per kg twice daily for 3 days; and thiabendazole (Mintezol), 25 mg per kg twice daily for 5 days—may be successfully employed to clear the upper intestinal tract of adult *T. spiralis.* However, as noted earlier, this phase (days 1 to 5) is largely unnoticed, and the disease therefore remains undiagnosed.

Mild systemic illness is self-limited and requires no treatment other than analgesics.

Patients with moderate systemic disease (significant muscle pain and tenderness, fever, periorbital edema) should be considered for benzimidazole therapy (mebendazole [Vermox] or thiabendazole [Mintezol]) to (1) reduce or eliminate continued larval production by ridding the intestinal tract of adult *T. spiralis* and (2) for their larvicidal activity. Mebendazole (Vermox)* is better tolerated but not as well absorbed as thiabendazole. Nevertheless, significant serum levels of mebendazole have been demonstrated, and there is evidence of larvicidal activity after

---

*Safety in its use during pregnancy has not been demonstrated.

oral doses of 5 mg per kg twice daily for 10 days. Nausea, diarrhea, and abdominal cramps are occasionally noted. Thiabendazole (Mintezol), 25 mg per kg twice daily for 5 days (maximal dose, 3 gm per day), is the only benzimidazole drug currently approved for the treatment of trichinellosis in the United States. Albendazole, 800 mg per day for 6 days, which is currently not available in the United States, is reported to be better tolerated and more effective in treating trichinellosis than is either mebendazole or thiabendazole.

In patients with severe disease, including high fever, marked muscle pain, periorbital edema, and one or more of the complicating organ involvements, corticosteroids (prednisone, 40 to 60 mg per day) may be required in order to reduce the host inflammatory response. Unfortunately, the immunoresponsiveness of the host may be similarly affected, permitting the adult worms to survive longer with greater larval production. Therefore, whenever corticosteroids are employed in the treatment of trichinellosis, a benzimidazole should be administered concomitantly.

PROPHYLAXIS

Because trichinellosis is a preventable disease, it is important that people be reminded that cooking to 170° F (77° C) or freezing to 5° F (−15° C) for 20 days is larvicidal. However, the arctic strain of *T. spiralis* is resistant to freezing. Smoking, salting, and drying of the meat does not alter transmission of the disease.

TULAREMIA

method of
CLAIRE B. PANOSIAN, M.D.
University of California, Los Angeles, School of Medicine
Los Angeles, California

Tularemia is a zoonosis found throughout the Northern hemisphere between the latitudes of 30 and 71 degrees. The causative agent is a small gram-negative coccobacillary bacterium, *Francisella tularensis,* which occurs in two main biovars. The predominant North American biovar, *F. tularensis tularensis,* is associated with rabbits, ticks, and deerflies and is highly virulent in humans. The second biovar, *F. tularensis palaearctica,* is associated with rodents and mosquitoes and is less virulent in humans. The organism is less commonly found in other wild mammals (such as deer, beaver, and coyote), domestic mammals (such as sheep, cattle, and cats), and a variety of birds, fish, amphibians, and environmental sources.

The transmission of *F. tularensis* to humans has traditionally been associated with direct handling of the tissues or body fluids of infected animal hosts, such as rabbits and muskrats; however, transmission also occurs via insect bite, animal bite, aerosol inhalation, and ingestion of contaminated water or the undercooked meat of a reservoir animal. In the United States, tularemia has been reported from all 50 states, but the majority of recent cases have occurred in Arkansas, Tennessee, Texas, Oklahoma, and Missouri. Individuals at increased risk for tularemia include hunters, trappers, and farmers. However, recent reports suggest a growing incidence of tularemia in children along with heightened awareness of tick-borne transmission in rural areas. The majority of infections occur during the summer months.

The clinical signs and symptoms of infection caused by *F. tularensis* reflect both the portal of entry and the possibility of bacteremic dissemination. When organisms are inoculated intradermally, as few as 10 bacilli can establish infection. After an average incubation period of 5 days, a local skin papule develops, followed by ulceration and regional adenopathy. Simultaneously, patients experience high fever, chills, and malaise. This form of disease is termed "ulcero-glandular," accounting for approximately 80% of all cases of tularemia. Other clinical categories of infection include oculoglandular (purulent eye involvement after conjunctival inoculation), oropharyngeal (exudative pharyngitis after ingestion of contaminated products), typhoidal (bacteremic illness without lymphadenopathy), pleuropulmonary (seen in 30 to 80% of typhoidal cases), and meningeal. A mild hepatitis commonly accompanies all forms of tularemia, and rash is seen in at least 20% of cases.

The diagnosis of tularemia is most often made serologically, either by a single positive titer of agglutinating antibody of 160 or higher or a fourfold rise in antibody. However, serologic reactions are usually negative during the first week of illness. An alternative means of diagnosis is by direct culture of blood, lymph node aspirate, sputum, or cerebrospinal fluid onto selected media. In most cases, the organism can be isolated and maintained on chocolate agar with cysteine supplementation. Microbiology personnel should always be alerted to the possibility of *F. tularensis* because the organism can create a hazardous infectious aerosol in the laboratory.

TREATMENT

Not all cases of tularemia require therapy, inasmuch as in some patients the infection has been retrospectively linked to a self-limited illness. However, any patient who is acutely ill with suspected tularemia should be treated promptly with empiric antibiotic therapy because diagnostic confirmation often lags by several days to weeks. With prompt use of antibiotics, the current rate of mortality from uncomplicated *F. tularensis* infection is 1 to 3%. Bacteremic cases with or without secondary complications such as pneumonia or meningitis are associated with a less favorable outcome.

The ideal therapy for tularemia has never been evaluated by means of a prospective controlled trial. Intramuscular streptomycin, 15 to 20 mg per kg per day in divided doses, has been effective in clinical practice and remains the drug of choice, although gentamicin (3 to 5 mg per kg per day intravenously or intramuscularly in divided doses) may be substituted. Oral tetracycline and chloramphenicol (30 mg per kg loading dose followed by 30 mg per kg per day in divided doses) have also been used successfully to treat tularemia, although clinical relapses have occurred when treatment extends less than 2 weeks. Late complications of tularemia include lymph node suppuration in up to half of patients presenting with a glandular syndrome, sometimes necessitating local aspiration or incision and drainage of affected nodes.

PREVENTION

There is no chemoprophylaxis recommended for the prevention of tularemia. Individuals with a high occupational risk are advised to take measures to prevent direct skin contact with potentially infected animals by use of protective clothing and gloves. Insect repellents should also be used to reduce bites by arthropod vectors such as ticks. A live attenuated vaccine of *F. tularensis* used only in experimental studies of laboratory workers protected against respiratory infection while producing a modified course of ulceroglandular disease; further information regarding the vaccine is available from the Drug Service at the Centers for Disease Control, Atlanta, Georgia.

NONTYPHOIDAL SALMONELLOSIS

method of
GARWIN B. SOE, M.D.
Kaiser Permanente Medical Center
Antioch, California

Infections caused by *Salmonella* produce great morbidity and mortality throughout the world. The genus *Salmonella* comprises non–spore forming, motile, gram-negative bacilli in the family Enterobacteriaceae. In biochemical tests, *Salmonella* will ferment glucose and mannose but not lactose or sucrose. However, in endemic areas, strains of *Salmonella* that ferment lactose have been identified.

The genus *Salmonella* traditionally has been divided into three species: *S. choleraesuis* and *S. typhi,* each containing one serotype, and *S. enteritidis* containing over 1800 serotypes. However, new DNA hybridization studies reveal that most strains are closely related genetically and can be grouped into six distinct subgroups, with virtually all human and animal disease–causing strains belonging to subgroup I. Most laboratories worldwide now report *Salmonella* by serotype name, with each serotype artificially treated as a species; e.g., *Salmonella* serotype Typhimurium is known as *Salmonella typhimurium.*

Infection is usually acquired by ingestion of contaminated food or water, but it can also be transmitted by contaminated "folk" medications such as rattlesnake capsules, mouth-to-mouth resuscitation, inadequately sterilized medical equipment, and platelet transfusions. Hospital personnel can carry the organism on hands or clothing, and fomites (dust, furniture, delivery suction apparatus) have been implicated. *Salmonella* can survive on fingertips for at least 3 hours.

Salmonellae have been isolated in all species, but are primarily pathogens of lower animals, which are the principal reservoir and source of *Salmonella* organisms that infect humans. A few serotypes are species specific, such as *S. typhi,* which only infects humans. Almost all known serotypes of *Salmonella* are pathogenic to humans.

Frequent outbreaks are reported from contaminated poultry products and from foods containing raw or undercooked eggs. *Salmonellae* are hardy organisms that survive refrigeration and can remain viable in eggs boiled 2 to 3 minutes. Beef and pork products account for about 13% of outbreaks. The largest outbreak, affecting over 16,000 persons, was due to multiple-antibiotic–resistant *S. typhimurium* contaminating pasteurized milk. Pet turtles and lizards and marijuana contaminated with animal manure have also been implicated as sources of human salmonelloses.

The incidence of *Salmonella* infections varies with the season, with peak incidence in warm weather months. In the United States, most infections are reported from July to November.

Host factors and the number and virulence of organisms influence the severity and location of infection. The acid pH (2.0) of the stomach will kill *Salmonella,* and large numbers (10^6 to 10^9) of organisms must be ingested to produce symptomatic infection.

Host defenses can alter the course of illness. Newborns and infants less than 1 year of age are most susceptible, probably due to the immaturity of humoral and cellular immune systems and the high frequency of fecal-oral contact. Severe recurrent *Salmonella* bacteremia in patients with acquired immunodeficiency syndrome (AIDS) and renal transplant recipients is probably due to impaired cell-mediated immunity. Major gastric surgery or achlorhydria predisposes to *Salmonella* infections. Children with sickle cell disease are prone to *Salmonella* osteomyelitis, because infarcted areas of gut, bone, and reticuloendothelial tissue furnish optimal environments for localization. Increasing resistance to *Salmonella* infections with increasing age is related to immunity produced by previous exposure to the organism, even though disease was not produced. Diabetic patients are at higher risk of infection due to decreased gastric acidity and anatomic neuropathy of the small bowel that reduces intestinal motility and prolongs the persistence of the organism in the gastrointestinal tract.

Salmonella produces a wide spectrum of illness. The clinical manifestations are usually classified as gastroenteritis, enteric fever (typhoid-like disease), bacteremia with or without focal extraintestinal infection, and the asymptomatic carrier state.

TREATMENT

Not all *Salmonella* infections need to be treated with antibiotics. In fact, antibiotics are known to prolong excretion of *Salmonella* in stool and can enhance susceptibility to intestinal infection in those given prophylactic antimicrobials to prevent "traveler's diarrhea."

The most frequently used antibiotics for treatment of salmonelloses are chloramphenicol (Chlormycetin), ampicillin, amoxicillin (Amoxil), and trimethoprim-sulfamethoxazole (TMP-SMX, Septra, Bactrim). The quinolone antibiotics ciprofloxacin (Cipro) and norfloxacin (Noroxin) are gaining popularity due to their activity against resistant organisms. The third-generation cephalosporins cefotaxime (Claforan) and ceftriaxone (Rocephin) are also effective but must be used parenterally.

Enterocolitis

The most frequently recognized syndrome is enterocolitis. The incubation period for *Salmonella* food poisoning is usually 8 to 48 hours. Initially nausea and vomiting occur, with abdominal cramps and diarrhea beginning a few hours later. Diarrhea usually persists for 3 to 4 days but can last longer than a week. Diarrhea ranges from a few loose stools to dysentery-like bloody stools with mucus. Fever greater than 38.9° C is present in 50% of patients and persists for only 1 or 2 days. Transient bacteremia occurs in 1 to 4% of patients. Signs and symptoms may mimic appendicitis and surgical peritonitis.

Management of enterocolitis involves control of symptoms such as pain, nausea, and vomiting with antipyretics and antiemetics. Antiperistaltic-antispasmodic agents such as loperamide and diphenoxylate are contraindicated because they can aggravate the illness. Correction of fluid deficits and electrolyte abnormalities with oral rehydration solutions is usually sufficient. In severe cases, intravenous hydration with saline and glucose solutions along with sodium bicarbonate or citrate may be necessary.

Antibiotics are generally not recommended, because studies have shown that they do not improve symptoms or shorten the duration of illness. However, recent studies have demonstrated a shortened clinical course and decreased duration of positive stool cultures with the use of ciprofloxacin, ofloxacin, and norfloxacin, but resistance can develop. The quinolone antibiotics are not recommended (i.e., not Food and Drug Ad-

ministration approved) for use in children, although they have been used in children as young as 1 year of age without adverse effects. At this time, antibiotics are not recommended for uncomplicated *Salmonella* enterocolitis. However, antibiotics are indicated in the following high-risk patients: (1) neonates less than 3 months old, (2) the elderly, (3) patients who are immunosuppressed (e.g., AIDS, lymphoproliferative disorders), (4) patients with cardiovascular abnormalities, (5) patients with significant bone or joint disorders, including surgically placed hardware, and (6) patients with sickle cell disease or other hemolytic blood dyscrasias.

In uncomplicated enterocolitis, one-third to one-half of patients will have positive stool cultures up to 3 weeks after onset of the illness, even though most are asymptomatic, but almost all have negative stools by 6 months after onset. The median duration of positive stools for children younger than 5 years of age is 7 weeks, while in older children and adults it is 3 to 4 weeks. The chronic carrier state (positive stool cultures for at least 1 year) is rare after nontyphoidal *Salmonella* enterocolitis.

Enteric Fever

Enteric fever is classically caused by *S. typhi* (typhoid fever), but it is also associated with *S. paratyphi A*, *S. schottmülleri* (*S. paratyphi B*), *S. hirschfeldii* (*S. paratyphi C*), and, rarely, other serotypes. Enteric fever caused by nontyphoidal *Salmonella* is called "paratyphoid fever."

The incubation period is usually 1 to 3 weeks. About 10% of patients have diarrhea initially. About 1 week later, a prolonged febrile course ensues, with fever increasing slowly along with malaise, anorexia, myalgia, arthralgia, cough, sore throat, and headache. During the second week of symptoms, constipation is more common than diarrhea, and abdominal tenderness and mental confusion may be seen. Splenomegaly (40 to 60% of patients), hepatomegaly (25 to 50%), and relative bradycardia for the degree of fever are also seen. Rose spots (slightly raised, discrete, irregular pink macules 2 to 4 mm in diameter that blanch on pressure) occur in crops of 5 to 15, last 3 to 4 days, then fade.

Clinical improvement in untreated enteric fever usually occurs between the second and fourth weeks. Complications such as intestinal perforation, intestinal hemorrhage, acute cholecystitis, pneumonia, and myocarditis appear during this period. Uncommon complications include pyelonephritis, prostatitis, and epididymitis. Urine cultures may be positive at this stage. If enteric fever does not resolve by the fourth or fifth week, metastatic infection or relapse can occur. Relapse occurs in 3 to 15% of patients whether or not antibiotics are used.

Chloramphenicol, 50 mg per kg per day (maximum 4 grams per day) in four divided doses, ampicillin, 150 to 200 mg per kg per day (maximum 12 grams per day) in four to six divided doses, or TMP-SMX, 5 mg per kg per dose of trimethoprim (maximum 160 mg) and 25 mg per kg per dose (maximum 800 mg) of sulfamethoxazole every 12 hours, is the standard parenteral antibiotic regimen for susceptible organisms. Oral therapy with amoxicillin, 100 mg per kg per day* (maximum 6 grams) in three divided doses, chloramphenicol, or TMP-SMX has been used in mild cases and after defervescence with parenteral therapy. Chloramphenicol and TMP-SMX should not be used in neonates and pregnant women. Duration of therapy is a minimum of 2 weeks, or 10 days after complete defervescence, whichever is longer. For resistant organisms, third-generation cephalosporins such as cefotaxime, 200 mg per kg per day (maximum 12 grams) in four divided doses, and ceftriaxone, 100 mg per kg per day (maximum 4 grams) in two divided doses, have been effective, along with ciprofloxacin, 10 mg per kg per dose (maximum 750 mg) twice a day. In patients with AIDS, indefinite prophylaxis with ciprofloxacin and norfloxacin has prevented relapse.

In patients with severe disease, who exhibit delirium, obtundation, stupor, coma, or shock, dexamethasone (initial dose 3 mg per kg, followed by 1 mg per kg every 6 hours for eight doses) in combination with antibiotic therapy appears to increase survival.

Fluid and electrolyte balance should be maintained. Aspirin is not recommended, because marked hypothermia can occur. Symptomatic treatment includes cold compresses and acetaminophen for fever. Patients should be monitored for abdominal complications, with surgical intervention if necessary.

Bacteremia and Focal Infections

This syndrome is characterized by intermittent high fever lasting for days to weeks without diarrhea. S. choleraesuis and S. typhimurium are the two most common isolates. Bacteremia can result in infected aneurysms, usually in the aortoiliac vessels, endocarditis, meningitis, brain abscess, endophthalmitis, pneumonia, empyema or lung abscesses, arthritis, osteomyelitis, splenic abscess, hepatic abscess, myonecrosis, soft tissue abscess, and orchitis. Salmonella bacteremia in AIDS patients is difficult to eradicate even with prolonged antimicrobial therapy.

*Exceeds dosage recommended by the manufacturer.

Salmonella meningitis is seen most often in neonates and infants as a complication of enterocolitis. Aortitis occurs in adults over 50 years of age, responds poorly to antibiotic therapy, and is associated with pre-existing heart disease, such as rheumatic heart disease or prosthetic valvular disease. Salmonella is the most common isolate in osteomyelitis in sickle cell disease. Salmonella osteomyelitis is a complication of total hip replacements. Splenic abscess occurs when subcapsular hematoma or splenic cysts are present. Hepatic abscess is rare, and has been associated with amebic abscess, echinococcal cyst, and hematomas. Cystitis and pyelonephritis result from colonization of the urinary tract from stool. Pulmonary abscess, pneumonia, and empyema are seen in the elderly and the immunocompromised, such as those with AIDS.

Treatment of infected aneurysm usually requires surgical excision, in addition to antibiotics. In patients who are not candidates for surgery, chronic antibiotic therapy with TMP-SMX or ciprofloxacin may suppress the infection. Endocarditis and bacteremia in AIDS patients require therapy with bactericidal drugs, such as ampicillin, amoxicillin, cefotaxime, or ceftriaxone. Ciprofloxacin and norfloxacin are effective in treatment of recurrent bacteremia in AIDS patients. After initial antibiotic therapy, zidovudine (AZT) alone can prevent relapse of bacteremia in AIDS patients. Zidovudine has in vitro activity against Salmonella.

The duration of antibiotic therapy varies with the type of infection. Bacteremia is usually treated for 14 days, whereas osteomyelitis or endocarditis requires a minimum of 4 to 6 weeks of therapy. Patients with AIDS should receive 3 to 4 weeks of therapy to prevent relapse but may require chronic suppressive therapy with ciprofloxacin or TMP-SMX. For meningitis, cefotaxime, 50 mg per kg (maximum 3 grams) every 6 hours for a minimum of 3 weeks, is the best choice.

Chronic Carrier State

The chronic carrier state, defined as persistence of positive stool culture for 1 year or longer, can follow acute infection, but occasionally occurs after asymptomatic ingestion of Salmonella organisms. Ninety-two percent of patients have positive stools 2 weeks after ingestion, 41% after 4 weeks, and 4.6% after 20 weeks. The chronic carrier state occurs in 0.2 to 0.6% of those infected with nontyphoidal salmonellas and 3% of those with typhoid fever. Age over 50 years, biliary tract disease, obstructive uropathy, tuberculosis, and schistosomiasis are predisposing factors. Chronic carriers are asymptomatic and are not prone to complications. Eradication of the carrier state is necessary to prevent spread of infection, particularly in food handlers and persons involved in caring for institutionalized patients and children. Chronic carriers can excrete 10^6 or more viable *Salmonella* organisms per gram of feces.

Ampicillin or amoxicillin, 4 to 6 grams per day in four divided doses for 4 to 6 weeks, is useful in those with susceptible organisms who do not have biliary tract disease. Probenecid, 2 grams per day in four divided doses, is often added. TMP-SMX, 160 mg of trimethoprim and 800 mg of sulfamethoxazole twice a day, is equally effective. Successful treatment has been obtained with ciprofloxacin, 750 mg twice a day for 28 days. Norfloxacin appears to be effective also, but clinical experience has been less extensive. Ceftriaxone, 2 grams per day parenterally for 3 days, has had success rates similar to those for prolonged oral regimens.

Cholecystectomy may be necessary to eradicate the chronic carrier state in those who relapse or cannot tolerate prolonged antimicrobial therapy.

Ciprofloxacin is not recommended in children; the drugs of choice are amoxicillin, TMP-SMX, parenteral ceftriaxone, or cefoperazone, although cefoperazone has not been as effective.

PREVENTION

There is no vaccine against nontyphoidal salmonelloses. The large number of *Salmonella* serotypes makes preparation of a single vaccine difficult, because immunity is serotype specific. Since *S. typhi* strains are antigenically homogeneous, typhoid vaccines are available.

In outbreaks of salmonelloses among health care workers and food handlers, ciprofloxacin, 500 mg twice a day for 5 to 7 days, eradicates the organism quickly in both asymptomatic and symptomatic individuals with positive stool cultures and prevents development of the carrier state.

TYPHOID FEVER

method of
JUAN ANTONIO TREJO Y PÉREZ, M.D.
Children's Hospital, National Medical Center,
Mexican Institute of Social Security
Mexico, D.F., Mexico

In recent years, there has been an impressive decline in the number of cases of typhoid fever in industrialized countries, attributable primarily to improvements in sanitation. Nevertheless, this infection remains highly endemic in many underdeveloped areas, with an annual incidence of more than 300 cases per 100,000 inhabitants.

Typhoid fever, produced by *Salmonella typhi*, is a severe disease with a high rate of complications. Humans are the only known reservoir for this enterobacteria, and infection implies direct or indirect exposure to a human source. *S. typhi* are ingested in contaminated food or water. The incubation period, which is usually 10 to 14 days but can vary from 7 to 21 days, is in general related inversely to the number of bacteria ingested.

The symptoms of enteric fever produced by *S. typhi* are nonspecific and at onset consist of fever, headache, abdominal pain, vomiting, muscle pain, and anorexia. By the end of the third week of illness, fever is prominent and continues to gradually increase to reach 40° C in the evening. The patient usually appears acutely ill, and other physical signs such as hepatomegaly and splenomegaly are noted in about 20 to 40% of patients. Rose spots can be detected in about 20 to 30% of patients, and about 10% have neuropsychiatric changes.

Definitive diagnosis is by isolation of *S. typhi* from blood or bone marrow. This latter source provides the best sample for isolation of the causative organism, and although less practicable than blood culture, bone marrow culture yields positive results in about 90% of patients with typhoid fever.

TREATMENT

Antimicrobial Therapy

The use of antimicrobial drugs has reduced death rates from 15 to 3% in areas where the disease is highly endemic. Selection of antimicrobial agents has been complicated by the emergence of *Salmonella* strains that are resistant to multiple antibiotics. Despite good in vitro activity of many antibiotics against this gram-negative bacilli, the clinical efficacy of some is unclear and others are only now being evaluated.

Chloramphenicol. Despite the emergence of chloramphenicol-resistant strains, this drug is still the antimicrobial of choice in most areas of the world. In 1972, an extensive epidemic caused by chloramphenicol-resistant *Salmonella* occurred in Mexico. However, the prevalence of these strains decreased to 3 to 6% in 1978, and only a few resistant strains have been isolated since then.

For adults the recommended dosage of chloramphenicol (Chloromycetin) is 3 grams per day in four divided doses. For children the dose is 50 to 100 mg per kg per day in four divided doses given orally or intravenously for at least 2 weeks. It is recommended that the total dosage not exceed 30 grams. Fever subsides quickly once treatment is started, and the temperature becomes normal within 3 to 5 days in most cases. Chloramphenicol is inexpensive and can be taken orally. However, relapses occur in 5% of patients, and 3% remain asymptomatic chronic carriers. Toxicity frequently takes the form of reversible dose-related bone marrow depression. A rare idiosyncratic reaction to chloramphenicol characterized by severe aplastic anemia occurs in 1 in 40,000 to 50,000 treatment courses; it is usually fatal.

Semisynthetic Penicillins. In view of chloramphenicol's hematologic toxicity many physicians prefer ampicillin (Omnipen) or amoxicillin (Amoxil) for treatment of typhoid fever. Both antimicrobials have been used with good results against *S. typhi,* although some strains are known to be resistant to both ampicillin and chloramphenicol. Ampicillin should be administered in doses of 100 mg per kg per day in four divided doses by mouth or intravenously for at least 2 weeks.

Amoxicillin is relatively well absorbed and should be administered in doses of 50 mg per kg per day in three divided doses for at least 2 weeks. Given orally, both drugs are less effective than chloramphenicol in producing a clinical response. Defervescence occurs within 6 to 7 days after starting therapy.

Recent studies have shown that intravenous ampicillin at high doses (200 mg per kg per day) is more effective than the oral form, with more rapid resolution of fever and a lower relapse rate. Ampicillin and amoxicillin are inexpensive and can be used in all age groups.

Furazolidone

Furazolidone (Furoxone) is an antibiotic with equivalent clinical efficacy to that of ampicillin; fever resolves within 6 to 7 days after starting therapy. There is evidence that this drug is well absorbed in the intestine and is active in vitro against isolates of *S. typhi.* Recommended doses* are a 2-week course of 10 to 15 mg per kg per day in four divided doses for children and 800 mg per day in four divided doses for adults. The cure rate is 85 to 95%, and relapse occurs in 3 to 5% of treated patients.

Furazolidone is inexpensive, can be used in all age groups, and does not cause severe adverse reactions. However, only the oral route is available and this limits its indications to uncomplicated typhoid fever or infection with *S. typhi* multiresistant to standard antibiotics.

Trimethoprim-Sulfamethoxazole

The combination in proportion of 1:5 is an acceptable alternative to chloramphenicol or ampicillin in the therapy of typhoid fever. The recommended dosage of trimethoprim-sulfamethoxazole (Bactrim, Septa) in adults is 320 to 640 mg of trimethoprim combined with 1600 to 3200 mg of sulfamethoxazole per day in two divided oral or intravenous doses for 14 days. For children, 8 mg of trimethoprim and 40 mg of sulfamethoxazole per kg per day in two divided doses for 14 days is recommended. Defervescence occurs within 6 to 7 days of the start of treatment. The failure rate is about 10%, and this antimicrobial has significant side effects such as anemia, rash, diarrhea, and Stevens-Johnson syndrome.

Third-Generation Cephalosporins and Aztreonam

Clinical experience with cefotaxime (Claforan), the most widely used third-generation cephalosporin for *S. typhi* infection, has shown it to be effective, with a low relapse rate. Two other cephalosporins of the same family, ceftriaxone (Rocephin) and cefoperazone (Cefobid), and the monobactam aztreonam (Azactam) have also been used successfully. Cure rates are 85% with cefotaxime, 92% with ceftriaxone, 93% with aztreonam, and 97% with cefoperazone. There have been no reported relapses related to this last antimicrobial; the other drugs have clinical efficacy like that of chloramphenicol. All four antibacterial drugs are very expensive and must be administered parenterally. These agents should be reserved for patients infected with multiresistant strains.

Quinolones

Clinical assays indicate that the quinolones are useful for the treatment of *S. typhi* enteric fever. Published data suggest good results with pefloxacin* (Peflacine) (1000 mg per day in two divided doses), ofloxacin (Floxin) (600 mg per day in two divided doses), and ciprofloxacin (Cipro) (1000 mg per day in two divided doses) for 5 to 10 days. Cure rates are high with these drugs, and relapses have not been reported. These agents are effective orally. Quinolones are very expensive and are not approved for use in children because of their potential to cause arthropathy. These antimicrobials should be considered as alternative therapy only for multiresistant strains of *S. typhi.*

Supportive Therapy

Supportive measures for patients with typhoid fever include maintenance of fluid balance and nutrition, preferably by mouth, although severely ill patients may need total parenteral nutrition. Fever is best controlled by physical measures,

---

*Exceeds dosage recommended by the manufacturer.

*Investigational drug in the United States.

since patients with typhoid fever frequently respond to antipyretics by developing hypothermia and transient hypotension.

Although corticosteroids can increase the relapse rate, some clinical assays suggest that critically ill patients can benefit from a short course of dexamethasone. The recommended dosage is an initial dose of 3 mg per kg followed by eight doses of 1 mg per kg every 6 hours intravenously.

Complications

Typhoid fever has been associated with two late complications: significant intestinal hemorrhage and perforation. Intestinal hemorrhage occurs in about 10% of patients and appears between the second and third weeks of illness. Severe anemia and shock can ensue, and plasma and blood transfusions may be required. Perforation of the terminal ileum, seen in about 3% of the patients, requires immediate surgical intervention, either laparotomy with primary closure or intestinal resection and drainage. Mortality is high and additional antimicrobial agents to chloramphenicol (amikacin plus metronidazole) are indicated.

Since bacteremia is an essential feature of typhoid fever, localized suppurative infection can develop anywhere in the body. These extraintestinal complications respond to basic antimicrobial treatment, although additional measures such as dexamethasone in meningitis may be required.

Relapses

S. typhi can survive within phagocytes, a circumstance that makes the intracellular penetration of antibiotics crucial for cure. Relapses should generally be treated with the same antimicrobial agent initially administered, although in some cases, alternative drugs must be employed.

Carrier State

There are two types of carrier states: (1) convalescent (patients continue to shed S. typhi for weeks or months), a self-limited condition that does not need treatment; and (2) chronic (patients continue to eliminate S. typhi after 1 year). The likelihood of becoming a chronic carrier increases with age and with the presence of biliary tract disease. There are two approaches to treating the chronic carrier state. Prolonged antibiotic therapy, usually with ampicillin, 4 to 6 grams per day plus 2 grams per day of probenecid, both divided in four oral doses for 6 weeks, eliminates S. typhi in about 95% of patients without gallbladder disease. In the presence of gallstones, the rate of failure is about 75%. Cholecystectomy is the treatment of choice in patients with gallbladder disease (gallstones or gallbladder dysfunction). If drug therapy alone fails, antibiotic treatment in combination with cholecystectomy usually results in cure.

PREVENTION

Control of typhoid fever depends on high standards of environmental sanitation, maintenance of an uncontaminated water supply, and good control of chronic carriers. Handwashing is of paramount importance in controlling person-to-person spread; salmonellae are easily removed by washing the hands with soap and water.

Trials with parenteral typhoid vaccines (acetone or heat-phenol inactivated S. typhi) have shown efficacy ranges of 79 to 93%. However, the immunity generated by available vaccines can be overcome easily when the inoculum is increased.

Use of live attenuated S. typhi (Ty21a strain) offers the possibility of a stable, easily administered oral typhoid vaccine free of the side effects of the parenteral vaccines. Two large-scale trials have been performed with this vaccine, but results have been contradictory. At this stage, the oral live vaccines seem to be about as effective as conventional parenteral whole cell vaccines but with fewer side effects. Vaccination should be considered for residents of epidemic areas and for persons traveling to countries where there is an appreciable risk of exposure to S. typhi. Booster doses every 3 years are recommended.

THE TYPHUS FEVERS

method of
BRUCE P. CHANDLER, M.D.
Anchorage Neighborhood Health Center
Anchorage, Alaska

The typhus fevers are diseases caused by obligate intracellular bacteria of the family Rickettsiaceae. The classic typhus fevers are (1) epidemic louse-borne typhus, caused by *Rickettsia prowazekii*, which includes the milder recrudescent typhus (Brill-Zinsser disease) that may occur in patients inadequately treated during initial illness, and (2) murine flea-borne (endemic) typhus, caused by *Rickettsia typhi*. A number of other rickettsial infections with similar clinical presentation and treatment are often considered among the typhus fevers. These include scrub typhus (mite-borne typhus), Q fever, ehrlichiosis, and the spotted fever group of tick- and mite-borne rickettsial infections.

The epidemiology of these diseases is summarized in Table 1. With the exception of epidemic louse-borne typhus, the rickettsial diseases exist in nature primarily as zoonoses of arthropods or mammals, and most

TABLE 1. **The Principal Vectors, Reservoirs, and Distribution of Human Rickettsial Diseases**

Disease	Etiologic Agent	Vector	Reservoir	Distribution
The Typhus Fevers				
Epidemic typhus				
Louse-borne	*Rickettsia prowazekii*	Body louse	Humans	Africa, Asia, Central America, South America, and Mexico
Flying squirrel	*R. prowazekii*	Squirrel flea	Flying squirrels	Eastern United States
Murine typhus	*R. typhi*	Rat flea	Rats, mice	Worldwide
Scrub typhus	*R. tsutsugamushi*	Mites	Mites	Asia, Australia
The Spotted Fevers				
Rocky Mountain spotted fever	*R. rickettsii*	Ticks	Ticks	North, Central, and South America
Boutonneuse fever	*R. conorii*	Ticks	Ticks	Europe, Africa, Middle East
Queensland tick typhus	*R. australis*	Ticks	Ticks	Australia
North Asia tick typhus	*R. sibirica*	Ticks	Ticks	Central Asia
Rickettsialpox	*R. akari*	Mites	Mice	Eastern United States, Russia, Africa, Korea
Others				
Q fever	*Coxiella burnetii*	Aerosols, contact with infected tissues or materials	Sheep, goats, cows, cats, ticks	Worldwide
Ehrlichiosis	*Ehrlichia canis*	Probably ticks	Unknown	North America

human disease results from incidental infection by arthropod vectors.

Humans are the primary reservoir for epidemic typhus, with transmission by the human body louse, *Pediculus humanus*. A reservoir of *R. prowazekii* identified in flying squirrels of the eastern United States has been associated with rare cases of human typhus infection. The probable vector for transmission to humans is the squirrel flea. This milder strain of *R. prowazekii* is genetically different from strains isolated in louse-borne epidemics in Europe and Africa.

The most common typhus fevers in the United States are Rocky Mountain spotted fever (RMSF), murine typhus, and Q fever. The severest of the spotted fevers, RMSF, is endemic throughout the United States; the majority of cases in recent years have occurred in the South Atlantic region. Epidemic louse-borne typhus and Brill-Zinsser disease are now extremely rare in the United States; foci of epidemic typhus remain in remote highland areas of eastern and central Africa, Central and South America, and Asia. There persists the potential for the importation of epidemic typhus and other typhus fevers by immigrants or travelers from endemic areas.

Environmental conditions that favor vector activity and human-vector contact are associated with increased incidence of human disease. Throughout history, epidemic louse-borne typhus has been associated with war and disaster, in which conditions of famine, lack of sanitation, and crowding favor the widespread cultivation of body lice required for transmission of the disease. The incidence of RMSF peaks in the summer when ticks are most active and human activity in tick-infested areas is highest. Similarly, murine typhus occurs commonly in habitats with rat and mouse infestation.

Humans generally are infected by bites, by rubbing infected insect feces into the skin, or by inhalation of infected material. An eschar at the site of inoculation is unusual with RMSF and epidemic and murine typhus, but it may be seen with scrub typhus, rickettsialpox, and other spotted fevers. Rickettsiae multiply locally at the site of inoculation and spread systemically by hematogenous dissemination. The proliferation of rickettsiae in the endothelial cells of small vessels produces a vasculitis responsible for much of the pathology seen with these diseases. Electrolyte imbalance, prerenal azotemia, hypovolemia, and shock may result from increased vascular permeability and extravasation of fluid. Thrombosis of vessels may cause gangrene of the skin and distal extremities. Cerebral dysfunction ranging from confusion to coma, interstitial pneumonitis, myocarditis, hepatic dysfunction, renal failure, and disseminated intravascular coagulation may be observed with severe disease.

After an incubation period of 3 days to 3 weeks, these infections generally manifest with the abrupt onset of fever, chills, an often excruciating headache, and muscle and joint pains. Especially with epidemic typhus and RMSF, initial malaise may quickly progress to prostration. Anorexia, cough, and photophobia are common, and a variety of other signs and symptoms may be reported. Cutaneous manifestations commencing 3 to 7 days after onset of illness are frequent, except with Q fever. The rash of epidemic louse-borne typhus usually begins as a maculopapular rash in the axillary folds and trunk and spreads centrifugally; that of RMSF typically appears on wrists and ankles and spreads centrally. With severe disease, the rash may progress to petechiae and hemorrhage.

The diagnosis of these diseases depends on a high degree of suspicion and astute clinical judgment, inasmuch as there are currently no laboratory findings that are diagnostic for the typhus fevers in the first week of illness. New laboratory methods, notably polymerase chain reaction and shell vial centrifugation culture,

TABLE 2. **Drug Treatment of the Typhus Fevers**

Drug	Oral Therapy	Intravenous Therapy	Maximal Total Daily Dose
Tetracycline	25–50 mg/kg/day, in 4 divided doses q 6 h	(tetracycline hydrochloride) 10–20 mg/kg/day, in 4 divided doses q 6 h	2 gm/day
Doxycycline	4.4 mg/kg/day, in 2 divided doses q 12 h	(doxycycline hyclate) 4.4 mg/kg/day, in 2 divided doses q 12 h	200 mg/day
Chloramphenicol	50 mg/kg/day, in 4 divided doses q 6 h	(chloramphenicol sodium succinate) 50 mg/kg/day, in 4 divided doses q 6 h	3 gm/day

show promise for the early diagnosis of rickettsial infections in the future. A serologic diagnosis may be made during the second or later weeks of illness by using the highly specific indirect immunofluorescent antibody (IFA) or complement fixation tests.

TREATMENT

The foundation of treatment for the typhus fevers is prompt antirickettsial therapy. In view of the fulminant course that may be seen with these diseases, especially with epidemic louse-borne typhus and RMSF, a case may prove fatal before a serologic diagnosis can be made if the initiation of treatment is delayed.

Compliant patients with mild illness may be treated as outpatients with oral antibiotics. Patients with more serious illness should be hospitalized for careful observation; full intensive care support may be required for severely ill patients. Attention should be directed to hemodynamic status and fluid regulation to ensure adequate organ perfusion. Patients unable to tolerate oral medication should receive intravenous antibiotics; oral therapy should replace intravenous therapy when feasible. High-dose corticosteroids have been used in the treatment of severely ill patients; however, their efficacy is unproven.

SPECIFIC TREATMENT

Tetracyclines and chloramphenicol remain the drugs of choice. Although these drugs are rickettsiostatic, not rickettsicidal, they are usually highly effective if given early and in adequate dosage. Clinical improvement is commonly noted within 24 hours after initiation of therapy; patients usually become afebrile within 72 hours. Alternative diagnoses should be considered if improvement is not noted within 72 hours. The usual course of treatment is 6 to 10 days; antibiotic treatment should be continued for at least 48 to 72 hours after defervescence. The one exception is with epidemic louse-borne typhus, in which a single dose of doxycycline is curative.

Chloramphenicol or doxycycline should be used in patients with diminished renal function; a reduction in chloramphenicol dosage may be required for patients with hepatic or renal dysfunction, and for infants and young children. Monitoring of plasma drug levels and hematologic parameters is advised for all patients receiving chloramphenicol. Chloramphenicol is recommended for pregnant women and children aged 8 years and younger, unless the relative benefits of treatment with tetracycline or doxycycline are clearly greater than the risks of dental staining and adverse bone development. Warnings and recommendations on drug labeling should be followed. Recommended dosages are presented in Table 2.

PREVENTION

Prevention of the typhus fevers involves public education concerning the risk of these diseases and their modes of acquisition. People should avoid tick-infested areas when it is feasible and should carefully inspect themselves for ticks after outside activity. An embedded tick should be carefully removed by using a slow pulling motion with forceps. Other preventive measures include the use of insect repellents and insecticides on skin and as clothing impregnants, as well as the elimination of rodent infestations in areas of human habitation. The treatment of clothing and bedding with the contact insecticide permethrin has been shown to offer highly effective protection against ticks, mites, and lice. Vector control with thorough delousing of patients and clothing is essential for interruption of outbreaks of epidemic typhus. Vaccines have been effective in the control of typhus epidemics but are not currently available. Suspect or documented cases of these diseases should be reported promptly to local or state health authorities.

WHOOPING COUGH
(Pertussis)

method of
HARRIS D. RILEY, JR., M.D.
Vanderbilt Children's Hospital, Vanderbilt
  University Medical Center
Nashville, Tennessee

Pertussis is an acute infection that affects children predominantly, but no age group is exempt. It is caused by *Bordetella pertussis,* a small, gram-negative, nonmotile bacillus with rather fastidious growth requirements. *B. pertussis* shares certain antigenic components with *Bordetella parapertussis* and *Bordetella bronchiseptica,* both of which (as well as adenoviruses) can cause respiratory disease resembling pertussis, but there is no evidence of cross-immunity with *B. pertussis.* After colonization of the respiratory tract, the bacteria produce at least five toxins that are responsible for the systemic manifestations of the disease. Humans are the only host.

After an incubation period of 2 to 10 days, pertussis classically presents in three distinct clinical stages. The initial, or catarrhal, stage is characterized by the nonspecific manifestations of an upper respiratory infection. This progresses to the paroxysmal stage, which is characterized by violent paroxysms of cough followed by a distinctive inspiratory whooping sound. This stage usually lasts only a few days, but in some cases it can linger for up to 2 or 3 weeks. In the convalescent stage, the patient gradually improves and the paroxysms are replaced by a chronic cough. Symptoms may last only 3 to 4 weeks, but in some cases the cough may last for months. The whoop may be absent in infants less than 6 months of age and in adults.

Pertussis is more dangerous than is usually believed, especially for infants and for children debilitated by underlying disease. The young infant is not protected by transplacental antibodies. Approximately 70% of all deaths from pertussis occur in the first year of life. Pertussis is highly communicable, with secondary attack rates of 80 to 90% in susceptible family members and 30 to 80% in those with less intimate exposure. As a rule, one attack confers immunity, but probably of a shorter duration than has generally been believed. Fifteen to 25% of immunized children will contract the disease on exposure, but in these patients the disease is usually much milder. In recent years, 6.5% of the cases have occurred in individuals 15 years of age or older. Laboratory confirmation (by culture or by fluorescent antibody techniques) is particularly important in atypical cases. Control of pertussis depends chiefly on immunization.

TREATMENT

General Measures

The patient should be isolated during the first 4 weeks of illness, which is the usual accepted period of communicability, or for 3 weeks from the onset of paroxysms, as this date usually can be set with more accuracy. Isolation serves not only to protect the patient from other infectious agents but also to prevent infection of susceptible contacts. In particular, patients with active or potentially active tuberculosis should rigidly guard against contact with pertussis. Nonimmunized children should be quarantined for 14 days following intimate exposure.

Hospitalization is usually indicated for children less than 2 years of age and always for patients with severe paroxysms or apnea. The importance of intensive care management with constant and resourceful nursing care cannot be overemphasized; in few other infectious diseases is it as crucial, and it can spell the difference between life and death. Nursing attendants should be equipped to institute mechanical lifesaving procedures such as suctioning and airway insertion. Choking attacks should be relieved by gentle suctioning at frequent intervals. Avoidance of factors that precipitate attacks of coughing, such as activity, excitement, and inhalant irritants, is important. Environmental temperature should be constant to reduce the paroxysm of coughing produced by sudden fluctuations, and humidification is often helpful. Oxygen is indicated for patients with respiratory complications or convulsions. Cough suppressants, expectorants, and sedatives should not be used.

It is important to maintain adequate nutrition and hydration. Small frequent feedings should be provided, and refeeding is important if vomiting is associated with the paroxysms. Parenteral supplementation is necessary if hydration or nutrition cannot be maintained by the oral route.

Strict respiratory isolation of infected patients is necessary to control the spread of pertussis. Uncomplicated pertussis is usually not accompanied by significant fever; its occurrence suggests the development of a secondary bacterial complication, usually of the respiratory tract.

Specific Therapy

Pertussis immune globulin (human) was at one time widely recommended both for treatment of patients with active cases and for prevention of pertussis in exposed susceptible individuals. However, its efficacy has not been scientifically established, and the results of controlled studies show little or no therapeutic benefit. As a result, it is no longer recommended.

No antimicrobial agent has been shown to be effective in modifying the severity or shortening the clinical course of the pertussis, and the role of such therapy is difficult to evaluate. In vitro,

B. pertussis is susceptible to a wide variety of antibacterial agents. Erythromycin, tetracycline, and chloramphenicol have been used on the thesis that they produce bacteriologic conversion of cultures to negative and render the patient noncontagious. Erythromycin estolate in a dose of 40 to 50 mg per kg per day in four divided doses administered for 5 days is the regimen of choice. When given in the preparoxysmal stage, it may abort the disease. Antibiotics may be useful in the face of complicating bacterial infections, and the choice of drug should be guided by microbiologic test results.

Favorable claims for the use of corticosteroids in pertussis have been advanced, but additional controlled studies are needed before they can be recommended.

Complications

Respiratory Tract. The most common and usually the most severe complication is pneumonia, which most often takes the form of an interstitial bronchopneumonia. It is usually caused by secondary invaders, most commonly *Haemophilus influenzae, Streptococcus pneumoniae,* and group A streptococci. *B. pertussis* has been shown on occasion to be the predominating microorganism. Although every attempt should be made to identify the causative organism, this is only infrequently productive, and antibacterial therapy must be based on clinical grounds. Ampicillin or erythromycin can be used, because they are effective to varying degrees against the most common causative pathogens. If the causative organism is isolated, antimicrobial therapy can be guided by the results of in vitro susceptibility tests.

Atelectasis is often recognized only on radiographic examination. If it does not subside spontaneously, bronchoscopic aspiration may be necessary to prevent the development of bronchiectasis. No child with pertussis should be released from medical surveillance until the lungs have been shown to be clear roentgenographically.

Otitis media is a frequent complication, particularly in infants. Emphysema usually resolves spontaneously after the acute illness but may lead to interstitial emphysema or pneumothorax.

Central Nervous System. Convulsions are relatively common and represent a serious complication of pertussis. There are probably several different causes, including asphyxia from severe paroxysms, petechial hemorrhages, subarachnoid bleeding, and the development of a diffuse encephalopathy. Convulsions should be treated with oxygen and with lumbar puncture to relieve increased pressure. Phenobarbital, 3 to 5 mg per kg per dose intramuscularly, is recommended because it does not ordinarily depress the cough reflex.

Other Complications. Hemorrhages, which are mechanical in origin and result from increased venous pressure and congestion associated with paroxysms, are relatively frequent. Epistaxis and subconjunctival hemorrhages are particularly common; intracranial bleeding can also occur.

Other complications include hernia and rectal prolapse associated with severe paroxysms and nutritional disturbances. Alkalotic tetany resulting from loss of acid gastric contents secondary to excessive vomiting should be treated with intravenous calcium gluconate. Digitalization should be done for the rare case of secondary cardiac failure.

PREVENTION

Because of the difficulty in diagnosis and the generally unsatisfactory therapy for the established disease, the control of pertussis lies in its prevention by means of active immunization. Vaccines are of no benefit, however, once clinical manifestations have begun. Five doses of diphtheria and tetanus toxoids with pertussis vaccine (DTP), given intramuscularly, are recommended. The first dose is usually given at about 2 months, followed by two additional doses at intervals of approximately 2 months. A fourth dose is recommended 6 to 12 months after the third dose, usually at 15 to 18 months of age, to complete the initial series. It can be given concurrently with other vaccines. A fifth dose is given before school entry (kindergarten or elementary school) at 4 to 6 years of age to protect these children from pertussis in ensuing years and to decrease transmission of the disease to younger children. A newly introduced acellular pertussis vaccine, which produces fewer untoward reactions, can be used for the fourth and fifth doses.

Management of Contacts

The dissemination of pertussis can be limited by decreasing the infectivity of the patient and by protecting close contacts. Oral erythromycin shortens the period of infectivity. Close contacts can be protected by active immunization and antibiotics. Those less than 7 years of age who have not received all five doses of diphtheria-tetanus-pertussis (DTP) or who have not received DTP within 3 years of exposure should be given a dose of vaccine. The value of chemoprophylaxis with erythromycin administered orally has never been conclusively demonstrated. It is usually recommended, however, that a 14-day course of erythromycin be provided to close contacts who are less than 1 year of age and to unimmunized close contacts less than 7 years of age. Passive immunization of susceptible, exposed contacts with human pertussis immune globulin is no longer recommended because there is no evidence that it alters the incidence or severity of the disease.

Section 3

The Respiratory System

ACUTE RESPIRATORY FAILURE

method of
STEPHEN S. LEFRAK, M.D., and
MICHAEL B. LIPPMANN, M.D.
The Jewish Hospital of St. Louis at Washington
University Medical Center
St. Louis, Missouri

Disruption of the complex interplay between the components of the respiratory system impedes gas exchange and alters the arterial oxygen tension (PaO_2), the arterial carbon dioxide tension ($PaCO_2$), or both. Dysfunction of the bellows (which consist of the respiratory centers and their efferent and afferent nerves, the respiratory muscles, and the chest wall) leads to an inappropriate rise in $PaCO_2$ with consequent acidosis and proportional decreases in PaO_2.

Disorders affecting the pulmonary airways and parenchyma interrupt normal ventilation/perfusion relationships and cause hypoxemia. $PaCO_2$ remains normal as long as the respiratory muscles are able to compensate for inefficient gas exchange by increasing minute ventilation ($\dot{V}_E$). When ventilatory demands outstrip the energy supply of the respiratory muscles, the muscles fatigue and are no longer able to generate sufficient $\dot{V}_E$ to maintain a normal $PaCO_2$ with ensuing hypercapnia and respiratory acidosis.

Severe dysfunction of any component of the respiratory system can cause respiratory failure, which is characterized by a PaO_2 of less than 50 mmHg while breathing room air at sea level or a $PaCO_2$ of greater than 50 mmHg and concomitant with a pH of less than 7.30.

INITIAL MANAGEMENT AND EVALUATION

The immediate goal of therapy is to correct life-threatening hypoxemia and respiratory acidosis. Therefore, regardless of etiology, the initial management of respiratory failure must be to provide (1) a patent airway, (2) adequate ventilation, and (3) supplemental oxygen. Oxygen must never be withheld from a patient in respiratory distress while awaiting measurement of arterial blood gases or during other diagnostic procedures. Even if mechanical ventilation is not indicated (to be discussed), oxygen is nevertheless administered. Intensive respiratory care is undertaken,

with frequent monitoring of clinical parameters and arterial blood gases. This care is best administered in an intensive care unit.

The decision to institute mechanical ventilation is based on (1) the patient's current clinical condition and the underlying disease process, (2) the adequacy of alveolar ventilation and bellows function, and (3) the severity and ease of correction of hypoxemia. Although arterial blood gas analysis is critical in the initial evaluation, the importance of the patient's clinical status must be stressed. Mechanical ventilation is supportive therapy that enables the patient to achieve chosen goals in obtaining definitive treatment (e.g., recovering function, returning home). This benefit of mechanical ventilation must be separated from its physiologic effects, which are to reduce the work of breathing and allow therapeutic manipulation of alveolar gas exchange. The use of mechanical ventilation to obtain physiologic effects without the possibility of benefit for the patient is inappropriate.

In general, mechanical ventilation is initiated immediately in patients with clearly inadequate ventilation and in those exhibiting a clear trend of deteriorating ventilation. Thus it is instituted (1) for apnea or agonal respiration; (2) for acute bellows failure (as occurs in drug overdose, myasthenia gravis, Guillain-Barré syndrome); (3) for acute lung failure in which the PaO_2 cannot be increased to 60 mmHg with a fraction of inspired oxygen (F_IO_2) of less than 0.50 (as in adult respiratory distress syndrome [ARDS]); (4) for acute deterioration of chronic bellows or lung failure when mental status is impaired, pH is less than 7.25, or PaO_2 is less than 30 mmHg (as in chronic obstructive pulmonary disease, kyphoscoliosis); (5) for respiratory failure associated with cardiovascular instability, multiple organ failure, or severe trauma; (6) for acute neuromuscular disease and impending respiratory failure characterized by a vital capacity of less than 1.0 liter or an inspiratory force of less than 25 cmH_2O; (7) for marked tachypnea (>40 breaths/minute) associated with any of the aforementioned conditions; and (8) before special procedures (bronchoscopy, pulmonary artery catheterization) when the patient's ventilatory reserve is in question.

150

OXYGEN THERAPY

Hypoxemia must be corrected with supplemental oxygen in order to avoid inadequate tissue oxygen delivery (hypoxia) and subsequent cell dysfunction and lactic acidosis. Superimposed anemia or low cardiac output exacerbates the hypoxia. The oxygen should be administered immediately to patients in respiratory distress. Although arterial blood for analysis may be obtained rapidly before oxygen administration, oxygen should not be withheld while the results of laboratory analysis are awaited. Further adjustments in F_IO_2, delivery apparatus, and oxygen flow rates are made through the use of blood gas data to obtain a PaO_2 of 60 mmHg, which usually ensures an oxyhemoglobin saturation of 90%. Therefore, little is to be gained from striving for a higher oxygen tension, especially if this requires exposing the patient to toxic concentrations of oxygen, progressive hypercapnia, or barotrauma from increased airway pressure. Nonhypercapnic patients should initially receive high inspired oxygen concentrations. This helps ensure a PaO_2 of 60 mmHg or higher and does not increase $PaCO_2$.

Oxygen therapy should never be withheld from hypoxemic and hypercapnic patients despite the risk of increasing alveolar carbon dioxide tension. However, in these patients, oxygen must be administered in a controlled manner, with an initial concentration of between 0.24 and 0.30. In these patients, the PaO_2 usually lies along the steep portion of the oxyhemoglobin dissociation curve. Small increases in PaO_2 result in relatively large increases in saturation and, therefore, an increase in oxygen delivery with little increase in $PaCO_2$. Close monitoring of arterial blood gases is required.

OXYGEN DELIVERY SYSTEMS

Oxygen may be delivered through a variety of systems. Low-flow oxygen (0.5 to 5 liters/minute) delivered through a flexible nasal cannula is the simplest and best tolerated system. A nasal cannula, however, does not afford precise control of the F_IO_2 which is dependent on oxygen flow rate and the patient's $\dot{V}_E$.

Venturi-type masks allow more precise control of the F_IO_2 between 0.24 and 0.50 regardless of oxygen flow rate or $\dot{V}_E$. These masks are less comfortable than nasal cannulas for the patient and must be removed for eating or expectorating. Tight-fitting masks equipped with partial or nonrebreathing reservoirs can deliver an F_IO_2 approaching 1.0 but are uncomfortable and difficult to fit to the face appropriately. Patients with hypoxemia refractory to high F_IO_2 concentrations delivered by face masks require intubation, institution of mechanical ventilation, and manipulation of mean airway pressure.

In addition to providing supplemental oxygen, other modalities such as bronchodilator drugs, chest physiotherapy, antibiotics, fluid management, and corticosteroids should be used when appropriate, as discussed in other articles in this book.

MECHANICAL VENTILATION

Mechanical ventilation provides a substitute for the patient's inspiratory muscles. Most mechanical ventilation today is positive pressure ventilation, in which a positive pressure is applied to the patient's airways via an endotracheal tube. This allows manipulation of peak and mean airway pressures so as to achieve adequate alveolar ventilation and oxygenation. Ventilators also allow regulation of supplemental oxygen and are equipped with timing mechanisms for initiating inspiration that provide an alternative to the patient's respiratory chemosensors and innervation of the inspiratory muscles. Four major parameters must be defined when mechanical ventilation is initiated and maintained: (1) F_IO_2, (2) $\dot{V}_E$, (3) mode of ventilation, and (4) positive end-expiratory pressure (PEEP) and mean airway pressure.

Concentration of Inspired Oxygen

An initial F_IO_2 of 1.0 virtually ensures an adequate PaO_2 even in the presence of marked intrapulmonary shunting. However, the goal is a PaO_2 of at least 60 mmHg, through the use of nontoxic oxygen concentrations. Therefore, further adjustments of the F_IO_2 are made on the basis of arterial blood gases. The F_IO_2 appropriate for achieving this may be calculated by using the ratio of alveolar oxygen tension (P_AO_2) to PaO_2 (P_AO_2/PaO_2). The P_AO_2 may be calculated by using the alveolar air equation

$$P_AO_2 = F_IO_2(P_B - P_{H2O}) - \frac{PaCO_2}{R}$$

where P_B is barometric pressure and P_{H2O} is partial pressure of water vapor. It may also be approximated by the "rule of sevens" (i.e., $700 \times F_IO_2 = P_AO_2$). The PaO_2 is obtained from arterial blood gases. Because the P_AO_2/PaO_2 remains relatively constant as F_IO_2 is changed, it can be used to decrease the F_IO_2 in order to obtain a desired PaO_2:

$$\frac{700 \times \text{current } F_IO_2}{\text{measured } PaO_2} = \frac{700 \times \text{new } F_IO_2}{\text{desired } PaO_2}$$

Prolonged exposures to F_IO_2 higher than 0.50 to 0.60 should be avoided. High F_IO_2 not only promotes atelectasis by washing out nitrogen, which stabilizes the alveoli, but also is toxic to the pulmonary parenchyma. Oxygen toxicity is characterized by worsening of oxygen transfer and diffuse pulmonary infiltrates. The occurrence of oxygen toxicity is directly related to the PaO_2 via the F_IO_2 and duration of exposure. Individual susceptibility varies, but exposure to an F_IO_2 higher than 0.6 for longer than 48 hours poses a significant risk. Mean airway pressure should be manipulated in order to avoid such high oxygen concentrations (see discussion of mean airway pressure).

Minute Ventilation

$\dot{V}_E$ is the product of tidal volume and respiratory rate. A tidal volume of approximately 10 mL per kg of ideal body weight at a rate of 10 to 15 breaths per minute is selected initially. The therapeutic goal is a pH of 7.35 to 7.45. The $\dot{V}_E$ required in order to achieve this goal varies among patients and depends on metabolic demands, dead space volume, and acid-base balance. Attempts to achieve "normal" values of $PaCO_2$ in patients with chronic carbon dioxide retention can lead to potentially life-threatening alkalosis and may make subsequent weaning difficult. Arterial blood gases obtained within minutes of initiation of mechanical ventilation serve to guide changes in tidal volume and respiratory rate to achieve a normal pH. The tidal volume delivered is a major determinant of the peak pressure attained by the ventilator. There is risk of barotrauma and further lung damage from subjecting the pulmonary parenchyma to either excess distention or excess pressure. In circumstances in which the damaged lung is nondistensible, the remaining normal lung may be at particular risk for this further injury. In such cases, peak pressures should be monitored and limited so as not to not exceed 50 cmH$_2$O and tidal volumes limited to 10 mL per kg (see complications).

Mode of Ventilation

This refers to the mechanism by which a mechanical ventilator initiates inspiration as well as the pressure and flow characteristics of the ventilator breath. Although many of the modes currently available are confusing, four modes are commonly employed: (1) control, (2) assist/control, (3) intermittent mandatory ventilation (IMV) or synchronized intermittent mandatory ventilation (SIMV), and (4) pressure-preselected modes. Each has benefits and drawbacks, and therefore no single mode is useful in all clinical situations.

In the control mode, the ventilator delivers a preset number of inspirations of a fixed tidal volume per minute, regardless of the patient's ventilatory efforts. The intrinsic timing of the ventilator initiates each inspiration. This is the mode of choice for apneic patients. It may also be necessary when the ventilator is operating at its pressure limit or when respiratory rates are rapid (>25 per minute).

Control may be accomplished by sedation with modest doses of morphine or diazepam (Valium) or with continuous infusion of fentanyl. On occasion, the patient may have to undergo drug-induced paralysis. If induction of paralysis is necessary, strict supervision and monitoring must be used, and the patient must never be left unattended. Concomitantly, the patient must be adequately sedated. Pancuronium (Pavulon) and vecuronium (Norcuron) are the long-term agents of choice. The initial intravenous dose is 0.8 mg per kg of body weight, followed by 0.1 to 0.4 mg per kg intravenously as needed to maintain control of ventilation. The other disadvantage of the control mode is that the patient cannot adjust the $\dot{V}_E$ to meet changing metabolic demands. Thus the $PaCO_2$ and the pH may fluctuate widely and require close monitoring.

In the assist/control mode, the patient triggers delivery of a fixed volume breath from the ventilator by spontaneously generating a negative pressure in the ventilator circuit. A backup (control) rate is set to ensure ventilation if apnea occurs. This rate should be approximately 80% of the spontaneous (assist) rate. Patients can adjust the $\dot{V}_E$ to match metabolic needs while the ventilatory muscles are relieved of some of the work of breathing. This allows the muscles to recover from fatigue and decrease oxygen consumption. The latter may result in improved tissue oxygenation in patients with shock, myocardial infarction, or severe oxygenation failure. However, severe respiratory alkalosis may develop in patients who are very agitated or in whom the underlying disease causes marked tachypnea (i.e., pulmonary edema, sepsis, pulmonary embolus, and so forth). When this occurs and if IMV cannot be used, controlled ventilation with sedation or even paralysis may be required in order to control respiratory rate in these patients.

With IMV, the $\dot{V}_E$ spontaneously achieved by the patient through an auxiliary gas flow through the ventilator circuit is augmented by a preset number of ventilator breaths of fixed volume. If the preset ventilator breaths are synchronized to occur only with the initiation of spontaneous inspiratory efforts by the patient, the mode is designated SIMV.

IMV and SIMV may decrease the risk of overventilation and thus reduce the need for sedation. However, inspiratory muscles that may be fatigued are not rested, and this mode should not be employed with initiation of mechanical ventilation; rather, it should be reserved for maintenance or weaning. Furthermore, if patients are unable to adequately supplement the preset $\dot{V}_E$, respiratory acidosis is likely to intervene. An additional hazard of IMV is that the work required to achieve an adequate $\dot{V}_E$ may place an intolerable burden on patients with impaired tissue oxygen delivery.

The pressure preset modes are pressure-support ventilation (PSV) and pressure-control ventilation (Pc). Although both entail a preselected pressure as a means of delivering a tidal volume by increasing transpulmonary pressure, there are significant differences between PSV and Pc. In essence, PSV is intended to serve as a support to spontaneous breathing and is similar to assist mode. The clinician selects a pressure that is maintained throughout the circuitry after initiation of inspiration by the patient. This allows the patient to receive a positive pressure augmented breath while retaining control of the length of the inspiratory cycle and its flow profile. IMV at a specified rate may also be selected. Because the tidal volume resulting from each pressure-supported breath is dependent on the impedance of the respiratory system, careful monitoring of tidal volume is necessary if PSV is chosen as a mode of ventilation. For this reason, in most instances, it should not be used in the initial phase of mechanical ventilation. The major use for this mode is in weaning, particularly in overcoming the resistance of endotracheal tubes (see the section on weaning). A hazard is that with most currently available ventilators, there is no control or backup rate for PSV, so that if respiratory drive decreases, life-threatening respiratory acidosis may rapidly supervene.

The Pc mode entails a flow and pressure pattern similar to that of PSV, but inspiration is time-cycled and preselected by the clinician rather than patient-cycled. It thus is a control mode entailing a predetermined pressure and duration of inspiration to deliver tidal volume. The tidal volume achieved is dependent on the preset pressure, the duration of inspiration, and the impedance of the thorax, lungs, and ventilator circuitry. Therefore, careful monitoring of exhaled tidal volume is required (see the section on acute lung failure).

Positive End-Expiratory Pressure and Mean Airway Pressure

When hypoxemia resulting from intrapulmonary right-to-left shunting is resistant to high F_IO_2, elevation of mean airway pressure frequently promotes improved oxygenation with less toxic concentrations of oxygen. Elevation of MAP should be employed when an F_IO_2 of more than 0.50 is required for maintaining a PaO_2 of 60 mmHg.

The two most frequently employed methods by which mean airway pressure is manipulated are PEEP and inverse ratio ventilation (IRV). On occasion both methods are employed simultaneously. "Inverse ratio ventilation" is a term that is applied when the normal ratio of inhalation time to exhalation time is reversed. Under normal circumstances, this ratio is usually 1:2 or 1:3. By prolonging inspiratory time and decreasing expiratory time during positive pressure breathing, mean airway pressure is increased and unstable airways are supported. PEEP raises functional residual capacity above closing volume by stabilizing terminal respiratory units that would otherwise collapse. Increases in mean airway pressure, however achieved, may also decrease the flow of blood distributed to the intrapulmonary shunt compartment by reducing cardiac output. Regardless of mechanism, the resultant increase in PaO_2 allows reduction of the F_IO_2 to less toxic levels. PEEP is generally applied first, and IRV is undertaken only when airway pressures become exceedingly high (see the section on complications). IRV may be undertaken by employing the volume mode of mechanical ventilation (Vc − IRV) or by using the pressure-preset, time-cycled Pc mode (Pc − IRV). In general, inspiratory-to-expiratory ratios exceeding 3:1 are rarely if ever required, and if adequate end-expiratory alveolar pressure is maintained, ratios should rarely exceed 2:1.

Increases in mean airway pressure, however applied, reduce cardiac output by decreasing venous return to the heart. In addition, changes in configuration of the interventricular septum, increases in right ventricular afterload, and other processes may reduce cardiac output when high levels of mean airway pressure are used. Such decreases in cardiac output may decrease tissue oxygen delivery despite an increase in PaO_2. Therefore when elevations of mean airway pressure are achieved either by PEEP or by IRV, pulmonary artery flotation catheters are critical for evaluating changes in cardiac output and oxygen delivery. Inotropic agents, packed red blood cell transfusions, and intravenous fluids may help augment tissue oxygen delivery under these circumstances. Renal function, as well as cerebral and splanchnic blood flow, may also be altered by PEEP and presumably by IRV. The renal dysfunction may occur independently of the decreased cardiac output and is characterized by decreases in both urine volume and sodium excretion.

COMPLICATIONS OF MECHANICAL VENTILATION

Potential complications of intubation and mechanical ventilation include upper airway trauma; aspiration of airway secretions or enteral feedings; nosocomial pulmonary infections; mechanical difficulties with the endotracheal tube, including prolapse of the balloon over the tip, obstruction by secretions, or displacement into the right main stem bronchus; and tracheal strictures or tracheoesophageal fistula resulting from prolonged intubation. Use of a well-stabilized endotracheal tube with a high-volume, low-pressure cuff reduces the risk of the last two complications. Airway secretions must be managed by ensuring adequate humidification of the inspired gas and by frequent chest physiotherapy, postural drainage, and suctioning. There is no firm evidence that a tracheostomy is associated with fewer long-term complications than endotracheal intubation. However, a tracheostomy facilitates oral intake, the patient's comfort, and the patient's ability to communicate.

Positive pressure mechanical ventilation can produce further lung injury as a result of increased airway and transpulmonary pressures. Barotrauma can produce pneumothorax, pneumomediastinum, interstitial emphysema, and air emboli and can even exacerbate acute lung injury. The last complication is of particular importance in patients who already have sustained an acute injury to their alveolar-capillary membrane. It is thought that the mechanism of further injury relates to overdistention of the ventilated lung. This occurs because the damaged lung does not participate in ventilation, and therefore the delivered tidal volume inflates the small amount of remaining lung, overdistending and injuring it. This concept has produced concern among clinicians about avoiding both excessive tidal volumes and extreme distending pressures. The exact limits to be placed on tidal volume or airway pressure are unclear. However, tidal volumes should usually not exceed 10 cmH_2O per kg of ideal body weight. When peak airway pressures in patients with nondistensible lungs approach 50 cmH_2O, consideration should be given to employing IRV, perhaps combined with pressure control. Another option would require ventilation with a smaller tidal volume and allowing the $PaCO_2$ to increase gradually. The latter alternative is also effective in patients with very high airway resistance, as in status asthmaticus.

An unintentional increase in end-expiratory pressure and mean airway pressure may occur during mechanical ventilation. This has been termed "dynamic hyperinflation," "auto-PEEP," and "intrinsic PEEP" by various observers. This unintentional PEEP escapes detection under ordinary monitoring circumstances as the exhalation valve opens to atmospheric pressure, and the proximal airway pressure manometer therefore records a 0-cmH_2O end-expiratory pressure, although the actual pressure is somewhat higher. PEEP can arise unintentionally if inspiration begins before the previous exhalation is completed. Factors that may produce this are therefore rapid respiratory rates, intrinsic or extrinsic airway obstruction, IRV, high V_E, and slow inspiratory flow rates. High levels of unintended and unmeasured PEEP can (1) decrease venous return and impair hemodynamic stability, (2) increase the work of breathing by increasing the pressure drop required to initiate the ventilator's inspiratory cycle, and (3) adversely effect measurement of wedge pressure by increasing alveolar pressure. Measurement of unintended PEEP requires that the expiratory port of the ventilator be occluded before the next inspiration and that the patient make no inspiratory efforts. The latter requirement is difficult to achieve and may require neuromuscular blocking agents. Therefore, it is frequently best to recognize the clinical circumstances under which unintended PEEP may occur, rather than to routinely monitor for it.

Patients requiring mechanical ventilation are subject to the same complications that any critically ill patient is at risk for, such as infection, malnutrition, thromboembolism, gastrointestinal bleeding, and cardiac dysrhythmias. The appropriate precautions and vigilance are required.

WEANING

Mechanical ventilation may be discontinued when the underlying conditions necessitating ventilatory support have significantly improved or dissipated. In such patients, removal may be accomplished promptly after a 1- to 2-hour trial of breathing through a T-piece with supplemental oxygen. Many patients who have exhibited maximal improvement in respiratory function but remain with significant deficits in bellows function or oxygenation require a more prolonged and gradual process, which has been called "weaning." Successful weaning requires not only that the respiratory system be capable of supporting ventilation and oxygenation but also that the general condition of the patient be close to optimal. Before weaning is initiated, (1) infection must be controlled, (2) cardiac output must be maximized and hemodynamic stability achieved,

(3) acid-base derangements must be corrected, (4) airway care and bronchodilation must be optimized, and (5) deficits in nutritional and metabolic status must be repaired.

Prediction of successful weaning of patients who remain with significant respiratory impairment is problematic. There are parameters that are useful when combined with clinical acumen and an understanding of their limitations. Spontaneous respiratory rate and tidal volume are perhaps the most generally useful. Patients who breathe rapidly with small tidal volumes are least likely to withstand withdrawal of support. Maximal inspiratory pressure and maximal voluntary ventilation (MVV) in 15 seconds are used to evaluate respiratory muscle strength and endurance, respectively. The $\dot{V}_E$ during quiet spontaneous breathing indicates metabolic demands and, indirectly, dead space volume. The forced vital capacity maneuver assesses airway function and respiratory muscle strength. The ease with which supplemental oxygen corrects hypoxemia enables the clinician to gauge the degree of ventilation/perfusion abnormality. Useful criteria are (1) a forced vital capacity of more than 10 to 15 mL per kg; (2) a spontaneous $\dot{V}_E$ of less than 10 liters per minute, which can be doubled during the MVV maneuver; (3) a maximal negative inspiratory pressure of more than 25 cmH_2O; (4) a ratio of respiratory rate to tidal volume (breaths per minute per liter) of less than 105; and (5) a PaO_2 of 60 mmHg while receiving F_IO_2 of less than 0.50. However, patients who fail these criteria may nonetheless be weaned successfully, and the entire clinical situation must be fully evaluated.

Although weaning may be accomplished by many techniques, each of which has theoretical advantages, none has been demonstrated to be more effective than another. It is important to stress that familiarity with one or two such techniques, and the application of them with the nursing staff and respiratory care team in a standardized manner, may be most consequential.

In patients with acute lung failure (as in ARDS) who have required manipulation of mean airway pressure and mode of ventilation, efforts are first directed toward (1) restoring inspiratory/expiratory ratios toward normal, (2) changing the mode from pressure control, if used, to assist/control or IMV, and (3) gradually lowering the F_IO_2 and PEEP until a PaO_2 of more than 60 mmHg is sustained by an F_IO_2 of less than 0.5 and a PEEP of 5 cmH_2O. Not only is it not necessary to decrease the applied PEEP below 5 cmH_2O, but it also may be desirable for all patients receiving mechanical ventilation to receive this level of end-expiratory pressure, which restores the lung volume lost in the supine position and prevents microatelectasis. After this has been achieved, weaning from ventilatory support may proceed as delineated.

The three most commonly used weaning techniques are T-piece, IMV, and PSV. The use of the T-piece has become increasingly restricted to patients who have fully recovered from a physiologic insult and who generally require only a short period of observation and measurement of arterial blood gases before extubation. In virtually all other circumstances, IMV is used, most frequently with PSV. Weaning is most often accomplished by decreasing the fixed or mandatory rate in the IMV mode until the patient is entirely self-supporting. In order to assist the patient in overcoming the resistance of the artificial airway, which can be considerable depending on its radius, PSV is employed. In this manner, the ventilator circuitry is pressurized during inspiration to a preset level, usually selected at 10 cmH_2O. This amount of pressure support may be sufficient to overcome the resistance of the artificial airway and avoid placing an additional load on already compromised inspiratory muscles.

Alternately, weaning may proceed with PSV as the primary ventilatory and weaning mode. In such circumstances, when the determination is made that a trial removal of ventilatory support may be accomplished, the ventilatory mode is changed to PSV by changing the ventilator setting and selecting the amount of pressure desired. This is usually 15 to 25 cmH_2O and should be sufficient to provide patients with the same tidal volume that they were previously receiving and a respiratory rate of less than 25 breaths per minute. The amount of preset pressure is gradually decreased as the patient becomes increasingly capable of assuming more of the ventilatory load. The criteria used for decreasing the pressure are maintaining the respiratory rate at <25 breaths per minute and periodic arterial blood gas measurements. Whichever method is chosen, the importance of a standardized approach to weaning, including the development and use of protocols, cannot be overemphasized.

Extubation is performed early in the day to optimize monitoring of the patient. After extubation, the patient is fitted with a high-humidity mask or face tent and is administered an F_IO_2 higher than that used with mechanical ventilation. Coughing is encouraged. Patients are observed and reintubated for progressive hypoxemia, progressive hypercapnia, acidosis, or laryngospasm not responsive to therapy.

ADULT RESPIRATORY DISTRESS SYNDROME

ARDS refers to acute lung failure ensuing from diffuse pulmonary injury resulting from a wide variety of insults. In ARDS, extravascular fluid accumulates as a result of alveolar epithelial injury. Both this and the increased cellularity of the alveolar capillary septum from the subsequent repair process result in (1) decreased pulmonary compliance, (2) collapsed terminal respiratory units, and (3) increased intrapulmonary shunt and dead space. These changes cause the tachypnea, intercostal muscle retraction, hypoxemia, and diffuse pulmonary infiltrates visible on chest roentgenograms.

Although treatment of the predisposing condition is paramount, management is primarily supportive. The fundamental goals are maintaining adequate tissue oxygen delivery and consumption, using nontoxic concentrations of oxygen, and avoiding deleterious increases in airway pressure. This almost uniformly requires increasing mean airway pressure and employing hemodynamic monitoring with a pulmonary artery balloon flotation catheter.

Mechanical ventilation is used to modulate mean airway pressure so as to ensure oxygenation with the least toxic oxygen concentration and to assist the inspiratory muscles to achieve an adequate $\dot{V}_E$ while simultaneously avoiding excesses of airway pressure. This frequently requires compromises. Initially, PEEP alone is used to increase mean airway pressure and to rapidly lower the F_IO_2 from 1.0 to less than 0.6 to achieve a PaO_2 of 60 mmHg. A $\dot{V}_E$ is selected by varying tidal volume to achieve a normal pH. The peak pressure and respiratory rate must be closely monitored in order to avoid both respiratory alkalosis and airway pressures in excess of 50 cmH$_2$O induced by the nondistensible lungs and the application of PEEP.

If airway pressures are excessive, or if adequate oxygenation cannot be achieved with a PEEP of less than 15 cmH$_2$O, the application of IRV, frequently with pressure control (Pc − IRV) may be used. The prolonged inspiration increases mean airway pressure and supports oxygenation by recruiting terminal respiratory units and preventing end-expiratory collapse or closure of unstable lung units. Excessive airway pressure is avoided by limiting the maximal pressure that can be achieved. The decelerating flow pattern achieved with pressure control may also improve gas exchange. Unintended PEEP frequently develops as a result of IRV, and monitoring is required in this situation. It is important to recognize that tidal volume in this mode is dependent on the pressure selected and on the compliance and resistance of the respiratory system, and thus careful observation is required. When initiating this mode, the clinician should choose a ratio of inspiration to exhalation of 1:1, a pressure limit to achieve a tidal volume no higher than 10 mL per kg ideal body weight, and approximately half the previously applied PEEP. Further changes are based on changes in arterial blood gases, in F_IO_2, and in hemodynamic parameters. It is almost never necessary to exceed a ratio of 1:1.7 or 1:2. Because of discomfort arising from the abnormal pattern of breathing, heavy sedation (frequently combined with respiratory muscle paralysis) is necessary.

Because of the large increases in mean airway pressure, which inhibits ventricular filling pressures and thus cardiac output, oxygen delivery and consumption must be monitored and optimized. The relationship between oxygen delivery and oxygen usage in this situation is complex. Normally, oxygen consumption remains constant despite wide variations in tissue oxygen delivery. Of course, marked decreases in delivery can be so great that eventually consumption is impaired. This occurs at very low levels of delivery, approximating 8 mL per minute per kg. In these situations, therapeutic intervention should be aimed at restoring cardiac output to normal, arterial oxygen saturation to 0.90%, and hemoglobin concentration to approximate 10 grams per dL. Data indicate that in ARDS, especially when complicated by shock, oxygen consumption increases with increasing oxygen delivery, reaching a plateau at a level higher than normal. Thus merely normalizing oxygen delivery or cardiac output in these patients is frequently *inadequate* therapy.

Oxygen delivery may be optimized by manipulation of cardiac output, arterial oxygen content, or hemoglobin concentration. There is little to be gained by increasing hemoglobin concentration beyond 7 to 10 grams per dL or by achieving a PaO_2 higher than 60 mmHg. Cardiac output is therefore the major determinant of oxygen delivery that may be effectively manipulated.

Cardiac output measurements must be interpreted in relation to oxygen consumption and delivery rather than to some categorization of "normal." Cardiac output should be maximized by monitoring arterial lactate concentration, oxygen delivery, and oxygen consumption. A clinical strategy is to measure arterial lactate concentration and, if it is higher than 2.2 mmol per liter, to effect an increase in oxygen delivery and evaluate the effect on oxygen consumption and lactate. This process may be repeated in an attempt to optimize oxygen delivery and consumption by using arterial lactate concentration as a marker of cellular hypoxia. When this concentration returns to less than 2.2 mmol per liter and oxygen consumption no longer increases, the cardiac output and oxygen delivery may be considered optimized.

This optimalization of cardiac output must be accomplished despite increases in mean airway pressure and the need to regulate intravascular volume within narrow limits in order to minimize extravascular lung water. Although maintenance of blood pressure and urine output of more than 30 mL per hour may be useful guides to volume management, the measurement of pulmonary artery occlusion pressure (PAOP) through the use of a balloon flotation pulmonary artery catheter may provide a more quantitative approach. To minimize pulmonary extravascular lung water, the PAOP should be maintained at the lowest level compatible with optimalization of cardiac output.

The use of vasoactive drugs such as dobutamine may be the agents of choice in balancing the need for maximal cardiac output with minimal volume loading. However, in addition to the usual constraints of ensuring accurate hemodynamic measurements, the use of the PAOP in patients with high mean airway pressures is often problematic. Falsely elevated PAOP measurements may result when (1) the catheter tip lies above the level of the left atrium, (2) exhalation is not passive and pleural pressure at end-exhalation is elevated, (3) pleural pressure is excessively increased by the elevated mean airway pressure, (4) the configuration of the cardiac ventricular septum is distorted by increased mean airway pressure, and (5) unintended PEEP is present and unmeasured. Thus an elevated PAOP in these patients must be interpreted with caution.

Successful management of these patients requires a holistic approach to the patient by the critical care team with meticulous attention directed at nutrition, circumvention or vigorous treatment of nosocomial infection, prevention and treatment of complications of mechanical ventilation, and avoidance or treatment of multisystem organ failure. Patients may be weaned as previously discussed.

ATELECTASIS

method of
WATTS R. WEBB, M.D.
Tulane University Medical School
New Orleans, Louisiana

The term "atelectasis" preferably is restricted to indicate an airless state in the lung without other pathologic changes. Thus the lung consolidated with pneumonia, drowned by pulmonary edema, or containing no air because of congestive atelectasis (the adult respiratory distress syndrome) is more properly designated by specific terms and does not constitute atelectasis in the pure sense of the term.

Atelectasis commonly has a segmental or lobar distribution but may develop as a diffuse process of microatelectasis. The first sign of developing atelectasis may be an area of bronchial breathing easily detected with a stethoscope, often appearing before fever, tachypnea, tachycardia, and hypoxemia become evident. The chest roentgenographic findings are patchy, focal, or segmental in distribution.

Atelectasis may be caused by (1) intrinsic or extrinsic airway obstruction, (2) compression of the lung, (3) inadequate alveolar ventilation so that all air within the alveoli is absorbed, or (4) loss or inactivation of the surfactant.

AIRWAY OBSTRUCTION

Atelectasis may be caused by intrinsic obstructions, such as a bronchial tumor, a foreign body, mucus, meconium, or a stricture of the bronchus. In these lesions, which are usually suggested by the presenting complaints, bronchoscopy is indicated as both a diagnostic and a therapeutic measure. Extrinsic compression of the trachea or bronchi can be caused by tumors, hyperplastic inflammatory or neoplastic lymph nodes, or vascular anomalies. Fortunately, many of the neoplastic lesions respond to irradiation therapy, and some of the inflammatory lesions respond to antibiotics. Infantile tuberculosis, for example, is particularly apt to cause distal atelectasis of a lobe or of an entire lung, but re-aeration is to be anticipated after therapy with antituberculosis drugs.

PULMONARY COMPRESSION

Pulmonary collapse may be caused by chest wall, diaphragmatic, or intrapleural lesions, such as thoracoplasty, pneumoperitoneum, pneumothorax, massive pleural effusion, or hemothorax. Overinflation of one portion of the lung (as a result of cysts) or of an entire lobe (e.g., as in congenital lobar emphysema) may cause compression and thereby atelectasis of the otherwise normal lung. Most conditions respond to appropriate surgical intervention.

The abdominal causes of atelectasis include acute gastric dilatation, generalized intestinal distention, and pneumoperitoneum. These conditions usually can be managed successfully by removing the peritoneal or gastrointestinal fluid and air.

INADEQUATE ALVEOLAR VENTILATION

Inadequate alveolar ventilation may be caused by (1) trauma, including that from operations (either because of associated pain or the inadequate bellows action of a flail chest), (2) various neurologic conditions (e.g., head injuries, congenital or birth defects, or myasthenia gravis), or (3) mere oversedation of a patient.

The primary therapy for fractured ribs consists of single or repeated paravertebral intercostal nerve blocks with local anesthetics—usually bipuvicaine (Marcaine)—and the stir-up regimen previously described. Constrictive bindings and external splinting of the chest have no place except as a first-aid measure. Ventilation is best ensured by internal pneumatic fixation by tracheal intubation and constant positive airway pressure (CPAP) and intermittent mandatory ventilation (IMV). CPAP increases the functional residual capacity (the air remaining in the lung at the end of quiet expiration) and opens up or prevents the development of small atelectatic areas that give rise to perfusion/ventilation abnormalities. The positive pressure needed usually is only 5 to 15 cmH$_2$O, although in very stiff lungs, higher pressures may be needed.

IMV allows the patient to breathe spontaneously while the respirator adds the requisite number of ventilations per minute to ensure adequate alveolar ventilation. Thus in patients with minimal or no spontaneous respiration, IMV may amount to completely controlled respiration. As the patient breathes more rapidly or deeply, he or she is gradually weaned from the IMV, as guided by the carbon dioxide tension.

Atelectasis in patients with neurologic conditions frequently is more difficult to treat because of the long-term nature or incurability of the underlying condition. Important considerations include adequate mobilization of the patient and careful nursing care to prevent aspiration. These patients often have depressed cough and gag reflexes. Feeding tubes are often needed, and if gastric emptying is delayed, gastric dilatation quickly develops. The tube passes through both esophageal sphincters, rendering them incompetent and thereby making regurgitation and aspiration common. Most often, it is advisable to perform a percutaneous endoscopic gastrostomy for decompression, with a feeding jejunostomy tube passed through the gastrostomy tube.

INADEQUATE SURFACTANT

Frequently there is loss or inactivation of surfactant (e.g., in inhalation of smoke or gases such as chlorine and ammonia) or aspiration of the acid gastric content (especially if the pH is less than 2). Management may necessitate bronchoscopy (for both diagnosis and therapy) and early use of CPAP and IMV. Minimal concentrations of oxygen should be used because of the toxic action of high concentrations of oxygen on surfactant and on the type II pneumocyte that produces surfactant. Artificial surfactant (colfosceril [Exosurf Neonatal]) by intratracheal instillation or nebulization is now effectively used in newborns with hyaline membrane disease. Its use in adult respiratory distress syndrome is beginning to be evaluated.

PNEUMONIA

Atelectasis is almost synonymous with pneumonia, because blood-borne bacteria are selectively deposited in the atelectatic lung. Antibiotics should be administered as soon as initial diagnostic measures have been performed. Initially, the antibiotic agent given should be effective against mouth organisms and gram-positive bacteria, particularly *Pneumococcus* and *Streptococcus* spp. A semisynthetic penicillin is most desirable because of its effectiveness and safety and because its limited spectrum of coverage does not promote the overgrowth of other bacteria. Cultures of cough specimens or tracheal aspirates should be performed daily, and the antibiotic coverage should be changed in accordance with the bacterial flora and sensitivity.

TREATMENT

More commonly, atelectasis is a postoperative or traumatic finding usually caused by retention of secretions, by blood, by aspirated material, or even by a misplaced endotracheal tube. Secretions accumulate because of ineffective or inadequate cleansing mechanisms: primarily, an inadequate cough. Important preventive and therapeutic measures include the following:

1. Adequate humidification of the inspired air to prevent inspissation of secretions. This usually requires a heated mist humidifier or an ultrasonic nebulizer. A so-called cold-stream humidifier can add only about half the moisture at room temperature needed to totally humidify air when warmed in the body to 37° C.

2. A stir-up regimen consisting of turning, deep breathing, and coughing at least every hour.

3. Insertion of a tracheal "cougher" (a small plastic catheter inserted percutaneously into the trachea at the first or second intertracheal ring) through which 2 to 10 mL of sterilized isotonic saline or a mucolytic agent can be injected as often as necessary. The most effective mucolytic agent to date for liquefying mucoid and purulent secretions is *N*-acetylcysteine (Mucomyst). This agent should be used as a 5% solution with the addition of bronchodilator to prevent bronchospasm that Mucomyst alone might stimulate.

4. Nasotracheal suctioning with the use of a sterile catheter and sterile gloves.

5. Bronchoscopy, which is particularly important in determining the presence of a foreign body or impacted material if the atelectasis persists or recurs.

6. Endotracheal intubation, either nasally or orally, which is valuable not only for repeated suctioning but also for assisted ventilation if needed.

7. Tracheostomy, used only after several days of intubation when it becomes apparent that intubation will be required for a further protracted period. A large tracheostomy tube, at least size 8 for a man and size 7 for a woman, should be used to ensure adequate airway size.

CHRONIC OBSTRUCTIVE PULMONARY DISEASE

method of
CHARLES G. ALEX, M.D., and
MARTIN J. TOBIN, M.D.
Edward Hines, Jr., Department of Veterans Affairs Hospital
Hines, Illinois

Chronic obstructive pulmonary disease (COPD) is a collective designation for chronic airway obstruction or airflow limitation caused by emphysema, chronic bronchitis, or some combination of these disorders.

At least 10 million Americans have COPD. Prevalence, incidence, and mortality rates for COPD increase with age, are higher among males than among females, and are higher among whites than among nonwhites. The single greatest risk factor for the development of COPD is cigarette smoking. Rates of obstructive airway disease, respiratory symptoms, and lung function abnormalities are higher among cigarette smokers than among nonsmokers. Recurrent or chronic respiratory infections and allergies are also predisposing factors for COPD. Alpha$_1$-protease inhibitor (API) deficiency is another risk factor for COPD, especially in emphysema. This deficiency accounts for approximately 1% of cases of COPD in the United States. Occupations in which atmospheres are polluted with dust or chemical fumes are associated with an increased incidence of chronic airway obstruction and increased rate of mortality from COPD.

Increased resistance to airflow during expiration characterizes COPD. Chronic bronchitis and emphysema are distinct disorders, the former limited to the conducting airways and the latter to the pulmonary parenchyma. Clinically, both processes often coexist in the same individual and may be associated with an asthmatic component seen as reversible airway obstruction on pulmonary function testing. Chronic bronchitis is typified clinically as a productive cough persisting for at least 3 months in a year and for at least 2 successive years. Airway obstruction must be documented and other infectious disorders ruled out. Patients with emphysema usually demonstrate progressive dyspnea and variable cough.

In chronic bronchitis, disease of the large and small airways increases airway resistance. Hypoxemia results because lung areas are underventilated for the degree of perfusion. In addition to airway obstruction, the hallmarks of emphysema are hyperinflation and reduced carbon dioxide diffusing capacity. The loss of elastic recoil limits airflow. Greater lung volumes develop in emphysema because of the loss of lung elastic recoil in the presence of a relatively unaltered chest wall recoil. Destruction of the alveolar-capillary interface results in a low diffusing capacity. Early in the development of emphysema, ventilation/perfusion relationships are affected proportionately, and gas exchange is preserved.

Pathologically, chronic bronchitis is characterized by hypertrophied and hyperplastic mucous glands, smooth muscle hyperplasia, cartilage atrophy, and mucosal inflammation of the large central airways. Similar involvement of the small airways with goblet cell hyperplasia and mucosal inflammation is considered an early marker of COPD. The small airways are the primary sites of obstruction in COPD. In emphysema, there is a permanent, abnormal enlargement of the airspaces distal to the nonrespiratory bronchioles, accompanied by destructive changes of the alveolar walls.

Pathogenetic mechanisms of COPD include protease-antiprotease imbalances. Cigarette smoke directly blocks the inhibitory capacity of API and promotes an excess of neutrophils through the attractant effects of alveolar macrophages. The neutrophils release elastases, which are capable of destroying the elastin structure of the lung. Cigarette smoking is also associated with goblet cell metaplasia and bronchiolitis, which contribute to airway obstruction.

TREATMENT

Bronchodilator use is the mainstay of therapy for COPD. Other aspects of care, including oxygen therapy, nutrition, pulmonary rehabilitation, preventive therapy with smoking cessation, and alpha$_1$-antitrypsin replacement for patients with deficient levels, are also important.

Pharmacologic Therapy

Several agents relieve airway obstruction, including sympathomimetics, anticholinergics, methylxanthines, and corticosteroids. Patients exhibiting marked improvement of airflow obstruction with bronchodilators probably have an asthmatic component to their disease and can achieve greater benefit from these agents. However, COPD patients with irreversible or "fixed" airflow obstruction demonstrated by pulmonary function testing may also respond substantially to bronchodilators and ultimately reduce the work of breathing.

Sympathomimetics. Inhalation of sympathomimetics or beta agonists is effective and usually provides the first- or second-line approach to therapy. Beta-adrenergic effects include $beta_1$ activity, which produces cardiac stimulation, and $beta_2$ activity, which produces bronchodilation and promotes mucociliary clearance. A disadvantage of $beta_2$ agonists is their effect on other muscle receptors that produces tremor. When they are given by inhalation, $beta_2$ selectivity is further enhanced, and the side effects of tachycardia, tremor, and slight hypoxemia are minimized. Commonly used $beta_2$ agonists include metaproterenol (Alupent, Metaprel), albuterol (Proventil, Ventolin), terbutaline (Brethaire), pirbuterol (Maxair), and bitolterol (Tornalate).

In stable patients with COPD, sympathomimetic agents inhaled from a metered-dose inhaler (MDI) are more effective than oral sympathomimetics. Proper instruction of patients on the use of MDIs is paramount. MDIs are usually given as two or three puffs three or four times per day, but several additional puffs or increased frequency may be necessary for acute exacerbations of COPD. Hypokalemia is a potential problem associated with higher doses of $beta_2$ agonists. If a patient with marked dyspnea is unable to use an MDI properly, sympathomimetics can be inhaled from a nebulizer. If a spacer device is used in combination with an MDI, bronchodilation is at least as great as that obtained with a nebulizer. Table 1 shows the commonly used dosages of sympathomimetics administered from MDIs or inhalant solutions that are available in the United States.

Anticholinergics. Anticholinergic agents are at least as potent as and usually superior to sympathomimetic agents, and thus they are suitable for first-line therapy. Patients with COPD may experience additional bronchodilation with anticholinergic agents, even after optimal bronchodilation with sympathomimetic agents or theophylline. Anticholinergics exert their effects by competitive inhibition of muscarinic cholinergic receptors, thereby relaxing bronchial smooth muscle. Because cholinergic tone tends to be heightened in COPD, anticholinergic agents usually are beneficial. Atropine, a tertiary ammonium compound, is available as a 1% solution of atropine sulfate and can be given by nebulizer in doses of 0.5 to 2.5 mg every 4 to 6 hours. However, the use of this agent as a bronchodilator has not been approved by the U.S. Food and Drug Administration, and side effects are common at this dosage.

Ipratropium (Atrovent), a synthetic quaternary ammonium compound, is approved for use in the United States. In clinical trials, inhalation of a single dose was as effective as albuterol in producing bronchodilation in patients with COPD. Adding nebulized ipratropium to albuterol further increased bronchodilation in these patients. A nebulized solution is not available in the United States, but trials are under way. The recommended dosage of the aerosol inhalant is two puffs (36 µg) every 4 to 6 hours, but this dose may be doubled or tripled to achieve maximal bronchodilation. Ipratropium is well tolerated, and its few side effects such as a mild cough and dry mouth make it an attractive first-line agent in the treatment of COPD. Glycopyrrolate (Robinul), although not approved for use as a bronchodilator in the United States, can be given as a nebulized preparation of 1 mg every 4 to 6 hours and may serve as a possible alternative to other anticholinergics.

Methylxanthines. Once thought to work by phosphodiesterase inhibition, methylxanthines (e.g., theophylline, aminophylline) appear to cause bronchodilation by some other mechanism, possibly by translocation of calcium ions in smooth muscle. Because of its narrow therapeutic range and weak bronchodilator effect in stable COPD patients, theophylline use is waning. For patients with acute exacerbations of COPD, the addition of intravenous aminophylline to a standard regimen of a beta agonist, a corticosteroid, and an antibiotic did not improve symptoms, spirometric results, or oxygenation. Theophylline can improve cardiac and diaphragmatic contrac-

TABLE 1. **Sympathomimetic Dosages for Metered-Dose Inhalers and Nebulized Solutions**

| Drug | Metered-Dose Inhaler | | Nebulization |
	Initial Dose	mg/Puff	
Albuterol	2–3 puffs q 4–6 h	0.09	0.3–0.5 mL 0.5% solution in 3 mL saline q 4–6 h
Bitolterol	2–3 puffs q 6–8 h	0.37	
Metaproterenol	2–3 puffs q 4–6 h	0.65	0.3 mL 5% solution in 2.5 mL saline q 4–6 h
Pirbuterol	2–3 puffs q 4–6 h	0.20	
Terbutaline	2–3 puffs q 4–6 h	0.20	

tility, diminish pulmonary vascular resistance, and stimulate central respiratory activity. Theophylline is usually relegated to third-line therapy as an oral, sustained-release preparation given in doses of 300 to 900 mg per day to stable COPD patients and as an intravenous preparation for severe, acute exacerbations of COPD.

Corticosteroids. Corticosteroids are considered beneficial for COPD patients with an asthmatic component or during an acute exacerbation. Methylprednisolone (Solu-Medrol) in a dose of 0.5 mg per kg of body weight given every 6 hours for 3 days has rapidly improved airway obstruction during acute exacerbations of COPD. It is prudent to reserve steroid treatment for patients with asthmatic symptoms or with persistent bronchospasm despite adequate therapy with sympathomimetics, anticholinergics, and theophylline. Because the long-term use of corticosteroids is fraught with adverse effects, their use should be minimized; burst therapy or inhaled steroid preparations should be used instead. Although there is recent evidence suggesting that chronic low-dose corticosteroid therapy may slow the progression of disease in patients with COPD, additional confirmatory studies are needed before this therapy can be recommended.

Antibiotics. The airways of a patient with chronic bronchitis provide a rich medium for bacterial colonization. Although viruses play a major role in the flare-up of bronchitis, colonizing organisms such as *Streptococcus pneumoniae, Haemophilus influenzae,* and *Moraxella catarrhalis* also have a pathogenic role. Antibiotics are good adjuncts to therapy during acute exacerbations of COPD. Selected antibiotic therapy should be administered intermittently for 7 to 10 days at a time. Recommended agents include ampicillin (500 mg every 6 hours), amoxicillin (500 mg every 8 hours), tetracycline (500 mg every 6 hours), trimethoprim-sulfamethoxazole (160/800 mg every 12 hours), or ciprofloxacin (500 mg every 12 hours). For repeated flare-ups, it is sometimes useful to vary the antibiotic. Prophylaxis is not advised.

Immunotherapy for influenza is recommended for all patients with COPD. In certain situations immediately after the onset of influenza A, amantadine (100 mg every 12 to 24 hours) can be given to reduce symptoms. Amantadine has no effect on influenza B infections. Pneumococcal vaccine is also recommended to prevent pneumonia in COPD patients, but its overall benefit has not been fully assessed.

Mucolytics and Expectorants. Excessive airway mucus is a common feature in patients with chronic bronchitis. The thick, tenacious sputum is often difficult to mobilize and contributes to airway obstruction and frequent coughing. Bronchial secretions can be diminished by using sympathomimetics and theophylline to enhance mucociliary clearance and corticosteroids to reduce airway inflammation. Mucolytics and expectorants aid in altering the rheologic properties of the bronchial mucus, but their overall efficacy remains unproven. Iodinated glycerol has some short-term benefit in COPD patients, but its long-term effects have not been evaluated. The expectorant guaifenesin appears to have no significant effect unless given in large doses. *N*-acetylcysteine (Mucomyst) acts as a mucolytic and can be administered as an aerosol, but it is rarely prescribed because it can produce severe coughing and bronchospasm. If coughing during a mild exacerbation of COPD is troubling and nonproductive, a trial of antitussive therapy (e.g., dextromethorphan) may be warranted.

Pulmonary Vasodilators. Pulmonary hypertension usually occurs as a result of chronic hypoxemia in patients with COPD. Oxygen administration remains the best therapy for pulmonary hypertension. Vasodilators, such as hydralazine, nitrates, calcium channel blockers, prostaglandins, and prostacyclin, can decrease pulmonary artery pressures, but they also cause systemic hypotension and have yielded variable results in patients with COPD. There is no practical role for these agents in the treatment of COPD.

Diuretics. The cautious use of diuretics is reserved for left ventricular failure or peripheral edema associated with cor pulmonale. Phlebotomy in a polycythemic patient with cor pulmonale is not recommended unless the patient maintains a severely elevated hematocrit (>55%) despite oxygen therapy.

Digitalis. The use of digoxin in COPD is controversial. It is best reserved for COPD patients with left ventricular compromise or atrial tachyarrhythmias.

Respiratory Stimulants. The safe use of respiratory stimulants in elderly COPD patients has not been substantiated and is not currently recommended.

Alpha$_1$-Antitrypsin Replacement Therapy. The protease-antiprotease hypothesis is based on the association of API deficiency and the development of emphysema. In patients with API deficiency, the rate of decline of pulmonary function is more rapid than in patients with COPD who have normal levels of API. However, not all API-deficient patients develop emphysema. Several alleles for the protease inhibitor have been demonstrated by various electrophoretic patterns. The homozygous null allele is completely API deficient, but patients with the homozygous Z allele have approximately 15% of normal API activity. A normal serum API level ranges from 180 to 280 mg per dL. Although costly, 60 mg per kg of active

API can be given intravenously as a weekly dose. The long-term effects of replacement therapy in the API-deficient population with emphysema are unknown.

Oxygen Therapy

Long-term oxygen therapy is the only form of treatment known to improve survival in hypoxemic COPD patients. It has also been demonstrated that patients given continuous oxygen therapy for longer than 19 hours each day exhibited the best overall survival. Oxygen improves the quality of life, pulmonary hemodynamics, and polycythemia. A patient with COPD who has received maximal medical management and who persistently has an arterial oxygen tension (PaO_2) of less than 55 mmHg is a candidate for continuous domiciliary oxygen therapy. A patient with a PaO_2 between 55 and 60 mmHg may benefit from oxygen therapy if there is associated cor pulmonale, polycythemia, or changes in mental status. Patients with COPD develop arterial oxygen desaturation during sleep, especially during rapid eye movement (REM) sleep. Nocturnal oxygen therapy in those prone to desaturation may improve the quality of sleep and minimize pulmonary arterial hypertension during periods of REM-induced hypoxemia. The administration of oxygen during exercise-induced hypoxemia may also be warranted. During acute exacerbations of COPD, oxygen administration is given by nasal prongs or face mask. Regional costs and preferences determine the source of oxygen (i.e., liquid, compressed gas, concentrator) and the method of delivery (i.e., reservoir cannulas, demand-delivery systems, transtracheal delivery).

Nutrition

Several factors contribute to the wasting syndrome of patients with COPD. Nutritional deficiencies decrease respiratory drive, respiratory muscle bulk, and strength. A diet high in carbohydrates may increase carbon dioxide production and place excessive demands on ventilation. This may precipitate hypercapnic respiratory failure. Although it seems logical to provide malnourished COPD patients with calories as a diet with adjusted fat-to-carbohydrate ratios, this approach has not been fully evaluated. If the patient cannot eat and is likely to require mechanical ventilation for more than 1 day, enteral feeding with a feeding tube should be initiated.

Pulmonary Rehabilitation

Rehabilitation should begin with education of the patient and behavior modification. Smoking cessation is encouraged through counseling, but nicotine given by gum (Nicorette) or transdermal delivery (Habitrol, Nicoderm, Nicotrol, Prostep) may be required in order to limit the symptoms of withdrawal. Pulmonary function may improve after patients with early COPD stop smoking. Other modalities of rehabilitation include chest physical therapy to assist secretion removal and exercise conditioning that may include inspiratory muscle training. Pulmonary rehabilitation programs have improved the quality of life and exercise capacity. Despite the success of these modalities, a standardized approach to rehabilitation has not been established.

Lung Transplantation

With improved immunosuppression, lung transplantation has become an option for selected patients with end-stage COPD. Originally, double-lung transplantation was advocated, but there has been increasing success with single-lung transplantation. Because of a lack of suitable donor organs and centers capable of performing this procedure, the availability of lung transplantation remains limited.

Management Options for COPD Patients

Several treatment options for the stable COPD patient are available. For mild or moderate disease, a sympathomimetic or anticholinergic MDI can be tried. For more severe disease, a sustained-release theophylline preparation can be added. Bronchodilators may be more effective if delivered as an aerosol with a spacer device or given as a nebulized preparation. In certain COPD patients, symptoms may persist, and a trial of corticosteroids is warranted. Exacerbations of COPD usually necessitate oxygen, more frequent doses of sympathomimetics and anticholinergics, and intravenous aminophylline and corticosteroids. Antibiotics are necessary if there is evidence of acute bronchitis or pneumonia. Other precipitating causes must be ruled out (e.g., congestive heart failure, pulmonary embolism, pneumothorax). Increased airway secretions also must be managed, and if the patient has cor pulmonale, oxygen therapy, diuretics, and possibly digoxin are necessary. In the event of severe respiratory failure in an end-stage COPD patient, any prior directive by the patient about life support must be respected. Intubation and mechanical ventilation may benefit patients with potentially reversible conditions, especially if there is respiratory muscle fatigue. Nasal continuous positive airway pressure may benefit some patients by minimizing respiratory muscle fatigue and avoiding intubation.

PRIMARY LUNG CANCER

method of
DAVID S. ETTINGER, M.D.
Johns Hopkins University School of Medicine
Baltimore, Maryland

Lung cancer is the leading cause of cancer-related deaths in the United States. It is estimated that 170,000 new cases will have been diagnosed in 1993 and 149,000 people will have died of lung cancer. Lung cancer incidence and mortality rates continue to climb, particularly in women.

Non–small cell lung cancer (NSCLC) accounts for approximately 75 to 80% of all cases of lung cancer, whereas small cell lung cancer (SCLC) constitutes 20 to 25% of all cases. The overall cure rate for patients with NSCLC is less than 10%. The poor survival rates reflect the advanced stage of the disease at diagnosis, high recurrence rates associated with surgery and radiation therapy, and the inability of systemic therapy (i.e., chemotherapy) to prolong survival significantly.

SCLC is a rapidly growing tumor with a propensity for early dissemination to distant sites. Although SCLC patients respond to both chemotherapy and radiation therapy, systemic chemotherapy is the cornerstone of therapy. In a small percentage of patients with limited-stage SCLC, the disease can be cured, whereas this cannot be done in patients with extensive-stage disease.

NON–SMALL CELL LUNG CANCER

The World Health Organization has recognized three major types of NSCLC: epidermoid (squamous) carcinoma, adenocarcinoma, and large cell carcinoma. Epidermoid carcinomas and adenocarcinomas each account for 30 to 35% of all lung cancers. The frequency of the latter appears to be increasing. Large cell carcinoma accounts for 15 to 20% of all lung cancers.

Surgical resection offers patients with NSCLC the best chance of cure. Unfortunately, only one-third of patients with NSCLC have resectable disease. Another one-third of patients have locally advanced disease that is not resectable, and the last third of NSCLC patients exhibit evidence of distant metastases. Whether a patient with NSCLC is a surgical candidate depends on the stage of the patient's disease.

Pretreatment Evaluation

The cornerstone of planning treatment for the patient with NSCLC is the correct staging of the disease. Staging of lung cancer is based on the TNM (tumor, node, metastases) classification of the American Joint Committee on Cancer (Table 1). All patients with NSCLC should undergo clinical diagnostic staging. Depending on the clinical stage, NSCLC patients who are believed to have surgically resectable disease should undergo pathologic staging, which is based on the histologic examination of tissue specimens obtained at surgery.

The clinical staging evaluation of a patient with NSCLC consists of a complete history and physical examination, complete blood count, blood chemistry studies, chest roentgenogram, and computed tomographic (CT) scans of the chest and abdomen. The CT scan is used to demonstrate evidence of liver and adrenal metastases. The use of magnetic resonance imaging is not routine for the evaluation of NSCLC. Bone, brain, and gallium scans are not ordinarily indicated in asymptomatic NSCLC patients.

Because surgery offers the patient with NSCLC the best hope of cure, it is necessary to perform certain invasive procedures to determine the resectability of a tumor by evaluating the mediastinal lymph nodes. These procedures include bronchoscopy with transbronchial needle aspiration or biopsy or both, mediastinoscopy, and sometimes limited thoracotomy. In general, patients with T4, N3, or M1 lesions (Stages IIIB and IV) have cancer that is nonresectable.

Studies of cardiac and pulmonary function are indicated if an NSCLC patient is considered a surgical candidate, especially for a pneumonectomy. A patient with a 1-second forced expiratory volume of less than 2.0 liters and a diffusing capacity of the lung for carbon monoxide of less than 60% are poor candidates for a pneumonectomy. Poor pulmonary function studies may not preclude surgery, but it may limit the type of resection that a patient can undergo.

An important part of the NSCLC patient's pretreatment evaluation is the assessment of the performance status. Not only is it of value for patients with localized disease who are being considered for surgery, but it is also an important prognostic factor for patients with advanced disease receiving chemotherapy. This prognostic factor is important in predicting the likelihood of a response or toxicity to therapy as well as duration of survival.

The Eastern Cooperative Oncology Group performance status (PS) scale is commonly used and is as follows: Patients with a PS score of 0 are asymptomatic; those with a PS score of 1 are symptomatic but fully ambulatory; those with a PS score of 2 have restricted activities but are out of bed more than 50% of the day; those with a PS score of 3 are bedridden more than 50% of the day; and those with a PS score of 4 are totally bedridden. Patients with a good performance sta-

TABLE 1. **Staging of Lung Cancer**

Definition of TNM

Primary Tumor (T)

TX	Primary tumor cannot be assessed, or tumor is proven by the presence of malignant cells in sputum or bronchial washings but not visualized by imaging or bronchoscopy
T0	No evidence of primary tumor
Tis	Carcinoma in situ
T1	Tumor 3 cm or less in greatest dimension, surrounded by lung or visceral pleura, without bronchoscopic evidence of invasion more proximal than the lobar bronchus (i.e., not in the main bronchus)
T2	Tumor with any of the following features of size or extent:
	More than 3 cm in greatest dimension
	Involves main bronchus, 2 cm or more distal to the carina
	Invades the visceral pleura
	Associated with atelectasis or obstructive pneumonitis that extends to the hilar region but does not involve the entire lung
T3	Tumor of any size that directly invades any of the following: chest wall (including superior sulcus tumors), diaphragm, mediastinal pleura, and parietal pericardium; or tumor in the main bronchus less than 2 cm distal to the carina but without involvement of the carina; or associated atelectasis or obstructive pneumonitis of the entire lung
T4	Tumor of any size that invades any of the following: mediastinum, heart, great vessels, trachea, esophagus, vertebral body, and carina; or tumor with a malignant pleural effusion

Regional Lymph Nodes (N)

NX	Regional lymph nodes cannot be assessed
N0	No regional lymph node metastasis
N1	Metastasis in ipsilateral hilar lymph nodes, including direct extension
N2	Metastasis in ipsilateral mediastinal or subcranial lymph node or nodes
N3	Metastasis in contralateral mediastinal, contralateral hilar, ipsilateral or contralateral scalene, or supraclavicular lymph node or nodes

Distant Metastases (M)

MX	Presence of distant metastasis cannot be assessed
M0	No distant metastasis
M1	Distant metastasis

Stage Grouping

Occult Carcinoma	TX	N0	M0
Stage 0	Tis	N0	M0
Stage I	T1	N0	M0
	T2	N0	M0
Stage II	T1	N1	M0
	T2	N1	M0
Stage IIIA	T1	N2	M0
	T2	N2	M0
	T3	N0, N1, N2	M0
Stage IIIB	Any T	N3	M0
	T4	Any N	M0
Stage IV	Any T	Any N	M1

Adapted from Definition of TNM and stage grouping. *In* American Joint Committee on Cancer's Manual for Staging of Cancer, 4th ed. Philadelphia, JB Lippincott, 1992, p 115.

tus (PS scores of 0 and 1) live longer and respond to and tolerate chemotherapy better than do patients with a poor performance status (PS scores of 3 and 4).

Surgery

The type of surgical resection used to treat a patient with lung cancer is determined by the pretreatment evaluation. The most common surgical procedures include wedge resection, segmentectomy, lobectomy, and pneumonectomy. Which type of surgical resection that is ultimately performed depends on the location of the tumor and the stage.

Wedge resection is used when a lesion is located peripherally and is less than 2 cm in diameter and there is no lymph node involvement (T1, N0, M0). The segmentectomy may be indicated for patients with lesions larger than 2 cm in diameter who have no lymph node involvement but cannot undergo a lobectomy because of poor pulmonary function. A lobectomy is performed in patients who have lung cancer with or without metastases to the lobar lymph nodes (T1, N0, M0; T2, N0, M0; T1, N1, M0; T2, N1, M0) in which an en bloc resection can be accomplished. A pneumonectomy is reserved for all other patients who have resectable disease (T2, N1, M0; T3, N0, M0; T3, N1, M0; any T, N2, M0). Chest wall involvement with cancer (T3, N0, M0) by itself may not preclude surgery. However, patients with clinical N2 disease do not in general benefit from surgery. The treatment of these patients with a combined-modality approach that includes surgery is being studied.

In general, 5-year survival rates correlate with the patient's stage of disease. Based on postsurgical staging, examples of 5-year survival rates are as follows: 69% for T1, N0, M0; 59% for T2, N0, M0; 54% for T1, N1, M0; 40% for T2, N1, M0; 44% for T3, N0, M0; 18% for T3, N1, M0; and 29% for any T, N2, M0. Patients with epidermoid carcinoma have a better survival rate than patients with adenocarcinoma and large cell carcinoma. Among patients undergoing surgical resection of lung cancer, the operative mortality rate is less than 5%.

Radiation Therapy

The administration of radiation therapy in the treatment of NSCLC has been termed either "definitive" or "palliative." Definitive radiation therapy—that is, therapy with curative intent—is reserved for patients with resectable lung cancer who for medical reasons are not candidates for surgery. The 5-year survival rate among these patients is approximately 20%. In patients with surgically inoperable lung cancer who receive definitive radiation therapy, the median duration of survival is less than 1 year; fewer than 10% of these patients survive for 5 years. High doses of radiation therapy (6000 cGy or more) are used for definitive therapy. However, such doses are associated with increased toxicity in comparison with the administration of lower doses of radiation therapy. The radiation therapy can be administered continuously until completion of the therapy or by a so-called split course, whereby patients are treated for 2 weeks, then given a 2-week break, and then treated for an additional 2 weeks. The former course of therapy is favored because it yields a higher local control rate.

Palliative radiation therapy is indicated for relief of symptoms caused by either the primary tumor or the metastases. Usually, lower doses of radiation therapy (i.e., 3000 cGy) are used.

Recent studies suggest that hyperfractionated radiation therapy (twice-a-day radiation therapy) may be better than standard radiation therapy. Studies evaluating this technique are ongoing.

Radiation therapy has been used in patients who have undergone surgical resection of the disease but are at high risk for local recurrence or metastases (Stages II and IIIA). Unfortunately, postoperative radiation therapy has not produced any survival benefits.

Chemotherapy

Most patients with NSCLC have inoperable disease at the time of presentation, and relapse occurs in the majority of patients who have undergone resection and patients who have not but have been treated with radiation therapy. Thus there is a potential role for effective chemotherapy in the treatment of NSCLC.

A number of drugs have produced responses in patients with NSCLC either as single agents or, more commonly, as part of combination chemotherapeutic regimens. More than 50 chemotherapeutic agents have been evaluated in phase II studies for the treatment of NSCLC. Of these agents, mitomycin (Mutamycin), cisplatin (Platinol), ifosfamide (Ifex), vinblastine (Velban), vindesine* (Eldisine), and etoposide (VePesid) have produced responses of 15% or greater in previously untreated NSCLC patients. Promising new agents include taxol, CPT-11,† navelbine,† and edatrexate.† Four of the commonly used chemotherapeutic regimens used to treat NSCLC are listed in Table 2.

---

*Investigational drug in the United States.
†Not commercially available in the United States.

TABLE 2. **Commonly Used Chemotherapeutic Regimens in the Treatment of Non–Small Cell Lung Cancer**

EP	
Etoposide (VePesid)	120 mg/m² IV, days 1, 2, and 3
Cisplatin (Platinol)	60 mg/m² IV, day 1
Repeat cycle every 3 weeks	
VP	
Vinblastine (Velban)	5 mg/m² IV a week for 5 weeks, then q 2 weeks
Cisplatin (Platinol)	120 mg/m² IV, day 1, q 4 weeks
EcP	
Etoposide (VePesid)	120 mg/m² IV, days 1, 2, and 3
Carboplatin (Paraplatin)	100 mg/m² IV, days 1, 2, and 3
Repeat cycle every 4 weeks	
MVP	
Mitomycin (Mutamycin)	8 mg/m² IV, days 1, 29, and 71
Vinblastine (Velban)	4.5 mg/m² IV, day 1; 2 mg/m² IV, day 8; 4.5 mg/m², days 15, 22, and 29 and q 2 weeks thereafter
Cisplatin (Platinol)	120 mg/m² days 1 and 29 and q 6 weeks thereafter

Abbreviations: EP, etoposide-cisplatin; VP, vinblastine-cisplatin; EcP, etoposide-carboplatin-cisplatin; MVP, mitomycin-vinblastine-cisplatin; IV, intravenously.

In general, objective tumor response to chemotherapy given to patients with NSCLC is associated with prolonged survival, in comparison with patients who show tumor progression after the administration of chemotherapy. However, the effect of chemotherapy on the quality or duration of survival in patients with NSCLC remains to be firmly established.

To fully evaluate the impact of chemotherapy on survival in patients with NSCLC, four factors should be considered. First, responses to chemotherapy in patients with NSCLC are usually partial responses and often are of limited duration (i.e., 2 to 6 months). Because these responses occur in fewer than 50% of patients, median duration of survival of the entire treatment group is not likely to be affected to a statistically significant degree by chemotherapy. However, a trend toward increased duration of survival among patients receiving chemotherapy as initial therapy has been observed. The administration of two to three cycles of chemotherapy is usually required in order to assess whether there is any antitumor response. Second, the rate of response to many chemotherapeutic regimens (20 to 25%) is similar to the percentage of patients who experience severe toxicity; therefore, although some patients benefit from therapy, this benefit may be offset by toxicity experienced by other patients. Third, patients with favorable prognostic factors, such as good performance status at initiation of treatment, tend to respond more favorably to chemotherapeutic regimens. There clearly appears to be a survival advantage for responders to chemotherapy over nonresponders. In addition, patients who are symptomatic because of NSCLC and who respond to chemotherapy may experience improvement in symptoms. Fourth, a consideration that often is not sufficiently emphasized is the psychological benefit that a patient may experience from receiving chemotherapy. This benefit may be very important for the patient's emotional well-being even though duration of survival may be only minimally prolonged.

To identify new active agents and to discover new combination chemotherapeutic regimens in the treatment of NSCLC that will produce higher remission rates and will have a significant impact on survival, further studies clearly are needed. But until this happens, both the physician and the patient must weigh the risks and benefits of chemotherapy available for the treatment of NSCLC (Table 3).

Combined-modality Therapy

The high local and distant metastatic recurrence rates associated with surgery and radiation therapy in NSCLC have led to use of combined-modality therapy. In general, adjuvant chemotherapy has been unsuccessful in prolonging survival in patients who have undergone surgical resection of lung cancer. At the present time, a national randomized adjuvant study is comparing radiation therapy with the concomitant use of chemotherapy and radiation therapy in NSCLC patients with Stages II and IIIA disease who have undergone surgical resection of the disease.

The standard treatment for patients with locally advanced NSCLC (Stages IIIA and IIIB) remains radiation therapy. However, the results of studies involving neoadjuvant chemotherapy followed by surgery or radiation therapy are encouraging, but this regimen cannot be recommended for standard use. These studies tend to report

TABLE 3. **Benefits and Risks of Chemotherapy for Metastatic Non–Small Cell Lung Cancer**

Benefits
Objective tumor response
Decrease in symptoms
Improved survival
Psychological
Risks
Toxicity associated with therapy
Treatment-related deaths
Costs and inconvenience of treatment
Increase in hospitalization time

Adapted from Simes RJ: Risk-benefit relationships in cancer clinical trials: The ECOG experience in non–small cell lung cancer. J Clin Oncol 3:462–472, 1985.

increases in antitumor response, median survival rates, and long-term survival in comparison with studies on the use of surgery and or radiation therapy alone.

An example of the former studies is a Cancer and Acute Leukemia Group B study, in which NSCLC patients (Stages IIIA and IIIB) were randomly chosen to receive radiation therapy (6000 cGy over 6 weeks) versus the administration of two cycles of chemotherapy (vinblastine and cisplatin) before the same radiation therapy. Among patients receiving the combined-modality therapy, there was an increase in the response rate (56% vs. 43%) and a significant increase in median survival (13.8 months vs. 9.7 months) in comparison with patients receiving the radiation therapy alone. However, more important was the increase in number of patients alive 1, 2, and 3 years among those who received the combined-modality therapy as opposed to those who received the radiation alone (55% vs. 40% at 1 year, 26% vs. 13% at 2 years, and 23% vs. 11% at 3 years).

SMALL CELL LUNG CANCER

SCLC is biologically and clinically different from NSCLC. Patients with SCLC usually have symptoms and signs for a short period of time before presentation because of the rapid growth of the tumor. SCLC is associated with a variety of neuroendocrine markers such as L-dopa decarboxylase, bombesin (gastric releasing peptide), and neuron-specific enolase. In addition, several paraneoplastic syndromes are found in SCLC patients and not in NSCLC patients. They include the syndrome of inappropriate secretion of antidiuretic hormone, Cushing's syndrome, and myasthenic (Eaton-Lambert) syndrome.

SCLC tumors are more sensitive to chemotherapy and radiation therapy than are NSCLC tumors. It has been recognized that mixed tumors may be more prevalent in SCLC patients than once thought. Although mixed small cell/large cell tumors are most common, other mixed tumors (e.g., small cell carcinoma/adenocarcinoma, small cell/epidermoid carcinoma) have been identified. These tumors may have to be clinically treated differently.

Pretreatment Evaluation

SCLC is usually divided into limited and extensive stages. Limited disease is defined as disease confined to one hemothorax with regional lymph node metastases, supraclavicular lymph node metastases, ipsilateral pleural effusions, or a combination of these (Stages I to III of the TNM staging classification). Usually the disease can be encompassed in a single radiation therapy port. Some investigators do not consider supraclavicular lymph node involvement and pleural effusion limited disease. Extensive disease is defined as disease that is not considered limited disease (Stage IV).

The pretreatment evaluation of a patient with SCLC is designed to determine whether the patient has limited or extensive disease. After it is established that the pathologic diagnosis is correct, the work-up for staging should include complete history and physical examination; complete blood cell count; CT scans of the chest, abdomen, and brain; bone scan; bone marrow aspiration; and biopsy. Because of the high incidence of distant metastases in SCLC patients, the CT and bone scans, bone marrow aspiration; and biopsy are warranted.

With the appropriate staging, 35 to 40% of all patients with SCLC are found to have limited disease, and 60 to 65% are found to have extensive disease. Which therapy is used to treat the patient with SCLC depends on the stage.

Chemotherapy

More than 10 drugs are active as single agents in the treatment of SCLC. The most commonly used are cyclophosphamide (Cytoxan), doxorubicin (Adriamycin), vincristine (Oncovin), etoposide (VePesid), and cisplatin (Platinol). Other agents used to treat SCLC are ifosfamide (Ifex) and carboplatin (Paraplatin). With so many active drugs and because combination chemotherapy has been found to be more effective than single agents, many different effective combination chemotherapeutic regimens have been developed to treat SCLC. Four of the commonly used induction chemotherapeutic regimens are listed in Table 4. The etoposide-cisplatin (EP) regimen for the treatment of SCLC patients appears to be the choice of most medical oncologists. Small cell lung cancer patients who are initially treated with CAV and in whom the disease becomes refractory to treatment can respond to EP, whereas the reverse is not true.

A major cause of the failure of effective combination chemotherapy to produce long-term remissions in patients with SCLC is the emergence of tumor cells resistant to the agents used in the various chemotherapeutic regimens. To overcome the development of drug-resistant cells, two alternating, equally active non–cross-resistant chemotherapeutic regimens as treatment for SCLC have been used. The National Cancer Institute of Canada, in a randomized trial involving SCLC patients with extensive disease demonstrated

TABLE 4. Commonly Used Chemotherapeutic Regimens in the Treatment of Small Cell Lung Cancer

CAV*	
Cyclophosphamide (Cytoxan)	1000 mg/m^2 IV, day 1
Doxorubicin (Adriamycin)	50 mg/m^2 IV, day 1
Vincristine (Oncovin)	1.4 mg/m^2 IV, day 1
Repeat cycle every 3 weeks	(maximal dose, 2.0 mg)
CAE	
Cyclophosphamide (Cytoxan)	1000 mg/m^2 IV, day 1
Doxorubicin (Adriamycin)	45 mg/m^2 IV, day 1
Etoposide (VePesid)	50 mg/m^2 days 1–5
Repeat cycle every 3 weeks	
EP†	
Etoposide (VePesid)	120 mg/m^2‡ IV, days 1–3§
Cisplatin (Platinol)	60 mg/m^2 IV, day 1
Repeat cycle every 3 weeks	
EcP	
Etoposide (VePesid)	120 mg/m^2‡ IV, days 1–3
Carboplatin (Paraplatin)	100 mg/m^2 IV, days 1–3
Repeat cycle every 4 weeks	

Abbreviations: CAV, cyclophosphamide-doxorubicin-vincristine; CAE, cyclophosphamide-doxorubicin-etoposide; EP, etoposide-cisplatin; EcP, etoposide-carboplatin-cisplatin; IV, intravenous.

*CAV alternating with EP may be used in patients with extensive disease.

†Thoracic radiation therapy may be used concurrently with EP in selected patients with limited disease.

‡Exceeds dosage recommended by the manufacturer.

§Etoposide can be given 240 mg/m^2 PO on days 2 and 3.

that CAV alternating with EP produced a higher response rate than did CAV alone, and overall survival time was statistically significant in favor of the alternating regimen. Unfortunately, however, the results of randomized studies have been conflicting.

Patients who are elderly ($\geq$70 years) or are medically unfit for aggressive therapy may benefit from single-agent therapy with etoposide, 240 mg/M^2 orally or 125 mg/M^2 intravenously on days 1 to 3 every 3 weeks, or carboplatin, 300 to 400 mg/M^2 intravenously on day 1 every 4 weeks.

What should be the duration of chemotherapy in the treatment of SCLC? Several studies have demonstrated that maintenance chemotherapy may only enhance toxicity and not increase survival rates among patients with SCLC. At the present time, the administration of six cycles of combination chemotherapy is the accepted standard in treating SCLC patients.

How intense should the chemotherapy be? The consensus is that the chemotherapy should be relatively intense; however, reported randomized studies comparing intensive to nonintensive therapy with the same drug combinations do not demonstrate an improvement in survival times when therapy has been intensive.

In general, SCLC patients with extensive disease who are treated with chemotherapy (1) have an approximately 20% chance that the disease will completely disappear clinically, (2) have a median length of survival of 10 months, and (3) are, unfortunately, dead within 2 years.

Radiation Therapy

In the early 1970s, radiation therapy was the predominant treatment for SCLC. With the development of effective combination chemotherapy to treat SCLC and the recognition that the disease disseminates early, chemotherapy, along with radiation, was given to SCLC patients as therapy.

In the early trials comparing radiotherapy plus chemotherapy with radiation therapy alone, the combined-modality therapy was superior in regard to lung relapses, response rates, and median survival times (3 to 6 months for radiation therapy alone, 9 to 12 months for radiation therapy plus chemotherapy).

Comparisons of combined-modality therapy with chemotherapy alone demonstrated similar response rates and median survival times, whereas 2-year survival rates were higher in SCLC patients with limited disease who were treated with the combined-modality therapy (17% vs. 7%). This difference was not seen in SCLC patients with extensive disease.

In combined-modality approaches (i.e., chemotherapy and radiation therapy) used in the treatment of SCLC, thoracic radiotherapy is given in one of three ways: sequential, alternating, or concurrent. The concurrent administration of thoracic radiation therapy and chemotherapy with the EP regimen is the preferred treatment for patients with limited-disease SCLC. The radiation dose used for local control of SCLC is 4500 cGy in 180-cGy fractions. If research indicates that multiple-dose fractionated thoracic radiation therapy is superior to standard thoracic radiation therapy in the treatment of limited-disease SCLC, it should replace the thoracic radiation therapy recommended earlier.

The role of radiotherapy in extensive disease SCLC is somewhat controversial. When it is used with chemotherapy to treat extensive disease SCLC, there may be a reduction in local chest failures; however, the overall response rates, median survival rates, and 2-year survival rates are essentially the same as those achieved with chemotherapy alone. The use of radiotherapy may be of value in patients with extensive-disease SCLC for palliation of symptoms, especially for brain metastases and superior vena cava (SVC) syndrome. A frequently used palliative radiotherapy dose schedule has been 3000 cGy in 10 fractions over 2 weeks. However, for the SVC syndrome, large daily doses such as 400 cGy are delivered in 3 days. With relief of symptoms, treatment of the SCLC patient can proceed with chemotherapy or by continuing thoracic radiation therapy with reduced daily fractions to 180 cGy and continuing treatment until the appropriate total dose is reached.

As the therapy for SCLC improves and the patients live longer, the chance that brain metastases will develop increases. Prophylactic cranial irradiation (PCI) in SCLC patients does reduce the chance for central nervous system relapse, however, with no improvement in survival rates. Moreover, it has become apparent that many patients who have received PCI and are long-term survivors suffer a variety of neuropsychiatric disorders. Because of this toxicity, many questions have been raised regarding the selection of appropriate SCLC patients to receive PCI.

Surgery

There has been renewed interest in defining the role of surgery as part of a combined-modality treatment approach in the treatment of limited-disease SCLC. At the present time, for Stage I disease, surgical resection of SCLC is justified when a thoracotomy is required to establish a tissue diagnosis. Well-staged patients with a small peripheral nodule and with a preoperative diagnosis of SCLC may also be candidates for surgical resection of the primary tumor. After the surgery, adjuvant chemotherapy should be administered for at least six cycles with or without thoracic radiation therapy. In other SCLC patients with Stage I or Stage II disease in whom surgical resection is being considered in combined-modality therapy programs, at least four cycles of chemotherapy should be given initially, followed by surgery in patients who responded to the chemotherapy. These patients should also receive thoracic radiation therapy.

In patients undergoing surgery after the administration of chemotherapy, as many as 20% of resected specimens may contain NSCLC or mixed SCLC/NSCLC. The best treatment for patients whose resected specimens contain NSCLC may, in fact, be the surgical resection.

At the present time, surgical resection for Stage III SCLC does not appear to be indicated.

COCCIDIOIDOMYCOSIS

method of
ANTONINO CATANZARO, M.D.
*University of California, San Diego, Medical
Center
San Diego, California*

Coccidioidomycosis is an infection that is acquired by the inhalation of the arthrospores of the fungus *Coccidioides immitis,* which are found in the soil of the southwestern United States and northern Mexico, as well as certain parts of Central and South America.

DIAGNOSIS

The immune response to *C. immitis* can be useful both in helping to make the diagnosis and in providing clues as to the extent of disease and the likelihood of a favorable response to therapy.

The delayed-type hypersensitivity (DTH) response to antigens (coccidioidin [CDN] and spherulin [SPN]) from the mycelial and spherule phases of *C. immitis* cells is an excellent stage to start. At the 1:100 dilution, both antigens are specific; at the 1:10 dilution, there is some cross-reaction with histoplasmosis. The issue about sensitivity is confounded by the fact that T cell dysfunction is a frequent concomitant of coccidioidomycosis, particularly in patients with severe disease. A positive skin test, particularly a conversion from negative to positive, is important information. However, a negative skin test is not conclusive, because many patients with multifocal coccidioidomycosis or with coccidioidomycosis in the presence of human immunodeficiency virus (HIV) infection have negative skin tests.

The serologic response is even more useful because it is almost always positive in patients with significant disease. The precipitin test (immunoglobulin M [IgM]) is positive early and stays positive for a few months. The complement fixation (CF) titer may take 3 to 4 months to reach its peak. The CF titer is also nearly always positive in patients with significant disease, and in general, the higher the titer, the stronger the indication for treatment. The converse is not always true: Patients with low titers, particularly those with miliary disease, may also be desperately sick.

Because the organism usually enters the body through the lungs, a chest roentgenogram is critical for determining the extent to which the infection has been localized. Dissemination beyond the pulmonary system can be determined by careful examination, concentrating on the skin, soft tissues, bones and joints, and the cerebrospinal fluid (CSF).

INDICATIONS FOR THERAPY

Primary Coccidioidomycosis. The initial response to *C. immitis* generally consists of symptoms such as cough, sore throat, headache, and fever. There is often a hyperemic rash. A pulmonary infiltrate, often with hilar adenopathy, may be found on the chest roentgenogram. This syndrome is usually self-limited and does not necessitate antifungal therapy. Unfortunately, in a few affected patients, progressive pulmonary or disseminated disease develops, and so management of these patients includes careful monitoring of clinical parameters to identify those who need antifungal treatment.

Persistent or Progressive Pulmonary Coccidioidomycosis. Choosing the patients in this group who need antifungal therapy can be challenging. Clinical findings are important; these include fever, weight loss, fatigue, cough, hemoptysis and weakness, the presence of DTH, and the amount of complement-fixing antibody to CDN, and of course the amount and type of changes noted on the chest roentgenogram. In patients who have undergone a period of observation, it is often possible to determine whether the infection is diminishing, is being focalized, or is progressing. Depending on the extent or amount of pulmonary tissue involved, the latter two situations may necessitate antifungal treatment. The author has used the period of 6 weeks as a cutoff for defining persistent pulmonary coccidioidomycosis. However, 3 months is a more conservative definition. The presence of pulmonary cavities or nodules, in general, does not influence the author's decision regarding antifungal therapy, inasmuch as these manifestations tend to follow their course regardless of antifungal therapy. The exception is the setting of dense consolidation around an enlarging cavity close to the pleura.

Disseminated Coccidioidomycosis. All patients with extrapulmonary active coccidioidomycosis must be treated with an antifungal medication. Such patients include those with miliary disease, as this presentation indicates widespread blood-borne disease, and even if no focus of infection is identified outside the lungs, it can be assumed that the capillary beds that cannot be visualized look as bad as the pulmonary capillary bed, which can be seen on the chest roentgenogram.

Coccidioidal Meningitis. This form of the infection is nearly always fatal without treatment. Despite the severity of this manifestation, symptoms can be unimpressive at the outset. In severe or multifocal cases, it is prudent to sample the CSF to be certain about the presence or absence of meningitis.

ANTIFUNGAL THERAPY

Amphotericin B. Amphotericin B (Fungizone) is the time-honored therapy for coccidioidomycosis. It is often called the gold standard of treatment; that statement comes from the fact that before amphotericin B was available, there was no effective therapy for cocci. Furthermore, for 20 years there was no alternative. As alternatives have become available, they have been compared with the established treatment, or gold standard. At this time, there are several antifungal therapies to consider. To date, none has been compared directly with another.

Amphotericin B is not absorbed from the gastrointestinal tract. Furthermore, its distribution into various fluids or tissues is not good. For this reason, it is administered intravenously, and when tissue penetration is needed, clinicians have often devised methods to administer it directly into a space (e.g., into CSF in meningitis, into a joint space in synovitis, and into the bone in osteomyelitis).

Administration. Intelligent use of this agent is imperative in order to minimize toxicity. Because of solubility problems, amphotericin B must be administered in 5% dextrose. The volume depends on the dose, site of administration, and the anticipated rate of infusion.

INTRAVENOUS INFUSION

If the infusion is being administered to an inpatient, the rate of infusion is not important. However, in an outpatient, a rapid infusion is important to the execution of the program. The author has found that an infusion over 45 minutes is well tolerated; that is, it is tolerated at least as well as an infusion over 4 hours. The author usually adds 1000 units of heparin to the intravenous solution to minimize the tendency for thrombophlebitis to develop at the site of infusion. Premedication helps to forestall general reactions of chills, fever, tremor, nausea, vomiting, and hypotension. The author usually administers by mouth an antipyretic such as aspirin or acetaminophen (Tylenol), an antihistamine such as diphenhydramine hydrochloride (Benadryl), and an antiemetic such as prochlorperazine (Compazine) or chlorpromazine (Thorazine). Renal effects include both glomerular and tubular toxicities. Tubular effects include wasting of potassium chloride and bicarbonate. Adverse consequences can be prevented by replacing these losses before the serum levels are depleted. The author always gives potassium chloride, 40 to 100 mEq per day starting with the first day of treatment, and monitors electrolytes carefully. Glomerular effects are more difficult to control, but maintaining more than adequate hydration is helpful. Finally, hydrocortisone, up to 50 mg, can be added to the intravenous solution to diminish the acute effects of intravenous amphotericin B. Doses of amphotericin B should be administered daily, starting with 1 mg and increasing to 5 mg, 15 to 20 mg, 25 to 35 mg, and 40 to 50 mg. The author tries not to exceed 50 mg per day in all but the biggest patients. Usually follow-up doses are administered daily until the patient is well enough to be treated at home. Then dosing is cut back to Mondays, Wednesdays, and Fridays. That dosing schedule is continued until the author believes that the disease is under control. At that point, dosing drops back to twice a week or, in some patients, once a week. The author aims for 1 gram total in mild cases of pulmonary disease or 3 grams total in severe cases of pulmonary or disseminated disease.

LOCAL INJECTION

Meningitis. Amphotericin B crosses the blood-brain barrier poorly and in quantities insufficient for the treatment of coccidioidal meningitis.* The drug may be administered directly by the following methods:

1. Percutaneous injection into the lumbar space. Amphotericin B injection into this space nearly always results in chemical arachnoiditis. When amphotericin B is administered in a hyperbaric solution, it can cause transverse myelitis.

2. Percutaneous injection into the cisterna magna. This can be accomplished by a midline or lateral cervical injection. This is the best way to get the drug where it is needed, but it can be dangerous, particularly if not done by a carefully trained physician.

3. Catheter delivery. Because of the pain and hazard associated with the percutaneous injections, several catheter systems have been devised: (1) In the Ommaya reservoir, a catheter is placed into the lateral ventricle with a small bladder just under the skin. Administration of amphotericin B into the bladder is easy. However, the diffusion of amphotericin B to the basilar meninges is not very good, particularly if circulation of the CSF out of the lateral ventricle is obstructed. (2) The ventriculoperitoneal shunt is often fitted with a bladder similar to the Ommaya reservoir. However, delivery of drug is even more difficult in patients with a shunt in place, because the obstruction is worse than in other patients, and the drug may actually be carried away to the peritoneal space when the shunt is opened. (3)

---

*This use of amphotericin B is not listed in the manufacturer's official directive.

The cisternal catheter is placed into the cisternal space, overcoming the objections listed earlier. Movement of the head on the spine is a challenge to this kind of hardware. The experience with this method, although limited, has been good. All catheters carry a risk of infection, particularly with *Staphylococcus epidermidis* and *Candida* spp.

4. Solution: intrathecal, 1 to 2 mL of 5% dextrose in water (10% in the case of hypertonic solution), to which has been added the following:

Amphotericin B, initial dose, 0.025 mg (with each administration, the dose is increased by 0.05 mg until a dose of 0.5 mg is reached).

Hydrocortisone, 25 mg.

The Azoles. This group of drugs includes several very strong alternatives to amphotericin B. Ketoconazole (Nizoral), of course, was the first orally absorbed azole to be demonstrated to be effective against cocci. However, its toxicity and erratic absorption relegate it to a secondary position at this time. The triazoles, fluconazole (Diflucan) and itraconazole (Sporanox), appear to be less toxic and at least as efficacious in controlling acute manifestations of cocci.

Fluconazole is currently approved by the FDA for the treatment of *Candida* and cryptococcal infections. However, studies by the National Institute of Allergy and Infectious Diseases (NIAID) Mycoses Study Group have clearly demonstrated that fluconazole is efficacious in treating coccidioidomycosis. Patients with chronic pulmonary disease (at least 3 months' duration), soft tissue disease, or bone and joint disease were treated initially with 200 mg per day. If they did not respond, the dose was increased to 400 mg per day. The mean duration of treatment was 18 months. Response rates were 58 to 90%.

Itraconazole has recently been released for the treatment of histoplasmosis and blastomycosis. However, studies by the NIAID Mycoses Study Group in patients with entrance criteria similar to those in the fluconazole study were treated with 100 to 400 mg of itraconazole per day. Of those who completed therapy, 57% achieved remission. However, the rates of drug intolerance and treatment failures were higher than with fluconazole.

There is not enough follow-up of these cases in either study to make a reliable statement about recurrence. However, this infection is marked by recurrence and exacerbations. A comparative double-blind study of fluconazole versus itraconazole is just now getting started.

Which Drug to Use? This is a tough question. To date, none of the drugs has been compared directly with another in the treatment of coccidioidomycosis. Coccidioidomycosis is such a protean disease and its course is so variable that to make comparison of these therapies by comparing the results in separate studies is not feasible. It is clear that amphotericin B, ketoconazole, fluconazole, and itraconazole are all active against *C. immitis*. The absorption, distribution, and toxicity of each compound define its use and limitations. At this time, the author believes that they rank as follows:

1. Fluconazole has a very low toxicity profile; efficacy appears to be very good. However, prolonged courses of treatment are needed.
2. Amphotericin B is considered the gold standard, but the author cannot confirm that its efficacy is greater than that of the newer drugs. However, in many patients he has confirmed its greater toxicity.
3. Ketoconazole offers the same basic action as the other azoles, but absorption is erratic and toxicity is common.
4. Itraconazole has recently been approved by the U.S. Food and Drug Administration for the treatment of blastomycosis and histoplasmosis. However, studies suggest that its efficacy is comparable with that of fluconazole for coccidioidomycosis. The author's experience with itraconazole is much more limited than that with fluconazole.

When Should Treatment Be Stopped? Coccidioidomycosis is a chronic infection. The disease is characterized by defects in T cell function. None of the antifungal agents is fungicidal. When amphotericin B was the only treatment available for coccidioidomycosis, the author thought that the role of antifungal therapy was to halt the proliferation of *C. immitis,* halt the production of factors that interfered with an effective host response, and allow the body to reconstitute the immune response and contain the fungus. At this point, it appears that the same is true of the use of the azoles. Therefore, the author recommends the use of amphotericin B or one of the azoles to halt the replication of the fungus. The drug should be maintained until

1. all evidence of active infection has disappeared; that is, no new lesions have appeared and the old lesions have cleared or have been reduced to the point that they are stable, and nonspecific signs of inflammation, such as fever, sweats, and fatigue and findings such as increased erythrocyte sedimentation rate, have disappeared.
2. complement fixation titers have diminished and stabilized; and
3. cell-mediated immunity has been reconstituted, as evidenced by delayed hypersensitivity response to coccidioidin or spherulin.

After these criteria are met, the author recommends that treatment continue a bit longer, for what might be called a consolidation period. A great deal of judgment is needed in using these criteria; they are guidelines.

HISTOPLASMOSIS

method of
LISA A. HAGLUND, M.D., and
GEORGE S. DEEPE, JR., M.D.
University of Cincinnati College of Medicine
Cincinnati, Ohio

Infection with the dimorphic fungus *Histoplasma capsulatum* is acquired by inhalation of mycelial fragments or microconidia that are deposited within terminal bronchioles and alveoli. Within days, the mycelial-phase elements transform into yeast cells. These forms spread via the lymphohematogenous route within phagocytes and invade the reticuloendothelial system. Thus most if not all cases of primary infection are disseminated. In tissues, yeast cells commonly evoke an inflammatory response that consists of caseating or noncaseating granulomas. Virtually all the clinical manifestations of histoplasmosis are caused by yeast cells.

Cases of histoplasmosis have been reported from each continent except Antarctica. In the United States, this fungal infection is endemic to the mideastern and south central regions. Variations in the prevalence of infection in these areas is most likely caused by the presence of hyperendemic foci. Point sources for infection include caves, chicken houses, bird roots, attics, and old buildings. Epidemics have been associated with mechanical disruption of infested areas by bulldozers or with renovation of old buildings.

Infection with *H. capsulatum* produces three distinct illnesses: acute pulmonary histoplasmosis (APH), chronic pulmonary histoplasmosis (CPH), and progressive disseminated histoplasmosis (PDH). APH often produces an influenza-like illness, but in some cases it is clinically inapparent. Severity of illness can be correlated directly with inoculum size. Each inhaled particle induces a small patch of bronchopneumonia. The primary lesions encapsulate, become necrotic in the center, and subsequently calcify.

CPH develops predominantly in older persons with structural lung damage such as obstructive lung disease. This form of histoplasmosis is characterized by weight loss, cough with abundant sputum production, and occasionally fever and hemoptysis. It is believed that the yeast-phase organisms proliferate in bullae and slowly induce additional destruction of the lung parenchyma. In some cases, *H. capsulatum* may spread via bronchi to the opposite lung.

In PDH, there is widespread involvement of the mononuclear phagocyte system by yeast cells. Two forms of PDH exist: The acute form is associated with high fever, weight loss, hepatosplenomegaly, pancytopenia, and coagulation disturbances. The chronic form is characterized by low-grade fever, hepatosplenomegaly, and mucocutaneous ulcers.

Both serologic tests and fungal cultures are useful in establishing the diagnosis of histoplasmosis. A complement fixation (CF) titer of 1:8 is considered positive, and a titer of 1:32 is strongly suggestive of active disease. A fourfold rise in CF titers over 4 to 6 weeks is indicative of active histoplasmosis. The immunodiffusion test is less sensitive than the CF test. The presence of an H precipitin band indicates active disease, whereas an M band signifies past or recent infection. Both may be present in acute disease.

In immunosuppressed patients, serologic tests may be of limited value. Histopathologic examination of tissues, particularly bone marrow or liver, is a useful adjunct. Tissues should be silver-stained in order to visualize yeasts. Culture of sputum and any tissue should be performed. The lysis-centrifugation blood culture system can detect *H. capsulatum* in patients with PDH in 1 to 2 weeks; this is better than other blood culture systems, which do not become positive for 3 to 6 weeks. There is an antigen detection system that is performed only in the laboratory of Dr. L. J. Wheat, Indiana University School of Medicine. It is especially useful in identification of patients with PDH and can be employed to follow the success of therapy (including human immunodeficiency virus [HIV]–infected patients).

TREATMENT OF ACUTE PULMONARY HISTOPLASMOSIS

Because APH is usually a self-limited illness, antifungal therapy is not required for most patients. Bed rest, antipyretics, and cough suppressants are effective for the influenza-like symptoms. Nevertheless, a few patients experience a prolonged illness (>3 weeks) that consists of fever, weight loss, chest pain, and cough. In these patients, antifungal therapy can hasten resolution of disease. Amphotericin B (Fungizone) should be given intravenously in a dosage of 50 mg per day or every other day, to a total dose of 500 mg to 1 gm, until the patient is well. Alternatively, this drug can be given until the patient is asymptomatic for 7 to 10 days. In children, 0.25 mg per kg of body weight of amphotericin B is given on the first day, followed by 0.5 mg per kg on day 2 and 1 mg per kg thereafter. Ketoconazole (Nizoral) may be administered at a dose of 400 mg per day for 3 to 6 months. However, resolution of illness is much more rapid with amphotericin B than with ketoconazole. There is little experience in treating the disease with the other azoles.

Certain sequelae may follow acute histoplasmosis. Examples include pericariditis, fibrosing mediastinitis, lymphadenitis, and arthritis. Pericarditis may be manifest approximately 6 weeks after acute exposure to *H. capsulatum*. Yeast cells rarely are detected in pericardium or pericardial fluid. This illness is treated with anti-inflammatory agents such as salicylates or nonsteroidal drugs. In uncommon instances, the severity of illness necessitates the use of corticosteroids. There is no role for antifungal treatment. If cardiac tamponade develops, pericardiocentesis is necessary. Pericardiectomy is indicated for constrictive pericarditis.

Fibrosing mediastinitis is a progressive illness that probably arises from an exuberant host response to the fungus. Proliferation of fibrous tissue leads to constriction of vital structures, including bronchi, the superior vena cava, and the pulmonary arteries. Optimal therapy for this disorder has not been determined. Amphotericin B, surgery, or corticosteroids or combinations thereof have been used but with disappointing results.

TREATMENT OF CHRONIC PULMONARY HISTOPLASMOSIS

Treatment of patients with cavitary lung disease or CPH should be instituted when there are thick-walled cavities, enlarging pneumonic lesions, progressive decline in pulmonary function, or persistent fever and weight loss. Ketoconazole, 400 mg once daily for at least 6 months, is curative in a high proportion of patients; in rare cases, higher doses of ketoconazole may be necessary. There is a paucity of clinical information on fluconazole or itraconazole, although it is likely that both would be efficacious. If disease progresses during oral therapy or if the patient is immunocompromised, amphotericin B should be substituted. The total amount of amphotericin B given should be 30 to 35 mg per kg of body weight. Surgical resection of involved lung tissue should be considered in patients with massive hemoptysis or in those who fail to respond to medical therapy.

TREATMENT OF PROGRESSIVE DISSEMINATED HISTOPLASMOSIS

PDH is fatal in more than 80% of untreated patients. Risk factors for the development of PDH are immunosuppressive drug treatment, lymphoreticular malignancy, infection with HIV, and age. It is uncommon for persons without known pre-existing immune defects to acquire PDH. Reactivation is the most frequent cause of PDH; less commonly, overwhelming primary infection produces symptoms of PDH. In endemic areas, PDH is diagnosed in 5% of patients with acquired immune deficiency syndrome (AIDS). However, PDH has been reported from non-endemic areas such as New York City and San Francisco (see next section).

Amphotericin B remains the treatment of choice for PDH in immunocompromised patients as well as in HIV-infected patients. In patients with PDH who are not otherwise immunocompromised, administration of 400 mg per day of ketoconazole for at least 6 months is generally as efficacious as amphotericin B. Both drugs effect cure rates greater than 90%. There are few data with the other imidazoles to recommend their use at this time. If a patient cannot tolerate ketoconazole or if there is progression of disease while a patient is taking this drug, amphotericin B should be used to a total dose of 30 to 35 mg per kg of body weight.

HISTOPLASMOSIS IN HIV-INFECTED PATIENTS

In HIV-infected patients from areas endemic for histoplasmosis, development of disseminated histoplasmosis, which is most likely a reactivation of remote primary histoplasmosis infection, has been well documented. The presenting features typically include fever, weight loss, and hepatosplenomegaly, but they can also include oral ulcerations, skin lesions, pneumonia, and cytopenias. Diagnosis should be vigorously pursued with tissue or bone marrow histologic examination and culture, and blood should be cultured by use of a method that maximizes fungal yield, such as the lysis-centrifugation blood culture system. Amphotericin B is the initial treatment of choice for HIV-infected patients. Total dose of amphotericin should be at least 2 grams. In HIV-infected patients, life-long suppressive therapy is necessary because there is a potentially high rate of relapse after therapy is ceased. Amphotericin B, ketoconazole, fluconazole, and itraconazole have been used in this role. One hundred milligrams of amphotericin B per week or 40 mg twice a week may be used. This regimen requires life-long intravenous therapy. The imidazoles (see next section) have the advantage of oral administration. The problem with ketoconazole is that it is poorly absorbed in HIV-infected patients who have hypochlorhydria. Thus itraconazole, 200 mg twice daily, may be preferred empirically for suppressive therapy. Fluconazole, 200 mg per day, although not a drug of choice for histoplasmosis, may also prove useful for suppressive therapy.

ANTIFUNGAL THERAPY

Amphotericin B

Amphotericin B (Fungizone) is a polyene antibiotic for which intravenous administration is required. This drug binds to membrane sterols, especially ergosterol, and increases permeability of fungal membranes, thus leading to loss of cell constituents and lysis of cells. The drug is insoluble in many solutions, including saline, and should be diluted in 5% dextrose and water at a concentration not to exceed 0.1 mg per mL. There is no loss of bioactivity if it is exposed to light. Although some clinicians begin with a test dose of 1 mg, the authors prefer to initiate therapy with 10 mg, which is infused over 2 to 4 hours. If tolerated, the dosage is increased by 10 to 15 mg per day until a maximal dose of 0.7 mg per kg is achieved. In adults, a dose of 50 mg given three times per week is generally well tolerated. Electrolytes, renal function, and hemoglobin should be checked two to three times weekly during the first 3 weeks of therapy and then once weekly until completion of therapy.

Adverse side effects of amphotericin B include fever, chills, headache, hypotension or hypertension, anorexia, and vomiting. These symptoms are observed frequently during the first few days of therapy and tend to subside thereafter. Fever, chills, and headache may be mitigated by premedication with acetaminophen (Tylenol), 650 mg orally in adults, and diphenhydramine hydrochloride (Benadryl), 25 to 50 mg orally or parenterally, 1/2 to 1 hour before amphotericin B administration. If symptoms persist despite these measures, slowing the rate of infusion may help. Parenteral meperidine (Demerol) or dantrolene (Dantrium) also may alleviate symptoms, but these drugs should be reserved for difficult cases. In addition, premedication with 10 to 25 mg of hydrocortisone (Solu-Cortef) may be added to alleviate side effects. Amphotericin B often causes phlebitis, especially if it is infused through peripheral veins. Addition of 1000 to 2000 units of heparin to the infusion is helpful in reducing phlebitis.

Renal dysfunction is the most serious toxic effect. The glomerular filtration rate is depressed in almost everyone who receives amphotericin B. Adequate hydration and salt intake help limit nephrotoxicity. Treatment should not be stopped until the creatinine or serum urea nitrogen level exceeds 3.0 mg per dL or 50 mg per dL, respectively. When the creatinine level falls to 2.5 mg per dL, the drug may be restarted. Moreover, because only a small fraction of amphotericin is excreted by the kidneys, the dosage regimen does not have to be modified in renal failure. A high percentage of patients experience hypokalemia secondary to renal tubular damage, and thus potassium supplementation often is necessary. This is especially true in patients receiving concomitant treatment with semisynthetic penicillins such as ticarcillin (Ticar). Amphotericin B also adds to the nephrotoxicity of cyclosporine (Sandimmune). Anemia, presumably from inhibition of erythropoietin production, is another side effect of amphotericin B. Transfusion usually is not required, and the hemoglobin level returns to pretreatment levels after completion of therapy. The anemia is presumed to result from direct marrow toxicity, inhibition of erythropoietin production, or both.

Ketoconazole

Ketoconazole (Nizoral) is an imidazole that inhibits ergosterol synthesis. Its advantages are that it is less toxic than amphotericin B and is administered orally. It is efficacious in the treatment of pulmonary, localized (e.g., infection of oropharynx, bone, lymph nodes), and disseminated histoplasmosis in immunocompetent patients. Resolution of infection appears to be slower than with amphotericin B. The combination of amphotericin B and ketoconazole does not offer any advantage over therapy with a single agent.

Twenty percent of patients complain of nausea, vomiting, and anorexia as side effects of ketoconazole (Table 1). These symptoms can be reduced by taking the drug in two divided doses rather than in a single dose or by taking the drug with meals or at bedtime. The drug is well absorbed from the gastrointestinal tract, but absorption is diminished by achlorhydria and by drugs that raise gastric pH, because the compound must be converted to the hydrochloride salt before it can be absorbed. Administration of ketoconazole either before or after meals, when gastric acidity is not buffered by food, enhances absorption. Ketoconazole blocks synthesis of testosterone, and high doses of the drug can produce oligospermia, gynecomastia, loss of libido, and loss of sexual potency. In addition, this agent inhibits cortisol secretion. To date, however, permanent hypoadrenalism has been reported in only one patient. Liver enzymes are elevated transiently in approximately 10% of patients, but there is symptomatic hepatic dysfunction in fewer than 0.1%. If jaundice or marked elevation of liver enzymes develops, ketoconazole must be discontinued; otherwise, fatal hepatic necrosis may result. Other drug interactions are discussed in the next sections.

Itraconazole

Itraconazole (Sporanox) is the newest of the azole antifungal compounds and is approved for use in histoplasmosis, including chronic cavitary pulmonary disease and disseminated, nonmeningeal histoplasmosis. Like amphotericin B, it is a highly lipophilic agent with little plasma protein

TABLE 1. **Characteristics of Available Imidazole Antifungal Agents**

Characteristic	Ketoconazole (Nizoral)	Itraconazole (Sporanox)	Fluconazole (Diflucan)
Route	PO, IV	PO	PO, IV
Peak serum concentration (μg/mL)	1.7–3.6	0.1	2.5–6.7
Half-life (hours)	8	15–40	20–30
Protein bound	99%	84–99%	11%
Requires HCl for absorption	Yes	Yes	No
Increased absorption with food	Yes	Yes	No
Adverse effects	GI upset; hepatitis; oligospermia; decreased steroid levels	GI upset; hypokalemia; impotence; liver function test abnormalities	GI upset; rashes; liver function test abnormalities
Drug interactions			
Phenytoin (Dilantin)	—	Increased phenytoin level, decreased itraconazole level	Increased phenytoin level
Warfarin (Coumadin)	—	—	Increased anticoagulation
Cyclosporine (Sandimmune)	Increased cyclosporine level	Increased cyclosporine level	Increased cyclosporine level
Carbamazepine (Tegretol)	—	Decreased itraconazole level	Increased carbamazepine level
Oral hypoglycemics	Increased hypoglycemic effect	Increased hypoglycemic effect	Increased hypoglycemic effect
Digoxin	—	Increased digoxin level	—
Terfenadine (Seldane)	Increased terfenadine level	Increased terfenadine level	—
Astemizole (Hismanal)	Increased astemizole level	Increased astemizole level	—
Rifampin, isoniazid	Decreased ketoconazole level	Decreased itraconazole level	Decreased fluconazole level
100-mg oral dose cost (AWP)	—	$4.92	$6.88
200-mg oral dose cost (AWP)	$2.32	—	$11.25

Abbreviations: PO = orally; IV = intravenously; HCl = hydrochloride; GI = gastrointestinal; AWP = average wholesale price.

binding. It is metabolized entirely by the liver. It is available in 100-mg capsules for oral administration only; no intravenous form is available yet.

Itraconazole absorption is quite variable; as with ketoconazole, an acidic environment is required. Absorption is impaired in the presence of a high gastric pH. Persons susceptible to this condition include the elderly, HIV-infected patients with hypochlorhydria, patients who have undergone ulcer operations, and patients taking antacids or H_2 blockers. Itraconazole capsules must be taken along with a meal to facilitate absorption; when taken on an empty stomach, serum levels are only one third of those achieved after the same dose is taken immediately after a meal. There is no experience yet with tube feedings, but the drug is not well absorbed when given through a nasogastic tube. Diarrhea has also been observed to interfere with absorption in some patients.

Transaminase elevations that are reversible on discontinuation of itraconazole have been described. The most common adverse reactions are nausea, vomiting, and rash, accompanying dosages up to 400 mg per day. These symptoms occur less frequently with itraconazole than with ketoconazole. Itraconazole-associated impotence and decreased libido have been reported. Reversible edema has also been observed. One case of reversible adrenal insufficiency occurred with high doses (600 mg per day). No dosage adjustment is necessary in the presence of renal insufficiency, and the drug is not removed from the body by either peritoneal dialysis or hemodialysis.

Drug interactions with itraconazole are summarized in Table 1. Two important drug interactions should be emphasized. Coadministration of terfenadine (Seldane) or astemizole (Hismanal) with itraconazole is contraindicated because this may result in increased levels of terfenadine or astemizole, which induce potentially fatal cardiac arrhythmias. Coadministration of rifampin or phenytoin (Dilantin) has been observed to profoundly decrease serum itraconazole levels by increasing itraconazole metabolism, thus resulting in loss of antifungal efficacy. This effect has also been observed with coadministration with phenytoin and H_2 antagonists. However, a small study of HIV-infected persons found that the pharmacokinetics of zidovudine (AZT) were not affected during concomitant administration of itraconazole.

Itraconazole is more efficacious in PDH than in CPH; this also true of amphotericin B, probably because of local factors in the cavitary pulmonary disease that interfere with antifungal therapy. For PDH in HIV-infected persons, itraconazole has been shown to be useful for both maintenance and suppressive therapy after induction with amphotericin B and for treatment of patients who are mildly to moderately ill with PDH.

Treatment should begin at a dose of 400 mg per day (200 mg twice daily). If there is any question of adequate absorption, serum itraconazole level can be measured, although this test is not generally available. Interpretation of the level depends on the method used; 200 mg per day has been used in studies for maintenance in PDH, with the same caveats regarding absorption and levels. There have been no studies in pregnant women, and itraconazole should be used in pregnancy only if the potential benefit outweighs the risks, as teratogenicity has been observed in rats experimentally.

Itraconazole should not be used in critically ill patients because absorption may be impaired. In the absence of food, absorption of the drug is drastically reduced. In addition, critically ill patients may receive agents that reduce gastric acidity, and this intervention may further impair absorption of the drug. Thus for several reasons, amphotericin B remains the drug of choice in patients with histoplasmosis who are extremely ill.

Fluconazole

Fluconazole (Diflucan) is a triazole antifungal agent with the same mechanism of activity as ketoconazole and itraconazole. Unlike these agents, however, it has low protein binding, it is distributed in the total body water, and 80% of administered drug is excreted unchanged in the urine. It is available in 50-, 100-, and 200-mg tablets for oral administration and in 200- and 400-mg injections for intravenous administration. Adverse effects associated with fluconazole include gastrointestinal irritation (anorexia, nausea, and vomiting), hepatitis (usually clinically inapparent transaminase elevations), and pruritic rashes; there has been one possible case of Stevens-Johnson syndrome. Chapped lips and alopecia have been observed with prolonged courses. To date, the interference with human steroidogenesis seen with ketoconazole has not been reported with either fluconazole or itraconazole.

For maintenance therapy of PDH, fluconazole is clearly less effective than maintenance amphotericin at lower doses (50 to 100 mg per day) and is currently being studied at higher doses (400 to 800 mg per day). Fluconazole will most likely not be a drug of choice for histoplasmosis.

DRUG INTERACTIONS WITH AZOLE ANTIFUNGAL AGENTS

The principal mechanism of action of the azole compounds is to preferentially inhibit cytochrome P-450 enzymes in fungal organisms. Because these enzymes are also present in mammalian cells, in which they play a key role in metabolic and detoxifying reactions, it is well known that this class of drugs interferes with metabolism of other compounds.

Plasma concentrations of azole antifungal agents are reduced when given concurrently with rifampin. Severe hypoglycemia has been reported in patients concomitantly receiving azole antifungal agents and oral hypoglycemic agents. These agents increase serum concentrations of cyclosporine; the dose of cyclosporine should be reduced by 50% when itraconazole is given, to avoid nephrotoxic levels of cyclosporine. Drug interactions with the addition of itraconazole include decreased metabolism and therefore toxic levels of digoxin, phenytoin, astemizole, and terfenadine. Fatal arrhythmias have been observed after toxic levels of astemizole and terfenadine have been reached. Fluconazole, even at low doses (100 mg per day), markedly potentiates the anticoagulant activity of warfarin (Coumadin); itraconazole may have the same effect. There is no information regarding cross-hypersensitivity among the azole antifungal agents.

BLASTOMYCOSIS

method of
CAROL A. KAUFFMAN, M.D.
Department of Veterans Affairs Medical Center
University of Michigan Medical School
Ann Arbor, Michigan

Blastomycosis is found most commonly in the southeastern, midcentral, and north central United States. The etiologic agent, *Blastomyces dermatitidis,* exists in the soil in a mycelial form and causes infection after it is inhaled into the alveoli. As expected, the predominant manifestations often are pulmonary, but the organism may disseminate to many sites, notably skin, bones, and the genitourinary tract. Both acute and chronic pulmonary and systemic infections may occur. The type of treatment depends on the extent of infection.

INDICATIONS FOR TREATMENT

Many patients with acute pulmonary blastomycosis have acute self-limited infection, which has resolved before the diagnosis is made. These patients do not require treatment. However, any patient with acute pneumonia that has not improved after several weeks should be treated. Patients with chronic nodular, cavitary, or mass-like infiltrates should receive therapy. Extra-pulmonary blastomycosis necessitates treatment even when the patient is not ill and has only isolated cutaneous lesions.

In rare patients, blastomycosis is life-threatening. It may take the form of adult respiratory distress syndrome, meningeal or intracerebral blastomycosis, or acute, overwhelming, disseminated disease. These patients obviously require immediate therapy. Recommended therapy for different forms of blastomycosis is listed in Table 1.

AMPHOTERICIN B (FUNGIZONE)

Before the 1980s, amphotericin B was standard therapy for all forms of blastomycosis. Cooperative multicenter studies conducted in the 1960s showed that a total of 2 grams of amphotericin B was effective for treatment of pulmonary and extra-pulmonary forms of blastomycosis.

Amphotericin B is administered intravenously in 5% dextrose in water, beginning with a 1-mg test dose so as to be certain that the patient does not have a serious arrhythmia or anaphylaxis. If the patient tolerates the test dose, the dose is increased by 10 mg each day to achieve a daily dose of approximately 0.5 mg per kg. If the patient is seriously ill, the dose can be raised more

TABLE 1. **Therapy for Blastomycosis**

Type of Infection	Therapy
Pulmonary	
Acute pneumonia, resolving in several weeks	No therapy
Acute pneumonia, progressing or not resolving in several weeks	Itraconazole
Chronic cavitary, nodular, or mass lesions	Itraconazole
Life-threatening pneumonia	Amphotericin B
Extrapulmonary	
Subacute or chronic cutaneous, bone and joint, or organ involvement	Itraconazole
Life-threatening disseminated infection	Amphotericin B
Central nervous system infection	Amphotericin B

quickly. The infusion is usually run over 4 hours, although shorter infusion times of 2 hours may be tolerated by some patients.

The main drawback to the use of amphotericin B is its significant toxicity. The most serious side effects associated with amphotericin B are renal insufficiency, hypokalemia, hypomagnesemia, anemia, and immediate reactions during the infusion, which include chills, fever, nausea, and vomiting. Immediate reactions vary from patient to patient; they may be totally absent or create significant distress. Infusion-related side effects may be averted with the pre-infusion use of ace-tominophen and diphenhydramine; intravenous meperidine (Demerol), 25 to 50 mg, may be required in order to stop serious rigors.

The serum creatinine, potassium, and magnesium levels should be monitored two or three times weekly. If the creatinine level rises higher than 3 mg/dL, the drug may have to be stopped for a few days and then given every other day. It appears that renal insufficiency is increased when patients are dehydrated; therefore, infusion of 500 mL of saline before amphotericin B administration may help decrease the nephrotoxicity of the drug. Renal tubular potassium and magnesium losses are common and often necessitate oral supplementation. In general, weekly blood counts are obtained to monitor anemia, which almost always occurs but rarely necessitates transfusion.

KETOCONAZOLE (NIZORAL)

In the mid-1980s ketoconazole became the drug of choice for non–life-threatening forms of blastomycosis. Cure rates of 84 to 89% in patients treated for at least 6 months were obtained in several trials with ketoconazole. Most patients with blastomycosis are treated for 6 months to 1 year, depending on their response to therapy. The usual dose is 400 mg, given orally with food once daily. If no response occurs, the dose can be raised to 600 or 800 mg daily. However, toxicity increases with the higher doses, and in most instances, itraconazole (Sporanox) is used instead of increasing the dose of ketoconazole. Gastric acidity is required for absorption of ketoconazole; therefore, the drug should not be given with H_2 blockers or antacids.

The side effects of ketoconazole include nausea, vomiting, and headaches. Hepatitis occurs in rare instances (approximately one in 15,000 patients), and effects from the suppression of testosterone secretion (gynecomastia, decreased libido, oligospermia) occur at higher doses.

Several important drug interactions occur with ketoconazole. When given with cyclosporine, warfarin, or phenytoin, toxic levels of those compounds may result. Ketoconazole should never be used with terfenadine (Seldane) or astemizole (Hismanal); serious arrhythmias have been reported in patients receiving these combinations. When rifampin and isoniazid are given with ketoconazole, serum levels of all three drugs are diminished to subtherapeutic levels.

ITRACONAZOLE (SPORANOX)

Itraconazole was released in 1992 and should become the azole of choice for treatment of non–life-threatening blastomycosis. A recent study conducted by the Mycoses Study Group noted success in 95% of 40 patients with blastomycosis who received 200 to 400 mg of itraconazole daily for at least 2 months. The drug is available in 100-mg capsules and requires gastric acidity for absorption; thus it should not be given with H_2 blockers or antacids. Most patients should be treated with a daily 200-mg dose. Itraconazole should be given with food once daily when a 200-mg dose is used and twice daily when 400 mg is used. Patients are usually treated for 6 months to one year, depending on the extent of disease and their response to therapy.

Itraconazole appears to be less toxic than ketoconazole. Side effects of itraconazole include nausea, vomiting, edema, and hypokalemia. In rare cases, hepatitis occurs, as noted with ketoconazole. At daily doses of up to 400 mg, suppression of testosterone or corticosteroid secretion does not occur. Higher doses than those approved by the U.S. Food and Drug Administration have been shown to suppress steroid synthesis.

Several important drug interactions occur with itraconazole. Increased cyclosporine and digoxin levels have been reported in patients receiving these drugs plus itraconazole; serum levels of these drugs should be monitored closely when they are used with itraconazole. Itraconazole should not be used with terfenadine or astemizole because of the occurrence of serious arrhythmias. When used concomitantly with phenytoin, carbamazepine, and especially rifampin, decreased serum levels of itraconazole, resulting in therapeutic failure, have been documented.

FLUCONAZOLE (DIFLUCAN)

Fluconazole is another oral azole currently approved for use in treating *Candida* and cryptococcal infections. It is not yet approved for therapy of blastomycosis or other endemic mycoses. Multicenter trials with fluconazole for the treatment of blastomycosis are currently ongoing. Initial studies showed that daily treatment with 200 mg of fluconazole was less efficacious than that previously noted with ketoconazole or itraconazole. Current trials are assessing the use of 400 and 800 mg of fluconazole for treatment of the endemic mycoses. Until these studies are finished, fluconazole should not be used for the treatment of blastomycosis.

Thus in general, most patients with blastomycosis should be treated with itraconazole. Those with severe disease should receive amphotericin B; after the infection is stabilized, therapy can be continued with itraconazole. Pregnant women should not be treated with azoles but can be treated with amphotericin B. When azoles are prescribed, drug interactions must be carefully assessed.

PLEURAL EFFUSION AND EMPYEMA THORACIS

method of
LOUIS KATTINE, M.D.
St. Patrick Hospital
Missoula, Montana

and

RANDALL K. WOLF, M.D., and
CREIGHTON B. WRIGHT, M.D.
The Jewish Hospital of Cincinnati
Cincinnati, Ohio

PLEURAL EFFUSION

The pleural cavity normally contains 1 to 5 mL of physiologic fluid. Pleural effusion is defined as a collection of fluid within the pleura in excess of what is present normally. Pleural effusion usually results from involvement of the pleura by underlying pulmonary or systemic disorders. In uncommon instances, pleural effusion may reflect primary pleural disease.

A multitude of disease states can lead to pleural effusion. Effusions may be divided into two groups: transudative and exudative. The type of pleural fluid present can be determined by the

TABLE 1. **Transudative Versus Exudative Effusions**

Characteristic	Transudate	Exudate
Color	Clear, serous	Cloudy, tan
White blood cell count	<1000/mL	>10,000/mL
Glucose	Normal	Low in certain conditions
Protein	<3 gm/dL	>3 gm/dL
Specific gravity	<1.016	>1.016
Lactate dehydrogenase	Normal	>67% of upper limit of normal
pH	Same as arterial	<7.20 suggests empyema

TABLE 2. Etiology of Transudative Pleural Effusions

Congestive heart failure	Constrictive pericarditis
Cirrhosis	Malignancy
Nephrotic syndrome	Atelectasis
Peritoneal dialysis	Urinothorax
Hypoalbuminemia	

characteristics listed in Table 1. Common causes of transudative effusion can be found in Table 2, those of exudative origin in Table 3. The mainstays of diagnosis include history, physical examination, and chest roentgenogram. The next step in the diagnostic evaluation of pleural effusion is usually thoracentesis. Patients who might not require diagnostic thoracentesis include those with a recurrent effusion of known etiology and those with uncomplicated congestive heart failure.

Analysis of pleural fluid from thoracentesis plays a key role in establishing the cause of pleural effusion. In approximately 75% of cases, results from the analysis of pleural fluid lead to diagnosis. Cost-effective tests that should be obtained on all specimens include total protein, lactate dehydrogenase (LDH), white blood cell count with differential, and either pH or glucose. Gram's and fungal stains as well as cultures should be obtained to identify infectious causes. Cytologic specimens should be obtained if malignancy is suspected or the etiology is unknown. Immunologic studies, amylase tests, or specific markers can be ordered on the basis of clinical

TABLE 3. Etiology of Exudative Pleural Effusions

Infectious
Bacterial
Parasitic
Tuberculous
Fungal
Viral

Immunologic
Lupus erythematosus
Rheumatoid
Connective tissue disease
Sarcoidosis
Postpericardiotomy syndrome

Malignancy
Carcinoma
Lymphoma
Mesothelioma
Leukemia

Iatrogenic

Other Inflammatory States
Pulmonary embolism
Uremia
Meigs' syndrome (effusion with ovarian tumor)
Radiation therapy
Pancreatitis

suspicion. In addition, fluid should be preserved (by using heparin and refrigeration) for future analysis after preliminary results are obtained.

Transudative effusions are the result of an imbalance in Starling's forces or of movement of fluid from the peritoneal cavity. Transudative effusions are usually associated with noninflammatory conditions, as noted in Table 2. Exudative effusions result from conditions that cause inflammation of the pleura and impaired lymphatic drainage, as noted in Table 3. Some fluid samples may have mixed characteristics.

Additional maneuvers include computed tomography (CT) and video thoracoscopy. Until recently, unguided pleural biopsy frequently followed thoracentesis or was added after nondiagnostic thoracentesis. This led to a diagnosis in 40 to 80% of the cases, depending on etiology: the percentage was higher in benign conditions and lower in malignant conditions. Since 1990 the authors have used video thoracoscopy as the next diagnostic and often therapeutic modality. The diagnostic yield with video thoracoscopy has been 100%. It is easy to use this method to visually inspect the pleural cavity as well as perform directed biopsies of the pleura, lung parenchyma, and nodal tissue. Thus video thoracoscopy has become the preferred secondary test after nondiagnostic thoracentesis and CT.

Treatment

Pleural effusions can be treated by various regimens according to characterization into one of three groups: complicated parapneumonic effusions (which are discussed later in the section on empyema thoracis), benign effusions, and malignant effusions. Benign pleural effusions usually respond to treatment of the underlying disease state; repeated thoracentesis or tube thoracostomy is reserved for patients with respiratory embarrassment.

Malignant effusions can present a significant therapeutic challenge. Treatment can be divided into two phases: drainage and obliteration of the pleural space. Drainage can be achieved by tube thoracostomy or by ultrasound- or CT-guided catheter placement. The latter two methods are especially useful for loculated collections. New, smaller, multiholed plastic catheters can be placed into the chest, producing less discomfort and providing good drainage. The authors currently prefer these methods to video thoracoscopy if initial drainage procedures do not prevent reaccumulation of the effusion.

Obliteration of the pleural space (pleurodesis) can be achieved by using chemical or mechanical pleural abrasion or resection of the pleura (pleurectomy). Chemical pleurodesis is usually performed by using a sclerosant such as bleomycin or sterile talc. Until it was withdrawn from the market, tetracycline was an effective and inexpensive sclerosant. Either talc or bleomycin may be used; however, talc is significantly less expensive. Obliteration of the pleural space can be performed effectively with talc insufflated into the pleural cavity. Malignant effusions secondary to a primary lung carcinoma have also been treated via pleural instillation of various chemotherapeutic agents (doxorubicin [Adriamycin], mitomycin C [Mutamycin], OK-432). These have been used in an attempt both to achieve sclerosis and to improve the quality of life. Currently, these methods must be considered experimental.

Open pleurectomy by thoracotomy, although very effective, is associated with significant rates of morbidity and mortality. Recurrent malignant effusions have been treated effectively with pleuroperitoneal shunts of the Denver type. More recently, video thoracoscopy has been used with good success in the treatment of these difficult recurrent effusions. With this technique, the pleural space can be drained, fibrous loculations divided, partial pleurectomy performed, and pleurodesis achieved. Pleurodesis can be accomplished through the thoracoscope by using a sclerosant, electrocautery, or laser. In the authors' practice, video thoracoscopy has been used since 1990 to treat patients with difficult recurrent malignant pleural effusions. All patients treated by this modality have had lysis of adhesions followed by talc pleurodesis. To date, all have remained free of recurrent, symptomatic pleural effusions. Video thoracoscopy offers the promise of results equal to those of surgical pleurectomy without the morbidity and mortality rates associated with the latter procedure. This is a distinct advantage in patients with a limited life expectancy.

EMPYEMA THORACIS

Empyema thoracis is defined as pus within the pleural space. Empyema fluid may grossly resemble pus or may be more watery and clear to yellow in color. Empyemas have the characteristics of an exudate: a specific gravity greater than 1.016, a protein content greater than 3 grams per dL, a low pH, a low glucose level, white blood cell counts greater than 10,000 per milliliter, and a positive Gram's stain and culture. The etiologies of empyema thoracis are listed in Table 4. Pyogenic pneumonia is by far the most common, accounting for 50% of all empyemas.

The bacteriology of empyema is complex. Before the development of antibiotics, *Pneumococ-*

TABLE 4. Etiology of Empyema Thoracis

Pyogenic pneumonia	50%
Lung abscess rupture	1–3%
Pulmonary tuberculosis	1%
Pulmonary mycotic infection	1%
Foreign bodies retained in bronchial tree	<1%
Secondary to generalized tuberculosis	1–3%
Secondary to trauma	3–5%
Secondary to surgery (esophagus, lung, mediastinum)	25%
Extension from subphrenic abscess	8–11%
Secondary to bronchopleural fistula of spontaneous pneumothorax	<1%
Secondary to parasitic infection	<1%
Miscellaneous	1%

cus and *Streptococcus* were the organisms most commonly isolated. With the advent of effective antibiotics and better culturing techniques, predominance has shifted toward gram-negative organisms such as *Pseudomonas, Escherichia coli, Klebsiella,* and *Enterobacter,* as well as anaerobes such as *Bacteroides, Fusobacterium, Peptococcus,* and *Clostridium.* Frequently, multiple organisms, including both aerobes and anaerobes, can be isolated concurrently. In children, however, *Staphylococcus* remains the organism most commonly isolated. Post-traumatic empyema reflects hospital flora. The most commonly isolated species include *Staphylococcus aureus, Pseudomonas, E. coli,* and *Enterobacter.*

The diagnosis of empyema can usually be established from the history and physical examination, chest roentgenogram, and thoracentesis. CT may be needed for access to loculated fluid collections. Bronchoscopy should be considered part of the evaluation of all patients with spontaneous empyema, to rule out endobronchial or endotracheal tumor or the presence of an inhaled foreign body.

Treatment

The treatment of empyema can be divided into two groups: spontaneous empyema and postsurgical empyema. Treatment of patients with spontaneous empyema is based on thoracentesis results. Thoracentesis fluid that is clear and watery may warrant tube thoracostomy in addition to intravenous antibiotics. Several characteristics of the pleural fluid are suggestive of infection within the pleural space and indicate the need for drainage: a pH of less than 7, a glucose level of less than 40, an LDH level of less than 1000, and a positive Gram's stain. At least one study has shown that pleural fluid with these characteristics can be treated effectively with antibiotics alone. At present, conservative therapy is still warranted; when pleural fluid is suggestive of infection, drainage should be added to antibiotic therapy.

Fluid that on thoracentesis is found to be grossly purulent is treated with both antibiotics and tube thoracostomy. Loculated empyemas may necessitate CT guidance for accurate catheter placement. In addition, streptokinase or urodinase may be instilled via the catheter to aid in the breakdown of loculations. Since 1990, the authors have frequently employed video thoracoscopy for lysing adhesions, removing debris, and performing decortication.

In acute empyema, the catheter can usually be removed slowly over a period of weeks to months as the disease process resolves. In the case of chronic empyema with a persistent cavity, more aggressive surgical intervention may be required. This may include rib resection, decortication, or the Eloesser procedure.

Postsurgical empyema often represents a difficult therapeutic challenge. Frequently, it is associated with a concomitant residual space and a bronchopleural fistula. Affected patients are initially treated with tube thoracostomy and intravenous antibiotics. If they remain unstable, more aggressive treatment is required, and the Eloesser procedure should be considered. In stable patients without a bronchopleural fistula, the residual space can be obliterated by muscle flap closure techniques after the cavity has been sterilized with tube thoracostomy and antibiotics. In stable patients with a persistent bronchopleural fistula, the fistula should be closed with a muscle flap and the residual cavity obliterated by thoracoplastic techniques.

PRIMARY LUNG ABSCESS

method of
SOL KATZ, M.D.
Georgetown University Hospital
Washington, D.C.

Lung abscess represents an area of pulmonary necrosis resulting from the aspiration and retention of infected secretions from the oropharynx. Thus the term "aspiration lung abscess" is more appropriate than "primary lung abscess." The source of this infected inoculum is especially the gingivodental crevices (in the presence of gingivodental infection) and the gastrointestinal tract. Normally, aspirated secretions are efficiently managed by cough, ciliary action, bronchial peristalsis from alternating contraction and relaxation of the bronchi, and alveolar macrophages. When these mechanisms are not fully effective, the aspirate laden with large numbers of organisms in saliva, in nasal,

oral, and nasopharyngeal secretions, and in blood or vomitus reaches the peripheral portion of the lung and establishes a localized zone of inflammation (pneumonitis) that progresses to necrosis and liquefaction. The process is usually pleura-based, and the pleural inflammation is manifested as a localized pleuritis, sterile pleural effusion, infected pleural effusion, or frank empyema. Aspiration infection is a continuum from pneumonia to cavitation to empyema.

PATHOGENESIS

The infected aspirate gravitates to the most dependent part of the bronchial tree, and the inaccurate term "bronchial embolism" readily explains the localization of aspiration lung abscess. When the patient is supine at the time of aspiration, the posterior segment of the upper lobes and the superior segment of the lower lobes are the sites encountered by the secretions as they descend along the posterior wall of the tracheobronchial tree. The basal segments are finally met. The more direct course of the right main bronchus explains the more frequent involvement of the right side.

Aspiration of infected secretions is more likely during suppressed levels of consciousness, as in head injury, alcoholism, seizure disorders, general anesthesia, cerebrovascular accidents, drug abuse, and motility or obstructive disorders of the upper gastrointestinal tract. Prolonged uncoordinated vomiting and disruption of defense barriers such as that caused by the use of nasogastric tube, endotracheal tube, or tracheostomy may encourage aspiration, as may dental procedures and difficult endotracheal intubation. Poor oral hygiene and periodontal disease increase the degree of bacterial contamination in the mouth and increase the likelihood of pulmonary infection when aspiration occurs.

Compromise of immunologic defenses, as in neutropenia, use of corticosteroids, cancer chemotherapy, and acquired immune deficiency syndrome (AIDS), may lead to lung abscess. Necrotizing pulmonary infection may result from direct spread from subphrenic abscess, bacteremia, and infection secondary to lung trauma. Bronchogenic carcinoma, presence of a foreign body, and bronchiectasis predispose to lung abscess by altering effective clearance of infected secretions. Aspiration of gastric contents results in a raging chemical pneumonitis from gastric acid and enzymes.

Many organisms may cause lung abscess, including anaerobes as well as aerobes. Careful studies with specimens obtained anaerobically along with appropriate anaerobic cultures have revealed that most community-acquired lung abscesses are polymicrobial and involve anaerobic bacteria. Confusion, inaccuracies, and contradictions have been overwhelming in the attempt to clarify the nosology and taxonomy of anaerobic bacteria. Although anaerobic lung abscesses often contain many genera, the predominant ones are organisms normally present in the gingival crevices and oropharynx that are then aspirated into the lungs.

The three most important anaerobic groups are anaerobic gram-positive cocci, *Bacteroides* spp., and *Fusobacterium* spp. *Peptostreptococcus* is the most common organism among the anaerobic gram-positive cocci. Organisms previously labeled *Peptococcus* are now classified as *Peptostreptococcus*. Organisms formerly labeled anaerobic or microaerophilic streptococci or facultative organisms are now officially classified as aerobic streptococci. Although these organisms grow optimally in an anaerobic environment, they are relatively aerotolerant, are classified as facultative aerobes, and therefore officially belong to the genus *Streptococcus*. Despite this designation, anaerobic techniques may be required for their exact isolation and characterization.

Bacteroides organisms are frequently isolated from anaerobic abscesses. Brown- or black-pigmenting *Bacteroides*, formerly called *B. melaninogenicus,* are now subdivided into eight species, the most important being *B. melaninogenicus* and *B. intermedius. B. fragilis,* a cause of intra-abdominal infection but not usually considered to be an oropharyngeal inhabitant, was previously reported to be present in 10 to 20% of cases of primary lung abscess. However, more recent studies implicate this organism in only 7% of cases, suggesting earlier errors based on taxonomic confusion. *Fusobacterium* makes up the third group of anaerobic organisms involved in lung abscess. *F. nucleatum* and *F. necrophorum* are the major species of this genus.

Aerobic bacteria are frequently the pathogens in hospital-acquired aspiration lung abscess and include the organisms associated with nosocomial infection. In these cases there is a progressive necrotizing pneumonia with cavitation. The bacteria encountered are *Staphylococcus aureus, Streptococcus pyogenes* (Group A streptococcus), other *Streptococcus* spp., and gram-negative bacilli such as *Klebsiella pneumoniae, Enterobacter* spp., *Serratia* spp., and *Pseudomonas* spp. On occasion, other gram-negative bacilli, such as *Proteus* spp. and *E. coli,* are cultured. Less commonly noted as examples of necrotizing cavitary pneumonia are *Nocardia* spp., *Pseudomonas pseudomallei, Haemophilus influenzae* (especially type B), and *Actinomyces* spp. Histoplasmosis, aspergillosis, and coccidioidomycosis may also resemble lung abscess. Of course, tuberculosis may (embarrassingly at times) resemble lung abscess. *Streptococcus pneumoniae*, especially types III and VIII, has occasionally been reported to cause lung abscess but many authors believe that this is an example of anaerobic infection superimposed on pneumococcal pneumonia. Mixed anaerobes and anerobes are also a feature of hospital-acquired aspiration lung abscess. Data suggest that there is no difference in the results of therapy between these cases and those treated as pure anaerobic infections.

The early phase of aspiration lung abscess is a localized area of consolidation with the roentgenographic appearance of pneumonia. On pathologic studies, this represents necrotizing pneumonitis. At times the area of consolidation is round and sharply defined, which aids in the early detection of lung abscess before liquefaction occurs. A few small highlights, indicating cavitation, then appear within the dense consolidation. Liquefaction progresses, and some of the purulent material is discharged through the communicating bronchus; air enters, and the specific sign of abscess—a fluid-containing cavity—appears.

There are several courses after this stage. The necrosis and liquefaction continue until cavitation replaces the entire area of consolidation. When the communicating bronchus is blocked by inflammation, by edema, and by exudate, the secretions accumulate, the air is absorbed, and the cavity becomes completely filled (blocked cavity). With good drainage, the secretions are evacuated, the fluid is reduced, and the pericavitary pneumonitis decreases. A diminution in cavity size and complete resolution of the surrounding infection follow. The draining ceases, and the lung may return to normal except for minor distortion of the vascular markings and linear fibrosis.

If the abscess does not disappear in 6 to 10 weeks, it is often because irreversible pulmonary changes have occurred. The chronic abscess is characterized by a rigid fibrous wall, pericavitary fibrosis, and bronchiectasis.

DIAGNOSIS

The diagnosis of lung abscesses is based on clinical, radiologic, and laboratory findings, including Gram's stain of sputum. About two-thirds of patients have foul sputum, which is considered pathognomonic of anaerobic infection. Because the usual organisms causing anaerobic abscesses are normally found in the mouth or oropharynx, cultures of expectorated sputum are contaminated by these organisms and therefore do not necessarily reflect the contents of the abscess. Appropriate specimens for anaerobic cultures are blood, pleural fluid, transtracheal aspirates, transthoracic lung aspirates, and bronchoscopic specimens collected with a shielded catheter or brush for quantitative cultures.

Positive blood cultures are obtained in fewer than 3% of proven anaerobic lung infections. Transthoracic needle aspiration provides accurate bacteriologic samples. There is the danger of pneumothorax and empyema when the lung abscess is not adherent to the pleura and when the aspirating needle has to traverse aerated lung before striking the abscess itself. With regard to specimens obtained bronchoscopically, the results are inconsistent even with a protected, shielded brush. Invasive techniques to obtain material for identification of anaerobes are not indicated when the manifestations of aspiration lung abscess are classic.

TREATMENT

Many antibiotics used alone or in combination have been successful, but three regimens have been rather consistently effective: penicillin G, clindamycin (Cleocin), and metronidazole (Flagyl) plus penicillin. When there is a bacteriologic complex infection with both multiple aerobic and anaerobic organisms, it is not necessary to identify each organism and establish antibiotic sensitivity in order to establish logical therapy. These organisms often live symbiotically, so that the elimination of the major culprits usually destroys the others, even those that are insensitive to the antibiotics being used.

Although penicillin given by mouth may produce a satisfactory outcome, using this route often results in a higher failure rate and slower response than does use of aqueous penicillin G in high dosage (12 to 20 million units daily) intravenously until there is clinical response. Foul sputum, when present, usually disappears in a few days, although cough and nonfoul sputum production often continue for longer periods. Fever and subjective improvement occur during the first week, but it takes 1 to 2 weeks longer for the temperature to become normal. The improvement in the chest films lags behind clinical improvement. After the acute phase of intravenous treatment, during which the toxic manifestations (e.g., cough, fever, heavy sputum production, malaise, sweats) subside, penicillin can be given orally as penicillin G, penicillin V, ampicillin, or amoxicillin, 500 to 750 mg four times a day. Oral therapy should be continued until there is complete clinical resolution and the chest film demonstrates complete resolution whether the manifestation is a stable fibrotic lesion or a small uninfected cavity. This second roentgenographic phase with clearing may be prolonged. The therapeutic process may last 4 to 10 weeks or, in some patients, longer.

Although penicillin is preferred by many physicians because it is safe, is inexpensive, and has a long favorable record, treatment may fail because of the presence of penicillin-resistant strains of Bacteroides and other organisms. In some studies, in vitro testing indicates that at least 15 to 30% of patients with anaerobic lung abscess harbor strains that are resistant to penicillin, despite the fact that a clinical response may occur as a result of elimination of sensitive organisms in a polymicrobial infestation. For this reason, the use of clindamycin is often favored at an intravenous dose of 600 to 900 mg every 8 hours until a clinical response occurs; at that point, oral clindamycin is given 300 mg three or four times a day until the criteria of stability have been achieved. Comparative studies of penicillin and clindamycin have shown that clindamycin has fewer failures, a lower frequency of relapses, a shorter mean duration of fever, and a shorter mean duration of putrid sputum. The major side effects of clindamycin therapy are diarrhea and pseudomembranous colitis.

When metronidazole is selected for therapy, it should not be used alone because it is frequently ineffective against aerobic and microaerophilic streptococci so often found in anaerobic lung infection. Metronidazole, 500 mg orally or intravenously every 6 hours combined with high-dose penicillin intravenously as described, or in clinically less severely ill patients, metronidazole by mouth plus oral penicillin, 500 to 750 mg four times a day, may be used throughout therapy. Metronidazole broadens the activity against the anaerobes that are penicillin-resistant. For patients who are penicillin-sensitive and who fail to respond to clindamycin, metronidazole with erythromycin, vancomycin, or chloramphenicol should be tried. For patients who fail to respond and who are not allergic to penicillin, imipenem-cilastatin (Primaxin), a new broad-spectrum beta-lactam agent, should be tried. In general, cephalosporins are somewhat unpredictable against anaerobes except cefoxitin (Mefoxin), cefoteten (Cefotan), cefmetazol (Zefazone), cefotaxime (Claforan), ceftizoxime (Cefizox), and cefoperazone (Cefobid). The antipseudomonad penicillins such as carbenicillin (Geocillin), ticarcillin (Ticar), mezlocillin (Mezlin), and piperacillin (Pipracil) may be more effective than penicillin because of the extraordinary high doses generally used.

Hospital-acquired aspiration lung abscesses are often caused by aerobic mixed gram-negative bacilli and S. aureus, in addition to the usual anaerobes. In this circumstance, the choice of antibiotic is best guided by identification of the causative organism and bacterial sensitivity data. Infection by S. aureus is treated with oxacillin (Prostaphlin), nafcillin (Nafcil) in high doses (2 grams every 4 hours) added to penicillin G, or clindamycin. For methicillin-resistant *S. aureus*, neither nafcillin nor clindamycin is useful, and intravenous vancomycin, 1 gram every 12 hours or 500 mg every 6 hours, is used. Gram-negative bacilli often require an appropriate aminoglycoside in addition to a third-generation cephalosporin such as cefotaxime (Claforan), ceftizoxime (Cefizox), ceftriaxone (Rocephin), cefoperazone (Cefobid), ceftazidime (Fortaz), or cefixime (Suprax) as determined by sensitivity testing. A diagnostic procedure (bronchoscopy and protected brush sampling, needle aspiration, pleural fluid tap) may be necessary for obtaining proper and appropriate specimens for culture and sensitivity studies.

As with an abscess anywhere in the body, appropriate treatment of lung abscess entails adequate drainage coupled with antibiotic treatment. Lung abscesses affect communicating bronchi and usually drain spontaneously, as shown by an air-fluid level on the chest roentgenogram and by improved drainage with chest physiotherapy, postural drainage, and inhaled bronchodilators to improve mucociliary clearance of secretions. Bronchoscopy may assist drainage, but its major role is to determine the presence of an obstructing lesion such as a foreign body, bronchial stenosis, or a neoplasm. Bronchogenic carcinoma with abscess should be suspected in the absence of fever, systemic symptoms, poor oral hygiene, or features that predispose to aspiration. An irregular cavity wall with mural nodules and the lack of an infiltrate surrounding the abscess are also suggestive of a malignant lung abscess.

Surgery is required in very few cases of lung abscess. The indications for surgery are clinical or roentgenographic deterioration despite good medical management; uncontrollable hemoptysis; benign or malignant bronchial obstruction; strong suspicion of necrotizing carcinoma; bronchopleural fistula with empyema; persistence of a significant cavity after 3 months of therapy in the presence of recurrent infection in that segment or lobe; and the presence of a large abscess cavity with continuing aspiration of the abscess contents to other parts of the lung. In patients who are critically ill and whose poor pulmonary reserve renders them an unacceptable surgical risk, pneumonotomy with incision and catheter drainage may be performed through an area of pleural symphysis under local anesthesia. The role of percutaneous needle or catheter drainage in treating all lung abscesses that fail to drain despite thorough medical therapy requires careful evaluation.

The prevention of lung abscess requires precautions to minimize the possibility of aspiration, particularly in feeble or confused patients and those with difficulty in swallowing. Special attention is necessary after feeding by gastric tube.

Histamine type II blockers and antacids are commonly used in intensive care settings in an attempt to prevent upper gastrointestinal bleeding caused by stress ulcers. This therapy may increase gastric pH and gastric and pharyngeal colonization with gram-negative bacilli. This may be avoided by the use of sucralfate (Carafate) instead of antacids and H_2 blockers.

The therapy of anaerobic abscess is incomplete unless there is adequate attention to periodontal disease and gingivitis to prevent recurrences.

OTITIS MEDIA

method of
PHILLIP H. KALEIDA, M.D.
University of Pittsburgh School of Medicine
Children's Hospital of Pittsburgh
Pittsburgh, Pennsylvania

Otitis media (OM) is one of the most common clinical problems encountered by providers of health care to children. Most children experience at least one episode of OM, and a substantial proportion (33% in one study) have multiple episodes.

Acute otitis media (AOM, or acute suppurative OM) refers to the recent onset of the symptoms or signs, or both, of middle ear infection. Acute perforation of the tympanic membrane with otorrhea may develop. Otitis media with effusion (OME, or secretory OM) is inflammation accompanied by liquid in the middle ear; it is commonly asymptomatic, except for hearing loss. Chronic OME can be defined as persistence of middle ear effusion for 3 months or longer. Recurrent AOM is defined as the occurrence of three or more episodes of AOM within a 6-month period, or four or more episodes within a 12-month period. Chronic suppurative otitis media (CSOM) refers to chronic otorrhea (longer than 6 weeks' duration) through a nonintact tympanic membrane; chronic mastoid inflammation is also regularly present.

CLINICAL EVALUATION

History

In cases of AOM the clinician can often elicit a history of otalgia (in young children, ear-pulling), irritability, or fever. Otalgia is the most specific sign. Fever may be present in as few as 25% of cases. Conductive hearing loss and, in a small proportion of children, vertigo may also develop during an episode of OM.

Physical Examination

Accurate diagnosis centers on pneumatic otoscopic examination. If necessary for adequate visualization of the tympanic membrane, cerumen should be removed from the external auditory canal. This can be performed with a curette under direct visualization by using the operating head of the otoscope. Some children need to be restrained for this purpose or even for satisfactory examination. After inspecting the pinna and the external auditory canal, the clinician should attempt to see the entire tympanic membrane because serious disease (e.g., cholesteatoma) may be present in less readily visible portions (posterior-superior quadrant and pars flaccida). The color, degree of translucency, position, and mobility of the tympanic membrane should be assessed. Absence of or impaired mobility of the tympanic membrane is the most important finding in determining the presence of middle ear effusion. The otoscopist should also note the presence of bubbles, air-fluid levels, and other pathologic conditions, such as tympanosclerosis, atrophic areas, retraction pockets, and cholesteatomas.

In AOM, the tympanic membrane typically appears erythematous or pale yellow (suggesting the presence of pus), opaque, full to the point of bulging, and poorly mobile. In OME, the tympanic membrane typically appears amber or sometimes bluish, opaque, retracted (or, less often, full), and poorly mobile.

In some cases, tympanometry may be performed as an adjunct to otoscopy.

BACTERIOLOGY

In general, aerobic bacterial cultures are positive in 75% or more of middle ear aspirates from children with AOM. *Streptococcus pneumoniae* (25 to 45%), *Haemophilus influenzae* (20 to 30%), *Moraxella catarrhalis* (8 to 20%), and *Streptococcus pyogenes* (3 to 4%) are the bacteria most commonly isolated. Approximately 20 to 33% of the *H. influenzae* (usually nontypable) and most of the *M. catarrhalis* middle ear isolates produce beta-lactamase. In the first 6 weeks after birth, gram-negative enterics and *Staphylococcus aureus* are isolated in 10 to 20% of cases. Enteric bacteria are usually isolated from neonates who have undergone nasotracheal intubation in an intensive care unit. Even in this age group, however, *S. pneumoniae* and *H. influenzae* are the bacteria most frequently isolated. In adults, *H. influenzae* is an important cause of OM.

In approximately 30% of cases of chronic OME, the pathogens found in AOM are isolated. Other bacteria (presumed nonpathogens) have been found in an additional 30% of cases. In CSOM, *Pseudomonas aeruginosa* and *S. aureus* are most likely to be isolated.

MANAGEMENT OF ACUTE OTITIS MEDIA

General Comments

Oral analgesics, usually acetaminophen (pediatric dose, 10 to 15 mg per kg per dose up to four to five times daily), can be used as needed. In rare instances, a narcotic analgesic may be required initially. In addition, warm compresses to the external ear and, if no perforation is present, ototopical analgesic drops (e.g., Auralgan) may be helpful.

Standard management of AOM in the United States includes a 10-day course of an oral antimicrobial agent. Table 1 displays dosage and other selected information regarding oral antimicrobial agents prescribed in the United States for treatment of OM. Because not all information and precautions about the use of these drugs can be provided in Table 1 or the accompanying text, the reader is referred to standard references for more details. Many of these agents can be associated with drug interactions, most notably erythromycin (with theophylline, carbamazepine, and so forth). In addition, some of these agents are not recommended for use in the first month (cefaclor) or 2 months (sulfonamides) after birth. Oral decongestants and antihistamines have not proved to be effective in hastening the resolution of middle ear effusion, at least in nonallergic children with OM.

First-Line Antimicrobial Agent

Amoxicillin. Because of its relative safety, efficacy, acceptability to patients, and low cost, amoxicillin is currently the drug of choice for treatment of AOM. It usually has good antibacterial activity against *S. pneumoniae, S. pyogenes,* and non–beta-lactamase–producing strains of *H. influenzae* and *M. catarrhalis.*

Second-Line Antimicrobial Agents

Indications for considering the use of a second-line antimicrobial agent in the treatment of AOM include (1) penicillin allergy (of course, amoxicillin-clavulanate cannot be used); (2) middle ear disease known to be caused by a beta-lactamase–producing pathogen; (3) otitis-conjunctivitis syndrome; (4) persistence of fever or otalgia attributable to OM after 48 to 72 hours of amoxicillin therapy; and perhaps (5) location in an area of the country where the prevalence of beta-lactamase–producing strains of middle ear pathogens is known to be very high. Cephalosporins should be used cautiously in patients with penicillin allergy. Each of the second-line antimicrobial agents offers certain advantages and disadvantages. The choice of one agent over another depends on the clinician's consideration of multiple factors: the age of the child (e.g., a neonate), underlying medical problems, bacteriologic factors (e.g., a high index of suspicion or documentation of a beta-lactamase–producing middle ear isolate), relative safety of the drug, frequency and types of side effects, anticipated compliance by the patient, acceptability to the patient, and cost.

TABLE 1. **Antimicrobial Agents for Otitis Media**

Name of Drug	Children		Adults		Comments*
	Daily Dose†	*No. Divided Doses*	*Single Dose*	*No. Doses*	
FIRST-LINE					
Amoxicillin	40 mg/kg	3	500 mg	3	Inexpensive
SECOND-LINE					
Amoxicillin clavulanate (Augmentin)	40 mg/kg	3	500 mg‡	3	More diarrhea than amoxicillin alone; expensive
Erythromycin ethylsuccinate– sulfisoxazole acetyl (Pediazole)	Erythromycin: 50 mg/kg Sulfisoxazole: 150 mg/kg	4	Erythromycin: 400 mg Sulfisoxazole: 1200 mg	4	Drug interactions; potential sulfonamide toxicity; moderately expensive
Trimethoprim-sulfamethoxazole§ (Bactrim, Septra)	Trimethoprim: 8 mg/kg Sulfamethoxazole: 40 mg/kg	2	Trimethoprim: 160 mg Sulfamethoxazole: 800 mg	2	Potential sulfonamide toxicity; convenient; inexpensive
Cefaclor (Ceclor)	40 mg/kg	3	500 mg	3	Serum sickness or erythema multiforme (1%); expensive
Cefixime (Suprax)	8 mg/kg	1	400 mg / 200 mg	1 / 2	Use only oral suspension; more frequent diarrhea; convenient; expensive
	Single Dose	*No. Doses*			
Cefuroxime axetil (Ceftin)	<2 years of age: 125 mg / 2–12 years of age: 250 mg	2/day / 2/day	500 mg	2	No oral suspension; convenient; expensive

*Most of these antimicrobial agents are associated with gastrointestinal side effects (usually diarrhea) and rash.
†In treatment of pediatric patients, adult dosages should not be exceeded.
‡Use 500-mg tablet rather than two 250-mg tablets.
§Also called co-trimoxazole.

Amoxicillin-Clavulanate (Augmentin). The combination of amoxicillin with clavulanate is an attractive second-line agent because amoxicillin, a penicillin, is presumed to be relatively safe and because clavulanate is a beta-lactamase inhibitor. The frequency of diarrhea may be lessened if the drug is given with food. The unused portion of the refrigerated reconstituted suspension should be discarded after 10 days.

Erythromycin Ethylsuccinate–Sulfisoxazole Acetyl (Pediazole). Products that combine a sulfonamide with a second antimicrobial agent provide acceptable alternatives for the treatment of OM in penicillin-allergic patients. Erythromycin may produce epigastric distress. Sulfonamide-containing drugs have been linked to Stevens-Johnson syndrome, blood dyscrasias, and, in patients with glucose-6-phosphate dehydrogenase deficiency, hemolysis.

Trimethoprim-Sulfamethoxazole (Bactrim, Septra). Trimethoprim-sulfamethoxazole does not provide adequate antibacterial coverage against *S. pyogenes*. In clinical situations in which this pathogen is not likely to be present, however, the drug offers convenient twice-a-day dosing.

Cefaclor (Ceclor). Cefaclor appears to have comparatively less antibacterial activity against beta-lactamase–producing isolates. Children are more likely to experience serum sickness or erythema multiforme reactions when receiving second or third courses of the drug. These concerns, combined with high cost, probably limit the usefulness of cefaclor in OM to relatively few situations.

Cefixime (Suprax). Because higher peak blood levels result, only the suspension of cefixime should be used to treat OM. Cefixime offers the convenience of once daily dosing. Reports to date suggest that the optimal role of cefixime may be for treatment of beta-lactamase–producing strains of *H. influenzae* and *M. catarrhalis*. Antibacterial activity against *S. aureus* does not appear to be adequate.

Cefuroxime Axetil (Ceftin). At present, there is no oral suspension of cefuroxime, and the tablet, when crushed, is bitter. Therefore, because most cases of OM occur in young children, there are relatively few clinical opportunities to consider use of this agent in OM. In addition, the drug is expensive.

Others. Other oral agents that could prove useful in the treatment of OM have been studied recently. However, at the time of this writing, experience, particularly in clinical settings, has been limited (e.g., loracarbef, cefprozil).

Tympanocentesis and Myringotomy

In patients with AOM, consideration should be given to performing tympanocentesis and myringotomy when an unusual pathogen is suspected (e.g., neonates [as discussed earlier] and immunodeficient patients), when a patient appears very ill or has a suppurative complication, when extreme otalgia is present, and when symptoms persist despite an adequate trial of a seemingly appropriate antimicrobial agent. If tympanocentesis or myringotomy is performed, specimens of middle ear fluid should be sent to the laboratory for culture and sensitivity testing.

MANAGEMENT OF OTITIS MEDIA WITH EFFUSION

As in AOM, oral antimicrobial agents have been shown to provide modest benefit in the treatment of OME. Consideration of antimicrobial treatment at the time of initial presentation of OME seems most appropriate when one or more of the following factors is present: (1) young age of patient (first several years of life); (2) pre-existing developmental delay or hearing deficit; (3) concurrent upper respiratory tract infection; (4) associated symptoms, such as otalgia or moderate or severe hearing loss attributable to the current episode; (5) anatomic abnormality (e.g., craniofacial malformation or cleft palate); (6) bilateral middle ear effusion; (7) a worrisome tympanic membrane finding (e.g., a new retraction pocket); (8) poor follow-up; and, perhaps, (9) a history of recurrent OM. It is reasonable to withhold antimicrobial therapy initially in some children, particularly those who are older (e.g., school-aged) and who meet none of the aforementioned criteria.

Follow-Up Visits

Middle ear effusion often persists for weeks or longer after initiation of treatment for AOM. Therefore, it is important to re-examine patients after each new episode of AOM or OME until the effusion has resolved.

MANAGEMENT OF CHRONIC OTITIS MEDIA WITH EFFUSION

When middle ear effusion persists for 2 to 3 months, a 10- to 14-day trial of a second-line antimicrobial agent is reasonable. (Most affected children have previously received a course of amoxi-

cillin for AOM.) If no improvement is seen after one or two such courses of treatment, referral to an otolaryngologist is appropriate. At present, more information is needed in order to determine which patients with chronic OME, if any, are likely to benefit from a trial of oral steroids without experiencing adverse effects.

Hearing should be assessed both in children with chronic OME and in children with recurrent AOM. In addition, in such children, the clinician should search for problems that may be contributory, such as the practice of bottle-propping, respiratory allergy, concurrent upper respiratory tract infection or sinusitis, anatomic abnormality (e.g., cleft palate, submucous cleft palate), nasopharyngeal tumor, and immunodeficiency. These problems can usually be uncovered by detailed history taking, careful physical examination, and, directed by these results, appropriate laboratory tests and, in selected cases, referral.

MANAGEMENT OF RECURRENT ACUTE OTITIS MEDIA

Children with recurrent AOM should be given a trial of prophylaxis with an oral antimicrobial agent. Amoxicillin, 20 mg per kg in a single nightly dose, or, in penicillin-allergic patients, sulfisoxazole (Gantrisin), 50 to 75 mg per kg in one or two divided doses, is usually recommended. The 1993 edition of the *Physicians' Desk Reference* states (without further comment) that trimethoprim-sulfamethoxazole is "not indicated for prophylactic or prolonged administration in otitis media at any age." The antimicrobial agent selected for prophylaxis should be continued for 3 to 6 months (usually during the colder weather months) or, in some cases, longer. Recurrences of AOM should be treated with an antimicrobial agent different from the prophylactic agent, which should be temporarily discontinued. If a patient develops a few such "breakthrough" episodes of AOM while on prophylaxis, especially within a short period of time, or if a patient is not compliant with medications, then referral to an otolaryngologist is appropriate. Children on prophylaxis should be examined at regular intervals (e.g., every 6 weeks) so that middle ear status can be documented and inquiry can be made about potential adverse effects of treatment.

MANAGEMENT OF CHRONIC SUPPURATIVE OTITIS MEDIA

Management of children with CSOM should begin with a trial of antimicrobial therapy with an oral second-line agent and ototopical drops. The physician should clean the external auditory canal before the start of ototopical therapy. Even though ototopical drops that contain potentially ototoxic agents (e.g., neomycin [Cortisporin, Coly-Mycin S Otic]) have been prescribed often, caution should be exercised, and perhaps even informed consent considered, when these agents are used in patients with nonintact tympanic membranes. When Cortisporin is prescribed for such patients, it is preferable to use the suspension rather than the solution because the latter may cause discomfort. If otorrhea does not resolve after such initial antimicrobial therapy, referral to an otolaryngologist is usually appropriate for further evaluation and treatment. Management often includes obtaining of cultures from the site of the perforation or tympanostomy tube, further investigation for underlying problems such as cholesteatoma, frequent aspiration of the ear, and ototopical and parenteral antimicrobial therapy.

ACUTE BRONCHITIS

method of
RICHARD B. BROWN, M.D.
Baystate Medical Center
Springfield, Massachusetts

Acute bronchitis represents two clinical syndromes: (1) acute infectious bronchitis that may occur in otherwise healthy persons of any age and (2) acute exacerbations of chronic bronchitis, more commonly seen in older persons (e.g., >65). Differentiation between these entities is important for management. Acute bronchitis in otherwise healthy persons usually manifests with the onset of a cough syndrome, often associated with other manifestations of upper or lower respiratory disease. Thus patients may, for example, have concurrent pharyngitis, laryngitis, or rhinitis. Constitutional symptoms are common, fever may be of any level, and cough is often productive. In some instances, such as viral influenza, bronchitis may be underemphasized because of other overriding complaints. Most cases are viral, and rhinovirus represents the most common agent associated with this syndrome. Table 1 depicts common etiologies of acute bronchitis, and the approximate percentage of cases in which this illness is likely to be noted.

Therapy for acute infectious bronchitis is supportive, with careful attention paid to hydration, relief of cough, and preservation of well-being. Antitussives such as dextromethorphan and codeine occasionally play a role but should not be employed if cough is productive. Antipyretics or anti-inflammatory agents are also often employed for symptom relief. Most patients improve within 1 week.

Potentially treatable causes of acute infectious bronchitis include *Mycoplasma pneumoniae, Chlamydia pneumoniae* (previously known as TWAR agent), *Bor-*

TABLE 1. Etiologies for Acute Infectious Bronchitis

Pathogen	Percentage*
Influenza, parainfluenza virus	95
Adenovirus	70
Respiratory syncytial virus	75
Rhinovirus	40–80
Coronavirus	40–80
Others	Variable
Organisms	
Mycoplasma pneumoniae	Most
Chlamydia pneumoniae	Many
Bordetella pertussis	95–100
Legionella pneumophila	Few

*Percentage of patients with selected pathogen whose disease is associated with acute bronchitis.

detella pertussis, and *Legionella pneumophila.* All are sensitive to erythromycin. The first two should be considered when cough is prolonged beyond 1 week or if the epidemiologic history is suggestive of these diseases. *B. pertussis* (whooping cough) should be considered in adults with prolonged afebrile nocturnal cough syndromes and can be confirmed by culture or antigen testing of nasopharyngeal specimens. The characteristic manifestation with whooping is rarely noted in adults. An uncommon syndrome associated with *L. pneumophila,* Pontiac fever, has been observed in rare cases. The manifestation is that of a self-limited influenza-like syndrome that is likely to remit spontaneously before erythromycin would be initiated. Bacteria such as *Streptococcus pneumoniae* and *Haemophilus influenzae* rarely are associated with acute infectious bronchitis.

TREATMENT

Most cases of acute infectious bronchitis should not be treated with antimicrobial agents. However, for disease that extends beyond 1 week or if there is a high probability of treatable illness, erythromycin, 250 to 500 mg daily for 10 to 14 days, is rational. The role for other antibiotics in treatment is not as well defined. Studies with tetracyclines (doxycycline) and trimethoprim-sulfamethoxazole have shown little benefit over placebo. For bronchitis associated with viral influenza, amantadine hydrochloride (Symmetrel) in doses of 100 to 200 mg daily for 5 days is sensible treatment in high-risk patients.

ACUTE EXACERBATIONS OF CHRONIC BRONCHITIS

Chronic bronchitis, defined as the production of sputum during most days for at least 3 consecutive months for at least 2 years, is most often associated with cigarette smoking. The likelihood of contracting this disease increases with the amount of smoking and can resolve with discon-

TABLE 2. **Antibiotics for Acute Exacerbations of Chronic Bronchitis**

Antibiotic	Dose
First-Line	
Amoxicillin (Amoxyl)	250–500 mg tid
Doxycycline (Vibramycin)	100 mg bid
Cefaclor (Ceclor)	250–500 mg tid
Trimethoprim-sulfamethoxazole (Bactrim, Septra)	160/800 mg bid
Cefuroxime axetil (Ceftin)	250–500 mg bid
Amoxicillin-clavulanate (Augmentin)	500 mg tid
Second-Line*	
Cefprozil (Cefzil)	500 mg bid
Cefpodoxime proxetil (Vantin)	200 mg bid
Loracarbef (Lorabid)	400 mg bid
Clarithromycin (Biaxin)	250–500 mg bid
Azithromycin (Zithromax)†	500 mg stat, 250 mg qd
Not Recommended‡	
Erythromycin	
Cefixime (Suprax)	
Quinolones (Cipro, Maxaquin, Oflox, etc.)	
Clindamycin (Cleocin)	
Penicillin V (Pen-Vee K, Veetids, etc.)	

*Generally newer products lacking convincing evidence of superiority over first-line agents.

†Course of therapy is 5 days.

‡Lack significant activity against at least one of common pathogens in acute exacerbations of chronic bronchitis.

tinuation of this habit. Acute exacerbations of chronic bronchitis (AECB) become clinically documented by increased cough, usually associated with a change in the amount, character, and color of sputum. Most commonly, patients note a change in sputum from mucoid or clear to green or yellow. Material becomes more viscous and copious. Hemoptysis is unusual. Mild constitutional symptoms may occur, but high fever is unusual. Some worsening of respiratory status is generally observed.

The degree of respiratory distress determines the need for hospitalization. Most patients can be treated in an ambulatory manner, and no specific laboratory testing is indicated. However, Gram's stain of expectorated sputum can provide useful information, primarily in differentiating between exacerbations that are allergy-related (in the presence of eosinophils) and those that are likely to be infectious (in the presence of polymorphonuclear leukocytes). Although the precise etiology of AECB remains controversial, many cases appear to be bacterial, and most should be treated with antibiotics.

TREATMENT

S. pneumoniae, H. influenzae (nontypeable, non-encapsulated), *Moraxella catarrhalis,* and other oral flora are generally implicated, and re-

cent data suggest a role in treatment for appropriate antimicrobial agents. At least 16% of strains of nontypeable *H. influenzae* and over 75% of those of *M. catarrhalis* produce beta-lactamases and are therefore resistant to ampicillin and amoxicillin. However, data demonstrating enhanced outcomes with agents that are beta-lactamase–stable are unavailable. Table 2 depicts useful antibiotics and doses; the choice of drug depends on host factors (e.g., allergy, concurrent medications, underlying diseases) and cost. Length of therapy is similarly controversial. Most physicians treat for 7 to 14 days, although some recent data suggest that courses of 3 to 5 days may suffice. According to recent information in a subpopulation of patients with AECB who were intubated in an intensive care unit, approximately 50% harbored no identifiable pathogens. The etiology of AECB is obscure, and antibiotics may not be indicated.

Prevention of AECB depends on discontinuation of smoking, judicious use of prophylactic antibiotics (generally doxycycline) in selected patients with chronic bronchitis and multiple exacerbations, and vaccination with both pneumococcal vaccine (once) and viral influenza vaccine (annually). There is no role for *H. influenzae* b (Hib) vaccine. Amantidine hydrochloride (Symmetrel) may be employed prophylactically to prevent viral influenza A in selected clinical circumstances.

BACTERIAL PNEUMONIA

method of
STEPHEN B. GREENBERG, M.D.
Baylor College of Medicine
Houston, Texas

Community-acquired pneumonia occurs in approximately 3 million persons per year in the United States and accounts for up to 500,000 hospital admissions. Pneumonia is the sixth leading cause of death in the United States and the third most common hospital-acquired infection. The elderly, immunosuppressed patients, and persons with underlying diseases are particularly susceptible to pneumonia. In patients with community-acquired pneumonia, common underlying diseases include chronic obstructive pulmonary disease (COPD), alcoholism, malignancy, heart disease, diabetes mellitus, chronic renal failure, and acquired immune deficiency syndrome (AIDS). These underlying conditions, as well as mechanical ventilation, also predispose patients to increased risk of nosocomial pneumonia.

ETIOLOGY

Bacteria must adhere to and colonize the upper airway to cause pneumonia. Aspiration of the adherent bacteria from the oropharynx is important in the pathogenesis of this infection. Exceptions to this mechanism include *Pseudomonas aeruginosa,* which can colonize the trachea directly, and *Mycobacteria tuberculosis* and *Legionella* spp., which reach the lung through inhaled airborne droplets. Outbreaks of pneumococcal pneumonia have occurred in closed or crowded populations, which suggests the possibility of aerosol colonization before the development of pneumonia.

The spectrum of organisms isolated from community-acquired pneumonias differs significantly from that of organisms isolated from nosocomial pneumonias (Table 1). Although the reported incidence from published series ranges widely, *Streptococcus pneumoniae* probably accounts for one- to two-thirds of community-acquired pneumonias. *Haemophilus influenzae, Staphylococcus aureus,* enteric gram-negative rods, and anaerobes account for the remainder of the bacterial isolates. Atypical agents such as viruses, *Mycoplasma pneumoniae,* chlamydia, Q fever, and *Legionella* spp. probably account for 15 to 30% of pneumonias in hospitalized patients. Even with the best and most recent diagnostic techniques, approximately 20% of cases have no identifiable pathogen.

Epidemiologic factors such as the patient's age, the season, the geographic location, and underlying conditions may help suggest a specific etiology.

Patients with COPD or a recent history of smoking are prone to infection with *H. influenzae, Moraxella catarrhalis,* and *Legionella* spp. Gram-negative aerobes are more commonly found in critically ill, debilitated, and alcoholic patients. *S. aureus* is isolated after influenzae virus infection and in intravenous drug users. Although pneumonia caused by *S. pneumoniae* can occur throughout the year, it peaks during the winter months. *Legionella* spp. and *Mycoplasma pneumoniae* are more commonly isolated in summer and fall. A history of environmental exposure to birds, rabbits, cattle, or water-heating units may be clues to infections such as psittacosis, tularemia, Q fever, or legionellosis.

Nosocomial pneumonias are caused predominantly by gram-negative organisms such as *P. aeruginosa, Acinetobacter calcoaceticus,* and *Klebsiella pneumoniae.* In 30 to 50% of cases, more than one organism is isolated in specimens from the lower respiratory tract.

TABLE 1. **Etiology of Community-Acquired and Nosocomial Pneumonias**

Agent	Community	Nosocomial
Streptococcus pneumoniae	33–67%	6%
Mycoplasma pneumoniae	9%	—
Haemophilus influenzae	7%	5%
Virus	7%	—
Legionella spp.	6%	—
Chlamydia spp.	6%	—
Staphylococcus aureus	3%	8%
Aerobic gram-negative bacteria	5%	80%

The mortality rate for hospital-acquired pneumonia approximates 50% and has not changed significantly since 1970.

DIAGNOSIS

Manifestations of acute bacterial pneumonia typically include sudden onset of fever, chills, cough productive of purulent sputum, and pleuritic chest pain. On physical examination, the patient is often acutely ill, febrile, and tachypneic. A new infiltrate appearing on chest x-ray is common.

In the elderly, nonrespiratory symptoms such as altered mental status, worsening of underlying COPD, and heart failure may be prominent. Patients requiring hospitalization for presumed community-acquired pneumonia are more likely to have a comorbid illness, to be over the age of 60, and to have experienced symptoms for less than 7 or more than 28 days. Possible aspiration, a history of lung disease, and involvement of more than one lobe are additional variables that help predict the need for hospitalization.

No clinical characteristics differentiate among the common bacterial pneumonias. Laboratory diagnosis involves obtaining sputum samples and blood cultures. Although peripheral leukocytosis with a leftward shift is common, leukopenia can also occur. Gram's stains of smears of sputum demonstrate polymorphonuclear leukocytes (PMNs) as a predominant cell type. An adequate sputum specimen contains fewer than 10 squamous epithelial cells and more than 25 PMNs per low-power field. For community-acquired cases, sputum cultures are not reliable. Sputum counterimmunoelectrophoresis for *S. pneumoniae* appears to be sensitive and specific, but it is not available everywhere. In ventilated hospitalized patients, quantitative bacteriologic methods involving bronchoalveolar lavage or protected bronchoscopy brushes are necessary for improving the rate of etiologic diagnosis of nosocomial pneumonias.

Chest x-ray findings are not specific or unique to any one bacterial species. Lobar or segmental infiltrates are common. With *S. aureus* and *S. pneumoniae,* parapneumonic effusions are common. Cavitation can be seen with *S. aureus, S. pneumoniae,* anaerobes, and *M. tuberculosis.* Bulging of the minor fissure in *K. pneumoniae* may be observed but is not unique to this pathogen.

TREATMENT

Before presumptive therapy for community-acquired pneumonia is initiated, the need for hospitalization should be assessed. Indications for admission are as follows:

1. A severe abnormality in a vital sign.
2. Altered mental status.
3. A complication such as meningitis, emphysema, or endocarditis.
4. Hypoxemia.
5. A comorbid illness such as alcoholism, COPD, or diabetes mellitus.
6. A severe abnormality in a laboratory finding.

One published series reported that the presence of more than one of the following risk factors was predictive of a complicated course and should be considered an indication for hospitalization:

1. Age greater than 65 years.
2. Comorbid illness.
3. Temperature greater than 38.3° C.
4. Immunosuppression.
5. High-risk etiology such as staphylococcal, gram-negative rod, aspiration, or postobstructive pneumonia.

Community-Acquired Pneumonia

Initial therapy should be guided by the most likely causative pathogen in a specific epidemiologic setting. In patients with no underlying risk factors who are not severely ill, macrolide antibiotics such as erythromycin (500 mg every 6 hours) or one of the new broad-spectrum macrolides (clarithromycin [Biaxin] or azithromycin [Zithromax]) should be effective (Table 2). Most bacterial pneumonias that follow influenza are still associated with *S. pneumoniae;* during influenza outbreaks, however, pneumonias should be treated initially with a penicillinase-resistant anti-staphylococcal penicillin such as nafcillin (Unipen), 1 gm every 4 hours. A second-generation cephalosporin, cefuroxime (Zinacef), 750 mg to 1.5 gm every 8 hours, is appropriate for patients with significant underlying disease who are at risk for infection with *H. influenzae, S. aureus, M. catarrhalis,* or *K. pneumoniae.*

In patients known to be immunosuppressed, initial therapy with broad-spectrum antibiotics should be started. A third-generation cephalosporin (ceftazidime [Fortaz, Tazidime]), 1 gm every 8 to 12 hours, or ticarcillin-clavulanate (Timentin), 3.1 gm every 6 hours, or imipenem-cilastatin (Primaxin), 500 mg every 6 to 8 hours, should provide adequate initial coverage. If *Legionella* or an atypical pneumonia is likely, the addition of erythromycin would be appropriate. The combination of erythromycin with a third-generation cephalosporin is often used as initial coverage

TABLE 2. **Presumptive Treatment of Community-Acquired Pneumonias**

Underlying Factor	Antibiotic
Normal host	Macrolide
Chronic obstructive pulmonary disease, alcoholism, elderly, nursing home patient	Second-generation cephalosporin and macrolide
Immunosuppression, recent hospitalization	Third-generation cephalosporin or imipenem-cilastatin and macrolide

pending laboratory results. Intravenous erythromycin has been linked to phlebitis, and oral preparations may produce significant gastrointestinal side effects.

Duration of treatment for most patients should be 5 to 7 days. If the initial response in a hospitalized patient is satisfactory, the patient can complete the antibiotic regimen at home. Patients with bacteremic pneumonia should receive parenteral antibiotics for at least 7 days before a change to an appropriate oral regimen is considered. Home intravenous antibiotic therapy can be useful in patients well enough to be discharged but in whom parenteral antibiotics are needed. Cephalosporins with a long half-life (e.g., ceftriaxone [Rocephin]), 1 gm every 12 to 24 hours, may be useful.

Nosocomial Pneumonia

No one antibiotic regimen has been reported to be significantly more effective than another. The high mortality rate is attributable to host factors as well as to the appropriate antibiotic choices. Gram-negative pathogens such as *Pseudomonas, Enterobacter,* and *Acinetobacter* spp. may be associated with a high mortality and a poor response to antibiotics. Presumptive therapy should include a third-generation cephalosporin such as ceftazidime, 1 gm every 8 hours, or cefotaxime (Claforan), 2 gm every 8 hours, plus an aminoglycoside such as gentamicin (Garamycin) or tobramycin (Nebcin), 5 to 7 mg per kg per day every 8 to 12 hours, on the basis of renal function. Other regimens could include imipenem-cilastatin, 500 mg every 6 hours; ticarcillin-clavulanate, 3.1 gm every 6 hours; or aztreonam (Azactam), 1 to 2 gm every 8 hours. Aztreonam has activity against only aerobic gram-negative organisms and not against gram-positive cocci or anaerobes. After a specific organism is microbiologically confirmed, the antibiotic regimen can be altered and narrowed to the least expensive and least toxic regimen.

The treatment of community-acquired and nosocomial pneumonias is determined by the epidemiologic clues in the history, by comorbid illnesses, and by host factors. Outpatient and inpatient treatment of community-acquired pneumonia are dependent on known risk factors for a complicated course, for increased morbidity, and for mortality. Bed rest, supplemental oxygen, and appropriate antibiotics are the cornerstones of treatment. The rate of mortality from nosocomial pneumonia, particularly in ventilated patients, remains high despite the excellent range of antibiotics available. Newer, innovative preventive measures and treatment interventions are being tested in order to lower this excessive mortality rate.

VIRAL RESPIRATORY INFECTIONS

method of
JANET ENGLUND, M.D., and
VERNON KNIGHT, M.D.
Baylor College of Medicine
Houston, Texas

Respiratory viruses are the most frequent causes of infectious illness of humans. The incidence of such illnesses is several times higher among infants than among adults, with a gradual reduction to adult levels by adolescence. The majority of these illness resolve in a week or more without sequelae, but otitis media in children and sinusitis in adults may complicate a small percentage of these cases. More serious and less frequent are infections that involve the lower respiratory tract. In infants and young children, the infection may consist of croup, tracheobronchitis, bronchiolitis, or pneumonia. Croup is often a discrete occurrence, whereas the others occur in various combinations. In older children and adults, the principal syndromes are laryngitis, tracheobronchitis, and bronchopneumonia. At all ages, underlying illness is associated with greater severity. In the aged or immunosuppressed patients, pneumonia is a common and often serious complication of lower respiratory tract viral infections. Secondary bacterial infections that follow viral infections may have severe sequelae.

The causes of acute respiratory illnesses in children, in decreasing order of frequency, are parainfluenza viruses, respiratory syncytial virus (RSV), influenza A and B, and adenoviruses. Less common are rhinoviruses, enteroviruses, herpesviruses, and coronaviruses. *Mycoplasma pneumoniae* causes illnesses that resemble those caused by viruses and is about as frequent as influenza virus. In adults, rhinoviruses cause about 40% of infections; the role of the other agents in such illnesses is consequently reduced. The rate of mortality from these diseases is low unless there is serious underlying illness. In immunocompromised patients, herpes simplex, cytomegalovirus, and herpes zoster may cause acute and chronic respiratory tract infections.

A conspicuous syndrome in children is viral croup characterized by laryngitis, barky cough, and, if severe, increased respiratory difficulty secondary to subglottic edema. Croup is caused mostly by parainfluenza viruses, adenoviruses, RSV, and occasionally influenza viruses and measles. Most patients with viral croup are under 3 years of age and rarely have high fevers or a toxic appearance. However, parainfluenza type 3 may cause high fever in a young child. No specific antiviral therapy is available, but most children with viral croup respond to inhalation of cold, damp air (e.g., when taken outside at night). On occasion, hospitalization is necessary. A cool mist tent with oxygen, if needed, and administration of aerosolized racemic epinephrine in saline are usually sufficient to decrease respiratory distress. In rare cases, a child may require intubation. The value of steroids in the treatment of viral croup has not been established.

Rapid viral diagnostic tests that can be performed on respiratory secretions are commercially available for RSV, parainfluenza, and influenza. Secondary bacterial infection is uncommon but is not necessarily ruled out by a positive result of a test for a viral agent. A diagnosis of acute measles, herpesvirus, or cytomegalovirus infections can be made by the presence of specific IgM antibody. Other viral agents require culture or paired serologic tests for diagnosis.

TREATMENT FOR SPECIFIC PATHOGENS

Acyclovir (Zovirax) is the drug of choice for infections in immunocompromised patients with either herpes simplex, varicella, or zoster infections. For such potentially serious infections, intravenous administration is preferable to oral preparations. The intravenous dosage is 750 mg per m^2 of body surface area (5 mg per kg) per day divided into three equal doses for herpes simplex infections. For varicella infections (either chickenpox or zoster), the intravenous dosage is 1500 mg per m^2 of body surface area (10 mg per kg) per day divided into three equal doses. Adequate hydration must be maintained, because the drug is excreted by the kidney and may precipitate in the tubules if renal blood flow is impaired. The dosage must also be adjusted downward for patients with impaired renal function.

Prophylaxis is also available for high-risk exposures to varicella, consisting of varicella-zoster immune globulin (VZIG). The dosage is 1 vial (125 units) per 10 kg of body weight (minimum of 125 units and maximum of 625 units). It should be administered intramuscularly soon after a known exposure and preferably within 48 to 96 hours for maximal benefit. Recent studies have demonstrated some clinical benefit in the treatment of chickenpox with oral acyclovir in otherwise healthy children and adults who received therapy within 24 hours of the diagnosis. Because of the higher incidence of varicella pneumonia and complications, the use of oral acyclovir, 800 mg five times daily, should be considered in adolescents and adults.

Influenza

Immunization against influenza A and B each fall is recommended for adults and children at high risk for severe influenzal disease. These people include patients with underlying cardiac or respiratory diseases or chronic disorders such as diabetes mellitus or renal diseases, residents of chronic care facilities and nursing homes, immunosuppressed patients, and healthy adults over 65 years of age. Household members in contact with patients at high risk for severe disease should also be immunized to decrease the risk of transmission to susceptible persons. For the same reason, health care personnel in direct contact with patients should receive annual immunization. In addition, children receiving chronic salicylate therapy should be vaccinated because of the possible increased risk for the development of Reye's syndrome.

Vaccine should be administered to children under 9 years of age in two doses for the first immunization and in one dose in subsequent years. For infants aged 6 months to 3 years, the dose is 0.25 mL given subcutaneously. For older children, the dose is 0.5 mL given subcutaneously. For adults and children over 9 years of age, a single 0.5-mL dose of whole or split virus vaccine given subcutaneously is sufficient. For maximal benefit, immunization should begin in the fall before the onset of the influenza season.

An alternative method of prophylaxis against influenza A virus is the daily use of oral amantadine (Symmetrel). This is not useful for influenza B prophylaxis. It can also be used as early therapy if begun at the onset of symptoms and continued for 2 to 7 days. The dosage for children is 4 to 8 mg per kg daily divided every 12 hours, not to exceed 150 mg in children under 9 years of age. For older children and adults, the dosage is 100 mg twice daily.

Measles

Although measles is a systemic exanthematous disease, respiratory involvement may be severe, especially in pregnant women, in whom severe pneumonia may occur. Bacterial complications of measles, particularly otitis media and bronchopneumonia, are not uncommon in normal hosts. In immunocompromised patients, severe progressive pneumonia may lead to death. Prevention is most desirable and is achieved with the use of measles vaccine (or combined measles-mumps-rubella vaccine) administered twice, once when the patient is 15 months old and a booster at school age. It can be given to younger infants (as young as 6 months) if there is a significant community outbreak, but such infants nevertheless require the two later doses at the recommended times. Pregnant women and seronegative immunocompromised patients with significant exposure can receive prophylaxis with serum immunoglobulin (0.5 mL per kg to a maximum of 15 mL) given intramuscularly.

Immunocompromised patients can also acquire a severe progressive pneumonia with the appearance of nodular infiltrates. No specific antiviral therapy for measles has been proved efficacious in well-controlled clinical trials.

Respiratory Syncytial Virus

Ribavirin aerosol is the only specific treatment for RSV infection. Controlled clinical trials showed a reduction in virus shedding and shortened illness in treated patients. Although it has not been approved for treatment of seriously ill intubated patients, a recent controlled study demonstrated its effectiveness without significant side effects or problems with its administration.

In 1991, the American Academy of Pediatrics recommended ribavirin aerosol for infants at high risk for severe complicated disease (e.g., those with congenital heart disease, bronchopulmonary disorders, or immune deficiencies); for infants under 6 weeks of age; and for infants severely ill with an arterial carbon dioxide tension ($PaCO_2$) of less than 65 mmHg or an increasing $PaCO_2$ before intubation. Ribavirin can be nebulized into a hood, tent, or mask from a solution containing 20 mg per mL of the drug dissolved in sterile water by an aerosol generator supplied by the manufacturer of the drug. The treatment is administered 12 to 18 hours daily for 3 to 7 days. Treatment with ribavirin aerosol should be monitored by experienced personnel in order to avoid the occasional occurrence of obstruction of tubing or obstruction within the respiratory tract resulting from precipitation of drug.

The use of aerosolized bronchodilators such as albuterol sulfate (Proventil) may be beneficial in certain patients with RSV-associated bronchospasm. Nebulized albuterol in saline can be administered by face mask or inhaler every 2 to 4 hours. Initial decreases in arterial oxygen tension, followed after approximately 30 minutes by improvement in oxygenation as measured by pulse oximetry, have been noted when this regimen is followed in some infants. Oral or intravenous bronchodilators (oral theophylline preparations and aminophylline drips) have been less effective in producing improvements in oxygenation and have more undesirable side effects: tachycardia, restlessness, and irritability. The use of corticosteroids in treatment of bronchiolitis has not been adequately evaluated.

SYMPTOMATIC TREATMENT

Other therapy for upper respiratory infections should consist of symptomatic treatment for rhinorrhea, cough, and fever, if present. Acetaminophen (Tylenol) is preferable to aspirin for fever control in children because of the association of aspirin administration with Reye's syndrome after viral infections, notably influenza and varicella. The dosage for children is 10 to 15 mg per kg per dose, given orally or rectally every 4 to 6 hours as needed; adults can take 325 to 650 mg per dose orally every 4 to 6 hours.

Topical treatment for rhinitis (0.25% or 0.50% phenylephrine hydrochloride [Neo-Synephrine]) is preferable to systemic therapy with drying agents such as pseudoephedrine (Sudafed) for children and adults, because there are fewer undesirable side effects such as drowsiness, reduced clearance of lower respiratory secretions, and jitteriness. However, topical agents should not be used for more than a few days because they may produce rebound mucosal edema and rhinitis (rhinitis medicamentosa). For young infants, saline nose drops and gentle suction with a bulb syringe should be sufficient; neither topical nor systemic agents should be employed, other than for fever control.

Antihistamines have little role in the treatment of acute respiratory viral infections. They do not decrease the risk of acquiring otitis media or sinusitis by decreasing nasopharyngeal secretions, nor do they hasten the resolution of middle ear effusion once otitis media has been effectively treated with antibiotics.

MYCOPLASMAL AND VIRAL PNEUMONIAS

method of
MICHAEL J. MOSKAL, D.O.
Broadlawns Medical Center
Des Moines, Iowa

MYCOPLASMA PNEUMONIAE

Discovered in 1944 as the Eaton agent, *Mycoplasma pneumoniae* is now recognized as the most common cause of community-acquired pneumonia, accounting for up to 20% of cases in the general population and as high as 50% in closed populations, such as college dormitories and military bases. *M. pneumoniae* can cause pneumonia in patients of all ages, but persons between the ages of 5 and 25 years appear to be at particular risk. Infection with this organism can be endemic and occur in all seasons, but, interestingly, epidemics occur at 4- to 7-year intervals, with a predilection for fall.

Infection is transmitted by respiratory droplet secretion. After invading the respiratory tract, *M. pneumoniae* must attach to the respiratory epithelium to cause disease. While remaining extracellular, it is able to initiate a series of events leading to inflammation, ciliostasis, and, finally, respiratory epithelial cell destruction.

After a 2- to 3-week incubation period, the onset of illness is heralded by a gradual prodrome of fever, malaise, myalgia, headache, and sore throat. Coryza is uncommon, which may be helpful from a differential diagnosis standpoint. A cough usually starts 3 to 5 days after symptoms begin. Initially described as nonproductive, it may become productive with time. Associated symptoms may include chills, nausea, vomiting, abdominal pain, and diarrhea. Rales are the most common physical finding, and wheezing may be present in up to 40% of affected children. Patients with hemoglobinopathies such as sickle cell disease are at high risk for severe disease.

The radiographic pattern of pneumonia associated with *M. pneumoniae* is often described as atypical, reticular, and interstitial, involving only the lower lobe of one lung field. In some cases, however, involvement is bilateral, occurs in any lung field, and is lobar in appearance. Small pleural effusions are demonstrated in 20% of cases, and hilar adenopathy is not uncommon.

The diagnosis of *M. pneumoniae* infection is based primarily on clinical suspicion. Immunoglobulin M (IgM) cold agglutinins, although not highly sensitive or specific, are helpful at titers higher than 1:32 and appear after the first or second week of illness. A rapid cold agglutinin screen can be performed at the patient's bedside by adding 0.4 mL of blood to a standard blue-topped prothrombin tube. After the tube is placed in ice water for 15 to 30 seconds, the tube is tilted and observed for the presence of coarse floccular agglutination of red blood cells, which is correlated with a cold agglutinin titer of 1:64 or higher. Complement fixation is readily available, but acute and convalescent titers are required. This test has been criticized for its lack of specificity. Culture requires special media with recovery, and identification often takes 2 to 3 weeks. New methods, particularly enzyme-linked immunosorbent assay (ELISA), DNA probe, and polymerase chain reaction, may aid rapid identification in the future.

Treatment

Because *M. pneumoniae* lacks a cell wall, penicillin and its derivatives and cephalosporins are ineffective antimicrobial agents. Erythromycin and tetracycline are effective antibiotics for the treatment of *M. pneumoniae* infection. Either drug can be given at a dose of 30 to 50 mg per kg daily in divided doses for 10 to 14 days. Tetracycline should be avoided in children under 8 years of age because of the drug's potential for permanently staining the teeth. Although neither drug eradicates the organism from the respiratory tract, it has been clearly shown that the duration of symptoms and clearance of pulmonary infiltrates are markedly reduced in treated patients.

Extrapulmonary Manifestations. Meningoencephalitis is the most common complication, occurring in up to 7% of hospitalized patients with pneumonia. However, a wide variety of other central nervous system derangements, such as transverse myelitis, ascending paralysis, and acute psychosis, have also been reported. Other nonrespiratory complications include Coombs' positive hemolytic anemia with IgM cold agglutinins directed against the I antigen of the red blood cells. The degree of hemolysis is usually subclinical, but significant anemia has been reported. Exanthems associated with *M. pneumoniae* range from a mild macular-papular rash to Stevens-Johnson syndrome. Pericarditis, myocarditis, congestive heart failure, and heart block have all been reported in association as well. More unusual complications include hepatic dysfunction, a rheumatic fever–like illness, and glomerulonephritis.

VIRAL PNEUMONIAS

Viral pneumonia is a leading cause of disease in adults and children; children under the age of 5 years are most often affected. Although a variety of viral agents can cause pneumonia, a majority are caused by respiratory syncytial virus (RSV); parainfluenzas I, II, and III; adenovirus; and the influenza viruses (Table 1).

RSV is the most common and is often a serious cause of viral pneumonia in children under 5 years of age. RSV epidemics usually occur from early winter to late spring and are heralded by increasing numbers of children presenting with coryza, anorexia, and a dry, tight, nonproductive cough. Fever is frequently absent. Auscultatory findings include rhonchi, fine rales, and, notably, wheezing. Infants are prone to severe disease, and respiratory distress, listlessness, and apnea may develop. Seriously ill patients may require mechanical ventilation. The overall rate of mortality approaches 2% and is higher in children with underlying conditions such as congenital heart disease, bronchopulmonary dysplasia, and cystic fibrosis.

Radiographic findings may be normal but usually show hyperexpansion with air trapping, infiltrates, and atelectasis. Secondary bacterial invasion must be considered when consolidation is present.

Diagnosis is based on the constellation of seasonal occurrence, clinical findings, radiographic features, and the detection of viral antigen in nasal washings. Several commercially available rapid immunoassay diagnostic methods detect RSV antigen with sensitivities of approximately 85% and specificities of 94 to 100%.

Treatment

Treatment is primarily supportive for the majority of patients and consists of humidified oxygen and fluids. Measurement of oxygen saturation with pulse oximetry is important in tachypneic ill children because the clinical assessment of oxygen desaturation is at best difficult. In fact, oxygen saturation levels of less than 90 to 95% may be the single best predictor of severity of illness. The use of bronchodilators is controversial but may be helpful in some cases. Albuterol inhalations at 0.01 to 0.03 mL per kg every 2 to 6 hours have been shown to improve oxygenation and decrease respiratory effort in some patients. Likewise, subcutaneous epinephrine, 0.01 mL per kg of a 1:1000 dilution, has also been demonstrated to be beneficial.

The efficacy of corticosteroids is questionable. Ribavirin (Virazole) has been shown to be benefi-

TABLE 1. **Common Causes of Viral Pneumonia: Representative Findings**

Characteristic	Parainfluenza	Respiratory Syncytial Virus	Adenovirus	Influenza
Age	<3 years	<5 years	All ages, military recruits, but majority <9 years	All ages
Season	I, II: fall III: year round	Winter–spring	Spring–summer	Winter–spring
Common Clinical Findings in Addition to Pneumonia				
Fever	≤25%	26–50%	76–100%	76–100%
Coryza	51–75%	76–100%	26–50%	26–50%
Pharyngitis	26–50%	≤25%	51–75%	51–75%
Cough	76–100%	76–100%	≤25%	76–100%
Conjunctivitis	≤25%	≤25%	51–76%	26–50%

cial in the treatment of RSV pneumonia but is reserved for children who are at high risk for significant morbidity and mortality (i.e., very young patients and those with serious underlying disease). Ribavirin is delivered directly to the respiratory tract via aerosol by oxygen mask, hood, mist tent, or endotracheal tube, depending on the severity of illness. Improvement is often noted within 24 to 48 hours after the drug is administered. Treatment duration is usually 3 to 7 days. Pregnant medical personnel and pregnant caretakers should avoid contact with ribavirin because of the potential for toxicity and teratogenicity to the fetus. Infants with documented RSV infection are at increased risk (33 to 50%) for recurrent wheezing episodes with future viral respiratory tract infections.

Parainfluenza viruses are better known for causing croup but are the second leading cause of viral pneumonia in children. Parainfluenzas I and II typically occur in the fall, often in an epidemic manner. Parainfluenza III occurs year round and accounts for the majority of cases of parainfluenza pneumonia. Ribavirin may be an effective antiviral agent in severe parainfluenza disease.

Adenovirus, a common cause of upper respiratory tract infection, has been estimated to cause 7% of viral pneumonias. Lower respiratory tract disease is usually mild in children and is associated with serotypes 3, 7, and 21. A fulminant course leads to death in rare instances. Because no pathognomonic features are associated with adenoviral disease, isolation of the virus is required for diagnosis.

Influenza can either be caused by type A or type B viruses. Type A infection usually occurs in winter to early spring in epidemics, and the epidemics last 4 to 8 weeks within a community. Because this organism shows frequent antigenic shifts, patients continue to be susceptible to it even though they have immunity to other serotypes. Type B influenza is a less frequent cause of disease and has demonstrated less antigenic drift. However, clinical manifestations are similar for each type. Persons older than 65 years, young infants, and debilitated patients are at highest risk for acquiring pneumonia. The pulmonary manifestations of this disease may be mild to severe, and it is not unusual for secondary bacterial infection to occur. The most common bacterial pathogens are *Streptococcus pneumoniae, Staphylococcus aureus,* and *Haemophilus influenzae.* Prevention may be the best means of treating this disease.

An up-to-date influenza A vaccine is available annually and is administered from midfall to early winter. Adults and children considered to be at high risk for severe influenza A disease (i.e., the elderly and patients with underlying conditions such as chronic pulmonary disease, clinically significant heart disease, hemoglobinopathies, symptomatic human immunodeficiency virus [HIV] infection, diabetes, and those individuals receiving immunosuppressive therapy) require priority and yearly vaccination. Vaccination is not routinely recommended for normal children at this time.

Initial management is dependent on the clinician's awareness of influenza outbreaks in the community and is initially supportive. Amantadine hydrochloride (Symmetrel) is active against influenza A (but not type B) and appears to benefit the clinical course of uncomplicated disease. It has also been useful as a prophylactic agent in patients exposed to type A disease (i.e., residents of nursing homes and of children's convalescent centers). The oral doses are 100 mg twice a day for adults (100 mg per day in patients over age 65) and 4.4 to 8.8 mg per kg per day (maximum 150 mg) in children 1 to 9 years of age. Children over 9 years can receive the adult dose. Treatment is started at the onset of symptoms and is continued for up to 7 days. Amantadine hydrochloride should be used with extreme caution in pregnant women and is contraindicated in nursing mothers. Ribavirin is also effective for influenza types A and B but should be reserved for critically ill patients.

LEGIONNAIRES' DISEASE AND PONTIAC FEVER

method of
PAUL H. EDELSTEIN, M.D.
University of Pennsylvania School of Medicine
Philadelphia, Pennsylvania

Legionnaires' disease is a type of pneumonia caused by *Legionella* bacteria, of which there are more than 35 species. The disease is the cause of about 1 to 5% of community-acquired pneumonias in adults but it is a very rare cause of pneumonia in normal children. Legionnaires' disease is a relatively common cause of nosocomial pneumonia, especially in immunocompromised patients. Because the disease occasionally causes epidemics, it has acquired an undeserved reputation for being especially lethal; if it is treated properly, the fatality rate is about the same as for pneumococcal pneumonia. Pontiac fever is a self-limited febrile systemic illness of several days' duration; its etiology is uncertain, but the disease is associated with exposure to *Legionella*-contaminated water.

DIAGNOSIS

Legionnaires' disease should be suspected in any adult with pneumonia. It is generally not possible to distinguish Legionnaires' disease on initial presentation from other causes of community-acquired pneumonia, on either clinical or roentgenographic grounds. Failure of the patient to respond to treatment with penicillin, cephalosporins, or aminoglycoside antibiotics should always lead to strong consideration of this disease, as should prior therapy with immunosuppressive doses of glucocorticosteroids, cyclosporine, or both. The only useful laboratory tests are those specific for Legionnaires' disease, such as sputum culture for *Legionella,* immunofluorescent detection of *Legionella* in sputum, DNA probe test of sputum for *Legionella,* detection of *Legionella* antigen in urine, and demonstration of *Legionella* antibodies in blood. If at all possible, culture diagnosis should be attempted in every suspected case of Legionnaires' disease. However, none of the specific tests is sensitive enough to exclude Legionnaires' disease in all situations. *Legionella* spp. are not detected on routine sputum culture. Isolation of *Pneumococcus, Haemophilus,* and even influenza virus from patients with pneumonia does not always rule out Legionnaires' disease, as co-infection with these agents may occur; in such patients, failure to respond to apparently appropriate therapy should lead to a search for Legionnaires' disease and, often, its empiric treatment.

TREATMENT

Specific Antimicrobial Therapy

Therapy for Legionnaires' disease differs from that of many other pneumonias because the bacteria are protected from normal host defenses and extracellular antibiotics by virtue of their presence and growth inside macrophages. Thus only antibiotics that enter and are active inside cells are effective against this disease. No prospective controlled clinical studies exist to guide therapy for this disease, and so the results of retrospective studies, case reports, and experimental studies are used to judge the potential effectiveness of therapy. Antimicrobial agents shown on this basis to be ineffective include cephalosporins (e.g., cefazolin [Ancef, Kefzol], ceftriaxone [Rocephin], and ceftazidime [Fortaz]), penicillins and penems (e.g., penicillin G, piperacillin [Pipracil], ampicillin, imipenem/cilastatin [Primaxin] ticarcillin/clavulanate [Timentin]), aminoglycosides (e.g., gentamicin and amikacin), monobactams (e.g., aztreonam), and lincosamides (e.g., clindamycin). The effectiveness of chloramphenicol is uncertain. Effective antimicrobial agents include the macrolides, fluoroquinolones, rifampin, trimethoprim-sulfamethoxazole, and tetracyclines. Animal model and in vitro studies show that the fluoroquinolone antibiotics are more active than is erythromycin, in that the former are bactericidal and the latter inhibitory only.

Within the macrolide group, clarithromycin (Biaxin) and azithromycin (Zithromax) appear to have advantages over erythromycin. Both of these new macrolides cause fewer gastrointestinal side effects than does erythromycin. Also, both of the newer macrolides are superior to erythromycin in nonhuman experimental studies. The very high tissue concentrations of azithromycin makes possible a short course of therapy. Prospective comparative human studies comparing erythromycin with newer or older drugs do not exist; thus the reason for the superior in vitro activity of the newer macrolide or fluoroquinolone antimicrobial agents is unknown. All of the newer macrolide and the fluoroquinolone antimicrobial agents are much more expensive than is erythromycin, and neither of the newer macrolide agents is available in intravenous form.

Because of the lack of comparative clinical antimicrobial agent efficacy studies for Legionnaires' disease, treatment of the disease is empiric (Table 1). The author gives erythromycin therapy alone to patients with mild disease. Although not always needed, intravenous erythromycin therapy is often advisable for the first several days of treatment until there has been a clinical response. No data exist regarding optimal dosage of erythromycin. The author gives the maximal tol-

TABLE 1. **Treatment of Legionnaires' Disease**

Antimicrobial Agent	Dosage
First Choice	
Erythromycin (E.E.S., Ilotycin)* ± rifampin (Rifadin)†‡	IV: 500 mg to 1 gm q 6 h PO: 500 mg of base equivalent q 6 h
Second Choices	
Azithromycin (Zithromax)§	PO: 500 mg on day 1, then 250 mg/day × 4 days
or	
Clarithromycin (Biaxin)‖	PO: 250 mg q 12 h
or	
Ciprofloxacin (Cipro)‖	IV: 400 mg q 12 h PO: 500 mg q 12 h
or	
Ofloxacin (Floxin)‖	PO or IV: 400 mg q 12 h
or	
Doxycycline (Vibramycin) ± rifampin†‡	IV: 200 mg q 12 h × 2 doses, then 200 mg q 24 h
or	PO: 200 mg once, then either 100 mg q 12 h or 200 mg q 24 h
Trimethoprim-sulfamethoxazole (Bactrim) ± rifampin†‡	PO or IV: 5 mg/kg of trimethoprim component q 8 h

Abbreviations: IV = intravenous; PO = orally.
*The only drug approved by the U.S. Food and Drug Administration for treatment of Legionnaires' disease.
†Rifampin (not given alone) given PO or IV; 600 mg q 12 h.
‡2 to 3 weeks.
§5 days.
‖2 weeks.
Modified from Edelstein PH: Legionnaires' disease, state of the art clinical article. Clin Infect Dis *16*:741–747, June 1993.

erated dose, 4 grams per day intravenously or 2 grams per day orally, and never gives less than 2 grams per day by either route. Rifampin* should be added in the case of more severe disease, such as multilobar pneumonia, respiratory failure, and extrapulmonary diseases such as *Legionella* endocarditis, or if the patient is severely immunosuppressed. The author gives rifampin for only the first 3 to 5 days of therapy, except in the case of poorly responsive disease, severe immunosuppression, or serious extrapulmonary disease.

An alternative to combined erythromycin and rifampin therapy is therapy with a fluoroquinolone antimicrobial agent* alone. The author routinely administers a fluoroquinolone antimicrobial agent alone to treat organ transplant patients with Legionnaires' disease because this class of antimicrobial agent does not interfere with cyclosporine metabolism, as does erythromycin and rifampin. Because the fluoroquinolone antimicrobial agents are not as effective as macrolide antimicrobial agents for the treatment of pneumococcal pneumonia and perhaps for *Chlamydia pneumoniae* pneumonia, these other diseases must be ruled out if therapy with a fluoroquinolone drug alone is used.

In the case of gastrointestinal intolerance of erythromycin, several alternative drugs exist. If the patient is able to absorb orally administered drugs, ciprofloxacin* (Cipro), ofloxacin* (Floxin), clarithromycin,* and azithromycin* are reasonable alternatives. Alternatively, intravenous or oral doxycycline* can be used, but it may be less effective than the newer macrolides or fluoroquinolone antimicrobial agents. The author generally treats patients with trimethoprim-sulfamethoxazole* only if the patient is already receiving the drug in high dosages for treatment of pneumocystis pneumonia and if there is a relatively low probability of concomitant Legionnaires' disease.

Clinical treatment failures have been reported for all antimicrobial agents for which there is sufficient experience. There exist no data to guide therapy in these circumstances. Anecdotes report success in these cases of changes in therapy to trimethoprim-sulfamethoxazole plus rifampin, doxycycline alone, pefloxacin (a fluoroquinolone agent not available in the United States) plus rifampin, and the addition of rifampin to an existing regimen. The first step is to initiate parenteral antibiotic administration, if the patient is receiving oral antibiotics. If the patient is already receiving parenteral erythromycin, substitution of parenteral ciprofloxacin or ofloxacin is advisable.

---

*Not approved by the U.S. Food and Drug Administration for this indication.

The duration of therapy is controversial, but the author prefers to give erythromycin therapy for 3 weeks because of the potential for relapse in some patients. Although experience is limited, a 5-day course of azithromycin is probably equivalent to a 3-week course of erythromycin. Also, 2 weeks' worth of either clarithromycin or fluoroquinolone antimicrobial therapies is probably sufficient. In the special cases of *Legionella* endocarditis or cavitary pulmonary disease, therapy is often given for 1 to 2 months.

Side effects of therapy can be troublesome. Erythromycin causes gastrointestinal intolerance in a high proportion of patients, whether given orally or intravenously; dose reduction is sometimes helpful in ameliorating this effect. On occasion, some erythromycin preparations cause less gastrointestinal distress than do others, but this reaction is highly individualized. Intravenous infusion of erythromycin is often painful or causes phlebitis; slowing infusion rates may be useful in this situation. In rare instances, deafness occurs in patients with renal failure who receive high-dosage erythromycin. This deafness appears to be reversible when the drug is stopped, and hearing is often restored when the dosage is reduced. Life-threatening cardiac arrhythmias have been very rarely reported in association with the intravenous infusion of erythromycin. Despite these rare serious side effects, erythromycin is an extremely safe, if not always well-tolerated, antibiotic. Doxycycline, ciprofloxacin, and ofloxacin also may cause gastrointestinal upset and in instances cause hepatitis (doxycycline), central nervous system disorders (fluoroquinolones), and phototoxicity (both). Ciprofloxacin or erythromycin may interfere with theophylline metabolism.

Response to Therapy

The first signs of response are often resumption of appetite, and of a general sense of well-being. Fever may persist for up to a week in immunocompetent patients, and for substantially longer in immunocompromised hosts; regardless, within a few days after the initiation of erythromycin therapy, the fever starts to decline. Chest roentgenographic abnormalities may persist for several weeks to months, and may even appear to worsen during the first few days of specific therapy; if the patient is improving otherwise, these changes can be ignored. Lung infiltrates may cavitate in patients who receive glucocorticosteroids in high dosages; prolonged antibiotic therapy is curative. Because cavitary lung infiltrates caused by other microorganisms may be seen in such patients, it is essential to confirm by culture or histopathologic study the diagnosis of Legionnaires' disease. The physical examination may also demonstrate extension of consolidation during the first few days of therapy; like the chest roentgenographic findings, this is not a cause for alarm if other clinical indicators demonstrate improvement.

Once a patient treated for Legionnaires' disease has become afebrile, it is rare for fever to recur; consideration should be given to poor oral absorption of antibiotics, development of metastatic infection, empyema thoracis, superinfection, and mistaken diagnosis. Clinical failures resulting from antibiotic resistance have not been reported. Empyema and soft tissue metastatic infections often require drainage. Relapse of Legionnaires' disease may occur, sometimes weeks after apparent cure, if the patient is receiving immunosuppressive therapy. Dual infection with *Legionella* and other pathogens occasionally occurs and sometimes accounts for therapeutic failures; these other pathogens have included *Cryptococcus, Aspergillus,* and *Pneumocystis* spp. and the usual respiratory tract pathogens such as *Pneumococcus, Haemophilus, and Mycoplasma* spp.

Case fatality rates vary according to age, underlying diseases, disease severity, and promptness of initiation of proper antibiotic therapy. Up to 95% of previously healthy patients with Legionnaires' disease are cured with the prompt initiation of specific antibiotic therapy. In contrast, only about 80% of previously ill, immunocompromised patients are cured after the initiation of prompt therapy. Respiratory failure portends a very poor prognosis. Without specific therapy, about 70 to 90% of previously healthy people recover. In some patients who have been cured of pneumonia, long-term sequelae develop. These include restrictive pulmonary disease, amnesia for the period of illness, persistent fatigue, and focal or global neurologic dysfunction; there appears to be no role for antibiotic therapy in the treatment of these complications. Glucocorticosteroids have been reported to be of use for the treatment of post-pneumonia pulmonary fibrosis in uncontrolled studies.

Pontiac Fever

No information exists regarding treatment for this disease. There is no evidence that antibiotic therapy influences the course of Pontiac fever, which usually resolves spontaneously over a period of several days. Symptomatic therapy may be indicated for treatment of fever, myalgia, and headache.

PULMONARY EMBOLISM

method of
JACQUES R. LECLERC, M.D.
Montreal General Hospital
McGill University
Montreal, Quebec, Canada

Pulmonary embolism is a serious and potentially fatal condition. Each year in the United States, it is responsible for the deaths of approximately 50,000 patients with an otherwise favorable prognosis and accounts for 300,000 hospitalizations. It is the third most common cardiovascular disease after ischemic syndromes and stroke.

NATURAL HISTORY

The immediate outcome of patients with pulmonary embolism is related to the size of the embolus and their underlying cardiopulmonary reserve. Most fatal emboli are caused by thrombi that obstruct more than 75% of the pulmonary circulation. Patients with underlying cardiopulmonary disorders may die of smaller emboli. Most deaths from pulmonary embolism occur shortly after the beginning of symptoms, too soon for the institution of effective treatment. Thus the only potentially lifesaving measure is the use of thromboprophylaxis. The subsequent outcome of patients with pulmonary embolism is determined by whether they receive effective treatment. Among patients who do not receive treatment, the mortality rate is approximately 30%. Most of these deaths are caused by recurrent embolization.

PATHOPHYSIOLOGY

Most pulmonary emboli originate from the deep venous system of the leg, mainly the proximal segment. The association between pulmonary embolism and deep vein thrombosis constitutes the fundamental principle of prophylaxis; that is, the prevention of lower extremity thrombosis will reduce the incidence of pulmonary embolism. Deep vein thrombosis in the calf is an infrequent source of pulmonary embolism. Without treatment, however, 20 to 30% of calf thrombi extend into the proximal veins. Other less common sources of emboli include the inferior vena cava; the renal, hepatic, and subclavian veins; and the right ventricle.

PREVENTION AND RISK FACTORS

The risk factors for pulmonary embolism are essentially the same as those for deep vein thrombosis (Table 1). Low-dose subcutaneous heparin (5000 units every 12 hours) is a time-honored method in abdominal surgery. Oral anticoagulants have been shown to be effective in major orthopedic surgery. They are given at a dose that maintains the prothrombin time (PT) at an international normalized ratio value of be-

TABLE 1. **Risk Factors for Venous Thromboembolism**

Clinical
Previous history of venous thromboembolism
Advanced age
Surgical/Obstetric Conditions
Orthopedic surgery
    Hip fracture
    Leg fracture
    Hip replacement
    Knee arthroplasty
General abdominal surgery
Gynecologic surgery
Neurosurgery
Kidney transplantation
Amputation
Post partum
Medical Conditions
Myocardial infarction
Stroke
Malignancy
Immobilized medical patients
Drugs
Chemotherapy
Oral contraceptives
Heparin induced thrombocytopenia
Laboratory
Antiphospholipid syndrome
Deficiencies
    Antithrombin III
    Protein C
    Protein S
Decreased fibrinolytic activity
Dysplasminogenemia
Erythrocytosis/thrombocytosis

TABLE 2. **Symptoms of Pulmonary Embolism and Their Possible Mechanisms**

Symptom	Possible Mechanisms
Dyspnea	Increased dead space ventilation
	Hypoxemia
	Perception of changes in lung mechanics and breathing pattern
Chest pain	
Pleuritic	Pleural inflammation adjacent to areas of lung hemorrhage
	Visceral pleural ischemia
Angina-like	Poor myocardial perfusion resulting from massive embolism
Hemoptysis	Intrapulmonary hemorrhage
Syncope	Low cardiac output
	Tachyarrhythmias
Apprehension	Increased sympathetic outflow resulting from hypoxemia
Wheezing	Focal edema
	Mediators released from thrombus or vessel wall
Nonproductive cough	Bronchial irritation
Palpitations	Raised cardiac output resulting from hypoxemia
Fever	Focal atelectasis
	Underlying deep vein thrombosis

tween 2.0 and 3.0. This method, however, requires careful laboratory monitoring. The efficacy and safety of low-molecular-weight heparin fractions have been demonstrated in orthopedic patients. Low-molecular-weight heparin is administered in a fixed-dose regimen without the need for laboratory monitoring. Low-dose heparin is the method of choice for immobilized medical patients. Intermittent pneumatic compression is the method of choice for patients in whom antithrombotic drugs are contraindicated (e.g., neurosurgery, hemorrhagic stroke, subarachnoid hemorrhage).

CLINICAL MANIFESTATIONS

The main symptoms of pulmonary embolism are listed in Table 2. The most common signs are tachypnea (respiratory rate ≥ 20 per minute), tachycardia (heart rate ≥ 100 per minute), increased pulmonary component of second heart sound, rales, fever ≥37.5° C), pleural rub, cyanosis, and hepatojugular reflux. The clinical manifestations of pulmonary embolism are influenced by several factors, including the number, size, and location of emboli; underlying cardiopul-

monary reserve; and the rate of resolution of emboli. The main syndromes of pulmonary embolism are shown in Table 3.

DIAGNOSIS

Testing

Clinical Assessment

The clinical diagnosis of pulmonary embolism is nonspecific because all of its symptoms and signs can be caused by other nonthrombotic dis-

TABLE 3. **Clinical Syndromes of Pulmonary Embolism**

Uncomplicated
Transient dyspnea with tachycardia and tachypnea

Congestive Atelectasis or Pulmonary Infarction
Dyspnea
Hemoptysis
Pleuritic pain

Massive
Apprehension
Angina-like chest pain
Syncope
Hypotension
Sudden death

Atypical
Arrhythmias
Bronchospasm
Fever
Isolated right-sided heart failure
Mental confusion
Paradoxical arterial embolism

orders (Table 4). This diagnosis is confirmed by pulmonary angiography in fewer than 50% of patients with clinical features of pulmonary embolism. Conversely, tests for the diagnosis of pulmonary embolism are insensitive in patients with mild or atypical features and when the disease is obscured by other processes (e.g., pneumonia, congestive cardiac failure).

The clinical assessment of patients with features of pulmonary embolism serves two purposes. First, a condition that simulates pulmonary embolism may be identified (e.g., chest wall pain, pericarditis, pneumothorax, myocardial infarction, respiratory tract infection). Second, it enables the practitioner to establish a clinical probability (i.e., before lung scanning) of pulmonary embolism.

Lung Scanning

Perfusion lung scanning is a sensitive tool for the detection of pulmonary embolism, and a normal result excludes this diagnosis. However, it is not specific for pulmonary embolism because other cardiopulmonary disorders may affect pulmonary blood flow and cause perfusion defects. Ventilation lung scanning is based on the theoretical principle that pulmonary emboli yield perfusion defects with normal gas entry, whereas other cardiopulmonary disorders should cause both perfusion and ventilation abnormalities. In routine practice, a probability of pulmonary embolism is assigned on the basis of size and distribution of perfusion defects, which are correlated with the ventilation scan and radiographic findings. A high-probability lung scan result (segmental perfusion defects with normal ventilation) carries an 85% certainty of embolism. All other lung scan abnormalities (intermediate or low probability) cannot either confirm or exclude the diagnosis of pulmonary embolism because they

TABLE 4. Differential Diagnosis of Pulmonary Embolism

Minor Pulmonary Embolism	
Pneumonia	Acute bronchitis
COPD	Musculoskeletal chest
Left-sided heart failure	wall pain
Atelectasis	Viral/immune pleuritis
Pleural effusion	Pericarditis
Bronchiectasis	Acute asthma
Hyperventilation	Lung cancer
Massive Pulmonary Embolism	
Acute myocardial	Septic shock
infarction	Pericardial effusion/
Pneumothorax	tamponade
Arrhythmias	Aortic dissection
Pulmonary edema	Exacerbation of COPD

Abbreviation: COPD = chronic obstructive pulmonary disease.

are associated with a 15 to 30% incidence of emboli. Thus additional investigation is required in patients with nondiagnostic scans.

Pulmonary Angiography

Pulmonary arteriography is the traditional reference method of resolving the dilemma of nondiagnostic lung scans. When performed by experts, it is a safe procedure with mortality and serious morbidity rates of 0.25% and 1.5%, respectively. The main drawbacks of arteriography are its invasive nature and the logistic problems associated with its routine use in all patients with nondiagnostic scans.

Assessment for Deep Vein Thrombosis of the Leg

The detection of deep vein thrombosis in patients with clinically suspected pulmonary embolism increases the likelihood of this diagnosis and provides a rationale for anticoagulant treatment. The three most accurate methods are contrast venography, impedance plethysmography, and compression ultrasonography. Impedance plethysmography and compression ultrasonography are useful for detecting proximal vein thrombosis but insensitive for calf thrombosis.

Ancillary Tests

No current ancillary tests reliably identify patients with pulmonary embolism. Patients with large emboli may have normal arterial blood gases, and the classical finding of hypoxemia and a widened alveolar-arterial oxygen gradient can be seen in many other cardiopulmonary disorders. Measurement of blood gases may assist in titrating supplemental oxygen for patients but should not be used to confirm or rule out pulmonary embolism. The most common electrocardiographic abnormalities in pulmonary embolism are sinus tachycardia and nonspecific features of right-sided heart strain. The classic $S_1Q_3T_3$ pattern occurs in no more than 10% of patients with pulmonary embolism. The electrocardiogram may be entirely normal in the presence of embolism. Acute myocardial infarction or pericarditis, which are sometimes alternative diagnostic possibilities, may be suggested by the electrocardiogram.

Chest x-ray abnormalities associated with pulmonary embolism include atelectasis, elevated diaphragm, pleural effusion, parenchymal infiltrates, and localized reduced vascular markings. As with blood gas measurements and the electrocardiogram, chest x-ray findings are not specific for embolism and may be normal in the presence of significant emboli. The main value of the chest x-ray is to assist in the interpretation of lung scanning and to demonstrate alternative diagnostic possibilities (e.g., pneumothorax, pulmonary edema, rib fracture, pneumonia).

Practical Diagnostic Approach

The first step is to perform a careful clinical evaluation (Fig. 1). Next, a ventilation/perfusion lung scan is performed. A normal and technically adequate perfusion scan rules out pulmonary embolism. A high-probability scan accompanying high clinical suspicion confirms the diagnosis of embolism. A high-probability scan with low clinical suspicion, however, carries less certainty of embolism (50 to 60%), and additional testing should be performed. The main difficulty of this diagnostic process is that most patients (70%) belong to the nondiagnostic scan category.

A number of approaches can be used in patients with nondiagnostic scans, depending on the clinical situation and the availability of tests. Noninvasive testing for leg deep vein thrombosis can be performed and the patient treated if the result is positive. The test is repeated serially if the initial result is negative. The approach of serial testing is based on the observation that patients have a favorable outcome in the absence of proximal vein thrombosis. Repeated noninvasive testing is not recommended for patients with serious cardiopulmonary disease, in whom recurrent embolization from calf vein thrombosis may worsen their condition. Contrast venography can

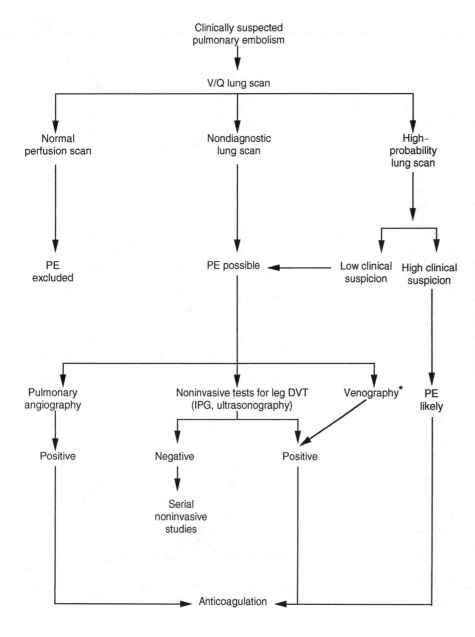

Figure 1. Diagnostic approach for patients with clinically suspected pulmonary embolism. *Abbreviations*: V/Q = ventilation/perfusion; PE = pulmonary embolism; DVT = deep vein thrombosis; IPG = impedance plethysmography. (*Pulmonary arteriography should be performed if venography results are negative.)

be used if noninvasive testing is not available or in patients with severe cardiopulmonary disease in whom angiography is more risky. The author favors angiography over testing for leg thrombosis when precise knowledge of the presence of embolism will influence either the nature (e.g., massive embolism, symptoms recurring during a course of therapeutic anticoagulation) or duration of treatment (e.g., suspected recurrent embolization). Pulmonary angiography also plays an important role in the investigation of patients with thromboembolic pulmonary hypertension.

Diagnosis During Pregnancy and Post Partum

The clinical diagnosis (Fig. 2) is no more reliable than in nonpregnant patients. Also, the physiologic dyspnea of pregnancy and such obstetric complications as amniotic fluid embolism, sepsis, and aspiration pneumonia may simulate pulmonary embolism. Adequate perfusion scanning can be obtained by using half the normal isotopic dose. Ventilation scanning is performed the following day to avoid interference from the per-

fusion scan. Lung scanning provides minimal radiation exposure to the fetus, and the risk involved with not performing these investigations far outweighs that of radiation. Venography should not be performed in view of the radiation risk to the fetus. Chest x-ray and pulmonary angiography should be performed with an abdominal shield. The use of serial noninvasive testing for leg thrombosis is not recommended because it has not been formally evaluated in this setting.

The diagnostic approach during the puerperium is the same as in nonpregnant patients except that nursing mothers should interrupt breast feeding for 48 hours after lung scanning studies.

TREATMENT

General Supportive Measures

Hypoxemic patients with pulmonary embolism, particularly with cardiorespiratory disorders, should have oxygen supplementation and those with pleuritic chest pain often require analgesics. Resuscitation of the hemodynamically compro-

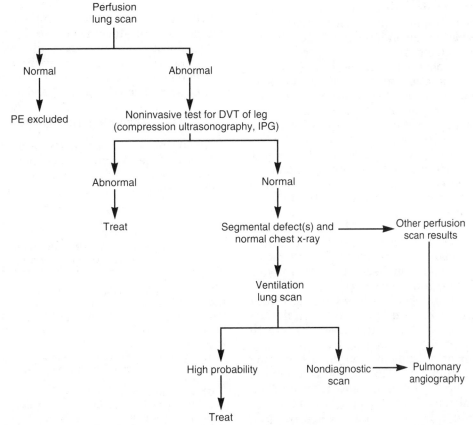

Figure 2. Diagnostic approach for clinically suspected pulmonary embolism during pregnancy. *Abbreviations*: PE = pulmonary embolism; DVT = deep vein thrombosis; IPG = impedance plethysmography.

mised patient should initially involve intravenous fluid boluses and vasopressor agents such as norepinephrine or dopamine.

Anticoagulant Treatment

The main goals of anticoagulant treatment are to prevent recurrent embolization and to treat the underlying deep vein thrombosis. Intravenous heparin is the initial drug of choice, in view of its rapid onset of action. It should be started as soon as the possibility of pulmonary embolism is considered, particularly if there is a delay in obtaining confirmatory studies. Heparin is initiated with a 5000-unit intravenous bolus followed by continuous infusion of at least 1200 units per hour. Treatment is monitored with the use of the activated partial thromboplastin time (APTT). The APTT should be maintained at 2.0 to 2.5 times the control value. A baseline APTT should be obtained, but the result should not be awaited before treatment is started. The first APTT is obtained 4 hours after the start of infusion and then every 6 hours until it is within the therapeutic range. It is then checked daily. For patients with major pulmonary embolism, the author recommends performing the first APTT one half-hour after the bolus dose because patients may exhibit a more rapid heparin clearance. A repeated bolus dose is given if the APTT is subtherapeutic. Hemoglobin measurement and platelet count should be obtained every other day.

The two most common adverse reactions of heparin are bleeding and heparin-induced thrombocytopenia. In the event of major hemorrhage, the effect of heparin can be reversed by protamine sulfate. Significant thrombocytopenia occurs in 2 to 5% of patients receiving therapeutic heparin. Heparin-induced thrombocytopenia is immune-mediated and can cause serious arterial or venous thromboembolic events. Heparin-induced thrombocytopenia warrants the cessation of heparin.

A period of oral anticoagulation is required after initial heparin treatment, to prevent recurrent venous thromboembolism. The author favors the use of warfarin sodium (Coumadin) over other vitamin K antagonists. The long half-life of this drug allows a more stable anticoagulation. Warfarin is started at an initial dose of 7.5 to 10 mg on the first day of heparin treatment. The effect of warfarin is monitored by performing daily prothrombin time. The goal of treatment is to maintain the prothrombin time at an international normalized ratio value of between 2.0 and 3.0. Heparin can be discontinued when the prothrombin time is within the therapeutic range for at least 2 consecutive days.

The optimal duration of oral anticoagulation for pulmonary embolism has never been established. The author treats patients for 3 months after a first episode. A longer treatment course is given to patients with recurrent embolism or those with a deficiency in antithrombin III, in protein C, or in protein S. It is good practice to repeat the perfusion scan before stopping oral anticoagulants; the result constitutes a useful baseline, should the patient return with recurrent symptoms of pulmonary embolism.

The outpatient administration of oral anticoagulants must be monitored regularly. Drugs that may alter the effect of warfarin should be avoided or administered with extreme caution. In the presence of major hemorrhage, the effect of warfarin can be reversed by the administration of vitamin K. The most common adverse reaction of warfarin is hemorrhage. Skin necrosis is a very rare complication of warfarin. Painful lesions typically develop in areas with high adipose tissue content during the first few days of treatment. These lesions rapidly become necrotic if warfarin is not discontinued.

The treatment of pulmonary embolism during pregnancy consists of the administration of intravenous heparin for 5 to 7 days, followed by subcutaneous heparin given in full therapeutic doses for the remainder of the pregnancy. Oral anticoagulants are teratogenic and are contraindicated. Subcutaneous heparin is best administered every 12 hours at a dose that maintains the APTT, obtained 6 hours later, within the therapeutic interval. Heparin does not cross the placenta.

Thrombolytic Therapy

Among patients with massive pulmonary embolism and persistent hypotension (i.e., systolic level < 100 mmHg), the mortality rate is 20 to 30% despite intravenous heparin. This is in stark contrast to patients with submassive embolism,

TABLE 5. **Contraindications to Thrombolytic Therapy**

Absolute
Active or recent internal bleeding
History of hemorrhagic stroke
Intracranial or intraspinal disease
Recent cranial surgery or head trauma

Relative
Major surgery, delivery or trauma in previous 10 days
Biopsy or invasive procedure at a noncompressible site in previous 10 days
History of nonhemorrhagic stroke
Gastrointestinal bleeding in previous month
Active peptic ulcer disease
Uncontrolled severe hypertension
Severe coagulation defects

TABLE 6. **Approved Thrombolytic Regimens for Pulmonary Embolism**

Streptokinase	
Loading dose	250,000 U over 30 min
Infusion	100,000 U/h × 24 h
Urokinase	
Loading dose	4400 U/kg over 10 min
Infusion	4400 U/kg/h × 12–24 h
Tissue Plasminogen Activator	
Infusion	100 mg over 2 h

among whom the mortality rate is less than 5% with adequate heparinization. Rapid removal of the thrombotic obstruction is necessary to restore cardiac output. Thrombolytic drugs are indicated in this setting in the absence of contraindications (Table 5). The approved thrombolytic regimens for pulmonary embolism are shown in Table 6. Anticoagulation in full doses is started after the thrombolytic agent is stopped, to prevent recurrent embolism.

The routine use of thrombolysis in nonmassive embolism is an area of controversy. A better preservation of pulmonary vascular blood flow would be potentially beneficial.

Vena Cava Filters

Patients in whom major bleeding develops during anticoagulant treatment are best treated by the insertion of a filter in the inferior vena cava. The best results have been obtained with the Kimray-Greenfield filter. This device is designed to trap incoming emboli without causing flow obstruction in the inferior vena cava. It is solidly anchored in the vein wall to avoid dislodgement and embolization of the device. It can be inserted via either the internal jugular or the common femoral vein.

Surgical Treatment

There is no indication for acute pulmonary embolectomy except possibly in patients with proven massive embolism in whom shock is refractory to resuscitation procedures and in whom there is a contraindication to thrombolytic therapy. A surgical team and cardiac bypass equipment must also be available immediately.

Surgery is indicated for patients in whom thromboembolic pulmonary hypertension develops. In approximately 0.1% of patients with pulmonary embolism, significant pulmonary hypertension develops over the ensuing years. These patients are amenable to surgical thromboembolectomy, but this procedure requires considerable technical expertise. Without surgery, these patients have a rather poor prognosis.

SARCOIDOSIS
method of
OM P. SHARMA, M.D.
*University of Southern California School of
Medicine*
Los Angeles, California

Sarcoidosis is a multisystem disorder of unknown cause. The disease most commonly affects young adults and frequently manifests with bilateral hilar lymphadenopathy, pulmonary infiltration, and eye and skin lesions. About 10 to 20% of patients have hypercalcemia. There is peripheral depression of delayed type hypersensitivity, imbalance of OK T4:T8 subsets, an influx of T4 helper cells to the sites of inflammation, hyperactivity of B cells, and immune complexes in the serum.

The course and prognosis of sarcoidosis are correlated with the mode of onset and clinical involvement. An acute onset with hilar adenopathy and erythema nodosum usually heralds a self-limited course of spontaneous resolution, whereas an insidious onset may be followed by relentless progressive fibrosis with diffuse pulmonary infiltration and skin lesions.

DIAGNOSIS

Any consideration for treating sarcoidosis should be preceded by obtaining the accurate diagnosis based on the following criteria: (1) compatible clinical or radiologic picture, or both; (2) histologic evidence of noncaseating granulomata either by an appropriate biopsy or by a Kveim-Siltzbach test; and (3) negative special stains and cultures (acid-fast bacilli, fungi, bacteria, protozoa) of tissue specimens. If all three steps are not performed, the diagnosis of sarcoidosis remains in doubt because clinical or radiologic features suggest too wide a differential diagnosis, and noncaseating granulomas may be induced by many bacteria, fungi, viruses, chemicals, and organic dust particles. Once the diagnosis is established, an attempt should be made to assess the activity, severity, and extent of the granulomatous process.

EVALUATION OF DISEASE ACTIVITY AND SEVERITY

During the 1980s, four new techniques useful in assessing the extent and severity of granulomatous inflammation and fibrosis emerged: determination of serum angiotensin-converting enzyme (SACE) levels, gallium 67 scans, bronchoalveolar lavage (BAL), and high-resolution computed tomography (HRCT). SACE, BAL analysis, and gallium 67 scans reflect different aspects of sarcoid activity. There is considerable uncertainty about how results of the three methods are correlated with each other. SACE does not accurately reflect activity of the disease as assessed by the BAL lymphocyte count. There is an approximate correlation between the results of gallium scanning and SACE activity but not between those of gallium lung scans and BAL lymphocyte counts. These findings are not surprising in view of the distinctive tissue sources of these markers: namely, the blood, the lung tissue, and the lavage fluid. HRCT is the most modern imaging technique, providing outstanding resolution of lung morphology. Much is yet to be learned about the usefulness of these and other, newer tests in assessing the activity of sarcoidosis. These tests are of little help in establishing the specific diagnosis of sarcoidosis.

NATURAL HISTORY

To evaluate the natural course of pulmonary sarcoidosis, patients must be selected and monitored while still in the early stages of the disease, without any type of treatment, for a long time. There are not many such studies. Smellie and Hoyle surveyed 125 patients with sarcoidosis for more than 2 years. Spontaneous radiographic improvement in a mean time of 1 year occurred in 71% of patients with hilar nodes and in 50% of those with pulmonary infiltration. The outlook was much better in patients with erythema nodosum. None of the patients who had experienced spontaneous remission experienced relapse. Pulmonary infiltration, if it persists for more than 2 years, is unlikely to remit without therapy.

The prognosis is poor in American blacks, particularly women, especially in those who at the time of the initial discovery have pulmonary infiltration and disease involving more than three organ systems.

TREATMENT

Pulmonary Involvement

Stage I. Asymptomatic patients with bilateral hilar lymphadenopathy with or without erythema nodosum but without extrapulmonary involvement should be left untreated. Patients with fever and joint pains respond to nonsteroidal anti-inflammatory agents. On occasion, prednisone, 15 to 20 mg per day, may be needed to control symptoms that do not respond to anti-inflammatory drugs. Symptoms of cough and dyspnea may be associated with airway obstruction—even in this early stage—and should be treated with corticosteroids. In a few of these cases, inhalational corticosteroids are found to be effective.

Stage II. Patients with bilateral hilar adenopathy and infiltration and symptoms (cough, dyspnea, chest pain, exercise intolerance) should be treated with corticosteroids.

Patients who are asymptomatic and have only mild impairment of lung function need only to be observed. However, if deterioration of lung function occurs over a period of 3 to 6 months, the treatment should be instituted.

Patients who are asymptomatic and have severe impairment of lung function should be treated. Serial chest radiographs and lung function measurement should be performed to establish the maximal response before the drug dosage is tapered to the maintenance level.

Stage III. Patients with diffuse pulmonary infiltration usually have symptoms along with lung function abnormalities and almost always need treatment.

Stage IV. Patients with extensive fibrosis and bullae formation respond poorly or not at all to corticosteroids and immunosuppressive therapy. However, the treatment should be given at least once to improve symptoms if possible. Some of these patients require lung transplantation. Bronchiectasis, hemoptysis, and aspergilloma are treated conservatively with appropriate antibacterial and antifungal agents.

Extrapulmonary Involvement

Indications for the treatment of extrapulmonary involvement are relatively straightforward. Ocular, neurologic, cardiac, and upper airway involvement almost always necessitate treatment with corticosteroids, often in higher doses (see Corticosteroid Therapy section) and for a long time. Glandular involvement, splenic enlargement, parotid swelling, and cutaneous lesions respond to modest doses (see Corticosteroid Therapy section). Asymptomatic hepatic involvement requires no therapy but regular follow-up evaluation must be provided.

Corticosteroid Therapy

Sarcoidosis is very sensitive to corticosteroids. The author administers 30 to 40 mg of prednisone daily in a single dose, gradually reducing to a maintenance level of 10 to 15 mg over a period of 6 months. Higher doses (60 to 80 mg daily) are needed to control severe ocular, neurologic, and myocardial lesions and malignant hypercalcemia. Relapse is common and is evidenced by reappearance of clinical signs, chest radiograph abnormality, impairment in lung function, or elevated levels of angiotensin-converting enzyme. If a relapse occurs, the dose is increased to the previously high level sufficient to control the recurrence. Although alternate-day regimen is effective in producing considerable reduction of side effects, daily treatment is recommended in order to ensure increased compliance by the patient. In selected cases with no extrapulmonary involvement, inhalational corticosteroids are useful.

Drugs Other Than Corticosteroids

Chloroquine* (Aralen) and methotrexate† are given to patients who either do not respond to prednisone or experience severe side effects. The author has used both these drugs in those two situations and also as the initial drug in treatment of chronic skin lesions. Chloroquine administration rarely leads to retinopathy; frequent eye examinations (every 3 months) are mandatory. In patients receiving methotrexate close monitoring of liver function is required. More information is needed about indications and precautions before they can be recommended as a part of the routine therapy for sarcoidosis.

SPECIAL SITUATIONS

Children

Sarcoidosis is not rare among children younger than 15 years of age. The younger children tend to have extensive, systemic disease, with a less favorable prognosis. Corticosteroids are indicated.

The Elderly

Sarcoidosis carries a low mortality rate, and many patients live with it into the later years. It is important to remember that a malignant disease of the lung, stomach, intestine, and even uterus may give rise to a granulomatous reaction in draining lymph nodes.

Pregnancy

Pregnancy has a favorable effect on the disease. Many patients improve and are able to discontinue or curtail corticosteroid therapy. The disease does not have any damaging effect on gestation or on the fetus. In a few patients, the disease worsens after parturition and responds well to corticosteroids.

Infection

The frequency of bacterial and viral infections in persons with sarcoidosis is not higher that in

---

*This use of chloroquine is not listed in the manufacturer's official directive.

†This use of methotrexate is not listed in the manufacturer's official directive.

the general population. Aspergilloma is the common fungal colonization in chronic fibrotic sarcoidosis.

Sarcoidosis, Malignancy, and Lymphoma

Sarcoid-like granulomatous lesions may be found in regional lymph nodes draining a carcinoma or even among the tumor cells at the site of the primary neoplasm. It is important that the local "sarcoid-reaction" be differentiated from the multisystemic sarcoidosis.

SILICOSIS

method of
JOHN E. PARKER, M.D.
*National Institute for Occupational Safety and
Health*
Morgantown, West Virginia

Silicosis, a fibrotic disease of the lungs, is caused by the inhalation, retention, and pulmonary reaction to crystalline silica. Despite knowledge of the cause of this disorder—respiratory exposures to silica-containing dust—this serious and potentially fatal occupational lung disease is tragically still seen in the 1990s in the United States and throughout the world. Silica, or silicon dioxide, is the predominant component of the earth's crust. The three important crystalline forms of silica are quartz, tridymite, and cristobalite. These forms are also called "free silica" to distinguish them from the silicates. The silica content in different rock formations, such as sandstone, granite, and slate, varies from 20% to nearly 100%. Occupational exposure to silica particles of respirable size (0.5 to 5 microns) is associated with mining, quarrying, drilling, and tunneling operations. Silica exposure is also a potential hazard to sandblasters, stonecutters, and pottery, foundry, ground silica, and refractory workers. The true prevalence of the disease is unknown, but more than 2 million workers in the United States are employed in trades that have been linked to the development of silicosis.

The precise pathogenic mechanism for the development of silicosis remains uncertain. Abundant evidence implicates the interaction between pulmonary alveolar macrophage and silica particles deposited in the lung. It is proposed that surface properties of the silica particle activate macrophages. These cells then release chemotactic factors and inflammatory mediators that result in a further cellular response by polymorphonuclear leukocytes, lymphocytes, and additional macrophages. Fibroblast-stimulating factors that promote hyalinization and collagen deposition are released. The resulting pathologic silicotic lesion is the hyaline nodule, containing a central acellular zone with free silica surrounded by whorls of collagen and fibroblasts, and an active peripheral zone composed of macrophages, fibroblasts, plasma cells, and additional free silica. Impaired macrophage function also plays a role in susceptibility to infectious organisms such as *Mycobacterium tuberculosis* and *Nocardia asteroides.*

There is mounting evidence that freshly fractured silica may be more toxic than aged silica; this characteristic is perhaps related to the presence of reactive radical groups on the cleavage planes of freshly fractured silica. This may be a pathogenic explanation for the observation of cases of advanced disease in both sandblasters and rock drillers, in whom exposures to recently fractured silica are particularly intense.

FORMS OF DISEASE: CLINICAL PICTURE

Chronic silicosis is often asymptomatic and manifests as a radiographic abnormality with small (<10-mm), rounded opacities predominantly in the upper lobes. A history of 15 years or more since onset of exposure is common. Pulmonary function testing may be normal or may show mild restriction. Less commonly, mild obstruction to airflow or reduced diffusing capacity may be present. Simple silicosis progresses to complicated disease in 20 to 30% of cases.

Complicated silicosis, also called progressive massive fibrosis, is more likely to manifest with exertional dyspnea. This form of disease is characterized by nodular opacities more than 1 cm in diameter on chest radiographs and commonly involve reduced carbon monoxide diffusing capacity, reduced arterial oxygen tension at rest or with exercise, and marked restriction on spirometry or lung volume measurement. Distortion of the bronchial tree may also lead to airway obstruction and productive cough. Recurrent bacterial infection not unlike that seen in bronchiectasis may occur. Weight loss and cavitation of the large opacities should prompt concern for tuberculosis or other mycobacterial infection. Pneumothorax may be a life-threatening complication, because the fibrotic lung may be difficult to reexpand. Hypoxemic respiratory failure with cor pulmonale is a common terminal event.

Accelerated silicosis may appear after more intense exposures of shorter (5 to 10 years') duration. Symptoms, radiographic findings, and physiologic measurements are similar to those seen in the chronic form. Deterioration in lung function is more rapid, and mycobacterial infection may develop in as many as 25% of patients with accelerated disease. Autoimmune disease, including scleroderma and rheumatoid arthritis, is seen with silicosis, often of the accelerated type. The progression of radiographic abnormalities and functional impairment can be rapid when autoimmune disease is associated with silicosis.

Acute silicosis may develop within 6 months to 2 years of massive silica exposure. Dramatic dyspnea, weakness, and weight loss are often the presenting symptoms. The radiographic findings of diffuse alveolar filling differ from those in the more chronic forms of silicosis. Histologic findings similar to pulmonary alveolar proteinosis have been described, and extrapulmonary (renal and hepatic) abnormalities are reported. Rapid progression to severe hypoxemic ventilatory failure is the usual course. Mycobacterial infection in acute silicosis is even more likely than in chronic or accelerated disease.

PREVENTION

There is no specific therapy for silicosis. Prevention remains the cornerstone of eliminating this occupational lung disease. Workers and employers should be educated with regard to the hazards of silica dust exposure and to measures for controlling exposure. The use of improved ventilation and local exhaust, process enclosure, wet techniques, personal protection (including the proper selection of respirators), and, where possible, industrial substitution of agents less hazardous than silica all reduce exposure.

Silicosis is a reportable disease in many states. If silicosis is recognized in a worker, removal from continuing exposure is advisable. Unfortunately, the disease may progress even without further silica exposure. In addition, finding a case of silicosis, especially the acute or accelerated form, should prompt notification of state or federal agencies, such as the Occupational Safety and Health Administration (OSHA), the Mine Safety and Health Administration (MSHA), and the National Institute for Occupational Safety and Health (NIOSH), to obtain workplace evaluation in order to protect other workers also at risk. NIOSH maintains a toll free number, 1-800-35-NIOSH, for occupational safety and health information and assistance with workplace health hazard evaluations.

TREATMENT

When prevention has been unsuccessful and silicosis has developed, therapy is directed largely at complications of the disease. Therapeutic measures are similar to those commonly used in the management of airway obstruction, infection, pneumothorax, hypoxemia, and respiratory failure complicating other pulmonary disease. The inhalation of aerosolized aluminum has historically been unsuccessful as a specific therapy for silicosis. Polyvinyl pyridine-N-oxide, a polymer that has protected laboratory animals, is not available for use in humans. Recent laboratory work with tetrandrine has shown in vivo reduction in fibrosis and collagen synthesis in silica-exposed animals treated with this drug. However, strong evidence of human efficacy is currently lacking, and this drug is not available in the United States. To date, the search for a specific therapy for silicosis has been unrewarding.

If obstructive airway disease with bronchospasm develops, bronchodilator therapy is indicated. Inhaled selective beta$_2$-adrenergic agents, such as albuterol (Ventolin, Proventil), two inhalations every 4 to 6 hours, may be helpful. Oral long-acting theophylline preparations, given twice daily, to achieve a blood level of 10 to 20 μg per mL may be beneficial alone or in combination with inhaled beta agonists.

Episodes of acute bronchitis, commonly caused by *Streptococcus pneumoniae* or *Haemophilus influenzae,* can be treated with ampicillin, 250 to 500 mg every 6 hours for 10 days. Tetracycline, erythromycin, and trimethoprim-sulfamethoxazole are also useful for treatment of initial or recurrent episodes of infectious bronchitis. If infection does not improve on empiric therapy, reevaluation with sputum Gram's stain, culture, and sensitivity tests should be performed. Pneumococcal and influenza vaccinations are recommended.

Airway secretions causing copious, tenacious sputum production and occasionally disabling cough should be managed with time-honored methods of adequate hydration, humidification, and postural drainage. Cessation of smoking is clearly important and must be strongly encouraged.

Tuberculosis is a common and serious complication, especially in complicated, accelerated, and acute silicosis. Patients with silicosis who have a significant tuberculin reaction but no clinical, bacteriologic, or radiographic evidence of active disease should be treated with isoniazid preventative therapy. Oral isoniazid, 300 mg daily, should be given for a minimum of 1 year. Some physicians recommend lifelong preventive therapy. Silicotic patients receiving glucocorticoids should also be given isoniazid preventive therapy.

The diagnosis of active tuberculosis infection in patients with silicosis can be difficult. Clinical symptoms of weight loss, fever, sweats, and malaise should prompt radiographic evaluation and sputum acid-fast bacilli strains and cultures. Radiographic changes, including enlargement or cavitation in conglomerate lesions or nodular opacities, are of particular concern. Bacteriologic studies on expectorated sputum may not always be reliable in silicotuberculosis. Fiberoptic bronchoscopy for additional specimens for culture and study may often be helpful in establishing a diagnosis of active disease.

Proven active tuberculosis and clinically suspected disease should be treated with isoniazid, 300 mg, and rifampin, 600 mg, daily for a minimum of 9 months. Many authorities recommend a third drug such as ethambutol, 15 mg per kg, as well as more prolonged courses. Antituberculous therapy should be guided by laboratory studies of sensitivity, especially in view of the recent recognititon of multidrug-resistant organisms. Initiation of therapy before bacteriologic confirmation is prudent in silicotic patients with clinical signs compatible with active tuberculosis. Careful long-term follow-up with chest radiographs, bacteriologic cultures, and clinical evaluation is imperative in view of numerous reports of recurrent pulmonary tuberculosis in silicotic patients after discontinuation of apparently adequate therapy.

Hypoxemia should be treated with supplemental oxygen to prevent the development of polycythemia, to delay or prevent development of pulmonary hypertension and cor pulmonale, and to improve exercise tolerance. The goal of oxygen therapy should be to elevate the arterial oxygen tension above 60 mmHg. Two to four liters per minute of oxygen by nasal cannula often achieves this level of arterial oxygenation. Measurement of arterial blood gases should guide the selection of flow rate. Portable and home oxygen systems for managing these patients are widely available.

Ventilatory support for respiratory failure is indicated when precipitated by a treatable complication. Pneumothorax, spontaneous and ventilator-related, is usually treated by chest tube insertion. Bronchopleural fistula may develop and surgical consultation and management should be considered.

Acute silicosis may rapidly progress to respiratory failure. In patients in whom this disease has resembled pulmonary alveolar proteinosis and severe hypoxemia is present, aggressive therapy has included massive whole-lung lavage with the patient under general anesthesia in an attempt to improve gas exchange and remove alveolar debris. Although appealing in concept, the efficacy of whole-lung lavage has not been established. Glucocorticoid therapy has also been used for acute silicosis; however, its benefit is still unproven. Prednisone has been used at dosages of 40 to 60 mg per day for 1 to 2 months and, if accompanied by evidence of clinical improvement, has been tapered to 15 to 20 mg per day and continued for 6 months to 1 year. Early, rigorous initial evaluation for tuberculosis and other mycobacterial infection cannot be overemphasized. Isoniazid given as described earlier while steroids are administered is recommended. Empiric therapy with two or three antituberculous drugs pending results of cultures for 6 weeks may be appropriate in the life-threatening acute form of disease.

Some patients with end-stage silicosis may be considered candidates for lung or heart-lung transplantation by centers experienced with this procedure. Early referral and evaluation for this intervention may be offered to selected patients.

The discussion of an aggressive and high-technology therapeutic intervention such as transplantation serves to dramatically underscore the serious and potentially fatal nature of silicosis, as well as to emphasize the crucial role for primary prevention.

HYPERSENSITIVITY PNEUMONITIS

method of
JORDAN N. FINK, M.D.
Medical College of Wisconsin
Milwaukee, Wisconsin

Hypersensitivity pneumonitis (HP), also known as extrinsic allergic alveolitis, is an immunologic inflammatory process of the lung resulting from exposure, sensitization, and re-exposure by inhalation to any of a wide variety of biologic dusts. The clinical features are both respiratory and systemic; immune responses to the offending agent can be demonstrated, and abnormalities can be detected in both the chest x-ray and pulmonary function. Histopathologic evaluation reveals an interstitial pneumonitis composed of lymphocytic infiltration of alveoli, septa, and pulmonary parenchyma; varying degrees of bronchiolitis obliterans lead to a fibrotic process. Farmer's lung, bird breeder's lung, and ventilation pneumonitis are the most frequent disorders: Summer-type HP appears to be unique to Japan. Numerous other HPs have been described, depending on the offending environment and sensitizing agent, as partially listed in Table 1. The diagnosis of HP requires the physician's suspicion, identification of the characteristic clinical responses, and establishment of the responsible agent or, at least, the responsible environment.

The clinical features of HP may occur in an acute, a subacute, or a chronic form, depending on the frequency, intensity, and duration of exposure as well as on the immune response of the patient. Acute HP commonly manifests as a flu-like illness with cough, dyspnea, malaise, myalgia, and fatigue associated with chills, sweats, and fever, which occur 4 to 8 hours after inhalational exposure, peak at 12 to 18 hours, and persist for up to 24 hours, although residual signs and symptoms may be present for days. The subacute form manifests with cough, dyspnea, anorexia, and weight loss with less of an acute flu-like syndrome. The chronic form is subtle; progressive dyspnea and cough may be present for months.

Depending on the temporal relationship between exposure and evaluation, the physical findings may be normal or may include bibasilar end-inspiratory rales in an ill-appearing patient. The signs may be present only transiently or may persist for weeks. With continued exposure, progression to end-stage fibrosis may occur. Chest x-ray evaluation demonstrates transient nodular infiltrations of the parenchyma or variable degrees of fibrosis. Pulmonary function evaluation detects a usually reversible restrictive defect and gas exchange defect with variable obstruction. Airway hyperresponsiveness may be present, likely caused by the airway inflammation that occurs. With progression of disease, the abnormalities become less reversible.

Immunologic evaluation of the patient reveals serum-precipitating antibody to the offending agent. Evaluation of the pulmonary milieu by bronchoalveolar lavage demonstrates marked lymphocytosis with a predominance of CD8 or suppressor-type T cells. Finally, purposeful challenge with exposure to the suspected environment or exposure to the offending agent in the laboratory induces an acute episode of HP, and removal from the environment usually results in complete clearing of the disorder unless permanent pulmonary parenchymal damage has occurred.

Thus the diagnosis may be established in most cases (1) if the history, physical examination, chest x-ray, and pulmonary function tests indicate interstitial lung disease, (2) if exposure to an offending agent occurs, and (3) if an immune response to that agent can be demonstrated. Evaluation of pulmonary cells obtained by bronchoalveolar lavage may be adjunct and preclude the need for lung biopsy. Purposeful inhalational exposure to the environment, which induces symptoms and pulmonary function changes, and avoidance of exposure, which results in resolution of the disorder, may be of value in establishing the diagnosis, although purposeful bronchoprovocation in the laboratory is considered by many investigators to be a research tool.

TREATMENT

The medical management of HP consists largely of control of the patient's behavior or offending environment to eliminate exposure to the inciting antigen. It may also involve occasional administration of glucocorticosteroids to hasten recovery or suppress inflammation while avoidance measures are being carried out.

Avoidance

The most effective treatment of HP is the patient's avoidance of the offending environment or agent. Removal of the patient from the environment or removal of the antigens from the patient's environment is ideal. For some patients such as bird fanciers, the need for alteration of the environment is apparent, but psychological attachment to the birds may be overwhelming and result in patients' resistance. In the case of occupational exposures, attempts at environmental controls should be instituted so as to result in the least economic distress to the patient as possible. Alteration of manufacturing processes,

TABLE 1. **Hypersensitivity Pneumonitis Syndromes**

Antigen	Source of Antigen	Disease
Thermophilic Actinomycetes		
Micropolyspora faeni	Moldy vegetable compost	Farmer's lung
Thermoactinomycetes candidus, T. vulgaris, T. sacharii	Moldy vegetable compost	Mushroom worker's lung
		Bagassosis
Thermoactinomycetes spp., *Amoeba* spp., thermophilic bacteria	Contaminated system	Ventilation pneumonitis
Fungi		
Alternaria spp.	Moldy wood pulp	Wood pulp worker's lung
Mucor stolonifer	Paprika dust	Paprika splitter's lung
Aspergillus clavatus	Moldy barley	Malt worker's lung
Pullularia spp.	Contaminated sauna	Sauna taker's lung
	Redwood dust	Sequoisis
	Moldy curtain	Shower curtain lung
Cryptostroma corticale	Moldy maple bark	Maple bark stripper's lung
Penicillium caseii	Cheese mold	Cheese worker's lung
Penicillium frequentans	Moldy cork	Suberosis
Trichosporon cutaneum	House dust	Summer pneumonitis
Saccharomonospora virdis	Dried leaves and grass	Thatched roof disease
Animal Proteins		
Aviary proteins	Avian dust	Bird breeder's lung
Bovine or porcine proteins	Bovine or porcine pituitary powder	Pituitary snuff lung
Insects		
Sitophilus granarius	Contaminated grain	Grain worker's lung
Reactive Chemicals		
Isocyanates	Chemical exposure	Isocyanate lung
Anhydrides	Chemical exposure	Anhydride lung

avoidance of specific areas in the work place that induce episodes of HP, or improving ventilation systems may be desirable but may not be economically feasible for the employer. The use of personal filtration devices is often only temporarily successful, inasmuch as the sensitized worker finds the devices too uncomfortable or obtrusive.

In some cases, alteration of the work place environment has been successful in controlling disease. Farmer's lung has been controlled by reducing the growth of thermophilic organisms through the use of 1% propionic acid on hay piles, by preventing composting of silage by keeping hay piles dry, and by using bottom-loading and -unloading silos. Contaminated air-handling systems have been cleaned or replaced with systems in which stagnant water collection does not occur and the environment conducive to microbiologic contamination is eliminated. Preventing maple logs from getting wet has eliminated cases of maple-bark stripper's disease, because the offending organism does not grow on dry logs.

When environmental controls are instituted, follow-up observation of the patient is essential. Careful history, chest x-ray, and pulmonary function testing are necessary and more important if there is subtle progression to irreversible disease. Unfortunately, in many cases, patients do not completely respond to environmental controls because the changes may not be sufficient, and a change in occupation becomes necessary.

Pharmacotherapy

Corticosteroids remain the primary therapy for HP. Systemic drug therapy is effective; inhaled drugs are not. Furthermore, there is no evidence that prophylactic administration of corticosteroids before exposure to antigen protects the patient from pulmonary inflammatory processes and impairment. Therefore, the drug should be used in conjunction with avoidance measures, not as sole therapy.

Corticosteroids are rarely needed in the acute explosive episodes of HP, which are limited in duration and associated with complete recovery. In the subacute form of HP, more intense symptoms occur, and signs and laboratory evaluations suggest more severe disease. Furthermore, the clinical episode may persist for days in spite of avoidance. Corticosteroids given intravenously in doses of 150 mg of hydrocortisone sodium succinate (Solu-Cortef) four times per day hasten recovery. Oxygen therapy may be of benefit during this time if respiratory distress is prominent. As the patient improves, prednisone, 1 mg per kg, may be given by mouth until clinical improvement is apparent and then tapered over the next 7 to 28 days. The duration of therapy is guided by the clinical response as monitored by physical examination and pulmonary function.

Patients with the chronic form of HP may need prolonged avoidance and corticosteroid therapy with frequent clinical evaluation to determine reversibility. Although many patients with this form may have irreversible pulmonary parenchymal damage, it may be useful to administer prednisone, 1 mg per kg for several months with frequent clinical evaluations. If improvement is evident, the drug may be given at the lowest dose that maintains function. Strict avoidance of antigen exposure is imperative in these patients. If the pulmonary impairment is irreversible, the long-term prognosis of the patient will not be improved by corticosteroids.

SINUSITIS

method of
JOSEPH L. LEACH, M.D., and
STEVEN D. SCHAEFER, M.D.
University of Texas Southwestern Medical School
Dallas, Texas

Simply put, sinusitis is an inflammation of the paranasal sinuses. Most inflammations of the sinuses affect the nose, and those of the nose affect the sinuses. The ostiomeatal complex is an area between the middle turbinate and the lateral wall of the nose where the majority of the paranasal sinuses drain. This is also the area in the upper respiratory tract where the most particle deposition from the inspired air takes place. Inflammation in the ostiomeatal complex may quickly lead to obstruction and inflammation of the sinuses.

Several factors may predispose to a sinus infection. Dry air, pollution, and medications have in common the ability to impair ciliary motility. Anatomic abnormalities, such as septal deviation, polyps, and foreign bodies may alter airflow or obstruct sinus ostia and lead to infection. Adenoidal hypertrophy, by restricting normal airflow within the nose, may lead to sinusitis in children. Diving or swimming can force bacteria under pressure into sinuses that are normally sterile. Alterations in the immune system such as allergy may adversely affect the normal mucosal environment of the sinuses. Acquired immune deficiency syndrome (AIDS) or other forms of immunodeficiency may predispose to rarer, opportunistic sinus infections. Loss of B and T cell regulation may result in a hyper-IgE state, producing symptoms much like those of allergic rhinitis. "Vaccine nonresponder state" is a newly described immunodeficiency manifesting in late childhood to adulthood. This should be suspected in patients with recurrent sinopulmonary infections.

ACUTE SINUSITIS

The most common types of acute rhinosinusitis are allergic and viral in etiology. Often, it is difficult to distinguish between the two types, although the patient's history may be of some help. Allergic rhinitis is usually seasonal in nature,

TABLE 1. Microbial Causes of Sinusitis

Acute

Viral
Rhinovirus
Influenza
Parainfluenza
Adenovirus

Bacterial
Streptococcus pneumoniae
Haemophilus influenzae
Moraxella catarrhalis
Streptococcus pyogenes

Chronic
Staphylococcus aureus
Haemophilus influenzae
Anaerobic organisms

and may be associated with itching and redness of the eyes. Viral rhinitis may be characterized by accompanying fever, malaise, and systemic symptoms. In addition, there may be a history of recent exposure to an infected person. Rhinovirus, influenza virus, adenovirus, and parainfluenza virus may all produce acute rhinosinusitis. The treatment of viral rhinosinusitis is nonspecific in the initial stages. It is best managed by adequate fluid intake and watchful waiting.

Acute bacterial sinusitis should be suspected in patients with congestion, thick and greenish nasal discharge, facial pain, and fever. The most commonly implicated organisms (Table 1) are *Streptococcus pneumoniae, Haemophilus influenzae, Moraxella catarrhalis,* and *Streptococcus pyogenes.* Amoxicillin (as a 10-day course) and a short course of decongestants are the recommended first-line therapy (Table 2). The recommended second-line antibiotics include trimethoprim-sulfamethoxazole (Bactrim, Septra), cefaclor (Ceclor), cefuroxime (Ceftin), and amoxicillin–clavulanic acid (Augmentin). If a patient fails to respond to therapy after 48 to 72 hours, consideration should be given to changing the antibiotics. Failure to respond to medical therapy is also an indication for aspiration of the maxillary sinus to obtain organisms for culture and sensi-

TABLE 2. Antimicrobial Therapy of Acute Sinusitis

Antibiotic	Recommended Oral Dose in Adults
Amoxicillin	500 mg q 8 h
Amoxicillin–clavulanate (Augmentin)	500 mg q 8 h
Cefaclor (Ceclor)	500 mg q 6 h
Cefuroxime (Ceftin)	250 mg q 12 h
Trimethoprim-sulfamethoxazole (160/800 mg) (Bactrim, Septra)	1 tablet q 12 h

tivity. Humidifiers and nasal saline irrigations may improve mucociliary function. Antihistamines are not recommended because they may cause further inspissation of secretions. Long-term (greater than 3 days) use of nasal decongestant sprays is to be condemned because tachyphylaxis may result.

A special case is acute frontal sinusitis, which manifests as pain, tenderness, and edema of the anterior cortex of the frontal sinus. Acute frontal sinusitis usually necessitates hospitalization with high-dose intravenous antibiotics and decongestants. Once the infection has subsided, and the danger of erosion into the cranial cavity has subsided, the patient may be discharged on a regimen of oral antibiotics. Should the anterior cortex of the sinus become soft, trephination of the sinus with otolaryngologic consultation is recommended. In some cases, osteomyelitis of the frontal bone results; *Staphylococcus aureus* is the most common organism responsible. Osteomyelitis of the frontal bone is diagnosed by technetium and gallium scans and usually necessitates prolonged courses of intravenous antistaphylococcal antibiotics.

CHRONIC SINUSITIS

There is no widely accepted definition of chronic sinusitis. Acute rhinitis may progress to a stage in which congestion and thick, green, purulent rhinorrhea persist for weeks to months (subacute sinusitis). Fever or facial pain, or both, may be present. *S. aureus, H. influenzae,* and anaerobes play prominent roles in chronic infections. Treatment consists of decongestants in short courses, antibiotics, and nasal saline irrigations. Antibiotics are generally not helpful in patients without fever, facial pain, or tenderness. In such instances, nasal saline irrigation, adequate oral fluid intake, and decongestants should suffice. Refractory cases should be considered for surgery, allergy management, or immunologic work-up. Aspiration of the sinuses may be indicated to detect a resistant organism. Referral to an allergist for allergen testing and/or computed tomographic (CT) scanning of the nasal sinuses may be appropriate in such cases. The scan may indicate areas of inspissated mucus, blockage of the nasal sinus drainage system, polyps, mucoperiosteal thickening, or other findings that are unlikely to respond to medical therapy alone. The preferred method of therapy for such cases at the authors' institution is functional endoscopic sinus surgery.

FUNGAL SINUSITIS

Fungal infections can range from mild infections resembling chronic sinusitis to severe life-threatening infections. Noninvasive fungal sinusitis is often found in patients after other infections or prolonged administration of antibiotics. *Aspergillus* and *Candida* species are commonly found in such instances. Symptoms may be similar to those seen with chronic sinusitis. Treatment may require surgical drainage of the sinuses. The prognosis is excellent.

The invasive form of fungal sinusitis tends to occur in transplant recipients, chemotherapy patients, or poorly controlled diabetics. *Aspergillus* and *Mucor* are two forms of fungi that tend to cause invasive disease in these situations. Symptoms include facial fullness, cranial neuropathies, and pain. Proptosis, facial swelling, and blood-tinged nasal discharge may also be seen. The examination typically reveals gray or black discoloration of the nasal mucosa. The diagnosis is confirmed by biopsy of the affected membranes. Treatment with amphotericin B, aggressive surgical management, and attempts to correct the underlying immunodeficiency may prevent death. Despite treatment, such infections carry a high rate of mortality.

Allergic fungal sinusitis is a recently described entity in which hyphae accumulate within the sinus cavity, producing a dense expansile mass. Many affected patients have a history of allergic rhinosinusitis punctuated by chronic sinusitis. Treatment is based on endoscopic removal of the inspissated mucus, opening of the sinus drainage pathways, postoperative use of copious saline irrigations, and administration of systemic or topical nasal steroids. A strain of *Bipolaris* spp. often grows in the mucus of patients with allergic fungal sinusitis.

COMPLICATIONS OF SINUSITIS

Because of the proximity of the brain and orbit, complications of sinusitis affecting these areas are sometimes seen. Children make up 70 to 80% of patients affected with orbital complications. Of these complications, the most common is preseptal (periorbital) cellulitis. This is recognized as edema of the upper and lower eyelids with associated erythema and fever. There is no proptosis or limitation of the extraocular muscles, and the vision is unaffected. The orbit itself is not tender. Responsible organisms include *H. influenzae* (most commonly), *S. aureus, Streptococcus pneumoniae,* and *S. pyogenes.* Treatment consists of high-dose intravenous antibiotics against the suspected organism. Intravenous cefuroxime in combination with a penicillinase-resistant penicillin (nafcillin, oxacillin) is recommended. A CT scan should be obtained to rule out more serious orbital complications.

Should the infection persist and spread beyond the orbital septum, orbital cellulitis results. This is characterized by proptosis, chemosis, edema, orbital tenderness and pain with eye movement, and erythema of the upper and lower eyelids. The extraocular muscle movement may be impaired, but the visual acuity is typically unaffected. Treatment with high-dose intravenous antibiotics is usually adequate. A CT scan should be obtained in these cases to rule out an area of loculated pus.

Subperiosteal abscess and orbital abscess are other manifestations of the aforementioned disease process. A subperiosteal abscess implies a collection of pus adjacent to the bony wall of the sinus. An orbital abscess is a pus collection within the orbital fat itself. A subperiosteal abscess is associated with downward and outward displacement of the globe. The visual acuity may or may not be impaired. Orbital abscess is difficult to differentiate from subperiosteal abscess because both entities may manifest with decreased extraocular muscle mobility, decreased vision, chemosis, tearing, and erythema and edema of the upper and lower lids. CT scans may indicate a low-density mass with gas-fluid levels and displacement of the medial rectus muscle. Both forms of abscess are surgical emergencies and necessitate immediate ophthalmologic and otolaryngologic consultation. Drainage of the pus is usually accomplished through an external ethmoidectomy approach, although the endoscopic approach has been used successfully for such cases.

The formation of pus at the posterior aspect of the orbit may produce orbital apex syndrome. This syndrome includes diminished vision and ophthalmoplegia caused by impingement on cranial nerves III, IV, and VI. There is also anesthesia of the globe and forehead caused by cranial nerve V involvement. If the infection travels posteriorly, the cavernous sinus may become infected. Cavernous sinus thrombosis is associated with bilateral orbital cellulitis. This may produce neuropathies of cranial nerves II, III, IV, V, and VI, as well as high fever, chills, and meningeal signs. *S. aureus* is the usual culprit. Treatment is with high-dose intravenous antibiotics.

Other intracranial complications include epidural abscess, subdural abscess, brain abscess, and meningitis. The common pathogens include *S. pneumoniae*, *H. influenzae*, and *S. aureus*. Treatment includes high-dose intravenous antibiotics, followed by surgical drainage of the affected sinuses. Epidural abscesses, subdural abscess, and brain abscesses are neurosurgical emergencies mandating appropriate referral if suspected.

STREPTOCOCCAL PHARYNGITIS

method of
JAMES W. BASS, M.D., M.P.H.
Tripler Army Medical Center
Honolulu, Hawaii

DIAGNOSIS

Numerous clinical studies have shown that experienced physicians are able to clinically differentiate patients who have streptococcal phayrngitis from those who have non-streptococcal pharyngitis with little more than 50% accuracy. Accordingly, throat culture has been considered the gold standard for laboratory confirmation of this diagnosis since the early 1950s. Because a delay in treatment of up to several days does not incur the risk of rheumatic fever and many authorities have taught that early treatment does not significantly alter the acute clinical course of the disease, delay in treatment for 24 to 72 hours until results of the throat culture may be known has been considered acceptable.

Recent well-controlled clinical studies have shown that early antibiotic treatment of children with streptococcal pharyngitis does significantly alter the acute clinical course of the disease. Also, tests that permit rapid laboratory-confirmed diagnosis of streptococcal pharyngitis by detecting group A carbohydrate–specific antigen directly on the throat swab have recently become available. These tests, called "rapid strep tests" (RSTs), require only minutes to perform, and in most studies results correlate well with those of the throat culture. These tests are quite specific, although they are not very sensitive; for this reason, most clinicians perform a throat culture at the same time to identify individuals who may have a false-negative RST.

Most individuals with streptococcal pharyngitis who receive early antibiotic treatment are afebrile and have marked symptomatic improvement within 24 hours. Early treatment decreases the incidence of suppurative complications and limits spread of the disease in the family and community. Throat cultures from antibiotic-treated patients are usually negative within 24 hours after initiation of treatment, so that the patients can be presumed to be noncontagious and return to school. Because both parents in many households in the United States currently work outside the home, early antibiotic treatment of children with streptococcal pharyngitis offers significant clinical, public health, social, educational, and economic benefits.

ANTIMICROBIAL TREATMENT

Penicillin remains the drug of choice for treatment of streptococcal infections. All strains of group A beta-hemolytic streptococci (GABHS) re-

The opinions or assertions contained herein are the private views of the author and are not to be construed as official or as reflecting the views of the U.S. Department of the Army or the U.S. Department of Defense. All material in this article is in the public domain.

main exquisitely sensitive to penicillin, and there has been no indication of emerging resistance to this drug. The optimal preparation and route of administration vary with clinical circumstances.

Oral Penicillin. In private practice settings, good compliance with oral treatment and results equal to those with intramuscular penicillin G benzathine can be achieved with parental counseling that emphasizes the need for the medication to be given for a full 10 days to eliminate the infecting organisms and prevent rheumatic fever. Oral penicillin G and penicillin V are equally effective, but the latter is preferred as it is acid-stable, is better absorbed, and produces predictably higher blood levels of penicillin. For children under 12 years of age, optimal oral penicillin treatment of streptococcal pharyngitis is achieved with a dose of 250 mg given twice daily for 10 days. For children over 12 years of age, adolescents, and adults, a dose of 500 mg twice daily for 10 days (a U.S. Food and Drug Administration–approved treatment regimen) is optimal. Higher doses or dosages more often than twice daily or for longer than 10 days do not produce higher cure rates. Because compliance in taking oral medications decreases with frequency of dosing and duration of treatment, dose intervals of more than twice daily and treatment periods for longer than 10 days should probably not be prescribed. In addition, twice-daily treatment can be more realistically achieved in school-aged children with working parents. A rational exception might be in the first 24 to 48 hours of treatment, during which doses may be given every 6 to 8 hours while the child remains sick and at home, in an effort to ensure an early bacteriologic cure and render the child noncontagious as early as possible.

Intramuscular Penicillin Preparations. In contrast to the circumstances outlined in which oral penicillin treatment is preferred, intramuscular penicillin G benzathine should be given to patients with streptococcal pharyngitis in areas where rheumatic fever is prevalent, particularly in poor and crowded inner city populations in which both medical care is episodic and compliance in taking oral penicillin cannot be relied on. These conditions apply in many pediatric populations in the United States and for most children in developing or Third World countries. In these circumstances, intramuscular penicillin G benzathine in a dose of 600,000 units for children weighing less than 27 kg (60 pounds) and 900,000 to 1,200,000 units for those weighing more than 27 kg provides optimal treatment. A significantly less painful and better accepted intramuscular preparation that contains 900,000 units of penicillin G benzathine and 300,000 units of penicillin G procaine within 2-mL volume has been shown to be effective for children. In addition to reducing the pain at the injection site, the procaine component produces higher initial penicillin blood levels; although this does not effect a more rapid clinical response than does straight penicillin G benzathine, it produces an earlier bacterial cure rate approaching 100% after 24 hours, presumably rendering the patient noncontagious and able to return to school. This 2-mL preparation offers optimal injection treatment for prepubertal children less than 12 years of age. For older children, adolescents, and adults, parenteral therapy is best achieved with 1,200,000 units of penicillin G benzathine.

Extended-spectrum oral penicillins, including ampicillin and ampicillin-like penicillins (amoxicillin and bacampicillin [Spectrobid]) as well as oral penicillinase-resistant penicillins (cloxacillin, dicloxacillin, and oxacillin) are all effective for treatment of streptococcal pharyngitis. Their use should be reserved for situations where they afford added benefit. They are generally more expensive and are associated with more untoward reactions, including skin rashes and gastrointestinal disturbances.

Alternatives to Penicillin. For patients who cannot take penicillin, erythromycin is considered the first alternative for oral treatment of streptococcal pharyngitis. The recommended erythromycin estolate dosage is 20 to 40 mg per kg per day in two to four divided doses, and the recommended erythromycin ethylsuccinate dosage is 40 mg per kg per day in two to four doses; both dosages are taken for 10 days. Erythromycin estolate given at 20 mg per kg per day in two divided doses has been shown to be well tolerated and equally effective as 250 mg of penicillin V given three or four times daily. Erythromycin ethylsuccinate must be given in a dosage of 40 to 50 mg per kg per day to be equally effective, and at this dosage it is better tolerated when given in four divided doses daily. Unlike most other oral antimicrobial agents, both of these oral erythromycin preparations are better absorbed and better tolerated when given with food rather than during fasting.

For children who cannot take penicillin or erythromycin, cephalexin or cephradine, 25 to 50 mg per kg per day in three to four divided doses, or cephadroxil, 30 mg per kg per day in two divided doses provides excellent treatment. Although oral cephalosporins are generally more expensive than oral penicillins, cephalosporin suspensions taste better and are significantly better accepted. Clindamycin, 25 to 40 mg per kg per day in three to four divided doses, is an acceptable alternative for patients who cannot take penicillins, cephalosporins, or erythromycin.

Oral second- and third-generation cephalosporins may be used to treat patients with streptococcal pharyngitis who also have otitis media (because of their additional activity against *Haemophilus influenzae* and *Moraxella catarrhalis*) and who cannot take penicillin drugs. Cefaclor (Ceclor), cefuroxime axitel (Ceftin), cefixime (Suprax), and cefpodoxime (Vantin) are acceptable for this purpose but they are quite expensive. Erythromycin-sulfisoxazole, 40 mg per kg per day of the erythromycin component, in four divided doses is an alternative under these circumstances, but trimethoprim-sulfamethoxazole is not because it is inadequate for treatment of GABHS infections.

RESPONSE TO TREATMENT

In children with streptococcal pharyngitis the clinical response to appropriate antimicrobial treatment is nearly always evident within 24 hours. Most children recover fully and become culture-negative within 1 to 2 days after initiation of treatment and can return to school. Persistence of high fever and severe symptoms beyond this period suggests the development of a suppurative complication or some other underlying disease.

FOLLOW-UP

Post-treatment follow-up throat cultures are not recommended for patients who remain asymptomatic. Exception to this policy should be made for patients who have had rheumatic fever or for other family members in the household who have had rheumatic fever. Every attempt should be made to eradicate GABHS from these patients and other household members in an effort to prevent further episodes of rheumatic fever.

CHRONIC CARRIERS

Nearly all treated patients remain culture-negative during the 10 days of treatment. However, if follow-up cultures are obtained during the 6-week period after treatment is completed, about 10 to 15% develop positive cultures for GABHS again, regardless of the type of treatment given. Most of these isolates are the same serotype as the initial isolate made before treatment was given, and they represent the asymptomatic chronic convalescent carrier state. This chronic carrier state usually persists for several months or more, regardless of whether the patient is re-treated or not, although cultures usually become negative during retreatment. In children who have classic streptococcal pharyngitis, are highly contagious, and are at significant risk of developing rheumatic fever if left untreated, throat cultures grow a heavy or almost pure culture of GABHS; in contrast, throat cultures of chronic carriers usually yield only a scant growth or a few colonies of GABHS. There is general agreement that chronic carriers are not a significant source of spread of infection or at risk of developing rheumatic fever. Therefore, there is no need or reason to seek detection of persons who only manifest the asymptomatic chronic convalescent carrier state of GABHS.

RELAPSES AND REINFECTIONS

Patients who develop symptomatic illnesses suggestive of streptococcal pharyngitis during the first 2 to 3 months after treatment and whose throat cultures are again positive for GABHS should be considered to have relapses or reinfections. Those with GABHS of the same serotype as the initial isolate before treatment should be considered to have relapses, and they should be re-treated. Those with a different serotype from the initial isolate should be considered to have reinfections; they too should be re-treated. Serotype information on GABHS isolates is difficult to obtain, expensive, time consuming, and not practical to be helpful in making decisions for management of these patients. It is not possible to clinically differentiate post-treatment symptomatic patients who have failed treatment or have reinfections from those who may be chronic convalescent carriers of GABHS and are symptomatic as a result of coincidental nonstreptococcal pharyngitis. Accordingly, all patients who have symptomatic illnesses suggestive of streptococcal pharyngitis and whose throat culture yields any growth of GABHS should be treated.

CONTACTS

Among members of the same household as index cases, there is a high incidence of secondary infection. From 30 to 50% of siblings and 10 to 20% of parents or adult household contacts are culture-positive for GABHS, and up to 50% of siblings develop symptoms of streptococcal pharyngitis within several weeks. These observations have led some treating physicians in the past to take cultures from all household members of index cases at the outset and to treat those who are culture positive in order to prevent "ping-pong" infection and reinfection in the household during and after the index case is treated. Most primary care physicians today, however, prefer to take cultures only from symptomatic household contacts and treat only those whose cultures are positive.

RECURRENT STREPTOCOCCAL PHARYNGITIS

Children who have frequent and recurrent bouts of culture-proven streptococcal pharyngitis are sometimes encountered as special management problems in pediatric clinic settings. If oral antibiotics were prescribed, compliance may be questioned, and consideration should be given for the use of intramuscular penicillin G benzathine for treatment. If other family members (usually siblings) are involved, intrafamilial spread of infection in a ping-pong manner may be suspected; consideration should be given to obtaining cultures from all household members and treating those with positive cultures for GABHS simultaneously in an effort to eradicate the organism from the household.

Recent studies present convincing evidence that the presence of beta-lactamase-producing organisms in tonsillar tissue may inactivate penicillin drugs and promote survival and persistence of GABHS in these tissues, leading to recurrent infection. If this is suspected, a trial of treatment with antimicrobial drugs that are not inactivated by penicillin-beta-lactamases, such as erythromycin, a cephalosporin, or clindamycin should be considered. Preliminary studies suggest that clindamycin may be most effective in this regard, and this drug is the most active against beta-lactamase-producing anaerobic organisms that are commonly found in tonsillar tissues. Recent reports contend that "tolerance" to penicillin by some strains of GABHS may be implicated in some cases of failure of penicillin treatment for streptococcal pharyngitis. These contentions require further verification. Meanwhile, the use of non-penicillin treatment regimens, including erythromycin and clindamycin, should obviate this possibility.

NON–GROUP A STREPTOCOCCAL PHARYNGITIS

Patients who have symptoms of streptococcal pharyngitis and whose throat cultures yield a significant growth of non–group A streptococci (usually groups C and G) pose a problem to the treating physician. Although it is agreed that these patients are not at risk of developing rheumatic fever if they do not receive antimicrobial treatment, there is controversy as to whether these organisms actually cause symptomatic streptococcal pharyngitis. There is also controversy as to whether the clinical illnesses in these patients are responsive to antimicrobial therapy. Most primary care physicians believe that non–group A beta hemolytic streptococci are a significant cause of streptococcal-like pharyngitis and that the clinical illness in these patients is responsive to penicillin treatment. Although clinical data specifically substantiating this belief are lacking, antimicrobial treatment is recommended for patients with symptoms of streptococcal pharyngitis and whose throat culture yields a significant growth of non–group A beta hemolytic streptococci. Because these organisms are usually sensitive to the same antimicrobial drugs that are effective against group A streptococci, the treatment regimens recommended for streptococcal pharyngitis caused by group A organisms are also recommended for non–group A organisms.

TUBERCULOSIS AND OTHER MYCOBACTERIAL DISEASES

method of
J. E. KASIK, M.D., Ph.D.
University of Iowa
Iowa City, Iowa

After a century of decline, there has been an increase in the incidence of tuberculosis in the United States in each of the last 5 years. This is unprecedented and alarming.

This increase is believed to have been produced by the advent of acquired immune deficiency syndrome (AIDS), increased immigration into North America from the Third World, homelessness, deinstitutionalization of the mentally ill, widespread drug abuse, and the dismantling of the previously existing, highly effective, antituberculous programs supported by various cities and states. The latter occurred in the name of economy and was based on the fallacious assumption that tuberculosis was no longer an important public health problem.

Tuberculosis has been and continues to be a serious problem in many areas of the world. It has been estimated that worldwide there are about 30 million new cases of tuberculosis annually and 3 million deaths. Many of these deaths occur because affected persons go untreated as the result of economic, social, or political conditions.

Another serious public health problem in this country has been the increasing incidence of multidrug-resistant mycobacteria. Although this problem has been limited to certain geographic areas (e.g., Southeast Asia) or certain populations (e.g., drug addicts, street people), it has been spreading from these populations to others, such as correctional officers, personnel in homeless shelters, and health care workers. In certain facilities, such as large urban hospitals, that care for many patients with tuberculosis, which is sometimes drug-resistant, it has been reported almost half of the front-line staff in contact with patients have had tuberculin skin test conversions, indicating that they have been infected.

EPIDEMIOLOGY

Infection with mycobacterium tuberculosis occurs as the result of inhalation of an infected droplet of sputa produced by coughing in a patient with active, cavitary pulmonary tuberculosis. The person infected is usually someone who lives in close contact with someone else who has active disease. The primary infection usually occurs in a respiratory area of the lung and spreads to the regional lymph nodes and, from there, throughout the body as subclinical miliary disease. With the development of immunity, the infection is usually controlled and becomes inactive, but the infection leaves a small foci containing live mycobacteria, which are quiescent. Reactivation of this foci can occur, frequently as the result of malnutrition, debilitation, immunosuppression, or other forms of stress. Hence active tuberculosis is associated with starvation, surgery, diseases such as Hodgkin's lymphoma and AIDS, immunosuppressive therapy, and immunosuppressive side effects of cancer chemotherapy.

Because tuberculosis is spread by person-to-person contact, the disease tends to appear in clusters, often among family members or other persons housed together.

The prevalence of active tuberculosis is directly proportional to the incidence of a positive cutaneous reaction to the purified protein derivative (PPD) of tuberculin in any population. A positive PPD skin test is a marker for latent tuberculosis and, in the absence of immunosuppression, a reliable indicator that the person with a positive test has viable mycobacteria within the body.

Control of the spread of tuberculosis depends on an aggressive approach to the diagnosis of active disease. The most hazardous situation involves the patient with a chronic cough who is treated with a variety of antibiotics by unsuspecting physicians who ignore the symptoms and signs of active tuberculosis. With the previous decline in the incidence of tuberculosis, there was a decline in the diagnostic skills and level of clinical suspicion needed to activate and initiate a vigorous program to diagnose the disease and prescribe appropriate chemotherapy.

Control of the spread of tuberculosis in hospitalized patients is achieved by promptly isolating patients with suspected tuberculosis in an appropriate, negative–air pressure room and appropriate masking of health care personnel involved in the care of the patient. The type of mask recommended is currently still unsettled because the degree of protection required, especially if the patient harbors drug-resistant mycobacteria, is unclear. The one settled point is that the flimsy, ill-fitting paper masks widely used in the past are inadequate and must be replaced by a mask that is leakproof, capable of removing particles as small as 0.5 μ in diameter, and capable of maintaining their integrity if wet by perspiration or saliva.

Another important factor to stress in preventing spread of tuberculosis is the well-documented control of infectiousness of tuberculosis by the prompt initiation of effective chemotherapy of tuberculosis. In patients with contagious tuberculosis, it has been shown that only a few weeks or even days of appropriate drug therapy lowers the risk of spread to others.

Education of patients will markedly reduce spread of disease almost at once. Teaching patients to cough into a disposable cellulose tissue and giving antitussive drugs markedly reduces the number of airborne infectious particles.

In the transport of patients with suspected tuberculosis, the patient should be masked, and movement throughout the hospital should be limited to travel for absolutely essential procedures. Such procedures as pulmonary function tests, sleep studies, or endoscopy should be withheld until the question of infectiousness has been settled.

DIAGNOSIS OF MYCOBACTERIAL DISEASES

The diagnosis of pulmonary tuberculosis and some forms of extrapulmonary tuberculosis depends on three primary factors:

1. A positive tuberculin skin test. Despite the many situations in which this test has little or no value, it is nonetheless a very important marker for both latent and active disease, when it is positive. Unfortunately, in patients with AIDS, in patients receiving immunosuppressive drugs, or in severely ill persons with widespread tuberculosis, the test may be negative despite the presence of active tuberculosis.

The usual strength of tuberculin used for diagnostic testing is 5 tuberculin units (TU). The old standard of a positive reaction to PPD was a reaction with 10 mm or more of induration. Since the advent of AIDS, more complicated rules have been needed to interpret the test (Table 1). The basis for these changes is an attempt to deal with the serious problem of the diminished reaction in immunosuppressed patients.

Another useful approach to this problem of the patient with a negative 5-TU test is to repeat the test by using 250 TU (second-strength PPD). This strength of PPD carries a higher incidence of false-positive results because exposure to atypical mycobacteria may produce a positive reaction to second-strength PPD. It has been shown that patients who have a negative reaction to intermediate-strength PPD and who are infected with mycobacteria can react to 250 TU. As a result, repeating the test with 250 TU may be useful, if interpreted intelligently.

The effectiveness of applying a number of other skin test antigens, such as mumps and *Candida,* to assess patient anergy, which is a widespread practice, has little documentation, and this procedure is no substitute for proper interpretation of the skin test. It is common to find patients who are nonreactive to the companion tests but have a vigorous reaction to PPD.

2. A suspicious chest x-ray. Pulmonary tuberculosis manifests on a chest x-ray as a fibronodu-

TABLE 1. **Drugs Commonly Used to Treat Tuberculosis and Their Side Effects**

Drug	Adult Dosage (per day)	Major Side Effects	Detection	Remarks
Isoniazid (INH)	300 mg	Peripheral neuritis, hepatitis, convulsions	Hepatic enzymes	For neuritis, vitamin B$_6$, 25–50 mg, as prophylaxis; hepatitis rare in persons under the age of 35 years
Ethambutol (EMB)	15 mg/kg	Optic neuritis	Visual acuity; red-green color discrimination	Ocular history and visual examination before use; discoloration of urine occurs
Rifampin	600 mg	GI disturbance, hepatitis, thrombocytopenia, rare renal damage, flu syndrome	Bilirubin, BUN, creatinine levels	
Pyrazinamide (PZA)	Weight 50–74 kg, 2 gm; >75 kg, 2.5 gm	GI disturbance, hepatitis, hyperuricemia, photosensitivity	Hepatic enzymes, uric acid	Hepatitis is dose related
Streptomycin (SM)	0.75–1.0 gm	Otic and vestibular toxicity, decreased hearing, vertigo, tinnitus	Gross hearing, audiograms	Side effects are more common in older patients (over 60); decrease dose or avoid drug if renal insufficiency exists

Abbreviations: GI = gastrointestinal; BUN = blood urea nitrogen.

lar infiltrate, usually in the apical posterior portion of the upper or lower lobe of the lung, with cavitation, often multiple. There is frequently upward retraction of the hila toward the lesion. An old pleural reaction or a calcified primary complex may be present.

Unfortunately, the classical x-ray manifestation of tuberculosis may be attenuated or even absent in immunosuppressed persons. Pulmonary filtrates with little or no fibrosis and lack of cavities can be found and can significantly mislead the physician.

3. Identification of mycobacteria. Mycobacteria have traditionally been identified by Ziehl-Neelsen staining of concentrates of sputa or other body fluids. Cultures of concentrated sputa is a much more sensitive way of identifying mycobacteria than smears, but results of this test should not be expected for 6 to 12 weeks, and an additional 4 to 6 weeks are needed for drug sensitivity studies to be completed.

The methods used for the identification of mycobacteria are at present in transition technologically, with considerable improvement in the length of time required to make a diagnosis. The polymerase chain reaction (PCR), when applied to mycobacteria, provides a rapid (48-hour) method of identifying small numbers of mycobacteria in sputa, urine, cerebrospinal or pleural fluid, and appropriately processed tissue specimens.

There has also been a marked improvement in the methods used to determine drug sensitivity in mycobacteria. Rapid automated radiometric detection of mycobacterial growth, as found in the BACTEC system, offers reliable drug sensitivity testing in approximately 1 week in a manner as reliable as the older, slower methods widely used at present.

TREATMENT (Table 1)

Isoniazid

Isoniazid (INH) was introduced into therapy in the early 1950s. It has only one use—therapy of mycobacteria infection—and in that role, it has been an almost ideal drug: It is cheap, highly effective, and bacteriocidal and carries a very low incidence of serious or even minor side effects. Because of its potency, it can be effectively administered only once a day, and less-than-perfect compliance with therapy is nevertheless usually associated with a favorable outcome of therapy.

The most common side effect of INH is drug-induced hepatitis with hepatocellular damage, but this complication is usually mild and reversible if the drug is discontinued. Mild elevations of levels of liver enzymes such as aspartate aminotransferase are fairly common, and if they are not severe or are continuing to rise or are associated with an elevated bilirubin level, the drug can be continued, with caution, because the test often returns to normal. Severe reactions, including fatalities, have occurred, however, when the drug was continued despite severe or progressive elevation of liver enzyme levels, an elevated bilirubin level, and resulting clinical jaundice. Other factors contributing to the toxicity of INH are pre-existing hepatic disease, alcohol abuse, and age. INH hepatic injury increases in frequency and severity with age. It is extremely rare in infants and children but common after age 35. As a result, INH in therapy can be used at any age, but it has been recommended that it not be used for prophylaxis in those persons over 35 except in unusual circumstances (e.g., patients with AIDS, latent or otherwise, with a positive reaction to PPD).

INH is metabolized mainly by hepatic conversion to the acetylated metabolite. The rate is genetically determined, and patients who are slow acetylators, as found in Asian populations, may have an increased rate of pyridoxine deficiency induced by free INH.

Rifampin

Rifampin is a broad-spectrum antibiotic used most often to treat tuberculosis. It carries a very low incidence of side effects; the usual side effect is a hypersensitivity reaction with hepatitis, joint pain, malaise, low-grade fever, and skin rash as major complaints. In contrast to INH-associated hepatitis, the hepatitis associated with rifampin precludes restarting the drug after hepatic function has returned to normal. Deaths have occurred in patients who had recovered from rifampin hepatitis when therapy with the drug was resumed.

Rifampin induces the hepatic microsomes involved in drug metabolism, and as a result, when rifampin therapy is initiated or discontinued, the levels of such drugs as theophylline, coumadin, steroids, digoxin, oral antihyperglycemic agents, and perhaps the oral contraceptives can change and produce serious complications of therapy. These drugs should be appropriately monitored when rifampin is used.

Rifampin induces a bright red-orange discoloration of the urine of recipients and may color breast milk, sweat, and tears. This is a harmless phenomenon that alarms uninformed patients.

Rifampin is bactericidal for susceptible mycobacteria and, although less potent than INH, is nonetheless a powerful antituberculosis agent. It is very commonly used as a companion drug with INH. Like INH, it is useful in treating all forms of tuberculosis, and it is now available parenterally as well as orally, permitting its use in unconscious patients.

Rifabutin (Ansamycin) is a semisynthetic derivative of rifampin that has been used almost exclusively, with limited success, for *Mycobacterium avium-intracellulare* complex (MAC) infection in patients with AIDS. Its properties and side effects are similar to those of rifampin.

Ethambutol

Ethambutol (Myambutol) is a chemotherapeutic agent used exclusively to treat tuberculosis as a companion drug with INH and rifampin. Although it is much less potent than INH or rifampin, it is very useful in preventing the emergence of drug resistance when used with these drugs. Ethambutol has been associated with retinal damage if used in doses of 25 mg per kg or higher. Lower doses (10 to 15 mg per kg) have a much lower incidence of the side effect.

Pyrazinamide

Pyrazinamide (PZA) is a very potent antituberculosis drug, at least as active as INH. Because this chemotherapeutic agent had an early and largely undeserved reputation of significant hepatic toxicity, it was never widely used in primary treatment regimens in the recent past. As a result, the incidence of drug resistance to PZA has been much lower than that to INH, and PZA is often used as a part of retreatment programs or other situations in which resistance to INH and rifampin is suspected. It is also useful in short-term therapy.

Oral PZA is a highly effective bacteriocidal agent and usually well tolerated.

Common side effects are gastrointestinal upset and inhibition of renal urate excretion with hyperuricemia and occasional clinical gout. Hepatic injury with elevation of levels of hepatic enzymes, hyperbilirubinemia, and clinical jaundice can occur. Acute fulminate hepatic necrosis has been reported. All of the hepatic side effects are dose-related, and it is important to avoid excessive doses of PZA (e.g., prescribing by weight in an obese patient). Prior liver damage may be another factor leading to an increased incidence of serious hepatic damage, as in alcoholism and hepatitis and perhaps, with age. The safety of PZA during pregnancy has not been established.

Streptomycin

Streptomycin has the distinction of being the first effective antituberculosis antibiotic. It was widely used at one time, but because it must be given by injection, it is expensive, and ototoxicity is associated with this antibiotic, it was largely superseded by other drugs, and its manufacture for human therapy was briefly discontinued. With the resurgence of tuberculosis, the drug has become available again.

Streptomycin is an injectable aminoglycoside. This limitation is sometimes an asset because it ensures compliance, and because of the difficulties and expense of administration, its use has been uncommon. As a result, less drug resistance has been associated with streptomycin, and this has made it one of the drugs often useful in the treatment of multidrug-resistant tuberculosis.

Ototoxicity is the most important side effect of streptomycin administration. The incidence of this complication is increased in older patients and in patients with pre-existing renal disease and is directly related to the cumulative total dose administered. If renal disease is present, the dose should be reduced, and it should be recalled that streptomycin may also produce damage of the eighth nerve in the fetus. Streptomycin also occasionally produces skin rashes, fever, and other symptoms of a hypersensitivity reaction.

Kanamycin and amikacin are other aminoglycosides used to treat drug-resistant tuberculosis; their advantages and disadvantages are similar to those of streptomycin. They do not have bacterial cross-resistance with streptomycin, but they do share its ototoxic properties. They are also renal toxic, and their use must be accompanied by monitoring the serum creatinine level.

Other Drugs

The drugs discussed here are not widely used for a variety of reasons, the most common being the frequency or severity of their side effects. As a rule, they are less effective than the standard drugs such as INH.

They are used to treat drug-resistant tuberculosis and occasionally for the treatment of atypical mycobacterial infections. It is advisable to use these drugs with consultation. When new drugs are added to an antituberculosis program, they should always be added in pairs (or more) to prevent the development of additional drug resistance. Adding a single drug to a failing program of chemotherapy of tuberculosis is a major error.

Para-aminosalicylic acid (PAS) is one of the oldest antituberculosis drugs. It is only weakly bacteriostatic but has value as a companion drug with the other more potent drugs such as INH or PZA. In this role, PAS prevents resistance to the primary drug. Its side effects are numerous but, fortunately, usually mild and reversible when the drug is discontinued. Loss of appetite, nausea, vomiting, gastritis, flatulence, and diarrhea are common (30%) and often lead to poor compliance with drug therapy. Hypersensitivity, in the form of fever, skin rash, and arthralgias may also occur, and in rare instances, leukopenia, thrombocytopenia, or agranulocytoses develop.

Capreomycin (Capastat Sulfate), a parenteral antituberculosis drug, has not been widely used. It is of value in retreatment programs of drug-resistant strains of *M. tuberculosis,* particularly in the early phases of retreatment. It has a number of potentially serious side effects, including ototoxicity, nephrotoxicity, reversible leukopenia, fever, skin rash, and hypokalemia. Neuromuscular blockade, similar to that sometimes seen with the aminoglycosides, has been reported.

Ethionamide (Trecator-SC) is another antituberculosis drug used almost exclusively in retreatment programs. It is orally effective with an impressive list of side effects. Gastric irritation has been reported in almost one-third of the patients who receive therapeutic doses of the drug, and the patient may lose weight when taking the drug because of induced anorexia. Other side effects include mental changes (i.e., confusion, depression), blurred vision, diplopia, vertigo, headache, neuropathy, and tremors. Hypersensitivity reactions, including fever and skin rash, and quasi-endocrine problems such as gynecomastia, menorrhagia, and impotence are occasionally seen. About 3 to 5% of the patients taking this compound may exhibit elevations of levels of hepatic enzymes, which clear when the drug is stopped. Some of these problems can be eliminated by the concomitant administration of pyridoxine (vitamin B_6), and hepatic enzyme levels should be monitored when this drug is used.

Cycloserine (Seromycin) is a broad-spectrum antibiotic that has only very limited use in tuberculosis because of its alarming central nervous system side effects. It is bactericidal, inhibiting cell wall synthesis. The drug should be used only in therapy of multidrug-resistant tuberculosis. Its side effects occur almost exclusively in the central nervous system: seizures, stupor, somnolence, personality changes, psychosis, and increased intracranial pressure. There is some evidence that large doses of pyridoxine (200 to 300 mg per day) can reduce the incidence and severity of these side effects. Alcohol increases the incidence of these side effects.

New Antituberculosis Drugs

Because of the increasing prevalence of multidrug-resistant tuberculosis and the alarming incidence of atypical mycobacterial infections as terminal events in patients with AIDS, there has been a renewed interest in developing new antituberculosis drugs.

Rifabutin is an orally effective semisynthetic member of the ansamycin family of broad-spectrum antibiotics. It is similar in structure and antibacterial spectrum to rifampin. Its side effects, including orange discoloration of body fluids, are similar to those encountered with rifampin. The major useful property of rifabutin is its activity, which is somewhat greater than that of rifampin, with some of the atypical mycobacteria, including MAC, a very difficult therapeutic problem. Rifabutin still has an ill-defined role with multidrug-resistant tuberculosis because its incidence of cross-resistance with rifampin awaits delineation.

Ciprofloxacin (Cipro) and ofloxacin (Floxin) are fluroquinolones, a well-established group of drugs of considerable usefulness for the treatment of gram-negative infections. Although the U.S. Food and Drug Administration has not approved their use in treating tuberculosis, there have been several reports of their effectiveness in atypical mycobacterial infections, a very difficult clinical problem.

The derivatives of erythromycin, azithromycin and clarithromycin, may be useful in the therapy of atypical mycobacterial infections. The infections with MAC in patients with AIDS has created a desperate need for drugs effective against this highly resistant organism. Although the new macrolides do not appear to be curative in this situation, they may suppress the infection, perhaps prolong life, and reduce symptoms.

Principles of Antituberculous Therapy
(Table 2)

If any of the three potent antituberculosis drugs—INH, rifampin, or PZA—is given alone, it has a beneficial effect in active tuberculosis. The numbers of mycobacteria diminish, the x-ray improves, and the patient has favorable clinical signs and symptoms. Unfortunately, this favorable course is often only temporary under these circumstances; within some months, drug-resistant organisms reappear and the disease re-emerges. This was the major problem first encountered when streptomycin was used alone in the earliest clinical trials of the treatment of tuberculosis.

The reasons for this sequence of events is straightforward. In pulmonary tuberculosis, the numbers of organisms found in the lung may be in the range of 10^8 bacteria. Among these billions of organisms, one in 10^5 to 10^6 organisms has an inherent resistance to INH, for example. As a result, if INH is used alone, the resistant organisms survive, multiply, and reestablish the infection, and the lung is now populated by organisms resistant to INH. Drug resistance in this context is an experiment in Darwinism with survival and dominance of the fittest in an adverse environment.

This outcome can be avoided by using several drugs. If one bacterium in 10^5 organisms is resistant to INH and one in 10^4 is resistant to streptomycin, the chances of encountering an INH-streptomycin–resistant organism is one in 10^9 bacteria, a very large number. This number should exceed the number of mycobacteria present, and therapy with these two drugs, if given for a sufficient period of time, should be successful. As a matter of fact, this theoretical prediction has been shown to be true by repeated clinical experiences. If three drugs are used, only one in 10^{14} organisms is resistant to all three.

In cavitary pulmonary tuberculosis, INH and ethambutol given together can be effective with an acceptably low rate of post-treatment recurrence even though ethambutol is a weak drug. To achieve this, the drugs must be given for a period of time sufficient to kill most of the mycobacteria (usually 18 months to 2 years). This was standard therapy for years. By adding another first-line, more bactericidal drug such as rifampin, the length of therapy can be reduced while an acceptable rate of recurrence is preserved.

As a result, therapy for pulmonary tuberculosis consists of two first-line drugs given for 1 year or less; this has a satisfactory outcome except in the most advanced disease. If three first-line drugs are used, even 6 months of therapy can have a favorable outcome.

If these concepts are put into perspective, it can be observed that the cost and side effects of the additional drugs, used in short-course chemotherapy, should be balanced against the different risks of a longer period of therapy with fewer drugs but with the attendant possibilities that the patient will discontinue the drugs or will be lost to follow-up.

Any clinician faced with the problem of initiating antituberculosis therapy must assess the reliability of the patient. Most patients who have had a poor outcome with treatment for tuberculosis have been unreliable, taking the drugs irregularly or failing to complete the course of treatment.

It must be stressed with the greatest emphasis that tuberculosis therapy is highly effective, safe, and reasonably free of side effects only if the patient complies with the prescribed regimen. The physician must be absolutely sure that the patient is following the program of treatment. Clinic visits, visiting nurses, social workers, and family members can be as important as properly prescribed drugs in ensuring a successful outcome to the therapy of tuberculosis.

TABLE 2. **Therapy of Pulmonary Tuberculosis in Adults (9 Months)**

Isoniazid	300 mg/day as a single daily dose
Rifampin	600 mg/day as a single daily dose
Ethambutol	15 mg/kg per day for first 60 days
Pyridoxine	25 mg/day is optional

Supervised intermittent therapy is one approach for the unreliable individual, and enforced hospitalization, or its equivalent, is another. These approaches represent a significant encroachment on the patient's civil rights, but in many instances, they appear to be the only way to prevent the spread of tuberculosis, often multidrug-resistant tuberculosis. Multidrug-resistant tuberculosis carries a very high mortality rate, especially among immunosuppressed persons, and is a serious health hazard for health care personnel.

Standard therapy for active pulmonary tuberculosis consists of INH, 300 mg per day; rifampin, 600 mg per day; and, if disease is extensive (bilateral, multicavitary, or several lobes involved), ethambutol, 15 mg per kg for the first 60 days of treatment. Total duration of therapy is 9 months in reliable, compliant patients who have a favorable clinical response.

If PZA (15 mg per kg; maximal dose, 2 grams) is added to ethambutol, INH, and rifampin, therapy can be shortened to 6 months if clinical indicators demonstrate satisfactory progress (i.e., sputum conversion, clearing, and improvement of chest x-ray). The PZA can also be discontinued after 2 months.

If the history or results of drug sensitivity tests suggest drug resistance, PZA must be continued for the duration of therapy, and streptomycin (1 gram daily or three times a week) in adults with normal renal function should be substituted for ethambutol.

Patients with demonstrated or suspected multidrug-resistant tuberculosis require consultation and careful evaluation. At present, many but not all such patients have organisms sensitive to PZA and streptomycin because these drugs have not been widely used in recent years, but this may not be true in the future. Multidrug-resistant tuberculosis must be treated for 18 months to 2 years with clear evidence of control of the infection.

Drug sensitivities must be obtained when mycobacteria are isolated for the first time and again periodically during therapy, especially if the patient is not doing well.

Patients with AIDS need at least 1 year of therapy and probably longer.

Miliary Tuberculosis and Other Extrapulmonary Infections

The same therapy used for pulmonary tuberculosis should be used for these infections. Some therapists advise a full year of treatment for renal, osseous, or lymph node infection.

Tuberculous Meningitis in Adults

In suspected tuberculous meningitis, the same initial therapy as for pulmonary tuberculosis is useful. However, there have been reports of tuberculous meningitis produced by drug-resistant organisms. These potentially disastrous infections usually occur in children from households in which a person who has been unsuccessfully treated for pulmonary tuberculosis resides. The physician who encounters a case of tuberculous meningitis should always inquire about this possibility and modify the chemotherapy to include two drugs different from those used in the treatment of the source case.

Another problem that occurs in tuberculous meningitis is what to do about the obtunded patient who cannot take oral medication. INH is available for intramuscular injection and can be used with streptomycin or injectable rifampin. PZA can be given by gastric tube after the tablets are pulverized.

Childhood Tuberculosis

Primary tuberculosis is treated with INH and rifampin. The usual dose of INH in children is 10 mg per kg per day (up to 300 mg) with rifampin (10 to 20 mg per kg per day, up to 600 mg per day). Duration of therapy is usually 9 months. If the child's contacts include persons with drug-resistant tuberculosis, two drugs never used by these contacts should be employed.

INTERMITTENT CHEMOTHERAPY

At present, there is a considerable body of data that indicates that intermittent chemotherapy has the same efficacy as continuous therapy and has an acceptable relapse rate. Usually the patient is given continuous therapy for 1 or 2 months, and this is followed by intermittent therapy two or three times a week for 8 to 10 months. The advantages of intermittent therapy that have been identified are reduced cost, the possibility for better supervision of patients, and perhaps better acceptance by patients.

A variety of treatment protocols have been shown to be effective. One of the simplest is the so-called Arkansas Protocol (Table 3), as modi-

TABLE 3. **Intermittent Therapy in Adults**

Isoniazid 300 mg/day
Rifampin 600 mg/day
Both are administered daily for the first 60 days, followed by twice weekly administration of the drugs for a total of 9 months. Ethambutol, 15 mg/kg/day can be added for the initial 60 days

fied. This protocol should not be used in patients suspected of having INH-resistant organisms, such as previously treated persons, immigrants from Southeast Asia, or patients with suspected atypical mycobacterial infections.

One group of candidates for intermittent therapy consists of persons who have an increased risk of noncompliance. These include alcoholics, drug abusers, and persons with social or psychological problems that make compliance with therapy a low priority. In these people, supervised therapy has been shown to be a successful alternative to long-term hospitalization. Supervision consists of witnessed administration of drugs and adequate, vigorous follow-up of patients who fail to accept their treatment program.

Prophylaxis (Table 4)

The advent of multidrug-resistant tuberculosis and AIDS and the interaction of these two problems has made the indications for the prophylaxis of tuberculosis more complicated. Indication for prophylaxis can be divided into two groups: highly recommended and optional. The optional choice is often based on the patient's age, risk of side effects, a history of liver disease, or social conditions.

The highly recommended group includes patients with positive PPD results (greater than 5 mm induration), those with AIDS, those with chronic immunosuppression produced by illness or malnutrition (i.e., chronic renal disease, poorly controlled diabetes mellitus, lymphoma), those taking certain drugs (high-dose steroids, anticancer therapy), and those with a history of active tuberculosis never treated with drugs. Other very important candidates in this group are persons in recent contact with a case of active tuberculosis, persons with recent skin test conversions, and persons who have a positive skin test who are under the age of 18 years. Prophylaxis should also be given to children who are or have been in recent contact with an infectious person until their status can be ascertained (e.g., allowing sufficient time [6 to 8 weeks] for skin test conversion).

Prophylaxis is optional in persons with a vigorous reaction to PPD (>15 mm) but who are free of other risk factors, in persons with a positive reaction (10 mm) who are from 18 to 35 years of age, and in members of certain high-risk social groups (i.e., incarcerated populations, drug users, and residents of nursing homes). Recent immigrants and hospital personnel with a positive skin test also need to be considered, especially if they are under 35 years of age. Nursing home patients are usually elderly and need monitoring of hepatic enzymes before therapy and monthly for the first 3 months.

Prophylaxis consists of INH, 300 mg (10 mg per kg in children) a day for 9 months. If the candidate for prophylaxis has been exposed to INH-resistant *M. tuberculosis,* rifampin, 600 mg per day (for adults), should be given.

Vigorous skin test reactors (PPD > 15 mm) who are otherwise healthy are also optional candidates for prophylaxis.

STEROIDS IN TUBERCULOUS INFECTIONS

Steroids have a mixed effect on tuberculosis. Although they inhibit delayed-type hypersensitivity and thus may activate a latent infection, they also ameliorate the symptoms of the disease. In combination with adequate chemotherapy, they have demonstrated value in patients with widespread disease with severe accompanying symptoms such as fever, malaise, anorexia, and debility. As a result, steroids are sometimes helpful in patients with widespread tuberculosis who are critically ill, if adequate chemotherapy is also given.

Steroids are also used in meningeal tuberculosis if there is impending or overt cerebrospinal fluid obstruction and hydrocephalus. Because of the serious nature of these complications, some clinicians advocate the use of steroids in all patients with tuberculous meningitis.

The usual drug used is prednisone (or equivalent drug), 20 to 30 mg twice daily in adults or 2 mg per kg per day in infants and children. After symptoms are controlled, the dose of drug can usually be reduced to the level that keeps the patient reasonably free of these problems. Steroids can be discontinued in about 4 weeks, in most instances.

In meningitis, therapy with steroids should be continued until signs of infection have cleared from the cerebrospinal fluid.

TABLE 4. **Tuberculosis Prophylaxis**

Mandatory (PPD > 5 mm)	Optional (PPD > 10 mm)
AIDS	Anyone under the age of 35 years
Immunosuppressive drugs	
Recent skin test converters	Recent immigrants
Presence of a lymphoma	Residents of long-term care facilities
Severe malnutrition	
Chronic renal disease	Health care workers
Diabetes mellitus pneumoconiosis	Other high-risk groups
IV drug abusers	
Incarcerated persons	
Institutionalized persons	

Abbreviations: PPD = purified protein derivative; AIDS = acquired immune deficiency syndrome; IV = intravenous.

PROBLEMS OF CONTACTS

The close contacts of a patient with active pulmonary tuberculosis must be skin tested and placed on prophylaxis at least until their status is determined. Close contacts are members of the household, co-workers in the immediate vicinity, and people who might also be confined with the source case in the same room for significant periods of time.

In childhood tuberculosis and in persons who have a recent skin test conversion with a normal chest x-ray or have extrapulmonary disease, infection of others is seldom a problem.

The physician treating tuberculosis must make use of the services of community agencies, such as the visiting nurse, to ensure adequate therapy of the patient at home and the identification and evaluation of contacts.

OTHER MYCOBACTERIAL DISEASES

Atypical Mycobacteria

Infections with *Mycobacterium kansasii* can be treated in the same manner as *M. tuberculosis* but for a longer period of time (i.e., 18 months). *Mycobacterium bovis* is also treated in the same manner as *M. tuberculosis*.

MAC infection is a much more difficult therapeutic problem. The manifestation of this infection often depends on the immunologic status of the patient. Patients with AIDS and T4 lymphocyte counts below 200 frequently develop disseminated disease, with positive blood cultures and sometimes positive direct smears of blood with acid-fast organisms. Response to therapy is at best marginal; therapy involves a multidrug program with several of the newer anti-infectives (i.e., ciprofloxacin, azithromycin), and the patient should be referred to a specialist for care and follow-up. This is also true for other atypical mycobacterial infections in patients with AIDS.

MAC infections in the presence of apparently normal immunity is often encountered in patients with pre-existing lung disease such as chronic obstructive lung disease, pulmonary fibrosis, or previous tuberculosis. Treatment with standard drugs plus PZA may be useful; a favorable response to therapy is seen in about 50% of such patients. Surgery, if possible, can be useful after initial chemotherapy (6 months).

Section 4

The Cardiovascular System

ACQUIRED DISEASES OF THE AORTA

method of
GEOFFREY S. COX, M.D.
Royal Melbourne Hospital
Melbourne, Australia

Surgery for aortic disease has advanced greatly since the first successful replacement of the infrarenal aorta by DuBost in 1951. With the development of cardiopulmonary bypass, and, more recently, profound hypothermia and circulatory arrest, surgical replacement of the entire aorta is now possible.

PREOPERATIVE ASSESSMENT

The risks of major aortic reconstruction are largely related to the coronary, pulmonary, and renal systems. Vascular surgery patients are usually elderly and exhibit varying degrees of disseminated atherosclerosis. Most patients have a history of tobacco abuse, and there is a high incidence of related diseases, including hypertension, diabetes mellitus, and chronic obstructive pulmonary disease.

As many as 60% of patients have coronary artery disease, with up to 30% having severe disease warranting intervention with coronary artery bypass or balloon angioplasty. Even in the absence of symptoms, and with a normal electrocardiogram (ECG), nearly 15% of patients will have significant coronary disease that may deserve treatment. All patients to undergo elective surgery should be evaluated, to reduce perioperative risk as well as to increase long-term survival. Exercise stress testing, with thallium myocardial imaging or echocardiography, may be inadequate because many elderly patients fail to achieve the predicted heart rate because of fatigue, claudication, or beta blockers. Although newer tests, including thallium/dipyridamole (Persantine) stress, dobutamine stress, and positron emission testing (PET scan), are now available, coronary arteriography remains the most reliable method to identify significant disease.

Pulmonary function tests, especially in those patients to undergo thoracotomy, will identify those at increased risk and may dictate the use of bronchodilator treatment or alternative surgical exposure. Pa-

tients with impaired renal function should be hydrated prior to angiography to avoid contrast-induced acute tubular necrosis. The serum creatinine concentration should be monitored and must return to baseline prior to surgery.

Intraoperatively, patients are monitored with central venous pressure lines, ECG monitors, and arterial lines. Those with poor ventricular function also benefit from the use of Swan-Ganz catheters. For patients who undergo suprarenal clamping, low-dose dopamine infusions and the use of cold renal perfusion may reduce the risk of renal failure.

MANAGEMENT

Abdominal Aortic Aneurysms

It is estimated that 3% of the population have this problem. Furthermore, the 5-year survival rate for untreated patients with aneurysms 5 or more cm in diameter is only 29%, with 63% of deaths due to rupture. Although the mortality rate following elective repair of abdominal aortic aneurysms is now only 1 to 2%, mortality following surgery for rupture is at least 50%, with many more patients dying before they reach the hospital. Therefore, aneurysms greater than 5 cm in diameter, as well as those 4 to 5 cm in low-risk patients, should be evaluated for elective repair.

Although diagnosis can be made with computed tomography (CT) scan, magnetic resonance imaging, and antiography, ultrasonography is an inexpensive and reliable method and can also be used for surveillance of small aneurysms. It has been advocated that all men over 50 years of age be screened for the presence of aortic aneurysms. Preoperative angiography may be performed routinely, or selectively in the presence of suspected visceral or iliac occlusive disease. As many as 20% of patients have associated occlusive disease of the renal or mesenteric arteries, which can be repaired during aneurysm resection.

Repair can be undertaken via a transperitoneal or extraperitoneal approach. This latter technique, through the left flank, is especially useful for difficult or recurrent aneurysms in the juxtarenal position. There is some evidence that it may also reduce respiratory complications in patients with chronic pulmonary disease. After replacement with a prosthetic graft of Dacron or polytetrafluoroethylene (PTFE), the aneurysm sac is used to isolate the graft from the adjacent duodenum and reduce the risk of aortoenteric fistula to 1%. With preservation of at least one hypogastric artery and reimplantation of the inferior mesenteric artery, when indicated, the incidence of ischemic damage to the colon is now also on the order of 1%. As a result of the routine use of cell-saver devices, as well as predonation of autologous blood, only one-third of patients now require homologous blood transfusion at the time of surgery.

Inflammatory aneurysms, which are suggested by chronic back pain, often in conjunction with low-grade fever and an elevated erythrocyte sedimentation rate, may be identified preoperatively on CT scan by a halo of lower intensity around the aortic wall. Because they are associated with retroperitoneal fibrosis, there is a higher risk of intraoperative injury to surrounding structures. Repair may be facilitated by the placement of ureteric stents, by supraceliac clamping of the aorta, or by extraperitoneal exposure.

Abdominal Aortic Occlusive Disease

Although limb-threatening ischemia is uncommon with aortoiliac occlusive disease alone, the exceptional patency rates associated with aortoiliac grafts warrant more aggressive treatment of claudication than usually is the case for femoropopliteal disease. Aortobifemoral grafts have a 5-year patency rate of greater than 90% and a 10-year patency rate of 80 to 85%. These patients often have associated coronary and cerebrovascular disease, although their claudication may prevent them from exhibiting the symptoms of angina or congestive failure. As is the case with aortic aneurysms, it is important to evaluate aortoiliac occlusive disease to reduce perioperative as well as long-term mortality and morbidity. In the presence of multilevel disease, it is necessary to correct inflow before performing infrainguinal reconstructions, if long-term patency is to be achieved.

There are now a variety of graft materials available for aortic replacement, including Dacron and PTFE. The proximal anastomosis should be performed in an end-to-end fashion to avoid subsequent aneurysmal degeneration of the infrarenal aorta and to facilitate closure of the retroperitoneum to minimize the risk of aortoenteric fistula. In any case, competitive flow, associated with end-to-side proximal anastomoses, usually results in thrombosis of the native circulation. A knitted graft often allows better compliance with calcified femoral arteries, and the distal anastomosis is performed in an end-to-side fashion to allow retrograde flow to perfuse the hypogastric arteries.

Alternatives to grafts include aortoiliac endarterectomy, as well as some endovascular techniques. Selected series of balloon angioplasty of stenoses or short occlusions of the iliac arteries have demonstrated patency rates of 70% at 2 years and 50% at 5 years. The results of newer methods, such as wall stents, are currently being evaluated.

Ascending Aortic Aneurysms

Ascending aortic aneurysms may be due to atherosclerosis, or the result of chronic aortic dissection. Syphilis, although a rare cause, should not be forgotten. All aneurysms greater than 5 cm in size should be evaluated for repair. Using cardiopulmonary bypass and mild hypothermia, the ascending aorta is replaced with a Dacron graft. Many patients with aortoannular ectasia will require synchronous replacement of the aortic valve. Bypass grafts to coronary arteries can be anastomosed to the graft without added difficulty. When indicated, the sinus segment can also be replaced with reattachment of the coronary arteries by direct reimplantation (Bentall) or with a Dacron side graft (Cabrol).

Transverse Aortic Arch Aneurysms

Aneurysms of the aortic arch can occur as isolated disorders or in association with aneurysms at other sites. They can represent extension of aneurysms of the ascending aorta or be part of a total aortic enlargement (mega-aorta). Surgical repair requires the reattachment of the great vessels, with temporary interruption of cerebral flow. Current techniques for repair entail the use of cardiopulmonary bypass, profound hypothermia, and circulatory arrest. With the patient cooled to 14° C, circulation is temporarily interrupted, avoiding the need for aortic clamping while the graft is sewn into place. Air is then carefully vented from the aorta and flow resumed. The patient is slowly rewarmed; large volumes of clotting factors are usually required in order to correct the coagulopathy induced by the low core temperatures. Blood flow can safely be arrested in this way for up to 60 minutes without cerebral ischemic damage.

Thoracoabdominal Aortic Aneurysms

Most often caused by atherosclerosis or chronic aortic dissection, these aneurysms involve both the thoracic and abdominal aorta and the ostia of branches to the kidneys, viscera, and spinal cord. Surgical repair includes reattachment of these branches in addition to excision and graft replacement of the aneurysm. The incidence of rupture is similar to that for aneurysms involving the infrarenal aorta, but with mortality rates for emergency surgery approaching 100%. All aneurysms greater than 5 cm in diameter should be evaluated for elective repair. Left untreated, the life expectancy for these patients is short, with a 5-year survival rate of less than 20%. With surgery, operative mortality rates of 9% and 5-year survival rates of better than 60% have been reported.

Surgical exposure requires a left thoracoabdominal incision, extraperitoneal dissection, and a double-lumen endotracheal tube to allow single-lung ventilation. Potential complications include renal failure, prolonged intubation and ventilation, postoperative bleeding, and spinal cord ischemia. The incidence of paraplegia is correlated with the extent of aortic replacement, the presence of chronic aortic dissection, and the duration of aortic cross-clamping. For patients having all of the descending thoracic and abdominal aorta replaced, this risk may be as high as 30%. In an attempt to reduce this complication, many techniques have been attempted, including cerebrospinal fluid drainage, identification and reimplantation of critical intercostal branches, and aortofemoral bypass. As yet, no method has objectively been shown to be of benefit.

Descending Thoracic Aortic Aneurysms

Repair of descending thoracic aortic aneurysms can be accomplished without the need for division of the diaphragm. The aorta is replaced with a tube graft, which can be beveled to incorporate patent intercostal vessels. The aortic occlusion time is short, and surgery is associated with a low incidence of renal insufficiency and spinal cord ischemic damage.

Acute Aortic Dissection

This disorder is usually associated with medial degeneration of the aortic wall. This may be associated with Marfan's syndrome or other collagen connective tissue disorders such as Ehlers-Danlos disease. Dissection is classified as acute if it has been present less than 30 days, or chronic if it has been present for longer. The dissection is also classified according to the site of intimal tear and to the degree of aorta involved. Using the DeBakey classification, Type I and Type II dissections begin just distal to the ostia of the coronary arteries and involve the ascending aorta. Type I dissections also extend into the thoracoabdominal aorta. Type III dissections begin just distal to the left subclavian artery and usually involve only the thoracoabdominal aorta, although on occasion they may extend in a retrograde fashion to involve the arch and ascending aorta. Rarely the primary intimal tear may be in the aortic arch or the subdiaphragmatic aorta. Iatrogenic dissection, caused by trauma from intra-aortic manipulation with endovascular devices, now occurs more frequently than in the past, but it does not seem to be associated with rupture and subsequent aneurysm formation.

Treatment is dependent on the type of dissection. Involvement of the ascending aorta is associated with a high incidence of rupture into the mediastinum or into the pericardium, resulting in cardiac tamponade, and with compromise of aortic valve function or coronary artery blood flow. Because of this, urgent surgical repair is recommended. Using cardiopulmonary bypass and moderate hypothermia, the aortic valve is repaired or replaced and then the ascending aorta is corrected with a Dacron graft. It is usually possible to retain the sinus segment, thus avoiding the need to reimplant the coronary arteries.

When only the thoracoabdominal aorta is involved (Type III), the initial treatment is medical. Systolic blood pressure is controlled at levels of 100 mmHg by using sodium nitroprusside (Nipride) infusion and intravenous beta blockers. Most patients treated in this way will respond. Surgery is indicated for continued pain despite adequate blood pressure control, aortic dilatation or rupture, or compromise of perfusion to distal branches. Surgical technique incorporates resection of the entry point, with redirection of flow into the true lumen, as well as replacement of aneurysmal segments of the aorta. All patients must be treated with antihypertensive medication for life, and the size of the aorta should be monitored with CT scan to detect the possibility of subsequent aneurysm formation.

Aortic Transection

Traumatic rupture of the thoracic aorta is one of the most common postmortem findings following high-speed motor vehicle accidents. Because of rapid deceleration and torsion of the thoracic aorta, complete or partial transection usually occurs just distal to the attachment of the ligamentum arteriosum. This is felt to be a point of relative fixation of the aorta, resulting in a shear force at this location. Death is most commonly instantaneous. In a small percentage of cases, the mediastinum will tamponade bleeding, although the situation is extremely unstable. Diagnosis is suspected by the recognition of a mediastinal hematoma, on the basis of mediastinal widening on chest x-ray, with deviation of the esophagus, trachea, or superior vena cava. This is confirmed by angiography and CT scan, which will identify the intimal tear. Although these patients often have other associated severe injuries, survival is dependent on urgent repair of the transection.

Via a left posterolateral thoracotomy, the aorta is repaired by either direct suture or with a short interposition graft. As with all thoracic aortic operations, there is the danger of ischemic damage to the spinal cord. Although the risk is low, some authorities feel it can be further reduced with the use of aortofemoral bypass at the time of aortic cross-clamping to maintain distal aortic perfusion. Results of surgery are largely dependent on the severity and prognosis of associated injuries.

In very exceptional circumstances, unrecognized ruptures present years later as calcified pseudoaneurysms. They can be regarded as similar to other thoracic aortic aneurysms, with treatment based on the size of the aneurysm.

Inflammatory Aortitis

The most common of these rare syndromes is Takayasu's arteritis. Of unknown etiology, it may affect the arch or visceral aorta, giving rise to occlusive disease of the brachiocephalic or visceral arteries and predisposing the patient to aneurysm formation. In the acute stage, manifested by a febrile illness and raised erythrocyte sedimentation rate, steroid treatment reduces the inflammatory reaction and arterial lesions may regress. In the chronic stage, surgery is always required for correction of symptomatic lesions. Bypass grafts should be based from uninvolved proximal aorta rather than from other branches, which may become affected as the disease progresses. Endarterectomy is rarely possible and is often associated with early recurrence.

ANGINA PECTORIS

method of
STEPHEN P. GLASSER, M.D.
University of South Florida
Tampa, Florida

Angina pectoris is the symptomatic expression of transient myocardial ischemia, a result of the imbalance between myocardial oxygen need (MVO_2) and supply. Chronic stable angina pectoris is a clinical syndrome of transient symptoms due to transient myocardial ischemia, usually precipitated by physical activity and relieved by rest. The classic presentation is substernal pressure, but many variations exist. When this classic presentation occurs in an individual at high risk for coronary artery disease the likelihood of underlying coronary atherosclerosis is greater than 90%.

PATHOPHYSIOLOGY

The prevailing theory holds that myocardial ischemia is a result of an increase in demand that cannot be met because of obstructive atherosclerotic plaque. More recently, increased coronary tone has been shown to be an equally important factor. During the 1980s, the factors that modulate coronary flow were further elucidated; dynamic changes in coronary luminal size that occur at the stenotic site as well as in the distal "ischemic bed" and the autoregulation of coronary blood flow by endothelial-derived factors and neurogenic activity were implicated.

In regard to the autoregulation of coronary blood flow, evidence suggests that normal coronary arteries dilate in response to exercise, autonomic stimulation, and a variety of chemical mediators (e.g., acetylcholine, histamine, arginine, and serotonin) that might be released from aggregating platelets. However, in contrast to normal coronary artery segments, stenotic segments may respond paradoxically with vasoconstriction. This aforementioned autoregulatory response results in part from a substance released from the endothelium known as EDRF (endothelium-derived relaxing factor) that acts in concert with other endothelium-derived relaxing and constricting factors.

The autoregulation of coronary blood flow is a complex phenomenon involving neural modulation, circadian variation, endothelial plasminogen receptors, and thromboxane in addition to the previously mentioned factors. This complexity and the clinical spectrum of ischemic disorders form the biologic foundation for the differing clinical manifestations and therapeutic responses in patients with myocardial ischemia and underlie the need for individualized therapy.

DIAGNOSIS

Once the diagnosis of angina has been properly made, extracardiac and ancillary cardiac factors must be addressed. These factors include comorbid disorders (e.g., anemia, thyrotoxicosis), cardiac stimulants (e.g., beta agonists, caffeine), and associated cardiac disorders (e.g., left ventricular dysfunction worsened by therapy). Anxiety in general or as response to chest pain should be treated when appropriate, using anxiolytic agents when indicated. It is now well documented that mental stress can exacerbate myocardial ischemia by inducing coronary vasoconstriction.

The diagnosis can be supported in some patients by exercise stress testing, but this test is also useful in risk stratification and in evaluating therapeutic response. A standard exercise tolerance test should be strongly considered for most patients with angina and all patients with persistent angina. (When the baseline electrocardiogram [ECG] precludes accurate ST segment analysis, radioisotope scanning should be considered.) Patients at high risk (in terms of altered survival) include those with marked ST segment depression during low exercise workloads (occurring in association with large nuclear perfusion deficits) and those who have greater than 60 minutes of ischemia during 24 hours of ambulatory ECG (Holter) monitoring (Table 1).

The cornerstone of therapy for all ischemic heart disease syndromes, but perhaps even more important for chronic stable angina pectoris, is risk factor modification. Studies support improvement in quality of life and exercise performance with a scheduled program of regular exercise with the potential (albeit more controversial outcome) of prolonged survival. In addition, aggressive lipid-lowering therapy has been shown to result in regression of atherosclerosis, as measured by serial quantitative angiography. Of some interest is that these regression trials have demonstrated modest reductions in the degree of obstruction (2 to 5% diameter reductions), but these reductions were associated with 30 to 50% reductions in the number of clinical events. Furthermore, these reductions in clinical events may occur within 4 months of lipid-lowering therapy.

MEDICAL THERAPY

There is increasing evidence that heart rate control is important in the majority of patients with ischemic syndromes and particularly in ischemic syndromes in which clinical indicators of "coronary tone–dependent" ischemia are absent (coronary tone–dependent ischemia is likely in patients with nocturnal, spontaneous, rest, or variable threshold angina). Thus, when a calcium

TABLE 1. **Ischemic Responses Associated with High Risk**

Exercise Tolerance Testing Criteria
Failure to complete >6.5 METS or to attain a heart rate >120 bpm
>2-mm ST-segment depression >6 min
ST-segment depression in multiple leads
Flat or declining systolic blood pressure response
ST-segment elevation
Exercise-induced ventricular tachycardia

Thallium-201 Testing Criteria
New defect at low workload
Increased lung uptake
Multiple defects
Enlargement of cardiac pool

Echocardiographic/MUGA Criteria
Ejection fraction <40%
Exercise-induced decrease in ejection fraction >5%
Multiple new defects

Ambulatory ECG Monitoring Criteria
>2-mm ST-segment depression
>60 min of ST-segment depression/24 h
>6 episodes of ST-segment depression/24 h

Abbreviations: METS = metabolic equivalents; MUGA = multiple gated acquisition.

antagonist is chosen as initial monotherapy, its effects on heart rate should be considered. Diltiazem or verapamil or a noncardioselective or cardioselective beta-adrenergic blocking agent (one that does not possess intrinsic sympathomimetic activity) might represent a reasonable first choice.

Nitrates

As antianginal agents, the nitrates, calcium antagonists, and beta blockers are equally effective, but the most controversial choice is nitrates. The issue of tolerance to or attenuation of the effects of the long-acting nitrates is the main focus of this controversy. Tolerance is predominantly an issue with the continuous use of nitroglycerin and is primarily assessed by exercise test walking time; attenuation does not occur (or occurs to a lesser degree) with the intermittent use of nitroglycerin. Tolerance to nitrates may not occur in all patients with angina, and exercise test walking time may not be an adequate measure of an antianginal agent's clinical utility. Also, some studies have suggested a disparity in an agent's ability to prolong exercise tolerance and either its antianginal or its anti-ischemic (as measured by ambulatory electrocardiographic monitoring) effect.

In terms of nitrate dosing, titration is necessary because first-pass metabolism is variable, resulting in broad optimal dose ranges, but for transdermal therapy the 10 and 15 mg per 24 hours (0.4 to 0.6 mg per hour) patches may be optimal. This is approximately equivalent to 3/4 to 1 inch of paste every 4 hours or 20 to 30 mg of isosorbide dinitrate every 8 hours. If a nitrate-free interval is utilized, a 10 to 12 hour period appears to be ideal (in terms of preventing the attenuation in exercise walking time). For oral isosorbide dinitrate therapy, eccentric dosing (e.g., 8 A.M.–2 P.M.–8 P.M.) on a three-times-a-day basis may prevent attenuation, although the actual duration of an adequate effect on exercise duration during this 24-hour period is actually quite short (as little as 6 of the 24 hours).

A major active metabolite of isosorbide dinitrate, isosorbide-5-mononitrate (IS-5-MN), a recent addition to the cardiologist's armamentarium, has the advantage of not being metabolized by the liver (i.e., has no "first pass" effect). This results in more predictable plasma levels with the potential for a more uniform effect over the dosing interval and greater ease of titration in comparison with other oral nitrates. Indeed, various sustained-release formulations of IS-5-MN are under development.

Calcium Antagonists

For calcium antagonist therapy, the optimal dose is titrated on the basis of clinical effect on angina frequency, exercise test performance, and ambulatory ECG (Holter) monitoring in conjunction with medication-induced side effects. Currently, there are no other ways of assessing therapeutic efficacy, and the use of exercise testing and ambulatory monitoring in this regard will be discussed later.

Currently, there are four classes of calcium channel blocking agents, all of which work by blocking the entry of calcium into the cell. However, calcium channel blocking agents differ (Table 2), and consideration of the ancillary properties of these agents helps in determining which agent should be selected for a given patient.

Beta-Adrenergic Blocking Agents

In most patients a reduction in resting heart rate (usually into the 50 to 55 beats per minute [bpm] range) serves as a guide to the effective dose of beta blockers. However, in a few patients (approximately 10%), resting heart rates may be in the 50s while exercise heart rates are relatively unaffected. Further dose increases will usually not further suppress resting heart rates but will limit the exercise heart rate.

We used a simple exercise squat test to assess the degree of beta blockade and found that this could be used as a screening tool for determining the need for further dose titration, often making the more expensive and time-consuming formal exercise test unnecessary. Specifically, after 60 seconds of squats, if the heart rate is greater than 120 bpm, adequate beta blockade is unlikely. Although all these drugs block beta-adrenergic receptors, other factors may be important in the choice of an agent for a specific patient. Thus, cardioselectivity (the ability to preferentially block beta$_1$ versus beta$_2$ receptors), intrinsic sympathomimetic activity (ISA) (the ability to block one type of beta receptor while stimulating the other), membrane-stabilizing activity (the added antiarrhythmic potential), and lipophilicity (the degree to which the agent penetrates the blood-brain barrier) may require consideration.

Combination Therapy

Combination therapy is, of course, used when patients remain symptomatic during therapy with a single agent. Common combinations include nitrates plus beta blockers, nitrates plus calcium antagonists, beta blockers plus calcium antagonists, or all three agents together. One must always be cognizant of drug interactions when combination therapy is utilized. For example, the concurrent use of beta-blocking agents and most calcium antagonists has a negative effect on left ventricular function. Sometimes low doses of two agents are used in the hopes of limiting side effects, while at other times titration to a maximal dose of one agent is achieved before a second agent is added. In occasional instances, a combination of two calcium antagonists (from different classes) is utilized, since different calcium antagonists presumably exert their calcium blocking effect by different mechanisms (i.e., binding to different receptors).

However, combination therapy does not always produce synergistic or even additive clinical benefits compared to the maximum tolerated dose of one agent. Combination therapy may be useful in reducing the anginal attack rate in patients who remain symptomatic despite optimal doses of one agent and in patients with relatively preserved left ventricular function (ejection fraction >40%). However, a patient's response to the addition of a second or third agent is less predictable than the response to initial therapy, and side effects will frequently be more severe. Finally, it is worth reemphasizing that drug efficacy as measured experimentally in clinical trials is largely assessed by the effect on exercise walking time on a treadmill, and this does not necessarily correlate with clinical efficacy as it relates to angina frequency

TABLE 2. **Comparative Effects of Nitrates, Beta Blockers, and Calcium Antagonists**

Effect	Nitrates	Beta Blockers	Calcium Antagonists			
			*Dihydropyridines**	*Verapamil*	*Diltiazem*	*Bepridil*
Coronary vasodilation	↑	0	↑	↑	↑	↑
Peripheral vasodilation	↑	↓ ↓	↑ ↑	↑	↑	0/ ↑
Myocardial contractility	0/ ↑	↓ ↓	↓ †		↓	0/ ↓
Heart rate	0/ ↑	↓ ↓	0/ ↑	0/ ↓	↓	↓
Arterioventricular nodal conduction	0	↓	0	↓	↓	↓

*Dihydropyridines approved for angina include nifedipine and nicardipine.
†Amlodipine may not decrease contractility.
↑ = increased effect; 0 = no effect; ↓ = decreased effect.

TABLE 3. **Randomized Trials in Coronary Artery Disease: Improved Survival with Surgery**

Disease Extent	Veterans Administration Study*	European Study†	Coronary Artery Surgery Study‡
Left main	Yes	Yes	Yes
Three-vessel disease			
Normal LVF	No	Yes	No
Reduced LVF	Yes	No data	Yes
Two-vessel disease	No	No	No
One-vessel disease	No	No data	No

*Data from the VA Coronary Artery Bypass Surgery Cooperative Study Group: Eleven year survival in the VA randomized trial of coronary bypass surgery for stable angina. N Engl J Med *311*:1333–9, 1984.

†Data from Vernauskas E, and the European Coronary Surgery Study Group: Twelve year follow-up of survival in the Randomized European Coronary Surgery Study. N Engl J Med *319*:1332–7, 1988.

‡Data from Coronary Artery Surgery Study (Alderman EL, Bourasso MG, Cohen LS, et al): Ten year follow-up survival and myocardial infarction in the Randomized Coronary Artery Surgery Study. Circulation *82*:1629–46, 1990.

Abbreviation: LVF = left ventricular function.

(or the frequency of silent ischemia for that matter).

In the patient with refractory chronic stable angina who is receiving combination therapy, several approaches are possible. After assessing relative dose levels of each agent and the way in which these levels were reached, one can begin by maximizing each dose or by employing "step down" therapy, discontinuing any one of the drugs first. Alternatively, one can discontinue all therapy (although a slower detitration of the beta blocker is appropriate) and reinstitute appropriate monotherapy. This practice is presumed to be safe and is the standard approach for almost all patients entering clinical trials of investigational drugs.

The Role of Exercise Testing and Ambulatory Electrocardiographic Monitoring

Although exercise testing has become routine for patients with angina pectoris, it is strongly recommended for patients with persistent angina. It can also be used sequentially to determine therapeutic response since daily activity is more difficult to quantitate. However, it should be appreciated that the exercise test may correlate poorly with daily activity and may not be a reliable way to judge the effect of therapy in an individual patient. In this regard, 24-hour ambulatory ECG monitoring may provide a more accurate picture of a patient's day to day ischemia but may not add any information regarding the patient's *symptomatic* response to therapy. Although questions remain regarding the use of ambulatory monitoring in the general angina population, its use in the patient with persistent angina is often warranted. It should be realized that exercise testing and ambulatory monitoring can give very different results, both about the ischemia itself and about the therapeutic response.

Interventional Therapy

There is no proof that the treatment of patients with chronic stable angina prolongs survival, but it does reduce the frequency and/or severity of angina in most patients. If we were to draw on experience with post–myocardial infarction patients, beta-adrenergic blocking agents would be chosen to prolong survival. However, the differing pathophysiology in acute myocardial infarction, postmyocardial infarction, and chronic stable angina patients makes extrapolation difficult. Acute myocardial infarction is most often the result of an acute occluding thrombus on a ruptured plaque, while in chronic stable angina, a slowly progressive atherosclerotic plaque with superimposed alterations in coronary tone is the predominant ischemic mechanism. In the post–myocardial infarction patient, the prevention of future plaque rupture and ventricular arrhythmia is most critical. Coronary revascularization has been shown to improve survival in certain subsets of patients—primarily those with left main coronary obstruction or three-vessel disease and impaired left ventricular function (Table 3). Beyond those indications, definitive data are lacking, and decisions relative to the use of mechanical revascularization are made based on other "high risk" indicators (see Table 1). The role of angioplasty and other catheterization techniques of revascularization in prolonging survival is unclear. In fact, the first report on the clinical efficacy of angioplasty in relieving angina showed at best only a modest benefit in symptoms, but with a higher adverse event rate as compared with medical therapy.

CARDIAC ARREST: SUDDEN CARDIAC DEATH

method of
JOHN W. BACHMAN, M.D.
Mayo Clinic and Mayo Foundation
Rochester, Minnesota

The term "sudden cardiac death" (SCD), as used in this article, refers to the unexpected natural cardiac arrest that occurs in an adult either instantly or up to 1 hour after the onset of symptoms. Although the term "death" is used, victims of SCD may survive if medical care is instituted in a timely manner. In the United States, SCD represents 30% of all nontraumatic and 50% of all coronary artery–related deaths. About 400,000 people die yearly, and one-third of the deaths are in the less than 65-year-old group. Since 1971, the number of persons having SCD has declined from 600,000 to 400,000. This decrease can be attributed to (1) use of preventive measures, (2) treatment and reduction of coronary risk factors, and (3) development of treatments for persons experiencing sudden death. Coronary artery disease is present in 80% of victims of SCD. The remaining victims have aortic rupture, cardiomyopathy, valvular heart disease, and electrical instability disorders, e.g., Wolff-Parkinson-White syndrome (Table 1).

Rhythms of SCD recorded by paramedics who arrive within 4 minutes of the event have shown the following: (1) ventricular fibrillation in more than 60%, (2) ventricular tachycardia in 7%, and (3) bradycardia rhythms in approximately 30%. Immediately prior to the arrest, complex ventricular rhythms are often noted. The mechanism of most sudden deaths is ischemia of the heart, which is modulated by increased sympathetic tone to produce ventricular arrhythmias. Although ischemia plays a role, only 40% of patients with SCD, if revived, show evidence of infarction. Typically, SCD occurs three times more often in males than in females. A summary of the characteristics of patients with SCD is shown in Table 2.

RISK FACTORS FOR SUDDEN DEATH

Risk factors for SCD include those for atherosclerotic heart disease such as smoking, hypertension, and hyperlipidemia. As the patients get older, the risk for SCD increases, and SCD incidence increases with each decade. Women's rates lag behind men's rates by 2 decades. There are, however, specific populations that have higher rates of SCD (see Table 2).

Previous SCD Victims Who Have Survived

This population has the highest risk of all groups for SCD. Recurrence rates for 2 years after the event range from 20% to 40%. If the victim had a myocardial infarction at the time of the arrest, the risk of recurrence is substantially less (e.g., 1-year and 2-year mortality rates of 0% and 14%, respectively, in an infarction group compared with rates of 32% and 43%,

respectively, in a noninfarction group). The victim who survives an event without infarction is clearly a candidate for some form of therapeutic intervention (discussed later).

Survivors of Acute Myocardial Infarction

The incidence of sudden death after myocardial infarction is about 10% per year. Subgroups at higher risk can be defined by the presence of ventricular ectopy or by ventricular function, signal-averaged electrocardiogram, electrical stimulation, or a combination of these factors. Left ventricular dysfunction after myocardial infarction is the major determinant for both total cardiac mortality and arrhythmic mortality. Patients with ejection fractions of less than 0.4 have a

TABLE 1. **Conditions Associated with Ventricular Arrhythmias and Sudden Cardiac Death**

Coronary artery disease
  Congenital
    Anomalous coronary vessels
  Acquired
    Atherosclerotic
      Pre-infarction (no myocardiac scar)
      Peri-infarction
      Post-infarction (scar ± aneurysm)*
  Coronary artery vasospasm
Cardiomyopathy
  Nonischemic dilated cardiomyopathy*
  Hypertrophic cardiomyopathy*
  Arrhythmogenic right ventricular dysplasia
  Hypertensive cardiomyopathy
Congenital cardiac anomalies
  Repaired tetralogy of Fallot
  Repaired transposition of the great arteries
Valvular abnormalities
  Aortic stenosis
  Mitral valve prolapse
Inflammatory or infiltrative conditions
  Myocarditis
  Sarcoid heart disease
  Amyloid heart disease
  Cardiac tumors
  Myocardial contusion
  Postinflammatory myocardial fibrosis
Long QT syndromes
  Congenital (idiopathic)
  Acquired (mainly drug induced)
Ventricular pre-excitation (Wolff-Parkinson-White) syndrome
Drug induced
  Antiarrhythmics (proarrhythmic effects)
  Cocaine
  Digitalis, tricyclic antidepressant toxic effects
Electrolyte derangements
  Severe hypokalemia
  Severe hypomagnesemia
Miscellaneous
  Ventricular aneurysms (congenital, post-infarction, post-trauma)
Idiopathic (no identifiable structural abnormality or predisposing condition)

---

*Most common predisposing causes of ventricular arrhythmias, cardiac arrest, and sudden cardiac death.

From Brooks R, McGovern BA, Garan H, and Ruskin JN: Current treatment of patients surviving out-of-hospital cardiac arrest. JAMA *265*:762–768, 1991. Copyright 1991, American Medical Association.

TABLE 2. **Common Characteristics of Patients with Sudden Death**

Age (yr)	55–60
Sex	Predominantly male
Primary rhythm	Ventricular fibrillation
Myocardial enzyme change	About 40%
Arteriosclerotic heart disease	Common
Onset	Without warning
Setting	In the community

2.4-fold increase in mortality. One-year mortality rates range from 5% for postinfarction patients with ejection fractions greater than 0.4 to 50% for patients with ejection fractions of 0.2.

The presence of ventricular ectopy in a patient who has had myocardial infarction is associated with an increased risk of sudden death. In a group of patients with complex ectopy found in a 1-hour monitoring period after an infarction, the rate of SCD was 2.6 times higher during a 5-year period. Complex ectopy has been associated with other risk factors, particularly left ventricular dysfunction, but it also is an independent risk factor. The Multicenter Investigation of the limitation of infarct size showed an incidence of SCD of 18% during an 18-month period if the patient had an ejection fraction of less than 0.4 and 10 premature ventricular complexes per hour. If the patient had only the ejection fraction factor, the incidence was 10%; if just the ectopy was present, the incidence was 8%; and if neither was present, the incidence was less than 2%. Ectopy, as an independent risk factor, is particularly valid in short-term prognosis, such as predicting SCD in the first year after a myocardial infarction. However, with the exception of trials of beta-adrenergic blockers, studies of antiarrhythmia drugs show no clear pattern of drugs helping to prevent SCD.

Signal-Averaging Electrocardiography

This noninvasive computerized method detects areas of slow regional conduction. The test is positive in up to 40% of patients after infarction. However, if the test is negative, the incidence of SCD is low (1% to 4% in a 1- to 2-year period). It can be combined with further testing to determine a prognosis or treatment.

There is significant variability in the results, after myocardial infarction, of electrophysiologic studies used for identifying patients at risk for SCD. They are helpful in identifying patients who are unlikely to benefit from antiarrhythmic therapies.

Other Risk Groups

Patients at high risk for sudden death include those with left main coronary artery disease, aortic stenosis, cardiomyopathies, and primary electrical disease of the heart such as Wolff-Parkinson-White syndrome. Some drugs and electrolyte abnormalities have also been associated with increased risk for SCD.

THE CHAIN OF SURVIVAL IN SCD

The American Heart Association has written about the "chain of survival" for improving outcomes for vic-

tims of SCD (Figure 1). More people can survive if a particular sequence of events occurs:

1. Recognition of the early warning signs of SCD
2. Activation of the emergency medical system (EMS)
3. Basic cardiopulmonary resuscitation (CPR)
4. Defibrillation
5. Intubation
6. Intravenous administration of medication

A weak link leads to a break in the chain and poor outcome. Strengthening only one link in the chain will not dramatically change survival unless the weakest links are also strengthened. Most EMS systems have defects in at least one link in the chain and as a result have had poor resuscitation rates. The following is a description of each link in the chain.

The Early Access Link

The time required to access a system begins from the moment an arrest occurs. A bystander must (1) recognize the arrest as an emergency, (2) locate a telephone and call for help, (3) talk with a dispatcher, and (4) have the dispatcher locate and activate the proper emergency vehicles. To strengthen this link, simplification of the access code is important: the 911 system is an ideal method for the public to access help. In those communities without a 911 system, especially those bordering systems with 911, stickers with local emergency numbers should be placed on or by telephones. In smaller communities, local civic groups may wish to educate their population about the emergency number through a sticker campaign. Physicians should ensure that patients at risk for SCD have emergency numbers next to their telephones and may wish to distribute emergency numbers to their new patients. Dialing 0 causes considerable delay because the operator must locate the appropriate EMS system. Public education programs that describe the warning signs of heart disease and "phone first" programs should be encouraged.

The Early CPR Link

The victim of SCD is better off if the witness to the arrest applies CPR. Numerous studies have shown

CHAIN *of* SURVIVAL

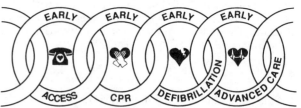

Figure 1. Sequence of events in emergency cardiac care is displayed schematically by the "chain of survival" metaphor. (From American Heart Association: Improving survival from sudden cardiac arrest: The "chain of survival" concept. Circulation *83*:1832–1847, 1991. By permission of the American Heart Association, Inc.)

that laypeople do not retain skills for performing CPR. Despite this, survival rates are doubled and neurologic sequelae are significantly decreased if bystanders try to apply CPR. Bystanders performing CPR are helping to keep the brain vital and the heart from deteriorating into asystole. Targeting people who are likely to witness SCD is important. These include emergency responders, relatives of high-risk patients, and medical personnel. The best survival rates come from systems in which first-responders arrive rapidly at the scene. In many communities, this may be fire personnel or police. In some rural areas, "Good Neighbor" programs ensure the rapid arrival on the scene of well-trained individuals in less than 4 minutes. For the early CPR link to be strong, CPR must be applied within 4 minutes of the arrest.

Early Defibrillation Link

The earlier defibrillation is applied to the victim of SCD, the better the outcome. A study involving medically supervised exercise programs with on-site defibrillators showed an 84% survival rate. Current thinking is that first-responders should use automated defibrillators. Automated defibrillators analyze the rhythm and deliver a shock. The machines are easy to use and have voice commands to tell the rescuer what to do. The shock is delivered up to 1 minute faster than with conventional machines. The International Association of Fire Chiefs has endorsed the concept and has started the initiative called RapidZap, which has as its goal the placement of automated defibrillators in all fire emergency response vehicles. As an added incentive to firefighters, the majority of sudden deaths in their occupation occur on the job near their vehicles. Rural areas have had less success. I authored two of the studies and feel that the lack of success has more to do with other links, specifically distance to arrest site, than with a lack of efficacy with early defibrillation. An effort has been made to furnish high-risk patients' family members with defibrillators. This is an evolving area, and its routine application outside of a study protocol is not advisable. Large public gatherings, such as at sports arenas or convention centers, are places where a first-responder team with a defibrillator can function well.

The Early Definitive Care Link

Endotracheal intubation and drugs provide additional chances for improved survival. In reviewing studies, it is difficult to tell which procedures make the most difference. King County's (Washington) experience shows that in communities in which only defibrillation was used, the survival rate was 16%. If the community also had paramedics arriving promptly at the site where a defibrillator was used, the survival rate increased to 29%. (Definitive care should arrive in less than 8 minutes.)

Summary

All links are important in the chain of survival (Figure 2). A fancy defibrillator is worthless if a community neglects access or attendants become less proficient in airway management. The goal remains CPR in 4 minutes and definitive care, primarily with defibrillation, in 8 minutes.

ISSUES OF PREHOSPITAL CARE

Medical Control

Personnel who perform defibrillation or provide drugs need to be supervised by a physician. Physicians may choose to develop protocols that can be followed at the scene. Physicians who arrive at the scene and are unfamiliar with EMS have two choices. They can (1) allow the responders to follow their protocols (certainly in an urban center where the paramedics have more experience than the average physician in handling cardiac resuscitation in the community) or (2) assume control (perhaps in rural areas, where emergency medical teams may not even see an arrest for periods of more than a year). When a physician is at the scene and takes control, he or she becomes responsible for that patient from the moment of intervention until control is turned over to other personnel at the hospital.

HIV Infection

There is widespread concern regarding the resuscitation of AIDS patients. Currently, the risk of contracting AIDS from administering CPR has not been documented. Saliva does not transmit the AIDS virus. There is a possibility that the HIV virus could be transmitted if there was an exchange of blood between the victim and the rescuer through open lesions or trauma to the buccal mucosa or lips. Other diseases of concern are tuberculosis, herpes, meningitis, and respiratory viral infections, which can be spread through mouth-to-mouth ventilation. Health care professionals who perform resuscitation frequently should have access to and be trained in the use of mechanical ventilation devices. Also, early endotracheal intubation should be encouraged. A shaped mouthpiece mask without one-way valves and handkerchiefs provides little barrier protection against infections. Lay rescuers are not obligated to provide CPR. Often there is a question of whether mannequins can pass on infection. The American Heart Association has guidelines specifying that students and instructors should not participate in CPR training with mannequins if they have dermatologic lesions on their hands or oral areas. Instructors should not allow participants to exchange saliva by performing mouth-to-mouth ventilation without barrier mouthpieces. Special plastic mouthpieces and specialized mannequins are now available that protect against the interchange of mucus.

CPR Retraining

Personnel involved in prehospital care need to be retrained frequently. In some rural areas, the average emergency medical team may see only one cardiac arrest every 5 to 8 years. To maintain CPR skills in rural areas, frequent practice and recertification are required.

Early Access
1. All communities should implement an enhanced 911 system.
2. All communities should develop education and publicity programs that focus on cardiac emergencies and a proper response by citizens.

Early CPR
1. Communities should continue to vigorously implement and support community-wide CPR training programs.
2. Community CPR programs should emphasize early recognition, early telephone contact with the EMS system, and early defibrillation.
3. Community CPR programs should develop and use training methods that will increase the likelihood that citizens will actually initiate CPR.
4. Communities should adopt more widespread and effective targeted CPR programs.
5. Communities should implement programs to establish dispatcher-assisted CPR.

Early Defibrillation
1. All communities should adopt the principle of early defibrillation. This principle applies to all personnel who are expected, as part of their professional duties, to perform basic CPR; they must carry an automated external defibrillator and be trained to operate it.
2. Health professionals who have a duty to respond to a person in cardiac arrest should have a defibrillator available either immediately or within 1–2 minutes.
3. Responsible personnel should authorize and implement more widespread use of automated external defibrillation by community responders and allied health responders.

Early Advanced Life Support
1. Advanced life support units should be combined with first-responding units that provide early defibrillation.
2. Advanced life support units should develop well-coordinated protocols that combine rapid defibrillation by first-responding units with rapid intubation and intravenous medications by the advanced cardiac life support units.

Figure 2. The Advanced Cardiac Life Support Subcommittee and the Emergency Cardiac Care Committee of the American Heart Association recommend that all communities take these actions to strengthen their chain of survival. *Abbreviations*: CPR = cardiopulmonary resuscitation; EMS = emergency medical service. (From American Heart Association: Improving survival from sudden cardiac arrest: The "chain of survival" concept. Circulation *83*:1832–1847, 1991. By permission of the American Heart Association, Inc.)

DO NOT RESUSCITATE

Under what circumstances should a person not be resuscitated? CPR should not be applied if (1) CPR would be futile in accord with the best interest of the patient, (2) the physician has already established with the patient that CPR would not be performed, or (3) the patient is incapable of rendering a decision about CPR but a surrogate has made the decision that the patient is not a candidate for CPR. A written do-not-resuscitate order, dated and signed by a physician, is needed in the hospital or nursing home setting. (See "Guidelines for the Appropriate Use of Do-Not-Resuscitate Orders," *Journal of the American Medical Association,* Volume 265, April 10, 1991, pp 1868–1871.)

MANAGEMENT OF CARDIAC ARREST

Techniques of CPR

The opportunity to learn CPR is widespread. People who have a greater chance of witnessing SCD, such as medical office personnel, hospital employees, and relatives of patients at risk for SCD, should be encouraged to learn CPR. Before dismissing a patient who has a cardiac condition, it is reasonable to discuss the need for relatives to know CPR. Also, relatives and people living with a victim at risk for SCD should be given specific instructions about how to access their EMS.

Understanding the technique of CPR is mandatory for physicians. A very brief review of this technique is provided in this discussion. However, in most communities in the United States, courses are available. Local hospitals that have intensive care units often have training for physicians to update their skills in basic life support.

To review, the witness to a cardiac arrest should confirm that the patient is unconscious and call for help (shake and shout). If unconsciousness is confirmed in an adult and no help is available, the EMS should be phoned. An airway is established by either the head tilt–chin lift method or the jaw-thrust maneuver. Apnea is confirmed by watching for chest motion or listening and feeling for expired air. This portion of CPR should take 5 seconds. Two mouth-to-mouth ventilations are applied, which should have enough volume to make the chest rise and fall. The carotid should be palpated; if there is no pulse, the diagnosis of cardiac arrest is made. If the victim is a child and the witness is alone, the EMS should be called.

Begin external chest compressions. Place the heel of one hand proximal to the xiphoid process of the lower half of the sternum. Place the other hand above this hand. Compress the chest smoothly with equal time for up-and-down strokes. The movement of the chest should be 4 to 5 cm. With one rescuer, the chest is compressed 15 times followed by two ventilations. If two rescuers are present, one rescuer ventilates the victim after every fifth compression. The rate of compression for one- and two-person rescue is 80 to 100 compressions per minute. A patient experiencing ventricular fibrillation can be taught to maintain consciousness for 90 seconds by repeated forceful coughing (cough CPR). If the witnesses of the arrest do not know CPR, dispatchers can provide instructions over the telephone. Such instruction can provide treatment to the victim comparable to that with other bystander CPR.

Airway Management

Airway management in the cardiac arrest victim is critical. In large emergency rooms, well-trained and experienced personnel can often intubate and ventilate a patient to the highest standard of care. However, in smaller emergency rooms or in the field, personnel may not be as well trained and equipment may not be handled in an optimum manner. The best suggestion is that inexperienced rescuers use simple equipment. For example, as director of a rural ambulance service, I removed all the airway equipment and replaced it with pocket masks for ambulance personnel and endotracheal equipment for physicians arriving at the scene. After an arrest, one of the people who had used the pocket mask for the first time said he didn't realize the chest should move up and down that much. Keep airway management simple. Use more sophisticated devices only with more experienced personnel.

Options Available to Rescue Personnel

Pocket Mask or Mouth-to-Mask Ventilation with a One-Way Valve. A simple plastic mask is almost impossible to misuse. The mask covers the mouth, the rescuer uses both hands to pull the mandible forward, and the rescuer blows into the mask and watches the chest move upward. An oxygen source can be attached to the mask. It is an excellent device to be used by rescuers who do not encounter arrests frequently or who are not usually involved in the initial management of an arrest.

Bag-Valve Mask. This can be a lethal weapon in the inexperienced user's hands. To work properly in the unintubated patient, three hands are really required—one to hold the mask in place, one to keep the head in the proper position, and one to squeeze the bag.

Manually Triggered, Oxygen-Powered Breathing Devices. These devices provide ventilation of 100% oxygen. When used by inexperienced rescuers, there are frequent problems with ventilation and gastric dilatation. Only those with a peak flow of 40 liters per minute should be used.

Dual-Lumen Airway Devices. The pharyngeal tracheal lumen airway and the esophagotracheal combitubes are modifications of the esophageal obturator airway. The esophageal obturator airway is a device that in theory places a balloon in the esophagus and lets air move into the trachea. In actuality, an operator could place the balloon into the trachea and create an unrecognized obstruction. The new devices are designed so that if the tube is inserted in the trachea or the esophagus, the patient still can be ventilated.

Transillumination Intubation. For blind intubations, transillumination techniques increase the odds of success. A tracheal tube has a rigid stylet with a light at the distal end. The tip of the tube is hooked under the epiglottis. If the tube is in the trachea, a bright circle of light can easily be seen in the midline. If the tube is placed in the esophagus, there is a diffuse color to the neck. Nasotracheal intubation can be made easier with transillumination.

Endotracheal Intubation. This is the definitive airway to be used in patients with cardiac arrests. Properly done, the endotracheal tube ensures an open airway to the lungs and eliminates the potential for gastric aspiration.

Use of Drugs and Order of Resuscitation

The best treatment for cardiac resuscitation is given by a well-trained team. The American Heart Association has a course that trains physicians, nurses, and paramedic staff in advanced cardiac life support. In this course, protocols are used so that each member of the team knows what steps should be taken. The protocols that were developed in 1992 are illustrated in Figures 3 through 8.

MANAGEMENT OF A PATIENT SURVIVING OUT-OF-HOSPITAL CARDIAC ARREST

Patients who have survived cardiac arrests and are stable should have an echocardiogram, followed in most cases by cardiac catheterization. These procedures provide information on the presence of valvular heart disease, cardiomyopathy, left ventricular function, and coronary anatomy. Most patients should undergo electrophysiologic testing in a drug-free state. A summary of treatment options is presented in Table 3. Drug

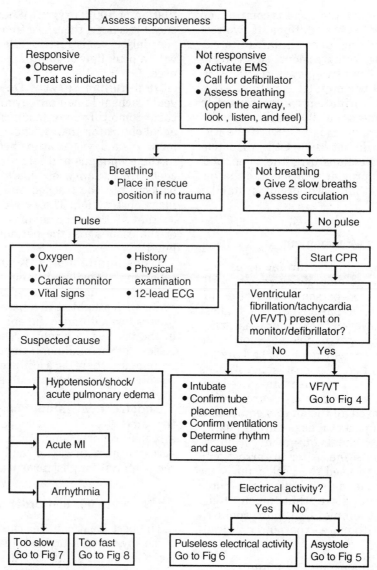

Figure 3. Universal algorithm for adult emergency cardiac care (ECC). (From Emergency Cardiac Care Committee and Subcommittees, American Heart Association: Guidelines for cardiopulmonary resuscitation and emergency cardiac care. Part III. Adult advanced cardiac life support. JAMA *268*:2199–2241, 1992. Copyright 1992, American Medical Association.)

therapy is checked for efficacy with repeat electrophysiologic testing when serum drug levels are optimum. The choice of drug depends on the response to intravenous drugs given at the initial electrophysiologic test and cardiac function. Those patients who are not candidates for drug therapy should have an implantable cardioverter-defibrillator. Empiric drug therapy has no place in the treatment of patients with recurring spontaneous or electrically induced rhythms. Patients with poor ventricular functions generally do not respond well to antiarrhythmia agents and may benefit most from implantable defibrillators.

Cardiac surgery for revascularization of coro-

nary artery disease may be recommended. Patients with left main coronary artery disease and three-vessel coronary artery disease have enhanced survival after operation.

The automatic implantable cardioverter-defibrillator was approved in 1985 by the Food and Drug Administration. In 1990, more than 4000 defibrillators were used in the United States. Shocks have been delivered to 33 to 50% of patients with these devices during the first 18 months. The manufacturer has data involving over 13,000 patients supporting a 5-year survival rate free from sudden death of 95%. The device will be used more in the future.

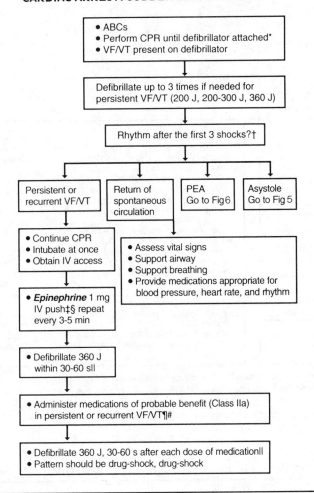

Figure 4. Algorithm for ventricular fibrillation and pulseless ventricular tachycardia (VF/VT). (From Emergency Cardiac Care Committee and Subcommittees, American Heart Association: Guidelines for cardiopulmonary resuscitation and emergency cardiac care. Part III. Adult advanced cardiac life support. JAMA *268*:2199–2241, 1992. Copyright 1992, American Medical Association.)

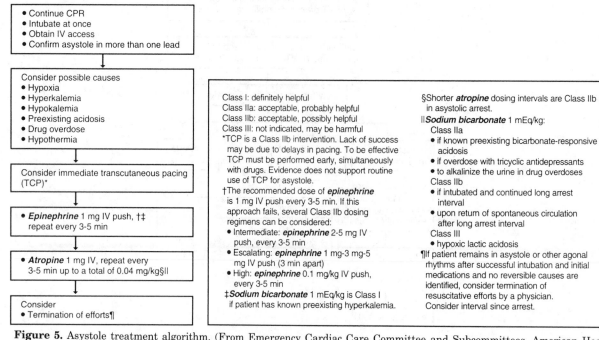

Figure 5. Asystole treatment algorithm. (From Emergency Cardiac Care Committee and Subcommittees, American Heart Association: Guidelines for cardiopulmonary resuscitation and emergency cardiac care. Part III. Adult advanced cardiac life support. JAMA *268*:2199–2241, 1992. Copyright 1992, American Medical Association.)

TABLE 3. **Treatment of Patients Surviving Out-of-Hospital Cardiac Arrest**

Anatomic Condition	Results of Electrophysiologic Testing	Treatment Options*
CAD	VF	Antiarrhythmia drugs or AICD ± revascularization
CAD	sMVT	Antiarrhythmia drugs or AICD ± revascularization; map-guided subendocardial resection ± antiarrhythmia drugs, AICD, and revascularization
CAD	No inducible sVA	AICD ± revascularization
Anomalous coronary vessels	sVT/VF	Revascularization ± antiarrhythmia drugs or AICD
NIDCM	sVT/VF	Antiarrhythmia drugs or AICD; cardiac transplantation
HCM	sVT/VF	AICD or antiarrhythmia drugs
AS	VT/VF	AVR ± antiarrhythmia drugs or AICD
MVP	sVT/VF	Antiarrhythmia drugs or AICD ± MVR
WPW syndrome	AF/VF	Surgical BPT division; transcatheter ablation
LQTS	± PVT	AICD and beta-adrenergic blocker; left cervicothoracic sympathectomy
No structural heart disease	sVT/VF	Antiarrhythmia drugs or AICD
. . .	No inducible sVA	AICD

*Patients receiving therapy (e.g., revascularization) directed at the underlying cardiac condition (e.g., coronary artery disease) require programmed ventricular stimulation prior to and following the surgical intervention to document responses. Patients whose arrhythmias remain inducible after cardiac surgery should be treated with drug therapy or an implantable cardioverter-defibrillator. In some patients, particularly those with poor left ventricular function, prophylactic placement of AICD electrode patches and/or sensing leads may be performed at the time of the initial surgical procedure to avoid a repeat thoracotomy in the event that an implantable cardioverter-defibrillator subsequently becomes necessary.

AF = atrial fibrillation; AICD = automatic implantable cardioverter-defibrillator; AS = aortic stenosis; AVR = aortic valve replacement; BPT = bypass tract; CAD = coronary artery disease; HCM = hypertrophic cardiomyopathy; LQTS = long QT syndrome; MVP = mitral valve prolapse; MVR = mitral valve repair or replacement; MVT = monomorphic ventricular tachycardia; NIDCM = nonischemic dilated cardiomyopathy; PVT = polymorphic ventricular tachycardia; s = sustained; VA = ventricular arrhythmia; VF = ventricular fibrillation; VT = ventricular tachycardia; WPW = Wolff-Parkinson-White syndrome.

From Brooks R, McGovern BA, Garan H, and Ruskin JN: Current treatment of patients surviving out-of-hospital cardiac arrest. JAMA *265*:762–768, 1991. Copyright 1991, American Medical Association.

PEA includes
- Electromechanical dissociation (EMD)
- Pseudo-EMD
- Idioventricular rhythms
- Ventricular escape rhythms
- Bradyasystolic rhythms
- Postdefibrillation idioventricular rhythms

- Continue CPR
- Intubate at once
- Obtain IV access
- Assess blood flow using Doppler ultrasound

Consider possible causes
(Parentheses=possible therapies and treatments)
- Hypovolemia (volume infusion)
- Hypoxia (ventilation)
- Cardiac tamponade (pericardiocentesis)
- Tension pneumothorax (needle decompression)
- Hypothermia (see hypothermia algorithm, Section IV)
- Massive pulmonary embolism (surgery, **thrombolytics**)
- Drug overdoses such as tricyclics, digitalis, β-blockers, calcium channel blockers
- Hyperkalemia*
- Acidosis†
- Massive acute myocardial infarction

- **Epinephrine** 1 mg IV push, *‡ repeat every 3-5 min

- If absolute bradycardia (<60 beats/min) or relative bradycardia, give **atropine** 1 mg IV
- Repeat every 3-5 min up to a total of 0.04 mg/kg§

Class I: definitely helpful
Class IIa: acceptable, probably helpful
Class IIb: acceptable, possibly helpful
Class III: not indicated, may be harmful
***Sodium bicarbonate** 1 mEq/kg is Class I if patient has known preexisting hyperkalemia.
†**Sodium bicarbonate** 1 mEq/kg:
    Class IIa
- if known preexisting bicarbonate-responsive acidosis
- if overdose with tricyclic antidepressants
- to alkalinize the urine in drug overdoses
    Class IIb
- if intubated and long arrest interval
- upon return of spontaneous circulation after long arrest interval
    Class III
- hypoxic lactic acidosis
‡The recommended dose of **epinephrine** is 1 mg IV push every 3-5 min.
  If this approach fails, several Class IIb dosing regimens can be considered.
- Intermediate: **epinephrine** 2-5 mg IV push, every 3-5 min
- Escalating: **epinephrine** 1 mg-3 mg-5 mg IV push (3 min apart)
- High: **epinephrine** 0.1 mg/kg IV push, every 3-5 min
§ Shorter **atropine** dosing intervals are possibly helpful
  in cardiac arrest (Class IIb).

Figure 6. Algorithm for pulseless electrical activity (PEA) electromechanical dissociation (EMD). (From Emergency Cardiac Care Committee and Subcommittees, American Heart Association: Guidelines for cardiopulmonary resuscitation and emergency cardiac care. Part III. Adult advanced cardiac life support. JAMA *268*:2199–2241, 1992. Copyright 1992, American Medical Association.)

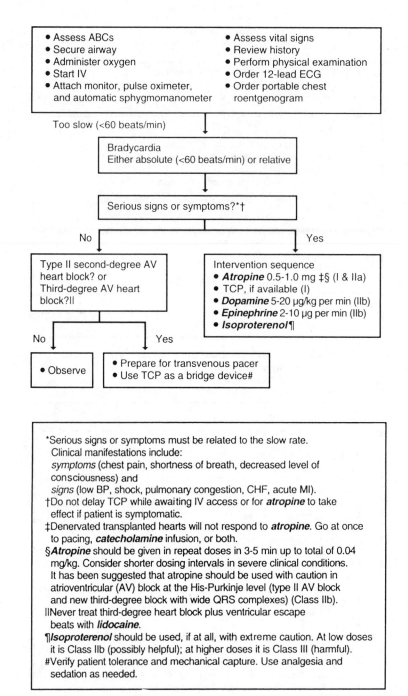

Figure 7. Bradycardia algorithm with the patient not in cardiac arrest. (From Emergency Cardiac Care Committee and Subcommittees, American Heart Association: Guidelines for cardiopulmonary resuscitation and emergency cardiac care. Part III. Adult advanced cardiac life support. JAMA *268*:2199–2241, 1992. Copyright 1992, American Medical Association.)

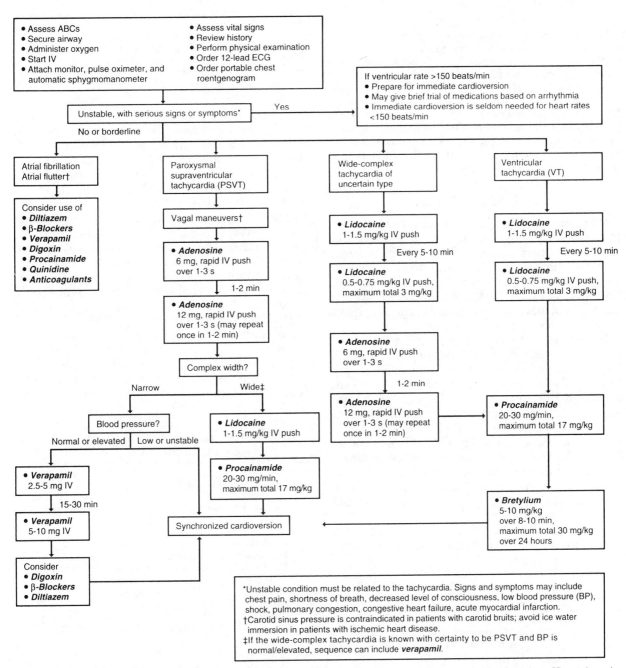

Figure 8. Tachycardia algorithm. (From Emergency Cardiac Care Committee and Subcommittees, American Heart Association: Guidelines for cardiopulmonary resuscitation and emergency cardiac care. Part III. Adult advanced cardiac life support. JAMA *268*:2199–2241, 1992. Copyright 1992, American Medical Association.)

ATRIAL FIBRILLATION

method of
JOHN H. McANULTY, M.D.
Oregon Health Sciences University
Portland, Oregon

While associated with increased mortality, atrial fibrillation is not a lethal rhythm. As therapy is selected, this should be remembered, because some drugs are more dangerous than the rhythm itself.

Atrial fibrillation is common. The incidence increases with age, and more than 2% of patients over age 60 have chronic persistent or intermittent atrial fibrillation. Because this arrhythmia is seen regularly by care providers, it is necessary to have an approach to management. In planning therapy, it is helpful to consider three phases of atrial fibrillation (Table 1).

THE ACUTE PHASE

When patients first develop atrial fibrillation, they are usually symptomatic as the result of a rapid ventricular response. Occasionally, the ventricular response is slow enough to cause few or no symptoms and urgent therapy is not needed. Rare patients have associated conduction system disease and develop long pauses, and emergent treatment for a bradycardia is required.

When the more typical rapid ventricular response is detected, urgent therapy is generally required to improve hemodynamics. There are two approaches to achieve this goal. One is synchronized DC cardioversion (Table 2). If the patient is severely symptomatic, is markedly hypotensive, and tolerates the rhythm poorly, this is the treatment of choice. The defibrillator paddles can be placed either in the anterior or posterior position or in the anterior and lateral positions with an equal chance of efficacy. To prevent skin burns and enhance efficacy, exposed metal should be covered with a conduction paste or defibrillator pads and the paddles should be applied flatly and firmly to the skin. Remember, *never cardio-*

TABLE 1. Therapeutic Considerations in Atrial Fibrillation

Acute Phase
  Control of ventricular rate
  Conversion to sinus rhythm

Subacute Phase
  Search for cause
  Consider cardioversion
  Address need for anticoagulation

Chronic Phase
  Prevent thromboemboli
  Control symptoms
    Control ventricular rate
    Maintain sinus rhythm

TABLE 2. Electrical Cardioversion

Resuscitation equipment available
Patent intravenous line
Adequate sedation
Anteroposterior paddle placement*
  No exposed metal
  Firm paddle pressure
DC energy
  Synchronized
  Initial energy 200 joules
  Subsequent energy 360 joules

*Anterolateral acceptable alternative.

vert an awake patient. Sedation to the level of unresponsiveness with diazepam (Valium), 2.5 to 5.0 mg increments every 3 to 5 minutes, or midazolam (Versed), 2.5 mg increments every 3 to 5 minutes. When the patient is asleep, the initial cardioversion should be performed with 200 joules (others recommend less), and if unsuccessful, repeated with 360 joules. If this is unsuccessful, urgent control of the ventricular rate should be achieved (see further on) with subsequent reconsideration of the need for repeat cardioversion. Emergency resuscitation equipment should be available, and after the procedure, the patient should be monitored until fully awake.

An alternative to cardioversion is rapid slowing of the ventricular rate (Table 3). In most patients with atrial fibrillation and a rapid ventricular response, the associated hypotension and symptoms are directly related to the increased rate.

TABLE 3. Drugs to Slow Conduction Through the AV Node and Control Ventricular Rate

Intravenous
  Calcium channel blockers
    Verapamil—5–10 mg over a minute; if rate control not adequate, repeat in 5 minutes; may be given every 2–4 hours
    Diltiazem, 20 mg IV
  Beta blockers
    Propranolol, 0.15 mg/kg given over 1–2 min
    Esmolol, 500 µg/kg bolus with maintenance drip of 50–200 µg/kg/min
    Metoprolol, 5 mg IV every 5 minutes × 3
    Labetalol, 20 mg IV over 2 min; repeat with 40 mg at 10 min if not effective
  Digoxin, 0.75 mg followed in 2–3 hours with 0.5 mg
Oral
  Calcium blockers
    Verapamil, 240–480 mg of sustained-release preparation qd
    Diltiazem, 90 mg of sustained-release preparation qd
  Beta-blocking agents
    Atenolol, 50–100 mg qd
    Propranolol (long acting), 160 mg qd
    Metoprolol (long acting), 50–100 mg qd
    Acebutalol, 400–800 mg qd
  Digoxin, 0.25–375 mg qd

Intravenous verapamil (Isoptin, Calan) (initial dose 5 mg followed by an additional 5 to 10 mg if there is no response in 5 minutes) is the drug of choice. Repeat 5- to 10-mg boluses can be given every 2 to 4 hours as needed for rate control. If this is unsuccessful, an intravenous beta blocker can be used. If there are concerns about the potential adverse effects of beta blockers, esmolol (Brevibloc) is the drug of choice—not because it offers better beta blockade, but because of its short half-life (see Table 2). Note that while adenosine (Adenocard) is the most effective atrioventricular (AV) node blocking agent available, it is not useful for the management of acute atrial fibrillation in that it (like the other AV node blockers) does not reliably convert atrial fibrillation, and its AV node blocking effect lasts for only 10 to 15 seconds. If there is no urgency about rate control, digoxin (Lanoxin) remains the drug of choice. Even when the other agents are used, it is appropriate to initiate digoxin therapy for long-term rate control.

Occasionally when a patient is hypotensive with signs of poor peripheral perfusion, it is not clear that it is safe to use verapamil or beta blockers because they potentially could exacerbate these conditions. Since it is the heart rate itself that is so often the cause of the hemodynamic instability, initial therapy with these drugs is still appropriate but with careful monitoring of the patient. If the hypotension worsens despite rate control, emergent cardioversion is indicated. Some have advocated the use of intravenous calcium prior to verapamil to prevent its hypotensive effect, but this has not been clearly demonstrated to be of value. Another calcium blocker, diltiazem (Cardizem) (initial 20 mg bolus), has been suggested as a way to decrease the initial hypotensive effect.

THE SUBACUTE PHASE

Once the ventricular response rate has been controlled and the patient is hemodynamically stable but atrial fibrillation persists, he or she can be considered to be in the subacute phase. A number of treatment issues should be considered. First, it is necessary to consider potentially reversible causes. Drugs (e.g., sympathomimetics, theophylline, occasionally tricyclic amines or phenothiazines), metabolic abnormalities, hormonal changes (particularly hyperthyroidism), and congestive heart failure should be identified and a decision made about treatment. Second, a cardioversion to normal rhythm should be considered. Reasons to proceed include the possibility that atrial fibrillation may somehow damage the heart, the possibility that a return to sinus rhythm will decrease subsequent thromboembolic complications, and the possibility that the patient will not feel well with atrial fibrillation despite rate control. While it is not clear that cardioversion is indicated in all patients, most will benefit from at least one attempt to return to sinus rhythm. Long-term duration of atrial fibrillation, the presence of severe associated heart disease, and a large left atrium all make return to chronic sinus rhythm somewhat less likely, but none are absolute contraindications to trying cardioversion at least once to achieve sinus rhythm.

The next major issue to consider in this phase is whether or not anticoagulation is required prior to the cardioversion attempt. There are no absolute rules, but in general, the worse the associated heart disease or the longer the patient has been in the rhythm, the greater the benefit from anticoagulation. It has never been clearly established that anticoagulation prior to cardioversion decreases the incidence of pericardioversion embolic events. Still, if it is feasible, it is best to give warfarin (Coumadin, Panwarfin) for 4 to 6 weeks prior to cardioversion. This anticoagulation prevents thrombus formation, and the 4 to 6 weeks of therapy allow any pre-existing atrial thrombi to either resolve or fibrose. If the patient has been in atrial fibrillation for a short period of time (1 to 2 days clinically) and/or if logistically it would be difficult to keep him or her in atrial fibrillation while an anticoagulation regimen is established, proceeding to cardioversion seems appropriate. A standard transthoracic echocardiogram is not helpful because it visualizes left atrial thrombi poorly. A transesophageal echocardiogram can be used in selected cases since it better demonstrates left atrial thrombi, but the test is expensive and inconvenient (for some) and carries some risks—all reasons not to use it on a routine basis. Cardioversion can be done on an outpatient basis; the patient is monitored until awake and not allowed to drive for 6 to 8 hours.

THE CHRONIC PHASE

Patients who remain in atrial fibrillation with reasonable rate control or in whom there is a reversion to sinus rhythm still enter the "chronic" phase of atrial fibrillation. While somewhat controversial, in most cases it is fair to assume that once a patient is an atrial fibrillation patient, he or she will always be an atrial fibrillation patient, and chronic management is required.

Stroke Prevention

Atrial fibrillation is associated with one serious complication—a thromboembolic event, in particular, a stroke. Stroke prevention should be addressed in all patients. When there is an associated severe dilated cardiomyopathy, mitral stenosis, or a prosthetic valve, warfarin therapy (Coumadin, Panwarfin) is required. In the remainder (and majority) of patients, those with so-called nonvalvular atrial fibrillation, five recent large studies have shown that the stroke rate is 5% per year without anticoagulation. All of the trials have shown that patients with chronic atrial fibrillation (whether persistent or intermittent) have a significant reduction in the incidence of strokes (0.5 to 2.0 strokes per year), with chronic warfarin therapy maintaining the prothrombin times in an international normalized ratio (INR) range of 2.0 to 4.5. One of the trials has shown that the benefit of aspirin, 325 mg per day, is equivalent to that of warfarin when the risk of strokes and of major bleeds with warfarin is considered.

Patients who have not had hypertension, who have no evidence of ventricular dysfunction or congestive heart failure, and who have not had a previous stroke have a particularly low risk of stroke, even in the presence of chronic atrial fibrillation, and an argument could be made for foregoing prophylaxis in this group. However, since aspirin is so safe and so inexpensive, it is recommended that all patients who have or have had atrial fibrillation take aspirin (325 mg) each day. In patients who have any of the aforementioned risk factors, antithrombotic therapy is more strongly recommended, and given its safety, ease of use, and low cost, one 325-mg aspirin tablet daily is recommended for them also, with therapy to continue for life. It is worth re-emphasizing that this recommendation for stroke prophylaxis is appropriate whether the patient is in sinus rhythm, in chronic atrial fibrillation, or vacillates between the two. If a stroke occurs, whether the patient is on aspirin or warfarin, reevaluation and alteration of treatment are required.

Rate Control

Whether the patient has atrial fibrillation or a normal sinus rhythm, pharmacologic rate control should be considered, particularly if the patient has demonstrated poor tolerance of a rapid rate (see Table 3). If sinus rhythm has been maintained for a year or longer, a strong argument can be made for stopping the drug. Digoxin is inexpensive, relatively safe, and often effective at a dose of 0.25 mg daily (0.75 to 1.25 mg for the first 24 hours). If it does not control the ventricular rate (50 to 80 beats per minute [bpm] at rest and below 150 bpm with exercise) once-daily verapa-

mil (240 mg) or a beta blocker (long-acting propranolol [Inderal LA], 160 mg once daily; atenolol [Tenormin], 50 mg once daily; acebutolol [Sectral], 400 mg once daily) can be added on.

Cardioversion

Another issue to be addressed in this chronic phase is whether or not it is necessary to try to convert atrial fibrillation to sinus rhythm (assuming that at least one attempt has been made in the past). In a patient with atrial fibrillation and good rate control who is totally asymptomatic, cardioversion is not necessary. If a patient is documented to have adequate rate control and still has symptomatic atrial fibrillation, an argument can be made for using an antiarrhythmic. Prospective trials have shown that patients who take an antiarrhythmic following cardioversion are more likely to remain in sinus rhythm for the next year than those who do not. Still, at the end of 1 year, atrial fibrillation returns in approximately 40 to 50% of patients on antiarrhythmic drugs. Again, however, the presence of symptoms despite reasonable rate control is a reason to consider drug therapy. However, all available antiarrhythmic drugs have a propensity to increase the mortality rate (by causing ventricular arrhythmias), and the risks must be balanced against the hoped-for clinical improvement. In addition, all antiarrhythmics have side effects and are expensive. Flecainide (Tambocor) has certain advantages that make it a good choice for initial therapy: it has to be taken only twice a day, it has few side effects, and it is as effective as any other drug in maintaining sinus rhythm. Flecainide should not be used in patients with congestive heart failure (it may worsen it) or in those who have had a myocardial infarction within the last 3 months. The standard drugs—quinidine, disopyramide, and procainamide—have well-recognized side effects, are not as effective in maintaining sinus rhythm, and also carry the risk of increased mortality. In preliminary studies, amiodarone (Cordarone) and sotalol have been shown to be effective. Hospitalization for 2 to 3 days is indicated when starting an antiarrhythmic drug in patients with severe left ventricular dysfunction; in others, drug therapy can be started at home and the patient can be brought back in a week for electrical cardioversion on the drug. If sinus rhythm cannot be achieved, another drug can be used or it may be necessary to just accept chronic atrial fibrillation.

Unusual Situations Related to Atrial Fibrillation

Occasionally, atrial fibrillation itself can be life-threatening. In the Wolff-Parkinson-White syndrome, the ventricular rate can be rapid enough to result in death. This problem should be considered when a patient presents to an emergency room with a particularly fast and irregular ventricular response rate (e.g., greater than 240 bpm with wide QRS complex beats). The AV node blocking agents are not only ineffective, but they may actually allow the heart to beat faster rather than slower if given during atrial fibrillation. When these patients are identified, urgent cardioversion is required and an expert in arrhythmia management should be consulted.

Newer forms of management for particularly refractory atrial fibrillation have been developed but rarely have to be applied. Surgical disruption of the atrium to alter the anatomic substrate required for atrial fibrillation is occasionally successful. On other occasions, when the ventricular response rate simply cannot be controlled, the AV node can be modified by using radiofrequency energy delivered through an intravenous catheter. This makes the patient pacemaker dependent, but occasionally this is preferable to the symptoms and limitations resulting from atrial fibrillation with a fast ventricular response.

PREMATURE BEATS

method of
A. DAVID GOLDBERG, M.D.
Henry Ford Hospital
Detroit, Michigan

Premature atrial and ventricular beats (extrasystoles) are very common. They are almost always asymptomatic and are often discovered incidentally during a medical examination. Patients with symptoms complain of palpitations or a feeling of skipped heart beats most often noticed during times of emotional stress or periods of quiet such as while resting in bed. Extrasystoles may be associated with tachycardias that, particularly if nonsustained (less than 30 seconds), may not be perceived by the patient. They may, however, cause angina, dyspnea, dizziness, syncope, or cardiac arrest depending upon the rate, duration, and underlying cardiac pathology.

The mechanisms of premature beats include reentry of the normal impulse associated with an area of slow conduction, abnormal automaticity, and the presence of afterpotentials. Many forms of cardiac and some noncardiac pathology can lead to extrasystoles. Atrial extrasystoles can be associated with atrial stretch due to mitral valve disease, left ventricular hypertrophy or failure, or pulmonary hypertension often caused by acute or chronic lung disease. Ventricular extrasystoles may be present in patients with congestive heart failure of any etiology and are frequently seen in patients with coronary artery disease, hypertension, or aortic valvular disease. In addition, metabolic disorders such as thyrotoxicosis and electrolyte abnormalities can initiate or aggravate arrhythmias. Many drugs provoke extrasystoles, especially theophyllines, caffeine, alcohol, tobacco, antiarrhythmic agents, and digoxin. Diuretics, often used in the treatment of heart failure and hypertension, can produce hypokalemia and hypomagnesemia and cause atrial and ventricular extrasystoles.

DIAGNOSIS

The diagnosis of an arrhythmia and the determination of its significance necessitate a complete medical history and physical examination. Symptoms such as angina, dyspnea, dizziness, and syncope may be caused by a tachyarrhythmia or bradyarrhythmia and indicate the clinical importance of the arrhythmia. Other cardiac and significant noncardiac disease such as thyrotoxicosis or pulmonary disease should be identified. Social and behavioral factors should be taken into account since palpitations are often secondary to emotional trauma. Hepatic and renal function should be assessed because many drugs used in the treatment of arrhythmias are metabolized by the liver or excreted through the kidneys.

While the 12-lead electrocardiogram (ECG) is necessary as part of the cardiac examination, it is unlikely, even with a 1-minute rhythm strip, to demonstrate an arrhythmia. Diagnosis and documentation are best achieved with an ambulatory ECG recorder (Holter recorder) for a 24- or 48-hour period. This technique is highly acceptable to patients because they are able to continue their normal daily activities. With the help of a diary it is possible to relate symptoms to the presence or absence of an arrhythmia. Because there is significant day-to-day variability in the frequency of arrhythmias, it is often necessary to repeat the Holter recording. A useful device for patients who have infrequent but prolonged arrhythmias is a solid-state event recorder that can be used by the patient to record up to 4 minutes of ECG tracings that can later be transmitted by telephone to a central site for analysis.

Because arrhythmias can occur with exercise, an exercise stress test should be considered for all patients with suggestive symptoms. This test can also help determine whether there is an ischemic substrate for the arrhythmia.

For patients with arrhythmias that are considered life-threatening, electrophysiologic stimulation studies may be considered. These tests require several days of hospitalization during which electrical stimulation of the heart is performed using intravenous catheters. Drugs can then be selected for their ability to suppress the electrically induced arrhythmia.

TREATMENT

Antiarrhythmic Drugs

Vaughn Williams classified the antiarrhythmic drugs based upon the predominant electrophysiologic property of each agent. While this has served as a useful classification, there is significant crossover since few drugs have an action that is confined to one class. No drug is specific to the cardiac conducting system and each has cardiac and noncardiac side effects.

Class I drugs interfere with the rapid sodium channel of the cardiac cells, causing a slowing of conduction of the stimulus in the heart. Drugs in this class are further divided into three subgroups according to the strength of this effect as well as their effect on repolarization. Quinidine, procainamide, disopyramide, and moricizine (Class IA) are moderately effective sodium blockers and delay repolarization. This latter effect can be observed on the ECG as a lengthening of the QRS complex and QT interval. The Class IB drugs lidocaine, mexiletine, and tocainide have a weak membrane-blocking effect and may normalize abnormal repolarization. No changes are seen on the ECG. The Class IC drugs flecainide and propafenone have the strongest effect on the sodium channels with no effect on repolarization. These drugs cause marked slowing of conduction with a prolonged PR interval and wide QRS complex.

All of the Class II drugs have the ability to block the beta-adrenergic receptors in the heart. The effect is primarily on the sinoatrial node, causing slowing of sinus rate, and on the atrioventricular node leading to slowing of supraventricular tachycardia and a reduction of the ventricular rate in atrial flutter and fibrillation. Although these drugs have only weak antiarrhythmic effects on ventricular tissue, they have significant clinical effects, particularly in the ischemic myocardium.

The Class III drugs bretylium and amiodarone (Cordarone) prolong repolarization. In addition, amiodarone possesses sodium channel, beta-adrenergic, and calcium channel blocking properties of other antiarrhythmic class drugs. These drugs also increase the ventricular fibrillation threshold in animals.

The calcium channel blocking drugs (Class IV) verapamil and diltiazem are effective only on the sinoatrial and atrioventricular nodes. These drugs cause sinus bradycardia, slow or stop supraventricular tachycardia, and reduce the ventricular response in atrial flutter and fibrillation. They have no effect on ventricular arrhythmias.

Side Effects

The most significant side effect of these drugs is their potential to cause lethal arrhythmias, such as torsade des pointes (polymorphic ventricular tachycardia), new or worsening monomorphic ventricular tachycardia, or sudden death. This proarrhythmic propensity is present in all the Class I and III drugs, but the frequency and significance can be defined only by long-term patient studies (discussed later).

Most of the drugs have negative inotropic potential and thus must be used with caution in patients with heart failure. In the Class I drugs, this effect is dependent on the strength of depression of depolarization. Disopyramide, flecainide, and propafenone have the greatest negatively inotropic activity. Class IB drugs have little effect on myocardial contractility. The beta blockers (Class II) and the calcium channel blockers (Class IV) are all negative inotropes and should be used with caution in patients with diminished cardiac reserve. Other side effects are listed in Table 1.

Ventricular Arrhythmia Suppression Versus Mortality

It has been a widely held belief that suppression of ventricular extrasystoles in patients with cardiac disease, especially post–myocardial infarction, reduces the incidence of sudden death. In the cardiac intensive care unit, it was recognized that many patients with acute myocardial infarction who develop primary ventricular fibrillation have warning ventricular extrasystoles, and the suppression of these arrhythmias with lidocaine rapidly became a standard of practice. There have been numerous placebo-controlled trials in which lidocaine was given to patients in either the prehospital or the hospital phase of acute myocardial infarction. Meta-analysis of the results demonstrates that although lidocaine reduces primary ventricular fibrillation by about one-third, in-hospital mortality appears to be, at best, unchanged and possibly increased in those treated with prophylactic lidocaine.

Treatment of potentially dangerous arrhythmias in other high-risk populations, especially following myocardial infarction, has not proven to be beneficial. The largest study, the Cardiac Arrhythmia Suppression Trial (CAST), was a multicenter study to determine the effects of suppression of ventricular extrasystoles in post–myocardial infarction patients with reduced left ventricular function and more than six ventricular extrasystoles per hour on a 24-hour Holter recording. After demonstration of suppression of the extrasystoles by antiarrhythmic therapy, patients were randomly assigned to medical therapy or placebo. In CAST, the two most effective drugs with the fewest noncardiac side effects, flecainide and encainide, were used. (The latter has since been withdrawn from commercial use by the manufacturer.) The study was terminated early due to an increase in mortality in the patients treated with either of the Class IC drugs. CAST II continued with the Class IA drug moricizine, a less effective antiarrhythmic agent. During the initial 2 weeks of titration with a low dose

TABLE 1. **Antiarrythmic Drugs**

Class	Drug	Trade Name	Efficacy		Side Effects	
			Atrial	*Ventricular*	*Cardiac*	*Noncardiac*
1A	Quinidine	Quinaglute, Quinidex, Cardioquin, etc.	+ +	+ +	Proarrhythmia, hypotension, asystole, CHF	Diarrhea, nausea, digoxin toxicity, hemolytic anemia, thrombocytopenia, headache, dizziness, tinnitus, rash, hypersensitivity
	Procainamide	Procan SR, Pronestyl	+ +	+ +	Proarrhythmia, hypotension, CHF, heart block	Agranulocytosis, lupus erythematosus, nausea, vomiting, rash, hypersensitivity reactions, headache, dizziness, psychosis
	Disopyramide	Norpace	+ +	+ +	Proarrhythmia, hypotension, CHF, heart block	Dry mouth, urinary retention, constipation, blurred vision, nausea, dizziness, rash
	Moricizine	Ethmozine	+	+	Proarrhythmia, hypotension, CHF, heart block	Dizziness, nausea, headache, nervousness
IB	Lidocaine	Xylocaine (IV)		+ +	Proarrhythmia, hypotension	Nervousness, confusion, drowsiness, tremors, convulsions, respiratory depression and arrest
	Mexiletine	Mexitil		+	Proarrhythmia	Nausea, vomiting, constipation, dizziness, tremor, coordination difficulties, blurred vision
	Tocainide	Tonocard		+	Proarrhythmia	Nausea, vomiting, dizziness, tremor, confusion, blurred vision, agranulocytosis
IC	Flecainide	Tambocor	+ + +	+ + +	Proarrhythmia, CHF, heart block	Dizziness, blurred vision, headache, nausea, tremor
	Propafenone	Rhythmol	+ + +	+ + +	Proarrhythmia, CHF, heart block	Dizziness, nausea, taste disturbance, constipation
II	Propranolol	Inderal	+ +	+	CHF, heart block, bradycardia, hypotension	Bronchospasm, Raynaud's phenomenon, sleep disturbance, fatigue
	Acebutolol	Sectral	+ +	+ +	CHF, heart block, bradycardia, hypotension	Bronchospasm, Raynaud's phenomenon, anxiety, sleep disturbance, fatigue
	Esmolol	Breviblock (IV)	+ +	+ +	CHF, heart block, bradycardia, hypotension	Bronchospasm, Raynaud's phenomenon, anxiety, sleep disturbance, fatigue
III	Amiodarone	Cordarone	+ + +	+ + +	CHF, heart block, proarrhythmia, bradycardia, hypotension	Fatigue, tremor, peripheral neuropathy, nausea, constipation, corneal microdeposits, photosensitivity, hypothyroidism, hyperthyroidism, pulmonary infiltrates, abnormal LFTs
	Bretylium	Bretylol (IV)		+ + +	Hypotension, proarrhythmia, bradycardia, transient hypertension, angina	Vertigo, dizziness
IV	Verapamil	Isoptin, Calan	+ +		Hypotension, proarrhythmia, bradycardia, CHF, heart block	Dizziness, constipation, headache, nausea
	Diltiazem	Cardizem	+ +		Hypotension, proarrhythmia, bradycardia, CHF, heart block	Dizziness, headache, constipation, edema, sleep disturbance

Abbreviations: IV = intravenous; CHF = congestive heart failure; LFT = liver function tests.

of moricizine there were 12 deaths or cardiac arrests compared with 3 in the placebo control group. Over the course of the next 2 years there was a trend toward increased mortality in the moricizine-treated group. Studies of other Class I drugs have had similar results. The use of mexiletine in post–myocardial infarction patients, regardless of the presence of ventricular arrhythmias, showed a trend toward worsening survival, and a study with disopyramide was inconclusive.

Studies comparing quinidine to other Class I drugs showed a worsened prognosis, which confirmed the impressions of cardiologists who, responding to a national questionnaire, ranked quinidine as the most proarrhythmic drug when given to patients with benign or malignant arrhythmias. The safety of quinidine has also been questioned when used to maintain sinus rhythm in patients with atrial fibrillation. Trials comparing the digoxin alone or with quinidine have confirmed improved maintenance of sinus rhythm but with a 1-year mortality rate of 2.9% compared to 0.8% on placebo.

Based on all these studies of Class I antiarrhythmic agents, it can be stated that extrasystoles can be suppressed, but this has not been shown to improve survival and may actually increase mortality.

The Class II antiarrhythmic drugs (beta blockers) have been extensively tested in both acute myocardial infarction and post–myocardial infarction patients. Results show that these drugs reduce mortality and the frequency of ventricular extrasystoles and tachycardia.

The use of the Class III drug amiodarone for prevention of sudden death in patients with ventricular arrhythmias is currently being investigated. The Class IV drugs verapamil and diltiazem have not been demonstrated to affect mortality.

Guidelines for Treatment of Premature Beats

Atrial premature beats are so common that they cannot be considered by themselves to constitute a significant risk factor. They may be present in patients with symptomatic atrial tachycardia, flutter, or fibrillation, but there are no data to suggest that treating the atrial premature beats will reduce the incidence of more significant arrhythmias. Because atrial premature beats are benign, drugs with proarrhythmic potential should be avoided. Treatment should be aimed at reassuring the patient and eliminating any potentially aggravating stimuli. In patients with no underlying cardiac pathology, lifestyle changes aimed at reducing stress, intake of caffeine, and use of tobacco should suffice. In patients with pulmonary disease, the goal should be reducing systemic use of theophyllines while attempting to maintain oxygenation.

Many symptomatic supraventricular tachycardias are amenable to ablation of the abnormal conducting pathways using catheter techniques. These procedures have evolved into safe, rapid therapy for many patients who have been incapacitated from the underlying cardiac disease or the drugs used for control. All patients with symptomatic supraventricular tachycardia should be referred to a cardiologist specializing in arrhythmias for this definitive treatment. However, if the patient's symptoms are only rarely bothersome, an atrioventricular node blocking drug should be sufficient. Treatment can be started with a beta blocker, the calcium channel blockers diltiazem or verapamil, or digitalis. Occasionally combination therapy will be required, with an increased risk of side effects. In selected patients it may be necessary to use amiodarone. Flecainide has recently been approved for treatment of supraventricular tachycardia and atrial fibrillation in patients with severe symptoms and no structural heart disease.

The treatment of ventricular extrasystoles depends on the underlying cardiac abnormality. All patients presenting with an acute myocardial infarction should be treated with a beta blocker unless there is a strong contraindication such as asthma, peripheral vascular disease, atrioventricular node block, or severe congestive heart failure. Patients should receive analgesia in a quiet environment, and plasma potassium and magnesium should be maintained in the normal range. During the early phase of an acute myocardial infarction, ventricular extrasystoles may presage ventricular fibrillation. Although lidocaine abolishes extrasystoles, the drug should not be used for prophylaxis of ventricular fibrillation but may be of benefit in patients with recurrent ventricular tachycardia. Bretylium, usually reserved for refractory ventricular tachycardia, is an alternative to lidocaine.

In the post–myocardial infarction patient, the role of ventricular extrasystoles to predict an increased risk of mortality has recently come under considerable challenge. In the placebo group of the CAST study, no clear relationship was seen between the frequency of extrasystoles and events. Other clinical factors associated with sudden cardiac death, including left ventricular dysfunction, coronary artery disease, and cardiac ischemia, need assessment and may require treatment. There is no good clinical rationale to treat ventricular extrasystoles. The beneficial effects on mortality and morbidity of beta blockers have been well established, and these drugs are indicated in all patients, irrespective of ventricular arrhythmia, for a period of at least 2 years. The dose should be adjusted to reduce the resting heart rate to less than 60 beats per minute or until side effects occur. Class I drugs should be avoided. If symptomatic or sustained ventricular tachycardia occurs, the patient should be referred to a cardiologist for consideration of revascularization, electrophysiologic studies, amiodarone, or an implanted antitachycardia device and defibrillator.

Patients with congestive heart failure often have extrasystoles and frequently demonstrate ventricular tachycardia. There is no study indicating an increase in mortality in patients with asymptomatic, untreated ventricular extrasystoles or nonsustained ventricular tachycardia. The primary aim of treatment is to maximize the therapy of the heart failure and correct or prevent electrolyte disturbances. Specific treatments that have been demonstrated to help these patients include afterload reduction with angiotensin-converting enzyme inhibitors such as enalapril (Vasotec), captopril (Capoten), or, if the patient cannot tolerate these drugs, hydralazine (Apresoline) and long-acting nitrates (e.g., Isordil, Nitrobid). For symptomatic patients, amiodarone may be effective in reducing ventricular tachycardia.

In the absence of heart disease and myocardial ischemia, extrasystoles are benign regardless of their frequency and quality. The optimal treatment is reassurance of the patient. Lifestyle changes may be necessary to reduce anxiety as well as to limit consumption of caffeine, alcohol, and tobacco. Because of their side effects and the proarrhythmic potential, Class I drugs are to be avoided. Class II beta blockers can be used to reduce symptoms in the occasional patient.

HEART BLOCK

method of
JOHN M. MILLER, M.D.
Temple University Hospital
Philadelphia, Pennsylvania

"Heart block" is a general term referring to a disturbance of impulse propagation from one part of the heart to another. Although usually pertaining to atrioventricular (AV) conduction, blocks may also occur between the sinus node and atrium (sinoatrial exit block of varying degrees, a type of so-called sick sinus syndrome), within the atria, as well as within the ventricles.

GENERAL CLASSIFICATION

AV block (AVB) has been conveniently categorized according to whether there is *prolonged conduction* (first-degree AV block), *intermittent conduction* (second-degree and high-grade block), or *no conduction* (third-degree block). The common anatomic locations of these types of block are shown in Table 1.

FIRST-DEGREE AV BLOCK (1° AVB)

Electrocardiographic (ECG) Features.
First-degree AVB, defined as a prolonged PR in-

TABLE 1. **Common Anatomic Locations of Atrioventricular (AV) Block**

	Anatomic Location of Block		
Abnormality	*AV Node*	*Intra-His Bundle*	*Infra-His Bundle*
First-degree AVB	+ + +	+	+
Second-degree AVB			
Type I	+ + +	+	−
Type II	−	+ +	+ +
High-grade	+ +	+ +	+
Third-degree AVB (complete AVB)	+	+ +	+ +

Abbreviations: + = occasional; + + = common; + + + = most frequent; − = rare.

terval (in excess of 0.20 second in adults, 0.18 second in children), is something of a misnomer; because each P wave is followed by a QRS complex, there is, strictly speaking, no "block." The PR interval can become extremely long in some cases (>0.40 second).

Clinical Settings/Pathogenesis. Because the site of the delay is usually the AV node (although it can be intra–His bundle), common causes of 1° AVB include medications (especially digitalis, beta blockers, and calcium channel blockers), increases in vagal tone, and ischemia or infarction of the inferior wall (which compromises blood supply to the AV nodal artery). First-degree AVB may also occur less commonly with acute myocarditis, as well as developing and progressing with normal aging.

Significance/Treatment. Because every P wave is followed by a QRS complex, 1° AVB has no particular significance of its own and requires no therapy. (With very long PR intervals, the mechanical efficiency of ventricular contraction could conceivably be adversely affected.) The importance of 1° AVB is confined to whatever risk exists of progression to higher degrees of AVB. Any medications implicated in causing 1° AVB should be eliminated if possible or the dosage decreased.

SECOND-DEGREE (2°) AV BLOCK

Second-degree AVB is characterized by *intermittency* of conduction: in most cases, the majority of P waves are followed by QRS complexes and an occasional, single P wave is blocked, leading to clusters of QRS complexes that are most easily recognized on a long rhythm strip. This so-called "group beating" is a hallmark of 2° AVB. The two common types of 2° AVB are distinguished by the manner in which block occurs—gradually (Mobitz Type I) or suddenly (Mobitz Type II). It is worth remembering that even in normal individuals, premature atrial beats may fail to conduct to the ventricles in the absence of any AV conduction system abnormality because they occur during the AV nodal refractory period; thus, diagnosis of 2° AVB requires a relatively regular atrial rhythm.

Type I 2° AVB

Also called "Wenckebach" block, this type of block occurs in a gradual manner.

ECG Features. A Wenckebach cycle consists of a series of P waves that are conducted to the ventricles following gradually lengthening PR intervals, until one P wave fails to conduct; the cycle then repeats, generally in a 3:2 or 4:3 ratio of P waves to QRSs. In the classical case, the R-R intervals during such a cycle gradually *decrease,* because although the PR is *increasing* from beat to beat, the absolute amount of increment progressively lessens on consecutive beats. In practice, this may be difficult to recognize because of only subtle changes in PR and R-R intervals. A more helpful diagnostic feature is that the last conducted PR interval (before the P that fails to conduct) is generally the longest PR in the cycle, whereas the PR interval of the first conducted beat in the new cycle is the shortest.

Clinical Settings/Pathogenesis. Many of the same factors that may cause 1° AVB are responsible for Type I 2° AVB: increased vagal tone (as during sleep), inferior wall ischemia/infarction, and medications such as digitalis, beta blockers, and calcium channel blockers. The location of the block is generally in the AV node, although lesions of the His bundle can occasionally be responsible.

Significance/Treatment. Type I 2° AVB is generally a benign disturbance, especially in the absence of organic heart disease, and requires no treatment; discontinuation of offending medications may be necessary. When inferior wall infarction is the cause, Type I 2° AVB is usually transient (lasting no more than 48 hours after the infarct) and either requires no treatment or responds to small doses of atropine. Rarely, temporary ventricular pacing may be needed if the ventricular rate remains marginal (i.e., <40 beats per min) despite atropine, if there is progression to complete heart block despite atropine, or if significant heart failure related to the arrhythmia is present.

Type II 2° AVB

In this less common subset of AV conduction disturbance, block occurs *suddenly* rather than after gradual prolongation of the PR interval.

ECG Features. In contrast to Type I block, the PR interval on all conducted beats is constant in Type II block, and sudden loss of conduction occurs without prior increments in the PR interval. There may be considerable difficulty distinguishing Type I from Type II block on the surface ECG, especially with relatively high conduction ratios (6:5 or greater), because the changes in PR intervals in Type I block may be very subtle. Bundle branch block is very commonly associated with Type II block, however, and if present may aid in differentiation.

Clinical Settings/Pathogenesis. Although bearing a superficial ECG resemblance to Type I block, the causes and importance of Type II block are much different. The location of the block is almost always in the His bundle or lower, and thus the status of AV conduction is more tenuous. Degenerative disease of the conduction system, anterior wall infarction, and injury to the His bundle at the time of aortic valve surgery are frequent causes of Type II block; less commonly, Class IA and IC antiarrhythmic drugs are implicated. Progression to complete heart block (with a very slow escape rhythm) may be sudden and permanent.

Significance/Treatment. Unlike Type I 2° AVB, the incidence of progression to complete heart block is high in patients with Type II 2° AVB—enough so that permanent pacing should be undertaken in these cases, even among asymptomatic individuals.

High-Grade AVB

ECG Features. This least common subset of 2° AVB is characterized by block of more than one P wave with a relatively constant P:QRS ratio, such as 3:1, 4:1, etc.

Clinical Settings/Pathogenesis. The location of the block may be either the AV node or the His bundle; features that aid in distinguishing the site of block include the presence of a narrow QRS complex, antecedent Wenckebach cycles, presence of beta or calcium blocking agents, and atropine responsiveness in cases of AV nodal block versus a wide QRS complex, lack of drugs that act on the AV node, and lack of atropine response in cases of block in the His bundle.

Significance/Treatment. The ventricular rate is generally slow enough in high-grade AVB that, unless there is some easily reversible cause (such as drugs worsening AV nodal conduction), permanent pacing is recommended in all cases.

Other Forms of Real and Apparent 2° AVB

More complicated forms of 2° AVB may occur during relatively fast atrial rhythms (atrial tachycardia and flutter), in which the conduction pattern appears to be relatively stable at 2:1 but with intermittent block of one or two additional P waves (i.e., predominant 2:1 conduction with periods of 3:1 or 4:1 conduction). This is generally caused by conduction abnormalities at two levels of the conduction system, most typically Type I 2° AVB at one level and Type II block at another. When 2:1 conduction occurs interspersed with periods in which there are two consecutive blocked P waves, Type I 2° AVB occurs at a more proximal level and Type II block more distally in the conduction system; if there are three consecutive blocked P waves in the pause, Type II 2° AVB occurs proximally and Type I block more distally. This form of conduction, which has been termed alternate-cycle Wenckebach periodicity because of the combination of Type I 2° AVB and 2:1 conduction, is quite uncommon and is generally observed only during atrial tachycardia or flutter. Because it is not in itself a manifestation of abnormal AV conduction under these circumstances, no specific treatment is required.

The ECG appearance of 2° AVB can occasionally be mimicked by the occurrence of so-called concealed His extrasystoles (CHE). These are premature depolarizations of the His bundle that occur prior to recovery of excitability of distal conduction system tissue (and thus no QRS complex results), and also penetrate the atrioventricular node (AVN) retrogradely to either collide with an oncoming sinus impulse or render the AVN refractory to a subsequent sinus impulse. This results in an occasional P wave that is unexpectedly not followed by a QRS, thus simulating Type II 2° AVB but in the absence of any true intrinsic conduction deficit. Because these CHEs are not directly manifested on the ECG (hence the name "concealed"), their existence must be inferred; occasional apparent junctional beats occurring prematurely (thus not "escape" beats) increase the likelihood that CHEs may be causing apparent AVB. The diagnosis can only be firmly made if His bundle recordings are obtained during invasive electrophysiologic studies showing nonpropagated premature His depolarizations that also result in a nonconducted P wave. Fortunately, this is a very uncommon abnormality and thus should not be a frequent cause of confusion; no treatment is needed for either the apparent AVB or the CHEs themselves.

COMPLETE (THIRD-DEGREE [3°]) HEART BLOCK (CHB)

CHB is defined as the absence of conduction of any atrial impulses to the ventricles, which are governed by an escape focus in the His-Purkinje system.

ECG Features. Atrial activity is present but has no influence on the occurrence of QRS complexes, which may be narrow or wide (depending on the level of the escape focus). Important diagnostic features of CHB include an atrial rate (sinus, atrial tachycardia, or atrial fibrillation) faster than the ventricular rate; a *regular* ventricular rhythm; and no alteration of the timing of QRS complexes regardless of when P waves occur.

Clinical Settings/Pathogenesis. CHB can be congenital (associated with a narrow, relatively rapid escape rhythm that can also accelerate with exercise), in which the block is almost always in the AV node. Acquired CHB can be due to either AV nodal or, more commonly, His bundle disease. In the former case, the QRS complexes of the escape rhythm are generally narrow and relatively fast (in the 50 to 60 per minute range); block within the His can also have a narrow QRS escape rhythm. Block occurring below the His is associated with a wider, slower escape rhythm.

Significance/Treatment. Generally, permanent pacing is required for patients with CHB because the ventricular rate is so slow; in some cases of CHB (especially congenital), however, pacing may not be necessary—that is, if the escape rhythm is fast enough and able to accelerate with exercise such that there is little diminution of functional capacity and scant risk of sudden death due to asystole.

FASCICULAR BLOCKS AND BUNDLE BRANCH BLOCK

The infranodal conduction system comprises the His bundle, which bifurcates into the left and right bundle branches; the left bundle itself soon bifurcates into anterior and posterior divisions, or fascicles (the left and right bundles are also fascicles). Any of these fascicles can become blocked, alone or in combination, generally as a result of age-related degenerative change or myocardial damage (infarction, infiltration, surgery). Isolated right bundle branch block (RBBB) is relatively common on routine ECGs and confers only a minimally increased risk for development of CHB; left bundle branch block (LBBB) may be associated with an even lower risk of progression to CHB, in that the ECG appearance of LBBB may not actually be anatomic block in the LBBB per se, but LBB delay or myocardial delay not due to LBB disease at all. The term *bifascicular block* refers to a combination of RBBB with either left anterior or left posterior fascicular block (LAFB and LPFB, respectively). The combination of RBBB and LAFB is the more common of these and is associated with a rate of progression to

CHB of up to 5% per year. This is not frequent enough to warrant prophylactic pacing in these patients to prevent sudden cardiac death due to the unexpected development of CHB, and in fact, several studies suggest that sudden death in patients with bifascicular block is more frequently due to ventricular tachyarrhythmias than is CHB. RBBB with LPFB, although much less common, nonetheless appears to advance to CHB more frequently (presumably because of the amount of myocardial damage necessary to produce this combination of lesions). *Trifascicular block* has been variously defined in the past, referring either to RBBB plus LAFB or LPFB, with additional 1° AVB (the third "fascicle"), or simultaneous RBBB, LAFB, and LPFB (i.e., CHB). The term "trifascicular block" is not a helpful distinction, except in the case of acute myocardial infarction (in which the presence of 1° AVB along with RBBB and LAFB or LPFB confers a greater risk of development of CHB).

AV CONDUCTION DISTURBANCES IN ACUTE MYOCARDIAL INFARCTION (AMI)

The development of conduction abnormalities in the setting of AMI represents a special case, in that (1) bradyarrhythmias leading to adverse hemodynamics may be quite poorly tolerated in this setting and (2) the acute injury to the conduction system may or may not result in lasting deficits that require a permanent pacemaker.

Temporary Cardiac Pacing in AMI

Several circumstances have been shown to result in a high enough risk of CHB during AMI to warrant temporary cardiac pacing (transcutaneous or transvenous). Most patients with inferior AMI will not require temporary pacing because the damage to the conduction system is generally confined to the AV node or proximal His bundle, and thus when CHB occurs, it has often been heralded by progression from a normal PR interval to 1° AVB followed by Type I 2° AVB, and may respond favorably to small intravenous doses of atropine. The rate of the escape rhythm in CHB is generally 45 to 60 beats per minute; this, combined with a relatively small loss of myocardial pump function, rarely results in a life-threatening situation. Temporary pacing may, however, be required if the heart rate in CHB is less than 40 beats per minute or is associated with hemodynamic deterioration.

In patients with anterior infarction, damage to the conduction system occurs more distally (His bundle, bundle branches). Development of CHB may be sudden (not preceded by gradual progression from 1° AVB to 2° AVB) and the escape rhythm usually has a rate greater than 40 beats per minute; this, combined with the loss of myocardial contractility with the AMI, can be life threatening. Thus, prophylactic temporary pacing may be used to prevent death due to sudden CHB if there is reason to believe CHB is likely to occur. The following conduction abnormalities have been associated with an increased risk of development of high-grade or complete heart block in anterior AMI: "new" RBBB, defined as either development of RBBB with the AMI or presence of RBBB in a patient without a prior ECG; "bilateral BBB," or block in two infranodal fascicles (RBBB + LAFB or LPHB, or LBBB [= LAHB + LPHB]); and 1° AVB. Each of these abnormalities alone confers approximately a 10% risk of developing higher degrees of AVB, whereas two of these together increase the risk to approximately 20%, and the occurrence of all three yields a risk of over 35%. Temporary pacing should be employed to prevent life-threatening bradycardia in patients with two or more of the above risk factors (approximately 20% risk of development of CHB).

Permanent Cardiac Pacing in AMI

There is much less agreement concerning the benefits of permanent pacing following AMI. Most workers feel that permanent pacing is indicated if transient high-grade or CHB has occurred in the setting of an anterior AMI or persists throughout the patient's hospital course in the setting of an inferior wall AMI. Persistence of new bundle branch block is viewed by some as an indication for permanent pacing. There is as yet no evidence that permanent pacing prevents sudden death following hospital discharge, which may in many cases be due to ventricular tachyarrhythmias rather than to CHB.

TACHYCARDIA

method of
ROBERT E. SPERRY, M.D., and
KENNETH A. ELLENBOGEN, M.D.
Medical College of Virginia
Richmond, Virginia

The tachycardias represent a diverse group of cardiac arrhythmias. Although by definition, any cardiac rhythm with a rate greater than 100 beats per minute (bpm) at rest is a tachyarrhythmia, this broad classification includes benign to potentially lethal and lethal arrhythmias. In general, it is useful to classify tachycardias as narrow (QRS duration <0.12 second) or wide complex (QRS duration >0.12 second), and additionally as either regular or irregular. This approach is helpful in establishing a diagnosis and instituting appropriate therapy for the arrhythmia (Fig. 1). This classification is shown in Table 1.

It is of paramount importance when first evaluating a tachyarrhythmia that the patient's clinical status—not the width of the QRS or tachycardia rate—be the primary focus. Both wide complex and narrow complex tachycardias may be associated with significant hemodynamic compromise, acute congestive heart failure, or angina, and this may be particularly true in patients with significant underlying cardiac or pulmonary disease and in the elderly. Patients with unstable tachyarrhythmias (narrow or wide complex) should undergo DC synchronized cardioversion after appropriate sedation with a short-acting benzodiazepine, such as midazolam (Versed), or with methohexital (Brevitol). Continuous monitoring of the patient's respiratory status and oxygen saturation and the ability to manage the patient's airway (i.e., intubation) are necessary should the need arise during cardioversion.

In evaluation of the patient who is stable during a tachyarrhythmia, an organized approach to diagnosis and treatment is essential. A rule the authors recommend *diagnosis first, treatment second*. For narrow complex tachycardias, the 12-lead electrocardiogram (ECG) can provide important information. An irregular rhythm without evidence of discrete P waves is indicative of atrial fibrillation or multifocal atrial tachycardia. A regular narrow complex tachycardia may be

atrial flutter, atrioventricular (AV) nodal reentrant tachycardia, AV reciprocating tachycardia (using an accessory pathway), intra-atrial reentrant tachycardia, ectopic atrial tachycardia, or less commonly junctional tachycardia. The presence of P waves, their morphology, and their relationship to the QRS are important diagnostic clues as well.

Although maneuvers to increase vagal tone such as coughing, a Valsalva maneuver, and carotid sinus massage have been used to terminate supraventricular tachycardias (with variable success, usually less than 20%), the authors find the administration of 6 mg of adenosine (Adenocard), or if unsuccessful 12 mg, as a rapid bolus injection given through a proximally located vein to be useful from both a diagnostic and a therapeutic standpoint. AV nodal reentrant tachycardia, AV reciprocating tachycardia, and some intra-atrial reentrant tachycardias will terminate with adenosine. For patients with atrial flutter, atrial fibrillation, or atrial tachycardia, block in the AV node with adenosine allows the identification of flutter and fibrillatory waves or an ectopic atrial rhythm. Methylxanthine agents (e.g., theophylline) are adenosine antagonists, and adenosine will be ineffective or very high doses will be required in patients taking these drugs. Caution should be used when administering adenosine to patients taking dipyridamole, which blocks the reuptake of adenosine from the circulation and thus potentiates its chronotropic and dromotropic effects.

Establishment of the mechanism for wide complex tachycardias is even more important. If the patient is stable, the 12-lead ECG is helpful in establishing a

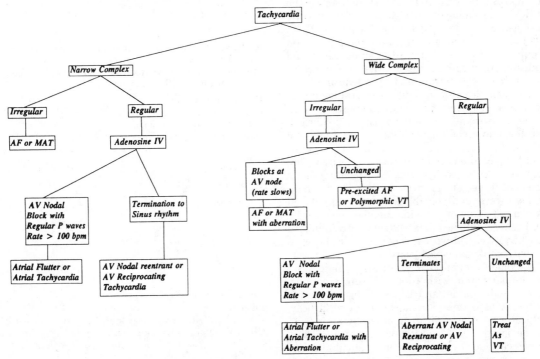

Figure 1. Diagnostic approach to patients with stable wide complex or narrow complex tachycardia. *Abbreviations:* AF = atrial fibrillation; MAT = multifocal atrial tachycardia; VT = ventricular tachycardia; AV = atrioventricular; bpm = beats per minute; IV = intravenous; BBB = bundle branch block.

TABLE 1. **Classification of Tachycardias**

Narrow Complex Tachycardias
Irregular
Atrial fibrillation
Multifocal atrial tachycardia
Regular
Atrial flutter
AV nodal reentrant tachycardia
AV reciprocating tachycardia (associated with WPW or using a concealed bypass tract)
Atrial tachycardia
Nonparoxysmal junctional tachycardia

Wide Complex Tachycardias
Irregular
Atrial fibrillation (aberrantly conducted)
Pre-excited atrial fibrillation (associated with WPW)
Torsades de pointes
Regular
Ventricular tachycardia
Aberrantly conducted supraventricular arrhythmias
Pre-excited antidromic reciprocating tachycardia (associated with WPW syndrome)

Abbreviations: AV = atrioventricular; WPW = Wolff-Parkinson-White syndrome.

diagnosis. Criteria that differentiate supraventricular tachycardia (SVT) with aberrant conduction from ventricular tachycardia are shown in Table 2. A helpful finding on the 12-lead ECG is a QRS duration of greater than or equal to 0.14 to 0.16 seconds (140 to 160 ms), which is more suggestive of ventricular tachycardia. If found on the 12-lead ECG, dissociation of the P waves from the QRS complex is diagnostic of ventricular tachycardia. If no clear P waves are seen on the surface ECG, an esophageal electrode can demonstrate the relationship of atrial activation to the surface QRS. In patients who are stable with a wide complex tachyarrhythmia, adenosine (Adenocard)* can be used to aid in diagnosis. Although in rare patients ventricular tachycardia has been terminated by adenosine (<2–3%, generally in patients without structural heart disease), significant slowing of the wide complex tachycardia (as with aberrantly conducted atrial fibrillation, atrial flutter, and atrial tachycardia) or termination of the tachycardia (e.g., aberrantly conducted AV nodal reentrant tachycardia or AV reciprocating tachycardia) rules out ventricular tachycardia as the arrhythmia mechanism. The use of the intravenous calcium channel blockers verapamil or diltiazem in patients in whom the mechanism of the wide complex tachycardia has not been established is strongly contraindicated and may be associated with hemodynamic collapse in patients with ventricular tachycardia.

Finally, whenever initiating antiarrhythmic drug therapy, in particular with Class IA (procainamide, quinidine, disopyramide) and Class III agents (amiodarone and sotalol), the patient should be electrocardiographically monitored for drug proarrhythmia (e.g., torsades de pointes, incessant ventricular tachycardia). Continuous cardiac rhythm monitoring should be per-

*This use of adenosine is not a U.S. Food and Drug Administration (FDA)–approved indication.

formed for a minimum of 24 hours to watch for QT prolongation during administration of Class IA agents. Patients should be monitored for at least 3 days when treatment with Class III agents (amiodarone and sotalol) is initiated.

TREATMENT

Narrow Complex Tachyarrhythmias

Atrial Fibrillation

Atrial fibrillation (AF) is the most common cardiac arrhythmia encountered in the adult population. Its incidence increases both with age and with the presence of other cardiac diseases. The arrhythmia may be paroxysmal or chronic. There are multiple underlying conditions associated with AF, as seen in Table 3.

Atrial fibrillation is likely due to a reentrant

TABLE 2. **Electrocardiographic Findings in Supraventricular Tachycardia with Aberrant Conduction vs. Ventricular Tachycardia**

Aberration
Triphasic contour in lead V_1 (rsR′) and V_6 (QRS)
V_1

V_6

Initial vector of the wide beat similar to that of the normally conducted beat
Initial beat(s) of the tachycardia are narrow, followed by widening of the QRS complex

Ventricular Origin
QRS duration >140 ms with RBBB morphology and >160 ms with LBBB morphology
Indeterminate (far right) axis deviation
Left "rabbit ear" taller in V_1 and QS or RS in V_6
V_1

V_6

AV dissociation
Fusion beats
Concordant QRS morphology in V_1-V_6 (positive or negative)
QR in V_6, QS in V_6 with an LBBB morphology, a broad R wave in V_1 (>40 ms), or rightward axis with negative QRS deflection in V_1>V_6

Abbreviations: RBBB = right bundle branch block; LBBB = left bundle branch block; AV = atrioventricular.

TABLE 3. Causes of Atrial Fibrillation

Associated with Underlying Heart Disease
Valvular disease, especially mitral stenosis and regurgitation
Hypertensive heart disease
Acute or chronic myocardial ischemia
Cardiomyopathies (dilated, hypertrophic, and restrictive)
Pericarditis seen postcardiotomy, postinfarction (including Dressler's), viral, neoplastic
Congenital heart disease (e.g., ASD)

Related to Underlying Disorders
Hyperthyroidism
Hypoxia due to pulmonary disease (acute or chronic)
Sympathomimetic amines (e.g., theophylline)
Other drugs (e.g., alcohol and caffeine)
Electrolyte imbalance
Alcoholic drinking binges

Abbreviation: ASD = atrial septal defect.

mechanism with atrial rates from 400 to 700 bpm and a variable ventricular rate modulated by the AV node. The symptoms associated with AF depend upon the ventricular rate and the presence of underlying cardiopulmonary disease.

In stable patients with acute onset of AF and a rapid ventricular response, the initial therapy should be directed toward heart rate control. Medications available for initial treatment include intravenous calcium channel blocking agents (diltiazem and verapamil), beta-blocking agents (esmolol [Brevibloc], propranolol, metoprolol, atenolol), and digoxin. In acute AF, the authors find that digoxin (Lanoxin) given as a loading dose (0.5 mg intravenously initially followed by 0.25 mg intravenously every 4 hours to a total dose of 1.0 to 1.5 mg) fails to adequately or promptly control heart rate in many patients. The dosage of digoxin should be decreased in the elderly and those with impaired renal function. The use of digoxin in patients with pre-excitation (Wolff-Parkinson-White syndrome) is contraindicated as it can facilitate conduction over the accessory pathway. Beta-blocking agents are the drugs of choice in those with AF due to hyperthyroidism. Unfortunately, many patients cannot tolerate intravenous beta blockers because of hypotension or underlying pulmonary disease. The authors' practice has been to use intravenous diltiazem (Cardizem) at an initial loading dose of 20 to 25 mg followed by a continuous infusion starting at 5 to 10 mg per hour. If there is no significant reduction (20% reduction from baseline) in heart rate within 15 minutes, a second intravenous loading dose of 25 mg may be given and the infusion rate increased to a maximum of 15 mg per hour. Intravenous diltiazem is generally well tolerated even in patients with congestive heart failure.

Once adequate rate control has been obtained

in patients who have had an acute episode of AF (duration less than 72 hours), DC cardioversion can be performed with an initial 200 joules and increasing to 360 joules if unsuccessful at lower energy. In patients who have been in AF for longer than 48 to 72 hours, 3 weeks of anticoagulation with warfarin sodium (Coumadin) should be administered before cardioversion, with dosage adjusted to maintain a prothrombin time 1.3 to 1.6 times control. Warfarin sodium should be continued for at least 2 to 3 weeks after cardioversion, since atrial mechanical contraction does not return to normal immediately following conversion and the incidence of embolic events remains high for some time after conversion. Intravenous procainamide (Pronestyl) or oral quinidine is useful for chemical cardioversion, particularly in those with acute-onset AF. Care must also be taken when initiating quinidine for attempted cardioversion or maintenance of sinus rhythm in patients without adequate rate control as quinidine has vagolytic action and can accelerate conduction through the AV node. In patients receiving digoxin, the dose should be reduced by 50% when initiating quinidine therapy as quinidine increases serum digoxin levels.

Class IA antiarrhythmics (procainamide 750 to 1000 mg every 6 hours, quinidine gluconate 324 to 648 mg every 8 hours, and disopyramide 100 to 200 mg every 6 hours) can be of benefit in maintaining sinus rhythm in some patients after DC cardioversion. However, caution must be used in patients with severely reduced left ventricular function as they are more likely to develop proarrhythmic side effects such as torsades de pointes (discussed further on) from these agents. Class IC antiarrhythmic agents (propafenone [Rythmol] and flecainide [Tambocor]) are highly effective in preventing recurrences of AF but should be avoided in patients with structural heart disease because of the increased risk of proarrhythmia. Amiodarone (Cordarone)* given in daily maintenance doses of 200 to 300 mg following a load of 400 mg twice daily for 7 days is highly effective in preventing recurrent AF and is well tolerated long term. Amiodarone should be reserved for patients who have failed conventional agents, because of its potential long-term side effects. Sotalol (Betapace), an antiarrhythmic agent with both beta blocking and Class III antiarrhythmic activity, is also highly effective in preventing episodes of paroxysmal AF. Typical doses range from 160 mg to 320 mg twice daily for sotalol.

Anticoagulation with warfarin sodium in patients with chronic AF (due to an inability to con-

---

*This use of amiodarone is not an FDA-approved indication.

vert them to sinus rhythm or an intolerance of antiarrhythmic agents) is in general well tolerated, even in the elderly. It has been shown to reduce the incidence of stroke by 40 to 70% (occurring in about 5% of patients per year with chronic AF). It is of particular importance in non-anticoagulated patients with mitral valve disease (especially mitral stenosis) in whom the incidence of embolic stroke is quite high. The warfarin sodium dose should be individualized in each patient to maintain a prothrombin time from 1.3 to 1.6 times control. Patients with rheumatic mitral valvular disease should be maintained at a more prolonged prothrombin time (1.5 to 2.0 times control). In those who cannot take warfarin sodium, aspirin has been shown to reduce the risk of stroke in chronic AF although the magnitude of its benefit is unknown.

In some patients, sinus rhythm cannot be restored, and rate control with AV nodal blocking agents cannot be achieved. These patients are candidates for radiofrequency ablation of the AV node with permanent pacemaker implantation.

Multifocal Atrial Tachycardia

Multifocal atrial tachycardia (MAT) is a second type of irregular narrow complex tachycardia. MAT is characterized on ECG by multiple (at least three) different P wave morphologies with a rate between 120 and 180 bpm. Because of its irregularity and the occasionally indistinguishable P waves, it may frequently be confused with AF. It is most commonly seen in patients with underlying pulmonary disease, especially in association with hypoxia, underlying infection, sympathomimetic agent administration, and metabolic imbalances. Treatment with Class IA agents and digoxin is ineffective in terminating the arrhythmia or in slowing AV nodal conduction. Beta blockers are generally not tolerated because of pulmonary disease, but calcium channel blockers may be helpful. The most effective treatment is correction of the underlying acute illness. Electrical cardioversion is not effective treatment for this arrhythmia because of its frequent recurrence.

Regular Narrow Complex Tachycardias

Atrial Flutter

Although less common than AF, atrial flutter is also a frequently encountered atrial arrhythmia. As with AF, underlying cardiac disease is common. A reentrant mechanism appears to be responsible for the arrhythmia in patients with classic flutter. The risk of clot formation in the atrium and the possibility of stroke are insignificant unless underlying structural heart disease (e.g., dilated cardiomyopathy, valvular heart disease) is present.

Atrial flutter has been categorized as Type I (negatively deflected P waves in the inferior ECG leads with rates from 230 to 350 bpm) and Type II (atrial rate 340 to 430 bpm), with Type I being more common. Because the AV node usually conducts atrial flutter with 2:1 AV block, this rhythm disturbance should always be considered when a regular tachycardia with a rate of 140 to 160 bpm is observed. Adenosine may be very useful in differentiating atrial flutter from other regular narrow complex tachycardias.

The treatment of atrial flutter depends upon the patient's underlying condition. In unstable patients, cardioversion with 50 to 100 joules is usually successful.

Slowing of the ventricular rate is helpful in stable patients and may be accomplished with calcium channel blocking agents, beta blockers, or digoxin. Once the heart rate is controlled, several options for treatment exist. Although many patients may be asymptomatic with just control of the heart rate, it is worthwhile to try conversion to normal sinus rhythm in most patients. Cardioversion is quite successful with 50 to 100 joules. Rarely, atrial flutter may be converted to AF by DC cardioversion and requires a second high-energy shock.

Type I, or common, atrial flutter also frequently responds to overdrive atrial pacing (pacing starting at approximately 125% of the atrial rate). This can be accomplished by inserting a transvenous atrial catheter or an esophageal electrode or by using temporary atrial pacing wires left in situ immediately after cardiac surgery. The ability to overdrive-pace atrial flutter is improved by using a Class IA agent (e.g., procainamide, quinidine, disopyramide) prior to pacing to slow the atrial rate.

Once sinus rhythm has been achieved, these patients frequently require antiarrhythmic agents to prevent recurrence. Class IA agents (procainamide sustained release tablets 750 to 1000 mg every 6 hours, quinidine gluconate 324 to 648 mg every 8 hours, or disopyramide 100 to 200 mg every 6 hours) are quite effective. Caution must be used, particularly in patients with reduced left ventricular function, when starting these agents. Antiarrhythmic therapy should be started in the hospital with continuous monitoring of the rhythm. Amiodarone is also quite effective for the treatment of atrial flutter but is again not used as a first-line agent due to its potential toxicity.

As with AF, the use of radiofrequency ablation of the AV node and permanent pacemaker placement is indicated in patients whose heart rate cannot be controlled by AV nodal blocking drugs or sinus rhythm cannot be maintained pharmacologically.

AV Nodal Reentrant Tachycardia

AV nodal reentrant tachycardia is the most common of a group of narrow complex arrhythmias referred to as paroxysmal supraventricular tachycardias (PSVT) (Table 4). This tachyarrhythmia is frequently seen in young to older female patients without structural heart disease. The rate of the tachycardia is usually between 150 and 250 bpm. It can be precipitated by exercise, sympathomimetic drugs, alcohol, or caffeine. The arrhythmia occurs because of the presence of two pathways of conduction in or near the AV node, the fast (normal) conduction pathway and a slow (abnormal) conduction pathway. An atrial premature beat may block conduction in the fast pathway with antegrade conduction over the slow pathway instead. Retrograde conduction up the fast pathway can then occur, and a reentrant circuit of antegrade slow and retrograde fast conduction results. Because retrograde conduction over the AV node is rapid, the reentrant atrial beat is usually concealed in the terminal portion of the QRS complex and not seen on the surface ECG. During an acute episode, patients may terminate their own tachycardia by vagal maneuvers or coughing. If this fails, adenosine is very effective for termination of the arrhythmia.

Calcium channel blockers (sustained-release verapamil, 240–360 mg every day; diltiazem, controlled delivery 240–300 mg daily), digoxin (0.125–0.250 mg daily), or beta-blocking agents are effective long-term treatment for the arrhythmia. In highly selected, otherwise drug refractory cases Class IC agents (flecainide and propafenone) have been used with good success; however, they should not be given to patients with structural heart disease. Long-term drug therapy in these patients is hampered by side effects (particularly with beta-blocking agents) and poor compliance due to the intermittent nature of the arrhythmia.

Radiofrequency ablation has emerged as the treatment of choice for young, otherwise healthy patients with recurrent episodes of AV nodal reentrant tachycardia, in preference to long-term drug therapy. Most centers now use techniques to localize and ablate the area of abnormal slow conduction while preserving normal AV nodal conduction. In centers experienced with the technique, the success rate of ablation is greater than 90%. The risk of complications is extremely low; the major one is complete heart block requiring permanent pacing, which occurs in fewer than 5% of patients.

Atrial Tachycardia

Atrial tachycardias are an uncommon cause of PSVT. The atrial tachycardia may be due to an automatic tachycardia or intra-atrial reentry. The P wave morphology and axis are typically different from those of the sinus beat. The atrial rate of the tachycardia is generally from 150 to 200 bpm. Block may occur in the AV node without effect on the atrial rate (particularly when associated with digitalis excess), causing atrial tachycardia with block.

Automatic atrial tachycardia is typically seen in those with underlying heart disease (e.g., acute myocardial infarction), metabolic disorders, in patients who are digoxin toxic (atrial tachycardia with block), and as a nearly incessant arrhythmia in pediatric and adolescent patients. The P wave morphology depends on the site of origin of the tachycardia in the atria, and the rate of the tachycardia ranges from 100 to 250 bpm. The tachycardia may show variation in rate and a "warm up" after initiation.

It is important to look for an underlying cause (e.g., digoxin toxicity) in adult patients that may be correctable. In patients who are not digitalis toxic, digoxin or beta blockers slow AV nodal conduction and thus the ventricular rate.

In pediatric and adolescent patients, the automatic atrial tachycardia will typically occur at least 50% of the time. It can result in a tachycardia-induced cardiomyopathy. Atrial mapping and radiofrequency ablation is the treatment of choice in this age group, with left ventricular function typically markedly improved afterward.

Intra-atrial reentry is another mechanism for some atrial tachycardias. Tachycardia rates range from 130 to 150 bpm. Some episodes of intra-atrial reentrant tachycardia have been terminated with adenosine. In adults, this arrhythmia is frequently associated with structural heart disease, and in children, with surgically corrected congenital heart disease. The pharmacologic treatment of these arrhythmias includes Class IA, IC, and III (amiodarone and sotalol) agents.

Junctional Tachycardia

Nonparoxysmal junctional tachycardia arises from the tissue in or near the His bundle. Since the inherent rate of the AV junctional tissue is 35

TABLE 4. **Types of Paroxysmal Supraventricular Tachycardias and Their Relative Frequencies**

AV nodal reentrant tachycardia (60%)
AV reciprocating tachycardia (25%)
Intra-atrial and sinus node reentrant tachycardia (10%)
Automatic atrial tachycardia (5%)

Abbreviation: AV = atrioventricular.

to 60 bpm, rates from 70 to 130 bpm are classified as junctional tachycardia. The arrhythmia mechanism is increased automaticity. It is frequently seen in conjunction with underlying heart disease (e.g., acute myocardial infarction or myocarditis) and in digitalis toxicity. In general, management focuses on identification and treatment of the underlying cardiac disease.

Tachycardias Associated with Accessory Pathways

The presence of one or more accessory pathways between the atrium and ventricle gives rise to different tachycardia mechanisms, as seen in Figure 2.

Conduction may occur in a retrograde-only fashion over the accessory pathway (AP). When there is no antegrade conduction over the accessory pathway, the PR interval and QRS duration on the 12-lead ECG during sinus rhythm will appear normal. The pathway may still be used for reentrant tachycardia, and these patients are said to have tachycardia due to a concealed accessory pathway. The tachycardia in patients with a concealed accessory pathway is retrograde through the accessory pathway and antegrade over the AV node (orthodromic SVT) with a nar-row complex (in the absence of aberration) (Fig. 2A). Because conduction is only in a retrograde fashion over the accessory pathway, antidromic tachycardia (Fig. 2B) and pre-excited atrial fibrillation (Fig. 2C) cannot occur in these patients.

The *Wolff-Parkinson-White syndrome* (WPW) is seen in patients with both antegrade and retrograde conduction over the accessory pathway. The diagnostic hallmarks of WPW are a short PR interval (<0.12 sec) and a wide QRS complex due to fusion of conduction over the AV node and accessory pathway. These patients may have an AV reciprocating (orthodromic) tachycardia or, less commonly, reentry occurring antegrade over the accessory pathway and retrograde through the AV node (antidromic tachycardia) (Fig. 2B). In addition, patients with WPW may conduct atrial fibrillation over the accessory pathway (pre-excited atrial fibrillation) (Fig. 2C).

Tachycardia Associated with a Concealed Accessory Pathway

In 30 to 50% of patients with paroxysmal supraventricular tachycardia (PSVT), a concealed accessory pathway (i.e., retrograde conduction only in the accessory pathway) is the cause of the tachycardia. As previously discussed, the 12-lead ECG in sinus rhythm is normal in these patients

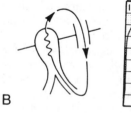
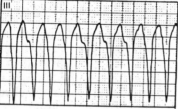

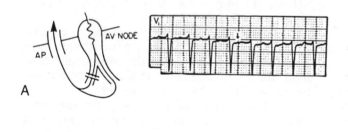

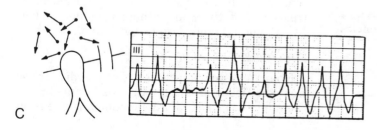

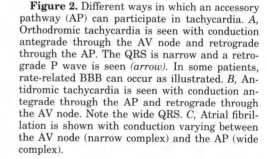

Figure 2. Different ways in which an accessory pathway (AP) can participate in tachycardia. *A,* Orthodromic tachycardia is seen with conduction antegrade through the AV node and retrograde through the AP. The QRS is narrow and a retrograde P wave is seen *(arrow).* In some patients, rate-related BBB can occur as illustrated. *B,* Antidromic tachycardia is seen with conduction antegrade through the AP and retrograde through the AV node. Note the wide QRS. *C,* Atrial fibrillation is shown with conduction varying between the AV node (narrow complex) and the AP (wide complex).

since antegrade conduction over the accessory pathway does not occur. Rates during tachycardia range from 150 to 300 bpm. Because retrograde conduction over the accessory pathway during tachycardia is longer than that seen in AV nodal reentry, a retrograde P wave seen on the surface ECG during tachycardia can help differentiate SVT due to a concealed accessory pathway from AV nodal reentry. During the tachycardia, antegrade conduction occurs over the AV node, and unless rate-related aberration occurs or pre-existing bundle branch block is present, the tachycardia will be narrow complex. The use of adenosine to terminate tachycardia is preferred for acute conversion by blocking antegrade conduction through the AV node.

Long-term pharmacologic therapy for patients with this tachyarrhythmia can include drugs that block the AV node, such as digoxin, verapamil, or propranolol, or drugs that block conduction over the accessory pathway (Class IA, IC, and III agents). We prefer using beta-blocking agents for AV nodal blockade. Class IA agents are highly effective for chronic suppressive therapy since they block accessory pathway conduction. They may also be given intravenously (procainamide) during acute episodes. The combination of an AV nodal blocking agent and a Class IA agent may be necessary in some patients to control the tachycardia. Infrequently, a Class IC or III antiarrhythmic agent may be necessary to control the episodes of tachycardia.

Results of radiofrequency ablation to destroy the accessory pathway are quite safe and effective in this group of patients (>90% successful), and this is considered the treatment of choice for otherwise healthy patients with frequent, symptomatic episodes requiring chronic drug therapy.

Tachycardia in Patients with WPW Syndrome

Patients with WPW have both antegrade and retrograde conduction over the accessory pathway, as previously described. WPW syndrome occurs in 0.1 to 0.5% of the population. It may be associated with other forms of heart disease; Ebstein's anomaly is the most common concurrent abnormality. While some patients with the syndrome may remain asymptomatic throughout their life, 25 to 70% have recurrent symptomatic tachycardia and a few may be predisposed to more serious arrhythmias (ventricular fibrillation and sudden death). Some patients may have multiple pathways present, each of which may participate in the tachycardia.

The major tachycardias seen with WPW syndrome include orthodromic SVT, antidromic SVT, pre-excited atrial flutter or fibrillation, and rapid atrial fibrillation with conduction over an accessory pathway degenerating to ventricular fibrillation.

Orthodromic SVT is the most common form of tachycardia in patients with WPW (Fig. 2A). Termination of orthodromic SVT in a patient with WPW is best accomplished with adenosine, 6 to 12 mg intravenously. In patients with recurrent episodes, intravenous procainamide may also be administered. Rapid antegrade conduction over the accessory pathway or a history of atrial fibrillation is a contraindication to digoxin or calcium channel blockers, as these agents can accelerate antegrade conduction over the accessory pathway (see later discussion). For chronic pharmacologic management of the arrhythmia, Class IA agents and, less frequently, Class IC or III agents may be used. If there is no response to monotherapy, beta-blocking agents may be added.

Atrial fibrillation is the second most common arrhythmia seen in patients with WPW. Most authors feel that this arrhythmia occurs more often in patients with WPW than in the general population, but the reasons are not completely understood. Patients with atrial fibrillation may conduct at a rapid rate over the accessory pathway. When conduction through the accessory pathway predominates, the ECG again will appear maximally pre-excited with an irregular, wide complex tachycardia (Fig. 2C). Digoxin or calcium channel blocking agents are contraindicated in patients with atrial fibrillation and pre-excitation on the ECG as these agents can enhance conduction through the accessory pathway, actually increasing the rate of the tachycardia and possibly leading to hemodynamic instability and ventricular fibrillation. Patients who are unstable in pre-excited atrial fibrillation should undergo DC cardioversion. In stable patients, intravenous procainamide (15 mg per kg loading dose infused over 30 minutes, followed by a continuous infusion at 2 mg per min) will slow conduction through the accessory pathway and frequently convert the arrhythmia to a sinus rhythm.

Antidromic (pre-excited) SVT occurs in only about 10% of patients with WPW. The reentrant pathway during tachycardia is antegrade through the accessory pathway and retrograde through the AV node (Fig. 2B). Because of this, the QRS complex is wide (maximally pre-excited) and it may be difficult to differentiate antidromic SVT from ventricular tachycardia on the surface ECG. Acute treatment of antidromic tachycardia is similar to that for orthodromic SVT (i.e., adenosine and/or Class IA agents intravenously). Chronic pharmacologic management is the same as for orthodromic tachycardia.

Ventricular fibrillation is an uncommon arrhythmia in WPW, occurring in those who conduct very rapidly (>240 bpm) over a single accessory pathway during atrial fibrillation or have multiple pathways. The rapidly conducted atrial fibrillation may then degenerate to ventricular fibrillation.

As with patients who have concealed accessory pathways, there is a high success rate (>90%) using radiofrequency ablation to eliminate the accessory pathway in patients with WPW. It is the treatment of choice in most young patients, with the alternative being chronic drug therapy. Surgical treatment, once frequently performed for this arrhythmia, is now rarely required.

Ventricular Tachyarrhythmias

Ventricular arrhythmias encompass a wide range of tachyarrhythmias, from benign episodes of nonsustained ventricular tachycardia (VT) to potentially lethal and lethal arrhythmias.

When evaluating patients with nonsustained ventricular arrhythmias, careful attention needs to be paid to the patient's symptoms. Eliciting a history of syncope or presyncope should alert the physician to the need for further investigation. Evaluation for the presence of underlying structural heart disease with echocardiography and stress-thallium testing is warranted in these patients to stratify them into low- and high-risk categories. The signal-averaged ECG can further help identify those patients at risk for sustained ventricular arrhythmias.

Patients who have an episode of sudden cardiac death (not associated with the early stage of acute myocardial infarction) represent the other end of the spectrum of ventricular arrhythmias. They may have sustained VT (>30 seconds) with or without ventricular fibrillation. An aggressive approach, including cardiac catheterization and invasive electrophysiologic procedures, is warranted in these patients as the likelihood of recurrence over a 2-year period is between 50 and 60%.

Nonsustained Ventricular Arrhythmias

Treatment of patients with nonsustained ventricular arrhythmias (greater than three beats) is one of the most controversial areas in cardiac electrophysiology. In patients with normal or only mildly depressed left ventricular function and a normal signal-averaged ECG, nonsustained VT carries at most a slightly increased risk of sudden cardiac death. However, in those with severely reduced left ventricular function due to coronary artery or other structural heart disease, frequent nonsustained VT is associated with an increased incidence of sudden death (20 to 25% over 1 year). "Suppressive therapy" for nonsustained VT (i.e.,

suppression of nonparoxysmal ventricular tachycardia on ambulatory Holter monitoring) in patients with known coronary artery disease using a Class IC (encainide or flecainide) and a Class IA agent (moricizine) was associated with an increased incidence of sudden cardiac death in the CAST (Cardiac Arrhythmia Suppression Trial) study, prompting its early termination. For this reason, the authors treat only patients with nonsustained VT who have documented symptoms with their episodes. In general, beta-blocking agents (metoprolol, atenolol, propranolol, nadolol) are used first, and if not effective, a Class IA agent may be substituted in selected patients. As discussed, the use of Class IA agents in patients with significantly impaired left ventricular function (ejection fraction <40%) may actually increase the risk of sudden death, and the benefits versus the risks of treatment must be carefully assessed in each patient.

Sustained Monomorphic Ventricular Tachycardia

Monomorphic VT (which can degenerate to ventricular fibrillation) is a common (60–70%) arrhythmic cause of sudden death in patients with structural heart disease (e.g., coronary artery disease). The mechanism for this arrhythmia is felt to be reentry around an area of ventricular myocardial scar. In patients who have experienced an episode of sudden cardiac death or syncope due to sustained VT, evaluation and management must address both the underlying structural heart disease and the arrhythmia. For this reason, we recommend cardiac catheterization in patients who have survived an episode of sudden cardiac death to evaluate the need for coronary revascularization, valve repair, or replacement and the presence of a ventricular aneurysm. Invasive electrophysiologic studies are then indicated to assess inducibility of the clinical arrhythmia(s). In patients who have sustained VT and coronary artery disease, electrophysiologic studies can be used to induce ventricular arrhythmias in 90 to 95% of these patients. Antiarrhythmic drug therapy can then be attempted using noninducibility of the clinical arrhythmia at follow-up study as an endpoint for successful therapy. With the use of these techniques, the risk of a recurrent episode of sudden death may be reduced from 50 to 60% over 2 years to 5 to 10% in those patients receiving effective drug therapy. Most laboratories start with Class IA agents (procainamide, quinidine, disopyramide), but these antiarrhythmics are able to suppress inducibility of ventricular arrhythmias in the electrophysiology laboratory in only 20 to 25% of patients. While Class IB agents (mexiletine [Mexitil]) alone have a low efficacy, combining one with a Class IA agent may increase the efficacy of ventricular arrhythmia suppression to 30 to 35%. The best available agents to suppress VT are the Class III antiarrhythmic agents (amiodarone and sotalol). These drugs suppress ventricular arrhythmias in 40 to 55% of patients with electrophysiologically guided therapy.

Since at best only 50% of VTs may be rendered noninducible with antiarrhythmic therapy, the use of implantable cardiovertor-defibrillator devices (ICDs) has increased dramatically. The ICD has a 95% 5-year efficacy rate in preventing recurrent sudden death in patients who have sustained VT. Newer ICD devices still undergoing investigation include both antitachycardia pacing capability (which can reduce the number of ICD discharges in some patients) and transvenous lead systems (which eliminate the need for thoracotomy to implant the device in most patients). Despite the use of ICD devices, a significant number of patients (40 to 50%) still require antiarrhythmic drug therapy to reduce the number of episodes or the rate of the VT. It is important to remember that although these devices markedly decrease the incidence of recurrent sudden death, they do not prevent patients from dying of progressive heart failure.

Torsades de Pointes

Torsades de pointes (twisting of the points) is a polymorphic VT frequently associated with QT prolongation from antiarrhythmic drug therapy (especially with Class IA agents), potassium or magnesium depletion, ischemia, or bradycardia (e.g., patients with complete heart block or, rarely, congenital long QT syndrome). Drugs that can cause QT prolongation include quinidine, procainamide, disopyramide, sotalol, amiodarone, phenothiazines, and tricyclic antidepressants. In addition, certain antihistamines (e.g., astemizole [Hismanal]) and agents such as ketoconazole (Nizoral) in conjunction with other QT-prolonging agents or electrolyte abnormalities have been associated with torsades de pointes.

Acutely, intravenous magnesium (1 to 3 grams intravenously) is used to shorten the QT interval in all patients except those in whom the cause of torsades de pointes is severe bradycardia. Atrial or ventricular pacing (90 to 100 bpm) will shorten the QT interval and is also recommended in these patients. Isoproterenol infusion may be helpful until a temporary pacing wire can be placed in some patients. Removal of the offending antiarrhythmic agent and correction of electrolyte abnormalities are essential.

Other Types of Ventricular Tachycardia

Rarely encountered types of VT also exist in association with right ventricular dysplasia, mitral valve prolapse, and bundle branch reentrant tachycardia as well as in patients with structurally normal hearts (primary electrical disease). While some of these tachycardias respond to traditional antiarrhythmic agents, radiofrequency ablation is recommended for others, especially those with right ventricular outflow tract tachycardia or bundle branch reentrant tachycardia. In patients who have catecholamine-sensitive VT and a structurally normal heart, beta blockers will suppress the arrhythmias in a significant percentage.

Ventricular Fibrillation

Ventricular fibrillation (VF) is a very rapid (400 to 600 bpm), and irregular ventricular arrhythmia associated with hemodynamic collapse and sudden death. VF can occur secondary to poor hemodynamic tolerance of ventricular tachycardia, acute myocardial infarction (MI), electrolyte imbalance, or drug proarrhythmia or less commonly as a primary ventricular arrhythmia. Defibrillation with 200 to 360 joules is necessary for conversion of the arrhythmia. Treatment of the underlying cause to prevent recurrence (e.g., electrolyte abnormalities, ischemia, hypoxia) is essential.

In patients who have VF within the first 48 to 72 hours of an acute myocardial infarction (MI), the chance of recurrent sudden death following MI is not significantly increased (especially in those with an inferior wall MI).

A small number of patients have primary VF in the setting of chronic coronary artery disease or other structural heart disease. ICD implantation is the treatment of choice for this group.

CONGENITAL HEART DISEASE

method of
STEVEN R. NEISH, M.D.
Fitzsimons Army Medical Center
Aurora, Colorado

In general, congenital heart disease is limited to only a few presentations. The most common are (1) a cyanotic newborn; (2) an infant with congestive heart failure, which is usually associated with a heart murmur; (3) an infant or a child with an asymptomatic heart murmur; and (4) an abnormal electrocardiogram (ECG) or chest roentgenogram that was obtained during screening before some therapeutic intervention.

Congenital heart disease is common, with an incidence of at least six to nine cases per 1000 live births. With current health care, at least 85% of newborns with congenital heart disease reach adulthood. Many require surgery or catheter intervention, but most are healthy after intervention. Some congenital heart defects are more common than others. The 10 most common defects make up 80% of all congenital heart defects. Those are (1) ventricular septal defect (VSD), (2) atrial septal defect (ASD), (3) pulmonic stenosis (PS), (4) aortic stenosis (AS), (5) coarctation of the aorta, (6) transposition of the great arteries (TGA), (7) patent ductus arteriosus (PDA), (8) tetralogy of Fallot, (9) atrioventricular (AV) septal defect, and (10) hypoplastic left heart syndrome.

VENTRICULAR SEPTAL DEFECT

By far the most common congenital heart defect is VSD. The manifestation of a VSD is dictated by the relative size of the interventricular communication and occasionally by the location of the defect. A small defect may occur with a characteristic systolic heart murmur in the neonatal period. Pulmonary vascular resistance and right ventricular pressure fall rapidly in the first few days of life in the normal newborn, and the murmur of a small VSD becomes manifest early. Newborns with a large VSD tend to have a delayed drop in pulmonary vascular resistance and right ventricular pressure. This minimizes the amount of excess flow through the pulmonary circulation in the first few days of life and therefore delays presentation. Infants with a large VSD tend to present between 2 weeks and 2 months of age. They may present with a minimally symptomatic holosystolic heart murmur or with varying degrees of pulmonary vascular congestion.

The ventricular septum is conventionally divided into four regions, and VSDs are classified according to the location of the defect. The most common VSD is the perimembranous VSD. A VSD in this location can be of any size. Small defects can close spontaneously. This occurs most frequently in the first few months of life, but it occasionally occurs as late as the second decade of life. These defects tend to close by incorporation of tricuspid valve tissue into the defect. Small VSDs that remain patent can provide the substrate for endocarditis. Also, small VSDs can cause chronic left ventricular volume overload. This is due to excess blood flow, which is pumped by the left ventricle through the VSD, the pulmonary circulation, and left atrium. Signs of left ventricular volume overload are indications for surgical VSD closure, even in an asymptomatic patient. On occasion, small perimembranous VSDs are associated with the development of progressive aortic valve insufficiency (AI). This is probably due to the absence of support at the commissure between the right coronary cusp and the noncoronary cusp. In addition, abnormal flow through the VSD may promote prolapse of the aortic valve into the VSD (Bernoulli's effect).

Most cardiologists recommend surgical closure if AI develops even if the VSD is small and seemingly hemodynamically insignificant otherwise. This may arrest the progression of AI.

A patient with a large perimembranous VSD usually presents in the first 2 months of life with a heart murmur and congestive heart failure caused by pulmonary overcirculation. On occasion, the onset of symptomatic heart failure may be delayed but usually is present by 4 months of age. The degree of heart failure is frequently sufficient to impair the infant's ability to feed normally and grow normally. The degree of pulmonary congestion can be ameliorated with a diuretic (usually oral furosemide [Lasix] in a total daily dose of 1 to 4 mg per kg per day in one to three divided doses). Although the mechanism of action is controversial, most pediatric cardiologists add digoxin (Lanoxin) (6 to 10 µg per kg per day in two divided doses) to the therapy if the pulmonary congestion is not adequately managed with diuretics alone. In rare cases, a symptomatic large VSD decreases in relative size during medical management. Usually, however, surgical VSD closure is required after 6 months of age. If surgery is delayed beyond 1 to 2 years of age, severe effects of chronic high pulmonary blood flow, high pulmonary artery pressure, or both may become manifest. These effects include marked growth failure, frequent pulmonary infections, left ventricular failure, and irreversible pulmonary hypertension (Eisenmenger's syndrome). If the VSD is repaired successfully in the first 1 to 2 years of life, however, the long-term effects of the VSD disappear, and mortality figures approach those of the normal population. Postoperative exercise tolerance is usually normal. Some patients never have the normal drop in pulmonary vascular resistance and therefore never develop excessive pulmonary blood flow. Pulmonary artery pressure is at systemic levels, and these patients require surgery in order to prevent the development of irreversible pulmonary vascular obstructive disease (Eisenmenger's syndrome). After surgery, the pulmonary vascular resistance and pulmonary artery pressure usually drop to normal during the first few postoperative months. One to two percent of patients suffer complete AV block at the time of surgical VSD closure and require placement of a permanent pacemaker.

The second most common location for a VSD is in the trabecular muscular septum. Defects in this location are almost as common as perimembranous VSDs in early infancy. They tend to close spontaneously in the first few months of life as the muscular ventricular septum grows and thickens. On occasion, muscular VSDs are associated with other congenital heart defects and complicate the hemodynamic disturbance brought on by each defect in a synergistic manner. In a minority of cases, a muscular VSD is an isolated defect and large enough to require surgical closure. The location of the defect can make the VSD difficult to close because it may be hidden by right ventricular trabeculations and by the location of the defect in the apex of the right ventricle.

Inlet muscular VSDs make up fewer than 10% of VSDs. Other names for this type of VSD are AV canal type VSD or endocardial cushion type VSD. Inlet muscular VSDs tend to be large. They do not close spontaneously. Often there is an associated cleft mitral valve. This type of VSD is similar to the VSD of an AV septal defect. Inlet muscular VSDs are more common in children with Down's syndrome. Surgical closure is usually required.

Supracristal or outlet muscular or juxta-arterial VSDs are the final type of VSD. In most ethnic populations, VSDs in this location make up only about 5% of all VSDs. In some Asian populations, however, they are the most common VSDs. It is unusual for this type of VSD to be as large as an isolated lesion. Supracristal VSDs do not close spontaneously. Frequently, progressive AI complicates the long-term course in this defect. The proposed mechanism is similar to AI in perimembranous VSDs but with valve support being inadequate at the commissure between the left and right coronary cusps. Bernoulli's effect is also thought to be operational. In both supracristal and perimembranous VSDs, the onset of AI is unusual before 2 years or after 10 years of age. In many cases, the AI is progressive and may progress in severity to the point at which aortic valve replacement is required. If AI is mild at the time of VSD closure, however, it tends to be stable in the postoperative period.

ATRIAL SEPTAL DEFECT

In almost every series, ASD is the second most common congenital heart defect. It is the most common defect to be diagnosed after infancy. The most common manifestations for ASD are an asymptomatic heart murmur or cardiomegaly on chest roentgenogram. Symptoms are unusual in the first decade of life and when they are present are often mild and subtle. The hallmark of diagnosis of an ASD by physical examination is the presence of fixed splitting of the second heart sound. By the fifth decade, if the ASD has not been closed, almost all patients are symptomatic. When symptoms arise, they are most commonly due to pulmonary vascular congestion (congestive heart failure), arrhythmias, and right ventricular failure. On occasion, symptoms are due to pulmonary vascular disease or paradoxical embolism. If surgery is performed before the onset of symptoms, preferably at 2 to 5 years of age, the natural history is similar to the natural history of patients without congenital heart disease. Sinus node dysfunction, supraventricular tachycardia, and atrial flutter have an increased incidence in postoperative ASD patients when compared with control patients.

There are four anatomic locations for an ASD. The most common type of ASD is the secundum or ostium secundum or fossa ovalis ASD. This defect occurs when there is an insufficient amount of secundum septum to cover the ostium secundum, a normal structure, in the primum atrial septum. Small defects almost universally close in infancy. Defects that are moderate or large after 1 year of age rarely close spontaneously. Because virtually all patients with an ASD become symptomatic with time, closure is almost universally recommended. In cases of only an isolated secundum ASD in otherwise normal children, surgical mortality is extremely rare. A device that can be delivered through a special catheter, the Lock Clamshell Occluder, is currently under investigation and may be available for nonsurgical ASD closure in the next few years.

Ostium primum ASDs, a type of AV septal defect, are the second most common type of ASD. Ostium primum ASDs do not close spontaneously. If not a part of a complete AV septal defect, and usually even if a part of an AV septal defect, ostium primum ASDs tend to be large. Usually the anterior leaflet of the mitral valve is cleft in association with an ostium primum ASD. In addition to a fixed split S_2 and the other findings of a secundum ASD, examination may reveal a murmur of mitral insufficiency. Symptoms tend to occur at a younger age than with secundum ASDs and tend to be more debilitating. Surgical repair of an ostium primum ASD is more difficult than a secundum ASD. This is because the mitral valve must be resuspended at the time of ASD closure. Postoperatively there may be mitral insufficiency or, less commonly, mitral stenosis. Mitral insufficiency may be progressive and may be severe enough to require a later operation for mitral valve repair or replacement. The postoperative course is usually benign but is dependent on the function of the mitral valve. Because of the cleft mitral valve, endocarditis prophylaxis around procedures should be continued indefinitely. Transcatheter closure techniques are not available for ostium primum ASDs because of the proximity of the defect to the AV valves.

Sinus venosus ASDs are located near the junction of the superior vena cava and the right atrium. This type of ASD also does not close spontaneously. Sinus venosus ASDs are frequently associated with anomalous connection of one or more pulmonary veins. The anomalous veins usually provide venous return from the right lung and connect to the right atrium or the superior vena cava. The anomalous pulmonary veins are typically in close proximity to the ASD and can be easily baffled into the left atrium at the time of ASD closure. Supraventricular arrhythmias are particularly common during long-term follow-up of this group of patients after surgery. Theories to explain this include absence of the normal sinus node and stitches and scarring in the region of the sinus node. Transcatheter closure techniques are not available for this defect because of proximity of the ASD to the pulmonary veins.

The least common type of ASD is a coronary sinus ASD. The orifice of the coronary sinus is a normal structure in the atrial septum. In patients with a coronary sinus ASD, however, the tissue that separates the coronary sinus from the left atrium is absent. This allows blood to pass from the left atrium into the right atrium. Surgical repair of this defect is more difficult than repair of a secundum ASD, and there are two options. The first is to close the defect in the atrial septum, which allows coronary sinus blood to return to the left atrium, creating a small right-to-left shunt. Alternatively, but more difficult surgically, one could create a new "roof" on the coronary sinus between the coronary sinus and the left atrium.

PULMONIC STENOSIS

PS is defined as obstruction to pulmonary blood flow and can exist in isolation or as a part of a complex of congenital heart defects, such as tetralogy of Fallot. When PS is a solitary lesion, it is usually pulmonary valve stenosis. It is useful to divide pulmonary valve stenosis into three categories according to severity—mild, moderate, and severe PS—based on the pressure gradient between the right ventricle and the pulmonary artery. Mild PS has a gradient of less than 30 to 40 mmHg. It is rare for mild PS to progress after the first few months of life, and in fact the gradient may decrease with growth. Physical examination reveals a systolic ejection click followed by a systolic ejection murmur, which is loudest at the left upper sternal border. The murmur radiates over the lung fields. ECG may be normal or may suggest right ventricular hypertrophy (right axis deviation of the frontal plane QRS axis, incomplete right bundle-branch block pattern). Many patients are asymptomatic, and the course is benign. Occasionally, mild exercise intolerance is present.

Moderate PS has a gradient less than 80 mmHg and right ventricular systolic pressure less than left ventricular pressure. A systolic thrill at the left upper sternal border and a right ventricular heave are usually present in addition to the ejection click and murmur. Occasionally there is cyanosis caused by right-to-left shunting of blood across the atrial septum (this occurs more commonly in neonates and in patients with severe PS). In the great majority of cases, there is right ventricular hypertrophy on ECG. The magnitude of the gradient frequently increases with time in moderate PS. Eventually the majority of patients with moderate PS become symptomatic, the most common symptom being exercise intolerance. This degree of obstruction causes right ventricular hypertrophy and right ventricular fibrosis, leading to right ventricular dysfunction. If the gradient is greater than 40 to 50 mmHg, cardiac catheterization and balloon pulmonary valvuloplasty are performed. Gradient relief with balloon valvuloplasty is good, and the gradient rarely returns.

In severe PS, the gradient is greater than 80 mmHg or the right ventricular pressure is equal to the left ventricular pressure or both conditions are present. Seventy-five percent of children with severe PS have symptoms, most typically exercise intolerance. If the valve is sufficiently abnormal (dysplastic), there may not be an ejection click. There is a thrill at the left upper sternal border associated with a harsh systolic murmur, which radiates to the lung fields. There is usually marked right ventricular hypertrophy on ECG. Usually balloon valvuloplasty relieves the gradient. If the valve is dysplastic, however, surgical valvotomy may be required. Regardless of the severity, after therapy, the long-term course of PS is usually benign.

AORTIC STENOSIS

Aortic valve stenosis is the most common form of obstruction to left ventricular outflow. Typically AS is due to a bicuspid aortic valve with an orifice that is too small to allow normal blood flow across the valve. About 1% of the general population have a bicuspid aortic valve, but only a few of these patients are diagnosed with AS in childhood. Natural history studies suggest that 50% of patients with AS die suddenly if surgery is not performed. Endocarditis occurred in 1% of patients with AS per year in the era before prophylactic antibiotics.

The most common manifestation for AS is an asymptomatic murmur noted at a routine examination. About 10% of patients with AS have congestive heart failure in the first year of life.

These patients usually present in the first 2 months with critical AS. At diagnosis, they have poor peripheral perfusion, decreased peripheral pulses, cyanosis, and respiratory distress. There may not be a murmur on cardiac examination because of low cardiac output. Often, however, there is an apical gallop, an ejection click, and increased precordial activity. Typically the ECG shows right ventricular hypertrophy. Chest roentgenogram shows cardiomegaly and pulmonary vascular congestion. Critical AS requires emergent therapy. Both surgical valvotomy and balloon valvuloplasty have been used to relieve the stenosis with similar results. Mortality rates for infants with critical AS remain significant.

Older patients are rarely symptomatic at the time of diagnosis. The most common symptom is limited exercise tolerance. Even with severe AS (left ventricle–aorta gradient >75 mmHg), however, only 30% of patients have excessive fatigue with exercise. Angina and syncope are more common in severe AS but still occur in fewer than 10% of patients. A systolic thrill is present in approximately 85% of patients with AS. Even patients with mild AS can have a thrill. The thrill is variably present in the suprasternal notch and at the right or left (or both) upper sternal borders. Up to 90% of patients have a systolic ejection click. The most common locations for the click are at the base of the heart at the left sternal border, the apex, and the right upper sternal border. The apical impulse is increased, especially with severe AS and marked left ventricular hypertrophy. ECG may be normal in mild AS. With progressive degrees of obstruction, there are progressive signs of left ventricular hypertrophy. With severe obstruction, there may be T wave changes in V6, suggesting left ventricular strain or ischemia. Chest roentgenogram is often normal. The most common abnormality is dilation of the ascending aorta, especially after infancy.

If there are no symptoms, intervention is usually reserved for patients with a gradient greater than 50 mmHg. If there are symptoms of heart failure or myocardial ischemia, intervention may be offered at gradients less than 50 mmHg. Both surgical valvotomy and balloon valvuloplasty can be successful in children and adolescents with AS. Many reports demonstrate gradient relief with balloon valvuloplasty that is equivalent to surgical valvotomy with more favorable morbidity and mortality. With either approach, stenosis can recur, or insufficiency can be created. On occasion, valve replacement is necessary. The risk of sudden death is lessened by successful intervention, but it remains above the normal population. If sufficient stenosis or insufficiency remains, activity should be restricted.

COARCTATION OF THE AORTA

Coarctation of the aorta is due to medial thickening of the proximal descending aorta. It is commonly associated with a bicuspid aortic valve. The presentation of coarctation depends on the severity of obstruction. A minority of patients present in the first few weeks. These patients have severe obstruction and present with congestive heart failure or even shock. In addition to discrete coarctation, they may have diffuse hypoplasia of the aortic isthmus. Other cardiac defects are frequently associated with neonatal coarctation, most typically VSD. Physical examination shows diminished lower extremity pulses and a differential in blood pressure between the right arm and the legs. A heart murmur may or may not be present. ECG shows right ventricular hypertrophy in many neonates. Chest roentgenogram may show increased pulmonary vascular markings.

Patients who present with coarctation after the neonatal period usually have more subtle signs and symptoms. Presenting signs and symptoms include diminished femoral artery pulses, upper extremity hypertension, and a heart murmur. The murmur of coarctation is variably present and is a murmur that peaks in late systole and extends into diastole. It is described as a delayed systolic murmur. It can be heard in the left infraclavicular area, in the back medial or below the left scapula, and in the left axilla. There also may be continuous murmurs over the chest wall due to arterial collaterals. Many patients have a systolic ejection click. The ECG may be normal or may show left ventricular hypertrophy, right ventricular hypertrophy, or biventricular hypertrophy. After infancy, the degree of left ventricular hypertrophy correlates with the severity of obstruction. Chest roentgenogram is typically normal, but there may be dilation of the ascending aorta and poststenotic dilation of the descending aorta. After the age of 5 years, rib notching owing to large arterial collaterals is frequently seen and correlates with more severe obstruction. The degree of obstruction tends to increase with time as intimal thickening develops in the area of the coarctation. Without intervention, 90% of patients with coarctation die by age 50 years. The primary causes of death are aortic rupture or dissection, endocarditis, congestive heart failure, and intracranial hemorrhage. Risks of morbidity and mortality from all of these causes lessen after successful repair.

If there is hypertension or congestive heart failure at presentation, intervention is recommended. In the neonatal period, an intravenous prostaglandin E₁ infusion helps to stabilize the patient with severe coarctation. Digoxin and diuretics help to alleviate pulmonary vascular congestion. Beta blockers help to normalize the blood pressure. Most cardiologists, however, recommend intervention directed at relieving the obstruction if there is heart failure or hypertension. Balloon angioplasty is effective in diminishing the gradient in most patients. In the early newborn period, balloon angioplasty is less effective. Surgical repair is also effective and is the treatment of choice if there is associated isthmic hypoplasia. Both approaches are complicated over the long term by return of obstruction and aneurysm formation.

TRANSPOSITION OF THE GREAT ARTERIES

TGA is the most common cyanotic lesion to be diagnosed in the first week of life. The pulmonary artery arises from the left ventricle, and the aorta arises from the right ventricle. The most common associated defect is a VSD. Often there is left ventricular outlet or subpulmonic obstruction. The degree of hypoxemia is usually critical and life-threatening. Physical examination at presentation may not suggest cardiac disease because a murmur may not be present. There is an increased right ventricular impulse and a single S_2. ECG shows right axis deviation and right ventricular hypertrophy. Chest roentgenogram is usually normal initially but eventually shows pulmonary congestion. Often newborns with this diagnosis can be stabilized temporarily with an intravenous infusion of prostaglandin E_1 which opens the ductus arteriosus to allow mixing between the systemic and pulmonic circulations. Further intervention is required in the first few days of life. Historically this was accomplished with a Rashkind balloon atrial septostomy. This procedure creates a large ASD, which allows mixing of systemic venous return with pulmonary venous return. Usually that was adequate to allow growth and development for a few months. After 3 to 6 months, a second procedure was required. The procedure of choice was usually an atrial baffle procedure known as the Mustard procedure or Senning procedure. Both procedures are complex atrial baffles that direct the systemic venous return to the mitral valve so that deoxygenated blood can pass into the left ventricle and pulmonary circulation, and the pulmonary venous return is directed into the right ventricle so oxygenated blood can be pumped into the aorta. Postoperative problems include baffle obstruction, sinus node dysfunction, atrial and ventricular arrhythmias, right ventricular dysfunction, and sudden death.

Now most infants who are born with TGA are managed differently. An arterial switch procedure is performed in the first few days or weeks of life. The pulmonary artery and the aorta are transected and removed from the left ventricle and right ventricle, respectively. The aorta is then reanastomosed to the native pulmonary root, and the coronary arteries are also transferred to the native pulmonary root. The pulmonary artery is reanastomosed to the native aortic root. Initially there was concern about the rate of operative mortality of this approach, but now the operative mortality is less than 5% in most active pediatric cardiac surgery centers. The intermediate-term follow-up of these patients is more benign than that of patients who have had an atrial baffle procedure.

PATENT DUCTUS ARTERIOSUS

PDA is always a normal finding during fetal life. Normally the ductus arteriosus constricts and functionally closes in the first few days of life. Persistent patency is more common in premature infants, infants with respiratory distress, and infants born at high altitude. Even though the ductus usually closes in the first 24 hours, a PDA is occasionally diagnosed as the cause of a heart murmur heard in the first few days or weeks of life. This can nevertheless be considered a normal variant. A PDA should be considered an abnormal structure only if it is present after the first 3 months or if it causes pulmonary vascular congestion.

Most commonly, a PDA is diagnosed in one of two situations. Most very-low-birthweight premature infants have a PDA that may need to be closed. Often this can be accomplished with intravenous indomethacin (Indocin). On occasion surgical ligation is necessary. The other common manifestation is an asymptomatic heart murmur in an infant or a child. This is typically a continuous murmur that is loudest in the left infraclavicular area. Occasionally there is an apical diastolic flow rumble. It is less common for a 3- to 6-week-old infant to present with a large PDA with congestive heart failure and failure to thrive. If the PDA is small, both the ECG and the chest roentgenogram are usually normal. A large PDA shows left ventricular hypertrophy and left atrial enlargement on ECG. Chest roentgenogram may show cardiomegaly and increased pulmonary vascular markings.

The natural history of an untreated PDA includes congestive heart failure in the very young or the very old, endocarditis, and rarely pulmonary vascular disease. If there is pulmonary vascular congestion, PDA closure is recommended at any age. If the PDA is asymptomatic, closure can be delayed until after the first birthday in most cases because many PDAs close spontaneously in the first year of life. The classical treatment is surgical ligation and division. There is now an investigational device that can be delivered through a catheter, the Rashkind PDA Occluder, which should be available in the next few years.

TETRALOGY OF FALLOT

The tetrad that makes up tetralogy of Fallot is overriding aorta, PS, VSD, and right ventricular hypertrophy. This is the result of deviation of the outlet ventricular septum into the right ventricular outflow tract. In some patients, the degree of deviation may be so significant that there is pulmonary atresia. Patients with tetralogy typically present in one of two ways. Most patients present with cyanosis sometime during infancy. The age at presentation depends on the adequacy of pulmonary blood flow. If there is critical obstruction to pulmonary blood flow, the cyanosis may be recognized in the first few hours of life.

More typically, the patient is suspected of having heart disease after discharge from the nursery sometime during the first few months. It is not unusual for presentation to be delayed until the age of 6 months. Usually there is a systolic heart murmur at presentation. In fact, the degree of cyanosis may be subtle, and the only abnormality noted at presentation may be a heart murmur. The typical heart murmur is a harsh systolic murmur that is loudest at the left upper sternal border, which radiates to the lung fields. The ECG shows right ventricular hypertrophy. Chest roentgenogram typically shows an abnormal cardiac shadow, *couer en sabot,* caused by right ventricular enlargement and absence of the main pulmonary segment. Pulmonary vascular markings are decreased. If the cyanosis is critical in a newborn, pulmonary blood flow can be increased with an intravenous infusion of prostaglandin E_1.

The approach to congenital heart disease was revolutionized in 1945 when A. Blalock and H. Taussig treated a patient with tetralogy of Fallot with a subclavian artery–to–pulmonary artery anastomosis. This augmented pulmonary blood flow and extended survival. This or a similar procedure is still used in some patients who require augmented blood flow in the first few months of life. Eventually, usually in the first 2 years of life, the VSD is closed, and the pulmonic stenosis is relieved surgically. The postoperative course is frequently benign, but it may be complicated by residual PS, pulmonary regurgitation, a residual VSD, right ventricular dysfunction, ventricular arrhythmias, and sudden death.

ATRIOVENTRICULAR SEPTAL DEFECT

AV septal defect, also known as AV canal defect or endocardial cushion defect, is an unusual defect among children with normal chromosomes, but it is the most common congenital heart defect among children with Down's syndrome. In a complete AV septal defect, there is a large inlet muscular VSD, an ostium primum ASD, and abnormalities of the tricuspid and mitral valves. All of these abnormalities are the result of one large, contiguous defect. These patients usually present similar to a patient with a large VSD and require surgery in infancy. In some patients, especially if there is Down's syndrome, the pulmonary vascular resistance may remain elevated, and there are minimal symptoms and few signs on physical examination. This group of patients develops early pulmonary vascular disease, but the pulmonary vascular disease is reversible if surgery is performed to correct the congenital heart defect in the first 6 to 12 months. For this reason, all patients with Down's syndrome should be seen by a pediatric cardiologist in the first few months.

Either the ASD or the VSD can be small in AV septal defect. This is known as a transitional or incomplete AV septal defect. The relative contribution of atrial and ventricular level shunting determines the presentation and course of an individual patient. Surgery for AV septal defect is more difficult than surgery for either a solitary ASD or VSD. Success of surgery is usually dependent on the adequacy of the repair of the mitral valve. Postoperative mitral insufficiency occurs commonly.

HYPOPLASTIC LEFT HEART SYNDROME

Hypoplastic left heart syndrome is a severe congenital heart defect that is characterized by marked left ventricular obstruction and a diminutive left ventricular chamber. The majority of patients have both aortic and mitral atresia or severe stenosis. Usually these patients are recognized before discharge from the nursery because symptoms arise early in life. Many patients with hypoplastic left heart syndrome are recognized prenatally on screening obstetric ultrasonography. The initial symptoms are usually due to pulmonary vascular congestion caused by increased left atrial and pulmonary venous pressure. There is usually cyanosis and respiratory distress in the first 1 to 2 days of life. As the patent ductus arteriosus closes, severe metabolic acidosis and shock occur. This is because all of the systemic blood flow must pass through the ductus arteriosus. Physical examination shows decreased peripheral pulses and perfusion, hepatomegaly, and respiratory distress. An apical gallop, a systolic murmur, and a diastolic rumble are variably present. ECG shows right axis deviation and right ventricular hypertrophy and may show diminished left ventricular forces. The chest roentgenogram usually shows cardiomegaly and increased pulmonary vascular markings.

Without intervention, 95% of these infants die in the first month, and there are only rare survivors beyond the first year. Initial therapy is directed at maintaining the patency of the ductus arteriosus with a prostaglandin E_1 infusion. There are two surgical options. The first is the Norwood procedure, which is a complex palliative procedure performed in two to three operations during the first 2 to 3 years of life. A second option, which has been adopted by more centers, is to offer cardiac transplantation. This procedure requires lifelong immunosuppression and is limited by the availability of donor organs.

ENDOCARDITIS PROPHYLAXIS IN CONGENITAL HEART DISEASE

Many surgical and dental procedures create bacteremia. In patients without heart disease, this is of no significance. In patients with congenital heart disease, however, the surface of the endothelium, endocardium, or both may be irregular and is predisposed to the development of endocarditis after an episode of transient bacteremia. One of the most important but frequently overlooked measures in preventing bacteremia associated with dental procedures is the maintenance of good dental hygiene. Antibiotics for endocarditis prophylaxis are recommended for most congenital heart defects. Antibiotic prophylaxis is probably unnecessary in secundum ASDs and 6 months after surgical repair of secundum ASD, VSD, or PDA if there is no residual shunt. (See the article "Infective Endocarditis.")

EXERCISE IN CONGENITAL HEART DISEASE

The issue of exercise in congenital heart disease raises many questions. Is exercise safe? How much exercise is safe? How much exercise is possible? Are there benefits of exercise specific to this population? In general, the safety and feasibility of exercise are dependent on the severity of the congenital heart disease that is present in an individual. This is particularly true after surgery or catheter intervention. If the hemodynamic status is near normal, as in a patient after surgery for an ASD or a VSD, exercise can usually be unlimited. Exercise testing in a controlled laboratory setting can be useful in assessing the re-

sponse to exercise. In patients who are likely to have residual hemodynamic abnormalities, such as those recovering from surgery for AS, TGA, or tetralogy, it is often prudent to restrict patients from high levels of competition. The benefits of long-term exercise in the congenital heart disease population are uncertain, although they do show a training effect from exercise.

MITRAL VALVE PROLAPSE

method of
ELLIOT CHESLER, M.D.
Veterans Administration Medical Center
Minneapolis, Minnesota

Names such as "floppy," "prolapsing," "systolic click-murmur syndrome," "anatomic MVP," "MVP syndrome," and "billowing mitral leaflet syndrome" refer to some anatomic or functional abnormality associated with myxomatous degeneration and prolapse of mitral valve leaflets. Prolapse detected by echocardiography, however, does not necessarily mean that the mitral valve is abnormal. For example, prolapse of normal thin leaflets may be found with left ventricular or papillary muscle dysfunction because of failure of chordal restraint in systole. Because the term "mitral valve prolapse" (MVP) is now widely accepted, it seems reasonable to restrict its use to the condition in which the clinical and echocardiographic features are compatible with those of a myxomatous mitral valve.

PATHOLOGY OF THE MYXOMATOUS VALVE

Myxomatous infiltration of the fibrous supporting layer weakens the mitral leaflets, leading to prolapse into the left atrium superior to the plane of the annulus. Usually the posterior leaflet is involved alone or at least more prominently than the anterior leaflet. The criterion for making a gross anatomic diagnosis is interchordal hooding of 4 mm or more, involving at least one-half of the anterior leaflet or two-thirds of the posterior leaflet. Fibrosis of the free aspect of the leaflets is a response to contact with an opposite prolapsing element or adjacent segment of the valve, and fibrosis of the left ventricular surface of the leaflets develops in response to stretching and tension. The chordae tendineae may be elongated and thickened, simulating rheumatic disease, but commissural fusion is absent.

Contact thrombosis may be found in two sites; one is on the atrial aspect of prolapsed units, and the other is situated between the posterior mitral leaflet and the left atrial wall (so-called angle lesion). Both are potential sources for systemic embolism.

Left ventricular endocardial friction lesions are formed as chordae make contact with subjacent left ventricular mural endocardium when the posterior leaflet prolapses. These lesions may coalesce, so that considerable portions of the base of the left ventricle become thickened and even calcified.

GENETICS AND EPIDEMIOLOGY

The myxomatous mitral valve is inherited as an autosomal dominant disorder. Most studies of the prevalence of MVP are based on findings of echocardiography. These studies have disadvantages, however, because some interchordal "hooding" is present in the normal mitral valve, and criteria for diagnosis of prolapse are variable. There is also considerable variation in interobserver and intraobserver interpretation. Epidemiologic studies based on loose echocardiographic criteria have reported the incidence of MVP in as much as 21% of the general population. The "true" incidence is probably in the vicinity of 4% of the general population. The prevalence is lower in childhood and adolescence but increases with advancing years. There is a higher frequency among elderly men, who also tend to have more severe mitral regurgitation and left ventricular dysfunction. The myxomatous valve is now a leading cause of mitral regurgitation in the United States. This is because of a decline in the incidence of rheumatic fever and a greater awareness of the condition by clinicians and pathologists. Some instances of "rheumatic" mitral regurgitation were actually myxomatous valves associated with secondary fibrosis, erroneously diagnosed as healed rheumatic or infective endocarditis.

ASSOCIATED ABNORMALITIES

An association with Marfan's and Ehlers-Danlos syndromes, pectus excavatum, straight back, scoliosis, and high-arched palate is established. MVP has also been described in association with many other cardiac and general medical conditions, but this is almost certainly fortuitous. Because MVP is identified in approximately 4% of the general population, coincidental association occurs when there is a high background prevalence of some other cardiac or noncardiac condition, such as mitral annular calcification or migraine.

CLINICAL FINDINGS

Symptoms

Most subjects are asymptomatic, and the condition is often diagnosed by detection of a nonejection click during routine physical examination of a young person. Exertional dyspnea, leading to symptoms of frank congestive heart failure, occurs in patients with a holosystolic murmur and significant mitral regurgitation, particularly when the chordae rupture.

Physical Examination

Occasionally there are some features of Marfan's syndrome or formes frustes thereof, i.e., high-arched palate, pectus excavatum, or scoliosis.

Auscultation

A high-pitched click in mid-systole is the keystone finding. It is heard in the region between the apex and the left sternal border and coincides with maximal excursion and tension on the posterior leaflet. Depending on volume changes in the left ventricle, the click may occur quite early in systole (Fig. 1). The murmur is late systolic and follows the click and also responds to maneuvers that change left ventricular volume. The intensity and character are variable, but it is best heard at the apex or left mid-precordium when mitral regurgitation is mild.

When myxomatous degeneration is severe and particularly when chordae rupture, the murmur becomes holosystolic and may have a loud vibratory "honking" quality simulating the murmur of aortic stenosis. The murmur is usually crescendo-decrescendo in shape and ends before the aortic component of S_2. S_3 is common, S_1 is of normal or increased intensity, and a mid-diastolic murmur is absent. These findings are quite different from rheumatic mitral regurgitation, in which S_1 is soft, the holosystolic murmur ends after S_2, and there is a significant mid-diastolic murmur.

Electrocardiography

The electrocardiogram is usually normal. The most commonly reported abnormality is flattening or inversion of the T waves in leads II and III and arteriovenous fistula. T wave inversion may occur spontaneously and independent of effort or may follow the patient's assumption of the erect position. The exact prevalence of these findings is unknown because of different selection criteria in various series. The Framingham study of the general population showed that persons with and without echocardiographic MVP were equally likely to have repolarization abnormalities. Left ventricular hypertrophy and left atrial enlargement are found when mitral regurgitation is significant.

Echocardiography

Invasive procedures are rarely indicated now because clinical and echocardiographic findings are so accurate. Both M-mode and two-dimensional techniques play a pivotal role in diagnosis and assessment of patients with MVP.

M-Mode Echocardiography

Mid-Systolic or Late Systolic Buckling. Sudden posterior displacement of the leaflets in mid-systole is quite characteristic of MVP, and there are few false-positive results.

Holosystolic "Hammocking." Holosystolic posterior displacement is not absolutely specific for MVP. False-positive results may occur when there is excessive cardiac movement in systole (e.g., pericardial effusion).

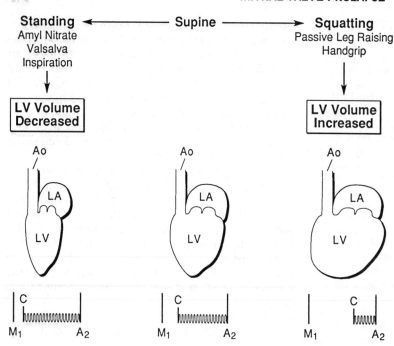

Figure 1. Effect of changes in left ventricular volume on timing of mid-systolic click (C) and late systolic murmur. *Abbreviations:* LV = left ventricle; LA = left atrium; Ao = aorta.

Two-Dimensional Echocardiography

The important changes are thickening of the leaflets and chordae with systolic displacement of segments of the valve into the left atrium above the plane of the saddle-shaped mitral annulus that has high points anteriorly and posteriorly. Because of this configuration of the mitral annulus, the mitral leaflets frequently appear to prolapse when viewed in the apical four-chamber view. Therefore, false diagnosis can be avoided by insisting that prolapse be visible in the long axis parasternal view. A calcified left atrial angle lesion above and calcified left ventricular endocardial friction lesion below the mitral annulus assist in diagnosis. When chordae rupture, there is (1) failure of leaflet coaptation, with the edges frequently observed in several views; (2) a whipping motion of the leaflet and attached chordae when a sizable portion of leaflet is detached; and (3) an eccentric jet demonstrated on color-flow Doppler imaging, depending on which chordae have ruptured. The transesophageal technique is particularly useful for defining anatomy more precisely.

COMPLICATIONS AND PROGNOSIS

The risk factors are infective endocarditis, mitral regurgitation, stroke, and sudden death. Infective endocarditis is a definite but infrequent hazard in patients with a late or holosystolic murmur. Progressive mitral regurgitation and congestive cardiac failure may supervene when chordae rupture. Elderly men are particularly prone to this complication and also to severe left ventricular dysfunction and its attendant risk of sudden dysrhythmic death as a result of long-standing mitral regurgitation. The incidence of systemic embolism is low, and the risk for sudden death among young people with mild mitral regurgitation and normal left ventricular function is minuscule. The prognosis is excellent, and few patients suffer complications. Pathologic studies comparing the age at death of patients with myxomatous valves with control autopsy material showed that patients with myxomatous valves lived longer.

MANAGEMENT

Effective management of patients with MVP requires a careful assessment of the clinical, electrocardiographic, and echocardiographic findings so that triage is appropriate.

Mitral Valve Prolapse Without Mitral Regurgitation

When MVP is discovered in asymptomatic subjects without clinical evidence of mitral regurgitation, even after provocative maneuvers (see Fig. 1), it should be strongly emphasized to patients that their prognosis is excellent, and every effort should be made to avoid engendering cardiac neurosis. Antibiotic prophylaxis is not necessary, but the physician should recognize that this does not completely solve the problem because patients who have intermittent murmurs may be at increased risk. Doppler evidence of mild mitral regurgitation is not a reason for prophylaxis because the technique is too sensitive. The majority of subjects remain asymptomatic for their lifetimes without complications.

Mitral Valve Prolapse with Mitral Regurgitation

Infective Endocarditis

This is a hazard for patients with MVP and a late systolic or holosystolic murmur. Thickened redundant leaflets identified by echocardiography and a predisposition to bacteremia through drug addiction or immunosuppression are additional strong reasons for meticulous antibiotic prophylaxis even when mitral regurgitation is mild.

PROCEDURES NECESSITATING ANTIBIOTIC PROPHYLAXIS

Dental Procedures. Patients should be educated to maintain the best possible dental hygiene. All dental procedures likely to result in gingival damage with bleeding, including routine cleaning by a dentist, should be preceded by antibiotic treatment. Flossing, brushing, rinsing with chlorhexidine gluconate (Peridex) mouthwash, and professional cleaning help reduce bacteremia before routine dental procedures. Dentures should be regularly checked for the presence of gingival ulceration. Shedding of primary teeth and adjustment of orthodontic appliances are not usually accompanied by *Streptococcus viridans* bacteremia, and prophylaxis is therefore unnecessary.

Upper Respiratory Tract Procedures. *S. viridans* bacteremia may follow bronchoscopy, tonsillectomy, and adenoidectomy, and prophylaxis is therefore recommended.

TABLE 1. **Recommended Standard Prophylactic Regimen for Dental, Oral, or Upper Respiratory Tract Procedures in Patients Who Are at Risk**

Drug	Dosing Regimen
	Standard Regimen
Amoxicillin	3.0 gm PO 1 h before procedure, then 1.5 gm 6 h after initial dose
	Amoxicillin / Penicillin-Allergic Patients
Erythromycin or	Erythromycin ethylsuccinate, 800 mg, or erythromycin stearate, 1.0 gm PO 2 h before procedure, then half the dose 6 h after initial dose
Clindamycin	300 mg PO 1 h before procedure and 150 mg 6 h after initial dose

Abbreviation: PO = orally.
From Dajani AS, Bisno AL, Kyung JC, et al. Prevention of bacterial endocarditis. JAMA *264:*2919–2922, 1990. Copyright 1990, American Medical Association.

TABLE 2. **Alternate Prophylactic Regimens for Dental, Oral, or Upper Respiratory Tract Procedures in Patients Who Are at Risk**

Drug	Dosing Regimen
	Patients Unable to Take Oral Medications
Ampicillin	Intravenous or intramuscular administration of ampicillin, 2.0 gm, 30 min before procedure, then intravenous or intramuscular administration of ampicillin, 1.0 gm, or oral administration of amoxicillin, 1.5 gm, 6 h after initial dose
	Ampicillin / Amoxicillin / Penicillin-Allergic Patients Unable to Take Oral Medications
Clindamycin	Intravenous administration of 300 mg 30 min before procedure and an intravenous or oral administration of 150 mg 6 h after initial dose
	Patients Considered High Risk and Not Candidates for Standard Regimen
Ampicillin, gentamicin, and amoxicillin	Intravenous or intramuscular administration of ampicillin, 2.0 gm, plus gentamicin, 1.5 mg/kg (not to exceed 80 mg), 30 min before procedure, followed by amoxicillin, 1.5 gm, PO 6 h after initial dose; alternatively, the parenteral regimen may be repeated 8 h after initial dose
	Ampicillin / Amoxicillin / Penicillin-Allergic Patients Considered High Risk
Vancomycin	Intravenous administration of 1.0 gm over 1 h, starting 1 h before procedure; no repeated dose necessary

Abbreviation: PO = orally.
From Dajani AS, Bisno AL, Kyung JC, et al. Prevention of bacterial endocarditis. JAMA *264:*2919–2922, 1990. Copyright 1990, American Medical Association.

Genitourinary and Gastrointestinal Procedures. These are important portals of infection in elderly men, and the organism is usually *Streptococcus faecalis*. Procedures include cystoscopy, urethral dilatation, prostatic massage, genitourinary and gallbladder surgery, and sclerotherapy for esophageal varices. Vaginal childbirth and hysterectomy also require prophylaxis.

ANTIBIOTIC REGIMENS

These follow the recommendations of the American Heart Association and are given in Tables 1 through 3.

Progressive Mitral Regurgitation

Signs of severe mitral regurgitation and heart failure supervene in a small proportion of patients with MVP, and men older than age 45 years are particularly prone to this complication. The average age of patients having mitral repair at our institution is 61 ± 2 years, and in most

TABLE 3. **Regimens for Genitourinary and Gastrointestinal Procedures**

Drug	Dosage Regimen
	Standard Regimen
Ampicillin, gentamicin, and amoxicillin	Intravenous or intramuscular administration of ampicillin, 2.0 gm, plus gentamicin, 1.5 mg/kg (not to exceed 80 mg), 30 min before procedure, followed by amoxicillin, 1.5 gm, PO 6 h after initial dose; alternatively, the parenteral regimen may be repeated once 8 h after initial dose
	Ampicillin/Amoxicillin/Penicillin-Allergic Patient Regimen
Vancomycin and gentamicin	Intravenous administration of vancomycin, 1.0 gm, over 1 h plus intravenous or intramuscular administration of gentamicin, 1.5 mg/kg (not to exceed 80 mg), 1 h before procedure; may be repeated once 8 h after initial dose
	Alternate Low-Risk Patient Regimen
Amoxicillin	3.0 gm, PO 1 h before procedure, then 1.5 gm 6 h after initial dose

Abbreviation: PO = orally.

From Dajani AS, Bisno AL, Kyung JC, et al. Prevention of bacterial endocarditis. JAMA *264*:2919–2922, 1990. Copyright 1990, American Medical Association.

cases the underlying pathology is myxomatous mitral valve, with or without rupture of chordae. Similar findings have been noted in larger surgical centers. Mechanisms for increasing mitral regurgitation include (1) increasing prolapse because progressive myxomatous degeneration weakens the leaflets; (2) dilatation of the annulus, which goes along with and may aggravate, in a vicious circle, increasing degrees of regurgitation; and (3) rupture of the chordae tendineae.

Patients with a holosystolic murmur and significant mitral regurgitation should be examined annually, particularly when there is echocardiographic evidence of marked leaflet redundancy and lengthening of chordae. Left ventricular function and internal dimensions should be carefully assessed at each visit. Afterload reduction with angiotensin-converting enzyme (ACE) inhibitors such as enalapril (Vasotec) in a dose of 2.5 to 10 mg twice a day may be useful in diminishing mitral regurgitation and preserving left ventricular function.

SURGICAL TREATMENT

Operation is indicated when the left ventricular end-systolic dimension exceeds 5.6 cm as measured by echocardiography. Although mitral anatomy, left atrial size, and functional status are important in predicting the outcome of operation, age and left ventricular ejection fraction are the crucial prognostic factors.

Repair is accomplished by excision of excess leaflet tissue (valvuloplasty) and annuloplasty or insertion of an annular ring. When monitored by transesophageal echocardiography, the results are excellent. Conservative repair has the obvious advantage of avoiding long-term anticoagulation, which is frequently risky in the elderly. In cases in which the valve anatomy is unsuitable for repair, replacement should be with a metallic or porcine valve.

Systemic Embolism

There is considerable evidence in the neurologic literature showing that MVP is associated with transient ischemic attacks or stroke in young patients. Although the exact mechanism for systemic embolism has not been documented, there are at least two sources for platelet, fibrin, and even cacific emboli: (1) contact thrombosis on surfaces of redundant leaflets and (2) angle lesion within the left atrium.

Antiplatelet treatment is recommended in patients who have had systemic embolism. Aspirin (160 to 320 mg) daily is effective. When embolism is recurrent, large, and associated with atrial fibrillation, warfarin (Coumadin) should be added.

Dysrhythmias

Atrial Dysrhythmias

Supraventricular tachycardia, atrial fibrillation, atrial flutter, and atrial ectopic beats are not specific for MVP but are a result of left atrial distention. They may complicate significant mitral regurgitation of any cause and should be treated in the same way: Pharmacologic cardioversion with Type Ia agents such as quinidine sulfate (Quinidex) or procainamide (Pronestyl) should be attempted and followed by synchronized DC cardioversion if the former fails. When atrial fibrillation persists, the ventricular response should be controlled with beta-blocking agents, such as atenolol (Tenormin) or metoprolol (Lopressor), or calcium channel blockers, such as verapamil (Isoptin) or diltiazem (Cardizem.)

Ventricular Dysrhythmias

It is the ventricular dysrhythmias, particularly high-grade ventricular ectopy and ventricular tachycardia, that have attracted so much attention and have been correlated with the risk of sudden death. It should be strongly emphasized, however, that sudden unexpected death resulting from dysrhythmia among young people with MVP is rare. Many cases of sudden death attributed to MVP were actually a result of drug toxicity, left ventricular dysfunction associated with long-standing mitral regurgitation, or an independent cardiomyopathy. In a recent review from the Pathology Branch of the National Institutes of Health, there were records of only 15 patients studied at necropsy who had died suddenly with MVP as the only explanation for death, and in their review of the literature, only an additional 39 cases had been reported elsewhere. Most victims were young women with little or no mitral regurgitation.

TREATMENT

The rare, small subset of patients who complain of dizziness, presyncope, or syncope and have high-grade ventricular ectopy should be fully evaluated. Left ventricular ejection fraction should be measured by two-dimensional echocardiography or radionuclide angiography because impaired left ventricular function of any cause carries a poor prognosis and a risk of sudden dysrhythmic death. Holter monitoring for 24 or 48 hours is useful for assessing severity of ventricular dysrhythmias when these are manifest on the resting electrocardiogram. When the resting electrocardiogram is normal and symptoms are infrequent, however, patient-activated event recorders are much more informative. Exercise electrocardiography is cost-effective only when symptoms are clearly related to exertion.

If ventricular dysrhythmia is excluded as a cause of syncope, vagal stimulation (carotid massage) and orthostatic tilt testing should be employed to exclude neurally mediated hypotension and bradycardia. The sensitivity of orthostatic tilt may be enhanced by isoprenaline infusion, which stimulates the mechanoreceptors in the left ventricle thought to be responsible for reflex, vagal-induced bradycardia and hypotension.

When serious symptomatic ventricular dysrhythmias such as nonsustained and sustained ventricular tachycardia are demonstrated, provocative electrophysiologic study to select an appropriate antidysrhythmic drug is indicated. Favorable experience has been reported with the use of sotalol (Betapace) a beta-blocking agent with antidysrhythmic activity, now available in the United States. Sotalol, as with all antidysrhythmic agents, must be used with caution in the presence of hypokalemia because it may lead to QT prolongation and torsades de pointes. The usual dose is 80 to 320 mg daily. Amiodarone (Cordarone) is highly efficacious in suppressing serious ventricular dysrhythmias, but because of its serious side effects it should not be used in long-term treatment of young patients. The maintenance dose is 200 to 400 mg daily.

Patients with disease refractory to or who suffer serious side effects from antidysrhythmic drugs should be considered for mitral valvuloplasty, which has proved effective in treating a few patients with intractable ventricular dysrhythmias. The mechanism may be relief of mechanical stimulation of the endocardium by elongated chordae of the posterior mitral leaflet, a notion supported by experiments showing that traction on papillary muscles may induce ventricular ectopy.

When carotid massage or orthostatic tilt reproduces syncope as a result of neurally mediated hypotension and bradycardia, left ventricular mechanoreceptor activity should be blocked with the use of a beta-blocking agent. Disopyramide (Norpace) is also effective because it has not only an anticholinergic effect that blocks vagal transmission but also a negative inotropic action that diminishes activity of the ventricular mechanoreceptors. The usual dose is 150 mg every 6 hours. The drug should be used with caution in elderly men because it frequently causes urinary retention.

Mitral Valve Prolapse Syndrome, Autonomic Dysfunction, and Somatization Disorder

A group of patients described as having "MVP syndrome" present with nonspecific symptoms, such as palpitation, fatigue, stabbing left inframammary pain, dizziness, and lightheadedness. These symptoms are indistinguishable from those occurring in "panic disorder with somatization," which affects 2 to 5% of the general population, 10 to 14% of patients in cardiologic practice, and 6 to 10% of patients in primary care clinics. The nature and severity of symptoms are unrelated to the degree of prolapse or mitral regurgitation. An association between anxiety state, panic disorder, agoraphobia, and autonomic dysfunction with a hyperadrenergic state and MVP has been described, but controlled studies have not supported these findings.

It is more likely that co-morbidity among highly symptomatic individuals is responsible and that many of the symptoms are a result of superimposed, or iatrogenic-induced anxiety in individuals who have been subjected to excessive medical attention. Many such patients respond to reassurance, and in some a beta-blocking agent, such as propranolol (Inderal) or metoprolol (Lopressor), has a useful anxiolytic effect by breaking up the vicious cycle of tachycardia aggravating anxiety. Patients presenting with anxiety neurosis or panic attacks and found to have coexisting MVP should receive appropriate professional psychotherapy.

CONGESTIVE HEART FAILURE

method of
WARD B. ROGERS, M.D., and
MARTIN J. FRANK, M.D.

Medical College of Georgia
Augusta, Georgia

Heart failure is defined by the inability of the ventricles to pump sufficient blood to meet metabolic demands of body tissues. The term "congestive heart failure" (CHF) is appropriate when there is accumulation of interstitial fluid in the lungs (left-sided heart failure) and the liver and extremities (right-sided heart failure). Because both sides of the heart are in series, severe left ventricular failure commonly results in right ventricular failure. Traditionally CHF has been typified by cardiomegaly, pulmonary congestion, and depressed left ventricular systolic function owing to primary myocardial diseases or owing to secondary causes, such as coronary, hypertensive, or valvular disease. Secondary disease is far more common. Approximately 6 million Americans have ischemic heart disease, which is responsible for about one-third (600,000) of all deaths in the United States annually. Moreover, about 10 to 15% of the estimated 37 million Americans with essential hypertension develop hypertensive cardiovascular disease caused by left ventricular hypertrophy, which is commonly associated with myocardial ischemia, even when epicardial arteries are normal.

DIAGNOSIS AND PATHOPHYSIOLOGY

Defining the nature of abnormal function is critically important for several reasons. First, noncardiac diseases of lungs, kidneys, or liver may mimic pulmonary or venous congestion. Second, both prognosis and therapy are distinctly different and dependent on the underlying cause and pathophysiology.

The pathophysiology of CHF can often be determined from a history, physical examination, chest radiograph, and electrocardiogram (ECG). Significant cardiomegaly and pulmonary venous congestion in chronic CHF without a loud heart murmur suggests failure arising from a dilated, hypokinetic left ventricle. With loud murmurs or absence of marked cardiomegaly, however, it is mandatory to evaluate valvular and ventricular performance by Doppler echocardiography, radionuclide angiography, or cardiac catheterization with ventriculography.

Diastolic Dysfunction

Recent technologic advances have shown that a significant minority of patients (especially those with hypertension or coronary disease) have normal or nearly normal systolic function but impaired diastolic relaxation, compliance, or both owing to left ventricular hypertrophy, ischemia, or fibrosis. In conditions such as hypertrophic cardiomyopathy, left ventricular function is hyperdynamic, but diastolic relaxation is impaired and permits adequate filling only with elevated atrial pressures, leading to pulmonary congestion. Diastolic heart failure should be suspected with pulmonary congestion with a normal-sized heart. Confirmation of elevated filling pressures with normal systolic function requires cardiac catheterization. Echocardiography is invaluable, however, because it noninvasively demonstrates left ventricular size and systolic function and may demonstrate left ventricular hypertrophy, left atrial enlargement, and augmented atrial contribution to left ventricular filling, which further support a diagnosis of diastolic left ventricular failure. It also helps exclude pericardial or mitral valve disease, which may impair left ventricular filling. Differentiation of diastolic from systolic failure is essential because therapy with inotropes or vasodilators may be ineffective or even detrimental in the former.

Valvular Disease

The relative importance of valvular disease as a cause of CHF continues to decline as the incidence of rheumatic heart disease declines. Nevertheless, severe mitral and aortic valvular disease must not be overlooked because surgical correction reverses CHF, improves symptoms, and prolongs life. The murmur of mitral stenosis may remain occult for some time but not severe mitral regurgitation or chronic aortic valve disease. A loud murmur in a patient with CHF should prompt evaluation by Doppler echocardiography to quantify severity and assess left ventricular size and function. Moderate mitral regurgitation (due to stretching of the annulus and supporting structures) is common in dilated cardiomyopathy, but severe regurgitation is uncommon. Aortic or mitral stenosis resulting in CHF and symptomatic, severe mitral and aortic regurgitation should be managed surgically before excessive left ventricular dilatation and dysfunction.

Coronary Artery Disease

Chronic coronary artery disease is a major cause of CHF and may produce CHF through systolic dysfunction, diastolic dysfunction, or both. Systolic failure results from loss of functioning myocardial tissue (hibernating muscle or scar) or impaired cardiac output owing to ejection of blood into an aneurysm or the left atrium as a result of mitral regurgitation. Stress myocardial perfusion imaging is useful in assessing the amount of viable and acutely or chronically ischemic myocardium. When large areas of myocardium are ischemic, beta-blocking or calcium channel–blocking drugs may improve congestive symptoms despite their negative inotropic properties. Revascularization procedures may similarly improve function. Coronary disease is often obvious because of a history or evidence on ECG of prior infarction or classic angina. In a sizable minority, however, particularly diabetics and the elderly, ischemia may be silent. When there is a clinical suspicion of coronary disease, rest symptoms are not present, and left ventricular function is normal, radionuclide or echocardiographic imaging during stress testing may be instrumental in demonstrating occult coronary ischemia.

MANAGEMENT

Management of CHF, particularly for patients who experience gradual progression of symptoms and disability, has become more complex since 1980 because of increasing availability of alternative drug regimens. A great majority of those with biventricular dilatation and CHF benefit from combined therapy with an inotropic drug (currently digitalis), diuretics, vasodilator drugs, and beta-blocking drugs. Beta-adrenergic blockade is particularly important in ischemic left ventricular dysfunction.

Digitalis

Current data suggest that this old remedy is still of benefit in patients with a dilated left ventricle and reduced stroke volume. The authors prefer digoxin as a solution, usually in a capsule (Lanoxicap) because bioavailability is 90 to 100% in comparison with 60 to 80% for a digoxin tablet, which may further be altered by diet and gut transit times. An initial loading with 0.4 to 0.6 mg is followed by increments of 0.1 to 0.2 mg to achieve a total dose of 0.8 to 1.0 mg in the first 24 hours for adults. Maintenance therapy, however, must be guided by renal function, which may be impaired in patients with CHF, particularly in the elderly, even though the serum creatinine level is normal. Safety can be enhanced by ensuring normal serum potassium and magnesium levels. Digoxin should be avoided in isolated diastolic dysfunction unless needed for atrial arrhythmia.

Diuretics

A moderate salt-restriction diet and one or more diuretics are often necessary to correct the sodium and fluid retention found in most patients with CHF. When patients have severe hepatomegaly and peripheral edema, reduced oral bioavailability owing to gut edema is often present, and the lowest effective dose of an intravenous loop diuretic (e.g., furosemide [Lasix], 20 to 40 mg) should be instituted. It may be necessary to titrate dosage upward to reduce pulmonary congestion and achieve a daily weight loss of 1 to 2 pounds in patients with significant fluid retention. Diuresis begins within 5 to 15 minutes of an intravenous dose of furosemide, and duration of action is 2 to 3 hours. If urinary output is measured for this interval and adequate diuresis is not achieved, the intravenous dosage should be doubled at 4 to 6 hour intervals until an adequate response is observed. Potassium-magnesium wasting can best be avoided by limiting administration to one or, at most, two daily doses, which permits cation retention for most of each day. When large doses of furosemide are necessary, complementary use of metolazone (Zaroxolyn), 2.5 to 5.0 mg orally ½ hour before furosemide, augments effect. After diuresis reduces gut edema, switch to oral furosemide, 20 to 40 mg more than the effective intravenous dose.

Adequacy of diuresis is best judged by daily weight measurements and strict measurement of intravenous and oral fluid intake and urine output. Also, neck vein distention can be watched. Examination of cervical veins in the semirecumbent position at 45 degrees from the horizontal rarely permits visualization of normal venous pulses greater than 2 cm above the clavicles, unless right-sided fluid retention is present. Moreover, if firm pressure exerted over the right upper quadrant further augments cervical vein filling, right-sided fluid retention is likely. When cervical veins are engorged above the clavicles while the patient is sitting, venous pressure is greater than 11 mmHg.

Vasodilators

Drugs that reduce impedance to left ventricular emptying through reduction in afterload are of great value in management of CHF. Currently the angiotensin-converting enzyme (ACE) inhibitors are most commonly used because of a greater improvement in quality of life and duration of survival than with the combination of hydralazine and nitrates. ACE inhibitors prevent the conversion of angiotensin I to angiotensin II. In patients with CHF, reduction in peripheral resistance and pulmonary venous pressure is accompanied by an increased stroke volume and renal blood flow. The latter may induce diuresis without any diuretic or permit a reduced dosage.

The effect of ACE inhibitors on blood pressure (BP) is hard to predict without an adequate understanding of the pathophysiology of CHF in a given patient. For example, patients with borderline pretreatment blood pressure (less than 120/80) on the basis of ischemic cardiomyopathy or mitral regurgitation might be anticipated to have a further BP decline after institution of ACE inhibitor therapy. Conversely, however, a decrease in the severity of mitral regurgitation or a reduced myocardial oxygen demand, owing to reduced left ventricular chamber dimensions, or both may improve left ventricular performance, with a resultant rise in BP.

A relatively common reason for hypotension after beginning ACE inhibitors is the simultaneous institution of an aggressive diuretic program, particularly in patients who do not experience an early improvement in left ventricular function. Hypotension can often be prevented by starting with a low dose of a short-acting ACE inhibitor, such as captopril (Capoten), 6.25 mg three times a day (half-life is 3 to 4 hours) for those with BP less than 120/80 mmHg and 12.5 mg three times a day for those with a higher BP. Significant, usually transient declines in BP of 20% or more, occurring at the first or an incremental dose, can be avoided by making these changes at bedtime. The authors increase dosage stepwise every 4 to 5 half-lives in nonhypotensive patients. When a daily dose of 150 mg of captopril has been reached, they switch to a longer acting ACE inhibitor, such as enalapril (Vasotec), lisinopril (Prinivil, Zestril), benazepril (Lotensin), or fosinopril (Monopril). These have a relative potency of 10 times that of captopril. Fosinopril (Monopril) appears to have an advantage in the elderly and in patients with hepatic or renal dysfunction because of its dual excretory route. Current evidence suggests that the greater the tolerance for ACE inhibitors, the better the long-term prognosis for compensated CHF. The authors have administered as much as 80 mg lisinopril per day.

Alternative vasodilators are useful for those who develop intolerable cough or angioedema. The authors' preliminary experience with doxazosin (Cardura), a once-daily selective alpha$_1$-adrenergic receptor blocker, has been encouraging. Caution must be used in patients with compromised liver function.

Beta-Blocking Drugs

Beta blockade for patients with severe left ventricular dysfunction owing to congestive cardiomyopathy was originally suggested in the mid-1970s. High levels of circulating catecholamines are cardiotoxic, induce vasoconstriction, increase plasma renin (ultimately angiotensin II), and down-regulate myocardial beta receptors. Also, rapid cardiac rates increase myocardial oxygen demand and reduce the diastolic filling period. Different benefits, however, might be anticipated in patients with congestive versus ischemic cardiomyopathy, particularly if the latter has a substantial mass of hibernating muscle. Reduction in ischemia may improve left ventricular size and function. In the absence of hibernating myocardium, beta blockade should be delayed until the patient has been stabilized with digoxin, diuretics, and vasodilators. The authors usually begin with 6.25 mg of metoprolol twice a day and increase to 12.5 mg in a few days if there are no adverse effects. Further increments are made monthly to a total of 75 to 100 mg. Some adjustment of diuretic therapy may be required initially. Most patients improve their physical capacity if they can tolerate 50 mg metoprolol or more per day. There is some evidence that drugs with intrinsic sympathomimetic activity (e.g., pindolol) may be better tolerated.

Acute Left Ventricular Failure

Patients presenting with acute pulmonary edema may have known cardiac disease or an acute illness, such as myocardial infarction. Pulmonary venous pressure is usually greater than 25 mmHg. Position patients at a 45-degree angle in bed and start oxygen with a 40% Venti-Mask. Morphine sulfate, 3 to 5 mg intravenously, given 1 mg per minute relieves anxiety and reduces the work of breathing. It is also sympatholytic, thereby lowering left ventricular filling pressures by venodilation and reducing peripheral resistance. The aforementioned dosage may be repeated once or twice to a total of 15 mg in 30 minutes, depending on body size, but must be used with great caution in those with hypotension or impaired pulmonary function. Serious side effects can be reversed by naloxone, 0.4 mg, which can be repeated at 2 to 3 minute intervals if necessary.

Furosemide is particularly valuable in pulmonary edema because, in addition to its diuretic effect, it is a venodilator and enhances pulmonary lymphatic drainage. These latter effects may occur before diuresis after 20 mg intravenously, which is an appropriate initial dose in normotensive patients without evidence of fluid retention. Higher doses can be used in patients who are hypertensive or have hepatomegaly and peripheral edema. If diuresis does not occur within 2 to 3 hours, the dose should be doubled and given intravenously. Ethacrynic acid (Edecrin), 25 mg intravenously, is an appropriate starting dose for those with known sulfonamide allergy.

In addition, nitroglycerin is valuable in managing pulmonary edema in patients without peripheral edema, particularly with evidence of myocardial ischemia or acute myocardial infarction. The authors prefer nitroglycerin to sodium nitroprusside because it is a more potent venous than arteriolar dilator, lowers pulmonary venous pressure more than peripheral arterial pressure, and has a wider safety margin in normotensive patients. The authors begin with a sublingual dose of 0.4 mg while the intravenous solution is being prepared. After following instructions for dilution in 5% dextrose solution, they begin an infusion of 10 μg per minute. The dosage may be increased in 5- to 10-μg-per-minute increments every 5 minutes, depending on vital signs and clinical response. If hypotension occurs and pulmonary edema remains uncontrolled, a balloon flotation catheter and an arterial line are inserted in order to monitor pulmonary capillary wedge pressure, thermodilution cardiac output, and systemic vascular resistance more carefully. The addition of dobutamine (Dobutrex), 2 μg per kg per minute, is appropriate if there is clear evidence of important left ventricular dysfunction. The dosage may then be adjusted upward every 3 to 5 minutes (maximum, 40 μg per kg per minute). In patients with acute myocardial infarction who were previously euvolemic, dobutamine may be preferable to diuretics as first-line therapy. Increases in heart rate greater than 10% of base line must be avoided in order to prevent extension of the infarct.

Hypotension alone in patients who are cerebrating, are urinating, and have warm extremities is usually not a problem if systolic pressures remain 85 mmHg or higher. With concomitant pulmonary congestion or shock, however, dopamine is preferable because dobutamine or amrinone may lower pressure further. In oliguric patients, low-dose dopamine (2 to 3 μg per kg per minute) may selectively improve renal blood flow and improve diuresis, but restoration of cardiac output and BP often require higher doses. Peripheral resistance increases along with the dose of dopamine, especially with 10 μg per kg per minute or more. This antagonizes cardiac contractility and may further impair vital organ perfusion. If hypotension can be corrected but requires large doses, addition of low doses of dobutamine, amrinone, or nipride may further improve cardiac output by blunting the vasoconstricting effect of high-dose dopamine. In patients with acute infarction complicated by pump failure and shock, intra-aortic balloon counterpulsation may be lifesaving if inotropic agents alone are ineffective. Such patients often are able to leave the hospital without marked failure if they can be supported acutely.

INFECTIVE ENDOCARDITIS

method of
ADNAN S. DAJANI, M.D.
Wayne State University School of Medicine
Detroit, Michigan

Infective endocarditis is a microbial infection of the endothelial surface (endocardium) of the heart, mainly involving native or prosthetic heart valves. Endocarditis can also involve the mural endocardium, intracardiac patches, and surgically constructed shunts. Infective endarteritis is a similar clinical condition involving arteries, including patent ductus arteriosus, the great vessels, aneurysms, and arteriovenous shunts.

Preexisting structural heart disease or defect is commonly present in patients who develop infective endocarditis. Endocarditis develops on injured endothelium and on damaged or abnormal heart valves where blood-borne adherent organisms lodge. Endothelial injury occurs from turbulent blood flow (e.g., valvular regurgitation or stenosis, congenital heart lesions) or from direct trauma (e.g., indwelling intravascular catheters, cardiovascular surgical procedures). Congenital heart disease and indwelling intravascular catheters and devices are common underlying conditions in patients in developed countries. Rheumatic valvular disease remains a major predisposing condition in many developing countries.

Surgical and dental procedures and instrumentation involving mucosal surfaces or contaminated tissues frequently result in transient bacteremia; however, only a limited number of bacterial species commonly cause endocarditis. Transient bacteremia may also occur without any identifiable antecedent event.

ETIOLOGIC AGENTS

Almost any microorganism may cause endocarditis; the great majority of such infections, however, are caused by a limited number of bacterial pathogens (Table 1). Overall, gram-positive cocci are the most common causative organisms, accounting for at least 90% of recoverable agents. Alpha-hemolytic (viridans) streptococci are the most common pathogens, particularly in cases of endocarditis that follow oral or dental procedures. Enterococci may cause endocarditis after gastrointestinal or genitourinary procedures. Groupable beta-hemolytic streptococci, nonenterococcal group D streptococci, and others may also cause endocarditis.

Staphylococci (*Staphylococcus aureus* and coagulase-negative staphylococci) may infect either native or prosthetic valves. Most cases of endocarditis caused by coagulase-negative staphylococci occur in patients with prosthetic valves. Staphylococcal endocarditis that follows corrective cardiovascular surgery usually occurs within 2 months of the surgical procedure.

Fungi (primarily *Candida* and *Aspergillus*), nosoco-

TABLE 1. **Etiologic Agents of Infective Endocarditis**

Organism	Approximate Percentage	
	Native Valve	Prosthetic Valve
STREPTOCOCCI		
Alpha-hemolytic	60	10–30
Enterococci	10	5–10
Pneumococci	1–2	<1
Beta-hemolytic	<1	<1
Others	<1	<1
STAPHYLOCOCCI		
Staphylococcus aureus	25	15–20
Coagulase-negative	<1	20–30
GRAM-NEGATIVE ORGANISMS		
Enterics	<5	<5
Pseudomonas spp.	<5	<5
HACEK*	<5	<1
Neisseria spp.	<1	<1
FUNGI		
Candida spp.	<1	5–10
Others	<1	<1

Haemophilus, Actinobacillus, Cardiobacterium, Eikenella, and *Kingella*

mial gram-negative rods, and other organisms may also cause postoperative endocarditis. Endocarditis that follows intravenous drug abuse can be caused by any of the aforementioned organisms and also by *Pseudomonas* spp. On occasion, *Chlamydia, Rickettsieae,* and viruses also cause endocarditis.

MICROBIOLOGIC ASSESSMENT

Symptoms and signs of infective endocarditis are often nonspecific, and it may be difficult to establish a clinical diagnosis. Endocarditis should be a serious consideration in a patient with an underlying cardiac defect who presents with unexplained fever or deterioration in cardiac function. Multiple blood cultures, both aerobically and anaerobically, should be obtained whenever possible. The author prefers obtaining at least three blood cultures, ideally from different peripheral sites. Repeat blood cultures should be obtained within a few days of starting antimicrobal therapy to document cessation of bacteremia. Also, blood cultures should be repeated once or twice within a few weeks of completion of therapy to detect a possible relapse.

TREATMENT

Selection of one or more appropriate antimicrobial agents is critical for the successful management of infective endocarditis. Preferred regimens include parenteral therapy, prolonged course, bactericidal agents, and synergistic combinations.

Table 2 outlines recommended therapeutic choices for the most common pathogens (gram-positive cocci). Highly penicillin-susceptible streptococci (minimal inhibitory concentrations [MICs] < 0.1 µg per mL) include most alpha-hemolytic streptococci, *Streptococcus bovis,* pneumococci, and group A streptococci. Aqueous crystalline penicillin G intravenously may be used alone for 4 weeks; shorter courses are not recommended. Gentamicin may be used in conjunction with penicillin; the aminoglycoside is used for the first 2 weeks, and penicillin is used for either 2 or 4 weeks.

Nutritionally deficient and relatively resistant streptococci with MICs between 0.1 and 0.5 µg per mL preferably are treated with a combination of penicillin for 4 weeks plus gentamicin for the first 2 weeks.

The usual penicillin MIC for *Streptococcus faecalis, Streptococcus faecium,* and *Streptococcus durans* is above 2 µg per mL. Because the combination of ampicillin and gentamicin is synergistic against enterococci, treatment of enterococcal endocarditis is best with this combination for 4 to 6 weeks.

Vancomycin is recommended for penicillin-allergic individuals. Treatment of streptococcal endocarditis with organisms that have MICs lower than 0.5 µg per mL can be with vancomycin alone for 4 weeks. Endocarditis caused by enterococci or other resistant streptococci should be treated with a combination of vancomycin and gentamicin for 4 to 6 weeks.

For methicillin-susceptible staphylococcal endocarditis, nafcillin or oxacillin is recommended. These two agents are comparable and preferred to first-generation cephalosporins. In patients who do not respond adequately to conventional therapy, rifampin may be used as a supplemental agent. It can be given orally or intravenously at a dose of 300 mg every 12 hours. Gentamicin may also be added initially for 5 to 7 days, particularly for prosthetic valve infections and in severe cases. Gentamicin should be avoided in instances of severe renal insufficiency. Vancomycin should be used for methicillin-resistant staphylococci (both *S. aureus* and coagulase-negative staphylococci) and in patients allergic to penicillins.

Endocarditis caused by gram-negative bacteria requires individualized antimicrobial regimens. The identity of the specific organism and its susceptibility pattern are essential for selecting an appropriate regimen. In general, gram-negative endocarditis should be treated for at least 6 weeks with parenteral antimicrobics. An extended-spectrum penicillin (e.g., ticarcillin or piperacillin) and a third-generation cephalosporin (e.g., cefotaxime or ceftriaxone), usually in combination with an aminoglycoside, are reasonable

TABLE 2. **Antimicrobial Treatment of Endocarditis Caused by Gram-Positive Cocci***

Organism	Antimicrobial Agent	Individual Dosage	Frequency of Administration	Duration
Streptococci				
	FOR PATIENTS NOT PENICILLIN-ALLERGIC			
Penicillin-susceptible (MIC <0.1 μg/mL)	Penicillin G *or*	2 million U	q 4 h	4 weeks
	Penicillin G and gentamicin	2 million U 1 mg/kg (max. 80 mg)	q 4 h q 8 h	2–4 weeks 2 weeks
Relatively resistant to penicillin (MIC >0.1–0.5 μg/mL)	Penicillin G and gentamicin	2 million U 1 mg/kg (max. 80 mg)	q 4 h q 8 h	4 weeks 2 weeks
Enterococci or other resistant streptococci (MIC >0.5 μg/mL)	Ampicillin and gentamicin	2 gm 1 mg/kg (max. 80 mg)	q 4 h q 8 h	4–6 weeks 4–6 weeks
	FOR PENICILLIN-ALLERGIC PATIENTS			
(MICs <0.5 μg/mL)	Vancomycin	30 mg (max. 2 gm)	q 6 h	4 weeks
(MICs >0.5 μg/mL)	Vancomycin and gentamicin	30 mg (max. 2 gm) 1 mg/kg (max. 80 mg)	q 6 h q 8 h	4–6 weeks 4–6 weeks
Staphylococci				
Methicillin susceptible	Nafcillin or oxacillin ± Rifampin ± Gentamicin	2 gm 300 mg (PO or IV) 1 mg/kg (max. 80 mg)	q 4 h q 12 h q 8 h	6 weeks 6 weeks 5–7 days
Methicillin resistant (including coagulase-negative staphylococci)	Vancomycin ± Rifampin ± Gentamicin	30 mg (max. 2 gm) 300 mg (PO or IV) 1 mg/kg (max. 80 mg)	q 6 h q 12 h q 8 h	6 weeks 6 weeks 2 weeks

Abbreviations: MIC = minimal inhibitory concentration; max. = maximum; PO = orally; IV = intravenously.
*See text for further details.

initial choices until the identity of the organism and its susceptibility pattern become available.

The prognosis in fungal endocarditis is poor, with high mortality and morbidity rates. Antifungal agents alone are usually inadequate; surgical intervention is often necessary. Amphotericin B is currently the agent of choice. A test dose of 0.1 mg per kg (maximum, 1 mg) is initially given, followed in 6 hours by 0.25 mg per kg. If this is well tolerated, the dose is increased by 0.25 mg per kg per day until the maintenance dose of 1 mg per kg per day is reached. A more rapid increase can be used in extremely ill patients. The minimal duration of therapy should be 6 to 8 weeks. Renal function and serum potassium concentrations should be carefully monitored. The therapeutic advantage of supplementing amphotericin B therapy with either 5-fluorocytosine (Ancobon) or rifampin has not been documented in clinical trials. Surgery is probably best performed after about 10 days of amphotericin B therapy.

Culture-negative endocarditis occurs in 5 to 15% of patients. Negative cultures may be due to previous antimicrobial therapy, fastidious or unusual organisms (fungi, *Rickettsieae, Chlamydia,* viruses, nutritionally deficient streptococci, *Brucella,* anaerobes), or right-sided endocarditis. The microbiology laboratory should be alerted to the possibility of these unusual pathogens, and serologic tests may be used to establish a diagnosis. Empirical therapy should be started with a peni-

cillinase-resistant penicillin plus an aminoglycoside. If response is adequate within the first week of therapy, the outcome is usually good. Duration of therapy should be for 6 weeks. Patients who remain febrile after 1 week of starting empirical therapy should be investigated thoroughly and treated on an individual basis.

SURGICAL THERAPY

Surgical intervention has become an important adjunct to medical therapy in the treatment of many cases of infective endocarditis. Excision of the infected tissue (vegetation) alone may be sufficient in some cases. In many patients with right-sided endocarditis, total tricuspid valvulectomy can be performed. For left-sided endocarditis, valve replacement is necessary. The decision for surgical intervention and the timing of such intervention must be individualized. Usual indications for surgery are (1) refractory congestive heart failure secondary to valvular malfunction, (2) uncontrolled infection despite appropriate antimicrobial therapy, (3) significant valvular obstruction, (4) demonstration of a large vegetation, (5) recurrent major emboli or a single major embolus, (6) most cases of fungal endocarditis, (7) most cases of prosthetic valve endocarditis, and (8) local suppurative complications.

PREVENTION

Infective endocarditis is associated with high rates of morbidity and mortality, and any meas-

TABLE 3. **Conditions for Which Prophylaxis Is Indicated**

Prosthetic heart valves and conduits*
Previous episode of infective endocarditis*
Systemic-pulmonary arterial communications
   Surgically constructed shunts*
   Unligated patent ductus arteriosus
Ventricular septal defects, isolated or associated with other heart defects
Left-sided valvular disease, congenital or acquired (includes mitral valve prolapse with regurgitation)
Hypertrophic cardiomyopathy
Most other congenital heart defects

*Patients at high risk for endocarditis.

ure that can prevent the disease is desirable. Endocarditis can be prevented by either repairing the underlying cardiac defect or reducing the likelihood of bacteremia in patients at risk.

Prophylactic antibiotics are recommended for individuals who are at risk to develop endocarditis (Table 3) when they undergo procedures that may induce bacteremia with organisms likely to cause endocarditis. Recommended prophylaxis regimens are based primarily on in vitro studies, clinical experiences, and experimental animal models. There are no adequate controlled clinical trials to validate the efficacy of such prophylaxis. Furthermore, endocarditis may occur despite appropriate antimicrobial prophylaxis.

In general, dental or surgical procedures that induce bleeding from the gingiva or from the mucosal surfaces of the oral, respiratory, gastrointestinal, and genitourinary tracts require prophylaxis. Such procedures include tooth extraction, professional dental cleaning, gum surgery, tonsillectomy and adenoidectomy, bronchoscopy with rigid bronchoscope, esophageal dilatation, cystoscopy, and urethral catheterization or urinary tract surgery if urinary tract infection is present. Prophylaxis is most effective when given perioperatively and in doses to ensure adequate serum concentrations during and shortly after a particular procedure.

Alpha-hemolytic streptococci are the most common cause of endocarditis that follows dental, oral, or upper respiratory tract procedures. Prophylaxis after such procedures should be directed specifically against these organisms, which are generally susceptible to penicillin, ampicillin, or amoxicillin (Table 4). The standard general prophylaxis regimen is recommended even in patients who are at high risk to develop endocarditis (see Table 3). On occasion, some physicians prefer a more stringent prophylactic regimen for these high-risk patients: ampicillin (2 gm) plus gentamicin (1.5 mg per kg; maximum, 80 mg) to be given intramuscularly or intravenously 30

TABLE 4. **Recommended Prophylaxis for Dental, Oral, or Upper Respiratory Tract Procedures**

Situation	Agent	Regimen
Standard general prophylaxis	Amoxicillin	3 gm PO 1 h before procedure, then 1.5 gm in 6 h
Unable to take oral medications	Ampicillin	2 gm IV or IM ½ h before procedure, then 1 gm in 6 h
Penicillin-allergic	Erythromycin*	1 gm PO 2 h before procedure, then 0.5 gm in 6 h
	or	
	Clindamycin	300 mg PO 1 h before procedure, then 150 mg in 6 h
Penicillin-allergic and unable to take oral medications	Clindamycin	300 mg IV ½ h before procedure, then 150 mg in 6 h

Abbreviations: PO = orally; IV = intravenous; IM = intramuscularly.
*Ethylsuccinate or stearate.
Modified from American Heart Association recommendations.

minutes before a procedure, to be repeated 8 hours after the initial dose. Penicillin-allergic patients who are at high risk may receive vancomycin (1 gm intravenously over 1 hour starting 1 hour before the procedure).

Bacterial endocarditis that follows genitourinary or gastrointestinal tract surgery or instrumentation is caused primarily by enterococci. Gram-negative bacilli may induce bacteremia after such procedures; however, endocarditis is

TABLE 5. **Recommended Prophylaxis for Genitourinary or Gastrointestinal Tract Procedures**

Situation	Agent	Regimen
Standard general prophylaxis	Ampicillin	2 gm IV or IM ½ h before procedure, then same dose in 6 h
	plus	
	Gentamicin	80 mg IV or IM ½ h before procedure, then same dose in 6 h
Penicillin-allergic	Vancomycin	1 gm IV over 1 h starting 1 h before procedure, then may repeat same dose in 8 h
	plus	
	Gentamicin	80 mg IV or IM 1 h before procedure, then may repeat same dose in 8 h
Low-risk	Amoxicillin	3 gm PO 1 h before procedure, then 1.5 gm in 6 h

Abbreviations: IV = intravenously; IM = intramuscularly; PO = orally.
Modified from American Heart Association recommendations.

rarely caused by these organisms. Prophylaxis is therefore directed primarily against enterococci (Table 5).

There are special situations in which the aforementioned recommendations may not apply. Surgical procedures through infected tissues require antimicrobial therapy directed against the most likely pathogen. Individuals who are receiving penicillin prophylaxis for prevention of recurrences of rheumatic fever may have alpha-hemolytic streptococci in their oral cavities that are relatively resistant to penicillins. In such cases, an agent other than amoxicillin (e.g., erythromycin or clindamycin) should be selected for endocarditis prophylaxis. Finally, prophylaxis is recommended for patients who undergo open heart surgery, but such prophylaxis should be aimed primarily against staphylococci. A first-generation cephalosporin or vancomycin is a reasonable choice and should be used only perioperatively and for a short duration.

HYPERTENSION

method of
HENRY R. BLACK, M.D.
*Rush–Presbyterian–St. Luke's Medical Center
Chicago, Illinois*

The latest (1988–1991) National Health and Nutrition Examination Survey (NHANES III) has estimated that 50 million Americans have hypertension. Although this figure is somewhat less than the 58 million suggested by NHANES II compiled in 1976–1980, high blood pressure (BP) remains the most common reason people in the United States see a physician and the risk factor that contributes the most to cardiovascular disease (CVD) morbidity and mortality.

The physician who treats hypertensives must decide how to classify and evaluate the patient with high BP and then how best to treat that individual. The reason we treat hypertension is clear. It is not simply to reduce BP but rather to reduce the morbidity and mortality associated with hypertension. Numerous well-controlled, long-term clinical trials have proved that antihypertensive therapy reduces death, especially from CVD, and prevents or delays the onset of cerebrovascular events, coronary artery disease (CAD), congestive heart failure (CHF), and aortic dissection. The data on whether renal functional decline and renal failure are prevented by treatment of hypertension are still incomplete. Recently the benefits of treatment of diastolic hypertension have been extended to the elderly regardless of age and to those older than 60 years of age with isolated systolic hypertension (ISH, ≥160/<90 mmHg).

The choices for antihypertensive therapy are vast, varying from lifestyle modifications to one or several of the more than 60 drugs and 20 fixed drug combinations

available (1993 *Physician's Desk Reference*). The problem for the practicing clinician is to choose which of these modalities is most appropriate for each individual patient. Hypertensives are a heterogeneous group. They are young or old, of different ethnic backgrounds, affluent or uninsured, and working or retired. Many are asymptomatic and otherwise healthy, whereas some are severely affected by the complications of high BP and related conditions. No one therapeutic solution works for all.

CLASSIFICATION

The Fifth Report of the Joint National Committee on the Detection, Evaluation and Treatment of Hypertension (JNC-V), published in 1993, proposed a new classification system for hypertension (Table 1). The committee thought that a new system was necessary because earlier reports (JNC I–IV) failed in two important ways. First, they did not take into account systolic blood pressure (SBP). We have known for decades that the levels of SBP correlated better with the complications of hypertension than did the levels of diastolic blood pressure (DBP), especially at levels considered "borderline" for SBP and definitely elevated for DBP. The recently published 12-year follow-up of the screenees in the Multiple Risk Factor Intervention Trial dramatically emphasized this point. CAD was equally likely to occur at SBP levels of 150 mmHg (previously called borderline ISH if DBP was <90 mmHg) and DBP levels of 98 mmHg (definite mild high BP) and at SBP of 170 mmHg (ISH) and DBP of 112 mmHg (moderate high BP). An SBP of only 130 to 139 mmHg doubled cardiovascular risk compared with less than 110 mmHg, whereas DBP needed to rise from between 70 and 74 mmHg to between 95 and 99 mmHg for cardiovascular risk to increase twofold. Second, the earlier classification system called those with DBP levels between 90 and 104 mmHg "mild" hypertensives. This designation implies that such a condition is benign and need not be taken seriously. We now know that 60% of the incremental risk of death and disability attributable to high BP occurs in patients with "mild" hypertension.

There was a third problem with earlier classifications, which was not completely rectified by JNC-V. There is no question that hypertensives with demonstrable target organ damage (TOD) (CAD, CHF, left

TABLE 1. **Classification of Blood Pressure for Adults Aged 18 Years and Older**

Category	Systolic, mmHg		Diastolic, mmHg
Normal	<130		<85
High normal	130–139		85–89
Hypertension			
Stage 1	140–159	*or*	90–99
Stage 2	160–179	*or*	100–109
Stage 3	180–209	*or*	110–119
Stage 4	≥210	*or*	≥120

Adapted from National High Blood Pressure Education Program Working Group report on primary prevention of hypertension. Arch Intern Med 153:186, 1993. Copyright 1993, American Medical Association.

ventricular hypertrophy [LVH]) renal insufficiency, hypertensive retinopathy, other cardiovascular risk factors (dyslipidemias, cigarette smoking, central obesity, and positive family history of premature CVD in particular) or co-morbid conditions, especially diabetes mellitus (DM), are at greater risk for cardiovascular events at all levels of BP than those not affected by these conditions. The more of these factors present, the higher the risk becomes, and the incremental effect is multiplicative rather than simply additive. It would be preferable to amend the stage based on BP by the letters A, for those without TOD, other risk factors, or co-morbidity, and B, when one or more of those conditions were present. The staging system is meant to provide a guide to prognosis and should distinguish those at greater risk from those whose BP level is not likely to be as much of a problem. A different classification for men and women is not necessary because the risks of a particular level of BP are essentially the same when other risk factors are taken into account, and different definitions of high BP are not necessary for adults of differing ages. For children younger than 18 years of age, we continue to use the 90th and 95th percentile by age to define hypertension.

EVALUATION

The evaluation of the hypertensive patient is directed at answering four questions:

1. What is the appropriate classification of the patient's hypertension?
2. Are there other risk factors or co-morbid conditions present?
3. Is there TOD?
4. Is there an identifiable (secondary) cause for hypertension in that patient?

In most patients, these questions can be answered without resorting to extensive laboratory testing or prolonged periods of observation.

BP should be measured by a properly trained individual using a well-functioning and properly calibrated sphygmomanometer, when the patient is in a somewhat or completely relaxed condition, usually after at least 5 minutes of rest. The measurements should be done in both arms at the first visit, and if the SBP readings differ by more than 10 mmHg, the arm with the higher readings should be noted and always used thereafter. Measurements should be made supine and standing to check for postural hypotension (a drop in SBP of >20 mmHg on assuming the upright position). Sitting BP should also be recorded and can be used thereafter unless the patient complains of symptoms suggesting reduced cerebral perfusion when standing. At least two and probably three readings should be taken, with the second two averaged and used as the BP for that visit. The patient should not be diagnosed as hypertensive until elevated readings are found after

three visits, each separated by at least a week. Patients with BP levels that would classify them as having Stage 3 or 4 hypertension may need to be considered hypertensive sooner and action taken. Those whose readings fluctuate greatly, especially if some readings are normal, may need additional observation and further measurements before the diagnosis of hypertension is definitely established. Some of these so-called labile hypertensives as well as patients who are hypertensive in the office but normotensive elsewhere ("white coat hypertensives") may be candidates for home BP measurements or for 24-hour ambulatory BP monitoring, to determine whether they are really hypertensive.

A complete history and physical examination should be done, directed at looking for TOD, other risk factors, co-morbid conditions, and features suggesting secondary hypertension. Only a few simple and inexpensive laboratory tests should be ordered in all hypertensive patients. These include tests looking for secondary hypertension (serum potassium, urinalysis, serum creatinine), other risk factors (lipid profile, including high-density lipoprotein [HDL] cholesterol and triglycerides [TG] because abnormalities of these components are common in hypertensives, and fasting glucose because hypertension, glucose intolerance, and Type II DM occur so often together, especially in obese individuals), and TOD (an electrocardiogram [ECG] or perhaps "limited" echocardiogram to determine if LVH is present). Although the ECG has long been the recommended way to determine whether a hypertensive patient has LVH, an ECG is not a sensitive test even with significant LVH, and recently it has been shown also to have poor specificity in African Americans. Other tests, such as a complete blood count and serum uric acid and calcium level determinations, are useful because they may discover important and treatable asymptomatic disease or because they may provide guidance in the choice of drug therapy.

If the history, physical examination, or the results of the routine laboratory studies suggest a secondary cause for the patient's hypertension, additional evaluation is often indicated. Some would argue that further testing for remediable hypertension would not be appropriate unless the patient would be a candidate for specific, often surgical, therapy should the disease be found. The pharmacologic approach to treating secondary forms of hypertension, however, is often also different from what is successful for primary (essential) hypertension, and so the clinician should attempt to diagnose these specific conditions if the risks of the testing are justifiably low.

TREATMENT

Lifestyle Modifications

Once the diagnosis of hypertension has been established, treatment should be instituted for all patients, although many do not need pharmacologic therapy at the start. Lifestyle modifications, the term now used for nondrug therapy, is an appropriate starting point in every patient. This type of treatment alone may be adequate in Stage 1 or 2 hypertensives if it reduces BP to goal level and if no TOD is present after a careful search. Whether the evaluation should include a limited echocardiogram is debatable. Although lifestyle modifications can lead to regression of an increased left ventricular mass, patients with LVH are at increased risk for CVD and thus warrant closer evaluation and follow-up should drug therapy not be prescribed.

A large number of lifestyle modifications have been evaluated as sole or adjunctive therapy for hypertension (Table 2). Of these, weight loss has consistently proved to be the most effective at lowering BP when compared with other nonpharmacologic strategies. The amount of weight loss necessary to lower BP need not be substantial. Several recently completed large, randomized, and properly controlled trials have reduced weight an average of 10 pounds (approximately 5% of total body weight) and maintained it over several years. BP was lowered in clinically significant amounts. Sodium restriction to approximately 100 mEq per day (2.3 grams of sodium or 6 grams of salt) also reduces BP, although not as much as weight loss, and may be effective only in sodium-sensitive individuals (the obese, elderly, African Americans, and non–insulin-dependent diabetics). Aerobic exercise and the reduction of excessive alcohol intake in those who drink four or more usual-sized drinks per day are also effective lifestyle modifications for treating hypertension, although usually not as good as weight loss or sodium restriction. Cigarette smoking should be stopped, not because BP will go down but because smoking is a powerful cardiovascular risk factor. Smokers as a group actually have a lower BP and tend to be less obese than nonsmokers, but neither of these factors should be used as an excuse for continuing to smoke.

Supplementing electrolytes, such as potassium, magnesium, or calcium, may be beneficial for a variety of reasons (vascular protection or osteoporosis, for example), but none of these treatments have been conclusively proved to lower BP and should not be recommended as specific antihypertensive therapy. Modification of macronutrients, such as increasing the intake of fiber and complex carbohydrates or fish oil or reducing saturated fat or protein, do not appear reliably to reduce BP, although these dietary modifications may also have other beneficial effects. Neither onion nor garlic, as food or in extract form, appears to lower BP. Finally, stress reduction makes patients feel better but cannot be counted on to reduce BP in most patients.

It is often not appreciated that lifestyle modifications are not necessarily inexpensive. Most successful programs used trained nutritionists who met with patients frequently, both individually and in groups. Furthermore, long-term adherence to substantive lifestyle changes is usually more difficult for most patients to do than it is to remember to take a pill or pills every day. Although lifestyle modifications are safe and some are quite effective, the data we have about the benefits of treating hypertension have come from studies using pharmacologic therapy. In fact, in the only long-term study available of the efficacy of lifestyle modifications (weight loss, sodium restriction, exercise, and alcohol reduction) compared with the combination of lifestyle modification and drugs (the Treatment of Mild Hypertension Study, TOMHS), combination therapy reduced BP and clinical events better than lifestyle modifications alone.

All patients should be instructed in how to lower BP without drugs. In those with uncomplicated (Stage 1A or 2A) hypertension, no other treatment may be needed if goal BP reduction (<140 mmHg systolic and <90 mmHg diastolic) is achieved and maintained. The clinician must be patient and give measures to alter lifestyle an adequate trial, perhaps as long as 6 months, before relegating them to simply an adjunctive role. In some instances, hypertensive patients may be able to avoid drug therapy completely, and many can delay the time when potentially dangerous and often expensive pharmacologic treatment is needed.

Once lifestyle modifications have been given an

TABLE 2. **Lifestyle Modifications**

Nutritional
  Weight loss
  Sodium (as chloride) reduction
  Potassium supplementation
  Calcium supplementation
  Magnesium supplementation
  Alteration in macronutrients
    Fish oil supplementation
    Fiber supplementation
    Protein reduction
  Garlic and onion supplementation
  Alcohol reduction
Isotonic exercise
Stress reduction
  Relaxation
  Biofeedback—generalized and specific

adequate trial and have failed to control BP or prevent TOD from developing, or if the initial level of BP is too high or the degree of TOD too extensive, drug therapy is indicated.

Pharmacologic Therapy

The proper selection of an antihypertensive regimen is one of the more frequent and difficult decisions that physicians regularly need to make. Happily we have a multitude of effective agents that reduce high BP and its associated complications.

There are a number of ways to classify antihypertensive therapy. Most prefer to divide the drugs first into those effective orally and useful for long-term treatment and those that work parenterally and are indicated only for the treatment of a hypertensive crisis. Both classes are then further divided by their primary pharmacologic action. A partial list is shown in Tables 3 and 4 along with the usual starting doses and dosing frequency for adults younger than age 60 and for adolescents. In patients older than age 60, the starting dose should be halved. For young children, in whom a secondary cause of hypertension has been carefully excluded, drug therapy has not been well studied and should be given only if lifestyle modifications have failed. Most agents useful in adults are safe and effective in children, with appropriate adjustment in dose.

The choice of the drug with which to begin therapy is of primary importance because approximately half of all patients respond and tolerate most of our rational options. If we choose wisely, our first choice will work and be the drug our patient remains on for the usually indefinite duration of therapy. So we must select a regimen that is affordable and interferes as little as possible with a patient's lifestyle and economic constraints. Because we have so many effective options, we must understand each patient's needs and plan treatment accordingly. In the author's view, there are nine factors we should consider when picking initial treatment and when adding to or altering it should our first choice fail (Table 5).

Efficacy

Because the objective of antihypertensive therapy is to reduce morbidity and mortality, JNC-V has properly distinguished between the drugs that have and have not been shown to reduce clinically measurable events and death in properly designed and conducted long-term clinical trials (Table 6). In addition to these clinical end points, there are a large variety of other end points, so-called surrogate end points, which may be altered by treatment. Therapy that affects parameters in a direction likely to be beneficial should, but does not necessarily, favorably affect clinical end points. To date, only thiazide diuretics, beta-adrenoreceptor blockers, alpha methyldopa, reserpine, hydralazine, and guanethidine have been used as therapy in clinical trials shown to reduce the complications of high BP. Only two of the classes, thiazide diuretics and beta-adrenoreceptor blockers, are reliably effective and well tolerated as monotherapy. Both are appropriate options with which to start antihypertensive treatment, and both have been recommended as initial therapy by JNC-V.

Other classes of drugs, especially angiotensin-converting enzyme (ACE) inhibitors and calcium entry blockers (CEBs), which were recommended as initial therapy by JNC-IV, and peripheral alpha$_1$ blockers and combined alpha and beta blockers, have been widely used. They reduce BP and surrogate end points in a substantial percentage of patients and do so as monotherapy without excessive adverse reactions or side effects. Drugs in these classes are appropriate choices for initial treatment of hypertension and were also recommended as such by JNC-V. These four classes of antihypertensives, however, have not yet been evaluated in long-term trials and have not as yet been shown to prevent clinical end points. Therefore thiazide diuretics and beta-adrenoreceptor blockers were considered by JNC-V to be the *preferred* choices for initial treatment. The others are appropriate alternatives if the physician has a reason not to select one of the preferred agents.

Adverse Reactions and Side Effects

There are two primary types of adverse reactions or side effects that occur with antihypertensive therapy, clinical and biochemical (Table 7). Clinical side effects are directly evident to the patient and often require stopping or reducing the dose of the supposedly offending agent. Biochemical side effects may lead to clinical side effects (hypokalemia from thiazide diuretics, for example, may be responsible for palpitations, nocturia, or muscle weakness), but usually biochemical abnormalities from antihypertensive therapy bother the physician more than the patient. The drugs recommended for initial therapy and monotherapy generally have a low incidence of clinical side effects, at doses that lower BP effectively when used alone. The biochemical side effects of these six classes of agents, however, are quite different. The drugs not recommended as initial therapy are either ineffective alone or substantially less well tolerated than those selected.

The importance of biochemical side effects is primarily that they may aggravate other risk fac-

TABLE 3. **Antihypertensives for Long-Term Treatment**

	Usual Starting Dose (in mg per pill or portion of pill)	Usual Maximum Dose (in mg per total daily dose)	Dosing Frequency (doses per day)
Diuretics			
Thiazides and related diuretics			
Hydrochlorothiazide	12.5–25	25–50	1–2
Chlorthalidone	12.5–25	25	1
Indapamide	2.5	5	1
Loop active diuretics			2
Furosemide	20	320–480	
Potassium-sparing diuretics			
Amiloride	5	20	1
Triamterene	37.5	150	1–2
Sympatholytics			
Beta-adrenoreceptor blockers without intrinsic sympathomimetic activity*			
Atenolol	25–50	100	1–2
Metoprolol	50	200	1–2
Nadolol	20	240	1
Propranolol	40	240–480	2
Beta-adrenoreceptor blockers with intrinsic sympathomimetic activity			
Acebutolol†	200	1200	1–2
Pindolol	10	60	2
Peripheral alpha$_1$-adrenoreceptor blockers			
Doxazosin	1	16	1
Prazosin	1	20	2
Terazosin	1	20	1
Alpha- and beta-adrenoreceptor blocker			
Labetalol	200	1200	2
Centrally acting alpha$_2$ agonists			
Alphamethyldopa	500	2000	2
Clonidine‡	0.1	1–2	2
Peripherally acting			
Reserpine	0.1	25	1
Guanethidine	10	100	1
Angiotensin-Converting Enzyme Inhibitors			
Benazepril	10	40	1
Captopril	25	150	2
Enalapril	2.5–5	40	1–2
Fosinopril	10	40	1
Lisinopril	5–10	40	1–2
Quinapril	10	40–80	1
Ramipril	1.25	20	1
Nondihydropyridines§			
Diltiazem	30	360–480	3–4
Verapamil	40	480	2–3
Dihydropyridines			
Amlodipine	5	10	1
Felodipine	5	20	1
Isradipine	2.5	10	2
Nicardipine‖	20	120	3
Nifedipine‖	10	120	3
Direct Vasodilators			
Hydralazine	10	300	2–4
Minoxidil	5	40	0.1

Selected Fixed-Dose Combinations

Hydrochlorothiazide/triamterene
Hydrochlorothiazide/amiloride
Hydrochlorothiazide/atenolol, nadolol
Hydrochlorothiazide/captopril, enalapril, or lisinopril
Hydrochlorothiazide/prazosin
Chlorthalidone/clonidine

*Long-acting formulations of propranolol and metoprolol are available. Atenolol and metoprolol are cardioselective and block beta$_1$ receptors more than beta$_2$ receptors.

†Acebutolol is cardioselective.

‡Clonidine is also available as a patch, which is effective for a week.

§Both agents are available in once or twice per day preparation and are marketed by more than one company. There may be differences in bioavailability and price, but there appear to be few differences in efficacy or side effects.

‖Nifedipine is available in a once-daily preparation, and nicardipine is available in a twice-a-day preparation.

Adapted from National High Blood Pressure Education Program Working Group report on primary prevention of hypertension. Arch Intern Med *153*:186, 1993. Copyright 1993, American Medical Association.

TABLE 4. **Antihypertensives for Hypertensive Crises***

	Starting Dose	Route of Administration
Sodium nitroprusside	0.25–10 µg/kg/min	IV infusion
Trimethaphan camsylate	1–4 mg/min	IV infusion
Labetalol	20–80 mg every 10 min, 2 mg/min	IV bolus IV infusion
Nifedipine	10–20 mg, repeat after 30 min	PO

*Multiple other drugs are occasionally useful in special situations or if preferred drug fails or is not tolerated. They include nitroglycerin (acute coronary ischemia); hydralazine (eclampsia); $MgSO_4$ (eclampsia); phentolamine (pheochromocytoma and other catecholamine excess states); clonidine (clonidine withdrawal); and diazoxide, enalaprilat, and parenteral alpha methyldopa.

IV = intravenous.

Adapted from National High Blood Pressure Education Program Working Group report on primary prevention of hypertension. Arch Intern Med *153*:186, 1993. Copyright 1993, American Medical Association.

tors, such as dyslipidemias, or increase the rate of clinical deterioration of a co-morbid condition, such as DM. Whether the minor and often short-term effects on total cholesterol, HDL-cholesterol, or TG from thiazide diuretics and beta-adrenoreceptor blockers are responsible for an increase in CAD remains to be proved. Whether hypokalemia from thiazide diuretics causes sudden death is unclear, and whether the glucose intolerance resulting from beta-adrenoreceptor blockers and thiazide diuretics has precipitated DM sooner or in patients who would otherwise not have become diabetic is by no means established. Although it is not certain that biochemical adverse reactions are clinically important, the author often treats a patient with dyslipidemia or DM with an alternative agent, as long as BP can be reduced successfully.

With the exception of ACE inhibitors, the frequency of clinical side effects tends to increase with increasing doses. Patients who develop an

TABLE 5. **Factors in the Choice of Antihypertensive Therapy**

Efficacy
   Clinical end points
   Surrogate end points
Safety
   Clinical side effects
   Biochemical side effects
Co-morbidity and other risk factors
Special populations
Dosage schedule
Drug interactions
Cost
Mechanism of action of the drug
Pathophysiology of the patient's hypertension

TABLE 6. **End Points for Antihypertensive Therapy**

Clinical End Points
Mortality from all causes
Cardiovascular mortality
Coronary artery disease
Cerebrovascular disease
Congestive heart failure
Progressive renal insufficiency and end-stage renal disease
Peripheral vascular disease
Aortic dissection
Progression to Stages 3 and 4 hypertension
Hypertensive crises

Surrogate End Points
Cardiac
   Left ventricular hypertrophy
   Systolic dysfunction
   Diastolic dysfunction
Renal
   Proteinuria
   Decline in glomerular filtration rate
Vascular
   Atherosclerosis
   Blood pressure
Metabolic
   Potassium
   Magnesium
   Uric acid
   Total cholesterol
   LDL cholesterol
   HDL cholesterol
   Triglycerides
   Insulin resistance
   Fibrinogen

LDL = low-density lipoprotein; HDL = high-density lipoprotein.

adverse reaction on high dose but who did well on a lower dose can often continue to be given that drug or a related compound if necessary. The primary problems with ACE inhibitors, cough and angioedema, tend to occur in a somewhat idiosyncratic fashion and are likely to occur with all drugs of this class and often at low doses. Thus reducing the dose or changing to a different ACE inhibitor is rarely helpful. Because other clinical side effects are unusual, ACE inhibitors can and should be increased to the maximum recommended dose before they are abandoned.

Co-Morbidity and Other Risk Factors

The presence of other risk factors and active clinical problems may exert a profound influence on the initial and subsequent choices for antihypertensive therapy. The appreciation that the drugs we prescribe to reduce BP can either improve or adversely effect other conditions provides the strongest argument for doing a thorough and careful evaluation before beginning therapy and for treating each patient with a regimen tailored to his or her individual needs.

TABLE 7. **Selected Important Adverse Reactions**

	Clinical	Biochemical
Diuretics		
Thiazides	Weakness	Hypokalemia
	Sexual dysfunction	Hyponatremia
	Diabetes mellitus	Hypomagnesemia
	Gout	Hyperglycemia
		Hypertriglyceridemia
		Hypercholesterolemia
		Hyperuricemia
		Hypercalcemia
		Reduction in HDL cholesterol
Loop active agents	Volume depletion	Same as thiazides except for hypercalcemia
Potassium-sparing agents	Gynecomastia and breast tenderness	Hyperkalemia (all)
	Sexual dysfunction	
	Menstrual irregularities (spironolactone only)	
Sympatholytics		
Beta-adrenoreceptor blockers	Fatigue	Hypertriglyceridemia
	Bronchospasm	Reduction in HDL cholesterol
	Intermittent claudication	Hyperglycemia
	Bradycardia and heart block	
	Systolic dysfunction	
	Sleep disturbances	
	Diabetes mellitus	
Peripheral alpha$_1$-adrenoreceptor blockers	Syncope	
	Orthostatic hypotension	
	Headache	
Alpha-, beta-adrenoreceptor blockers	Syncope	
	Orthostatic hypotension	
	Headache	
Central alpha$_2$ agonists	Sedation	
	Dry mouth	
	Orthostatic hypotension	
	Fatigue	
	Rebound hypertension	
	Liver toxicity (alpha methyldopa)	
	Hemolytic anemia (alpha methyldopa)	
	Rash (clonidine patch)	
Peripherally acting sympatholytics	Orthostatic hypotension	
	Retrograde ejaculation (guanethidine)	
	Lethargy	
	Depression (reserpine)	
	Dizziness (reserpine)	
	Dyspepsia	
Angiotensin-converting Enzyme Inhibitors	Cough	Hyperkalemia
	Angioedema	
	Renal failure	
Calcium Entry Blockers		
Nondihydropyridines	Bradycardia	
	Heart block	
	Constipation (verapamil)	
	Headache (diltiazem)	
Dihydropyridines	Headache	
	Dizziness	
	Edema	
	Palpitations	
Direct Vasodilators	Palpitations	
	Edema	
	Headache	
	Hirsuitism (minoxidil)	

HDL = high-density lipoproteins.
Adapted from National High Blood Pressure Education Program Working Group report on primary prevention of hypertension. Arch Intern Med *153*:186, 1993. Copyright 1993, American Medical Association.

DYSLIPIDEMIAS

Patients with high BP and lipid abnormalities probably should not be treated with drugs that may worsen their particular dyslipidemia. This is an important consideration because nearly one-half of all hypertensive patients also have an abnormal lipid profile. Although it has not yet been possible to prove that the small changes in serum lipids caused by some antihypertensives are harmful, it is certainly prudent to choose an equally effective drug that is lipid neutral or select one that may even improve the lipid profile in such patients. Peripheral alpha$_1$-adrenoreceptor blockers, for example, reduce total cholesterol and low-density lipoprotein (LDL) cholesterol approximately 8 to 10%, reduce TG 15%, and raise HDL cholesterol 10 to 15%. Although these alterations are modest, the overall cardiovascular risk of a patient whose lipids are changed in this fashion is clearly improved. ACE inhibitors do not affect serum lipids, although some studies have shown favorable effects similar to those seen with peripheral alpha$_1$-adrenoreceptor blockers. CEBs of both the dihydropyridine and nondihydropyridine type are lipid neutral.

Thiazide diuretics in large doses (50 to 100 mg of hydrochlorothiazide or chlorthalidone) at least temporarily raise total cholesterol and LDL-cholesterol (approximately 5 to 10%) and may lower HDL-cholesterol (2 to 4%). TGs are increased 15 to 30%. The effects with smaller doses are considerably less. Beta-adrenoreceptor blockers without intrinsic sympathomimetic activity (ISA) lower HDL-cholesterol (10%) and raise TG (20%). Total cholesterol and LDL-cholesterol are unchanged. Beta-adrenoreceptor blockers with ISA and combined alpha- and beta-adrenoreceptor blockers are lipid neutral. Other sympatholytics tend not to affect the lipid profile, whereas direct vasodilators, such as hydralazine, improve it (raise HDL-cholesterol and lower total cholesterol, LDL-cholesterol, and TG), even in combination with thiazide diuretics.

GLUCOSE AND INSULIN

Antihypertensive drugs also affect glucose metabolism and do so in a fashion similar to lipids. Peripheral alpha$_1$-blockers and captopril improve peripheral insulin sensitivity, whereas other ACE inhibitors and CEBs are neutral. Both thiazide diuretics and beta-adrenoreceptor blockers without ISA adversely affect insulin sensitivity and may worsen glucose tolerance. Occasionally these classes of drugs precipitate DM. There are little data on other classes of antihypertensives. Although, as stated in JNC-V, no classes of antihypertensives are contraindicated in diabetics, the author strongly believes that agents with adverse effects on glucose and insulin should be avoided in the diabetic or in a patient thought to be at high risk of developing diabetes.

LEFT VENTRICULAR HYPERTROPHY

LVH is a common consequence of hypertension and a robust independent risk factor for CVD and mortality. Although comparative data are still incomplete, it appears that all classes of antihypertensives, with the possible exception of direct vasodilators, reduce left ventricular mass if BP is lowered. In two prospective and well-controlled studies, TOMHS and a recently completed Veterans Administration trial, representatives from most commonly used classes of antihypertensives reduced left ventricular mass equally well. Thiazide diuretics were the most effective.

SYSTOLIC AND DIASTOLIC DYSFUNCTION AND CONGESTIVE HEART FAILURE

In patients with CHF caused by systolic dysfunction, diuretics, ACE inhibitors, and possibly amlodipine would be good choices for antihypertensive therapy. For patients with significant diastolic dysfunction, nondihydropyridine CEBs, especially verapamil, or beta-adrenoreceptor blockers provide a distinct advantage.

OTHER CONDITIONS

The presence of certain other co-morbid conditions also influences the selection of an antihypertensive agent. Patients with bronchospasm should not, for example, be treated with beta-adrenoreceptor blockers, and patients with gout should not receive thiazide diuretics. Patients with renal insufficiency usually need loop active diuretics to achieve the often necessary reduction in plasma volume. Preliminary studies have suggested that ACE inhibitors and perhaps nondihydropyridine CEBs may slow the decline in glomerular filtration rate in patients with renal insufficiency and so may be the best choice for these patients. Before using an ACE inhibitor, bilateral renal artery stenosis or stenosis of an artery to a single kidney should be excluded, or else serum creatinine and serum potassium levels must be watched extremely closely. Hypertensives with angina pectoris should be given beta-adrenoreceptor blockers or a CEB, and those who have sustained a myocardial infarction benefit from a beta-adrenoreceptor blocker without ISA and possibly should continue on an ACE inhibitor if one was given at the appropriate time after the acute myocardial infarction. Smokers may not respond to nonselective beta-adrenoreceptor blockers (propranolol, nadolol [Corgard], pindolol [Visken]), and obese patients may do especially well with thiazide diuretics because their hypertension is often salt sensitive. Patients who wish to exercise are often unable to perform at maximum capacity if treated with beta-adrenoreceptor blockers without ISA. Patients with migraine headaches are helped by beta-adrenoreceptor blockers, whereas those with peripheral vascular disease or cardiac conduction defects may be harmed by these drugs. Nondihydropyridine CEBs should also be avoided in patients with cardiac conduction defects.

SPECIAL POPULATIONS

The choice of antihypertensive therapy is often influenced by whether a patient is a member of a particular demographic group or by the severity or lack of responsiveness of a patient's hypertension or by whether the patient is pregnant.

Demographic Considerations

African Americans and Other Ethnic Minorities

Some classes of antihypertensives reduce BP more or less effectively in certain ethnic groups. Thiazide diuretics, for example, are more effective in African Americans than they are in whites, whereas ACE inhibitors and beta-adrenoreceptor blockers work better in whites than in African Americans. Peripheral alpha$_1$-adrenoreceptor blockers, combined alpha- and beta-adrenoreceptor blockers, and CEBs are as effective in African Americans as they are in whites. What is often forgotten is that many African Americans respond quite well to ACE inhibitors and beta-adrenoreceptor blockers, and those drugs can and should be used if other factors would favor selecting them rather than thiazide diuretics or CEBs. The response rate in Hispanics to particular antihypertensives is usually intermediate between that seen in whites and African Americans. Asians respond as do whites but often require lower doses.

Age

All classes of antihypertensives lower BP effectively in older persons, albeit at lower doses than is necessary in young and middle-aged hypertensives. Certain drugs and classes of drugs, however, should be used cautiously in older patients. These include peripheral alpha$_1$-adrenoreceptor blockers, dihydropyridine CEBs, and some sympatholytics. These drugs may cause or exacerbate postural hypotension, which is common in the elderly usually owing to baroreceptor dysfunction. Beta-adrenoreceptor blockers and nondihydropyridine CEBs may aggravate subtle or subclinical cardiac contraction abnormalities or precipi-

tate systolic dysfunction and CHF. Verapamil frequently causes constipation and may not be well tolerated in older patients. Some believe that cough from ACE inhibitors is more common in the elderly, especially elderly women, than it is in younger patients.

The treatment of hypertension in adolescents is similar to adults. Less is known about the efficacy of newer agents in young children, and so the therapeutic approach tends to rely on agents that have been available longer.

Gender

There is no evidence of any difference in response to antihypertensives in men and women.

Pregnancy

In pregnant women with pregnancy-induced hypertension, alpha methyldopa and hydralazine have been the mainstays of treatment for decades and remain so. There is some favorable experience with atenolol and nifedipine but little else with other drugs. Diuretics should be used cautiously in the second and third trimester or if preeclampsia is suspected. Pregnant women with essential hypertension can generally stay on what has been successful before pregnancy. ACE inhibitors are contraindicated in pregnancy.

Hypertensive Crises

The proper management of hypertensive crises requires rapid and accurate diagnosis and careful selection of treatment. Hypertensive emergencies are those conditions that require BP to be reduced within minutes. For hypertensive urgencies, the reduction can proceed over hours. For both types of crises, the clinician must seriously avoid excessive BP reduction and try only to prevent acute TOD. The ideal drug with which to treat a hypertensive emergency is one that is effective parenterally, virtually always works, has an almost instant onset, and has a very short duration of action. The drug should be easy to titrate and not cause cerebral or cardiac dysfunction. The ideal drug for a hypertensive urgency would be one that is orally active and almost always effective, but the onset and duration of action can be longer than the drugs used for emergencies. Drugs useful for the urgent treatment of hypertension should also not cause dysfunction of vital organs and ideally should be appropriate choice for long-term therapy, although this feature is not critical. Table 8 lists selected hypertensive crises and appropriate and inappropriate choices for treatment.

TABLE 8. **Hypertensive Crisis Emergencies**

	Drug of Choice	Acceptable Alternatives	Contraindicated
Central nervous system			
Hypertensive encephalopathy	Sodium nitroprusside	Trimethaphan camsylate Labetalol Diazoxide	
Intracranial hemorrhage			
Cerebrovascular accident			
Cardiac			
Acute left ventricular failure	Sodium nitroprusside	Trimethaphan camsylate	Labetalol
Acute coronary ischemia	Nitroglycerin	Labetalol Sodium nitroprusside	
Unstable angina	Nitroglycerin	Labetalol	
Vascular			
Aortic dissection	Trimethaphan camsylate	Sodium nitroprusside and propranolol	Hydralazine
Eclampsia	MgSO$_4$	Hydralazine	
Pheochromocytoma	Phentolamine		Beta-adrenoreceptor blockers
Urgencies			
Stage 3 or 4 hypertension with imminent or mild TOD damage	Nifedipine (oral short-acting preparation)	Captopril Clonidine Labetalol	

TOD = target organ damage.
Adapted from National High Blood Pressure Education Program Working Group report on primary prevention of hypertension. Arch Intern Med *153*:186, 1993. Copyright 1993, American Medical Association.

Refractory Hypertension

A refractory hypertensive is a patient whose BP remains elevated (>140 mmHg SBP or 90 mmHg DBP) on the maximum dose of two or more appropriately chosen antihypertensive drugs. The most common reasons why patients are resistant to treatment are related to either physician or patient behavior. The physician, for example, may not be prescribing the right drugs or may not be giving them in adequate doses. He or she may fail to recognize that a particular patient has secondary hypertension, which often fails to respond well to conventional therapy, or may not appreciate that a patient with renal disease needs a loop active diuretic, whereas a patient with normal renal function responds better to a thiazide. Or the physician may be giving another drug, such as a nonsteroidal anti-inflammatory agent (NSAID), which may interfere with the antihypertensive effect of the drug chosen to reduce BP. Patient-related behavior can also result in apparent unresponsiveness to therapy. In fact, in most studies, medication noncompliance was the most common reason for refractory hypertension. Obese patients may not respond as well to antihypertensive treatment. Also, patients may be ingesting excessive alcohol or using over-the-counter medications, such as sympathomimetic amines or nasal decongestants, which may raise BP or interfere with the action of what would otherwise be a successful regimen. The measurement of BP may not accurately reflect the patient's true status because he or she may have office or "white coat" hypertension. The measurement may be artifactually high because of excessively sclerotic arteries (pseudohypertension), or it may have been done too soon after caffeine or nicotine intake. If otherwise clinically indicated, the physician should search for these problems in any patient who fails to respond to treatment as anticipated. In the event that none of these or other reasons for refractory hypertension are found, additional drugs may be needed, or a higher BP or treatment may have to be accepted.

DOSAGE SCHEDULE

There are two elements of dosage scheduling that need to be considered when prescribing antihypertensive therapy. One is the ability of patients to comply with the regimen, and the other is the need to treat hypertension for all 24 hours of the day and night. Patients are much more likely to take their medications as prescribed if the agent is effective once or, at most, twice a day (see Table 3). The compliance with any therapy falls dramatically once more than three pills per day of any kind are needed, and so all unnecessary elements of a treatment regimen should be stopped. Fixed-dose combinations that provide the right amounts of the desired agents can be used to reduce the number of pills ingested daily.

Recently we have become aware that a more

than expected percentage of myocardial infarctions and ischemic strokes occur in the hours from 6 A.M. to noon or within 1 hour of awakening. One of the possible explanations as to why the early morning hours are particularly risky relates to our understanding of the pattern of BP during a 24-hour period. BP tends to be at its lowest level in both normotensives and hypertensives from midnight to 4 A.M., at which time it rises and peaks near noon. It gradually falls until 2 to 4 A.M. when, coincident with increased secretion of cortisol and catecholamines, BP begins to rise again. Some believe that this rise in BP predisposes to plaque rupture and results in a greater frequency of cardiovascular events. Thus, it is appropriate to select drugs that we are sure will work for 24 hours or to give shorter-acting agents, including those that have a duration of action of 18 to 20 hours (e.g., atenolol or enalapril), twice rather than once per day. Recently the Food and Drug Administration has become much stricter about approving a drug for once-daily use, and so those agents recently released with that designation indeed have a 24-hour duration of action.

DRUG INTERACTIONS

The selection of initial therapy for hypertension must be done with the understanding that perhaps as many as half of the patients treated may not reach goal BP on that agent alone. Certain combinations of antihypertensives are particularly effective, such as thiazide diuretics with beta-adrenoreceptor blockers or with ACE inhibitors. Thiazide diuretics with other sympatholytics or peripheral alpha$_1$-adrenoreceptor blockers are also quite effective, as is the combination of thiazides with hydralazine in the elderly. Dihydropyridines, especially nifedipine, and beta-adrenoreceptor blockers are a useful combination, as are CEBs and ACE inhibitors. There is still some doubt as to whether CEBs and thiazide diuretics are effective in combination, although most recent studies have shown additional BP control when these drugs are used together. The antihypertensive action of all antihypertensives may be reduced by NSAIDS or oral contraceptives, and so both of these classes of drugs should be avoided in hypertensive patients unless absolutely necessary.

COST

Cost considerations are playing an increasingly important role in the pharmacologic management of hypertension. No regimen, no matter how carefully selected and appropriate, will work if the patient cannot afford to buy it. Thiazide diuretics and beta adrenoreceptors, for which generic preparations are available, tend to be the least expensive options for initial therapy, although reserpine is the least expensive antihypertensive available. There are generic preparations of prazosin and some CEBs, but none of the less expensive formulations are effective once or twice a day. On the average, CEBs are the most expensive, followed by ACE inhibitors; peripheral alpha$_1$-adrenoreceptor blockers; nongeneric beta-adrenoreceptor blockers including labetalol; and finally sympatholytics, direct vasodilators, and thiazide diuretics. Many of the newly marketed ACE inhibitors and CEBs are less expensive than older brands, and many cost the same for all dose levels.

The "cost" of antihypertensive therapy, however, is more than just the price of the drug. There are pharmacy fees to fill the prescription, which are often the same regardless of the cost of the drug. There are office visits to check the response to treatment, and there are blood tests to evaluate if any adverse biochemical events have occurred. And there is the vast potential for excessive cost should one choice of treatment not be as effective as another at preventing the complications of hypertension. All of this should be considered when we try to estimate the real cost of therapy.

Unfortunately, the information we need to compare the long-term benefits and costs of our many options is not yet available, and it is not known whether using more expensive drugs, which have theoretical advantages over older and cheaper agents, would actually save us money in the end, even though they are more costly at the point of service.

MECHANISM OF ACTION OF THE DRUG

Pathophysiology of the Patient's Hypertension

If we really understood exactly how drugs worked and precisely why an individual patient was hypertensive and if we could easily and safely ascertain that information, treating high BP would be simple. Attempts to profile patients, either biochemically using plasma renin activity (PRA), for example, or hemodynamically, are intellectually appealing but would be too expensive to do in all patients and would not always provide the necessarily definitive information we need to predict the response to therapy in a particular patient. Although it is true that African Americans and the elderly tend, on the average, to have low or suppressed PRA, many do not, and many who do will respond to drugs, such as beta-adrenoreceptor blockers or ACE inhibitors, which are less effective, on the average, in hypertensives with low PRA. Although it is true that hypertensive elderly tend to have a modestly decreased plasma volume compared with younger hypertensives, thiazide diuretics are not only effective but also very well tolerated in older patients. Although it is true that ACE inhibitors usually suppress the endocrine renin-angiotensin system, the antihypertensive effect is still evident even as plasma angiotensin II levels return to pretreatment levels. This is compelling evidence that there is either a tissue site of action for these drugs or that other mechanisms must play a role in how they lower BP. All effective antihypertensives, not only CEBs, reduce intracellular calcium concentrations, which may be the primary pathophysiologic abnormality in essential hypertension.

Despite the fact that we cannot precisely determine the mechanism of action of our drugs or why a particular patient has high BP, our empirical approach to management has dramatically reduced the rate of stroke and CAD in the United States since 1965–1970, when we began treating hypertension aggressively. Our approach has paid great dividends.

SUMMARY AND RECOMMENDATIONS

Although there are numerous options and many sources for error, the successful pharmacologic treatment of a hypertensive need not be too complicated, nor should it be oversimplified. Once the diagnosis has been established and the routine evaluation and any more complex testing believed to be necessary are completed, lifestyle modifications should be initiated and given adequate time and encouragement to work, unless clinical considerations (Stage 3 or 4 hypertension, serious TOD, or co-morbidity) mandate immediate drug therapy. Drug treatment is appropriate in all hypertensives who do not reach goal BP after an adequate trial of nondrug therapy.

The following steps are recommended in choosing a regimen and altering it until satisfactory control is achieved:

1. Deal first with cost. If the patient is unable to afford any but the least expensive drugs, price becomes the primary issue.

2. Ascertain whether or not other risk factors or co-morbidity is present. For patients who have DM or glucose intolerance or dyslipidemias, agents that do not adversely affect these parameters become preferable. For patients with gout or asthma or with systolic or diastolic dysfunction, the options are limited accordingly.

3. Find out what clinical adverse reactions the patient would find most troublesome, and avoid agents likely to cause these problems. For some patients, fatigue or sexual dysfunction would be intolerable, whereas others would not find such side effects particularly disturbing.

4. Consider demographic issues and make the selection with a higher probability of success should options be available.

5. Start with the lowest effective dose and plan to see the patient within 2 to 4 weeks unless the severity of the hypertension or other problems warrants follow-up sooner. Do appropriate biochemical monitoring when necessary.

6. Increase the dose if goal BP has not been reached, even when there has been only a minimal response to the first dose. Do not increase the first dose or any dose prematurely. Give each dose adequate time to be fully effective. If intolerable side effects have occurred and are likely to be drug related, stop that agent and switch to your next alternative.

7. Continue the process of dose titration and monitoring until the maximum recommended dose has been reached. Stopping before full dose leads to the situation in which the patient is treated with multiple agents at subtherapeutic doses when only one or two is necessary.

8. Should the first choice fail to reduce the patient's BP to the predetermined goal, the author prefers to add a drug of a different class. Alternatively an appropriate fixed-dose combination can be used if one is available that provides the dose of initial choice and the proper starting dose of the next selection. Others recommend stopping the first drug and switching to another agent of a different class, so-called sequential monotherapy.

9. The author proceeds to titrate the second drug the same as the first, once again up to full dose with appropriate monitoring, before doing anything further.

10. Should the two-drug combination fail, a specific cause for refractory hypertension should be sought.

11. Should none be evident, the author would add a third agent and continue the same as with the first two choices. One of these agents should always be a diuretic appropriate to the patient's level of renal function.

12. Plan to see the patient at least every 3 months to be sure control is sustained.

13. If control is achieved for 18 to 24 months, consider slowly reducing the doses of one or more components of the regimen, especially if the patient has made substantial adjustments in lifestyle.

14. Plan to do a re-evaluation similar to the

initial evaluation annually and more frequently for certain parameters.

15. Reinforce the need for compliance and always question carefully about adverse reactions.

Although some patients do not completely respond to this approach even with all of the many effective treatment options available, most come under or close to control. Those who do can anticipate substantial long-term benefit with an extended life expectancy and a much reduced risk of strokes, CAD, CHF, and probably renal failure and dementia as well. Although treating high BP can be costly and at times difficult, the rewards make it worthwhile.

ACUTE MYOCARDIAL INFARCTION

method of
MARK A. THOMPSON, M.D., and
ALLAN M. ROSS, M.D.
George Washington University Medical Center
Washington, D.C.

Myocardial infarction is a disease of the twentieth century. Little was known about this entity before the clinical presentation of myocardial infarction was described by Herrick in 1912. With the increasing incidence of coronary artery disease came an increasing array of diagnostic tools, beginning with the electrocardiogram (ECG) in the 1920s and continuing with the clinical use of cardiac enzymes in the 1950s. As recently as the early 1960s, however, myocardial infarction treatment had varied little from Herrick's time: complete bed rest for several weeks augmented with digoxin and diuretics if there were signs of congestive heart failure (CHF). The development of the cardiac care unit (CCU) in 1962 heralded a new era of cardiac care: a newfound ability to decrease myocardial infarction mortality by recognizing and treating potentially fatal arrhythmias.

Despite the availability of thrombolytic therapy (streptokinase) as early as 1959, general use did not begin until the early 1980s, after DeWood rekindled the old notion that coronary thrombosis was the major final event in acute myocardial infarction, a concept that had been common in Herrick's time but had lost some following in the 1970s when pathology reports failed to identify thrombus consistently in autopsy cases of myocardial infarction. When Rentrop in 1981 confirmed DeWood's observation of coronary thrombosis in the vast majority of patients with acute myocardial infarction by immediate catheterization and showed effective lysis by intracoronary administration of streptokinase, the thrombolytic era officially began.

Now in the 1990s, reperfusion therapy is considered standard care for acute myocardial infarction. Although the in-hospital mortality rate for acute myocardial infarction in the pre-CCU era had been 30 to 40%, this rate fell to 15 to 20% following standard critical care monitoring and has since fallen to 7 to 10% since the institution of thrombolytic therapy. Currently there is a parallel interest in acute catheterization and angioplasty as the primary method of treatment of myocardial infarction. The standard use of direct angioplasty is not, however, likely to supersede the use of thrombolytic therapy, given the limited availability and logistical difficulties of this procedure.

Economic concerns will be a large priority in the next decade, as the health care costs in the United States continue to escalate and the yearly cost of treating patients with myocardial infarction surpasses the $100 billion mark. New therapies will be judged not only on efficacy, but also on economic efficiency. It will prove to be a complicated but rewarding time for those involved in the care of patients with myocardial infarction.

ATHEROGENESIS AND PATHOPHYSIOLOGY OF ACUTE MYOCARDIAL INFARCTION

The cause of atherogenesis was presciently theorized by Virchow in the late 1800s to be intimal damage, inflammation, and thrombosis. Others refined these ideas until a unified theory emerged centered on a "response to injury" tenet, which best fits our understanding of the pathogenesis of atherosclerosis.

Superficial atherosclerotic "fatty" streaks may appear in childhood and represent the first gross changes in the disease. These early atherosclerotic lesions progress to elevated fibrous plaques by the third and fourth decade, then progress to complex, eccentric, ulcerated, and hemorrhagic plaques by the fifth and sixth decade, culminating in plaque rupture or intraplaque hemorrhage and coronary occlusion.

Endothelial injury provides the basis for atherogenesis. The fragile endothelium is damaged or denuded by hypertension, elevated low-density lipoprotein (LDL) cholesterol, diabetes, smoking, and other factors. Simple denudation exposes vascular collagen, which triggers circulating platelet adhesion and aggregation and a cascade of growth factor release, including thromboxane A_2, prostacyclin, platelet-derived growth factor (PDGF), a potent stimulator of smooth muscle cell proliferation, and other factors. Smooth muscle cell and monocyte proliferation, along with lipid accumulation under the influence of these growth factors, leads to the atherosclerotic lesions already described.

Coronary atherosclerosis is responsible for 97% of all myocardial infarctions, the remainder being due to coronary vasospasm and other rare entities. The actual precipitating event in acute myocardial infarction is thrombus formation at the site of an atherosclerotic plaque, either because of plaque rupture with a large amount of collagen exposed and platelet adhesion, or because of subintimal plaque hemorrhage with anatomic change in the plaque morphology, which leads to decreased blood flow, stasis, and thrombus formation. Coronary arteriography performed during acute myocardial infarction reveals visible thrombus formation in the vast majority of cases. Those without visible thrombus frequently have partially occlusive eccentric or ruptured plaque, and the presumption is occluding thrombus has spontaneously lysed. The eccentricity and complexity of an atherosclerotic lesion is directly related to its incidence of plaque rupture or hemorrhage and hence thrombus formation and coronary occlusion.

The pathophysiology of unstable angina and "non-Q" or nontransmural infarcts is identical to that of transmural infarct with one major exception: duration and completeness of occlusion. Patients with unstable angina who have coronary angioscopy, or direct visualization of the coronary artery lumen, have visible thrombus in every case. Alternating thrombus formation and lysis occur in these patients at such a rate that the magnitude of ischemia is not long enough to produce necrosis or infarction. Similarly, angioscopy of patients with nontransmural infarcts shows the same thrombus formation at the site of underlying atherosclerotic lesions, with the time of total thrombotic occlusion being greater than that of unstable angina but less than transmural infarction, such that only subendocardial necrosis results.

The knowledge of this ubiquitous presence of coronary thrombosis, with its ebb and flow of formation and lysis, is extremely important when considered in the arena of treatment of all acute ischemic syndromes. The use of antiplatelet drugs (aspirin), anticoagulants (heparin, hirudin), and thrombolytics (recombinant tissue plasminogen activator [rt-PA], streptokinase) and the timing of these agents become more understandable when considered in the context of the underlying pathophysiology.

Sudden death as a result of acute myocardial infarction is almost always due to ventricular fibrillation (VF) induced by the electrical instability of the ischemic/infarction zone. VF is most common either at the immediate onset of coronary occlusion or at the time of coronary reperfusion (reperfusion arrhythmia). Given the known oscillation of coronary occlusion/reperfusion even in acute myocardial infarction, it is ironic that sudden death as a result of myocardial infarction can occur at a time when blood flow *returns* to the infarcted region following a period of occlusion.

Finally, the episodic nature of coronary occlusion in acute myocardial infarction helps explain why reperfusion strategies of thrombolytic therapy or mechanical reperfusion employed fairly late in the course of acute myocardial infarction show long-term benefit. In experimental animals, total ligation of a coronary artery results in complete and irreversible damage in less than 2 to 3 hours. Clinical trials, however, have shown benefit with reperfusion strategies even if treatment is delayed 12 hours or more after onset. Those patients who benefit likely have transient total occlusion with periods of partial or complete flow restitution even during the infarct process, which "protects" the myocardium from irreversible damage until much later than the 2 to 3 hours shown experimentally.

Risk Factors

Factors that increase the risk of coronary artery disease are well established. A family history of coronary artery disease, a prolonged and heavy smoking history, the presence of diabetes or hypertension, and an elevated LDL cholesterol level each lead to an increased risk of coronary artery disease. Male gender, older

than 50, type A personality, and estrogen lack in women also increase this risk.

Hemostasis and Thrombosis

Any educated, logical approach to the management of a clinical condition that has thrombosis as its primary inciting force requires at least a basic understanding of the pathophysiology of bleeding and clotting. It has been said that the definition of thrombosis is simply hemostasis in the wrong place at the wrong time. Although a thorough review of hematology is not the goal here, a simplified explanation helps to clarify the reasoning behind different therapeutic treatment strategies.

Hemostasis (or thrombosis) is based on two hematologic systems: platelets and the coagulation system. Unactivated platelets adhere immediately to subendothelium, which has been exposed because of damage or loss to the endothelial cell layer. Platelets then release chemotactic factors, which bring leukocytes and more platelets to the damaged area. This event is termed "primary hemostasis" and is the first line of defense against hemorrhage after vascular injury.

The secondary hemostatic system, or coagulation system, is simultaneously activated during vascular injury. Thrombin is formed through the interaction of several plasma factors, which in turn converts fibrinogen to fibrin. Fibrin strands then combine with and strengthen the platelet plug. These two systems work in concert to provide adequate hemostasis, or inappropriate thrombosis, following vascular injury.

Conversely, clot lysis (fibrinolysis) is regulated by an equally sophisticated system centered on plasmin. Plasmin is an enzyme that effectively digests fibrin clots and is formed by the activation of its precursor, plasminogen, which is conveniently incorporated into fibrin clots. The main endogenous activators of plasminogen are urokinase and t-PA. An active inhibitor of this process is plasminogen activator inhibitor (PAI-1).

Both the hemostatic systems and the fibrinolytic system are fully activated during acute myocardial infarction. Interference of one system over another with hematologically active substances can drastically tip the scales in favor of either thrombosis or hemorrhage.

Aspirin inhibits platelets irreversibly by inhibiting cyclooxygenase, which in turn inhibits the production of thromboxane A_2, a potent platelet activator. 7E3 is a monoclonal antibody that blocks the GPIIB-IIIA platelet receptor, effectively preventing platelet aggregation. Heparin binds and activates antithrombin III, preventing thrombin formation. Hirudin is an irreversible thrombin inhibitor. Warfarin (Coumadin) is a vitamin K antagonist that blocks the production of thrombin. Each of these agents can have a drastic effect on the hematologic processes that are so integral to acute myocardial infarction.

The pathophysiology of acute myocardial infarction is a complex interaction of physical and humoral factors centering on acute coronary artery thrombosis occurring in a damaged atherosclerotic lesion.

DIAGNOSIS

The classic patient description of acute myocardial infarction is that of crushing substernal chest pressure or pain with radiation to the neck and left arm associated with nausea, vomiting, diaphoresis, and a sensation of impending doom, lasting more than 30 minutes and less than 12 hours. Unfortunately, this classic description is found only in a small minority of patients. It is difficult to rely on patient history to make a definitive diagnosis of acute myocardial infarction. Most emergency room visits for chest pain are noncardiac, and even most cardiac causes are not acute myocardial infarction. Thus the history should be used as a rapid screening process to categorize patients with possible acute myocardial infarction so additional appropriate testing can be obtained quickly.

The Multicenter Chest Pain Study in 1991 identified features that predicted the presence of acute myocardial infarction in more than 6000 patients evaluated for chest pain in the emergency room. The only features found to be associated with a higher probability of acute myocardial infarction were symptom duration of greater than 1 hour but less than 48 hours, previous history of angina or acute myocardial infarction, age older than 40, and radiation of pain to the neck or left arm. Features associated with a lower probability of acute myocardial infarction were pain radiation to back, abdomen, or legs; stabbing character of pain; and reproduction of pain with palpation.

In a related study by Pozen in 1984, six characteristics were found to be "critical" to the diagnosis of acute myocardial infarction or unstable angina: (1) pain in chest or left arm; (2) pressure, pain, or discomfort in chest as "most important" symptom; (3) history of acute myocardial infarction; (4) history of nitroglycerin prescription; (5) ST elevation or depression greater than 1 mm on ECG; and (6) T waves inverted greater than 1 mm or peaked on ECG.

Two trials have underscored the difficulty of diagnosing acute myocardial infarction by history alone. The MITI trial of prehospital thrombolytic therapy involved 2472 patients with possible acute myocardial infarction by history; only 18% actually developed acute myocardial infarction. The thrombolysis early in acute heart attack trial (TEAHAT) of prehospital thrombolysis randomized patients with the cardiologist-determined clinical diagnosis of acute myocardial infarction; only 59% had confirmed acute myocardial infarction.

When taking the history, several critical noncardiac diagnoses must be considered and excluded, both because of the morbidity of the condition if not recognized and because of the iatrogenic morbidity of incorrect acute myocardial infarction therapy in a patient with another condition. For instance, aortic dissection is suggested by the description of a ripping or tearing sensation in the back in the presence of hypertension. Pulmonary embolus is highlighted by pleuritic pain and severe dyspnea. Pericarditis is characterized by positional and pleuritic pain.

Because of the standard use of thrombolytic therapy in acute myocardial infarction, a standard part of the history taking should include investigation of contraindications to thrombolytic therapy. Any history of stroke, severe hypertension, recent surgery, or gastrointestinal bleeding should be carefully elicited.

Despite the lack of sensitivity and specificity of the clinical history in acute myocardial infarction, it still remains the cornerstone of diagnosis. It is the history on which all further diagnostic studies are based. No patient with any symptoms suggestive of this diagnosis should fail to have an ECG and additional studies if indicated. Conversely, an extensive history is unnecessary and often delays appropriate therapy; therefore a directed history should take less than 10 minutes to obtain.

Physical Examination

Similar to the history, a brief, directed physical examination should be obtained in all patients with suspected acute myocardial infarction. The physical examination may be normal in the presence of acute myocardial infarction, but abnormalities are frequently seen in those at greatest risk. Abnormal vital signs of tachycardia, bradycardia, hypotension, or tachypnea suggest a large myocardial infarction with increased morbidity. The presence of rales or ventricular gallop suggests congestive heart failure and also predicts greater morbidity. Cardiac murmurs, although unusual in this setting, suggest acute cardiac decompensation because of mitral regurgitation or ventricular septal rupture.

The physical examination should also be directed toward likely alternative diagnoses. The presence of a pericardial friction rub suggests pericarditis, whereas unilateral absence of breath sounds suggests pneumothorax. Differential blood pressures in each arm, absent lower extremity pulses, or the murmur of aortic insufficiency should suggest aortic dissection.

Finally, as with the history, the physical examination should be directed toward contraindications of thrombolytic therapy. Normal neurologic status, the absence of active bleeding, and the absence of severe hypertension should be documented before administering thrombolytic therapy.

Laboratory Tests

The standard 12-lead ECG is the most important and most definitive test in the diagnosis of acute myocardial infarction. The ECG is sensitive; 70 to 90% of patients with more than 1 mm ST elevation in two contiguous leads and consistent history have acute myocardial infarction. Unfortunately, it is less specific, and as many as 60% of patients with acute myocardial infarction do not have these classic ECG changes.

The location of ST elevation on the ECG predicts the culprit coronary artery occlusion. Right coronary artery occlusion most commonly causes inferior ST elevation, left anterior descending artery occlusion causes anterior or apical ST elevation, and circumflex artery occlusion causes lateral or inferior ST elevation.

If an initial ECG is nondiagnostic in a patient with suspected acute myocardial infarction, the ECG should be repeated a brief time later. Episodic ST elevations are common in the early hours of acute myocardial infarction and may be present on a follow-up ECG even if absent initially. The need for frequent repeat ECG tracings in equivocal diagnostic cases cannot be overemphasized.

Cardiac muscle cells are rich in creatine kinase MB (CK-MB) isoenzyme. CK-MB is currently the best confirmatory blood test in the diagnosis of acute myocardial infarction. The detection of elevated levels of CK-MB in the bloodstream is dependent on two processes. Local acidosis can cause the myocardial cell sarcolemma to become permeable to intracellular macromolecules. Second, frank cellular membrane disruption can lead to release of all intracellular components into the bloodstream. Because of this, CK-MB levels may be normal in the early hours of myocardial infarction, before frank cellular necrosis has occurred. CK-MB plasma levels peak 10 to 18 hours after coronary occlusion. An earlier and greater magnitude peak can be seen following coronary reperfusion. Abnormal CK-MB elevation can occur in the absence of diagnostic ECG evidence of acute myocardial infarction and can retrospectively confirm the diagnosis. Similarly, absence of significant CK-MB elevations when drawn serially excludes acute myocardial infarction even in the presence of an abnormal ECG. New rapid assays for CK-MB allow efficient assessment of patients with prolonged chest pain in the emergency room setting. A normal CK-MB level in a patient with 8 hours of continuous chest pain effectively rules out acute myocardial infarction in this setting. Finally, antimyosin antibodies may provide an even earlier method of enzymatic confirmation of acute myocardial infarction.

The majority of patients with acute myocardial infarction need no more than an appropriate history and confirming ECG to begin appropriate therapy. Occasionally, however, other methods may be necessary if both ECG and history are nondiagnostic. An echocardiogram can pick up wall motion abnormalities, but it has two major drawbacks when used in the diagnosis of acute myocardial infarction. It cannot distinguish a new defect from an old defect and hence is frequently not helpful in patients with a prior infarct. In addition, it is not sensitive, and a patient with a small acute myocardial infarction may not have a significant wall motion abnormality on echocardiography.

Rest thallium imaging can also effectively identify areas of infarction, although it cannot identify between old and new infarcts, and it also cannot distinguish between infarcted and ischemic tissue.

The general algorithm given in Figure 1 can help confirm the diagnosis of acute myocardial infarction in situations when the history and ECG are nondiagnostic.

1. If the clinical history is suggestive of acute myocardial infarction and the ECG is diagnostic, sublingual nitroglycerin is given, and the ECG is repeated in 5 minutes. If it remains diagnostic, even if symptoms improve, acute myocardial infarction is confirmed.

2. If the history is suggestive and ECG is diagnostic but nitrates bring immediate relief of symptoms and the ECG returns to normal, vasospasm is confirmed, and the patient can be observed closely in a CCU setting and semielective catheterization scheduled.

3. If the history is suggestive, the clinical status is stable, but the ECG is nondiagnostic, we obtain a bedside echocardiogram and repeat the ECG several times. If the clinical status is unstable, we perform immediate cardiac catheterization.

4. If the history is not suggestive but the ECG appears diagnostic, we carefully assess for alternative diagnoses, obtain a bedside echocardiogram, and treat as acute myocardial infarction only if no other diagnosis seems possible and echocardiography reveals a wall motion abnormality. We alternatively perform immediate catheterization in these patients.

5. If neither the history nor ECG are diagnostic, acute myocardial infarction is unlikely, and alternative diagnoses should be entertained.

Prehospital Diagnosis

In the past 10 years, a new push has been made to diagnose and treat acute myocardial infarction as early as possible. Many major thrombolytic trials have confirmed the survival advantage of very early thrombolytic treatment (within

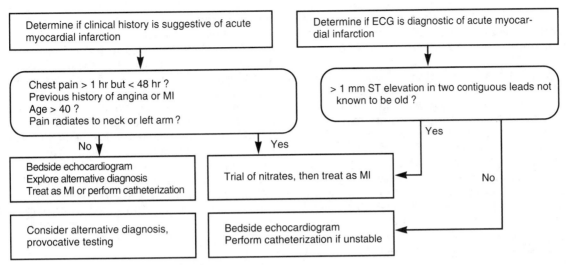

Figure 1. Diagnosis of acute myocardial infarction.

the first hour of symptoms) in these patients. Unfortunately, significant time delays of patient recognition, transfer to the hospital, emergency room assessment, and definitive diagnosis have made the average time from onset of symptoms to treatment several hours. Trials have been performed assessing the efficacy of diagnosis and treatment of acute myocardial infarction before arrival at the hospital.

In general, the difficulties of prehospital diagnosis and treatment of acute myocardial infarction are the risk of misdiagnosis and inappropriate therapy with thrombolytics in patients without acute myocardial infarction. These risks must be compared with the survival advantage of early thrombolytic therapy in those with myocardial infarction.

The GREAT study in 1992 was a Scottish randomized, double-blind, placebo-controlled trial of at-home treatment of acute myocardial infarction with the thrombolytic agent APSAC (anisoylated plasminogen streptokinase activator complex) (Eminase) compared with standard emergency room treatment. Three hundred patients with the clinical diagnosis of acute myocardial infarction were seen at home by general practitioners and given the first vial of study drug, either APSAC or placebo. The second vial was then administered on hospital arrival. Home treatment resulted in a 50% decrease in mortality (8 vs. 16%), and most patients were treated within 2 hours after the onset of symptoms. The lag time between home treatment and hospital treatment was 130 minutes. More than 75% of patients in the trial had confirmed acute myocardial infarction.

In the United States, physician-staffed ambulances are uncommon. The accepted method of

prehospital acute myocardial infarction diagnosis here is likely to be fax transmission of the ECG to an emergency room physician. This has been shown not only to be a safe means of initiating prehospital thrombolytic therapy, but also to facilitate emergency room triage in patients who do not receive prehospital thrombolysis. Hospital delay to treatment has been improved by 30 to 60 minutes in patients with the prehospital transmission of a diagnostic ECG.

Prehospital diagnosis of acute myocardial infarction is feasible and accurate and appears to facilitate hospital triage and therapy without delaying the transfer time to the hospital. Prehospital treatment of acute myocardial infarction is also feasible and accurate and appears to be associated with a low risk of adverse events. Further data are necessary, however, to assess the amount of clinical benefit and to determine whether prehospital treatment will become the standard of care.

THROMBOLYTIC THERAPY

The cornerstone of treatment of acute myocardial infarction is thrombolytic therapy. It is an established, effective therapy that limits myocardial necrosis, preserves left ventricular function, and reduces mortality. Not to use thrombolytics or other means of reperfusion in eligible acute myocardial infarction patients is considered substandard medical care.

Despite the excellent data in support of thrombolytic therapy, only 30% or less of patients with acute myocardial infarction currently receive this therapy. Of the remaining 70%, only 20% have true contraindications or equivocal ECG findings. Many clinicians still withhold thrombolytic therapy in older patients and in those seen later in the course of acute myocardial infarction, despite the compelling data to support therapy in these groups.

Every subgroup of patients with acute myocardial infarction benefits from thrombolytic therapy. Patients with inferior wall myocardial infarction, prior bypass surgery, prior myocardial infarction, or left bundle-branch block (LBBB) benefit from thrombolytics. Patients older than age 75, although excluded from many earlier trials, do have a higher complication rate with thrombolytic therapy, but their mortality reduction is so much greater that the overall survival benefit is actually highest in this age group. A patient in the GUSTO trial was over 100 years old and received thrombolytic therapy without complications.

Patients who present more than 6 hours after symptom onset were frequently excluded from early trials, but the recent LATE study unequivocally showed a significant survival advantage of thrombolytic therapy even when given up to 12 hours after the onset of acute myocardial infarction symptoms. This study randomized 5700 patients who presented more than 6 hours after acute myocardial infarction onset to either thrombolytic therapy (rt-PA) or placebo. Those patients who received rt-PA within 12 hours had a significant 27% decrease in mortality compared with placebo.

Contraindications to thrombolytic therapy have become streamlined over the past few years. Former "contraindications" of advanced age, any hypertension, and presentation after more than 6 hours have been abolished. The only current major contraindications to thrombolytic therapy are (1) active internal bleeding, (2) suspected aortic dissection, (3) prolonged or traumatic cardiopulmonary resuscitation, (4) recent head trauma or known intracranial neoplasm, (5) hemorrhagic retinopathy, (6) pregnancy, (7) systolic blood pressure greater than 180 mmHg, (8) history of cerebrovascular disease, and (9) trauma or surgery within 2 weeks that could be a source of rebleeding.

Several well-designed megatrials over the last 10 years have sought to better define the efficacy of thrombolytic therapy. GISSI-I (1986) showed a significant mortality reduction in patients who received streptokinase compared with placebo for acute myocardial infarction (10.7% with streptokinase vs. 13% for controls). The beneficial effect was related to the time to treatment; those treated within 1 hour of the onset of symptoms had the greatest benefit, a 47% reduction in mortality. ISIS-2 (1988) confirmed this in 17,187 patients and found aspirin to have an additive effect on mortality reduction. TIMI-1 in 1985 showed

higher early infarct artery patency with rt-PA than streptokinase, but neither GISSI-2 (1990) nor ISIS-3 (1991) showed any survival benefit of rt-PA over streptokinase. A criticism of those two studies was the lack of routine intravenous heparin, which has been shown to improve the short-term patency rate of rt-PA. The recent GUSTO trial (1993) compared accelerated dosing rt-PA, streptokinase and intravenous heparin, streptokinase and subcutaneous heparin, and a combination of rt-PA and streptokinase in 41,021 patients. rt-PA was found to reduce mortality by 14% more than did streptokinase or the combinations, and this mortality reduction correlated with higher coronary artery reperfusion (patency), as assessed by angiography in the rt-PA group.

A large amount of media and literature attention has been directed toward deciding the "best" thrombolytic agent. Although determining which agent saves the most lives is clearly important, the differences in mortality between agents is an order of magnitude less than the difference between giving and not giving a thrombolytic. It must be emphasized that the most lifesaving decision is whether to administer a thrombolytic agent, not which one. Additionally, time is of the essence in achieving mortality reduction. Several trials have shown a remarkable survival advantage in patients who received any thrombolytic agent within the first hour or two of symptoms.

With that said, there are subtle differences between agents that may influence one's decision. Alteplase, an rt-PA (Activase), is a fibrin-specific recombinant DNA product, now often given in a "front-loaded" fashion, 15 mg intravenous bolus followed by 50 mg over 30 minutes, then 35 mg over 60 minutes (100 mg over 90 minutes). This agent provides a high early patency rate but is relatively short-acting and may be more dependent on adjunctive intravenous heparin to maintain patency. Streptokinase is a nonspecific thrombolytic that costs substantially less per dose than rt-PA and has a longer half-life but achieves a lower early artery patency than rt-PA. In patients who present late, the early artery patency may be much lower than with rt-PA. Streptokinase is given 1.5 million units over 30 to 60 minutes. Because of its longer half-life, however, the reocclusion rate may be lower with this agent. Hypotension and allergic reactions are more common with streptokinase. Because streptokinase produces antibodies that can render repeat doses of streptokinase ineffective or cause an allergic reaction, it should not be repeated in the same patient within 2 years of the initial dose. APSAC is a streptokinase analogue that is given as a 30-mg intravenous bolus over 5 minutes. It is otherwise similar to streptokinase except for its increased cost, and its main advantage is ease in administration.

The most serious complication of thrombolytic therapy is intracranial hemorrhage. This feared complication occurs in only 0.5 to 1.0% of patients but is more common with more aggressive adjunctive anticoagulation, in women, in patients with low body weight or severe hypertension, and in the elderly. There is also evidence to suggest that the frequency of intracerebral hemorrhage is marginally higher in rt-PA–treated than in streptokinase-treated patients.

The overall recommendation for use of thrombolytic therapy is to use it immediately in every patient with the clinical history suggestive of acute myocardial infarction (Table 1) and ST elevation in two contiguous ECG leads, without major contraindications to thrombolytic therapy, who presents within 12 hours of symptom onset. APSAC may be most useful when ease of administration is a high priority. Streptokinase may be most useful if adjunctive anticoagulation with intravenous heparin cannot be carefully controlled or if cost is a major concern. rt-PA may be most useful in patients who present very early or, alternatively, very late in the course of acute myocardial infarction and in those who have previously received streptokinase or APSAC.

CONJUNCTIVE THERAPY

Although thrombolytic administration is the cornerstone of medical treatment for acute myocardial infarction, adjunctive medical therapy is required to achieve the highest complete and sustained artery patency and the lowest mortality. Described next are the accepted adjunctive therapies and future directions in adjunctive therapy.

The role of concomitant heparin in the initial treatment of acute myocardial infarction has become increasingly clear over the last few years. The HART investigators and others have shown that early, effective anticoagulation with heparin maintains rt-PA–induced coronary artery patency much more effectively than aspirin alone. In fact, subgroup analyses have shown that patients with therapeutic heparin administration, as measured by activated partial thromboplastin time (APTT), have an extremely high artery patency approaching 95% following rt-PA administration. The need for routine adjunctive heparin anticoagulation for streptokinase-treated patients is more controversial.

The extent of anticoagulation with heparin varies between individual patients and therefore must be carefully titrated by APTT. In the GUSTO trial, for example, patients received 5000 units of heparin bolus followed by 1000 units per hour constant infusion and titrated every 6 hours to maintain an APTT of 60 to 85 seconds for at least 48 hours.

Although heparin is an effective antithrombin agent and effectively helps maintain coronary artery patency following thrombolysis, it has some potential drawbacks. First, it requires a cofactor, antithrombin III, to exert its antithrombin effects. Second, its anticoagulant effects are quite variable between patients and are somewhat difficult to maintain accurately over time.

Hirudin is a new investigational antithrombin agent, which does not require antithrombin III and is easier to titrate. The preliminary results of TIMI-V, which randomized patients to either heparin or hirudin with rt-PA for acute myocardial infarction, showed a 50% decrease in death or reinfarction and less bleeding complications with hirudin. Hirudin showed less APTT variability over time and was easier to maintain in the therapeutic range. Hirudin may soon replace heparin as standard adjunctive therapy in acute myocardial infarction.

Aspirin is the only adjunctive agent that has unequivocally been shown to reduce mortality alone or in conjunction with thrombolysis in patients with acute myocardial infarction. The ISIS-II study showed that acetylsalicylic acid (ASA) reduced mortality by one-quarter and was just as effective as streptokinase alone in patients with acute myocardial infarction. ASA had an additive effect, however, when administered with streptokinase, and this combination reduced mortality 42% in this study.

TABLE 1. **Thrombolytic Therapy in Acute Myocardial Infarction**

Agent	Dose	Comments
Streptokinase (Streptase) (Kabikinase)	1.5 million U IV over 30–60 min	Thrombolytic agent with lower short-term patency rates than rt-PA but less expensive
APSAC* (Eminase)	30 mg IV bolus over 5 min	Thrombolytic agent related to streptokinase. Advantage is ease of administration
rt-PA† (Activase)	10 mg IV bolus, then 50 mg IV over first h, then 40 mg IV over next 2 h	Standard regimen. High short-term patency but more expensive than other thrombolytics
rt-PA	15 mg IV bolus, then 50 mg IV over 30 min, then 35 mg over 1 h for 100 mg total	"Front loaded" regimen used in GUSTO. Higher early patency rate than standard regimen

*APSAC = anisoylated plasminogen streptokinase activator complex.
†rt-PA = recombinant tissue plasminogen activator.
IV = intravenous.

The first ASA dose is given in a chewable form starting concurrently with thrombolysis and continued once daily for at least 1 month. Although the optimal dose has not been established, it seems reasonable to administer 160 mg per day. In patients allergic to ASA, it may be reasonable to use ticlopidine, a new platelet inhibitor that is commercially available.

New antiplatelet agents being vigorously investigated include 7E3, an antibody to the platelet receptor GPIIA/IIIB, which prevents platelet aggregation, thereby accelerating clot lysis and eliminating reocclusion. Clinical trials are under way to determine if the addition of this agent improves thrombolysis in patients with acute myocardial infarction.

Nitroglycerin has been used for many years in the treatment of acute myocardial infarction. A mortality reduction with nitroglycerin, however, has been shown only in patients who did not receive thrombolytic therapy. The ongoing ISIS-4 and GISSI-3 trials may provide mortality data for nitroglycerin use in the thrombolytic era. Nonetheless, nitrates improve compromised hemodynamic conditions and have platelet inhibitory effects. Recently two small studies have suggested that intravenous nitroglycerin may decrease infarct size in patients given thrombolytic therapy. Because of this suggestive but inconclusive data, we usually administer intravenous nitroglycerin for 24 to 48 hours to patients with acute myocardial infarction, particularly those with hypertension or left ventricular dysfunction.

Several early studies have shown that beta blockade improves survival following acute myocardial infarction. Most of these data, however, were collected in the prethrombolytic era. True mortality reduction has been more difficult to show in patients receiving thrombolytic therapy, but there is suggestive evidence to recommend routine beta blockade in conjunction with thrombolytic therapy. Beta blockade has been shown to reduce the incidence of reinfarction, recurrent angina, and long-term cardiac mortality.

No clinical trials to date have shown an overall beneficial effect of calcium channel blockade on mortality in patients with acute myocardial infarction. Diltiazem has been shown to decrease recurrent infarction and angina following non-Q myocardial infarction, and many clinicians have extrapolated these data to include patients who reperfuse following thrombolytic therapy. It should be emphasized, however, that no clinical trial has confirmed this extrapolation, and routine use of calcium channel blockers in the setting of acute myocardial infarction should be discouraged until such data are available.

Several studies have sought to investigate whether angiotensin-converting enzyme (ACE) inhibitors decrease mortality in acute myocardial infarction, but most involved patients did not receive thrombolytic therapy. The CONSENSUS-II trial randomized 6000 patients to either ACE inhibitor or placebo, but only half had received thrombolytic therapy. There was no difference in mortality at 3 months. The ongoing GISSI-3 and ISIS-4 trials may provide further data. Until then, routine administration of ACE inhibitors is not recommended, although these agents may be helpful in the subsets of patients with large infarcts, heart failure, or hypertension.

Warfarin reduces the incidence of reinfarction, thromboembolic events, CHF, and death following acute myocardial infarction. The risk of major bleeding, however, increases. The benefits therefore are at least partially offset by the morbidity associated with bleeding. The WARIS randomized trial of long-term anticoagulation following myocardial infarction in 1214 patients showed a 25% mortality reduction in patients taking warfarin, but little benefit was seen in patients with prior myocardial infarction or diabetes. Oral anticoagulation should probably be administered only to patients with large anterior infarcts and left ventricular thrombus, patients with left ventricular aneurysm, and patients with markedly diminished residual left ventricular function. Routine administration following acute myocardial infarction is still controversial.

Magnesium salts cause coronary vasodilation, have antiplatelet effects, and have antiarrhythmic properties. Recently the LIMIT-2 study, which randomized 2300 patients to either intravenous magnesium (8 mmol over 5 minutes followed by 65 mmol over 24 hours) or placebo in patients with acute myocardial infarction, showed a significant 24% mortality reduction in those patients receiving magnesium, confirming several smaller studies. The administration of intravenous magnesium as a bolus and constant 24-hour infusion to raise serum magnesium levels to twice-normal values should now be seriously considered in the routine care of patients with acute myocardial infarction.

The routine care of patients with acute myocardial infarction should include thrombolytic therapy in patients without contraindications and adjunctive therapy commonly including heparin, aspirin, nitroglycerin, beta blockers, and magnesium. ACE inhibitors, warfarin, and calcium channel blockers should be considered only on a case-by-case basis.

For patients with acute myocardial infarction who are deemed unsuitable for reperfusion therapy or who have the diagnosis confirmed too late for acute reperfusion therapy, the treatment should consist of medical therapies shown to reduce mortality in the era before routine thrombolytic use. These therapies include the routine use of beta blockers, intravenous nitroglycerin, aspirin, and perhaps ACE inhibitors (Table 2). There will continue to be a role for these agents in the primary treatment of acute myocardial infarction because a significant minority of patients will have some contraindication to acute reperfusion therapy, or will have the diagnosis of acute myocardial infarction made later in the disease process, either because of patient delay or nondiagnostic criteria on hospital presentation.

ROLE OF PERCUTANEOUS TRANSLUMINAL CORONARY ANGIOPLASTY IN ACUTE MYOCARDIAL INFARCTION

Although thrombolytic therapy has been widely accepted in the management of acute myocardial infarction, its limitations include serious bleeding complications, coronary artery patency rates of only approximately 75%, a high rate of reocclusion and recurrent ischemic events, and the relatively limited number of patients who are eligible for treatment.

Because of these drawbacks, several studies have examined the role of percutaneous transluminal coronary angioplasty (PTCA) in the setting of acute myocardial infarction. PTCA has several potential advantages over thrombolytic therapy. The procedure can be performed on patients with contraindications to thrombolytic therapy. PTCA

can be a "rescue" therapy for failed thrombolysis or can be routinely used following thrombolysis to improve residual coronary stenoses.

First, delayed routine PTCA following thrombolytic therapy has no benefit over thrombolysis alone, as definitively shown in the TAMI and TIMI-II trials. Second, TAMI-V showed that rescue PTCA, or PTCA following angiographically proven failed thrombolysis, decreased adverse events, including recurrent ischemia, compared with conservative therapy. Finally, the recent PAMI trial of primary, or direct, angioplasty in myocardial infarction randomized 395 patients with acute myocardial infarction to either routine thrombolytic therapy or immediate PTCA without thrombolysis. In the PTCA subgroup, recurrent ischemic events were reduced by two-thirds, in-hospital mortality was slightly lower, and intracranial bleeding was less than in the thrombolytic subgroup.

With these results, one can consider primary angioplasty an acceptable alternative therapy to thrombolysis in patients with acute myocardial infarction. Whether primary angioplasty becomes an increasingly used mode of therapy in acute myocardial infarction remains to be established by further randomized studies. Logistical considerations and the limited availability of this procedure within 30 to 60 minutes of diagnosis make the routine use of this therapy unfeasible in most hospitals. Primary PTCA is currently recommended in patients with contraindications to

TABLE 2. **Commonly Used Adjunctive Agents in Acute Myocardial Infarction**

Agent	Dose	Comments
Aspirin	160 mg PO at time of initial presentation and every day thereafter	Reduces rethrombosis and recurrent myocardial infarction
Beta blockade (metoprolol)	5 mg IV bolus q 5 min ×3, then 50 mg PO q 6 h for 48 h, then 100 mg PO bid	Contraindicated with hypotension or bradycardia, severe left ventricular dysfunction, atrioventricular block. Hold additional doses if hypotension or bradycardia develops. Especially effective for reflex tachycardia or hypertension
Heparin	5000 U IV bolus followed by 1000 U/h	Begun concomitantly with thrombolytic. Titrate to APTT = 60–85 s. Continue for 24–48 h
Magnesium sulfate	8 mmol IV over 5 min, then 65 mmol over 24 h	Benign therapy shown to reduce mortality. Side effects include flushing and bradycardia
Morphine sulfate	2–5 mg IV every 5–30 min and as needed	Excellent analgesic/anxiolytic. Decreases preload and afterload. Decreases myocardial oxygen demand. May cause hypotension
Nitroglycerin	0.4 mg sublingual followed by 5–10 μg/min IV infusion	Rate can be increased in 10-μg increments to 100 μg/min to control symptoms or to decrease mean blood pressure by 10%
Oxygen	2–4 L/min by nasal cannula	Administered to all patients during initial hours of treatment. Higher flow rates may be necessary in patients with congestive failure or frank hypoxia
Warfarin	10 mg every day for 3 days, then 2.5–5 mg/day	Indicated for severe left ventricular dysfunction to prevent mural thrombus. Titrate to PTT 1.5–2.0 × control

PO = orally; IV = intravenous; APTT = activated partial thromboplastin time; PTT = partial thromboplastin time.

thrombolysis and in patients in cardiogenic shock. Rescue PTCA should be considered in high-risk patients who are thought clinically to have failed thrombolysis. Routine delayed PTCA is not recommended in patients without evidence of recurrent ischemia following acute myocardial infarction.

Logistics make the use of emergent coronary artery bypass graft surgery (CABG) for the treatment of acute myocardial infarction unwieldy. The small subgroup of patients, however, with acute myocardial infarction who are hemodynamically unstable and have coronary anatomy unsuitable for PTCA can be considered for emergent CABG. In addition, patients who develop recurrent ischemia following acute myocardial infarction and have coronary anatomy unsuitable for PTCA should be routinely considered for CABG. The mortality rate for elective CABG following acute myocardial infarction is very low.

SHOCK

Shock, or hypotension in the setting of inadequate end-organ perfusion, is generally divided into two categories in the acute myocardial infarction patient. The first category is that of hypovolemic hypotension. Acute myocardial infarction patients frequently are relatively hypovolemic, and their cardiac output may be compromised without significant left ventricular dysfunction. Treatment with intravenous fluid is both simple and effective and should be initiated in any patient thought to be hypovolemic. The absence of rales, jugular venous distention, or signs of pulmonary congestion in a hypotensive patient with acute myocardial infarction suggests hypovolemia as a cause, and pulmonary artery catheter measurements should be considered in any acute myocardial infarction patient with hypotension. The pulmonary capillary wedge pressure is generally a good indicator of left ventricular filling pressure, and if this value is less than 12 to 18 mmHg, an intravenous fluid bolus should be administered. Only if the filling pressure is above 18 mmHg should the second category of shock be considered, that of cardiogenic shock.

Hypovolemic shock can also be seen in patients with acute right ventricular infarction. Up to one-third of patients with inferior infarcts have right ventricular involvement. Dyspnea and signs of left heart failure are uncommon, but jugular venous distention and hypotension are frequent. ECG may reveal ST elevation in right precordial leads. Pulmonary artery catheterization typically reveals disproportionately high right-sided filling pressures with normal or low left-sided filling pressures and a depressed cardiac output. As in hypovolemia, the treatment of choice is rapid intravascular fluid expansion with normal saline solution up to a measured central venous pressure of 15 to 20 mmHg.

True cardiogenic shock is characterized by persistent hypotension and a poor cardiac index (<1.8) in the presence of adequate left ventricular filling pressures (>18 mmHg) and occurs in 7 to 10% of all patients with acute myocardial infarction. It is generally caused by severe left ventricular dysfunction and occurs with large infarcts with damage to greater than 40% of the left ventricle. Untreated, the condition is deadly, with an in-hospital mortality of 85 to 95%. Initial therapy consists of intraaortic balloon pump placement to increase coronary flow and decrease afterload, which improves cardiac output and peripheral perfusion. Coronary reperfusion, however, is the mainstay of treatment and when achieved acutely with PTCA has been shown in several studies to decrease the short-term mortality to 40 to 50%. Reperfusion with thrombolytic therapy is not routinely recommended in this setting because coronary artery patency is achieved in only a minority of patients.

Other pharmacologic treatments for cardiogenic shock include morphine, dopamine, and dobutamine (Dobutrex). It should be emphasized, however, that this condition is almost invariably fatal without coronary revascularization. Any treatment protocol for cardiogenic shock should include intraaortic balloon pump, cardiac catheterization, and emergent PTCA as the first line of therapy. Patients whose anatomy is not amenable to PTCA should be considered for emergent CABG. Only with coronary revascularization do hemodynamic parameters normalize and mortality improve.

Other causes of cardiogenic shock should be considered in the evaluation of the hypotensive patient with acute myocardial infarction. A loud holosystolic murmur along the left sternal border suggests an acute ventricular septal defect (VSD), which occurs 1 to 7 days after acute myocardial infarction, is more frequent with anterior than inferior myocardial infarction, and is associated with a worse prognosis following inferior myocardial infarction because it frequently involves the posterior left ventricular wall. The diagnosis is confirmed by echocardiogram. Untreated, acute VSD carries a mortality rate of 80 to 90%, and all patients should be considered for emergent surgical repair. An intraaortic balloon pump may temporize an unstable patient while awaiting surgery.

The abrupt onset of heart failure, cardiogenic shock, and a holosystolic apical murmur with radiation to the axilla suggests acute mitral regurgitation owing to papillary muscle rupture. Similar to VSD, papillary muscle rupture usually occurs 1 to 7 days after acute myocardial infarction, is confirmed by echocardiogram, is temporized with intraaortic balloon pump, and carries a high mortality without emergent mitral valve surgery.

Rupture of the left ventricular free wall is a rare complication of acute myocardial infarction. It usually occurs 1 to 7 days after acute myocardial infarction and is more common after the first infarction and with hypertension and after the late administration of thrombolytic therapy. Most patients develop immediate electromechanical dissociation and die rapidly. Approximately 30% develop symptoms of pericardial tamponade with increased venous congestion and decreased cardiac output. If the diagnosis is made promptly, definitive surgical repair can be performed. The remainder form a false aneurysm, which becomes "walled off" by pericardial tissue and may not cause symptoms for long periods. If the condition is recognized, however, confirmation with angiography or echocardiography should be promptly followed by surgical resection because spontaneous rupture is common.

Left ventricular aneurysms occur when a large region of ventricular myocardium becomes permanently dyskinetic after acute myocardial infarction. Although scar formation is expected following a completed acute myocardial infarction, true aneurysms occur in only 7 to 15% of patients. Most occur after anterior acute myocardial infarction, and 35 to 50% develop a mural thrombus owing to stasis of blood in that area. Patients with ventricular aneurysms should be treated with warfarin to prevent thrombus formation and its sequelae of systemic embolic events because embolization is clinically apparent in 5 to 7% of patients with mural thrombi.

As described earlier, a true aneurysm should be distinguished from a false aneurysm. A true aneurysm is formed by the outpouching of myocardial tissue and myocardial scar, and rupture is rare. A false aneurysm is formed by subacute myocardial rupture and formation of a thick-walled pericardial sac, which is continuous with the left ventricular cavity, and rupture is common. Resection of a true left ventricular aneurysm is reserved for patients with refractory arrhythmias, embolic events despite anticoagulation, or refractory heart failure.

ARRHYTHMIAS IN ACUTE MYOCARDIAL INFARCTION

The major decline in the death rate following acute myocardial infarction occurred during the era of arrhythmia recognition and treatment. Although perhaps more emphasis is now placed on coronary reperfusion strategies, arrhythmia recognition and treatment are still a primary part of acute myocardial infarction therapy. Some rhythm abnormality occurs in up to 96% of all patients with acute myocardial infarction. Both bradyarrhythmias and tachyarrhythmias can complicate acute myocardial infarction.

The most common bradyarrhythmia in acute myocardial infarction is sinus bradycardia, seen in 25% of patients, most commonly with inferior infarctions and frequently associated with transient hypotension. The cause is usually increased vagal tone or treatment with beta-adrenergic blockers. Sinus bradycardia rarely requires specific treatment but when associated with hypotension or hypoperfusion should be treated with atropine and, if ineffective, temporary pacing.

Bradycardia owing to atrioventricular (AV) block occurs in 15 to 25% of patients with acute myocardial infarction. First-degree block, characterized by a prolonged PR interval greater than 0.2 second, occurs in 4 to 14% of patients with acute myocardial infarction and requires no therapy. Second-degree block, Mobitz type I (Wenckebach) is characterized by progressive PR interval prolongation followed by a nonconducted P wave, then a normally conducted P wave with a normal PR interval. It occurs in 4 to 10% of patients, most commonly with inferior infarction, generally resolves within 24 to 48 hours, and requires no specific therapy unless the ventricular response is slow enough to produce symptoms. Mobitz type II second-degree heart block, in contrast, usually occurs following anterior acute myocardial infarction, is characterized by nonconducted P waves following a constant PR interval, and is associated with a higher morbidity and progression to complete heart block. Mobitz II block is much less common than Mobitz type I block, occurs below the level of the AV node, and is a manifestation of significant myocardial necrosis. For this reason, prophylactic temporary pacing should be instituted in patients with anterior myocardial infarction and Mobitz II block, and if the block is still evident after 1 week, permanent pacing should be instituted.

Third-degree (complete) heart block occurs in 2 to 5% of patients with acute myocardial infarction, is characterized by AV dissociation usually with a slow ectopic ventricular rate of 30 to 40 beats per minute, and occurs more commonly in inferior infarctions. When it occurs during anterior infarctions, it is usually permanent, requires permanent pacing, and is associated with a high 1-year mortality. When it occurs during inferior infarctions, it is usually temporary, although it may take up to 2 weeks to resolve and does not carry a significantly increased 1-year mortality.

Most peri-infarct bradyarrhythmias, particularly those associated with inferior wall infarcts, respond promptly to intravenous atropine. It should be noted, however, that occasional individuals actually experience progressive AV block with anticholinergic therapy.

Premature ventricular contractions (PVCs) occur frequently following acute myocardial infarction and do not require treatment. Couplets, triplets, multifocal PVCs, and short runs of nonsustained ventricular tachycardia are effectively treated with intravenous lidocaine, although no survival advantage has been shown with lidocaine in this setting. Many clinicians do not treat these nonmalignant ventricular arrhythmias because they rarely progress to life-threatening arrhythmias and can effectively be treated with cardioversion or defibrillation if they do and because lidocaine has potentially serious adverse effects. Lidocaine is not recommended in the routine prophylactic treatment of acute myocardial infarction. In addition, long-term prophylaxis of PVCs with oral antiarrhythmics, such as flecainide (Tambocor) and encainide (Enkaid), following acute myocardial infarction has been shown in the CAST study to increase mortality drastically, and these agents are contraindicated for this purpose.

Sustained ventricular tachycardia in the presence of maintained systemic pressure should be treated with intravenous lidocaine. Sustained ventricular tachycardia with systemic hypotension should be treated with DC cardioversion followed by lidocaine infusion. If lidocaine is ineffective, procainamide, bretylium, or intravenous amiodarone can be considered.

Ventricular fibrillation should immediately be treated with DC defibrillation. It is important to note that successfully treated ventricular fibrillation during acute myocardial infarction carries no higher incidence of morbidity or mortality than in patients without ventricular fibrillation.

A variety of supraventricular arrhythmias occur in patients with acute myocardial infarction. Most are a consequence of hypokalemia, hypomagnesemia, hypoxemia, mitral valve disease, pericarditis, severe left ventricular dysfunction, or rarely atrial ischemia or infarction. Premature atrial contractions are benign, may be related to left atrial hypertension owing to left ventricular dysfunction, and do not require treatment. Paroxysmal supraventricular tachycardia occasionally causes symptoms or hypotension and is usually effectively treated with intravenous adenosine, 6 mg bolus, or intravenous verapamil, 5 mg. Atrial flutter occurs in 2 to 4% of patients with acute myocardial infarction and can be treated by slowing the ventricular rate with verapamil, diltiazem, or short-acting beta blockade or by restoring sinus rhythm with cardioversion or overdrive atrial pacing. Atrial fibrillation occurs in 5 to 8% of patients with acute myocardial infarction and is treated similarly to atrial flutter in the acute myocardial infarction situation. Sinus tachycardia is commonly seen after acute myocardial infarction and may signify substantial ventricular damage, but fever, anxiety, and hypovolemia are other easily correctable causes.

One of the main reasons for prompt treatment of tachyarrhythmias during acute myocardial infarction is to minimize myocardial oxygen requirements. Tachycardia increases myocardial oxygen demand and can potentially increase infarct size if not quickly treated.

A summary of the commonly used antiarrhythmic agents in acute myocardial infarction is given in Table 3.

BUNDLE-BRANCH BLOCK

Some type of bundle-branch block occurs in 12 to 20% of patients with acute myocardial infarc-

TABLE 3. **Commonly Used Antiarrhythmic Agents in Acute Myocardial Infarction**

Agent	Dose	Comments
Adenosine	6 mg rapid IV bolus, then 12 mg if no response	For the treatment of supraventricular tachycardia. Can cause transient atrioventricular block
Atropine	0.5 mg IV bolus, repeated every 5 min up to 2 mg	Effective for symptomatic sinus bradycardia or Wenckebach and for morphine-induced nausea/vomiting
Lidocaine	1 mg/kg IV bolus; 0.5 mg/kg may be repeated up to 4 mg/kg, then 2–4 mg/min infusion	Indicated for frequent, multifocal, or closely coupled premature ventricular contractions, nonsustained VT, or for sustained VT and VF, in association with defibrillation and cardiopulmonary resuscitation as indicated. Toxic effects include nausea, drowsiness, dizziness, confusion, slurred speech
Procainamide	1–2 mg/kg bolus q 10 min to max 1000 mg, then 2–4 mg/min	Second-line therapy for ventricular arrhythmias after lidocaine. Must follow procainamide serum levels

IV = intravenous; VT = ventricular tachycardia; VF = ventricular fibrillation.

tion. LBBB, left anterior hemiblock (LAHB), and LAHB with right bundle-branch block (RBBB) occur in equal frequency. Isolated RBBB is uncommon; left posterior hemiblock (LPHB) rare. Patients with new LBBB or bifascicular block (RBBB + LAHB) and acute myocardial infarction should receive prophylactic temporary pacing because of their frequent progression to third-degree block. All patients with bundle-branch block have an increased 1-year mortality, probably reflective of the large infarct size frequently seen in these patients. Patients with persistent bundle-branch block and first-degree block or persistent bundle-branch block and transient advanced AV block should be considered for permanent pacing.

GENERAL HOSPITAL CARE

Although coronary reperfusion strategies are the cornerstone of therapy in acute myocardial infarction, general hospital care should not be neglected. General measures should be directed toward decreasing oxygen demand and continuous monitoring for arrhythmias. Therefore, complete bed rest with continuous ECG monitoring and frequent nursing assessment for hemodynamic instability or signs of recurrent ischemia is recommended in a CCU setting for 48 to 72 hours. Less intensive monitoring can then be continued for 5 to 7 days in a "step-down" unit that provides continuous ECG monitoring. Ambulation can be initiated after 2 to 4 days of bed rest, with careful assessment for signs of recurrent ischemia.

Cardiac enzymes should be obtained every 6 to 8 hours for the first 24 to 36 hours of the hospital stay and with any episodes of prolonged ischemia. An ECG should be obtained daily and with any clinical episode that might represent recurrent ischemia.

Nasal oxygen should be administered to all patients during the acute phase of treatment, and intravenous morphine is useful to minimize myocardial oxygen demand and decrease discomfort. General comfort measures should not be neglected, including stool softeners and antianxiety medications, when indicated.

Pulmonary artery (Swan-Ganz) catheterization is indicated in patients with severe or progressive heart failure or with cardiogenic shock or progressive hypotension. It may be helpful in hypotensive patients who do not respond to a fluid bolus or in patients with signs of pulmonary congestion.

Arterial pressure monitoring is useful in hypotensive patients and those receiving vasopressor agents and is required in those in cardiogenic shock. It is not necessary, however, in the routine care of the myocardial infarction patient and may

unnecessarily contribute to bleeding complications with thrombolytic therapy. Patients who have an uncomplicated course can be discharged 5 to 7 days after admission. The predischarge evaluation is discussed subsequently.

RISK STRATIFICATION

After the patient is stabilized following the acute management period of acute myocardial infarction, the most important evaluation is that of risk stratification, i.e., identification of that subset of patients at highest risk of reinfarction and death following acute myocardial infarction. Patients shown to be at highest risk after acute myocardial infarction include those with a large region of myocardial damage, spontaneous or provocative ischemia, abnormal signal-averaged ECG, and ventricular ectopy. It is of paramount importance then to identify each of these risk factors in each patient to determine which specific therapies should be considered. The goal of proper risk stratification is not only to provide prognostic information, but also to assist in choosing appropriate and specific mortality-reducing therapies.

Risk stratification needs to be addressed in three phases of the hospital course: on initial presentation, during the early in-hospital stay, and before discharge (Fig. 2). The first stage involves identification of patients who receive thrombolytic therapy but fail to reperfuse and those who do not receive thrombolytic therapy because of contraindications or other reasons and are at highest risk. Unfortunately, there is no fail-safe method to identify patients who do not reperfuse following thrombolytic therapy. Abrupt relief of pain, normalization of ST changes, reperfusion arrhythmias such as accelerated idioventricular rhythm or bradycardia, and improvement in hemodynamics frequently herald reperfusion, although reperfusion occasionally occurs without any of these signs. Therefore patients with large infarctions (as determined by ECG, echocardiogram, or clinical signs of significant left ventricular dysfunction) and continued pain or ECG evidence of ischemia in the hours following thrombolysis may benefit from a diagnostic catheterization to establish the status of the infarct-related artery. As mentioned in a previous section, emergent PTCA in a stenosed but patent artery with normal flow is associated with increased morbidity and is not recommended in the early stages of acute myocardial infarction. PTCA of an occluded artery following failed thrombolysis ("rescue" PTCA) has been shown in some studies to improve recurrent ischemic events and may benefit these patients. Because

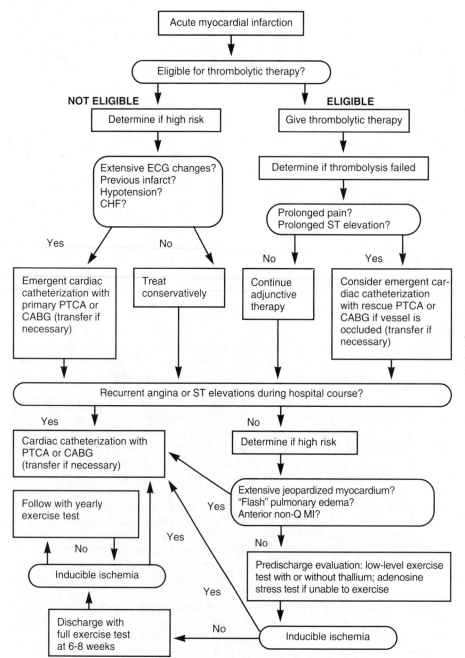

Figure 2. Risk stratification after acute myocardial infarction. Adapted from AHA/ACC Joint Task Force Guidelines for the early management of patients with acute myocardial infarction, 1990.

early PTCA is associated with increased procedure-related morbidity, however, the decision to perform rescue PTCA should be individualized and perhaps limited to those patients with large infarcts seen early in the course of acute myocardial infarction.

In patients who have contraindications to thrombolytic therapy, those at high risk are best treated with emergent primary angioplasty. Those with extensive ECG changes, as determined by amplitude of ST elevation or the pres-

ence of anterolateral or inferoposterior involvement, and those with previous infarction, hypotension, congestion (rales), or severe pain are considered high risk. Those at low risk and those in whom the risks of intervention are elevated may best be treated conservatively.

Treatment of high-risk patients at a center without facilities for PTCA presents a dilemma to the physician. The ACC/AHA Task Force recommends that patients with ongoing ischemia, hemodynamic instability, or resistant arrhythmias after thrombolytic therapy be immediately transferred to a tertiary care facility capable of performing emergency PTCA.

Those patients with acute myocardial infarction but contraindications to thrombolytic therapy should be transferred to a tertiary care facility when the risk for potential myocardial salvage outweighs the risk of transportation and intervention. Suitable candidates include those with hemodynamic instability or large infarctions seen early in the course of acute myocardial infarction.

The second phase of risk stratification occurs between 24 hours and 5 days and involves identification of patients with ongoing ischemia. Patients should be carefully evaluated for the presence of recurrent ST changes, recurrent angina or anginal equivalent, episodic hemodynamic instability, pulmonary edema, or mitral regurgitation. These patients as well as those with a prior infarction are at increased risk of reinfarction and death and benefit most from revascularization. Therefore, early cardiac catheterization and angiography are recommended in patients with any of these attributes. Patients with a non-Q myocardial infarction may also be at greater risk of reinfarction and recurrent angina, and some have recommended early angiography in this population. The data are conflicting, however, and the routine use of angiography in this group without evidence of ischemia is not currently endorsed.

The third phase of risk stratification occurs during predischarge evaluation. This evaluation is designed to identify patients with provocative ischemia or electrical instability. Approximately three-fourths of all cardiac deaths within 1 year after acute myocardial infarction are due to an arrhythmia, and one-fourth are due to myocardial failure. Unfortunately, although the presence of complex ventricular ectopy following acute myocardial infarction has long been identified as a poor prognostic factor, there currently exist few treatment options. Some oral antiarrhythmic agents have been shown in the CAST study to increase the mortality rate in patients with asymptomatic ventricular ectopy after acute myocardial infarction. Decreased heart rate variability, as determined by Holter monitoring, is also a poor prognostic factor, presumably reflecting decreased vagal tone, increased sympathetic tone, or both.

The signal-averaged ECG is a simple technique to identify patients at high risk for sudden death or symptomatic ventricular ectopy following acute myocardial infarction. The presence of late potentials or low-amplitude depolarizations following the QRS complex have been associated with a 10-fold increase in arrhythmic events in patients with ejection fractions less than 0.40 following acute myocardial infarction. Whether all patients with an abnormal signal-averaged ECG following acute myocardial infarction should undergo a more vigorous evaluation for complex arrhythmias is controversial. Several ongoing studies are investigating this approach, but until further data become available, empirical electrophysiologic study or antiarrhythmic therapy in the asymptomatic patient is not routinely recommended.

To identify patients with provocative ischemia, low-level exercise treadmill testing has traditionally been performed before discharge in the postacute myocardial infarction patient. Many patients, however, cannot perform the test, and the test may be contraindicated in patients at high risk. Concomitant thallium imaging increases the sensitivity of exercise testing, but it is unclear whether this affects long-term prognosis. In patients who cannot exercise, adenosine or persantine thallium is equally effective at identifying patients at risk. Patients with provocative ischemia should undergo angiography and revascularization when appropriate.

It should be emphasized, however, that the presence or absence of provocative ischemia following acute myocardial infarction does not necessarily predict recurrent ischemic events. The decision to perform angiography and revascularization is frequently made on the basis of other prognostic factors.

The ACC/AHA Joint Task Force published an algorithm in 1990 to help risk-stratify patients after acute myocardial infarction. In essence, all patients with evidence of reperfusion should have a predischarge evaluation, and in most cases, patients found to be at high risk should have angiography. Those found to have significant coronary stenoses in vessels supplying viable myocardium have a lower mortality following surgical revascularization. Similar data for PTCA are not currently available, but small observational studies suggest that the mortality rate after PTCA in this population is low.

After discharge, patients can gradually increase activity levels over a period of 6 to 8 weeks if they feel well. A routine symptom-limited (maximum) stress test should be performed at this time both for prognostic value and to provide assurance to the patient that normal activity levels can be resumed. The asymptomatic patient with a normal maximal stress test can then be followed every 4 to 6 months with a yearly stress test to assess for inducible ischemia.

Perhaps the most important issues after discharge are physical reconditioning and risk factor modification. Patients who smoke, are sedentary, or have elevated cholesterol levels are at increased risk of accelerated atherosclerosis and should be carefully counseled to quit smoking, begin a supervised exercise program, or begin a low-cholesterol diet. Cardiac rehabilitation programs are designed to improve exercise tolerance gradually in post–myocardial infarction patients in a supervised setting and should be routinely recommended. Pooled clinical trials have shown a significant reduction in mortality in those randomized to exercise training. Smoking patients may benefit from a formalized smoking cessation program or topical nicotine therapy. The National Cholesterol Education Program recommends that patients with a cholesterol level greater than 200 or LDL cholesterol level greater than 130 following acute myocardial infarction initiate a low-cholesterol diet. If after 6 months levels continue to be elevated, lipid-lowering medications are then recommended. Lipid modifications have been shown to slow the progression of atherosclerosis and decrease cardiac mortality.

Psychological factors should not be ignored in the post–myocardial infarction setting. Acute cardiac events create anxiety and depression in both patients and family members. Medical restrictions on even the most routine of activities, such as driving, climbing stairs, lifting, and sexual activity, create a psychologically stressful environment. Fear of recurrent cardiac events may become a significant impediment to the resumption of a full and active lifestyle. Cardiac rehabilitation programs, besides improving exercise capacity, have been shown to improve confidence levels and sense of well-being significantly after acute myocardial infarction. It is important to encourage patients to resume normal activity levels after acute myocardial infarction, and a supervised exercise program is an effective means of achieving this.

CORONARY REHABILITATION

method of
L. KENT SMITH, M.D., M.P.H.
Arizona Heart Institute
Phoenix, Arizona

Coronary rehabilitation is a unique array of services for the patient with diagnosed coronary artery disease that includes, but is not limited to, exercise training and is designed to ensure maximum possible attainment of functional capacity, risk factor, psychosocial, and economic status. Traditionally coronary rehabilitation programs have dealt with patients recovering from an acute cardiac event, most specifically, myocardial infarction or coronary artery bypass surgery and percutaneous transluminal coronary angioplasty (PTCA). In recent years, these services have been ex-

tended to include patients with other cardiovascular disorders (e.g., congestive cardiomyopathy, cardiac transplantation, peripheral arterial disease, and heart valve replacement). Formal, structured coronary rehabilitation programs offer an array of services provided to the patient by a multidisciplinary team of health care professionals. This team is headed by a physician with special interest and training in cardiovascular rehabilitation and is often composed of nurses, exercise physiologists, nutritionists, physical or occupational therapists (or both), and vocational rehabilitation specialists. In the past few years, rehabilitation of the patient with coronary artery disease has been critically evaluated by several important organizations, and the value and benefit of the programs have been well accepted. These evaluations have been carried out by the health care financing administration (HCFA) of the federal government, the American Heart Association, the American College of Cardiology, and the American College of Physicians. Each of these organizations has issued extensive reports on the rehabilitation of coronary artery disease patients.

COMPONENTS OF THE CORONARY REHABILITATION PROGRAM

The unique feature of a rehabilitation program is the exercise component. A comprehensive program, however, now includes many other important components that characterize the multidisciplinary approach to rehabilitation of the patient with coronary artery disease. It is helpful to understand the components of the rehabilitation program by describing them in the order in which they are offered to a patient with coronary artery disease. This order begins with the evaluation or intake phase and then proceeds to the prescription and delivery of the services themselves. Finally, documentation of the outcome of the services allows for a critical determination of the risks and benefits of a rehabilitation program in the patient with coronary artery disease.

The evaluation or intake phase has as its cornerstone the assessment of the patient's pathophysiologic status. The traditional use of the graded exercise test is the hallmark of the initial evaluation of the patient with manifest coronary artery disease. In the last decade, prognostic value of a graded exercise test has been well established. A markedly ischemic electrocardiographic response to exercise testing (2 mm or greater ST depression, particularly if in several electrocardiographic leads and occurring at a relatively low workload of the exercise test) places a patient in a high-risk prognostic category. Twenty percent 1-year fatality is not uncommon in patients manifesting this type of graded exercise test result following recovery from an acute myocardial infarction. These patients are often recommended to undergo coronary angiography with the hope of identifying and correcting coronary lesions that underlie the ischemic response. Carefully monitored and supervised cardiac rehabilitation, however, can be carried out in this high-risk category of patient. The initial intake and evaluation of a patient's cardiovascular physiology may also include a measure of ventricular dysfunction. A drop of systolic blood pressure of 20 mmHg or more with progressive workload on graded exercise testing may define the patient with serious left ventricular dysfunction. A more quantifiable evaluation can be obtained with radionuclide exercise evaluation, exercise echocardiography, or both. Patients who manifest significant left ventricular dysfunction also carry a high 1-year mortality rate at times exceeding 20%. Nevertheless, emerging new data (see later) have established that patients with left ventricular dysfunction can safely participate in and benefit from supervised cardiac rehabilitation efforts. The evaluation process for entering a rehabilitation program also includes documentation of the coronary artery disease risk factor status of a patient. This status would include a determination of the lipid profile, presence and degree of glucose intolerance, determination of current or past cigarette smoking habits, documentation of overweight and a determination of percent body fat, and an assessment of the patient's psychosocial status. The entire evaluation or intake information then becomes the basis for an appropriate and individualized prescription for the patient to follow to optimize the benefits of rehabilitation while minimizing the potential risks.

The prescription of the multidisciplinary components of the rehabilitation program is then carried out. The exercise component can occur in either a supervised or a nonsupervised setting depending on the risk factor status of the patient as determined during the evaluation phase. It has been determined by both the American College of Cardiology and the American College of Physicians that about one-quarter of patients involved in a coronary rehabilitation program are of sufficiently high risk to require a formal structured program with supervision and electrocardiographic monitoring. These high-risk patients include those who manifest considerable ischemia during the intake graded exercise test, show high-grade ventricular ectopy during exercise, have significantly diminished left ventricular function, and are unable to self-monitor exercise intensity.

The exercise prescription addresses five key features. The most important, in terms of individualization, is the intensity of the training effort. In general, the target heart rate at which the patient exercises ("dose" of exercise) should be approximately 70% of the heart rate that the patient could safely achieve during graded exercise testing without manifesting an ischemic response or significant ventricular ectopy. In patients whose heart rates are not altered by drug therapy, it is often possible to teach the patient to equate a certain subjective feeling of exercise intensity to the target heart rate level. Coronary rehabilitation programs often use a rating system known as the Borg scale to assist patients in achieving a training intensity appropriate for their exercise prescription. In the early weeks of exercise training, patients are encouraged to work at a level of 13 or 14 on the Borg scale, advancing up to 17 or 18 once this higher level of intensity can be shown to be safely achieved (Table 1). With shorter hospital stays, even in patients undergoing coronary artery bypass surgery, the activity or exercise component of coronary rehabilitation can safely begin in low-risk patients in the first 24 to 48 hours of hospitalization. The initial, or baseline graded, exercise test, however, often does not occur until 2 to 3 weeks after a myocardial infarction or coronary bypass surgery. Patients undergoing PTCA can have the exercise test much sooner if they are clinically stable. Once the exercise test has occurred, the exercise prescription can be individualized and the training component started. Often a follow-up graded exercise test is carried out toward the conclusion of the initial phase of a coronary rehabilitation program, which classically lasts for 8 to 12 weeks. A revision of the exercise prescription then occurs based on the follow-up exercise test result.

For patients who are found to be low risk, a

TABLE 1. **Borg Rating of Perceived Exertion Scale**

Grade	Description
6	No exertion at all
7	Extremely light
8	
9	Very light
10	
11	Light
12	
13	Somewhat hard
14	
15	Hard (heavy)
16	
17	Very hard
18	
19	Extremely hard
20	Maximal exertion

From Borg GV. An introduction to Borg's RPE scale. Ithaca, NY, Mouvement Publications, 1985. © Gunnar Borg, 1985.

nonsupervised program can safely occur, provided that the patient understands to limit the intensity of exercise training to the level deemed to be safe based on the graded exercise test result. Further, transtelephonic systems for documenting the electrocardiogram response to home exercise have been evaluated and found to be effective.

The nonexercise components of a coronary rehabilitation program are also based on the intake evaluation data. Often patients with manifest coronary artery disease have unfavorable metabolic parameters. Diet or pharmacologic therapy (or both) to optimize the metabolic status of patients should be carried out. In formal rehabilitation programs, this is often a shared responsibility of the dietician, physician, and nurse. Active involvement by the patient's spouse and family members may lead to a greater degree of compliance and a more optimum result as well. Many patients recovering from an acute coronary event often manifest anxiety and depression. Behavioral counseling may then be recommended to the patient to address these issues. The vocational status of the patient is also assessed during the evaluation phase, and when appropriate, vocational counseling becomes a part of the overall coronary rehabilitation program.

OUTCOMES OF CORONARY REHABILITATION

As with any therapy, a critical evaluation of the potential risks needs to be done. The most extensive information regarding the safety of cardiac rehabilitation involves patients participating in programs after an acute myocardial infarction. This evaluation of cardiovascular complications of outpatient programs involved more than 50,000 patients participating at 167 randomly selected coronary rehabilitation centers. This study documented the occurrence of cardiac arrest at a rate of 1 per 110,000 patient hours and a mortality rate of 1 per 784,000 patient hours. There was no difference in the occurrence of cardiovascular complications among programs of various size or programs that used constant versus intermittent electrocardiographic monitoring of the exercise sessions. Other information, however, regarding cardiovascular complications has established that cardiac arrest most often occurs during the warm-up or cool-down phases of the training program as compared with the time the patient is working at his or her training heart rate. This underscores the importance of a high level of vigilance for the patient during the entire period within the rehabilitation program location. Furthermore, the physician responsible for a coronary rehabilitation program should be available within the facility where the coronary rehabilitation program is being carried out and should be able to respond quickly to a cardiovascular emergency. Both HCFA and the American Heart Association, however, have determined that the physician need not be present in the room where the exercise training is being carried out.

The functional capacity of patients undergoing coronary rehabilitation improves by 25 to 30% after the traditional 8 to 12 weeks of a rehabilitation program. This has been documented to occur in patients who are older than age 65 as well as in patients who manifest compromised left ventricular performance. This improvement in functional capacity occurs in patients who participate in cardiac rehabilitation programs after a myocardial infarction as well as patients who have had coronary artery bypass surgery. An equally beneficial training effect is seen in patients with stable angina pectoris who have not had an acute event. Furthermore, patients who participate in coronary rehabilitation following PTCA have been shown to improve their functional capacity. Regarding the important issue of restenosis following PTCA, however, there are reports that this has no beneficial effect in reducing the rate of restenosis as well as a single report of a reduction in restenosis rates in a group of patients undergoing coronary rehabilitation training (17% restenosis rates at 3 months) compared with a nontraining group, which showed the more usual rate of restenosis of 40%. Clearly this single report requires confirmation but could represent an important additional benefit of coronary rehabilitation training following PTCA.

Improvements in lipoprotein levels have been achieved in patients participating in coronary rehabilitation programs. This seems especially the case with patients who enter programs with undesirably low high-density lipoprotein (HDL) cholesterol levels. Dietary intervention alone carried out during 12 weeks of exercise training significantly increases HDL cholesterol level. This has been achieved in patients who are participating in programs after recovery from myocardial infarction as well as patients having undergone coronary artery bypass surgery. Furthermore, there has been a desirable reduction in plasma triglyceride levels. Pharmacotherapy has resulted in an even greater improvement in lipid profiles.

In the subgroup of patients with impaired left ventricular dysfunction and congestive heart failure, there has been increasing evidence regarding the beneficial effects of coronary rehabilitation. Several studies have now documented improved functional capacity in these patients. This appears to occur, however, as a result of the beneficial effects of training on the skeletal muscle metabolism and not as a result of improved left ventricular function. Specifically sequential echocardiographic assessment of left ventricular function has shown no improvement as a result of exercise training in patients with diminished left ventricular ejection fraction at baseline. With only one exception in the literature, however, it appears that functional capacity is improved with no detrimental effect on left ventricular ejection fraction.

A further recent extension of cardiovascular rehabilitation to a specific patient group includes patients who are recovering from aortic valve replacement. Patients randomly allocated to a training group showed increased functional capacity after 12 weeks of rehabilitation compared with a control group. Furthermore, return to gainful employment was greater in those patients participating in the training program. Another new patient group who have had evaluation of the beneficial effects of rehabilitation are those with peripheral arterial disease. This group of patients showed less impairment owing to claudication and resultant increase in walking distance on completion of the program. Furthermore, more than 80% of the patients became ex-smokers and showed significant reduction in serum cholesterol and triglyceride levels. In addition, patients with non–insulin-dependent diabetes were randomly allocated to a training or a nontraining group. The training group showed significant improvement in functional capacity and improvement in systolic blood pressure and resting heart rate as a result of the rehabilitation program. Glycosylated hemoglobin was decreased, as were triglyceride levels.

Women with coronary artery disease have not been the subject of extensive evaluation and studies in the medical literature. This pertains to the issue of coronary rehabilitation as well. It appears that women are less often referred to coronary rehabilitation programs and when referred drop out at a higher rate than their male counterparts. Furthermore, it has noted that men are better able to tolerate the physical training component of rehabilitation and are found to be less anxious and less depressed than women entering rehabilitation programs. Women who do enter and complete coronary rehabilitation programs, however, show the same degree of improvement in functional capacity as do men.

The important outcome of improved return to work after cardiac rehabilitation in patients having experienced a myocardial infarction remains controversial. Newer studies show both an improvement in return to work in some cases and no such improvement in others. Many other nonphysiologic factors appear to play an important role in the patient's decision to return to work.

Randomized trials of coronary rehabilitation in Europe and the United States have recently addressed the important issue of improvement in thallium myocardial perfusion by comparing training and nontraining groups. There was a consistent documentation of improved thallium myocardial perfusion in patients participating in supervised exercise programs three times per week for up to 12 months. In the European study, this is associated with improvement in lipoprotein parameters as well. In that same European study, sequential coronary angiography was carried out at baseline and 1 year, and regression of coronary atherosclerotic lesions was reported in 39% of the intervention group compared with only 8% of the control group. This important beneficial effect requires confirmation but remains an exciting finding.

Finally, metaanalysis of 22 randomized, controlled studies evaluating no rehabilitation versus coronary rehabilitation in patients having experienced an acute myocardial infarction documents improved morbidity and mortality. Specifically the 1- to 3-year reduction in total mortality, cardiovascular mortality, and fatal reinfarction rates of 20 to 25% has been established by comparing the rehabilitation group with the nonrehabilitation group. The best results appear to have occurred in programs that are multidisciplined and offer more than exercise trainng in the array of rehabilitation services.

PERICARDITIS

method of
JAMES B. YOUNG, M.D.
Baylor College of Medicine
Houston, Texas

Pericarditis is a reasonably common disease process that challenges the diagnostic wit of primary care physicians. From a pathophysiologic perspective, the difficulty results from acute or chronic inflammation of the pericardial sac. This generally causes a chest pain syndrome. Because patients with chest pain frequently present to their internist or family physician, the nuances of pericarditis must be understood and the condition kept in a differential diagnosis. It is also important to remember that inflammatory conditions of the pericardium are frequently accompanied by an effusive process. This difficulty can be life-threatening, depending on the volume and rapidity of fluid build-up.

PERICARDIUM

The pericardial sac is a fibrous structure with mesothelial cell lining that suspends the heart in the mediastinum. Normally about 50 mL of clear fluid is present. This fluid is rich in phospholipids that reduce friction between the heart and mediastinal contents during heart beat and body motion. There is some evidence that the pericardium modulates efferent cardiac sympathetic nerve stimulation and electrophysiologic properties of the heart; however, the major function of this structure likely relates to anatomic issues. Specifically, excessive cardiac motion with body movement is controlled, and a barrier is created between the heart and other mediastinal organs and the lungs. This may be particularly important when malignancy or infection exists in structures contiguous with the heart. This also explains why certain conditions, such as carcinoma of the lung or pneumococcal pneumonia, often cause pericarditis. Although individuals with congenital absence of the pericardium do not have manifest circulatory difficulties, the pericardium does play a role in cardiac filling and emptying dynamics. Specifically, excessive acute cardiac dilatation is prevented, and diastolic coupling of right and left ventricular filling is effected.

ETIOLOGY OF PERICARDITIS/PERICARDIAL EFFUSION

Table 1 summarizes most, but not all, of the causes of pericarditis. As can be seen, they range from common maladies, such as adenovirus, mumps, and pneumococcal pneumonia, to more obscure difficulties, such as autoimmune diseases and tuberculosis. Because pericarditis rarely represents a process affecting the pericardium alone, it is important to diagnose underlying diseases promptly and accurately because ther-

TABLE 1. **Etiology of Pericarditis/Pericardial Effusion**

Viral infections (coxsackie, adenovirus, echovirus, mumps, mononucleosis, varicella, hepatitis, acquired immunodeficiency syndrome)
Acute bacterial infection (pneumococcus, staphylococcus, streptococcus, *Neisseria* gonorrhoeae, *N. meningitidis*, *Legionella*)
Fungal infections (histoplasmosis, coccidioidomycosis, *Candida* spp, blastomycosis)
Tuberculosis
Unusual infections (*Nocardia*, Lyme disease, toxoplasmosis, mycoplasma, amebiasis, actinomycosis, echinococcosis)
Uremia (de novo, dialysis associated)
Neoplastic diseases (lung cancer, breast cancer, melanoma, leukemia, lymphoma, Hodgkin's disease)
Myocardial infarction (acute evolving infarction, Dressler's syndrome)
Inflammatory disease states (systemic lupus erythematosus, rheumatoid arthritis, acute rheumatic fever, scleroderma, polyarteritis nodosa, sarcoidosis, amyloidosis, inflammatory bowel disease)
Radiation injury
Drug reactions (hydralazine, procainamide, phenytoin, isoniazid, phenylbutazone, dantrolene, doxorubicin, methysergide, cyclophosphamide)
Myxedema
Dissecting aortic aneurysm
Chylopericardium
Trauma (blunt, penetrating, cardiac catheterization complications)
Idiopathic

TABLE 2. **Differentiating Ischemic from Pericardial Pain**

Pain Characteristics	Angina/Infarct	Pericarditis
Location	Precordial	Precordial
Radiation	Shoulder, arms	Scapular region
Description	Pressure, burning, oppression	Sharp, stabbing, dull ache
Pleurisy	No	Yes
Fever	Unusual	Common
Posture related	No	Yes (worse supine)
Effort related	Yes	No
Time course	Minutes–hours	Hours–days
Related to concomitant diseases	Not usually	Frequently

apy of the primary difficulty is mandatory if pericarditis is to be cured. Whenever a chest pain syndrome accompanies situations listed in Table 1, pericarditis should be considered. Often young patients present with a history of chest pain suggesting pericarditis, pericardial friction rub, and diagnostic electrocardiogram for pericarditis, yet do not have an obvious primary disease process. These patients are usually labeled as having idiopathic pericarditis, but a careful review of history or serial viral titer measurements frequently implicate a preceding viral infection.

DIAGNOSIS OF PERICARDITIS/ PERICARDIAL EFFUSION

Chest pain is the most frequent symptom of acute pericarditis. Because angina pectoris caused by coronary heart disease also produces a chest pain syndrome, it is important to try to differentiate these two conditions. Table 2 lists several characteristics of both ischemic and pericardial pain. Acute pericarditis generally presents with the insidious onset of sharp or stabbing precordial chest discomfort that often has a pleuritic component to it and is positional (worse supine). The pain may be described as dull and aching and is persistent over many hours and days. It is not exertional in character. Radiation to the back (especially the scapular region) is common and noted in particular with inspiration. Low-grade fever is frequently reported, as is malaise, and this likely represents underlying inflammatory perturbations.

As mentioned, pericarditis is often caused by other concomitant diseases, and symptoms specific to conditions noted in Table 1 should be sought. For example, arthralgias and claudication might suggest systemic lupus erythematosus or polyarteritis nodosa. Patients may also complain of palpitations or cardiac arrhythmias. Because post–myocardial infarction pericarditis usually appears several days after the infarct, recurrent chest pain in this setting is not always ischemic in origin, and careful evaluation of the patient is required to differentiate pericarditis from ischemia with angina pectoris. Use of certain drugs that can cause pericarditis must always be considered. This is an often overlooked cause of this malady.

Physical findings in patients with pericarditis are generally caused by either pericardial inflammation or effusion resulting in hemodynamic disturbances. A pericardial friction rub often is present, although it may be transient and difficult to hear. Significant pericardial effusion can cause elevated venous pressure, a paradoxical inspiratory fall in systemic blood pressure or pulse pressure (>10 mmHg) and tachycardia. Shock becomes apparent, sometimes suddenly, when effusions grow to such a size that cardiac filling and thus emptying become impaired. It is critically important to determine presence of a pericardial effusion early so progression to cardiac tamponade can be prevented.

An electrocardiogram should be scrutinized. Diffuse ST segment elevation, particularly with PR segment depression, indicates pericarditis. Focal Q waves with ST segment elevation and T wave inversion point toward myocardial infarction. Atrial and sometimes ventricular arrhythmias may be seen, as has been noted. When large effusions are present, low QRS voltage is sometimes apparent, and electrical alternans, or rhythmic inspiratory progressive diminution of QRS voltage, should be of concern because of the likelihood of incipient cardiac tamponade. A chest x-ray may not be helpful when looking for small pericardial effusions, but large ones can cause cardiomegaly. Further, chest radiography gives insight into concomitant pathology, such as pneumonia or possible pulmonary malignancy. Echocardiography is the most practical method (considering diagnostic accuracy, cost, and availability) to detect and size pericardial effusions. It should be performed in every patient suspected of having pericarditis. Computed tomographic scans of the chest or magnetic resonance imaging of the heart are alternative methods of assessing pericardial pathology.

When other concomitant diseases are suspected or known to be present, disease-specific tests and evaluation must be ordered. This is particularly important when an infectious cause of pericarditis is a possibility.

TREATMENT

Because the development of an effusion with subsequent tamponade is possible, hospital admission during initiation of therapy for pericarditis is not inappropriate. Table 3 lists the major difficulties associated with pericarditis and pericardial effusions. Pain syndromes, purulent effusions with sepsis, cardiac tamponade, and pericardial constriction are the most frequent problems requiring subsequent therapeutic attention. The pain of acute pericarditis generally responds well to the anti-inflammatory medica-

tion aspirin (650 mg every 3 to 4 hours). Other nonsteroidal anti-inflammatory drugs may be equally effective. Indomethacin (25 to 50 mg four times daily) is reserved for more severe pain syndromes because of the frequency of gastrointestinal difficulties encountered with this drug. Steroids should be reserved for patients with pain syndromes persisting after 48 hours of treatment despite adequate doses of nonsteroidal anti-inflammatory drugs. Chronic pain syndromes, or recurrent, relapsing pericarditis, should also be treated with a course of steroids. One approach is to give prednisone (approximately 1 mg per kg) daily for 1 week, beginning a slow dose taper (5 mg per day) when symptoms have abated. Rarely is the combination of prednisone and a nonsteroidal agent justified because of the significant risk of gastrointestinal difficulties. Chronic pain syndromes may require pericardiectomy to achieve symptom relief. Selection of patients for this operation may be difficult, and all other causes of chest pain must be excluded. Further, removal of the entire pericardium is required for the operation to be successful.

As mentioned previously, treatment must be focused on concomitant disease processes as well if associated pericarditis is to be resolved. This is particularly important if purulent pericarditis is present. Care must be taken in these patients to prescribe appropriate antimicrobials, while draining the effusion and avoiding steroid administration. Anticoagulants should be discontinued, if at all possible, when pericarditis is diagnosed because of the risk of increasing effusion size (hemorrhage) and precipitating cardiac tamponade. Patient management is particularly problematic, therefore, in patients with prosthetic heart valves or early post–myocardial infarction when thrombolytics have been used. If absolutely necessary, anticoagulation should be accomplished with continuous intravenous heparin infusion so clotting times can be precisely monitored. Serial echocardiography is important to assess progression or regression of effusion size.

Atrial arrhythmias are common in patients with pericarditis with premature atrial contractions, atrial flutter, and atrial fibrillation responding to anti-inflammatory therapy and digoxin administration. Unless the syndrome is treated first with anti-inflammatory agents, electrical cardioversion of atrial flutter and fibrillation is rarely successful in the long term.

TABLE 3. **Potential Difficulties of Pericarditis/ Pericardial Effusion**

Acute pain syndrome
Chronic pain syndrome
Purulent effusion with sepsis
Cardiac tamponade
Chronic constrictive hemodynamic syndrome

MANAGEMENT OF PERICARDIAL EFFUSIONS

It must be re-emphasized that all patients with pericarditis should undergo echocardiography to determine presence and size of pericardial effusion. Echocardiographic evidence of cardiac tamponade (inspiratory atrial or ventricular chamber collapse) must be excluded if conservative medical management of effusions is pursued. Large effusions, effusions with evidence of tamponade, and possible purulent effusions must be tapped expeditiously. Also, when cause of an effusion is in doubt, pericardiocentesis can be helpful. One should remember that asymptomatic pericardial effusion is most frequently secondary to concomitant ailments. When a large effusion is encountered, an indwelling drainage catheter can be left in place for at least 24 hours. Frequently with treatment, the rate of fluid production is dramatically slow. Having a tube in place generally prevents tamponade, allows estimation of speed of fluid build-up and, if necessary, provides access for installation of sclerosing, chemotherapeutic, or anti-infective agents.

If a patient with pericarditis and known effusion becomes tachycardic, hypotensive, or tachypneic, cardiac tamponade may be occurring. Volume expansion with isotonic fluid given rapidly may initially stabilize the situation, while preparations for urgent pericardiocentesis are made. Sometimes isoproterenol or dopamine therapy is helpful. This approach is designed to increase cardiac filling pressures and augment contractility, thereby countering the effects of external compression of the heart by the pericardial fluid. This form of therapy is temporary, however, and more definitive pericardial drainage procedures must be planned. In chronic effusions that cannot be controlled with ordinary medical therapy or therapy directed at the underlying problem (such as a malignancy), surgically resecting a portion of the pericardium and creation of a "window" allow fluid to drain into a pericardial space and prevent recurrent tamponade.

Chronic pericarditis may cause a concomitant effusive process. Sometimes occult constrictive hemodynamics can be unmasked during cardiac catheterization and hemodynamic evaluation with rapid volume expansion. In any event, one must be absolutely certain that a patient's symptoms and functional limitation are, for the most part, related to constrictive or effusive-constrictive pericarditis. Certain intrinsic myocardial diseases (such as hemochromatosis, cardiac amyloidosis, or sarcoidosis) can produce restrictive hemodynamic physiology with symptoms and findings similar to chronic constrictive pericarditis. Patients should not, therefore, be referred for pericardiectomy without endomyocardial biopsy having been performed that excludes infiltrative myocardial processes.

PERIPHERAL ARTERIAL DISEASE

method of
JAMES C. STANLEY, M.D.
University of Michigan Medical School
Ann Arbor, Michigan

CHRONIC ARTERIOSCLEROTIC OCCLUSIVE DISEASE OF LOWER-EXTREMITY ARTERIES
(Table 1)

Arteriosclerotic macrovascular occlusive disease commonly affects the extremity arteries in the elderly. This disease, like that affecting the coronary and carotid circulations, may have a dominant genetic cause, but is more likely to develop in smokers, diabetics, patients with lipid disorders, and hypertensives. Rheologic factors are also important, in that severe disease is usually most evident at origins and branchings of arteries, with lesser degrees of disease affecting the intervening segments. Fortunately, such focal disease is more easily treated by operation or catheter angioplasty than diffuse disease.

Men are affected with lower-extremity arteriosclerotic occlusive disease twice as often as women. Clinical symptoms evolve when the tissue's metabolic needs exceed the oxygen delivery capacity of the blood flow. Claudication is the usual first manifestation, representing reproducible pain in a muscle group precipitated by a fixed degree of walking, with relief following a brief period of rest. An advanced form of ischemia that occurs when the occlusive process is more extensive and collateral vessels are insufficient is rest pain. This is classically manifested by pain in the distal foot (metatarsalgia) occurring at night. The reduced cardiac output during sleep causes mean perfusion pressures to fall below critical capillary closing pressures, resulting in severe tissue ischemia. Actual tissue loss and gangrene are the

TABLE 1. **Chronic Lower-Extremity Arteriosclerotic Occlusive Disease**

Male:female ratio 2:1
Clinical manifestations
  Claudication (calf discomfort most common; ankle:brachial index 0.6; 5% progress to gangrene)
  Rest pain (nocturnal metatarsalgia; ankle:brachial index 0.25; impending tissue loss likely)
  Gangrene (ankle:brachial index 0.1; amputation inevitable)
Nonoperative treatment for nondisabling claudication; walking exercise program beneficial in 80%
Treatment for disabling claudication or rest pain; percutaneous catheter angioplasty or bypass grafting (most often aortobifemoral, femoropopliteal, or femorotibial reconstructions)

most serious manifestations of this disease. However, only 5% of individuals with claudication not subjected to therapeutic interventions eventually develop extremity gangrene over a 5-year period.

Pallor, decreased muscle mass, and loss of secondary skin appendages reflect chronically reduced extremity blood flow, but these are often inconsistent findings among these patients. Although diminished pulses may be evident, a more objective means of quantitating impaired blood flow is to compare the posterior tibial or dorsalis pedis arterial blood pressure with that of the brachial artery. In normal individuals the ratio established by this comparison, the so-called ankle:brachial index, is usually 1.0 or slightly greater. Pressures are established by the use of Doppler instrumentation. The typical triphasic Doppler waveform associated with normal blood flow is lost as the occlusive state progresses, first to a biphasic waveform and then to a monophasic waveform. A decrease in the index to the 0.6 range is typical of claudication, and rest pain ensues with indices in the 0.25 range. Impending or actual gangrene is a frequent accompaniment once the index is 0.1 or less. Arteriography facilitates planning of operative treatment, but in general should not be viewed as a primary diagnostic test. In fact, simple Doppler ankle:brachial pressure measurements and waveform assessments usually can define the extent and location of clinically relevant disease.

Nonoperative therapy should be offered to the majority of patients with lower-extremity arteriosclerotic occlusive disease. Control of severe hyperlipoproteinemias, cessation of smoking, and control of hypertension are important in these patients. Pentoxifylline (Trental), a drug that increases red blood cell deformability, has been advocated as a means of increasing a patient's tolerance to impaired extremity blood flow. Although there are a few studies with statistical evidence that this may be the case, this drug has not proved to be very useful clinically. Similarly, vasodilators have no value in treating symptomatic lower-extremity occlusive disease. The most efficacious nonoperative treatment has been an active exercise program, in the form of relatively vigorous walking for as little as 20 minutes twice a day. This physical activity facilitates the evolution of collateral vessels and reduces the severity of claudication in 80% of patients.

Percutaneous transluminal balloon angioplasty is useful in treating select patients with lower-extremity arteriosclerotic occlusive disease. This involves vessel plaque fracture and is most successful in treating focal lesions, especially those affecting the iliac artery. It is less valuable for treating femoral, popliteal, or tibial artery occlusive disease. Complications attending balloon angioplasty occur in fewer than 10% of cases, with initial successes occurring in more than 75% of these patients. Unfortunately, percutaneous balloon angioplasty is durable treatment in only half of these cases because of re-stenosis. Improvement in the outcome of transcatheter treatment by use of laser and atherectomy devices awaits further advances in existing technology.

Surgical therapy for peripheral vascular occlusive disease affecting the lower extremities is justified only among patients manifesting disabling claudication, rest pain, or tissue loss. Various operations are possible, depending upon the site of disease. Arteriosclerosis of the lower extremities may be categorized as to the anatomic location of the most severe obstructions, being divided into patients exhibiting: (1) Leriche's syndrome; (2) generalized aortoiliac occlusive disease; and (3) femoral-popliteal or tibial-peroneal occlusive disease.

Leriche's syndrome is associated with thrombotic obliteration of the terminal aorta, occurring as a result of severe focal arteriosclerotic disease. Men with Leriche's syndrome most often have lower-extremity fatigue (not claudication), lower-extremity muscular atrophy and trophic skin changes, pallor of their legs and feet, and inability to sustain an erection. A similar clinical pattern is seen in women, excluding erectile dysfunction. Most patients are in the 35-to-60-year age range. Treatment consists of an aortobifemoral bypass with a synthetic vascular graft. This can be undertaken with a mortality rate of less than 2% and a 5-year graft patency rate of 95%.

Generalized aortoiliac arteriosclerotic occlusive disease (so-called inflow disease because it affects inflow of blood into the lower extremities) usually involves patients in the 60-to-70-year age group. Lower-extremity claudication is more common than tissue loss, with the latter often occurring as a consequence of additional tandem occlusive lesions in the distal extremity arteries. Treatment usually encompasses an aortobifemoral bypass. This procedure can be undertaken with a 2 to 3% operative mortality rate and a 5-year graft patency rate approaching 90%. Aortoiliac endarterectomy provides a similar outcome, but is more technically difficult to perform than a bypass with a synthetic graft. In high-risk patients with serious cardiac disease, alternative therapies include extra-anatomic revascularizations in the form of axillobifemoral or femoral-femoral bypasses. The operative risks are reduced with these extra-anatomic reconstructions. In the case of axillofemoral bypasses, the long-term patency rates are less than with direct aortic reconstructions.

Femoral-popliteal and tibial-peroneal arteriosclerotic occlusive disease (so-called outflow disease because it affects the vascular outflow within the lower extremity) is most often manifest by calf or foot claudication due to superficial femoral or infrapopliteal arterial disease, respectively. Rest pain and tissue loss are more likely to accompany diseases of outflow vessels than aortoiliac disease. Treatment usually entails an autologous saphenous vein bypass either as a reversed conduit or in the in situ position. Although these procedures involve dissections only within the subcutaneous tissues, operative mortality is in the 3 to 5% level. Cardiac events are the most serious complications attending these operations. In this regard, individuals with both occlusive and aneurysmal lesions of the aorta or distal arteries should undergo preoperative cardiac assessments by noninvasive means to ensure the absence of precarious coronary artery disease that if untreated might compromise the patient's subsequent care.

ACUTE EMBOLIC OCCLUSIVE DISEASE OF LOWER-EXTREMITY ARTERIES
(Table 2)

Acute embolic occlusions of the aorta and distal arteries must be differentiated from acute thromboses of pre-existent atherosclerotic occlusive lesions. The latter usually occur in patients with antecedent histories suggesting chronic extremity ischemia. Patients with extremity embolism often present acutely with the "five p's": pain, pallor, paresthesias, paralysis, and pulseless extremities. The discomfort and color changes invariably occur distal to the site of occlusion, with collateral vessels affording adequate circulation in the region of the actual arterial obstruction.

Macroembolism is most often due to arteriosclerotic heart disease and associated atrial fibrillation. In this situation, stagnant blood within the upper chamber of the heart may clot and subsequently become dislodged into the circulation. Ventricular aneurysm thrombus and endocardial clot accompanying transmural myocardial infarctions are less common sources of emboli. The site of embolic obstruction is the aorta in 10% of patients, the femoral artery in 40%, and the popliteal artery in 20% of cases. Mortality associated with peripheral arterial embolism ranges from 10 to 15%, usually due directly to the coexisting cardiac disease, not limb ischemia. Treatment involves advancing a Fogarty balloon catheter beyond the embolic occlusion and extracting the obstructing material and associated thrombus. This usually can be accomplished under local anesthesia. Limb salvage is 85 to 90% in these circumstances. In order to lessen the likelihood of recurrent embolism, all patients presenting with acute embolic disease should be immediately anticoagulated with heparin and subsequently maintained on long-term anticoagulant therapy with warfarin (Coumadin).

Atheroembolism is an important second form of extremity embolism. In these individuals, dislodged debris from aneurysms or extensive occlusive lesions becomes entrapped in small distal arteries with diameters of 50 to 200 μm. This frequently causes severe pain and may cause focal cutaneous infarctions. Occasionally a ruborous-blue appearance of a digit occurs due to sluggish capillary blood flow; this is referred to as the "blue toe" syndrome. Treatment of atheroembolism is controversial. Most physicians prescribe antiplatelet agents as a means of lessening recurrent embolism. However, some physicians believe that it impairs the stability of the fibrous cap over soft heterogeneous atheromatous plaques and increases subsequent embolism. If multiple episodes of atheroembolism are associated with tissue loss, then elimination of the embolic source by aneurysmectomy or bypass and exclusion of the offending vessel are justified.

ANEURYSMS OF THE AORTA AND THE FEMORAL AND POPLITEAL ARTERIES
(Table 3)

Aortic aneurysms may be related to acquired or genetic defects in elastin metabolism and collagen cross-linking. Nevertheless, most of these aneurysms exhibit arteriosclerosis. Arteriosclerosis is probably a secondary event in aortic aneurysms, but once present, clearly contributes to further vessel wall weakening. Among these aneurysms, the ascending aorta is involved in 5% of cases, the descending thoracic aorta in 12%, the thoracoabdominal aorta in 2.5%, and the infrarenal aorta in 80%. The iliac arteries are also involved in 20% of the latter lesions. Men are affected four times as often as women.

The diagnosis of an aortic aneurysm should be considered when the lateral aortic pulsations on physical examination or radiographic evidence of calcifications of the aortic walls suggests such a

---

TABLE 2. **Acute Lower-Extremity Embolic Occlusive Disease**

Source of macroemboli: atrial fibrillation 90%
Site of obstruction: femoral artery 40%, popliteal artery 20%, aortic bifurcation 10%
Prophylactic early (heparin) and long-term (warfarin) anticoagulation
10 to 15% mortality from underlying cardiac disease
Treatment: balloon catheter embolectomy with 85–90% limb salvage

TABLE 3. **Aneurysmal Disease**

Aortic Aneurysms

Male:female ratio 4:1

Location: ascending aorta 5%, descending aorta 12%, thoracoabdominal aorta 2.5%, infrarenal abdominal aorta 80%

Associated femoral-popliteal artery aneurysms 2%; associated lower-extremity occlusive disease 20%

Most aneurysms are asymptomatic

Rupture rate of 20–30% over 2–3 yr with 5-cm diameter (emergent operative mortality for ruptured aneurysm: 45–55%)

Treatment: elective aneurysmectomy, 95–98% survival

Femoral Artery Aneurysms

Male patients: bilateral 70%

Associated aortic aneurysms 85%; associated popliteal artery aneurysms 45%

Thrombotic occlusion or distal embolization 15%

Treatment: elective aneurysmectomy and interposition grafting

Popliteal Artery Aneurysms

Male patients: bilateral 45%

Associated aortic aneurysms 60%; associated popliteal artery aneurysms 40%

Thromboembolism resulting in amputation 33%; thrombosis resulting in claudication 33%

Treatment: elective aneurysmectomy or aneurysm exclusion and bypass

---

lesion. In regard to the latter, a lateral abdominal radiograph is more useful than an anteroposterior (AP) abdominal radiograph. Certain imaging studies objectively document the presence and size of an aortic aneurysm. Ultrasonography is currently the best way to screen for these lesions. Computed tomography and magnetic resonance imaging are more costly, but provide additional anatomic information regarding the extent of an aneurysm and involvement of its branches. Arteriography should not be used for diagnosis of an aortic aneurysm. In many cases, intramural thrombus may result in the angiographic appearance of a relatively normal aortic lumen. Arteriography should be restricted to preoperative planning of surgical therapy in these patients.

Most aortic aneurysms are asymptomatic, often recognized as painless pulsatile masses during routine physical examination. With expansion, they may be associated with back or flank pain. Lower-extremity pain is not a manifestation of an uncomplicated aortic aneurysm. However, in 20% of these cases coexistent lower extremity occlusive disease may produce extremity discomfort. Coincidental femoral and popliteal artery aneurysms affect 2% of patients with aortic aneurysms. This generalized form of aneurysmal disease is usually observed in men.

Rupture of aortic aneurysms appears related to size. Aneurysms 5 to 6 cm in diameter carry a 20 to 30% risk of rupture over a 2- to 3-year period, whereas aneurysms greater than 6 cm in diameter have a slightly greater than 40% risk of rupture. Aneurysms 4 cm in diameter may still rupture, but have a less clearly defined natural history. Many 3- to 4-cm aneurysms are followed with serial ultrasonography or some other form of imaging.

Operation is recommended for all aortic aneurysms 5 cm or larger and those whose diameter growth exceeds 4 mm over a 12-month period. Operative treatment usually entails aneurysmectomy and interposition aortic or aortoiliac grafting with a synthetic vascular prosthesis. Surgical mortality for elective treatment of aortic aneurysms is in the 2 to 5% range. Once patients have symptomatic aneurysms, the operative mortality increases to 7 to 15%. The mortality accompanying treatment after rupture ranges from 45 to 55%. Abdominal aortic aneurysmectomy is lifesaving. Those individuals undergoing elective resection have 1-, 3-, and 5-year survival rates of 77%, 64%, and 48%, respectively; individuals not subjected to operative intervention have survival rates at these same time periods of 55%, 30%, and 18%, respectively. Approximately 35% of patients with abdominal aortic aneurysms not subjected to surgical treatment succumb from later aneurysmal rupture.

Femoral artery aneurysms occur almost exclusively in men. The etiology of these aneurysms is poorly defined, but may be related to a collagen cross-link defect. Most femoral artery aneurysms exhibit arteriosclerotic changes, but these are thought to represent a secondary process rather than a cause of these lesions. They usually present as a discreet pulsatile groin mass. Most importantly, 85% of patients with these femoral artery lesions have associated aortic or aortoiliac aneurysms. Femoral artery aneurysms are bilateral in approximately 70% of individuals, and associated popliteal aneurysms occur in 45% of patients. Femoral artery aneurysms rarely rupture but often have large quantities of mural thrombi that in approximately 15% of cases progress to arterial occlusion or result in distal embolization. All femoral artery aneurysms greater than 3 cm in diameter are appropriately treated by excision and arterial reconstruction with interposition synthetic or autologous vein grafts. Smaller aneurysms may be followed cautiously.

Popliteal artery aneurysms are associated with aortic aneurysms in nearly 60% of patients and exhibit concomitant femoral artery aneurysms nearly 40% of the time. Popliteal artery aneurysms are bilateral in 45% of cases. These lesions invariably occur in men. Like other aneurysms, their cause may be linked to a genetic defect in collagen metabolism, although arteriosclerosis is a common histologic finding. Popliteal artery aneurysms are limb threatening, with local thrombosis or distal embolism leading to irreparable tissue injury and amputation in a third of cases. Another third of patients have symptomatic leg and foot occlusive disease. The remaining third are asymptomatic at the time of aneurysm recognition. Rupture is an exceedingly rare complication of a popliteal artery aneurysm. Most of these aneurysms should be treated operatively. Standard surgical care includes an interposition or bypass graft procedure with exclusion of the aneurysm. The latter eliminates subsequent embolic dislodgement of thrombus from the aneurysm. Although femoral and popliteal artery aneurysms are limb threatening but not life-threatening, they are frequently associated with life-threatening abdominal aortic aneurysms.

DEEP VENOUS THROMBOSIS OF THE LOWER EXTREMITIES

method of
JOHN D. CORSON, M.B., Ch.B.
Department of Surgery
The University of Iowa Hospitals and Clinics
Iowa City, Iowa

Deep vein thrombosis (DVT), pulmonary embolism, and the postphlebitic syndrome are major health problems that can be reduced by DVT prophylaxis. Because a variety of different patient populations are at risk of developing DVT and its complications, prophylaxis should be a priority for all physicians regardless of their specialty. Surprisingly prophylaxis is still underused despite the availability of effective methods for DVT prevention.

ETIOLOGY

Usually several factors play a role in development of DVT. The observation made by Virchow in 1856 that the slowing of the bloodstream was an etiologic factor for DVT remains an important concept. Hypercoagulability and venous endothelial injury are other factors of etiologic significance.

Patients with decreased mobility are at increased risk of developing DVT. A paraplegic patient or a person with a paralyzed or immobilized limb is at increased risk for the development of DVT, as are bedridden medical patients, especially those with congestive heart failure, stroke, or a hypercoagulable state. Although all surgical patients are at risk of DVT, it has become clear that certain patients are at higher risk than others (Table 1). Additional factors may further increase the DVT incidence in the moderate-risk group. Elderly patients with hip fractures and the increasing number of individuals undergoing hip or knee prosthetic replacement are a large, high-risk group for developing DVT.

In association with venous stasis, activation of blood coagulation occurs after trauma or surgery. A small number of patients who develop DVT have a primary hypercoagulable disorder, which is usually an inherited abnormality of a single component of the hemostatic system. These patients usually present with the onset of one or more well-documented thromboembolic events before the age of 35 and also have a family history of idiopathic thromboembolism or intrauterine fetal demise. Patients with primary hypercoagulability often have an unusual location or presentation of their venous thrombosis. These patients may be refractory to conventional treatment or develop early recurrences after discontinuation of prolonged oral anticoagulant therapy. These primary hypercoagulable states include antithrombin III deficiency, protein C or S deficiency, dysplasminogenemia, hypoplasminogenemia, homocystinuria, or the presence of lupus anticoagulant. Patients with erythrocytosis, thrombocytosis, or paraproteinemia with hyperviscosity are also at an increased risk. Most commonly, a hypercoagulable state is secondary to a general condition, such as pregnancy or malignancy. In such conditions, the cause of the hypercoagulable state is multifactorial and not related to a specific single abnormality. In pregnancy, there are hormonal changes associated with increased blood viscosity as well as impaired flow in the pelvic veins owing to compression by the enlarged uterus. The association between venous thromboembolism and estrogen-containing oral contraceptives is well known. The use of lower-dose estrogen preparations decreases the risk of DVT. The degree of risk for DVT while on oral contraceptives is, however, less clearly defined but is higher than with other forms of contraception.

Patients with neoplasms who are undergoing major abdominal or gynecologic surgical procedures are at high risk for DVT. Patients with adenocarcinoma seem to be especially vulnerable, possibly because mucinous tumors secrete extracts that activate Factor X or because of chronic, low-grade intravascular coagulation; depressed levels of protein C; or elevated levels of fibrin monomer. Chemotherapeutic agents may further increase the risk of DVT in persons with a malignancy. The high incidence of DVT in these patients may be secondary to hematologic or vascular changes, decreased mobility, or dehydration. Other debilitated patients, such as those with active inflammatory bowel disease, are also at increased risk for DVT.

Endothelial injury from direct venous trauma or intravenous infusion of a sclerotic agent may cause DVT. Endothelial tears have been noted to occur in veins secondary to venodilatation caused by various anesthetic agents. The exact clinical significance of these findings has not yet been determined. Regional anesthesia may be associated with less risk of DVT and should be used if possible when a patient is judged to be at high risk for DVT.

A history of DVT is associated with an increased risk for a new venous thrombosis, especially in the previously affected extremity, probably owing to endothelial damage, venous obstruction, or incomplete recanalization. Additionally, the initial risk factors for DVT may be unchanged.

TABLE 1. **Risk Categories in Surgical Patients**

Risk Category	Risk of Venous Thromboembolism (Assessed by Objective Tests)		
	Calf-Vein Thrombosis (%)	Proximal Vein Thrombosis (%)	Fatal Pulmonary Embolism (%)
High risk	40–80	10–30	1–5
General and urologic surgery in patients over 40 years with recent history of DVT or PE			
Extensive pelvic or abdominal surgery for malignant disease			
Major orthopedic surgery of lower limbs			
Moderate risk	0–40	2–10	0.1–0.7
General surgery in patients over 40 years lasting 30 minutes or more and in patients below 40 years on oral contraceptives			
Low risk	<10	<1	<0.01
Uncomplicated surgery in patients under 40 years without additional risk factors			
Minor surgery (i.e., less than 30 min in patients over 40 years without additional risk factors			

DVT = deep venous thrombosis; PE = pulmonary embolism. From Nicolaides AN, et al: Prevention of venous thromboembolism. Int Angiol 2:151–159, 1992.

PREVENTION

DVT is a preventable disease, and despite recommendations for the prevention of DVT, apathy and skepticism among the medical community remain concerning the use and benefits of prophylactic regimens. Significant mortality and morbidity could be averted both by maintaining a high index of suspicion for the early diagnosis of DVT and by the appropriate use of venous prophylaxis. One recent study found that only 32% of patients at risk for DVT received any form of venous prophylaxis. This finding may partly be explained by the individual physician's infrequent exposure to a patient with a fatal pulmonary embolus and the perceived high risk of bleeding complications with the use of antithrombotic drugs for prophylaxis. It should be stressed that although the use of antithrombotic drugs for prophylaxis is associated with an increased incidence of postoperative hematomas and other bleeding complications, major hemorrhagic events are uncommon.

The recognition and stratification of DVT risk is the key to successful DVT prophylaxis. A patient-oriented approach for risk assessment, as shown for surgical patients in Table 1, is a satisfactory scheme for clinical use. These risks have been more fully evaluated and studied in surgical rather than medical patients.

A combination of prophylactic techniques can often be used. Measures to avoid venous stasis are important. Encouragement to dorsiflex the feet actively while resting with the limbs elevated when in bed limits venous stasis. Early mobilization, which means that the patient walks actively on a regular basis, is an important and inexpensive form of prophylaxis. Graduated compression stockings should be worn. Sitting passively in a chair for long periods of time should be avoided. A combination of simple measures such as leg elevation and support stockings has been shown to provide benefit and provide adequate prophylaxis in low-risk patients.

Subcutaneous, small, fixed doses of heparin have been shown to be effective in significantly reducing the risk of DVT and work by augmenting the antithrombotic effect of antithrombin III. This prophylactic method has been used successfully in medical patients with acute myocardial infarction, congestive heart failure, and paralysis owing to thrombotic stroke. This regimen has also been shown to be beneficial in patients undergoing general, thoracic, or gynecologic operations. In contrast, the use of fixed-dose heparin for patients with orthopedic conditions has been disappointing; it does not reduce the incidence of DVT to an acceptable clinical level. There is no need to monitor the level of inhibition of the activated partial thromboplastin time (APTT) when using subcutaneous low fixed-dose heparin for prophylaxis. An adjusted-dose heparin regimen that maintains an APTT of 1.3 to 1.5 times control (adjusted-dose heparin) has been shown to be effective prophylaxis in orthopedic and other high-risk patients.

Fractionated heparins (low-molecular-weight heparins ([LMWHs] [Normiflo]) and heparinoids appear to have significant promise because they seem to be more effective than unfractionated heparin for prophylaxis. Also, they appear to have therapeutic benefit for venous prophylaxis even in high-risk patients.

Low-molecular-weight dextran has been shown

to be beneficial for DVT prophylaxis by lowering blood viscosity and inhibiting platelet aggregation. The large volume of fluid infused, however, is frequently a limiting factor, especially in patients with recent myocardial ischemia or pre-existing congestive failure.

Oral anticoagulants are another alternative for prophylaxis in high-risk general surgical and orthopedic patients. There is an increased incidence, however, of major bleeding when warfarin is begun preoperatively. The patient's inability to take warfarin postoperatively limits its use for prophylaxis in high-risk abdominal surgery patients and other patients undergoing procedures in whom oral intake may be unpredictable. Additionally, there is the need for close monitoring of the prothrombin time in these patients. "Mini-dose" warfarin begun a few weeks before an elective operation may be an alternative method of successful prophylaxis for low-risk or moderate-risk patients. "Low-dose" warfarin may be used for moderate-risk or high-risk patients. Yet another alternative approach is "two-step" warfarin therapy, in which a small dose is given preoperatively and is then increased postoperatively as the risk of bleeding decreases. The various drugs and regimens useful for DVT prophylaxis are listed in Table 2.

If there is any increased risk of bleeding or when anticoagulation is contraindicated after neurosurgical or ophthalmic surgery, alternative methods of prophylaxis must be used. Intermittent pneumatic compression (IPC) is as effective as the use of fixed-dose heparin in moderate-risk patients. Activation of the fibrinolytic system by IPC may be of more benefit than improving venous efflux from the extremity. Attention to details in the use of these devices is important, as also is nursing and patient compliance. Patients in intensive care units and trauma, urologic, or neurosurgical patients seem well suited to this form of prophylaxis. IPC devices may also be used to augment prophylaxis in high-risk patients who are also on a prophylactic drug regimen. Although uncomfortable to wear, IPC devices have no significant complications.

DIAGNOSIS

An accurate initial diagnosis of DVT is extremely important. The mislabeling of a patient as having DVT may have significant implications in regards to future treatment or prophylaxis. In women, it may influence therapeutic decisions during pregnancy or the puerperium or when considering estrogen use for contraception or postmenopausal symptoms. In addition, clinicians should be concerned about the risks associated with the use of anticoagulants, which may further escalate if invasive therapy is recommended after a bleeding complication. These risks cannot be justified if the diagnosis of DVT is incorrect. In addition, a number of conditions may be worsened by the indiscriminate use of anticoagulation to treat "suspected DVT" without first confirming the diagnosis with objective noninvasive testing. A patient with a tender, painful, swollen calf owing to an intramuscular hemorrhage may respond poorly to anticoagulation and may develop major and avoidable complications. Hence objective noninvasive vascular diagnostic testing is mandatory before a patient is treated for suspected DVT.

The clinical diagnosis of DVT lacks specificity and has a low sensitivity. Equivalent diagnostic accuracy can be provided by the flip of a coin. Physical signs of swelling, pain, and erythema are notoriously unreliable. The signs of Louvel, Mose, Lisker, Lowenberg, Peabody, and Homan are of historical interest, but they have no prac-

TABLE 2. **Optional Drug Regimens for the Prevention of Venous Thromboembolism in Patients at Risk**

Agent	Administration	Comments
Heparin		
"Fixed" dose	10,000–15,000 U subcutaneously daily divided into bid or tid dosages	Low- or moderate-risk patients
"Adjusted" dose	Subcutaneous heparin given bid or tid, adjusted to keep APTT:	
	32–36 s (high-normal range) *or* 1.3–1.5 × control	High-risk patients Hip surgery patients
Warfarin (Coumadin)		
"Mini" dose	1 mg daily starting 3 weeks before surgery	Low- or moderate-risk patients
"Low" dose	Sufficient dose to achieve PT of 1.3–1.5 × control	Moderate- or high-risk patients
Two-step	Preoperatively: Sufficient dose to increase PT up to 3 s Immediately postoperatively: Raise dose to increase PT to 1.5 × control	High-risk patients

APTT = activated partial thromboplastin time; PT = prothrombin time. Modified from Rakel RE (ed): Conn's Current Therapy 1992. Philadelphia, WB Saunders Co, 1992, p 291.

tical value in the modern era. A careful history and physical examination, however, may elucidate another cause for the patient's leg symptoms, such as cellulitis, hematoma, or a Baker's cyst, thus obviating the need for further diagnostic venous studies.

In contrast to DVT, superficial thrombophlebitis presents as a tender, reddened, indurated cord over the involved superficial vein. It is a common complication of varicose veins. Superficial thrombophlebitis can usually be treated symptomatically with an oral anti-inflammatory agent. These patients do not require bed rest or anticoagulation unless there is associated DVT. Patients with superficial thrombophlebitis should undergo a noninvasive duplex study to exclude associated DVT and to assess the extent and level of thrombotic involvement of the superficial vein. Serial noninvasive studies are helpful in monitoring any progression of superficial thrombophlebitis with extension into the deep venous system. Patients without varicose veins, who have episodic bouts of superficial thrombophlebitis, should be evaluated further to exclude an underlying condition, such as Behçet's syndrome, Buerger's disease, a hypercoagulopathy, or a paraneoplastic syndrome.

The standard for the diagnosis of DVT has been ascending phlebography. It is highly accurate provided that the study is technically adequate and strict diagnostic criteria are adhered to. Phlebography provides equal sensitivity and specificity at both the calf and the thigh levels. It is, however, invasive, expensive, associated with occasional serious contrast allergy problems, and, in a small percentage of patients, it is a cause of DVT. Physiologic, noninvasive tests are appealing because they do not have the aforementioned problems of phlebography. Impedance plethysmography, phleborheography, and Doppler techniques have some limitations, however. Although these techniques are reliable and highly accurate for the diagnosis of symptomatic occlusive thrombi in the deep veins above the knee, they miss nonocclusive thrombi or thrombi in duplicate veins. They are unreliable for the diagnosis of thrombi in calf veins, and unfortunately these techniques provide no information on the location and extent of thrombosis. They are not useful for DVT surveillance in high-risk patients.

Color duplex scanning is emerging as the standard diagnostic technology for DVT and has largely replaced ascending phlebography and the other noninvasive physiologic tests. A real-time, color-coded, Doppler flow map is superimposed on the B-mode image and provides a two-dimensional image of the tissue being studied. For above-knee thrombi, the sensitivity and specificity approach 100%. B-mode imaging may be diffi-

cult to use over the iliac veins. Hence Doppler-derived flow patterns in the proximal veins are important to aid in the diagnosis of occlusive thrombi above the inguinal ligament. Duplex scanning can also diagnose nonocclusive thrombi, which previously might have gone undetected. Color flow significantly facilitates examinations of calf veins. A sensitivity of 94% and a specificity of 81% have been reported for symptomatic patients with thrombi in calf veins, and a sensitivity of 78% and a specificity of 96% have been reported for asymptomatic patients with calf vein thrombi. Portable duplex units can be easily taken to critical care areas if the patient is not able to be transported to the vascular laboratory. A well-trained, experienced technologist is essential to achieve results with a high sensitivity and specificity, especially for the diagnosis of thrombi in the calf veins.

Computed tomography and magnetic resonance imaging studies can detect venous thrombi, especially when they occur in unusual locations. Future studies will help define their clinical role. It is unlikely that they will replace color duplex scanning for lower extremity DVT diagnosis.

TREATMENT

Once the diagnosis of DVT is confirmed by objective testing, treatment must be tailored to the requirements of each patient and depends on a variety of factors, including the ability to use anticoagulants safely, any history of thromboembolic problems, the presence of co-morbid conditions, and the site and extent of the DVT. Patients should initially be placed at bed rest, and the lower limbs should be elevated. The patient begins to ambulate once symptoms subside. External support to the limb with carefully applied Ace wraps that may be adjusted throughout the day as needed should be provided. A customized, graduated compression stocking is not fitted until the swelling of the limb stabilizes, which is usually when the patient is seen as an outpatient a couple of weeks after discharge.

The mainstay of treatment is anticoagulation. Aggressive treatment is required to avert the early complication of PE and the late complication of the postphlebitic syndrome. The following regimen provides immediate protection against thromboembolism and minimizes the risk of DVT recurrence. An intravenous bolus of heparin is given at a dose of 100 units per kg of body weight and is followed by a continuous infusion starting at 1000 units per hour and continued for at least 7 to 10 days. The APTT is checked 4 to 6 hours after the initial bolus dose. The aim of the continuous heparin infusion is to keep the APTT 1.5 to 2 times control. Heparin requirements may vary depending on the weight, age, and nutritional status of the patient and the extent of the thromboembolic process. Traditionally warfarin (Coumadin), in a starting oral dose of 10 mg per day for two days, is initiated after 5 days of heparin therapy. The warfarin dose is adjusted by the results of the one-stage prothrombin time. The heparin is continued until a therapeutic warfarin dose is found. Oral anticoagulants should be continued for at least 3 to 6 months depending on the extent of the DVT and the presence of risk factors. Accurate dosing with warfarin requires some experience because the anticoagulant effect of warfarin is delayed. Older patients, those with hepatic insufficiency, and those with vitamin K depletion are more sensitive to warfarin. The dose is monitored by the one-stage prothrombin time, and the goal is to maintain an international normalized ratio (INR) between 2.0 and 3.0. Nomograms may be helpful to facilitate accurate oral anticoagulation dosing. In an effort to shorten hospitalization, it has been suggested that warfarin could be started within 48 hours of the onset of heparin therapy, which should be continued for at least 5 days. This method has become our preferred approach recently. Theoretical arguments against this approach include the risk of propagation of a poorly adherent thrombus owing to a suboptimal heparin dose because warfarin also elevates the APTT. Also, "therapeutic" prothrombin times may be obtained after a few days, while the patient remains at risk of thrombosis because of continued elevation of intrinsic pathway clotting factors. Additionally, one of the earliest effects of warfarin is to decrease proteins C and S, thereby promoting extension of thrombus. Recent comparative studies suggest that these are theoretical rather than practical problems. Significant cost savings can be achieved by starting warfarin early. This method also shortens the total duration of heparin infusion and hence may reduce the incidence of heparin-related complications.

Before initiating anticoagulant therapy, baseline prothrombin time and APTT studies should be obtained. Abnormal prolongation of either or both of these studies suggests the need for a more extensive hematologic work-up. An elevated APTT suggests either an abnormality of the intrinsic pathway or the presence of a circulating anticoagulant. This can make heparin dosing unreliable unless either thrombin times or plasma heparin levels are used. Occasional patients may develop signs of heparin resistance. A consultation with a hematologist or vascular surgeon is valuable when heparin resistance is found because serious sequelae may develop unless appropriate action is taken. Platelet counts should be monitored every 48 to 72 hours during heparin therapy to detect the development of heparin-induced thrombocytopenia (HIT), which can result in serious thrombotic problems. The HIT syndrome should be suspected in any patient whose platelet count falls to 50% of the baseline value. Heparin therapy should be discontinued once a diagnosis of HIT is made.

Patients with isolated calf vein thrombosis (CVT) are a special group and are being diagnosed more frequently owing to the increased use of color duplex scanning for DVT diagnosis. Most patients with CVT can be treated conservatively and followed using serial noninvasive testing. Anticoagulation can be given to those individuals who demonstrate propagation of clot or evidence of pulmonary embolism. This recommendation is based on a review of 735 patients with isolated CVT, in whom the frequency of thrombotic propagation and pulmonary embolism are 10% and 3.4% in those patients not treated with anticoagulants and 5.6% and 2.3% in patients administered anticoagulants. If a patient with CVT cannot undergo serial noninvasive studies, he or she should be fully anticoagulated for at least 6 weeks. Recurrent DVT presenting as CVT should be treated with full anticoagulation.

When a patient has recurrent DVT, it is important to check on patient compliance and make sure sufficient medication has been taken to maintain an appropriate level of anticoagulation. Patients with underlying hypercoagulopathy secondary to disease states, such as malignancy, which place them at continued risk for DVT, are best managed by long-term oral anticoagulation, unless the risk of bleeding exceeds the risk of recurrent DVT. One recurrent episode of thromboembolism should be treated with anticoagulants for 1 year, unless there is a serious underlying disease increasing DVT risk and necessitating lifetime anticoagulation. Patients with more than one recurrent episode may require lifetime anticoagulation.

Fractionated heparins (LMWHs) and heparinoids appear to have some potential patient benefits for DVT treatment owing to less thrombocytopenia and an improved antithrombotic to hemorrhagic ratio. They are as effective and safe as a continuous infusion of unfractionated heparin for the treatment of established DVT and can be given in a once-daily dose subcutaneously, which opens up the possibility of treating DVT on an outpatient basis. It is anticipated that these agents will eventually be available in the United States if further studies validate the current available data.

Pregnant patients, patients with DVT recurrence or embolus despite adequate documented

TABLE 3. Indications for Insertion of a Vena Caval Filter

Absolute Indications

DVT or documented thromboembolism in a patient who has a contraindication to anticoagulation

Recurrent thromboembolism despite adequate anticoagulation

Complications of anticoagulation forcing therapy to be discontinued

Immediately after pulmonary embolectomy

Failure of another form of caval interruption demonstrated by recurrent thromboembolism

Relative Indications

High-risk patients with a large free-floating iliofemoral thrombus demonstrated on venography

Patient with a propagating iliofemoral thrombus despite adequate anticoagulation

Chronic pulmonary embolism in a patient with pulmonary hypertension and cor pulmonale

Patient who has more than 50% of the pulmonary vascular bed occluded and who would not tolerate any additional thrombus

Presence of recurrent septic embolism

From Greenfield LJ, Whitehill TA: New developments in caval interruption: Current indications and new techniques for filter placement. *In* Veith FJ (ed): Current Critical Problems in Vascular Surgery, Vol 4. St. Louis, Quality Medical Publishing, Inc, 1992, pp 113–121.

therapeutic anticoagulation, patients who cannot get their prothrombin time monitored to adjust warfarin dosage, or those who cannot take warfarin can be treated by subcutaneous heparin given every 12 hours to maintain an APTT 1.5 to 2 times control when measured 6 hours after injection. Once the correct dosage is found, the patient does not need to be monitored by an APTT except during pregnancy, when the dosage requirements may change.

DVT patients who were previously refractory to anticoagulation or in whom anticoagulation was contraindicated used to be treated surgically by the use of a variety of techniques involving ligation, plication, or sieving the vena cava. These techniques, however, were associated with significant morbidity and have been superseded by transvenous filter placement. Long-term experience with a transvenous stainless steel filter developed by Greenfield has shown this device to be associated with limited morbidity, excellent long-term caval patency, and a low incidence of pulmonary embolization. This device is usually placed in the vena cava just below the renal veins. Occasionally suprarenal or superior vena caval placement may be required. Currently a variety of newer percutaneously directed caval

devices are being studied. The titanium Greenfield filter with modified hook, which can be introduced through a No. 12 French carrier-catheter, is currently our preferred device. Indications for vena caval filter placement are listed in Table 3. The availability of newer percutaneous devices may prompt expansion of the indications for filter placement beyond those listed, especially for prophylaxis in high-risk patients. Further studies are needed to determine the wisdom of altering the indications for filter placement. Anticoagulation should, if possible, be continued in patients who require a filter in the presence of DVT so that the incidence of post-thrombotic complications may be lowered.

Iliofemoral venous thrombectomy, although popular in Europe, is rarely used in the United States. In an attempt to reduce an unacceptably high rethrombosis rate, a femoral arteriovenous fistula is now fashioned at the completion of venous thrombectomy to maintain venous patency. The use of venous thrombectomy in the United States is mainly reserved for patients with phlegmasia cerulea dolens who fail to show clinical improvement on standard therapy.

Systemic intravenous thrombolysis has been suggested as therapy for recent lower extremity DVT to recanalize the occluded deep veins rapidly and preserve valvular function. Young patients with recently diagnosed proximal DVT may be suitable candidates for systemic thrombolysis. Data confirming the ability of thrombolysis to preserve valvular function, however, are limited. Additionally, patients with significant clot in the iliofemoral system, especially those with phlegmasia cerulea dolens who are at danger of limb loss, may benefit from thrombolytic therapy given directly into the venous thrombus via a catheter. A transjugular approach is preferred.

Patient education is important to limit the late lower extremity sequelae of DVT. A customized stocking should be fitted and used long term and always renewed when wearing out. Early treatment of venous stasis ulceration may obviate significant later problems.

Recent studies suggest that a patient's increased risk of DVT will continue for up to a month following hospital discharge after surgery. Hence further continuation of venous prophylaxis should be considered in all high-risk patients after they leave the acute care hospital.

Section 5

The Blood and Spleen

APLASTIC ANEMIA

method of
JOEL M. RAPPEPORT, M.D.
Yale University School of Medicine
New Haven, Connecticut

Aplastic anemia is characterized by peripheral blood pancytopenia and hypocellular bone marrow depleted of hematopoietic progenitors. The disorder is heterogeneous in both severity and etiology and may have at different times in its course variable degrees of neutropenia, thrombocytopenia, and anemia with reticulocytopenia. Aplastic anemia occurs in both females and males of any age, with an estimated 1000 to 2000 new cases seen in the United States yearly. Since treatment options differ, it is important to establish whether the patient's disorder is congenital or acquired. The two most common congenital forms are Fanconi's aplastic anemia and dyskeratosis congenita. Onset of aplasia may not occur in these syndromes until late adolescence or early adulthood.

Various etiologic factors have been associated with aplastic anemia, only some of which have a clear relationship. Idiosyncratic drug reactions are seen with chloramphenicol, sulfonamides, anticonvulsants, phenylbutazone, and gold, among others. While most chemotherapeutic agents cause pancytopenia, only a few, including the nitrosoureas and busulfans, result in irreversible aplasia. A number of infections have been implicated in the etiology of aplasia, including hepatitis types A, B, C, and non-A, non-B, non-C. Aplasia can complicate hepatitis of varying severity, including asymptomatic cases, and usually occurs as the clinical syndrome is resolving. A few cases have followed infectious mononucleosis. Marked pancytopenia is noted in patients with acquired immunodeficiency virus (AIDS), but whether this aplasia is associated with the human immunodeficiency virus (HIV) or some combination of viruses and therapy is unclear. A variety of environmental toxins and chemicals, including benzene-containing compounds and insecticides, used both in industry and the home have been linked with impaired hematopoiesis. Significant irradiation of the bone marrow can result in aplastic anemia in circumstances in which the total hematopoietic compartment is exposed; reversibility is related to the total dose of exposure. A curious relationship exists between the rare clonal disorder paroxysmal nocturnal hemoglobinuria (PNH) and aplastic anemia, with 20 to 30% of patients with PNH developing aplastic anemia, while 10 to 20% of patients with long-standing aplastic anemia subsequently develop PNH.

The pathophysiology of aplastic anemia involves three phenomena, the most frequent of which is a loss of pluripotential hematopoietic stem cells. Secondly, pluripotential stem cells may be present but unable to differentiate. Finally, microenvironmental defects may exist whereby normal hematopoiesis cannot be supported. These defects may include abnormalities in stromal cells, decreased production of growth factors, and immunologically mediated hematopoietic suppression. The assignment of one of these processes to a given case is both difficult and time consuming, although identification may aid in determining appropriate therapy. Since hematopoiesis is usually re-established following marrow transplantation, the frequency of stromal defects is probably low. In most patients measurable growth factors are elevated, and therefore growth factor deficiency is not common. However, one must reserve judgment about as yet unknown growth factors that influence the hematopoietic pleuripotential stem cell. Finally, a large body of data supports the concept of immune suppression of hematopoiesis being operative in a significant number of cases.

DIAGNOSIS AND LABORATORY FEATURES

Prompt establishment of the correct diagnosis is an essential element of treatment. Aplastic anemia is a pancytopenia with variably decreased peripheral blood cellular elements. The total white cell count can be low or normal, but the absolute granulocyte count is always decreased, sometimes to zero. On the other hand, the lymphocyte number may be normal. The platelet count is also reduced. Anemia is present, with normochromic, often macrocytic red blood cells, reflecting stress erythropoiesis. The *corrected* reticulocyte count is inappropriately low. Bone marrow aspiration often yields a "dry tap," but biopsy reveals markedly diminished to absent hematopoietic cells without evidence of an infiltrative process of either hematopoietic or nonhematopoietic origin. Empty stroma and fat are noted. The myeloid and megakaryocytic lines are most severely affected, with occasional niduses of erythropoiesis present. Residual eosinophils, mast cells, plasma cells, and lymphocytes may be noted.

Of importance from both a prognostic and therapeutic point of view is the differentiation of mild aplastic anemia from severe aplasia. In severe aplastic anemia, any two of the following three parameters are present: neutrophils below 500×10^9 per liter, platelets below 20×10^9, and a corrected reticulocyte count of less than 1%. In severe aplasia the bone marrow biopsy is markedly hypocellular with less than 25% cellularity. Patients with aplastic anemia must be closely watched, since the patient's disease may change from mild to severe aplasia and vice versa. The blood count is monitored as an indication of the response to therapeutic interventions. HLA typing of the patient and family should be undertaken not only for possible bone marrow transplantation, but also for platelet transfusion, should alloimmunization occur.

CLINICAL FEATURES

The clinical features of aplastic anemia are a direct consequence of the pancytopenia. Anemia results in increasing fatigue and pallor. Thrombocytopenia can present as petechiae and purpura and can cause epistaxis, bleeding from the gums, and menorrhagia. Fever and sepsis are associated with neutropenia, and infectious complications become increasingly important during the course of the illness. Lymphadenopathy and hepatosplenomegaly are not usually present. Patients with mild aplastic anemia may have no symptoms other than fatigue, whereas repeated life-threatening hemorrhages and infectious complications mark the course of severe aplastic anemia. Patients with severe aplasia may have a rapid fulminate course resulting in death in weeks to months; patients with mild aplasia can have a protracted course over years. Long-term survivors may have to face the consequences of iron overload from frequent red cell transfusions as well as an increased risk of a myelodysplastic syndrome, acute nonlymphocytic leukemia, or paroxysmal nocturnal hemoglobinuria.

TREATMENT

Aplastic anemia is a hematologic emergency that requires both general and specific therapeutic interventions. In the arena of general therapy, the following measures should be instituted. At presentation, the patient's hematologic status should be determined. Exposure to potential etiologic agents must be immediately stopped. In the case of mild aplasia, a course of watchful waiting with the hope of spontaneous recovery may be most appropriate.

Judicious blood transfusion is the mainstay of therapy. Initial transfusions can influence the ultimate outcome, either by alloimmunizing the patient to future platelet transfusions or by enhancing graft rejection in a marrow transplant. The patient's serologic status for cytomegalovirus (CMV) should be determined; if negative, only CMV-negative blood products should be transfused. The need for platelet transfusions should be determined by the patient's clinical status as well as the platelet count. Should the patient become alloimmunized to random platelet transfusions, HLA-matched platelets should be administered. If at all possible, family-derived platelets should be avoided if bone marrow transplantation is under consideration. Transfused erythrocytes and platelets should be leukocyte depleted. Currently, there are extremely few indications for granulocyte transfusions.

Other preventive measures include suppression of menses in females to prevent life-threatening menorrhagia. Avoidance of exposure to infection should be attempted, particularly by patients with severe neutropenia. Protocols vary from center to center, but attention should be paid to mouth care, adherence to a low-bacteria diet, and avoidance of exposure to respiratory infections. Prophylactic antibiotics remain controversial. Fever should be managed aggressively with careful examination, adequate cultures, and broad-spectrum therapy until a specific organism is identified.

Hematopoietic Growth Factors

Specific therapeutic interventions to restore hematopoiesis include (1) stimulation of residual bone marrow with androgens or a variety of lymphokines, (2) immunosuppressive therapy, and (3) bone marrow transplantation.

A variety of androgens have been administered in an attempt to increase hematopoiesis. While patients with mild aplasia may respond to androgen therapy, controlled randomized studies have demonstrated no effect in severe aplastic anemia.

Trials of recombinant growth factors have been undertaken, most often with granulocyte colony-stimulating factor (G-CSF) and granulocyte-macrophage colony-stimulating factor (GM-CSF). In pharmacologic doses, G-CSF can increase circulating granulocytes and monocytes, particularly in patients with residual hematopoiesis, but little to no effect is noted on platelet or red cell production. Similar responses are seen with GM-CSF. In both cases the responses last only as long as the drug is administered; there is little long-term effect on the course of aplastic anemia. In combination with antibiotics, these agents may be of use in the treatment of infectious complications.

Utilizing knowledge of normal hematopoiesis, clinical trials are currently under way of combinations of growth factors and of growth factors that might be effective in stimulating more primitive progenitors.

Immunosuppressive Therapy

A variety of immunosuppressive therapies have improved the overall survival of patients with severe aplastic anemia. The biologic agents antilymphocyte globulin (ALG) and antithymocyte globulin have improved survival from approximately 20% to 35 to 75%, but only a few patients achieve complete recovery. Experience with these agents is important given their unique immediate and long-term side effects. Cyclosporine alone or in combination with ALG is effective. Some patients failing to respond to one immunosuppressive drug may respond to another. Responses may take weeks to months, and patients must be adequately supported during this period. Some patients who have had recurrence of disease following an initial response have responded to subsequent courses of immunosuppression. While conventional doses of corticosteroids are ineffective and deleterious, high-dose methylprednisolone in the range of 20 mg per kg per day has been effective.

Bone Marrow Transplantation

The definitive treatment in most cases of severe aplastic anemia is replacement of absent or defective hematopoietic stem cells through bone marrow grafting. When the donor is an HLA identical sibling, engraftment can be achieved in most cases. However, overall survival is related to clinical status, transfusion history, and patient age (80% of untransfused patients younger than 19 years old are long-term survivors, compared with 40% of patients older than 30 years). Transfusion prior to transplantation adversely affects success, and therefore initial consideration of transplantation is critical. Unlike other therapeutic maneuvers, bone marrow transplantation can achieve complete correction of hematopoiesis; however, deaths can occur from transplant-related complications. For patients without an HLA-identical sibling donor, transplantation can be performed with marrow from one-antigen–mismatched family members. Although some success has been achieved, an increased incidence of graft rejection has been noted. Similarly, transplantation of tissue from matched unrelated donors identified from donor registries has been less successful, but this may in part be due to the length of time necessary to identify the donor. As registered donors increase and searches become more efficient, success rates should improve. At present, bone marrow transplantation is the definitive treatment for appropriate patients with severe aplastic anemia, and initial evaluation and treatment of the patient must be undertaken with this in mind.

IRON DEFICIENCY ANEMIA
method of
CRAIG S. KITCHENS, M.D.
University of Florida
Gainesville, Florida

Iron deficiency anemia is a global problem but is found primarily in developing nations due to the shortage of iron-rich food and the high incidence of gastrointestinal blood loss from parasites. Iron deficiency anemia in the United States affects 0.2% of adult men, 2% of postmenopausal women, and 3% of premenopausal women.

Iron deficiency is more common in pediatric practice. Because both human and cow's milk contain inadequate amounts of iron, infants can easily become iron deficient. This can be prevented by iron supplementation. A "physiologic" form of iron deficiency can develop during the period of rapid growth in adolescence.

In adults, iron deficiency anemia is not a specific diagnostic entity, but rather a manifestation of some underlying clinical situation that causes blood loss, chiefly through the gastrointestinal or genitourinary tract. As these underlying conditions may be extremely serious, adults with iron deficiency anemia require a thorough diagnostic work-up.

Body iron is carefully maintained by a stingy homeostatic system (Figure 1). Life depends on iron, yet excessive iron can be detrimental. The average man has 3500 to 4500 mg of total body iron, the majority (2500 mg) of which circulates in the form of hemoglobulin, leaving 1000 to 2000 mg stored in the reticuloendothelial system (RES). Women have a smaller amount of storage iron and consequently less total body iron. Very small amounts of iron (4 mg) circulate in the plasma in the form of transferrin, which is normally 30 to 40% saturated with iron. This transport molecule shuttles iron between nascent red cells in the bone marrow and body stores. Transferrin turns over its load of iron several times a day. Ferritin is in equilibrium with RES iron; and levels parallel the quantity of stored iron. Small amounts of iron are also contained in a more steady state in either myoglobin (250 mg) or respiratory enzymes (10 mg). Approximately 20 cc of effete red cells are degraded daily in the RES, and iron from the released hemoglobin is extremely efficiently cannibalized by the RES. In turn, an equal amount of iron is deposited daily into 20 cc of newly developed red cells. This represents iron equilibrium. If red cells are lost in other ways, such as with blood donation, menstruation, hemorrhage, or intravascular hemolysis, that iron is lost from the system.

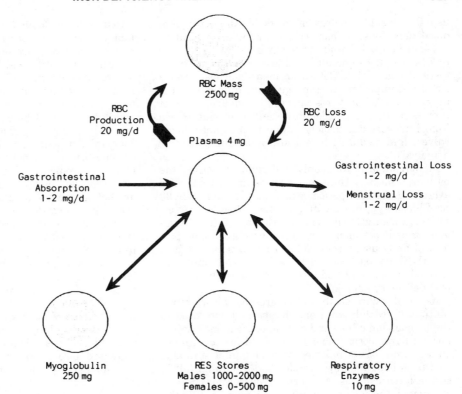

Figure 1. Iron homeostasis. *Abbreviations:* RBC = red blood cells; RES = reticuloendothelial system.

Normally, 1 to 2 mg per day of iron are lost, the majority from shedding of normal cells from the gastrointestinal tract, with smaller amounts from the genitourinary tract and skin. Women additionally lose 30 cc of red cells through menstruation, representing an additional 1 mg per day of iron loss. Balancing these losses is the iron gained from food. The average American daily diet contains 10 to 20 mg of iron. The gastrointestinal system is rather inefficient in absorbing iron; only about 10% is absorbed in normal situations, representing 1 to 2 mg of iron absorption per day.

Understanding this homeostatic system is important in the diagnosis and management of iron deficiency anemia. Physiologic iron loss is balanced precariously by an equal gain from gastrointestinal absorption. However, absorption of dietary iron cannot keep pace with greater blood loss; which explains why storage iron and total body iron are higher in males and non-menstruating females than in menstruating females. Delivery of a full-term infant depletes a woman of an additional 250 to 300 mg of iron. Because pregnant women lose iron to the growing fetus and have such limited iron stores, iron supplementation is generally prescribed during pregnancy.

Physiologic iron absorption from the gastrointestinal tract requires adequate stomach acid and a normal mucosal surface at the site of iron absorption, namely the upper small intestine. Surgical operations that decrease gastric acidity can result in both continued blood loss and decreased iron absorption. Additionally, the Bilroth II operation decreases anatomic sites of iron absorption.

Such a tightly regulated homeostatic system allows little margin for perturbation. Accordingly, small, slow, but persistent leakage of blood frequently results in profound iron deficiency over time. Gross hematuria, hematachezia, menometrorraghia, hematemesis, and melena are easily identified as primary causes of acute blood loss anemia; however, if not corrected, they can also result in iron deficiency anemia. More subtle is the iron deficiency from microscopic hematuria or daily loss of blood in the gastrointestinal tract in amounts too small to cause either melena or a positive stool guaiac test (most such tests for occult blood do not become positive until at least 5 cc to as much as 20 cc of blood are lost daily from the gastrointestinal tract). It is grossly underappreciated that gastrointestinal bleeding of this quantity can result in profound iron deficiency anemia over time even in the face of repeated negative stool guaiac tests. Common causes of this type of blood loss include tumors, polyps, inflammatory bowel disease, hiatal hernia, and gastritis. Surgical procedures for the treatment of peptic ulcer disease can result in small channel ulcers that are detected only with great difficulty. An increasingly common cause of blood loss is the ingestion of one aspirin a day to prevent cardiovascular disease. Both aspirin and other nonsteroidal anti-inflammatory drugs can cause significant increases in "guaiac-negative" gastrointestinal blood loss.

In adults, iron deficiency anemia has many causes, but diet is *not* one. Because only a minute amount of total body iron comes from food, a diet low in iron in and of itself cannot result in iron deficiency. It would take literally years of no intake of dietary iron to cause iron deficiency. However, a diet low in iron can induce or intensify anemia in association with ongoing blood loss. Inquiry into the cause of acute blood loss will usually reveal a history of gross bleeding, frequent blood donations, or menorrhagia. Studies evaluating cases of idiopathic iron deficiency have found that 60 to 70% are due to occult blood loss from the gastrointestinal tract, 25 to 35% from menstrual loss, and a small but important percentage from chronic iron loss in the urine. Urinary loss can result from urinary tract tumors or from hemoglobinuria and hemosiderinuria from intravascular hemolysis due to prosthetic heart valves, IgM-mediated hemolysis, or microangiopathic hemolysis.

Menorrhagia is commonly underappreciated by the patient, who may think her periods are normal. The average menstrual period results in approximately 30 cc of blood loss, representing 30 mg of iron loss. Average American women use approximately 8 to 12 tampons or pads per menstrual period with a common pattern of daily usage being 3-3-2-1 on days one to four. Clearly daily patterns such as 8-8-6-5-2-1 imply increased menstrual blood loss, which can explain occult iron deficiency anemia.

As blood is chronically and progressively lost, iron is continually withdrawn from storage and deposited in the hemoglobin of new red cells in order to maintain a normal hematocrit (Table 1). As blood loss continues, storage iron loss is reflected by depletion of stainable iron from bone marrow samples and a parallel fall in serum ferritin levels. As storage iron becomes totally exhausted, the serum iron falls below normal and total transferrin increases (reflected by the total iron-binding capacity [TIBC]), resulting in a decrease in total percent saturation of transferrin to less than 10%. If blood loss is not corrected and iron is not replenished, altered red cell production is evidenced by smaller red cells (microcytosis) and a fall in mean corpuscular volume (MCV). Abnormal red cell morphology and altered red cell indices (measured with electronic counting devices) are not usually observed until the hematocrit falls to 30 to 35%. If anemia worsens and the hematocrit falls into the 25 to 30% range, red cells become hypochromic as manifested by a fall in the mean corpuscular hemoglobin concentration (MCHC). As anemia worsens (hematocrit of 15 to 25%), anisocytosis and poikilocytosis are indicated by a widening in the red cell distribution width (RDW). As anemia becomes severe (hematocrit <15%), bizarre, misshapen, fragmented, and tattered red cells containing only rims of hemoglobin are seen. Such intense anisocytosis and poikilocytosis can lead one to reject iron deficiency anemia as the diagnosis. These late findings are also accompanied by a decrease in red cell survival as the cells become brittle and noncompliant. These steps in progressive chronic iron deficiency are reflections of forced erythropoiesis in an iron-depleted environment; they are not seen with rapid blood loss anemia, (e.g., massive hemorrhage).

The body has limited responses to falling iron stores. Whereas platelet counts increase in mild to moderate iron deficiency (and actually fall in extreme iron deficiency anemia), it is doubtful that the increased platelet count improves hemostasis. The gastrointestinal tract does become slightly more efficient in absorbing normal amounts of food iron, increasing from a baseline efficiency of approximately 10% to as high as 20 to 30%; however, this often proves to be insufficient in the face of blood loss of more than 10 to 15 cc per day as increased absorption results in only 10 mg of iron absorption per day, which produces only 10 cc of red cells.

CLINICAL MANIFESTATIONS

Symptoms of iron deficiency are usually quite mild. (Symptoms of hypovolemia will not be discussed here, as those signs and symptoms are due to reduced blood volume from acute blood loss.) Mild iron deficiency does not produce symptoms. Iron deficiency alone requires a hematocrit of 25% or lower to cause symptoms. Whereas persons with hematocrits of 32% may be fatigued, listless, and otherwise symptomatic, it is not the anemia that causes the symptoms. With more severe anemia, (i.e., hematocrit of 10 to 20%), patients may tire more easily, but only with activity. With very severe anemia (i.e., hematocrit below 10%) marked dyspnea on exertion may be seen as well as lassitude and confusion, and there may be a slightly widened pulse pressure and minimal tachycardia at rest. Examination may also show pallor. Ridging and spooning of the fingernails sometimes accompany severe anemia. The tongue may be smooth but not to the degree seen in pernicious anemia. A peculiar habit that is nearly specific for iron deficiency is pica. Patients may eat dirt, clay, starch, or especially ice. This symptom abates with iron replacement.

DIAGNOSIS

The diagnosis of iron deficiency anemia requires an anemic state. Serum iron and percent saturation of transferrin will usually be low. Microcytosis and hypochromia are seen only in more

TABLE 1. **Sequence of Events in Progressive Iron Loss**

Events	Approximate Corresponding Hematocrit
Normal	
Normal iron stores	Normal
Iron Deficiency	
Decreasing tissue iron stores; decreasing serum ferritin	Normal
Absent tissue iron stores; serum ferritin <10 ng/mL	Normal
Falling serum iron; increasing TIBC; percentage saturation <10%	Normal
Iron Deficiency Anemia	
Microcytosis	30–35%
Hypochromia and microcytosis	25–30%
Anisocytosis and poikilocytosis	15–25%
Severe anisocytosis and poikilocytosis	<15%

Abbreviation: TIBC = total iron-binding capacity.

severe anemia. Serum ferritin levels in iron deficiency anemia are usually below 50 ng per mL. Iron deficiency can be confused with the so-called "anemia of chronic disease" in which not only iron levels but also TIBC levels may be low, resulting in only borderline percent saturation with higher ferritin levels. Not uncommonly, the two diseases coexist. In complex cases, bone marrow examination for stainable iron will serve as the final arbiter: in anemia due to iron deficiency, stainable iron stores will not be present, whereas in anemia of chronic disease, iron stores are present or even increased. Other causes of microcytic hypochromic anemia include the thalassemias, hemoglobin H disease, hemoglobin E disease, lead poisoning, or any of several disorders resulting in so-called "sideroblastic anemia."

One can have iron deficiency without anemia, and in fact substantial percentage of menstruating women have depleted iron stores without anemia. Similarily, persons with polycythemia vera who are treated by repeated phlebotomy are intensely iron deficient but not anemic.

Once iron deficiency with anemia has been established, the source of blood loss should be identified. This can almost always be accomplished by diligent history taking and physical examination.

As previously mentioned, even if repeated stool guaiac tests are negative, radiographic or endoscopic diagnosis or both are in order for refractory cases.

TREATMENT

The first therapeutic goal is identifying the source of blood loss and correcting it. This will not be discussed further.

The second therapeutic goal is replenishment of iron. It must be stressed that the treatment for iron deficiency is iron replenishment, not blood transfusion. It can be argued that transfusion is appropriate when iron deficiency is accompanied by acute, ongoing blood loss, such as active gastrointestinal bleeding. However, the patient who is not acutely bleeding rarely, if ever, requires blood transfusion regardless of the hematocrit level. Symptoms of iron deficiency based on anemia alone occur only when the hematocrit is in the range of 25% and patients are frequently encountered with hematocrits in the 10% range who are virtually asymptomatic.

The cheapest and most efficient way to replace iron is with iron salts, such as ferrous sulfate. A 300 mg tablet of iron sulfate provides 60 mg of elemental iron. Iron tablets can cause gastrointestinal upset, dyspepsia, constipation, and diarrhea and are often not well tolerated initially. This can usually be overcome by prescribing one tablet per day for several weeks followed by two tablets per day and finally three or even four per day as tolerated. Maximal absorption of medicinal iron is achieved by taking the tablets before meals, a practice that may increase gastrointestinal side effects. Offering the pills with meals decreases side effects but also decreases iron absorption. Other tablet forms of iron are available but differ from iron sulfate only in being more expensive.

Liquid iron is occasionally better tolerated than tablet iron although it may stain clothing and teeth.

The body responds to iron deficiency by making gastrointestinal absorption of food iron somewhat more efficient. Unfortunately, absorption of medicinal iron is inversely related to the dose: the larger the dose of medicinal iron, the smaller the net percentage of absorption. Taking four tablets of 300 mg of iron sulfate results in 240 mg of elemental iron being available in the gastrointestinal tract, and if 15% is absorbed, approximately 30 cc per day of red blood cells can be produced. Clearly, iron loss may be faster than 30 mL per day, which would result in a situation of continued iron loss despite iron replacement. This demonstrates that gastrointestinal absorption of iron is the limiting step in production of red cells. In situations in which blood loss chronically exceeds iron absorption, parenteral iron will allow more iron to be deposited in the bone marrow with greater red cell production. Although parenteral iron is not without side effects, it does present fewer risks than multiple transfusions.

The response to treatment is not as brisk as that seen in either folate or vitamin B_{12} deficiency, and patients who are responding may not be perceived as doing so. Response usually occurs after about 1 week of therapy and is manifested by only a modest (i.e., 4 to 6%) increase in the reticulocyte count. Because iron deficiency is a chronic condition, therapy must be long-term. It may require 1 to 3 months before the hematocrit is normal and even longer if blood loss is concomitant with iron replenishment. When the hematocrit has been normalized, iron therapy should continue for an additional 3 months in order to replenish iron stores.

Failure to respond to treatment can have several causes. The first is incorrect diagnosis. If a patient fails to respond, one should consider other disorders in the differential diagnosis. The second and most common cause of nonresponse is failure to comply with therapy. Taking tablets 3 to 4 times per day for up to 6 months can be trying, particularly for patients who are only mildly symptomatic. Noncompliance can be confirmed by pill counts or frank discussions with the patient. Compliance can also be ascertained by the discoloration of stools seen with oral iron therapy. Once patients understand the mechanism of iron replacement, compliance usually improves. Another cause for failure is an ongoing illness that decreases the bone marrow's ability to produce blood; this can occur with chronic infections, inflammatory processes, or malignancies. Continued blood loss in excess of iron replenishment is another reason for failure of the hematocrit to increase. There is usually evidence of blood loss with a falling hematocrit in the face of reticulocytosis. Failure of the gastrointestinal tract to absorb the iron is occasionally seen in patients who have surgically altered gastrointestinal tracts, malabsorption, or achlorhydia.

AUTOIMMUNE HEMOLYTIC ANEMIA

method of
PETER B. RINTELS, M.D., and
JAMES P. CROWLEY, M.D.
Rhode Island Hospital
Providence, Rhode Island

Hemolysis is a normal physiologic process by which senescent erythrocytes are removed from the circulation after an average 120-day life span. Autoimmune hemolytic anemia (AIHA) occurs when this life span is significantly shortened by pathologic antibodies. Since antibody binding to red blood cells (RBCs) may be incidental, the diagnosis of AIHA requires that (1) the RBC life span is shortened (i.e., hemolysis is occurring) and (2) that hemolysis is immune mediated.

Normal bone marrow supported by an adequate erythropoietin response can increase its production of erythrocytes tenfold, and usually accelerated hemolysis is compensated for by an increase in the reticulocyte count. In AIHA, this response is highly variable, however, and the increase may be only twofold in up to 30% of cases. Since the reticulocyte count is expressed as a percentage of circulating erythrocytes, one must correct for the reduction in hematocrit (hct) level as well as for the early release of reticulocytes from stressed marrow, which doubles their life span in the circulation from 1 to 2 days. Thus, the "reticulocyte index" is calculated as

$$\text{current HCT/normal HCT} \div 2$$

A more direct measure is the absolute reticulocyte count, calculated as

$$\% \text{ reticulocytes} \times \text{RBC/mm}^3$$

It should be greater than 100,000/mm³ in AIHA.

Other evidence for increased RBC destruction includes elevation of lactate dehydrogenase fractions 1 and 2, elevation of indirect (unconjugated) bilirubin, and reduction in serum haptoglobin, which is rapidly removed by the monocyte-macrophage system after binding of circulating free hemoglobin. Haptoglobin

levels are low when median RBC survival falls below 23 days and should be absent if it is below 17 days. Haptoglobin, however, is an acute phase reactant and may be spuriously normal if stimulated by the inflammatory reactions that can accompany AIHA. The "gold standard" for establishing accelerated RBC destruction is the 51-Cr red cell survival study, which may be helpful in ambiguous circumstances such as chronic lymphocytic leukemia, in which nonhemolytic antibody binding, marrow failure, and inflammatory changes can make the diagnosis of AIHA difficult.

The immune component of accelerated RBC destruction is established by the Coombs' test, which can be rapidly performed by any blood bank. In the direct Coombs' test (also referred to as the direct anti-globulin test [DAT]), anti-human IgG and anti-human C3d are incubated directly with the patient's RBCs to establish the presence of membrane-bound IgG or C3d, the latter most often indicating prior IgM binding. (IgM does not bind avidly to RBC membranes and is washed off in the standard Coombs' procedure; consequently, it is not detected directly by standard techniques.) In the indirect Coombs' test, the patient's serum is incubated with a panel of donor cells of defined antigen specificity, then with anti-human IgG. Its purpose is to detect and define the specificity of any circulating alloantibody that may have been acquired during prior transfusion or pregnancy. The lack of any antigen specificity in the indirect Coombs' test is strong evidence for the presence of an autoimmune process. Table 1 outlines the findings of the Coombs' test in most commonly encountered clinical settings.

Immune hemolytic anemias are generally classified as either warm or cold antibody type, depending on the temperature at which the antibody binds most avidly to the RBC. With important exceptions, warm antibodies are usually IgG, cold antibodies IgM. Other types include drug-induced immune hemolysis and paroxysmal cold hemoglobinuria (Table 2).

WARM ANTIBODY AUTOIMMUNE HEMOLYSIS

Physiology

Warm antibody AIHA is an isolated (idiopathic) abnormality in 20 to 80% of cases in different series. Secondary AIHA is usually seen in the setting of a lymphoproliferative disorder or another autoimmune syndrome such as systemic lupus erythematosus (SLE). Especially in older patients, AIHA can herald the presence of a lymphoproliferative disorder, and patients should have thorough evaluation and follow-up. The Coombs' test is positive in 18 to 43% of patients with human immunodeficiency virus (HIV) infection, usually attributable to nonspecific antibody deposition attributed to hypergammaglobulinemia. In rare cases, unequivocal hemolysis responsive to standard therapy has been documented in some patients, however.

The cause of AIHA is not known. The illness

TABLE 1. **Interpretation of Coombs' Test**

Direct Coombs' Test	Indirect Coombs' Test	IgG	C3	Usual Scenario/Comments
+	+	+	—	No antigen specificity (often "panagglutinin"): Warm antibody autoimmune hemolysis* Alpha-methyldopa (Aldomet) type drug-induced hemolysis Antigen specificity New alloantibody: delayed hemolytic transfusion reaction Autoantibody: warm antibody autoimmune hemolysis with antigen specificity
+	—	+	—	Drug-induced hemolysis mediated by drug absorption— penicillin prototype (C3 rarely positive) Warm AIHA with low-titer free serum antibody
+	+	+	+	Common in lupus-associated AIHA; seen in roughly 30% of warm AIHA
+	—	—	+	Cold agglutinin disease Drug-induced hemolysis mediated by immune complex— quinidine prototype.
—	—	—	—	Coombs'-negative hemolysis. Consider microangiopathy, G6PD deficiency, unstable hemoglobin, etc. Rarely IgA immune-mediated; possibly very low-titer IgG-mediated

*Indirect Coombs' test may be negative in 20% of warm AIHA due to low serum antibody titer.

appears to be associated with loss of suppression of naturally occuring autoreactive B lymphocytes, either as part of a global tendency toward autoantibody formation (SLE) or in relation to immune dysfunction associated with a lymphoproliferative disorder. In the latter case, the antibody responsible for the hemolysis is not a byproduct of the malignant clone but rather is a polyclonal abnormality associated with a broader disorder of immune regulation. The IgG autoantibody can be either antigen specific or nonspecific. The most

TABLE 2. **Classification of Immune Hemolysis**

Warm antibody
  Idiopathic (usually polyclonal antibody)
  Secondary
    Lymphoproliferative disorders (CLL, non-Hodgkin's lymphoma, etc.)
    Nonlymphoid malignancy (rare)
    Idiopathic autoimmune disorders (systemic lupus erythematosus, rheumatoid arthritis, pernicious anemia, autoimmune thyroiditis)
    HIV infection (rare)
Cold antibody
  Idiopathic (usually monoclonal antibody)
  Secondary
    Lymphoproliferative disorders
    Infections (Epstein-Barr virus, cytomegalovirus, *Mycoplasma pneumoniae*)
Drug-induced
  Drug absorption mechanism (penicillin prototype)
  Immune complex mechanism (quinidine prototype)
  True autoantibody induction (alpha-methyldopa [Aldomet] prototype)
Paroxysmal cold hemoglobinuria (Donath-Landsteiner antibody)

Abbreviations: CLL = chronic lymphocytic leukemia; HIV = human immunodeficiency virus.

common specificity is to the Rh system or to antigens within it.

Membrane-bound IgG does not injure RBCs directly but rather induces either phagocytosis or cytolysis by binding to monocyte/macrophage Fc receptors, primarily in the spleen. Partial phagocytosis of the RBC membrane is responsible for the creation of the microspherocytes seen on the peripheral blood smear in warm AIHA. At least three macrophage Fc receptors exist. In vitro, FcRI most avidly mediates RBC destruction. In vivo, however, evidence suggests that binding to FcRII and FcRIII initiates the process. The degree of interaction of the RBC with the macrophages is highly dependent on the subclass of IgG on the RBC surface (IgG3 > IgG1 > IgG2 >> IgG4). IgG3 is a potent mediator of hemolysis and can induce RBC destruction at low antibody densities. In contrast, IgG4 binding may not mediate hemolysis at all. Clinically, IgG1 is most commonly found on the RBCs of patients with warm AIHA, followed by IgG3. The amount of RBC-bound antibody does not correlate well with the degree of hemolysis in groups of patients but is likely to be relevant in an individual patient followed over time.

Diagnosis

Signs and symptoms of warm antibody AIHA are the nonspecific manifestations of anemia, which include fatigue, exertional dyspnea, and exacerbation of angina in susceptible patients. The physical examination may demonstrate pallor, pale conjunctivae, and mild jaundice. Splenomegaly is found in approximately one-third of patients. Signs and symptoms of a coexisting autoimmune or lymphoproliferative disorder should also be sought.

Findings consistent with hemolysis should be present, as described previously. The blood smear should demonstrate polychromasia and microspherocytes. Rarely, AIHA coexists with immune thrombocytopenia, an association referred to as Evan's syndrome. It is imperative that the diagnosis of Evan's syndrome be made only when the hemolysis is immune. The presence of Coombs'-negative hemolysis and thrombocytopenia is strongly suggestive of thrombotic thrombocytopenic purpura (TTP), especially if microangiopathic changes (i.e., schistocytes) are present on the peripheral blood smear. Such patients require urgent treatment as described elsewhere.

The direct Coombs' test should be positive, revealing IgG and less commonly (about 30%) C3d on the RBC surface. In 2 to 5% of patients with AIHA the direct Coombs' test is negative, possibly because the pathologic antibody is IgA or IgM, the antibody does not bind avidly, or the number of antibodies is too small to detect by standard agglutination techniques. The indirect Coombs' test may be negative if the amount of free serum antibody is low; this occurs in about 20% of patients. Antibody detected by the indirect Coombs' test often lacks a definable antigen specificity, which implies that it is an autoantibody.

Treatment

The goals of therapy are twofold: (1) to reduce transfusion dependence and (2) to minimize long-term side effects of treatment. Prednisone, 1 to 2 mg per kg per day orally, will suppress hemolysis in 80% of patients with primary AIHA and in 60% with secondary AIHA, initially by inhibiting macrophage function and subsequently by decreasing autoantibody production. Higher doses and intravenous therapy are no more effective. Responding patients will usually show a benefit by 7 days, but full responses may require 4 to 6 weeks. Therapy is then tapered over a 3-month period with careful observation for recurrent hemolysis. Only about 20% will be successfully weaned from steroid therapy; and an equal number may be maintained on low doses (10 to 15 mg per day). Osteoporosis prophylaxis should be given to postmenopausal women on maintenance steroid therapy.

Patients who do not respond to or cannot tolerate steroids are candidates for splenectomy. A cholecystectomy is also indicated if stones are present. Between 50 and 80% of splenectomized patients will be able to reduce or stop prednisone altogether. RBC survival studies to document splenic destruction of RBCs are not sufficiently predictive of a response to warrant their routine use prior to splenectomy. The authors advise patients undergoing splenectomy to receive pneumococcal vaccine before surgery and to use penicillin or an equivalent empirically for febrile episodes after surgery. Splenic irradiation (2000 cGy) has been tried with apparent success in one reported patient who could not undergo splenectomy.

Therapy for patients who can tolerate neither steroids nor splenectomy is problematic. Danazol, 200 mg three times daily, is the most benign therapy. An attempt to taper can be made at 3 to 6 months. Immune suppression with azathioprine, 80 mg per M^2 per day, or cyclophosphamide, 60 mg per M^2 per day—both orally—may benefit approximately 60% of such patients. Treatment is continued for 3 months and the dose titrated according to the response and the degree of marrow suppression. Cyclophosphamide* (Cytoxan, Neosar), is associated with significant long-term side effects, including sterility, bladder toxicity, and risk of second malignancy, which must be discussed with the patient prior to initiating this treatment.

Intravenous immunoglobulin† (IVIG) therapy, 2 grams given over 2 to 5 days, has been helpful in some patients, most notably those with malignancy. The benefit typically lasts 21 to 28 days and maintenance therapy of 0.4 mg per kg every 3 weeks is usually required to maintain the effect. In some series, however, only one-third of patients responded, and doses of up to 5 grams per kg were required. IVIG works in part by blockading macrophage Fc receptors but appears to have immune modulating effects as well. IVIG's main drawback is expense. Cyclosporine‡ (Sandimmune), 4 to 6 mg per kg per day, has also been reported beneficial but poses risks from immune suppression and nephrotoxicity.

Postsplenectomy searches with sulfa-colloid or, more sensitively, with tagged heat-damaged RBCs will occasionally identify an accessory spleen. The dangers of reoperation are significant because of the risk of pancreatic injury, and the success rate is only about 50%.

Transfusion

The hazards of transfusion therapy in patients with AIHA are often overstated but remain sig-

---

*This use of cyclophosphamide is not listed in the manufacturer's official directive.

†This use of intravenous immunoglobulin is not listed in the manufacturer's official directive.

‡This use of cyclosporine is not listed in the manufacturer's official directive.

nificant. The autoantibody will not destroy transfused RBCs any faster than the patient's own and therefore does not directly place the patient at risk for catastrophic intravascular hemolysis. However, a nonspecific autoantibody that agglutinates all cells on the indirect Coombs' test will obscure the identification of potentially significant alloantibodies acquired during pregnancy or prior transfusion. Up to 40% of patients with AIHA may have such alloantibodies, many of which can cause severe hemolytic reactions.

Several strategies have been used to contend with this problem. In some cases, it is possible to perform serial absorptions of the patient's serum with his or her own RBCs and decrease the titer of autoantibody enough so that it no longer interferes with the crossmatch. Preservation of pretransfusion RBCs for future absorptions is wise, since this procedure must be performed on native erythrocytes. Transfusion of blood that is lacking the most dangerous antigens is always wise, both to minimize the risk of a reaction and to prevent the subsequent formation of hazardous alloantibodies. Antibodies to Kidd, Kell, and Duffy antigens fix complement and pose the highest risk.

Lastly, an "in-vivo crossmatch" can be performed. In this procedure, transfusion is begun with 10 to 15 cc of RBCs over 30 minutes, at which time a specimen is drawn and examined for free hemoglobin. If the results are negative and the patient has tolerated the transfusion well, it is continued.

COLD ANTIBODY-MEDIATED HEMOLYSIS

Physiology

"Cold" antibodies, so named because they bind RBCs most avidly at 4° C, are usually referred to as "cold agglutinins." Cold agglutinins are most commonly of the IgM class, although IgG and IgA cold antibodies have been described. IgM antibodies are immunoglobulin pentamers, hence they agglutinate RBCs at much lower titers than IgG. Indeed, the observation of obvious agglutination on a routine blood smear is often the first indication that a cold agglutinin is present.

The ability of IgM antibodies to mediate hemolysis, however, depends on their ability to bind RBCs at physiologic temperatures. The highest temperature at which IgM binds is referred to as the "thermal amplitude" (above this temperature they fall off) and correlates well with the degree of clinical hemolysis. For patients at "room temperature," the temperature of blood in the acral circulation falls to 28 to 31° C. Consequently, cold agglutinins with thermal amplitudes below 28° C

may be clinically insignificant except in cold weather.

The interaction of IgM with RBC membranes does not damage them directly; rather antigen binding by IgM makes available the binding site for C1q, the initiator of the classical complement cascade. In most cases, the cascade proceeds to the creation of the C3 convertase (C4,2a), with the result that C4b and C3b remain covalently bound to the RBC membrane. RBC-bound C3b interacts with phagocytic cells in the liver and can cause sphering and RBC destruction in a manner analogous to IgG-mediated hemolysis by the spleen. Alternatively, C3b is degraded to C3d or C3dg, which is physiologically inactive and actually protects RBCs from phagocytosis. This variability of outcomes of complement interaction with RBCs explains in part why cold agglutinin hemolysis is usually mild.

Cold agglutinins are typically seen in two settings: (1) in older patients, in association with a lymphoproliferative disease, in which case the IgM is monoclonal, and (2) secondary to infection, most commonly with *Mycoplasma pneumoniae* or Epstein-Barr virus (EBV), in which case it is polyclonal. In some older patients, "idiopathic" monoclonal IgM cold agglutinins can appear in the absence of a detectable lymphoproliferative disorder, a situation analogous to "monoclonal gammopathy of unknown significance" (MGUS). Most cold agglutinins are directed against antigens of the I/i system, an oligosaccharide antigen associated with the ABO blood group, and glycophorin, a membrane glycoprotein. I is usually found on mature RBCs, i on cord blood and reticulocytes. I specificity is more common in patients with cold agglutinins that are idiopathic, secondary to a lymphoproliferative disorder, or secondary to mycoplasma; hence, these antibodies are more likely to be pathogenic. EBV-related cold agglutinins usually have i specificity.

Diagnosis

Patients can present with nonspecific signs of anemia or the predisposing illness, (e.g., lymphoproliferative disorders or infection with EBV or mycoplasma). Acrocyanosis, attributed to sludging of agglutinated red cells in cooler peripheral vessels, may also be found. A history of Raynaud's phenomenon can often be obtained.

Nonspecific indicators of hemolysis should be present, as previously discussed. RBC agglutination in the test tube or the blood smear is often obvious, and microspherocytes may also be present. When agglutination is present on the smear, the mean corpuscular volume will appear spuriously high because the automated counter cannot distinguish individual RBCs. This can cause miscalculation of the hematocrit, but the directly measured hemoglobin will be correct. The direct Coombs' test should be positive for C3d. The cold agglutinin titer should be greater than 1/64 but is usually much higher and can help discriminate between cold agglutinin disease and drug-mediated hemolysis associated with immune complexes. Low-titer cold agglutinins can be found incidentally in most people and are not pathologic.

Treatment

In many cases, cold agglutinin disease is sufficiently mild that no treatment is warranted, especially if it is infection related and therefore likely self limited. As always, reversible causes of bone marrow failure should be corrected. Erythropoietin (Epogen, Procrit), may be helpful if renal function is compromised and may obviate more toxic therapy. It may be sufficient, too, to offer commonsense advice about keeping warm, especially the extremities; this is also true for hospitalized patients, particularly in the intensive care unit. Steroids are usually ineffective but are helpful often enough to be worth a limited trial; patients with low titer–high thermal amplitude cold agglutinins are most likely to respond. Splenectomy is rarely indicated (as expected), but may be considered for the rare steroid-resistant patient. Pulsed cyclophosphamide or chlorambucil has been helpful in some instances. There is a recent report of benefit from interferon therapy, 3 MU 3 to 5 times per week. Because IgM is located 80% intravascularly, plasmapheresis or exchange may be transiently helpful in urgent situations. Crossmatching for transfusion is usually not a problem, since warming eliminates agglutination by most cold antibodies. Transfusions should be given with a blood warmer.

DRUG-INDUCED IMMUNE HEMOLYSIS

A careful drug history is part of any evaluation for immune hemolysis. Some drugs, most notably beta-lactam antibiotics, can induce nonspecific protein deposition, including immunoglobulin, on RBCs. This can be detected by a Coombs' test and should not be confused with true drug-induced hemolysis.

Drug-induced hemolysis is generally felt to have three mechanisms:

1. Penicillin prototype—neoantigen formation by drug binding to the RBC membrane. The onset is usually after 7 days of treatment; sooner in previously sensitized patients. The Coombs' test shows positive direct IgG, rarely positive direct C3d, and the indirect Coombs' test is negative in the absence of preincubation with the offending drug.

2. Quinidine prototype—formation of drug antibody immune complexes that bind RBC membranes, fix complement, and initiate hemolysis as described for cold agglutinins. The drug itself binds RBCs weakly. Recent evidence has challenged the notion that the interaction of antibody with the RBC membrane is nonspecific in this situation. The direct Coombs' test is positive for C3d and negative for IgG. The indirect Coombs' test is negative. Hemolysis may be severe with low-dose drug exposure.

3. Alpha-methyldopa (Aldomet) prototype—induction of warm autoantibodies. The mechanism of antibody induction is not known. Levo-dopa and some unrelated medications have also been implicated. This form of drug-induced hemolysis is indistinguishable by Coombs' test from warm AIHA. The Coombs' test is positive in 11 to 36% of patients taking alpha-methyldopa over 3 to 6 months, but hemolysis occurs in fewer than 1%. Hemolysis is usually mild and resolves over days to weeks. Interferon has recently been implicated in autoantibody induction.

PAROXYSMAL COLD HEMOGLOBINURIA

This rare entity was more commonly seen prior to the introduction of effective therapy for syphilis. It is now usually associated with childhood exanthems, if a precipitant is identified. Clinically, massive paroxysmal hemolysis is seen with cold exposure, which may be associated with fever, dark urine, and back and abdominal pain. Hemolysis is induced by the Donath-Landsteiner antibody, a cold-reacting IgG antibody typically directed against P group RBC antigens that fixes complement and induces lysis at physiologic temperatures. The diagnosis is made by the biphasic Donath-Landsteiner test, in which the patient's serum is incubated with RBCs at 4° C and then warmed to 37° C with induction of hemolysis. Therapy is mainly avoidance of cold exposure. Steroids for acute attacks are of uncertain value.

NONIMMUNE HEMOLYTIC ANEMIA

method of
BARBARA L. ASSELIN, M.D., and
GEORGE B. SEGEL, M.D.
University of Rochester
Rochester, New York

The hemolytic anemias are a diverse group of disorders that can be congenital or acquired and acute, episodic, or chronic. Hemolysis results from accelerated destruction of red cells and a consequent shortened red cell life span. It usually is accompanied by a compensatory increase in erythropoiesis, which is manifested as a reticulocytosis. The red cells can be destroyed either within the circulation (intravascular hemolysis) or outside of the circulation (extravascular hemolysis). Hemolytic anemias can be further classified as resulting from extracellular factors, primarily acquired, or cellular abnormalities, primarily inherited. This chapter describes a treatment approach for nonimmune hemolytic anemias other than sickle cell anemia and thalassemia major, which are discussed elsewhere in this text.

CLINICAL MANIFESTATIONS

The diagnosis of hemolysis is suggested by reticulocytosis in the absence of bleeding or administration of hematinic therapy. Hemolysis does not always result in anemia, because normal marrow can compensate for premature destruction by increasing the production of red cells approximately by six to eightfold. When the rate of hemolysis exceeds the capacity for compensation, anemia is observed. The mean cell volume is usually normal or somewhat increased secondary to the reticulocytosis. Other nonspecific features that commonly accompany hemolysis are indirect hyperbilirubinemia, increased serum lactic dehydrogenase, decreased serum haptoglobin, and splenomegaly. In some hemolytic syndromes, hemolysis can be primarily intravascular, and if severe, hemoglobinemia and hemoglobinuria can result.

DIAGNOSIS

The clinical presentation and initial diagnostic studies should indicate the need for further evaluation, possible consultation, and definitive treatment. Even in patients with life-threatening anemia, a complete history, physical examination, and limited laboratory evaluation should be performed prior to transfusion. If it becomes necessary to transfuse the patient prior to establishing the diagnosis, anticoagulated blood in both citrate and heparin, as well as serum, should be obtained before transfusion to permit later diagnostic testing as outlined in Table 1.

TREATMENT

The causes of nonimmune hemolytic anemia and an outline of the recommended therapies are shown in Table 1. Guidelines for the longitudinal care of patients with hemolytic anemias are presented in Table 2.

General Therapeutic Procedures

Transfusion

Transfusion for chronic hemolytic anemias usually is not instituted until the hemoglobin falls below 6 to 7 grams per dL. Aside from thalassemia major and sickle cell disease, most nonimmune hemolytic anemias do not require chronic transfusion, although occasionally patients with red cell membrane disorders, such as hereditary spherocytosis and pyropoikilocytosis, or enzyme disorders, such as pyruvate kinase deficiency, require transfusion support until splenectomy is performed (see Table 1). The need for transfusion must be weighed against the potential complications, which include infection with hepatitis B or C, human immunodeficiency virus, cytomegalovirus, or Epstein-Barr virus, transfusion reactions, development of alloantibodies, and iron overload.

Packed red cells are the preferred transfusion product. The use of leukocyte-poor red cells reduces the likelihood of nonhemolytic, febrile transfusion reactions and alloimmunization to HLA antigens and should be used for patients with a history of febrile or other allergic transfusion reactions or those who require frequent transfusions. Premedication with antipyretics, antihistamines, or glucocorticoids also can be helpful in preventing allergic transfusion reactions. Red cell antigen phenotyping is recommended for patients who are to receive multiple transfusions, since typing is unreliable after transfusion therapy is started. This information can be used to provide antigen-matched red cells to prevent or circumvent sensitization to minor blood group antigens.

Transfusion may be required for acute episodes of anemia resulting from aplastic crises, acute hemolysis in glucose-6-phosphate dehydrogenase deficiency, or unstable hemoglobins or any of the extracellular defects (see Table 1). The packed red cells should be administered cautiously to avoid precipitating hypervolemia and heart failure. Simple transfusion of 2 units of packed red cells in adults or 10 mL per kg in children increases the hemoglobin at least 2 grams per dL and increases the oxygen-carrying capacity in uncomplicated anemia. A diuretic such as intravenous furosemide can be administered midway through the total transfusion, or smaller, repeated transfusions can be given if volume overload becomes a problem. Alternatively, a partial volume exchange transfusion permits safe, rapid correction of the red cell volume in severe anemia (hemoglobin less than 5 grams per dL) and is tolerated well even in extremely ill patients. This involves removing whole blood (hemoglobin concentration very low) and replacing it with packed

TABLE 1. **Hemolytic Anemias and Their Treatment**

Diagnosis	Defect	Laboratory Tests	Treatment
Cellular Defects MEMBRANE DEFECTS			
Hereditary spherocytosis	Cytoskeletal protein defects Frequently involves spectrin, ankyrin, protein 3	Spherocytes on blood film Negative Coomb's test eliminates immune hemolysis Increased incubated osmotic fragility, corrected by glucose Abnormal cytoskeletal protein analysis	1. If Hb >10 gm/dL and retic <10%—no treatment 2. If severe anemia, poor growth, aplastic crises, and age <2 years—transfusion 3. If Hb <10 gm/dL and retic >10% or massive spleen—splenectomy, preferably >age 6 but earlier if necessary 4. Folic acid 1 mg qd
Hereditary elliptocytosis	Cytoskeletal protein defects Frequently involves spectrin, protein 4.1, glycophorin C	Elliptocytes on blood film Red cells mildly heat sensitive Abnormal cytoskeletal protein analysis	1. Mild types—no treatment 2. Chronic hemolysis—transfusion and splenectomy as recommended for spherocytosis (above) 3. Folic acid 1 mg qd
Hereditary pyropoikilocytosis	Cytoskeletal protein defects Abnormality in α-spectrin	Extreme variation in red cell size and shape on blood film Thermal sensitivity— fragmentation at 45° C for 15 min	1. Transfusion and splenectomy as recommended for spherocytosis (above) 2. Folic acid 1 mg qd
Hereditary stomatocytosis	Cytoskeletal protein defects Decreased protein 7.2b Abnormal red cell cation and water content	Stomatocytes on blood film	1. Response to splenectomy variable 2. Folic acid 1 mg qd
Paroxysmal nocturnal hemoglobinuria	Primary acquired marrow disorder Red cells unusually sensitive to complement-mediated lysis	Ham test, sugar water test Marrow aspirate and biopsy to assess cellularity	1. Folic acid 1 mg qd 2. Mild cytopenias—no treatment 3. Chronic hemolysis and other cytopenias—prednisone 60 mg qd initially, then taper if possible, and switch to a qod regimen 4. Iron for secondary iron deficiency 5. Androgens—halotestin 10–30 mg qd
ENZYME DEFICIENCIES G6PD deficiency	A⁻ type: age-labile enzyme Mediterranean type: no enzyme activity in circulating red cells	G6PD assay	1. Avoid oxidant stress to red cells 2. Transfusion if acute anemia is symptomatic
Pyruvate kinase deficiency	Decreased or abnormal enzyme	PK assay—decreased V_{max} or rarely low affinity (high Km) variant	1. If severe anemia with symptoms, poor growth, and age <2 years— transfusion 2. Splenectomy >age 6 but earlier if necessary 3. Folic acid 1 mg qd

red cells (hemoglobin concentration > 18 grams per dL).

Splenectomy

Since the spleen is the most common site of red cell sequestration, its removal can result in a significant improvement in red cell survival in disorders such as hereditary spherocytosis wherein splenic sequestration and splenic trapping are primarily responsible for the hemolysis. The benefits of splenectomy must be weighed against possible postoperative complications. The major risk is bacterial sepsis caused by encapsulated organisms such as *Streptococcus pneumoniae, Haemophilus influenzae,* and *Neisseria meningitidis.* Because of the already heightened risk of sepsis in infancy and early childhood, the authors normally delay splenectomy until the child is older

TABLE 1. **Hemolytic Anemias and Their Treatment** *Continued*

Diagnosis	Defect	Laboratory Tests	Treatment
HEMOGLOBINOPATHIES Unstable hemoglobins	Amino acid substitution (usually β-chain), loss of heme from molecule, or disruption of hemoglobin secondary structure	Basophilic stippling on blood film Heinz body preparation Hb electrophoresis Thermal instability—hemoglobin precipitates at 50° C for 1 hr Alteration in oxygen affinity	1. Avoid oxidant stress to red cells 2. Folic acid 1 mg qd 3. Rarely severe anemia may require transfusion and if chronic, splenectomy
Extracellular Defects ANTIBODIES FRAGMENTATION HEMOLYSIS DIC, TTP, HUS	Direct damage to red cell membrane	Fragments on blood film	1. Treat underlying condition 2. Transfusion, but transfused cells also will have shortened life span
Extracorporeal membrane oxygenation			
Prosthetic heart valve			1. Folic acid 1 mg qd 2. Iron for secondary iron deficiency
Burns—thermal injury	Direct damage to red cell membrane	Spherocytes on blood film	1. Supportive 2. Transfusion
HYPERSPLENISM	Effects of sequestration, ↓ pH, lipases and other enzymes, and macrophages on red cells	Thrombocytopenia and neutropenia	1. Treat underlying condition—cytopenias usually mild 2. Splenectomy if complicating other anemia, e.g., thalassemia major 3. Folic acid 1 mg qd
PLASMA FACTORS Liver disease	Alteration in plasma cholesterol and phospholipids	Target cells or spiculated red cells on blood film Abnormal liver function tests	1. Treat underlying condition 2. Transfusion, but transfused cells also will have shortened life span 3. Folic acid 1 mg qd
Abetalipoproteinemia	Absence of apolipoprotein β Vitamin E deficiency and heightened sensitivity to oxidative damage	Acanthocytes on blood film Absent chylomicrons, VLDL and LDL	1. Vitamins E, A, K, and D 2. Folic acid 1 mg qd 3. Dietary restriction of triglycerides
Infections	Toxic effects on red cells	Associated symptoms and signs Cultures	1. Antibiotics 2. Supportive
Wilson's disease	Effect of copper on red cell membrane, usually self-limited	Spherocytes on blood film Copper, ceruloplasmin Penicillamine challenge and urine copper excretion	1. Penicillamine 2. Supportive 3. Transfusion if acute anemia is symptomatic

Abbreviations: retic = reticulocyte count; G6PD = glucose-6-phosphate dehydrogenase; DIC = disseminated intravascular coagulation; TTP = thrombotic thrombocytopenic purpura; HUS = hemolytic uremic syndrome; VLDL = very low-density lipoproteins; LDL = low-density lipoproteins.

than 6 years. Occasional patients will require earlier splenectomy because of an excessive transfusion requirement, aplastic crises, or delayed growth. Under these circumstances the authors avoid splenectomy before age 2 and continue to transfuse the patient for additional time if possible.

Depending on their age, splenectomized patients should be immunized with pneumococcal vaccine (Pneumovax 23 or equivalent, 0.5 mL in-

tramuscularly), *H. influenzae* B conjugate vaccine (HibTITER or equivalent, 0.5 mL intramuscularly), and meningococcal vaccine (Meningovax or equivalent, 0.5 mL subcutaneously). Children are given all three immunizations prior to splenectomy and are reimmunized every 3 to 5 years with pneumococcal vaccine until the age of 10 years. Adults are given the pneumococcal and meningococcal vaccines, but reimmunization is not recommended. The efficacy of these vaccines

TABLE 2. **Longitudinal Care for Patients with Chronic Hemolytic Anemia**

Monitor hemoglobin and reticulocyte count
Folic acid supplementation: 1 mg per day
Iron supplementation (only if secondary iron deficiency is
    documented):
    Adults 300–900 mg per day (60–180 mg elemental iron)
    Children 6–8 mg per kg per day of elemental iron
If fever or intercurrent illness, check hemoglobin and
    reticulocyte count every 2 days until illness resolves
If anemia severe (hemoglobin <8 gm/dL):
    Chest x-ray to evaluate heart size every 2 years after age
        10
    ECG, echocardiogram if cardiomyopathy or myocardial
        ischemia suspected
Post splenectomy
    Verify immunization with pneumococcal vaccine, *H.
        influenzae* vaccine, meningococcal vaccine
    Repeat pneumococcal vaccine:
        Children—every 3–5 years until age 10
        Adults—not recommended
    Penicillin prophylaxis (penicillin VK or equivalent):
        Age ≤5 years—125 mg twice daily
        Age >5 years and adults—250 mg twice daily
    If fever ≥38.5° C:
        Evaluate with physical examination, complete blood
            count, reticulocyte count, blood cultures
        Treat with intravenous antibiotics

in protecting splenectomized patients from sepsis is not absolute, since not all strains are represented in the inoculum and some strains are less immunogenic than others.

In addition to vaccination, prophylactic penicillin, penicillin VK or equivalent is given after splenectomy to protect against pneumococcal sepsis (see Table 2). The need for continued antibiotic prophylaxis for adults is controversial since the incidence of postsplenectomy sepsis is lower in adults than in children. However, adults can succumb to postsplenectomy sepsis, and therefore the authors recommend continuing penicillin prophylaxis. Following splenectomy, all patients regardless of age, immunization status, or compliance with prophylaxis should be cautioned to seek medical attention if they develop a fever greater than 38.5° C. Administration of intravenous antibiotics is indicated until a bacterial source for infection is ruled out by blood culture.

Bone Marrow Transplantation

Bone marrow transplantation from an HLA-matched sibling has been used successfully to treat several disorders that involve intrinsic red cell defects, primarily thalassemia major, sickle cell anemia, and paroxysmal nocturnal hemoglobinuria. This therapy remains investigative, and although the mortality has been less then 5% in thalassemia major and sickle cell anemia, there is significant morbidity from acute and particularly chronic graft-versus-host disease. The best

candidates for bone marrow transplantation are minimally transfused children.

Therapy for Specific Disorders

Membrane Defects

There are three major inherited red cell membrane disorders: hereditary spherocytosis, hereditary elliptocytosis, and hereditary stomatocytosis.

The spherocytes in *hereditary spherocytosis* are destroyed almost exclusively in the spleen: thus, splenectomy cures the hemolysis associated with this disorder. After splenectomy, the spherocytosis and increased osmotic fragility persist, but the anemia, hyperbilirubinemia, and reticulocytosis resolve. There is controversy about whether all patients with hereditary spherocytosis should have their spleens removed. It has been the authors' practice *not* to remove the spleens of patients who are growing normally and have hemoglobin concentrations greater than 10 grams per dL and a reticulocyte count of less than 10% (see Table 1). Their management includes folic acid supplementation and periodic re-evaluation. For patients with more severe anemia and reticulocytosis (hemoglobin less than 10 grams per dL, reticulocytes greater than 10%), the authors recommend splenectomy at age 6 to avoid the heightened risk of postsplenectomy sepsis at younger ages (see General Therapeutic Procedures: Splenectomy and Table 1).

Hereditary elliptocytosis comprises a group of inherited disorders that have in common the presence of elliptical red cells on the blood film. Hereditary elliptocytosis is heterogeneous in terms of severity of hemolysis, red cell morphology, and underlying molecular defects. A particularly severe variant is hereditary pyropoikilocytosis, which more often affects African Americans. Splenectomy has been helpful in severely affected patients. The criteria for and timing of splenectomy are similar to those for hereditary spherocytosis (see Table 1).

Hereditary stomatocytosis includes a heterogeneous family of hereditary hemolytic anemias. Response to splenectomy is variable and may not correct the hemolysis, which can result in severe thrombocytosis and a hypercoagulable state. Chronic red cell transfusion therapy to suppress hemopoiesis decreases the platelet count and the hypercoagulable tendency. It is best to avoid splenectomy in these patients.

Paroxysmal nocturnal hemoglobinuria is an *acquired* stem cell disorder that affects the membranes of red cells, granulocytes, and platelets. It is associated with chronic intravascular hemolysis, a tendency toward thrombosis, and occasionally aplastic anemia. In this disorder, red cells are particularly sensitive to complement lysis, and this usually produces chronic rather than episodic intravascular hemolysis. Hemolysis in some patients has responded to glucocorticoids or androgens (see Table 1). Folic acid is administered to prevent secondary megaloblastic anemia, and iron is given if there is secondary iron deficiency from renal losses. Marrow transplantation from a histocompatible donor is the treatment of choice if pancytopenia develops. Alternatively, antithymocyte globulin (ATG) and cyclosporine may be effective as in aplastic anemia.

Enzyme Defects

The most common enzyme defect, *glucose-6-phosphate dehydrogenase (G6PD) deficiency,* is a sex-linked condition that involves decreased activity of a major enzyme of the red cell hexose monophosphate shunt. There are more than 300 different G6PD variants, and their phenotypic clinical manifestations differ widely among different genotypes. The A⁻ variety is present in 10% of the African American male population. Hemolysis occurs in the A⁻ variety only with a severe oxidative insult from certain drugs, such as primaquine or high-dose aspirin. Normal doses of aspirin or sulfonamides usually do not cause symptoms. In the absence of an oxidant stress there is no hemolysis. Patients with other varieties of G6PD deficiency (e.g., Mediterranean) may be more susceptible to agents precipitating acute hemolysis, and others actually may have a chronic hemolytic anemia.

Patients with G6PD deficiency should avoid medications known to precipitate hemolysis. A number of medications, toxins, and conditions associated with hemolytic episodes are shown in Table 3. Ingestion of fava beans provokes hemolysis in some G6PD deficiency syndromes but not in others. When drug-induced hemolysis is suspected, prompt withdrawal of all potentially involved medications is indicated and may be all that is required for treatment. In the A⁻ variant, hemolysis is limited, and the medication could be continued if essential to the treatment of another problem.

Defects in the red cell glycolytic pathway, the other major glucose metabolizing pathway, are rare. The most common of these rare conditions is erythrocyte *pyruvate kinase deficiency.* This disorder is usually associated with chronic hemolysis that can vary from completely compensated, asymptomatic hemolysis to severe, transfusion-dependent, life-threatening anemia. Splenectomy may be helpful in treating the more severe anemias that result from such enzymopathies (see Table 1).

TABLE 3. **Agents Precipitating Hemolysis in Glucose-6-Phosphate Dehydrogenase Deficiency**

Medications
Antibacterials
    Sulfonamides
    Trimethoprim-sulfamethoxazole
    Nalidixic acid
    Chloramphenicol
    Nitrofurantoin
Antimalarials
    Primaquine
    Pamaquine*
    Chloroquine
    Quinacrine
Others
    Acetophenetidin*
    Vitamin K analogues
    Methylene blue
    Probenecid
    Acetylsalicylic acid
    Phenazopyridine
Chemicals
  Phenylhydrazine
  Benzene
  Naphthalene
Illness
  Diabetic acidosis
  Hepatitis

*Not available in the United States.

Hemoglobinopathies

The major hemoglobinopathies, including sickle cell disease and thalassemia syndromes, are discussed in other articles in this text.

Unstable hemoglobins result from an amino acid substitution that alters the stability of the hemoglobin molecule so that it is easily denatured. Most patients have well-compensated hemolysis, and treatment is not required. Episodes of infection and exposure to oxidant drugs can precipitate heightened hemolysis. The primary treatment is avoidance of oxidant drugs (see Table 3). Splenectomy has been of variable benefit (see Table 1), but it is not recommended in patients with high oxygen-affinity variant hemoglobins.

Extracellular Defects

Immune hemolytic anemias are discussed elsewhere in this text. Therapy for other hemolytic anemias that result from extracellular factors depends on the nature of the underlying disease. Secondary red cell destruction usually resolves with treatment of the primary condition.

Treatment of Complications of Hemolysis

Hypoplastic or Aplastic Crises

Patients with chronic hemolysis are at risk for aplastic crises, characterized by a transient failure of red cell production and precipitous fall in hemoglobin, potentially resulting in a serious life-threatening anemia. These crises often are preceded by viral illnesses, most commonly caused by parvovirus B19, which infects erythropoietic precursors and inhibits their growth. Both the hemoglobin concentration and the reticulocyte count need to be evaluated since an early decrease in reticulocytes heralds the inevitable fall in hemoglobin. Such aplastic crises may be life-threatening and must be considered when patients with hemolysis are evaluated for febrile illnesses. Transfusion often is necessary to prevent high-output cardiac failure while awaiting erythroid marrow recovery.

Hemolytic Crises

Increased hemolysis characterized by a transient intensification of jaundice, a modest increase in spleen size, and a rise in the reticulocyte count is commonly associated with febrile illnesses in patients with an underlying hemolytic anemia. Severe hemolytic crises with marked jaundice, severe anemia, nausea and vomiting, and tender splenomegaly are relatively rare but may require transfusion.

Folic Acid Deficiency

Patients with hemolytic anemias have an increased requirement for folic acid to support the accelerated production of red cells. When the dietary intake of folic acid is inadequate to support increased erythropoiesis, a megaloblastic anemia can be superimposed on the existing hemolytic anemia, causing a decreased reticulocyte count, a further reduction in hemoglobin concentration, and an increase in mean cell volume. The administration of 1 mg per day of folic acid prevents megaloblastic anemia in patients with chronic hemolysis (see Table 1).

Gallbladder Disease

Gallbladder disease with cholelithiasis (pigment stones) is the most common complication of chronic hemolysis, frequently appearing in children as young as age 3. The incidence is 40 to 50% between ages 10 and 40 years and rises steadily thereafter. It is not known how many patients with pigment gallstones will develop symptomatic gallbladder disease or obstruction. Cholecystectomy is recommended only for patients who develop cholecystitis or biliary obstruction. At the time of cholecystectomy, the spleen should also be removed in conditions in which splenectomy is of known benefit (e.g., hereditary spherocytosis). This will help prevent the subsequent development of common duct stones.

Complications of Severe Chronic Anemia

Complications of severe chronic anemia (hemoglobin <7 grams per dL) include poor growth, limited exercise tolerance, cardiomegaly with cardiomyopathy, expansion of the marrow space with skeletal deformities (e.g., frontal bossing and fractures), and extramedullary hemopoiesis. These complications are rarely seen even in the severe anemias such as thalassemia major because "hypertransfusion" as currently practiced in chronic transfusion programs maintains the hemoglobin at greater than 10 grams per dL.

Secondary Iron Deficiency

Hemolytic syndromes associated with intravascular hemolysis, hemoglobinemia, hemoglobinuria, and hemosiderinuria produce a renal loss of iron, often sufficient to result in secondary iron deficiency. Appropriate treatment consists of iron supplementation with ferrous sulfate (see Table 2). Hemolytic anemia associated with extravascular hemolysis does not increase the dietary iron requirement due to reutilization of iron released from hemolyzed red cells, and iron therapy is not usually indicated.

PERNICIOUS ANEMIA AND OTHER MEGALOBLASTIC ANEMIAS

method of
RONALD A. SACHER, M.D., and
JOSEPH EVERS, M.D.
Georgetown University
Washington, D.C.

The megaloblastic anemias are a group of disorders characterized by the presence of hypersegmented neutrophils and oval macrocytes in the blood or the presence of megaloblasts in the bone marrow. "Megaloblast" is a descriptive term referring to the abnormal red cell precursors found in the bone marrows of patients with these anemias. Appropriate therapy of megaloblastic anemia requires an understanding of the differential diagnosis and laboratory evaluation of other causes of anemia with macrocytic red blood cells. The most common causes of megaloblastic anemia include pernicious anemia (cobalamin deficiency) and folic acid deficiency.

Cobalamin deficiency is almost always due to vitamin B_{12} malabsorption. Pernicious anemia is the usual cause and is likely due to a lack of intrinsic factor, the essential cofactor needed for vitamin B_{12} absorption in the terminal ileum. Intrinsic factor is normally produced by the parietal cells of the gastric mucosa and is deficient in any condition depleting this production, such as atrophic gastritis or gastrectomy. Occasionally, dietary deficiency (veganism) and malabsorption states

TABLE 1. **Five Clinical "P"s of Pernicious Anemia**

> Pancytopenia
> Peripheral neuropathy
> Posterior spinal column neuropathy
> Pyramidal tract signs
> Papillary (tongue) atrophy

or bacterial overgrowth with organisms requiring intestinal vitamin B_{12} for their metabolism may produce a vitamin B_{12} deficiency.

In contrast, deficiency of folic acid is nearly always due to a dietary deficiency. Stores of folic acid are only sufficient for 3 months and can be rapidly depleted in conditions of increased folate demand, such as pregnancy, rapid growth, rapid cell turnover (e.g., hemolytic anemias), poor folate intake, and alcoholism. Occasionally, folic acid deficiency may occur with other malabsorption states or with selective interference by drugs such as birth control pills and anticonvulsants.

CLINICAL FEATURES

Clinical features, though not specific, are often helpful in differentiating pernicious anemia from folic acid deficiency. Table 1 lists the five clinical "P"s of pernicious anemia helpful with this distinction. Macrocytic anemia occurring with alcoholism or in a postpartum state is more likely to be due to folic acid deficiency. Ultimately, however, cobalamin (vitamin B_{12}) deficiency and folate deficiency are confirmed only by laboratory assay.

LABORATORY FINDINGS

Macrocytosis occurs when the mean cell volume (MCV) is greater than 100 fl. Erythrocytic macrocytosis can easily be determined with the aid of an automatic electronic particle counter, which gives an accurate and reproducible value for the MCV. The finding of macrocytic indices does not automatically imply megaloblastic anemia, as can be seen from Table 2. An elevated MCV, however, is an abnormal finding and may precede by months or years the onset of a megaloblastic anemia. Megaloblastic anemia may be masked in the presence of complicating infections, inflammatory disease, or iron deficiency.

Spurious macrocytosis can occur, and an elevated

TABLE 2. **Differential Diagnosis of Macrocytosis**

Actual
Megaloblastic anemias
Liver disease
Reticulocytosis
Myeloproliferative diseases (leukemia, myelofibrosis)
Multiple myeloma
Metastatic disease of bone marrow
Hypothyroidism
Aplastic anemia
Drugs (cytotoxic agents, alcohol)
Spurious
Autoagglutination/cold agglutination disease

MCV must be corroborated by examination of the peripheral blood smear. The peripheral blood smear findings are invaluable in differential diagnosis. The earliest sign of megaloblastic anemia reflected in the peripheral blood is hypersegmentation of the polymorphonuclear leukocytes. Red cell morphology can help distinguish the macrocytosis of liver disease (round macrocytes), megaloblastic anemia (oval macrocytes), reticulocytosis (basophilic round macrocytes), and acute leukemias. In general, however, a bone marrow examination is essential to establish the presence of megaloblastic anemia, although the bone marrow examination cannot distinguish vitamin B_{12} deficiency of pernicious anemia from folic acid deficiency.

DIAGNOSTIC WORK-UP

The initial laboratory evaluation for vitamin B_{12} deficiency always includes a complete blood count with examination of the peripheral smear. If megaloblastic anemia is suspected, a serum vitamin B_{12} level is then obtained. In the nontransfused patient, bone marrow examination at this time can be particularly useful, showing megaloblastic maturation. If vitamin B_{12} deficiency is now thought to be likely, a Schilling test should be done to demonstrate the lack of intrinsic factor versus other malabsorptive states. This test determines vitamin B_{12} absorption using the urinary excretion of radiolabeled vitamin B_{12} after an oral dose given with or without intrinsic factor. Initially a parenteral loading dose of vitamin B_{12} (1000 µg) is administered so that when vitamin B_{12} is absorbed a significant amount is subsequently excreted in the urine. This dose, however, can correct the laboratory and hematologic evidence of megaloblastosis. Recently, assays for methylmalonic acid and total homocystine have become available. These amino acids are increased in vitamin B_{12}–deficient states because enzymes responsible for their conversion are vitamin B_{12}–dependent. In symptomatic patients, these levels are increased two to three times normal. Likewise, levels are increased in asymptomatic patients. These amino acid levels may be elevated before the falling vitamin B_{12} levels and diagnostic bone marrow morphologic findings are recognized.

TREATMENT

Immune-Mediated Vitamin B_{12} Deficiency (Pernicious Anemia)

Therapeutic aims are directed at reversing the immediate sequelae of the disorder, such as the pancytopenia and neurologic abnormalities (initial treatment), and toward maintenance of the remission and prevention of relapse (maintenance treatment).

Initial Treatment

The aim is to correct the deficiency and to replenish the stores. Because the disorder is caused by vitamin B_{12} malabsorption in most cases, parenteral vitamin B_{12} supplementation is given, using preferentially the intramuscular or subcutaneous routes. After injection, significant amounts of the vitamin are excreted in the urine; therefore, initial therapy should be several large doses (100 to 1000 μg) of vitamin B_{12}. Every-other-day injections replenish stores more rapidly than daily injections, although no established regimen works better than the others. Our approach is to administer a series of seven 1000-μg injections of vitamin B_{12} every other day over a period of 2 weeks. Patients or family members can be taught to inject the vitamin themselves. Following this, we usually continue with weekly injections over the next 4 weeks to ensure replacement of the vitamin stores and then monthly for life. It is not clear whether larger and more frequent doses of vitamin B_{12} are needed in patients with neurologic damage; however, in these patients, we give the same schedule of vitamin B_{12} as aforementioned; however, after a 2-month period of weekly injections, we then continue giving therapy every 2 weeks for a period of 6 months, and from that point on, one injection every month for the lifetime of the patient. There are, of course, no hard data on duration of initial therapy, but one tends to administer more aggressive treatment to patients with neurologic dysfunction.

The clinical response to initial therapy is often dramatic. Rapid reversal of pancytopenia and mucosal changes can occur with even minimal doses (as low as 1 μg). The patients often describe a sense of well-being, and within a week the mucosal changes reverse. Hematologic response is frequently noted after 3 days, with improvement in the hemoglobin 5 to 7 days after treatment. Disappearance of macrocytic red cells and correction of the MCV may take several weeks. During initial therapy, it is advisable to monitor serum potassium levels because rejuvenation of new cells may produce hypokalemia due to movement of plasma potassium into the rapidly proliferating hematopoietic cells. Patients who are on diuretic therapy and have an initial hypokalemia, patients with a history of cardiac disease, and those on digitalis therapy should be carefully monitored.

Coexistent iron deficiency or marginal bone marrow iron stores can limit the recovery and should be treated with 300 mg ferrous sulfate three times a day.

Maintenance Treatment

The second aim of vitamin replacement therapy is to maintain the vitamin stores so that relapse does not occur. Good clinical remission can be maintained even with partial repletion of the stores. Following repletion of the stores and in situations in which the underlying disease is irreversible, as in pernicious anemia, lifelong maintenance therapy is then administered. Our program for maintenance is to administer monthly injections of 1000 μg of cyanocobalamin, the most widely used and inexpensive form of vitamin B_{12} available in the United States. Another preparation, hydroxocobalamin, is more physiologic and has a longer biologic half-life than cyanocobalamin and may be given by intramuscular injection every 3 months. It is more expensive but does have the advantage of being retained longer after injection than cyanocobalamin.

Although patients may be instructed in self-administration of the injections, they should be evaluated at least once or twice a year by a physician. I see my patients at least annually, at which time they have a general examination and complete blood count. Clinical evaluation includes three serial stool guaiac determinations because there is a 2 to 3% incidence of carcinoma of the stomach in patients with pernicious anemia. Evaluation of thyroid studies in patients with suggestive symptoms is also performed, because there is an association between pernicious anemia and autoimmune thyroid disorders.

The need for continuous monitoring should be stressed to the patients, because lifelong therapy is essential. Proper patient education requires reinforcement of this fact, inasmuch as relapse in pernicious anemia is not uncommonly seen.

Other Vitamin B_{12} Deficiency States

Treatment of nonpernicious vitamin B_{12} deficiency anemia obviously depends upon the underlying cause. Patients who have had their source of intrinsic factor removed, such as those who have had a gastrectomy, also require lifelong therapy. Our program for these patients and for those who have had an ileal resection is identical to the management of patients with pernicious anemia. The diet of vegan patients who are deficient in vitamin B_{12} because of negligible intake can be supplemented by small amounts of oral cyanocobalamin. Doses of 25 μg daily may be sufficient. Alternatively, these patients may be given injections of cyanocobalamin every 6 months.

Folic Acid Deficiency

The clinical findings in folic acid deficiency are similar to those in pernicious anemia, except for the important observation that these patients lack any neurologic symptoms. The laboratory findings are also similar to those in pernicious anemia, with the complete blood count, peripheral blood smear, and bone marrow examination being indistinguishable from those in the vitamin B_{12}–deficient states. The diagnosis is usually made following determination of a low serum folate level. This test should be interpreted with caution. Serum folate levels can be normal in the presence of low folate stores, especially immediately following folate intake. A red blood cell folate level can be obtained and is more sensitive for assessing folic acid deficiency in these circumstances.

Treatment of folic acid deficiency, which usually occurs as a result of decreased dietary intake, is aimed at reversal of the initial effects of the deficiency, replenishment of folate stores, and maintenance of sufficient dietary intake to ensure adequate folate nutrition.

Folate absorption occurs throughout the small intestine. Megaloblastic anemia from folic acid deficiency responds readily to oral folate doses as low as 100 to 200 µg. In general, however, larger doses are administered and are usually sufficient to correct deficiency even in malabsorption states. Most available preparations contain 1 mg of folic acid, but in situations of severe malabsorption, doses of between 2 and 5 mg of folate can be given daily. Our general approach is to give 1 mg of folic acid daily except in situations of severe malabsorption, when we administer 3 mg daily. In these cases, we ensure that vitamin B_{12} deficiency is not coexistent and may initially administer 1000 µg of vitamin B_{12} monthly until such time as the malabsorption state is corrected. Replenishment of folate stores can be achieved within several weeks of oral therapy. If the underlying cause can be reversed, maintenance therapy is not indicated.

No significant primary toxicity from folate treatment has been reported. Its use in vitamin B_{12}–deficient patients can, however, precipitate subacute combined degeneration of the spinal cord; thus, one must exclude vitamin B_{12} deficiency in patients with folate deficiency.

In any patient with nutritional deficiency, the need for folate replacement must be emphasized. Patients should be educated about foods rich in folate, such as green leafy vegetables, and about the fact that folic acid is a labile vitamin and can easily be destroyed by overcooking or boiling.

In pregnancy, relative folic acid deficiency can occur despite apparently adequate normal blood levels when there is an enhanced requirement for both mother and fetus. Prevention and treatment of megaloblastic anemia of pregnancy can be accomplished with 1 mg of folic acid daily administered throughout pregnancy and during the period of lactation.

Alcoholics pose a special problem because poor nutrition is compounded by poor compliance and because alcohol per se is an antagonist to biologic folate cofactors. We treat these patients with higher doses, such as 5 mg of folate daily, inasmuch as compliance is the major limiting factor and the side effects of megavitamin therapy are negligible.

Other individuals requiring folate supplementation include patients requiring long-term hemodialysis and those with disorders of increased cellular turnover, such as chronic hemolytic states. These patients are indoctrinated as to the necessity of receiving 1 mg of folate daily as lifelong therapy.

Patients taking drugs that decrease normal folate absorption (birth control pills, phenytoin) may require folate supplementation (1 mg daily) if they develop evidence of folate deficiency. Folinic acid (citrovorum factor) is a reduced form of folic acid that bypasses the antifolate activity of the chemotherapeutic agent methotrexate. It is usually administered parenterally to "rescue" systemic antifolate effects of the drug, enabling higher "antimitotic" doses to be given.

Severe Megaloblastic Anemia
Acute Management

Transfusion therapy is rarely indicated because many patients do not exhibit overt hemodynamic decompensation (inasmuch as anemia is slowly progressive) and because response to the appropriate vitamin replacement is usually rapid and symptoms can be controlled by bed rest. Furthermore, "shotgun" therapy with B_{12} and folate pending diagnostic laboratory studies is usually unnecessary. However, patients with deteriorating neurologic signs or altered mental status should receive 1000 µg of intramuscular vitamin B_{12} immediately.

In the severely anemic patient with circulatory distress or in the elderly patient with cardiac or neurologic dysfunction, transfusion may be essential. These patients invariably have an increased plasma volume. Therefore, packed red cell transfusions should be administered slowly (3 hours per unit) with intravenous diuretics (e.g., furosemide) and potassium supplementation. Hypokalemia has been observed during the initial recovery phase following vitamin replacement therapy, particularly in these patients.

THALASSEMIA

method of
GEORGE PHILLIPS, Jr., M.D., and
RUSSEL E. KAUFMAN, M.D.
Duke University
Durham, North Carolina

The human hemoglobin protein is the major oxygen-carrying protein in the human body. This protein is a tetramer composed of two members of the α-globin family and two members of the β-globin family. During development, different hemoglobins are produced to meet the different physiologic needs of the developing fetus. Fetal hemoglobin (hemoglobin F), the major hemoglobin produced during fetal development, contains two α-globins and two γ-globins. It is replaced at birth with hemoglobin A, the major adult hemoglobin, in which β-globins are substituted for the γ-globins. The β-globin gene resides on chromosome 11 and is present in two copies in the diploid genome. Two α-globin genes reside on chromosome 16, and the α-globin gene is therefore present in four copies in the diploid genome. The products from the two gene families are usually produced in equal amounts. Thus abnormalities in either the α- or the β-globin gene family can cause an imbalance in the production of globin protein, which can result in decreased production of hemoglobin. Red cells in individuals with these abnormalities are smaller (microcytic) and have less hemoglobin protein in their cytoplasm (hypochromasia). Anemia results from a combination of decreased production and increased destruction of red cells.

Thalassemias, disorders resulting from imbalance in globin chain production, are classified according to the globin chain that is diminished in production, e.g., α-thalassemia or β-thalassemia. The emergence of clinical manifestations corresponds to the developmental stage when the affected globin chain is normally expressed. The α-chain mutants affect hemoglobin synthesis beginning in the second trimester, whereas mutations in β-globin genes are not fully manifested until approximately 6 months postnatally when the β-globin gene is fully expressed. This globin chain production imbalance produces erythrocytes with low hemoglobin content and a tendency to undergo destruction in the marrow and spleen.

In addition to the classification based on the involved globin chain, the thalassemias are also classified by clinical severity. In the most severe form, *thalassemia major,* greatly decreased synthesis of β-chains produces a severe, life-threatening anemia. Individuals with thalassemia major require transfusion therapy on a regular basis. Less severe forms of the disease, *thalassemia intermedia* and *thalassemia minor,* result from a moderate reduction in globin-chain synthesis. Given the simultaneous occurrence of α- and β-thalassemia or of thalassemia and another hemoglobinopathy, such as sickle cell disease, there is a wide spectrum of clinical disorders associated with thalassemias.

DIAGNOSIS

α-Thalassemia

The α-globins are the products of four α-globin genes per diploid genome. Four distinct clinical syndromes are associated with defects involving one or more of these genes. Not surprisingly, the greater the number of abnormal α-globin genes, the more severe the disorder. These syndromes range in clinical severity from a silent carrier state (one gene deletion) to a severe intrapartum

anemia that results in stillbirth (all four genes defective). Intermediate clinical syndromes include α-thalassemia 1, in which two α-globin genes are defective, resulting in a mild microcytic anemia, and hemoglobin H disease, in which three genes are defective. This form of thalassemia produces a severe microcytic anemia with hemoglobin concentrations around 7 gm per dL. Hemoglobin H is a tetramer of β-globin chains that can be identified by its characteristic rapid mobility during hemoglobin electrophoresis. In addition to producing hemoglobin H, newborns with α-thalassemia due to three defective globin genes and fetuses with four defective globin genes will also form γ-globin tetramers, termed Hb Barts. Because most forms of α-thalassemia are due to deletion of α-globin genes, these conditions can usually be diagnosed by α-globin gene-mapping studies of the patient's DNA.

β-Thalassemia

The β-thalassemia syndromes vary widely in clinical severity; the most common forms are thalassemia minor and major. β-*Thalassemia minor* produces a mild to moderate microcytic, hypochromic anemia with targeting of the erythrocytes. The HbA_2 level is moderately elevated (3.8 to 8%) in most cases, while increased levels of fetal hemoglobin (2 to 10%) occur in approximately half the cases. β-*Thalassemia major* is a severe anemia characterized by markedly hypochromic erythrocytes that have numerous inclusions and show marked variations in size and shape. Fetal hemoglobin usually constitutes a large percentage of the total hemoglobin. The diagnosis can be confirmed by measuring β-globin chain synthesis in the reticulocytes, although the presence of β-thalassemia trait in both parents is usually adequate to establish the diagnosis when the hematologic and clinical pictures are appropriate. Laboratory techniques available in most hemoglobin reference laboratories allow the determination of the precise molecular defects by direct analysis of the patient's DNA with a combination of polymerase chain reaction DNA amplification and hybridization with allele-specific probes. This approach is particularly valuable if prenatal diagnosis is to be performed during subsequent pregnancies from the affected partners.

α-Globin chains are synthesized during fetal and adult development for incorporation into fetal hemoglobin ($α_2$, $γ_2$) and hemoglobin A ($α_2$, $β_2$). Since α-globin chains are a component of fetal and adult hemoglobins, deficient synthesis is manifest during both fetal and adult life. Defective β-chain synthesis, on the other hand, is not clinically apparent until 3 to 6 months after birth, when hemoglobin A replaces fetal hemoglobin. Patients with β-thalassemia major then develop a progressively severe anemia, with hemoglobin values usually falling to less than 7 grams per dL.

Blood transfusion is usually required for survival in over 80% of patients with β-thalassemia major. Impaired growth and development and susceptibility to serious infections characterize the first several years of life for these children, and long-term complications may become apparent by 5 years of age. The spleen can progressively enlarge in response to the large burden of thalassemia and transfused erythrocytes, and transfusion requirements gradually increase as the first signs of hypersplenism become apparent. Eventually most patients will require splenectomy as thrombocytopenia and leukopenia develop.

The severe anemia associated with β-thalassemia is a potent stimulus for erythroid marrow proliferation. Marrow expansion may fill most of the marrow space and cause extensive skeletal changes. Long bones become osteoporotic and easily broken, and cranial bones can thicken, producing disfiguring facial changes. Extramedullary marrow proliferation can produce spinal cord compression or visceral masses, which can be painful or interfere with other organ functions.

An additional response to the severe anemia is increased gastrointestinal iron absorption, which contributes to the already great transfusional iron burden and can play a significant role in the eventual severe iron toxicity. Iron overload is one of the greatest threats to the individual with β-thalassemia major. Iron deposition in the heart can produce cardiac failure and life-threatening arrhythmias, and chronic damage to hepatocytes results in cirrhosis and altered hepatic function. Likewise, endocrine gland function, especially of the pituitary and adrenals, may be impaired, leading to serious metabolic disturbances that may be recognized only at times of stress, such as surgery or serious infection. Tissue iron toxicity is probably mediated in part by free radical damage. The highly reactive free radicals produced by ionized iron are scavenged by antioxidants, including vitamins E and C, resulting in low serum and tissue levels of these micronutrients.

TREATMENT

β-Thalassemia Minor

No therapy is required for the mild anemia associated with β-thalassemia minor. Supplemental iron should not be given unless the patient has proven iron deficiency, and treatment should stop once iron stores are replenished. The role of micronutrient supplementation in β-thalassemia minor remains to be elucidated.

β-Thalassemia Major

β-Thalassemia major is treated primarily by transfusion of red blood cells. Achieving goals of maintaining an optimal hemoglobin level and preventing or delaying long-term complications requires an individualized program of transfusions, iron chelation, and surveillance for the development of skeletal, endocrine, and cardiac abnormalities. Most of the therapeutic guidelines for β-thalassemia major also can be applied to a milder form of homozygous β-thalassemia termed β-*thalassemia intermedia*. These patients may not be dependent on transfusions but can still develop many of the complications associated with β-thalassemia major, particularly skeletal changes. The decision to transfuse depends in large part on the patient's capacity to undertake the following comprehensive program.

Transfusion Therapy. Prior to the 1960s, transfusion schedules were predicated on the goal of limiting iron accumulation since this was the major cause of early mortality. Hemoglobin values were generally maintained between 8 and 10 grams per dL. Studies in the 1960s demonstrated that hypertransfusion programs, in which hemoglobin concentration was maintained above 10 grams per dL, resulted in more normal growth and development and fewer skeletal changes. More frequent transfusions were required, however, and the iron burden increased. Coupled with iron chelation therapy, more aggressive transfusion programs were initiated, which maintained hemoglobin above 12 grams per dL. These "supertransfusion" programs generally required no great increase in the rate of transfusion once the patient was transfused and maintained at the higher hemoglobin level. This is probably explained by the reduction of the greatly expanded blood volume seen prior to initiation of "supertransfusion." Gastrointestinal iron absorption is also suppressed. Most centers now use an aggressive transfusion program, although numerous factors can affect this decision.

To reduce the frequency of febrile and urticarial transfusion reactions, washed, frozen, thawed packed cells should be used when available. Accurate records of transfusion requirements will help document the development of hypersplenism. The desired hemoglobin level can usually be obtained by transfusion on an outpatient basis two to four times per month. The anticipated transfusion requirement for most supertransfusion programs is less than 250 ml per kg per year for an individual without hypersplenism. Requirements can increase greatly following the development of hypersplenism. Experimental programs using apheresis and separation techniques allow the infusion of blood enriched with young erythrocytes (neocytes) and depleted of aged erythrocytes; total transfusion requirements are reduced because of the increased survival of transfused cells. The transfusional iron burden is also decreased because of the removal of aged erythrocytes, which have a short survival following transfusion.

IRON OVERLOAD. The successful transfusion programs have produced significant iron burdens in most individuals with thalassemia. The excess iron is toxic in part due to its promotion of the generation of free radical species, which produce oxidative damage to proteins and DNA. Aggressive iron chelation therapy can prevent heavy iron loading and probably many of the associated complications.

A number of parameters are used in deciding whether to undertake iron removal therapy: serum iron, iron-binding capacity, serum ferritin, quantitative iron from liver biopsy, and computed tomography and magnetic resonance imaging of the liver have all been used. However, it has been suggested that individuals with thalassemia who have received 30 units of transfused blood and are expected to continue on a regular transfusion program should be considered for an iron removal program.

Effective iron excretion can be achieved by the daily subcutaneous continuous infusion of deferoxamine (Desferal) via a small portable pump. Patients with significant iron stores excrete 15 to 60 mg of iron daily when given 20 to 40 mg per kg per day of deferoxamine. Infusions last 10 to 12 hours and can be continued overnight. Pruritus, swelling, and pain at the injection site reduce the likelihood of long-term compliance, but these complications can be prevented in many cases by adding 0.1 mg of hydrocortisone to each milliliter of deferoxamine at the time of infusion. Use of cold towels or diphenhydramine (Benadryl) cream can reduce the discomfort once the local reaction has developed. Patients unable to use this route of administration can receive parenteral deferoxamine via subcutaneous ports or Hickman catheters.

Excretion of iron is enhanced by the administration of ascorbic acid along with deferoxamine. However, when ascorbic acid is administered in high doses, cardiotoxicity frequently develops. Therefore, the dose of ascorbic acid should not exceed 100 mg per day. This therapy should be reserved for individuals who have significant increases in urinary iron excretion with, or are deficient in, vitamin C.

Among the numerous complications of deferoxamine therapy are auditory impairment, visual impairment, decline in renal function, pulmonary complications, and local irritation. Therefore, it is suggested that individuals receiving this drug should have at least annual auditory and visual testing.

Vitamin E is another potent antioxidant that is frequently present in low amounts in the serum of transfused thalassemia individuals. Replacement of vitamin E has not been demonstrated to reduce the toxicity of iron overload. Furthermore, in this disease, replacement therapy does not have any significant effect on erythrocyte survival, although it may reduce the rate of deferoxamine-induced iron excretion. Studies are in progress to determine the role of vitamin E in thalassemia.

Splenectomy. Hypertransfusion programs have greatly reduced the incidence of hypersplenism in early childhood and, consequently, the need for early splenectomy. However, splenectomy may be required in later childhood. It is suggested that the transfusion index (the total volume of packed red cells received in a year divided by the mid-year weight in kilograms) should be the criterion: when the index exceeds 160 mg per kg per year, splenectomy should be considered. Vaccination for *Pneumococcus* and *Haemophilus influenzae* should be considered before splenectomy. Occasionally, the spleen becomes large and painful in the absence of overt hypersplenism and may require removal. Daily prophylactic administration of penicillin V (125 mg daily) is also recommended after splenectomy. In the event of unexplained fever in the splenectomized patient, parenteral administration of broad-spectrum antibiotics is indicated because of the serious threat of overwhelming sepsis.

Complications of Iron Overload

Cardiac Complications. Histologic studies on cardiac tissue from patients with iron overload in β-thalassemia indicate that the preferred sites of early deposition of iron are the pericardium and the myocardium. This pattern parallels the clinical events. Pericarditis is a frequent and early event and atrial arrhythmias are common complications of the pericarditis. Within several years of the onset of pericarditis, most patients develop ventricular ectopy, including ventricular tachycardia. Cardiac rhythm disturbances usually herald the onset of myocardial contraction dysfunction with its poor prognosis. Echocardiography and radionuclide cineangiography in patients without clinical evidence of pump failure demonstrate thickening of the ventricular wall and impaired ejection fractions with exercise. Symptoms of cardiac failure usually develop within 2 to 3 years of the onset of cardiac signs unless the iron loading is reversed.

The treatment of these conditions is primarily symptomatic. Pericarditis is best managed with bed rest, analgesics, and anti-inflammatory drugs such as indomethacin and ibuprofen. Atrial arrhythmias can be suppressed with digoxin, propranolol, or calcium channel blocking drugs. Ventricular arrhythmias are more difficult to manage and may be impossible to eliminate. In such cases, a reasonable goal is suppression of ventricular premature beats to a symptomatically tolerable level. Agents of choice are those active against ventricular arrhythmias in other conditions. However, therapy must be highly individualized and portable monitoring devices may be needed.

The onset of congestive heart failure is ominous. In the early stages, symptoms of volume expansion and pulmonary congestion can be managed with salt restriction, diuretics, and digoxin. In later stages of heart failure, pulmonary congestion may decrease, but the patient may complain of severe fatigue and experience wasting of skeletal muscle in a pattern typical of biventricular cardiac failure. These patients are prone to develop ascites since they have coexisting hepatic disease. In some patients, agents that reduce afterload have been useful.

Hepatic Complications. Most patients who have β-thalassemia and are on a transfusion program have some degree of hepatomegaly. Hepatic enzymes may be mildly elevated chronically and are greatly increased only with hepatitis or other causes of significant hepatocyte damage. The synthetic capacity of the liver is impaired only after extensive iron damage has occurred, although prothrombin times may be moderately prolonged. This can usually be corrected with injections of vitamin K. Iron chelation therapy is effective in reversing many of the hepatic complications of iron loading. Unlike the heart, the liver has remarkable regenerative capacity. As in most hemolytic anemias, biliary disease from the formation of pigmented stones is an almost certain complication and should be managed surgically when appropriate.

Endocrine Complications. Virtually all endocrine glands accumulate iron when total body stores increase. However, the extent of endocrine dysfunction is highly varied. Often the first sign of iron overload, failure of sexual maturation is due to impaired gonadotropin release rather than target organ failure. Early iron deposition in the adrenals is in the zona glomerulosa, although mineralocorticoid regulation is seldom impaired. Later in the course of disease, the corticosteroid response to ACTH becomes blunted, and the patient's skin may take on the slate gray cast typical of ACTH hypersecretion. Adrenal crisis can occur during times of severe stress unless adrenal insufficiency is recognized and appropriate replacement therapy given. Pancreatic endocrine function is frequently impaired late in the illness, and insulin therapy is usually required to treat the diabetes mellitus. Subclinical deficiencies of thyroid and parathyroid function have been reported but are usually not a problem. The most important aspect of management of endocrine abnormalities is early recognition. Therapy in all cases is by appropriate hormonal replacement.

Bone and Skeletal Disease

Facial disfiguration is frequently the greatest concern of patients with β-thalassemia. Fortunately, this has become much less a problem since the initiation of aggressive transfusion programs. Extramedullary hematopoiesis can have serious consequences in patients with the thalassemic syndromes, especially when it occurs in the spinal canal, causing spinal cord compression. If the proliferation of erythroid tissue cannot be controlled with transfusion therapy, local radiation therapy may prove useful.

Experimental Therapy

Bone Marrow Transplantation. The success of marrow transplantation in children with aplastic anemia and leukemia has raised hopes for the correction of other hematologic disorders, including the thalassemias and hemoglobinopathies. Marrow transplantation should be considered for the transfusion-dependent child less than 16 years of age when there is an HLA-identical donor and the recipient has relatively little end-organ dysfunction.

Genetic Manipulation. Recent studies of gene organization and regulation suggest new avenues for treatment of these diseases. The principal goals of genetic manipulation are replacement of adult hemoglobin synthesis with fetal hemoglobin synthesis or substitution of the dysfunctional β-globin gene with a normal β-globin gene. Studies are in progress to determine the feasibility of these approaches.

Pharmacologic Manipulation of Fetal Hemoglobin Synthesis

The severity of β-thalassemia is greatly reduced in individuals with coexisting conditions that increase fetal hemoglobin synthesis, such as hereditary persistence of fetal hemoglobin. Pharmacologic agents that affect DNA methylation (5-azacytidine) or cell cycle kinetics (hydroxyurea or cytosine arabinoside) have increased fetal hemoglobin synthesis in patients with β-thalassemia major or sickle cell disease in well-controlled clinical trials. Recently, butyrate compounds have shown similar effects and may offer a greatly reduced long-term risk of toxicity. These therapies are considered experimental and should not be undertaken outside of controlled trials, although they offer great hope for management of patients with severe disorders of hemoglobin synthesis.

PREVENTION OF β-THALASSEMIA

In general, parents at risk for having a child with thalassemia major can be easily identified by simple laboratory measurement of erythrocyte parameters such as the mean corpuscular volume. In the past, couples who were heterozygous for thalassemia trait had few options other than limiting the size of their family. However, the development over the past 10 years of methods for prenatal detection of hemoglobin variants and thalassemias in utero underscores the importance of recognition of β-thalassemia minor and the need to properly inform individuals with this condition of their risk of having a child with β-thalassemia major. Many couples at risk have chosen to undergo antenatal diagnosis and termination of pregnancy when the fetus is deemed likely to have β-thalassemia major. This approach was limited by the unacceptable fetal wastage associated with sampling of fetal blood, but current techniques have reduced the risk to the fetus and increased the accuracy of diagnosis. These techniques require direct examination of DNA derived from fetal cells in the amniotic fluid or the chorionic villus. Two approaches are used to determine if the fetus carries the defective globin genes. The original method of DNA analysis utilized restriction of endonuclease polymorphisms linked to the defective β-globin gene on the chromosomal DNA of the parents to determine whether the β-thalassemic globin gene had been transmitted to the fetus. With this technique, more than 95% of affected fetuses can be identified with less than a 0.1% chance of inadvertent fetal wastage. Current technologies allow direct examination of the β-globin genes and the determination of the specific defects.

Further advances in reproduction biology offer the possibility of in vitro fertilization and DNA analysis at the blastocyst stage to determine the presence of the thalassemia genotype. Most centers performing antenatal diagnosis can precisely determine the molecular defect in the β-globin gene by direct examination of the DNA sequence.

In developed parts of the world, use of these techniques should lead to a great reduction in the incidence of the severe form of the disease. Simplification and standardization of these techniques are essential to their use in underdeveloped regions of the world in which thalassemia is common.

SICKLE CELL DISEASE

method of
PAUL F. MILNER, M.D.
Medical College of Georgia
Augusta, Georgia

The sickle cell diseases are inherited hemolytic anemias in which some or all of the normal hemoglobin A is replaced by the mutant hemoglobin S (Hb S). About 1 in 12 people of African descent in the Americas carry the sickle cell trait (A/S), but it is also present in Greeks, Italians, Turks, Saudi Arabians, and members of certain tribes in the Indian subcontinent. Subjects who have sickle cell trait are not anemic and have a normal life expectancy. Between 25 and 40% of their hemoglobin is Hb S. Under normal circumstances, their red cells do not sickle or hemolyze. About 3% of A/S subjects, however, have episodes of painless hematuria, which if prolonged, may require treatment. At high altitudes (above 8000 feet), nausea and splenic pain can occur.

Sickle cell anemia (S/S) comes about through the inheritance of two Hb S genes, one from each parent. About 2.5% of African Americans carry another mutant hemoglobin, Hb C, and about 1% carry a gene for β-thalassemia. Interaction between these hemoglobin genes and Hb S gives rise to heterozygotes such as Hb S/C and Hb S/β-thalassemia (S/β⁰thal, S/β⁺thal). These subjects have varying degrees of anemia and symptoms of sickle cell disease. Interactions between Hb S and other rare abnormal hemoglobins are seen from time to time, with phenotypic expression similar to that of the more common heterozygotes.

At birth the red cells of the S/S infant contain mainly fetal hemoglobin (Hb F). Within a few months, these red cells are replaced by cells containing mainly Hb S, but a few red cells containing about 15 to 30% Hb F (F-cells) usually persist into adult life. In some S/S patients, however, many F-cells persist into adult life. As these cells are much less likely to sickle, these patients experience less hemolysis, milder anemia, and fewer complications. This phenotype is quite common among patients in Saudi Arabia, the Indian subcontinent, and the Senegal area of Africa. About 15% of S/S patients in the United States have this phenotype.

About 30% of African Americans also carry a hemoglobin defect known as α-thalassemia-2. One of the two active α-globin genes on chromosome 16 is deleted (αα/α−) in heterozygotes and (α−/α−) in homozygotes. Subjects with Hb A and this defect have a microcytic red cell morphology without anemia. Patients with sickle cell anemia and α-thalassemia have a somewhat different clinical course from that of the usual S/S patient. Definitive identification of α-thalassemia requires DNA analysis, but it can often be suggested by the low mean corpuscular volume (MCV), a milder degree of anemia, and a stronger physique. Finally, a few S/S patients of African descent have both an α-thalassemia gene and high levels of fetal hemoglobin associated with a relatively mild disease that may not be diagnosed until the late teen or early adult years. Sickle cell anemia of this type is common in eastern Saudi Arabia and India.

GENERAL MANAGEMENT

Infants and Children

Ideally, infants should be diagnosed at birth, but the child or young adult may not have been tested. If the type of sickle cell disease is uncertain, hemoglobin electrophoresis and quantitation of Hb F should be done at the initial visit. It is important to inquire as to recent blood transfusion, as this will confuse the result. A full blood count with reticulocyte count, chemistry profile, and urinalysis should be obtained and repeated as necessary at future visits.

Regular check-ups should be carried out at intervals that will depend, to some extent, on the course of the disease and the frequency of symptoms. Parents should be educated about the nature of the disease and how to detect complications, particularly acute ones. They should be able to take a temperature, palpate the spleen, and suspect a worsening anemia and should be instructed to report any acute change in the child's condition immediately. The National Association for Sickle Cell Disease, Inc.* publishes a useful pamphlet on sickle cell disease in childhood entitled "How to Help Your Child to Take It in Stride."

Nutritional Supplements

Folic acid, 1 mg per day, should be prescribed for children to prevent deficiency, but extra vitamins are unnecessary and iron is contraindicated unless a deficiency has been clearly established.

Immunization and Pneumococcal Prophylaxis

The usual course of inoculations should be given, including *Haemophilus B* conjugate and hepatitis B. Blockage of the splenic microcirculation by sickled red cells produces hyposplenia, which renders infants vulnerable to pneumococcal septicemia. Morbidity and mortality have been greatly reduced by the institution of daily oral penicillin therapy. The dose is 150 mg penicillin V in liquid form twice a day. This should be continued to age 3 years, when polyvalent pneumococcal vaccine should be given. Some pediatricians continue prophylaxis to age 5 years with amoxicillin, 250 mg chewable tablets twice a day.

Splenic Sequestration

The spleen is usually palpable in infants and small children but may become acutely enlarged due to rapid sequestration of sickled blood. As the acute anemia can be rapidly fatal, this is an emergency requiring admission to the hospital and prompt blood transfusion.

*3460 Wilshire Boulevard, Suite 1012, Los Angeles, CA 90010-2273.

Osseous Complications

The hand-foot syndrome, a painful swelling of the hand or foot caused by infarction of bone marrow in metacarpal or metatarsal bones and phalanges, is common between the ages of 6 months and 2 years. It resolves spontaneously in about a week. In older children and adults, infarcts in other long bones can cause pain and swelling of an arm or leg. Osteomyelitis, usually caused by salmonellae, should be ruled out. It is much more common in Africa than in North and South America. Osteonecrosis is discussed further on.

Aplastic Crises

Aplastic crises are caused by viral infections, particularly with the human parvovirus B19. The patient, usually a child under 18 years who may be recovering from an infection, presents with profound anemia and a fall in the reticulocyte count to below 1%. Although this is not an emergency, the child should be admitted to the hospital for observation and, usually, a blood transfusion. Spontaneous recovery in a week to 10 days is the rule, and recurrence is extremely rare.

Stroke

Stroke, resulting from blockage of the internal carotid artery or its branches, affects about 5% of S/S children. The treatment is a program of exchange transfusions to lower the proportion of Hb S to less than 50% and maintain it at that level throughout childhood. This prevents a second stroke and helps neurologic recovery. There is mounting evidence that investigation of the cerebral circulation by transcranial Doppler ultrasonography can predict the onset of stroke, which might then be prevented by starting the child on a chronic transfusion program. It is important to institute a program of iron chelation with deferoxamine concomitant with the transfusion regimen.

Pain Control at Home

Almost half of S/S patients, and most S/C and Sβ+thal patients, rarely experience pain severe enough to require hospital treatment. However, episodes of pain lasting several days involving the lower back, chest, and long bones are not uncommon and can be treated at home. Acetaminophen with 30 mg of codeine, or 5 to 7.5 mg of hydrocodone, is usually sufficient. For more severe pain, which may keep the patient in bed, oxycodone in the form of Percodan Demi for children, or 5 mg (Percocet, Percodan) for older children or adults, every 4 to 6 hours, may be necessary. More localized bone or joint pain is best treated with nonsteroidal anti-inflammatory drugs. Indomethacin, 25 mg three times a day for a few days, is very effective. Knee effusions respond well to rest and analgesics and should not be tapped unless septic arthritis is suspected.

About 14% of S/S children younger than 10 years and about 30% of teenagers develop gallstones. Abdominal pain requires investigation by ultrasonography of the upper abdomen. Laparoscopic cholecystectomy has greatly reduced the incidence of postoperative complications and the need for intraoperative transfusion. Children improve after surgery, gain weight, and have fewer hospital admissions.

Transition to Adulthood

From about age 8 years into the teens, the frequency of crises and symptoms may decrease, only to recur with greater intensity after puberty. The onset of puberty and of the adolescent growth spurt are often late, and menarche and bone age may be delayed by 4 to 5 years in some cases. Once the growth spurt occurs, the child may return to the same height percentile or a slightly higher one. Although normal or decreased weight for height is usual, some teenage S/S children are obese.

Children should be encouraged to lead a normal life and attend school. Teachers should be aware that the child's physical activity is restricted by anemia and pain and needs to urinate frequently. Home-bound teaching should be arranged when necessary. Competitive sports should be avoided, but regular exercise should be encouraged. Swimming seems to precipitate pain attacks and is best avoided. It is important to encourage a healthy lifestyle with an optimistic outlook, particularly in adolescence. Few adult patients are unable to work if their occupation is sedentary. Manual work that requires strenuous physical exertion is not suitable for most S/S patients.

The late teen or early adult years are a good time to discuss the clinical complications that can occur and answer any questions the patient or relatives may have regarding life expectancy. The long-term prognosis for most patients is good if they receive adequate continuing care.

Avascular Necrosis

Patients should be counseled to report any unusual symptoms, such as persistent pain in the hip or shoulder, so that an early diagnosis of osteonecrosis can be made. Despite a seemingly normal hip x-ray, magnetic resonance imaging may show early necrosis of the femoral head. Further deterioration of the joint, which might later require total hip replacement, can be avoided by early core decompression of the femoral head, a relatively simple procedure.

Proliferative Retinopathy

The young adult with Hb S/C, S/β+ thalassemia, or S/S α-thalassemia with a relatively high hematocrit should be referred to an ophthalmologist familiar with retinal disease so that proliferative retinopathy can be diagnosed and treated before complications arise. These patients should be re-examined at least every 2 years.

Contraception and Pregnancy

Oral contraceptives are not contraindicated in sickle cell disease. The low-estrogen preparations should be prescribed, but some patients may prefer medroxyprogesterone (Depo-Provera) or levonorgestrel (Norplant), particularly if sickle cell symptoms occur with the menses, which is often the case.

Maternal mortality is now very low (less than 0.5%) and even the more symptomatic S/S patients can have a successful pregnancy, but they should be considered at high risk, especially for fetal complications. Prophylactic exchange transfusions are contraindicated but blood transfusion may be necessary if the Hb falls below 7 grams per dL. All blood given should be matched for the major antigens, as delayed transfusion reactions are common in this population and can cause fetal death. First-trimester miscarriages are still common. Contrary to anecdotal reports, most Hb S/C women have an uneventful pregnancy and delivery. Teenage pregnancy should be avoided.

Priapism

Attacks of priapism in boys and young men are distressing but can usually be managed conservatively. These attacks are usually self limited but may occur frequently. Priapism sometimes responds to nifedipine, 10 mg in repeated doses, and some patients find that a nitroglycerine patch, 0.2 to 0.4 mg per hour, applied in the early evening, will prevent nocturnal attacks. If an attack persists for more than 6 hours, the patient should be admitted to the hospital, and if it continues for more than 24 hours despite conservative measures, a urologist should be consulted. Most of these patients have relatively high Hb and hematocrit levels, and there is no convincing evidence that blood or exchange transfusion aborts the attack. A corpora spongiosa/cavernosa shunt through the glans penis (the Winter procedure) is often effective and may need to be repeated. Subsequent erectile function is usually not affected. Repeated attacks of priapism can result in thickening and gross enlargement of the penis, which remains semierect. Impotence can be treated by penile implants.

Ankle Ulcers

Ankle ulcers occur in about 6% of young adult and older S/S patients and can be very resistant to treatment. It is essential to eradicate infection, and this can be achieved by instructing the patient to bathe the ulcerated area with a dilute hypochlorite solution (one tablespoon of Clorox added to a quart of water) twice a day and to apply a gauze pad soaked in the same solution. Ointments containing proteolytic enzymes (Elase, Travase, Colaginase) are useful for dissolving thick sloughs but are fairly expensive. Other ointments and topical antibiotics, except chloramphenicol, are best avoided. When the area is clean, zinc cream or Unna's boot can be applied. Duoderm has recently been used successfully to promote healing. Blood transfusions given over several months may be advantageous, especially in older patients with more severe anemia. As a last resort skin grafting may be needed along with blood transfusion. Recurrence is often a problem and grafting may have to be repeated. Chronic pain from ankle ulcers can be controlled with sustained-release morphine (MS Contin), 30 mg every 8 hours as necessary.

Painless Hematuria

Gross, painless hematuria is most often encountered in patients with either Hb S/C or sickle cell trait. It is caused by necrosis of the tip of a renal papilla and prolonged by the action of urokinase in the urine. Although the hematuria may continue for several weeks, it seldom requires hospitalization and may cease spontaneously. It is important to rule out more serious causes by appropriate urologic investigations. Treatment with ε-aminocaproic acid (EACA) (Amicar), 5 grams three times a day, combined with rest in a horizontal position, is usually effective. EACA should not be given parenterally or in higher oral doses because of the risk of blood clots in the renal pelvis.

Acute Pain Crisis

The onset of a vaso-occlusive crisis is usually abrupt with intense pain, often in the back, ribs, sternum, and extremities. Pain tends to come in waves every few minutes but may be fairly continuous. Contrary to popular belief, pain crises in adults are seldom associated with infection; even severe infections, such as pneumococcal sepsis, may not be associated with painful symptoms. Mild fever may be present initially in children but is unusual in adults, although a swinging fever may develop later and indicate a complication such as lung infiltration. An increase in the white cell count (up to 25,000 per mm^3) with increase in polymorphs can be due to bone marrow infarction alone. The hemoglobin and hematocrit may be high initially, compared with steady state

values, only to fall below these as the crisis progresses.

Treatment

Treatment is usually initiated in the emergency room. Patients who show improvement over 6 to 8 hours may be discharged with oral analgesics. If improvement does not occur by then, or if fever is present, patients should be admitted to the hospital.

The main aim of treatment is to correct dehydration and provide adequate pain relief. Prior to seeking medical help, the patient will probably have tried to combat the pain with increased fluid intake and oral analgesics. An intravenous line should be placed and 5% dextrose (D_5W) administered at a rate of about 5 mL per kg per hour (250 to 300 mL per hour for the average adult). After diruresis has occurred, 0.45% NaCl in D_5W can be used. There is no difficulty with water excretion, so large infusions are quickly excreted. Continuous infusion of 0.9% NaCl, however, can produce fluid overload because of impaired excretion of sodium.

A high fever should be treated with intravenous antibiotics until blood culture results are available, but fever is often caused by bone marrow infarction alone and may respond to acetaminophen. Blood transfusion is usually not necessary for treatment of anemia per se, but may be beneficial if there is an infection or an expanding lung infiltrate with the possibility of hypoxia. Oxygen should be provided as indicated by blood gas analysis, but it is not necessary routinely in an uncomplicated pain crisis.

Narcotic analgesics should be used in adequate doses. The intramuscular route is best avoided in these patients because frequent administration causes tissue fibrosis and poor absorption of the drug. Patient-controlled analgesia (PCA) pumps are now widely used; they provide more continuous pain relief with less total narcotic use. Morphine, 0.1 to 0.15 mg per kg every 3 to 4 hours, is the best narcotic for children. Meperidine (Demerol) is popular with both doctors and patients, but prolonged use at high dosages can lead to accumulation of a toxic metabolite, normeperidine, which causes seizures. Buprenorphine (Buprenex), an agonist/antagonist analgesic, is useful in the emergency room. Given intravenously, a dose of 0.3 mg will usually provide relief for 4 to 6 hours. Patients who habitually take oral oxycodone, however, may develop tolerance to this preparation. Drugs of the nalorphine type such as nalbuphine (Nubain) may cause unpleasant sensations of withdrawal in patients who habitually take oral oxycodone and are best avoided. Hydromorphone (Dilaudid) is contraindicated because of its high addictive potential. As the patient improves, the dose of narcotic should be reduced, keeping the interval the same. Whatever schedule is used, it is important to gain the patient's confidence and provide effective pain relief from the outset.

Antidepressants, such as amitriptyline (Elavil), 25 mg orally three times a day; or hydroxyzine (Vistaril), 50 mg orally three times daily, are useful adjuncts to treatment of pain in these patients. A caring, supportive, and optimistic attitude toward the patient helps to allay the anxiety that most sickle cell patients feel when they go into crisis. The patient should be switched to an oral preparation such as MS Contin, 30 mg every 8 hours, or oxycodone, 5 mg every 4 hours, prior to discharge.

Most pain crises are short lived with recovery within about a week, but occasionally they can be very severe, with extensive bone marrow infarction. It is important to follow each patient closely with daily laboratory blood tests and, if necessary, arterial blood analysis. Fat embolization from infarcted necrotic bone marrow can cause rapid development of disseminated intravascular coagulation, a rare complication with a high mortality. It is therefore important to monitor the platelet count and order coagulation tests if it falls dramatically. Patients have been saved by prompt exchange transfusion and intensive care. The use of heparin is controversial.

Surgery and Anesthesia

Patients should be admitted 24 hours before surgery and intravenous fluids started at 1.5 times maintenance requirements if oral fluids are to be restricted. Blood transfusion is not necessary preoperatively for minor surgery or laparoscopic cholecystectomy if the hemoglobin is above 7 grams per dL. For major surgery, an exchange of a least 50% should be considered to raise the hematocrit to about 35%. Great care must be taken to match the patient's antigens to avoid a delayed transfusion reaction. The most common postoperative complications are atelectasis and pulmonary infarction. Both can be prevented by physiotherapy and the use of an incentive spirometer.

Future Therapy

Bone marrow transplantation is already being performed successfully with low mortality in infants and children with sickle cell anemia, but a tissue match is possible in only about 18% of patients. Ethical questions arise because the prognosis in any given case is uncertain, and less drastic therapy can still improve the quality of life and life expectancy.

Hydroxyurea (Hydrea),* 15 to 25 mg per kg, has been used in adults to increase Hb F and F-cells. It improves well-being and reduces sickling and hemolytic anemia. A placebo controlled drug trial is under way to see whether this drug can significantly reduce the frequency of vaso-occlusive crises. Other agents, such as butyrate, are being investigated and soon there may be several agents available to provide a better quality of life for these patients.

---

*This use of hydroxyurea is not listed in the manufacturer's official directive.

NEUTROPENIA

method of
ROBERT L. BAEHNER, M.D.
University of Southern California School of Medicine
Childrens Hospital of Los Angeles
Los Angeles, California

Neutropenia is defined as an absolute granulocyte count (AGC) of less than 1500 granulocytes per mm³. The AGC is calculated as follows:

ACG = neutrophils + bands × total white cell count

Depending on the AGC, neutropenia may present with severe infection or as an isolated laboratory finding. Neutropenia can occur alone or in combination with other hematologic abnormalities suggestive of more generalized marrow disease, such as aplastic anemia or leukemia. The family history, association with other disease or cancer therapy, degree and duration of neutropenia, and ability to handle infection should be considered in the evaluation and management of neutropenia.

CLINICAL PRESENTATION

In the absence of infection, there are no signs or symptoms associated with neutropenia itself. The degree of neutropenia will determine the probability of infectious complications such as sepsis, periodontal disease, or skin, mouth, or gastrointestinal ulceration. A history of recurrence of fever every 19 to 30 days is suggestive of cyclic neutropenia.

DIFFERENTIAL DIAGNOSIS

Isolated neutropenia can be either acquired or congenital. Certain congenital neutropenias are due to marrow failure, but most are benign and immune in origin. Patients with the latter type do well despite very low absolute neutrophil counts. Acquired neutropenia can be due to marrow failure, as in the case of drug toxicity; increased margination of neutrophils to the microvasculature, as in complement activation or severe burns; or peripheral destruction, as in hypersplenism or immune neutropenia. An important correctable, although rare, cause of neutropenia is vitamin B_{12} or folate deficiency. In the newborn, neutropenia is a sign of sepsis. Primary or metastatic marrow malignancy can present with neutropenia; however, other hematologic abnormalities are usually present as well. Transient neutropenia can follow viral infection or immunization.

EVALUATION

In the absence of any clinical findings or history, isolated mild neutropenia requires only observation. Medications known to be associated with neutropenia should be stopped. Most postviral neutropenias resolve within 4 to 8 weeks. The blood count should be followed weekly until recovery and with each subsequent febrile episode until it is clear that the neutropenia is not recurrent. If anemia or thrombocytopenia develops in conjunction with the neutropenia, bone marrow aspiration should be performed immediately. If the neutropenia is persistent, bone marrow aspiration and biopsy, determination of vitamin B_{12} and folate levels, collagen vascular evaluation, and a serum antineutrophil antibody assay should be performed. Twice weekly blood counts for 6 weeks are required to rule out cyclic neutropenia. Epinephrine or steroid stimulation tests and serum lysozyme determinations are sometimes done but are of no help in establishing a diagnosis or selecting treatment.

TREATMENT

Supportive Management

Supportive management of the neutropenic patient depends upon the degree of neutropenia, the cause, and the patient's past history of ability to handle infection. Because it is not possible to predict the duration or progression of neutropenia at first presentation, management must be much more aggressive than in the case of chronic neutropenias. The absolute granulocyte count can be used as a guide (Table 1). There is rarely room for clinical judgment in the management of patients with absolute neutrophil counts below 250 per mm.[3] If these patients have significant fever (>38.5° C), they must be admitted to the hospital and appropriate cultures obtained, then placed on empiric broad-spectrum parenteral antibiotics. Common bacterial causes of febrile episodes in neutropenic patients include gram-negative bacilli and cocci (*Pseudomonas aeruginosa, Escherichia coli, Klebsiella* species) and gram-positive bacilli and cocci (*Staphylococcus aureus* and *epidermidis, Streptococcus pneumoniae, pyogenes,* and *viridans* group, *Enterococcus faecalis, Coryne-bacterium* species). In the clinical setting of prolonged periods of neutropenia, concomitant polymicrobial and sequential infections are not uncommon. Systemic fungal infections, especially

TABLE 1. **Clinically Significant Absolute Neutrophil Counts**

Neutrophil Count (granulocytes/mm³)	Significance
>1000	Normal host defenses against infection
500–1000	At some increased risk; will still show signs of infection; may have chronic periodontal disease
200–500	Some protection but at great risk for infection; may not show signs of infection; usually treated with antibiotics parenterally in the hospital
<200	At marked risk of overwhelming infection; few signs of inflammation; must be hospitalized and empirically treated with antibiotics

candidiasis and aspergillosis, often occur during the course of broad-spectrum antibiotic therapy. Such a large armamentarium of highly effective antibiotics is currently available that it is difficult to recommend a specific antibiotic or combination of antibiotics. Based on the *1990 Guidelines for the Use of Antimicrobial Agents in Neutropenia Patients with Unexplained Fever* by the Infectious Diseases Society of America, the following regimens are suggested.

In patients without renal impairment, combinations of an aminoglycoside (gentamicin, tobramycin, or amikacin, 2.5 mg per kg every 8 hours), and an antipseudomonal carboxy- or ureido-penicillin (piperacillin [Pipracil], ticarcillin with [Ticar] or without [Timentin] clavulanic acid, azlocillin [Azlin], or mezlocillin [Mezlin], 350 mg per kg every 4 hours), or an aminoglycoside with a third-generation antipseudomonal cephalosporin (ceftazidime [Fortaz, Tazidime], or cefoperazone [Cefobid]), 30 to 50 mg per kg every 8 hours, are effective. Serum levels of the aminoglycoside should be monitored and doses adjusted as needed to achieve the following therapeutic concentrations: peak, 5 to 8 μg per mL; trough, 2 μg per mL or less.

In patients with renal impairment, combinations of a third-generation cephalosporin, such as ceftazidime or cefoperazone, 30 to 50 mg per kg every 8 hours, and a ureido-penicillin, such as piperacillin or mezlocillin, 350 to 500 mg per kg every 4 hours, are effective.

In patients in whom coagulase-negative staphylococci, methicillin-resistant *Staphylococcus aureus, Coryne bacterium* species, or alpha-hemolytic streptococci are suspected (e.g., those with indwelling central venous catheters), vancomycin can be added later if gram-positive bacteria are isolated in culture or if no response is obtained from the initial antibiotics after a few days. In the author's opinion, this limits the number of patients receiving the drug therapy, reduces the costs of treatment, and minimizes adverse drug reactions and development of antimicrobial resistance. If the cultures are negative and the fever has resolved, antibiotics can be discontinued after 3 to 5 days. If a source of infection is documented, specific therapy should be instituted, and it may need to be continued longer than in the non-neutropenic patient. Granulocyte transfusions may be of limited use in patients who have blood culture–proved gram-negative sepsis. For patients who remain febrile and neutropenic for more than a week, a systemic fungal infection should be diligently sought: common sites include the lower esophagus, chest, and sinuses. Amphotericin B infusions starting at 0.1 mg per kg per dose in 0.1 mg per ml 5% dextrose water to a maximum of 1 mg per kg per dose should be infused over 2 to 6 hours on a daily basis. If a systemic fungal infection is identified, the course of antifungal therapy will be determined by the extent and response of disease. It is suggested that if after 2 weeks of daily doses of amphotericin B no discernible lesions can be found by clinical evaluation, chest radiograph, endoscopy, and computed tomography (CT) of abdominal organs, the drug can be stopped.

In treating children with benign congenital neutropenia, it is not always necessary to be as aggressive as one would for neutropenias of equal degree due to other causes. The child should be hospitalized and treated with parenteral antibiotics during the first few episodes of fever. If the child responds well to therapy, hospitalization will not be mandatory for future episodes, even though the granulocyte count may be below 250 per mm^3. Because most of these patients have immune-mediated neutropenia, a trial of high-dose intravenous gamma globulin, 400 mg per kg per day for 3 days, may result in a transient increase in the neutrophil count and is indicated for more serious infections such as pneumonia, osteomyelitis, or cellulitis. Steroid therapy (prednisone, 2 mg per kg per day) could also be used to raise the neutrophil count, but has obvious disadvantages in the case of acute infection.

Standard reverse isolation procedures are of no benefit in these patients and probably hinder good care. Rectal examination and rectal thermometers should be avoided. Insistence on excellent dental care with regular professional cleaning and good oral hygiene is important.

Specific Treatment

During the past several years, remarkable progress has been made in the use of recombi-
nant human colony-stimulating factors. Granulocyte colony-stimulating factor (G-CSF) and granulocyte-macrophage colony-stimulating factor (GM-CSF) currently are approved for use in the treatment of neutropenia associated with cancer chemotherapy and bone marrow transplantation. Patients with a variety of malignancies who receive GM-CSF after standard doses of chemotherapy have demonstrated significant reductions in the duration of leukopenia. Use of GM-CSF after high-dose chemotherapy with or without bone marrow rescue appears to hasten recovery of a normal white blood count and reduce infective complications. Definitive data are not yet available to guide dosage for most potential indications, but dose ranges of 0.3 to 10 μg per kg per day of GM-CSF appear appropriate. Subcutaneous injection is convenient and generally tolerated except for local site inflammation. However, the intravenous route may be used and is preferred for bone marrow transplantation enhancement. In cases of severe neutropenia resulting in significant clinical morbidity, such as congenital neutropenia (Kostmann's syndrome), cyclic neutropenia, and acquired idiopathic neutropenias, G-CSF administration has resulted in a dose-dependent increase in the levels of circulating neutrophils and a significant reduction in the number of infections. Dose levels of G-CSF required to achieve clinical success vary from 1 μg per kg per day to 20 μg per kg per day given either intravenously or subcutaneously. Sequential combinations of other bone marrow growth factors such as interleukin-3 and GM-CSF appear to have synergistic action in some cases of bone marrow failure, reducing the risk of neutropenia, associated infections, and thrombocytopenic bleeding. Clinical trials employing other combinations of bone marrow growth factors are underway.

Side effects of G-CSF include bone pain, which can be controlled by analgesics, and rarely vasculitis. G-CSF is contraindicated in patients with known hypersensitivity to E. coli–derived proteins. Caution should be exercised in using G-CSF in any malignancy with myeloid characteristics. In order to avoid potential complications of excessive leukocytosis, a complete blood count is recommended twice a week during therapy. Side effects of GM-CSF include fluid retention, pleural effusion, pericardial effusion, respiratory symptoms, cardiac arrhythmias, and renal and hepatic dysfunction. Although rare, these side effects are potentiated by pre-existing organ dysfunction. GM-CSFs are contraindicated in patients with excessive leukemic myeloid blasts in the bone marrow (≥10%) or peripheral blood and in those with known hypersensitivity to GM-CSF yeast-derived products or any component of the product. Transient rashes and local injection site reactions have occasionally been observed, but no serious allergic or anaphylactic reactions have been reported. If the absolute neutrophil count exceeds 20,000 per mm³ or if the platelet count exceeds 500,000 per mm³, GM-CSF administration should be stopped. Biweekly monitoring of the CBC with differential should be performed to preclude development of excessive counts.

G-CSF is marketed as Neupogen (Filgrastion) by Amgen, Inc. GM-CSF is marketed as Prokine (Sargramostim) by Immunex and distributed by Hoechst-Roussel Pharmaceuticals, Inc.

HEMOLYTIC DISEASE OF THE NEWBORN
(Fetal Isoimmunization)

method of
YVONNE GOLLIN, M.D., and
JOSHUA A. COPEL, M.D.
Yale University School of Medicine
New Haven, Connecticut

Isoimmunization is the most common cause of hemolytic disease of the newborn, followed by infection, hereditary red blood cell membrane and enzyme defects, and chronic fetomaternal hemorrhage. With isoimmunization, maternal sensitization to dissimilar fetal antigens during an index pregnancy places subsequent pregnancies at risk. Paradoxically, it is this *physiologic* immunologic response to foreign (fetal) cells in one pregnancy that creates a *pathologic* environment in later gestations. The D (Rh) antigen in the Rhesus system is the most frequent cause of red blood cell isoimmunization and, therefore, of hemolytic disease of the newborn. The availability of anti-D immunoglobulin (Rhogam) prophylaxis has dramatically decreased the incidence of hemolytic disease of the newborn resulting from Rh sensitization. Rh isoimmunization represents one of the few diseases in obstetrics for which prophylaxis is available.

HISTORY

The association between jaundice and hydrops was first noted by a midwife in the seventeenth century who delivered a set of affected twins. It was not until the 1930s, however, that jaundice, hydrops fetalis, and anemia were linked to the presence of increased erythroblasts in the fetal circulation. Maternal antibodies to fetal hemoglobin were initially thought to cause the hemolytic anemia seen in the newborn period. With the discovery of Rhesus antigens on the surface of the red blood cell, antibodies against the Rh factor, not hemoglobin, were implicated in the pathogenesis of hemolytic disease of the newborn. Transplacental passage of fetal red blood cells was later established as the inciting event necessary for maternal sensitization and the resultant cascade of immune responses.

Since the discovery of the Rhesus blood group, many other "atypical" antigens have been identified that can also cause hemolytic disease of the newborn. The following discussion will focus on Rh incompatibility, the most common cause of hemolytic disease of the newborn, but these principles can be extrapolated to alloimmunization caused by the other, atypical blood groups.

ETIOLOGY

Prior to the advent of a rapid method to type and crossmatch blood, isoimmunization to the ABO and Rhesus antigens occurred when women were emergently transfused with unmatched blood. Currently, isoimmunization resulting from transfusions occurs against "atypical" antigens that are rarely tested for in the United States. This has led to a decrease in the overall incidence of Rh isoimmunization resulting from blood transfusions and a relative increase in the percentage of cases occurring secondary to atypical antigens, such as Kell and Duffy.

Escape of fetal red blood cells into the maternal circulation is the mechanism by which a pregnant woman can become sensitized to a fetal antigen. Fetomaternal exchange occurs with increasing frequency with advancing gestation: it has been reported in 7, 16, and 29% of cases in the first, second, and third trimesters, respectively, and in over half of all deliveries. The surface of the fetal red blood cell does not display antigens until after the seventh week of gestation, theoretically precluding maternal sensitization prior to that time. Fetomaternal exchange also occurs in pathologic situations such as spontaneous abortion, ectopic pregnancy, and abruptio placenta. In addition, several obstetric procedures that necessitate disruption of the placental barrier can augment or initate fetomaternal exchange, including chorionic villus sampling, amniocentesis, percutaneous umbilical blood sampling, external cephalic version, induced abortion, and manual removal of the placenta. Quantitative detection of fetal cells in the maternal circulation is possible with the Kleihauer-Betke technique, which elutes adult hemoglobin from the cell but leaves the fetal erythrocyte intact.

The Rhesus system antigens (D, C, c, E, and e) are highly immunogenic and are responsible for the majority of cases of isoimmunization that occur subsequent to fetomaternal exchange.

PATHOPHYSIOLOGY

Hemolytic disease of the newborn secondary to alloimmunization occurs with exposure of the mother to incompatible red blood cells. This occurs either by transfusion in the nonpregnant state or via fetomaternal exchange during pregnancy. A maternal immune response to the foreign red blood cells occurs in most cases, but is not universal. The formation of maternal IgG antibodies that cross the placenta can place a fetus in jeopardy of anemia. However, a fetus will be affected only if its red blood cells carry the surface antigen to which the maternal antibody is directed. The type of cell carrying the antigen can affect the severity of anemia. If the cell is an erythrocyte, destruction can lead to severe anemia; significant hemolysis is less likely if the antibody is directed against ABO antigens, as these are present on many different cell surfaces throughout the body and the effect of the antibody is diluted. Moreover, ABO antibodies are often IgM, precluding transplacental passage. Antibodies to antigens located exclusively on red blood cells, such as D, Kell, and Duffy, can result in a profound anemia and ultimately lead to hydrops and fetal death.

Immune Response

Central to the pathophysiology of isoimmunization is the maternal immune response. If fetomaternal exchange of dissimilar cells occurs but does not result in a maternal immune response, subsequent pregnancies are not placed at risk. The initial studies in Rh-negative men who were given 1 unit of Rh-positive blood revealed that 90% became sensitized, suggesting that sensitization, although dose dependent, is not an obligatory consequence of exposure.

The initial maternal immune response results in the production of IgM, whose large size (molecular weight approximately 900,000) precludes transplacental passage and consequent fetal effects. Later, IgG antibody is produced, and its small size (molecular weight approximately 160,000) permits passage across the placenta. The production of IgG is greatly augmented if additional episodes of fetomaternal exchange occur (anamnestic response).

Controversy exists regarding the predictive value of the immune response, as reflected by the IgG titer, in the initially sensitized pregnancy and subsequent gestations. A high titer in the first sensitized pregnancy is generally regarded as a poor prognostic sign and indicative of an increased risk of fetal hemolysis. Measurement of the titer in subsequent pregnancies is felt by some investigators not to be clinically useful.

CLINICAL MANIFESTATIONS

Maternal exposure to dissimilar fetal red blood cells, the formation of IgG antibody, and transpla-

cental passage of this antibody all occur in the "maternal-placental" compartment. Additional steps required in the development of hemolysis must then occur within the fetus. In Rh isoimmunization, the maternally derived anti-D antibody crosses the placenta and attaches to the Rh antigen on the surface of the fetal red blood cell. By chemotaxis, coated red blood cells attract macrophages, which also attach themselves to the red cells, causing damage to the membrane. The antibody, blood cell, and macrophage form rosettes, which are trapped in the reticuloendothelial system and gradually lysed. As a result of destruction of the fetal red blood cells, extramedullary hematopoietic sites in the liver, spleen, intestines, kidneys, adrenals, and placenta begin to increase red cell production in an attempt to compensate. Hypertrophy of erythropoietic cells leads to compression and destruction of the normal hepatic cells, impairing the synthesis of albumin and other proteins. This results in a decrease in the fetal intravascular oncotic pressure. Hepatomegaly and splenomegaly contribute to the development of portal hypertension and ascites. "Hydrops," which usually occurs when the fetal hematocrit is below 15%, refers to the presence of ascites, placentomegaly, polyhydramnios, and pericardial and pleural effusions. Polyhydramnios is one of the earliest signs of significant fetal anemia.

TREATMENT

Prenatal Management

Information important in the management of the isoimmunized pregnant patient can be obtained noninvasively by review of the prior obstetric history, measurement of maternal antibody titer, and ultrasound assessment of the fetus. Invasive techniques, such as amniocentesis and percutaneous umbilical blood sampling, provide both quantitative (hematocrit) and qualitative (blood type) assessment of fetal risk. Use of these invasive techniques is often dictated by the findings of the noninvasive methods.

A poor obstetric history mandates the need for close surveillance and early testing. The severity of anemia, the need for exchange transfusion in the neonatal period, and the gestational age at which significant fetal anemia develops are generally the same or worse in subsequent pregnancies. Typically, a woman with a previous hydropic infant will require intervention and close surveillance in a later pregnancy.

As noted previously, the maternal antibody titer has generally been thought to correlate with the severity of fetal disease in the first sensitized pregnancy but is less reliable in later gestations.

Historically, a titer greater than 1:8 has been considered the critical antibody titer and an indication for invasive fetal testing.

Ultrasound evaluation can provide definitive information regarding a severely affected fetus, as the sonographic diagnosis of hydrops is unequivocal. However, fetuses affected to lesser degrees or those on the verge of becoming hydropic cannot *reliably* be distinguished by ultrasound. Nevertheless, polyhydramnios can precede the development of other signs of hydrops. Ultrasound is also used for biophysical profile testing to evaluate fetal condition.

Liley, in the 1960s, was the first to use amniocentesis for the evaluation of Rh isoimmunization. In the setting of hemolysis, bilirubin is released from the fetal red blood cell and is thought to reach the amniotic cavity via tracheal secretions. Liley measured the concentration of bilirubin in amniotic fluid spectrophotometrically at 450 nm and plotted the difference in absorbance (delta optical density [OD] 450) on a semilogarithmic scale in relation to gestational age. The concentration of bilirubin in amniotic fluid normally decreases with advancing gestational age; an elevated or rising bilirubin in a sensitized pregnancy is presumptive evidence of fetal hemolysis.

Amniocentesis has traditionally been performed at or after 25 to 26 weeks of gestation to assess the severity of isoimmunization. The desire to predict the severity of fetal disease at an earlier gestational age has prompted some centers to extrapolate Liley's graphs to the late second trimester. A recent study substantiated this approach by demonstrating that chloroform extraction of bilirubin allowed reliable assessment of the affected fetus in the late second trimester. After the initial amniocentesis, the need for serial amniocenteses depends on the absolute delta OD value or trend. The presence of hydrops, regardless of the delta OD titer, mandates immediate fetal blood sampling and probable transfusion.

Percutaneous umbilical blood sampling (PUBS) provides a direct measurement of fetal hematocrit and allows typing of fetal red blood cells. With this method, fetuses with a blood type identical to the mother's can be identified, obviating the need for further testing. For example, when the paternal genotype is heterozygous at the D locus (i.e., Dd), fetal blood sampling can identify Rh-negative fetuses (dd) that have inherited the d antigen from both parents. These fetuses do not require further evaluation, while Rh-positive fetuses may need repeat blood sampling or amniocentesis.

In addition to its value in the assessment of fetal blood type, PUBS is also used to transfuse an anemic fetus or to determine the hematocrit of a fetus whose delta OD value is climbing or is in Zone III of the Liley graph. If the fetal hematocrit is less than 30%, a transfusion is usually performed.

The placental cord insertion is the preferred sampling site because laceration of the cord is less likely than if the abdominal cord insertion is used, and it is easier to sample than a free loop of cord. Once fetal access has been obtained and the fetal hematocrit assessed, pancuronium or another neuromuscular blocking agent is often injected into the umbilical vein if a transfusion is planned to immobilize the fetus temporarily. The amount of O-negative, irradiated blood to be transfused depends upon the estimated fetoplacental blood volume, initial fetal hematocrit, hematocrit of the donor blood, and the desired fetal hematocrit. Repeat transfusions are usually carried out at 1.5- to 2.5-week intervals, depending on the exit hematocrit. In general, transfusions are not performed after 34 weeks of gestation.

Once a patient has been found to be immunized (i.e., a positive antibody screen), the antibody titer should be determined. In a first-sensitized pregnancy, measurement can be done on a monthly basis and invasive testing averted if the titer remains low (<1:8). A titer greater than 1:8 warrants amniocentesis or PUBS to determine the fetal condition. The timing of the procedure in patients found to be sensitized for the first time depends on the level of the titer. For minimally elevated titers, amniocentesis is performed between 25 and 26 weeks of gestation and is repeated at 1- to 3-week intervals, depending on the delta OD 450 value. Amniocentesis or PUBS can be performed earlier if the titer is markedly elevated.

In subsequently sensitized pregnancies, in contrast, the antibody titer is generally not predictive of fetal risk and invasive testing is routinely recommended. The timing of this testing, however, is dependent on the titer as well as the obstetric history. A patient with a benign obstetric history and low titer can be managed with amniocentesis later in gestation. If there is a history of erythroblastosis fetalis or a high titer, PUBS can be performed as early as 18 weeks. This management scheme optimizes early identification of the fetus in need of a transfusion. The advantages of PUBS over amniocentesis include a direct hematocrit measurement and the ability to type fetal blood. Fetal blood typing obtained by cordocentesis (PUBS) distinguishes Rh-positive from Rh-negative fetuses, with the latter group not requiring further testing.

Neonatal Management and Outcome

The prognosis for infants with hemolytic disease secondary to isoimmunization differs depending on the presence of hydrops. The corrected survival rate is 96% for nonhydropic fetuses and 60 to 70% for hydropic fetuses. In an effort to evaluate factors causing decreased survival in hydropic infants, one group of investigators examined the changes in indices of red blood cell concentration that occur with transfusion. They suggested that lower pretransfusion hematocrits and higher relative increases in post- over pretransfusion hematocrits are significant contributing factors to fetal death after in utero transfusion. The prognosis for nonhydropic fetuses successfully treated by intrauterine transfusion is excellent, with no adverse sequelae noted on long-term follow-up.

Neonatal management is based on principles similar to those influencing management in the antenatal period with several exceptions. Elevated bilirubin concentrations, cleared from the fetus by the placenta, are critically important in the neonate because the immature liver may not be an adequate substitute for the placenta. The neonate is sensitive to elevated bilirubin levels, which can cause severe sequelae such as kernicterus. In addition, the hydropic neonate, in contrast to the hydropic fetus, requires ventilatory management, which may be difficult due to pleural effusions and edema of the airways and chest wall. Finally, careful follow-up of the neonate is indicated since late anemia can develop because of persistent anti-D antibody. Infants who undergo numerous intrauterine transfusions may develop a hyporegenerative anemia.

Infants who have been transfused in utero may not require a transfusion in the neonatal period. In general, if the hematocrit is greater than 35% and the bilirubin level is normal, a transfusion is not necessary. Exchange transfusion is usually used to lower the bilirubin concentration.

PREVENTION

Hemolytic disease of the newborn secondary to Rh isoimmunization is, for the most part, preventable. The development of anti-D (Rh) immunoglobulin in the late 1960s heralded a new era in preventive medicine. Once Rh immune globulin became commercially available, the incidence of sensitization to the D antigen dropped precipitously. Its efficacy was demonstrated in earlier clinical trials in male prisoners in which a 300-μg dose was found to prevent isoimmunization for transfusions of up to 30 mL of Rh positive blood.

Indications for Rh immune globulin therapy in a nonsensitized Rh (D)-negative pregnant woman are listed in Table 1 and include spontaneous and iatrogenic causes of fetomaternal exchange. The

TABLE 1. **Indications for Rh Immune Globulin Therapy**

Indication	Dose Rh Immune Globulin (μg)
Threatened abortion	
<12 wk	50
>12 wk	300
Spontaneous abortion	
<12 wk	50
>12 wk	300
Ectopic pregnancy	50
Chorionic villus sample	300
Amniocentesis (second or third trimester)	300
Abdominal trauma (second or third trimester)	300
Fetal blood sample*	300
Delivery	300†

*Determination of fetal blood type recommended if fetal blood sample is performed in Rh-negative woman for indications other than Rh status of fetus. Rh immune globulin can then be given based on fetal Rh type.

†Cord blood should be sent for Rh typing to determine appropriateness of Rh immune globulin. Kleihauer-Betke test may be useful to ensure that an adequate dose of Rh immune globulin is administered (20 μg/mL red cells). Larger doses may occasionally be necessary if a large fetomaternal hemorrhage occurs.

authors give it routinely in all Rh-negative pregnancies at 28 weeks, since the incidence of fetomaternal transfusion is greatest in the third trimester. Rh immune globulin is also administered postpartum if the infant is Rh positive.

After the introduction of Rh immune globulin, the incidence of isoimmunization in Rh-negative women delivering Rh-positive infants decreased from 8 to 1.6% with postpartum administration alone, and to 0.11% with combined antepartum and postpartum prophylaxis. Now, most cases of D sensitization occur because of failure of Rh immune globulin administration or because of a fetal-to-maternal bleed in excess of 30 mL of whole blood, the latter occurring in only 0.23% of cases of fetomaternal hemorrhage.

There are two potential dangers inherent in the use of antepartum prophylactic Rh immune globulin: fetal hemolysis from transplacental passage of the IgG molecules, and transmission to mother or fetus or both of infectious agents contained in the preparation. The latter is also of concern with postpartum prophylaxis. Significant fetal hemolysis has not been reported in the literature with the administration of Rh immune globulin at 28 weeks, probably because of the large volume of distribution in maternal plasma and the extravascular space. Regarding the risk of infection, since the immunoglobulin is derived from pooled donors, the possibility of hepatitis and, recently, human immunodeficiency virus transmission has been cited. However, the cold alcohol fractionation technique used to prepare

Rh immune globulin adequately eradicates both viruses.

Currently, there is no preventive mechanism available for the subgroup of isoimmunization caused by atypical antigens.

Over the last 50 years, the pathogenesis of hemolytic disease of the newborn resulting from immunization to the D antigen in the Rh system has been elucidated and methods of diagnosis and treatment have been extensively studied. The development of anti-D globulin facilitated a rapid decline in the incidence of fetal anemia and erythroblastosis fetalis occurring from Rh isoimmunization. Despite these advances, Rh sensitization still complicates pregnancies and can result in significant perinatal morbidity. The Rh-immunized pregnancy is best managed in a perinatal facility that provides expertise in percutaneous umbilical blood sampling and intrauterine transfusion. Delivery of the neonate with hemolytic disease secondary to Rh disease should be effected in a tertiary care center.

Although severe hemolytic disease of the newborn usually results from Rh incompatibility, it can also occur with sensitization to atypical antigens such as Kidd, Kell, and Duffy. However, mild hemolytic disease in the newborn period is most often secondary to a major blood group incompatibility, especially in group O individuals with IgG antibodies. Hyperbilirubinemia in a neonate with an uncomplicated antenatal course should arouse suspicion of hemolytic disease secondary to ABO alloimmunization.

HEMOPHILIA AND RELATED CONDITIONS

method of
JEANNE M. LUSHER, M.D., and
INDIRA WARRIER, M.D.
Wayne State University School of Medicine
Detroit, Michigan

Hemophilia A (factor VIII deficiency) and hemophilia B (factor IX deficiency) are hereditary bleeding disorders that are transmitted as X-linked recessive traits and thus affect males almost exclusively. Hemophilia A and B are clinically indistinguishable but can easily be differentiated by factor VIII and factor IX activity assays. In hemophilia A, the factor VIII procoagulant moiety is deficient or abnormal while other components of the factor VIII system (factor VIII-related antigen and von Willebrand factor) are normal. Hemophilia has a wide range of clinical severity, but affected males within a family almost always have the same degree of impairment. In general, the severity of clinical bleeding manifestations correlates well with the factor VIII activity value, assay values of less than 0.02 units per

mL (2%) being associated with spontaneous hemorrhage into joints and soft tissues. Levels of 2 to 5% are associated with moderately severe disease, while levels of 6 to 50% occur in mild disease.

Hemophilia B is characterized by subnormal factor IX activity, which may reflect a quantitative or qualitative abnormality in the factor IX molecule. While the factor VIII complex has a molecular weight of about 1.5 million daltons, the human factor IX molecule is considerably smaller, having a molecular weight of 60,000 daltons. As in hemophilia A, a factor IX assay value of less than 2% is generally associated with a clinically severe bleeding tendency (spontaneous bleeding into joints and soft tissues).

It is apparent that both hemophilia A and hemophilia B are heterogeneous conditions. At least six different subtypes of hemophilia B have been described. While all have low levels of factor IX activity, the degree of clotting factor deficiency varies, and several of the subtypes have other laboratory evidence of abnormalities of the factor IX molecule. Within a given kindred, however, there does not appear to be heterogeneity.

While accurate statistics are unavailable, the estimated incidence of hemophilia in the United States is 1 in 10,000 individuals, or 1 in 5000 males. Hemophilia A is approximately four times as frequent as hemophilia B.

Von Willebrand's disease (vWD), first described in Scandinavia in 1926 by Ehrich von Willebrand, is the most common of the hereditary bleeding disorders, affecting an estimated 1% of the population. However, vWD is a very heterogeneous disorder, and clinically significant vWD is far less common than 1%. Von Willebrand factor (vWf) is a large, complex, multimeric adhesive glycoprotein that has two very important functions in hemostasis: it serves as an adhesive bridge between platelets and areas of vascular damage, and it binds to and stabilizes factor VIII in the circulation. Thus, if normally functioning vWf is absent or low, the bleeding time will be prolonged and the affected individual will have mucous membrane bleeding (such as menorrhagia, epistaxis, gum bleeding, and gastrointestinal bleeding) and prolonged bleeding from minor cuts or other trauma. Additionally, on laboratory testing, factor VIII may be quite low as it is not being stabilized by vWf and thus undergoes rapid proteolytic destruction.

There are three major types of vWD, and each is genetically and phenotypically heterogeneous. In most populations, type I (classic) vWD is the most common form and is characterized by subnormal levels of normally functioning vWf. The type II variants (IIA, IIB, IIC, etc.) are characterized by qualitative abnormalities in vWf. Types I and II are usually inherited in an autosomal dominant fashion. Type III vWD is the severe form, characterized by absent or nearly absent vWf. Type III vWD is relatively rare and results from the inheritance of two genes for vWD. In addition to having significant mucous membrane bleeding, affected individuals often bleed into joints and soft tissues.

In classic (Type I) vWD, clinical severity varies considerably. Most affected individuals have only a mild to moderate bleeding tendency, and a negative history for excessive bleeding is not uncommon. On the other hand, some patients have epistaxis, menorrhagia, and other bleeding problems throughout life. A large number of mutations in the vWf gene have recently been characterized, and new ones continue to be described.

Among the type II variants, the most commonly encountered by far is IIA; IIB is the next most common. From a therapeutic standpoint, it is important to distinguish IIA and IIB. Both are characterized by a decrease in the concentration of high-molecular-weight vWf multimers in plasma. Since the largest vWf multimers are the most important hemostatically, persons with a selective loss of high-molecular-weight multimers have prolonged bleeding times and mucous membrane bleeding due to defective platelet plug formation. In vWD type IIA, not only the high but also the intermediate weight multimers are absent from plasma. The defect in IIB is characterized by an increased affinity of vWF binding to platelets and absorption of the high-molecular-weight multimers from plasma. Thrombocytopenia is variable but often occurs with increases in vWf release (and subsequent platelet clumping) as seen with inflammation, stress, and pregnancy and following administration of desmopressin acetate (1-deamino-8-D-arginine vasopressin) (DDAVP).

Although far less common than hemophilia A, hemophilia B, or vWD, hereditary deficiencies or abnormalities of other clotting factors also exist. While some of these (e.g., factor XII deficiency) are not associated with a bleeding tendency, congenital deficiencies or abnormalities of fibrinogen, prothrombin, and factors V, VII, X, and XIII (and sometimes XI) do cause bleeding. The majority of these uncommon conditions are inherited in an autosomal recessive manner.

TREATMENT

Hemostatic Abnormalities

Replacement Therapy

In general, if a person with a hereditary coagulation disorder is bleeding and treatment is indicated, he or she should receive an intravenous infusion of the clotting factor that is deficient. While through the mid-1960s only whole plasma was available, high-purity, viral attenuated plasma-derived clotting factor concentrates have become the mainstay of treatment for hemophilia B and severe or moderately severe vWD. For hemophilia A, in addition to high-purity plasma-derived concentrates, recombinant factor VIII preparations are also available, while for mild hemophilia and type I vWD the synthetic agent DDAVP is the treatment of choice.

Fresh-Frozen Plasma. Fresh-frozen plasma (FFP) is still useful in several situations. In the relatively rare hereditary deficiencies of prothrombin and factors V, VII, X, XI, and XIII, cessation of hemorrhage can generally be achieved with FFP in a dosage of 10 mL per kg. Although an estimated 15% of activity is lost in the process of freezing and thawing plasma, an average unit of FFP of 230 mL still contains approximately 200 units of activity for each of the clotting factors. (One unit of clotting factor activity is defined as the amount present in 1 mL of fresh plasma, e.g., 1 unit of factor VIII activity is the amount present in 1 mL of fresh plasma.)

Cryoprecipitates. Prepared from single units of plasma, cryoprecipitates contain approximately 50% of the factor VIII activity, von Willebrand factor activity, and fibrinogen that was present in the unit of plasma initially. Thus, a single donor bag of cryoprecipitate should contain approximately 100 units of factor VIII activity and 0.25 to 0.30 grams of fibrinogen, in a volume of about 10 mL. While formerly regarded as the treatment of choice for vWD, as it contains vWf in addition to factor VIII, cryoprecipitate is now considered less desirable than either DDAVP or the virally attenuated concentrates that are rich in vWf. Cryoprecipitates are still used for hypofibrinogenemia and afibrinogenemia. The main disadvantages of cryoprecipitates are that they must be stored in a deep freeze, they are somewhat difficult to reconstitute and administer, and bags of cryoprecipitates vary considerably in their factor VIII content. Perhaps most importantly, they are not subject to viral attenuation processes.

Factor VIII Concentrates. These are produced by several different manufacturers in the United States and Europe and are the mainstay of treatment for hemophilia A. Plasma-derived and recombinant (r) factor VIII preparations are available.

Plasma-Derived Factor VIII Concentrates. These are available in varying degrees of purity (generally referred to as intermediate, high and ultra pure, the latter being immunoaffinity purified). Each lot of concentrate is prepared from a large volume of starting plasma that has often been obtained from plasmapheresis of as many as 20,000 donors. All manufacturers of plasma-derived clotting factor concentrate use one or more viral-attenuation processes in the preparation of these products. Also, it should be noted that donor screening procedures include not only self-deferral but also laboratory testing for seropositivity to human immunodeficiency virus type 1 (HIV-1), HIV-2, hepatitis B virus (HBs Ag and Ab and HB core Ab), and hepatitis C virus (HCV). Such improved methods of donor screening and viral attenuation (pasteurization, solvent-detergent treatment, steam treatment, as well as loss of virus in purification steps), have resulted in much safer factor VIII concentrates than were available in the 1980s. It is noteworthy that *none* of the factor VIII concentrates currently marketed in the United States has been implicated in seroconversion to HIV-1, HIV-2, or hepatitis A,

B, or C. However, it is also noteworthy that none of the current viral-attenuation methods appears to kill human parvovirus B19.

Plasma-derived factor VIII concentrates are easy to store, reconstitute, and infuse, and each bottle is labeled with the number of factor VIII units contained. Advantages of immunoaffinity purified factor VIII over the less pure preparations include smaller vial size, ease of reconstitution, and in several studies, better maintenance of cellular immunity in HIV-infected hemophiliacs.

Recombinant Factor VIII Concentrates. Currently marketed by two manufacturers in the United States, recombinant factor VIII (rF VIII) preparations are produced in well-established mammalian cell lines (Chinese hamster ovary cells and baby hamster kidney cells) that are transfected with a gene encoding for human factor VIII. Both rF VIII preparations have been well studied and appear to be quite effective and safe. The main therapeutic advantage of rF VIII over plasma-derived factor VIII is the added margin of viral safety.

Factor IX Concentrates. There are two types of factor IX concentrates: *complex* concentrates, which contain all of the vitamin K–dependent clotting factors (II, VII, IX, and X), some in partially activated form; and *coagulation factor IX* concentrates, which are highly purified factor IX. Both types are plasma derived and both are subjected to viral depletion processes. None of the currently marketed products has been implicated in transmission of HIV-1, HIV-2, or hepatitis viruses. While factor IX complex concentrates (often referred to as prothrombin complex concentrates) have been the mainstay of treatment for hemophilia B, these products can cause disseminated intravascular coagulation (DIC), deep venous thromboses, and pulmonary embolism. Thus one must be aware of their thrombogenic potential (described later in Complications of Treatment). The newer, highly purified coagulation factor IX concentrates appear to be far less thrombogenic and are recommended for any person with hemophilia B who is undergoing surgery, who has a large intramuscular hemorrhage or crush injury, who has significant liver dysfunction (with resulting lower levels of antithrombin III and protein C and difficulty clearing clotting intermediates from the circulation), who has a history of thrombotic complications, or is a neonate. Additionally, since thrombotic complications can occur in other clinical situations, many physicians now recommend coagulation factor IX products for all persons with hemophilia B.

Over the past two decades, factor IX complex concentrates (either standard or purposely activated) have been widely used to treat bleeding episodes in persons (with hemophilia A or B) who have developed inhibitor antibodies to factor VIII or factor IX (see the following section Inhibitors).

Antifibrinolytic Therapy. Epsilon aminocaproic acid (EACA) and tranexamic acid are antifibrinolytic agents that act by inhibiting plasminogen activation. These antifibrinolytic agents are useful adjuncts in certain specific situations when one desires to prevent lysis of a clot that has already formed as a result of specific factor replacement therapy. Their primary use in the hereditary clotting disorders has been in the management of bleeding in the oral cavity (e.g., due to dental extractions or other oral surgical procedures or tongue or mouth lacerations). One can usually prevent or at least decrease rebleeding and the amount of factor replacement needed in such situations by the addition of EACA in a dosage of 75 mg per kg every 6 hours orally, or tranexamic acid, 25 mg per kg every 8 hours. The antifibrinolytic agent should be continued for 7 to 10 days. Since there is at least a theoretical risk of enhanced thrombogenicity if an antifibrinolytic agent is given concurrently with factor IX complex concentrate, patients can use a high-purity coagulation factor IX product *or* tranexamic acid as a mouthwash rather than systemically.

Other Agents. In normal persons, and in those with only mild deficiencies, *estrogen preparations* raise the circulating levels of several coagulation factors (including factors VII, VIII, IX, and X and vWf). Various estrogen-containing preparations have proved clinically useful in women with vWD who have menorrhagia.

DDAVP, a synthetic analogue of the antidiuretic hormone 9-arginine vasopressin, is the treatment of choice for persons with classic (type I) vWD and for those with mild or moderate hemophilia A whenever an approximate threefold increase in factor VIII or vWf will be sufficient to control bleeding. Intravenous infusion (or highly concentrated intranasal spray) of DDAVP, in a dosage of 0.3 µg per kg, produces a marked, transient increase in factor VIII/vWf activity in normal persons as well as in those with quantitative (type I) variants of vWD or mild hemophilia A. In persons with measurable amounts to start with, there is a two to tenfold (average threefold) increase in factor VIII over the baseline value, with a half-life of 6 to 8 hours. This drug indirectly effects release of factor VIII and vWf from storage sites. Thus, in severe (type III) vWD there is no vWf to be released, and in persons with a functionally abnormal form of vWf (type II variants), the abnormal form will be released.

Drug-Induced Platelet Dysfunction

Joint or soft tissue hemorrhage in hemophilia (or other hereditary coagulopathy) is often painful. If aspirin or an aspirin-containing compound is taken to relieve pain, the bleeding tendency may worsen as aspirin interferes with platelet function. (Aspirin inhibits platelet aggregation, an effect mediated by inhibition of prostaglandin synthesis and due to an irreversible inhibition of platelet cyclooxygenase.) Thus in persons with a coagulation disorder, aspirin-containing agents should be avoided. Acetaminophen is recommended for relief of mild pain or fever.

Among other drugs that interfere with platelet function are antihistamines, phenothiazine, and nonsteroidal anti-inflammatory agents such as indomethacin.

Complications of Treatment

Risk of Viral Transmission. In using blood components, clotting factor concentrates, and synthetic agents, one must be aware of the potential complications of their use. Fresh-frozen plasma (FFP) and cryoprecipitate are obtained from single units of blood (rather than from thousands of donors); thus, until recent years these products were considered safer than commercially prepared clotting factor concentrates. However, FFP and cryoprecipitates are not subjected to the rigorous viral inactivation methods now employed in the production of clotting factor concentrates. Despite greatly improved donor screening methods, there remains a very slight risk of hepatitis (or other blood-borne virus) transmission with the use of FFP, cryoprecipitate, and other blood components. Current estimates of HCV risk are 1:2000 to 1:6000 per unit of blood transfused.

While none of the currently marketed clotting factor concentrates has been implicated in seroconversion to HIV-1, HIV-2, or viral hepatitis, it is known that human parvovirus B19 is still being transmitted by viral-attenuated factor VIII and factor IX concentrates. Parvovirus B19 seldom causes severe disease; however, the realization that this virus is not destroyed by state-of-the-art viral-attenuation methods raises the possibility of contamination of plasma-derived products by more virulent viruses.

HEPATITIS AND HIV/AIDS. It is now known that essentially all clotting factor concentrates prepared from plasma collected in the United States between 1979 and 1984 were infected with HIV. Approximately 90% of persons treated with factor VIII concentrates and 55% of those receiving factor IX complex concentrates prepared from plasma collected during this period became infected with HIV. Many of them have now succumbed to acquired immunodeficiency syndrome (AIDS) or have varying degrees of HIV-related symptoms.

Although not suffering the devastating consequences of AIDS, a very high percentage (more than 85%) of hemophiliacs treated with clotting factor concentrates prepared through the mid-1980s became infected with HCV. It is estimated that approximately 50% of these patients now have chronic HCV infection; some have proceeded to end-stage liver disease and death.

Thrombogenicity. This remains a potential complication associated with the use of factor IX complex concentrates (prothrombin complex concentrates [PCC]). The risk is greatest in immobile recipients who have undergone orthopedic surgical procedures, those who have sustained crush injuries (with release of thromboplastic materials into the circulation), those with large intramuscular bleeds (e.g., iliopsoas or thigh), neonates, and those with significant hepatocellular disease (who are likely to have low levels of antithrombin III, and suboptimal clearance of clotting intermediates from the circulation). However, DIC and thromboembolic complications can occur in other situations as well, and many physicians now prefer to use the high-purity coagulation factor IX products, which appear to be considerably less thrombogenic than PCCs. The increased thrombogenicity associated with PCCs has been attributed to zymogen overload (increasing levels of factors II, VII, and IX, which the hemophilia B patient already has in adequate amounts) and small amounts of activated factors (e.g., factor Xa) that are present in PCCs.

Acute Myocardial Infarction. This complication has occurred in at least 30 hemophiliacs with inhibitor antibodies who were receiving relatively large, repeated doses of factor IX complex concentrates (PCCs) for treatment of bleeding. Many of these patients were young (15–22 years of age), and among those who died, myocardial transmural hemorrhage was the most consistent pathologic feature. The pathogenesis of this phenomenon is not entirely clear. The risk of this serious and often fatal complication can be decreased by avoiding repetitive, large (>75 units per kg) doses of PCC in inhibitor patients (i.e., if three or four doses of PCC are insufficient to control an acute hemarthrosis, it is unlikely that further doses will be effective and they may be hazardous).

Potential Complications of DDAVP. The synthetic vasopressin analogue DDAVP is remarkably safe if certain precautions are kept in mind. One must remember that DDAVP is a potent antidiuretic agent. While normal feedback mechanisms are such that persons who have received DDAVP do not feel thirsty and decrease their own fluid intake for a time, hyponatremia and water intoxication have been described in a number of patients. Those at greatest risk are neonates and infants, the very elderly, and persons of any age who are being given intravenous fluids postoperatively without careful monitoring of fluid and electrolyte balance. Most reported instances of water intoxication have been in very young children; thus DDAVP is not recommended for children under 2 years of age.

Other Side Effects. Somewhat more common but less serious side effects of treatment with plasma, cryoprecipitate, and plasma-derived clotting factor concentrates include urticaria, rashes, headache, and low-grade fever. The purer the factor VIII or factor IX product, the less likely any of these will occur.

Regional Comprehensive Care for Hemophilia and von Willebrand's Disease

In 1976, a network of federally funded, regional comprehensive hemophilia diagnostic and treatment centers was established in the United States. At each center, a team of experts provides periodic assessments and makes recommendations to the patients and to their local health care providers. In addition to the internist and pediatric hematologist, comprehensive care team members include hemophilia nurses, social workers, a physical therapist, orthopedic surgeon, dentist and dental hygienist, genetics counselor, psychologist, and in some instances, a vocational counselor and nutritionist as well.

Since the devastation of the hemophilia community by AIDS, many hemophilia centers now have a close working arrangement with one or more infectious disease specialists. Additionally, hemophilia physicians, nurses, and social workers have by necessity become knowledgeable in dealing with the many problems caused by HIV infection.

At the comprehensive hemophilia centers, patient education, home treatment (self-infusion) training, vocational planning, and prophylaxis are stressed, including exercises and attention to dental hygiene. Carrier detection and genetic counseling are offered, and routine laboratory testing includes surveillance for inhibitor antibodies to factor VIII (or IX), hepatitis testing, and longitudinal CD4 determinations. A booklet listing the federally funded hemophilia centers, as well as other hospitals providing comprehensive hemophilia care, can be obtained from the National Hemophilia Foundation, Soho Building, Suite 303, 110 Greene St., New York, NY 10012. The National Hemophilia Foundation's Hemophilia and AIDS/HIV Network for the Dissemination of Information (HANDI) provides current information for physicians and patients and their families concerning a wide variety of issues, including treatment protocols and drugs for HIV/AIDS. A HANDI Information Specialist can be reached by calling 1-800-42-HANDI.

Home Infusion Programs

During the early 1970s, the concept of home care for hemophilia rapidly gained in popularity and acceptance. Most hemophilia centers now have programs to teach hemophiliacs or their parents not only the techniques of self-infusion but also when to self-treat, how to determine the proper dosage of concentrate, and when to call the center personnel. Advantages of home treatment include (1) prompt initiation of therapy for an acute bleeding episode, (2) greater independence, (3) less time lost from school or work, and (4) fewer costly visits to the emergency room. Prompt home treatment of acute hemarthroses has decreased the incidence of chronic joint disease. Children 11 or 12 years of age are usually eager to learn the techniques of self-infusion, while a parent of a child 3 years of age or older can generally be taught to start and administer the infusion of clotting factor.

Treatment of Hemophilia A

Although interest in starting all children with severe hemophilia on prophylaxis to *prevent* joint hemorrhage is now considerable, clotting factor concentrates are generally used only for acute bleeding episodes. The most common indications for treatment are acute joint hemorrhage (hemarthrosis) and bleeding into a muscle mass. When such bleeding begins, early treatment will reduce complications (such as chronic joint disease) as well as the total amount of clotting factor needed for treatment of the episode. Treatment consists of factor VIII replacement and rest of the affected part. Factor VIII replacement is achieved by infusion of factor VIII concentrates, prepared from human plasma or by recombinant techniques. The label on each bottle of concentrate indicates the amount of factor VIII it contains. In calculating the dosage of factor VIII, it can be assumed that 1 unit of factor VIII per kg of body weight will raise the recipient's factor VIII level by 0.02 unit per ml (2%). Thus, if a severely affected hemophiliac with a baseline factor VIII level of less than 0.01 unit per ml received 20 units of factor VIII per kg, one would expect an immediate postinfusion factor VIII level of 0.40 unit per ml (40%).* The half-life of factor VIII is 8 to 12

---

*One should not discard any "extra" factor VIII (i.e., above the calculated amount) in a vial. If the patient's calculated dose of factor VIII is 860 units and the bottle contains 950 units the entire amount should be infused.

hours; however, it may be less if the recipient is febrile or has had a major bleed (situations that activate the coagulation system).

Hemarthrosis. Acute hemarthrosis is the most common indication for treatment. *Prompt treatment is of the utmost importance!* Untreated or inadequately treated acute hemarthroses eventually result in progressive, chronic joint disease that can be extremely disabling.

Each episode of acute hemarthrosis results in synovial inflammation that can become chronic if repeated joint hemorrhages are not promptly treated. Chronic synovitis leads to (1) increased proliferation of the inflamed synovium, which is very vascular, thus making more frequent hemorrhages likely; (2) destruction of cartilage and gradual resorption of bone with cyst formation; (3) instability of the joint, resulting in more frequent bleeding into the joint and surrounding soft tissues; and (4) chronic joint pain, with subsequent disuse atrophy of surrounding muscles and even greater joint instability.

Acute hemarthroses most frequently involve the knee, elbow, and ankle, although bleeding into the shoulder, hip, and wrist can also occur. Joint bleeding can be spontaneous or result from trauma. Recurrent bleeding without obvious trauma can occur in a particular joint, presumably because of the synovial irritation and increased vascularity resulting from earlier hemorrhage into the joint.

The early symptoms of joint bleeding can generally be recognized by the patient. Most describe a peculiar sensation or minimal discomfort or tingling in the joint before actual pain and swelling develop. *Treatment with clotting factor should be given at this time.* If joint bleeding goes untreated, pain and joint swelling increase and there is progressive limitation of motion of the joint. By this time the joint hemorrhage is far advanced and synovial inflammation will have begun.

Treatment consists of *clotting factor replacement* and immobilization or *rest* of the affected joint. The recommended dosage of factor VIII is shown in Table 1. In general, the earlier an acute hemarthrosis is treated, the less clotting factor is required. Thus, if a patient with hemophilia on home treatment treats himself at the earliest symptoms of bleeding into the joint, cessation of bleeding will generally be attained with half the dosage of concentrate required for a hemorrhage of several hours' duration that has resulted in a very painful, distended joint. Rest of the affected joint during the acute phase of bleeding is also important. For an elbow hemorrhage a sling is often helpful. In a small child with an extensive hemarthrosis of the knee, a light-weight splint may be helpful. This is usually not necessary for early joint hemorrhages, however, as response to

clotting factor concentrates is generally rapid. Immobilization should not be continued for more than a few days, because of the danger of muscle atrophy. Ice packs provide symptomatic relief from pain associated with an acute hemarthrosis.

Joint Aspiration. Aspiration is seldom indicated, and should be reserved for acute joint distention associated with severe pain. (Although this situation was commonly encountered prior to the 1970s, relatively few painfully distended joints are seen now, as most acute hemarthroses are treated early.) When joint aspiration is indicated, it should be done with careful attention to aseptic technique and only after infusion of clotting factor concentrate.

As described previously, frequent recurrent hemarthroses can result in disuse muscle atrophy; thus physical therapy is important. Isometric exercises are often quite useful in preventing atrophy of the quadriceps group, thus lessening the chance of reinjury to the knee. High-top padded hiking boots provide stability and lessen the chances of ankle injury. Occasionally, a long leg brace may be indicated for stabilizing and protecting a chronically swollen, severely affected knee.

In the case of frequent, recurrent episodes of bleeding into a single joint (referred to as a "target joint"), a *prophylactic regimen* of every-other-day clotting factor concentrate may stop the cycle and allow healing of the inflamed synovium. Such prophylaxis, once begun, should be continued for at least a month and often considerably longer. If chronic synovitis is problematic, with continuous boggy swelling and rebleeding, synovectomy may be helpful. Synovectomy can now be performed by arthroscopic as well as by nonsurgical techniques (radionuclide synovectomy).

Muscle Hemorrhage. Intramuscular hemorrhage is the second most common indication for replacement therapy with clotting factor concentrates. As in the case of acute hemarthroses, pain and limitation of motion of the affected part usually occur. A longer course of replacement therapy is often necessary for a severe intramuscular hemorrhage than for joint hemorrhage. Clotting factor concentrates should be given every 12 hours until the affected muscle mass begins to soften and pain has disappeared. Several days of treatment are often required.

Whereas intramuscular bleeding in such areas as the calf or forearm is quite visible, with tense swelling and tenderness, the symptoms and signs of an iliopsoas hemorrhage are generally limited to ill-defined pain in the groin, flexion of the thigh, and pain on extension of the thigh. A large iliopsoas hemorrhage can cause displacement of the kidney and ureter, anemia from contained hemorrhage, and compression of the femoral nerve. Hospitalization with clotting factor concentrate

TABLE 1. **Recommended Dosages of Factor VIII for Severe and Moderately Severe Hemophilia A**

Type of Bleeding	Dosage Factor VIII (U/kg)	Repeat Doses Factor VIII (U/kg)	Ancillary Treatment
Acute hemarthrosis			
Early	10	Seldom necessary	
Late (painful, with limitation of motion)	20	20 q 12 h	
Intramuscular hemorrhage	20–30	20 q 12 h (usually requires several days of treatment)	
Life-threatening situations* Intracranial hemorrhage Major trauma Major surgery	50	25–30 q 12 h or, preferably, continuous infusion of factor VIII (see text)	
Other serious bleeding*			
Tongue or neck bleeding with potential airway obstruction	40–50	20–25 q 12 h	
Severe abdominal pain	30–40	20–25 q 12 h	
Tongue and mouth lacerations*	20	20 q 12 h	EACA or tranexamic acid; sedation in small child
Extraction of permanent teeth	20	20 q 12 h as necessary to control bleeding	EACA or tranexamic acid beginning day before extractions; continue 7–10 days
Painless spontaneous gross hematuria	None		Increased PO fluids

*These conditions should be treated in a comprehensive hemophilia center. If the patient is first seen in another hospital, initial treatment should be given, and the hemophilia center should be contacted and the patient transferred.

EACA = epsilon aminocaproic acid.

given every 12 hours for a period of several days is indicated.

Oral Bleeding. Tongue and mouth lacerations occur most often in the toddler age group but are occasionally seen in older children or adults. While clotting factor concentrate should be given to all, ancillary management depends on the age of the patient and the size and extent of intraoral injury. An infusion of clotting factor concentrate causes local clot formation, but it is difficult to maintain an intact clot in this moist environment, particularly on the tongue. In small children, cessation of hemorrhage and healing of the wound can best be achieved by hospitalization, with (1) heavy sedation, (2) clotting factor concentrate every 12 hours (or by continuous infusion), (3) no oral intake and maintenance with intravenous fluid, and (4) the use of an antifibrinolytic agent such as tranexamic acid or epsilon aminocaproic acid (EACA), to prevent clot lysis. Three to five days of hospitalization may be required for management of a tongue laceration in a small child. In an older child or adult with a similar lesion, outpatient management consists of clotting factor concentrates, an antifibrinolytic agent, and continued attention to prevent clot dislodgement. Cold, clear liquids followed by a soft diet are recommended. Local application of orahesive gauze may also be useful. (The orahesive gauze sheets are cut to the desired size, then placed firmly over the wound.) EACA or tranexamic acid should be continued for 7 to 10 days, or until healing appears complete.

Hematuria. Gross hematuria can follow a blow or other injury to the kidney, in which case clotting factor concentrate is indicated. However, gross hematuria more commonly occurs spontaneously. Especially in children, one should rule out other possible causes of painless, gross hematuria such as acute glomerulonephritis. If other underlying causes are excluded, it has been the authors' practice to allow the patient to continue usual activities and to drink extra fluids until hematuria stops, usually within 2 to 7 days. If it persists beyond that time, one or two doses of clotting factor concentrate can be given, but antifibrinolytic agents should be avoided, as ureteropelvic obstruction by clots can occur. While some recommend bed rest or corticosteroids for the management of gross hematuria, these measures are not of proven benefit.

Surgical Procedures. If the patient with hemophilia A does not have an inhibitor (see the next section), surgery can generally be accomplished without undue risk as long as there is careful planning and cooperation among surgical, medical, and laboratory personnel. Preoperative planning is essential and should include testing for an inhibitor, which can develop at any age and makes surgery hazardous. One should also ensure that an adequate supply of clotting factor concentrate is on hand for the entire postoperative period. Clotting factor replacement should begin 45 minutes to 1 hour preoperatively. Following the initial bolus dose, factor VIII is given by continuous infusion, thus avoiding peaks and troughs. Although administration of factor VIII at the rate of 3 units per kg per hour will generally result in a factor VIII level of 50%, daily assays should be performed to ensure that adequate levels are being maintained. Replacement therapy should be continued for 7 to 10 days postoperatively for most major surgical procedures. A longer period of treatment (often 4 to 6 weeks) is required for extensive orthopedic procedures. When the patient is ready for discharge, factor VIII can be given at home by intravenous bolus every 12 to 24 hours. Surgery should be undertaken only in a hospital that has a hemophilia center, a reliable coagulation laboratory, a major blood bank, and an appropriate rehabilitation team for postoperative management. A notation taped on the front of the patient's chart should indicate that no intramuscular injections are to be given and that all aspirin-containing compounds must be avoided.

For *oral surgical procedures,* EACA or tranexamic acid is begun 1 day preoperatively and continued for 10 days postoperatively (in a dose of 75 mg per kg every 6 hours for EACA, or 25 mg per kg every 8 hours for tranexamic acid). As for other surgical procedures, preoperative screening for inhibitors is mandatory. Clotting factor concentrate should be given 45 minutes to 1 hour preoperatively and continued every 12 hours for 1 or 2 days or longer, depending on the extent of the procedure and the appearance of the local lesion.

Inhibitors. Inhibitors (antibodies) develop in 10 to 15% of patients with hemophilia A and 1 to 2% of those with hemophilia B. Most inhibitors develop in early childhood. The inhibitor is an antibody that acts specifically against factor VIII (or factor IX) procoagulant activity. While some patients develop inhibitors in low titer (and can thus continue to be treated with factor VIII concentrates), many are high-titer antibody formers.

In those with high-titer inhibitors, bleeding episodes do not respond to usual treatment with factor VIII, as the inhibitor antibody will bind and inactivate the infused factor VIII. Over the past two decades, most have recommended either "standard" or "activated" factor IX complex concentrates (PCC). Dosage is 75 factor IX units per kg, which is higher than that used for hemophilia B. The precise mechanism of action of PCC in stopping bleeding in inhibitor patients remains uncertain, but it appears that one or more of the *activated* clotting factors present in PCC acts as a substitute for factor VIII (or factor IX) in the clotting sequence. The response to PCC (either standard or activated) is not nearly as good in patients with inhibitors as is the response to factor VIII in a hemophiliac without an inhibitor. However, for lack of a readily available, more effective form of treatment for inhibitor patients, most hemophilia centers use PCC as first-line treatment for acute hemarthroses and early intramuscular bleeding or other soft tissue bleeding (Table 2). As noted earlier, acute myocardial infarction has occurred in young (15–22 years of age) inhibitor patients who received repetitive large doses of PCC. Thus, if a hemarthrosis or soft tissue hemorrhage fails to respond to three or four doses of PCC, therapy should stop.

A highly purified porcine factor VIII concentrate, Hyate:C,* has been used extensively in the United Kingdom since the late 1970s and was licensed for use in the United States in 1986. Since there is some degree of species specificity in factor VIII inhibitors, factor VIII inhibitors developing in humans generally destroy human factor VIII to a greater extent than factor VIII from another species. Inhibitor patients who are likely to respond can be selected on the basis of in vitro testing for cross-reactivity of their inhibitor to Hyate:C; however, in general, patients whose inhibitor levels to human factor VIII are less than 50 Bethesda units (BU) usually respond well to Hyate:C. The recommended starting dose of Hyate:C is 50 to 100 units per kg, with subsequent doses determined by the recipient's factor VIII response. While side effects of Hyate:C are uncommon, there is a risk (albeit slight) of anaphylaxis since it is a foreign species protein. Most physicians have limited their use of Hyate:C to more serious hemorrhagic episodes, such as head trauma, acute surgical emergencies, or other life- or limb-threatening situations, and in most instances it has proved to be highly effective. Thrombocytopenia is occasionally seen following Hyate:C administration; therefore, it is recommended that platelet counts be monitored during its use.

Although not licensed by the United States Food and Drug Administration at the time of this writing, another potentially useful agent for treatment of bleeding in inhibitor patients is rFactor VIIa,† a safe and often effective treatment modality currently available on a compassionate use basis for inhibitor patients who have not responded to PCC and are not candidates for porcine factor VIII (because of cross-reactivity).

In addition to such attempts to control bleeding episodes, there has been considerable interest in "immune tolerance induction" regimens to eradi-

---

*Porton Products, Ltd., Agoura Hills, California.
†Novo Nordisk, Copenhagen, Denmark.

TABLE 2. **Recommended Treatment for Hemophiliacs with Inhibitor Antibodies***

Type of Bleeding	Product¶	Initial Dose	Repeated Doses¶	Comments
Acute hemarthrosis, soft tissue hemorrhage	PCC or APCC	75 U/kg	75 U/kg 12 h if necessary	Do not exceed 3 or 4 doses†
Large intramuscular hemorrhage‡,§ (e.g., iliopsoas, thigh)	Hyate:C (porcine factor VIII) or APCC†	50–100 U factor VIII/kg 75 U/kg	Over at least several days; dosage determined by recipient's factor VIII response in the case of Hyate:C	Bed rest; monitor platelet count
Life-threatening situations‡,§ Intracranial hemorrhage Acute surgical emergencies Major trauma Tongue or neck bleeding with potential airway obstruction	Hyate:C or APCC †	50–100 U factor VIII/kg 75 U/kg	Over at least several days; dosage determined by receipient's factor VIII response in the case of Hyate:C	
Tongue and mouth lacerations‡	APCC	75 U/kg	75 U/kg	Do not exceed 3 or 4 doses Antifibrinolytic agent (consider mouthwash of tranexamic acid) Sedation, NPO in small child

*Refers to "high responder" inhibitor patients. In contrast, patients who form inhibitor antibodies in low concentration only (<10 BU) can often be treated successfully with factor VIII.

†If the patient fails to respond to three or four doses of PCC or APCC, it is unlikely that further doses will be effective and they *may* be hazardous. At least 20 instances of acute myocardial infarction have been documented in association with repetitive doses of PCC in inhibitor patients.

‡These patients should be treated in a comprehensive hemophilia center. If first seen in another hospital, initial treatment should be given, and the hemophilia center should be contacted and the patient transferred.

§If there will be a delay in obtaining and preparing Hyate:C, start with an APCC (e.g., Immuno's FEIBA or Baxter/Hyland's Autoplex) until Hyate:C is available.

¶If the patient's bleeding fails to respond to APCC and Hyate:C, or if it is known that the patient will *not* respond to APCC and Hyate:C, another therapeutic option is Novo Nordisk's rFVIIa (can be obtained on a compassionate use basis if not yet licensed).

Abbreviations: PCC = prothrombin complex concentrate; APCC = activated prothrombin complex concentrate.

cate the inhibitor. A variety of regimens have been tried; some employ daily doses of factor VIII alone, while others use cytotoxic drugs, corticosteroids, or intravenous gamma globulin in combination with daily doses of factor VIII. A growing number of patients have been successfully treated with such immune tolerance regimens, although treatment failures have occurred.

Treatment of Hemophilia B

Clinical manifestations of hemophilia B (recurrent episodes of bleeding into joints and soft tissues) are indistinguishable from those of hemophilia A. Consequently, recommended management of hemorrhage in hemophilia B is generally identical to that for hemophilia A, but a different type of concentrate is given at a different dosage. The pharmacologic properties of factor IX concentrates used for replacement therapy in hemophilia B differ significantly from those of factor VIII in hemophilia A. This difference is due mainly to the smaller molecular weight of factor IX, which permits increased diffusion from intravascular to extravascular sites; as a result, a larger dose must be given to achieve the same factor level in the circulation. While a dose of 1 unit per kg of factor VIII raises the recipient's

factor VIII level by 2% (0.02 unit per mL), the same dosage of factor IX raises the factor IX level by only 1% (0.01 unit per mL). The circulating half-life of factor IX is 18 to 24 hours, approximately twice that of factor VIII, which allows less frequent dosing (factor IX every 12 to 24 hours, versus factor VIII every 8 to 12 hours). As in hemophilia A, the recommended dosage of factor IX depends on the nature and severity of the bleeding episode (Table 3). One should aim for a minimum factor IX level of 20% for most hemorrhagic episodes, although larger doses are recommended for life- or limb-threatening bleeding and surgery. Dosing should be repeated every 12 to 24 hours as necessary to maintain hemostasis, and factor IX levels should be monitored to ensure adequacy of therapy during treatment of life-threatening bleeding episodes.

Until recently, many hemophilia centers avoided elective surgical procedures in patients with hemophilia B because of the risk of DIC and thromboembolic complications following intensive use of factor IX complex concentrates. However, in December 1990 the first of two highly purified coagulation factor IX concentrates was licensed for use in the United States. These coagulation factor IX concentrates (Alpha Therapeutics' AlphaNine and Armour's Mononine) ap-

TABLE 3. **Recommended Dosage Schedules for Severe and Moderately Severe Hemophilia B**

Type of Bleeding	Initial Dosage and Source of Factor IX (U/kg)	Repeat Dose and Source of Factor IX (U/kg)	Ancillary Treatment
Acute hemarthrosis			
Early	20 (PCC or coagulation F IX)	None	
Late (painful, with limitation of motion)	30 (PCC or coagulation F IX)	20–25 q 12 h	Ice pack, splinting may be helpful
Intramuscular hemorrhage	30–40 (coagulation F IX)	30 q 12 h (usually requires several days of treatment)	
Life-threatening situations*	40–50 (coagulation F IX)	20–25 q 12 h	
Intracranial hemorrhage			
Major trauma			
Major surgery			
Other serious bleeding*			
Tongue or neck bleeding with potential for airway obstruction	40 (coagulation F IX)	20 (coagulation F IX) q 12 h	
Severe abdominal pain			
Tongue and mouth lacerations* or extraction of permanent teeth	30 (PCC or coagulation F IX)	20 (PCC or coagulation F IX)	Tranexamic acid or EACA (if PCC is used, tranexamic acid should be in mouthwash form) Sedation, NPO in small children
Painless spontaneous gross hematuria	None		Increase PO fluids

*These conditions should be treated in a comprehensive hemophilia center. If the patient is first seen in another hospital, initial treatment should be given, then the hemophilia center should be contacted and the patient transferred.

Abbreviations: PCC = prothrombin complex concentrates; coagulation F IX = high-purity (and less thrombogenic) factor IX concentrates; EACA = epsilon aminocaproic acid.

pear to be far less thrombogenic than factor IX complex concentrates and are recommended for use in any person with hemophilia B who is undergoing surgery. They are also recommended for persons with hemophilia B who have sustained a large intramuscular hemorrhage or crush injury, for neonates, and for those with significant hepatocellular dysfunction (i.e., any risk situation for excessive thrombogenicity if a factor IX complex concentrate is used). While factor IX complex concentrates are still used to treat persons with hemophilia B who do not fall into one of these high-risk categories, thrombotic complications can occur on occasion in *any* recipient of factor IX complex, and some physicians are now recommending the use of coagulation factor IX concentrates for all hemophilia B patients.

With the availability of viral-attenuated factor IX concentrates, fresh-frozen plasma is no longer recommended for persons with mild hemophilia B who require infrequent treatment. As is true of all currently marketed factor VIII concentrates, none of the currently marketed factor IX concentrates has been implicated in any instance of HIV-1, HIV-2, or hepatitis transmission.

For *oral surgical procedures,* or other bleeding in the oral cavity (e.g., tongue or mouth lacerations), an antifibrinolytic agent should be used as adjunctive treatment. In order to prevent increased thrombogenicity, one should avoid the concomitant use of factor IX complex concentrates and an antifibrinolytic agent given systemically. One can use either (1) a coagulation factor IX concentrate with EACA or tranexamic acid given systemically or (2) a factor IX complex concentrate with tranexamic acid in mouthwash form.

Bleeding episodes in hemophilia B patients with inhibitors are usually treated with factor IX complex concentrates in a dose of 75 units per kg. However, response to treatment is generally suboptimal as compared with that in a noninhibitor patient. Porcine factor VIII is *not* indicated in hemophilia B patients with inhibitors, but recombinant factor VIIa (rF VIIa) (available on a compassionate use basis) may be effective.

Attempts to induce immune tolerance in hemophilia B patients with inhibitors should include one of the high-purity coagulation factor IX concentrates (rather than repeated doses of a factor IX complex concentrate).

Treatment of von Willebrand's Disease

Although von Willebrand's disease (vWD) is the most common of the hereditary disorders of hemostasis, relatively few patients require treatment. Many have minimal bleeding problems that are self limited or can be controlled by local measures. However, those with moderately severe or severe bleeding may require periodic treatment.

The goal of treatment in vWD is correction of the hemostasis defect, particularly correction of the factor VIII deficiency and the prolonged bleeding time. For persons with type I (classic) vWD, the synthetic vasopressin analogue DDAVP is the treatment of choice. When given intravenously in a dosage of 0.3 μg per kg, persons with type I vWD will generally have a rapid two to tenfold (average threefold) increase in factor VIII, an average two to threefold increase in vWf, and transient correction of the bleeding time. DDAVP is variably effective in vWD type IIA. Each patient requires a test dose to determine individual responsiveness prior to treatment of bleeding or for surgical coverage. The drug is diluted in 30 to 50 mL normal saline solution just prior to use and is then infused over 15 minutes. In most patients with mild to moderate type I vWD, the increase in factor VIII/vWf obtained following DDAVP is sufficient to stop hemorrhagic episodes and to provide adequate hemostasis during and following minor surgical procedures and oral surgery. As noted previously, hyponatremia and water intoxication can occur if certain precautions are not observed. Although not licensed in the United States at the time of this writing, a highly concentrated intranasal spray formulation of DDAVP has been shown to be quite effective for outpatient or home use.

Replacement therapy with plasma-derived products may be indicated when normal hemostasis must be maintained for several days, as for major surgical procedures. A clotting factor concentrate rich in vWF or cryoprecipitates should be used for bleeding patients with type II variants, for those with type III (severe) vWD, and for very young children (less than 2 years of age). Now that (virally) safer factor VIII concentrates are available, those concentrates providing sufficient vWf activity are preferable to cryoprecipitates (as the latter are not subjected to viral-attenuation processes). While clinical experience with viral-attenuated factor VIII/vWf intermediate-purity concentrates produced by different manufacturers is limited, several products are usually effective in vWD. In general these are the factor VIII concentrates that contain the intermediate-molecular-weight vWf multimers and variable amounts of the high-molecular-weight multimers, (e.g., Behring's Humate P and Miles' Koate HP). An almost pure vWf concentrate produced by Behring is currently undergoing prelicensure clinical trials in the United States; this vWf concentrate contains the most hemostatically active high-molecular-weight multimers of vWf.

For surgical procedures, correction of factor VIII deficiency appears to be more important than correction of the bleeding time. On the other hand, normalization of the bleeding time appears to be quite important in mucosal bleeding, particularly of gastrointestinal origin. Although no studies of dosage for vWD are available and thus treatment remains empirical, a set of recommendations has been published by the World Federation of Hemophilia's Committee on von Willebrand Disease. The authors' recommendations, which are quite similar, appear in Table 4. As is true for hemophilia A and B, an antifibrinolytic agent (EACA or tranexamic acid) should be used as adjunctive treatment for bleeding in the oral cavity.

As noted briefly earlier, a not yet licensed highly concentrated intranasal spray preparation of DDAVP (150 μg per spray) has been shown to be nearly equivalent to the intravenous form of

---

TABLE 4. **Recommended Treatment for von Willebrand's Disease**

For most minor bleeding episodes, minor surgery, and dental extractions in type I vWD
 DDAVP* in dosage of 0.3 μg/kg; repeat every 12–24 hours if necessary (for bleeding in oral cavity, also use an antifibrinolytic agent for 7–10 days to prevent rapid clot lysis)
For situations in which DDAVP cannot be used (or is not effective†): replacement therapy with plasma-derived clotting factor concentrates rich in von Willebrand factor should be used.
 For major surgery: Maintain factor VIII level ≥50% for 7–10 days (usually accomplished with 20–40 U/kg once daily)
 For minor surgery: Maintain factor VIII level ≥50% for 1–3 days; then maintain factor VIII level >20–30% for additional 4–7 days
 For dental extraction(s): Single large infusion to obtain a postinfusion peak of 50–60%. Also use an antifibrinolytic agent (tranexamic acid or EACA) for 7 days, starting the day before extraction
 For spontaneous or traumatic bleeding: Treatment as for hemophilia A

*Note cautions in text concerning hyponatremia and water intoxication. Do not use in children <2 years of age.
†If hemostasis cannot be maintained with DDAVP in vWD type I; in children <2 yrs; in Type II variants and type III vWD.
Abbreviations: vWD = von Willebrand's disease; DDAVP = desmopressin acetate; EACA = epsilon aminocaproic acid.

the drug in terms of response. The authors have found the intranasal spray formulation to be ideal for home use for menorrhagia, epistaxis, and other minor bleeding episodes.

PLATELET-MEDIATED BLEEDING DISORDERS

method of
DOREEN B. BRETTLER, M.D.
The Medical Center of Central Massachusetts
Worcester, Massachusetts

In primary hemostasis, platelets form a vascular plug after an initial injury and then provide a surface that promotes blood coagulation. Once a vessel is injured, the platelets adhere to subendothelial components and collagen in the vessel wall, a function that is enhanced by von Willebrand factor. Subsequently, aggregation between platelets occurs. This reaction is mediated by thrombin, released adenosine diphosphate (ADP), and thromboxane A_2, a product of arachidonic acid metabolism created when platelets are stimulated. Platelet secretion of serotonin, adenosine triphosphate, calcium from dense granules and fibrinogen, factor V, and von Willebrand factor from alpha granules occurs in response to the same stimuli that cause aggregation and stimulates more aggregation. Platelet membranes contain multiple glycoprotein receptors that bind various proteins, such as von Willebrand factor, fibrinogen, ADP, and thrombin. Inherited bleeding disorders that are platelet mediated are most often due to qualitative defects involving membrane glycoprotein deficiencies or abnormalities of the granules. Acquired platelet-mediated disorders may be qualitative or quantitative.

CLINICAL PRESENTATION AND TESTING OF PLATELET-MEDIATED BLEEDING

Patients with platelet-mediated bleeding disorders will most often present to their primary care physician with increased bruising, mucocutaneous bleeding, or both. Epistaxis, gingival bleeding, and menorrhagia may also be presenting complaints, and petechiae and ecchymoses may be found on examination. However, some patients will be asymptomatic with a decreased platelet count found only on a routine complete blood count. Before a work-up is instituted for thrombocytopenia, pseudothrombocytopenia must be ruled out. This is caused by platelet clumping secondary to the anticoagulant used in the tube, most often EDTA. If the smear shows platelet clumps, the test should be done again using tubes that contain a different anticoagulant, such as citrate.

In addition to the platelet count two clinical tests are done routinely to evaluate platelet function: bleeding time and platelet aggregation. The bleeding time (BT) is dependent on platelet number as well as their ability to adhere and aggregate. There are various methods used to measure the bleeding time, but most laboratories currently use a modified Ivy method, in which a commercial disposable spring-loaded blade is released when a trigger is pressed. A single incision 6 mm long and 1 mm deep is made on the forearm. At 30-second intervals, blood from the incision is absorbed on filter paper discs until bleeding stops. The bleeding time will almost always be prolonged if the platelet count is very low or the platelets are qualitatively abnormal. Up to 7 minutes is considered normal, but each laboratory has its own range. However, conditions unrelated to platelet number or function can also prolong the bleeding time, such as collagen defects (Ehlers-Danlos syndrome), poor skin quality, and subcutaneous edema, and the bleeding time should be interpreted accordingly.

Platelet aggregation tests are carried out to assess platelet function. They are most helpful when the bleeding time is prolonged with a normal platelet count. The ability of platelets to aggregate with ADP, thrombin, epinephrine, and collagen or to adhere with ristocetin is assessed in an aggregometer.

TREATMENT

Inherited Disorders of Platelet Function

In these disorders, a specific membrane receptor on the platelet is absent or dysfunctional or the alpha or the dense granules may be absent. Several of these disorders may also have associated thrombocytopenia. Most of them are quite rare.

Bernard-Soulier syndrome, inherited as an autosomal recessive trait, usually presents in infancy or early childhood with ecchymosis or gingival bleeding. In adulthood, gastrointestinal bleeding or menorrhagia may be present. The bleeding time is prolonged, usually over 20 minutes. The platelet count may be decreased markedly, and the platelets appear large on the blood smear. The platelets are unable to adhere to the subendothelial matrix mediated by von Willebrand factor because the platelet membrane lacks the glycoprotein Ib/IX, which is a von Willebrand factor receptor. The platelets aggregate poorly with ristocetin compared to normal platelets but respond normally to other agonists including ADP, epinephrine, and thrombin. If the patient is hemorrhaging, platelet transfusions are the best treatment. Desmopressin acetate (DDAVP) may shorten the bleeding time and should be tried.

Glanzmann's thrombasthenia is inherited as an autosomal recessive trait and seen in populations in which consanguinity is frequent. It presents with mucocutaneous bleeding. Bleeding times are markedly prolonged, although the platelet counts and morphology are normal. These platelets do not aggregate with ADP or epinephrine, although they may aggregate normally with thrombin. They are structurally abnormal, having a deficiency of glycoprotein IIb/IIIa complexes, which serve as receptors for both fibrinogen and von Willebrand factor, proteins necessary to support platelet aggregation. Treatment is instituted only for hemorrhages and is limited to transfusion of normal platelets. In contrast to Bernard-Soulier syndrome, DDAVP has no role in treatment.

Additional deficiencies of the platelet membrane are still being discovered but continue to be rare. If a patient presents with mucocutaneous bleeding and a prolonged bleeding time, sophisticated analysis of the glycoprotein receptors on the platelet may be performed by specific laboratories.

Storage pool deficiencies encompass a variety of inherited defects of either the platelet granules or the secretory mechanism. Patients can present with mucocutaneous bleeding or increased postoperative blood loss. The platelet count is normal, but the bleeding time is prolonged. On platelet aggregation tests, the second-wave aggregation caused by epinephrine and ADP may be absent and response to collagen decreased. Because aspirin and nonsteroidal anti-inflammatory drugs can cause very similar defects, patients should discontinue all such drugs before testing.

Alpha granule deficiency (gray platelet syndrome) presents with a mild bleeding diathesis, moderate thrombocytopenia, and a prolonged bleeding time. Dense granule deficiency also occurs in *Hermansky-Pudlak syndrome* (oculocutaneous albinism) and *Chédiak-Higashi syndrome*. Platelet counts and morphology are usually normal and the bleeding time is usually prolonged.

In all the platelet release defects, if bleeding is severe, DDAVP at doses of 0.3 µg per kg intravenously is the treatment of choice. If DDAVP is not efficacious, a transfusion of normal platelets can be tried. It should be noted that in approximately 25% of patients who are found to have a prolonged bleeding time, no defect is identified. If it is necessary to shorten the bleeding time, as for surgery, a therapeutic attempt using DDAVP should be made.

Acquired Disorders of Platelet Function

Drug-Induced Platelet Dysfunction

Drug-induced platelet dysfunction is probably the most common type of acquired platelet disorder. Cyclooxygenase is an enzyme involved in converting arachidonic acid, found in abundance in the platelet membrane, to thromboxanes. Thromboxanes enhance platelet aggregation by causing granule release. Even at lower doses, aspirin irreversibly inactivates cyclooxygenase for the life of the platelet, thus inhibiting platelet aggregation, especially the second wave. Patients taking aspirin may have prolonged bleeding times and a slight increase in the risk of bleeding during surgery. Platelet aggregation studies may show a decreased secondary wave of aggregation. In general, patients should stop aspirin intake 4 to 6 days prior to undergoing major surgery. Nonsteroidal anti-inflammatory drugs also inhibit cyclooxygenase but not irreversibly. Thus, bleeding times may be prolonged and platelet aggregation affected, but if the drug is stopped for 2 to 3 days, platelet function should normalize. Ticlopidine (Ticlid), a new drug that is effective in the prevention of stroke in patients with previous transient ischemic attacks, is a more potent inhibitor of platelet aggregation than aspirin, interfering in vitro with ADP-induced aggregation.

Chronic Renal Failure

Bleeding times may be prolonged in uremic patients; however, this may be associated with the anemia of renal failure. As the anemia is corrected with blood transfusions, or more recently erythropoietin, the bleeding time normalizes secondary to the rheology of red cell and platelet interaction. In addition, the prolonged bleeding times in uremia is thought to be secondary to abnormal platelet–vessel wall interactions, although the exact mechanisms have not been elucidated. Empirically, both conjugated estrogens and DDAVP at a dose of 0.3 µg per kg intravenously shorten the bleeding time in uremic patients.

Liver Cirrhosis

Patients with liver disease also have prolonged bleeding times. As in renal disease, it is not clear whether the prolonged bleeding time is due to platelet abnormalities or to the underlying disease. Patients with liver disease may be thrombocytopenic secondary to hypersplenism. Abnormalities in the multimeric structure of von Willebrand factor may also occur. DDAVP has been shown to shorten bleeding times in patients with cirrhosis and should be tried if normalization of the bleeding time is a prerequisite for surgery.

Cardiopulmonary Bypass

Surgical patients on cardiopulmonary bypass may have abnormal platelet function, perhaps caused by the membrane oxygenator in the extracorporeal circulation. Thrombocytopenia can also occur secondary to hemodilution and sequestration. In some series, platelet dysfunction was thought to cause excessive bleeding, which seemed to diminish with the use of perioperative or postoperative DDAVP.

Quantitative Disorders of Platelets

The platelet count is considered decreased when it falls below 150,000 cells per mm^3, but the smear should be examined whenever there is an unexpected drop in the platelet count, since the platelets may clump with the anticoagulant. Thrombocytopenia can be secondary to increased destruction, which may be immune mediated or due to decreased production or sequestration.

Increased Platelet Destruction

Drug-Induced Thrombocytopenia

Most drug-induced thrombocytopenia is immune mediated. Quinidine or quinine can cause thrombocytopenia, which may be severe, with counts less than 10,000 per mm^3. Occurring approximately 2 weeks after ingestion, it is mediated by a drug-dependent IgG that binds to the platelet in the presence of the drug. The drug should be stopped as soon as thrombocytopenia is discovered. The platelet count will rebound within 7 to 10 days. Steroids have not been shown to be helpful in these cases, but intravenous gamma globulin (IVIG), 400 mg per kg for 4 days, can be used if there is an acute need to obtain an increased platelet count.

Gold-induced thrombocytopenia has been seen in patients with rheumatoid arthritis. It occurs in 1 to 5% of patients receiving gold therapy, appears to be HLADR3 associated, and is found mainly during the first 20 weeks of treatment. It is immune related, resolving when the drug is stopped.

Heparin-induced thrombocytopenia is a widespread problem since heparin is a commonly utilized drug. It occurs in patients who are receiving therapeutic or prophylactic heparin and even in those having heparin flushes for indwelling intravenous lines. Approximately 5 to 10% of patients receiving heparin develop thrombocytopenia, usually 5 to 15 days after administration begins. This side effect is more prevalent with bovine than with porcine heparin. It is caused by an IgG antiheparin antibody. In about 20% of patients who develop thrombocytopenia while on heparin, arterial or venous thrombosis or both occur, paralleling the fall in the platelet count. Thrombosis is thought to be secondary to platelet activation and release caused by the binding of the antibody-heparin immune complex to the platelets. Patients receiving heparin should have daily platelet counts, and the drug should be discontinued if thrombocytopenia is noted. If the underlying thrombosis needs treatment, alternatives such as warfarin, an inferor vena cava filter, or dextran should be considered. Ancrod, a derivative of snake venom that causes hypofibrinogenemia, has also been utilized at doses of 2 units per kg intravenously over 6 to 12 hours until warfarin becomes effective. Patients with heparin-induced thrombocytopenia should not be rechallenged with heparin unless absolutely necessary. Whether thrombocytopenia will be induced by the new low-molecular-weight heparins is now under study.

An abbreviated list of drugs causing thrombocytopenia is given in Table 1. If a patient develops thrombocytopenia while on multiple drugs, all drugs should be discontinued if possible, since it may be difficult to determine which particular drug is the causative one.

Idiopathic Thrombocytopenic Purpura

Idiopathic thrombocytopenic purpura (ITP) occurs most often in people between the ages of 20 to 50 and is three times more common in females than males. Although in children it may be associated with an acute viral infection, such a history is rarely obtained in adults. The patient may be asymptomatic or signs of mucocutaneous bleeding may be present. Platelet counts are usually below 100,000 and may be as low as 1000 to 2000 per mm^3. On peripheral smear, the platelets may be large. The hemoglobin and white blood cell counts are usually normal. Other disorders such as disseminated intravascular coagulopathy, sepsis, thrombotic thrombocytopenic purpura, systemic lupus erythematosus, drug-induced thrombocytopenia, and more recently, human immunodeficiency virus type 1–induced thrombocytopenia must be ruled out. Bone marrow examination shows normal to increased megakaryocytes, and if obtained, an antiplatelet antibody test may be positive. However, since the sensitivity of this test is poor, a negative result does not rule out the diagnosis. The disease is caused by an IgG autoantibody directed against Gp IIb/IIIa or other membrane glycoproteins. Treatment should be instituted if the platelet count falls below 30,000 to 50,000 per mm^3.

High-dose corticosteroids (prednisone 1 to 2 mg per kg per day orally) are usually the treatment of choice and should not be considered a failure until they have been given for 4 to 6 weeks. They will both decrease autoantibody production and interfere with binding of the antibody to macro-

TABLE 1. **Commonly Used Drugs That Can Cause Thrombocytopenia**

Heparin
Gold
Quinine/quinidine
Antibiotics
Sulfa drugs
High-dose penicillin/cephalosporins
Procainamide
Valproic acid

phage receptors. The platelet count will increase in most patients over 7 to 10 days, but only a small proportion of patients will achieve remission. Splenectomy should be considered in patients who are steroid dependent; the response rate is 60 to 80%. Danazol (Danocrine), a synthetic androgen/progesterone, at doses of 200 mg three to four times a day orally, will also increase the platelet count. Side effects include masculinization and hepatic toxicity. Intravenous gamma globulin (IVIG), 400 mg per kg per day intravenously for 4 days or 2 gm per kg per day for 2 days, has also been successful in this disease. However, the rise in platelet count is usually transitory, making IVIG most useful when a rapid increase in the platelet count is necessary. Platelet transfusions are ineffective in elevating platelet counts and in general should not be used. If a patient with ITP who has had a splenectomy becomes thrombocytopenic again, both steroids and danazol can induce long-term remissions.

Human immunodeficiency virus (HIV-1) can induce thrombocytopenia that mimics ITP, and patients presenting with ITP should be questioned about risk factors for HIV-1 and tested if appropriate. Studies have shown that HIV-1 can induce autoantibodies against platelets as well as directly affect megakaryocyte production of platelets. Steroids and splenectomy have been successful in this setting, but fears of causing more immunosuppression have limited their use. IVIG has been used with good results, although elevation of platelet counts may be temporary. Anti-Rh factor (RhoGAM), given either intramuscularly or intravenously, also increases platelet counts in thrombocytopenic HIV-1 seropositive individuals and is much cheaper than IVIG. More recently, zidovudine has been shown to elevate platelet counts in this group, and it should be considered when CD4 lymphocyte counts fall below 500 cells per mm³.

Posttransfusion Purpura

While the previously discussed diseases are caused by an autoantibody, posttransfusion purpura is caused by an IgG alloantibody that is seen 1 week after transfusion of red cells or other blood products. The antibody is directed against the PlA1 antigen on platelets in most cases and occurs in the small percentage of PlA1-negative patients who are receiving PlA1-positive platelets. The syndrome is thought to occur in previously sensitized individuals such as those with prior pregnancies or who have received blood transfusions. Thrombocytopenia may last as long as 1 month. Treatment is problematic. Plasmapheresis to remove the IgG antibody has been successful in some cases, and IVIG has had some efficacy, especially in combination with corticosteroids.

TABLE 2. **Treatment of Thrombocytopenia**

Treatment		Disease
Platelet transfusions	*Effective:*	TP due to decreased production, qualitative platelet disorders
	Ineffective:	TP due to immune-mediated destruction (e.g., ITP)
High-dose steroids	*Effective:*	ITP, HIV-1–induced TP
	Ineffective:	Drug-induced TP
Intravenous gamma globulin	*Effective:*	ITP, HIV-1–induced TP, drug-induced TP
	Ineffective:	Production defects or sequestration
Danazol	*Effective:*	ITP
Desmopressin (DDAVP)	*Effective:*	In some qualitative platelet disorders
	Ineffective:	In TP due to increased destruction or decreased production

Abbreviations: TP = thrombocytopenia; ITP = idiopathic thrombocytopenic purpura; HIV-1 = human immunodeficiency virus type 1.

Decreased Platelet Production

These disorders are covered in greater detail in other articles in this volume. The acute leukemias, infiltrative diseases of the bone marrow, and nutritional disorders such as vitamin B_{12} and folate deficiency can all cause thrombocytopenia and must be ruled out with appropriate blood tests and physical and bone marrow examination. Excessive alcohol intake can also cause thrombocytopenia by suppressing platelet production in the bone marrow.

Massive hemorrhage can cause thrombocytopenia secondary to the dilutional effects of replacement with banked blood that has few viable platelets and the inability of the body to rapidly produce more platelets. Platelet concentrates should be administered after each 10 to 12 units of blood transfused to avoid this problem.

Increased Platelet Sequestration

The spleen normally acts as a reservoir for platelets and contains a large exchangeable pool (about 30% of the total platelet mass in a normal-sized spleen and up to 90% in an enlarged spleen). Thrombocytopenia can occur in splenomegaly of any origin, but usually in conjunction with leukopenia, anemia, or both. The thrombocytopenia is rarely severe and symptoms of mucocutaneous bleeding are not present. If the spleen is not palpable, diagnosis may require imaging studies. Splenomegaly can occur secondary to numerous disorders, such as congestion from liver disease, lymphoma, storage diseases, and infections. Splenectomy is rarely the treatment of choice unless it is done for diagnosis or for relief of pain or early satiety. Since patients are rarely symptomatic, the underlying cause of splenomegaly should be found and treated.

Treatments for the various types of thrombocytopenia are summarized in Table 2.

DISSEMINATED INTRAVASCULAR COAGULATION

method of
ALISON MOLITERNO, M.D., and
WILLIAM R. BELL, M.D.
The Johns Hopkins University School of Medicine
Baltimore, Maryland

Disseminated intravascular coagulation (DIC) is a clinical syndrome that is the result of pathologic activities of the coagulation and fibrinolytic systems. DIC is not a primary disease entity, but rather a consequence of an underlying severe systemic illness.

DIC is a progressive biologic process that induces alterations in platelets and fibrin formation. Most commonly, DIC is manifested by bleeding; less frequently, it presents as thrombosis, and even more infrequently as simultaneous bleeding and thrombosis. Examination of pathologic material reveals the deposition of microthrombi in the vasculature.

PATHOGENESIS

The pathogenesis of DIC has been studied extensively, yet many of the mechanisms responsible for the clinical and laboratory features of this illness are not understood. Normally hemostasis is precisely regulated by opposing forces of activators, inhibitors, and mechanisms for the clearance of activated factors. Entrance into the circulation of a procoagulant, such as a thromboplastic substance from damaged or abnormal tissue, induces activation of the coagulation and fibrinolytic systems and promotes the aggregation of platelets. DIC may be promoted through the release of substances from an inflammatory response or from the breakdown of vascular endothelium or of substances from infective organisms. In addition, excessive activation of the coagulation system can result in the depletion of any or all of the coagulation factors.

Although the clinical scenarios vary, the common agent in the production of DIC can be understood by the deregulation of thrombin and plasmin. Thrombin is essential to the formation of microthrombi, in that it cleaves fibrinogen to form fibrin, which is then cross-linked by factor XIII, which itself is activated by thrombin. Thrombin also activates factors VIII and V, which provide positive feedback via the coagulation cascade to produce additional thrombin. Thrombin also promotes platelet aggregation and activates protein C, an agent that degrades activated factors V and VIII.

Supported in part by NIH research grant HL 36260 from the NHLBI of the National Institutes of Health, Bethesda, MD.

Plasmin is a proteolytic enzyme capable of digesting fibrin and fibrinogen, thereby releasing many fragments. The degradation products interrupt fibrin polymerization and thereby normal coagulation. In addition, by binding to the platelet glycoproteins Ib and IIb-IIIa, the degradation products alter platelet function.

Regulation of these opposing forces is complex. Tissue factor activates factors VII and VIIa, generating thrombin via the extrinsic pathway. Tissue plasminogen activator released from endothelial cells and factor XII via the intrinsic pathway both stimulate plasmin generation. The relative activities of thrombin and plasmin create the spectrum of presentations of DIC: from thrombus formation without bleeding to excessive fibrinolysis and hemorrhage.

ASSOCIATED CONDITIONS

DIC is a consequence of a severe, usually systemic illness. It can be associated with any illness, but most commonly with sepsis, malignancy, trauma, obstetric complications, and hepatic disease.

DIC has been reported as a consequence of infection with bacteria, fungi, viruses, spores, rickettsia, and protozoa. It is more commonly reported in conjunction with gram-negative than with gram-positive organisms, possibly due to the effects of endotoxin on the coagulation cascade.

When associated with malignancy, DIC is more commonly a late complication. Carcinoma of the lung, pancreas, stomach, and prostate are most frequently reported with DIC. Prostatic neoplasms contain large amounts of thromboplastin; patients with this disease may have extended courses of DIC. Malignancy heralded by recurrent, migrating thrombosis of both the arterial and venous systems is characteristic of the Trousseau syndrome, a type of DIC in which the presenting feature is often thrombosis. Laboratory evidence of DIC can be demonstrated in the majority of Trousseau-related cases. Why thrombosis alone is observed in some patients with Trousseau syndrome is unknown.

Obstetric complications such as toxemia, retained placenta, premature separation of the placenta, placenta previa, septic and induced abortion, postpartum hypertensive renal failure, and retained dead fetus have all been reported to induce DIC. The clinical course of DIC in these cases is marked by abrupt onset with severe widespread hemorrhage and prompt improvement once the underlying condition is ameliorated. It has been postulated that tissue thromboplastin is released from the uterus into the maternal circulation, thereby activating the coagulation cascade and depleting clotting factors.

As the major producer of coagulation factors and inhibitors, as well as the route of clearance of activated factors via the Kupffer cells, liver failure is associated with the loss of coagulation regulation. True DIC can exist concomitantly with severe liver disease, and laboratory distinction of the two states is difficult. Clearly, liver disease both lowers the threshold for and perpetuates the course of DIC. Illustrating this point are the many reports of DIC after placement of a peritoneovenous shunt for control of intractable ascites.

CLINICOPATHOLOGIC FEATURES

The most common clinical presentation of DIC is frank bleeding or a tendency to bleed. When present, the hemorrhage is widespread via the skin, mucous membranes, trachea, gastrointestinal tract, genitourinary tract, and central nervous system. Prompt appearance of ecchymoses after venipunctures, neurologic examination with a reflex hammer, or sphygmomanometry is also characteristic, as is excessive oozing from intravascular line sites, nasogastric tube erosions, or venipuncture sites. In addition to hemorrhage, physical findings of acral cyanosis and pallor are present.

The major pathologic findings of DIC at postmortem examination are fibrin thrombi, large and small vessel thrombosis, marantic endocarditis, hemorrhage, and the consequences thereof. The kidney, lungs, liver, adrenal glands, gastrointestinal mucosa, brain, and pituitary gland are most frequently involved.

Although unexpected exsanguination into a body cavity can cause death, more commonly death is due to pulmonary failure, septicemia, cardiogenic shock, acute tubular necrosis, or hepatic failure. In the majority of cases, death is attributable to the underlying illness.

LABORATORY DIAGNOSIS

There is no single test for the diagnosis of DIC, but there are several that taken together identify its presence. Similarly, serial measurements can indicate trends that support the diagnosis.

Examination of the peripheral blood smear must be undertaken as the first step in the diagnostic process. First, the blood smear provides an accurate assessment of thrombocytopenia, which nearly always accompanies DIC. The platelet counts usually range from 40,000 to 75,000 per mm^3. Second, the blood smear provides the only means with which to assess the red blood cell morphology. Although not specific for DIC, microangiopathic changes of the red cells are frequently present. In addition, the blood smear can provide critical information regarding the underlying illness such as the toxic granulations and Döhle bodies of sepsis or the target and spur cells of liver failure.

Although thrombin and plasmin generation can be measured via thrombin-antithrombin III and plasmin-α_2-antiplasmin complexes, these are not routinely available. For clinical purposes, the activities of plasmin and thrombin are most commonly ascertained by indirect measures. Plasmin activity is assessed by both the absolute value and the temporal trends of fibrinogen, fibrinogen-fibrin degradation products (FDP-fdp), and fragment D-dimer. Fibrinogen may be elevated in malignancy or inflammatory states, but if DIC is present it will eventually fall as a consequence of plasmin activity. Classically, in severe DIC, the plasma fibrinogen concentration is markedly reduced, often in the range of 10 to 50 mg per 100 mL plasma. As the plasminogen/plasmin system is the only endogenous system that digests fibrinogen and fibrin, elevation of the degradation products indicates excessive activity of the fibrinolytic system and lends support to the diagnosis of DIC. Routine assays for FDP-fdp do not discriminate between fragments of fibrinogen and fibrin. To this end, the D-dimer assay has been applied. The D-dimer is a fragment released by the digestion of polymerized or cross-linked fibrin and as such may reflect both thrombin and plasmin activity. Comparisons of the two assays reveal that the D-dimer may be more specific for DIC while the FDP-fdp is more sensitive.

Although frequently reported as good screening tests for the diagnosis of DIC, the prothrombin time, the activated partial thromboplastin time, and the thrombin time frequently are not helpful, as the results may be normal in DIC. Many investigators have reported the utility of specific coagulation factor assays. Since there is excessive activity of the fibrinolytic system in this disease process, it is not surprising to find reduction in levels of factors II, V, VIII, IX, X, XI, XII, and XIII. However, the time required for performance of these tests renders them impractical for diagnosis in this illness.

One of the simplest and most helpful tests that can be performed at the bedside is a single-tube clotting time. This is done by placing 1 mL of whole blood in a clean glass tube and gently tilting it every 30 seconds until a visible clot forms. Normally, a clot will form within 10 minutes. The tube can then be secured to a wall and observed. If sufficient platelets are present, clot retraction will occur within 1 hour. If the fibrinolytic system is activated, clot dissolution can be observed as the clot becomes a lumpy liquid. This test provides qualitative information regarding coagulation, platelet number and function, and fibrinolysis.

In summary, the laboratory studies needed to establish the diagnosis of DIC can be chosen selectively by the realization that this process results in simultaneous activation of the coagulation, platelet, and fibrinolytic systems. As is often the case, the initial set of studies may not be confirmatory, and serial measurements may be needed before the diagnosis is established.

TREATMENT

To identify and eradicate the primary illness is of paramount importance in the treatment of DIC. If the inciting agent and other comorbidities are not addressed, the likelihood of successful therapy is negligible. Secondary processes such as tissue ischemia, hypovolemia, hypotension, hypoxemia, and electrolyte and acid-base disturbances must be managed aggressively.

Often DIC is revealed in hospitalized patients by perturbations in daily laboratory measurements in the absence of clinical manifestations. While its presence may be suspected or even documented, the greater effort is spent in treating the primary condition rather than the DIC itself. This is generally an acceptable approach. However, controversy ensues once bleeding occurs.

Faced with abnormal coagulation measurements and significant bleeding, it is reasonable to attempt replacement of depleted coagulation factors with those found in fresh-frozen plasma (FFP). FFP has the advantage of supplying many factors at once with the disadvantage of presenting the risk of volume load.

Cryoprecipitate is useful mainly in circumstances in which the fibrinogen level is extremely low. The role of platelet transfusion is often questionable. Certainly in the setting of bleeding and severe ($<10,000/mm^3$) thrombocytopenia transfusion is warranted. If a 1-hour post-transfusion platelet count does not show an adequate increment (5 to 10,000 increase per unit platelet transfused), then further infusion is not likely to be useful. Theoretically, repletion of plasma proteins will provide the substrate required to generate more FDP-fdp, and through these inhibitors further derange coagulation. However, there are no clinical data to support the notion that platelet, FFP or cryoprecipitate transfusions accelerate the course of DIC.

In an attempt to treat the DIC primarily, control of both the coagulation and fibrinolytic systems has been employed. Heparin has long been considered a useful therapeutic agent for DIC. Heparin binds to antithrombin-III and promotes its anticoagulant action. The heparin-antithrombin-III complex has a neutralizing effect on thromboplastin and therefore could be helpful if the DIC is induced by thromboplastic-like substances. The clinical benefit of heparin is well known in the Trousseau syndrome; recurrence or treatment failure despite therapeutic anticoagulation with warfarin should lead the physician to suspect a DIC-type process. Heparin sensitivity and warfarin resistance can occur if the inciting agent is a thromboplastic material as opposed to a vitamin K–dependent protein. DIC associated with acute promyelocytic leukemia is another disease entity where heparin is routinely employed. In this case heparin improves the laboratory manifestations of DIC but whether there is a clear clinical benefit has yet to be proved. Heparin has been reported to reduce the necrosis associated with purpura fulminans and to alleviate the bleeding associated with amniotic fluid embolism and the dead fetus syndrome. Other presentations of DIC generated by alternate mechanisms may not respond to heparin therapy, and its use could aggravate the bleeding tendency. Therefore, a trial of heparin is recommended only if the clinical situation deteriorates despite supportive and replacement measures.

Interest in the use of epsilon aminocaproic acid (Amicar) to control fibrinolysis has grown. Aminocaproic acid inhibits fibrinolysis by preventing conversion of plasminogen to plasmin. Combined therapy with aminocaproic acid and heparin could potentially control both coagulation and fibrinolysis. However, the use of aminocaproic acid alone in DIC cannot be advised as widespread thrombosis can occur.

Finally, much interest in antithrombin III and protein C has been generated. Many investigators have found both protein levels to be low in DIC. Replacement of these proteins has been attempted as primary therapy with some reported success, but controlled studies are necessary to establish a clear clinical benefit.

Because of the variety of presentations and the context of the underlying illness, it is difficult to delineate specific strategies and regimens for the treatment of DIC. Therapy must be employed on a patient-to-patient basis and always within the framework of aggressive treatment of the underlying illness.

THROMBOTIC THROMBOCYTOPENIC PURPURA–HEMOLYTIC UREMIC SYNDROME

method of
WILLIAM R. BELL, M.D., and
MICHAEL STREIFF, M.D.
The Johns Hopkins University School of Medicine
Baltimore, Maryland

Thrombotic thrombocytopenic purpura–hemolytic uremic syndrome (TTP-HUS) is a devastating illness characterized by microangiopathic hemolytic anemia, thrombocytopenia, renal and neurologic dysfunction, and fever. Although originally these two entities were considered separate syndromes, many authorities feel that they are two different manifestations of the same pathologic process. Therefore, we refer to these syndromes as a single illness throughout this review.

CLINICAL FEATURES

TTP-HUS is a rare illness with an estimated frequency of one case for every 45,000 to 50,000 hospital admissions. The median age at diagnosis is 35 years, but affected neonates as well as nonagenarians have been reported. Women are affected slightly more often than men (M:F ratio 2:3), and whites are affected more often than blacks. Typically, patients present within 1 to 2 days of the appearance of the initial manifestations, most commonly neurologic difficulties, easy bruising, and abdominal discomfort. Other complaints include malaise, weakness, fatigue, nausea, vomiting, and fever. Some patients experience a viral-like upper respiratory or gastrointestinal illness prior to diagnosis.

The principal clinical findings are microangiopathic

hemolytic anemia and thrombocytopenia, which are often severe. Forty percent of patients have hemoglobin concentrations below 6.5 mg per dL and 56% have platelets counts below 20,000 per mm³. Lactate dehydrogenase and total bilirubin are usually elevated, reflecting a brisk intravascular hemolytic process. Critical to the diagnosis of TTP-HUS is the peripheral blood smear, which is characterized by numerous fragmented red blood cells of all types, polychromasia, frequent nucleated red blood cells and large platelets in decreased numbers. Without this picture, the diagnosis must be questioned.

Neurologic abnormalities are common and include headaches, confusion, aphasia (particularly expressive aphasia), seizures, and coma. Renal involvement occurs in the vast majority (88%) and can be as minimal as microscopic hematuria or elevations of the blood urea nitrogen and creatinine. Less commonly, significant uremia develops, and this manifestation is much more common in the HUS variant of the TTP-HUS continuum. Fever occurs in approximately 90% of patients at some time during their illness, although only 18 to 25% present with it. It is thought to be due to microcirculatory involvement of the hypothalamus or the generation of endogenous pyrogens.

Cardiopulmonary and endocrine disturbances are infrequently clinically significant. Likewise, screening coagulation studies are usually normal or minimally abnormal. In nearly 50% of patients, mild to moderate laboratory evidence of disseminated intravascular coagulation (DIC) is present, but not to a degree where confusion with the syndrome of DIC would result.

Although TTP-HUS is classically associated with a pentad of symptoms (hemolytic anemia, thrombocytopenia, central nervous system abnormalities, fever, renal dysfunction), only approximately 77% of patients develop all of these abnormalities during their illness. The clinical course of TTP-HUS is often marked by one or more relapses after successful treatment, usually within the first 2 months after diagnosis, and the rare patient will experience a relapse beyond this period. With aggressive treatment, most adults with TTP-HUS who achieve a remission have no permanent adverse sequelae. In contrast, children not infrequently have residual renal dysfunction. Although most cases of TTP-HUS follow an acute course, a minority of patients develop a chronic relapsing variant characterized by multiple relapses over many years.

The diagnosis of TTP-HUS should never be made hastily. Disseminated intravascular coagulation, Evans' syndrome, paroxysmal nocturnal hemoglobinuria, malignant hypertension, pre-eclampsia, eclampsia, postpartum renal failure, systemic lupus erythematosus, HELLP syndrome, scleroderma, subacute bacterial endocarditis, polyarteritis nodosa, and purpura fulminans all share some of the clinical features associated with TTP-HUS and must be excluded in the differential diagnosis.

PATHOLOGY

The characteristic pathologic finding in TTP-HUS is disseminated hyaline thrombosis of the terminal arterioles and capillaries. Inflammation is usually not present and the venous system is typically spared. These thrombi consist predominantly of platelets and adherent fibrin. The kidneys, pancreas, heart, adrenals, and brain are the most heavily involved sites, while the liver and lungs tend to be spared. In the past, various organs, including the skin, bone marrow, gingiva, and kidneys, were biopsied to confirm the diagnosis of TTP-HUS. However, because of the nonspecific nature of the pathologic findings in this illness, we feel that these procedures should be performed only when true diagnostic confusion exists.

PATHOGENESIS

The clinical findings of TTP-HUS are thought to result from diffuse endothelial injury leading to the formation of platelet-rich thrombi in the microcirculation, causing hypoperfusion and organ dysfunction. Why certain organs are more heavily involved than others is not understood. Red blood cells are mechanically disrupted as they traverse the partially obstructed capillaries, producing an abrupt and profound hemolytic anemia. Thrombocytopenia results from thrombocytolysis and possibly the consumption of platelets during the formation of these thrombi.

Early investigators suggested that immunologically mediated endothelial damage was responsible for this illness; however, subsequent investigation has failed to support this suggestion. Others have implicated platelet aggregating factors in the pathogenesis of TTP-HUS, but replication of their experimental results has proved difficult. Ultra-large von Willebrand factor multimers, which have been detected in the plasma of some patients with chronic relapsing TTP-HUS, have also been proposed as a possible cause. However, similar multimers have been found in many other diseases associated with endothelial damage (e.g., scleroderma, vasculitis, *Rickettsia rickettsii* infection), and they probably represent a marker of disease activity rather than the critical initiating pathogenic event. Prostacyclin deficiency and elevated levels of soluble thrombomodulin, thrombospondin, calpain, and PAI-1 are other abnormalities that have been documented in TTP-HUS, and in all likelihood they also are secondary phenomena.

It is evident that investigative efforts have been successful in documenting many of the pathologic events that occur in TTP-HUS. However, none of these findings appears to be sufficient to explain the origin of this process and the critical trigger of this devastating illness remains to be identified.

ASSOCIATED CONDITIONS AND EXPOSURES

TTP-HUS has been associated with a myriad of different diseases, medications, toxins, and infections, perhaps because of its unknown etiology (Table 1). In most cases these associations are probably fortuitous rather than pathogenic; however, a few exceptions do exist. Considerable evidence appears to support a causal link between *Escherichia coli 0157:H7* infection in children and the development of TTP-HUS. Less impressive but still persuasive evidence supports a

TABLE 1. **Conditions and Exposures Associated with TTP-HUS**

Diseases	Malignancies
Ankylosing spondylitis	Acute myelogenous
Graves' disease	leukemia
Immune thrombocytopenic	Cholangiocarcinoma
purpura	Colon adenocarcinoma
Polyarteritis	Gastric adenocarcinoma
Polymyositis	Hodgkin's disease
Rheumatoid arthritis	Non-Hodgkin's lymphoma
Sjögren's syndrome	Plasma cell dyscrasia
Systemic lupus	
erythematosus	**Toxins**
Ulcerative colitis	Bee sting
	Carbon monoxide poisoning
Pregnancy	Chloronaphthaline in
	varnish
Drugs	Dog bite
Bleomycin	
Cisplatin	**Infections**
Cyclosporin A	*Aeromonas hydrophila*
FK 506	*Aspergillus*
5-Fluorouracil	*Bacteroides*
Influenza vaccine	*Campylobacter jejuni*
Iodine	Coxsackie B virus
Mitomycin C	*Escherichia coli* 0157:H7
Oral contraceptives	Herpes simplex virus
Oxophenarsine	Human immunodeficiency
Penicillamine	virus
Penicillins	Influenza A
Quinine	*Legionella pneumophila*
Rifampin	Measles
Sulfonamides	Meningococcemia
Ticlodipine	Microtatobiote
Triple antigen and TAB	Mononucleosis
vaccine	*Mycoplasma*
Vinca alkaloids	*Streptococcus pneumoniae*

Abbreviation: TAB = typhoid salmonella paratyphi, types A and B.

connection between mitomycin C and TTP-HUS. Pregnancy also appears to predispose to this illness. Perhaps each of these disorders results in endothelial damage leading to TTP-HUS, but the exact sequence of pathogenic events remains unknown.

TREATMENT

Therapy for TTP-HUS, because of its fulminant course and unknown etiology, has often been applied in a haphazard and desperate fashion. Corticosteroids, splenectomy, plasma infusion, plasmapheresis exchange, antiplatelet agents, vincristine, heparin, thrombolytic therapy, intravenous immunoglobulin G, and prostacyclin have all been used in various combinations. Not surprisingly, accurate response rates for many of these treatments remain unknown.

Currently, plasma exchange (plasmapheresis and replacement with fresh-frozen plasma) appears to be the therapeutic modality of choice. Response rates as high as 91% have been reported. Our current approach to this disease is as follows. Patients who have no neurologic symptoms (except minimal headache) and moderate hematologic and renal involvement (hematocrit >20%, platelet counts >10,000 per mm^3, creatinine levels <5 mg per dL) are treated initially with high-dose intravenous corticosteroids (methylprednisolone, 200 mg intravenously every day). If clinical deterioration occurs, neurologic symptoms develop, or improvement is not seen within 48 hours, then aggressive daily plasmapheresis (65 to 140 mL per kg per day) is initiated. The clinical condition is monitored by daily physical examinations and assessment of hemoglobin/hematocrit values, platelet and reticulocyte counts, and lactate dehydrogenase and creatinine concentrations. Peripheral blood smears are performed every 3 days to assess schistocytosis and platelet number. Patients with hematocrit values below 20% receive transfusions to raise the hematocrit to 25% or more prior to plasmapheresis. Platelet infusions are not given, no matter how severe the thrombocytopenia, because occasional patients have deteriorated dramatically following their administration.

Patients refractory to standard plasma exchange receive plasma volume expansion by transfusion of fresh frozen plasma or whole blood, and consideration is given to vincristine sulfate (Oncovin), 1.4 mg per M^2 not to exceed 2.0 mg intravenously on days 1, 4, 7, and 10. After remission is achieved, steroids and plasmapheresis are tapered. Relapses are treated in the same manner as initial presentations. After discharge, patients are continued on a gradual steroid taper and followed in the hematology clinic for a minimum of 1 year.

We have not been impressed with the efficacy of splenectomy or antiplatelet agents in the treatment of this disease. Most investigators feel that responses to splenectomy are more likely due to the blood and plasma administered perioperatively than to the procedure itself. Antiplatelet agents often cause bleeding complications and have only rarely been associated with remissions when used alone. Although isolated success using intravenous gamma globulin G and prostacyclin has been reported, these therapies must be evaluated in a prospective, randomized manner before general application can be recommended. Heparin and thrombolytic therapy, with only the rarest exceptions, should not be used for TTP-HUS because they are ineffective and can potentially cause disastrous bleeding complications.

TTP-HUS, once a uniformly fatal illness, is now eminently treatable with early recognition and aggressive therapy. Current research is directed at identifying the elusive trigger of this catastrophic process so that more specific and safer therapies can be developed.

HEMOCHROMATOSIS

method of
LAWRIE W. POWELL, M.D., Ph.D.
Queensland Institute of Medical Research
Herston, Brisbane, Queensland, Australia

Hemochromatosis is the most common autosomal recessive disease in humans. Homozygosity for the hemochromatosis allele occurs in about 3 per 1000 persons of central and northern European ancestry. The hemochromatosis gene lies very close to the HLA-A locus on the short arm of chromosome 6. It is now considered likely that all *primary* iron overload in Caucasian populations (i.e., not associated with thalassemia major, sideroblastic anemia, or multiple blood transfusions) is probably due to homozygosity for hemochromatosis. Identification of the gene and knowledge of the gene product will be a significant advance in the diagnosis and management of the disease.

Clinical and Laboratory Findings

The complications of hemochromatosis are due to prolonged excessive iron accumulation. Symptoms include weight loss, weakness, fatigue, joint pain, palpitations, and impotence. Common physical findings include gray-bronze pigmentation of the skin, hepatomegaly, enlargement and tenderness of the metacarpophalangeal joints and knees, decreased body hair, and testicular atrophy. About 60% of symptomatic subjects with hemochromatosis have diabetes mellitus, and some 25% have arthritis (chondrocalcinosis).

The role of alcohol ingestion in the development of iron overload has been clarified by recent genetic studies. Iron and alcohol have a synergistic effect, and cirrhosis develops earlier in patients with hemochromatosis who drink to excess. However, significant iron overload occurs only in those homozygous for the disease.

The most common laboratory findings are elevated serum iron concentration, transferrin saturation, serum ferritin concentration, glucose concentration, and hepatocellular enzymes. Other abnormal serologic test results include decreased plasma testosterone in men and decreased plasma estradiol in women. Hypogonadism usually is of the secondary hypogonadotrophic type (i.e., associated with markedly decreased concentrations of luteinizing hormone and follicle-stimulating hormone in the blood).

Diagnosis

A high index of suspicion has traditionally been required for the early diagnosis of the disease, especially in subjects under 40 years of age with unexplained cardiomyopathy or endocrinopathy. However, the widespread use of biochemical screening tests in standard physical examinations has led to increased diagnosis of the disease in the precirrhotic stage. Individuals with elevated transferrin saturation and serum ferritin concentration should undergo liver biopsy, because definitive diagnosis requires demonstration of excess paren-

chymal iron *and increased hepatic iron concentration* (HIC). Because of an age-related rise in liver iron concentration in homozygous subjects, calculation of the *hepatic iron index* (HIC ÷ age) has proved useful in distinguishing between heterozygotes and young homozygotes who should be treated (Table 1). Liver biopsy is important in defining the extent of tissue injury (fibrosis and/or cirrhosis) as well as the degree of iron overload. Indeed, the demonstration or exclusion of cirrhosis is vital to the management of the individual case.

Computed tomography and magnetic resonance imaging are of limited diagnostic value, especially in the early detection of the disease.

Since the responsible gene is known to be located close to the HLA-A locus on chromosome 6, HLA typing can be used to track the inheritance of the disorder in affected pedigrees. Thus, HLA typing is of value in identifying siblings who are HLA identical to an affected brother or sister and who are likely to develop hemochromatosis themselves (putative homozygotes). However, HLA typing cannot be used to screen the general population for hemochromatosis because the genetic locus for hemochromatosis is sufficiently separate from the HLA-A locus for genetic recombination to have recurred with time, such that different HLA-A alleles (not only HLA-A3) may be found in association with hemochromatosis in different kindreds.

Prognosis

The prognosis of hemochromatosis depends on the extent of the disease at diagnosis. Patients diagnosed before the development of hepatic cirrhosis and diabetes and adequately treated can expect a normal life span. However, hepatic cirrhosis is associated with a lifelong risk of development of primary hepatocellular carcinoma, and these patients should undergo periodic screening.

Treatment

The most important treatment for hemochromatosis is phlebotomy therapy, conducted in two

TABLE 1. **Diagnostic Criteria**

Screening Tests

Blood Tests Reflecting Iron Stores
Transferrin saturation >60%

Elevated Serum Ferritin Concentration
>350 μg/L in men
>150 μg/L in women

Proof of Diagnosis

Liver Biopsy
Assessment of stainable hepatocellular iron
 (grades 3 or 4)
Hepatic iron concentration (μmols Fe/gm dry wt)

Hepatic iron index: $\dfrac{\text{Iron concentration}}{\text{Age}}$

>2 indicative of homozygous state
<2 heterozygote, normal, or alcoholic liver disease

phases (Table 2). The first phase of iron depletion therapy is achieved through rapid-sequence phlebotomy. This entails the withdrawal of 1 to 2 units (500 mL each) of whole blood each week until iron-limited erythropoiesis and low values of transferrin saturation and serum ferritin concentration are demonstrated.

The second phase of phlebotomy therapy continues for the rest of the individual's life. This entails withdrawal of 1 unit of whole blood every 3 to 6 months to prevent reaccumulation of excessive body storage iron. Monitoring of body iron stores is done by periodic measurement of the serum ferritin concentration, which correlates well with liver iron storage in the absence of inflammatory disease (e.g., arthritis), in which it is elevated as an acute-phase protein. Thus, one should aim to keep the hematocrit normal and serum ferritin level under 100 μg per liter.

Men with hemochromatosis may require 30 to 130 units of phlebotomy to deplete their excessive storage iron, whereas women usually require only 10 to 50 units. Management of hepatic failure, diabetes, cardiac failure, and arthritis in hemochromatosis differs little from conventional management of these conditions. Loss of libido and changes in secondary sex characteristics may be partially or entirely reversed by intramuscular testosterone (testosterone proprionate, 250 mg every 3 weeks) or gonadotropin therapy.

It is important to identify and treat individuals with hemochromatosis by aggressive, effective phlebotomy therapy as soon as possible after the diagnosis of iron overload is made. Undertaking phlebotomy without prior liver biopsy is inadvisable since an accurate prognosis cannot be given and underlying cirrhosis will remain a possibility.

The question frequently is raised about heterozygosity versus homozygosity in an individual who has only a moderately elevated serum ferritin concentration and hepatocellular iron levels. This can usually be resolved by family and HLA studies (where possible) and by liver biopsy with determination of the hepatic iron concentration and hepatic iron index. When genuine doubt exists, careful follow-up with sequential estimation of serum ferritin and transferrin saturation will

TABLE 2. Management Guidelines

Rapid-sequence phlebotomy to deplete iron stores
Lifelong maintenance phlebotomy program to maintain normal hematocrit and low to normal serum ferritin concentration
Ultrasound and alpha-fetoprotein in phlebotomized individuals to screen for malignant hepatoma in individuals found to have cirrhosis on initial biopsy
Family screening, especially of siblings, to detect and treat early disease

usually resolve the question since homozygous subjects usually develop progressive iron accumulation if iron intake is adequate.

Because hemochromatosis is a common disorder in Caucasians, homozygous-heterozygous marriages are not uncommon. For this reason, parents and children of an individual who has hemochromatosis should also be evaluated for elevated transferrin saturation and serum ferritin concentration. Relatives who have elevated transferrin saturation and serum ferritin concentration are likely to have hemochromatosis and should undergo liver biopsy and phlebotomy therapy when appropriate.

HEMOSIDEROSIS

Increased organ iron stores (hemosiderosis) can be caused by transfusion of red blood cells, intramuscular or intravenous injection of iron, and possibly by medicinal iron abuse for many years, particularly in individuals who have anemia associated with ineffective erythropoiesis (e.g., thalassemia major). Heavy iron overload in individuals who do not possess two HLA-linked hemochromatosis genes can lead to organ injury similar to that seen in hemochromatosis homozygotes.

Treatment

Most individuals with severe anemia and iron overload cannot tolerate phlebotomy therapy. They can, however, be treated with an injectible iron chelator, deferoxamine (Desferal). As deferoxamine circulates in the body, it binds iron. The resultant deferoxamine-iron complex is water soluble and is excreted mainly in urine and also in bile.

Deferoxamine-induced excretion of iron is greatest when deferoxamine is administered as a continuous intravenous infusion. This method is cumbersome, and most individuals with hemosiderosis can be treated with nightly subcutaneous infusions of deferoxamine while sleeping. This is done with a portable pump that is connected to a syringe and tubing whose fine-gauge needle is inserted into the subcutaneous layer of the abdominal wall or the thigh. The needle and the pump are removable so the individual can remain active during the day. Iron depletion therapy by this method is expensive, but there is no alternative to deferoxamine therapy for many patients.

The effectiveness of deferoxamine therapy can be assessed by measuring serum ferritin concentration before therapy and at 2- to 6-month intervals during therapy. A rising serum ferritin concentration during therapy indicates that iron stores are increasing faster than the deferoxamine can remove iron.

The usual dosage of deferoxamine is 1 to 2 grams administered subcutaneously over 8 to 10 hours at night. Some individuals may require a higher dosage (3 to 4 grams each night) that exceeds the manufacturer's recommendation.

Deferoxamine has been associated with rash, itching, and pain or swelling with redness at the infusion site. Cataract formation has been linked to deferoxamine therapy and may be seen on slit-lamp examination. However, the risk of cataract formation is smaller than the risk of vital organ injury from massive iron overload.

The use of deferoxamine to chelate aluminum or iron in patients on chronic hemodialysis has been associated with opportunistic infections, especially *Yersinia* infections and mucormycosis. It seems likely that both deferoxamine (acting as a siderophore to enhance growth of the microorganisms) and an underlying host immunologic defect are involved in the pathogenesis of these infections. This problem occurs only in patients undergoing chronic hemodialysis.

HODGKIN'S DISEASE: CHEMOTHERAPY

method of
DAVID J. STRAUS, M.D.
Memorial Sloan-Kettering Cancer Center
New York, New York

The treatment of Hodgkin's disease is one of the success stories in medical oncology. Extended-field radiation therapy (EF RT), introduced over 30 years ago by Kaplan, was a major advance in the treatment of patients with early-stage disease. DeVita and colleagues began the use of combination chemotherapy with the MOPP trial (nitrogen mustard [Mustargen], vincristine [Oncovin], procarbazine [Matulane], and prednisone) for patients with advanced Hodgkin's disease in the mid-1960s, which was the second major advance in treatment. More recently, combination chemotherapy, either with RT (combined modality treatment) or alone, is being used in the treatment of early-stage Hodgkin's disease.

HISTOPATHOLOGY AND STAGING

Currently, the Rye modification of the Lukes and Butler histopathologic classification is in use throughout the world. The hallmark of Hodgkin's disease is the *Reed-Sternberg cell,* a large binucleate cell with single distinct nucleoli, in the proper histopathologic setting. *Lymphocyte predominance* is characterized by an abundance of small lymphocytes with occasional, often atypical Reed-Sternberg cells of the lymphocytic-histiocytic

variety. It is associated with a favorable prognosis, although late relapses may occur. *Nodular sclerosis* is the most common histologic subtype in North America and Western Europe. There is often abundant fibrosis in the node dividing tumor nodules containing inflammatory cells and the lacunar cell variant of Reed-Sternberg cells. *Mixed cellularity,* characterized by a pleomorphic cellular infiltrate of plasma cells, eosinophils, lymphocytes, histiocytes, and Reed-Sternberg cells, is the second most common histologic subtype in North America and Western Europe and is more frequent in poorer parts of the world and in older patients. In *lymphocyte depletion,* there is a paucity of cellular elements and an increased reticular network. It is the rarest histologic subtype and may be confused with non-Hodgkin's lymphomas, particularly T-cell types. It is associated with advanced age, systemic symptoms, and retroperitoneal nodal and extranodal involvement and has the worst prognosis.

The current staging classification was established by the Ann Arbor workshop in 1971 (Table 1). "Clinical staging" refers to all staging procedures short of staging laparotomy; "pathologic staging" refers to the findings at staging laparotomy during which splenectomy, liver biopsies, and biopsies of retroperitoneal nodes are performed. Staging procedures include chest x-ray, bipedal lower extremity lymphangiography, liver/spleen scanning, complete blood count with platelet and differential counts, bone marrow aspiration and biopsy, serum liver biochemistries including alkaline phosphatase and 5'-nucleotidase, and erythrocyte sedimentation rate. Computed tomography (CT) of the abdomen shows enlarged retroperitoneal and pelvic lymph nodes. Some involved nodes may not be enlarged, but may appear abnormal on lymphangiography. Mesenteric node involvement at presentation is much less common in Hodgkin's disease than in the non-Hodg-

TABLE 1. **Ann Arbor Staging Classification for Hodgkin's Disease**

Stage	Characteristics*
I	Involvement of a single lymph node region (I) or of a single extralymphatic organ or site (I_E).
II	Involvement of two or more lymph node regions on the same side of the diaphragm (II) or localized involvement of an extralymphatic organ or site and of one or more lymph node regions on the same side of the diaphragm (II_E).
III	Involvement of lymph node regions on both sides of the diaphragm (III), which may be accompanied by localized involvement of an extralymphatic organ or site (III_E), or by involvement of the spleen (III_S), or both (III_{SE}).
IV	Diffuse or disseminated involvement of one or more extralymphatic organs or tissues, with or without associated lymph node enlargement. Involvement of the liver or bone marrow is always considered Stage IV.

*Unexplained increase in temperature (>38° C [100.5° F]), night sweats, and/or weight loss (>10% of body weight) in the 6 months preceding diagnosis are defined as systemic symptoms and denoted by the suffix letter B. Asymptomatic patients are denoted by the suffix letter A.

kin's lymphomas. The accuracy of lymphangiography in determining the presence or absence of Hodgkin's disease in retroperitoneal and pelvic nodes approaches 90% in experienced hands.

If there are abnormalities on the liver/spleen scan, deviations from normal in serum liver biochemical studies, lymphangiographic or CT evidence of retroperitoneal or pelvic nodal disease, or systemic B symptoms (see Table 1, note), a liver biopsy should be performed. Slight elevations of serum alkaline phosphatase may be seen without liver involvement. Laparoscopy with direct visualization of the surface of the liver and biopsy of suspicious areas increases the diagnostic yield over that of blind percutaneous needle biopsy. Gallium scanning may be useful for following mediastinal disease, but it is associated with a significant number of false-negative and false-positive results. CT of the chest may show disease, particularly retrosternal disease, missed by a plane chest x-ray. Patients with involved lymph nodes in the lung hilum may have small lung nodules seen on chest CT but not on plane chest x-ray.

TREATMENT

Chemotherapy

MOPP. The doses and schedule for MOPP are shown in Table 2. MOPP is usually administered for a minimum of six cycles, or two cycles beyond the achievement of a complete remission (CR). In the experience of the National Cancer Institute, among patients with mainly stage III and IV disease, 84% achieved a CR and 66% of these have remained free of disease for more than 10 years.

ABVD. Table 2 shows the doses and schedule for doxorubicin (Adriamycin), bleomycin (Blenoxane), vinblastine (Velban), and dacarbazine. In patients with Stage IIA, IIB, or IIIB disease, the group at the National Tumor Institute in Milan achieved CR in 92.4% of patients, with 87.7% remaining in remission 7 years, after six cycles of

ABVD and RT, a result that was somewhat better than that with MOPP and RT in a randomized trial. The results of a randomized trial by the Cancer and Acute Leukemia Group B suggested that ABVD alone may be superior to MOPP alone in patients with poor-risk Stage IIIA, IIIB, or IV disease.

MOPP/ABVD. The groups at Memorial Sloan-Kettering Cancer Center (MSKCC) and the National Tumor Institute in Milan introduced alternating monthly MOPP and ABVD, two potentially non–cross-resistant chemotherapy combinations. The group at MSKCC achieved a CR in approximately 80% of patients with Stage IIB, IIIB, and IV disease, 80% of whom remained in remission 10 years after eight or nine cycles of MOPP alternating monthly with ABVD along with involved-region RT (2000 to 3000 cGy). Similar results were achieved in some patients with six to eight cycles of MOPP/ABVD hybrid along with involved-field RT by the group at the Cancer Control Agency of British Columbia in Vancouver. In this regimen, nitrogen mustard (6 mg per M^2 intravenously) and vincristine (1.4 mg per M^2, maximum 2 mg intravenously) are administered on day 1. On day 8, doxorubicin (35 mg per M^2 intravenously), bleomycin (10 units per M^2 intravenously), and vinblastine (6 mg per M^2 intravenously) are given. Procarbazine, 100 mg per M^2 orally, is administered on days 1 through 7 and prednisone, 40 mg per M^2 orally, on days 1 through 14. As with the other combination regimens, the cycle is repeated every 28 days. Several randomized and nonrandomized studies have shown better results with alternating monthly MOPP/ABVD or hybrid regimens than with MOPP. As mentioned, one study suggests that this may be due to an effect of ABVD.

Combined Modality Treatment

As discussed, ABVD, MOPP/ABVD, and MOPP/ABV hybrid have often been given along with RT. In analyzing the results of alternating monthly chemotherapy regimens at MSKCC, it was found that all initially involved lymph nodes that were not irradiated were at risk as sites of relapse regardless of whether or not they were initially bulky. Thus, RT to all initially involved lymph nodes is now being administered in combination with MOPP/ABVD in patients with advanced Hodgkin's disease at MSKCC.

Chemotherapy and Combined Modality in Early-Stage Disease

Results at least as good as those achieved with EF RT have been achieved with MOPP either alone or in combination with RT. Pathologic staging is not necessary for patients treated with chemotherapy or combined modality treatment since

TABLE 2. **Chemotherapy Regimens for Hodgkin's Disease**

Agent	Dose (mg/M²)	Days and Route
MOPP		
Nitrogen mustard	6	1 and 8 IV
Vincristine (Oncovin)	1.4	1 and 8 IV
Procarbazine	100	1–14 PO
Prednisone	40	1–14 PO
Repeat every 28 days		
ABVD		
Doxorubicin (Adriamycin)	25	1 and 15 IV
Bleomycin	10*	1 and 15 IV
Vinblastine	6	1 and 15 IV
Dacarbazine (DTIC)	375	1 and 15 IV
Repeat every 28 days		

*Dose in μ/M².
Abbreviations: IV = intravenously; PO = orally.

adequate chemotherapy seems to eradicate sub-diaphragmatic splenic or other disease detectable only by staging laparotomy.

Several trials have been reported using potentially less toxic regimens than MOPP. The group at Stanford reported excellent results in pathologically staged patients with favorable Stage I, II, and IIIA disease using six cycles of VBM (vinblastine, 6 mg per M² intravenously, bleomycin, 10 units per M² intravenously, and methotrexate, 30 mg per M² intravenously) administered on days 1 and 8 of each 28-day cycle along with involved-field RT. The group at MSKCC has successfully employed eight courses (four cycles) of TBV (thiotepa, 35 mg per M² intravenously, vinblastine 6 mg per M² intravenously to a maximum of 10 mg, and bleomycin, 2 units subcutaneously daily on days 4 to 10) along with involved-region RT in clinically staged IA and IIA disease. The same group is currently investigating six cycles of ABVD with or without RT in patients with clinically staged IA, IB, IIA, IIB, and IIIA Hodgkin's disease without bulky disease.

Combined modality treatment is recommended over RT alone for patients with bulky Stage I or II disease (mediastinal mass greater than one-third the thoracic diameter or peripheral nodes greater than 10 cm). Combined modality treatment or chemotherapy is also recommended for patients with Stage I and II disease with other unfavorable prognostic features such as an elevated erythrocyte sedimentation rate (>50 mm per hour for Stage IA or IIA or greater than 30 mm per hour for Stage IB or IIB patients).

Toxicity

There is a 14-fold increased risk of secondary myelodysplasia or acute leukemia with six or more cycles of MOPP-type chemotherapy containing an alkylating agent of a class similar to nitrogen mustard and procarbazine and a fivefold increased risk with less than six cycles. An increase in sterility is seen in women over the age of 30 years with MOPP-type chemotherapy; women under 25 years rarely become infertile with this regimen, although they may undergo early menopause. Because most males become azoospermic after six cycles of MOPP, sperm banking prior to chemotherapy is recommended for men in their reproductive years. ABVD and VBM may have less potential for leukemogenesis and production of sterility than MOPP-type chemotherapy.

Current Treatment Recommendations

1. *Clinical Stages I and II without bulky disease*: six cycles of ABVD with involved-region RT (e.g., mantle for supradiaphragmatic disease) is a treatment option.

2. *Clinical Stages I or II with bulky disease*: Chemotherapy (six cycles of ABVD) with involved-region RT is recommended.

3. *Clinical or pathologic Stage IIIA*: Chemotherapy (six cycles ABVD) with involved-region RT is recommended.

4. *Stage IIIB*: Chemotherapy and involved-region RT (six cycles ABVD, eight cycles MOPP/ABVD or MOPP/ABV hybrid) is recommended.

5. *Stage IV*: Chemotherapy with involved-region RT to all involved lymph node sites is recommended. MOPP/ABVD or MOPP/ABV hybrid is standard. ABVD alone may also be acceptable.

HODGKIN'S DISEASE: RADIATION THERAPY

method of
JOACHIM YAHALOM, M.D.
Memorial Sloan-Kettering Cancer Center
New York, New York

Over the last three decades, advances in radiation therapy (RT) and the advent of combination chemotherapy have resulted in the cure of more than 75% of all newly diagnosed patients with Hodgkin's disease (HD). HD is sensitive to radiation and to many chemotherapeutic drugs, and for the majority of patients there is more than one effective treatment. The longest experience with the cure of HD has been with RT, and radiation alone has remained the treatment of choice for most patients with early-stage HD. As the most potent single agent for treatment, RT also plays an important role in the management of advanced-stage HD and in salvage programs as an adjunct to combination chemotherapy.

It has become clear that effective treatment of HD is complex and requires the skills of a multidisciplinary team during staging of the disease and subsequent treatment. Additionally, the use of a modern, high-quality radiotherapy facility staffed with an experienced team has been shown to significantly affect the treatment results.

STAGING

Precise definition of the extent of nodal and extranodal involvement during the staging of HD is critical for the selection of the proper treatment strategy. Detailed documentation of the extent of disease will also assist in delineating the radiation fields, evaluating the response to therapy, and monitoring for potential relapse. The staging classification that is currently used for HD was adopted at the Ann Arbor Conference held in 1971 (Table 1). The following definitions are suggested to clarify and update the Ann Arbor classification:

TABLE 1. **Ann Arbor Staging System
for Hodgkin's Disease**

Stage

Stage I: Involvement of a single lymph node region (I) or of a single extralymphatic organ or site (I_E)

Stage II: Involvement of two or more lymph node regions on the same side of the diaphragm (II), or localized involvement of an extralymphatic organ or site and one or more lymph node regions on the same side of the diaphragm (II_E)

Stage III: Involvement of lymph node regions on both sides of the diaphragm (III), which may also be accompanied by localized involvement of an extralymphatic organ or site (III_E) or by involvement of the spleen (III_s) or both

Stage IV: Diffuse or disseminated involvement of one or more extralymphatic organs and tissues with or without nodal involvement

Systemic Symptoms

A Asymptomatic

B Presence of (1) unexplained loss of 10% of body weight in the 6 months preceding diagnosis, (2) unexplained fever with temperature greater than 38.5° C, or (3) drenching night sweats

1. *Type of staging*: Clinical staging (CS) refers to information that has been obtained without a staging laparotomy, whereas patients who undergo a staging laparotomy are considered to be pathologically staged (PS).

2. *E lesion or Stage IV*: The designation E is used when a well-localized extranodal lymphoid malignancy arises in or extends to tissues beyond, but adjacent to, major lymphatic aggregates. This lesion can be encompassed in a curative RT field. Stage IV refers to disease that is diffusely spread throughout an extranodal site such as the liver.

3. *Bulky mediastinal disease*: Bulky mediastinal disease is defined as a mediastinal mass width greater than one-third of the maximal chest diameter as measured on a posteroanterior chest radiograph. Patients with a bulky mediastinal involvement have a higher risk of relapse after radiotherapy or chemotherapy alone compared to treatment with both modalities.

4. *Stage III*: This stage can be subdivided into Stage III_1 and Stage III_2. Patients with Stage III_1 disease have subdiaphragmatic involvement limited to the spleen, splenic hilar lymph nodes, celiac nodes, and porta hepatis nodes. Stage III_2 refers to involvement of the para-aortic, pelvic, or mesenteric nodes. Favorable Stage IIIA patients are those who had a staging laparotomy that confirmed PS III_1 disease with an uninvolved or only minimally involved spleen (<five nodules).

The presence of typical systemic symptoms (B symptoms) also affects the prognosis of HD. When obtaining the history, attention should be paid to the presence or absence of unexplained fever, drenching night sweats, or significant weight loss—the B symptoms. In our experience, the presence of generalized pruritus is also a serious adverse prognostic symptom.

In addition to a careful physical examination, the following laboratory studies are important. Blood studies include a complete blood count, erythrocyte sedimentation rate (ESR) and liver function tests. Abnormalities should lead to careful evaluation for the presence of disease in bone marrow, liver, or bone. The ESR has some prognostic importance and is useful as an indicator of potential relapse. In all patients, a bone marrow biopsy is obtained for pathologic examination.

Evaluation of the Neck

In addition to a thorough physical examination of the head and neck, computed tomography (CT) with intravenous contrast or magnetic resonance imaging will contribute to detailed mapping of abnormal lymph nodes in the neck. This information may influence the design of the radiation fields in patients with suspicious involvement of the upper neck.

Evaluation of the Chest

The standard chest x-ray provides basic information regarding the extent of disease in the chest. We also perform routine thoracic CT scans of the chest in all patients. The incremental data on thoracic involvement obtained with CT of the chest are important for the design of the radiation field and for assessment of response. Since the thoracic CT scan can remain abnormal for a long period after completion of therapy, evaluation of pretreatment involvement and response to therapy is assisted by a gallium scan, a sensitive indicator of disease above the diaphragm, particularly when a dose of 10 mc and single photon emission computed tomography (SPECT) are employed. A negative gallium scan in follow-up supports the supposition that there is no active disease after completion of treatment even in the presence of residual abnormality on the CT scan.

Evaluation of the Abdomen and Pelvis

CT scan and bipedal lymphography are essential complementary imaging studies for the evaluation of the abdomen and pelvis. Lymphography accurately evaluates the opacified retroperitoneal and pelvic lymph nodes and is helpful in the design of radiation fields and in assessing the response to therapy. The celiac, splenic hilar, porta hepatis, and mesenteric nodes are not opacified during lymphography and are best evaluated with a CT scan. Unfortunately, even modern imaging studies fail to detect abdominal disease (mostly splenic involvement) in approximately 20 to 30% of patients with CS Stage I-II HD. Hence, surgical staging by laparotomy is appropriate if the findings will influence the subsequent treatment plan; that is, if radiotherapy alone is contemplated. Selected patients (CS IA female patients and CS IA males with lymphocyte-predominant histology and CS IA patients with mediastinal involvement only) have a very low likelihood of subdiaphragmatic disease and are acceptable candidates for treatment with RT alone based solely on their clinical stage. Laparotomy should be omitted in patients who have Stage I or II disease and who will receive chemotherapy as part of the treatment program (i.e., children or patients with bulky mediastinal disease).

During the staging process and prior to possible laparotomy, the patient should receive a pneumococcal vaccine (Pneumovax), and the option of sperm banking should be presented to male patients.

RADIATION THERAPY

Proper irradiation technique requires the use of linear accelerators that produce 6 to 10 MV photons and have a source-to-skin distance of 120 to 150 cm to permit the delivery of a relatively homogenous dose to large fields. Careful treatment planning is based on the imaging information obtained during the staging process. Simulation is performed on a simulator that duplicates the features of the treatment unit and should be done with the patient in the treatment position with appropriate immobilization devices. Port film verification is obtained on a weekly basis and the patient clinical set-up is checked regularly.

Radiation Fields

Successful therapy with radiation alone requires treatment of all clinically involved lymph nodes and all nodal and extranodal regions at risk for subclinical involvement. The HD radiation fields were designed to conform to the philosophy of treatment beyond the immediately involved area, while accounting for normal tissue tolerance and the technical constraints of field size. To avoid excessive toxicity, the radiation fields are treated sequentially, the total dose is fractionated, and the irradiated volumes are carefully tailored with individualized cerrobend blocks. When patients require separate treatment of adjacent regions, the calculation of field separation is exceedingly important to avoid overlap at the spinal cord.

The Mantle Field

The radiation field that covers most lymph node areas above the diaphragm is called the "mantle." Extending from the base of the mandible to the diaphragm, the mantle field covers the submandibular, cervical, supraclavicular, infraclavicular, axillary, mediastinal, and hilar nodal areas. Individually contoured cerrobend blocks shield the lungs and the cardiac apex. In addition, depending on anatomy and disease location, supplementary blocks are placed over the humeral heads, occiput, and mouth posteriorly and anteriorly. We also insert half-value layer blocks to shield the larynx anteriorly and the cervical cord posteriorly throughout the treatment course. If high cervical lymph nodes (above the thyroid notch) are involved, the preauricular nodes are treated prophylactically to a dose of 3000 to 3600 cGy.

The Subdiaphragmatic Fields

The classic subdiaphragmatic radiation field for HD is the inverted Y, which includes the major lymph node regions from the diaphragm to the femoral area. Sequential treatment to the mantle and inverted Y fields is termed "total lymphoid irradiation" (TLI). When TLI is indicated, we often divide the inverted Y field into two fields that are administered sequentially with a 2-week break in between to allow bone marrow recovery. The upper field, called the "para-aortic field," includes all the para-aortic lymph nodes between the aortic bifurcation and the bottom of the mantle field. The para-aortic field is normally positioned to encompass the lateral transverse processes of the lumbar vertebrae unless imaging or surgical data indicate more extensive disease. This field also includes the spleen and the splenic hilar nodes. If the spleen has been removed, only the splenic pedicle is included. Attention should be paid to the location of the kidneys, as they may be partially included in the field and proper shielding can decrease the irradiated renal volume. The inferior border of the para-aortic field is placed at the bottom of the L4 vertebral body.

The pelvic field encompasses the iliac, inguinal, and femoral nodes. The superior border is at the level of L5, matched with an appropriate gap to the bottom of the para-aortic field. A customized cerrobend block shields the midline structures that are not at risk. The large central block covers the bladder, rectum, and centrally transposed ovaries in women and the testes in male patients. We use a double-thickness midline block and a scrotal shield to decrease the dose to the testes or centrally placed ovaries to 3 to 8% of the fractionated total dose. Iliac wing blocks are placed to spare bone marrow.

Often, it is not necessary to treat the pelvic lymph nodes, and only the mantle and the para-aortic fields are irradiated in sequence. The treatment is then termed "subtotal lymphoid irradiation" (STLI).

Dose Considerations

When radiation alone is used for the treatment of HD, the standard total dose to each field is 3600 cGy delivered in daily fractions of 180 cGy over a period of 4 weeks. In patients who receive radiation as their only treatment, treatment is intensified in clinically involved areas by the addition of an individually tailored boost of 540 cGy to 900 cGy in three to five fractions to bring the total dose to these areas to 4140 to 4500 cGy. Patients who receive radiation to this field as consolidation after chemotherapy receive a total dose of 3000 to 3600 cGy in fractions of 150 to 180 cGy.

We use opposed anterior and posterior fields that are evenly weighted, and both fields are treated daily. Special clinical situations may require treatment of the entire cardiac silhouette to a dose of 1500 cGy. When irradiation of the whole lung is considered, treatment with partial (37%) transmission blocks allows concomitant low-dose irradiation of the lungs during full-dose mantle field irradiation. When whole liver irradiation is considered, the use of a partial (50%) transmission liver block during the para-aortic field will keep the dose below the radiation tolerance of the liver.

Treatment Recommendation by Stage

Pathologic Stages I and II

For most patients with pathologic Stage (PS) IA and IIA disease, radiation therapy is the treatment of choice. Over 20 years of experience with this method of treatment has shown it to be effective and safe. Following a staging laparotomy, treatment includes mantle field irradiation to a dose of 3600 cGy, followed by a boost of 540 to 900 cGy to clinically involved areas. This is followed by prophylactic para-aortic field irradiation to 3600 cGy. With subtotal lymphoid irradiation, approximately 75 to 80% of PS I and II patients will enter complete remission (CR) and never have a relapse. The remaining 25% generally enter CR but later relapse. Most of these relapsing patients, however, are subsequently cured with combination chemotherapy, so that the overall cure rate (10-year actuarial survival) for PS I and II patients is about 90%.

About 20% of patients with Stage I and II disease present with B symptoms (see Table 1). After pathologic staging, patients with PS IB and IIB disease who do not have bulky mediastinal involvement can be managed effectively with subtotal lymphoid irradiation alone. A staging laparotomy is essential, however, because Stage IIIB disease should never be treated with irradiation alone; rather it should be managed primarily with systemic chemotherapy followed by irradiation of the involved sites.

If chemotherapy is planned from the onset, then staging laparotomy is not necessary. The cure rates for PS I–IIB patients treated with radiation alone or CS I–IIB patients treated with combined modality therapy are high, with a 10-year actuarial survival of approximately 90%.

Clinical Stages I and II

Selected patients with very favorable presentations can be managed with radiation alone without a staging laparotomy (see under Stag-

ing). In these patients, the spleen should be irradiated as part of the para-aortic field.

An alternative treatment for patients whose early stage was not confirmed by a staging laparotomy is chemotherapy followed by mantle irradiation. We have induced a response with six courses of ABVD (doxorubicin [Adriamycin], bleomycin [Blenoxane], vinblastine, [Velban], and dacarbazine [DTIC]) followed by mantle irradiation to a dose of 3600 cGy. However, the long-term experience with such a combined modality approach for early clinically staged patients is still limited. Careful monitoring of pulmonary and cardiac function during and after treatment is essential.

Stage I and II with Bulky Mediastinal Disease

Patients with bulky mediastinal Hodgkin's disease often have a poor outcome when treated with single modality therapy, so in most instances they receive combined modality therapy. Chemotherapy is administered first in order to decrease the mediastinal mass and permit the use of more limited radiotherapy fields. We use six cycles of ABVD chemotherapy followed by mantle field irradiation to a total dose of 3600 cGy as our standard treatment in this situation. In the mediastinum, we irradiate the prechemotherapy tumor volumes to a dose of 1800 cGy and then cone down with additional 1800 cGy to the postchemotherapy mediastinal volumes. Although most patients with bulky mediastinal Hodgkin's disease are managed most effectively with combined modality therapy, the use of irradiation alone is reasonable in patients who have bulky disease by measurement but in whom the disease is restricted to the superior mediastinum, without involvement of adjacent organs. In these patients, careful delineation of the treatment volume with the use of treatment planning CT scan and evaluation of the treatment volume after 1800 cGy with the application of a shrinking field technique minimize the volume of lung irradiated. In carefully selected patients with bulky mediastinal disease, well-planned and executed irradiation is as effective as combined modality therapy.

Stage IIIA

For most patients with Stage IIIA HD, the recommended treatment is chemotherapy followed by irradiation of the initially involved sites. Only patients with favorable PS IIIA disease are acceptable candidates for radiotherapy alone. Therefore, patients in whom abdominal or pelvic involvement has been clearly detected by a CT scan or a lymphogram do not require further surgical staging. We achieved encouraging results by combining ABVD with subsequent mantle and para-aortic/splenic field irradiation to a dose of 3000 to 3600 cGy in patients with CS IIIA disease. We add a pelvic field only when this area is clinically involved. The 5-year relapse-free survival rate with this program is approximately 90%.

Stages IIIB, IVA, and IVB

In Stages IIIB and IV, the primary treatment modality is clearly combination chemotherapy. However, subsequent to effective chemotherapy, adjunctive radiotherapy has an important role in decreasing the relapse rate in advanced-stage patients who have attained a complete response with chemotherapy. In our experience, most of the relapses in patients with advanced-stage disease occur in unirradiated nodal sites that were originally documented to be involved with HD.

This predictable pattern of relapse is not limited to bulky sites alone, but to all sites of clinically detectable disease. Studies at Memorial Sloan-Kettering Cancer Center (MSKCC) and other institutions have demonstrated a significant improvement in disease-free survival and in overall survival for patients who received adjuvant radiation therapy to all sites of initial involvement compared to patients who received chemotherapy alone or received postchemotherapy irradiation to only selected sites. We advocate detailed delineation of all sites of disease prior to the initiation of chemotherapy in patients with Stage III and IV disease to assist in defining the irradiated volumes. Following induction of response with six to eight courses of effective chemotherapy such as ABVD or MOPP*/ABVD the patients are rigorously restaged to confirm CR. Those in CR receive radiation to all originally involved sites. In general, the treatment fields design follows the same outline described for primary irradiation fields. The fields are treated sequentially to a total dose of 3000 to 3600 cGy.

Salvage Therapy in Refractory or Relapsed Disease

The majority of HD patients who relapse after radiation alone are treated successfully with combination chemotherapy. On the other hand, patients with advanced stage disease who remain refractory to chemotherapy or relapse within the first year after completion of chemotherapy have a poor prognosis with standard-dose chemotherapy salvage regimens. At MSKCC we developed

*Mechlorethamine, vincristine, procarbazine, and prednisone.

a salvage program for previously unirradiated patients who failed to respond to multiple chemotherapy regimens. This treatment program incorporates accelerated hyperfractionated total lymphoid irradiation (TLI) with high-dose chemotherapy followed by autologous bone marrow transplantation. This program yielded promising results, with 50% of the patients remaining free of disease at a median follow-up of 3 years.

Special Considerations in the Treatment of Children

The cure rate of children with Stages I and II HD is excellent. However, prepubertal children who have not completed their growth may develop intraclavicular narrowing and a decreased crown-to-rump height following mantle and para-aortic irradiation. In prepubertal children, treatment with chemotherapy and low-dose involved or extended-field irradiation is the preferred approach. The cure rate is approximately 90%, and with low-dose irradiation the effect on growing bones and muscles is minimal.

Side Effects and Complications

Acute Side Effects

Expected transient side effects during mantle irradiation can include localized hair loss in irradiated areas, mild pharyngitis, mouth dryness, change in taste, dry cough, mild dysphagia, nausea and loss of appetite, mild skin reaction, and fatigue, and loss of energy. Generally, these side effects can be managed symptomatically and subside gradually after the completion of radiation therapy.

The main side effects of subdiaphragmatic irradiation are loss of appetite, nausea and vomiting, mild diarrhea, and urinary frequency. These reactions are usually mild, can be minimized with standard antiemetic medications, and disappear shortly after the completion of treatment.

Subacute Side Effects

Fatigue and loss of energy are common symptoms during and after irradiation. Although most patients are able to continue their routine activities during treatment, it often takes 6 months after completion of treatment for the patient to regain full baseline energy level.

Patients with HD have a propensity to develop herpes zoster infection within 2 years after treatment. Usually the infection is confined to a single dermatome and is self limited. If the cutaneous eruption is identified promptly, systemic acyclovir (Zovirax) will limit the duration and intensity of the infection.

Lhermitte's sign develops in approximately 15% of patients receiving mantle irradiation. The syndrome is characterized by an electric shock sensation radiating down the backs of both legs when the head is flexed. It generally occurs 6 weeks to 3 months after completion of mantle therapy and resolves spontaneously after a few months. It may be secondary to transient demyelinization of the spinal cord and is not associated with late or permanent damage to the cord.

Radiation pneumonitis occurs in fewer than 5% of patients, more often in those who had extensive mediastinal disease. Symptomatic management may be adequate, but some patients require corticosteroids. Acute pericarditis occurs in 2 to 5% of patients; it has become rare with modern radiation techniques. It can be managed with nonsteroidal anti-inflammatory agents, and symptoms usually subside within a few weeks.

Late Complications

Late complications include hypothyroidism, sterility, pulmonary fibrosis, cardiac damage, transverse myelitis, growth abnormalities in children, and secondary malignancies.

Subclinical hypothyroidism develops in about one-third of patients after mantle irradiation. This is detected by elevation of the sensitive thyroid-stimulating hormone (TSH). Thyroid replacement with L-thyroxine is recommended, even for asymptomatic patients, to prevent overt hypothyroidism and decrease the risk of benign thyroid nodules.

Irradiation of the pelvis may have deleterious effects on fertility and gonadal function. Irradiation of the mantle and para-aortic fields alone does not increase the risk of sterility. However, chemotherapy, particularly the MOPP regimen, has detrimental effects on the fertility of almost all men and most women.

With modern irradiation techniques, constrictive pericarditis and symptomatic pulmonary fibrosis are very rare complications of mantle irradiation. Mediastinal irradiation is associated with an increased risk of coronary heart disease. Recent long-term observations of morbidity patterns of survivors of HD indicate that mediastinal irradiation carries an increased risk of coronary heart disease. To minimize this complication, patients should be monitored and advised about the control of other established risk factors for coronary heart disease such as smoking, hyperlipidemia, hypertension, and poor dietary and exercise habits. Development of a second cancer is a well-recognized hazard for patients cured of HD. Secondary acute nonlymphocytic leukemia (ANLL) is clearly evoked by certain chemotherapy regimens (e.g., MOPP or MOPP-like combinations) with or without radiotherapy. Secondary solid tumors were observed after RT alone, chemotherapy alone, and combined modality therapy. The most frequent solid tumors reported after HD are lung cancer, breast cancer, stomach cancer, and melanoma. Patients cured of HD are also at high risk of late (10 to 15 years) development of non-Hodgkin's lymphoma. Cigarette smoking should be strongly discouraged because the increase in lung cancer after mantle irradiation has been detected mostly in smokers. The increase in breast cancer is inversely related to the age at HD treatment: in women irradiated after the age of 30 years, no increase in the risk of breast cancer was found. Breast cancer is curable in its early stages, and early detection has a significant impact on survival. Breast examination should be part of the routine follow-up program for women cured of HD, and routine mammography should begin about 8 years after treatment of HD.

ACUTE LEUKEMIA IN ADULTS

method of
HANS W. GRÜNWALD, M.D.
Queens Hospital Center
Jamaica, New York

The prognosis of acute leukemia in adults is not yet as good as that achieved by newer treatments in children. However, enormous strides have been made in the last few years with intensive induction and postremission combination chemotherapy and the use of bone marrow transplantation in selected patients. With currently available therapeutic measures, the projected cure rate for acute leukemia (predicted from the freedom from relapse rate in the first 2½ years) is expected to be 25 to 40% of all adults, and in selected subsets of patients with good prognostic features, the cure rate may be as high as 50 to 60%. In addition to the introduction of more intensive treatment regimens, improved results can be ascribed to better supportive care and the increasing use of newer methods to identify therapeutically pertinent disease characteristics. Nowadays, it is essential to ascertain not only cytochemical markers of the leukemic cells but also their biochemical, immunologic, and especially cytogenetic characteristics. These studies are frequently complemented by the investigation of molecular alterations at the DNA level utilizing well-defined probes.

Under investigation but still controversial is the use of growth factors (CSFs) in acute leukemia. On the one hand, they may prove beneficial in enhancing recovery from severe cytopenias induced by cytotoxic chemotherapy; on the other hand, they may stimulate regrowth of the leukemic cells that carry receptors for such growth factors. Other major advances that may yield a higher proportion of cures of acute leukemia include (1) the identification of minimal residual disease after completion of intensive postremission therapy using immunologic and molecular markers and (2) the eradication of residual disease by biological response modifiers (interleukins, interferons, growth factors, and other cytokines) singly, in combination, or even combined with cytotoxic chemotherapeutic agents. These investigational advances require that as many patients as possible participate in clinical trials. All new patients with acute leukemia should first be evaluated for entry eligibility on investigational protocols. Patients can be treated off protocol if they are not eligible or if they refuse to participate. The intensive therapy needed both during remission induction and during postremission consolidation is associated with a high rate of complications and even significant mortality. Therefore, all treatment should be done in a major medical center capable of providing the needed supportive measures for such critically ill patients.

ACUTE MYELOID LEUKEMIA

Clinical and Laboratory Findings

The clinical manifestations of acute myeloid leukemia (AML) are related mostly to bone marrow failure. The lack of erythropoietic activity, manifested by anemia of varying severity, causes fatigue, palpitations, lightheadedness, and dyspnea on exertion. The lack of megakaryocytic activity, manifested by thrombocytopenia, leads to purpura and mucosal bleeding. The lack of normal myeloid maturation, manifested by granulocytopenia, frequently leads to infections, often of life-threatening nature. Common infections at presentation include pneumonia, perirectal abscesses, sinusitis, and otitis, but fever and bacteremia without a localizing site of infection are also common.

Some patients with hyperleukocytosis (greater than 80,000 myeloblasts per μL) have central nervous system (CNS) symptoms characterized by confusion and even loss of consciousness (cerebral leukostasis) or pulmonary symptoms characterized by dyspnea and inadequate gas exchange (pulmonary leukostasis). Caution must be used in the interpretation of the results of an arterial blood gas specimen obtained in a patient with high leukocyte counts. The laboratory report may suggest extreme hypoxia, but this pseudohypoxia is due to in vitro oxygen consumption by the white blood cells (WBCs) ("leukocyte oxygen larceny"). This laboratory abnormality can be avoided by adding fluoride to the heparin in the syringe loaded with arterial blood, thus arresting glycolysis. Many such patients with high leukocyte counts have been inappropriately intubated and placed on respirators.

Some patients with myelomonocytic or monocytic AML may present with severe gingival hyperplasia, marked tendency to gum bleeding, and skin or subcutaneous infiltrates.

Patients with promyelocytic AML frequently have serious hemorrhagic manifestations and consumption coagulopathy (disseminated intravascular coagulation [DIC]) due to release of proteolytic (thrombin-like) enzymes into the circulation. These patients require close monitoring, including all evaluation of coagulation parameters. Such patients benefit from the administration of heparin in addition to fresh frozen plasma, cryoprecipitate, or both.

Prognostic Factors

Patients with a history of cytopenias due to marrow dysplasia (myelodysplastic syndrome), or of exposure to aromatic hydrocarbons such as benzene, or of treatment with alkylating chemotherapeutic agents (secondary myeloid leukemias) have a low remission induction rate (approximately half that of comparable patients with de novo AML), and when achieved, these remissions are rarely durable. Thus, in younger patients (<40 years of age) with secondary AML and an HLA-matched sibling donor, early bone marrow transplantation should be considered.

Age is the second important prognostic feature in AML. The complete remission (CR) rate and the cure rate are higher in younger patients. In spite of the poorer prognosis in the elderly, CR can be achieved even in the eighth and ninth decades of life, and treatment with curative intent should always be offered to the elderly provided they understand the risks involved. The risk-benefit ratio must be clearly presented so that an informed decision can be made concerning treatment.

Certain subsets of patients with AML using the FAB classification (based on morphology and cytochemical features of the leukemic cells; e.g., M4 with marrow eosinophilia, M3 hypergranular promyelocytic) have a better prognosis. These rare patients can often be identified by the characteristic cytogenetic abnormality, and therefore, it is better to rely on the karyotype for therapeutic decisions after CR has been achieved (postremission therapy). Chromosome analysis (karyotyping) is one of the best methods to identify subsets of AML that have a higher probability of prolonged remissions and cures. Such subsets include chromosomal inversions and translocations such as inv 16, t(15;17), t(8;21). Chromosome analysis is also the best way to identify subsets of AML with a poor prognosis such as trisomy 8, abnormalities or loss of chromosome 5 or 7, abnormalities of chromosome 11q, or multiple translocations or trisomies. These abnormalities predict not only a short remission, but also refractoriness to standard remission induction chemotherapy. More intensive regimens incorporating high-dose cytarabine may be warranted for such patients.

Finally, immunophenotypic markers can identify patients with poorer prognoses. Those whose blasts have the CD34 antigen on their surface (an antigen of early hematopoietic progenitors) have a high probability of being refractory to conventional induction chemotherapy and trials with a more intensive regimen are warranted.

ACUTE LYMPHOBLASTIC LEUKEMIA

Clinical and Laboratory Findings

Most patients with acute lymphoblastic leukemia (ALL) present with manifestations of bone marrow failure: anemia, thrombocytopenia (with characteristic purpura and mucosal bleeding), and granulocytopenia (with infections of all kinds). In addition, such patients often have bone pain and tenderness and generalized lymphadenopathy, splenomegaly, or both. Fever at presentation can be due to the high leukemic cell turnover but should always be considered to be of infectious origin until exhaustive investigations prove negative.

Prognostic Factors

Age is a very important prognostic factor in ALL. Young adults have a cure rate of about 70%, whereas in the elderly the prognosis of ALL is not much better than that for AML (i.e., 20%).

The initial white blood cell count is a major prognostic factor in ALL. Patients with leukocytosis above 50,000 per μL readily achieve a CR, but usually have an early relapse. Such patients require more intensive postremission therapy or bone marrow transplantation.

The morphology of the leukemic blasts in peripheral blood and bone marrow smears can identify the Burkitt type (FAB L3) ALL. Such blasts are characteristically large, with deep blue cytoplasm and with cytoplasmic vacuoles. This type of ALL has a much lower CR rate than the L1 and L2 varieties and warrants the use of different and more intensive therapeutic regimens. Burkitt-type leukemia can also be identified by the surface immunoglobulin of the blast cells, a characteristic of B cells, and by the characteristic chromosomal translocations [t(8;14) or t(8;22)] involving the *c-myc* oncogene on chromosome 8.

Chromosome analysis in ALL also can yield important prognostic clues. One or more translocations, especially t(4;11) and t(9;22), indicate a high probability of early relapse after a remission has been attained. This justifies more intensive postremission chemotherapy or allogeneic bone marrow transplantation if a suitable donor is available.

INITIAL EVALUATION

Initial evaluation of the patient with acute leukemia begins with a complete history and physical examination. Next the peripheral blood and bone marrow smears are examined to determine the morphology and classification of the leukemia. The bone marrow aspirate and biopsy tissue stained with Wright/Giemsa stain yield the exact cytologic type and subtype (AML or ALL and its FAB class) in 80 to 90% of patients. It is also essential to perform a full cytochemical panel on the blood and marrow smears, an assay for terminal deoxynucleotidyl transferase (TdT), immunophenotyping, and cytogenetic analysis of the bone marrow cells. This serves not only to confirm the morphologic classification but also to identify the prognostic subtypes mentioned previously.

Also part of the initial evaluation is analysis of the coagulation system, including prothrombin time (PT), activated partial thromboplastin time (APTT), plasma fibrinogen level, and serum fibrin degradation product (FDP) assay. These tests can identify the consumption coagulopathy (DIC) present in most patients with acute promyelocytic leukemia (AML FAB M3) and in some patients with myelomonocytic and monocytic leukemia (FAB M4 and M5).

Renal, hepatic, pulmonary, and especially cardiac function should also be assessed, since most antileukemic drugs are excreted by the kidneys or detoxified by the liver and are potentially toxic to these organs. Cardiac dysfunction diagnosed before treatment is begun can obviate the use of anthracyclines, which can lead to potentially fatal cardiac insufficiency in patients with poor cardiac function.

Multiple cultures should be obtained from blood, excreta and various mucosae prone to colonization by bacteria, fungi, and viruses (pharynx, nose, and rhinopharynx). Such cultures should be obtained not only in patients with suspected infection and fever but also in asymptomatic and afebrile patients, in order to predict the causative microorganism in infections occurring later in the patient's course (surveillance cultures).

Finally, histocompatibility (HLA) typing should be performed in every new patient, not only to identify potential bone marrow donors among the patient's siblings (or even from the unrelated donor data banks), but also to provide HLA-matched platelet transfusions if and when the patient becomes refractory to unmatched platelet transfusions due to alloimmunization. It is usually not possible to HLA type the patient when alloimmunization is detected, because there usually are few or no leukocytes in the peripheral blood to type as a result of cytotoxic chemotherapy.

TREATMENT

Although chemotherapeutic drugs should be started as soon as possible after the diagnosis of AML or ALL, it is rarely necessary to initiate such treatment as an emergency and there is usually sufficient time to perform all the aforementioned pretreatment evaluations. Biochemical, hemostatic, or other abnormalities should be corrected before initiation of cytotoxic chemotherapy. Hyperleukocytosis (greater than 80,000 blast cells per μL), however, constitutes a medical emergency requiring immediate leukapheresis (removal of leukocytes by blood centrifugation at the bedside) and rapid initiation of cytotoxic chemotherapy to avoid pulmonary or cerebral leukostasis, which can be fatal.

Before chemotherapy, patients with acute leukemia should be hydrated and given allopurinol (Zyloprim), 300 mg per day orally, to prevent hyperuricemia and urate nephropathy. Optimally, the allopurinol should be started 36 hours before the initiation of cytotoxic chemotherapy and continued for a total of 10 days. Thereafter, the risk of urate nephropathy is minimal, and the frequency of cutaneous hypersensitivity to the drug increases.

Venous access for the duration of treatment and the period of severe cytopenia that follows should be assured prior to initiation of treatment. Many patients have adequate peripheral veins to permit administration of all required drugs and blood products, but some eventually develop venous access problems during induction chemotherapy. Therefore, it is common to centrally implant a Silastic (Hickman or Broviac) catheter that is externally accessible. Alternatively, a port can be attached to the catheter and remain permanently under the skin (requiring a noncoring needle to access). Venous access is also possible with a peripherally inserted central line (PIC line), which does not require use of operating room facilities for insertion but can remain in place for only 3 to 6 weeks.

Infection control prior to cytotoxic chemotherapy is accomplished with appropriate antiviral, antifungal, or bactericidal antibacterial agents. The use of bacteriostatic antibiotics *must* be avoided, since they are ineffective in granulocytopenic patients and may antagonize bactericidal antibiotics.

Finally, severe anemia and thrombocytopenia are corrected by packed red blood cell (RBC) and platelet transfusions. Fresh-frozen plasma and heparin are given to correct the hemostatic abnormalities of the consumption coagulopathy. All blood cell transfusions (RBCs and platelets) should incorporate a WBC-retaining filter to minimize exposure to allogeneic HLA antigens and thus reduce the risks of eventual platelet refractoriness and presensitization for eventual bone marrow transplantion. For the same reason, family members deemed suitable for allogeneic bone marrow transplantation should *not* be used as donors for RBC or platelet transfusions.

If evidence of a consumption coagulopathy is detected (prolonged PT and PTT, increased FDP, prolonged thrombin time, decreased factors I, II, V, and VIII), prompt heparinization in addition to administration of fresh-frozen plasma or cryoprecipitate or both reduces the incidence of fatal hemorrhage. Heparin should be started with a bolus of 8000 to 10,000 units intravenously, followed by a continuous infusion of 1000 units per hour during the first 48 hours, thereafter reduced to 700 units per hour. The heparin infusion is continued until all evidence of intravascular coagulation activity disappears (normalization of FDP and factors I, II, V and VIII).

Chemotherapy

Acute Myeloid Leukemia

The majority of patients with AML of all types (FAB M1 through M7) respond to standard induction combination chemotherapy with cytarabine (Cytosar-U) and an anthracycline given in the 7 + 3 regimen: cytarabine is given as a continuous intravenous infusion of 100 to 200 mg per M^2 per day for 7 days, and daunorubicin (Cerubidine), 45 mg per M^2 per day as a slow intravenous bolus

for the first 3 days. An alternative anthracycline with a therapeutic spectrum similar to that of daunorubicin is idarubicin (Idamycin) given at a dose of 12 mg per M^2 per day as a slow intravenous bolus for 3 days. These doses are given irrespective of the initial blood count, since the goal is to achieve temporary marrow aplasia to be followed by normal marrow regeneration (achievement of a complete remission). However, if initial liver function tests demonstrate major impairment (bilirubin >3 mg per dL, alanine aminotransferase (ALT) >3× normal), the doses of both drugs should be reduced by half and the cytarabine infusion stopped after 5 days if the results of liver function tests have not improved by then. Antiemetics such as ondansetron (Zofran), metoclopramide (Reglan), or prochlorperazine (Compazine) can be used liberally.

Patients over the age of 70 years should have their anthracycline dose decreased by 33% (30 mg per M^2 per day for 3 days of daunorubicin or 8 mg per M^2 per day for 3 days of idarubicin). Patients with a history of coronary artery disease or heart failure or who have a decreased cardiac ejection fraction on MUGA scan can be given mitoxantrone (Novantrone) instead of daunorubicin (lower risk of heart failure) at a dose of 12 mg per M^2 per day, given as a 1-hour intravenous infusion for the first 3 days, together with the 7-day cytarabine infusion. A bone marrow examination is performed on the day immediately following the conclusion of the cytarabine infusion to assess the extent of cytoreduction. If the marrow cellularity on biopsy has not decreased to 20% or less and the proportion of leukemic blasts has not decreased by 80% or more, it is unlikely that a complete remission will result. Additional chemotherapy consisting of 3 days of mitoxantrone, etoposide (VePesid), or high-dose cytarabine (at dosages discussed later for refractory or recurrent AML) may then be considered, but at the cost of increased toxicity (e.g., mucositis, pancytopenia of greater duration).

An exception to these recommendations is presented by acute promyelocytic leukemia (FAB M3), in which the day 7 bone marrow may still be markedly hypercellular with a predominance of leukemic promyelocytes, yet the patient has a good chance of achieving complete remission with this single course of chemotherapy (slow leukemic depopulation of the marrow).

Daily blood counts during and after induction chemotherapy are essential to measure the cytoreduction. Platelet count monitoring guides the administration of platelet transfusions, and packed RBC transfusions are given depending on hemoglobin levels. Frequent measurement of serum electrolytes is needed to detect the occurrence (fortunately rare) of tumor lysis syndrome.

A second postinduction bone marrow aspiration and biopsy should be performed 1 week after completion of the course of chemotherapy, to help in deciding whether a second course is needed. If the proportion of leukemic blasts in the aspirate remains above 5% and the cellularity on biopsy is over 10%, a second course of the same drugs used initially should be given. However, the duration of the second chemotherapy course should be shorter, with a 5-day infusion of cytarabine and two daily doses of the anthracycline (at the same daily doses given for the first course [5 + 2 regimen]). If the bone marrow cellularity is less than 10%, but the majority of cells are blasts, it is advisable to wait 3 to 5 days and repeat the bone marrow aspiration and biopsy, since it is virtually impossible to differentiate between residual leukemia and very early marrow regeneration. A subsequent marrow biopsy can reveal further lineage differentiation (appearance of promyelocytes, myelocytes, and even metamyelocytes) indicative of early regeneration. A persistently leukemic marrow shows a further increase in blasts. If after a second course of cytarabine plus anthracycline (5 + 2 regimen), the marrow remains leukemic, one should characterize the leukemia as "refractory" to the induction chemotherapy.

Refractory or Relapsed AML. Patients refractory to induction chemotherapy or who relapse after having attained a complete remission require more intensive induction chemotherapy, usually with the high-dose cytarabine (HIDAC) regimen consisting of 1 to 3 grams of cytarabine per M^2 every 12 hours for 6 days (a total of 12 doses) given as a 75-minute infusion each. Since cytarabine at these high doses concentrates in tears and can cause keratitis, it is important to wash the eyes with saline or artificial tears at least six times per day. Patients must also be closely monitored for cerebellar toxicity involving coordination and speech, and the drug must be discontinued at the first sign of ataxia or slurred speech. Less common toxicities of high-dose cytarabine include hemorrhagic enterocolitis and noncardiac pulmonary edema.

After the 6 days of cytarabine infusions, bone marrow aspiration and biopsy are performed: if the marrow still shows more than 20% leukemic blasts, it is advisable to give 3 days of mitoxantrone, 12 mg per M^2 per day as a 1-hour infusion.

An alternative regimen for refractory or relapsed AML is mitoxantrone (Novantrone) and etoposide (VePesid): etoposide is given as a 5-day continuous infusion of 150 mg per M^2 per day, and mitoxantrone is given as above (12 mg per M^2 per day) for the first 3 days. If, after completing this 5-day regimen, the marrow shows reduction but not disappearance of the leukemic blasts,

a second 5-day course of these two drugs can be administered. Normal hepatic function is needed for detoxification of these drugs, and they should thus not be used if the patient has abnormal liver function tests (ALT $>3\times$ normal, bilirubin >3 mg per dL).

Postremission Consolidation. Once complete remission has been achieved (normal bone marrow, reticulocyte, platelet, and granulocyte counts), and the patient is deemed free of infections and aftereffects of the induction chemotherapy (attainment of a near-normal performance status), postremission therapy is planned. In recent years, very intensive postremission consolidation chemotherapy has achieved long relapse-free survival (and thus possible cure) in some patients. The intensity of treatment is similar to or greater than that used for remission induction. Such treatment, however, can produce life-threatening toxicities. Most patients can be treated on an ambulatory basis (the need for regular platelet transfusions requires an ambulatory transfusion center). Furthermore, since most patients remain markedly neutropenic for 10 to 30 days following each consolidation course, they are advised to avoid external sources of infection (e.g., crowds, animals, vases with stagnant water) and to come to the hospital for prompt initiation of antibiotic therapy at the first evidence of fever or infection. Complete blood counts to monitor hemoglobin and leukocyte and platelet counts are performed every other day (until recovery of adequate granulocyte and platelet levels), and blood biochemical monitoring is done weekly.

Drugs used for consolidation are the same as those used in induction and are given at similar or higher doses. Thus, a first consolidation course may consist of cytarabine and an anthracycline used in the 7 + 3 induction regimen. The patient should also receive at least one course of the HIDAC (high-dose cytarabine) regimen. A third consolidation course might consist of etoposide plus mitoxantrone (as described previously for refractory or relapsed AML). The total number of consolidation courses ranges from three to six, depending on the patient's tolerance to the drugs, the rate of recovery from each course of consolidation (if hematologic depression lasts longer than 3 weeks, the probability of very prolonged or even irreversible cytopenias after an ensuing course increases), and the initial prognostic category (patients at high risk for relapse should receive the highest possible number of consolidation courses).

Bone Marrow Transplantation. Patients at very high risk for early relapse (high initial WBC count or other sign of high leukemic burden, such as very high lactate dehydrogenase level, trisomy 8, abnormalities of chromosome 5 or 7) should be considered for a bone marrow transplant if they attain a complete remission. Young patients (<45 years of age) with an HLA-matched sibling should receive an allogeneic transplant from that sibling. For patients between 45 and 60 years of age, or for patients without an appropriately matched sibling, autologous marrow transplant should be considered. This procedure involves harvesting bone marrow shortly before a planned consolidation chemotherapy course. The marrow is subjected to in vitro purging (using either drugs or antibodies with complement) and frozen.

Peripheral blood stem cell harvesting can also be done when the WBC count is increasing after a course of chemotherapy. These patients are subjected to repeated blood cell pheresis, then given a preparative regimen of high-dose cyclophosphamide (Cytoxan), plus total body irradiation (or busulfan) followed by infusion of the thawed marrow (and, if available, peripheral blood) cells.

Acute Lymphoblastic Leukemia

The majority of patients with acute lymphoblastic leukemia (ALL) achieve a remission following vincristine and prednisone. Significant increases in both the rate and duration of remission can be attained by the addition of anthracyclines, L-asparaginase, and alkylating agents. The present recommended remission induction regimen for adults with ALL consists of the following drugs: cyclophosphamide (Cytoxan) 1 gram per M^2 by slow intravenous injection once; vincristine (Oncovin), 2 mg by slow intravenous injection weekly for four doses; prednisone, 100 mg per day orally for 21 days (no need to taper); daunorubicin (Cerubidine), 45 mg per M^2 per day by slow intravenous injection for 3 days; and L-asparaginase (Elspar) 6000 units per M^2 intramuscularly (subcutaneously if the platelet count is below 50,000 per μL) every 4 days for six doses. For patients over the age of 65 years, the cyclophosphamide dose is reduced to 700 mg per M^2, the daunorubicin decreased to 30 mg per M^2, and the duration of prednisone administration reduced to 10 days. Blood counts are performed daily to monitor cytoreduction and to evaluate the need for RBC and platelet transfusions. Bone marrow aspiration and biopsy are performed 4 weeks after the start of chemotherapy. If the leukemic blasts have not disappeared, an alternative induction regimen with teniposide, cytarabine, and prednisone should be initiated. If the marrow on day 28 shows disappearance of the leukemic blasts but is not yet normal, an additional week to 10 days off chemotherapy may reveal the signs of remission (normalization of marrow, reticulocyte, granulocyte, and platelet counts).

Once remission has been documented, central nervous system (CNS) prophylaxis is given with 15 mg of intrathecal methotrexate (be careful to use preservative-free drug) every week for 4 weeks combined with cranial radiation (24 Gy). During this 4-week period, the patient is also given 6-mercaptopurine (6-MP) (Purinethol), 60 mg per M^2 daily by mouth, and methotrexate, 20 mg per M^2 weekly by mouth. Blood counts are done at least twice weekly, and the dosage of 6-MP and methotrexate is reduced if cytopenia occurs. Liver function tests should also be closely monitored, and the dosage of both drugs reduced if abnormalities are seen.

After completion of CNS prophylaxis, and only if and when the blood counts and blood chemistries are normal, an intensive 2-month course of consolidation chemotherapy is initiated as follows: cyclophosphamide, 1 gram per M^2 intravenously on weeks 1 and 5; cytarabine, 75 mg per M^2 per day subcutaneously for 4 days on weeks 1, 2, 5, and 6; 6-MP, 60 mg per M^2 per day orally during weeks 1, 2, 5, and 6; vincristine, 2 mg intravenously per week on weeks 3, 4, 7, and 8; and L-asparaginase, 6000 units intramuscularly (subcutaneously if the platelet count is below 50,000 per μL) twice weekly on weeks 3, 4, 7, and 8. Patients usually require frequent platelet and occasional RBC transfusions during this period of consolidation, but treatment can be accomplished on an outpatient basis if an ambulatory transfusion and chemotherapy unit is available. If at the start of week 5 there is persistent thrombocytopenia or neutropenia (below 50,000 and 1000 per μL, respectively), the scheduled chemotherapy should be postponed for 1 week.

After completion of this intensive consolidation chemotherapy, repeat bone marrow aspiration and biopsy are performed to confirm continued remission. Then the 2-year maintenance phase is initiated, consisting of 6-MP, 60 mg per M^2 by mouth daily; methotrexate, 20 mg per M^2 by mouth weekly; vincristine, 2 mg intravenously monthly; and prednisone, 80 mg per day for 5 days every month (starting on the day of vincristine administration). Blood counts are performed weekly and blood chemistries biweekly. If significant cytopenia or liver dysfunction occurs, the maintenance chemotherapy is dose-reduced or temporarily withheld until acceptable values are achieved.

Patients with prognostic indicators for early relapse (e.g., initial WBC count of 50,000 per μL or higher, t(9;22) or t(4;11) translocations) may be considered for allogeneic bone marrow transplantation after achieving a remission if an HLA-compatible donor is available.

Patients with B-cell ALL (Burkitt-type leukemia, FAB-L3) can be treated with shorter and more intensive lymphoma-like induction chemotherapy followed by CNS prophylaxis, without a prolonged maintenance phase. The regimen includes the use of high-dose cyclophosphamide and methotrexate (with leucovorin reversal) plus vincristine, dexamethasone, cytarabine, etoposide, and doxorubicin.

Supportive Care

In addition to the proper chemotherapeutic agents, all other aspects of the patient's care must be optimal. The major reason for failure to achieve complete remission is the death of the patient due to complications of the disease or chemotherapy. Primary resistance to chemotherapy is infrequent.

A most important clinical consideration is the assurance of adequate hemostasis; thrombocytopenia associated with acute leukemia or resulting from the use of cytotoxic drugs is the most common cause of hemorrhage. Platelet transfusions have markedly reduced morbidity and mortality from bleeding and should be given whenever the platelet count is 20,000 per μL or less, although hemorrhage can occur even with higher levels. Some patients may have very low platelet counts (below 10,000 per μL) without bleeding. Patients who require an invasive intervention (e.g., Hickman catheter insertion, lumbar puncture) should have their platelet count increased to 50,000 per μL with platelet transfusions. The presence of consumption coagulopathy (DIC) as manifested by prolonged PT, PTT, elevated FDP or decreased fibrinogen in addition to thrombocytopenia mandates the administration of both platelets (to raise the platelet count above 30,000 per μL) and fresh-frozen plasma or cryoprecipitate or both to restore normal hemostatic function. In addition, heparin given to such patients (as described previously) has proven helpful in this situation. Finally, prolongation of PT and PTT well into the course of treatment can occur in some patients, probably as a consequence of vitamin K deficiency due to poor oral food intake or prolonged antibiotic therapy, which alters the intestinal flora. Hemostatic function must be monitored and supplementary vitamin K given as needed.

After a few weeks of treatment, some patients become totally refractory to platelet transfusions as shown by a lack of increase in platelet count 1 hour after completion of the transfusion. This is usually due to HLA alloimmunization and can be overcome by using HLA-matched platelets for transfusion. The use of filters, which remove WBCs from all transfused blood products (RBCs and platelets), from the start reduces (but does not eliminate) the incidence of HLA alloimmunization. This not only decreases the incidence of platelet refractoriness, but also reduces the risk of graft rejection after bone marrow transplantation.

The main cause of morbidity and mortality in patients with acute leukemia is infection, both during induction chemotherapy and later during the intensive consolidation phases of treatment. Prophylactic antibacterial therapy with a quinolone such as ciprofloxacin (Cipro) or with trimethoprim-sulfamethoxazole (Bactrim), and antifungal prophylaxis with fluconazole (Diflucan) have not yet been proven to decrease the risk of such infections. However, it is advisable to initiate such therapy as soon as the granulocyte count falls below 500 per μL, in spite of the risk of drug-resistant infection.

Fever in the neutropenic patient requires prompt and aggressive attention. Cultures for bacteria, fungi, and viruses should be obtained from all potential sites of infections. Immediately thereafter, treatment with broad-spectrum bactericidal antibiotics such as a semisynthetic penicillin (e.g., piperacillin [Pipracil]) and an aminoglycoside (e.g., gentamicin [Garamycin]) should be initiated. For the possible cutaneous entry of hospital bacteria, such as methicillin-resistant *Staphylococcus aureus,* or catheter colonization by *Corynebacterium* of the JK subtype, the addition of vancomycin (Vancocin) is recommended. If the patient remains febrile after 72 hours of such triple antibiotic therapy, antifungal therapy with amphotericin B (Fungizone) should be started on an empiric basis. Therapy of infections is guided and modified according to results of cultures obtained prior to the initiation of the antibiotic therapy.

Viral infections, although uncommon, must also be addressed. Serology for herpes simplex virus and cytomegalovirus should be obtained prior to the start of induction chemotherapy. Changes are then monitored during febrile episodes if mucosal lesions suggesting herpes simplex appear. Treatment with intravenous acyclovir (Zovirax) may be highly effective. Cytomegalovirus can cause interstitial pneumonia as well as esophagitis, enterocolitis, and hepatitis, all of which can be treated with gancyclovir (Cytovene).

Psychosocial Issues

Sensitive counseling and repeated explanation of all planned phases of treatment are important for patients with acute leukemia and their families, who are not prepared for the major alterations in lifestyle that the disease and its treatment will cause. An excellent source of information for both patient and family is a patient with a similar diagnosis who has already undergone treatment similar to the one planned, who can provide the information in terms easily understood by lay persons.

Once induction chemotherapy has induced a complete remission and the patient has returned home, contact with patients with successfully treated hematologic neoplasms (such as the Candlelighters) has helped patients to make the adjustments required by the disease and its therapy more tolerable. These groups are led by a trained professional and provide the wherewithal for physical and psychologic adjustment. The availability of a social worker and a psychiatrist with oncologic orientation as team members helps greatly in patient management.

ACKNOWLEDGMENT

I am grateful to Dr. Fred Rosner, Director of Medicine at Queens Hospital Center, for his invaluable editorial aid.

ACUTE LEUKEMIA IN CHILDHOOD

method of
NORMAN J. LACAYO, M.D., and
GARY V. DAHL, M.D.

*Lucile Salter Packard Children's Hospital at
    Stanford*
Palo Alto, California

There are two primary types of acute leukemia, acute lymphocytic leukemia (ALL) and acute nonlymphocytic leukemia (ANLL). Leukemia cells are classified according to a morphologic scheme called the FAB (French American British) classification. Using morphologic, cytochemical, immunologic, and cytogenetic criteria, approximately 80% of cases are classified as ALL and 20% as ANLL.

Currently, laboratory investigators are identifying biologic differences in leukemic cells not previously appreciated under the microscope alone. This genetic and molecular information will shed light on the differences in cure rate and help investigators to tailor treatment for different subtypes of leukemia.

The treatment and cure rate for acute leukemia of childhood has improved greatly in the last 20 years. This has been accompanied by advances in the classification of acute leukemia, more effective chemotherapeutic agents, new and improved antibiotics for infectious complications, and safer supportive care with blood products.

For ALL, risk-specific treatment schemata have been developed based on the patient's clinical and biologic characteristics. Criteria at the time of diagnosis such as age, leukocyte count, central nervous system involvement, leukemia cell immunophenotype, ploidy group, and karyotype are used to select appropriate therapy. For ANLL similar characteristics are important.

The Pediatric Oncology Group (POG) has elected to use clinical and biologic characteristics to guide the selection of therapy for ALL. Separate treatment protocols are used for patients with B-precursor ALL, T-cell ALL, B-cell ALL, infant ALL, and ANLL. This approach is based on the differences in drug sensitivities, differences in the risk of relapse, and rate of proliferation of the leukemic cells of these different phenotypes.

CLINICAL MANIFESTATIONS

Acute leukemia commonly presents with signs and symptoms caused by replacement of normal marrow with leukemic cells up to 10^{12}. Clinically, pallor, petechiae (or signs of bleeding), and fever, along with hepatosplenomegaly and adenopathy are the most frequent findings on physical examination. Laboratory findings usually include anemia, thrombocytopenia, elevated white blood cell count, and neutropenia. Additionally, elevated uric acid and lactate dehydrogenase (LDH) are frequently noted. Usually at the time of diagnosis abnormalities in at least two of the three bone marrow–derived cell lines are found, with blasts identified in the peripheral blood smear. Suspicion of leukemia warrants a prompt referral to a center with experience in pediatric oncology, since the evaluation of a new patient now includes quantitative and qualitative tests for biologic features that are prognostically important.

DIAGNOSIS

The diagnostic work-up (Table 1) starts with review of the medical history and a thorough examination. The blood smear is promptly reviewed for the identification of peripheral blasts. The most important laboratory data are hemoglobin count, white blood cell count and differential, platelet count, and electrolyte, uric acid, creatinine, and LDH levels. In addition, alanine aminotransferase (ALT), total bilirubin, prothrombin time (PT), partial thromboplastin time (PTT), fibrinogen, and immunoglobulin measurements and urinalysis are helpful. A varicella titer is obtained if there is no history of chickenpox.

TABLE 1. **Diagnostic Work-up**

Medical history and physical examination
Blood smear review
Hgb, WBC, differential, platelets
Electrolytes, uric acid, phosphorus, calcium, creatinine, ALT, total bilirubin, alkaline phosphatase, LDH, glucose, amylase
Urinalysis
PT, PTT, fibrinogen
Immunoglobulins, varicella titer
CXR (PA and lateral) and KUB or renal ultrasound if specifically indicated
Bone marrow aspirate: cell morphology with cytochemical stains, immunophenotype, DNA ploidy, cytogenetics, and storage for future studies

Abbreviations: Hgb = hemoglobin; WBC = white blood cell count; ALT = alanine aminotransferase; LDH = lactate dehydrogenase; PT = prothrombin time; PTT = partial thromboplastin time; CXR = chest x-ray; PA = posteroanterior; KUB = kidney-ureter-bladder.

A chest radiograph (posteroanterior and lateral) is obtained as part of the initial evaluation. Abdominal flat plate or ultrasonography is optional to determine kidney size. A bone marrow aspirate and frequently a bone marrow biopsy are obtained to determine cell morphology, cytochemical staining characteristics, immunophenotype, cytogenetics, and DNA ploidy. In the initial bone marrow examination, determination of the leukemia cell karyotype is of utmost importance for diagnosis and follow-up of acute leukemia; approximately 60 to 80% of ANLL and more than 90% of ALL cases are now found to exhibit clonal chromosome abnormalities. The need for this information at diagnosis mandates referral of patients to specialized pediatric oncology centers.

Usually, a diagnosis can be made within 24 hours. During the period of evaluation before the diagnosis is certain it is important to address psychosocial issues and offer the family support from the medical, nursing, and social work staff. The family should be reassured that acute leukemia is frequently curable and that almost all patients go into remission.

TREATMENT

Complications and Initial Management

Infection, metabolic abnormalities, hyperleukocytosis, anemia, and bleeding are the most serious problems complicating the initial management of the newly diagnosed child with acute leukemia. These clinical problems are most often the result of leukemic infiltration of the bone marrow and other organs. The greater the leukemic burden, manifested by high white blood cell count and enlarged liver, spleen, kidneys, or lymph nodes, the greater the clinical difficulty in managing a patient during the initial phases of therapy (Table 2).

Fever

More than 50% of patients with acute leukemia present with fever greater than 38.5° C. Fever caused by leukemia itself is rare; it more likely indicates a serious infection. In a patient with leukemia, fever should be considered to be due to infection until proven otherwise. Untreated infection can progress quickly and terminate fatally. If severe neutropenia exists (less than 500 neutrophils per mm³), it is necessary to look for sites of infection. If none are found, blood and urine cultures are obtained and antibiotic therapy is initiated with broad-spectrum coverage for gram-negative and gram-positive organisms. We begin patients on ceftazidime (Tazidime, Fortaz), 50 mg per kg given intravenously every 8 hours. Cultures are repeated periodically if the fever persists. No change in coverage is made if the patient is stable and defervesces and cultures remain negative. If fever persists for more than 72 hours or the patient's condition indicates a

TABLE 2. **Initial Management**

Anemia	Transfuse if in high-output heart failure with 5 ml per kg of packed red blood cells
Bleeding	Transfuse 0.2 U per kg of platelets; evaluate for disseminated intravascular coagulation
Hyperleukocytosis	Hydration 2.4–3 L per M²; allopurinol, alkalinization; leukapheresis if respiratory or CNS symptoms
Fever	Blood cultures; careful examination for source; antibiotics to cover gram-negative and gram-positive organisms
Hyperkalemia	Kayexalate, sodium bicarbonate, calcium gluconate, insulin, and glucose
Hyperuricemia	Allopurinol, 100 mg per M² tid
Hyperphosphatemia	Aluminium hydroxide, 100–150 mg per kg per day
Hypocalcemia	Calcium gluconate, 100–200 mg per kg per dose, if symptomatic
Renal failure	Hemodialysis

need for broader antibiotic coverage, an aminoglycoside (amikacin or tobramycin) is added. Vancomycin, 10 mg per kg intravenously every 6 hours, is added only if gram-positive organisms are cultured; levels must be monitored to prevent renal toxicity. Resistant bacteria and disseminated fungal infections need to be considered if the patient does not improve clinically. Antibiotic use varies among institutions based on their own experience with patterns of resistance. Some medical centers use two or three antibiotic regimens as initial therapy for fever and neutropenia. Early institution of antifungal therapy may be necessary for patients who continue to be febrile from 5 to 7 days on good antibiotic coverage.

Tumor Lysis Syndrome

Uric acid nephropathy, manifested by elevated uric acid and creatinine with low urine flow, can occur before chemotherapy is given or develop once chemotherapy is started. Patients with large tumor burdens at diagnosis are more likely to have this complication. As therapy is started, biochemical abnormalities develop that can also lead to renal failure. This constellation of problems is referred to as acute tumor lysis syndrome. Lysis of blasts releases potassium, purines, and phosphorus, resulting in hyperkalemia, hyperuricemia, and hyperphosphatemia with secondary hypocalcemia.

To prevent these complications we measure creatinine, blood urea nitrogen, uric acid, electrolytes, calcium, and phosphorus on admission and every 6 hours thereafter until the risk of tumor lysis syndrome has subsided. We institute vigorous hydration starting at 2400 to 3000 ml per M^2 per day with 5% dextrose and 0.2 normal saline and sodium bicarbonate ($NaHCO_3$), 20 to 40 mEq per liter to keep urine pH above 6.0. If urine output is less than 2 to 3 mL per kg per hour, diuretics (i.e., Lasix) may be needed. Hydration will assure good urine output and kaliuresis once therapy is begun. Allopurinol is started at 100 mg per M^2 three times a day to prevent hyperuricemia.

Mild hyperkalemia can be treated with Kayexalate, 1 gram per kg administered orally and mixed with sorbitol. Severe hyperkalemia, with a serum potassium level greater than 7.0 to 7.5 mEq per liter should be treated with sodium bicarbonate, calcium gluconate, and insulin with glucose. If these methods fail, hemodialysis is indicated to prevent cardiac arrythmias.

Hyperuricemia can lead to renal failure by precipitation of uric acid in renal tubules. Renal failure can result in increasing hyperkalemia, which in turn can cause cardiac arrythmias. The release of phosphorus from blasts causes hyperphosphatemia. When the level exceeds the calcium and phosphorus solubility, calcium phosphate can precipitate and cause hypocalcemia and may further worsen renal damage. In the case of severe hyperphosphatemia, alkalinization should be discontinued and aluminum hydroxide, 100 to 150 mg per kg per day in three divided doses, should be considered. Acetazolamide (Diamox), 5 mg per kg per dose repeated two to three times over 24 hours, can be used to keep urine pH above 7.0 if $NaHCO_3$ needs to be discontinued. Severe symptomatic hypocalcemia can be treated with intravenous calcium gluconate, 100 to 200 mg per kg per dose.

Hyperleukocytosis

Complications from hyperleukocytosis are rare, but more common in ANLL than in ALL. Stasis can develop with white blood cell counts greater than 100,000 cells per mm^3. The increased viscosity of blood and poor deformability of blasts impair blood flow in the microcirculation and greatly increase the risk of thrombotic and hemorrhagic complications.

Hyperleukocytosis in acute leukemia is associated with a risk of intracranial hemorrhage. Central nervous system (CNS) leukemic involvement can result in visual blurring, papilledema, and headache as well. Hyperleukocytosis can impair pulmonary function, and tachypnea, dyspnea, and hypoxia can be seen. Once the diagnosis is confirmed, our approach to hyperleukocytosis is hydration with 3 or more liters per M^2 per day of intravenous fluid administered with $NaHCO_3$ for

alkalinization and allopurinol daily prior to and during the first few days of induction. Leukopheresis can be used to reduce the blood cell count if renal compromise develops; however, its effect is temporary and it may not prevent sludging in the microcirculation.

Anemia

The degree of anemia depends on the duration and type of disease. Leukemia involving a large cell burden gradually crowding out normal hematopoeitic precursors in the bone marrow for weeks can lead insidiously to severe anemia. T-cell leukemia, characterized by more bulky extramedullary disease, may present with mild anemia, since many times the thymus is the site of origin with later spread to the marrow. If there is any evidence of cardiac failure or respiratory compromise not secondary to hyperleukocytosis, the patient undergoes transfusion with 10 mL per kg of irradiated and cytomegalovirus (CMV)-negative packed red blood cells over 4 hours. If the patient presents with severe anemia (hemoglobin less than 6 mg per dL), we transfuse with 5 mL per kg of packed red blood cells over 4 hours every 6 to 8 hours until the hemoglobin level approaches 8 mg per dL. Unless there is a history of significant bleeding in leukemia, anemia usually has had a chronic onset, and most patients have adapted to a low oxygen-carrying capacity. Therefore, less stringent criteria for transfusion may be used if the patient is hemodynamically stable in order to avoid exposure to blood products. The majority of patients are not transfused prior to referral to oncology centers.

Bleeding

Bleeding is usually a result of thrombocytopenia, a coagulopathy due to infection- or leukemia-associated disseminated intravascular coagulopathy (DIC). Initial evaluation should include evaluation of the platelet count, PT, PTT, and fibrinogen. If thrombocytopenia is the etiology, transfusion of 0.2 units of irradiated, CMV-negative platelets per kg (4 to 6 units per M^2) should increase the platelet count by 75,000 platelets per μL. We empirically transfuse patients to keep the platelet count above 15,000 platelets per μL if bleeding is a problem. Patients with ANLL are at higher risk of a hemorrhagic complication. DIC is frequently associated with promyelocytic (M3 by FAB) and monocytic (M5 by FAB) subtypes. Initial therapy of M3 ANLL with all-trans-retinoic acid may abrogate the bleeding problem. Frequent transfusions with platelets and fresh-frozen plasma can help control the DIC-related bleeding until specific therapy has a chance to work.

Acute Lymphocytic Leukemia

Most children with ALL have B-precursor ALL (85%). This subtype has the best prognosis (75% of patients in remission over 5 years). Those whose leukemic cells are positive for CD-10 antigen (CALLA+) have an even better prognosis. Approximately 14% have T-cell ALL, a subtype more frequently found in male teenagers with white blood cell counts above 100×10^9 per liter and anterior mediastinal masses on chest radiography. Occasionally, superior vena cava syndrome can develop. These children respond reasonably well to treatment but have a somewhat worse prognosis, with approximately 55% in remission after 5 years. B-cell ALL with surface immunoglobulin represents only 1% of ALL and these rare children are presently being treated with Burkitt's non-Hodgkin's lymphoma directed therapy. Approximately 60% of these children are in remission over 5 years.

The Pediatric Oncology Group (POG) classifies ALL by age, white blood cell count, CNS involvement, DNA index, and karyotype. Patients are grouped into standard or high-risk categories. Infants and patients with T-cell and B-cell ALL are considered to have biologically different diseases and are treated with different regimens.

The treatment for ALL is divided into three components: induction, consolidation or intensification, and maintenance. During these three stages, the CNS is treated with intrathecal chemotherapy.

In the POG treatment plans, therapy for B-precursor ALL, T-cell ALL, and infant ALL are different; the therapy plan for the more frequently seen B-precursor ALL patient follows.

Induction

Induction therapy involves a multidrug regimen designed to induce remission. Prednisone, 40 mg per M^2 orally divided into three doses daily for 28 days; vincristine (VCN), 1.5 mg per M^2 intravenously weekly for 4 weeks with a maximum dose of 2.0 mg; and L-asparaginase (L-Asp), 6000 IU per M^2 intramuscularly twice a week for 3 weeks is standard therapy. For patients considered to be at high risk, a fourth drug, daunorubicin (Cerubidine), 30 mg per M^2 intravenously once a week for 3 weeks, is added. CNS prophylaxis is given with intrathecal methotrexate (MTX), cytosine arabinoside (Ara-C), and hydrocortisone (HDC). The doses are adjusted according to age, and the patient is treated once during the first month if the cerebrospinal fluid (CSF) does not reveal leukemic involvement at the time of diagnosis. If leukemia is present the patient is treated weekly for a month and until the CSF is clear of blasts for 2 consecutive weeks. The complete remission rate is over 97%, and in most group studies, disease-free survival is now greater than 70%. During induction therapy the patient and family are instructed on the appropriate therapy, risk, and consequences of infections in immunocompromised patients. Prophylactic therapy with trimethoprim-sulfamethoxazole (TMP-SMX), 150 mg per M^2 divided twice a day for 3 consecutive days every week, is initiated to prevent infection with *Pneumocystis carinii*. Another issue discussed during induction therapy is the advantage of central venous access. If the consolidation regimen is to be intense, it will require ready venous access for chemotherapy and supportive care.

Consolidation

After 1 month of induction therapy the bone marrow and CSF are evaluated to establish whether the patient is in remission. If the bone marrow has less than 5% blasts, one proceeds with consolidation chemotherapy. The aim of this phase is to continue to eradicate a large proportion of the leukemic blasts that remain undetected after induction therapy. Combinations of agents known to be effective are used. Currently the POG randomizes standard risk patients to three groups: (1) intravenous intermediate-dose MTX and high-dose 6-mercaptopurine (6-MP); (2) intravenous intermediate-dose MTX alone; and (3) oral MTX and intravenous high-dose 6-MP. These courses alternate every other week with intramuscular MTX and oral 6-MP.

Patients at high risk for relapse are randomized separately to two regimens: 12 courses of intravenous intermediate-dose MTX plus intravenous 6-MP versus 12 courses of alternative intensive chemotherapy combinations (6-MP/MTX, VM-26/Ara-C, VCR/prednisone/PEG–L-asparaginase/daunorubicin/Ara-C). CNS therapy continues with a schedule of intrathecal MTX, Ara-C, and HDC. The duration of consolidation therapy is 30 weeks. Once this is completed, maintenance therapy is initiated.

Maintenance Therapy

Maintenance therapy is given for a duration of 2.5 years from diagnosis. It consists of MTX, 20 mg per M^2 intramuscularly weekly, and 6-MP, 50 mg per M^2 orally daily. Intrathecal therapy with MTX, Ara-C, and HDC continues every 3 months for the first year only. Drugs used in the treatment of ALL are summarized in Table 3.

Blood counts and chemistries are done periodically during consolidation and maintenance therapy to monitor for toxicity as doses and schedules may need to be modified to fit patient tolerance. Surveillance bone marrow aspirates are not done.

TABLE 3. **Drugs Used to Treat Acute Leukemia**

Drug	Adverse Reactions
Vincristine (Oncovin)	Alopecia, neuritic pain, constipation, difficulty in walking, peripheral neuropathy, leukopenia, severe cellulitis if extravasated
Prednisone (Deltasone)	Immunosuppression, increased appetite and weight gain, Cushing's syndrome, myopathy, mood changes, hyperglycemia, relative adrenocortical insufficiency in times of stress
L-Asparaginase (Elspar)	Anaphylactic reactions, decreased protein synthesis (including coagulation factors), pancreatitis, hyperglycemia
6-Mercaptopurine (Purinethol)	Myelosuppression, hepatotoxicity, immunosuppression
Methotrexate (Amethopterin)	Stomatitis, myelosuppression, immunosuppression, photosensitivity, hepatic fibrosis
Doxorubicin (Adriamycin)	Myelosuppression, cardiac toxicity, alopecia, nausea and vomiting, stomatitis, gastrointestinal ulceration, severe cellulitis if extravasated, hypersensitivity reactions
Cytosine arabinoside (Cytosar-U)	Myelosuppression, nausea and vomiting, stomatitis
VP-16/VM-26 (Etoposide/Teniposide)	Nausea and vomiting, diarrhea, fever, hypotension, allergic reactions, alopecia, peripheral neuropathy, mucositis, hepatic damage with high doses
Thioguanine (Lanvis)	Nausea and vomiting, bone marrow depression, hepatic damage, stomatitis
5-Azacytidine (Mylosar)	Severe nausea and vomiting, diarrhea, fever, drowsiness, hepatic damage, muscle pain and weakness, prolonged bone marrow suppression, possible cardiotoxicity

Other Lymphocytic Leukemias

Infants with ALL are treated with a very intense treatment regimen using multiple courses of marrow hypoplasia–inducing drug combinations. Treatment is difficult to administer and the frequency of relapse is very high. Children less than 1 year of age at diagnosis tend to have very high white blood cell counts, specific high-risk chromosome translocations, and CNS involvement.

Treatment for T-cell ALL is identical to treatment given for T-cell non-Hodgkin's lymphoma. The approach is to combine patients with T-cell ALL and lymphoblastic lymphoma on the same protocol; experience has proven that these treatments are more effective.

Relapse

Patients who are in remission must be monitored closely for relapse. Relapse (recurrent leukemia) can occur in the marrow, extramedullary sites (testis, CNS, eye), or a combination of sites. Patients who relapse in the marrow while receiving maintenance chemotherapy or within 6 months of stopping treatment are difficult to treat. Although remission can be achieved with chemotherapy, subsequent remission and survival are usually short in the majority of these children. Bone marrow transplantation (BMT) offers an improved prognosis: 35 to 60% of children with marrow relapse on therapy or within 6 months of stopping therapy can be cured. Isolated extramedullary relapse on therapy can be effectively treated with chemotherapy alone in 30 to 40% of children and up to 80% with BMT.

Bone Marrow Transplantation

Despite the fact that approximately 70% of children with ALL can be cured with current chemotherapy regimens, there remains a significant group of patients at high risk of treatment failure. Patients who are identified as likely to fail therapy should be considered for BMT. The identification of leukemia cell biologic characteristics at the time of diagnosis helps to identify these patients.

Finding the Philadelphia (Ph) chromosome t(9;22)(q34;q11) at diagnosis is the worst prognostic feature. Three to 5% of children are Ph+ at diagnosis, and there are only rare survivors with conventional therapy. Presently children with Ph+ ALL on POG protocols are undergoing BMT from HLA-identical donors as soon as they achieve complete remission. The translocation t(4;11) carries an outlook similar to that for Ph+ patients for certain age groups. Many t(4;11) patients are now undergoing BMT but it is too early to say if such aggressive therapy improves survival in these children. Failure to achieve complete remission with initial induction agents should be considered an indication for BMT as initial treatment. The fact that most children do not have a matched related donor available has led to the use of purged autologous and matched unrelated BMT for patients who relapse. Leukemic relapse rates are higher with autologous transplants.

Acute Nonlymphocytic Leukemia

Although more than 85% of children with ANLL achieve remission, fewer than 40% enjoy event-free survival on chemotherapy trials. Identification of active chemotherapeutic agents has led to higher remission induction rates. Drugs most commonly used for induction therapy include daunorubicin, Ara-C, and 6-thioguanine (6-

TG). Unfortunately most patients, even those on intensive experimental chemotherapy regimens, relapse within the first 12 to 18 months.

The current approach to the treatment of ANLL is to prolong the duration of the initial remission with early intensification using chemotherapy or BMT to improve survival. The POG is currently evaluating a prospective comparison of patients randomized to an intensive multi-agent regimen or to autologous BMT early in first complete remission. DAT (daunorubicin, 45 mg per M^2 per day for 3 days; Ara-C, 100 mg per M^2 by continuous infusion for 7 days; and 6-TG, 100 mg per M^2 orally per day for 7 days) induction is completed in 7 days. The bone marrow is evaluated on day 15, and if it is hypocellular, the second induction course is delayed for a week or until recovery. If the marrow is normocellular and absolute neutrophil count is greater than 750 cells per mm^3 and platelet count is greater than 100,000 per μL or the blast count is more than 5% and less than 15%, one proceeds with a second induction course of HDA_6 (high dose Ara-C 3 gm per M^2 every 12 hours for six doses).

All patients who achieve complete remission and have an available matched sibling donor are offered allogeneic BMT before randomization. Patients with no available donor are randomized. First, they are given further consolidation with a course of VP/Az (VP-16 250 mg per M^2 intravenously for 3 days followed by 5-azacytidine 300 mg per M^2 intravenously for 2 days) and then assigned randomization to autologous BMT, with ex-vivo marrow purging with 4-hydroperoxycyclophosphamide, or six additional cycles of consolidation chemotherapy with alternating non–cross-resistant drug combinations given every 3 to 4 weeks. These drug combinations include VP/Az, HDA_6 with daunorubicin, HDA_6 alone, and DAT. Drugs used in the treatment of ANLL are listed in Table 3.

In summary, approaches to the treatment of postremission ANLL have included intensive chemotherapy, allogeneic bone marrow transplantation, and autologous bone marrow transplantation after ex-vivo purging. Better supportive care is decreasing the mortality and morbidity secondary to BMT, making it a more viable option. Currently, we recommend that patients in first remission and with an available matched related donor undergo bone marrow transplantation. Matched related donor transplants offer a lower risk of leukemic relapse than autologous transplants after purging and a longer disease-free survival than further intensive chemotherapy.

Management During Remission

Outpatient management during remission frequently involves care directed from centers that specialize in the care of pediatric oncology patients. The referring physician can provide much of the remission maintenance therapy in the office setting. The most frequent problems encountered during therapy are caused by chemotherapy-induced myelosuppression and other drug-related toxicities.

Infection

Fever and neutropenia are common in patients with acute leukemia. By convention, a patient is febrile and neutropenic when an oral temperature greater than 38.5° C or three successive temperatures greater than 38° C develop and there are fewer than 500 neutrophils per mm^3. If fever and neutropenia occur, patients are admitted to the hospital and started on an empiric broad-spectrum antibacterial regimen. This approach has dramatically decreased the morbidity and mortality due to infection. In most cases the infectious etiology of fever is not determined even though multiple cultures are obtained.

Patients with indwelling intravenous (Hickman or Broviac) catheters are treated with additional empiric antibiotic coverage for gram-positive organisms initially or later depending on cultures (usually *Staphylococcus epidermidis*). Generally, a blood culture is obtained from the catheter and from a peripheral venipuncture.

Broad antibiotic coverage is continued until the neutrophil count is above 500 per mm^3. If a specific organism is isolated and sensitivities are determined, antibiotic coverage can be more specific but never less than broad spectrum. In some patients with acute leukemia, granulocyte colony-stimulating factor (G-CSF) has been used to shorten the duration of neutropenia, as it has only rarely been shown to stimulate proliferation of leukemic cells in vivo. Although G-CSF and granulocyte-macrophage colony-stimulating factor (GM-CSF) are not yet used as standard therapy for patients with leukemia, they are increasingly being accepted into clinical practice.

If neutropenia and fever persist after 5 to 7 days and no bacterial organism has been isolated, antifungal therapy (usually amphotericin B) is initiated. This can be added earlier if indicated by the patient's clinical course.

Patients presenting with fever but a neutrophil count greater than 500 per mm^3 should be carefully evaluated. However, antibiotic therapy is not required unless it is warranted by the degree of illness. If the source of fever is identified on examination (e.g., otitis media or pneumonia), it should be treated appropriately. If no etiology can be found, a blood culture can be obtained and the patient watched closely without antibiotic therapy.

During the last decade, new and potent broad-spectrum antibiotics and antifungal agents such as third-generation cephalosporins, extended-spectrum penicillins, fluoroquinolones, fluconazole (Diflucan), and itraconazole (Sporanox) have been introduced. These drugs may further reduce the morbidity and mortality caused by infection.

Prophylactic use of TMP-SMX to prevent *Pneumocystis carinii,* a frequently fatal interstitial pneumonitis, is given 3 consecutive days a week to all patients with acute leukemia while they are undergoing chemotherapy.

There is an increased risk of fungal infections due to the use of more aggressive chemotherapy and broad-spectrum antibiotics. Amphotericin B (Fungizone) continues to be the agent of choice for fungal infections. The empirical use of fluconazole to prevent fungal infection is being tested to determine its efficacy as a prophylactic agent.

The viral infection of most concern is varicella. Patients exposed to varicella should receive zoster immunoglobulin within 72 hours of exposure to attenuate or prevent disease. Immunocompromised patients with disseminated varicella can suffer severe pneumonia, hepatitis, and encephalitis. With the availability of acyclovir (Zovirax), the morbidity from disseminated varicella has decreased. Patients who contract varicella on or within 3 months of stopping therapy should be given intravenous acylovir in the hospital setting. Herpes zoster can be treated with oral acyclovir in an outpatient setting unless it involves the eye, in which case intravenous acyclovir is needed as well as consultation with an ophthalmologist to direct local therapy.

Immunizations as part of health care maintenance should continue. Live viral vaccines are contraindicated during treatment and up to 6 months after therapy has been completed. Diphtheria-pertussis-tetanus vaccine can be given safely during therapy; it may have to be repeated 6 months after the end of therapy, however, if the immune response was not sufficient.

Myelosuppression

Marrow supression is common during treatment and is followed by blood counts to indicate whether adequate doses of chemotherapy are being given. Significant anemia and thrombocytopenia require treatment with transfusions of packed red blood cells and platelets. Low blood counts can be a sign of early relapse, intensive therapy, infection, or a marrow proliferative abnormality. Modification of the dosage of chemotherapeutic agents may be necessary to prevent long periods of myelosuppression.

Drug Toxicities

Numerous agents can cause reversible and irreversible renal and hepatic toxicity. Schedules and doses of chemotherapeutic agents may have to be modified or held until hepatic and renal function returns to normal. Management of chemotherapy extravasation is presented in Table 4.

Long-Term Treatment Sequelae

As more patients survive childhood leukemia due to successful treatment regimens, the challenge is to eliminate the long-term side effects of therapy without compromising its efficacy. In the case of leukemia, the recent success and effectiveness of intrathecal and intravenous therapies have led to the elimination of preventive meningeal irradiation for most children. Most children no longer require anthracyclines (daunorubicin) or alkylating agents (cyclophosphamide), so cardiac and bladder toxicity are much less common.

The increased cure rate for ALL has been paralleled by an increased incidence of second cancers. These second malignancies can be grouped into three categories: (1) CNS tumors, (2) leukemias and lymphomas, and (3) other neoplasms. Radiation therapy and leukemogenic antineoplastic drugs are contributing factors. Cranial irradiation and the epipodophyllotoxins (VM-26 or VP-16) are known to increase the risk of brain tumors and secondary acute nonlymphocytic leukemia, respectively. To increase the cure rate while reducing toxicity, other means of CNS prophylaxis have been emphasized and different schedules of VM-26/VP-16 administration utilized.

For those involved in long-term care of successfully treated patients, late effects of therapy will have an increasingly prominent role in their practice. The risk of second malignancy after ALL is 5% with long-term (15 to 20 years) follow-up

---

TABLE 4. **Prevention and Treatment of Chemotherapy Extravasation**

---

1. When placing a line, avoid the antecubital fossa. The dorsum of the hand should be the first choice. The forearm is acceptable.
2. Stop the flow immediately if extravasation is suspected. Keep the needle in place.
3. Aspirate as much of the infiltrated drug as possible.
4. Remove the needle.
5. Inject specific antidote. For vincristine (Oncovin) use hyaluronidase (Wydase). Use a 27-gauge needle, point toward center of extravasated area. Give ¼ of antidote with each needle stick at 12, 3, 6, and 9 o'clock. Change needle after each injection. If there is no specific antidote, use hydrocortisone, 50–100 mg subcutaneously. ʟ ɘe will depend on the size of the infiltrate.
6. Apply a film of 1% hydrocortisone cream over the affected area.
7. Apply ice packs. Cold should be used for all vesicants and irritants except for vincristine and VP-16/VM-26, which should be treated with heat.

---

after diagnosis; however, a 5% incidence of secondary ANLL alone has been reported with some new therapies. Clearly, careful selection of therapy and serial comprehensive follow-up of all children off therapy are important to identify and treat late effects.

Growth delay is another significant side effect of treatment for leukemia. Children receiving chemotherapy often grow poorly if at all during treatment due to the direct effects of the chemotherapy or complicating infections, but "catch-up" growth usually occurs once therapy is discontinued. Pituitary function is affected if patients have CNS involvement or receive CNS radiation therapy. Close follow-up of neuroendocrine abnormalities primarily involving the hypothalamic-pituitary axis is needed since early detection makes successful intervention more likely. Growth hormone deficiency is a frequent complication. Replacement therapy will increase growth velocity, but most children will not attain the normal height for their age. Intellectual deficits affecting visual-spatial and verbal memory have been identified. Children may benefit from evaluation for learning disabilities if school performance is compromised.

In young children it is important to follow height, weight, and growth velocity. In patients who have received craniospinal irradiation, a thorough back examination should be done to evaluate for scoliosis. If there is any indication of gonadal dysfunction, testosterone, follicle-stimulating hormone, and luteinizing hormone should be evaluated. If anthracyclines have been used in treatment, one should monitor cardiac function periodically with chest films, electrocardiography, and echocardiography to evaluate left ventricular ejection and shortening fractions. In some studies, up to 50% of patients receiving anthracyclines had evidence of cardiac dysfunction. Long-

TABLE 5. **Resources for Parents**

Cancer Hotline: 1-800-FOR-CANCER
The Candlelighters Childhood Cancer Foundation
7910 Woodmont Avenue
Suite 460
Bethesda, Maryland 20814
1-800-366-2223

The Leukemia Society of America, Inc.
Local chapters available
600 Third Avenue
New York, NY 10016
1-212-573-8484

The American Cancer Society
Local chapters available
1599 Clifton Road, N.E.
Atlanta, GA 30329
1-404-320-3333

term survivors should be evaluated annually with a complete blood count with differential and platelets. A testicular examination is important since it is a common site of relapse. In women a Pap smear and mammography should be performed according to standard guidelines.

Most centers that see large numbers of children following successful therapy continue to see these patients regularly for many years so that late effects of therapy can be prevented or identified and treated.

Equally important is the evaluation of the psychosocial issues related to surviving cancer. These issues may involve family and occupational difficulties, and medical insurance problems. Psychosocial stabilization and psychosocial management of parents and their children after a diagnosis of cancer are complex. *Your Child Has Cancer: A Guide to Coping* by Joan Taksa Rolsky, M.S.W., published by the Committee to Benefit the Children, St. Christopher's Hospital for Children, Philadelphia, Pennsylvania (1992), presents a thorough discussion of how to approach psychosocial issues during diagnosis and treatment (Table 5).

CHRONIC MYELOID LEUKEMIA

method of
RICHARD T. SILVER, M.D.
New York Hospital–Cornell Medical Center
New York, New York

Chronic myeloid leukemia (CML) is a chronic myeloproliferative disorder of a pluripotent stem cell with a specific cytogenetic abnormality—the Philadelphia (Ph) chromosome—that involves myeloid, erythroid, megakaryocyte, and occasionally B lymphoid cells. Recent advances in cell biology and molecular genetics have yielded much new data regarding this disease. Advances in marrow transplantation and the effects of recombinant interferon-alpha have been significant, although their roles in the overall treatment of the disease remain to be determined.

CML is characterized by two phases. The "benign" or "chronic" phase, which usually lasts about 3 years, terminates in a second more acute or abrupt illness, called the "accelerated," "terminal," or "blast" phase.

In the chronic phase, symptoms and signs usually develop insidiously and include fatigue, anemia, progressive splenomegaly, and leukocytosis. The white blood cell (WBC) count approximates 200,000 per µL. The myeloid cells in the peripheral blood show all stages of differentiation, but the myelocyte predominates. Basophils and eosinophils are prominent. More

This study was supported in part by grants from the United Leukemia Fund, Inc., and the Cancer Research and Treatment Fund, Inc.

than half the patients have platelet counts above one million per μL. A slight degree of anemia is common.

Terminal chronic myeloid leukemia can develop at any time during the course of CML, but usually after a median interval of 36 to 48 months. A number of criteria can be used to define this relatively abrupt change in disease status, the most reliable being the presence in the peripheral blood, bone marrow, or both of myeloblasts and promyelocytes exceeding 30% of the differential distribution. This occurs in about 70% of cases. In the absence of frank blast crisis, other criteria include fever of undetermined origin, increasing splenomegaly, a rising WBC count, basophilia, an increased degree of anemia and thrombocytopenia, and refractoriness to previously effective therapy such as busulfan and hydroxyurea. High blast cell counts can lead to pulmonary leukostasis and hemorrhage. The median survival after blastic transformation is approximately 3 months.

The blast crises are divided into two general types, myeloid and lymphoid. A lymphoid blast crisis occurs in 20 to 30% of patients. The cells often seem to resemble those in acute lymphocytic leukemia and contain terminal deoxynucleotidyl transferase (TdT). This transferase is found mainly in poorly differentiated normal and malignant lymphoid cells of T cell and B cell origin and is lost as these lymphocytes differentiate and mature.

The basic mechanism whereby chronic phase disease is transformed into blast phase is not understood. Although additional cytogenetic abnormalities are seen as patients enter the blast phase, these may not necessarily be causally related to the transformation.

CYTOGENETIC AND MOLECULAR ABNORMALITIES

A brief understanding of the cytogenetic and molecular abnormalities in CML must be appreciated in order to understand response to treatment.

The Philadelphia chromosome, the hallmark of CML, appears following reciprocal translocation of cytogenetic material from chromosomes 9 and 22. These cytogenetic abnormalities are mirrored by the formation of a unique molecular abnormality, resulting in the formation of the fusion bcr-abl oncogene, which gives rise to a hybrid mRNA, which is subsequently translated into a 210kD protein, instead of the normal 145kD protein. This abnormal 210kD protein expresses abnormal tyrosine kinase activity, and this kinase may be involved in cellular abnormalities of growth, regulation, and differentiation.

TREATMENT

Chronic Phase

The cardinal therapeutic principle in treating CML is that initially the great majority of patients respond to many drugs and even radiation therapy. Although the quality of life in CML may be improved by such treatment, no evidence exists that survival is prolonged by conventional agents. This is because neither the Philadelphia chromosome nor the bcr-abl molecular abnormality is affected significantly by conventional drugs. Although many agents are effective in the chronic phase, none are superior to either busulfan or hydroxyurea, which remain the agents most frequently used other than interferon.

Busulfan

Busulfan (Myleran) is an alkylating agent. The standard initial daily dose is 4.0 to 6.0 mg per M^2 (0.06 to 0.1 mg per kg) orally with a maximal dose of 8.0 mg. The dose of busulfan is gradually reduced as the white blood cell count falls by 50%, and it should be discontinued when the WBC count falls to less than 15,000 per μL. A rapid decrease in the platelet count in relation to the WBC count requires prompt dose modification. In some patients, specific cytostatic effects may be slow to appear. Additional treatment is sometimes required after the WBC count is normalized if the platelet count remains substantially elevated, although a new agent, anagrelide, may be effective in such cases (see further on).

Continuous or intermittent therapy with busulfan has been employed to maintain the WBC count in the range of 15,000 per μL. Although this does not affect survival, it may reduce morbidity. Since prolonged remissions may be seen after the induction course, I prefer to wait for the white blood cell count to return to 75,000 to 100,000 per μl before restarting busulfan after the first induction course. Refractoriness to busulfan is most uncommon in the chronic phase of CML and usually signifies impending terminal phase disease.

Busulfan has significant side effects. Bone marrow hypoplasia is usually dose related but may be idiosyncratic. Busulfan can cause exfoliative cytologic abnormalities of sputum, urine, and cervical secretions suggestive of a coexistent neoplasm. In this event, busulfan should be discontinued to determine whether the cytologic abnormalities disappear. Other common toxic effects include amenorrhea, increased skin pigmentation, a wasting syndrome with features of Addison's disease, cataracts, "busulfan lung," and endocardial fibrosis.

Hydroxyurea

Because of the side effects associated with busulfan, many hematologists use hydroxyurea (Hydrea) instead. This S-phase specific inhibitor of ribonucleotidase can be used in a fashion similar to busulfan. The drug is started in a dose of 5 to 15 mg per kg per day orally, depending upon the WBC count, then tapered as for busulfan as the WBC count, platelet count, or both fall. The same principles of maintenance therapy are applicable to hydroxyurea. Side effects, which occur less frequently than with busulfan, include minor stomatitis, nausea and vomiting, and a maculopapular rash. Unlike busulfan, hydroxyurea must be given continuously to maintain remission.

Blast Phase

No substantial progress has been made in the treatment of blast phase disease. We and others have tested a large series of drugs and drug regimens, including those used for acute leukemias, without success. In view of this, I prefer to use a combination of agents that can be given on an outpatient basis. A combination of hydroxyurea, 6-mercaptopurine (Purinethol), and prednisone in patients (especially patients who have not received prior therapy with hydroxyurea) yields a response rate of approximately 30%. This modest improvement in response is characterized by a mean remission duration of about 7 months, compared with 2 or 3 months for patients with no response. Although vincristine/prednisone with or without other drugs is especially useful in lymphoid blast crises, in my experience, survival is not significantly increased over that in myeloid blast crisis even with "tailored" chemotherapy. These results suggest that therapeutic responsiveness in blast crisis depends on the inherent sensitivity of the blast cells rather than on the effectiveness of the therapeutic regimen. Hospitalized patients with myeloid blast crisis can be given an anthracycline and intravenous cytosine arabinoside in the same dosage as used in de novo acute myeloid leukemia.

Treatment of Elevated Platelet Counts

Within recent years, we have observed a significant number of patients with CML who developed refractory thrombocytosis resistant to both hydroxyurea and busulfan that was associated with significant thrombotic and hemorrhagic complications. A new agent, anagrelide, a quinazolin derivative still undergoing phase III trials, is highly effective in reducing the platelet count in patients with CML who are resistant to hydroxyurea, busulfan, or both. (This agent is also effective against the thrombocythemia associated with other myeloproliferative diseases.) Using a dose of approximately 0.5 mg four times a day, a significant fall in platelet counts can occur within 4 to 6 weeks. (This drug is currently distributed by special permission by Roberts Pharmaceutical Company, Eatontown, N.J.)

Interferon

The fact that interferons have a wide variety of biological activities, including antiproliferative and oncogene regulatory activity, certainly warranted their trial in CML. Sufficient evidence has accrued both in this country and in Europe to indicate that in a small but significant percentage of patients recombinant interferon-alpha (rIFNα) can correct the characteristic cytogenetic and molecular abnormalities of CML. Overall, about 20 to 25% of patients (particularly those defined as "good-risk" patients) treated for 1 to 2 years with a dose of 5 million units per M^2 per day subcutaneously can expect a beneficial cytogenetic and molecular response that is associated with prolonged survival. In some patients, rIFNα results in Ph-negative marrows, but the more sensitive molecular abnormality persists. Preliminary evidence suggests that these patients may also have a significantly improved survival time.

The side effects of rIFNα are not trivial, and therefore, not all patients can tolerate it for long periods although they obviously should be encouraged to do so. In addition to leukopenia and thrombocytopenia, nonhematologic effects include fever, chills, malaise, headache, anorexia, joint pain, myalgia, various types of neuropathy, changes in mood and concentration, and abnormalities of liver enzymes can occur. Nevertheless, dose intensity with rIFNα is important because for unknown reasons it is necessary to produce leukopenia of 2000 to 3000 per µL in order to obtain a cytogenetic response. Thus, from the standpoint of clinical management, it is wise to warn patients of these complications. Over time these side effects usually abate.

Although recombinant interferon-gamma (rIFNγ) shares many of the functional properties of rIFNα, significant differences exist. Although several therapeutic trials have demonstrated some activity of rIFNγ, even in patients resistant to rIFNα, the side effects are similar to those of rIFNα but much more severe, which limits its clinical usefulness.

The addition of chemotherapy to rIFNα has also been investigated in the expectation of a synergistic effect. This is an experimental procedure and cannot be recommended for general use at the present time.

Bone Marrow Transplantation

Although marrow transplantation in CML has attracted much interest, only 10% of patients are eligible for this procedure; age and histocompatibility requirements eliminate the majority of CML patients. In order for marrow transplantation to be successful, the patient should be relatively young, preferably under 40 years old and closer to 30 years. (However, some centers will accept patients up to the age of 55.) Induction and conditioning regimens include high-dose cyclophosphamide, total body radiation, and modifications such as high-dose cytosine arabinoside, etoposide, and busulfan. A discussion of the advantages and disadvantages of these therapeutic approaches is beyond the scope of this paper.

The question of *when* to perform marrow transplantation is not a simple one. Most hematologists recommend that any patient with CML who has a normal identical twin to serve as a donor should be considered for marrow transplantation regardless of age or stage of disease. Yet, results of HLA-identical sibling transplants in CML indicate a 3-year disease-free survival rate of only 40 to 70% because of a 20% relapse rate. For patients with an allogeneic match, the mortality in the first 1½ years after treatment is about 30%. Further, the poor quality of life in patients who develop graft-versus-host-disease who survive (nearly half) has not been emphasized. Patients under the age of 40 with an HLA-matched donor should certainly be considered for transplantation although whether or not such patients should initially receive a 1-year trial of interferon if in a good-risk category has not been resolved. (I prefer to do this.) It is hoped that additional information and experience will provide answers to these questions.

NON-HODGKIN'S LYMPHOMA

method of
JOSEPH M. CONNORS, M.D.
University of British Columbia
Vancouver, British Columbia, Canada

Human lymphocytes come in a variety of subtypes that vary greatly in site of origin, rate of growth, function, life span, usual tissues of residence, and apparent purpose. It is, then, no surprise that the illnesses derived from them are protean. It is necessary to appreciate this inherent variation in order to understand the different manifestations of lymphocytic diseases known as non-Hodgkin's, or malignant, lymphomas. That different types of lymphoma can be present in the same patient at the same or different times adds to this complexity. Thus, much of the task of understanding the lymphomas and planning their rational treatment depends on recognizing patterns and groupings that allow reasonable prediction of natural history and response to treatment. The best approach is to identify the usual behavior of several common subtypes and then add the additional observations useful for detailed understanding of special sites of presentation, patterns of spread, typical complications, and individual responses to treatment.

DIAGNOSIS

The diagnosis, prognosis, natural history, and response to treatment of malignant lymphomas all depend on identification of the specific subtype of lymphoma present and determination of the extent of disease. This first step, identification, requires an ample tissue sample, preferably from an involved lymph node, which is carefully examined by an experienced hematopathologist. Frozen and fixed tissue should be analyzed with a variety of standard and immunohistochemical stains, complemented as necessary by flow cytometric, cytogenetic, and molecular genetic techniques. The result should be a diagnosis of a specific subtype of lymphoma, and if this cannot be done, rebiopsy should be strongly considered.

Histologic Classification

The most widely used classification scheme in North America for the malignant lymphomas is the Working Formulation (WF), developed initially as a means of interconverting several older schemes, but now often used as the primary system. In its original formulation, the WF divided the ten common subtypes of lymphoma into three groups; low, intermediate, and high grade. It has become clear that one of the subtypes, immunoblastic lymphoma, is better grouped with the intermediate than with the high-grade lymphomas as was proposed in the original WF. The subgrouping shown in Table 1 reflects this modification of the WF and arranges the lymphomas in practical sets according to natural history, prognosis, and response to treatment. The WF does not take the B or T cell immunophenotype directly into consideration; however, most pathologists are influenced by this information because it has become clear that virtually all cases of follicular lymphomas and small noncleaved Burkitt's lymphoma are of B cell origin and lymphoblastic lymphoma is similarly almost always of T cell origin. Although some authorities have found that T cell origin may confer a poorer prognosis, this has little importance in North America for two reasons. First, fewer than 15% of lymphomas here are of T cell origin and, second, the most careful comparisons, in which groups of patients have been matched for age, stage, histologic subtype, and

TABLE 1. **Classification of Malignant Lymphomas: A Practical Modification of the Working Formulation**

Group	Subtype	Frequency (%)
Low grade	Follicular small cleaved cell	16
	Small lymphocytic	6
	Follicular mixed small and large cell	6
Intermediate	Follicular large cell	3
	Diffuse small cleaved cell	6
	Diffuse mixed small and large cell	5
	Diffuse large cell	26
	Immunoblastic	9
High grade	Lymphoblastic	1
	Small non–cleaved cell	
	Burkitt type	1
	Non–Burkitt type	1

treatment, have failed to show any difference in outcome.

Several gaps in the WF have been recognized. Mantle cell lymphoma, also called lymphocytic intermediately differentiated lymphoma, appears to be a distinct subtype with a prognosis and clinical behavior most similar to those of diffuse small cleaved-cell lymphoma. Ki-1 positive anaplastic large cell lymphoma is a type of diffuse large cell lymphoma that stains with an antibody originally thought specific for the Reed-Sternberg cells of Hodgkin's disease. This type of lymphoma has a predisposition for cutaneous and soft tissue involvement and a response to treatment similar to that of the usual large cell lymphomas. HTLV-I–associated lymphoma is a T-cell lymphoma with a tendency to involve skin, bone, bone marrow, and the central nervous system (CNS) and to cause hypercalcemia and to be resistant to standard treatments. Mycosis fungoides and the related Sézary syndrome are cutaneous T cell lymphomas with a typically slowly progressive course culminating in fatal visceral involvement. Splenic lymphoma with villous lymphocytes is a rare lymphoma, probably of B cell origin, with a quite indolent course. Polylobulated lymphoma is a B cell–derived large cell lymphoma with a relatively favorable natural history and good response to multiagent chemotherapy.

About 10% of patients with lymphoma present with apparently different histologic subtypes within one lymph node (composite) or at different sites (discordant). The combination of a mixed or large cell lymphoma at a nodal or extranodal site plus small cleaved cell lymphoma in the bone marrow is common among these patients. About one half of these discordances are trivial, such as follicular mixed at one site and follicular small cleaved cell lymphoma at another, but the other 5% are major (e.g., diffuse large cell and small cleaved cell lymphoma) and require management as though two separate diseases are present. Finally, approximately 5% of lymphomas defy subclassification and fall into a not-otherwise-specifiable category. Despite these inadequacies, the WF is quite useful for most lymphomas and facilitates rational prognostication and treatment.

Staging

In addition to specific histologic subtype, the other major factor affecting treatment outcome for patients with malignant lymphoma is extent of disease. Table 2 shows the minimal testing required to identify the extent or stage of the disease. HIV antibody testing

TABLE 2. Basic Staging Evaluation for Patients with Malignant Lymphoma

History with attention to constitutional symptoms
Examination with attention to lymph node or abdominal organ enlargement
Complete blood counts
Serum creatinine, liver transaminases, lactate dehydrogenase, calcium, protein electrophoresis
Chest radiograph
Bone marrow biopsy and aspiration
Computed tomography of abdomen and pelvis

TABLE 3. A Practical Staging System for the Malignant Lymphomas

Limited	Advanced
Ann Arbor stage I or II and	Ann Arbor stage III or IV or
No B symptoms* and	B symptoms or
No tumor greater than 10 cm in largest diameter	Any tumor greater than or equal to 10 cm in largest diameter

*Fever, night sweats, or more than 10% weight loss.

should be performed in all patients with intermediate or high-grade lymphoma, and the serum uric acid level should be determined if a high tumor burden is present.

Additional testing may be selectively useful. Cerebrospinal fluid, pleural, or peritoneal cytology may reveal disease if symptoms or effusions suggest involvement. Spinal cord compression and soft tissue presentation are best evaluated with magnetic resonance imaging (MRI). Gallium and bone radionuclentide scanning may help localize additional disease and should be performed if bone pain is present or if the existence of additional sites of involvement will affect treatment planning. Contrast studies of the gastrointestinal (GI) tract, including a small bowel followthrough, should be performed when disease presents in the upper aerodigestive tree and will reveal occult involvement in 10 to 20% of such cases. A reciprocal risk of oropharyngeal involvement is present when lymphoma manifests in the stomach or small intestine. It is imperative that the necessary staging evaluation be conducted expeditiously, especially in the presence of intermediate or high-grade lymphoma, because of the potential for rapid evolution or spread of disease even in a matter of weeks. The staging evaluation should be stopped as soon as sufficient information is available to formulate a rational treatment plan.

The usual staging system for malignant lymphoma is the Ann Arbor system, which was borrowed from Hodgkin's disease. It is attractive because of its simplicity and familiarity, but it is only partially applicable to diseases such as the lymphomas that frequently spread widely and hematogenously early in their clinical evolution. The Ann Arbor stage is best viewed as part of the assessment of disease extent to be augmented by additional measures of tumor burden and biologic aggressiveness such as tumor bulk, constitutional symptoms, lactate dehydrogenase levels, and special sites of spread such as the testicles, skin and CNS. A practical, easily applied division of the lymphomas into two broad stages, limited and advanced, is shown in Table 3. Armed with the the histologic subtype and simplified stage, a clinician can anticipate the usual natural history and plan a rational treatment approach for most patients with malignant lymphoma.

TREATMENT

Three major factors must be considered when treatment is planned for malignant lymphoma:

TABLE 4. **Basic Treatment Strategies for Malignant Lymphoma**

Subgroup	Stage	Frequency	Age	Treatment
Low grade	Limited	10%	All	Radiation therapy
	Advanced	90%	All	Chemotherapy
Intermediate	Limited	30%	All	Brief chemotherapy plus radiation therapy
	Advanced	70%	<70 y	Multiagent chemotherapy
			>70 y	Individualized chemotherapy
High grade	All	100%	<60 y	Intensive chemotherapy ± bone marrow transplantation + CNS treatment
			>60 y	Palliative chemotherapy

Abbreviation: CNS = central nervous system.

histologic subtype, stage, and age of the patient. The basic strategy for treatment assignment is shown in Table 4; within this general framework specific individualized plans can be developed in more detail. Regardless of the final plan adopted, certain sites of presentation require special additions to the staging evaluation or treatment strategy; these are shown in Table 5. In general, they should be added to the basic plan of treatment already formulated. In our experience, involvement of the paranasal sinuses or the peripheral blood with intermediate or high-grade lymphoma carries a risk of approximately 50% for leptomeningeal involvement and should always prompt a course of intrathecal chemotherapy once the patient is otherwise in a complete remission. When lymphoma is localized to a testicle or an epidural mass, the risk of CNS disease is low and special measures are not needed, although at least one cerebrospinal fluid cytologic examination should be performed. On the other hand, when disease is more widespread and additional sites are involved along with the testicle or epidural soft tissue or whenever the bone marrow is involved with large cell lymphoma, risk of spread to the leptomeninges is high and a course

of intrathecal chemotherapy is required. Bone marrow involvement with low-grade lymphoma is rarely associated with CNS disease; however, similar involvement with intermediate- or high-grade disease carries a 5 to 25% risk of CNS spread and should prompt strong consideration of intrathecal chemotherapy. Lymphoma in the stomach or small intestine may be associated with abrupt hemorrhage or perforation. This risk is eliminated by local resection, which should be attempted unless it is likely to lead to long-term toxicity or substantial delay in initiation of additional treatment. Attention to all of these special cases is necessary if the clinician wishes to optimize therapeutic outcome.

Low-Grade Lymphomas

Only about 10% of patients with low-grade lymphomas present with limited stage disease. The rest typically have widespread nodal or extranodal involvement. Extranodal disease is seen most frequently in the bone marrow, GI tract, liver, or soft tissue about the upper aerodigestive tract, occasionally in the conjunctiva or lungs, and rarely in skin, muscle, bone, visceral organs

TABLE 5. **Special Additions to Staging or Treatment of Malignant Lymphoma Dependent on Site of Presentation**

Site	Problem/Implication	Response
Waldeyer's ring	GI involvement	Upper GI series and small bowel follow-through
GI tract	Waldeyer's ring involvement	Otolaryngologic examination
Paranasal sinuses	Leptomeningeal spread	Intrathecal chemotherapy
Epidural mass	Leptomeningeal spread	Consider intrathecal chemotherapy
Testicle	Opposite testicle spread	Full scrotal irradiation
	Leptomeningeal spread	Consider intrathecal chemotherapy
Retina, choroid	Opposite eye, brain spread	CNS imaging, consider whole body irradiation
Brain	Retina, choroid spread	Include posterior orbit in irradiation
Bone marrow, peripheral blood	Leptomeningeal spread	Intrathecal chemotherapy if intermediate or high-grade histologic type
Stomach or small intestine	Hemorrhage or perforation	Resection, but only if this can be accomplished with minimal toxicity

Abbreviations: GI = gastrointestinal; CNS = central nervous system.

other than the liver, the CNS, or gonadal or connective tissue. Treatment depends on extent of disease.

The 10% of patients with low-grade lymphomas who have apparently localized disease after standard clinical staging have an excellent prognosis if treated with involved-field irradiation. At our institution, more than 50% of such patients have remained in remission 10 years after diagnosis and few relapses have occurred after 3 years. Those patients with initially localized lymphoma that recurs after irradiation should be managed similarly to those with advanced disease at presentation.

The 90% of patients with low-grade lymphomas found to have advanced disease at diagnosis have a relatively good short-term prognosis. Median survival is age dependent but is usually in excess of 8 to 10 years in reported series. However, the large majority of these patients eventually die of lymphoma despite available treatments. Improved approaches are obviously needed and such patients should be encouraged to enter well-designed clinical trials of new regimens. Because advanced low-grade lymphoma usually pursues an indolent course, is currently not known to be curable, often responds to minimally toxic treatment, and is frequently encountered in patients who are frail due to age or co-morbid illness, it is reasonable to manage patients who cannot enter a clinical trial with a goal of long-term palliation. Such an approach employs observation when the disease is asymptomatic and not threatening to progress in an area of strategic importance, such as next to a ureter where it may cause obstruction. Cosmetically unacceptable or slowly progressive symptomatic disease should be treated with involved-field irradiation if localized or single-agent chlorambucil or cyclophosphamide if widespread. The addition of a corticosteroid may speed the response or quiet associated immunological problems such as immune-mediated hemolytic anemia. Eventually disease will progress despite these measures, and regimens more suitable for initial treatment of intermediate-grade lymphoma become necessary. No treatment approach, even ones based on intensive highly toxic multiagent or high-dose chemotherapy with or without irradiation, has been proven to be superior to conservative measures combining watchful waiting with escalation of treatment as demanded by the disease.

Patients with advanced low-grade lymphoma often develop a more aggressive type of lymphoma secondary to their continued low-grade disease, an event often referred to as transformation. About 5% of patients (the group with discordant lymphoma) will have already developed such transformation at initial diagnosis. Within 5 to 10 years after diagnosis, about 10% of patients with small lymphocytic lymphoma and 50% of those with follicular lymphoma develop clinically evident transformation, and even higher proportions do so by the time of death. Certain characteristic changes often accompany transformation, and patients should be carefully monitored for their appearance: (1) isolated disproportionate progression of a single site of disease; (2) new localized symptomatic disease, especially associated with pain; (3) rapid rise in serum lactate dehydrogenase level; (4) spread of disease to unusual sites such as the CNS, pleura, connective tissues, or skin; (5) hypercalcemia; (6) sudden appearance of fever, night sweats, or weight loss exceeding 10% of the baseline value, especially at times when apparent tumor burden is low or unchanged. Any of these findings, especially if coincidental, should prompt a search for biopsiable material to confirm the change. Fine-needle aspiration biopsy, virtually useless for initial diagnosis, is well suited to detect transformation. If proven or strongly suspected, transformation should prompt initiation of an approach suitable for intermediate-grade lymphoma based on apparent extent of the transformed or discordant disease.

Judicious use of observation, low-toxicity chemotherapy, and irradiation and escalation to multiagent chemotherapy for transformed or otherwise refractory disease can provide a patient with an advanced low-grade lymphoma years of comfortable survival. It is reasonable to hope that treatments currently under investigation, including high-dose chemotherapy with hematopoietic growth factor and stem cell transplantation, monoclonal antibodies with or without linked toxins, biologic agents such as interferon or the interleukins, and the promising new purine analogues such as fludarabine (Fludara) and chlorodeoxyadenosine, will have a major impact over the next decade. Until then the artful application of available treatments will remain a challenging but rewarding area of oncologic practice affording patients useful and prolonged palliative support.

Intermediate-Grade Lymphoma

Most intermediate-grade lymphomas are variants of diffuse large cell lymphoma: diffuse mixed small and large cell, diffuse large cell cleaved, noncleaved, and not subclassifiable and immunoblastic lymphoma. All of these have similar sites of presentation, natural histories and responses to treatment. Although the much less common subtypes of follicular large cell and diffuse small cleaved cell lymphoma may have a course more similar to that of low-grade lymphoma, they at least at times resemble diffuse large cell lymphoma. Because diffuse large cell lymphoma is potentially curable, all patients with an intermediate-grade lymphoma should be considered for treatment with intent to cure.

About 30% of patients with intermediate-grade lymphoma have apparently localized disease at initial evaluation. However this limited extent is only apparent. Treatment with a purely local modality such as involved-field irradiation is followed by relapse rates exceeding 50 to 75%. All such patients should receive initial treatment with multiagent chemotherapy. The best tolerated approach for most patients combines a brief course of multiagent chemotherapy with one of the regimens in Table 6, given for 6 to 12 weeks and followed by involved-field irradiation. Because the irradiation will control the localized disease, the chemotherapy is needed only to treat the occult micrometastatic component. Thus, chemotherapy can be kept quite brief and within the tolerance of even frail or elderly individuals. At our institution the relapse-free and disease-specific survivals in this patient subgroup approach 90%.

Two special subgroups within this set of patients with limited stage disease should be recognized and treated with chemotherapy alone. First are those with disease at a site that would require irradiation of most of the salivary glands including both parotids. Irradiation risks permanent xerostomia and should be avoided in favor of a more prolonged course of chemotherapy if feasible. The second group is composed of those patients whose lymphoma was completely resected at the time of the initial diagnostic biopsy. The only danger to them is distant recurrence and, therefore, they require only brief chemotherapy.

Advanced-stage large cell lymphoma can be cured only with multiagent chemotherapy. Table 6 lists the regimens commonly in use in North America. Results from prospective comparative evaluations of CHOP, M-BACOD, ProMACE-CytaBOM, MACOP-B, and VACOP-B* have now shown that, given with attention to maintenance of dose intensity and optimal supportive care, all of these regimens are equivalent in efficacy and toxicity. Clinicians should choose among them on the basis of cost, duration of treatment, and familiarity with the commonly associated toxicities. Patients treated with these regimens have a likelihood of cure directly related to tumor burden and host tolerance for toxicity. Several studies of prognostic variables have shown that tumor-associated variables such as stage and lactate dehydrogenase level and host-associated factors such as age, constitutional symptoms, and performance status determine outcome. Seventy to 80% of younger fit patients with low tumor burden can be cured using these regimens. Patients with multiple factors indicating poor prognosis are unlikely to be cured with these or any other described regimens and should be enrolled in experimental protocols if at all possible.

A minority of patients who have advanced diffuse large cell lymphoma with favorable prognostic factors and most of those with a poor prognosis fail to enter a complete remission or relapse. Presently most such patients can be offered only palliative short-term control of disease using such secondary regimens as DHAP, ESAP, or MINE† or even single-agent chemotherapy with or without local irradiation. Selected younger patients who develop a relapse with disease that still responds to standard-dose chemotherapy can be offered treatment with high-dose chemoradiotherapy and hematopoietic stem cell transplantation with the expectation that as many as 30% may be cured. Whether these results are superior to what can be achieved with optimal standard-dose chemotherapy plus irradiation in these highly selected patients is open to question and is being addressed by an important European study. When progressive intermediate lymphoma develops any time during or after initial multiagent chemotherapy, it usually proves refractory to available approaches and the best treatment emphasizes palliative measures aimed at achieving symptomatic relief.

High-Grade Lymphomas

Lymphoblastic and small non-cleaved cell Burkitt type lymphomas are uncommon types

TABLE 6. **Chemotherapy Regimens Commonly Used for Intermediate-Grade Lymphomas**

Regimens

Common: CHOP, M-BACOD, ProMACE-CytaBOM, MACOP-B, VACOP-B
Usually secondary: DHAP, MINE, ESAP

Agents

A, H	doxorubicin (Adriamycin), hydroxydaunorubicin
B	bleomycin (Blenoxane)
C	cyclophosphamide (Cytoxan)
Cyta	cytosine arabinoside (Cytosar-U)
D	dexamethasone (Deadron)
E, V	etoposide (VP-16) (VePesid)
I	ifosfamide (Ifex)
M	methotrexate
N	mitoxantrone (Novantrone)
O	vincristine (Oncovin)
P	prednisone (exception: cisplatin (Platinol) in DHAP
Pro	procarbazine (Matulane)
S	methylprednisolone (Solu-Medrol)

*See Table 6 for names of individual drugs.
†See Table 6 for names of specific drugs.

usually seen in children and young adults. These lymphomas are characterized by rapid growth, early dissemination, frequent involvement of the bone marrow and CNS, and remarkable sensitivity to chemotherapy. The non–Burkitt variant of small non–cleaved cell lymphoma is seen more often in older individuals and probably behaves more like large cell lymphoma than the other two high-grade lymphomas. At our institution, such individuals are treated in a fashion identical to that which we use for diffuse large cell lymphoma with comparable results. However, some authorities feel strongly that this group should receive treatment as intensive as that reserved for the Burkitt type variant.

Treatment of patients with lymphoblastic and Burkitt type lymphomas can result in extremely rapid tumor lysis and metabolic overload, especially in the presence of high tumor burden, high pretreatment lactate dehydrogenase level, renal dysfunction, or leukemic phase disease. All patients with lymphoblastic or Burkitt type lymphoma should begin treatment as soon as possible after diagnosis, preferably within 48 hours, whether or not their staging evaluation is complete. Patients at high risk for tumor lysis syndrome should be treated in the hospital with frequent monitoring of serum electrolytes, creatinine, phosphate, and uric acid and vigorous intravenous fluid infusion, allopurinol, urinary alkalinization, and prompt hemodialysis if alarming metabolic deterioration occurs. All patients with lymphoblastic or Burkitt type lymphoma are at high risk for CNS involvement and should receive treatment with at least intrathecal chemotherapy.

Lymphoblastic lymphoma is a T cell lymphoma most frequently seen in young men and often associated with a mediastinal tumor and bone marrow and CNS involvement. Regardless of apparent stage, patients should be treated with regimens appropriate for acute lymphoblastic leukemia. Although some authorities advocate separating patients into good- and poor-risk subgroups, we have not found that useful at our institution where we have been unable to identify a group with better than 50% likelihood of cure with any standard dose protocol. Given the young age of most of these patients we prefer intensive chemoradiotherapy for all with hematopoietic stem cell transplantation, preferably from an HLA-matched donor or, if none is available, using purged autologous bone marrow.

Burkitt type lymphoma is rare in North America. Occasionally patients present with quite localized asymptomatic, low-bulk disease and can be treated effectively with regimens that emphasize higher than usual doses of cyclophosphamide. Most patients have advanced, rapidly progressing disease at diagnosis and should be treated with a regimen of high-dose chemoradiotherapy and hematopoietic stem cell transplantation similar to that used in lymphoblastic lymphoma.

Special Problems

HIV-Related Lymphoma

The AIDS epidemic has not surprisingly been associated with a parallel epidemic of intermediate- and high-grade lymphomas in the same population. This was predictable due to the immunologic compromise caused by HIV-mediated destruction of helper T cells. These lymphomas are of B cell origin and are usually aggressive, often involve extranodal sites, especially the CNS, GI tract, liver, lung, and bone marrow, and are difficult to treat. The major obstacle to effective treatment is the coincident immunologic compromise, which often leads to recurrent infection, malnutrition, deterioration of liver, lung, and other organ function, and impaired hematopoiesis. Patients with HIV-related lymphoma who have normal or only minimally impaired performance status should be treated the same as similar patients without HIV infection, with additional careful attention to prophylaxis of bacterial, viral, and pneumocystis infection. Those with compromised performance status should be treated palliatively.

Primary CNS Lymphoma

Primary lymphoma of the brain usually presents as a space-occupying lesion or global cerebral deterioration. It is seen in about 5% of patients with HIV-related lymphoma and in 1% of all lymphomas. Only rarely does it spread outside of the CNS, but involvement of the choroid or retina is seen in a substantial minority. Standard treatment includes whole-brain and posterior orbital irradiation, but results to date have been unsatisfactory. Long-term survival is seen in fewer than 20 to 30% of patients. Newer protocols testing addition of chemotherapy are in progress.

CUTANEOUS T CELL LYMPHOMA

method of
STANFORD I. LAMBERG, M.D.
Johns Hopkins University School of Medicine
Baltimore, Maryland

Cutaneous T cell lymphoma (CTCL), composed of mycosis fungoides (MF) and its variant, Sézary syndrome (SS), is a malignancy of thymus-derived helper lymphocytes, usually CD4+ in phenotype. Males are affected twice as often as females, and races are affected equally. The average age of onset is 55, although cases do occur in young adults and even children. Occupational exposure to heavy manufacturing or chemicals is associated with an increased risk of CTCL, and family members of patients appear to have a higher than expected frequency of other leukemias or lymphomas.

DIAGNOSIS

In most cases, CTCL begins with subtle lesions that are clinically and pathologically only suggestive of the disease. The first lesions most commonly appear on the lower part of the trunk. Most patients with CTCL have pruritus; itching is especially severe in SS.

In this so-called premycotic phase, the eruption often resembles a common benign disorder, such as psoriasis or atopic eczema. Other more distinctive patterns include poikiloderma atrophicans vasculare, characterized by patches of telangiectasias, atrophy, and pigmentation resembling radiation dermatitis; alopecia mucinosa, patchy hair loss associated with an inflammatory mucinous infiltrate around hair follicles; and large plaque parapsoriasis, usually seen as scaly, pink to dusky, sometimes slightly infiltrated patches. When MF is more advanced, individual plaques become thickened, reddish brown, flat, annular, or serpiginous; and with SS erythroderma develops, accompanied by thickened facial features, enlarged lymph nodes, and large numbers of circulating atypical lymphocytes. When this occurs, histologic sections of skin obtained by biopsy usually show numerous atypical lymphocytes with convoluted nuclei near and within the epidermis as well as clusters within the epidermis (Pautrier's microabscesses).

STAGING

The TNM (Tumor-Node-Metastasis) classification system, modified for CTCL, is most commonly used to describe the extent of disease (Table 1). The presence or absence of those features that have been found to be associated with a differing clinical course and prognosis should first be determined; they can then be used to stage the disease and select therapy. The only clinical variables found to be significantly associated with survival in CTCL are the extent of T (skin) involvement and N (peripheral lymph node) enlargement. Obtaining a peripheral lymph node biopsy is generally not done in early patch/plaque disease, especially if the nodes are not palpable, since such lymph nodes are rarely positive, showing only dermatopathic lymphadenitis. Histologically proven lymph node involvement as well as extracutaneous lymphoma in blood (B) or viscera (M) suggests further shortening of survival and may affect treatment selection.

Tests recommended for evaluation and staging of patients with CTCL are listed in Table 2. A distinction is made in the table between tests known to have prognostic significance, which can be justified as a routine and those more suitable for patients on a research protocol. For example, computed tomographic scans,

TABLE 1. TNM Classification of Cutaneous T Cell Lymphoma (CTCL)

Classification	Description
T:	*Skin**
T0	Clinically and/or histopathologically suspicious lesions
T1	Limited plaques, papules, or eczematous patches covering less than 10% of the skin surface
T2	Generalized plaques, papules, eczematous patches covering 10% or more of the skin surface
T3	Tumors, one or more
T4	Generalized erythroderma
N:	*Peripheral Lymph Nodes†*
	a) Clinical
N0-8	The number of sites of palpable peripheral lymph nodes.
	b) Combined Clinical and Pathologic:
N0	No clinically or palpably abnormal peripheral lymph nodes, pathology negative for CTCL
N1	Clinically abnormal peripheral lymph nodes, pathology positive for CTCL
N2	No clinically abnormal peripheral lymph nodes, pathology positive for CTCL
B:	*Peripheral Blood*
B0	Atypical circulating cells not present or less than 5 per cent
B1	Atypical circulating cells present in 5 per cent or more; total WBC, total lymphocyte counts and number of atypical cells per 100 lymphocytes recorded
M:	*Visceral Organs*
M0	No involvement of visceral organs
M1	Visceral involvement (must have confirmation of pathology; organ involved should be specified)

*Pathology of T1–4 is diagnostic of a CTCL. When characteristics of more than one T exist, all are recorded and the highest is used for staging, e.g., T4(3).

†Cervical (left + right = 2), epitrochlear (1), submandibular (1). Total possible = 8.

which are nearly always negative even in advanced disease, are not justifiable as a routine evaluation procedure.

TREATMENT

Optimal therapy for CTCL has not yet been established. Long remissions and possible cures have been claimed in patients with early disease, but present modes of treatment are not curative for patients with visceral involvement. A recent National Cancer Institute study confirmed the widely held impression that late-stage patients with extensive plaques, tumors, or erythroderma do worse when treated aggressively, usually because of increased susceptibility to superinfection. Left unanswered was the question of whether aggressive (multimodal topical and systemic) therapy or conservative (topical modality)

TABLE 2. **Recommended Evaluation Procedures**

	Routine	Investigational
History and physical examination	X	
Skin biopsy	X	
Complete blood count, serum chemistries, liver function tests, renal function tests, uric acid, serum calcium	X	
Peripheral smear to determine the absolute lymphocyte count and percentage of Sézary cells	X	
Chest radiograph	X	
Scans and/or biopsies of organs when history or physical examination suggests abnormalities	X	
Lymph node biopsy	X (see text)	X
Liver biopsy		X
Bone marrow biopsy		X
Abdominal ultrasound/CT scans		X

therapy is better for patients with early patch/plaque disease because there were too few patients in this group to provide meaningful data.

Development of optimal schedules for present therapies and investigation of new forms of therapy cannot occur unless patients with CTCL are entered into ongoing treatment protocols whenever possible. Most studies permit the referring physician to participate in the continuing care of the patient. Information on studies in progress can be obtained by calling the Cancer Information Service, National Cancer Institute, Bethesda, MD at 1-800-4CANCER.

At present, topical therapy is used for disease considered to be confined to the skin and systemic therapy for disease proven to involve the viscera, including lymph nodes and blood. Total skin electron beam radiation is the most aggressive of the topical options but is the most likely to induce remissions and even "cures." The addition of adjuvant therapy, such as interferons,* in early stages is controversial, with most of its advocates among the European investigators.

Early MF Apparently Confined to the Skin: T_1 and $N_{(any)}$ or T_2 and N_{0-1} (M_0)

Photochemotherapy

PUVA (long-wavelength ultraviolet light [UVA] combined with oral psoralen [P])† suppresses early thin lesions in the majority of cases, espe-

cially if the pathology is only "suspicious" for CTCL. Indeed, in some of these cases the skin may remain clear following a course of therapy but these may represent only cases of parapsoriasis en plaque, rather than CTCL. Control of patients with thickened MF plaques or tumors with definite CTCL pathology is unlikely with this therapy alone, and such patients require frequent maintenance light treatments to maintain control.

Topical Mechlorethamine (Nitrogen Mustard, Mustargen, HN_2)

Topical application of nitrogen mustard* can yield excellent response rates (60 to 90%). In about 10% of patients, the skin remains clear after therapy is stopped, but these are early-stage patients with questionable histologic evidence of CTCL. For thicker plaques and definite histologic evidence of CTCL, sustaining remission usually requires continued use of the agent. Although there is no bone marrow suppression or other systemic toxicity associated with topical HN_2, epidermal neoplasms appear at a severalfold higher rate than is expected, and about a third of users eventually become allergic to the agent.

Instructions. The metal cap of a 10-mg vial of nitrogen mustard [Mustargen]† is removed by the patient and the contents mixed just before use in 1 to 2 oz of water. Standing in a bathtub before bedtime, the patient applies the entire volume from head to toe with a 2-inch nylon brush, reserving a small amount to be further diluted for painting in the intertriginous areas. If the skin is dry and itchy, a teaspoonful of glycerin may be added to the solution. On arising, patients should bathe and can apply an emollient, such as Eucerin.

Nitrogen mustard also can be used in an ointment form (5 × 10-mg vials of Mustargen dissolved in a small amount of absolute or 95% ethanol and mixed into a pound of Aquaphor). The aqueous form may be used to induce the remission and the ointment form for maintenance, particularly with patients who experience excessive dryness from the liquid form. However, no efficacy studies comparing the preparations have been conducted.

Treatment is carried out daily until clearing is complete, which may take several months to a year or even longer. Therapy should then be continued for 6 to 24 months, perhaps at a decreased frequency, and then discontinued. In many patients, lesions clear except for one or a few

---

*This use of interferons is not listed in the manufacturer's offical directive.

†This use of PUVA agent is not listed in the manufacturer's official directive.

---

*This use of nitrogen mustard is not listed in the manufacturer's official directive.

†This use of Mustargen is not listed in the manufacturer's official directive.

patches; such patients seem to require continuous therapy to maintain control. If allergy develops, desensitization can be accomplished in about 50% of patients by using graded increases of diluted HN_2; this is generally managed by dermatologists with prior experience with the agent.

Topical Carmustine (BCNU)

Although less frequently used than HN_2, topical BCNU* is an effective alternative. It is particularly useful for patients who became allergic to HN_2 and who still have early stage disease. However, local irritation and telangiectasias, which usually are persistent, frequently develop, and, because the drug is absorbed, there is a risk of delayed (after 6 weeks) reversible bone marrow depression with decreased leukocytes and platelets.

Instructions. Supply the patient with a stock solution by prescribing a 100-mg vial of BCNU dissolved in 50 ml of absolute or 95% ethanol to be stored at home in the refrigerator. For use, 5 ml of the stock is added to about 60 ml of water and painted on the entire body once daily, as with HN_2. Because of the potential for bone marrow suppression, treatment should continue for only 6 to 8 weeks. If the response is incomplete, this course can be followed immediately by treating individual lesions with the undiluted alcoholic stock solution up to twice daily (up to 70 mg or 35 mL/week), or following a 6-week rest period, the patient can be retreated using twice the concentration (10 mL stock per 60 mL water) for another 6 to 8 weeks. The cycle of treatment can be repeated as necessary to suppress visible lesions.

Complete blood counts, including platelet counts, should be obtained every 2 to 4 weeks during and for 6 weeks after total body and intensive local applications.

Total Skin Electron Beam (TSEB) Radiotherapy

Mycosis fungoides is radiosensitive, and conventional orthovoltage radiation therapy has been used for decades. Total skin electron beam radiation has a distinct advantage over orthovoltage radiation; the penetration of electrons, being particles, can be controlled to reach depths as shallow as a few millimeters, whereas orthovoltage radiation passes deeply into tissues. Thus a large surface dose can be given with electron beam radiotherapy without deep tissue injury or bone marrow suppression.

Most patients in early stages will achieve a complete remission, and substantial numbers (up to a third) will remain free of lesions and, perhaps, cured. TSEB also is useful for later stage disease but must be combined with adjuvant chemotherapy, such as topical HN_2 or low-dose methotrexate, to maintain clearing, as recurrences are common. In late stages, TSEB is less useful, as palliation is only temporary.

Therapy usually is fractionated over 6 to 10 weeks to a total of about 3000 to 3600 cGy. All portions of the body must be treated; a higher recurrence rate was found in patients who elected scalp shielding to prevent hair loss. Acute side effects, which usually subside in a month, include skin edema, erythema, and fissuring. Hair, nails, and sweat glands usually return to normal in 3 to 6 months. The treatment is costly ($5,000 to 10,000). Most large cities have medical centers that offer TSEB.

Later Stage MF with Poorer Prognostic Signs, Although Apparently Confined to the Skin: T_2 and N_2 or T_3 (M_0) (B_0)

Cure is not yet achievable for disease of this extent. These patients respond only partially to PUVA or topical chemotherapy alone, and tend to relapse when radiation therapy is used alone. Generally, some form of radiation therapy (orthovoltage and/or electron beam) is used to induce clearing of thick plaques or tumors, and additional topical or systemic therapy is used to maintain the remission. Maintenance therapy usually is topical HN_2, particularly if the patient recently received TSEB, as PUVA is difficult to administer in that setting. An alternative adjunctive therapy is low-dose oral methotrexate* (25 to 50 mg/week in a single dose).

Late Stage CTCL with Visceral Involvement, Failure of Previous Therapy, or Sézary's Syndrome

Treatment in this stage is palliative. As aggressive systemic chemotherapy can shorten survival of patients with late-stage disease, immunomodulators, such as interferons, extracorporeal photopheresis (if there are significant numbers of circulating Sézary cells), or low-dose single-agent systemic chemotherapeutics seem more useful.

Systemic Chemotherapy

Single drugs that have been effective in some cases include methotrexate,* systemic nitrogen mustard,† cyclophosphamide, and chlorambucil.‡

---

*This use of BCNU is not listed in the manufacturer's official directive.

*This use of methotrexate is not listed in the manufacturer's official directive.

†This use of nitrogen mustard is not listed in the manufacturer's official directive.

‡This use of chlorambucil is not listed in the manufacturer's official directive.

High doses of methotrexate (500 mg per M²) followed by citrovorum factor (25 mg every 8 hours for six doses) have been used to induce remissions in more advanced cases, although resolution of cutaneous tumors usually requires radiotherapy as well. As above, maintaining the remission usually requires continuation of the drug at lower doses, generally 25 to 75 mg per week of methotrexate in a single weekly oral dose.

Therapies undergoing clinical trials include 2′-deoxycoformycin (pentostatin), thymopentin, cis-retinoic acid, fludarabine phosphate, FK506, T cell monoclonal antibodies tagged to cytotoxic agents, tretinoin, and autologous bone marrow transplantation after sublethal radiation and chemotherapy.

Extracorporeal Photopheresis

Extracorporeal photochemotherapy holds promise in the treatment of patients with significant numbers of circulating atypical lymphocytes. In this procedure, the patient's centrifugally separated white blood cells are exposed to UVA in the presence of psoralen and then infused back into the patient. Whether because of a direct cytotoxic effect on the lymphocytes or because of an additional anti-idiotype antibody reaction induced by lymphocyte damage, substantial reduction in the numbers of circulating atypical cells is seen in most patients. Furthermore, skin lesions often improve, presumably due to movement of atypical cells from the skin into the circulation where they can be targeted. Side effects are minimal, but the treatment, given in the hospital over 1 to 2 days monthly, is expensive and not widely available. Adjuvant therapy with interferons may improve the response rate. Continuing trials are being performed, but extracorporeal photopheresis has been approved by the FDA for treatment of CTCL.

Interferons

Interferons, especially recombinant interferon alfa-2a (Roferon-A)* and interferon-gamma (Actimmune),† are proving useful as primary treatment in early-stage CTCL and in combination with radiation, retinoids, or PUVA in later stages. Most patients have an objective response, and up to 20% appear to have a full remission. Although low doses have been tried, most patients require the maximum tolerated dose (15 to 50 million units per day or every other day given intramuscularly or subcutaneously) for maximal response. Patients are expected to develop fever and a flu-like illness for a few days and most have persistent fatigue and anorexia. The degree of leukopenia is the dose-limiting side effect, but recovery is rapid and systemic infections are rare. Intralesional interferon also is useful for individual tumors.

Pruritus

Pruitus is a common, sometimes overwhelming, problem for patients with CTCL. Moderate relief may be gained with systemic antihistamines, such as hydroxyzine, 25 mg orally every 4 hours as needed, and topical emollients, such as Eucerin, or topical corticosteroids, such as betamethasone, fluocinonide, or triamcinolone, in either cream or ointment form applied as needed or overnight under plastic wrap occlusion.

MULTIPLE MYELOMA

method of
MEHDI FARHANGI, M.D.
University of Missouri–Columbia School of Medicine
Columbia, Missouri

Multiple myeloma (MM), presenting predominantly as destructive bone disease, is due to B cell malignancy. Traditionally, the neoplastic cells have been thought of as late, terminally differentiated B cells (plasma cells) that avidly synthesize and secrete immunoglobulin. Recent studies indicate that the neoplastic clone extends to cellular elements with early B cell phenotypic expression. Some tumor cells may bear T cell and myeloid markers. There is ample evidence that the neoplastic process extends to the circulating blood lymphocytes.

The incidence of MM is rising in most of the industrialized world. In the United States, there were an estimated 12,500 cases in 1992, making it the most common hematologic malignancy after non-Hodgkin's lymphoma. There is a high correlation between disease incidence and increasing age with a median age at presentation of 62 to 65 years in most reported series. The incidence is higher in blacks. The etiology of MM is unknown, although in a minority of patients radiation, chronic antigenic stimulation, genetic factors, and chemical exposure in farming and the metals, plastics, rubber, petroleum, and asbestos industries have been incriminated.

LABORATORY STUDIES

A serum monoclonal immunoglobulin (MIg) or a urinary monoclonal light-chain [Bence-Jones (BJ)] protein can be demonstrated in all but 1 to 2% of patients. On electrophoresis, these monoclonal proteins manifest as

---

*This use of interferon-alfa-2a is not listed in the manufacturer's official directive.

†This use of interferon-gamma is not listed in the manufacturer's official directive.

TABLE 1. **Differential Diagnostic Criteria**

Features	MM	SMM	MGUS
Bone marrow plasma cells (%)	>10	>10	<10
Osteolytic lesions	Present	Present	Absent
MIg (gm/dL)	>3.0	>3.0	<3.0
BJ (gm/24 h)	≥0.5	<0.5	<0.5
β_2 Microglobulin	Elevated	Normal range	Normal range
Plasma cell labeling index (%)	>0.5	<0.5	<0.5
Symptoms: bone pain, anemia, renal failure, hypercalcemia	Present	Absent	Absent

Abbreviations: MM = multiple myeloma; SMM = smoldering multiple myeloma; MGUS = monoclonal gammopathy of undetermined significance; MIg = monoclonal immunoglobulin; BJ = Bence-Jones protein.

very tight bands and appear as peaks on densitometer tracings. Because of incoordinate synthesis of light- and heavy-chain immunoglobulins by the malignant plasma cells, BJ protein is excreted in the urine in over 50% of patients. In 25% of cases the BJ protein is the sole monoclonal protein. Therefore, both serum and urine should be analyzed.

The subtype of MIg (IgG, IgA, rarely IgM, IgD, IgE) and of BJ protein (K,L) should be determined by immunofixation or immunoelectrophoresis. The amounts of serum MIg and urinary BJ proteins correlate well with body tumor load, and they can be quantitated periodically during the course of treatment by electrophoresis.

Bone marrow aspiration and biopsy and bone x-rays, but not bone scintigram, are necessary to establish the diagnosis. A near absence of osteoblastic reaction makes bone scintigraphy of doubtful value. The serum beta$_2$ microglobulin level is quite useful for prognostication. The bone marrow plasma cell labeling index, if obtainable is another independent prognostic indicator.

DIAGNOSIS

Multiple myeloma must be differentiated from monoclonal gammopathy of undetermined significance (MGUS). Also due to B cell clonal expansion, MGUS is a benign, or at most a premalignant, condition. To avoid unjustified treatment in patients with MGUS, the diagnosis of MM must be unequivocal. Moreover, a subset of MM patients who have indolent disease, the so-called smoldering multiple myeloma (SMM), may not require treatment and should be identified. Table 1 provides criteria for the differential diagnosis.

PROGNOSIS

Classification of MM patients into three groups (Table 2) provides a measure of survival predictability, with Stage III patients having the shortest life expectancy. The presence of renal failure alters prognosis in a dramatic way. As noted earlier, elevation in the serum beta$_2$ microglobulin level and the marrow plasma cell labeling index indicates a poor prognosis. Newer studies have shown that elevated serum lactic dehydrogenase, DNA hypodiploidy, and plasmablastic cellular morphology each identifies a subset of patients with poor prognosis.

TREATMENT

General Management

Bone resorption in MM is due to increased osteoclastic activity, which in part is mediated by interleukin-1 (IL-1B) and tumor necrosis factor (TNF) produced by the malignant cells. Increased bone resorption leads to development of bone pain in 70% of patients at the time of diagnosis. Pathologic fracture and hypercalcemia are other consequences.

Bone Pain

Acetaminophen and codeine at frequent intervals are often adequate, but at times, narcotic analgesics may be required. The palliation of well-localized pain can be accomplished by the judicial use of radiation. Care must be taken to avoid bone marrow failure due to the use of unnecessarily large radiation fields and irradiation of multiple sites to the detriment of early tumoricidal chemotherapy. Prosthetic devices (lumbar corsets, back braces) can assist early ambulation,

TABLE 2. **Staging Criteria for Multiple Myeloma**

Stages	Corresponding Laboratory Features
I	All of the following must be present: Hb >10 gm/dL Ca <12 mg/dL No or solitary osteolytic lesion MIg: IgG <5.0 gm/dL, IgA <3.0 gm/dL BJ: <0.4 gm/24 h
II	Fulfilling criteria fitting neither those above nor those below
III	One or more of the following must be present: Hb <8.5 gm/dL Ca >12 mg/dL Advanced osteolytic lesions MIg: IgG >7.0 gm/dL, IgA >5.0 gm/dL BJ: >12.0 gm/24 h
Substage A:	BUN <30 mg/dL, creatinine <2.0 mg/dL
Substage B:	BUN >30 mg/dL, creatinine >2.0 mg/dL

Abbreviations: Hb = hemoglobin; Ca = calcium; MIg = monoclonal immunoglobulin; BJ = Bence-Jones protein; BUN = blood urea nitrogen.

particularly in patients with spinal instability. The long-term use of such devices, however, should be discouraged to avoid acceleration of bone resorption in the immobilized segment. Radiculopathy, often associated with paroxysmal exacerbation of pain and muscle spasm, can be very troubling and unresponsive to analgesics alone. Adequate pain medication together with diazepam and the use of braces are recommended.

Hypercalcemia

Mild hypercalcemia (<12 mg/dL) can be treated with isotonic saline diuresis to produce a 24-hour urine volume of 3 liters or more. Furosemide (Lasix), 40 to 80 mg once or twice daily, can be used to avoid volume overload. Prednisone, 1.0 to 1.5 mg per kg per day, is quite effective in the treatment of hypercalcemia associated with MM. Together with saline diuresis it should be the first choice for patients with moderate to severe hypercalcemia. Patients failing to respond to prednisone and isotonic saline diuresis can be treated with pamidronate (Aredia), 60 to 90 mg as a single intravenous infusion over 24 hours, or etidronate (Didronel), 7.5 mg per kg in 250 mL saline intravenously for 3 to 5 days. Salmon calcitonin in a dose of 200 to 400 Medical Research Council (MRC) units subcutaneously every 12 hours together with prednisone, 40 to 60 mg per day, is also recommended.

Renal Failure

Among several causes of renal failure in MM (e.g., hypercalcemia, infection, hyperviscosity, amyloidosis), the myeloma kidney (cast nephropathy) caused by nephrotoxic BJ proteins accounts for the majority of cases. Myeloma kidney is at times precipitated by fluid depletion due to diarrhea, vomiting, nephrotoxic antibiotics, nonsteroidal anti-inflammatory drugs, and radiocontrast materials used in angiography and pyelography. Avoidance of these precipitators and maintenance of adequate fluid intake appear justified. Hemodialysis may be required if symptomatic renal failure due to myeloma kidney proves irreversible after adequate diuresis. Chronic hemodialysis is particularly rewarding in patients who have previously responded to cytotoxic chemotherapy. Repeated plasmapheresis is reported to produce renal functional improvement by some authors, but others have not found it useful.

Neurologic Complications

Myelopathy due to spinal cord compression must be ruled out by careful neurologic examination in patients with back pain. Magnetic resonance imaging, myelography, or computed tomographic scanning should be employed in suspected cases. External beam radiation may prevent catastrophic paralysis in patients with incipient myelopathy. Occasionally, myelopathic paralysis can be reversed if radiation and dexamethasone (4 to 8 mg four times daily) are administered less than 24 hours after onset.

Meningeal myelomatosis is a rare complication occurring mostly in patients with advanced disease. Intrathecal methotrexate or cytosine arabinoside and brain irradiation can be beneficial. The demonstration of MIg in the spinal fluid is not adequate for the diagnosis; malignant cells must also be present.

Hyperviscosity

In contrast to macroglobulinemia, the hyperviscosity syndrome occurs uncommonly in MM. By virtue of their molecular structure the IgA and IgG3 paraproteins can occur as polymers, and this accounts for most of the hyperviscosity in MM. A serum-to-water viscosity ratio of greater than 6 at 37° C (normal 1.4 to 1.8) is almost always associated with hyperviscosity syndrome.

Plasmapheresis is the mainstay of treatment. By using a continuous flow cell separator, theoretically all circulatory blood can be processed in 2 to 3 hours. Patients exhibiting central nervous system manifestations, bleeding, or cardiovascular symptoms attributable to hyperviscosity should be treated. Pheresis is performed daily or on alternate days with 1 to 2 liters of plasma processed each day until symptomatic improvement is attained.

Rapid removal of large volume of plasma can cause orthostatic hypotension and cardiac arrhythmias. Moreover, since plasmapheresis requires the administration of heparin and citrate, the possibility of hypocalcemia and heparin-associated thrombocytopenia should be borne in mind. The depletion of coagulant proteins is another potential complication. Use of fresh-frozen plasma and replacement of plasma volume using human albumin may reduce the risks.

Chemotherapy

The choice of chemotherapy agents is somewhat controversial. Since the 1960s, it has been established that melphalan (Alkeran) and prednisone (M&P) produces objective response in 50 to 60% of patients. The median survival has been prolonged from 9 to 11 months in the prechemotherapy era to 30 to 40 months currently. Several randomized studies have shown that polychemotherapy using four or five drugs produces higher response rates, particularly in patients with Stage III disease, without increasing survival

TABLE 3. **Drug Regimens for Multiple Myeloma**

M&P

    Melphalan 0.15 mg/kg, PO, for 7 days
    Prednisone 20 mg PO, three times daily for 7 days
    Repeat this treatment every 6 weeks
    Increase daily dose of melphalan by 2 mg in the next
        cycle until midcycle cytopenia is produced

VBMCP

    Vincristine 1.2 mg/M^2 IV, day 1
    Carmustine 20 mg/M^2 IV, day 1
    Cyclophosphamide 400 mg/M^2 IV, day 1
    Melphalan 8 mg/M^2 PO, days 1–4
    Prednisone 40 mg/M^2 PO, days 1–7 and 20 mg/M^2 PO,
        days 8–14
    Repeat this treatment every 5 weeks

VMCP–VBAP

  VMCP

    Vincristine 1 mg/M^2 IV*, day 1
    Melphalan 6 mg/M^2 PO, days 1–4
    Cyclophosphamide 125 mg/M^2 PO, days 1–4
    Prednisone 60 mg/M^2 PO, days 1–4
    Alternate VMCP with VBAP (see below) every 3 weeks

  VBAP

    Vincristine 1 mg/M^2 IV*, day 1
    Carmustine 30 mg/M^2 IV/1 h, day 1
    Doxorubicin 30 mg/M^2 IV, day 1
    Prednisone 60 mg/M^2 PO, days 1–4

ABCM

  AB

    Doxorubicin 30 mg/M^2, day 1
    Carmustine 30 mg/M^2 IV, day 1
    Alternate AB with CM (see below) every 3 weeks

  CM

    Cyclophosphamide 100 mg/M^2 PO, days 1–4
    Melphalan 6 mg M_2 PO, days 1–4

VAD:

    Vincristine 0.4 mg continuous IV infusion, days 1–4
    Doxorubicin 9 mg/M^2 continuous IV infusion, days 1–4
    Dexamethasone 40 mg PO, days 1–4, 9–12, 17–20
    Repeat cycles every 28 days

Abbreviations: PO = by mouth; IV = intravenously.
*Maximum, 1.5 mg.

when compared with the M&P regimen. Polychemotherapy programs have been associated with greater toxicity, and a recent meta-analysis of the randomized studies confirmed these empirical conclusions. Table 3 describes the M&P regimen and common polychemotherapy regimens, such as VBMCP, VMCP-VBAP, and ABCM.* In view of the fact that polychemotherapy regimens produce a better and faster response but with greater toxicity, Stage III patients with better performance status might be treated with such programs, with M&P administered to all others.

The role of interferon in the treatment of MM remains to be established. Given as a single agent in otherwise untreated patients, it produces brief remission in one third of the patients,

*See Table 3 for names of specific agents.

a result which is inferior to that obtained with M&P and polychemotherapy. Thus far, when administered in combination with chemotherapy, interferon does not prolong survival, although a pilot study showed more complete responses when interferon was combined with the VBMCP regimen. The final answer awaits the completion of the ongoing randomized study by the Eastern Cooperative Oncology Group.

Maintenance Treatment

In responders, a plateau phase occurs that is characterized by stable levels of MIg and BJ protein, continuation of symptom-free status, and hematologic improvement. In approximately 10% of patients treated with M&P and a higher percentage receiving polychemotherapy, the myeloma proteins become nondetectable and the percentage of bone marrow plasma cells drops into normal range (complete responders). The plateau phase is associated with low levels of serum beta$_2$ microglobulin and a low plasma cell labeling index.

The necessity of continuing chemotherapy during the plateau phase has been questioned. In fact, treatment can be terminated and resumed when signs of disease progression appear without reducing life expectancy. Based on work by the Italian Myeloma Study Group, the administration of interferon during the plateau phase causes prolongation of the first remission, but does not increase overall survival.

Advanced Phase Disease

Three sets of patients fall into this group. The first consists of patients who have relapsed after a period of unmaintained remission. Such patients stand a good chance of responding to primary chemotherapy, particularly if the interval has exceeded 6 months. The second set of patients are those who have become refractory to chemotherapy after an initial response. At this phase of disease, the biologic signs of aggressive disease, such as extraosseous plasmacytoma, hypercalcemia, plasma cell leukemia, and a lymphoma-like myeloma associated with elevated serum lactic dehydrogenase, can be identified in some patients. Thus far, the VAD regimen (Table 3) appears to be most effective in patients refractory to M&P and polychemotherapy. A response rate of 40 to 60% with a median survival of 1 to 1½ years has been reported. The treatment requires hospitalization, and toxicity can be severe. High-dose corticosteroids alone are occasionally effective.

The third set of patients are those who exhibit refractoriness from the onset. Such unresponsiveness is an ominous prognostic signal, since response to alternate regimens is unrewarding. An objective response to the VAD regimen is seen in 40% and to high-dose glucocorticord in 30% of such patients.

Radiation Therapy

As mentioned previously, radiation therapy can play a useful role in the palliation of well-localized bone pain. In advanced disease when all cytotoxic treatments have been exhausted, the technique of hemibody radiation can be employed for pain relief. However, fatal myelotoxicity can follow hemibody radiation, and therefore this treatment modality should be reserved for symptom relief in terminally ill patients.

A curative dose of radiation should be administered to patients who present with solitary plasmacytoma in whom a careful examination of the skeleton by bone x-rays and bone marrow aspiration and biopsy fails to show the spread of disease.

High-Dose Chemotherapy with Syngeneic, Allogeneic, and Autologous Bone Marrow Transplantation

Because of the advanced age of most myeloma patients, the problem of graft-versus-host disease (GVHD), and the risk of infection, only a limited number of patients have undergone bone marrow transplantation. Two of seven patients who received syngeneic bone marrow transplantation have lived 7 and 14 years, suggesting that bone marrow transplantation with high-dose chemotherapy can be rewarding. The European Bone Marrow Transplantation group has reported the largest series of patients receiving allogeneic bone marrow transplantation after total body irradiation and cyclophosphamide (Cytoxan) with or without other drugs. The percentage of complete responders has been high (43%), and patients who received one-drug therapy prior to transplantation had a particularly good success rate (60%). Unfortunately the transplantation-related mortality has also been high (40%).

Because of the advanced age of many patients with myeloma and the lack of suitable donors, high-dose chemotherapy with purged or unpurged autologous bone marrow is being tried in a few centers. High-dose melphalan, total body irradiation, or other drug regimens were employed prior to the administration of autologous bone marrow. It has been estimated that 10 to 30% of patients with refractory disease will achieve a complete remission. The use of peripheral stem cells for grafting is also being studied.

Thanks to the progress made in the treatment of MM over the last three decades, improved duration and quality of life can be expected in the majority of patients.

POLYCYTHEMIA VERA

method of
KAUSHIK A. SHASTRI, M.D., and
GERALD L. LOGUE, M.D.
State University of New York at Buffalo
Buffalo, New York

Polycythemia vera, a disease that occurs more often in persons of middle age or older, is a clonal malignancy of hematopoietic stem cells. This disease is closely linked to the other three myeloproliferative disorders arising at the stem cell level, namely, chronic myelogenous leukemia, essential thrombocythemia, and agnogenic myeloid metaplasia. Polycythemia vera often undergoes transition to myeloid metaplasia or may terminate into acute leukemia. In a few cases, essential thrombocytosis precedes the polycythemia. In polycythemia vera, erythropoiesis is autonomous and independent of erythropoietin stimulation; therefore, erythropoietin levels are suppressed. The expanded red cell mass from the abnormal clone signals for a reduction in erythropoietin secretion, which further hampers the proliferation of the remaining normal erythroid progenitors.

The increased blood viscosity from an enlarged red cell mass gives rise to headaches, dizziness, and visual disturbances. The sluggish flow of viscous blood and increased hemoglobin concentration can lead to peripheral cyanosis and overall ruddy appearance. Splenic enlargement is almost always present in polycythemia vera, a feature that distinguishes it from secondary polycythemia. Increased gastric acid secretion stimulated by increased histamine release and mucosal ischemia caused by hyperviscosity lead to increased incidence of peptic ulcers in polycythemia vera. Generalized itching, especially after showering or bathing, although not very common, is a distinctive complaint. This symptom has generally been attributed to histamine release from the increased basophils. However, one study found correlation between the increase in the number of skin mast cells and itching, and not with the number of circulating basophils. The increased cellular turnover in polycythemia vera leads to hyperuricemia and increased incidence of gout, renal stones, and nephropathy. Fatigue, generalized weakness, and mild fever result from an overall hypermetabolic state.

Thrombotic as well as hemorrhagic complications occur due to hyperviscosity, thrombocytosis, platelet dysfunction, and increased interaction between platelets and vascular endothelium. Thrombosis accounts for one-third of the deaths in polycythemia vera. The vessels generally involved are the cerebral, coronary, and abdominal vessels. Polycythemia vera is one of the most common predisposing causes of hepatic vein thrombosis (Budd-Chiari syndrome).

During the later stages of the disease, bone marrow

fibrosis and myeloid metaplasia occur. This stage of disease is known as spent polycythemia or post polycythemic myeloid metaplasia and occurs with the same incidence in patients treated with myelosuppressive therapy as with phlebotomy alone. These patients are at an increased risk of developing acute leukemia. The fibrosis is reactive in nature and the fibroblasts are not a part of the malignant clone. Myeloid metaplasia with extramedullary hematopoiesis in the spleen and liver can cause extensive enlargement of these organs. The enlarged spleen causes hypersplenism with pancytopenia and is prone to infarctions. This stage of disease is usually accompanied by abnormalities seen on peripheral blood smear such as the tear drop and other misshapen red cells, nucleated red cells, immature white cells, and thrombocytopenia.

Acute leukemia is part of the natural history of polycythemia vera and occurs with a frequency of 1 to 2% in patients treated with phlebotomy alone. This incidence approaches 10 to 15% in patients treated with alkylating agents. The acute leukemia is usually of acute nonlymphocytic variety, is abrupt in onset, and is generally less responsive to chemotherapy than the de novo acute nonlymphocytic leukemia.

DIAGNOSIS

In the differential diagnosis of erythrocytosis, it is important to distinguish absolute polycythemia, in which there is an increase in the red cell mass, from relative polycythemia, in which the red cell mass is normal but the plasma volume is contracted.

Table 1 shows causes of absolute polycythemia. When an increase in the red cell mass occurs due to the autonomous production, it is called polycythemia vera. Secondary polycythemia, which is far more common, occurs due to increased erythrocyte production as a result of excess erythropoietin stimulus as in hypox-

emia, abnormal hemoglobins, or tumors producing erythropoietin. A very common but often underappreciated cause of mild erythrocytosis is smoker's polycythemia. It has been estimated that increased hematocrit values occur in up to 3% of all cigarette smokers. This elevation of the hematocrit in smokers is due to an absolute increase in the red cell mass and is reversible upon cessation of smoking. Cigarette smokers have carboxyhemoglobin levels that range from 3 to 20% (normal levels <0.5%). Increased levels of carboxyhemoglobin stimulate erythropoietin primarily through tissue hypoxia produced by decreased oxygen carrying capacity. Carboxyhemoglobin determinations provide the diagnosis but should preferably be done in the evening when concentration is highest, after daytime smoking.

The Polycythemia Vera Study Group proposed the diagnostic criteria and classifications according to their relative significance into:

Category A:
1. Increased red cell mass (males $\geq$36 mL per kg; females $\geq$32 mL per kg)
2. Normal arterial oxygen saturation ($\geq$92%)
3. Splenomegaly

Category B:
1. Thrombocytosis (platelets $\geq$400 $\times$ 10^9 per liter)
2. Leukocytosis (white count $\geq$12 $\times$ 10^9 per liter in absence of fever or infection)
3. Elevated leukocyte alkaline phosphatase score over 100 in the absence of fever or infection
4. Elevated serum vitamin B_{12} level over 900 pg per mL or unbound vitamin B_{12} binding capacity over 2200 pg per mL.

The diagnosis of polycythemia vera may be made with reasonable certainty if (1) all the criteria from category A are present or (2) the combination of an elevated red cell mass and normal arterial oxygen saturation is present with any two criteria from category B.

While these criteria serve as useful guidelines, they are not foolproof. Measures to exclude secondary polycythemia should be undertaken in all cases, unless the diagnosis is obvious. A smoker who also has alcoholic liver disease may meet all the criteria despite not having polycythemia vera. On the other hand, many patients with early polycythemia do not meet the criteria. Additionally, up to 10% of patients with polycythemia vera have developed significant iron deficiency prior to the diagnosis and usually present with thrombocytosis and normal red cell mass with microcytosis. Correction of iron deficiency may be necessary to establish the diagnosis of polycythemia vera.

TABLE 1. Causes of Increased Red Cell Mass

Primary polycythemia
  (polycythemia vera) (erythropoietin decreased)
Secondary polycythemia
  Increased erythropoietin production
    Appropriate
      Hypoxemia as a result of:
        (1) Pulmonary disease
        (2) High altitude
        (3) Right-to-left cardiac shunts
      Abnormal oxygen delivery
        (1) Hereditary high-affinity hemoglobins
        (2) Carboxyhemoglobinemia (smokers)
    Inappropriate
      Neoplasia
        Hepatoma, hypernephroma, adrenal and ovarian
          carcinomas
        Large uterine fibroids
        Cerebellar hemangioblastomas
      Non-neoplastic conditions
        Renal cysts
        Hydronephrosis
        Post–renal transplantation
  Increased sensitivity to erythropoietin
    Administration of androgens

MANAGEMENT

Polycythemia vera is a disease that is easily treatable but that leads to permanent disability or death if therapy is deferred or inadequate. Untreated polycythemia vera is a serious disease with a median survival of less than 2 years. Despite the malignant nature of the disease, meticulous patient management and control of disease produces a life expectancy that does not differ from that of the age-matched population without polycythemia vera. The major goal of therapy for polycythemia vera is the normalization of hematologic parameters, particularly the hematocrit. If this can be achieved, most of the early complications can be avoided.

Phlebotomy

Phlebotomy is the preferred treatment for younger patients. In the initial phases of treatment, 500 mL of blood is removed twice a week until a hematocrit of about 45% is achieved. Removal of this amount of blood during each venesection does not require replacement with intravenous fluids if adequate oral hydration is maintained. Older patients or patients with cardiovascular disease should have 300 to 350 mL of blood removed per session. Removal of 1 unit of blood results in a loss of 250 mg of iron. Because most patients with polycythemia vera have depleted bone marrow iron stores, clinical iron deficiency soon sets in after initiation of the phlebotomy program. The hematocrit remains controlled due to lack of iron and microcytosis; consequently, patients require fewer phlebotomies; some patients require as few as three or four phlebotomies per year. Iron supplements should not be given to patients with polycythemia vera because it would only increase the need for more phlebotomies. The nonhematologic effects of chronic iron deficiency state, such as chronic fatigue, dysphagia, soreness or burning of the tongue, fissures at the corners of the mouth, pica, and koilonychia, are generally not problematic in these patients. However, should they become intolerable, judicious iron supplementation with more frequent phlebotomies may have to be employed.

Myelosuppressive Therapy

Inasmuch as alkylating agents have been associated with increased risk of leukemia in patients with polycythemia vera, their use is no longer recommended. In the Polycythemia Vera Study Group experience, the risk factors that could be identified for thrombosis were previous history of thrombosis, age older than 70 years, and the phlebotomy program itself. Because of the increased risk of thrombosis associated with age, patients older than 70 years are most effectively treated with myelosuppression and supplemental phlebotomy. Although there are no conclusive data, most physicians would treat excessive thrombocytosis in this disease (in excess of 1 million per μL) with myelosuppressive therapy. Excessive and symptomatic splenic en-largement, poor veins, bone tenderness, and intractable pruritus are other indications for addition of myelosuppressive therapy.

Hydroxyurea (Hydrea) is a nonalkylating myelosuppressive agent specific for the inhibition of the cells in the S phase of the cell cycle. Its apparent mechanism of action is a decrease in DNA synthesis by inhibition of ribonucleoside diphosphate reductase. Hydroxyurea has not been found to be leukemogenic in other disease states. Although its lack of leukemogenicity in polycythemia has not been definitely confirmed, in a series of 51 patients with polycythemia vera treated with hydroxyurea for a median duration of 5 years, the incidence of leukemia was similar to that in patients treated with phlebotomy alone. The usual starting dose is 1 gram, given orally every day with careful monitoring of blood counts at least once per week. When the platelet counts return to normal range, the dose is reduced to the lowest levels possible. This could range from 500 mg per day to 500 mg two to three times per week. Because hydroxyurea results in a megaloblastic blood picture with increased mean corpuscular volume (MCV), its effect on hematocrit is slower, and initially supplemental phlebotomies are required. Toxicity of this agent is minimal at doses employed for polycythemia vera and is limited to gastrointestinal intolerance, occasional rash, or fever. If there is no response in the spleen size or blood counts, the dose may be increased to 1.5 grams per day and then subsequently reduced when desired hematologic parameters are achieved. Unfortunately, sustained remission is not usually possible with discontinuation of hydroxyurea. Hence, the drug usually has to be continued indefinitely, and strict patient compliance is vital to the success of this modality of treatment.

Radioactive phosphorus (sodium phosphate P 32), is a strong beta-ray–emitting agent that, when given intravenously, is concentrated to some degree in the mitotically active cells in the bone marrow, liver, and spleen. As with alkylating agents, its use in polycythemia vera is associated with increased incidence of leukemia. In addition, it has also been associated with an increase in the incidence of nonhematologic malignancies. It should therefore be used only in elderly patients requiring myelosuppressive therapy but not responding to hydroxyurea. Hence, radioactive phosphorus is rarely used. After an initial dose of 2.5 mCi per M^2 intravenously, maximal suppression of marrow proliferation, reduction in spleen size, and normalization of hematologic indices occurs in 10 weeks. A second small dose of 1.5 mCi per M^2 may be required 12 to 16 weeks after the initial injection in order to achieve optimal control. Responsive patients may have a remission lasting 6 to 24 months.

Other Treatment Considerations

Because of the relative success of alpha-interferon in chronic myeloid leukemia, its use in polycythemia vera has been of recent interest. An added theoretical attraction of interferon therapy is its ability to inhibit the fibroblast-stimulating platelet-derived growth factor. Thus, the use of alpha-interferon may prevent the development of myelofibrosis, part of the natural history of polycythemia vera. The experience with this agent is still very limited, but a few patients treated with this agent appear to have had an adequate control of hematocrits after 6 months without subsequent phlebotomies. The initial dose employed in this disease ranges from 3 to 5×10^6 units, three to five times per week, with subsequent reduction to achieve the minimal dose required to sustain continued response. Early side effects associated with alpha-interferon include flu-like symptoms such as fever, fatigue, and muscle and bone pain. Reported late toxic reactions that occur during chronic therapy include fatigue, dry skin, weight loss, and neurotoxicity. More experience in a clinical trial setting is needed before interferon can be recommended as a first-line therapy for polycythemia vera.

Aspirin and dipyridamole (Persantine), when used in conjunction with phlebotomy, have failed to reduce the incidence of thrombosis in patients with polycythemia vera and have caused an increase in hemorrhagic complications. Therefore, long-term prophylactic use of these agents is not recommended. Use of platelet-antiaggregating agents may be considered during transient attacks of digital, cerebral, or cardiac ischemia. All of these situations, however, require myelosuppressive therapy to normalize hematologic parameters.

Anagrelide is a member of the quinazolin series of compounds with a powerful antiaggregating effect on platelets. During studies in humans, anagrelide was found to produce thrombocytopenia in doses that were far below those required for its antiaggregating effects on platelets. In a large clinical trial, daily use of anagrelide reduced platelet counts in 40 of the 47 evaluated patients who had polycythemia vera. The median duration of response was 7.7 months in these patients. This drug does require daily administration, since platelet counts returned to pretreatment levels within 4 days of discontinuation of the drug. The more frequent side effects include fluid retention, papitations, headaches, dizziness, nausea, and diarrhea. When commercially available, this agent may be useful in treating thrombocytosis associated with polycythemia vera.

For patients with elevated uric acid levels, allopurinol (Zyloprim), 300 mg per day, is given to prevent the complications of hyperuricemia. This generally needs to be given only during the initial phase of therapy, and once the disease is under control, it may be stopped.

Pruritus related to the release of histamine may be relieved by oral cyproheptadine (Periactin) in doses of 8 to 16 mg per day, as needed. Phlebotomy does not relieve pruritus, but half of the patients on myelosuppressive therapy get relief from this symptom.

Treatment of Late Complications

Treatment of spent phase (myelofibrotic stage) of polycythemia vera is extremely difficult and at times frustrating. For the anemia, evidence of iron or folate deficiency should be sought and corrected if found. Androgens may stimulate erythropoiesis and should be tried; however, the response is slow and therapy should be continued for at least 6 months. Splenomegaly is associated with expansion of plasma volume and in some patients, anemia may be dilutional. Massive splenomegaly may respond to hydroxyurea, and radiation therapy to the spleen in small doses is occasionally helpful. Splenectomy may benefit selected patients with hypersplenism. However, splenectomy in patients with postpolycythemic myeloid metaplasia is associated with significant mortality, with increased incidence of excessive hemorrhage and infections.

Treatment of acute leukemia developing in patients with polycythemia vera is disappointing. As with patients who have other secondary leukemias, these patients have a very poor survival. Another contributing risk factor is the older age of these patients. In younger patients, with good performance status, conventional chemotherapy schedules for acute leukemia can be attempted. In others, supportive therapy with transfusions and antibiotics for infections may be appropriate.

Surgery in Patients with Polycythemia Vera

Performance of surgical procedures on patients with uncontrolled polycythemia vera carries excessively high morbidity and mortality. Hence, elective surgery should not be performed until hematologic control is achieved and maintained for at least 4 months. If emergency surgery is necessary, the patient should be phlebotomized rapidly to attempt to achieve a near normal hematocrit. Following both emergency and elective surgery, the patient should be mobilized as early as possible to prevent thrombotic complications.

Pregnancy and Polycythemia Vera

Polycythemia vera occurs infrequently during childbearing years. Spontaneous abortions and pre-eclampsia have been reported to occur more frequently in these patients. Expansion of plasma volume and suppression of erythropoiesis due to high estrogen levels may lead to normalization of hematocrit during pregnancy and thus obviate the need for specific therapy. Judicious phlebotomy during pregnancy may be used to keep hematocrit values around 45%.

Choice of Therapy

Appropriate management of patients with polycythemia vera is rewarding because the benefits conferred by proper treatment are dramatic in terms of improved survival and well-being. Most patients can be treated with phlebotomy alone. Myelosuppressive therapy with hydroxyurea may be added for patients older than 70 years of age, those with excessive thrombocytosis, those with prior history of thrombosis, and those with symptomatic splenomegaly.

THE PORPHYRIAS

method of
GEORGE H. ELDER, M.D.
University of Wales College of Medicine
Cardiff, United Kingdom

The porphyrias are a group of disorders of heme biosynthesis in which characteristic clinical symptoms occur in association with overproduction of heme precursors. Each porphyria results from a partial deficiency of one of the enzymes of heme biosynthesis (Table 1). Two main types of illness characterize the porphyrias: acute neurovisceral attacks and skin lesions. The former are always associated with overproduction of the porphyrin precursors porphobilinogen (PBG) and 5-aminolevulinic acid (ALA). The latter are caused by photosensitization through deposition of porphyrins in the skin. All the porphyrias, except some forms of porphyria cutanea tarda (PCT), are inherited but clinical penetrance of the autosomal dominant disorders is low; probably no more than 10% of those who inherit the enzyme deficiencies ever have clinical symptoms. Patients with the more severe forms may wish to join support groups such as those provided by the American Porphyria Foundation or, in the United Kingdom, the Research Trust for Metabolic Diseases in Children.

THE ACUTE PORPHYRIAS

The clinical features of acute porphyria are identical in acute intermittent porphyria (AIP), variegate porphyria (VP), and hereditary coproporphyria (HC) and are neurologic in origin. Almost all patients have severe abdominal pain, often accompanied by pain in the back and extremities, nausea, vomiting, and constipation. Peripheral neuropathy develops in about 60% of patients who are ill enough to require hospitalization and may progress to respiratory paralysis. Mental confusion, often with hallucinations, is common and there may be convulsions, sometimes associated with hyponatremia. Tachycardia and mild hypertension are frequently seen.

The diagnosis is established by demonstrating increased PBG excretion (Table 1). Further investigation to determine the type of porphyria can wait until after treatment has been started. Acute porphyria is very rare before puberty, has its peak incidence between the late teens and midthirties, and is commoner in women. Attacks vary greatly in severity and frequency; many patients have only a single acute illness, others may suffer frequent reccurrence or have repetitive premenstrual attacks. Recovery after attacks is usually complete; probably fewer than 5% of attacks that require hospitalization end fatally. Attacks can occur spontaneously, but most are precipitated by drugs, alcohol, reduced caloric intake (dieting, acute illness), or endocrine factors. Lists of drugs that are unsafe (barbiturates, most anticonvulsants, sulfonamides, griseofulvin, oral contraceptives and many others) and those that are safe in the acute porphyrias are given in "The Porphyrias" in Scriver, Beaudet, Sly, and Valle's *The Metabolic Basis of Inherited Diseases* (6th ed., New York, McGraw-Hill, 1989, pp 1305–1365) and in Adverse Drug Reaction Bulletin, No. 129, April 1988.

Early diagnosis and consequent early treatment are important. Initially, any drugs or other potential precipitating factors should be stopped. Two specific treatments are available: carbohydrate loading and intravenous hematin. Both suppress ALA and PBG formation in the liver, and the latter replenishes hepatic heme. Patients should be advised to increase their carbohydrate intake by taking sweetened drinks (e.g., glucose polymers) as soon as they feel an attack coming on; newly diagnosed patients should similarly be given carbohydrates (through a nasogastric tube if there is nausea and vomiting), to achieve an intake of around 400 grams per day. Intravenous infusion of carbohydrate (20% levulose, up to 2 liters per day) is required if hematin is not available and the attack worsens.

Hematin should be administered as soon as

TABLE 1. **The Main Types of Porphyria**

Porphyria	Defective Enzyme	Main Clinical Features	Laboratory Diagnosis	Inheritance
ALA-dehydratase deficiency	ALA-dehydratase	Neurovisceral	↑ ALA (urine)	Autosomal recessive
Acute intermittent porphyria (AIP)	Porphobilinogen deaminase	Neurovisceral	↑ PBG→ALA (urine)*	Autosomal dominant
Congenital erythropoietic porphyria (CEP)	Uroporphyrinogen III synthase	Cutaneous	↑ Uro- and coproporphyrin I (urine) ↑ Coproporphyrin I (feces)	Autosomal recessive
Porphyria cutanea tarda (PCT)	Uroporphyrinogen decarboxylase	Cutaneous	↑ Uroporphyrin and 7-5 carboxylic porphyrins (urine) ↑ Isocoproporphyrin (feces)	Complex (20% autosomal dominant)
Hereditary coproporphyria (HC)	Coproporphyrinogen oxidase	Neurovisceral ± cutaneous	↑ PBG>ALA, coproporphyrin (urine) ↑ Coproporphyrin III (feces)*†	Autosomal dominant
Variegate porphyria (VP)	Protoporphyrinogen oxidase	Cutaneous ± neurovisceral	↑ PBG>ALA (urine) ↑ Proto>coproporphyrin (feces)	Autosomal dominant
Erythropoietic protoporphyria (EPP)	Ferrochelatase	Cutaneous	↑ Free protoporphyrin (erythrocytes)	Autosomal dominant

*PBG may polymerize to porphyrin and other compounds in urine (red-brown color).
†In VP and HC, PBG and ALA are increased only during acute neurovisceral attacks.
Abbreviations: ALA = 5-aminolevulinic acid; PBG = porphobilinogen.

possible to all patients admitted with acute symptoms, unless there are clear signs of clinical improvement. Two preparations are available: lyophilized hematin (Panhematin, Abbott Laboratories) and heme arginate (Normosang, Huhtamaki Oy Leiras, Turku, Finland). The latter is more stable and may produce fewer side effects, but it is not licensed for use in the United States. Both should be used immediately after solubilization (addition of albumin may help to stabilize Panhematin). The dose is 2 to 4 mg per kg body weight given intravenously over a period of about 15 minutes into either a large peripheral vein (if possible, a different one each day) or through a central venous line to decrease the risk of thrombophlebitis. Infusion should be repeated once or twice daily until symptoms improve, up to a maximum of 7 days. Most patients given Normosang, 3 mg per kg per day) improve within 5 days. Hematin can produce transient coagulation abnormalities and should not be used with anticoagulants.

Other treatment is symptomatic. Pain can be controlled by nonopioid analgesics but is usually severe enough to require intramuscular pethidine (meperidine), which should be given as required.

Concurrent administration of chlorpromazine or promazine and nursing in a quiet, darkened room may help to decrease the need for analgesics and control distress and agitation. In patients who have frequent attacks or chronic pain between attacks, efforts should be made to avoid prolonged use of addictive analgesics. Nausea and vomiting may respond to phenothiazines or cyclizine hydrochloride and severe constipation to neostigmine. Tachycardia and hypertension should be controlled with propranolol. Patients with progressive neuropathy or cardiovascular instability should be monitored (expiratory peak flow rate, ECG) to predict any need for assisted ventilation and to avoid precipitation of cardiovascular collapse by paroxysmal tachycardias. Severe hyponatremia, possibly caused by excessive secretion of antidiuretic hormone, may be exacerbated by intravenous fluid therapy which, if required for dehydration, should be carefully controlled. Hyponatremia usually responds to fluid restriction. Seizures are best treated with diazepam.

Prevention of acute attacks is the other important aspect of the management of acute porphyrias. Relatives of patients should be screened by a specialist laboratory (measurement of erythrocyte PBG deaminase and/or DNA analysis is required for AIP) to identify genetic carriers. Affected individuals should then be advised to avoid known precipitants, particularly drugs. One way of doing this is to give them a list of drugs that are known to be safe in acute porphyria and suggest that they take no others unless given medical advice to the contrary. They should also wear a bracelet or necklace or carry a card saying that they have porphyria. For patients who have recurrent premenstrual attacks, suppression of ovulation with luteinizing hormone–releasing hormone analogues may be effective.

CUTANEOUS PORPHYRIAS

Skins lesions can be prevented or controlled by avoiding direct sunlight by staying indoors, wearing appropriate clothes, or using reflectant sunscreen creams with high UVA protective efficacy, such as Uvistat Ultrablock cream (SPF30) (Windsor),* which are cosmetically more acceptable than older preparations.

Erythropoietic Protoporphyria

Patients with erythropoietic protoporphyria (EPP) have acute photosensitivity, which usually starts in early childhood. An unpredictable minority develop irreversible hepatic failure secondary to accumulation of protoporphyrin in the liver.

In addition to avoiding sunlight, skin damage can be minimized by building up a protective layer of beta-carotene, which blocks photodamage by acting as a singlet oxygen trap. In adults, the optimal serum carotene concentration of 6 to 8 mg per liter is achieved by an oral dose of 10 to 180 mg of beta-carotene per day. At this concentration the skin turns orange-yellow. No toxic effects have been reported but some patients find it unpleasant to take or cannot tolerate the skin discoloration, and not all find it beneficial. Alternative treatments under evaluation include oral N-acetylcysteine.

Liver failure is difficult to predict. All patients should be monitored by half yearly or yearly biochemical tests of liver function and investigated further if abnormalities persist or worsen. Further accumulation of protoporphyrin in the liver may be slowed if its enterohepatic circulation is interrupted with oral cholestyramine or activated charcoal, but the only successful treatment for established hepatic failure is liver transplantation.

Porphyria Cutanea Tarda

Porphyria cutanea tarda (PCT) is the commonest form of porphyria. The skin lesions (bullae, fragility, hypertrichosis, pigmentation) usually occur in association with liver damage caused by alcohol, other types of liver disease, or estrogen preparations for contraception or other purposes. Most patients have hepatic siderosis.

On diagnosis, provoking agents such as alcohol should be avoided, although the treatments suggested will still be effective if they are not. PCT responds to two specific treatments that are ineffective in other cutaneous porphyrias: depletion of body iron stores by phlebotomy and low-dose chloroquine. Phlebotomy of 1 unit of blood is carried out every week or two until iron stores are depleted, as judged by a fall in transferrin saturation to 15% or hemoglobin to 11 to 12 gram per dL, or by decreased serum ferritin concentration. This usually requires about 8 to 12 phlebotomies and may precede any clinical improvement or substantial decrease in porphyrin excretion. Full remission, which may last for years, usually follows within about 6 months. For PCT in patients undergoing chronic hemodialysis, erythropoietin, with or without phlebotomy, may deplete hepatic iron stores and produce remission.

Alternatively, PCT can be treated with oral chloroquine (125 mg twice weekly for adults, less for children). This usually produces clinical improvement in about 4 months but should be continued until urinary uroporphyrin excretion decreases to around 100 μg per day, which usually takes at least 10 months.

Both treatments are similarly effective. Venesection ensures compliance but may be unsafe in ischemic heart disease, difficult to perform, or poorly tolerated. Drawbacks to chloroquine are poor compliance and potential hepatotoxicity, although there is no evidence to suggest that liver damage in PCT is worsened. During remission, patients can be monitored by measuring urinary uroporphyrin excretion, and treatment can be restarted if concentrations reach around 1000 μg per liter.

Congenital Erythropoietic Porphyria

Congenital erythropoietic porphyria (CEP) (Table 1) is a rare disorder in which skin lesions develop soon after birth and may progress to severe photomutilation. Hemolytic anemia of varying severity is common. A milder, late-onset form also occurs.

Management requires strict avoidance of sunlight and prompt treatment of secondary skin infections. Hypertransfusion and intravenous infusion of hematin to suppress porphyrin production are not practical for the long term. The use of oral activated charcoal to trap porphyrin in the gut remains under evaluation. Treatment of the hemolytic anemia may require splenectomy and repeated transfusion. Prenatal diagnosis of the infantile form is both feasible and justified.

---

*Not available in the United States.

THERAPEUTIC USE OF BLOOD COMPONENTS

method of
CATHY CONRY-CANTILENA, M.D., and
HARVEY G. KLEIN, M.D.
National Institutes of Health
Bethesda, Maryland

Transfusion therapy has changed over the last decade since the acquired immunodeficiency syndrome (AIDS) was determined to be transmissible by transfusion. The general public and the average physician appear more aware of the risks of blood transfusion despite the fact that blood is safer than ever before. Caution is desirable if it means that more thought is given to specific use of appropriate blood components and to suitable alternatives, but concerns should not interdict or delay transfusion when it is indicated.

Currently, the estimated risk for exposure to the human immunodeficiency virus (HIV) is small, approximately one case per 225,000 units transfused. Since testing for the hepatitis C virus began in 1990, the risk for acquiring hepatitis has fallen to less than 1% per transfusion episode. Potential for exposure to a variety of other organisms remains (such as malarial parasites and trypanosomes); however, in the United States, life-threatening infection as a result of blood transfusion is fortunately rare.

Other adverse effects of blood transfusion include a variety of allergic reactions and volume overload. (These adverse effects are discussed in greater detail in the following article, "Adverse Reactions to Blood Transfusion.") Red blood cell (RBC) alloimmunization occurs with a frequency of approximately 1% per unit transfused. Febrile transfusion reactions, while common, are of limited clinical importance. Hemolytic transfusion reactions occur infrequently (1 per 6000 units transfused). Fatal transfusion reactions are even less likely (1 per 100,000); most are the result of clerical error, especially in emergency situations.

Transfusion must be justified on an individual basis to minimize risk and maximize benefit. Suitable alternatives and adjunctive therapy should be sought for specific clinical situations to avoid unnecessary blood use.

BLOOD COLLECTION AND STORAGE

Almost all blood in the United States is collected from volunteer donors who are meticulously screened. All components are tested (currently with seven tests) to minimize the risk of transfusion-transmitted disease. Volunteer donors provide approximately 450 mL of whole blood (WB) collected into sterile plastic bags containing a citrated anticoagulant/preservative solution. For this reason calcium-containing solutions should not be mixed with stored blood or it will clot. To simplify separation, WB is collected into a system of sterile bags, and components are prepared by centrifugation. Fresh WB is separated into RBCs, platelets, and plasma. RBCs can be stored for up to 42 days or further processed. Platelets from single units of blood are referred to as "random donor" platelets and can be stored at room temperature for up to 5 days. Four to ten units are "pooled" immediately prior to transfusion. Plasma can be refrigerated as liquid plasma or frozen ($-18°$ C) within 6 hours of collection for future use to provide fresh-frozen plasma (FFP). Cryoprecipitate (antihemophilic factor, or CRYO) can subsequently be harvested from FFP. Derivatives of plasma, such as albumin and immune serum globulin are prepared by commercial manufacturers from pools of thousands of plasma units using cold ethanol precipitation.

WHOLE BLOOD AND RED BLOOD CELLS

Whole blood (WB) is indicated for actively bleeding patients who have lost 30% or more of their blood volume. It provides both oxygen-carrying capacity and blood volume expansion. Since WB can be refrigerated for weeks, platelets and granulocytes contained in WB units are not clinically functional.

WB can be used in "massive transfusion" settings such as severe trauma or rapid, unanticipated operative blood loss. In emergency situations or exsanguination in which the patient's blood type is unknown, non–crossmatched group O WB can be administered while cross-matching of compatible units is underway. Crystalloid and colloid infusions should be started immediately to support intravascular volume expansion and tissue perfusion. Rapid infusion of refrigerated RBCs can lower the body temperature; therefore, use of an in-line blood warmer may be advisable.

As mentioned, WB is indicated when volume expansion and increased oxygen-carrying capacity are required. The plasma portion generally contains therapeutic doses of most clotting factor proteins except for labile factors V and VIII; however, even these proteins are present in reduced amounts. While massive transfusion with banked blood dilutes out platelets, use of WB can retard the loss of plasma coagulation factors by dilution. WB can also be employed for neonatal exchange transfusion but should be less than 7 days old to minimize potassium load and provide adequate RBC 2,3-diphosphoglycerate content. There are few other indications for fresh WB. One unit of WB should increase hemoglobin 1 gram per dL in the average adult. For pediatric patients, 3 mL of WB per kg should produce an incremental increase in hemoglobin of 1 gram per dL.

RBCs (given with or without crystalloid and

colloid solutions) increase oxygen-carrying capacity and are indicated for most situations in which blood loss results in symptomatic anemia. "Standing orders" using hemoglobin levels as the only guide for transfusion should be avoided; the "transfusion trigger" should be tailored to an individual patient's needs. A hemoglobin level of 8 grams per dL may be adequate, provided there is no impairment of tissue oxygenation. In young individuals or those with chronic anemias, other physiologic compensatory mechanisms (such as increased cardiac output and improved oxygen delivery to tissues) can reduce the need for RBCs. However, patients who cannot appropriately increase cardiac output due to underlying disease may require transfusion to raise the hemoglobin level enough to ensure adequate tissue oxygenation.

The usual dose for RBCs is the same as that for WB. One unit of RBCs is infused through 170-μ filter to remove particulate debris, generally over 1 to 2 hours or as tolerated with careful monitoring for adverse effects. Acetaminophen can be given to the patient as premedication to prevent nonhemolytic febrile reactions. Addition of solutions other than normal saline can cause hemolysis or agglutination of RBCs and should be undertaken with caution. Chronic transfusion therapy results in iron overload, and chelation therapy should be considered for patients who have received more than 50 RBC transfusions.

Saline Washed Red Blood Cells

The purpose of washing RBCs with normal saline is to remove plasma. As an added benefit, washing reduces the number of white blood cells (WBCs) by about 80%. Although washing is not the most efficient method of leukocyte removal, it can help to prevent both febrile and allergic transfusion reactions. Saline washing of RBCs using automated equipment can remove 99% of the plasma with a small amount of RBC loss. Since washing of RBCs violates the sterility of the closed storage system, washed RBCs must be transfused within 24 hours. Transfusion of blood or components that contain IgA can cause anaphylaxis in IgA-deficient recipients. Therefore, washed RBCs may be indicated in this situation when IgA-deficient or autologous blood is unavailable. Washed RBCs for patients with paroxysmal nocturnal hemoglobinuria have been advocated, but group-specific RBCs transfused through a leukocyte reduction filter (as described later) are sufficient in most cases.

Leukocyte-Reduced Red Blood Cells

Leukocyte-reduced (leuko-reduced) RBCs by definition contain less than 80% of the original WBC content, which is usually sufficient to prevent febrile reactions. Reduction can be achieved by removal of a buffy coat layer by centrifugation, saline washing, or microaggregate filtration. Newly developed leukocyte-removal RBC filters can effect a 3-log reduction in the number of WBCs per unit while retaining more than 85% of the RBCs in the original unit. Use of such leuko-reduced RBCs ($<5 \times 10^6$ WBC) appears to decrease the rate of HLA alloimmunization and may eliminate transmission of such cell-associated viruses as HTLV-1 and cytomegalovirus. Leuko-reduced components may be advantageous for previously minimally transfused patients who require lengthy transfusion support during chemotherapy or for transplant patients. Expense limits more widespread use of these filters.

Frozen Deglycerolized Red Blood Cells

RBCs can be frozen using glycerol as a cryoprotectant and stored at temperatures below $-65°$ C for 10 years or longer. After being thawed and washed to remove glycerol, these frozen RBCs are essentially plasma free and leuko-reduced. Additionally, freezing does not alter their survival or functional characteristics. Freezing, thawing, and washing must be performed by trained staff to prevent hemolysis, and thawed and washed units must be used within 24 hours of deglycerolization. If postthaw washing is incomplete, osmotic lysis of transfused cells can result in hemoglobinuria. Indications are limited to patients with rare blood types, autologous storage, and neonatal transfusion.

PLATELETS

Platelets are transfused to effect hemostasis or to prevent bleeding in patients with low levels of circulating platelets or qualitative platelet dysfunction. An individual "unit" of platelets is prepared from WB and contains at least 5.5×10^{10} platelets in 50 to 70 mL of plasma. Six to eight units can be pooled to provide a standard dose of "random donor" platelets for administration to an average adult. Platelets should be administered within 4 hours of pooling. Single-donor apheresis platelets collected with automated instruments should contain more than 3×10^{11} platelets (about 8 units) in 200 to 300 mL of donor plasma. A variety of instruments can collect platelets by centrifugation with little WBC contamination but not with sufficient reliability to prevent alloimmunization to HLA antigens. HLA-compatible single-donor platelets are the components of choice for patients who have acquired HLA alloantibodies and immune platelet refractoriness (see further on).

There are a variety of indications for platelet transfusions. Patients with platelet counts of less than 20,000 per μL may be predisposed to bleeding. Prophylaxis of spontaneous hemorrhage via platelet concentrate transfusion may be advisable, especially if the patient is febrile or has infection or if the platelet count has been falling rapidly. With platelet counts of less than 10,000 per μL, the risk of serious spontaneous hemorrhage is great and prophylactic platelet transfusion is often prudent. For patients with platelet counts in the 20,000 to 50,000 per μL range, excessive bleeding during invasive procedures can be prevented by prophylactic use of platelet concentrates. For major operative procedures, platelet counts in the 50,000 to 100,000 per μL range are desirable and should be maintained for several days. During massive transfusion, platelets may be required to thwart the dilutional "washout" of platelets; 6 units of platelets for every 10 to 20 units of RBCs is a useful rule of thumb, but usage should be monitored with platelet counts. For patients with adequate platelet numbers but qualitative platelet defects, platelets can be administered along with pharmacologic therapy (such as DDAVP for uremic patients) for bleeding episodes. Rough guidelines for platelet dosage are as follows: For an adult, one unit of random donor platelets should increase the platelet count five-10,000 per μL. For infants and small children, the same dose should increase platelet counts by seventy-five to 100,000 per μL. More precise platelet increments can be calculated with the following formula for "corrected count increment":

$$\frac{\text{Post–platelet increment} - \text{Pre–platelet increment}}{\text{Number of platelets transfused} \times 10^{11}} \times \text{body surface area (M}^2\text{)}$$

A patient can be considered platelet refractory when a dose of platelets less than 24 hours old fails to result in a corrected increment of greater than 5000 per μL on two occasions. Good practice includes monitoring the effectiveness of platelet transfusions with a post-transfusion platelet count drawn 15 to 60 minutes after platelet infusion. Factors that contribute to poor platelet increments include fever, sepsis, disseminated intravascular coagulation, hypersplenism, platelet autoantibodies, and poor-quality platelet concentrate, as well as platelet and HLA alloimmunization to HLA- and platelet-specific antigens. If a serum screen is positive for HLA alloantibodies, subsequent avoidance of these HLA antigens using HLA-typed single-donor apheresis platelet concentrates can improve platelet increments. Platelet crossmatching, while employed in some centers, is not yet a standardized laboratory technique. The use of ABO-compatible platelet concentrates generally results in better yields and therefore is preferable but not required. Out-of-group plasma can be minimized by volume reduction of the platelet concentrate when necessary.

Rh_o (D) sensitization can occur if Rh positive platelets are given to an Rh-negative recipient as a result of the small number of RBCs that are transfused in each bag. Anti-Rh_o (D) hyperimmune globulin can be given in standard doses (300 μg per 15 mL RBCs transfused) to prevent the formation of anti-D in Rh-negative recipients. This is especially important in Rh-negative women of childbearing age.

Leukoreduction of platelets with high-efficiency filters can decrease the rate of HLA alloimmunization and probably cytomegalovirus (CMV) infection when CMV-negative donors are not available. Platelets can be washed and frozen but these are not standard techniques for platelets as they are for RBCs.

GRANULOCYTES

Granulocytes are collected by apheresis and have been traditionally used for severely granulocytopenic patients with gram-negative infections. One "unit" of granulocytes contains approximately 0.8 to 3.5 × 10^{10} granulocytes, about 1/40th the number of cells a normal individual mobilizes for infection. Since granulocyte concentrates contain a large number of RBCs (hematocrit, 20 to 30%), the granulocyte unit must be crossmatch compatible. Because granulocytes lose function rapidly after procurement, they should be transfused as soon as possible after collection, and certainly within 24 hours.

Modern antibiotics have made granulocyte transfusions less valuable, although they are still useful for patients with severe neutropenia (absolute neutrophil count <500 per μL) and sepsis or continued fever despite appropriate antibiotic therapy or for progressive local infection. They are also used as adjunctive therapy in neonatal sepsis. The utility of granulocyte therapy in fungal infections is unknown. Prolonged courses (weeks) of granulocytes reportedly help patients with chronic granulomatous disease and documented infection. One unit of granulocytes should be infused over 2 to 4 hours. Once begun, daily infusions are given for a minimum of 4 days.

Adverse effects of granulocyte transfusions are common and include fever, chills, and shortness of breath. Respiratory distress can be related to HLA alloimmunization with pulmonary sequestration of granulocytes. In view of the severe reactions and the likelihood that granulocytes will not migrate to sites of infection in an alloimmune recipient, development of HLA alloimmunization is a contraindication to further granulocyte transfusion therapy. If amphotericin B therapy is also required, it should be temporally separated from granulocyte transfusion, since pulmonary compromise has been reported with their concomitant administration. WBC concentrates from CMV-positive donors are likely to transmit CMV. The large number of lymphocytes poses a risk for transfusion-associated graft-versus-host disease in susceptible recipients. Since hazards of granulocyte transfusion can be significant, the potential benefits should be weighed carefully before a course of therapy is undertaken.

PLASMA

Refrigerated liquid plasma contains all the stable clotting factors. Labile clotting factors V, VIII, and von Willebrand factor diminish in plasma that is stored at 1 to 6° beyond 6 hours. Clotting factors are present at an average level of 1 unit per mL, and fibrinogen levels average 1 to 2 mg per mL. The indications for liquid plasma transfusion are similar to those for FFP, except for states in which the labile factors are deficient. FFP contains factors V and VIII and all clotting factors (approximately 1 unit per mL); levels of all the coagulation proteins can vary somewhat with each unit of FFP. A hemostatic dose for infusion is 10 to 15 mL per kg. To prevent allergic responses to plasma infusion, particularly urticaria, diphenhydramine (Benadryl), 25 to 50 mg, can be used as premedication.

Plasma has been considered the most misused blood component. Therapeutic guidelines for FFP use were established at a National Institutes of Health consensus conference in 1984. FFP should not be used for volume expansion, wound healing, or nutritional supplementation. Indications for appropriate use include specific clotting factor deficiencies when specific concentrates are unavailable or unsafe; traumatic or operative blood loss requiring massive transfusion with documented coagulopathy and bleeding; bleeding or invasive procedures when a coagulopathy exists as a result of liver dysfunction; rapid reversal of warfarin therapy; and treatment of thrombotic thrombocytopenic purpura in conjunction with plasma exchange. Plasma therapy should be monitored by assessment of prothrombin time, partial thromboplastin time, or specific factor levels when appropriate. Plasma infusions will not reverse the anticoagulation induced by heparin.

CRYOPRECIPITATED ANTIHEMOPHILIC FACTOR

Cryoprecipitated antihemophilic factor (CRYO) is the cold insoluble portion of plasma remaining after FFP is thawed. It contains clotting factor VIII (FVIII), von Willebrand factor, factor XIII, fibrinogen, and fibronectin. The yield of FVIII is 40 to 60% (80 to 120 units). Fibrinogen levels are usually 150 to 250 mg per bag of CRYO. Fibronectin has no standard clinical uses as yet. Each "bag" has a volume of 15 to 20 ml. The usual therapeutic dose of CRYO requires the thawing and pooling of 10 to 20 bags, which will provide an average adult with approximately 2 grams of fibrinogen and 2000 units of the other coagulation proteins.

CRYO has been used to control bleeding in patients with hemophilia A or von Willebrand's disease, although factor concentrates are generally safer today. Factor XIII and fibrinogen deficiencies, while rare, respond to CRYO replacement. CRYO has also been reported to be effective in controlling bleeding in uremic patients with platelet dysfunction. Many physicians use a combination of CRYO and platelet transfusion to support patients with disseminated intravascular coagulation until the underlying disease process is controlled. CRYO does not contain factor IX and is ineffective for patients with hemophilia B (Christmas disease). "Fibrin glue" is prepared for topical hemostasis by mixing CRYO with thrombin directly at the site of bleeding.

Although CRYO contains concentrated FVIII, the protein can be further purified; however, yield is sacrificed at the expense of purity. FVIII concentrate is commercially available as a lyophilized product. It is obtained by fractionation of pooled plasma from thousands of donors, and in the past recipients had a high risk of contracting a transfusion-transmitted disease. Current manufacturing processes, including heat treatment, have probably eliminated the risk of HIV and hepatitis transmission.

FVIII content is expressed as units per mg protein on the label. After reconstitution, FVIII concentrate is administered at 10 to 20 units per kg for episodes of acute bleeding or for bleeding prophylaxis in hemophilia A. Specific doses can be adjusted based on clinical need, degree of deficiency, and plasma level to be obtained. FVIII half-life is approximately 10 hours. It can be given as a constant infusion perioperatively. Approximately 10% of patients with hemophilia A who have been treated with clotting factors develop FVIII antibodies that can inhibit the activity of FVIII concentrate. Immunosuppression and desensitization strategies have had limited success in these patients; however, commercially available anti-inhibitor complex has been effective in some patients with FVIII antibodies who require treatment.

Factor IX concentrate or prothrombin complex (PTC) is available as the lyophilized preparation of clotting factors II, VII, IX, and X; the units for each protein are specified on the label. PTC is used in congenital clotting factor deficiencies with clinical bleeding and, specifically, factor IX deficiency (hemophilia B). The half-life of factor IX is 18 to 24 hours. PTC is well-known for its thrombogenic properties. As with FVIII concentrate, the risk of acquiring HIV infection or hepatitis is diminished by heat treatment of this blood product. Recombinant factors have proven safe and effective, and recombinant FVIII has been licensed, but cost has limited its widespread use.

IRRADIATION OF BLOOD

Transfusion of immunologically competent T lymphocytes can initiate graft-versus-host reaction in susceptible patients. Transfusion-associated graft-versus-host disease (TA-GHVD) has a reported mortality exceeding 90%. Cellular blood components contain varying numbers of lymphocytes, therefore leuko-depletion alone is probably not sufficient to prevent TA-GVHD. Irradiation of blood or blood components with 25 Gy (2500 rads) is sufficient to prevent activity of immunocompetent lymphocytes. Patients at high risk for development of TA-GVHD whose blood should be irradiated prior to transfusion include bone marrow transplant recipients, premature neonates and fetuses, and patients with congenital immunodeficiency syndromes (subacute combined immunodeficiency disease and Wiskott-Aldrich syndrome), acute and chronic leukemias, lymphomas, several other malignancies, and patients receiving directed blood donations from relatives. Irradiation does not prevent febrile reactions or transfusion of infectious agents, nor do the blood components carry risk of radiation injury to the recipient. Despite severe immune compromise, AIDS patients have not yet been reported to develop TA-GVHD and are not currently restricted to receiving irradiated blood components.

ALTERNATIVES TO ALLOGENEIC TRANSFUSION

Pre-donation of the patient's own (autologous) whole blood is desirable when an elective operative procedure is planned and the patient's health does not preclude blood donation. Autologous blood is the safest blood. Several studies suggest that "directed" blood donation (blood from friends and relatives of a specific patient) may carry a greater risk of infectious complications than donations from volunteers; directed donations are a form of allogeneic donation and should not be confused with autologous blood. Autologous blood may be refrigerated or stored frozen for future use for rare donor types. Autologous blood should not be transfused simply because of its availability but should be used as indicated just as allogeneic transfusions. Other methods used to minimize perioperative allogeneic blood use are intraoperative blood salvage, preoperative hemodilution, and postoperative blood salvage techniques. Intraoperative salvage is most useful when large-volume loss is anticipated (open heart surgery, orthopedic procedures) and postoperative salvage may not save enough to be practical.

Human serum albumin is a fractionation plasma component. Viral inactivation is accomplished by treating this product for 10 hours at 60° C. Albumin is available as 5% and 25% solutions and is the active component of plasma protein fraction (PPF). Approximately 96% of the albumin solution is albumin; the remaining 4% is globulin. In contrast, PPF contains approximately 83% albumin, the rest consisting of alpha and beta globulins. Albumin is responsible for providing the majority of plasma's colloid oncotic pressure and remains predominantly in the intravascular space after administration; therefore, its primary use is as a volume expander. Support of intravascular volume is particularly important in burn patients and in patients with hypotension and shock. Albumin can be used as a replacement solution after plasmapheresis. Crystalloid solutions are usually used as adjunctive therapy when albumin is administered. PPF has been reported to cause hypotensive reactions thought to be secondary to the presence of prekallikrein activator, and there is no reason to prefer it to albumin.

Blood substitutes are commonly used in clinical practice to provide volume expansion and intravascular oncotic pressure. Most often, albumin solutions are used for this purpose. Hydroxyethyl starch, pentastarch, and low-molecular-weight dextran are less frequently used colloids. Dextrans interfere with platelet function and have been associated with an increased bleeding tendency. Candidate RBC substitutes that could provide oxygen-carrying capacity include perfluorochemicals and modified hemoglobins, but as yet, no RBC substitute has proven safe and effective.

ADVERSE REACTIONS TO BLOOD TRANSFUSION

method of
RICHARD NEWMAN, M.D.
University of California, Irvine, Medical Center
Orange, California

As with other treatment modalities in medicine, a risk/benefit assessment must be performed in arriving at a decision of whether or not to transfuse blood or any of its components—platelets, white cells, cryopre-cipitate, and fresh frozen plasma. In order to perform this assessment, physicians must be knowledgeable about the potential adverse consequences of blood transfusion and their relative frequencies so as to intelligently discuss these risks with patients (Table 1). In addition, physicians must know these risks so that if an adverse reaction does occur, they can institute immediate and potentially lifesaving therapy.

Transfusion reactions can be classified as either acute—within 24 hours of transfusion—or delayed—occurring days, weeks, months, or years later, and as either hemolytic or nonhemolytic, with potentially life-threatening consequences observed with either type (Table 2).

ACUTE HEMOLYTIC REACTIONS

Acute hemolytic transfusion reactions are most frequently due to ABO incompatibility between patient and donor. They can occur after infusion of any blood product (red cells, white cells, platelets, or fresh frozen plasma). Usually, the donor red cells have an antigen (A or B) not found on the patient red cells, although rarely the reverse can be true (i.e., patient red cells have an antigen not found on donor red cells, and the donor plasma has an antibody). Less commonly, acute hemolytic reactions are seen when a patient has an antibody to a donor red cell antigen such as Rh, Kell, Kidd, and Duffy. Rarely, acute hemolytic reactions are seen in patients with paroxysmal nocturnal hemoglobinuria, an acquired hemolytic anemia due to a red cell membrane defect predisposing a patient's cells to lysis by activated complement C5b-9. Due to this defect, these red cells are prone to lyse when patients are transfused; what would be considered negligible complement activation in a normal individual due to recognition of another individual's white blood cells, platelets, and plasma proteins is enough to lyse the red cells of these patients. Consequently, these patients are usually transfused only with washed red cells.

Symptoms of an acute hemolytic transfusion reaction can include any of the following: heat or pain at the site of infusion, fever, chills, lower back pain, chest pain, abdominal pain, nausea, and a feeling of apprehension or impending doom. Signs of this reaction include hypotension, hemoglobinuria, renal failure, and a generalized bleeding diathesis. The severity of the reaction is proportional to the amount of incompatible blood given; hence, whenever a potential reaction is suspected, the transfusion should be immediately stopped, although normal saline should be kept flowing in the patient's intravenous line. The blood bank should be immediately notified of this reaction because where there is one patient getting a wrong unit of blood, there may be another patient about to get a wrong unit because of a clerical mix-up.

To analyze whether a reaction has occurred, blood samples are drawn from the patient and sent to the blood bank. In the laboratory, the patient's serum is checked visually for hemoglobin (i.e., pink or red color) and a direct Coombs' test on ethylenediaminetetra-acetic acid (EDTA)-anticoagulated blood is performed in order to detect antibody coating of the patient's red blood cells.

The three most dangerous sequelae of an acute hemolytic transfusion reaction are renal failure (associated with a 50% mortality rate), shock, and disseminated intravascular coagulation (DIC). To counteract hypotension and minimize the risk of renal failure, intravenous saline should be administered in an attempt to keep urine output at 100 mL per hour. If a pressor is

TABLE 1. **Classification of Transfusion Reactions by Frequency per Unit Transfused**

	Frequency
Acute	
Febrile	1/200
Urticarial	1/200
Fluid overload	?
Immunologically mediated pulmonary edema	1/10,000
Acute hemolytic	1/25,000
Septic shock	
Yersinia enterocolitica	1/40,000
Other bacteria	1/360,000
Anaphylactic hypotensive	1/150,000
Paroxysmal nocturnal hemoglobinuria	Rare
Other (air embolism, citrate toxicity, hyperkalemia, hypothermia)	Unknown
Delayed	
CMV seroconversion	1/14
Viral hepatitis	1/1000
HTLV I infection	1/60,000
Delayed hemolytic	1/2,500
Malaria	Rare
AIDS (HIV-1)	1/100,000
Leukemia (HTLV I)	Rare
Graft-versus-host disease	Rare
Post-transfusion purpura	Rare

Abbreviations: CMV = cytomegalovirus; HTLV = human T lymphotropic virus; AIDS = acquired immunodeficiency syndrome; HIV = human immunodeficiency virus.

TABLE 2. **Classification of Transfusion Reactions by Type**

Acute hemolytic
   ABO incompatibility
   Other red cell antigens
   Paroxysmal nocturnal hemoglobinuria
Acute nonhemolytic
   Respiratory distress
     Fluid overload
     Immunologic mediated pulmonary edema
     Bacterial contamination of donor blood
     Anaphylaxis
     Air embolism and microembolism
   Cardiac arrhythmia
     Hypothermia
     Potassium toxicity
     Citrate toxicity
   "Mild" reactions
     Febrile
     Urticarial
Delayed hemolytic
Delayed nonhemolytic
   Infectious diseases
     Viral hepatitis
     Cytomegalovirus
     HIV-1 and 2
     HTLV I
     Malaria
     Other infectious diseases
   Graft-versus-host disease
   Post-transfusion purpura

Abbreviations: HIV = human immunodeficiency virus; HTLV = human T lymphotropic virus.

required, dopamine is the pressor of choice because at low dosage (<2 μg per kg per minute), its effect is to increase renal blood flow, whereas other pressors decrease renal perfusion; above 20 μg per kg per minute, renal vascular dilation and increased perfusion may not be seen. Intravenous furosemide (Lasix), 20 to 40 mg, repeated as necessary, should also be used. DIC with renal vascular obstruction is also believed to contribute to renal failure; however, the use of heparin to counteract DIC remains somewhat controversial, especially in a patient who may be perisurgical or postsurgical with major bleeding. Consequently, early prophylactic heparin (loading dose 5000 units, followed by approximately 1000 units per hour, targeting an activated partial thromboplastin time [APTT] of 1.5 to 2.5 times control) is reserved for cases in which there has been an infusion of more than about 1 unit of ABO-incompatible red cells, because ABO incompatibility reactions tend to be the most severe. Heparin should be continued for 6 to 24 hours. Close monitoring of coagulation parameters is advised, and treatment of excessive bleeding with platelets, cryoprecipitate, and/or fresh frozen plasma should be guided by laboratory testing.

ACUTE NONHEMOLYTIC REACTIONS

Respiratory Complications

Fluid Overload

This is one of the more common adverse consequences of blood transfusion, especially in infants and the elderly, although reliable statistics on its incidence are not generally available. Patients susceptible to fluid overload may require slow transfusion of 1/2 unit of packed red cells over up to 4 hours; premedication with furosemide may also be required. Blood issued from the blood bank should never be transfused over more than 4 hours because of the risk of bacterial growth at room temperature in a glucose-rich medium in which red cells are suspended. If fluid overload does develop, the transfusion should be stopped and furosemide administered. In severe cases unresponsive to conservative management, phlebotomy and rotating tourniquets may be of value.

Immunologically Mediated Pulmonary Edema

This condition is clinically similar to fluid overload, although it occurs much less frequently. It is usually due to an anti–white cell antibody (often an anti–human leukocyte antigen [HLA] antibody) in donor blood (usually from a multiparous female) with a specificity toward an antigen on the patient's white cells. The result is leukoagglutination with obstruction of blood flow and release of toxic granulocyte products that damage the endothelial barrier and cause postcapillary vasoconstriction with increased pulmonary vascular resistance. Chest x-ray frequently is often indistinguishable from that seen with fluid overload, but the patient's fluid "in and out" record is balanced and pulmonary capillary wedge pressures are normal. Diagnosis requires a clinical suspicion of this entity. Treatment, in addition to respiratory support, includes one to two large doses of corticosteroids (30 mg per kg body weight of methylprednisolone sodium succinate or 90 mg per kg of hydrocortisone). Laboratory confirmation of the diagnosis is usually slow and effectively retrospective and requires analysis of donor plasma for antigranulocyte and/or antilymphocyte antibodies.

Bacterial Contamination of Donor Blood

Severe hypotension, chills, fever, respiratory difficulty, nausea, vomiting, and hemoglobinuria can be associated with bacterial growth in transfused donor blood. Mortality is high, and death often occurs within 6 to 12 hours. Gram-negative rods that prefer growth at cold temperatures or use citrate are often the culprit, and since 1987 *Yersinia enterocolitica* has been the most common cause, with a 70% mortality rate. Fortunately, this is an uncommon occurrence. A Gram's stain of the implicated blood product (from the blood bag, *not* the blood bag segment) will assist in the diagnosis. Treatment includes intravenous antibiotics and, if hypotension is present, dopamine.

Anaphylaxis

These rare reactions, characterized classically by wheezing and respiratory distress, are usually found in patients who are IgA deficient and have formed anti-IgA antibodies during prior transfusion or pregnancy. Anaphylaxis usually begins before 10 mL of blood have been infused. Other signs include flushing, hypotension, back pain, chest pain, abdominal pain, and nausea. Treatment includes intravenous epinephrine (0.5 mg, or 5 mL of a 1:10,000 solution for adults, repeated every 5 to 10 minutes as needed), O_2, fluids, steroids (with a peak effect at 6 hours), and vasopressors if shock is present. Prevention requires use of autologous blood, washed red cells, or red cells from an IgA-deficient donor.

Air Embolism and Microembolism

Both of these conditions can cause post-transfusion respiratory distress, although the incidence is low, and the existence of the latter has not been proved by controlled studies. Air embolism is most likely to occur when blood is infused under pressure while using an open system, such as is found with some older intraoperative blood salvage pumps that do not have traps to catch air collected with recovered blood. The conscious patient may experience chest pain and dyspnea, whereas the unconscious patient may manifest this complication by shock and respiratory deterioration. Treatment includes placing the patient in the left lateral Trendelenburg position to trap air in the right ventricle until it eventually dissolves.

Microembolism by microaggregates of white cells has been thought by some to occur in patients receiving large quantities of stored blood in less than a 24-hour period. Although in the United States, special in-line 170-μ filters are standard in blood infusion sets, they cannot trap smaller aggregates of white cells believed by some to cause this complication. This complication can be prevented by the use of a 20- to 40-μ micropore filter.

Cardiac Arrhythmias

Hypothermia

Blood is normally stored at 4° C. When large quantities of blood are rapidly infused, and particularly when the blood is administered through a central line, the core body temperature of the patient can drop and cardiac arrhythmia can result. Blood-warming devices constructed specifically for transfusion can help prevent this complication. These devices are also of value when transfusing patients with cold autoimmune hemolytic anemias such as cold agglutinin disease and paroxysmal cold hemoglobinuria.

Potassium Toxicity

Marked electrocardiographic (ECG) changes can be seen when the serum potassium level is more than 8 mmol per liter. It is also known that stored packed red cells can have a plasma potassium level of 44 to 84 mmol per liter, depending on the particular storage solution used. Nevertheless, hyperkalemia is an unlikely complication of blood transfusion unless the patient is already hyperkalemic due to an underlying disorder such as renal failure.

Citrate Toxicity

Excessive citrate can bind and reduce concentrations of free ionized calcium in the plasma, thereby causing ventricular fibrillation, hypotension, tetany, muscle contractions, perioral numbness, or nausea. Maintenance of circulatory volume is important to reduce the effects of excessive citrate, especially because it promotes metabolism of citrate by the liver. Rarely is calcium infusion required to counteract its effects, even in massively transfused patients; however, patients with liver disease or hypothermia may have increased risk of citrate toxicity. If calcium infusion is instituted, caution should be exercised, as it can cause cardiac arrhythmias. Calcium supplementation is indicated when ECG changes characteristic of hypocalcemia are encountered. Typical treatment consists of 5 to 10 mL of 10% calcium gluconate, given through a line in which blood products are *not* infusing.

"Mild," Nonhemolytic Reactions

Febrile Reactions

Febrile reactions occur in approximately 2% of transfused patients. These reactions are defined as a rise of temperature of at least 1° C that is not associated with a patient's primary disease. They are usually due to antibodies toward donor white cells, and they require a history of prior transfusion or pregnancy for primary sensitization. They usually occur within 2 hours of completion of blood infusion, and they may be associated with chills. Because fever may at times be the only indication of an acute hemolytic transfusion reaction, the infusion of blood should be halted, and the patient's physician should be notified.

The physician should assess whether the fever existed prior to the transfusion; if not, a transfusion reaction should be called, the blood bank should be notified, and blood samples should be drawn to rule out hemolysis. If the patient had fever prior to transfusion, clinical judgment should be exercised; if there is any suggestion that fever during transfusion may be indicative of hemolysis (e.g., temperature higher than previously charted, chills not previously present, or shaking chills), a transfusion reaction work-up should also be instituted.

For those patients in whom febrile reactions are severe or repeated, prevention is attained by usage of either washed red cells or filtered red cells and platelets.

Urticarial Reactions

Urticarial reactions characterized by erythema, hives, and itching occur in about 2% of transfused patients. They do not require a history of prior transfusion or pregnancy for manifestation of symptoms. Unless unusually severe, they can be treated with diphenhydramine (Benadryl) (25 to 50 mg intravenously in adults) after stopping the infusion of blood. After 15 to 30 minutes, if symptoms subside, the same donor unit can be slowly restarted. If on subsequent occasions, reactions occur despite premedication with diphenhydramine, washed red cells and washed or reduced-volume platelets can be utilized because the symptoms are a consequence of a reaction to donor plasma proteins.

DELAYED HEMOLYTIC REACTIONS

Delayed hemolytic reactions generally occur about 5 to 7 days after transfusion, although they have been observed up to 21 days after transfusion. They are usually asymptomatic, but they do have the potential for being acute, fulminating, and clinically indistinguishable from an acute hemolytic reaction. Virtually all cases have resulted from an anamnestic, secondary response to an antigen to which the patient has previously been exposed by transfusion or pregnancy. Of note, the quantity of antibody produced during the primary sensitizing event is usually below detectable levels. Some antibodies that have been associated with these reactions include anti-Fy^b, anti-Jk^a, anti-E, anti-C, anti-D, and anti-K. These usually asymptomatic reactions generally come to attention unexpectedly while the laboratory is searching for compatible blood for transfusion.

DELAYED NONHEMOLYTIC REACTIONS

Infectious Disease

Viral Hepatitis

Non-A, Non-B Hepatitis. The most frequent cause (90%) of post-transfusion hepatitis is non-A, non-B viruses, the most common of which is hepatitis C. Current estimates suggest that less than 1% of transfused patients develop viral hepatitis, and the risk of a patient becoming infected is 0.1% per unit transfused. Infection by this small RNA virus is characterized by a lifelong viremia, although 75% of the time the infection remains clinically unrecognized. The time from infection to seroconversion ranges from 6 weeks to 1 year. Nonetheless, individual cases can become severe and fulminant.

Diagnosis of non-A, non-B hepatitis requires elevation of liver function enzymes (alanine aminotransferase [ALT]) with a negative history for other causes of liver dysfunction (e.g., alcohol use) and negative tests for other causes of hepatitis (hepatitis A, B, and D viruses, cytomegalovirus [CMV], and Epstein-Barr virus). Diagnosis of hepatitis C is indicated by the presence of antibody to hepatitis C.

Chronic sequelae of non-A, non-B hepatitis include chronic hepatitis (50%), cirrhosis (20%), and hepatocellular carcinoma and liver-related fatality (5%).

Randomized studies have suggested a decreased severity of non-A, non-B hepatitis in exposed patients when immune serum globulin is utilized. When a patient has been inadvertently exposed to a transfusion of blood with a test suggestive of non-A, non-B hepatitis, immune serum globulin should be given.

Hepatitis B. Hepatitis B comprises about 10% of the cases of post-transfusion hepatitis, with an average incubation time of 11 to 12 weeks. Potential sequelae are similar to those of non-A, non-B hepatitis, although the risk of fulminant disease and of hepatocellular carcinoma may be greater.

There are no controlled studies examining the efficacy of passive and active immunization for hepatitis B in patients exposed to large volume transfusions contaminated with hepatitis B. Nevertheless, as this treatment has been shown to be efficacious in neonates born to hepatitis B–positive mothers, it seems reasonable to administer as soon as possible after known hepatitis B exposure a dose of 5 ml of hepatitis B immune globulin and a series of three prophylactic intramuscular injections in the deltoid (0, 1, and 6 months) of hepatitis B vaccine.

Hepatitis A and D. Hepatitis A and D so rarely cause post-transfusion hepatitis that they should not be regarded as primary transfusion-related hepatitis viruses.

Cytomegalovirus

The estimated risk of CMV infection per unit transfused is between 2.5% and 12%. Transmission requires transfusion of a blood product containing white cells (most likely B lymphocytes). After infection, antibodies to CMV appear an average of 17 days after onset of clinical symptoms and signs.

Although in most patients, CMV infection is not considered dangerous, significant morbidity and mortality can be seen in immunosuppressed transplant patients and in premature neonates weighing less than 1250 grams. Clinical manifestations include pneumonia, hepatosplenomegaly, hepatitis, and various cytopenias. In adults, gastrointestinal inflammation (colitis, gastritis, esophagitis), arthralgias, arthritis, encephalitis, and retinitis can also be seen. In neonates, serious morbidity may occur in 50% of infected infants, and 40% may die; in adult transplant patients, mortality has been estimated to be 60 to 85%, and death is more often seen in patients with severe graft-versus-host disease.

Because of the risk of serious morbidity and mortality, all CMV-negative premature neonates weighing less than 1250 grams and all CMV-negative transplant candidates should be given only CMV-negative blood.

Human Immunodeficiency Virus 1 and 2 (HIV-1 and 2)

The risk of HIV-1 from transfusion has been estimated to be between 1 in 36,000 and 1 in 225,000; only rare cases of HIV-2 have been reported in the United States. Antibodies to HIV-1 proteins and glycoproteins usually develop within 6 to 10 weeks after transfusion, although in some patients this can take more than a year. In patients who receive HIV-positive blood, 50% develop acquired immune deficiency syndrome (AIDS) within 7 years of transfusion.

Human T Lymphotropic Virus I (HTLV I)

HTLV I is the causative agent of adult T cell leukemia/lymphoma, tropical spastic paraparesis, and HTLV I–associated myelopathy. It can be transmitted by white cells in an infected donor's blood. Clinical infection may follow an asymptomatic period ranging from 6 months to more than 10 years, with most infections remaining subclinical. Although the risk of infection from transfusion is about 1 in 60,000, the actual risk of clinical disease is less than 1 in 1,500,000.

Malaria

Between 1972 and 1981, 26 cases of post-transfusion malaria were documented in the United States. In four cases, the outcome was fatal.

Other Infectious Diseases

Syphilis. In early syphilis, when spirochetes can be transmitted by blood transfusion, blood screening tests are often negative; in fact, only 25% of patients with primary syphilis have a reactive serologic test. By the time the serologic test becomes positive, spirochetemia has usually cleared. Consequently, serologic tests for syphilis play only a minor role in protecting the blood supply. Nevertheless, syphilis infection from blood transfusion is a rare event.

Brucella. Brucella is a rare complication of blood transfusion.

Lyme Disease. Transfusion-related cases of Lyme disease (*Borrelia burgdorferi*) have not yet been reported, but the potential is there. It is a disorder that begins with a characteristic skin lesion (erythema chronicum migrans) that later progresses to neurologic, joint, and cardiac manifestations.

Parasitic Infections. Parasitic infections other than malaria are also rarely reported. These include cases of Chagas' disease, toxoplasmosis, and babesiosis.

Noninfectious Consequences

Graft-Versus-Host Disease

This is a rare complication of blood transfusion in which donor blood lymphocytes attack patient tissues. Cases have been reported in patients with primary immunodeficiency syndromes; neonates with hemolytic disease of the newborn, alloimmune neonatal thrombocytopenia, or prematurity; acute leukemia; lymphoma; and solid tumors. Several cases of graft-versus-host disease have recently been reported in immunocompetent patients receiving transfusion from HLA-identical donors (often first-degree relatives). No cases have yet been reported in patients with AIDS. The acute graft-versus-host disease syndrome occurs 4 to 30 days after transfusion and has a 90% mortality. The chronic graft-versus-host disease syndrome starts more than 100 days after transfusion and also has a high mortality. The clinical syndrome may include fever, skin rash, hepatitis, diarrhea, and pancytopenia.

This complication can be prevented by using gamma-irradiated blood, and some authors have recommended that the following patient groups receive only irradiated blood: neonates receiving intrauterine transfusion (including all subsequent transfusions); genetically immunodeficient patients; patients with Hodgkin's disease; and patients receiving bone marrow transplantation.

Post-Transfusion Purpura

Post-transfusion purpura is characterized by sudden, dramatic thrombocytopenia 5 to 10 days after blood transfusion in a patient with a history of prior transfusion or pregnancy. Most cases are seen in parous women whose platelets are P1^{A1} antigen negative. Laboratory work-up in this condition is negative for autoimmune thrombocytopenic purpura, microangiopathic hemolytic anemias (i.e., thrombotic thrombocytopenic purpura and hemolytic uremic syndrome), disseminated intravascular coagulation, sepsis, and drug-induced thrombocytopenia.

Post-transfusion purpura is usually unresponsive to platelet transfusion. Both plasmapheresis and intravenous gamma globulin (400 mg per kg per day for 1 to 10 days) have been found to be effective therapies. High-dose corticosteroids (2 mg prednisone per kg) are also often used.

Section 6

The Digestive System

CHOLECYSTITIS AND CHOLELITHIASIS

method of
R. SCOTT JONES, M.D., and
BRIAN T. JONES, M.D.
University of Virginia Health Sciences Center
Charlottesville, Virginia

The incidence of gallstones is roughly 8 to 10%, or 20 million people in the United States, being found in women twice as frequently as in men. Symptoms of cholelithiasis can result from intermittent obstruction or spasm of the cystic duct, obstruction with subsequent ischemia and possible infection, or the passage of stones through the common bile duct and ampulla of Vater. It is estimated that nearly one-half to two-thirds of those people with gallstones remain asymptomatic. Those that are symptomatic, however, come to the attention of the primary care physician or surgeon, who may then present to the patient a variety of therapeutic options.

PATHOGENESIS

Gallstones are categorized by their primary composition. Cholesterol stones account for more than 75% of the stones in patients in the United States. Cholesterol stones are formed as a result of supersaturation of bile with cholesterol, resulting either from an increased cholesterol production or from a decreased production of phospholipids (primarily lecithin) or of bile acids. Some conditions interfere with the ileal absorption of bile acids, including short bowel syndrome, inflammatory bowel disease, and certain rapid weight-loss programs, and are associated with cholesterol stone formation. Supersaturation combined with gallbladder dysmotility and altered absorptive function allows cholesterol crystal formation.

Pigment stones constitute less than 25% of the stones found in patients in the United States; however, they form the majority of stones in patients in other parts of the world, particularly in Asian countries. Pigment stone formation results from the altered dissolution of unconjugated bilirubin. It is associated with hemolytic diseases, such hereditary spherocytosis and sickle cell anemia, in addition to occurring in patients with prosthetic heart valves. Other conditions associated with pigment stones include cirrhosis, long-term gallbladder stasis, and infected bile.

CLINICAL PRESENTATIONS

Roughly one-half of patients with cholelithiasis are symptomatic. In those who are not symptomatic, the risk of developing symptoms over 10 to 20 years ranges from 10 to 40%. At present, there are no asymptomatic groups in whom cholecystectomy is recommended routinely. Once symptoms do occur in a patient with previously asymptomatic gallstones, however, definitive treatment should be recommended because the incidence of complications rises significantly.

Chronic Cholecystitis

Chronic cholecystitis is characterized by repeated episodes of biliary colic, usually self-limited and not requiring hospitalization. Biliary colic classically presents as sharp epigastric or right upper quadrant abdominal pain that is often described as feeling like a belt tightening around the upper abdomen. Occasionally this pain is referred to the substernal or the right chest region or right scapular region. These symptoms may occur after eating fatty or heavy meals and may be accompanied by excessive eructation or flatulence. Painful symptoms are usually limited to a time period of less than 6 hours. Physical findings are minimal, with little to no tenderness on abdominal palpation. After repeated attacks, the gallbladder may be shrunken and contracted. Occasionally hydrops of the gallbladder results from prolonged cystic duct obstruction, producing a palpable, mildly tender mass. Porcelain gallbladder (i.e., the presence of a calcified wall from chronic inflammation) is another unusual finding that is associated with an elevated risk of gallbladder cancer.

The diagnosis of chronic cholecystitis is confirmed by this clinical picture plus the presence of gallstones on either ultrasound scan or oral cholecystogram and perhaps negative findings on other studies, such as upper gastrointestinal contrast studies or endoscopy. In the patient with classic symptoms of biliary colic but no documented cholelithiasis, a nuclear study with technetium99m–labeled iminodiacetic acid (IDA) combined with cholecystokinin may be used to determine gallbladder ejection fraction. An abnormal ejection fraction has been shown to correlate with symptom relief after cholecystectomy in these patients.

Complicated Gallstone Disease

The complications of gallbladder disease may be the first manifestation of cholelithiasis and may be associated with significant mortality and morbidity. Acute cholecystitis is the most common complication of chronic gallbladder disease and occurs in approximately 25% of patients with chronic symptomatic cholelithiasis. Gallstones are present in 90 to 95% of patients with acute cholecystitis. Acute acalculous cholecystitis is another and potentially lethal complicated presentation of gallbladder disease. Gangrene of the gallbladder and septicemia may occur in acute cholecystitis, as may perforation, intra-abdominal abscess, and hepatic abscess. Choledocholithiasis may complicate cholelithiasis, resulting in cholestasis and hepatic insufficiency, cholangitis, liver abscess, or gallstone pancreatitis. Fistula formation may occur between the gallbladder and the common duct or between either of these structures and adjacent bowel from the erosive and inflammatory action of stones. Finally, gallbladder cancer is associated cholelithiasis; however, a cause-and-effect role has not been proved.

Acute Cholecystitis

Three factors contribute to the development of acute cholecystitis: obstruction, ischemia, and infection. Obstruction of the cystic duct by stone is present in at least 90% of cases. Ischemia may result from the congestion and swelling of the gallbladder and cystic duct region with venous and lymphatic hypertension restricting arterial flow. Infection with enteric pathogens may be present in up to two-thirds of patients with acute cholecystitis; however, it is thought that this is a secondary factor after obstruction and stasis have already occurred.

The clinical history of acute cholecystitis usually includes repeated attacks of biliary colic as described earlier. Occasionally the only differentiating factors between biliary colic and acute cholecystitis are the duration or severity of symptoms. Nausea and vomiting frequently accompany the pain. Findings on physical examination are more remarkable with acute cholecystitis. The patient appears more ill and may even appear septic. Jaundice or scleral icterus may be present. Significant abdominal tenderness, in the epigastrium or right upper quadrant, occasionally with guarding or rebound tenderness is present. A positive Murphy's sign is elicited when pain is perceived during deep inspiration as the gallbladder descends to impact the examiner's fingers under the right costal margin. A palpable mass representing an enlarged, tender gallbladder may be present in 20% of patients with acute cholecystitis. The presence of light or clay-colored stools or dark urine should be noted.

Laboratory studies reveal leukocytosis and occasionally an elevation in amylase or bilirubin or other liver enzymes (particularly alkaline phosphatase). Abdominal x-rays are important in the initial work-up to exclude other causes of abdominal pain and may also demonstrate radiopaque stones (found in approximately 10%) or air in the biliary tree representing a fistulous communication with the gastrointestinal tract. Ultrasonography has approximately a 95% accuracy in detecting gallstones in suspected patients. Ultrasonography may also show associated features, such as gallbladder wall thickening or pericholecystic fluid, common bile duct dilatation, or evidence of pancreatitis. Nuclear imaging with technitium99m–labeled IDA confirms the diagnosis of acute cholecystitis gallbladder by nonfilling of the gallbladder.

TREATMENT

Temporizing measures for the patient with biliary colic include primarily the avoidance of symptom-producing foods. Of questionable efficacy is the use of anticholinergics, such as dicyclomine hydrochloride (Bentyl) or Donnatal. In the setting of acute cholecystitis, pain control with a nonmorphine analgesic, bowel rest, intravenous hydration, and antibiotics if fever or leukocytosis is present are indicated. More aggressive resuscitative measures may be necessary in patients with cholangitis, hepatic abscess, or pancreatitis. Additionally, a careful evaluation for other systemic diseases is necessary for preoperative assessment.

Cholecystectomy

Cholecystectomy remains the standard treatment of symptomatic cholelithiasis. When performed electively, cholecystectomy is associated with an overall mortality rate of approximately 0.5%. This mortality rate increases in the presence of acute cholecystitis; age older than 65 years; the presence of concomitant diseases including cirrhosis and diabetes mellitus, choledocholithiasis, pancreatitis, depressed immune function; and with acute acalculous cholecystitis. Cholecystectomy may be performed early in the course of acute cholecystitis with good result. The presence of jaundice or pancreatitis, however, increases the likelihood that common bile duct exploration will be required. Even when unsuspected, choledocholithiasis may be present in up to 8% of patients undergoing cholecystectomy. After routine cholecystectomy through a right upper quadrant incision, patients typically are hospitalized 2 to 5 days and return to work in 4 to 6 weeks.

Recently advances in laparoscopic technology and technique have allowed laparoscopic cholecystectomy to become the preferred mode of surgical management of gallstone disease. Laparoscopic cholecystectomy offers the advantages of markedly reduced postoperative pain, decreased hospitalization, and earlier return to full activity and employment. The cost has not been sufficiently improved owing to the cost of operative instruments. Complications, particularly common bile duct injury, appear to occur more frequently with the laparoscopic approach; however, only early reports are available at present. Contraindications to laparoscopic cholecystectomy are constantly evolving. Peritonitis, advanced cholecystitis (gangrene or perforation), cholangitis, portal hypertension, and serious bleeding disorders are current contraindications to the laparoscopic approach. Morbid obesity, acute cholecystitis, a history of prior abdominal surgery, suspected common bile duct stones, and pregnancy were once considered contraindications. Several reports of successful laparoscopic cholecystectomy in these groups of patients, however, have been presented.

At present, laparoscopic cholecystectomy is certainly an acceptable treatment by a surgeon well trained in both the open cholecystectomy technique and laparoscopy in a patient with uncomplicated cholelithiasis. More complicated clinical situations, such as jaundice, may be approached but may require advanced laparoscopic skills.

Medical Therapy

Gallstone dissolving agents may be used in certain groups of patients with noncalcified cholesterol stones. Oral agents presently used include chenodeoxycholic acid (chenodiol [Chenix]) and ursodeoxycholic acid (ursodiol [Actigal]). These agents are bile acids that allow dissolution of cholesterol gallstones by decreasing cholesterol synthesis and increasing the bile acid pool. These agents require a functioning gallbladder because they are excreted in the bile and must get into the gallbladder via the cystic duct. Best results are obtained with 2- to 3-mm floating stones as demonstrated on either ultrasound scan or oral cholecystogram and in the nonobese. Side effects include hepatotoxicity and diarrhea but are less common with ursodeoxycholic acid. Complete dissolution of gallstones was noted in only 14% of patients after 2 years of therapy in a study with chenodeoxycholic acid.

Direct contact dissolving agents include methyl tertiary-butyl ether (MTBE) and mono-octanoin, the latter being used mostly in the dissolution of common bile duct stones. Use of MTBE requires percutaneous access to the gallbladder; dissolution usually occurs in less than 15 hours of contact application. It is not necessary to have a functioning gallbladder. Complications from its usage include duodenitis, hemolysis, and anesthesia. Peritoneal leakage can result in hemorrhagic peritonitis. The recurrence rate of gallstones after MTBE therapy is up to 20%.

The patients eligible for gallstone dissolving therapy constitute only about 20% of those with symptomatic cholelithiasis. Gallstone dissolving therapy is currently being recommended in patients who are not satisfactory operative candidates and also is used in conjunction with lithotripsy methods.

Extracorporeal shock wave lithotripsy has been applied to gallstones with mixed success. Stones that are larger than 5 mm and noncalcified or that have a thin calcified rim with an overall aggregate of less than 3 cm in stone have been evaluated with extracorporeal shock wave lithotripsy in both Europe and the United States. Results in the United States have not been promising; stone clearance with lithotripsy and ursodeoxycholic acid therapy combined has been only 20 to 50%. Biliary colic complicates this form of management in approximately 35% of patients; however, cholangitis and pancreatitis have not been frequent complications. Recurrence after 12 months in one study has been reported at 10%. Currently lithotripsy is not approved by the Food and Drug Administration in the United States. Ongoing studies are necessary to document its efficacy.

CIRRHOSIS

method of
STEPHEN D. ZUCKER, M.D., and
JOHN L. GOLLAN, M.D., PH.D.
Harvard Medical School
Boston, Massachusetts

Cirrhosis of the liver is prevalent in the United States, representing the fifth most common cause of all deaths and the third leading cause of death in individuals aged 25 to 65 years. It is a pathologic process characterized by diffuse hepatic fibrosis with nodular parenchymal regeneration. Liver fibrosis is the result of hepatocellular injury and necrosis, with subsequent collapse of hepatic lobules, formation of diffuse fibrous septa, and nodular regrowth of hepatocytes. Because the liver has a limited range of responses to injury, the ultimate histologic pattern observed in cirrhosis is similar, regardless of the underlying cause. Alcoholic (previously Laennec's) cirrhosis is the most common form of chronic liver disease both in the United States and in Europe, followed by chronic viral hepatitis, caused by either the hepatitis B or hepatitis C (formerly non-A, non-B) virus. In the past, 10 to 30% of cases were labeled cryptogenic, although recent data suggest that the majority of these patients may actually have chronic hepatitis C infection. A more comprehensive list of causes of cirrhosis is provided in Table 1.

The prognosis for patients with cirrhosis depends on the extent of hepatic dysfunction and the nature of the underlying disorder. Although generally believed to be

TABLE 1. **Etiology of Cirrhosis**

Drugs and Toxins
Alcohol
Alpha-methyl dopa (Aldomet)
Methotrexate (Rheumatrex)
Isoniazid (INH)
Nitrofurantoin (Macrodantin)
Perhexiline maleate*
Oxyphenisatin*
Amiodarone (Cordarone)
Trichloroethylene

Infections
Chronic hepatitis B (+/− delta hepatitis)
Chronic hepatitis C
Congenital syphilis

Cholestatic Liver Disease
Primary biliary cirrhosis
Chronic extrahepatic biliary obstruction
Sclerosing cholangitis
Biliary atresia
Graft-versus-host disease

Metabolic Disorders
Hemochromatosis
Wilson's disease
Alpha$_1$-antitrypsin deficiency
Galactosemia
Hereditary tyrosinemia
Hereditary fructose intolerance
Glycogen storage diseases
Mucopolysaccharidoses

Venous Outflow Obstruction
Budd-Chiari syndrome
Chronic right heart failure
Constrictive pericarditis
Veno-occlusive disease

Miscellaneous
Autoimmune chronic active hepatitis
Cystic fibrosis
Sarcoidosis
Jejunoileal bypass
Indian childhood cirrhosis
Neonatal hepatitis
Agnogenic myeloid metaplasia and myelofibrosis
Cryptogenic cirrhosis

*Not available in the United States.

TABLE 2. **Staging of Liver Disease**

Child's Classification			
Parameter	*Class A*	*Class B*	*Class C*
Bilirubin (mg/dl)	<2.0	2.0–3.0	>3.0
Albumin (gm/dl)	>3.5	3.0–3.5	<3.0
Ascites	None	Easily controlled	Poorly controlled
Encephalopathy	None	Mild	Advanced
Nutritional status	Excellent	Good	Poor

Pugh's Modification *Points*			
Parameter	1	2	3
Encephalopathy (grade)	None	1–2	3–4
Ascites	Absent	Slight	Moderate
Bilirubin (mg/dl)	<2.0	2.0–3.0	>3.0
Albumin (gm/dl)	>3.5	2.8–3.5	<2.8
Prothrombin time (sec prolonged)	1.0–4.0	4.0–6.0	>6.0

Class A: 5–6 points; Class B: 7–9 points; Class C: 10–15 points

irreversible, hepatic fibrosis has been observed to regress in selected patients receiving long-term treatment for Wilson's disease and hemochromatosis. Patients with compensated cirrhosis have a 6-year survival that approaches 55%; however, the survival rate falls to 20% when cirrhosis is decompensated. The Child's classification system (Table 2) serves as a useful short-term prognostic guide in cirrhotic patients. Pugh and colleagues proposed a modification of the Child's classification that replaces nutritional assessment with the prothrombin time and assigns point scores for each component depending on the severity. With increasing score, the median survival time decreases from 6.4 years to 2 months.

TREATMENT

Once the diagnosis of cirrhosis is established, treatment has focused on elimination of the offending hepatotoxic agent and aggressive management of complications as they develop. In an attempt to retard or reverse the fibrotic process, a variety of therapies have been evaluated (Table 3). Although many of these treatments are well established, the precise role of medical therapy in many forms of liver disease remains poorly defined.

Abstinence is the single most effective therapy for patients with alcoholic liver disease, and a marked improvement in survival is evident in cirrhotic alcoholics who abstain from further alcohol intake. It seems prudent to advise any patient with cirrhosis, regardless of the cause, to avoid known hepatotoxins (e.g., alcohol, acetaminophen) in an effort to minimize further hepatic injury. In addition to alcohol, all cirrhotic patients should refrain from eating raw shellfish or any other activity that would place them at risk for contracting viral hepatitis. It also is reasonable to administer the hepatitis B vaccine to patients seronegative for hepatitis B surface antibody.

Inasmuch as fibrosis is the major histologic feature of cirrhosis, it has been postulated that administration of penicillamine (Cuprimine, Depen), which inhibits the cross-linkage of collagen, may benefit patients with chronic liver disease. Although this medication is effective in the treatment of Wilson's disease (as a result of efficient chelation and detoxification of copper), controlled trials revealed no significant clinical improvement in patients with cirrhosis owing to causes other than copper overload. The combination of colchicine and probenecid (ColBENEMID) interferes with microtubular function and transcellular movement of collagens and increases collagenase production. Several studies suggest an improvement in both survival and liver histology in cirrhotic patients treated with this drug. If future studies confirm these results, oral colchicine may become a useful therapy for patients with mild to moderate cirrhosis.

It has been proposed that hypoxic liver injury, accentuated by a hypermetabolic state, leads to the hepatocellular damage and fibrosis associated with alcohol abuse. Propylthiouracil (PTU), an antithyroid medication, has been applied to the treatment of alcoholic liver disease in an attempt to reduce hepatic hypermetabolism. Although not limited exclusively to individuals with cirrhosis, a recent 2-year study revealed a significant reduction in the mortality of patients with alcoholic liver disease receiving PTU (150 mg twice daily). Because PTU has the potential for toxicity (e.g., hypothyroidism, hepatotoxicity), however, further trials are necessary before this drug can be recommended for routine use in the treatment of patients with alcoholic liver disease.

Numerous studies evaluating the use of corticosteroids in the treatment of cirrhosis have been reported. The results of these trials indicate that prednisone has a limited, albeit specific, role in the management of cirrhosis. Those patients who benefit from corticosteroid therapy have evidence of active disease on liver biopsy (extensive piecemeal necrosis, marked inflammation), relatively compensated cirrhosis (no ascites), and evidence of immunologic abnormalities (positive antinuclear or smooth muscle antibodies [or both]). Individuals with decompensated cirrhosis, particularly when caused by alcohol or viral hepatitis, have a worse prognosis with prednisone therapy. In this latter group, protein catabolism, infectious complications, and other side effects induced by corticosteroids far outweigh any potential benefit. Moreover, prednisone appears to heighten the risk of upper gastrointestinal hemorrhage from peptic ulceration and esophageal varices in patients with ascites or alcoholic liver disease.

It is postulated that the intrahepatic accumulation of bile acids in patients with primary biliary cirrhosis, and possibly other chronic cholestatic disorders, contributes to liver injury. Thus, it has been suggested that replacement of hydrophobic (i.e., potentially hepatotoxic) bile acids by the more hydrophilic ursodiol (Actigall) will reduce or arrest further hepatic damage. Ursodiol also may function as an immune mediator by inhibiting the expression of histocompatibility antigens on biliary epithelial cells. Preliminary trials have demonstrated improvement in both symptoms and biochemical parameters following the administration of ursodiol (300 mg twice daily) to patients with primary biliary cirrhosis, sclerosing cholangitis, and graft-versus-host disease. Ursodiol also may improve liver histology and prolong survival in patients with primary biliary cirrhosis. Initial case reports of the use of methotrexate (Rheumatrex) in the management of precirrhotic primary biliary cirrhosis and sclerosing cholangitis also have been encouraging. Owing to the potential toxicity of this drug, however, it cannot be recommended until the results of carefully controlled trials are available.

TABLE 3. **Medical Therapy for Common Causes of Cirrhosis**

Cause	Therapy
Alcoholic cirrhosis	Abstinence
	?Corticosteroids (limited indications)
	?Propylthiouracil
	?Colchicine
	?Polyunsaturated lecithin
Viral hepatitis B or C	Alpha-interferon
Hemochromatosis	Phlebotomy
	Deferoxamine (in the setting of anemia)
Autoimmune hepatitis	Corticosteroids
	Azathioprine
Primary biliary cirrhosis	Colchicine
	Ursodiol
	?Methotrexate
Sclerosing cholangitis	?Ursodiol
	?Methotrexate
Wilson's disease	Penicillamine
	Triethylenetetramine dihydrochloride (trientine)
Cystic fibrosis	?Ursodiol
Graft-versus-host disease	?Ursodiol

Preliminary studies of alpha-interferon (Intron A) suggest that this compound inhibits fibrogenic activity in the liver. In addition, alpha-interferon possesses antiproliferative properties and is the only agent with demonstrated efficacy against chronic viral hepatitis. At either a daily dose of 5 million units or 10 million units 3 times a week subcutaneously over a 4-month period, alpha-interferon results in the disappearance of serum hepatitis B virus DNA and hepatitis B$_e$ antigen in more than one-third of patients with chronic hepatitis B. Although serum transaminase levels normalize in nearly 45% of treated patients, long-term histologic follow-up is not yet available. Liver function tests also improve in one-half of patients with chronic hepatitis C receiving a 6-month course of 3 million units of alpha-interferon three times per week. Unfortunately, in contrast to hepatitis B, the relapse rate is well over 50% in successfully treated hepatitis C patients. Guidelines for retreatment and maintenance therapy in patients with relapsing hepatitis C remain to be established. Long-term studies also are necessary to determine if alpha-interferon is capable of inhibiting or reversing hepatic fibrosis in patients with chronic hepatitis.

Investigators are focusing on the role of non-parenchymal liver cells (i.e., lipocytes, Kupffer, and endothelial) in the generation of hepatic fibrosis. Monokines (e.g., interleukin 1, tumor necrosis factor, transforming growth factor β_1), which are produced by Kupffer cells, have been shown to stimulate lipocyte (Ito cell) proliferation and collagen deposition. Thus, the progression from hepatic injury to fibrosis may be perpetuated by cytokine-mediated interactions between nonparenchymal cells. It is likely that novel therapies employing various cytokine inhibitors will emerge from this exciting area of research.

MANAGEMENT OF COMPLICATIONS OF CIRRHOSIS

Because current medical therapy is ineffective in preventing all but a few specific forms of cirrhosis, treatment has focused on the management of the complications of this disorder (Table 4). Significant advances have occurred with regard to understanding the underlying pathophysiology of the various complications of cirrhosis, and, as a result, the number of available therapeutic alternatives has expanded dramatically over the past several years.

Portal Hypertension

The most common cause of portal hypertension in the United States is cirrhosis of the liver, and

TABLE 4. **Complications of Cirrhosis**

Portal hypertension
  Esophageal varices
  Congestive gastropathy
  Hypersplenism
Hepatic encephalopathy
Ascites
  Spontaneous bacterial peritonitis
  Umbilical hernia (spontaneous rupture)
Hepatorenal syndrome
Coagulation abnormalities
Hepatocellular carcinoma
Pulmonary dysfunction
Hepatic osteodystrophy
Cholelithiasis
Pericardial effusion
Impaired reticuloendothelial system function

30 to 60% of patients with cirrhosis manifest a significant degree of portal pressure elevation. Portal pressures above the normal range of 7 to 14 mmHg may have serious clinical consequences, including gastrointestinal hemorrhage, hypersplenism, encephalopathy, and ascites.

Esophageal Varices

The subject of esophageal varices is thoroughly discussed in the article, "Bleeding Esophageal Varices."

Hypersplenism

"Hypersplenism" is the term used to describe the depression of one or more of the hematologic cell lines in the circulating blood caused by splenic enlargement and sequestration. Portal hypertension secondary to cirrhosis is the most common cause of congestive splenomegaly. Approximately 70% of cirrhotic patients develop splenic enlargement, which occasionally can be massive. Depression of various hematologic cell lines can exacerbate the risk of hemorrhage, infection, or alcohol-related bone marrow suppression. Hypersplenism secondary to cirrhosis, however, rarely reduces blood counts to the extent that splenectomy is required. In addition, increased blood flow through an enlarged spleen is insufficient to augment portal hypertension to any significant degree. Thus, splenectomy alone is inadequate surgical therapy for portal hypertension. In the rare case when splenectomy is indicated in a patient with cirrhosis, surgery should be planned so as to facilitate concomitant correction of the underlying portal hypertension with a portacaval, mesocaval, or splenorenal shunt.

Hepatic Encephalopathy

The term "hepatic encephalopathy" covers a broad spectrum of neuropsychiatric disturbances that occur in patients with impaired liver function. It is thought to result from metabolic derangements because the potential exists for complete reversal of symptoms, and there is a paucity of histologic lesions in the central nervous system on postmortem examination. Manifestations of hepatic encephalopathy range from mild alterations in mental status to coma and are divided into four clinical stages (Table 5). Although hyperammonemia is present in the majority of patients, it is not uniformly observed; thus, the serum ammonia level should never be used as the sole diagnostic indicator of hepatic encephalopathy. More than 95% of cirrhotic patients who present with hepatic encephalopathy have a cause for their decompensation other than progression of their underlying liver disease. Common precipitating insults include infection (viral or bacterial), gastrointestinal hemorrhage, azotemia or electrolyte abnormalities (usually secondary to diuretic therapy), cardiovascular disease, tranquilizer ingestion, or alcohol consumption. The basic therapeutic approach to patients with hepatic encephalopathy involves oral protein restriction, gut cleansing, and the administration of lactulose. The majority of patients respond to these measures (in conjunction with management of the inciting event), and the mental status examination usually returns to baseline within 24 to 72 hours. Failure to respond generally indicates inadequate treatment of the cause of the neurologic decompensation or heralds the terminal phase of the underlying liver disease.

Dietary modifications used in the management of hepatic encephalopathy are designed to minimize the absorption of ammonia and other nitrogenous products of bacterial metabolism from the gastrointestinal tract. Protein restriction is indicated only in cirrhotics who manifest encephalopathy because many patients with liver disease have poor nutrition and may actually benefit from high protein intake. When protein restriction is required, typical outpatient diets permit only 40 to 60 grams of protein per day, which approaches the limits of tolerance. Patients with Stage III or IV hepatic encephalopathy should have little or zero oral protein intake. Paradoxically it is precisely those cirrhotic patients who should reduce oral nitrogen intake that exhibit marked protein-calorie malnutrition. Encephalopathy can be avoided by simply by-passing the gastrointestinal tract, providing nitrogenous support through the administration of standard amino acid solutions, either via a central vein as part of a total parenteral nutrition regimen or via a peripheral vein as a supplement to an oral diet. Hence, patients who require more than 1 to 2 days of a zero protein diet should receive parenteral protein supplementation. As encephalopathy abates, oral feeding can be reinstituted, with a stepwise increase in dietary protein. Cirrhotic patients appear to tolerate vegetable protein better than animal protein, owing to the lower ammoniagenesis and significant laxative effects of the former. Branched-chain, enriched, or other "hepatic" diets are generally unnecessary except in rare circumstances. Increased dietary fiber also may reduce the risk of hepatic encephalopathy by increasing the elimination of nitrogen contained in fecal bacteria.

Oral administration of lactulose (Cephulac) is the treatment of choice for chronic hepatic encephalopathy. Lactulose is a synthetic disaccharide that is not hydrolyzed by the intestinal mucosa. Oral lactulose reaches the cecum unchanged, where it is metabolized by the colonic flora. It is believed to improve encephalopathy by several mechanisms: (1) induction of an osmotic diarrhea decreases the amount of time available for the production and absorption of toxins; (2) acidification of the colon impairs ammonia absorption; (3) suppression of colonic bacteria reduces intestinal ammonia generation; and (4) stimulation of ammonia incorporation into bacterial proteins results in increased fecal nitrogen excretion. The usual starting dose for lactulose is 15 to 30 mL orally three times a day. The dose is subsequently titrated to maintain two to four loose bowel movements daily. Side effects, such as diarrhea, cramps, and flatulence, are generally mild. In patients who are unable to receive oral lactulose owing to ileus or bowel obstruction, the syrup may be diluted in 2 to 3 volumes of water and 1 liter administered every 6 hours as a retention enema. Serum chemistries should be care-

TABLE 5. **Staging of Hepatic Encephalopathy**

Stage	Symptoms	Signs	Electro-encephalogram
I	Disordered sleep Euphoria/ depression Loss of affect	±Asterixis Mild tremor Impaired handwriting	Normal
II	Moderate confusion Disorientation Drowsiness	Asterixis Alaxia Hypoactive reflexes	Abnormal
III	Marked confusion Incoherent speech Sleepy but arousable Stuporous	Asterixis Hyperactive reflexes Clonus	Abnormal
IVa	Coma Poor muscle tone	Asterixis not testable	Abnormal
IVb	Unresponsive to noxious stimuli	Hypoactive reflexes Decerebrate/ decorticate posturing	

fully monitored for evidence of electrolyte disturbances during enema therapy.

Antibiotics also are useful in the treatment of hepatic encephalopathy by reducing the intestinal bacteria content and thereby decreasing ammonia production. Neomycin sulfate (Mycifradin, Neobiotic), in a dose of 1 to 2 grams twice daily, is the prototype antibiotic used in the management of encephalopathy. Metronidazole (Flagyl, Protostat), 250 mg two to three times daily, also has been shown to be effective. Although infrequent, potentially serious side effects, such as nervous system toxicity and antibiotic-associated colitis, have been associated with the use of these medications, making them a second-line therapy after lactulose. Carbidopalevodopa (Sinemet) and bromocriptine (Parlodel) have been used in the treatment of encephalopathy; however, more extensive testing is necessary before these drugs can be recommended. Preliminary studies using benzodiazepine receptor partial inverse agonists appear promising.

Ascites

The presence of detectable fluid in the peritoneal cavity is common in cirrhotic individuals. In patients with chronic liver disease, ascites results in significant morbidity and predisposes to several potentially lethal complications, including peritonitis and respiratory compromise. The reported 2-year survival rate for cirrhotic patients who develop ascites is approximately 40%. Cirrhosis is the most common cause of ascites and is implicated in nearly 75% of all cases. Ascites may either appear suddenly or accumulate insidiously over the course of months. The acute onset of ascites generally results from a precipitating insult and should prompt a systematic evaluation to determine the cause. Most commonly, an alcoholic binge or poor compliance with a prescribed dietary or diuretic regimen underlies the rapid reaccumulation of ascitic fluid; however, ascites may present suddenly in association with any additional impairment in hepatocellular function. Intravascular volume depletion (e.g., hemorrhage), bacterial peritonitis or other infection, hepatotoxic medications, or hepatocellular carcinoma all may acutely precipitate ascites in cirrhotic patients. Acute thrombosis of the portal vein owing to pancreatitis, diverticulitis, or other intra-abdominal infections may result in ascites formation in patients with underlying impaired hepatic function, typically in the setting of hypoalbuminemia. The insidious onset of ascites in patients with cirrhosis heralds a poor prognosis. This usually reflects the fact that such patients have no clearly rectifiable precipitant of the ascites, and the accumulation of fluid is indicative of progressive worsening of the underlying liver disease.

Paracentesis should be performed in any cirrhotic patient who exhibits clinical deterioration. Diagnostic paracentesis can be performed safely, even in the presence of a coagulopathy, when aseptic technique is used, a small (21-gauge) needle is employed, and surgical scars are avoided. We prefer a midline approach between the umbilicus and symphysis pubis, with the patient in a supine position with the head of the bed elevated. The patient should void immediately before the procedure or have a urinary catheter in place. A "Z-track" technique for needle insertion minimizes the risk of an ascitic fluid leak postprocedure. Evaluation of fluid obtained by paracentesis should include a chemistry profile (total protein, albumin, triglyceride), cell count and differential, amylase, cytologic analysis, and cultures. Although the ascitic fluid in cirrhotics is typically transudative (protein <2.5 to 3.0 grams per dL), about 20% of these patients have a protein content higher than 2.5 grams per dL. Subtraction of the ascitic fluid albumin concentration from the serum albumin concentration (S-A gradient) may provide a more reliable indicator of portal hypertension than the absolute protein content of the ascites. A difference between the serum and ascites albumin concentration of greater than 1.1 grams per dL is highly suggestive of portal hypertension (e.g., cirrhosis, fulminant hepatic failure, massive liver metastases, Budd-Chiari syndrome, right-sided heart failure, myxedema), whereas a low S-A gradient (<1.1 grams per dL) generally indicates a cause of ascites unrelated to portal hypertension (e.g., peritoneal carcinomatosis, tuberculous peritonitis, pancreatic or biliary ascites, nephrotic syndrome). A cell count and cultures are helpful in ruling out an infectious process.

There is no definitive evidence that the presence of ascites per se necessitates therapy. Defined indications for the treatment of ascites include significant patient discomfort, respiratory compromise, a large umbilical hernia, or recurrent bacterial peritonitis. Aside from these circumstances, the extent of medical management of ascites remains a matter of clinical judgment. Sodium restriction is considered the cornerstone of therapy for ascites. Cirrhotic patients require significant curtailment of sodium intake (250 to 500 mg per day) to obtain clinical benefit. About 10 to 20% of patients who maintain a strict low-salt diet achieve complete resolution of ascites without any additional therapy. The need for fluid restriction is more controversial, although it is probably unnecessary unless significant hyponatremia (i.e., serum sodium <125 mEq per liter) is present. Unfortunately, the majority of cirrhotics who are compliant with a low-sodium diet require the addition of diuretics to achieve resolution of their ascites. In contrast to edema fluid, ascites can be absorbed by the peritoneum into the intravascular compartment only at a limited rate (about 900 mL per day), regardless of the volume of urine excreted by the kidneys. More rapid diuresis occurs only at the expense of intravascular volume. Hence, it is recommended that a diuretic regimen should not induce a weight loss exceeding 0.5 to 0.75 kg per day unless peripheral edema is present, in which case a rate of 1 to 2 kg per day is acceptable. Exceeding this rate of fluid excretion risks intravascular volume depletion, with resultant azotemia and hypotension. Daily morning measurement of the patient's weight is the best guide to the efficacy of diuretics. Mental status evaluation should be performed, and serum electrolyte, blood urea nitrogen, and creatinine levels should be monitored frequently to screen for potential complications, especially during initiation of or alterations in therapy. The development of azotemia, hyponatremia, or worsening encephalopathy is a relative contraindication to the continued use of diuretics at the prescribed dose.

Spironolactone (Aldactone), an aldosterone antagonist, is the first-line diuretic in the treatment of cirrhotic ascites. It is effective in controlling ascites in 40 to 75% of cirrhotics and has several notable features: (1) It is a mild diuretic that leads to a gentle, gradual diuresis; (2) elevated serum aldosterone levels are believed to contribute to the excessive sodium retention observed in cirrhosis; (3) as a potassium-sparing diuretic, it counteracts the potassium depletion that occurs in cirrhosis; (4) despite the predominant hepatic clearance of the drug, liver disease does not appear to prolong the circulating half-life significantly; and (5) in contrast to loop diuretics, spironolactone does not require tubular secretion, frequently making it more efficacious than the former in cirrhotic patients. The usual starting dose of spironolactone is 25 to 50 mg three or four times daily. Owing to a prolonged onset of action, dosing changes should be made only after 3 to 4 days of monitoring on a stable regimen. Increments of 100 to 200 mg per day, up to a maximum of 400 mg per day, may be required before a diuresis is obtained. Development of significant gynecomastia, hyperchloremic metabolic acidosis, or hyperkalemia may necessitate discontinuation of the drug. Other potassium-sparing diuretics that may be substituted for spironolactone include triamterene (Dyrenium) in a dose of 50 mg twice daily (up to a maximum of 300 mg per day), or amiloride (Midamor), 5 mg twice daily (up to 20 mg per day).

The use of combined diuretic therapy should be limited to patients who fail to respond to an optimal regimen of dietary restriction and potassium-sparing diuretics. Such patients generally exhibit enhanced proximal renal sodium reabsorption, so the addition of a more proximal-acting agent, such as hydrochlorothiazide (HydroDIURIL), 50 mg daily, or furosemide (Lasix), 10 to 20 mg daily, to the medical regimen effectively enhances diuresis. Gradually increasing doses of hydrochlorothiazide (200 mg per day maximum) or furosemide (240 mg per day maximum) may be administered to refractory patients. Dose increments above these levels are unlikely to be effective. In general, proximally acting diuretics should always be administered in conjunction with a diuretic that blocks distal tubular function, such as spironolactone. Careful monitoring of renal function and serum electrolytes is imperative when using combination therapy.

Up to 90 to 95% of patients with cirrhosis experience resolution of their ascites on a stepwise diuretic regimen, as outlined. Those with refractory or "intractable" ascites have a poor prognosis, with the majority of patients dying within 6 months. Recently, large-volume paracentesis with albumin (or dextran) infusion, 6 to 8 grams per liter of fluid removed at a rate of 2 mL per minute, has been shown to be effective in patients with refractory ascites. Compared with diuretic therapy, paracentesis mobilizes ascites much more rapidly and significantly shortens the duration of hospitalization, without any increase in the rate of complications or hospital readmission. As long as albumin is administered concomitantly, all of the ascites present may be completely mobilized within 1 to 2 hours (in some cases more than 20 liters) without adverse hemodynamic consequences. Thus, large-volume paracentesis, although not a substitute for dietary or diuretic therapy, is useful both in the management of refractory ascites and as an adjunct in the treatment of massive or tense ascites.

Rarely patients with cirrhosis and refractory ascites who are severely disabled by rapidly reaccumulating intra-abdominal fluid despite repeated large-volume paracentesis may be candidates for peritoneovenous shunting. The technique involves surgical placement of a mechanical device that transfers fluid from the peritoneal cavity to the superior vena cava. A mechanical valve maintains unidirectional flow from the intraperitoneal to the intrathoracic compartment. Contraindications to this procedure include decompensated liver disease, hepatic encephalopathy, congestive heart failure, recent variceal hemorrhage, and peritonitis. Complications are common and include infection, shunt failure, a disseminated intravascular coagulation (DIC)–

like syndrome, and mesenteric fibrosis with bowel obstruction (long term). The procedure has a 10 to 15% operative mortality, and 25% of patients die within a month. Although successful peritoneovenous shunting may improve the quality of life in cirrhotic patients with refractory ascites, controlled studies have not adequately demonstrated a survival benefit. There have been anecdotal reports of successful management of refractory ascites with the use of transjugular intrahepatic portosystemic shunting (TIPS); further trials are awaited before this procedure can be recommended.

Spontaneous Bacterial Peritonitis

Spontaneous bacterial peritonitis (SBP) is a primary infection of ascitic fluid that occurs in patients with severe liver disease in the absence of a demonstrable cause of peritonitis or intraabdominal abscess. It is caused by spontaneous bacteremia with resultant seeding of the ascites, which serves as an excellent culture medium. Patients with SBP may present with fever, abdominal pain or tenderness, unexplained encephalopathy, deteriorating renal or hepatic function, worsening ascites, or general failure to thrive. Owing to the protean manifestations, the gravity of the condition, and the importance of early initiation of therapy, one should have a low threshold in performing early diagnostic paracentesis in patients with ascites. Routine paracentesis reveals a 10 to 27% prevalence of SBP on hospital admission in patients with cirrhosis and ascites.

The diagnosis of SBP is made (and treatment should be initiated immediately) if the cell count from the ascitic fluid reveals more than 250 polymorphonuclear leukocytes (PMN) per mm^3 or when cultures from the paracentesis are positive. Although organisms are observed on Gram's stain of the ascitic fluid in up to 60% of patients with SBP, the bacterium identified is frequently not in agreement with the culture results. Thus, the Gram's stain should not be used as the sole criterion for antibiotic selection. All cultures should be processed by inoculating 10 mL of ascitic fluid into each of two sets of aerobic and anaerobic blood culture bottles. The sensitivity of this technique for documenting peritonitis is greater than 90%, which is double that attained by conventional ascitic fluid culture methods. Cultures of blood should be obtained in addition to, but not in place of, paracentesis because bacteremia is demonstrated in only 50% of patients. SBP is nearly always caused by a single pathogen (Table 6).

Empirical antibiotics should be initiated before the availability of culture results in any patient with clinical or laboratory evidence of SBP. The

TABLE 6. **Organisms Isolated from Ascitic Fluid in Patients with Sontaneous Bacterial Peritonitis**

Organism	% of Total Isolates
Gram-Negative Bacteria	85
Escherichia coli	55
Klebsiella pneumoniae	10
Other isolates:	
Salmonella spp	
Enterobacter cloaci	
Pseudomonas spp	
Neisseria spp	
Aeromonas sobria	
Proteus spp	
Citrobacter	
Acinetobacter	
Campylobacter spp	
Serratia	
Gram-Positive Bacteria	12
Enterococcus	5
Other isolates:	
Streptococcus pneumoniae	
Staphylococcus aureus	
Miscellaneous streptococcal spp	
Anaerobic Bacteria	3
Bacteroides	2
Other isolates:	
Clostridium spp	
Lactobacillus	
Fungi	<1
Candida albicans	

combination of ampicillin (Omnipen) and gentamicin (Garamycin) has been the generally recommended therapy, although recent data suggest that the third-generation cephalosporin cefotaxime (Claforan), 2 grams intravenously every 6 hours, is more efficacious and has fewer side effects (e.g., nephrotoxicity). The mortality from SBP is reduced from essentially 100% to 20% by the rapid institution of antibiotic therapy. Unfortunately, even if treatment is successful, there is a high rate of recurrence (about 50% within 1 year). It has been recommended that, when feasible, patients be kept free of ascites to minimize the risk of recurrence of SBP, although little data exist to support this notion. Recent studies suggest that the prophylactic use of the antibiotic norfloxacin (Noroxin), 400 mg once daily in cirrhotic patients with a history of SBP, to achieve selective gram-negative intestinal decontamination, markedly reduces the risk of recurrence. It is premature, however, to recommend long-term norfloxacin for all patients following an episode of SBP until concerns about the emergence of resistant organisms and the cost effectiveness of this approach are addressed.

Umbilical Hernias

Umbilical hernias occur in up to 20% of patients with cirrhosis and ascites, compared with a 2% prevalence in the general population. Although it is a relatively uncommon event, the spontaneous rupture of an umbilical hernia in a patient with ascites (Flood's syndrome) is fatal in more than one-third of cases. Common complications of a ruptured umbilical hernia include hypotension, peritonitis (usually due to *Staphylococcus aureus*), and renal insufficiency. Rupture tends to occur in patients with chronic ascites (average duration 22 months), decompensated hepatic disease, and ulcerated hernias. Treatment includes intravenous antibiotics, hemodynamic stabilization, and supportive care. All patients with a ruptured umbilical hernia should undergo surgical repair because mortality is quadrupled when managed by medical therapy alone. In patients with nonincarcerated hernias, immediate closure of the skin over the hernia under local anesthesia is recommended, with consideration of peritoneovenous shunt placement if medical management of the ascites subsequently fails. Although most cirrhotics with ascites and umbilical hernias do not require therapy, patients with an ulcerated hernia should undergo large-volume paracentesis and should have pressure dressings maintained to prevent rupture. Surgical placement of a peritoneovenous shunt should include repair of a concomitant umbilical hernia, because of the high risk of incarceration postoperatively.

Hepatorenal Syndrome

Although at risk for any of the usual causes of acute azotemia, cirrhotic patients are susceptible to a unique form of renal failure for which a specific cause still has not been identified: the hepatorenal syndrome. There are no histologic abnormalities noted in the kidneys on postmortem examination of patients with hepatorenal syndrome, and these organs have been used successfully for renal transplantation. The syndrome typically occurs in patients with advanced cirrhosis and is almost invariably progressive, with mortality rates approaching 90%. The onset may be insidious, or it may be precipitated by an acute reduction in effective blood volume following gastrointestinal hemorrhage, sepsis, vigorous diuretic therapy, paracentesis, or surgery. An early decline in glomerular filtration is often overlooked in cirrhotic patients because they frequently do not exhibit the rise in serum blood urea nitrogen (BUN) or creatinine levels that is usually observed in renal failure. Decreased hepatic production of urea and creatine (the precursor of creatinine) and diminished muscle mass owing to poor nutrition are primarily responsible for the lack of typical laboratory features of renal dysfunction.

The hepatorenal syndrome is characterized by oliguria (<500 mL of urine per day) and a slowly progressive rise in the serum BUN and creatinine concentrations. Patients have a strikingly low urinary sodium concentration (<10 mEq per liter) and fractional excretion of sodium (<1%). These laboratory findings, in the setting of a normal urinalysis, help to differentiate the hepatorenal syndrome from acute tubular necrosis, although the latter actually is a more common cause of renal failure in patients with liver disease. The prognosis for patients with hepatorenal syndrome is poor, with the majority dying within 3 weeks of the onset of renal failure. Death is frequently due to a complication of cirrhosis, such as gastrointestinal hemorrhage or hepatic coma. Care should be taken to avoid agents that reduce renal perfusion or are directly nephrotoxic, such as nonsteroidal anti-inflammatory drugs (which inhibit prostaglandin synthesis), diuretics, and certain antibiotics (i.e., gentamicin, neomycin). Volume expansion results in only transient improvement in renal hemodynamics without any impact on final outcome. The use of colloid, whenever possible, rather than crystalloid, however, slows the rate of intra-abdominal fluid accumulation. The role of hepatic transplantation in the management of hepatorenal syndrome is unclear, although it may be appropriate in selected patients.

Coagulation Abnormalities

The liver is the primary site of synthesis of all coagulation proteins except von Willebrand's factor. It also produces most of the circulating protease inhibitors, such as antithrombin III and α_2-antiplasmin, which modulate the coagulation cascade. Primary fibrogenolysis is observed in cirrhosis owing to increased levels of circulating plasminogen activator, which is normally cleared by the liver. In addition, diminished bile salt secretion results in malabsorption of fat-soluble vitamins, thereby further impairing the synthesis of vitamin K–dependent clotting factors. Concomitant thrombocytopenia due to hypersplenism and alcohol-induced bone marrow suppression as well as qualitative platelet function abnormalities serves to exacerbate the bleeding tendency in cirrhotic patients. Thus, it is not surprising that coagulation abnormalities are detectable in 80 to 90% of patients with cirrhosis and commonly contribute to the development and perpetuation of hemorrhage in these individuals.

The prothrombin time (PT) is the simplest and most reliable index of hemostatic abnormalities in patients with liver disease. There is little indication for treatment of coagulation abnormalities in cirrhotic individuals unless (1) there is evidence of active hemorrhage, (2) the patient is considered to be at high risk for bleeding, or (3) an invasive procedure is contemplated. All cirrhotic patients with evidence of bleeding and a prolonged PT should be treated with intramuscular vitamin K_1 (AquaMEPHYTON, Konakion), which is administered in a daily dose of 10 mg over 3 consecutive days. Because anaphylaxis and death have been associated with the intravenous administration of vitamin K_1, this mode of drug delivery is not generally recommended. Vitamin K corrects coagulopathies secondary to malabsorption (i.e., bile salt deficiency) or malnutrition, but it has little effect in patients whose bleeding tendencies are predominantly a result of hepatocellular dysfunction. Fresh frozen plasma serves as an adequate source of Factors V, VII, VIII, X, and XI as well as prothrombin and facilitates the emergent correction of coagulation abnormalities. It is administered in a dose of 2 units intravenously every 2 to 3 hours until bleeding ceases or the PT is corrected to within 3 seconds of normal. Platelet transfusions are indicated in cirrhotics with active bleeding, even in the face of normal platelet counts, owing to a high prevalence of qualitative platelet function abnormalities. Desmopressin (DDAVP) a vasopressin analog, transiently increases the levels of Factor VII and von Willebrand's factor and reduces bleeding time and partial thromboplastin time. Desmopressin is administered in a dose of 0.3 µg per kg body weight diluted in 50 mL of sterile saline, as a slow intravenous infusion over 30 minutes. Cryoprecipitate is not particularly useful in the management of hepatic coagulopathies because it is an effective source of Factors VIII and XIII only.

HEPATIC TRANSPLANTATION

Orthotopic liver transplantation has become an accepted therapy for end-stage chronic liver disease. In adult patients with cirrhosis undergoing hepatic transplantation, liver disease is most commonly the result of primary biliary cirrhosis, alcohol cirrhosis, or cryptogenic cirrhosis. Although alcoholic liver disease has been considered a relative contraindication to hepatic transplantation, recent studies suggest that, using a multidisciplinary approach, the outcome in alcoholic cirrhotics is similar to that for patients with other forms of liver disease. Nevertheless, many programs require a period of abstinence ranging from 3 to 12 months before alcoholic individuals are considered candidates for transplantation. Individuals older than 50 years of age have a survival rate that has been shown to be comparable to that of younger patients. The use of transplantation in patients with cirrhosis owing to hepatitis B virus infection remains controversial as a result of the high incidence of aggressive recurrence postoperatively. Available data suggest, however, that recurrence of hepatitis C following hepatic transplantation follows a more benign course.

The optimal timing for transplantation in patients with chronic liver disease is often difficult to define. It is clear that patients who present with catastrophic complications from florid hepatic failure have a poorer outcome following transplantation than individuals with more compensated liver disease. In addition to the expense, however, hepatic transplantation has numerous inherent risks and requires long-term immunosuppressive therapy as well as prolonged medical follow-up. Perioperative mortality is currently around 10 to 20%. Thus, liver transplantation should be viewed as an exchange of one disease state (liver failure) for another (transplantation), rather than a definitive "cure." Only after a vigorous trial of medical therapy has been unsuccessful should consideration be given to hepatic transplantation for a cirrhotic patient. For those patients with serious disability from progressive and refractory liver failure and its complications, liver transplantation offers the possibility of long-term survival with an excellent quality of life.

PREGNANCY AND CIRRHOSIS

Because most women with cirrhosis who are of childbearing age have associated amenorrhea, it is relatively uncommon for cirrhotic patients to conceive. There appears to be no significant adverse effect of pregnancy on cirrhosis, so chronic liver disease per se is not an indication for termination of pregnancy. Unfortunately, women with cirrhosis have a high rate of spontaneous abortion (30%) and premature delivery. The approach to the management of the pregnant patient with cirrhosis is similar to that for nonpregnant patients. Except for known teratogens, it is imperative that specific therapy for the underlying liver disease be continued throughout the pregnancy, especially in the case of Wilson's disease, because discontinuation of treatment may lead to fulminant hepatic failure. There appears to be no undue risk to the fetus from penicillamine, trientine (Syprine), azathioprine (Imuran), or steroid therapy. The administration of spironolactone should be avoided because it crosses the placenta and is excreted in breast milk.

BLEEDING ESOPHAGEAL VARICES

method of
STEPHEN D. ZUCKER, M.D., and
JOHN L. GOLLAN, M.D., PH.D.

Harvard Medical School
Boston, Massachusetts

The portal vein carries blood from the spleen, stomach, small and large intestine, gallbladder, and pancreas to the liver (Fig. 1). Any increase in intrahepatic or extrahepatic resistance to portal blood flow induces an elevation in portal venous pressure. It also has been proposed that a massive increase in portal blood flow can cause a rise in portal pressure, although current evidence suggests that the contribution of increased portal flow to the pathophysiology of portal hypertension is negligible. An increase in portal pressure above the normal range of 5 to 10 mmHg may have serious clinical consequences, including gastrointestinal hemorrhage, hypersplenism, ascites, and encephalopathy. The leading cause of portal hypertension in the United States is cirrhosis of the liver; however, there are a number of other less common noncirrhotic causes of increased portal pressure (Table 1).

Spontaneous portosystemic collaterals develop in patients with established portal hypertension in an attempt to decompress the portal system (Table 2). The collaterals that result in the greatest clinical problems are gastroesophageal varices, which represent dilated submucosal vessels that channel splanchnic venous

TABLE 1. **Classification of Portal Hypertension**

Site of Increased Resistance	Cause
Prehepatic	Portal vein thrombosis
	Splenic vein thrombosis
Intrahepatic	
Presinusoidal	Sarcoidosis
	Schistosomiasis
	Congenital hepatic fibrosis
	Metastatic cancer
	Primary biliary cirrhosis
	Sclerosing cholangitis
	Myeloid metaplasia
	Toxins (e.g., vinyl chloride, arsenic)
	Nodular regenerative hyperplasia
	Idiopathic portal hypertension
Sinusoidal	Cirrhosis (most causes, including alcoholic and viral)
Postsinusoidal	Budd-Chiari syndrome
	Veno-occlusive disease
Posthepatic	Congestive heart failure
	Constrictive pericarditis
	Tricuspid regurgitation
	Inferior vena cava obstruction (e.g., web)

blood from the high-pressure portal system to the low-pressure azygous and hemiazygous veins. Gastrointestinal hemorrhage from esophageal varices is the major life-threatening consequence of portal hypertension, which occurs in more than 40% of patients with cirrhosis. Variceal hemorrhage is due to rupture of the vessel as a result of increased intravascular pressures and thinning of the overlying parenchyma, rather than erosion of the esophageal mucosa by acid-peptic digestion or the trauma of swallowing food. Thus patients with portal venous pressures exceeding 11 to 12 mmHg and those individuals with large varices are more prone to develop bleeding. Varices also may occur at other sites, such as the small intestine (particularly the duodenum), the rectum, an ileostomy site, or peritoneal adhesions (postoperative), and collectively are the cause of massive hemorrhage in approximately 2% of patients with intrahepatic portal hypertension. It traditionally has been estimated that 40 to 50% of cirrhotic patients die within 6 weeks of a variceal bleed, although recent data suggest that the mortality from

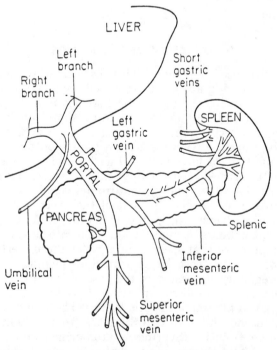

Figure 1. Anatomy of the portal venous system. (From Sherlock S: Diseases of the Liver and Biliary System, 7th ed. Oxford, England, Blackwell Scientific Publications, 1985, p 135.)

TABLE 2. **Location of Portosystemic Collaterals in Portal Hypertension**

Location	Examples
Transition zones between squamous and columnar epithelium	Gastroesophageal junction
	Anus
	Ileostomy
Obliterated fetal circulation in the falciform ligament	Umbilical and periumbilical veins
Retroperitoneal channels originating from the splenic circulation	Splenorenal and splenoadrenal collaterals
Retroperitoneal organs	Duodenum
	Colon (ascending, descending)
	Spleen

variceal hemorrhage has been reduced significantly as a result of new and more aggressive therapeutic modalities.

ACUTE MANAGEMENT OF BLEEDING ESOPHAGEAL VARICES

All patients with suspected variceal hemorrhage should be hospitalized, and supportive measures should be instituted promptly (Table 3). The approach to these patients should include monitoring in an intensive care setting and the administration of intravenous fluid and blood products (packed red blood cells, platelets) through one or two large-bore intravenous lines, as appropriate. Any coagulation abnormalities should be corrected with fresh frozen plasma and vitamin K. Care should be taken to avoid overexpansion of plasma volume, which may increase portal pressures and exacerbate variceal hemorrhage. Moreover, the rapid infusion of large volumes of crystalloid frequently results in the development of peripheral edema, ascites, and hyponatremia in cirrhotic patients.

A nasogastric tube should be inserted promptly to determine the rate of bleeding and facilitate gastric lavage. Lavage should be performed with room temperature (rather than iced) saline or tap water because cold temperatures not only impair clotting, but also unnecessarily lower the core body temperature. If bleeding is brisk or numerous clots are noted, the nasogastric tube may be replaced with a larger caliber Ewald tube. This maneuver facilitates the more rapid and complete removal of blood from the stomach, thereby affording a clearer view during the subsequent emergent endoscopy. Although variceal hemorrhage ceases spontaneously in nearly 60% of patients, it is not possible to predict those patients who will continue to bleed. Hence, any cirrhotic patient with evidence of ongoing or recurrent hemorrhage requires emergent endoscopy both for diagnosis and for therapy. It is important to note that more than 30% of patients with known esophageal varices and upper gastrointestinal hemorrhage have a source of bleeding other than varices and thus require an alternative therapeutic approach.

If variceal bleeding is confirmed by endoscopy, pharmacologic therapy with vasopressin* (antidiuretic hormone [Pitressin]) should be initiated promptly. Vasopressin induces vasoconstriction of the splanchnic arteries, thereby decreasing portal venous flow and thus portal pressure. It is administered intravenously via a continuous infusion of 0.2 units per minute following a bolus of 20 units in 100 mL of 5% dextrose. The rate may be increased hourly by 0.1 to 0.2 unit per minute until bleeding ceases, a maximum dose of 1.0 unit per minute is achieved, or adverse effects are noted. The overall short-term efficacy of vasopressin in patients with acute variceal hemorrhage is approximately 50%. Its use, however, is frequently limited by adverse effects, which include nausea, vomiting, abdominal cramps, myocardial ischemia, bradycardia, pulmonary edema, and mesenteric infarction. The concomitant administration of nitroglycerin, intravenously, sublingually, or transdermally, has been shown to reduce the systemic vasoconstrictive side effects and enhance the hemodynamic effects of vasopressin on the portal system. In patients with ongoing hemorrhage and hemodynamic instability, the use of nitroglycerin requires careful monitoring, with the intravenous route of administration affording the best hemodynamic control. Dosing typically begins at 40 μg per minute and is increased gradually until adverse symptoms are controlled, the systolic blood pressure falls significantly, or a maximum dose of 400 μg per minute is attained. Alternatively, sublingual nitroglycerin, given every 30 minutes for up to 6 hours, may be used. Selective intra-arterial infusion of vasopressin offers no advantage over intravenous administration and introduces the added risks associated with catheter placement. Alternative intravenous agents, such as the synthetic vasopressin analog terlipressin (Glypressin), administered as a 1-mg bolus every 4 hours following a 2-mg loading dose, or somatostatin (octreotide),† as a continuous infusion of 250 μg per hour following a 250-μg bolus, appear to be at least as effective as and less toxic than vasopressin in controlling variceal hemorrhage. Further controlled trials, however, are needed before these medications can be recommended routinely.

TABLE 3. **Management of Acute Variceal Hemorrhage**

Initial Management
Supportive measures
   Nasogastric tube with gastric lavage
   Intensive monitoring
   Intravenous fluid and blood products
   Correction of coagulopathy
Intravenous vasopressin
Endoscopic sclerosis or band ligation
Salvage Therapy (If Initial Management Is Unsuccessful)
Balloon tamponade (Minnesota tube)
Transjugular intrahepatic portosystemic shunt
Esophageal transection
Emergent surgical portosystemic shunting
Transhepatic catheter embolization

*This use of vasopressin is not listed in the manufacturer's official directive.

†This use of somatostatin is not listed in the manufacturer's official directive.

The rate of acute recurrence of variceal bleeding is exceedingly high once pharmacologic therapy is tapered; hence emergent endoscopic sclerotherapy generally is advocated as the primary definitive treatment for acute variceal hemorrhage. In experienced hands, endoscopic sclerosis is successful in controlling active variceal bleeding in 70 to 80% of patients following a single injection session, and this rate approaches 90 to 95% with an additional sclerotherapy session. Once hemorrhage is controlled, the remaining variceal channels should be sclerosed, and diagnostic panendoscopy should be completed to exclude the possibility of other synchronous lesions. Although sclerotherapy induces fibrosis and ultimately obliterates the injected varix, it does nothing to lower portal pressure acutely. Hence, vasopressin should be continued for at least 24 hours after successful sclerotherapy before being tapered gradually.

Endoscopic band ligation of esophageal varices represents a novel approach to the management of acute variceal hemorrhage. This technique involves the ligation of varices by the application of small, elastic O-rings. Recent studies indicate that endoscopic ligation is equally as effective as endoscopic sclerotherapy for the control of active variceal bleeding. Furthermore, initial studies suggest that band ligation is associated with fewer complications as compared with sclerotherapy. The major drawback of variceal ligation is the reduction in the endoscopist's field of vision as a result of the attachment of the ligating device. Moreover, because only one O-ring can be loaded at a time, the placement of an overtube is required to facilitate the repeated withdrawal and insertion of the endoscope. If further studies support the promising initial results, however, endoscopic ligation of varices may replace sclerotherapy as the principal treatment method for acute variceal hemorrhage.

If sclerotherapy (or band ligation) is unsuccessful, bleeding may be controlled by direct tamponade using a four-lumen balloon tube (modified Sengstaken-Blakemore or Minnesota tube). Placement of the tube by either a nasogastric or orogastric route acutely arrests variceal hemorrhage in more than 90% of patients. Owing to the 60% rebleeding rate after removal of the tube and the significant incidence of serious complications (15%), however, a more definitive procedure should be performed within 12 hours of tube insertion. Aspiration pneumonia and esophageal perforation, which are the primary complications associated with the use of the Minnesota tube, culminate in the death of nearly 6% of patients. Hence, balloon tube tamponade should be performed only by trained physicians and only when uncontrolled variceal hemorrhage has been documented endoscopically. The patient's stomach should be emptied and the airway protected by endotracheal intubation before tube insertion to reduce the risk of aspiration, particularly in those individuals with altered consciousness. After preliminary inflation of the gastric balloon with 50 mL of air, the position of the tube must be confirmed radiographically before further therapeutic inflation to 150 mL. The Minnesota tube then is withdrawn until firm resistance is encountered at the esophagogastric junction, and 1 pound of pressure is applied to maintain tension on the tube. If bleeding persists, the esophageal balloon is inflated to between 35 and 40 mmHg, and the pressure is monitored continuously by an attached pressure gauge. Inflation of the esophageal balloon for periods longer than 24 to 36 hours significantly increases the risk of necrosis and consequent perforation of the esophagus. Deflation of the esophageal balloon for brief periods of time at 12-hour intervals may reduce the risk of perforation.

For patients in whom the aforementioned therapeutic maneuvers fail to control variceal bleeding, emergent surgical intervention with portocaval shunting or esophageal transection warrants consideration. Although portocaval shunts are more effective than sclerotherapy in preventing recurrent variceal hemorrhage in decompensated cirrhotic patients, the high operative mortality in the emergency setting (up to 50%) and the unpredictable occurrence of postoperative encephalopathy make this a procedure of last resort. The use of a staple gun to transect the esophagus is a relatively simple alternative emergent measure that appears to control ongoing variceal bleeding as effectively as sclerotherapy. In the absence of a more extensive subsequent devascularization operation, however, recurrence of varices within a few months is common.

The introduction of the transjugular intrahepatic portal systemic shunt (TIPS) represents a novel angiographic alternative to surgical shunting procedures in patients with refractory variceal hemorrhage. This procedure, which requires only local anesthesia, appears to be particularly promising in patients with severe (Child's class C) cirrhosis, whose mortality rate associated with emergency shunt operations exceeds 50%. TIPS involves the creation of an intrahepatic communication between hepatic and portal vein branches via a transjugular approach (Fig. 2A). The newly created tract is dilated with a balloon (Fig. 2B), and an expandable metal stent then is inserted to maintain patency (Fig. 2C, D). This procedure effectively creates a functional side-to-side portocaval shunt within the hepatic parenchyma and has been shown to reduce portal pressures by an average of 40 to 50%. A recent study

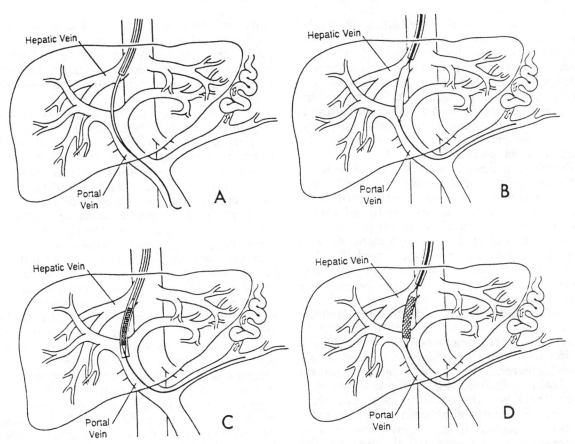

Figure 2. Transjugular intrahepatic portosystemic shunting. *A,* Right jugular venous access is obtained with a 16-gauge transjugular needle and No. 10 French sheath. The hepatic parenchyma is punctured from the right hepatic vein to the proximal right portal vein, and a No. 5 French catheter is introduced to permit measurement of portal venous pressure. *B,* An 8-mm balloon catheter is expanded across the hepatic parenchymal tract. *C,* A 30-mm-long Palmaz stent mounted on an 8-mm balloon catheter is advanced across the parenchymal tract within a No. 10 French vascular sheath. *D,* After withdrawal of the sheath, the stent is deployed by fully expanding the balloon. The residual portosystemic gradient is measured, and shunt position and patency are confirmed by splenoportography. (From Zemel G, et al: Technical advances in transjugular intrahepatic portosystemic shunts. RadioGraphics *12:*617–619, 1992.)

in patients with Child's class B or C cirrhosis and variceal bleeding refractory to endoscopic sclerotherapy demonstrated a relatively low 13% mortality, 20% risk of rebleeding, and 13% incidence of encephalopathy associated with the TIPS procedure. Although preliminary, these data indicate that TIPS represents a relatively safe and effective modality for portal decompression, which may be particularly well suited for the control of variceal hemorrhage in cirrhotic patients who are at high risk for surgery or are awaiting liver transplantation. If confirmed, these findings suggest that TIPS may virtually eliminate the need for portocaval shunting or esophageal transection in the management of acute variceal bleeding.

The use of transhepatic catheter embolization of varices for the short-term control of hemorrhage is controversial. Rebleeding following this procedure is frequent, owing to persistence of the underlying portal hypertension. Furthermore,

portal vein thrombosis and gastrointestinal ischemia and necrosis are not uncommon complications. In patients who have undergone partial portal decompression, however, either by selective shunting or by the use of small-caliber portocaval shunts, there may be a role for transshunt coronary vein embolization for the control of variceal rebleeding.

LONG-TERM MANAGEMENT OF ESOPHAGEAL VARICES

Owing to the 70% likelihood of recurrent bleeding in untreated patients with a history of variceal hemorrhage and the high mortality associated with each bleeding episode, long-term therapy is generally recommended in patients who have had an initial episode of variceal bleeding. Repeated sclerotherapy is the most commonly used long-term treatment for variceal hemorrhage. It effectively eradicates esophageal varices in the vast majority of patients and significantly reduces the incidence of recurrent bleeding once all of the visible varices have been eliminated. This form of therapy, however, requires prolonged follow-up, and although the complication rate for long-term sclerotherapy is low, the risk of esophageal ulceration, stricture, or even perforation increases progressively with the number of sessions.

Following an acute episode of variceal bleeding, patients typically undergo a second sclerotherapy session within 1 week. Endoscopic sclerosis is repeated at 3- to 4-week intervals until all varices are obliterated, at which point follow-up examinations are conducted every 3 to 6 months. Using this approach to sclerotherapy, a marked reduction in the number of subsequent bleeding episodes per patient is achieved, although there is only a small decrease in the actual number of patients who develop an additional hemorrhagic event. In fact, almost 50% of patients who undergo long-term sclerotherapy for esophageal varices have at least one additional bleeding episode. Moreover, there appears to be no significant survival benefit from long-term endoscopic sclerosis. There is a theoretical concern, supported only by anecdotal clinical experience, that obliteration of esophageal varices by long-term sclerotherapy may increase portal pressure and thereby induce the development of gastric varices. These venous channels occur primarily in the cardia and fundus of the stomach and can bleed in much the same manner as their esophageal counterpart. Unfortunately, in contrast to esophageal varices, sclerotherapy is ineffective in controlling either acute or recurrent hemorrhage from gastric varices. It also has been suggested that patients undergoing long-term sclerotherapy may be at increased risk for bleeding from congestive gastropathy (see discussion later in this article).

A recent study comparing repeated endoscopic band ligation with sclerotherapy for the management of patients with cirrhosis and bleeding esophageal varices noted a significantly lower incidence of treatment-related complications associated with the former procedure (2% vs. 22%). Specifically the risk of esophageal strictures, pneumonia, and peritonitis was reduced in the patients undergoing band ligation. Over a mean follow-up period of 10 months, the mortality rate in the band ligated group (28%) was significantly lower than in the patients who underwent sclerotherapy (45%). There also was a trend toward fewer rebleeding episodes (36% vs. 48%) and a lower mean number of treatments required for the eradication of varices (4 ± 2 vs. 5 ± 2) in the banded patients. If these findings are confirmed,

endoscopic ligation likely will replace sclerotherapy as the therapy of choice for the long-term management of esophageal varices. In addition, trials evaluating the combined use of band ligation and low-volume sclerotherapy are currently under way.

Portal-to-systemic shunt operations (Fig. 3) are the most successful procedures for preventing recurrent hemorrhage from esophageal varices. Shunting generally is reserved for patients who do not respond to sclerotherapy. Some centers advocate elective portosystemic shunting as primary therapy for low-risk cirrhotic patients, despite reported operative mortality rates that approach 10%. In addition, the risk of shunt-induced hepatic encephalopathy is a concern (20%), and this complication may be incapacitating in some cases. The selective distal splenorenal shunt (Fig. 3F) is most often recommended, owing to both a slightly diminished incidence of associated encephalopathy and a lower likelihood of interfering with a potential subsequent hepatic transplantation. As with sclerotherapy, there is no definitive evidence for improved survival in cirrhotic patients who undergo shunt placement. Except in the rare patient with isolated splenic vein thrombosis, there is no role for splenectomy alone in the management of bleeding varices. In patients with cirrhosis, hepatic transplantation is the only form of therapy that addresses the underlying liver disease and should be considered when variceal hemorrhage recurs despite appropriate therapy. Although controversial, hepatic transplantation in patients with alcoholic cirrhosis has been demonstrated to be quite effective when combined with aggressive psychosocial support.

Reduction of portal pressure by oral beta-blocking agents, such as propranolol* (Inderal), has been shown in several studies to reduce the incidence of bleeding from esophageal varices significantly. Despite a reduction in the risk of recurrent variceal hemorrhage, however, there is a lack of evidence that beta-blocker therapy alone improves survival in cirrhotic patients. Drug side effects and poor compliance, especially in alcoholics, are significant problems. Typical regimens begin with 20 mg of oral propranolol twice daily. If this is tolerated, the patient is converted to an equivalent once-daily dose of a long-acting propranolol preparation (Inderal LA), which is increased gradually until a 20 to 25% reduction in baseline heart rate is achieved, or until a maximum dose of 320 mg per day is reached. Several trials have demonstrated that propranolol alone

---

*This use of propranolol is not listed in the manufacturer's official directive.

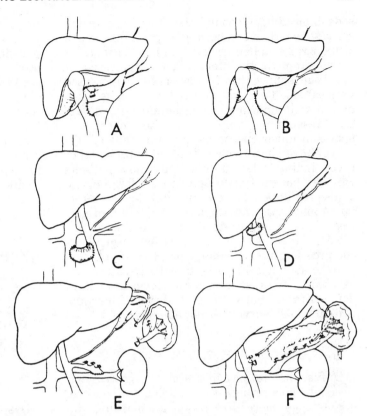

Figure 3. Surgical portosystemic shunting procedures. *A,* End-to-side portocaval shunt; *B,* side-to-side portocaval shunt; *C,* mesocaval interpositional H-graft; *D,* portocaval interpositional H-graft; *E,* central splenorenal shunt; and *F,* selective distal splenorenal shunt. (From Terblanche J, et al: Controversies in the management of bleeding esophageal varices. N Engl J Med *320:*1396, 1989. Reprinted by permission of the New England Journal of Medicine, vol. 320, p. 1396, 1989.)

is less effective than sclerotherapy in preventing rebleeding. Hence, few physicians would recommend propranolol as the sole therapy for the long-term management of variceal bleeding except in the uncommon situation when both sclerotherapy and surgical intervention are unacceptable. Preliminary studies, however, suggest that the administration of propranolol in conjunction with sclerotherapy or endoscopic band ligation is more effective than endoscopic therapy alone in the prevention of rebleeding from esophageal varices. Further clinical trials are necessary to define the precise role of combined endoscopic and beta-blocker therapy.

PROPHYLACTIC THERAPY FOR THE PREVENTION OF FIRST VARICEAL HEMORRHAGE

The use of prophylactic therapy to prevent the first episode of variceal hemorrhage remains an area of controversy. Because nearly two-thirds of patients with cirrhosis and varices never develop bleeding, the treatment of all patients with varices results in unnecessary intervention in the majority of cases. A recent meta-analysis of trials using prophylactic beta-blocker therapy in patients with cirrhosis and esophageal varices suggested that the oral administration of twice-daily

propranolol or once-daily nadolol* (Corgard), significantly reduced the risk of first variceal hemorrhage, particularly in patients with medium-sized to large-sized varices or with a hepatic vein pressure gradient above 12 mmHg. Both of these medications were administered in doses ranging from 80 to 320 mg per day and were titrated so as to reduce resting heart rate by 25%. Although there was a trend toward reduced mortality, no statistically significant survival advantage was demonstrated for patients receiving prophylactic beta-blocker therapy. Furthermore, treatment was associated with a 20% rate of noncompliance and a 10% incidence of significant complications, including asthma and hypotension. It remains to be seen whether a selected group of patients with portal hypertension will demonstrate improved survival rates with prophylactic oral beta-blocker therapy.

The role of prophylactic esophageal sclerotherapy is unclear, with some studies showing improved survival and others actually demonstrating an increased mortality in treated patients. Currently there is no compelling evidence for the use of prophylactic sclerotherapy in the management of esophageal varices before the first epi-

---

*This use of nadolol is not listed in the manufacturer's official directive.

sode of bleeding. Ongoing studies are designed to address whether a subgroup of patients at high risk for variceal hemorrhage can be identified, for which prophylactic intervention is indicated. It has been shown that the presence of increased variceal size (>5 mm) and red color signs, such as red wale markings (longitudinal dilated venules resembling whip marks) and cherry-red spots, on upper endoscopy are important predictors of future hemorrhage. It is unknown whether these findings adequately identify those patients who will benefit from prophylactic sclerotherapy. It also remains to be determined if there is a role for prophylactic endoscopic band ligation of varices, given its lower rate of complications.

There appears to be no place for surgical decompression in the primary prophylaxis of variceal hemorrhage in patients with cirrhosis and esophageal varices. Several controlled trials have demonstrated that although the risk of bleeding is diminished, survival is not enhanced.

CONGESTIVE GASTROPATHY

Diffuse or focal bleeding from the gastric mucosa, which can range from insidious to massive, accounts for more than 5% of all bleeding episodes in cirrhotic patients. A variety of structural changes are observed in the stomach of portal hypertensive patients, including numerous mucosal vascular ectasias, thickened arterioles, submucosal edema, and arteriovenous communications. The pathogenesis of these vascular changes has been variably ascribed to the direct effect of portal hypertension, increased splanchnic blood flow, and local disturbances in vascular tone regulation. Recent studies suggest that in patients with cirrhosis the prevalence of gastric mucosal abnormalities approaches 70%. The term "congestive gastropathy" has been coined to describe these abnormalities, which on endoscopy may vary in appearance from a mild diffuse hyperemia or reticular pattern ("watermelon stomach") to a more severe form consisting of a granular mucosa with discrete punctate red spots. The 5-year actuarial risk of overt hemorrhage in patients with cirrhosis and endoscopic evidence of severe congestive gastropathy approaches 75%, as compared with a 7% risk in those individuals without observable gastric mucosal abnormalities.

Individuals with portal hypertension who develop significant bleeding from the gastric mucosa rarely respond to medical or surgical therapy aimed at reducing gastric acid secretion. Hence, H_2-blockers, sucralfate (Carafate), and antacids generally are ineffective in these patients. In contrast, recent studies suggest that propranolol, at a dose sufficient to reduce the resting heart rate either by 25% or to 55 beats per minute, significantly decreases the incidence of recurrent bleeding from gastric lesions in patients with congestive gastropathy. Portosystemic shunting also has been shown to be effective in controlling refractory nonvariceal hemorrhage from portal hypertensive gastropathy in cirrhotic patients. The role of TIPS in patients with congestive gastropathy is undefined, and owing to the high operative mortality, gastrectomy should be avoided except as a treatment of last resort.

DYSPHAGIA AND ESOPHAGEAL OBSTRUCTION

method of
MORRIS TRAUBE, M.D.
Yale University School of Medicine
New Haven, Connecticut

DIAGNOSTIC APPROACH

Dysphagia, or difficulty in swallowing, can be analyzed in terms of two main phases of swallowing (1) transfer from the mouth into the esophagus and (2) transit along the esophagus into the stomach.

Transfer from the mouth to the esophagus is the more complex of the two phases, being highly dependent on coordinated muscular movements, which are in turn affected by multiple cranial nerves. This tight control is necessary to prevent the movement of food into the respiratory tree as well as to propel food into the pharynx and proximal esophagus. Once in the esophagus, bolus transit occurs via peristaltic contractions. Finally, at the distal esophagus, the lower esophageal sphincter, normally protecting the esophagus from reflux of gastric material, must relax in response to swallowing, thereby removing the barrier for the food bolus and allowing entry into the stomach.

The history still remains helpful in the diagnosis of dysphagia. For example, slowly progressive symptoms suggest a motor disorder, such as spasm or achalasia, rather than mechanical obstruction. The rapid onset of dysphagia during weeks to months, along with substantial weight loss, suggests a neoplasm of the esophagus. A long history of heartburn followed by slow progression of dysphagia suggests a benign stricture. Dysphagia for both liquids and solids suggests a motor disorder; dysphagia for solids alone suggests mechanical obstruction, such as a stricture;

and dysphagia that is worse for liquids than solids suggests a proximal disorder, usually neurologic in origin, such as cricopharyngeal dysfunction. If dysphagia is accompanied by odynophagia, or painful swallowing, mucosal disease, such as severe reflux esophagitis or infectious esophagitis, as is so common today with acquired immune deficiency syndrome (AIDS), is suggested. The presence of risk factors, such as smoking, alcohol, or previous caustic ingestion, increases suspicion for a carcinoma of the esophagus.

The physical examination may be useful in the evaluation of dysphagia. Evidence of marked weight loss may suggest cancer. Telangiectasia or sclerodactyly may indicate systemic sclerosis, and oral candidiasis may suggest involvement of the esophagus by the same organism. The general examination may show absence of a gag reflex or presence of fasciculations, indicating neurologic disease. The patient may be asked to swallow some water and show immediate coughing, again suggesting neurologic dysfunction leading to aspiration.

Despite the widespread use of endoscopy, the barium x-ray remains the best overall study for the evaluation of dysphagia and should almost always be done. A complete study, which can be altered to the situation, includes both single-contrast and double-contrast examinations and careful attention to fluoroscopy, particularly with video. The single-contrast esophagogram is the best study for evaluating various anatomic abnormalities, such as stricture or ring, whereas the double-contrast esophagogram offers more information regarding the mucosa, such as small ulceration. Videofluoroscopy is most important in the evaluation of the oropharyngeal phase of swallowing but is also valuable in the evaluation of esophageal motor abnormalities. Occasionally it is advantageous to give a solid bolus, such as a barium tablet, to help reveal an abnormality, such as a lower esophageal ring or stricture. This technique helps not only to identify the lesion, but also to show arrest of the bolus at the lesion and relate the symptoms to the anatomic abnormality.

Endoscopic examination usually follows the radiographic one. Endoscopy yields further information regarding inflammatory and infectious disorders of the esophagus. It helps to categorize and grade the effects of reflux as well as to diagnose specific fungal and viral infections of the esophagus. Along with biopsy, it is more commonly helpful in evaluating masses, which are generally malignant, and in evaluating strictures, most of which are benign. Although a negative endoscopic examination is gratifying, the physician must recognize that dysphagia may result from abnormalities not well evaluated by endoscopy, such as extrinsic compression of the esophagus and, more commonly, motility disorders.

If an extrinsic disorder, such as cancerous lymph nodes, a large thyroid, or a tortuous aorta from atherosclerosis, is suspected, special studies are in order. These include computed tomographic (CT) scan, barium with fluoroscopy, or a thyroid scan. More commonly, however, when radiographic and endoscopic studies are negative, a motility disorder is responsible, and the diagnostic study of choice is esophageal manometry. Such studies may confirm a diagnosis of achalasia, esophageal spasm, systemic sclerosis, or other less well-described motility disorders.

Acute obstruction is seen with foreign body ingestion. Most nonfood foreign body ingestions are in children, and most food impactions are in adults, usually in those with underlying esophageal disease, such as a lower esophageal ring or stricture. These patients may have a sense of choking, distress, or sialorrhea. Although plain films of the chest are helpful, particularly in children, the diagnosis is usually made by other means. Unless there is strong concern for a proximal lesion or for perforation, the diagnostic method of choice is endoscopy; radiographic studies make a subsequent endoscopic examination, with its therapeutic potential, more difficult.

OROPHARYNGEAL DYSPHAGIA

Although the majority of patients with oropharyngeal dysphagia have common neurologic disease, such as cerebrovascular disease, it is imperative to consider specific disorders because only these may have disease-specific therapy. The patient with parkinsonism may improve with L-dopa and the patient with myasthenia gravis with cholinesterase inhibitors, such as pyridostigmine (Mestinon). The patient with hypothyroidism may respond to thyroid replacement, as may the patient with polymyositis to steroids. The patient with a Zenker's diverticulum may respond to cricopharyngeal myotomy, as long as the diverticulum is also removed if large.

Unfortunately, most patients have common neurologic disease such as stroke, for which there is no specific therapy. Nevertheless, the patient may benefit from various dietary and behavioral approaches. Such patients have more trouble with liquids than with solids and may benefit nicely from changing the consistency of the food to a paste. Retraining to swallow can be undertaken as well, usually with the help of a speech pathologist with interest in dysphagia. The patient may be taught to use those muscles or movements that help to propel the bolus forward. Often patients with acute stroke and dysphagia are treated with percutaneous endoscopic gastrostomy for purposes of feeding. In some cases, improvement over time allows the patient to ingest at least some food. Less commonly, patients may undergo cricopharyngeal myotomy, particularly if there is intact oropharyngeal sensation and control of tongue and pharyngeal movements. With the greater ease of gastrostomy, such intervention, with frequently poor results, should be undertaken only rarely.

PRIMARY ESOPHAGEAL MOTOR DISORDERS

Achalasia

Achalasia is characterized by loss of peristalsis and by relaxation of the lower esophageal sphincter in response to swallowing. All treatments are designed to reduce the functional obstruction at the sphincter. The patient may benefit from calcium channel blockers, which reduce the resting sphincter pressure. The best agent is nifedipine (Procardia), which has the greatest effect on the sphincter. The best result is obtained when the patient bites the 10-mg nifedipine capsule and swallows the contents 30 minutes before meals. If there are no side effects, such as headache or flushing, the dose may be increased to two or three capsules before each meal. Unfortunately, patients usually have only partial or short-lived results, and such treatment is recommended only in patients who cannot undertake more definitive treatment.

Some have recommended bougienage, but the results are only transient, and the procedure should be limited to those who cannot tolerate more. A large-size bougie, such as No. 48–54 French Maloney, may be passed without the need for initial passage of smaller sizes. It is recommended that this be done under fluoroscopy or over a wire, such as with the Savary system, in view of the lack of peristalsis, the hold-up at the sphincter, and commonly the tortuous nature of the esophagus.

Most patients with achalasia should undergo pneumatic dilation of the esophagus. Various dilators have been used, but currently the most commonly used is the Microvasive Rigiflex achalasia dilator. The author prefers to use the 40-mm dilator unless there is prior myotomy, concomitant medical conditions, or if the patient is a child, which would lead to the use of the 35-mm dilator. The procedure is done in the fluoroscopy suite, with the patient premedicated as for routine endoscopy. Atropine, 0.5 to 1.0 mg, is given intravenously to decrease salivary secretions dur-

ing the procedure. The endoscope is inserted into the esophagus, and any residual food or secretions are suctioned out. If a large amount of food is present, the scope should be removed and a large Edlich or similar tube used to lavage and clean the esophagus. Endoscopic examination of the esophagus should indicate that there is no mass or stricture, but some inflammation secondary to stasis may be seen. A retroflexed view of the fundus is carried out to exclude a tumor and secondary achalasia. With the scope in the stomach, a guidewire is placed through the scope, and the scope is then removed. The dilating balloon is then passed over the wire, with fluoroscopy being used to indicate proper placement. When the balloon is at the level of the sphincter, insufflation will lead to a "waist" appearance. A pressure of about 5 pounds per square inch is maintained for about 1 minute. If discomfort is too great or if there is rapid and complete ablation, the pressure is released. If the patient can tolerate it and there is only partial ablation, the procedure is repeated after several minutes. It is common to see some blood on the dilator on removal. As long as the patient is monitored all day long, it is not necessary to perform contrast studies of the esophagus routinely to exclude perforation, a complication that occurs approximately 5% of the time. Close watching may indicate pain or fever, at which time a contrast study that may indicate perforation should be performed. Small perforations may be treated by antibiotics, but most are treated surgically by repair, at which time myotomy is also performed.

Patients who do not respond to several pneumatic dilations should be offered Heller myotomy, with success rates of about 80%, somewhat more than with pneumatic dilation.

Esophageal Spasm

Esophageal spasm is a disorder in which there is an increased percentage of simultaneous waves, with some preserved peristalsis. It is probably overdiagnosed but may nevertheless be a cause for dysphagia. Although various drugs are used, none has been established in blind studies to be effective. Nevertheless, some patients may respond to various drugs, such as anxiolytics, nitrates (either oral nitrates or sublingual nitrates on an as-needed basis), or calcium channel blockers such as diltiazem (Cardizem) or nifedipine. Rather than treat long term with drugs of suboptimal efficacy, it appears more reasonable to this author to treat with bougienage, even if the effect may not be more than placebo. If there is no tortuosity to the esophagus and if a barium study leads to suspicion of no other disorder, it is fine to pass a large bougie, such as a No. 48 French Maloney, directly without moving up from smaller sizes. On other occasions, it would be appropriate to perform such dilation over a wire.

Rarely patients with dysphagia from esophageal spasm may also have lower esophageal sphincter dysfunction that may not respond to bougienage but may respond to pneumatic dilation, performed in a manner similar to that in achalasia described earlier. Even rarer is the patient with dysphagia who responds to neither medical nor dilation treatment and who could be a candidate for long esophagomyotomy. This myotomy involves the distal half of the esophagus and thereby differs from the Heller myotomy of achalasia, which involves only the sphincteric area.

Nonspecific Motor Disorders

In contrast to achalasia and spasm, the nutcracker esophagus has normal peristalsis but an increased mean contraction amplitude in the distal esophagus. This disorder as well as other nonspecific disorders is more common in the population of patients with noncardiac chest pain. Many of these patients, however, also complain of dysphagia. As for spasm, there is no evidence that the disorder responds to pharmacologic therapy or to bougienage. Nevertheless, if dysphagia is a key symptom, bougienage may be tried, as for spasm.

Systemic Sclerosis

The esophagus is the most commonly involved gastrointestinal organ in patients with systemic sclerosis. Progressive muscle atrophy and fibrosis lead to loss of peristalsis as well as reduction of sphincter pressure. As a secondary phenomenon, these lead to substantial gastroesophageal reflux and its complications, such as esophageal stricture. Unfortunately, no medication, including the newer prokinetic agents, can restore the esophageal function toward normal. Despite this pessimism, there is a role for other medical treatment. The patient should be advised to chew his or her food well and to take in liquids with food. If there is heartburn, certainly treatment for reflux is indicated, and such patients should receive full doses of H_2-blockers (e.g., ranitidine [Zantac], 150 mg twice daily) or the proton pump inhibitor omeprazole (Prilosec), 20 mg per day, depending on the severity of the symptoms. Even if symptoms are less troublesome, if radiographic or manometric studies show severe motor dysfunction, such as complete loss of contraction, prophylactic therapy is indicated.

Before assuming that dysphagia results from the motor dysfunction alone, one must exclude superimposed disorders. A barium study or an endoscopic one should be undertaken to exclude strictures, an esophageal ring, or both. If these are present, they should be treated as would any stricture or ring, as described later. Such treatment may be required only several times or may be required on an ongoing maintenance basis.

MECHANICAL OBSTRUCTION

Esophageal Rings

The most common cause of dysphagia is the lower esophageal ring, or the Schatzki ring, which sits at the border of the esophagus and stomach. It is almost always seen with a hiatal hernia, so that the ring is just proximal to the hernia. Typically patients have dysphagia that is rather intermittent and for solids only. Once the diagnosis is confirmed by radiographic or endoscopic means (or both), the treatment approach is straightforward: dilation of the ring. Because the goal is rupture, the approach should be abrupt dilation rather than progressive stretching. If the radiographic and endoscopic studies have shown no tortuosity of the esophagus, it is appropriate simply to pass a large bougie through the esophagus into the stomach, and this may be anywhere from No. 48 to No. 60 French. It is not necessary to use fluoroscopy, but if the patient has no relief of symptoms, a repeat dilation should be performed under fluoroscopy to verify entrance of the bougie into the stomach. If the dilation is performed at the end of an endoscopic procedure, the dilation may be performed over a wire placed endoscopically, but this is generally not necessary. A lack of response to dilation may occur because of associated motor dysfunction or from lack of rupture of the ring by the dilation. Under such circumstances, repeat radiographic and manometric studies would be necessary to sort out the possibilities. Treatment of the lower esophageal ring by dilation is usually done once or twice, but late recurrences are possible. Nevertheless, a continuous program of dilation is not necessary, a situation that differs from that of esophageal strictures.

Esophageal Strictures

The diagnosis of an esophageal stricture is made by the initial barium x-ray or by endoscopy. In any event, endoscopic examination is warranted to allow for biopsy to exclude cancer. The endoscopic examination also allows for therapeutic dilation.

The size of the endoscope can be used to determine the size of the lumen of the stricture. If the lumen is at least No. 38 French in size, it is unnecessary to perform the dilation over a wire, and simple passage of the bougie is sufficient. For dilating strictures, the tapered Maloney bougies are used. Bougies of successively larger sizes, in 2-French increments, are passed. The physician notes and measures the resistance of the stricture to passage of the dilator. Although the "rule of threes" has been variably interpreted, this author generally takes the conservative approach and limits the dilations to a total of three with mild to moderate resistance.

Guided dilations should be performed rather than simple bougienage under certain circumstances, such as long strictures, angulation of the esophagus, or the presence of esophageal diverticula. Even more common, tight strictures, usually defined as a lumen smaller than No. 38 French, are also dilated by guidance. This author prefers the Savary dilator, which is passed over a wire, which is passed through the endoscope. For proximal lesions or for tight lesions not allowing passage of even the pediatric scope, this should be done with fluoroscopy as well. If the scope can be passed through the stricture or if the wire can be seen easily to pass the short area of stricture into the normal esophagus and stomach, fluoroscopy is not mandatory. Nevertheless, caution should be used to make sure that the wire is not coiling in either esophagus or stomach; less experienced clinicians would do best to use fluoroscopy.

Repeated dilation is often necessary, and this can be done several days to 1 week after the initial procedure. Depending on the response, the intervals can be lengthened and the patient can be observed by symptoms. There is no demonstrable benefit to routine x-ray or endoscopy simply to determine patency.

On occasion, the stricture is somewhat angulated, very tight, or both, making placement of a wire difficult. Under such circumstances, the newer small balloon dilators passed through the scope can be used. Generally the Savary system is preferable, however, and the need for the balloons is rather uncommon.

Neoplasms

Malignant dysphagia is usually related to squamous cell carcinoma or adenocarcinoma, the latter of which is often secondary to Barrett's esophagus. The approach is similar to that of benign strictures of the esophagus. Experience indicates that most neoplasms of the esophagus can be dilated in a manner similar to benign strictures. Such dilations may be undertaken while the patient is receiving other therapy, such as external radiation therapy. Details of the various modalities, such as surgery or chemotherapy, may be read elsewhere, but it is often appropriate to try to obtain patency of the lumen early on, so nutritional adequacy is guaranteed. Although some have advocated other therapies, such as tumor probes or laser ablation, this author finds the need for them rather infrequent. Likewise, esophageal prosthesis placement has only a limited role, particularly because dilations over a wire are easier today than years ago. It nevertheless is valuable in the treatment of neoplastic tracheoesophageal fistula, in that the prosthesis can seal off the fistula.

Miscellaneous Disorders

Having excluded the primary motor disorders and organic obstruction, one can appropriately discuss various miscellaneous disorders.

Most common is nonobstructive dysphagia in patients with gastroesophageal reflux disease. This is related to motor dysfunction of the esophagus, with either secondary spasm or nonpropulsive low-amplitude contractions. Such dysmotility has no primary therapy, but aggressive antireflux treatment should be given. It is possible that prolonged medical treatment can improve the dysphagia, and this is also seen after surgical treatment by fundoplication.

Particularly in the era of AIDS and immunosuppression from organ transplantation, the physician often sees patients with dysphagia and odynophagia from infections of the esophagus. *Candida* esophagitis responds readily if the patient is not immunosuppressed. This can be treated by nystatin (Mycostatin) ("swish and swallow"). If oral tablets are preferred, ketoconazole, 200 mg once per day, is sufficient, although double the dose may be necessary in the presence of immunosuppression, particularly in patients with AIDS in whom absorption of the agent is diminished. A newer alternative is fluconazole (Diflucan), and this may be preferred in the setting of AIDS. Herpes simplex esophagitis may also cause dysphagia and odynophagia. In the immunocompetent patient, it is not necessary to give specific antiviral treatment because the infection usually clears within days. This is not the case in the immunocompromised, who should receive acyclovir (Zovirax), which can be given orally or intravenously, as needed. Increasingly recognized is cytomegalovirus, particularly in patients with AIDS, and such patients should receive ganciclovir (Cytovene), although the long-term prognosis in such patients is poor. Prophylactic treatment with ganciclovir is also indicated once the acute infection has been treated.

ACUTE OBSTRUCTION AND FOREIGN BODIES

The diagnosis of esophageal foreign body is made by the history and confirmed by either radiographic or endoscopic means, preferably by the latter. The treatment is usually endoscopic removal, although other medical means may be tried. What should not be tried is enzymatic therapy, such as meat tenderizer, because this may cause necrosis of the esophageal wall. While arrangements are made for endoscopic removal, it may occasionally bear fruits to try pharmacologic therapy. Some have tried nifedipine in a dose of 10 mg taken sublingually, whereas others have tried sublingual nitrates. This author prefers the intravenous injection of glucagon, 0.5 mg, a dose that can be repeated in 10 minutes. It is only a rare patient, however, who suddenly recognizes relief of the food obstruction. Blind passage of a bougie to push the bolus into the stomach is not recommended, and it is not preferable to use Foley catheters to remove the impacted food. Patients with foreign body impaction in the esophagus are best treated by endoscopic removal. If the lesion is proximal, such procedures are usually done under general anesthesia and with the rigid esophagoscope of the otorhinolaryngologist. The procedure in small children is also generally best performed under general anesthesia. Under other circumstances, the procedure can be done in the endoscopy suite with standard conscious sedation and the use of flexible endoscopes. Generally the rule is to pull rather than to push the foreign body into the stomach. The object can be grabbed with a snare and retrieved through the mouth. It is wise to use an overtube, so the respiratory tree is protected, in that the object is surrounded by the overtube. An overtube should also be used if the bolus is easily fragmented, requiring repeated removal and insertion of the endoscope with attached snare. Although such procedures may be lengthy, it is rare not to be able to remove a foreign body. In general, foreign body removals entail greater risk than other types of endoscopy and should be performed only by experienced physicians. Finally, endoscopy may show the cause of obstruction, such as a stricture or ring; dilation may be done immediately unless there is marked friability from the impaction.

DIVERTICULA OF THE ALIMENTARY TRACT

method of
GARY SPIEGELMAN, M.D.
Fort Sanders Park West Medical Center
Knoxville, Tennessee

and

JAMIE S. BARKIN, M.D.
University of Miami, School of Medicine
Miami, Florida

Diverticula may be seen throughout the alimentary tract and are anatomic outpouchings through its wall. The majority are false diverticula or pseudodiverticula and represent herniation of the mucosa and submucosa through the bowel wall. Congenital or true diverticula are less common and represent herniation of all layers of the gut wall. Although the majority of diverticula are clinically silent, they may become symptomatic, and complications may occur throughout the gastrointestinal tract.

ESOPHAGEAL DIVERTICULA

Esophageal diverticula generally occur in three regions: (1) immediately above the upper esophageal sphincter (Zenker's), (2) in the mid-esophagus (traction), and (3) immediately above the lower esophageal sphincter (epiphrenic). All of these are false, acquired diverticula, presenting with symptoms later in life, and are commonly associated with esophageal motility disturbances.

ZENKER'S DIVERTICULUM

This proximal diverticulum is an acquired, single, false diverticulum of variable size that originates between the pharynx and proximal esophagus. It is a globular sac located posterior between the esophagus and spine in the midline. The pathophysiology probably involves increased intraluminal pressure combined with functional obstruction at the cricopharyngeal level. The obstruction is thought to be secondary to motor incoordination between the cricopharyngeus, which functions as the upper esophageal sphincter, and the pharynx. This causes protrusion of mucosa between the oblique fibers of the inferior pharyngeal constrictor and the transverse fibers of the cricopharyngeus. A small Zenker's diverticulum is often asymptomatic but may present with mild dysphagia. As the sac enlarges enough to retain food debris, patients may also complain of pulmonary aspiration, regurgitation of undigested food and saliva, foul-smelling breath, or gurgling in the throat. As the diverticulum grows, it may progressively compress and obstruct the esophagus during the course of a meal.

The diagnosis may be suggested by history but is usually confirmed by x-ray contrast studies. Endoscopy should be done under direct visualization to avoid perforation and emergent surgical repair.

Surgical intervention is indicated when significant symptoms are present. The preferred technique for a large diverticulum is cricopharyngeal myotomy and one-stage diverticulectomy. If the diverticulum is small, a myotomy alone is usually curative.

MID-ESOPHAGEAL DIVERTICULA

Diverticula located in the mid-esophagus, also known as traction or parabronchial, were thought to occur secondary to fibrous adhesions from tuberculous mediastinal lymph nodes. Adhesions are rarely seen in autopsy studies, whereas a wide variety of motility disturbances are commonly found, including vigorous achalasia, diffuse spasm, and nonspecific disorders. Midesophageal diverticula are generally small and asymptomatic, requiring no therapy unless tuberculosis is present. Rarely symptoms, such as dysphagia, or complications, including bleeding, perforation, pericarditis, or fistula formation, may occur. If the diverticulum is thought to be responsible for the symptoms, evaluation should include barium swallow, endoscopy, and manometry. Therapy is simple excision along with treatment of secondary complications.

EPIPHRENIC DIVERTICULA

Lower esophageal diverticula are acquired and usually occur in adults. They involve a herniation of the mucosa and submucosa through the supporting musculature, occur within 10 cm of the gastric cardia, and are usually asymptomatic. There is a strong association with a variety of esophageal motor abnormalities and the presence of hiatal hernia. Symptoms may be present in up to 20% of patients and include obstruction, retention, or regurgitation of undigested food or saliva. The diagnosis is commonly made by x-ray contrast studies, and further evaluation with endoscopy and manometry is essential to rule out associated inflammatory or motility disorders. Treatment in symptomatic cases is surgical diverticulectomy and should include esophageal myotomy or hiatal hernia repair if motility disorders or hiatal hernias are present.

INTRAMURAL DIVERTICULOSIS

Tiny flask-shaped outpouchings in the upper esophagus are uncommonly found in barium studies in patients complaining of dysphagia. They are often associated with a smooth stricture of the upper esophagus and may be complicated by superimposed candidal infection. These pseudodiverticula represent dilated ducts draining submucosal glands. Treatment includes dilation of the stricture and treatment of the candidal infection if present.

DIVERTICULA OF THE STOMACH

Gastric diverticula are rare, predominantly asymptomatic, and associated with few complications. The majority are single diverticula located high on the posterior wall of the fundus approximately 2 cm below the esophagogastric junction and 3 cm from the lesser curvature. These true, congenital diverticula are generally asymptomatic but on occasion cause halitosis or regurgitation of food. Approximately 15% of gastric diverticula are prepyloric and acquired as a result of antecedent peptic, granulomatous, or neoplastic disease, and 10% are found in the mid-stomach. The majority of diverticula are incidentally found on x-ray or endoscopic studies. The most common symptom is dyspepsia, which may be unrelated to the diverticulum, and complications, such as hemorrhage and perforation, rarely occur. Endoscopy may be required to differentiate between a diverticulum and ulcer. There is no relationship between gastric and colonic or small bowel diverticula. Treatment is unnecessary unless the patient presents with a complication.

SMALL INTESTINAL DIVERTICULA
Duodenal Diverticula

Duodenal diverticula are seen in up to 5% of barium studies and autopsy series of the upper gastrointestinal tract and are classified as either extraluminal or intraluminal. Extraluminal diverticula are outpouchings of mucosa and submucosa through a weak area of the bowel wall, and two-thirds are located on the medial aspect of the second duodenum with 2.5 cm of the ampulla of Vater. Coexistent colonic diverticulosis is present in up to 30% of patients. The vast majority are asymptomatic and require no therapy. Rare complications include duodenal obstruction, bacterial overgrowth with associated malabsorption, perforation, and hemorrhage. Patients with periampullary diverticula have an increased incidence of choledocholithiasis and pancreatitis. This may be explained by bacterial overgrowth and a dysfunctional ampulla of Vater leading to an ascending infection with bacterial flora and subsequent deconjugation of bilirubin with stone formation. Obstruction of the common bile duct or pancreatic duct may result from external compression by a duodenal diverticulum and result in cholangitis or pancreatitis. Endoscopic retrograde cholangiopancreateography with or without sphincterotomy is technically more difficult if the ampulla lies within the diverticula.

Intraluminal diverticula are rare and result from congenital webs or membranes localized to the second portion of the duodenum. These diverticula arise from a membrane that attaches to a part of the circumference of the lumen and result from incomplete recanalization of the duodenal anlage during development. Coexistent anatomic abnormalities occur in up to 40% of patients. Symptoms may include bloating, early satiety, crampy abdominal discomfort, or nausea and vomiting. Duodenal obstruction followed by pancreatitis is the most common complication, whereas cholangitis and possible peptic ulceration are less commonly seen.

Treatment is indicated for symptomatic duodenal diverticula. In patients with obstructive symptoms or intractable pain in the absence of other pathology, surgical excision of extraluminal diverticula is indicated. Emergent excision may be required in patients with hemorrhage, perforation, bowel obstruction, or biliary tract obstruction. Symptomatic intraluminal diverticula have been excised both surgically and endoscopically. During surgical procedures, careful definition of the biliary and pancreatic ducts is essential.

Diverticula of the Jejunum and Ileum

Diverticula of this region have been described in up to 1% of small bowel series. They are more frequent in later life and often multiple in number when present. These are acquired or false diverticula with protrusion of mucosa and submucosa through the mesenteric border of the small bowel. Jejunal diverticula are more common and larger than those found in the ileum. The vast majority are asymptomatic and require no therapy. Possible complications include malabsorbtion secondary to bacterial overgrowth, diverticulitis, hemorrhage, incomplete bowel obstruction, and benign pneumoperitoneum. Bacterial overgrowth may present with signs of malabsorption, including diarrhea, steatorrhea, and macrocytic anemia secondary to vitamin B_{12} malabsorption. Intestinal pseudo-obstruction may be present as a result of an associated scleroderma, visceral myopathy, or neuropathy in which there is an increased incidence of diverticula. Diagnosis of bacterial overgrowth may be suspected by clinical signs of malabsorption, but confirmatory diagnostic tests should be performed if available. Small bowel intubation with sampling and quan-

titative culture provides the most accurate diagnosis.[14] C-labeled xylose breath tests or a Schilling test after antibiotic therapy are alternate diagnostic methods. Treatment with one or more courses of broad-spectrum antibiotics (tetracycline, metronidazole [Flagyl], erythromycin) is usually successful. Surgical therapy is limited to severe complications, such as obstruction, bleeding, and perforation, and involves resection of the involved segment with end-to-end anastomosis.

Meckel's Diverticulum

Meckel's diverticula are the most common congenital abnormalities of the gastrointestinal tract, occurring in 1 to 3% of the population. They are remnants of the omphalomesenteric (vitelline) duct, which connects the primitive gut to the yolk sac in early fetal life. Failure of obliteration most commonly results in a Meckel's diverticulum, with or without a fibrous connection to the umbilicus. Meckel's diverticula are true diverticula, containing all layers of the intestinal wall, and are usually located on the antimesenteric border of the ileum within 100 cm of the ileocecal valve. The average diverticulum is 3 cm in length, and approximately half contain heterotrophic mucosa (gastric mucosa in >60%). Complications include bleeding, obstruction, and perforation. Bleeding is the most common complication in children and is strongly associated with the presence of heterotrophic acid secreting gastric mucosa and adjacent ulceration of ileal mucosa. The bleeding is classically acute, episodic, and painless. Adults are more likely to present with melena, whereas children usually present with hematochezia. Chronic anemia secondary to occult blood loss is uncommon. Obstruction is the most common complication in adults and may occur with or without a fibrous band connected to the umbilicus. Obstruction may result from a variety of causes, including entanglement of the small bowel within a fibrous cord, entrapment of an ileal loop with a mesodiverticular band, intussusception, volvulus, incarceration within an inguinal or femoral hernia (Littre's hernia), or chronic Meckel's diverticulitis. The third most common presentation is an inflammatory process that presents with peritoneal signs and is often confused with appendicitis. Diverticulitis, peptic ulceration of ileal mucosa, and foreign body impaction in the diverticular lumen are frequent causes of the inflammation. Carcinoids, sarcomas, and benign mesenchymal tumors rarely occur in Meckel's diverticula.

Visualization of a Meckel's diverticulum may be difficult, especially in adults. Routine small bowel series are insensitive, and enteroclysis improves the diagnostic yield. Meckel's scanning with technetium 99m is useful if bleeding from a diverticulum is suspected. A positive scan requires a diverticulum, which contains at least 1.8 cm^2 of gastric mucosa, and its diagnostic yield may be enhanced by prior administration of pentagastrin and cimetidine. Angiography in the setting of bleeding may be diagnostic by demonstrating a branch of the ileocolic artery representing bleeding from a remnant of the right vitelline artery.

Treatment in adults is reserved for symptomatic diverticula. A surgical diverticulectomy or a resection of the ileal segment containing the diverticulum with end-to-end anastomosis is performed. In adults, a Meckel's diverticulum found incidentally should be removed from patients with (1) a history of unexplained gastrointestinal bleeding or abdominal pain; (2) a narrow diverticular neck, which may predispose to complications; (3) a palpable mass within the diverticulum; (4) a fibrous band tethering to the umbilicus, which may predispose to volvulus or obstruction; or (5) a diverticulum with a vitelline artery, which lacks a mesentery.

COLONIC DIVERTICULA

Colonic diverticula are the most common diverticula of the alimentary tract, occurring in about 15% of the population of developed countries. Geographic, cultural, and dietary factors appear to play a large role in the development of colonic diverticula. The worldwide prevalence of diverticular disease is only 1% but gradually increases as the population moves to a westernized lifestyle. A low-fiber diet in an aging population is thought to be the cause of diverticular disease in westernized countries. Colonic diverticula are uncommon before the age of 40 and increase in westernized countries from a frequency of 5% in the fifth decade to 50% in the ninth decade. Of those affected, approximately 20% develop symptoms and signs of illness, 10% require hospitalization, and 0.5% require surgery.

The vast majority of colonic diverticula are false diverticula or pseudodiverticula representing herniation of mucosa, submucosa, and mesentery mucosa through the muscular layers of the colon at points where nutrient arteries pass through to the submucosa. Nearly all diverticula emerge in parallel rows between the mesenteric and lateral taenia. The number and size of diverticula vary, but the sigmoid colon is involved most commonly in 95% of cases, followed by more proximal involvement in continuity to the sigmoid. Spastic diverticulosis is the most common varia-

tion and is characterized by marked wall thickening with indentation of the lumen by overtrapping folds of circular muscle separated by narrow haustra through which the diverticula protrude. In 30% of cases, numerous diverticula without circular muscle thickening are present in the sigmoid and more proximal regions. Rarely diverticula may be present only in the right colon. True diverticula are uncommon, usually solitary, and located in the cecum or proximal right colon.

Eighty percent of patients with diverticulosis are asymptomatic, with its incidental diagnosis made during radiography, laparotomy, or endoscopy. Crampy left lower quadrant or midline abdominal pain is the most common symptom, which results from spastic diverticulosis. Its duration varies from hours to days and may be accompanied by diarrhea, constipation, or flatulence. The pain is often worse after eating and may be relieved after defecation or passage of flatus. Physical findings include left lower quadrant tenderness without peritoneal signs or fever, and laboratory evaluation reveals a normal leukocyte count and sedimentation rate. Diagnosis is often confirmed by the demonstration of diverticula and muscle thickening during barium enema or endoscopy. These symptoms may easily be confused with those of irritable bowel syndrome, which may be present combined with diverticula, but despite improvement with similar therapy, their pathophysiology appears to be unrelated.

Treatment is aimed at relieving symptoms and preventing complications. Therapy includes the gradual introduction of fiber into the diet to increase stool bulk. Dietary supplementation with vegetable fiber (at least 10 to 25 grams per day of unprocessed wheat bran) has been shown to relieve pain and other symptoms, increase stool mass, and decrease the sigmoid intraluminal pressure. Alternative fiber sources include potatoes, legumes, leafy vegetables, and fruit as well as psyllium, methylcellulose, or related products. Antispasmodics available in the United States have not been shown to provide significant relief. If analgesics are temporarily needed, the drug of choice is meperidine. Opiates such as morphine should be avoided because of related increases in intraluminal pressure and distention of diverticula. Antibiotics are not indicated in uncomplicated diverticular disease.

COMPLICATIONS

Bleeding

Diverticular bleeding occurs in up to 10% of patients with diverticulosis and usually presents with painless blood per rectum of varying significance. Microscopic studies have demonstrated the bleeding source to be a minute rupture of an intramural arterial branch on the wall adjacent to the diverticular lumen. Inflammation is not essential in the pathogenesis of bleeding. Severe hemorrhage from diverticula is the most common cause of life-threatening lower gastrointestinal bleeding in the elderly. In those cases, right colonic diverticula are demonstrated to be the source in approximately 70%. It should be noted that right colon arteriovenous malformations may be present along with diverticuli and be responsible for the bleeding.

Clinical features include the sudden passage of a variable amount of bright red blood with or without clots or maroon or, less likely, melanotic stools. Bleeding may be intermittent or continuous over several days and stops spontaneously in 80% of cases. Hypotension or signs of hypovolemia may be present during the acute bleeding. Recurrent bleeding occurs in one-fourth or more of patients and with higher rates after a single recurrence.

Therapy includes intravenous fluid or blood transfusions, exclusion of an upper tract bleeding source with nasogastric lavage or upper endoscopy, and possible sigmoidoscopy to exclude non-diverticulum distal sources. The latter may be severely limited by the presence of blood in the lumen limiting the visualization of mucosa. If bleeding appears to continue, nuclear bleeding scans with technetium 99m–labeled red blood cells are indicated to identify the presence and location of active bleeding. Labeled red blood cells are preferable to sulfur colloid because they allow for repeated scanning within 24 hours without reinjection of the marker. If active bleeding is detected, selective angiography is initiated to localize the bleeding. If a site of active diverticular bleeding is identified, vasopressin is selectively infused to the bleeding diverticular site at a rate of 0.2 to 0.3 unit per minute and tapered over 36 hours. Initial cessation of hemorrhage is achieved in up to 90% of patients, but rebleeding may occur in up to 50% of patients after the vasopressin is stopped. Selective angiographic embolization of the bleeding site is an alternative therapy but includes a risk of bowel infarction. In patients with active bleeding who do not respond or rebleed despite angiographic intervention, surgical segmental resection of the bleeding portion of colon is indicated. Diverticular bleeding stops spontaneously in the vast majority of patients. In these cases, colonoscopy, after a full bowel preparation, should be performed to determine the potential sources of bleeding. Subtotal colectomy is the surgical procedure of choice in patients with recurrent bleeding, diverticulosis as the sole ab-

normality on colonoscopy, and negative angiograms.

Diverticulitis

Diverticulitis is the most common complication of diverticular disease. The initial pathologic findings are inflammation in the diverticular wall at its apex secondary to inspissated fecal material. Inflammation then spreads, causing peridiverticulitis, which may lead to necrosis or microperforations or macroperforations with fecal contamination of the surrounding tissues. Frequently only a single diverticulum is involved. The most common location is in the sigmoid colon. Peridiverticulitis usually remains contained within the mesentery, fat, and surrounding tissues. If a microperforation occurs, a small paracolonic abscess may form, which may become more extensive with repeated episodes. After a single macroperforation, a larger abscess may form and travel longitudinally and re-enter the colonic lumen or rupture into adjacent structures and form fistulas. Free perforation into the peritoneum with widespread peritonitis is a rare, life-threatening complication.

Diverticulitis clinically presents with the acute onset of persistent left lower quadrant pain, which may be accompanied by chills and leukocytosis with a left shift. These symptoms may be accompanied by sepsis, anorexia, nausea, vomiting, change in bowel habits, abdominal distention, or dysuria. Physical examination demonstrates left lower quadrant tenderness with possible peritoneal irritation or a palpable mass. The diagnosis may be made by the aforementioned clinical findings during the acute setting and later confirmed by radiologic or endoscopic findings. A gently performed, single contrast study, using thin barium or gastrograffin to demonstrate the presence of diverticulitis, can be performed in the acute stage but is generally reserved for later in the course, secondary to the risk of disruption of a localized perforation with peritoneal soilage. Radiographic criteria include demonstration of contrast material outside the colon or diverticulum, a paracolic mass, a colonic fistula, or a segment of narrow colon with normal mucosal pattern. Flexible sigmoidoscopy with minimal air insufflation can demonstrate diverticula and acute mucosal inflammation but should be avoided in the acute phase to avoid further complications. Computed tomography (CT) is the diagnostic procedure of choice in the acute phase of diverticulitis and is virtually risk free. CT stages the extent of inflammation and determines the presence of a peridiverticular fluid collection, which may require percutaneous or surgical drainage. CT when compared with barium enema has limitations in its ability to differentiate diverticulitis from spastic colon. CT is superior in its ability to distinguish the extent of more severe and complicated disease. The author's initial diagnostic test in a patient with suspected diverticulitis is CT, and if the diagnosis is still in question, a contrast enema is performed for confirmation. The differential diagnosis of diverticulitis includes a complicated colon cancer, inflammatory bowel disease, and ischemic colitis. Elective endoscopy is often indicated after the acute setting has resolved to confirm the diagnosis of diverticulosis and exclude other lesions.

Complications of diverticulitis include intra-abdominal abscess, fistulas, bowel obstruction, and generalized peritonitis. Intra-abdominal abscess is suggested by persistent fever and leukocytes despite antibiotics and is best confirmed and defined by CT scan. Fistulas most commonly involve the bladder but may also involve the small bowel, uterus, vagina, or the skin. They are suspected by symptoms of pneumaturia or fecaluria, or passage of stool or flatus through the vagina. Coloenteric fistulas are usually asymptomatic. Diagnosis is confirmed by contrast studies or endoscopy. Bowel obstruction may occur during the acute setting and usually resolves spontaneously as the inflammatory process improves. Generalized peritonitis rarely complicates an acute uncontained diverticular perforation and requires urgent surgical intervention.

Antibiotics and bowel rest are the mainstay of treatment in uncomplicated diverticulitis. *Bacteroides fragilis* and *Escherichia coli* are the most common implicated organisms. Mild disease is defined by direct abdominal tenderness in the left lower quadrant, low-grade fever, and the absence of peritoneal signs and may be treated with a 5- to 7-day course of oral antibiotics (e.g., first-generation cephalosporin or amoxicillin/clavulanate [Augmentin]) and 2 to 3 days of clear liquid diet. Hospitalization is indicated for patients with severe pain, peritoneal irritation, or temperature greater than 101°F. In hospitalized patients, intravenous antibiotics, after cultures of the blood are collected, are given for 7 to 10 days. Commonly used antibiotics include second- or third-generation cephalosporins, ticarcillin/clavulanate (Timetin) or ampicillin/sulbactam (Unasyn). Patients are given nothing by mouth, nutrition is initiated with elemental diets or total parenteral nutrition. CT scan is used to guide therapy. Diverticulitis limited to the bowel wall or small diverticular abscesses contained by the pericolonic mesentery are treated with bowel rest and intravenous antibiotics. Larger abscesses are drained percutaneously with CT guidance before elective surgical resection of the involved segment to al-

low a one-stage procedure. Patients with diffuse peritoneal soiling and irritation require urgent surgical intervention. In the emergent setting, surgery includes a diverting colostomy with or without resection of the diseased segment, extensive peritoneal lavage, and either a mucous fistula or Hartmann's pouch. A two- or three-stage procedure is indicated in these patients to re-establish continuity at the bowel. Elective surgery is generally curative and is indicated in patients with recurrent disabling attacks of diverticulitis, fistulous disease, persistent partial obstruction, or after a single severe episode of complicated diverticulitis. An extensive bowel preparation and one-stage procedure is preferred with primary resection and anastomosis. The resection should include all of the involved segment of bowel. The proximal margin should include all thickened muscle, while the distal margin is extended to the nonperitonealized rectum.

ULCERATIVE COLITIS

method of
PAUL M. CHOI, M.D., and
STEPHAN R. TARGAN, M.D.
Cedars–Sinai Medical Center
Los Angeles, California

Ulcerative colitis is a chronic inflammatory disease of the colon and rectum. The cause of ulcerative colitis is not yet known, although hereditary, environmental, and immunologic factors are thought to be important in its pathogenesis. Most studies show that men and women are equally susceptible. The peak age at onset of ulcerative colitis is between the second and third decades of life, but it can affect individuals of any age. Epidemiologic studies indicate that the risk of the development of ulcerative colitis is higher among whites, especially among Jews. Over the past several decades, its overall incidence in the Western hemisphere appears to have stabilized.

The most common symptom associated with ulcerative colitis is frequent bloody diarrhea. Other common symptoms include tenesmus, urgency, and cramping abdominal pain. In patients with severe colitis, systemic symptoms, such as fever, tachycardia, and weight loss, are also seen. These patients often demonstrate evidence of anemia, hypoalbuminemia, and leukocytosis. Patients should be monitored carefully for the development of toxic megacolon and free perforation. Stricture is a complication of ulcerative colitis that can occur relatively late and may harbor unsuspected carcinoma. Extraintestinal complications are frequent and include arthritis, ankylosing spondylitis, pericholangitis, primary sclerosing cholangitis, erythema nodosum, pyoderma gangrenosum, and uveitis.

DIAGNOSIS

The diagnosis of ulcerative colitis requires exclusion of other specific causes of colonic inflammation. Infectious agents, including *Campylobacter, Shigella, Salmonella, Clostridium difficile,* and *Entamoeba histolytica,* should be ruled out with appropriate stool cultures and examinations. Other causes of colitis that can mimic ulcerative colitis include ischemic colitis, radiation enteritis, diverticulitis, microscopic and collagenous colitis, and colitis induced by nonsteroidal anti-inflammatory drugs (NSAIDs). These conditions need to be ruled out with appropriate history taking and diagnostic evaluations. Crohn's colitis must be excluded before a firm diagnosis of ulcerative colitis can be made. This at times requires a combination of colonoscopic, histopathologic, and radiologic evaluations. The diagnosis can remain indeterminate, however, in up to 15% of patients with inflammatory bowel disease.

TREATMENT

Although the cause of ulcerative colitis remains unknown, the role of chronic inflammation in its pathogenesis is well established. Recent studies have identified multiple potential cellular and molecular components of inflammation that may be important in the development of specific "targeted" therapies. In addition to currently available medical therapies (discussed subsequently), other classes of drugs that hold exciting promises are currently under active investigation. These potential novel therapies include inhibitors of T cell activation and leukotrienes, antagonists of cytokines, and agents that modulate reactive oxygen metabolites.

Aminosalicylates

Sulfasalazine

Sulfasalazine (Azulfidine) has a proven efficacy in the management of patients with ulcerative colitis. It is the initial therapy of choice in the treatment of patients with mild to moderately active disease and in maintenance of remission. Orally administered sulfasalazine reaches the colon intact, where the azo bond is cleaved by colonic flora, thereby releasing sulfapyridine and 5-aminosalicylic acid (mesalamine or 5-ASA). Mesalamine is the therapeutically active moiety of the drug. Although the exact mechanism of its action remains uncertain, its efficacy may be related to inhibition of the cyclooxygenase and lipoxygenase pathways and ability to scavenge oxygen radicals.

The major limitation in the use of sulfasalazine is the intolerance and allergic reaction that can affect up to 30% of treated patients. Reasons for poor tolerance include dyspepsia, nausea, vomiting, and headaches. These problems can be minimized if the drug is introduced in a low dose of 0.125 to 0.5 gram daily and gradually increased to 0.5 to 1.0 gram four times daily. Frequent dyspeptic symptoms may be reduced by taking the drug with meals, by using an enteric-coated formulation of the drug, or by combining it with an antacid. Headache can usually be managed with the addition of acetaminophen. Hemolysis, agranulocytosis, hepatotoxicity, pneumonitis, oligospermia, rashes, and folate deficiency are known rare side effects. Sulfasalazine has clearly been implicated in rare exacerbations of acute bloody diarrhea. This side effect is unusual in that it appears to be related to the aminosalicylate rather than to the sulfapyridine component of the compound. In fact, sulfapyridine, which appears to have little or no therapeutic effect, is responsible for most of the adverse effects associated with the use of sulfasalazine.

Mesalamine

Because of the side effects of sulfasalazine, a variety of newer aminosalicylate preparations have been developed over the past few years. These formulations enable the patient to take mesalamine without also taking sulfapyridine. In addition, newer delivery systems of mesalamine permit aminosalicylate to reach the colon at relatively high concentrations without the loss from absorption in the small bowel. These novel delivery systems include substitution of sulfapyridine with alternative carrier molecules (olsalazine, balsalazide*), a pH-dependent release system (Asacol, Claversal*, Salofalk*), and a time-dependent release formulation (Pentasa). These preparations show therapeutic efficacy comparable with that of sulfasalazine when administered in equimolar concentrations of mesalamine. Although side effects are less frequent, dyspepsia, alopecia, and secretory diarrhea (with olsalazine) have been reported.

Asacol and olsalazine (Dipentum) are currently available in the United States for use in the treatment of patients with ulcerative colitis. The usual dose for Asacol is 2.4 grams per day and for olsalazine is 1.0 gram per day, given in divided doses. Many patients may require higher doses for optimal therapeutic response. Because of their relatively high cost, the use of these medications should be reserved for patients unable to tolerate sulfasalazine or for patients with resistant disease requiring a higher dose of mesalamine.

*Not available in the United States.

Topical Mesalamine

Topical therapy for distal colitis with 5-ASA enema (left-sided colitis) and suppository (proctitis) has the advantage of achieving a high local concentration of aminosalicylate in the distal colon with minimal systemic toxicity. In addition, patients who do not improve with topical corticosteroids may respond to this therapy. Enemas containing 5-ASA (Rowasa) are usually administered as a 4-gram retention enema nightly, and suppositories are given (0.5 gram) either twice or three times a day. Adverse effects are minimal and include perianal irritation and trauma secondary to insertion. Although short-term response can be high, patient compliance or acceptance can be a greater problem than with oral formulations. In addition, long-term remission usually requires either long-term maintenance therapy or institution of concurrent oral aminosalicylate.

Corticosteroids

Corticosteroids remain a cornerstone in the management of patients with acute ulcerative colitis. They are, however, not efficacious in the maintenance of remission. Because of the considerable side effects associated with their use, corticosteroids should be reserved for patients whose condition fails to respond or who are unable to tolerate aminosalicylates and for individuals with severe or fulminant colitis.

Topical Corticosteroids

Local corticosteroid therapy may be useful in the treatment of patients with active left-sided disease. They can be given as a retention enema, hydrocortisone, 100 mg given once or twice a day, or as a rectal foam, hydrocortisone acetate (Cortifoam), 90 mg given once or twice a day. They may also be useful in patients with pancolitis who have severe distal disease and severe symptoms. Unfortunately, systemic absorption of topical corticosteroids can be high, particularly with prolonged therapy, resulting in systemic toxicity. Newer corticosteroid enema preparations have been designed to minimize this problem. These agents retain local anti-inflammatory activity but have reduced systemic absorption or undergo extensive first-pass hepatic clearance. These topical corticosteroids with diminished systemic effects are under active clinical investigation and include beclomethasone dipropionate, budesonide, prednisolone metasulfobenzoate, and tixocortol pivalate.

Oral Corticosteroids

For moderate to severe active ulcerative colitis, oral corticosteroids are indicated. They are usually given as prednisone in the range of 20 to 60 mg per day as a single oral dose for 2 to 4 weeks. When the relief of symptoms has been attained, the dose can be tapered gradually. Because the most frequent cause of failure of corticosteroids is a tapering program that is either too rapid or premature, care should be exercised to avoid this pitfall. The optimal regimen for tapering, however, can vary considerably depending on the patient and the severity of the disease and therefore needs to be individualized. In the meantime, maintenance therapy with aminosalicylates should be initiated to facilitate the tapering process. In patients whose condition is refractory or who are chronically dependent on corticosteroids, considerations should be given for therapy with immunosuppressive agents or surgery.

Parenteral Corticosteroids

Intravenously administered corticosteroids should be considered in patients with severe to fulminant ulcerative colitis. These patients are usually severely ill and require hospitalization. They need to be monitored carefully for the development of toxic megacolon and silent perforation. Intravenous corticosteroids are given as either hydrocortisone, 300 mg, or methylprednisolone, 40 to 60 mg per day in divided doses. When symptoms have stabilized, corticosteroids should be changed to an oral formulation, and sulfasalazine is added. In patients whose condition fails to respond to the intravenous regimen by 7 to 10 days, surgery or a rapid-acting immunosuppressant (cyclosporine) may be considered.

Immunosuppressive Drugs

Azathioprine/6-Mercaptopurine

The purine analogues, azathioprine (Imuran) and 6-mercaptopurine (Purinethol), have corticosteroid-sparing effects and may be useful in the induction and maintenance of remission in patients with refractory ulcerative colitis. The usual starting dose is 0.5 to 1.5 mg per kg per day. This dose should be reduced by at least 50% in patients taking allopurinol because the latter prolongs the half-life of the former. Azathioprine and 6-mercaptopurine are slow-acting drugs that may require up to 3 to 6 months of treatment before clinical efficacy becomes apparent. Frequently described toxicities include pancreatitis, leukopenia, drug-induced hepatitis, and hypersensitivity reaction. They are usually reversible when the drug is discontinued. Of greater concern, however, is the risk of the development of neoplasms. Although a definite increase in the risk for neoplasm has not been established, it would be prudent to avoid their use in patients who are pregnant or who are at an increased risk for the development of a neoplasm. This may be particularly true in patients with ulcerative colitis of long duration who have a viable option of a surgical cure.

Cyclosporine

Cyclosporine (Sandimmune) is an immunosuppressant that suppresses the immune response by inhibiting the production of cytokine by helper T cells. A preliminary report suggests that it may have a role in the treatment of patients with severe active ulcerative colitis and whose disease is refractory to intravenous corticosteroids. This study suggests that treatment with intravenous cyclosporine has a rapid response time and may be able to prevent colectomy. A variety of adverse effects have been reported with its use, primarily in the transplant literature. They include hypertension, renal and hepatic dysfunction, hyperkalemia, hirsutism, gingival hypertrophy, and lymphoma. Additional studies on its efficacy and safety in patients with ulcerative colitis are currently underway. In patients for whom therapy with cyclosporine is indicated, it is recommended that they be referred to specialized centers with extensive experience.

SUPPORTIVE MEASURES

Patient education is an important component in successful long-term management of individuals with ulcerative colitis. Education should include specific instructions about the nature of the disease, its clinical spectrum and complications, and reasonable expectations for therapy. Patients should be encouraged to become enrolled in Crohn's and Colitis Foundation of America (CCFA) and be involved actively with the support group activities.

Supportive Medications

Antidiarrheal medications can be helpful in the treatment of mild diarrhea and rectal urgency associated with ulcerative colitis. The usually prescribed medications include diphenoxylate sodium with atropine (Lomotil) and longer acting loperamide (Imodium). An infectious cause should be ruled out before therapy is initiated to avoid stasis and prolonging the carrier state. In addition, these agents are contraindicated in severe colitis because they can predispose to the development of toxic megacolon.

Anticholinergic agents may be useful in reducing abdominal cramps and rectal urgency. These agents include tincture of belladonna, clidinium bromide, dicyclomine hydrochloride, and propantheline bromide. Similar to antidiarrheal agents, their use should be avoided in severe colitis because they can also precipitate toxic megacolon.

Nutritional Support

A nutritionally balanced diet with minimal restriction should be recommended for most patients with ulcerative colitis. Primary nutritional therapies with elemental diet or total parenteral nutrition and bowel rest have not shown beneficial therapeutic effects. In severely malnourished patients, however, supplementation with enteral or parenteral nutrition may be necessary. In individuals with known lactose intolerance, instructions for a lactose-free diet should be given for improved bowel function. Patients may benefit from calcium supplementation, particularly when osteoporosis is evident or they require long-term corticosteroid therapy. Folate supplementation may be indicated for patients taking sulfasalazine as long-term maintenance therapy. For patients with chronic blood loss, iron supplementation may be necessary.

SURGICAL THERAPY

Indications for surgery in ulcerative colitis can be subdivided into emergent and elective indications. Emergency colectomy may be required for toxic megacolon and severe fulminant colitis. Elective surgery is often necessary in patients whose disease fails to respond to medical therapy or who have unacceptable side effects of therapy, usually from prolonged requirement of high doses of corticosteroids. Other elective indications include findings of high-grade dysplasia and carcinoma, symptomatic stricture, and, in children, growth retardation despite maximal nutritional and medical therapy.

Three major types of colectomy are performed. The standard operation is proctocolectomy with conventional ileostomy. This procedure is associated with the lowest rate of complication and is the surgical treatment of choice in emergent situations. Its major drawback is that the patient has an ileostomy and is incontinent. The continent ileostomy is composed of an ileal loop reservoir with a nipple valve. It has the advantage that an external appliance is not required. The pouch, however, must be emptied at regular intervals by catheterization. In addition, valve malfunction is a frequent late complication, and the rate of revisional surgery can be high. The ileal pouch–anal anastomosis has the advantage of anal continence and cosmetic appeal. The results are superior in individuals younger than 50 years of age. Complications include leakage from the anastomosis, bladder and sexual dysfunction, and pouchitis. Because of technical difficulty and a steep learning curve, both continent ileostomy and ileal pouch–anal anastomosis are best performed by an experienced surgeon.

SPECIAL MANAGEMENT CONSIDERATIONS

Pregnancy

Because ulcerative colitis frequently affects patients of childbearing age, concerns regarding its effect on pregnancy are common. Ulcerative colitis does not appear to affect fertility adversely. The use of sulfasalazine in male patients, however, may be associated with reversible oligospermia. Pregnant women with active ulcerative colitis have more frequent fetal complications, regardless of drug treatment. Thus it may be advisable to postpone pregnancy until remission of the disease is achieved. Pregnancy in patients with active ulcerative colitis, however, is not an indication for therapeutic abortion except in rare instances in which the life of the mother is threatened. The effect of pregnancy on the course of ulcerative colitis does not appear to be appreciable.

The management of pregnant women with ulcerative colitis is similar to that of nonpregnant patients. The use of corticosteroids and sulfasalazine does not appear to affect the fetus adversely. However, because sulfasalazine interferes with folic acid absorption in the small bowel, and it is important in fetal development, folate supplementation may be prudent in pregnant women taking sulfasalazine. Because immunosuppressants and metronidazole are known teratogens in animals, they are best avoided or discontinued in patients planning to conceive. In addition, radiographic studies should be minimized, particularly during the first trimester.

Colorectal Cancer

Colorectal cancer is the most frequent malignant complication in patients with ulcerative colitis. The increased cancer risk in ulcerative colitis is well established and is thought to be dependent on the duration and extent of disease. Some consider early age at onset of disease and concomitant presence of primary sclerosing cholangitis as additional independent risk factors. It is not yet known whether long-term therapy with immunosuppressive agents can result in a higher rate of malignant complications.

For patients with extensive colitis of 8 to 10 years, periodic colonoscopic surveillance with multiple biopsies is currently recommended. Because of concerns regarding the effectiveness of the current biopsy technique, recently proposed modifications have included adjustments of the sampling interval and timing of colonoscopy to use better the rectosigmoid predominance of neoplasia and the duration-dependent increase in cancer risk. Patients with low-grade dysplasia should undergo repeat studies. All patients with confirmed high-grade dysplasia, or dysplasia-associated lesion or mass are strongly advised to undergo colectomy. A recent study suggests that cancer surveillance may allow the detection of carcinoma at an earlier stage and improve the survival of patients with cancer.

CROHN'S DISEASE

method of
CHRISTOPHER W. IVES, M.D.
Louisiana State University School of Medicine
New Orleans, Louisiana

and

CHESLEY HINES, JR., M.D.
Southern Baptist Hospital
New Orleans, Louisiana

Crohn's disease is a chronic transmural inflammatory process that can involve any part of the gastrointestinal tract from the mouth to the anus and affects primarily younger rather than older patients. The cause of this disease still remains unknown, but theories as to its pathogenesis include immunologic processes, dietary factors, infectious agents, and even psychological influences. There is no cure for this often debilitating disease, and treatment goals are aimed at inducing remission from acute flares; minimizing and treating such complications as abscesses, fistulas, and intestinal perforation; and maintaining patients' nutritional status during their lifelong bout with this disorder.

TREATMENT

The typically encountered signs and symptoms are those seen in acute flares of Crohn's disease and include abdominal pain, fever, anorexia, nausea, vomiting, and diarrhea (which is not usually grossly bloody). The mainstay of medical therapy remains corticosteroids and sulfasalazine, alone or in combination.

Corticosteroids

The National Cooperative Crohn's Disease Study published in 1979 demonstrated a positive response to a course of prednisone in symptomatic patients. Since that time, corticosteroids have been used effectively. They should be administered initially at a dose of 20 to 40 mg of oral prednisone per day or at an equivalent intravenous corticosteroid dose when oral intake is contraindicated, as in suspected obstruction and perforation. The corticosteroid dose is then tapered over several weeks to months with a goal of getting the patient off the medication. As most clinicians know, however, many patients remain on maintenance doses of corticosteroids to control their symptoms. Because corticosteroids have never been demonstrated to maintain remission and because their use is fraught with many notorious side effects, every attempt possible should be made to wean patients off these medications if possible. To control left-sided Crohn's colitis and proctitis, topical corticosteroids in enema form are often helpful. There are several hydrocortisone enema and foam preparations that deliver from 80 to 100 mg of hydrocortisone and are given in a retention form overnight for a period of 2 to 3 weeks. In an attempt to minimize the systemic side effects of corticosteroids, short-acting oral and topical corticosteroids are being developed and studied. Although not available at this time, these drugs, such as budesonide, tixocortal pivalate, and beclomethasone dipropionate, undergo extensive first-pass metabolism by the liver and have many potential advantages. For patients who require long-term corticosteroid usage, alternate-day dosing is a reasonable approach, although no studies have demonstrated the efficacy of this regimen in Crohn's disease specifically. Corticosteroids are not contraindicated in the pregnant patient with Crohn's disease.

Aminosalicylates

Sulfasalazine (Azulfidine), composed of sulfapyridine and 5-aminosalicylate (5-ASA) linked together by an azo bond, has been used in the treatment of inflammatory bowel disease for almost 50 years. It is the 5-ASA portion, released when colonic bacteria split the azo bond, that is thought to be responsible for the anti-inflammatory effects of sulfasalazine. Although the exact mechanism of action is unknown, sulfasalazine is effective in the treatment of Crohn's colitis and ileocolitis. It is not effective in disease of the small bowel. Side effects, which are many and due to the sulfapyridine component, include headache, dyspepsia, nausea, anorexia, fever, rash, hemolytic anemia, leukopenia, pancreatitis, hepatitis, thrombocytopenia, reversible oligospermia, and a lupus-like syndrome. Sulfasalazine

should be initiated at a dose of 1 to 2 grams per day and increased as tolerated to 2 to 4 grams per day in evenly divided doses, preferably after meals. Because the drug competes with folate for receptor sites, long-term use should be supplemented with 1 mg per day of folate. Sulfasalazine is not contraindicated in pregnancy.

Because of the many side effects of the sulfapyridine component and because 5-ASA is rapidly broken down by the low pH of the stomach, recent attempts have been successfully made at delivering a sulfa-free aminosalicylate to the lower gastrointestinal tract. Several topical and oral aminosalicylates are now available, and although approved by the Food and Drug Administration (FDA) only for use in ulcerative colitis, they may be helpful in treating Crohn's colitis and ileocolitis. Topical mesalamine (Rowasa) is available as either an 8-hour overnight retention enema (4 grams per 60 mL aqueous suspension) or as a rectal suppository (500 mg twice a day) for 3 to 6 weeks. Topical mesalamine is most effective in treating distal colitis and proctitis. Olsalazine (Dipentum) is an oral agent joining two molecules of mesalamine by an azo bond that is split by colonic bacteria. Supplied as 250-mg capsules, a total daily dose of 1 gram in two divided doses may be effective in treating Crohn's colitis and ileocolitis, although it is approved by the FDA only for maintenance of remission in ulcerative colitis. Oral mesalamine (Asacol), using an acrylic coating that delays release until a pH of 6 to 7 in the distal ileum is encountered, has recently been released and approved by the FDA for use in ulcerative colitis. Given as two 400-mg tablets orally three times a day for 6 weeks, this drug may also be effective in treating Crohn's colitis and has the theoretical advantage of being more effective in ileal disease. Awaiting approval and release is another oral mesalamine agent (Pentasa), which uses a coating of ethylcellulose microgranules that break down in the small intestine. These newer agents should be reserved for those patients with Crohn's disease who cannot tolerate sulfasalazine and who have disease limited to the colon or terminal ileum. Sulfasalazine also has a slight cost advantage. There is no benefit in combining sulfasalazine with one of the newer 5-ASA agents.

Immunosuppressive Agents

The purine analogues, azathioprine (Imuran) and its metabolite, 6-mercaptopurine (Purinethol), have been shown to be effective in a corticosteroid-sparing role. Their use may enable discontinuation or significant dosage reduction in Crohn's patients who are steroid dependent or who suffer from side effects of long-term steroid use. They may also be successfully used in patients who have failed conventional therapy trials or who have had surgery and are failing medical therapy for recurrent disease. Either drug may be started at a dose of 50 mg per day and increased to 100 mg per day over several days and continued for up to 1 year. A disadvantage is the delayed onset of action, which is approximately 3 months. After 1 year, an attempt at discontinuation should be made. Side effects, which are often more tolerable than those of corticosteroids, include anemia, leukopenia, fever, rash, pancreatitis, arthralgias, alopecia, hepatitis, and susceptibility to opportunistic infections. These drugs should not be used during pregnancy.

Cyclosporine* (Sandimmune) also has been shown to have a steroid-sparing role in Crohn's disease with the advantage of an onset of action in 1 to 2 weeks. Serious side effects include nephrotoxicity and hypertension. Immunosuppressives should be considered only after thorough consultation with the patient and a gastroenterologist experienced with their use.

Metronidazole

Metronidazole (Flagyl) can be effective in treating Crohn's colitis and ileocolitis in patients who have failed a course of more traditional medical therapy. Noteworthy is metronidazole's efficacy in promoting healing of fistulas and other perineal complications. Although not approved by the FDA for this use, it is often given in a dose of 10 to 20 mg per kg per day for 1 to 2 months. It is unknown how metronidazole exerts its effects in Crohn's disease; however, it is thought to be different from any antibiotic mechanism. Metronidazole can also be used in combination with anti-inflammatory agents, such as corticosteroids and any of the 5-ASA preparations. Metronidazole should not be used in the first trimester of pregnancy. Significant side effects include seizures, peripheral neuropathy, and a disulfiram-like reaction when the drug is used in conjunction with alcohol.

NUTRITIONAL SUPPLEMENTATION

Controversy still remains regarding the efficacy of intravenous versus an elemental diet in the induction of remission and treatment of active Crohn's disease. There are investigations supporting the efficacy of both regimens. In the case of total parenteral nutrition and bowel rest, it is unknown whether the positive effects are

secondary to the nutrition, bowel rest, or a combination of the two. As for elemental diets, their unpalatability usually requires that they be given by way of a nasogastric tube, making compliance a problem. Because most Crohn's patients are malnourished to some degree, nutritional support is at least warranted to maintain and improve nutritional status and to attempt to maintain a positive nitrogen balance. If nonobstructive disease is present, a trial of an elemental diet should probably be attempted. If obstructive disease is suspected, the patient should receive some form of intravenous nutrition either as total parenteral nutrition via a central line or as peripheral intravenous alimentation. Elemental diets should be initiated at lower concentrations and gradually increased as tolerated so as to avoid abdominal pain that may be caused by the diet's hyperosmolarity. Many patients may require nutritional support either enterally or parenterally for prolonged periods, if not for life. Such long-term supplementation has been demonstrated to improve quality of life. One popular method of delivering adequate nutrition is to allow the patient to eat any desired and tolerable foods during the day, supplemented with enteral nutrition by way of a nasogastric tube at night. Elemental diets have been particularly effective in inducing remission in children with Crohn's disease. They are also particularly helpful in preventing growth retardation in children, a problem that can be secondary to the chronicity of the Crohn's disease itself or to side effects of long-term corticosteroid use.

SUPPORTIVE THERAPY

In acute Crohn's disease, adequate hydration with intravenous fluids and electrolyte replacement is necessary. This is particularly true in the setting of diarrhea, bowel obstruction, prolonged emesis, and suspicion of sepsis. If obstruction, perforation, or abscess has been ruled out, antidiarrheal agents may be used with caution (i.e., loperamide, codeine, Lomotil). If abscess or perforation is suspected, broad-spectrum antibiotics should be initiated after appropriate cultures have been taken.

The chronicity of Crohn's disease necessitates a strong support system consisting of thorough patient education and a strong physician-patient relationship. This can help prevent or alleviate some of the fears, anxieties, frustrations, and eventual depression that may occur. Even with a strong support system, psychiatric intervention may occasionally be warranted.

SURGERY

If possible, surgery should be avoided because it does not necessarily offer a cure for Crohn's

---

*This use of cyclosporine is not listed in the manufacturer's official directive.

disease, which recurs in 50 to 60% of postoperative patients. Surgery, consisting of a resection of involved bowel, should be reserved for those patients who are unresponsive to medical therapy, who have an abscess or fistula refractory to medical therapy, or who have an intestinal obstruction or perforation.

IRRITABLE BOWEL SYNDROME

method of
JAIME ZIGHELBOIM, M.D., and
NICHOLAS J. TALLEY, M.D., PH.D.
Mayo Clinic and Mayo Foundation
Rochester, Minnesota

The irritable bowel syndrome (IBS) is the most common gastrointestinal disorder encountered in clinical practice and is characterized by abdominal pain associated with a chronic disturbance of defecation. It is estimated that 15% of persons in the general population have IBS, but only a minority ever consult a physician.

DIAGNOSIS

Patients with IBS usually present with chronic or recurrent abdominal pain. The pain is often in the lower abdomen but may occur in any location, and it is typically related to defecation. Usually the patient also complains of variable constipation, diarrhea, urgency, or alternating constipation and diarrhea. The standard medical history, if well enough structured, can strongly suggest that IBS, rather than organic disease, is the diagnosis. Six symptoms can help discriminate IBS from organic bowel disease: relief of pain with bowel movements, more frequent stools with the onset of pain, looser stools with the onset of pain, visible abdominal distention, fecal passage of mucus, and a feeling of incomplete rectal evacuation. It has been shown that the more of these symptoms that are present, the greater the probability that the diagnosis is IBS. Based on clinical and epidemiologic studies, specific symptom criteria for IBS have now been developed (Table 1).

Certain symptoms may suggest that an underlying organic process is more likely (e.g., weight loss, prominent vomiting, or overt bleeding). Extraintestinal complaints, including headaches, backaches, and fatigue, are common in patients with IBS; however, if the gastrointestinal symptoms are not dominant but merely constitute one aspect of a multitude of health complaints, a diagnosis of psychiatric disease (e.g., depression or somatoform disorder) should be considered. Abdominal pain that has been present for more than 6 months, is unremitting, and is unrelated to bowel habit should raise the suspicion of a chronic pain syndrome rather than IBS.

Physical examination is usually normal in patients with IBS except for the occasional presence of multiple abdominal scars resulting from negative exploratory surgery. Localized mild abdominal tenderness may occur in patients with IBS; abdominal wall pain, however, should be suspected if tenderness persists or worsens on tensing the abdominal muscles. The presence of fever, an abdominal mass, or blood in the stools should prompt the clinician to search for an organic cause, such as infection, inflammatory bowel disease, or malignancy.

It is important to make a positive diagnosis of IBS whenever possible based on symptoms and to avoid performing expensive, inconvenient, invasive, and even potentially dangerous tests. The diagnostic evaluation on first presentation should usually be limited to include a hematology and chemistry group, erythrocyte sedimentation rate (ESR), stool examination for blood, and flexible sigmoidoscopy. These tests are normal in IBS, and any abnormalities (e.g., anemia, elevated ESR, proctitis) would point toward another diagnosis. With this simple approach, the clinician is able to rule out most other chronic conditions that could be confused with IBS.

Lactose-containing products should be avoided for 2 weeks because lactose intolerance may be confused with IBS, particularly in patients whose predominant complaints are diarrhea, bloating, and flatulence. This is more practical than performing a lactose tolerance test, unless the patient does not adhere to the lactose-free diet. Some specific situations may warrant additional testing. In patients with chronic, watery diarrhea, colonic biopsies to rule out lymphocytic or collagenous colitis are indicated. Stools should also be examined for ova and parasites. If clinically suspected, thyroid function tests may be obtained to rule out hyperthyroidism or hypothyroidism. Patients older than 40 years of age, particularly with new-onset constipation or diarrhea, should have a barium enema or colonoscopy to exclude a colonic neoplasm. In patients who have undergone repeated diagnostic testing in the past, careful review of previous evaluations is often all that is necessary.

MANAGEMENT

The underlying pathophysiology of IBS remains poorly understood, but it is probably a multifactorial disorder; more than one mechanism may be disturbed in different individuals. Disordered small bowel and colonic motor func-

TABLE 1. **Diagnostic Criteria for the Irritable Bowel Syndrome**

Definition
Continuous or recurrent symptoms for at least 3 months of:
  Abdominal pain or discomfort relieved with defecation or associated with a change in the frequency or consistency of stool
                                              and
  An irregular (varying) pattern of defecation at least 25% of the time (3 or more of the following):
    Altered stool frequency
    Altered stool form (hard or loose/watery stool)
    Altered stool passage (straining, urgency, or feeling of incomplete evacuation)
    Passage of mucus
    Bloating or feeling of abdominal distention

Other Clinical Features Against an Organic Explanation
Age at onset <40 years
Symptoms are longstanding
Symptoms are not steadily progressive
Absence of:
  Rectal bleeding
  Nocturnal symptoms (awaking patient)
  Rapid weight loss
  Vomiting
  Fever

tion, abnormal visceral perception to balloon distention in the gut, and psychological dysfunction have all been described in IBS. Patients with IBS have been observed in some cases to have painful cramps that coincide with the passage of high-amplitude pressure waves through the small bowel. Motor activity in the colon in IBS often shows excessive responses to various normal stimuli, such as a fatty meal. Patients with predominant diarrhea have been found to have an accelerated gut transit and a greater number of fast colonic contractions. In contrast, some patients with predominant constipation have fewer high-amplitude propagated colonic contractions and slower colonic transit. Approximately 50% of IBS patients have been reported to have excessive sensitivity to balloon distention in the rectum. The management of the patient with IBS therefore needs to be individualized (Table 2).

Patients with IBS who present for medical care (who represent only a minority of IBS sufferers in the community) have as a group a higher prevalence of somatization, anxiety, and depression compared with IBS "nonpresenters." Unreported sexual abuse may also be linked to IBS. Patients who present with organic bowel disease, however, have in general a similar degree of psychological disturbance. Furthermore, IBS "nonpresenters" are psychologically no more disturbed than other persons in the general population. Therefore, it is unlikely that psychological factors cause IBS, but they may coexist with IBS, promoting health care seeking and enhancing symptom severity.

General Principles

Reassurance

The first step in the management of the patient with IBS is to reassure him or her that the symp-

toms are real, that they are not life-threatening, and that they do not lead to cancer or other serious disease. It is also useful to explain that IBS is probably a disorder of the gastrointestinal nervous system and that exaggerated gut responses to normal stimuli (e.g., eating or emotion) occur in IBS. The physician should always try to determine why the patient having chronic symptoms has presented on this occasion and allay any unwarranted fears. Patients are often relieved to learn that the condition does not presage serious illness, require surgery, or shorten life expectancy. It should be emphasized that IBS is a common problem. In addition, the potential chronic and recurring nature of the disorder needs to be explained, although some patients spontaneously lose their symptoms for prolonged periods. The more realistic goal of learning to "cope" with the symptoms of IBS, rather than "cure," needs to be

TABLE 2. **Management Strategy in Irritable Bowel Syndrome**

General Principles
Reassurance
Explanation
Advice about precipitating factors
Exploration of psychological issues
Dietary advice (high fiber, antigas diet)
Follow up patient at least once to determine the response to treatment and to reinforce the general principles

Drug Therapy (Specific Symptoms)
Constipation—bulking agents, avoid laxatives
Diarrhea—bulking agents, loperamide, cholestyramine
Abdominal pain—bulking agents, anticholinergics

Refractory Patient
Antidepressants
Psychotherapy
Behavioral therapy

instilled. Advice on avoiding precipitants of symptoms (e.g., certain foods, alcohol, coffee) and reducing anxiety or life stress (where possible) can help moderate the severity of the complaints in many cases. A careful review of the patient's current medications is important because some drugs can aggravate constipation (e.g., calcium channel blockers, nonsteroidal anti-inflammatory drugs) or induce diarrhea (e.g., magnesium-containing antacids, antibiotics, quinidine, or theophylline).

Diet

Dietary intervention is the mainstay of therapy for IBS. The typical American diet provides only about 12 grams of fiber per day. A high-fiber diet with an intake of 20 to 30 grams of fiber per day is recommended for IBS patients with either predominant constipation or diarrhea. Although it is preferable that this goal be accomplished by increasing the amount of dietary fiber (Table 3), patients frequently are unwilling or unable to change their diet and often prefer to use commercially available fiber supplements (Table 4). These products are available in powder, tablet, or wafer forms; they should be started with a single daily dose and increased if necessary to three times a day gradually, adding one extra daily dose every 5 to 7 days during the first 2 to 3 weeks of treatment, to avoid side effects such as bloating and flatulence. The powder form must be mixed thoroughly with at least one glass (280 mL) of water or other beverage (except milk); patients often do not tolerate or dislike the taste of the powder mix, so the use of the tablet or wafer

TABLE 3. **Foods High in Dietary Fiber**

Food	Portion Size
6–7 gm of Fiber per Serving	
All Bran	¼ cup
40% Branflakes	1 cup
Raisin Bran	1 cup
Wheat Bran	¼ cup
Dried beans, cooked	½ cup
4–5 gm of Fiber per Serving	
Grape-Nuts	½ cup
Shredded Wheat	1 cup
Wheat Germ	¼ cup
Blackberries, fresh	1 cup
Currants, fresh	1 cup
Guava	1 medium
Okra, cooked	½ cup
Sweet potato, cooked	½ cup
Black-eyed peas, cooked	½ cup
Chickpeas (garbanzo beans), cooked	½ cup
Lentils, cooked	½ cup
Lima beans, cooked	½ cup

Adapted from Anderson JW: Plant Fiber in Foods, 2nd ed. Lexington, KY, HCF Nutrition Research Foundation, Inc., 1990.

TABLE 4. **Examples of Commonly Used Commercially Available Fiber Products**

Product	Form	Fiber Content
Metamucil		
Psyllium	Powder	3.4 gm/dose*
Psyllium	Wafers	3.4 gm/wafer
Fibercon		
Polycarbophil	Tablets	0.5 gm/tablet
Fiberall		
Polycarbophil	Tablets	1.0 gm/tablet
Psyllium	Wafers	3.4 gm/wafer
Psyllium	Powder	3.4 gm/tsp
Citrucel		
Methylcellulose	Powder	2.0 gm/tbsp

*Regular and sugar-free—tsp; orange and strawberry flavor—tbsp.

form may achieve better compliance in some patients.

Patients who complain of bloating and flatulence should avoid carbonated beverages and reduce the quantity of air that is swallowed by eating slowly. Certain foods, such as legumes, beans, cabbage, and lentils, may cause "gas" because of their complex carbohydrate content that is unabsorbed in the small bowel and fermented by colonic bacteria. Empirical use of simethicone (Mylicon), either alone or with activated charcoal (Flatulex, Charcoal Plus) tablets, three or four times a day is probably not useful in reducing intestinal gas, although anecdotally a minority of patients do benefit. Sorbitol-containing drinks and medication syrups should be avoided, particularly in patients with diarrhea. Empirical "elimination diets" are not indicated, and we do not recommend additional dietary restrictions in most cases.

Medications

Because IBS is a heterogeneous disorder, it is not surprising that drug therapy is often ineffective. Indeed, there is no compelling evidence that any therapeutic agent is truly efficacious over placebo in IBS, primarily because the trials have been poorly designed. When reassurance, diet, and bulking agents fail, we use drug therapy, targeted at treating specific symptoms.

Placebo Effect

The placebo response in IBS is remarkably high, ranging from 20% to in excess of 70% in controlled trials, but it should not be forgotten that similar placebo responses can occur in organic disease. Indeed, spontaneous symptomatic improvement in IBS may be erroneously attributed to the coincidental use of a particular drug or other intervention.

Abdominal Pain

Antispasmodics are the most commonly used agents for the treatment of pain in IBS. Although randomized controlled trials have not offered any convincing evidence of their overall efficacy in IBS, antispasmodics may be helpful in individuals who predominantly complain of postprandial pain, diarrhea, or both because of their anticholinergic actions on the gut. There are a variety of agents available in the United States (Table 5), including hyoscyamine (Levsin, Levsinex), tincture of belladonna, dicyclomine (Bentyl), and propantheline bromide (Probanthine). In general, these drugs should be administered 30 to 60 minutes before meals. This approach may help reduce the impact of the neurohumoral-induced gastrocolic response on sensitized colonic smooth muscle, which could be responsible for the exaggerated colonic contractions and postprandial symptoms seen in some IBS sufferers. It is important to monitor for anticholinergic side effects, such as dry mouth, blurred vision, and urinary retention, and to reduce the dose if necessary. We do not recommend routine use of preparations that also contain small amounts of benzodiazepines (e.g., chlordiazepoxide with clidinium bromide [Librax]) because they have not been shown to be superior to anticholinergics alone and because of their potential for sedation and habituation. Barbiturate-containing compounds should not be prescribed.

Constipation

Long-term use of stimulant laxatives (e.g., Dulcolax, Senokot, Peri-Colace) for constipation should be discouraged because of their potential harmful effects (e.g., water and electrolyte losses, drug dependence). Patients who use these drugs on a long-term basis frequently are unable to discontinue them and may develop refractory constipation that does not respond to intensive bowel retraining and high doses of dietary fiber. For patients with resistant constipation, lactulose or milk of magnesia may be beneficial. New "prokinetic" drugs, such as cisapride, may have a role in the treatment of constipation-predominant

IBS. Metoclopramide (Reglan) is not useful for constipation.

Diarrhea

For patients with predominant diarrhea, loperamide (Imodium) at a dose of 2 to 4 mg, three to four times a day, is the pharmacologic agent of choice and is preferred over diphenoxylate, codeine, or other narcotics that cross the blood-brain barrier. Loperamide slows intestinal transit, enhances intestinal water and ion absorption, strengthens rectal sphincter tone, and may also be of benefit in the occasional patient with bile acid–induced diarrhea by allowing more contact time between the bile acids and the intestinal epithelial surface. It should be started at low doses and titrated upward according to the patient's response.

A few patients with refractory diarrhea may have idiopathic bile acid malabsorption. The true prevalence of this disorder is unknown. A therapeutic trial with cholestyramine (Questran),* which acts as a bile acid–binding agent, at a dose of 2 grams every 6 hours, is reasonable if other therapy has failed; this dose should be increased to 4 grams every 6 hours before it is deemed ineffective.

A small number of patients with IBS do not have true diarrhea but on close questioning actually are suffering from fecal incontinence; this may respond to loperamide or biofeedback therapy.

Refractory Patients

General Approach

A subset of patients with IBS have intractable symptoms that impair their quality of life. They exhibit abnormal illness behavior, often with a history of "doctor shopping." Believing that a serious disease is being overlooked, they often frustrate their physician's attempts to care for them by insisting on unneeded diagnostic studies and

---

*This use of cholestyramine is not listed in the manufacturer's official directive.

TABLE 5. **Anticholinergic Medications Commonly Prescribed for Patients with Irritable Bowel Syndrome**

Medication	Form	Dose
Levsin (hyoscyamine)	Tablet, elixir, drop	0.125–0.25 mg*
Levsinex (hyoscyamine)	Timed-release capsule	1–2 tablets twice daily
Tincture of belladonna drops	0.1 mL = 2 drops	0.2–0.75 mL*
Bentyl (dicyclomine)	Tablet, capsule, and syrup	20–40 mg*
Probanthine (propantheline)	Tablets (7.5 and 15 mg)	1 tablet*

*Before meals and at bedtime.

treatments. The physician in such a case must avoid performing unnecessary tests and should emphasize more realistic goals aimed at improving the patient's general well-being and functional status rather than symptomatic cure. Patients with severe chronic abdominal pain may benefit from referral to a pain treatment center. Referral for formal psychiatric evaluation is usually indicated only if major psychiatric disease is suspected.

Psychopharmacologic Agents

Antidepressant agents should be reserved for patients with intractable IBS who have failed other interventions and for patients with evidence of underlying depression in addition to IBS. The mechanism of action of these drugs in IBS is not well understood. Some antidepressants may improve symptoms in part because of their anticholinergic actions. They may also provide relief simply by enhancing the patient's overall sense of general well-being rather than by improving gastrointestinal symptoms per se. There does not appear to be any advantage of a particular drug in terms of effectiveness; however, amitriptyline (Elavil) is associated with a high incidence of anticholinergic side effects, whereas desipramine (Norpramin) and trazodone (Desyrel) are much less prone to do so. Trazodone has the advantage of being less sedating and having fewer cardiovascular effects (postural hypotension, arrhythmias) when compared with the older tricyclic antidepressants. Other drugs, such as fluoxetine (Prozac), act by blocking neuronal uptake of serotonin, which may induce central analgesia. All these agents are preferably started at low doses and titrated upward. Most may be given once a day (preferably at night, except for fluoxetine which should be given in the morning). Therapeutic effects may not be evident for at least 3 to 4 weeks. Some examples are shown in Table 6. If successful, antidepressant therapy should be continued for 6 months and then tapered and the clinical response observed to determine if medication can be discontinued.

Psychotherapy and Behavioral Treatments

Short-term psychotherapy may be effective in a subset of patients with IBS, especially those who are refractory to pharmacologic interventions alone. Patients who respond better to this approach include those with variable, periodic symptoms that can be linked to environmental stresses or emotional difficulties (most commonly marital and other relationship problems). Patients who do poorly with psychotherapy are those who have chronic, constant pain that has been present for many years and patients who are resistant to the idea that psychological factors might be involved in their illness. Diarrhea and abdominal pain have been noted to respond better to this treatment than constipation or abdominal distention.

Behavioral treatments may be useful in helping patients to reduce anxiety associated with certain situational or physiologic stressors. Relaxation training can be particularly useful. In biofeedback, skeletal muscle activity is monitored as the patient learns to control an unconscious physiologic function (such as the internal rectal sphincter muscle). Biofeedback may be particularly useful in patients who have constipation because of a pelvic floor disorder or in patients with IBS who also have fecal incontinence.

HEMORRHOIDS, ANAL FISSURE, AND ANORECTAL ABSCESS AND FISTULA

method of
PETER A. TUXEN, M.D.
St. Joseph's Medical Center
Stockton, California

Although patients often describe any abnormality of the anorectal region as "hemorrhoids," the accurate diagnosis can be suspected from a concise medical history and then confirmed by careful physical examination. Table 1 correlates anorectal symptoms with a likely diagnosis.

The proctologic examination is facilitated with nursing assistance and preparation of necessary equipment beforehand. Good lighting is essential, and the patient should be placed in a comfortable position. The lateral, left-side-down position with the buttocks over the edge of the examining table and the prone jackknife position are both convenient. After spreading the buttocks, the perianal skin should be inspected for any asymmetry,

TABLE 6. **Examples of Commonly Used Antidepressant Drugs in Irritable Bowel Syndrome**

Generic Name*	Trade Name	Usual Daily Dose (mg)
Amitriptyline	Elavil	25–100
Desipramine	Norpramin	25–100
Doxepin	Sinequan	25–100
Imipramine	Tofranil	25–100
Nortriptyline	Pamelor	25–100
Trazodone	Desyrel	100–150 (in divided doses)
Fluoxetine	Prozac	20–40 (once/day)

*All except fluoxetine are available generically.

TABLE 1. **Correlation Between Anorectal Symptoms and Diagnosis**

Diagnosis	Symptoms			
	Bleeding	Pain	Swelling	Drainage
Internal hemorrhoids	+		+	±
Thrombotic hemorrhoids		+	+	
Anal fissure	+	+		
Perianal abscess		+	+	
Fistula in ano	±			+
Colorectal neoplasm	+			

protrusion, drainage, or discoloration. The perianal skin can then be slightly everted to help expose a possible anal fissure. Both the perianal skin and the contour of the sphincter should be gently palpated to detect spasm, localized tenderness, and induration. Next a digital examination of the anal canal and rectal ampulla should precede anoscopy and sigmoidoscopy. Colonoscopy and barium enema are important and useful, especially when colorectal neoplasia is suspected, but these examinations can usually wait until a painful emergency has passed.

HEMORRHOIDS

Hemorrhoids are normal, elastic, vascular cushions of tissue lining the lower rectum and anus. Patients seek treatment when hemorrhoids become enlarged and produce symptoms. Clinically hemorrhoids may be divided between *external* (those below the mid-anal canal and covered by sensitive skin) and *internal* (those swellings originating above the mid-anal canal and covered with insensitive mucous membrane). Hemorrhoids typically present in three circumferential locations: left lateral, right posterior, and right anterior.

Although hemorrhoids have many causes, one common factor is usually excessive straining. Therefore, all treatment programs should include a high-fiber diet supplemented with psyllium seed preparations (Konsyl or Metamucil), methylcellulose (Citrocil), stool softeners (Surfak, Colace), and adequate fluids to counteract the inertia of hard, dry feces. Hemorrhoid suppositories, creams, and ointments may have a salutary affect. Frequent, warm sitz baths provide prompt but temporary relief of acute symptoms in all cases.

External Hemorrhoids

Acute Thrombosis

Sudden onset of a painful swelling near the anus is usually a thrombosed hemorrhoid or peri-

anal hematoma. The swelling is usually smooth, bluish in color, single, tender, and less than 1.0 cm in size. Sometimes swellings may become much larger and multiple.

The best treatment for a simple thrombosis is frequent sitz baths and soothing topical ointments. This is effective because the pain usually subsides after the first few days, and the swelling resolves completely in several weeks.

Surgical treatment may be recommended in the following situations: (1) prompt diagnosis in the first 48 hours after onset in the patient with unbearable pain and (2) hemorrhoid surface has ulcerated so bleeding is a problem. Excision is preferred to incision and drainage, and the clinic is an appropriate location for performing excision. Local anesthesia (bupivacaine with adrenaline via a No. 27 gauge needle) is administered around the base of the swelling so an ellipse of skin can be taken from the top of the lesion along with the contents of the hemorrhoid. If the hemorrhoid is larger than 1.0 cm, the dead space created by the excision should be closed with a catgut suture to prevent delayed hemorrhage. When multiple or large thromboses occur, hemorrhoidectomy in an operating room may be necessary.

Chronic Skin Tags

These protuberances are usually the result of recurrent attacks of acute hemorrhoids resulting in stretching and hypertrophy of the skin. Occasionally a firm, rubbery, hypertrophied *anal papilla* enlarges to the point where external prolapse occurs. Uncomplicated skin tags produce few or no symptoms. There is no medical treatment to shrink chronic skin tags. Patients request the removal of skin tags and fibrotic anal polyps because of their physical presence and because there is difficulty cleaning between these protuberances. Surgery is done in the clinic under local anesthetic, and each skin ellipse is closed subcutaneously with fine catgut or polyglycolic suture.

Perianal Dermatitis

Perianal itching and burning are not symptoms of hemorrhoids but rather indicate skin irritation or damage that is usually the result of overzealous perianal wiping and cleaning. Often the skin appears normal or slightly inflamed, but in reality the protective epidermis has been traumatized and abraded by toilet paper. Induration and redness suggest specific infection. When chronic skin damage is visible, the condition is referred to as *pruritus ani*. Chronic skin damage is more difficult to treat, but nearly all cases of dermatitis can be improved by educating the patient to avoid excessive wiping, scratching, and overmedication of the anal skin. This allows the damaged epithelium to mature, heal, and protect itself from normal moisture and feces. The patient should receive suggestions that include gentle washing of the skin in the shower or sitz baths twice daily (especially after a bowel movement) and careful drying of the skin plus the wearing of a flattened cotton wafer in the perianal crease to absorb moisture and prevent abrasion and chafing. Occasionally a short course of 1% hydrocortisone cream can reduce acute itching. Medicated powders (Balmex baby powder or Desitin) or plain cornstarch may be helpful.

Internal Hemorrhoids

The most common manifestation of symptomatic internal hemorrhoids is painless, bright red bleeding. Inspection and digital examination are not much help for internal hemorrhoids because the average internal lesion is not visible or palpable unless there is significant prolapse. With air insufflation, sigmoidoscopy flattens out the soft cushions during routine examination and may miss internal hemorrhoids. A short, wide-mouthed, self-illuminated anoscope, however, when gently and carefully inserted into the rectum, is useful for both diagnosis and treatment. It should be withdrawn slowly, carefully, and sometimes withdrawn more than once with the patient straining slightly. The redundant vascular cushion now begins to reveal itself. This in effect reproduces the process of defecation, and an examiner can now see the loose, congested vascular cushion begin to swell, prolapse, and even bleed as it follows the anoscope outward. The degree of internal hemorrhoids should be assessed and therapy recommended (Table 2). Elimination of symptomatic redundant tissue, fixation of loose mucosa, and general streamlining of the anorectal junction are the treatment goals.

Most bleeding grade I hemorrhoids can be treated medically with improved diet and bowel habit. Sclerotherapy (submucosal injection of 0.3 mL of a sclerosing agent, such as 5.0% phenol in sterile peanut oil) is useful for recurrent bleeding in small, vascular hemorrhoids without significant prolapse. Sclerotherapy is inexpensive, effective, and safe.

For grade II internal hemorrhoids, an elastic band ligation is ideal because the redundant tissue can be pinched off through ischemic necrosis. The resulting inflammation fixates the adjacent mucosa to the muscular side wall of the rectum. A one-handed suction rubber band ligator is quick, easy to use; and avoids taking too much tissue. Patients do better if they are given a written instruction sheet alerting them to the unpleasant side effects and complications. For example, pressure sensation may exist for a day or two. The treatment can also cause delayed hemorrhage, perianal thrombosis, and rarely infection. Other outpatient treatments for grade II internal hemorrhoids include infrared coagulation and bipolar coagulation, but both require purchase of special equipment (expensive compared with banding), and there are no proven advantages.

Grade III hemorrhoids can be treated by elastic banding as well as some of the other methods described. As the hemorrhoids become larger and more difficult to reduce, however, approaching fixed mucosal prolapse (grade IV), surgical hemorrhoidectomy is best. Individuals who are properly selected for hemorrhoidectomy benefit tremendously and are among the most grateful and satisfied patients. Cryosurgery and laser surgery have the support of a few enthusiasts, but neither method has proven advantages to justify the significantly higher cost.

ANAL FISSURE

The anal canal fissure, a split or linear ulcer, is located often in the posterior midline and less often in the anterior position. Few conditions, besides fissure, produce the typical severe pain associated with each bowel movement. Bleeding is sometimes present. Fissure may be difficult to prove because the diagnostic examination is impaired by tenderness and spasm. Useful clues during examination in this situation include an edematous skin tab at the lower margin of the anal canal ("sentinel pile") and involuntary spasm noted during gentle pressure on the anal opening. Often the lower edge of the fissure can be visualized by everting the anoderm, or it can be palpated as a rough and reproducibly tender spot during digital examination.

Initial treatment includes frequent warm or hot sitz baths, rest, and reassurance. This is im-

TABLE 2. **Classification of Internal Hemorrhoids by Degree and Recommended Treatment**

Degree	Definition	Treatment
First	Bleeding without prolapse	Sclerotherapy IRC
Second	Bleeding and prolapse but spontaneous return	Rubber band ligation Sclerotherapy IRC
Third	Prolapse requires manual reduction	Rubber band ligation Surgery
Fourth	Fixed mucosal prolapse	Surgical hemorrhoidectomy

IRC = infrared coagulation.

portant because the onset of a fissure often follows a disruptive life event, such as major surgery, pregnancy, or a stressful change at work or school. The exact cause varies, but often the patient recalls a large and painful bowel movement. In addition to the sitz baths, the patient should be placed on bulk laxatives (psyllium powder), a high-fiber diet, and stool softeners. A lubricating local anesthetic ointment (Anusol) or a glycerin suppository is sometimes helpful just before the anticipated painful bowel movement. The author has had little or no success with steroid creams and foams.

Surgery should be considered when anal fissures fail to heal with medical therapy, relapse recurrently, or are associated with significant anal stenosis. Occasionally the patient's acute pain is so severe that he or she cannot wait. It is appropriate to examine such patients under general anesthesia or under local anesthesia with or without conscious sedation using intravenous midazolam (Versed) or diazepam (Valium). Sometimes the procedure can be done in the clinic or office using local anesthetic alone. Bupivacaine with 1:200,000 epinephrine is administered through a No. 27 gauge needle circumferentially along the anal canal with the operating speculum in place. The fissure is inspected but usually not disturbed, unless there is a significant undermining recess that traps stool or if there is a sizable prolapsing, hypertrophied, fibrotic anal papilla. In these cases, minor tissue excision is good, but actual fissurectomy has little importance in the modern treatment of anal fissure. Instead unilateral *partial internal* sphincterotomy is performed so the hypertrophied band of internal sphincter is partially divided, allowing the anus to enlarge gradually. A No. 11 or No. 15 scalpel blade is inserted through a stab wound or through an open incision under direct vision to divide the light-colored, internal sphincter fibers subtotally. A few minutes of gentle pressure is applied to the sphincterotomy site to create a slight depression and to allow hemostasis. If under anesthesia a taut band or hypertrophied sphincter is not readily apparent, the author often does a gentle dilatation only and then reassesses the patient for further medical therapy. Postoperative care, as in all rectal procedures, includes multiple daily sitz baths for a few weeks plus psyllium and a high-fiber diet. Recovery from surgery and fissure symptoms is surprisingly prompt. Complications are infrequent but can include minor incontinence, superficial fistula, and occasional bleeding. Recurrence after sphincterotomy is rare.

Pitfalls of anal fissure treatment include operating on patients with Crohn's disease (lateral and multiple fissures), undiagnosed malignant anal ulcers, and patients with fissures and stenosis from prior excisional hemorrhoidectomy. These cases require biopsy and consultation.

ANORECTAL ABSCESS

Anorectal abscess is a common and painful bacterial infection near the anus. The bacteria that cause abscess usually originate in the normal fecal flora and enter the perirectal tissues through the anal canal glands. Less frequently, skin infection may lead to perianal abscess or hidradenitis suppurativa.

Abscess should always be suspected whenever a patient complains of constant or progressively worse, throbbing pain over several days. Usually swelling and induration are present, but typical symptoms alone should lead the physician to perform an examination with the patient under anesthesia. Fluctuance is a reliable but late indicator of abscess. Drainage is the proper surgical treatment of abscesses at all stages, and antibiotics have little or no place in their management. If there is significant doubt, a No. 16 or 18 gauge needle can be inserted into the site of maximal pain and tenderness to aspirate pus, following which the surgeon may then insert the scalpel with greater confidence.

In most cases, the office or clinic setting is an appropriate place for abscess drainage. 1.0% lidocaine (with epinephrine) is infiltrated with a No. 30 gauge needle. An extra few minutes is allowed because local anesthetic is slow to take affect on the inflamed tissues. A No. 11 scalpel is used to make a 1.0-cm stab wound. Placement close to the anus may reduce the length of a subsequent fistula. The stab wound is gently enlarged with a small mosquito clamp to allow free egress of pus. Irrigation may be helpful. Packing is generally not a good idea, unless it is done to control hemorrhage. Instead insert a small Penrose drain or a short mushroom catheter into the cavity so that only 1.0 cm protrudes. The drain usually falls out during sitz baths in a few days, but the mushroom may be left longer and occasionally irrigated. The patient should be brought back in a few days to assess adequacy of drainage and then for a more complete examination in a few weeks to assess for fistula. Fistula is the expected outcome of perirectal abscess drainage in about one-half of cases. Recurrent abscess is a good indication that fistula therapy is needed. Simultaneous abscess drainage and fistula surgery require ideal circumstances and considerable experience to avoid sphincter injury.

FISTULA

A fistula is a chronic inflammatory tunnel through which a bacterial anorectal abscess has spontaneously or surgically drained. Purulent seepage through a *secondary opening* is the usual presenting symptom. This suggests an inadequately drained abscess, a significantly large connection to the anal crypt source (the *primary opening*), or both. Fistulas may produce other symptoms, including discomfort, bleeding, and localized itching. An occasional fistula may have no symptoms. The treatment of symptomatic fistula is surgical.

Successful outcome depends on good exposure, judicious use of anesthesia, and complete unroofing (drainage) of the entire fistula tract. Superficial fistulas, in which the tract is palpable and the probe can be passed effortlessly to the anal primary opening, are treated in the office with the patient under local anesthesia. When any uncertainty exists as to the difficulty of the fistula or the involvement of significant sphincter, general anesthesia is preferred, so gentle, accurate exploration is possible. Situations involving significant amounts of anal sphincter, in which postoperative incontinence is possible, should be referred for consultation with a surgeon. Occasionally an apparently simple fistula is operated on, but despite one's best effort, the primary opening cannot be located. In this situation, the author recommends laying open the apparent tract below the anal sphincter and then terminating the operation by packing. Sometimes these situations heal owing to the improved drainage. Avoid creation of a new primary opening and false passages.

Following a surgical operation, postoperative care includes sitz baths and a small gauze pad to absorb drainage and separate the wound edges. The patient may be checked every few weeks to be sure that the skin edges do not bridge and reform the fistula.

Hydradenitis suppurativa, an indolent sweat gland infection, affects the perianal skin with subcutaneous fistulas. Physical examination reveals single or multiple purulent openings and painless darkening of the perianal skin. Undermining of the skin can be quite extensive. Simple but sometimes wide excision of the skin overlying the infection under local anesthesia in the office usually allows healing.

GASTRITIS

method of
FRANZ GOLDSTEIN, M.D.
Jefferson Medical College and Lankenau Hospital
Philadelphia, Pennsylvania

Gastritis is a commonly entertained diagnosis, both by practitioners of medicine and by the lay public. Yet the term "gastritis" is virtually meaningless unless defined precisely. Patients often complain of gastritis when they wish to describe a wide variety of gastrointestinal symptoms that may or may not originate in the stomach. Radiologists tend to refer to gastritis when the gastric fold pattern is nonspecifically abnormal. Folds seen on barium x-rays may appear enlarged and evoke a diagnosis of hypertrophic gastritis, or they may be flattened and evoke a diagnosis of atrophic gastritis. With double contrast x-ray technique, fine mucosal erosions can be detected and may suggest an x-ray diagnosis of erosive gastritis. It should be remembered that gastritis signifies an inflammation of the stomach that cannot be reliably diagnosed by x-ray and that any abnormal gastric fold pattern should be investigated and the diagnosis confirmed by endoscopy and biopsies. Endoscopically a number of gastric fold patterns have been described that may suggest various forms of gastritis. In superficial erosive gastritis with or without hemorrhagic features, the endoscopic picture may be the only and most reliable diagnostic abnormality because, strangely, this type of gastritis does not correlate with histologic features of gastritis. In most instances, though, it is the biopsy of gastric mucosa and at times a full-thickness biopsy of the gastric wall that are essential for a precise and accurate diagnosis. The collaboration between endoscopist and pathologist in arriving at a diagnosis is important because endoscopic, clinical, and histologic correlations are often necessary to arrive at the correct diagnosis. This is particularly so because there is no parallelism between the four aspects cited: the clinical picture to be described in more detail, the x-ray appearance, the endoscopic appearance of the stomach, and histologic features.

The clinical correlates of gastritis tend to be epigastric symptoms of pain, distress, nausea, and fullness, often affected in some way by eating and at times relieved by antacids and by drugs neutralizing or reducing the secretion of gastric acid. Belching, gaseousness, and indigestion are other clinical correlates often used. Gastritis, histologically verified, often causes no symptoms. In some countries and increasingly in the United States, nonulcerative dyspepsia has become a frequent diagnosis to denote a similar set of symptoms, but this term, despite its present popularity, lacks clear or specific meaning.

There are numerous causes of gastritis in addition to the various forms of gastritis. Attempts have been made for at least 100 years to classify gastritis with no overwhelming success. The most recent effort was unveiled at the 1990 World Congress of Gastroenterology in Sydney, Australia, produced by a predominantly European group of investigators and dealing primarily with the classification of chronic nonspecific gastritis. The classification has not met with uniform acceptance and is far too complex to present here in detail. In simplified terms, gastritis can be classified into an acute and chronic form and then subclassified by cause when this can be determined. The acute form is characterized histologically by the presence of neutrophilic inflammatory cell infiltrates, whereas chronic gastritis is characterized by chronic inflammatory cell infiltrates. Chronic active gastritis denotes a form of gastritis with both chronic and acute inflammatory cells. One unusual exception already hinted at is the acute erosive or even hemorrhagic gastritis associated with nonsteroidal anti-inflammatory drug (NSAID) use so obvious on endoscopy yet not diagnosable by histologic means because of the absence of inflammatory changes. There are few if any counterparts to such a situation in other areas of medicine.

Among the specific causes of both acute and chronic gastritis are various infections, including viruses, bacteria, fungi, and parasites, and various chemical agents, including corrosive alkali, acid, concentrated alcohol, and a variety of noxious drugs. Among the latter, the standouts are aspirin and all NSAIDs, which cause erosive or hemorrhagic gastritis all too frequently.

Many of the causes that can lead to acute gastritis can also produce chronic gastritis, among them some drugs; thermal stimuli; alkali and acid injuries; strong alcohol; therapeutic radiation, and possibly injury by certain foods—for instance, spiced pickles. Among chronic infectious causes should be mentioned the rare, but lately once again increasingly frequent, syphilis and tuberculosis of the stomach. There is a form of gastritis that is closely related to peptic ulcer disease. Granulomatous gastritis is occasionally encountered as part of Crohn's disease or other granulomatous diseases or may appear to be an isolated phenomenon. Hypertrophic gastritis has been recognized for more than 100 years since Ménétrier's description of several conditions characterized by large gastric folds or nodules. Some experts would limit the term "Ménétrier's disease" to those cases of hypertrophic gastritis associated with protein-losing enteropathy. The exact cause of hypertrophic gastritis is not known, but it can be associated with normal, excessive, diminished, or no acid secretion. Some patients progress slowly through stages from hypertrophic to atrophic gastritis with immunologic factors usually present in atrophic gastritis. Antibodies to parietal cells and to intrinsic factor can be found in such patients, and antibodies to the latter are particularly seen in patients who have progressed to pernicious anemia.

Atrophic gastritis and other forms of gastritis are often divided into a diffuse type and a type I, or A, and type II, or B, form. The gastric antrum is spared in type I gastritis typical of pernicious anemia, whereas type II gastritis involves preferentially the gastric antrum. Diffuse gastritis involving the entire stomach is sometimes referred as type III or C gastritis. In type I gastritis, the lack of acidity is usually combined with high levels of serum gastrin produced by the G cells of the unaffected gastric antrum. This type of gastritis may progress to intestinal metaplasia and occasionally to gastric carcinoma. Hypertrophic gastritis also car-

ries a higher risk of immediate or delayed gastric malignancy. With the advent of computed tomography scanning, a thickened gastric wall observed on scanning is suspect for submucosal infiltration by either lymphoma or carcinoma. A full-thickness surgical biopsy is often needed in such cases to make the initial differential diagnosis between hypertrophic gastritis and submucosal neoplasm. Even when the condition is initially found to be benign, patients with hypertrophic and atrophic gastritis should be kept under surveillance for future development of gastric carcinoma, although specific recommendations for the type of surveillance or frequency of endoscopic biopsies and cytology are lacking.

The most exciting development in our understanding of gastritis has been the discovery by Marshall and colleagues in the mid-1980s of the presence of bacterial organisms in the stomach, especially the gastric antrum, in association with a chronic active gastritis. The organism was initially named Campylobacter pylori and subsequently renamed Helicobacter pylori. It is found in the vast majority of patients with antral gastritis and in most patients with peptic ulcer, both duodenal and gastric. There are preliminary data to suggest that the prolonged presence of Helicobacter gastritis may lead to gastric carcinoma. H. pylori is typically absent in some specific forms of gastritis, such as pernicious anemia, Ménétrier's disease, eosinophilic gastritis, and others and is not found in tissues other than gastric mucosa. H. pylori is found in 20 to 90% of various populations, depending on age and social and hygienic status.

Symptoms of gastritis caused by H. pylori are often vague and similar to symptoms already referred to but are similar to symptoms produced by other gastric conditions, including gastric ulcer or gastric malignancy, and gastritis can exist without symptoms. The prolonged presence of epigastric distress or pain in the absence of x-ray findings of ulcer or neoplasm and unresponsive to antiulcer treatment is especially suggestive of H. pylori gastritis.

Confirmation of the diagnosis and presence of H. pylori is usually dependent on endoscopy and biopsy, with radiographs playing a progressively smaller part. The presence of Helicobacter organisms is important to determine. This can be done by a variety of means. The author prefers gastric biopsy and staining with Giemsa stain, which facilitates visualization of the typical curved bacilli with their delicate flagellae attached to mucous cells. Other stains can be used, including the originally recommended Warthin-Starry silver impregnation stain, which is accurate but more complex. Culture of the organisms is possible and has great specificity but low sensitivity. Culture permits determination of antibiotic sensitivities not yet widely used. Indirect methods include immunologic and enzyme-linked immunosorbent assay (ELISA) tests, which are most useful for epidemiologic studies but are less reliable to determine an individual's current status. Indirect methods may also use the high urease concentration of H. pylori and hence its ability to split urea into carbon dioxide and ammonia. The CLO test requires a piece of gastric tissue to be placed on plates with indicator dye that changes color from yellow to red with a rise in pH owing to the release of ammonia. The release of carbon dioxide can be documented with breath tests after feeding labeled urea to test patients and analyzing their breath for C^{13} with a mass spectrometer or for C^{14} with a beta counter. Neither method is widely available and requires research settings. Recently methods have also been recommended to test biopsy material by cytologic means, but insufficient data are available at present to substitute this potentially more rapid testing for the probably more reliable histologic method.

TREATMENT

Once the diagnosis of gastritis and the type of gastritis are established, treatment logically follows. In many acute forms of gastritis, the offending agent, e.g., NSAIDs, simply has to be removed or allowed to disappear spontaneously for the condition to clear. In acid-peptic disorders, the use of histamine II receptor antagonists or omeprazole is most helpful. Any specific gastritides should be treated by specific means directed at the cause. It would seem that the majority of patients with true gastritis suffer from *Helicobacter*-related gastritis, and this is where most of the emphasis has been placed lately. The precise details and doses of treatment are still evolving. It is clear, however, that two or three agents are necessary to obtain a high percentage of eradication of *Helicobacter* and healing of gastritis. Treatment usually consists of administration of a bismuth compound and one or two antibiotics. In the United States, only bismuth subsalicylate is available (as Pepto-Bismol). This can be given in the form of tablets or liquid, usually for 2 weeks in a dose of 1 tablespoon or 2 tablets four times a day, each containing 262 mg of the compound per tablet or tablespoon. Simultaneously and also for 2 weeks, one or two antibiotics are added, with metronidazole being the mainstay in a dose of 1 to 1.5 grams a day in divided doses for 1 to 2 weeks. Preferably tetracycline or amoxicillin should also be used for 2 weeks in a dose of 250 to 500 mg four times a day with precautions and warnings to the patient about possible side effects from each one of these components. Long-term treatment with Pepto-Bismol is not indicated because of potential neurotoxicity, but 80 to 90% of patients have long-lasting healing with a single course of the aforementioned triple treatment. The addition of H_2 blockers or of omeprazole (Prilosec) does not interfere with the eradication of *Helicobacter* and may be used concomitantly if deemed clinically necessary, especially if an ulcer is also present. In other countries, bismuth subcitrate (DeNol) has been preferred in place of Pepto-Bismol, but this drug is not available in the United States.

Another form of gastritis is bile reflux gastritis, which is seen most commonly in patients with prior gastric surgery but also in patients with prior biliary tract surgery, particularly cholecystectomy, and occasionally without antecedent surgery. If bile and accompanying intestinal juices containing digestive enzymes enter the stomach in substantial quantities, they are noxious to the gastric mucosa and can produce a severe form of gastritis and gastric metaplasia. Treatment is not totally satisfactory, and no drugs are available to "neutralize" the noxious effects of the biliary/alkaline reflux. Prokinetic drugs that enhance antegrade esophageal and gastric peristalsis and hence gastric emptying have found some favor, but the only currently available drug in the United States for this purpose is metoclopramide (Reglan), which has a high central nervous system side effect profile and is not tolerated by at least 25% of patients. Cisapride is in the process of approval in the United States, has purely prokinetic effects without central nervous system side effects, and should prove to be a useful adjunct in the treatment of bile reflux gastritis. Surgical diversion of bile from the stomach can be resorted to in severe cases, but even this approach can produce serious gastric stasis problems.

ACUTE AND CHRONIC HEPATITIS

method of
WILLIAM SIEVERT, M.D.
Monash University
Melbourne, Victoria, Australia

Viral hepatitis is a systemic viral infection whose primary biochemical, histologic, and clinical manifestations relate to the altered function of liver cells owing either to the direct effects of the virus or to an immunologic attack on virally infected hepatocytes. The majority of both acute and chronic viral hepatitis is caused by the hepatitis viruses A, B, C, D, and E. Acute hepatic inflammation may be due uncommonly to infection with cytomegalovirus or Epstein-Barr virus.

HEPATITIS A VIRUS

Hepatitis A virus (HAV) is an RNA virus first identified in the feces of human volunteers in 1973. HAV has only one serotype (an important factor in vaccine development), and replication is probably limited to liver cells. Infection is primarily by the fecal-oral route, hence transmission between family members, between institutionalized subjects, or from common-source outbreaks is frequent (Table 1). There are well-documented episodes of transmission by blood transfusion, but these account for fewer than 1% of cases. The

TABLE 1. **Risk Factors for Hepatitis A Virus Infection**

Contact with a person in the late incubation period

Travel to a high prevalence area (e.g., to North Africa or the Middle East)

Contact with young children with inapparent infection (e.g., day care centers)

Individuals residing or working in institutions with close living conditions

Intravenous drug use

---

infectivity of saliva, urine, or semen is low, and transmission by these routes is not clinically important. Vertical transmission of HAV has not been described.

HAV has an incubation period of 3 to 6 weeks. The virus appears in feces toward the end of the incubation period and peaks just before the onset of symptoms, an increase in alanine aminotransferase (ALT), and the appearance of anti-HAV immunoglobulin M (IgM). Thus, the greatest risk of transmission occurs before the disease is clinically apparent. Acute hepatitis A is characterized by a typical viral prodrome with anorexia, nausea, vomiting, low-grade fever, and fatigue. Clinical manifestations vary with age: Young children generally have a mild, anicteric illness (and may harbor an unrecognized source of infection), whereas most HAV infection in adults is icteric. Complete recovery should occur within 1 to 2 months, although occasionally patients may develop a prolonged cholestatic phase or relapse after initial resolution. Hepatitis A never causes persistent infection or chronic liver disease, although it may rarely be a cause of fulminant hepatic failure.

The diagnosis of acute hepatitis A depends on demonstration of hepatitis A IgM antibodies in serum. Hepatitis A immunoglobulin G (IgG) appears in the convalescent phase and confers lifelong immunity against HAV infection. The treatment of acute hepatitis A is symptomatic with the common sense recommendations for adequate rest; a low-fat, high-carbohydrate diet; adequate fluid intake; and avoidance of alcohol while liver function tests remain abnormal. Hospitalization is required for inability to maintain hydration orally or development of an altered consciousness state. A prolonged prothrombin time is an important indicator of seriously impaired hepatic function.

Methods to prevent spread to household and other close contacts include adequate hygiene (especially hand washing) and postexposure prophylaxis with immune serum globulin (ISG). ISG prophylaxis is recommended for all household and intimate contacts at a dosage of 0.02 to 0.06 mL per kg. Age and pregnancy are not contraindications. If ISG is administered within 2 weeks of exposure, HAV infection is prevented in most people, although these individuals are not immune to future HAV infection. In approximately 20% of subjects, subclinical HAV infection occurs, but clinical symptoms are ameliorated and longterm immunity (passive/active immunization) occurs. Preexposure prophylaxis should also be considered for travelers to high prevalence areas. For travel of less than 3 months' duration, 0.02 mL per kg is recommended. For prolonged travel, travelers should be screened for anti-HAV IgG and, if not immune, receive 0.06 mL per kg every 4 to 6 months. A vaccine for HAV has recently been developed, and initial studies show it to be safe and effective after three or fewer injections. The individuals most likely to benefit from vaccination are travelers to endemic areas, workers in day care centers, those residing in institutions with close living conditions, and those in the military.

HEPATITIS B VIRUS

This small DNA virus chronically infects an estimated 300 million people worldwide. Circulating virus exists as a double-shelled structure with hepatitis B surface antigen (HBsAg) providing an outer coat around an internal core composed of the viral DNA (hepatitis B virus [HBV] DNA), a DNA polymerase, and a polypeptide from which both hepatitis B core antigen (HBcAg) and hepatitis B "e" antigen (HBeAg) are derived. HBcAg is found only in infected liver cells and, in contrast to HBeAg, does not circulate in blood. The presence of HBV DNA and HBeAg in the blood is a marker for active viral replication and reflects a greater degree of infectivity.

The highest levels of HBV are found in blood, and therefore transmission of the virus is mainly parenteral or by the so-called inapparent parenteral route. Although infected semen and saliva may transmit the virus, there is no evidence that urine, breast milk, sweat, tears, or feces is infective. Transmission of HBV occurs in several important ways (Table 2).

The majority of adults with acute HBV infection do not develop a clinical illness but have a silent subclinical course with complete recovery. About 25% develop overt hepatitis, and of these a tiny fraction (1% or less) develop fulminant hepatitis, which carries a high mortality rate. Therefore, 90 to 95% of patients with acute HBV infection go on to full recovery and subsequent immunity. Approximately 5 to 10% develop chronic HBV infection. Patients with chronic HBV infection are often categorized into healthy carriers (those with no discernible liver disease,

TABLE 2. **Risk Factors for Hepatitis B Virus Infection**

Parenteral transmission includes transfusion of blood or blood products, needle stick injuries (e.g., accidental injury in health care workers or by sharing needles in intravenous drug abuse), or other percutaneous exposure such as tattoos or acupuncture

It is important to remember that hepatitis B is a sexually transmitted disease. Both heterosexuals with multiple partners and male homosexuals (especially with anal receptive intercourse) are at risk of HBV infection

Maternal-neonatal (vertical) transmission of HBV is common in areas with a high prevalence of HBV infection. Mothers who are HBeAg positive or who develop acute HBV in the third trimester of pregnancy are more likely to infect their infants at the time of birth. Vertical transmission is not accompanied by clinical illness, and the majority of infected neonates become chronic HBV carriers unless preventive measures are taken

Household members of others in close contact with chronic HBV carriers are at risk of infection. This nonsexual method of spread is presumably by the "inapparent parenteral" route from exposure to virus containing bodily fluids from a chronic HBV carrier

Abbreviations: HBV = hepatitis B virus; HBeAg = hepatitis B "e" antigen.

about 80%) and those with chronic hepatitis, both groups being at risk of developing hepatocellular carcinoma.

The incubation period for HBV ranges from 40 to 140 days. In the early, replicative stage, high titers first of HBsAg and then HBeAg are found in serum followed by the onset of symptoms of hepatitis and high ALT measurements, reflecting intense lysis of liver cells. As the infection resolves over days to weeks, first HBeAg and then HBsAg disappear from the blood, and specific antibody appears. The earliest appearance is that of the IgM class of antibody against HBcAg (IgM anti-HBc) followed by the IgG class of anti-HBc. The presence of IgM anti-HBc and HBsAg in serum is diagnostic of acute HBV infection. Following clearance of HBsAg from serum, which may take several weeks, specific antibody (anti-HBs) appears; this antibody is protective and confers lifelong immunity to further HBV infection.

Detection of HBsAg in serum for more than 6 months defines chronic HBV infection. HBsAg may persist for years; annually less than 1% of patients spontaneously clear HBsAg. Anti-HBc is detectable in high titer in chronic HBV infection, most of which is of the IgG class. Protective anti-HBs is not found; instead the persistence of viral replication markers (HBeAg, HBV DNA) for months to years is the rule. In many patients after years of chronic infection, the virus ceases active replication and becomes integrated into the host genome. This event is characterized serologically by the disappearance of HBV DNA

and HBeAg and the appearance of anti-HBe and is often accompanied by a transient rise in ALT and worsening of symptoms. Subsequently ALT often normalizes, and symptoms subside for an indefinite period, although a few patients may undergo spontaneous reactivation. Unfortunately, HBeAg seroconversion may occur only after permanent liver damage has occurred.

Worsening liver disease in a chronic HBV carrier may be the result of reactivation of HBV; coincident infection with HAV, hepatitis D virus (HDV), or hepatitis C virus (HCV); or toxicity owing to alcohol or medications.

Epidemiologic studies have demonstrated a 300-fold increase in the risk of developing a hepatocellular carcinoma in patients with chronic hepatitis B infection compared with noninfected patients. This risk appears to increase with duration of infection, which probably reflects the eventual integration of the HBV genome into the host genome and the greater recognition of this disease in populations with endemic infection. Hepatoma most often develops in a patient with coexisting inactive cirrhosis.

Six to 12 monthly surveillance programs in patients with chronic hepatitis B, especially men who acquired the infection in childhood, include ultrasonography and measurement of alpha-fetoprotein. The value of such an approach in improving survival by identifying early, surgically resectable lesions is controversial.

Treatment of Hepatitis B Infection

The management of acute hepatitis B is supportive. Patients with mild disease may be treated at home with bed rest during the symptomatic period. In the first weeks of infection, when HBsAg and HBeAg are present in high titer, patients are infectious. Toothbrushes and razor blades should not be shared, and patients should be reminded that hepatitis B can be spread by sexual intercourse. Generally the resolution of symptoms and abnormal liver function tests correlates with the disappearance of HBsAg; these tests should be followed until results are negative or normal, indicating that the patient is no longer infectious. Specific therapy with interferon (or other antiviral therapy) is not indicated for patients with acute hepatitis B.

In counseling patients with chronic hepatitis B, education regarding the nature and prognosis of the disease, risk and manner of spread of infection to others, and the need for vaccination of intimate contacts and family members is important.

Specific treatment of chronic HBV infection with corticosteroids and antiviral agents, such as adenine arabinoside (vidarabine [Vira-A]), has been ineffective or in some cases resulted in deterioration. Recently recombinant interferon-alpha$_{2a}$ has been approved for the treatment of chronic hepatitis B. The usual regimens involve from 5 to 10 million units given subcutaneously three times each week for 4 to 6 months. Side effects include flu-like symptoms, neutropenia, thrombocytopenia, and mood changes. Interferon has shown the best response in patients with a relatively short duration of HBV infection, raised pretreatment ALT, and low HBV DNA levels. A response to treatment (defined as symptomatic, biochemical, and histologic improvement with seroconversion of HBeAg to hepatitis B "e" antibody [HBeAb]) occurs in approximately 40 to 50% of patients, although cure of HBV infection (loss of HBsAg) occurs in only 10%. Eventual loss of HBsAg, however, has been documented in patients followed for several years after an initial response to interferon therapy. Patients should be carefully selected for treatment, given the side effects and cost of therapy. In general, treatment of healthy HBV carriers (normal liver function tests, no markers of active viral replication) is not appropriate, and significant deterioration in patients with advanced liver disease may occur as a result of interferon treatment.

Prevention of Hepatitis B Infection

Universal vaccination may lead to eventual control and prevention of hepatitis B. Strategies for vaccination and passive immunization with hepatitis B immune globulin (HBIG) should be considered in preexposure and postexposure prophylaxis (Table 3).

HEPATITIS D VIRUS (DELTA HEPATITIS)

This defective virus exists as a core of RNA, which expresses hepatitis D antigen (HDAg), surrounded by an outer core of HBsAg. Infection with HDV occurs only in patients who are also infected with HBV. The virus is transmitted parenterally, with approximately 5% of HBsAg carriers worldwide being infected. In Western societies, patients at risk for HBV infection, such as intravenous drug users, are most likely to be infected with HDV.

Simultaneous infection with both HDV and HBV, termed "co-infection," has a variable clinical course because HDV growth is dependent on the number of HBV-infected liver cells. Because most HBV infection resolves and HDV cannot survive without the help of HBV, most co-infected patients do not develop chronic liver disease. In-

TABLE 3. Prevention of Hepatitis B Virus Infection

Infants born to HBV-infected mothers (especially those mothers developing acute hepatitis B late in pregnancy or who are HBeAg positive) should receive 0.5 mL of HBIG within 12 h of birth followed by the first dose of hepatitis B vaccine within 7 days of birth. Further doses of HBV vaccine should follow at 1 and 6 months

Preexposure immunization with recombinant hepatitis B vaccine should be considered in high-risk groups:
  Health care personnel with regular blood contact (laboratory technicians, dentists, nurses, physicians)
  Intimate contacts and household members of patients with chronic hepatitis B infection
  Persons at risk of sexual exposure: homosexual men, prostitutes, promiscuous heterosexuals
  Patients regularly requiring blood products: renal dialysis and transplant patients, thalassemics, and hemophiliacs
  Institutionalized residents

Postexposure prophylaxis should be considered in:
  Persons who receive needle stick, other percutaneous, mucous membrane, or sexual exposure to a person with chronic HBV infection
  HBIG (0.05 mL/kg) should be given preferably within 24 h followed by a course of hepatitis B vaccine (3 injections). In those recipients who have been previously vaccinated, a single booster dose of HBV vaccine is sufficient. A combination of HBIG and HBV vaccine is generally recommended for sexual, but not household or casual, contacts of patients with acute hepatitis B

Abbreviations: HBV = hepatitis B virus; HBeAg = hepatitis B "e" antigen; HBIG = hepatitis B immune globulin.

fection with HDV in a chronic HBV carrier, termed "superinfection," has a more severe course and commonly leads to chronic liver disease. The presence of a large number of chronically HBV-infected hepatocytes is fertile ground for further HDV replication. Superinfection may transform mild chronic hepatitis B into more active chronic liver disease with cirrhosis. Fulminant hepatitis D may occur after either co-infection or superinfection.

Serologic diagnosis is possible by testing for HDAg or anti-HDV in an HBsAg-positive patient. In co-infection, HDAg circulation is usually brief, disappearing with the loss of HBsAg. In superinfection leading to chronic delta hepatitis, HDAg usually persists in serum, and some diminution of HBsAg titers occurs as HBV replication is suppressed.

Interferon therapy has been only partially successful in HDV infection with frequent relapse after cessation of therapy. Immunization against hepatitis B prevents hepatitis D infection, although there is little to offer the HBsAg-positive patient for protection against HDV.

NON-A, NON-B HEPATITIS

Chronic liver disease of presumed viral origin, not due to infection with HAV, HBV, or HDV, was termed non-A, non-B hepatitis in 1975. Non-A, non-B hepatitis was thus a diagnosis of exclusion based on epidemiologic factors and the exclusion of other known causes of chronic liver disease. Two forms were recognized, a *parenterally transmitted* disease, which developed following blood transfusion or in patients with a history of intravenous drug use and shared needles, and an *enterically transmitted* disease, which was seen mainly in outbreaks of hepatitis in India, Africa, Asia, and Mexico. The agents of both diseases have now been characterized: Parenterally transmitted NANB hepatitis is largely due to infection with hepatitis C virus (HCV) and the enterically transmitted disease is due to the hepatitis E virus (HEV).

HEPATITIS C VIRUS

The characterization of the HCV genome in 1989 through the use of sophisticated molecular biologic techniques plus the development of an assay for antibodies against the virus has resulted in an explosion of information. HCV is now recognized as the cause of most post-transfusion non-A, non-B hepatitis as well as sporadic non-A, non-B hepatitis not associated with an obvious route of transmission. Routine screening for HCV in donated blood has dramatically reduced the incidence of post-transfusion HCV infection.

The ability to detect HCV is still in its infancy in comparison to available testing for HBV. The original enzyme-linked immunosorbent assay (ELISA) tests for antibody against a nonstructural protein, whereas more recent ELISAs incorporate both structural and nonstructural proteins. The recombinant immunoblot assay (RIBA) is a supplementary test that is based on the same recombinant viral proteins as the ELISA. Direct detection of the virus in liver tissue or serum is possible by using the polymerase chain reaction (PCR), which can detect tiny amounts of viral RNA. There is as yet no "gold standard" test for HCV detection.

Antibody against HCV is usually not detectable during the acute phase of the illness but generally appears within 6 months of the initial infection, although delays in seroconversion up to 1 year have been reported. The antibody is not protective but simply indicates exposure to the virus. There is not always a good correlation between presence of antibody detected by ELISA or RIBA and the presence of virus detected by PCR; whether this relates to resolution of infection, intermittent viremia, or alteration in antibody production or detection is unclear.

The risk of acquiring HCV is greatest after exposure to infected blood or blood products; sexual exposure or needle stick injury is less effective in transmitting the virus (Table 4).

Perinatal or vertical transmission of HCV is uncommon, although some studies have shown the presence of virus by PCR in antibody-negative infants. Similarly, spread of HCV by inapparent parenteral transmission to household members is rare. Studies of heterosexual transmission of HCV have shown anti-HCV in from 0 to 7% of partners of HCV-positive subjects.

The mean incubation period for post-transfusion non-A, non-B hepatitis ranges from 6 to 12 weeks. The clinical course of acute HCV infection is usually mild, with jaundice in approximately 25%. Characteristically there is fluctuation of ALT values, which makes determination of resolution difficult. In contrast to HBV infection, which resolves in more than 90% of patients, HCV infection becomes chronic in 50% of patients, whether it is acquired parenterally or sporadically. Of these chronically infected patients, 50% have mild disease, whereas the rest develop chronic active hepatitis, and 10 to 25% of these progress to cirrhosis. The development of cirrhosis seems to occur over many years and is linked to age at exposure and the degree of liver damage on initial biopsy, so older patients with chronic active hepatitis are at greater risk. It does appear that HCV-related cirrhosis is clinically less severe than that from alcohol, although long-term data on mortality are scarce. A number of studies have linked chronic HCV infection with cirrhosis to the development of hepatocellular carcinoma. Acute HCV (acute non-A, non-B hepatitis) is treated symptomatically and supportively in the same manner as acute HAV or HBV infections. The use of interferon in acute HCV infection has been studied in only a small number of patients.

A large number of studies have evaluated interferon as therapy for chronic hepatitis C. In general, patients treated have had evidence of chronic active hepatitis on biopsy and elevated ALT levels with symptoms of fatigue. After 1 to 3 months treatment with 3 million units three times weekly of interferon, 40 to 60% of patients respond with a diminution or normalization of ALT values, resolution of symptoms, and im-

TABLE 4. **Risk Factors for Hepatitis C Virus (HCV) Infection**

Risk Factor	% Anti-HCV Positive
Post blood transfusion	90
Intravenous drug use	70–90
Hemophilia	50–90
Hemodialysis	10–20
Homosexual men	5
Health care workers	1

provement in liver histology. Once therapy is discontinued, half of these patients relapse, so a long-term response is seen in only 25% of patients. Recent studies suggest that such a long-term response is associated with virologic cure.

HEPATITIS E VIRUS

Enterically transmitted non-A, non-B hepatitis has been reported in epidemics from India, Asia, Africa, Mexico, and the former Soviet Union. The etiologic agent is an RNA virus that has been named HEV. Transmission of this virus is usually fecal-oral or by contaminated water with outbreaks that often involve thousands of cases. The illness has a mean incubation period of 6 weeks and is usually self-limited with no progression to chronic liver disease. Persons between ages 15 and 40 years are most vulnerable to infection. A striking feature of HEV infection is a high (20%) mortality rate in pregnant women. Recently a specific antibody test for HEV has been developed that confirms that most patients with enterically transmitted non-A, non-B hepatitis in the countries noted are infected with HEV.

MALABSORPTION SYNDROMES

method of
AMITABH CHAK, M.D., and
JOHN G. BANWELL, M.D.
Case Western Reserve University
Cleveland, Ohio

Intestinal malabsorption is somewhat of a misnomer in that it encompasses impaired luminal digestion, translocation, and absorption as well as the inadequate delivery of nutrients. Moreover, patients with malabsorption often do not have "classic" symptoms of chronic diarrhea with bulky, greasy, foul-smelling stools that may be improved by dietary fat restriction. Thus, the clinician should be aware of the symptoms and signs of a variety of nutrient deficiencies. Any evaluation for suspected malabsorption should proceed in a logical, stepwise manner. Subsequent therapy should combine treatment of the specific intestinal cause with repletion of nutrients.

PATHOGENESIS

It is helpful to break down the syndrome of malabsorption into three categories, based on the predominant mechanism: (1) defective luminal digestion, (2) decreased mucosal absorption, and (3) impaired delivery to the tissues. Digestion is primarily impaired by processes that alter the effective action of pancreatic enzymes or bile salts. Decreased output of pancreatic enzymes or inactivation of enzymes by high gastric acid output leads to maldigestion of fat, carbohydrate, and protein. Low concentrations of luminal bile salts may be a result of cirrhosis, biliary disease, impaired ileal uptake, precipitation of bile salts by excess gastric acid, or deconjugation of bile salts by bacteria. The result is impaired emulsification and fat maldigestion. Following intraluminal digestion, nutrient absorption requires further processing by brush border enzymes and adequate contact of the digested nutrients with an intact intestinal mucosa to achieve translocation. Defects of specific brush border hydrolases (e.g., lactase) produce malabsorption of specific nutrients (lactose). Inflammatory or infectious processes may cause diffuse mucosal damage, leading to a global malabsorption. Decreases in intestinal absorptive surface, whether by noninflammatory diseases (celiac sprue, tropical sprue) that cause flattening of intestinal villi or by extensive surgical resection, can result in malabsorption. Malabsorption is also present when nutrients have reduced contact with the absorptive surface, as a result of rapid intestinal transit (short bowel syndrome), intestinal bypass (fistulous or surgical), or infection (giardiasis). After absorption by enterocytes, fats are incorporated into chylomicrons, which are delivered into the lymphatic system. A defect in the production of chylomicrons (abetalipoproteinemia) or obstruction of the lymphatic system causes a postabsorptive "malabsorption" of fat. Obstruction or inflammation of the lymphatic system may also lead to intraluminal leakage of protein (protein-losing enteropathy).

CLINICAL FEATURES

Various symptoms and signs are clues to the presence of malabsorption. Diarrhea, attributable to the fluid-secretory stimulus of unabsorbed deconjugated bile salts and long-chain free fatty acids and to the osmotic effect of unabsorbed dietary carbohydrates, is often present. A selective bile salt malabsorption causes a watery diarrhea, whereas more global malabsorption is characterized by steatorrhea. Patients often have significant weight loss because of anorexia and fecal loss of calories. Malabsorption of protein may result in hypoalbuminemia with edema and ascites. Anemia is commonly related to deficiencies of iron, folate, or vitamin B_{12} but can also occur with chronic deficiencies of vitamin E or B_6. Malabsorption of fat-soluble vitamins produces a variety of clinical syndromes. Thus, bone pain (osteomalacia) or tetany (hypocalcemia) suggests vitamin D malabsorption; ecchymoses and purpura (hypocoagulability) suggest vitamin K deficiency; night blindness may indicate vitamin A deficiency; and neurologic symptoms, especially spinocerebellar ataxia, may be from a lack of vitamin E. Peripheral neuropathy may be a sign of vitamin B_{12} or thiamine deficiency. Amenorrhea and infertility, related to hormonal disturbances, are often seen. Skin manifestations of malabsorption include glossitis, cheilosis, and stomatitis with iron, folate, vitamin B_{12}, niacin, or riboflavin deficiency; a scaly dermatitis with zinc or essential fatty acid deficiency; and hyperkeratosis with vitamin A deficiency.

DIAGNOSTIC EVALUATION

Evaluation of a patient with suspected malabsorption depends on a detailed history. Characterization of stools in terms of the number of bowel movements, volume, appearance, presence of blood and fat, and response to food restriction may help distinguish noninflammatory versus inflammatory intestinal pathologic processes. Response to specific food items should be elicited because this may indicate a food intolerance (lactose, fructose, sorbitol). Bouts of severe abdominal pain may point to pancreatic disease, whereas severe ulcer-type symptoms suggest the presence of a gastrinoma. Details of endocrine disorders (diabetes, thyroid disease, and hypoadrenocortical disease) should be elicited. Connective tissue diseases (scleroderma, polyarteritis nodosa) may indicate a motility disorder. Chronic liver and biliary disease may suggest bile acid deficiency. The extent of any previous surgery of the stomach and small bowel must be defined. Location and dose of previous radiation therapy are important in assessing the risk of radiation enteritis. Recent or past travel history may indicate an infectious or parasitic cause. Given the increasing incidence of acquired immune deficiency syndrome (AIDS), all patients should have an assessment of risk factors (drug abuse, homosexuality, transfusions). Such information obtained from the careful history is an important guide to the sequence of diagnostic tests.

Specific interventions should be tried before instituting intensive investigations. Given the high prevalence of lactase deficiency, adolescents and most adults presenting with symptoms of abdominal bloating, cramping, flatulence, and chronic diarrhea should be placed on a reduced-lactose diet. Hydrogen breath tests with oral carbohydrate challenge should be reserved for patients who do not respond to a lactose-free diet and in whom the diagnosis of disaccharidase deficiency is still suspected.

Patients with suspected malabsorption should have a complete blood count; sedimentation rate; prothrombin time; and serum for levels of cholesterol, albumin, calcium, carotene, transaminases, bilirubin, and alkaline phosphatase drawn. Low levels of carotene, cholesterol, and albumin are observed more often with diffuse mucosal diseases than with luminal diseases. Anemic patients need to have serum analyzed for levels of iron, folate, and vitamin B_{12}. An elevated prothrombin time from vitamin K malabsorption should normalize after vitamin K repletion. A high alkaline phosphatase from bone may be evidence of vitamin D deficiency and should be worked up with parathyroid hormone and vitamin D levels.

If the history and these initial laboratory tests are indicative of a malabsorption syndrome, the first test should be a qualitative microscopic examination of a fecal specimen. The presence of fat droplets on a heated and acidified fecal smear containing Sudan stain identifies malabsorption of lipid and confirms steatorrhea. At the same time, it may be convenient to examine stool for leukocytes and acid-fast organisms. Routine cultures should be done, and three specimens should be examined for ova and parasites. If the qualitative stool examination for fat is repeatedly positive and other features strongly suggest malabsorption, quantitative stool collection is rendered unnecessary. Otherwise, a 72-hour stool collection on a diet of at least 50 grams of fat per day may be necessary but often is difficult to obtain accurately. Fecal fat excretion of less than 6 grams per day excludes the diagnosis of fat malabsorption; a markedly elevated stool fat (>25 grams per day) is encountered in pancreatic exocrine deficiency, severe mucosal disease, and short bowel syndromes.

After evidence for malabsorption is obtained, the next step is to distinguish between mucosal and luminal diseases by obtaining absorptive tests (D-xylose excretion or vitamin B_{12} [Schilling] tests). Normal D-xylose excretion rules out diffuse mucosal disease, and an abnormal Schilling test, in the absence of pernicious anemia, then favors ileal disease or small bowel bacterial overgrowth. If bacterial overgrowth is suspected, noninvasive breath tests (fasting and postglucose hydrogen excretion) may be useful in detecting bacterial fermentation in the small bowel but are not highly specific. Small bowel bacterial overgrowth can reliably be diagnosed by obtaining aerobic and anaerobic cultures via a small intestinal tube that has been fluoroscopically (or endoscopically) positioned. Pancreatic calcifications on a radiograph are highly suggestive of chronic pancreatitis. D-Xylose excretion is normal in patients who have malabsorption secondary to chronic pancreatic disease. The Schilling test may or may not be diminished. Pancreatic insufficiency may be validated by the bentiromide (Chymex) test. This test assays pancreatic enzyme output by measuring the amount of product (paraaminobenzoate) excreted into the urine after oral intake of a specific substrate (N-benzoyl-L-tyrosyl-p-aminobenzoic acid) for chymotrypsin. Endoscopic retrograde cholangiopancreatography (ERCP) may show changes of chronic pancreatitis with a 90% sensitivity but cannot quantify enzyme output. Mucosal disease of the small bowel is suspected when D-xylose excretion is abnormal. Alpha$_1$-antitrypsin content of the stool may be a useful measure of protein exudation associated with bowel wall inflammation or intestinal lymphangiectasia. Contrast studies of the small bowel (small bowel follow-through or enteroclysis) may demonstrate focal mucosal disease, strictures, fistulas, mass lesions, or small bowel diverticuli. Endoscopy is the preferred means for obtaining biopsy specimens of the small bowel, inasmuch as it affords an opportunity to visualize the duodenal mucosa, and to obtain fluid for parasitologic examinations. In certain select cases, one may still need to obtain a biopsy specimen of more distal small bowel by other means (colonoscopy with ileoscopy, peroral Crosby capsule, or laparotomy). Abdominal computed tomography (CT) scans may be useful in delineating a cause for lymphatic obstruction (retroperitoneal tumors or fibrosis).

CAUSES OF MALABSORPTION SYNDROMES

Defective Luminal Digestion

Bacterial Overgrowth

Small bowel bacterial overgrowth is defined by the presence of greater than 10^5 per mL aerobic and anaerobic bacterial organisms in luminal fluid of fasting bowel. Motility disorders (intestinal pseudo-obstruction, scleroderma) and structural abnormalities of the small bowel that favor stasis, such as blind loops (afferent loop of gastroenterostomy), fistulas, or jejunal diverticula, allow the proliferation of this flora. Immunodeficiency disorders of B and T cell function are also associated with small bowel bacterial overgrowth. Major clinical manifestations are diarrhea and steatorrhea, abdominal pain, anorexia, and bloating. Patients may be deficient in the fat-soluble vitamins D, A, and E; vitamin K levels are generally normal because vitamin K is produced by bacteria. Vitamin B_{12} deficiency from bacterial utilization is common. Treatment should be directed toward correcting underlying conditions. Thus, if feasible, one should operatively manage afferent loops, fistulas, strictures, or diverticula. Broad-spectrum antibiotics, such as trimethoprim-sulfamethoxazole (Bactrim DS) twice daily; tetracycline, 250 mg four times a day; or metronidazole (Flagyl), 250 mg three times a day, should be given in short courses of 2 to 4 weeks. Courses of antibiotics may be alternated. Metoclopramide (Reglan), 10 mg three times a day, may be useful for some motility disorders. Nightly subcutaneous injections of 50 µg of octreotide* (Sandostatin) may be tried in patients with scleroderma. Nutritional supplementation is

___
*This use of octreotide is not listed in the manufacturer's official directive.

of importance, and initial treatment may require parenteral hyperalimentation. Deficiencies of vitamins B_{12}, D, A, and E need to be corrected.

Pancreatic Exocrine Insufficiency

Although a lack of pancreatic enzymes causes malabsorption of all nutrients, the clinical problem is primarily due to steatorrhea, which occurs when lipase output is less than 10% of normal. The most common cause for pancreatic exocrine insufficiency is chronic pancreatitis, which can be secondary to alcohol, hypertriglyceridemia, trauma, or hereditary pancreatitis. There is generally a long history of recurrent bouts of abdominal pain before the onset of steatorrhea and diabetes. Other diseases that result in ineffective pancreatic enzyme output are pancreatic carcinoma or ampullary tumors, cystic fibrosis, and rarely somatostatinoma.

Treatment consists of oral supplementation with pancreatic enzymes. Clinical response may help confirm the diagnosis. The goal of therapy is to deliver 30,000 units of lipase per meal to the duodenum. This can be achieved by using any of a number of different enzyme preparations (Viokase, Ilozyme, Kuzyme HP, Cotazym-S, Pancreatin, Creon, or Pancrease). One difficulty is that pancreatic enzymes are inactivated in the stomach by acid and pepsin. Enteric-coated preparations are not useful because the size of the pill prevents it from being delivered effectively into the duodenum with the meal. Pancrease and Creon, preparations coated with a pH-dependent polymer, can be effective in patients with low gastric pH but are expensive. Therapy should be started with about two tablets of a high-potency enzyme preparation taken with each meal but may require up to eight tablets per meal to be effective. If this is ineffective one can reduce acid degradation by use of H_2 receptor antagonists or proton pump inhibitors.

Zollinger-Ellison Syndrome

More than half of the patients with gastrinomas have diarrhea, which may precede the onset of peptic symptoms of pain, bleeding, and perforation. Manifestations of the disease are secondary to gastric acid hypersecretion. Diarrhea is of a mixed secretory and osmotic type. The secretory component is related to the large volume of gastric secretion, whereas steatorrhea is secondary to the inactivation of pancreatic enzymes by acid, the precipitation of bile salts, and the acid-induced damage to the mucosa of the upper small bowel. A fasting gastrin level of greater than 1000 pg per mL in the presence of gastric acid (pH <3) is virtually diagnostic; with lower levels of hypergastrinemia, provocative testing with intravenous secretin (2 units per kg) should generate at least a 200 pg per mL rise in the gastrin level. Symptoms of the syndrome can usually be controlled by using high doses of acid suppressants, which can be titrated to achieve nearly complete acid suppression as judged by a 24-hour pH probe. On average, one needs about 250 mg of famotidine (Pepcid), 1.2 grams of ranitidine (Zantac), 3.6 grams of cimetidine (Tagamet), or 60 mg of omeprazole (Prilosec) per day. Omeprazole, a proton pump inhibitor, is the treatment of choice because it has had higher success rates. If medical therapy is unsatisfactory, total gastrectomy may be undertaken as a last resort. With improved techniques (venous sampling for gastrin, intraoperative ultrasonography) for localizing the gastrin-secreting tumor, curative resection may be possible in as many as 30% of the cases. Chemotherapy has only a limited role in reducing the tumor mass.

Disorders of Intestinal Mucosa

Celiac Sprue (Gluten Enteropathy)

Celiac sprue, also known as gluten enteropathy, is an immunologic disorder of the small bowel mucosa observed in children and adults. Exposure of the small intestine to antigenic components of certain cereal grains in susceptible persons causes subtotal or total villous atrophy with reactive crypt hyperplasia. This is usually most marked in the proximal small bowel but can involve the whole small bowel in prolonged disease. In childhood, the disease presents with diarrhea, impaired growth, and nutrient deficiencies. Clinical presentation of the disease in adults is highly variable. Patients may have gastrointestinal complaints of abdominal distention; excessive flatus; large, bulky, foul-smelling stools; and weight loss; others may have nonspecific complaints of weakness and fatigue. Patients may present with anemia from iron or folate deficiency. Other celiac sprue patients may be symptomatic from deficiency of a fat-soluble vitamin or vitamin B_{12}. Diagnosis is made by demonstrating the characteristic histology on small bowel biopsy specimen. Therapy consists of instituting a gluten-free diet, that is, avoiding any products containing wheat, rye, barley, or oats. Cereals such as corn, rice, buckwheat, sorghum, and millet are not pathogenic and may be substituted. Clinical improvement is generally seen after several days on a gluten-free diet, whereas restoration of normal histologic architecture takes weeks to months. The diagnosis can be confirmed by demonstrating villous blunting on rechallenge with gluten. This is especially necessary for children, in whom an erroneous diagnosis could impose a gluten-free diet for life. When sprue does not respond to a gluten-free diet, it is important to ensure that the patient has been compliant with the diet before ruling out other diseases. Recurrence of symptoms in long-standing quiescent sprue may signal the development of a complication of the disease (T cell lymphoma, intestinal ulceration, or collagenous sprue).

Idiopathic Chronic Ulcerative Jejunoileitis

Chronic ulcerative jejunoileitis is a disease that is clinically and histologically similar to celiac sprue except that it does not improve with gluten withdrawal and is unresponsive and severe in its course. It may develop spontaneously, and in patients with long-standing sprue, it may progress to lymphoma. Despite a frequent lack of clinical response to a gluten-free diet, patients should be initially treated in this manner. Multiple small bowel biopsy specimens of the jejunum should be examined for evidence of lymphoma. If lymphoma is not present, 10 to 40 mg prednisone per day may ameliorate symptoms.

Tropical Sprue

Visitors to and residents of certain areas of the tropics (Indonesia, Southeast Asia, Puerto Rico) develop a small bowel malabsorptive disorder with diffuse villous damage, lengthened crypts, subepithelial fat, and an inflammatory infiltrate in the lamina propria, histologically similar to celiac sprue. This disease may be associated with secondary contamination of the small intestine by coliform bacteria. Disease onset may be acute, with watery diarrhea, or chronic. Eventually symptoms of anorexia, weakness, and weight loss develop. The D-xylose test is usually abnormal, and steatorrhea is present. Vitamin B_{12} malabsorption, which is secondary to bacterial uptake and terminal ileal disease, is present in all cases. Impaired hydrolysis of the polyglutamate derivatives of folate leads to folate deficiency. Treatment with 5 mg of folate daily or 1000 μg of subcutaneous or intramuscular vitamin B_{12} every week produces prompt remission of the anemia and anorexia. Some patients with early disease may be cured by this therapy alone. More advanced and chronic disease requires additional treatment with antibiotics, such as tetracycline, 250 mg four times a day, or trimethoprim-sulfamethoxazole twice a day. Chronic disease may need treatment for up to 6 months. Repeat courses of therapy may be beneficial in relapses.

Giardiasis

Giardia lamblia, a common protozoan parasite found throughout the world, is transmitted either through contaminated water or via a fecal-oral route. Trophozoites released from ingested cysts under the influence of gastric acid colonize and multiply in the proximal small intestine. These trophozoites adhere to the brush border, leading to prolonged malabsorptive diarrhea by an unclear mechanism. It is important to examine repeated stools and duodenal aspirates to detect the presence of the organism. The most effective treatment for giardiasis is quinacrine (Atabrine), 100 mg four times a day, or metronidazole, 250 mg three times a day for a 7- to 10-day course.

Infiltrative and Inflammatory Diseases of the Small Bowel

Infections of Small Bowel

Whipple's disease is a rare systemic, multiorgan bacterial disease of middle-aged men with predominant involvement of the gut and its lymphatic drainage. Whipple's disease should be suspected in patients with symptoms of weight loss, diarrhea, and steatorrhea, along with symptoms of arthralgia, lymphadenopathy, chest pains, or central nervous system disturbances. A diagnostic small bowel biopsy demonstrates clubbed villi with the lamina propria infiltrated with macrophages and bacteria that stain with periodic acid–Schiff (PAS) both within and outside the phagocytic cells. Treatment should be initiated with 1.2 million units of intramuscular procaine penicillin G plus 1 gram of intramuscular streptomycin daily for 2 weeks, followed by trimethoprim-sulfamethoxazole twice a day for 1 year. If the patient is allergic to sulfonamides, oral penicillin VK, 250 mg four times a day for 1 year, can be used. Chloramphenicol, 250 mg four times a day for 1 year, should be given when there is no therapeutic response. Patients may also require supplementation with folate, vitamin B_{12}, fat-soluble vitamins, and iron. A prolonged course with an antibiotic that penetrates the blood-brain barrier is essential to prevent subsequent central nervous system relapses.

A similar infiltrative disorder of the small intestine with PAS-positive bacteria and macrophages occurs with *Mycobacterium avium-intracellulare* infection associated with AIDS. The disease can be differentiated from Whipple's disease by the acid-fast staining of the mycobacterial organisms. Therapy with a combination of three antituberculous drugs (clofazimine [Lamprene], 150 mg daily; ethambutol [Myambutol], 25 mg per kg daily; rifampin [Rifadin], 300 mg daily; ciprofloxacin [Cipro], 250 mg twice a day; or amikacin [Amikin], 7.5 mg per kg every 12 hours) may be tried.

Immunodeficiency and immunocompromised states favor colonization of the small bowel with various protozoa (see heading "Malabsorptive Syndromes and AIDS") that cause malabsorptive diarrhea. Effective antimicrobial therapy for cryptosporidia and microsporidia is unavailable. *Isospora belli,* detectable in stool, is responsive to trimethoprim-sulfamethoxazole twice a day for 2 weeks.

Parasitic infestation of the small bowel with *Strongyloides stercoralis* may cause malabsorption and weight loss in residents of the southern United States, Latin America, Africa, and Asia, who acquire it from contaminated soil. Eosinophilia is common, and the larva may be identified in stools and duodenal aspirates. Thiabendazole (Mintezol), 25 mg per kg twice a day for 2 days, is generally effective therapy. Patients who are immunocompromised may have disseminated disease, requiring repetitive 5-day courses.

Other conditions, such as primary or secondary amyloidosis and macroglobulinemia, may be associated with infiltration of the small intestine. Diffuse involvement of arterioles or all layers of the small bowel wall may result in malabsorption in these conditions.

Immunoproliferative Small Intestinal Disease

Immunoproliferative small intestinal disease (alpha-chain disease, Mediterranean lymphoma) is a diffuse infiltrative disease seen in residents of and immigrants from impoverished Mediterranean countries that is characterized by an intense lymphoplasmacytic infiltrate. Chronic disease may progress to development of a diffuse B cell lymphoma. If it is recognized in the early prelymphomatous phase, treatment with tetracycline can revert histology to normal. In developed countries, primary small bowel lymphomas are uncommon but are observed in association with celiac sprue and AIDS.

Crohn's Disease

Nearly all patients with active small bowel Crohn's disease have diarrhea secondary to the inflammation. Malabsorption can occur from a variety of causes. Crohn's patients with surgical resection or severe disease of the terminal ileum may have either a bile salt diarrhea or frank steatorrhea secondary to decreased levels of bile salt. Strictures of small bowel and enteroenteric fistulas may accompany small bowel bacterial overgrowth. A diagnostic work-up should include a small bowel series and colonoscopy with ileoscopy to evaluate for structural abnormalities and extent of disease. Treatment of active jejunoileitis is generally 40 to 60 mg of prednisone per day for several weeks. Azathioprine or 6-mercaptopurine at a dose of 1.5 to 2 mg per kg per day may be useful as adjuvant therapy but exerts an effect only after 3 to 4 months. Metronidazole, 250 mg three times a day, has definite benefits but is more useful for perianal disease. Antimotility agents (diphenoxylate/atropine [Lomotil], three times a day, or loperamide [Imodium], 2 to 4 mg four times a day) should be used with caution, especially when colonic disease is present. High-protein, high-calorie supplements are generally useful. Patients with steatorrhea from ileal disease often need to restrict fat and oxalate in their diet and often need monthly parenteral vitamin B_{12}. Patients with fistulas or strictures may require surgery. Parenteral hyperalimentation before surgery in patients with chronic malnourishment diminishes perioperative morbidity.

Eosinophilic Gastroenteritis

Hypersensitivity to allergens in food has been proposed to be the cause of eosinophilic gastroenteritis, but evidence is limited. Steatorrhea and protein-losing enteropathy, secondary to mucosal inflammation, can occur in 10 to 30% of patients. The peripheral blood smear generally has a low eosinophil count. Stool examination may show Charcot-Leyden crystals. A barium study of the small bowel may show a diffuse, nodular mucosal pattern or intraluminal masses. Because of the patchy nature of the disease, diagnosis is made by obtaining multiple small bowel biopsy specimens at different levels. The mucosa demonstrates eosinophilic infiltration. Treatment is generally successful with 20 to 40 mg of prednisone a day. Courses may be repeated. Antihistamines have also been used with limited success.

Radiation Enteritis

Radiation injury to the small bowel may be acute or late. Acutely malabsorption is often observed when radiation treatment of uterine or ovarian tumors involves pelvic exposure of the ileum. Symptoms usually resolve within a few weeks after the radiation treatments end. Late manifestations of radiation injury usually occur 6 months to 1 year following radiation but can manifest many years later. A minimal injurious dose is 4500 rad, with doses greater than 6000 rad causing serious injury. This late form is primarily an ischemic disease of large vessels leading to formation of strictures, fistulas, and abscesses. Patients can develop malabsorption from bacterial overgrowth secondary to abnormal small bowel motility or fistulas. Diagnosis is usually made by barium studies. Repetitive courses of antibiotics (see earlier section entitled "Bacterial Overgrowth") are useful for malabsorption. Sulfasalazine and steroids have little efficacy, al-

though nonsteroidals may be effective. Surgery may be needed to treat strictures and fistulas. Patients who have extensive small bowel damage may require home parenteral hyperalimentation.

Rare Disorders Associated with Impaired Delivery of Nutrients

Abetalipoproteinemia

Abetalipoproteinemia is a rare, heterogeneous, congenital, autosomal recessive childhood disorder of apoprotein B synthesis or processing in enterocytes. It is characterized by low cholesterol, low triglycerides, and low apoprotein B in the plasma. The intestinal mucosa fails to synthesize and secrete chylomicrons, resulting in engorgement of cells with lipid droplets. Along with fat malabsorption, there is malabsorption of fat-soluble vitamins. Treatment involves restriction of fat and supplementation of fat-soluble vitamins. Medium-chain triglycerides, which can be absorbed into plasma without incorporation into lipoproteins, may be used to meet caloric requirements.

Intestinal Lymphangiectasia

Intestinal lymphangiectasia can be congenital or can be secondary to retroperitoneal carcinoma, lymphoma, retroperitoneal fibrosis, Whipple's disease, tuberculosis, sarcoidosis, constrictive pericarditis, and congestive heart failure. Obstruction to lymphatic drainage, associated with this condition, results in steatorrhea and protein-losing enteropathy. Patients may develop chylous ascites. On endoscopy, one may see white duodenal spots. Multiple jejunal biopsy specimens are necessary to demonstrate the characteristic, dilated lacteals. Barium studies and an abdominal CT scan are necessary to evaluate for secondary causes. In the congenital form, malformed lymphatics may be demonstrable by lymphangiography. Treatment should be directed at the specific cause when possible. Restriction of fat in the diet and supplementation with short-chain and medium-chain triglycerides may cause a relief of lymphatic pressure. This may lead to a decreased protein loss and an increase in serum albumin.

Disorders of Mixed Etiology

Short Bowel Syndrome

Resection of portions of small bowel can have variable effects, depending on the region and length of small bowel removed. Patients with more than three-quarters of their small bowel removed always have major problems with malabsorption. The ileum is able to adapt and carry out functions of jejunum if the jejunum is resected. The jejunum, however, is not able to absorb vitamin B_{12} or conjugated bile salts. Thus, removal of 60 to 100 cm of terminal ileum causes bile acid–induced colonic fluid loss, whereas removal of greater than 100 cm of ileum leads to severe bile salt malabsorption, diarrhea, and steatorrhea. Removal of the ileocecal valve favors bacterial overgrowth of the small bowel. Resections of small bowel can also be accompanied by gastric hypersecretion.

Treatment depends on the cause of malabsorption. Antimotility agents (see the article "Crohn's Disease") may be effective in increasing transit time. Cholestyramine (Questran) is effective in cases of bile acid malabsorption associated with limited ileal resections. Acid suppression with H_2 blockers or omeprazole is often needed in the immediate postsurgical phase and in those patients in whom gastric hypersecretion persists. Courses of antibiotics (see "Bacterial Overgrowth") may be needed in patients with bypass loops or resected ileocecal valves. Following large resections, severe diarrhea on oral nutrition may need to be treated with total parenteral nutrition. Generally the oral route can be used for partial nutritional support. Elemental or polymeric diet can be started, and the diet can be advanced as the small bowel adapts. A low-oxalate diet in patients with ileal resection may help avoid the formation of kidney stones. Patients with chronic malabsorption should usually be on a high-carbohydrate diet with approximately 30 grams of fat per day. They should also receive fat-soluble vitamins, 1500 mg of calcium per day, monthly vitamin B_{12} injections (for ileal resections), and oral or intramuscular iron. Some patients are maintained on home total parenteral nutrition. Surgical procedures, designed to increase transit time, are not satisfactory and should be considered only when a long trial of medical therapy fails. Small bowel transplantation is as yet unsuccessful.

Malabsorptive Syndromes and AIDS

Chronic diarrhea and weight loss are extremely common in patients infected with the human immunodeficiency virus (HIV). Diarrhea can be divided into two types. A small bowel malabsorptive-type diarrhea is characterized by three to eight large-volume, nonbloody, nonpainful bowel movements, whereas a colitic-type diarrhea is characterized by several small-volume, slightly bloody bowel movements associated with fever and abdominal tenderness. Most patients with small bowel–type diarrhea have D-xylose malabsorption. They often have abnormal villous architecture. Along with stool cultures and parasite examination, it is important to obtain small bowel biopsy specimens for histology, cytology, viral culture, and occasionally electron microscopy to identify small bowel infectious processes (giardiasis, mycobacterium, cytomegalovirus, cryptosporidia, isospora, and microsporidia). A malabsorptive state without an identifiable pathogen may be found in up to 30% of AIDS patients and has been termed AIDS enteropathy. Symptomatic treatment is often unsatisfactory. Octreotide at doses of 50 to 500 µg subcutaneously every 8 hours has been found to be effective in approximately 30 to 60% of patients who have not responded to antimotility agents. Weight loss in patients with AIDS can be severe and is often difficult to treat. Although malabsorption may play a role, other causes, including anorexia and hypercatabolism due to fevers and systemic infections, are probably more important. Most patients should receive high-protein supplementation, with restriction of fat in those with steatorrhea. Weight gain, however, is difficult to achieve. AIDS enteropathy may improve when patients are started on azidothymidine (Zidovudine).

ACUTE PANCREATITIS

method of
DAVID B. ADAMS, M.D.
Medical University of South Carolina
Charleston, South Carolina

Acute pancreatitis has a broad clinical spectrum with multiple causes and varying presentations. The pathogenesis of acute pancreatitis, related to acinar cell injury, is poorly understood. Management strategies are based on early diagnosis and supportive care of associated organ dysfunction.

PATHOGENESIS

Pancreatic acinar cells, which secrete digestive enzymes, compose 95% of the exocrine pancreas. The ductal and centroacinar cells secrete water and electrolytes and compose the other 5%. The pathogenesis of acute pancreatitis is related to intracellular and interstitial enzyme activation. Ischemia related to regional hypoperfusion and a microcirculatory insufficiency are important factors related to the development of pancreatitis. Models of experimental pancreatitis that are pertinent to the clinical setting are produced by maximum stimulation of the pancreas by a cholecystokinin (CCK) analogue, cerulein, and blockage of zymogen granule secretion, which leads to zymogen granule fusion with intracellular lysosomes and activation of the zymogen proenzyme, trypsinogen. Ninety-five percent of the cases of acute pancreatitis are related to alcohol abuse and cholelithiasis. Other causes include hyperlipidemia, trauma, shock, vasculitis, tumor, duodenal obstruction, drugs, and viral infections. Frequently the cause of acute pancreatitis cannot be determined.

The pathogenesis of alcohol-related pancreatitis is due to stimulation of exocrine pancreatic secretions and partial ampullary obstruction. Increased pancreatic ductal permeability and precipitation of pancreatic proteins are observed experimentally. Acinar and capillary endothelial injury may also be related to elevated free fatty acids associated with alcohol intake. Gallstone pancreatitis is associated with impaction of small gallstones in the terminal duct when the distal bile duct and pancreatic duct share a common channel, leading to elevated pancreatic ductal pressure. Drugs implicated in the cause of acute pancreatitis include azathioprine, hydrochlorothiazide, furosemide, tetracycline, estrogen, clonidine, steroids, and sulfonamides.

DIAGNOSIS

Diagnosis of acute pancreatitis is based on history, physical examination, laboratory tests, and radiographic findings. The majority of patients with acute pancreatitis seek medical help because of the development of acute epigastric pain radiating into the back and associated with nausea and vomiting. Frequently the patient may sit upright and lean forward to seek relief of pain. Serum amylase and serum lipase are the most valuable laboratory tests in diagnosing acute pancreatitis. There are a variety of causes of elevated serum amylase, and the serum lipase has been noted to have greater sensitivity and specificity in the diagnosis of acute pancreatitis. Serum amylase assays, however, are readily available in most laboratories and are used more frequently than assays for lipase. Measurement of amylase isoenzymes, urinary amylase, and peritoneal fluid amylase occasionally may be helpful when the diagnosis is obscure. Other disorders associated with an elevated total serum amylase include nonpancreatic biliary tract disease, intestinal obstruction, mesenteric infarction, perforated peptic ulcer, ruptured ectopic pregnancy, acute appendicitis, ruptured aortic aneurysm, and salpingitis. Impaired amylase excretion may be present in renal failure. Patients with salivary gland disorders (mumps and parotitis) may have elevations of serum amylase that can be differentiated from pancreatic amylase based on isoenzyme studies. Miscellaneous causes of elevated serum amylase include ketoacidosis, pregnancy, pneumonia, cerebral trauma, or burns. Plain abdominal radiographs and upper gastrointestinal contrast series have been supplanted by ultrasonography and computed tomography (CT) in the diagnosis of acute pancreatitis.

CLINICAL COURSE AND PROGNOSIS

The early phase of acute pancreatitis lasts from 1 to 3 days and is associated with vasomotor instability and hypoperfusion. In the middle phase of severe pancreatitis, which lasts from days to a week, pancreatic edema and inflammation may progress to necrosis. Associated early organ dysfunction may occur. In the late phase of severe pancreatitis, which occurs after the first week, infection, sepsis, and multisystem organ failure may develop. The cause of death in early pancreatitis is related to shock and in rare cases to adult respiratory distress syndrome (ARDS). Modern fluid resuscitation techniques have eliminated the early deaths related to shock; however, ARDS continues to be problematic and is an ominous development.

Because acute pancreatitis is an inhomogeneous disease with a wide clinical spectrum, numerous measurements of severity have been examined to improve management strategies. Most commonly used are Ranson's early prognostic signs of acute pancreatitis (Table 1). The relationship between Ranson's prognostic signs and morbidity and mortality noted in Table 2 has improved in recent reported experiences. Because Ranson's scoring system requires 48 hours of observation and may underestimate the influence of chronic medical comorbidity, the Apache II severity of disease classification has been used successfully in grading prognosis of acute pancreatitis. CT has also been useful in classifying acute pancreatitis. Five CT categories of pancreatitis that have prognostic significance in predicting abscess development have been defined by Ranson (Table 3). The risk of abscess development in CT Grades A and B was zero. With CT Grade C or D and fewer than three of Ranson's positive prognostic signs, it was 4.5%; in CT Grade E or CT Grade C or D and three or more prognostic signs, the risk of abscess was 56.7%. The mortal-

TABLE 1. **Ranson's Eleven Early Objective Signs Used to Classify the Severity of Pancreatitis**

At Admission or Diagnosis
Age older than 55 years
White blood cell count more than 16,000/mm³
Blood glucose more than 200 mg/dL
Serum lactic dehydrogenase more than 350 IU/L
Serum glutamic oxaloacetic transaminase more than 250 IU/L

During Initial 48 Hours
Hematocrit fall greater than 10 percentage points
Blood urea nitrogen rise more than 5 mg/dL
Serum calcium level less than 8 mg/dL
Arterial PO_2 less than 60 mmHg
Base deficit greater than 4 mEq/L
Estimated fluid sequestration more than 6000 mL

TABLE 2. **Relationship Between Ranson's Prognostic Signs and Mortality and Morbidity**

Demographic	0–2	3–4	5–6	7–8
Number of patients	347	67	30	6
Mortality, no. (%)	0	11 (16)	12 (40)	6 (100)
No. (%) dead or severely ill >7 days in intensive care unit	13 (3.7)	27 (40)	28 (93)	6 (100)

ity of patients who develop abscess with acute pancreatitis is approximately 20 to 60%. It is important to remember that prognostic indices are only a statistical method for identifying high-risk patient groups and that individual patients need not conform.

MANAGEMENT

Medical therapy used in the management of acute pancreatitis has included intravenous fluid administration, giving the patient nothing by mouth, nasogastric suction, H_2 blockers, somatostatin, antibiotics, and peritoneal lavage. Accurate replacement of fluid losses is the keystone of therapy. In a prospective study, nasogastric suction has been observed to have no influence on the clinical outcome and is useful chiefly to prevent vomiting when patients have moderate to severe pancreatitis with an associated ileus. H_2 blockers are beneficial in preventing gastric mucosal ulceration but do not appear to alter the course of pancreatitis. Octreotide acetate* (Sandostatin), an 8–amino acid, long-acting synthetic analogue of the native hormone somatostatin, is a potent inhibitor of pancreatic exocrine secretion, and it has been postulated to be of value in the treatment of acute pancreatitis. In randomized prospective studies, however, there has been no demonstrated reduction of mortality with use of the native or synthetic hormone.

The use of prophylactic antibiotics in acute pancreatitis is controversial, and although no clear benefit has been shown, many think that

*This use of octreotide acetate is not listed in the manufacturer's official directive.

TABLE 3. **Features Used to Classify Findings on Early Computed Tomography**

CT Grade	Features
A	Pancreas and peripancreatic tissues radiographically normal
B	Pancreatic enlargement alone without inflammatory changes in peripancreatic tissues
C	Inflammatory changes confined to the pancreas and peripancreatic fat
D	One peripancreatic fluid collection
E	Two or more peripancreatic fluid collections

antibiotics may diminish septic complications in patients with severe pancreatitis. Broad-spectrum antibiotic coverage to include gram-negative and anaerobic organisms has been employed based on observations of organisms cultured in pancreatic abscesses and evidence that indicates that intestinal bacterial translocation may be related to the development of pancreatic abscesses in acute pancreatitis.

The use of short peritoneal lavage over 48 to 96 hours has been observed to diminish early systemic complications of acute pancreatitis but does not decrease late pancreatic septic complications and overall mortality. Long peritoneal lavage, however, which is instituted within 48 hours of hospitalization and carried out over a 7-day period, has been observed to diminish septic complications and mortality in severe acute pancreatitis. After placing a peritoneal dialysis catheter under local anesthesia within 48 hours of hospitalization, an isotonic-balanced electrolyte solution containing 15 grams per liter dextrose, adding 8 mEq potassium, 1000 units USP heparin, and 250 mg ampicillin to each 2 liters of dialysate, is infused under gravity for 15 minutes, left for 30 minutes, and then drained by gravity. The cycle is repeated hourly for 7 days. Guidelines for medical management of acute pancreatitis are presented in Table 4.

Surgical complications of acute pancreatitis include pancreatic necrosis, pancreatic abscess, and pancreatic pseudocyst. Serum markers of pancreatic necrosis include C-reactive protein, polymorphonuclear leukocyte elastase, phospholipase A, and phospholipase B. Nonenhancement of the pancreas on a contrast-enhanced CT scan has been called the "gold standard" of pancreatic necrosis. It is known, however, that hypoperfusion may occur during pancreatitis, and therefore nonenhancement does not mean definite necrosis. Pancreatography performed following recovery from massive pancreatic necrosis has shown normal ductal anatomy of the entire pancreas in many instances. Management of pancreatic necrosis and infection is controversial. Debates about surgical management of necrosis and infection relate to the timing and extent of operations.

Early diagnosis and surgical drainage of infected pancreatic and peripancreatic fluid collections have been the cornerstone of therapy for pancreatic abscesses for many years. Recently it

TABLE 4. **Medical Management of Acute Pancreatitis**

Mild Disease
Hospital observation
NPO
Intravenous fluids (D5LR)
Monitor input and output
Narcotic analgesic (meperidine hydrochloride [Demerol], 50–
  100 mg intramuscularly every 3 h as needed or
  intravenously with patient-controlled analgesic pump)

Moderate Disease
Same as above
Nasogastric suction
Foley catheter
H_2 blockers with antacid supplement to keep gastric aspirate
  pH >5
Contrast-enhanced CT scan if clinical deterioration or no
  improvement within 72 h

Severe Disease
Same as above
Intensive care unit monitoring
Arterial line
Intravenous antibiotics (imipenem + cilastatin [Primaxin]
  500 mg intravenously every 6 h)
Total parenteral nutrition
Nystatin swish and swallow 30 ml PO every 8 h
Consider long peritoneal lavage
Careful monitoring Ca^{2+}, PO_2, glucose
CT scan every 5–7 days if no improvement to assess for
  nonenhancement of pancreas, fluid collections

Abbreviations: NPO = nulla per os (nothing by mouth); D5LR =
lactated Ringer's solution with 5% dextrose; CT = computed tomography.

has been shown, however, that patients with Apache II scores less than 10 and fewer than three of Ranson's signs can be successfully treated with percutaneous catheter drainage. Patients who have complex, multiloculated abscesses; inaccessible abscess cavities; and abscesses associated with bleeding complications are not suitable candidates for percutaneous catheter drainage. In the past, mortality rates for pancreatic abscesses have ranged from 20 to 60%, and more recently mortality rates as low as 10% have been reported.

Pancreatic pseudocysts, collections of pancreatic exocrine secretions in or adjacent to the pancreas contained within a fibrous wall, are a complication of acute pancreatitis and may require surgical management. Asymptomatic pancreatic pseudocysts less than 5 cm in diameter that develop subsequent to a bout of acute pancreatitis may be followed expectantly. Symptomatic or large cysts may erode into adjacent structures, leading to life-threatening complications, and may require operative internal drainage or external drainage procedures. CT-directed percutaneous catheter drainage also has been found to have a valuable role as an adjunct or alternative in the management of pancreatic pseudocysts.

The management of pancreatic necrosis is controversial. Although most surgeons agree that infected pancreatic necrosis requires wide operative débridement and drainage, many think that non-infected pancreatic necrosis can be managed expectantly.

Indications for operative management of acute pancreatitis include uncertain diagnosis (rare with evaluation with CT scan) and clinical deterioration despite optimal support of septic complications. Although the therapy of acute pancreatitis in many instances is supportive, mortality over the past decade has decreased from 25 to 5%. Management in the intensive care unit and early recognition and treatment of associated surgical complications are responsible in large measure for the improved mortality rate.

CHRONIC PANCREATITIS

method of
WILLIAM O. RICHARDS, M.D., and
JOHN L. SAWYERS, M.D.
*Vanderbilt University School of Medicine
Nashville, Tennessee*

Chronic pancreatitis is a persistent inflammatory lesion of the pancreas that does not resolve once the etiologic factor has been removed, thus differentiating it from acute pancreatitis, which regresses when the etiologic factor is removed. Clinically it can be difficult, however, to differentiate chronic and recurrent acute pancreatitis. If periods of inflammation persist and cause a progressive destruction of the gland with loss of endocrine and exocrine function, it is recognized as a form of chronic pancreatitis. The Marseilles-Rome classification defines chronic pancreatitis as the presence of chronic inflammatory lesions characterized by the destruction of exocrine parenchyma and fibroses and in the later stages by destruction of endocrine parenchyma. The incidence of chronic pancreatitis in autopsy reports ranges from less than 1 to 5%.

ETIOLOGY

Alcoholic Pancreatitis

Alcohol is the major etiologic factor involved in creation of chronic pancreatitis in Western societies (Table 1). Autopsy series indicate that the risk is 45 to 50 times less in nondrinking individuals, and there is a linear relationship between the risk of developing

TABLE 1. **Causes of Chronic Pancreatitis**

Alcohol	Ductal obstruction
Tropical or nutritional	Pancreas divisum
Hereditary	Idiopathic
Hyperparathyroidism	

chronic pancreatitis and daily consumption of alcohol. Ingestion of a high-fat, high-protein diet appears to increase the risk of developing alcohol-induced pancreatitis.

The pathophysiology of alcohol-induced chronic pancreatitis is not clear largely because there are no animal models to duplicate the human situation. What is known is that alcohol does increase pancreatic secretion of proteases, enzymes, amylase, and lipase. One theory suggests that there is an abnormality in the production, intracellular transport, and discharge of digestive enzymes, which causes autodigestion and results in protein precipitation, particularly in the secondary ducts of the peripheral pancreas. Precipitation of calcium carbonate forms calculi within the ductal system and leads to increased pressure within the pancreatic ducts. This theory explains the findings frequently seen in early chronic pancreatitis, in which there is involvement of the secondary pancreatic ductal system rather than involvement of the main pancreatic duct. As stones form in the main pancreatic duct, there is progressive dilation of the duct, which is associated with increased pressure.

Tropical or Nutritional Pancreatitis

This is a form of chronic pancreatitis described in adults and in some African and Asian countries. Patients present with malnutrition, diabetes, and disseminated pancreatic calcifications. The exact cause of this disease is unclear but may be associated with childhood malnutrition and consumption of nutritional toxins.

Hereditary Pancreatitis

Chronic hereditary pancreatitis appears in childhood usually between the ages of 10 and 12 years and is inherited through an autosomal dominant gene. It is equally represented in men and women and is an uncommon cause of chronic pancreatitis. There is increased risk of ductal adenocarcinoma developing in this population. This type of pancreatitis should be suspected when two or more family members develop recurrent pancreatitis in absence of other causes.

Hyperparathyroidism

Chronic pancreatitis can be caused by untreated hyperparathyroidism that is caused by the potent stimulation of pancreatic enzyme secretion with precipitation of calcium within the ducts of the pancreas. The incidence of this disease process, however, is decreasing rapidly and is likely to constitute no more than 1 to 2% of patients with chronic pancreatitis. This is probably because the routine measurement of calcium during medical evaluation has reduced the incidence of chronic untreated hyperparathyroidism.

Pancreatic Ductal Obstruction

Obstruction of the pancreatic duct by scars from previous trauma or tumors leads to chronic pancreatitis characterized by atrophy of the acinar cells with fibro-

sis and dilation of the ductal system. These patients frequently develop pseudocysts and respond well to surgical relief of obstruction. Endocrine and exocrine insufficiency develops 8 to 10 years after the onset of pancreatitis if the obstruction is not alleviated.

Pancreas Divisum

This anatomic anomaly is caused by failure of the dorsal and ventral pancreatic ducts to fuse. Drainage of the main pancreatic duct is through the minor papilla. Clinical significance of pancreas divisum has been a hotly debated topic; however, patients with idiopathic pancreatitis undergoing endoscopic retrograde cholangiopancreatography (ERCP) have a much higher incidence of pancreatic divisum than patients with biliary disease also undergoing ERCP. This suggests that pancreas divisum may be an etiologic factor in some patients with chronic pancreatitis. At least some physicians have suggested that stenosis of the accessory papilla is a necessary cofactor in the development of obstructive pancreatitis. Many centers are developing expertise in endoscopic diagnosis and management of this anomaly through placement of a stent into the minor papilla to allow unobstructed drainage of the main pancreatic duct. If this procedure helps, endoscopic or operative sphincterotomy alleviates recurrent pancreatitis in many patients.

Idiopathic Pancreatitis

Although alcoholic pancreatitis is the most common form afflicting patients in Western culture, the second major cause of chronic pancreatitis is idiopathic. There appear to be two distinct types: a juvenile type with onset around 18 years of age and a type that affects an older age group with a peak at 60 years of age. Presentation of the juvenile type is typically with pain, whereas the elder age group presents with exocrine insufficiency, diabetes, and diffuse pancreatic calcification. Before labeling the patient with idiopathic etiology, however, a thorough evaluation should exclude all other possibilities, including gallstones and hyperlipidemia.

CLINICAL MANIFESTATIONS

Pain

The vast majority of patients with chronic pancreatitis in Western cultures have abdominal pain as a distinct clinical problem (Table 2). As many as 15% of

TABLE 2. **Clinical Presentation**

Pain
Malnutrition
Endocrine/exocrine insufficiency
Complications
Pseudocysts
Splenic vein thrombosis
Common bile duct stricture
Fistula causing ascites and/or pleural effusion
Infection (abscess)

patients, however, do not have any pain associated with chronic pancreatitis. The patients with alcohol-induced chronic pancreatitis are more likely to have pain than patients with idiopathic chronic pancreatitis. Pain is often brought on shortly after ingestion of a meal. Typically patients describe a dull constant pain that radiates to their back.

Malnutrition

Patients with chronic pancreatitis and pain frequently reduce their calorie intake for fear of increasing their pain. This has been the generally recognized reason for weight loss, although endocrine and exocrine insufficiency also contributes to weight loss.

Endocrine/Exocrine Insufficiency

Enzyme secretion must be reduced to less than 10% of normal before malabsorption occurs in patients with chronic pancreatitis and is an end-stage phenomenon in patients with chronic pancreatitis. Malabsorption from exocrine insufficiency is better tolerated than malabsorption secondary to mucosal disease such as sprue. There is generally less fecal water, and thus the patient's stool is more bulky and formed than in other diarrheal states. Absorption of fat-soluble vitamins (K,A,D,E) is fairly well preserved, so vitamin deficiency is rarely observed because of fat malabsorption.

Endocrine insufficiency to some degree is identifiable in the majority of patients with chronic pancreatitis, although need for insulin is relatively rare.

COMPLICATIONS

The initial presenting symptom may be a complication of pancreatitis.

Pseudocysts

Pancreatic pseudocyst is a collection of pancreatic secretions outside of the ductal system enclosed by a fibrous capsule. This complicates 25% of patients with chronic alcoholic pancreatitis and is more commonly found in the body of the pancreas than in the head or the tail. Pain is a frequent symptom of pancreatic pseudocyst, with diagnosis usually determined by computed tomography (CT) or ultrasonography. Complications can ensue from large pseudocysts: Hemorrhage from erosion into a major vessel occurs in 5% of patients with chronic pseudocysts and accounts for nearly 50% of all deaths related to chronic pancreatitis. Acute rupture of the pseudocyst can result in peritonitis, hypotension, and shock secondary to sequestration of fluid into the peritoneal cavity. If the leak occurs more slowly over time, ascites forms secondary to the pancreatic enzymes. Pseudocysts can also rupture into an adjacent segment of intestine or become secondarily infected with all the sequelae of bac-

terial infection. Although complications can occur with any pseudocyst, those less than 4 cm in diameter can be safely observed with serial ultrasound studies or CT examinations.

Splenic Vein Thrombosis

Splenic vein thrombosis complicates 3 to 5% of patients with chronic pancreatitis. Bleeding from gastric varices and thrombocytopenia caused by the hypersplenism are usually life-threatening. Accurate diagnosis of this particular type of portal hypertension is essential because portosystemic shunting does not reduce the gastrosplenic hypertension, whereas splenectomy cures the patient of the bleeding.

Common Bile Duct Stricture

Stricture of the intrapancreatic portion of the common bile duct can progress to cause obstructive jaundice, and if left uncorrected, biliary cirrhosis results. Strictures result from progressive fibrosis of the surrounding gland, and once there is persistent elevation of alkaline phosphatase (twice normal) and dilation of the common bile duct (>10 mm), surgical bypass is indicated.

DIAGNOSIS

Diagnosis is usually made by history and confirmatory studies, including a plain abdominal film showing calcifications, CT revealing calcifications and dilated duct, and ERCP again identifying changes of pancreatic duct dilation and areas of stenosis. Serum enzymes (amylase, lipase, trypsin), although often elevated during an acute exacerbation of chronic pancreatitis, offer little prognostic or diagnostic information other than identification of acute exacerbations of the chronic pancreatitis.

TREATMENT

Treatment is aimed to (1) control pain, (2) prevent and treat pancreatic exocrine insufficiency, and (3) prevent the sequelae of complications in chronic pancreatitis.

Dissolution of Pancreatic Duct Stones

Many patients with chronic pancreatitis and dilated ductal systems have stones that contribute to the blockage of pancreatic ducts and to the pain experienced by the patient. Removal of stones by extracorporeal shock wave lithotripsy, endoscopic sphincterotomy combined with mechanical removal, or oral dissolution with high doses of citrates has recently come in vogue for treatment. Early reports of pain relief after successful removal of stones are encouraging, but it remains to be seen if results are long lasting or can be duplicated by other investigators.

Abstinence from Alcohol Ingestion

It has been a long-held dictum that abstinence from alcohol intake reduces the toxic effects of alcohol on the pancreas and provides pain relief in the majority of patients. There are a significant number of patients, however, with alcoholic pancreatitis who, once they have the onset of chronic alcoholic pancreatitis, do not become pain free on abstinence from alcohol. Certainly every attempt to encourage the patient to cease alcohol intake is strongly advised.

Analgesics

The most prominent symptom of chronic pancreatitis is pain. Most patients with chronic pain presenting to the physician's office for relief have already found nonnarcotic analgesics insufficient for control of their pain. Many patients with chronic pancreatitis need prescriptions for narcotic analgesics, although this should be tempered with a work-up to identify treatable causes of continued pancreatitis or pain.

Celiac Plexus Blocks

Fluoroscopic-guided percutaneous celiac plexus blocks have been helpful in many patients' pain secondary to pancreatic cancer. It seems to be less useful, however, in patients with benign disease and a longer life span. Most patients do not benefit, and those that have initial pain relief almost always develop recurrent pain within 3 months.

Enzyme Treatment for Pain Control

At least three double-blinded studies have indicated good results in pain relief in patients treated with pancreatic enzyme supplementation. Pain is created because exocrine pancreas is hyperstimulated to make up for the decreased enzyme secretion. Ingestion of exogenous enzymes inhibits the stimulation of pancreatic enzyme secretion, which reduces the pain experienced by the patient. There is little to lose by a trial of pancreatic enzyme supplementation in patients who have pain as a prominent portion of their disease process but do not have surgically correctable ductal obstruction.

Surgical Treatment

There is good evidence to suggest that patients with dilated pancreatic ducts have elevated pancreatic ductal pressures and that creation of a lateral side-to-side pancreaticojejunostomy (Puestow procedure) using a Roux-en-Y limb reduces these pressures. Recent studies suggest that not only can pain be alleviated, but also the progression of pancreatic exocrine and endocrine insufficiency can be interrupted. Once destruction of endocrine and exocrine function has occurred, drainage procedures do not influence function. Aggressive treatment to drain obstructed pancreatic ducts must be considered before destruction of the gland. Surgical attempts at sphincteroplasty or Duvall procedures (end pancreaticojejunostomy) have not been successful in long-term follow-up, largely because of inadequate drainage and recurrent elevated ductal pressures and stones.

Resectional Surgery

Removal of 60 to 95% of the body and the tail of the pancreas results in the alleviation of pain in most patients; however, it is done only as a last resort because this frequently results in endocrine and exocrine insufficiency. In the alcoholic patient, morbidity and mortality from poor control of the diabetes are high. Pancreaticoduodenectomy has been performed when complications of chronic pancreatitis are particularly severe in the head of the gland and the body of the gland is relatively spared. When done for benign disease, the surgical mortality should be less than 1%. A modification of the standard Whipple procedure is usually performed in which the antrum and pyloric mechanism is maintained, thus creating a pyloric-sparing Whipple procedure. The pyloric-sparing Whipple procedure prevents the sequelae of dumping, and patients have fewer nutritional complications than the patients who have had gastric resections performed. It is unclear as to how many patients go on to have continued pancreatitis present within the body and tail of the gland, requiring further resectional therapy for their chronic pancreatitis. During resection and when there is no evidence of splenic vein thrombosis, the spleen can be preserved.

Pseudocysts

Pancreatic cysts associated with chronic pancreatitis seldom resolve spontaneously and are considered to be mature cysts with a thick enough wall to permit internal drainage, which usually results in resolution of the cyst. Cysts in the head of the pancreas may be drained into the duodenum or by Roux-en-Y cystojejunostomy.

Cysts in the tail of the pancreas if adherent to the stomach may be drained by cystogastrostomy.

Internal drainage is preferred to external drainage and is usually associated with less morbidity.

Not all cysts need to be managed by drainage. Cysts smaller than 4 cm in asymptomatic patients or those with minimal symptoms usually do not need to be drained. Unfortunately, resolution of a pseudocyst by drainage does not always relieve the patient's pain because of persistence of the underlying disease.

Thorascopic Splanchnicectomy

Patients with small duct disease and pain may benefit from sectioning the left splanchnic nerves. The approach is through the left side of the chest with videoscopic control. Early reports are enthusiastic and claim pain relief in 80% of patients. For the 20% that do not obtain pain relief with the sectioning of the left splanchnic nerve, the right splanchnic nerves can be cut, and almost all patients have pain relief. Although long-term follow-up is necessary, the early results are promising. Furthermore, the procedure, because of the minimally invasive techniques, results in a short hospital stay, reduced postoperative pain, and markedly reduced postoperative recovery.

PROGNOSIS

Patients with alcoholic chronic pancreatitis have a high mortality rate with or without surgery. Continued alcoholism, malnutrition, and drug addiction complicate treatment and increase mortality in the alcoholic population, whereas there is a slightly better prognosis in nonalcoholic patients. Comparison of treatment in these patients is almost impossible because of the multitude of confounding factors—etiology, continued alcohol intake, patient compliance, and hospital (county, private, or Veterans Administration).

PEPTIC ULCER DISEASE

method of
JAMES L. ACHORD, M.D.
University of Mississippi Medical Center
Jackson, Mississippi

Although the frequency of hospital admissions for peptic ulcer disease has progressively decreased throughout the world during the past 50 years, the rate of admissions for complications of this disease has not changed. The decrease in this male-predominant disease has been accompanied by a slight increase among women, narrowing the male-to-female ratio. The prevalence of gastric ulcers has not changed, and peptic disease remains a common cause of discomfort and time lost from work. Its complications are serious and sometimes life-threatening. The effectiveness of therapy has improved considerably during the past 20 years, with no sacrifice of safety. The drugs are so safe that physicians tend to use them for symptoms that only remotely suggest ulcerative diseases. Little benefit can be expected from this approach.

PATHOGENESIS

Peptic ulcer disease represents an imbalance between protective mechanisms and the aggressive factors of an environment that is normally hostile to living cells. The intrinsically aggressive factors are hydrochloric acid and pepsin. The protective factors include the mucous layer and epithelial barrier to acid diffusion, the secretion of bicarbonate in the submucosa of the stomach into the lumen of the duodenum, blood flow, and epithelial regeneration. Prostaglandins provide cell protection by mechanisms that are not understood. Ulceration of the mucosa may result from markedly excessive acid secretion, as in gastrin-secreting tumors (i.e., Zollinger-Ellison syndrome). Much more common are factors that interfere with one or more of the protective mechanisms, including direct epithelial cell destruction (e.g., *Helicobacter pylori,* aspirin and other nonsteroidal anti-inflammatory drugs [NSAIDs], concentrated alcohol), failure to replace damaged cells (e.g., severe systemic disease, starvation, malnutrition) interference in prostaglandin production (e.g., NSAIDs), alteration of the character of the mucus layer (e.g., NSAIDs, *H. pylori*), or reduction in bicarbonate secretion (e.g., acidosis, smoking).

Although glucocorticoid drugs appear capable of reactivating quiescent ulcer disease, they are no longer considered ulcerogenic. These steroids are commonly used in patients with severe systemic diseases and with other medications, either of which may be associated with ulceration of the mucosa of the gut. Prophylaxis against ulcer disease solely because of steroid treatment is not recommended.

H. pylori is now recognized as an important factor in ulcer disease. Some investigators think that in view of the mandatory presence of acid and the absence of other ulcerogenic factors, peptic ulcer disease does not occur without *H. pylori. H. pylori* was first described as a pathogen in the stomach in 1983, and there have been many confirming studies since then. The spiral organism is found beneath the gastric mucous layer, attached to and sometimes between gastric mucosal cells in humans and nonhuman primates only. It protects itself from the low pH of the gastric lumen by its position beneath the mucous layer and by metabolizing urea with urease to produce ammonia, thus surrounding itself with a more alkaline and hospitable microenvironment. The organism injures epithelial cells and incites a local inflammatory reaction; histologic gastritis is evident in most persons infected. It alters the character of gastric mucus, causing it to be more permeable to hydrogen ions.

Family studies indicate that the infection is spread from person to person by fecal-oral transmission. Its wide distribution and high prevalence suggest that it is ubiquitous in the environment, perhaps in some water supplies. The organism is known to survive for at least 1 year in water at 4° C in a dormant state. The prevalence of infection increases with age. In the United States and similarly developed countries, approximately 20% of persons in their twenties and 40% or more of those over 50 years of age are infected. In countries with poor public sanitation and less than ideal water supplies, the population becomes infected at a very early age; 80% or more of those in their twenties are infected. H. pylori may be the most common human pathogen in the world. After 20 to 40 years of infection, gastric atrophy, long considered a premalignant condition, results. Therefore, if a poulation is infected early and if carcinogens are ingested, the rate of gastric cancer is higher than in populations in which infection with H. pylori comes later in life. In several surveys in different countries throughout the world, approximately 90 to 95% of patients who have documented duodenal ulcers and about 60% of those with gastric ulcers are harboring H. pylori.

H. pylori can be seen on biopsy and can be detected by tests for the urease that it produces. Immersing a biopsy specimen in a gel containing urea and a pH indicator causes a color change within minutes if H. pylori urease is present. Breath tests are used to detect ^{13}C or ^{14}C from ingested urea. The organism stimulates IgG serum antibodies, the titer of which slowly falls if the organism is eradicated. Because the organism lives only on gastric cells, its relevance to duodenal ulcers seems puzzling. It is known, however, that gastric cells commonly occur in the duodenum as gastric metaplasia or heterotropia.

These data have led to the hypothesis that H. pylori is a major cause of duodenal ulcers, but there are several problems with this hypothesis. Many people are infected with H. pylori, but only a few develop duodenal ulcers. In contrast, almost everyone with a duodenal ulcer has H. pylori infection. Extrapolation of data suggests that about 1 in 5 or 10 infected persons in the United States develops a symptomatic ulcer. Therefore, other factors must also be present before H. pylori can be responsible for the crater. Although rapid healing of the ulcer can be achieved with acid-blocking agents alone, it is possible to accelerate ulcer healing by eradicating H. pylori at a rate that is comparable with the rates achieved with H$_2$-blocking agents. Furthermore, the recurrence rate of duodenal ulcers after healing with the blocking agents is about 60 to 80% within 1 year, although most are asymptomatic and found only in studies in which endoscopy is routinely and periodically performed. In contrast, eradication of H. pylori results in a dramatically lower relapse rate of symptomatic and asymptomatic ulcers.

Infection with H. pylori shows no sexual predilection, but duodenal ulcer disease occurs predominantly in males. Men have gastric metaplasia in the duodenum at a rate that is about three times higher than for women. There is also dichotomy in the United States in the peak-age incidence (i.e., third and fourth decades of life) of duodenal ulcers and the peak prevalence (i.e., sixth decade and later) of H. pylori infection. Although the rate of infection with H. pylori in prepubescent children is less than 5%, H. pylori is detectable in children with duodenal ulcers or at least one of their parents as often as in adults with ulcers (>95%).

In the current concept of the pathogenesis of peptic ulcer disease, ulcers are the result of H. pylori damage to the mucus and to the superficial epithelium of the stomach and duodenum in concert with interference in intrinsic protective mechanisms, making the lining susceptible to erosion by acid and pepsin. The situation in the case of H. pylori is analogous to ulcers associated with aspirin and aspirin-like compounds, which increase the permeability of the mucosal barrier to acid and pepsin and injure the epithelium. The ulcers associated with NSAIDs are predominantly gastric, and those associated with H. pylori are predominantly duodenal. H. pylori does not cause a crater to form unaided; peptic ulcer disease remains a multifactorial problem.

TREATMENT

Gastritis

Although acute gastritis may produce vague and nonspecific symptoms that are almost always self-limited, chronic gastritis without ulcer formation, including that caused by H. pylori, rarely causes symptoms. Epigastric symptoms should be investigated, if persistent, and not ascribed to "gastritis" unless a histologic diagnosis of one of the uncommon forms, such as eosinophilic gastritis, is obtained. Functional symptoms respond as well to antacids as to the more expensive antiulcer drugs.

Duodenal Ulcer

A diagnosis of duodenal ulcer by symptoms is only moderately reliable and then only if the physician adheres to a rigid definition of indicators. These include epigastric pain on an empty stomach, and the pain should disappear or at least markedly improve within 10 to 15 minutes after eating (i.e., pain–food–relief pattern) or taking acid-neutralizing tablets or solution. The pain is usually absent until the stomach is again empty. Pain seldom exists on awakening in the morning, but it may awaken the patient about 2 hours after retiring. Over an interval of years, ulcerative pain occurs episodically, is variably bothersome for several weeks, and spontaneously disappears. It seldom persists without relief for longer than 2 or 3 months but recurs once or twice each year. The healing rate of duodenal ulcers in the placebo controls of careful studies was about 85% in 8 to 12 weeks. Symptoms are often "uncharacteristic," and ulcers often produce no symptoms until a complication, such as hemorrhage, occurs. An accurate diagnosis requires endoscopic examination. Radiologists seem unwilling to make a firm diagnosis of an ulcer, usually adding the qualifying statement that "endoscopic confirmation (or evaluation) is suggested."

For patients with a pattern of symptoms that suggest duodenal ulcer, a therapeutic trial of one of the H_2-blocking drugs and adjunctive measures is both justified and cost effective. Relief of symptoms should occur within 1 to 3 days, and this success should be followed by a full course of treatment for 4 to 6 weeks with a presumptive diagnosis of duodenal ulcer. If symptomatic relief is not obtained within approximately 7 days, the medication should be discontinued and definitive diagnostic measures undertaken.

When an objective diagnosis of duodenal ulcer is made, adjunctive measures that underlie effective treatment should be instituted before drugs are considered. Probably the most important of these is to ensure that no aspirin compounds or NSAIDs are being taken. Other ulcerogenic drugs should be discontinued, if possible, at least temporarily. A patient who is a smoker should be informed that smoking slows healing and increases relapse rates; it should be discontinued. Diet is no longer considered important in the cause or the treatment of duodenal ulcer. Customary advice is to eat a balanced diet of three regularly scheduled meals each day. Any food that does not cause symptoms may be included. Spicy foods need not be excluded if they are part of the patient's normal diet. In the author's view, emotional stress usually has little or no influence on the disease. Mood-altering drugs are rarely indicated. Alcoholic beverages may be ingested in modest amounts but should be taken with or followed by a meal.

Effective compounds in the treatment of duodenal ulcer can be divided into those that neutralize gastric acid, inhibit its secretion, or provide some mucosal protection. At this time, routine treatment for *H. pylori* infection is not recommended (see last paragraph of this section). Neutralizing compounds (i.e., antacids) are effective but must be taken frequently; they have been supplanted by other drugs, except for symptomatic relief. Drugs that inhibit acid secretion include the anticholinergic agents, those that occupy histamine receptor sites unique to the stomach, and those that block the secreting mechanism (the proton pump) on the luminal surface of acid-secreting cells. Anticholinergic drugs are relatively weak inhibitors of acid secretion and are no longer used for this purpose. They do, however, add to the inhibiting properties of the H_2-blocking drugs. Compounds that offer local or cytoprotection include sucralfate (Carafate) and prostaglandin analogues. Rates of healing achieved with sucralfate are not significantly at variance from those obtained with the H_2-blocking drugs, but this drug has never been popular because of its interference with absorption of simultaneously administered drugs, its tendency to cause constipation (especially in older patients), and the necessity for taking it four times a day (1 gram/dose). Prostaglandin analogues are effective only in antisecretory doses and are not recommended for treatment.

The H_2-blocking drugs currently available are cimetidine (Tagamet), ranitidine (Zantac), famotidine (Pepcid), and nizatidine (Axid); others are in development. All of the H_2-blocking drugs are equally effective and remarkably safe. The cheapest should be used for the usual case. Because these drugs all have variable tendencies to inhibit the hepatic drug-metabolizing P-450 enzymes, caution should be exercised when they are administered to patients already receiving multiple drugs. The major load of unopposed gastric acid secretion occurs during sleeping hours. It has been shown by several carefully controlled studies that the healing rate of a duodenal ulcer is as good when a single large dose of an H_2-blocking drug is given after the evening meal as when the same amount is given in divided doses during daytime hours. The usual dose is 800 mg of cimetidine, 300 mg of ranitidine, 40 mg of famotidine, or 150 mg of nizatidine. Pain relief is usually obtained within 1 to 3 days. At these equivalent doses, healing rates are about 80% in 4 weeks and more than 90% in 8 weeks for all the blocking drugs. Treatment is usually given for 6 weeks for uncomplicated disease.

The newest class of drugs is the H^+/K^+ATPase inhibitors (omeprazol). These compounds are extremely effective blockers of acid secretion. They inhibit the enzyme responsible for the secretion of acid from the luminal side of the parietal cell. Whereas binding of the H_2 receptors by the blocking drugs is fairly loose, omeprazole binds irreversibly, and new receptors must be produced by a cell before secretion can resume. Unlike the H_2-blocking drugs, omeprazole causes a significant increase in serum gastrin. Because of the trophic effects of this hormone and the demonstration that rats develop gastric carcinoid tumors when they are made severely and chronically hypochlorhydric with omeprazole, prolonged use in humans is not recommended, although no clear association between carcinoid tumor and omeprazole use has been reported for humans. Healing rates of duodenal ulcers by omeprazole are faster than with any other currently available drug, and pain relief is slightly faster, but these findings have little clinical relevance and do not seem to justify a greater expense in the usual case. Unlike the H_2-blocking drugs, omeprazole is destroyed by gastric acid, and the formulation should not be pulverized and administered through a nasogastric tube.

Treatment of *H. pylori* is indicated for any duodenal ulcer that promptly recurs (as defined by symptoms) after treatment with H_2-blocking drugs or that is complicated by bleeding, obstruction, or persistence (see Problems in Treatment section).

Gastric Ulcer

One of the most common etiologic factors for ulcers is the ingestion of aspirin or other NSAIDs. If these compounds are being used primarily for pain relief, their use should be strongly discouraged. Because differentiating benign gastric ulcers from ulcerated malignancies is extremely difficult, careful and continuing diagnostic evaluation is necessary. An experienced radiologist can differentiate between benign and malignant ulcerations with 85 to 90% accuracy; therefore, endoscopy is not considered mandatory if both the radiologist and the attending physician agree that the crater is benign. Many radiologists are unwilling to commit themselves to the diagnosis, and if there is any doubt, endoscopy and biopsy are required. All gastric ulcers (but not gastric erosions) should be followed to 6 months after complete healing. This can be done by a confident and experienced radiologist, but it is usually done by endoscopy to allow biopsy. Extensive biopsy specimens should be obtained from all quadrants of the margin and the base of the ulcer; six or eight samples should be removed at every procedure.

Gastric acid secretion, mandatory for the development of benign gastric ulcers, is commonly lower than in duodenal ulcer disease. Nocturnal acid secretion is not significantly different from that in normal persons. Single bedtime doses of H_2-blocking drugs are not as effective as in treating duodenal ulcer and are not recommended. Most gastroenterologists recommend H_2 blockers two or four times daily in a total daily dose equivalent to single bedtime doses used in duodenal ulcer. A single morning dose of 20 mg of omeprazole is also effective. The duration of treatment required for more than 80% of gastric ulcer to be healed is usually 12 weeks. Endoscopy is recommended 12 weeks after the original diagnosis. Because larger craters take longer to heal, slavish adherence to the dictum that any gastric ulcer that does not heal in 12 weeks should be surgically resected is often unreasonable; healing should, however, be progressive under treatment. Failure to heal may be caused by an underlying gastric malignancy, but the most common reason that a benign gastric ulcer has not healed in 12 weeks is an initial large size. If healing has been progressive and all biopsy specimens are benign,

continued treatment and periodic evaluation is justified, even if the ulcer is smaller but still present after 12 weeks. Because ulcerated gastric malignancies may escape careful investigation, surgery is indicated for an ulcer that shows little or no progressive healing despite adequate therapy.

Problems in Treatment

Treatment-Resistant Ulcers. Ulcers that are resistant to treatment may be defined as those that do not heal after the recommended treatment program, that recur promptly after treatment, or that recur during maintenance therapy as documented by endoscopy. Treatment-resistant ulcers should prompt a search for gastrin-producing tumors (i.e., Zollinger-Ellison syndrome) by obtaining a measurement of serum gastrin level after fasting.

Ulcers heal more slowly and recur sooner and at significantly higher rates in patients who continue to smoke than in nonsmokers. Persistent use of aspirin or NSAIDs is a common cause of failure to heal or prompt recurrence of gastric or duodenal ulcers. Poor compliance with prescribed medication produces poor results. Physicians may forget that many patients are noncompliant because of the cost of medication, not because they are obstinate. It is better that a patient take a suboptimal drug than not take the optimal but more expensive one. In chronically debilitated patients, ulcer craters heal poorly, just as do all epithelial wounds.

Most ulcers that do not heal in the expected interval of adequate treatment respond to the same dose for a longer interval. Occasionally, larger doses of blocking drugs or omeprazole are required.

Maintenance Therapy. The 1-year symptomatic recurrence rate for duodenal ulcer is at least 60% in nonsmokers and significantly higher in smokers. The endoscopic recurrence rate is about 20% higher in both cases. Because complications in asymptomatic recurrent ulcers of the duodenum are uncommon, the author uses the disappearance of symptoms as the basis for assuming the crater has healed. Neither radiographs nor endoscopy are recommended to be certain the duodenal ulcer has healed. Radiographs can be quite misleading because the re-epithelialized healed crater can be mistaken for an unhealed ulcer. Physicians must treat the patient, not the radiograph. The considerable expense of another endoscopic procedure is not justified despite the known disassociation between symptoms and the presence of a crater. However, symptoms of duodenal ulcer that persist despite treatment indicate the need for another endoscopic evaluation.

Symptomatic recurrence of an endoscopically or radiographically documented duodenal ulcer shortly after an apparently successful regimen should be treated with 4 to 8 more weeks of full therapy (without endoscopy), followed by triple therapy for *H. pylori* as noted earlier. Renewed efforts should be made to have the patient stop smoking and another search made for possible ulcerogenic drugs.

The 1-year recurrence rate of benign gastric ulcer is approximately 40%. Maintenance therapy usually requires the same dose of drug as in the treatment of the acute gastric ulcer. Chronic, indolent, benign gastric ulcer that does not heal over a period of months despite adherence to a program that is usually successful was described many years ago. Although the newer treatments have produced a dramatic decrease in their number, chronic indolent gastric ulcer is still seen occasionally, usually in elderly or chronically debilitated patients. A nonhealing ulcer raises the specter of an undiagnosed ulcerated gastric carcinoma, and most clinicians recommend resection. Because the rate of infection with *H. pylori* in gastric ulcer is only approximately 60%, in comparison with more than 90% in duodenal ulcer, it is not clear which of them should be treated with triple therapy for *H. pylori*.

Most duodenal and benign gastric ulcers that do not heal in the expected interval respond to extended treatment. Because failure of the duodenal ulcer to heal correlates with basal acid output, increasing the amount of H_2-blocking drug and administering it twice a day rather than once is often successful. It is seldom helpful to add another class of drug to the regimen. Recalcitrant ulcers should be treated for *H. pylori* before a surgical procedure is considered.

Helicobacter pylori. Resident *H. pylori* is easily suppressed by bismuth compounds and antibiotics, but it is difficult to eradicate. Permanent eradication requires 2 weeks of bismuth subsalicylate (1 tablespoon or 2 tablets four times daily) combined with 2 weeks of amoxicillin (Polymox) or tetracycline (Sumycin; 500 mg four times daily) simultaneously with metronidazole (Flagyl; 500 mg four times daily). The cure rate with this regimen is more than 90% (Am J Gastroenterol 87:1716, 1992). Reinfection is common if the prevalence in the surrounding population is high. The emergence of resistant strains has been documented. Risks of treatment, predominantly antibiotic-associated diarrhea or pseudomembranous colitis, have led to a conservative approach in the selection of patients to be treated. Currently, only certain patients are considered for therapy of *H. pylori*: those with proven, recurrent

duodenal ulcer disease that has necessitated prolonged suppression with H_2-blocking agents; those who have had complications of duodenal ulcer, such as bleeding or perforation, and have had recurrent symptomatic disease; and those who are being considered for surgical procedures because of intractability or complications.

Patients with symptoms that suggest duodenal ulcers but in whom no ulcers are found at endoscopy (e.g., non-ulcer dyspepsia) have not been shown to have *H. pylori* infection at a rate different from that in the general population and do not appear to respond to treatment for it.

Stress-Related Mucosal Disease. The acute mucosal damage associated with intense metabolic stress is most commonly superficial (e.g., erosions) but is occasionally deep enough to cause an ulcer (i.e., through the muscularis mucosae). The lesions are always multiple, do not cause subjective complaints, and occur in the acid-secreting portion of the stomach (i.e., antrum). Stress-related mucosal disease (SRMD) is characteristic of burns (e.g., Curling's ulcer) and central nervous system (CNS) trauma (e.g., Cushing's ulcer). They are seen in most severely ill patients in intensive care units, especially those who require artificial ventilation; those suffering from sepsis, shock, or trauma; those undergoing major surgical procedures (especially when done as a life-saving measure); and those with multiple-organ failure. They are rarely seen in patients undergoing elective, relatively routine surgical procedures. Approximately 20% evidence any bleeding, and perhaps 5% bleed heavily. The importance of SRMD lies in the 5% of patients with bleeding sufficient to require hemodynamic support with blood transfusions. In this group, the reported mortality rate is 60 to 80% and sometimes higher. This rate is directly related to the fact that bleeding occurs in patients who are already severely ill with an underlying problem. Mortality rates attributable to coexisting disease processes tend to multiply, rather than be additive.

Bleeding from SRMD responds poorly to endoscopic cautery. Like most bleeding erosions or ulcers, the evidence strongly suggests that treatment with H_2-blocking drugs does not stop hemorrhage. The best approach is prevention of bleeding. Intravenous infusion of H_2-blocking drugs reduces the occurrence of hemorrhage from levels of 20% or more in placebo-treated patients to levels of 5% to 15%. Continuous infusion demonstrably increases the intraluminal gastric pH to levels above 4. At this level, acid concentration is constantly above the level required to activate pepsinogen to its proteolytic form, pepsin. Cimetidine infusions at the rate of 37.5 to 50 mg per hour or ranitidine in doses of 6.25 mg per hour are highly effective. Although the U.S. Food and Drug Administration has not specifically approved this use of other H_2-blocking agents, many clinicians use them in a similar manner. Bolus injections also reduce bleeding rates, but the data indicating that intermittent elevations of the intragastric pH are as effective as constant elevations are not convincing. These drugs can be advantageously added to hyperalimentation solutions. Data from investigations of sucralfate and of frequent intragastric administration of antacids, although demonstrating effectiveness, are not as impressive as are the studies of the H_2-blocking drugs. There is no acceptable evidence to incriminate consistently high pH as a predisposing cause of aspiration pneumonia.

The H_2-blocking drugs are commonly given in situations in which there is no evidence that SRMD is a likely complication. Examples are routine, uncomplicated surgery, minor burns, renal failure treated with dialysis, CNS disease without coma, and soft tissue injury without sepsis or shock. This use is unjustified and adds unnecessarily to medical costs.

NSAID-Induced Mucosal Disease. About 25% of patients taking NSAIDs for inflammatory musculoskeletal disease complain of upper gastrointestinal symptoms. The greatest predictor of symptoms is previous symptoms on taking these drugs. About 40 to 50% of patients complaining of symptoms have gastric erosions at endoscopy. However, it is difficult to predict mucosal injury by the presence or absence of symptoms, especially in the elderly, who make up a large percentage of users. Among large groups of patients on these drugs who underwent endoscopy without regard to symptoms, approximately 40% had at least gastric erosions or ulcers and 15% had duodenal lesions. Multiple examinations over time while the drugs are still being taken show that erosions come and go. They rarely cause bleeding. Endoscopy is not routinely indicated because therapy will not be changed.

NSAID-induced symptoms or demonstrated injury should first prompt a review of the necessity for these compounds. If there is no evidence of an inflammatory process and the drugs are being taken primarily for pain relief, nonsalicylate pain relievers should be substituted. A reduction in dose is sometimes effective, because the injury is related to dose. Taking the medication with meals is sometimes helpful, and enteric-coated aspirin is sometimes better tolerated. Although there are some claimed differences in their propensity for producing mucosal lesions, there is little to recommend one NSAID over the other. Despite statements to the contrary, parenteral nonsteroidal drugs also injure the gastric mucosa if given for longer than 3 days. Treatment with H_2-

blocking drugs after discontinuation or reduction of the dose of NSAIDs usually produces rapid resolution of symptoms. Misoprostol (Cytotec) provides very poor symptomatic relief. Patients who develop iron deficiency anemia while taking NSAIDs should have upper endoscopy without regard to epigastric symptoms. If the upper endoscopy does not reveal significant lesions, the colon should be examined, because these patients are in the age group that is at relatively high risk for colon carcinoma. For patients with frank gastric ulceration due to NSAIDs that would be difficult or impossible to stop, omeprazole or misoprostol should be prescribed. For those with frank duodenal ulcers, an H_2-blocking drug or omeprazole should be prescribed. Consideration should be given to temporarily stopping NSAIDs while frank ulceration is being treated.

It is not recommended that every patient placed on NSAIDs receive prophylactic therapy. Risk factors that may prompt prophylactic therapy include a history of ulcer disease, especially if there is a history of an ulcer complication, and age (>65 years old). Older patients seem more likely to develop severe complications of NSAID-induced disease than are younger ones. The H_2-blocking drugs are appropriate for patients with a history of duodenal ulcer, and misoprostol is appropriate if a gastric ulcer is in the history. Either can be used for prophylaxis if the only risk factor is age.

Indications for Surgery

Surgical procedures for duodenal ulcer are largely confined to patients with acute complications, such as perforation or bleeding that fails to respond to conservative management. Persistent or chronic recurrent gastric outlet obstruction due to scarring at the pylorus accounts for other cases. In view of the effective medical therapy available, elective surgery is rarely needed to control unremitting symptomatic disease. Patients with recalcitrant pain without endoscopically proven ulcer disease should not be submitted to ulcer surgery.

The frequency of surgery for gastric ulcer remains higher than the rate for duodenal ulcer. This reflects a realistic concern for the possibility that the crater represents an ulcerated malignancy, rather than an unhealed benign ulcer, despite multiple biopsies.

It is better for the patient to undergo a procedure with less alteration of the anatomy, such as a selective vagotomy with or without a pyloroplasty rather than a resection, even though such procedures are accompanied by a higher recurrence rate of ulcer disease. Alimentary tract surgeons have shown that severe and debilitating postgastrectomy syndromes are considerably less frequent with the lesser procedures, and it is uncommon to see severe dumping syndromes in the patients treated with conservative methods.

TUMORS OF THE STOMACH

method of
THEODOR B. GRAGE, M.D., Ph.D.
University of Minnesota Hospital
Minneapolis, Minnesota

The astonishing fivefold decline in gastric cancer in the United States during the last 50 years, from 25 to 5 per 1000 persons in the general population, has been attributed to improved diets. High rates of gastric cancer continue to be observed in Japan, the Scandinavian countries, parts of Latin America, and China. In the United States, blacks, Indians, and Hawaiians continue to have high rates of this disease. High intake of salt, of certain fish, and of complex carbohydrates, nitrates, and a low intake of animal fat and protein, fresh fruits, and fresh green leafy vegetables are observed in the high-risk group.

Pathologists and epidemiologists now recognize two distinct forms of adenocarcinoma. The essential morphologic element is cell cohesion. With cohesion, cells remain attached to each other and form glandular elements, as in other intestinal cancers. This is called the "intestinal type." Without cohesion, cells independently infiltrate the gastric wall without forming a discrete mass. This is called the "diffuse type." In areas of high gastric cancer incidence, the intestinal type predominates, and for that reason, it has also been called the "epidemic type." In populations with dramatic decreases in the gastric cancer incidence, the frequency of the intestinal type has decreased. The diffuse type has not changed in frequency. The intestinal type is more common in males and older patients. It is better differentiated and has a better prognosis than the endemic type, and it is frequently preceded by a prolonged precursor process, such as chronic gastritis, intestinal metaplasia, and dysplasias.

Unfortunately, most patients in the United States do not become symptomatic until the disease is advanced. Early gastric cancer involving only the mucosa and submucosa has only vague symptoms. Screening endoscopy in Japan has raised the percentage of patients presenting with early gastric cancer to 35 to 40% of all gastric cancers seen, but in the United States, fewer than 10% of patients with gastric cancer are seen at this stage. Surgical treatment at this early stage provides a 5-year survival rate of 90% or more.

As the cancer advances, symptoms of anorexia, weight loss, postprandial fullness, and indigestion appear. Pain is common, appearing ultimately in more than 90% of patients, and it can mimic peptic ulcer disease. Any patient with anorexia, weight loss, anemia, or dysphagia should be suspected of having a gastric cancer and should undergo gastroscopy. Mass screening in the United States is not cost effective, but identification and examination of high-risk groups (e.g., previous gastrectomy for benign disease, chronic gastritis, pernicious anemia) is important.

On physical examination, findings are positive only for patients with advanced disease, such as metastases to the cervical nodes, a rectal shelf, abdominal mass, Krukenberg tumor, hepatomegaly secondary to metastatic disease, or ascites.

Laboratory investigation may reveal anemia, occult blood in the stool, or abnormal liver function studies and hepatic metastases. Thorough endoscopic examination coupled with modern staining techniques, biopsy, washings, and brushings have become the "gold standard" in the diagnosis of gastric carcinoma, with an accuracy rate of more than 90%.

Barium contrast radiologic examination of the stomach with air contrast may give information about the extent of disease or differentiate a polypoid mass from an ulcer crater. With diffuse infiltration of the gastric wall, the stomach appears stiff and nondistensible. Unfortunately, radiologic examination does not have the accuracy of endoscopic examination and may miss early, superficial cancers, which are highly curable.

Computed tomography (CT) of the abdomen can determine the extent of disease, such as extension beyond the gastric wall or nodal and hepatic metastases.

TREATMENT

Adenocarcinoma

The only effective treatment of adenocarcinoma of the stomach is surgical resection. In the United States, a radical subtotal gastrectomy with a Billroth II reconstruction is the method of choice for cancers involving the distal two-thirds of the stomach. The resection includes removal of the omentum and the node-bearing areas along the lesser and greater curvatures. This operation may encompass resection of organs directly infiltrated by tumors, such as the transverse colon, pancreas, or left lateral edge of the liver.

Total gastrectomy with adjacent lymphadenectomy is reserved for tumors involving most of the stomach. In Europe, there is increasing enthusiasm for total gastrectomy in most patients with resectable cancer, although improvement in long-term survival must be determined. Operative morbidity and mortality rates are substantially higher with total gastrectomy, as are postoperative nutritional problems.

For tumors in the upper one-third of the stomach, usually around the esophagogastric junction, a proximal gastrectomy and resection of the lower two-thirds of the esophagus with an esophagogastrostomy high in the chest is an excellent and relatively safe operation. It provides extra longterm palliation and occasional cures. Unfortunately, carcinomas in this area are often of the diffuse type, are poorly differentiated with a high percentage of signet cell rings, and carry a poor prognosis, even with the most radical approach.

In general, the author does not favor preoperative needle biopsy of the liver if the CT scan suggests hepatic metastases. Almost every patient with a diagnosis of gastric carcinoma should undergo a thorough abdominal exploration for possible cure and to alleviate problems of bleeding, perforation, and obstruction.

Japanese surgeons have become increasingly aggressive in the surgical treatment of gastric carcinoma, with enviable results. Radical resection of the stomach includes an extensive lymphadenectomy from areas of potential spread, such as the celiac axis lymph nodes; nodes along the common hepatic artery, splenic hilus, splenic artery, and hepatoduodenal ligament; retropancreatic nodes; and nodes in the mesenteric root. However, 30 to 35% of resected cancers in Japan are the early-stage tumors, and most gastric cancers are the well-differentiated intestinal type, which affects surgical success rates. Nevertheless, a rigorous evaluation of the more radical resection is needed in the United States.

Despite improvements in the rates of resectability, morbidity, and mortality after gastric resection, the overall results of surgical treatment in this country have not changed in 30 years, and the results are dismal. Of 100 random patients with newly diagnosed gastric cancer, 15 have tumors that are nonoperable as a result of extensive metastatic spread, poor surgical risk, or refusal of surgical treatment. Of the remaining 85 patients, only half have tumors resectable for cure, with an operative mortality of 5 to 10%, and only 25% of those undergoing resection are alive and free of disease after 5 years. The other half may undergo palliative procedures, such as resection, bypass, or biopsy only. Thus, only 10 of the original 100 patients are alive and well 5 years after the diagnosis.

Chemotherapy in the form of single agents or combination therapy, such as 5-fluorouracil, doxorubicin (Adriamycin), and mitomycin C (Mutamycin), has achieved temporary partial responses in 20 to 40% of patients. Most responses are short-lived and have rarely resulted in prolongation of life. Adjuvant chemotherapy after curative resection has not resulted in reproducible improvement in most large-scale studies. However, intensive efforts are being made to improve the dismal results of surgical treatment by the use of chemotherapy.

Primary Lymphomas

Primary malignant lymphomas represent approximately 5% of all gastric neoplasms. Tumors usually involve the distal part of the stomach and may be rather large and bulky. Patients with malignant lymphoma of the stomach usually have fewer signs and symptoms than do patients with equally large adenocarcinomas of the stomach. Lymphoma patients possess reasonably good nutritional status and rarely have the anemia seen in patients with adenocarcinoma. Surgical treatment is similar to that for adenocarcinoma of the stomach. Postoperative radiation therapy is increasingly part of the treatment for primary malignant lymphomas of the stomach. Overall results are excellent; more than 50% of the patients are alive and free of disease after 5 years.

Benign Tumors

Benign tumors of the stomach represent approximately 5 to 7% of all neoplasms of the stomach and usually produce few symptoms. They may ulcerate and bleed and may lead to vague epigastric distress and fullness. The tumors include adenomatous and hyperplastic polyps, which are usually benign. The diagnosis can be made by endoscopy, and unless a polyp is larger than 2 cm in diameter, no treatment is necessary. Larger benign polyps should be excised. Progression to malignancy is uncommon. Leimyomas of the gastric wall represent about 40% of all benign tumors, and local excision is curative.

TUMORS OF THE COLON AND RECTUM

method of
THEODORE J. SACLARIDES, M.D.
Rush–Presbyterian–St. Luke's Medical Center
Chicago, Illinois

Colon and rectal cancer is the second most common malignancy in the United States, affecting 5 to 6% of American-born persons. Approximately 150,000 new cases are diagnosed annually in the United States; about half of these patients die of the disease. In women, only breast and lung cancers cause more deaths; in men, only lung cancer causes more deaths. In general, cancer of the colon and rectum affects elderly persons, the mean age being 67 years. Approximately 8% of cases, however, are diagnosed in patients under the age of 40, and in these instances the disease may follow a more virulent course.

SCREENING

Despite improvements in anesthesia, surgical technique, and supportive care, the cure rates for colorectal cancer have not changed appreciably over the last several decades. Early diagnosis, therefore, is extremely important in that prognosis is directly correlated with transmural penetration and lymph node metastases. Screening patients at average risk, as well as the ability to identify high-risk groups, should be part of the armamentarium of every physician.

Digital Examination

The digital examination should be an integral part of every examination, especially in patients reporting a change in bowel habits. Aside from examination of the rectum, assessment of prostate size, smoothness, and homogeneity can be obtained as well. The mid- and lower rectum can be examined for any space-occupying lesions, and the presacral space can be palpated for any nodal metastases or tumor fixation. The only drawback to a routine digital rectal examination is the false sense of security that a normal finding would give a physician treating a patient whose symptoms mandate a more thorough examination.

Proctosigmoidoscopy

The flexible sigmoidoscope enables the physician to examine more of the distal colon (up to 60 cm) than does the rigid proctoscope (25 cm), and hence the diagnostic yield is perhaps greater. For screening asymptomatic patients for colorectal cancer, current recommendations are for a flexible sigmoidoscopy at ages 50 and 51; if both examination findings are normal, the procedure should be repeated at 3-year intervals. In the presence of Hemoccult-positive stools, or if a high-risk patient is identified on historical grounds, proctosigmoidoscopy alone is insufficient; in these instances, a double-contrast barium enema or colonoscopy is the preferred examination.

Colonoscopy

Colonoscopy is currently the most accurate diagnostic tool for colorectal neoplasms. Furthermore, colonoscopy has therapeutic potential for many benign-appearing lesions. Colonoscopy should be advised for patients with Hemoccult-positive stools and for screening high-risk patients such as those with a personal history of colorectal tumors, those with a family history of polyposis or colorectal cancer, or those who have had chronic ulcerative colitis. Colonoscopy is also recommended for patients in whom a cancer or polyp was recently diagnosed on proctosigmoidoscopy; in these instances, synchronous proximal lesions are frequently identified. Colonoscopy is not recommended as a screening tool in low-risk patients.

Colon Radiography

Double-contrast barium enemas provide a less invasive, less expensive means of assessing the colon in symptomatic or high-risk patients. Although the diagnostic yield is less than that for colonoscopy, the two tests are not competitive in nature; rather, they are complementary. In some instances, colon x-rays may be preferable: for example, if the colon is angulated,

fixed, or tortuous, endoscopy may be painful, hazardous, or unlikely to examine the entire colon by reaching the cecum. Also, an obstructing or perforating cancer is perhaps more safely assessed with a water-soluble contrast enema than with endoscopy.

Fecal Occult Blood Tests

Fecal occult blood (FOB) tests utilize the peroxidase-like capability of hemoglobin to convert a quinone into a blue-colored substrate in the presence of hydrogen peroxide. Fecal occult blood tests provide the most cost-effective means of screening low-risk patients for tumors of the colon and rectum. Test results, however, may be altered by certain dietary factors, such as red meats, vitamin C, and fruits and vegetables that possess peroxidase capability. Large population-based studies in which FOB tests were used as a screening device have found that among patients with positive results, adenomas are subsequently found in 30 to 40% and cancers in fewer than 10%. In these studies, a higher percentage of early cancers were found; however, survival rates appear to be unaltered.

PREMALIGNANT CONDITIONS

Familial Adenomatous Polyposis

Inherited as an autosomal dominant trait, familial polyposis occurs in 1 of every 7,000 live births. The disease is characterized by carpeting of the colon and rectum by hundreds to thousands of adenomas, and it usually develops after puberty. Colorectal cancer develops in virtually 100% of patients by the age of 40 if left untreated. The average age at death from cancer is approximately 42 years. Extracolonic manifestations, such as osteomas, sebaceous cysts, desmoid tumors (Gardner's syndrome), or central nervous system tumors (Turcot's syndrome), may develop. Screening family members at risk helps identify asymptomatic patients at an early age. Among patients in whom the diagnosis is made after symptoms of hematochezia develop, approximately one-third already have cancer.

Screening should commence at puberty, and because colon polyps rarely develop in the absence of rectal polyps, screening is accomplished with annual sigmoidoscopy. If sigmoidoscopy reveals polyps, colonoscopy and biopsy are performed to verify that the polyps are adenomas (rather than hamartomas), and upper endoscopy should be performed to rule out gastric or duodenal polyps. Once the diagnosis is made, surgery is advised. Options include colectomy with ileorectal anastomosis, colectomy with rectal mucosectomy and ileoanal anastomosis, and proctocolectomy with either a Brooke ileostomy or a Koch continent ileostomy. If an ileorectostomy is chosen, the rectal remnant must be examined with proctoscopy at 6-month intervals; fulguration of any remaining rectal polyps is then performed.

Chronic Ulcerative Colitis

In approximately 5% of patients with chronic ulcerative colitis, cancer develops. There are subsets of patients, however, who are at especially high risk, and these include patients with disease of long duration and those in whom the disease involves the entire colon. The risk of cancer increases after 7 years of disease and is estimated to increase at a rate of 2% per year after 10 years of disease. In contrast to patients with pancolitis, patients with ulcerative proctitis do not have an appreciably higher risk of cancer. Other factors that are thought to be associated with a higher cancer risk include chronically active disease and the onset of disease in youth.

Obtaining random biopsy specimens of the colon during colonoscopy has been recommended for patients with long-standing disease. Biopsy samples are then assessed for dysplasia, which is thought to be a marker for malignancy developing elsewhere in the colon. Such assessment requires a pathologist skilled in distinguishing dysplasia from inflammation and for several reasons is not a totally failsafe means of detecting which patients will develop cancer. Dysplasia does not always precede cancer, is not always evenly distributed throughout the colon, and may be reversible. Despite these drawbacks and because there is a lack of other effective screening measures, biopsies for dysplasia continue to be performed. If surgery is necessary, options are similar to those for polyposis.

Crohn's Disease

The risk of cancer is higher in patients with Crohn's colitis, although the risk does not approach that seen in patients with ulcerative colitis. The risk seems to be highest in surgically bypassed segments of bowel and in patients with long-standing disease. There are currently no established recommendations for cancer surveillance in patients with Crohn's disease.

Hereditary Nonpolyposis Cancer Syndromes

A familial tendency to develop cancer has been noted in certain kindreds and is distinct from the polyposis syndromes. Lynch syndrome I is specific for colorectal cancer, and it has been noted that within affected families, the average age of patients in whom cancer develops is approximately 44 years. There is a higher proportion of right-sided cancers and greater frequencies of synchronous (18%) and metachronous (40%) colorectal cancers. Screening family members at risk should be performed with colonoscopy and should commence at an early age. Lynch syndrome II includes a higher risk of breast, ovarian, endometrial, and gastric cancers in addition to colorectal cancer. If surgery is necessary for a newly diagnosed colon cancer, consideration should be given to performing a subtotal colectomy (because of the higher incidence of metachronous colon cancers) as well as a hysterectomy and oophorectomy in a woman beyond childbearing age.

Polyps

Colorectal polyps with malignant potential are tubular adenomas, tubulovillous adenomas, and villous adenomas. Tubular adenomas are the most common type, constituting 75% of all polyps, only 5% of which are cancerous. Tubulovillous adenomas constitute 15% of polyps, 22% of which are malignant. Corresponding figures for villous adenomas are 10% and 40%. The incidence of malignancy also varies with polyp size; polyps less than 1 cm are rarely malignant, whereas larger polyps have a higher chance of harboring an occult invasive cancer.

Most polyps do not produce symptoms and are discovered incidentally during colon x-rays or screening endoscopic examinations. On occasion, polyps may produce occult blood loss, anemia, hematochezia, diarrhea, or, rarely, electrolyte disturbances from the secretion of a potassium-rich mucus. Once diagnosed, polyps should be removed; however, the technique chosen depends on polyp size and morphology.

Colonoscopic snare polypectomy is the procedure of choice for most polypoid lesions if they are accessible with a colonoscope and the lesion in question is not excessively large or broad based. Most pedunculated polyps and smaller sessile polyps are easily removed in this manner. Piecemeal excision is often required for larger sessile adenomas. The risk of perforation after colonoscopic polypectomy is usually less than 1%.

If cancer is found within a polyp, decisions regarding further management are based on polyp morphology and the extent of cancer invasion. For example, a flat villous adenoma with invasive cancer should be treated with a segmental bowel resection unless the polyp was located in the distal rectum, in which case a transanal local excision could be performed. A pedunculated polyp with cancer, in contrast, has a much lower chance of associated lymph node metastases and therefore could be managed simply by endoscopic polypectomy if the cancer was localized to the polyp head. If invasive cancer was found penetrating down to the base of the stalk, however, segmental resection is advised. Other ominous histologic features that mandate segmental resection are poor differentiation and venous or lymphatic invasion.

TREATMENT

Principles of Surgery

Colon Cancer

After a thorough history, physical examination, and complete evaluation of the colon with either colonoscopy or colon x-ray, surgery may be undertaken. The presence of known metastatic disease is not a contraindication to surgical resection of the primary tumor if at least a 6-month survival is anticipated. Furthermore, significant palliation of bleeding, pain, or obstruction can be obtained even in the presence of metastatic disease.

The primary tumor and the associated mesentery that bears the regional lymphatic channels should be resected. On occasion, a tumor is found to invade neighboring viscera such as the small bowel, bladder, ovaries, or uterus, and these organs should be removed en bloc. A subtotal colectomy with ileorectal anastomosis is advised when there are multiple synchronous colon cancers, when there are a cancer and multiple adenomatous polyps found in disjoint colon segments, or in a patient with a hereditary nonpolyposis cancer syndrome.

Occasionally a surgeon must operate on a patient with a completely obstructing tumor. In such instances, a preoperative bowel preparation is usually not possible, and performing an anastomosis with a dilated stool-laden colon is hazardous. A temporary colostomy is usually necessary in such instances; alternatives include a subtotal colectomy with ileorectal anastomosis, intraoperative colonic lavage followed by primary anastomosis, or placement of an intraluminal colonic stent to protect the anastomosis. Each case should be individualized, and the decision as to which option to choose must take into consideration bowel wall viability and edema, the presence of an associated perforation, and overall stability of the patient.

Rectal Cancer

Evaluation and preparation for patients with rectal cancer are similar to those for patients with colon cancer; however, because there are more surgical options available for rectal cancer patients, a preoperative assessment for metastatic disease should be routinely performed. For example, transanal fulguration of a rectal cancer rather than a laparotomy and radical resection could be chosen for a patient with unresectable liver or pulmonary metastases.

The type of operation is determined by the location of the tumor within the rectum, the ability to obtain the necessary 2-cm distal margin of normal rectum, and the body habitus of the patient. Lesions located in the upper third of the rectum (between 10 and 15 cm) are resected and intestinal continuity reestablished by either a stapled or hand-sewn anastomosis. In this way, the sphincter is preserved and there is minimal, if any, disturbance of intestinal function. Lesions located in the mid-third of the rectum (between 5 and 10 cm) can be treated in a similar manner if the body habitus of the patient and the skill of the surgeon permit a safe low pelvic anastomosis. If this is not possible, a coloanal anastomosis (suturing the colon directly to the anal canal after removal of the rectum) is another option for sphincter preservation. Last, an abdominoperineal resection, which necessitates a permanent colostomy, can be performed for midrectal cancers if the anastomotic techniques just described are not possible. Cancers in the distal rectum (0 to 5 cm) generally are removed by an abdominoperineal resection because the distal margin above the sphincter and below the tumor is inadequate to permit the preservation of anorectal function.

Approximately 5 to 10% of rectal cancers can be treated with local (transanal) means while a high cure rate is maintained. Strict preoperative selection criteria must be satisfied before local therapy is undertaken: namely the lesions must be minimally invasive, be well-differentiated, have no penetration of the vascular or lymphatic channels, and be no larger than 3 to 4 cm. Preoperative endorectal ultrasonography may help select which tumors can be treated thus. Electrocoagulation with a needle-tip coagulator eradicates a tumor down to its base and thus maintains rectal patency. Five-year survival rates of 50 to 60% have been reported, and operative complications are few. High-dose contact radiotherapy performed during multiple sessions can eradicate a superficial carcinoma. The radiation is delivered transanally through a specially designed rectoscope. The depth of penetration is only approximately 6 mm; therefore, proper selection of patients is essential if this is to be applied with curative intent. A full-thickness transanal excision with a 5- to 10-mm rim of normal mucosa is preferred because it allows for a more thorough histologic assessment; further decisions regarding radical surgery or external radiation can be made on the basis of histologic and morphologic features of the tumor.

Adjuvant Therapy

Colon Cancer

There is no evidence to suggest that preoperative radiation or chemotherapy offers a survival benefit for colon cancer. Patients with lymph node metastases (Duke's type C) have significantly improved survival if postoperative 5-fluorouracil is given in conjunction with levamisole.

Rectal Cancer

Preoperative radiation therapy and chemotherapy have been used in an attempt to improve the resectability of locally advanced rectal cancers. Such a treatment regimen has been shown to downstage a tumor and to lower local recurrence rates. However, an improvement in survival has not been consistently reported. Postoperative radiation therapy alone similarly lowers local recurrence rates without an appreciable effect on survival. When postoperative radiation therapy is combined with chemotherapy for patients in whom tumors had either transmural penetration or lymph node metastases, significant improvements are noted in overall survival and disease-free survival.

Treatment of Metastatic Disease

Because there are no effective chemotherapeutic regimens that when given alone can cure metastatic colorectal cancer, surgery should be considered for selected patients with metastatic disease. The primary tumor must be controlled or controllable; resection of the metastatic burden must be anatomically feasible with preservation of normal function postoperatively; the cancer must not have spread into multiple organ systems; and the patient must have an acceptable operative risk. If these selection criteria have been met, surgery may be undertaken.

Liver Resection

Approximately 20% of patients are found to have liver metastases at the time of laparotomy for the primary tumor; ultimately, metastases occur in 70% during the course of the disease. If left untreated, virtually all patients die within 2 years. Five-year survival rates of approximately 30% have been observed after liver resection for metastatic disease. In general, resection is to be avoided if both lobes of the liver are involved, if the porta hepatis is involved, and if there are more than four nodules within the liver.

Thoracotomy

In approximately 10 to 15% of patients, pulmonary metastases develop during the course of the illness; unfortunately, in most cases the cancer is disseminated, and rarely is it limited solely to the lungs. Only 1 to 2% of patients with a history of colorectal cancer ever undergo thoracotomy. Five-year survival rates as high as 47% and a median survival length of 24 to 42 months have been noted after thoracotomy for metastatic disease. Patients with solitary nodules and those with longer disease-free intervals between resection of the primary tumor and thoracotomy seem to fare better. Despite these favorable results, cancer recurs in the lungs in most patients, usually with dissemination to other organ systems as well. Death is still most likely caused by recurrent colorectal cancer.

Follow-Up

Carcinoembryonic Antigen (CEA)

Although CEA levels are not useful as a means for screening patients for colorectal cancer, elevated levels obtained postoperatively may herald recurrence of cancer before the development of symptoms. A baseline preoperative level should be obtained; an elevated level is more frequently associated with subsequent recurrence of cancer. Postoperatively, CEA levels should be measured at 2 to 3-month intervals for the first 2 years. If levels are elevated, further evaluation with endoscopy, chest radiographs, and/or computed tomographs of the abdomen are in order.

Endoscopy

Colonoscopy is recommended 1 year after surgery to detect recurrences, as well as metachronous cancers or polyps, along suture lines. True isolated suture line recurrences without disease elsewhere are rare; recurrence in the tumor bed or pelvis with subsequent erosion through the anastomosis is more common. Colonoscopy should be repeated at 2 to 3-year intervals as long as each examination is normal.

Chest Radiographs

Chest x-rays should be obtained at 6-month intervals and continued for approximately 5 years because the appearance of pulmonary nodules may be delayed. If plain radiographs reveal one or more nodules, further studies with linear or computed tomography are required in order to inspect for calcifications within the nodule and to detect additional nodules elsewhere in the lung.

Computed Tomograms of the Abdomen

Abdominal computed tomographic scans are generally not routinely obtained unless symptoms, physical examination, or elevated CEA levels suggest a recurrence.

Other Cancers

Cancer surveillance for other tumor types should not be forgotten. Women should undergo mammograms, pelvic examinations, and Pap smears at the appropriate time intervals, and men should undergo prostate examinations.

INTESTINAL PARASITES

method of
MARTIN S. WOLFE, M.D.
Traveler's Medical Service
Washington, D.C.

Intestinal protozoa and helminths constitute major disease problems worldwide. Because they are ubiquitous, they must always be considered in dealing with the disease problems of populations in both the developing and developed world. Intestinal parasites may be contracted in the United States by, for example, campers and hikers drinking untreated stream water; those served by certain small community water supplies; children in day care centers; male homosexuals; and institutionalized individuals. Imported infections can be present in Americans returning from travel or residence in the developing world and in immigrants and refugees from developing countries. It is important to consider the possibility of an intestinal parasitic infection in such persons before embarking on a time-consuming and costly medical work-up. The proper performance of certain relatively simple and inexpensive laboratory procedures can often lead to the finding of an intestinal parasite as the explanation of a perplexing symptom complex. This can then be treated in a straightforward manner, usually with results highly gratifying to both patient and physician.

Most of the drugs described here are licensed and commercially available in the United States. Some are currently licensed for some indications but not for others. A few foreign-made drugs are not approved in the United States but may be obtained from the Parasitic Disease Drug Service of the Centers for Disease Control in Atlanta, Georgia (telephone 1-404-639-3670).

Summaries of drug therapies for intestinal protozoa and helminths are given in Tables 1 to 4.

PROTOZOAN INFECTIONS

Giardia lamblia

This is the most common pathogenic intestinal protozoa diagnosed in the United States, particularly affecting campers and hikers, male homosexuals, and children and staff in day care centers. *G. lamblia* is contracted in both temperate and tropical areas worldwide. Although not all those infected are symptomatic, the majority have some of the following typical symptoms: foul diarrhea and flatulence, abdominal distention, weight loss, fatigue, and malabsorption.

The most effective drug is quinacrine hydro-

chloride (Atabrine). Cure rates of 90 to 95% are usually reported. Common side effects include gastrointestinal discomfort, headache, and dizziness. Less frequent but more disturbing side effects include yellow discoloration of the skin and sclerae, vomiting, fever, exfoliative dermatitis, and toxic psychosis (1.5% incidence). Tolerance in young children may be improved by placing the ground-up portion of the tablet required in a gelatin capsule. In 1993 the manufacturer became unable to obtain certain raw materials needed to produce quinacrine, and the drug is difficult if not impossible to obtain, both in the United States and abroad.

Metronidazole (Flagyl) remains unapproved for giardiasis in the United States, but it is frequently prescribed. Although somewhat less effective than quinacrine, it is generally better tolerated. Side effects may include nausea; metallic taste; dark urine; possible *Candida* overgrowth on the skin, on mucous membranes, and in the intestine; and a disulfiram-like effect when taken with alcohol. Authors of a number of reviews consider the risk to humans of carcinogenicity and mutagenicity to be low, if not negligible, but have recommended that physicians must decide whether benefit from the drug outweighs the potential risk.

Furazolidone (Furoxone) is an antibiotic whose

TABLE 1. **Drug Therapy of Intestinal Protozoan Parasites***

Parasite	Drug	Adult Dose†	Pediatric Dose†	Availability
Giardia lamblia	Metronidazole	250 mg tid × 7 days	5 mg/kg tid × 7 days	Flagyl (Searle) (tablets)
	or Quinacrine Hcl	100 mg tid × 5 days	2 mg/kg tid × 5 days	Atabrine (Winthrop) (tablets)
	or Furazolidone	100 mg (tablet) qid × 7 days	1.25 mg/kg qid × 7 days (suspension)	Furoxone (Roberts) (tablets and suspension)
Dientamoeba fragilis	Paromomycin	500 mg tid × 7 days	30 mg/kg/day in 3 divided doses × 7 days	Humatin (Parke-Davis) (capsules)
	or Iodoquinol	650 mg tid × 20 days	40 mg/kg/day in 3 divided doses × 20 days	Yodoxin (Glenwood, Inc.) (tablets)
	or Tetracycline	500 mg qid × 10 days	10 mg/kg qid × 10 days (max 2 gm/day) above age 8 years	
Balantidium coli	Iodoquinol	As per *D. fragilis*	As per *D. fragilis*	
	or Tetracycline	As per *D. fragilis*	As per *D. fragilis*	
Isospora belli	Trimethoprim-sulfamethoxazole (TMP-SMX)	160 mg TMP/800 mg SMX qid × 10 days, then bid × 3 weeks	—	Bactrim (Roche) (tablets) Septra (Burroughs-Wellcome) (tablets)
Cryptosporidium	Spiramycin‡	3 gm/day in divided doses for 2 to 4 weeks	—	Rovamycin (Rhone-Poulenc Montreal) (tablets)
Blastocystis hominis	Iodoquinol	As per *D. fragilis*	As per *D. fragilis*	
	or Metronidazole	As per *G. lamblia*	As per *G. lamblia*	

Entamoeba histolytica is discussed in a separate article.
†All recommended drugs given by mouth.
‡Not approved in the United States. Permission to use this drug must be obtained from the U.S. Food and Drug Administration.

TABLE 2. **Drug Therapy of Intestinal Helminths—Part One**

Parasite	Drug	Adult Dose*	Pediatric Dose*	Availability
Ascaris lumbricoides	Mebendazole or	100 mg bid × 3 days	Same as adult dose (>2 years)	Vermox (Jannsen) (tablets)
	Pyrantel pamoate	11 mg/kg single dose (max 1 gm)	Same as adult dose (max 1 gm)	Antiminth (Pfizer) (suspension)
Trichuris trichiura	Mebendazole	As per *Ascaris*	As per *Ascaris*	
Hookworm *Necator americanus*	Mebandazole or	As per *Ascaris*	As per *Ascaris*	
Ancylostoma duodenale	Pyrantel pamoate†	As per *Ascaris*	As per *Ascaris*	
Enterobius vermicularis	Mebendazole or	100-mg single dose; repeat in 2 weeks	Same as adult dose (>2 years)	
	Pyrantel pamoate	11 mg/kg single dose; repeat in 2 weeks	Same as adult dose	
Strongyloides stercoralis	Thiabendazole or	25 mg/kg bid × 2 days (max 3 gm/day)	Same as adult dose	Mintezol (Merck, Sharp and Dohme) (suspension and tablets)
	Mebendazole†	As per *Ascaris*	As per *Ascaris*	
Trichostrongylus spp.	Thiabendazole† or	As per *Strongyloides*	As per *Strongyloides*	
	Pyrantel pamoate† or	As per *Ascaris*	As per *Ascaris*	
	Mebendazole†	As per *Ascaris*	As per *Ascaris*	

*All recommended drugs given by mouth.
†Considered an investigational drug for this purpose by the U.S. Food and Drug Administration.

major indication for use in the United States is for giardiasis. It is the only one of the three available anti-*Giardia* drugs produced in suspension form, making it particularly useful in young children. Cure rates have ranged from 77 to 92%. Side effects may include vomiting, diarrhea, nausea, fever, and skin rash. Furazolidone can produce a disulfiram-like reaction with alcohol; it is a monoamine oxidase inhibitor; and it may cause mild hemolysis in patients with glucose-6-phosphate dehydrogenase deficiency.

Tinidazole (Fasigyn) is not available in the United States, but in reports from abroad, a single 2-gram dose has been found to be more effective and better tolerated than metronidazole, a related nitromidazole product.

Dientamoeba fragilis

Formerly thought to be an ameba, *D. fragilis* is now considered an ameba-like flagellate occurring only in a labile trophozoite form. Although considered a nonpathogen by some authors, in recent years correlation has been found with infection and intermittent diarrhea, abdominal pain, anorexia, and in some cases eosinophilia. It is being increasingly recognized in diagnostic parasitology laboratories in the United States, especially when stained slides are made from specimens collected in preservative. Tetracycline and iodoquinol (Yodoxin) are often mentioned as the drugs of choice, but careful review of the litera-

ture indicates that cure rates are not high with these drugs. Paromomycin (Humatin) is more effective, although this drug may cause diarrhea and other intestinal side effects.

Balantidium coli

This ciliated parasite has a worldwide distribution, and infection is particularly common in pigs, which are the main reservoir of infection to humans. *B. coli* is very rarely diagnosed in the United States. The drug of choice is iodoquinol or tetracycline.

Isospora belli

This sporozoan parasite also has a worldwide distribution, but is uncommonly diagnosed. It has recently been recognized as an opportunistic infection in immunosuppressed individuals and in male homosexuals. Trimethoprim-sulfamethoxazole has been found to be curative.

Cryptosporidium

This coccidial parasite has in recent years been increasingly recognized as a cause of diarrhea in humans. It is a cause of highly lethal fulminant diarrhea in patients with acquired immune deficiency syndrome (AIDS). *Cryptosporidium* has also been recognized in immunologically normal children and adults in various parts of the world,

TABLE 3. **Drug Therapy of Intestinal Helminths—Part Two**

Parasite	Drug	Adult Dose*	Pediatric Dose*	Availability
Tapeworms				
Taenia saginata	Niclosamide or	Single dose/4 tabs (2 gm) chewed thoroughly	11–34 kg: single dose/ 2 tabs (1 gm) >34 kg: single dose/3 tabs (1.5 gm)	Niclocide (Miles) (tablets)
Taenia solium	Paromomycin†	1 gm q 15 minutes × 4 doses	11 mg/kg q 15 min × 4 doses	Humatin (Parke-Davis) (capsules)
Diphyllobothrium latum and *pacificum* *Dipylidium caninum*	or Praziquantel†	15 to 20 mg/kg once	Same as adult dose	Biltricide (Miles)
Hymenolepis nana	Niclosamide or	Single 2-gm/dose × 6 days	As above for other tapeworms, single dose daily × 6 days	
	Praziquantel†	15 to 20 mg/kg once	Same as adult dose	
Cerebral *Cysticercus cellulosae*	Praziquantel†	50 mg/kg/day in 3 divided doses × 14 days	Same as adult dose	
Schistosomiasis				
S. mansoni	Praziquantel† or	40 mg/kg in 2 divided doses for 1 day	Same as adult dose	Biltricide (Miles) (tablets)
	Oxamniquine	Caribbean and South American strains: 15 mg/kg single dose African strains: 15 mg/kg bid × 2 days	Same as adult dose	Vansil (Pfizer) (tablets)
S. japonicum	Praziquantel	60 mg/kg in 3 divided doses for 1 day	Same as adult dose	
S. mekongi	Praziquantel	As per *S. japonicum*	As per *S. japonicum*	
S. intercalatum	Praziquantel	As per *S. mansoni*	As per *S. mansoni*	
S. hematobium	Praziquantel	40 mg/kg in 2 divided doses for 1 day	Same as adult dose	

*All recommended drugs given by mouth.
†Considered an investigational drug for this purpose by the U.S. Food and Drug Administration.

TABLE 4. **Drug Therapy of Intestinal Helminths—Part Three**

Parasite	Drug	Adult Dose*	Pediatric Dose*	Availability
Intestinal flukes				
Fasciolopsis buskii *Heterophyes heterophyes* *Metagonimus yokogawi*	Praziquantel†	25 mg/kg tid for 1 day	Same as adult dose	
Liver flukes				
Clonorchis sinensis *Opisthorchis viverrini*	Praziquantel†	25 mg/kg tid for 1 day	Same as adult dose	
Fasciola hepatica	Bithionol† (capsule) or	30 to 50 mg/kg on alternate days × 10–15 doses	Same as adult dose	Parasitic Disease Drug Service, Centers for Disease Control, Atlanta, Georgia
	Praziquantel†	25 mg/kg tid for 1 day	Same as adult dose	
Paragonimus westermani	Praziquantel† or	25 mg/kg tid for 1 day	Same as adult dose	
	Bithionol†	As per *F. hepatica*	As per *F. hepatica*	

*All recommended drugs given by mouth.
†Considered an investigational drug for this purpose by the U.S. Food and Drug Administration.

after community water-borne outbreaks, in travelers, and in day care centers in the United States. In these individuals, infections are either asymptomatic or self-limited after about 7 to 21 days. A satisfactory drug has not yet been identified. A few patients have had relief of diarrhea with negative stool examinations and upper intestinal biopsy at the end of a 4-week course of spiramycin (Rovamycin). Permission to use this drug must be obtained from the U.S. Food and Drug Administration. Treatment is primarily symptomatic and includes adequate fluid and nutritional support. In a few cases, successful reversal of the underlying immune deficiency has cleared the parasites. Somatostatin (Octreotide), paromomycin (Humatin), and azithromycin (Zithromax) are being investigated for treatment of severe diarrhea in AIDS patients.

Microsporidiosis

An increasingly recognized cause of chronic diarrhea and weight loss in homosexual men is *Enterocytozoon bienuesi*. Early cases were diagnosed by intestinal biopsy, examined under light microscopy and confirmed by electron microscopy. Recently, diagnosis has been possible with direct fecal smears stained with a modified trichrome stain. At this time, no effective treatment is available. Partial remission has been achieved with metronidazole and octreotide. Albendazole has been found to cause degenerative changes in the organism and to control diarrhea, and it appears to be a useful palliative treatment.

Cyanobacterium-Like Bodies (CLB)

Cyanobacteria are considered by many researchers to be coccidian parasites resembling large cryptosporidia. Outbreaks and individual cases in immunocompromised persons and normal travelers have been described. Symptoms include malaise, explosive watery diarrhea, cramps, and nausea, which have lasted for up to 4 weeks with cycles of relapses and remissions. There is currently no published or anecdotal information on drug treatment of this infection.

Blastocystis hominis

This is a commonly diagnosed parasite whose pathogenicity is not well established. It is frequently found in small numbers in asymptomatic individuals and necessitates no treatment. In one careful study of symptomatic persons with *B. hominis* infection, most were harboring another difficult-to-recognize pathogenic protozoa. When *B. hominis* is present in large numbers in the absence of other pathogenic organisms in a symptomatic patient, treatment might be indicated. Drugs used include iodoquinol and nitroimidazoles, but no drug has been proven regularly effective, and no well-controlled studies have been reported.

Nonpathogenic Protozoa

A number of nonpathogenic amebae and flagellates are frequently found on stool examination, indicating fecal contamination of the host. If intestinal symptoms are present, further search should be made for recognized pathogens. These nonpathogens include *Entamoeba hartmanni, Entamoeba coli, Endolimax nana, Iodamoeba bütschlii, Chilomastix mesnili, Trichomonas hominis, Enteromonas hominis,* and *Retortamonas intestinalis. Entamoeba histolytica* is discussed in a separate article.

HELMINTHIC INFECTIONS
Ascaris lumbricoides (Roundworm)

A number of safe and effective drugs are available for this infection. Mebendazole (Vermox) for 3 days is well tolerated and approximately 98% effective. Pyrantel pamoate (Antiminth) in a single dose is also highly effective, but side effects may be more common. When *Ascaris* is present with another intestinal helminth, it should preferentially be treated first because some drugs can cause *Ascaris* worms to migrate to aberrant locations.

Trichuris trichiura (Whipworm)

This is perhaps the commonest intestinal helminthic infection and is often associated with *Ascaris*. Most infections seen in the United States are asymptomatic, but all infections can be treated with mebendazole. Cure rates are about 70%, but there is a 98% egg reduction rate. In severely infected children in developing countries, rectal prolapse and anemia may be caused by *Trichuris* and a 0.2% hexylresorcinol retention enema* can be administered.

Hookworm Infections

A distinction must be made in temperate areas between (1) hookworm infection or carrier state and (2) the less common hookworm disease with anemia. Hookworm infection may be treated with antihelminthic drugs alone, but hookworm dis-

---

*Not commercially available in the United States.

ease with anemia must also be treated with iron supplements and, in severe anemia, with transfusions. Mebendazole for 3 days is effective against both common species of hookworm, *Necator americanus* and *Ancylostoma duodenale*. Pyrantel pamoate is an alternative.

Enterobius vermicularis (Pinworm)

This is a cosmopolitan infection, found more commonly in middle-class children in the United States than in children in developing countries. Although pinworm infection is usually a scourge of children, adults—particularly parents of infected children—can also be infected. Single-dose treatments, repeated in 2 weeks, with mebendazole or pyrantel pamoate are highly effective and well tolerated. It is acceptable practice to treat the entire family when at least one member is known to be infected. Attempts should be made to prevent reinfection by such measures as keeping nails short, showering every morning, and wearing snug-fitting undergarments. More heroic measures, such as soaking night clothes and bed linen in ammonia (or boiling these) and scrubbing or disinfecting floors and toilet seats, are usually doomed to failure owing to the hardiness of the eggs and their frequent reintroduction into the household.

Strongyloides stercoralis

This parasite can live for 30 to 40 years in an infected host, because of its unique autoinfection cycle leading to self-perpetuating infection. The continued presence of this parasite poses a potential threat of lethal dissemination by hyperinfection if the infected individual becomes immunosuppressed or is treated with cancer chemotherapy, radiation therapy, or corticosteroids. *S. stercoralis* must be considered in anyone who has been in an endemic area and has an otherwise unexplained eosinophilia and/or periodic diarrhea and intestinal discomfort, urticaria, creeping eruption in the area of the buttocks and thighs, and possibly pulmonary complaints. The currently available treatment of choice is thiabendazole (Mintezol) in a 2-day course. Although highly effective, this drug is often not well tolerated, particularly in adults, and can cause nausea, vomiting, dizziness, and rarely angioneurotic edema. Mebendazole, an alternative treatment, is better tolerated but less effective. Albendazole and ivermectin, newer broad-spectrum antihelminthics (not yet available in the United States), have shown good effect against *S. stercoralis* in studies elsewhere. In disseminated strongyloidiasis, thiabendazole should be continued for at least 5 days.

Trichostrongylus Species

This parasite is particularly common in Iran, Korea, and Indonesia and may be the cause of a high eosinophilia and gastrointestinal symptoms in some infected patients. Thiabendazole, in doses used for strongyloidiasis, is the drug of choice. Pyrantel pamoate and mebendazole are alternative drugs.

Tapeworm Infections

Taenia saginata (the beef tapeworm), *Taenia solium* (the pork tapeworm), *Diphyllobothrium latum* and *pacificum* (fish tapeworms), and *Dipylidium caninum* are best treated with a single dose of niclosamide (Niclocide). An alternative drug is paromomycin (Humatin). Praziquantel (Biltricide) is an effective single-dose treatment but is not yet approved in the United States for use against tapeworms. *Hymenolepis nana* (the dwarf tapeworm) and the much less common *Hymenolepis diminuta* necessitate a 6-day course of niclosamide or a single dose of praziquantel.

Tissue invasion of the brain or muscles with *Cysticercus cellulosae*, the larval form of *T. solium*, can now be treated with praziquantel, on an investigational basis. Corticosteroids should be given concomitantly to counter any increased cerebral pressure caused by destruction of cysts. Albendazole has been used effectively abroad but is not yet licensed in the United States. Praziquantel is not recommended for ocular cysticercosis.

Schistosomiasis

The most common form of intestinal schistosomiasis seen in the United States is *Schistosomiasis mansoni*. Rare cases of *S. japonicum* from East Asia, *S. mekongi* in refugees from Southeast Asia, and *S. intercalatum* from Central Africa may also be seen. The treatment of choice for all these species, as well as for urinary schistosomiasis (*S. hematobium*), is praziquantel in a single-day course. This drug is now approved in the United States for treatment of all forms of schistosomiasis; it is effective and well tolerated, and all patients with active schistosomiasis infection should be treated. Oxamniquine (Vansil) is an alternative drug for *S. mansoni*. Somewhat higher doses of oxamniquine are required for the African strain than for the Caribbean strain.

Intestinal Flukes

Fasciolopsis buskii, Heterophyes heterophyes, and *Metagonimus yokogawi* are very rare parasites in the United States. All can be treated with praziquantel, which is currently an investigational drug in the United States for these parasites.

Liver Flukes

Clonorchis sinensis and *Opisthorchis viverrini* infections are not uncommon in refugees from and natives or residents of the Far East and Southeast Asia. *Fasciola hepatica* is rarely reported in the United States. Eggs of *Paragonimus westermani,* the lung fluke, may be found in the stool, and this parasite may in rare cases cause cerebral lesions. Praziquantel, investigational in

the United States also for these parasites, is the drug of choice for all except *F. hepatica*; bithionol, also investigational, is more effective for *F. hepatica.*

Follow-Up Examinations

In all patients receiving treatment for intestinal parasites, three stool examinations for ova and parasites should be examined by direct and concentration methods and stained slides, approximately 4 weeks after completion of treatment, as a check for cure.

Metabolic Disorders

DIABETES MELLITUS IN ADULTS

method of
JAMES W. ANDERSON, M.D.
Veterans Administration Medical Center
Lexington, Kentucky

and

MIRIAM OLIVEROS DE ANGULO, M.D.
University of Caraboro
Valencia, Venezuela

Diabetes affects over 13 million Americans and costs over $23 billion in direct and indirect costs. About 90% of diabetic patients in the United States are adults with non–insulin-dependent (Type II) diabetes, and 60 to 80% of these are obese. Type II diabetes is inherited, and the genetic diathesis ranges from 25% for Caucasians to 50% for Native Americans. Obesity, high-fat diets, low-fiber intake, and lack of exercise enhance expression of this condition. A major challenge of diabetes management is enabling patients to make important lifestyle changes.

Diabetes is diagnosed by finding at least two fasting plasma glucose values exceeding 140 mg per dL or random glucose values above 200 mg per dL with symptoms of diabetes. Oral glucose tolerance tests should not be performed for the diagnosis of diabetes in nonpregnant persons and are rarely indicated in clinical practice except during pregnancy. Because diabetes is diagnosed, on average, 4 years after the onset of significant hyperglycemia, any random plasma glucose level above 150 mg per dL should alert the practitioner to the possibility of diabetes and trigger measurements of fasting glucose levels.

Therapeutic objectives for management of Type II diabetes are (1) to achieve and maintain normal metabolism and biochemistry and (2) to prevent microvascular and macrovascular (atherosclerotic) complications. *Practical goals* for Type II patients are (1) to alleviate symptoms such as polyuria and blurred vision, (2) to maintain health and well-being, and (3) to prevent chronic complications.

TREATMENT

Maintaining good glycemic control reduces risk for complications of diabetes. Goals of glycemic control should be individualized. In general, fasting plasma glucose levels should be less than 140 mg per dL and postprandial plasma glucose levels should be less than 200 mg per dL (Table 1). These levels usually correspond to a hemoglobin A_{1C} (glycohemoglobin) level of less than 7.0% (15% above the upper limit of normal for laboratory).

Good glycemic control should be achieved without significant hypoglycemia or substantial weight gain. Type II patients are less susceptible to hypoglycemia than insulin-dependent patients, and hypoglycemia is usually not a problem unless they have gastric emptying problems, malabsorption, or renal failure. Weight gain, however, seems to be inevitable when glycemic control in Type II patients changes from poor to good. A weight gain of about 1% of body weight is related to rehydration and restoration of normal metabolism. Further weight gain appears related to hyperinsulinemia. Whether good to excellent glycemic control at the expense of significant weight gain reduces risks for atherosclerotic cardiovascular disease is unclear.

Monitoring Glycemic Control

Self-monitoring of blood glucose (SMBG) represents a significant advance in diabetes management. SMBG enables diabetic persons to get involved in self-management and assume responsibility for glycemic control. Glucose monitors are inexpensive and provide accuracy that is not possible with visual readings. Most Type II diabetic persons should perform SMBG at least once daily. For patients who achieve good to excellent control by using diet and exercise, monitoring 3 days

TABLE 1. **Assessment of Glycemic Control**

Measurement	Normal	Acceptable	Poor
Fasting plasma glucose	<115	<140	>200 mg/dL
Postprandial plasma glucose	<140	<200	>235 mg/dL
Glycosylated hemoglobin	<6	<7	>10%

weekly is adequate. For insulin-treated patients, SMBG at least twice daily is essential. For excellent glycemic control, SMBG must be performed four times daily, before meals and bedtime.

Dietary Modification

Diet is the cornerstone of management of Type II diabetes. Most diabetic patients eat too much fat and protein and too little carbohydrate and fiber. Diabetes associations in Western countries have, by consensus, a recommendation that diabetic patients get 50 to 60% of energy from carbohydrates, 12 to 15% from protein, and less than 30% from fat, and about 40 grams of fiber daily (Table 2). Diets may include more fat if the additional fat is monounsaturated.

Lean Patients

After diagnosis of Type II diabetes, a patient should be referred to a dietitian or an experienced nutritionist for instruction in a diabetes diet incorporating the features outlined in Table 2. *Energy requirements* are about 12 kcal per pound of actual body weight for most men and about 11 kcal per pound of body weight for most women. Energy expended in aerobic exercise and physical activity is added to these requirements. Type II diabetic patients should have three meals per day, those taking insulin should have a bedtime snack, and some insulin-treated patients need midmorning and midafternoon snacks.

Fat is the major problem in the diet of diabetic patients. Most diabetic patients eat substantially more fat than the average American despite recommendations to consume less than 30% of energy from fat. Excessive fat intake contributes to weight gain, produces resistance to insulin action with resulting hyperinsulinemia, and increases low-density lipoprotein (LDL) cholesterol.

Complex carbohydrates and fiber offer major benefits for diabetic individuals. Foods rich in carbohydrates and fiber promote weight maintenance; enhance insulin sensitivity, thereby reducing hyperinsulinemia; and lower LDL cholesterol

levels. These foods are rich in vitamins, minerals, and antioxidants. Sucrose, fructose, and other sugars can be included in reasonable amounts.

Most Americans consume 150% of recommended amounts of *protein* per day and diabetic persons use even more protein. High protein intake is often accompanied by high saturated fat intake, thereby enhancing risk for coronary heart disease. High-protein diets may contribute to osteoporosis and accelerate development of renal disease.

Alcohol if used should not exceed 10 drinks per week; one serving is 4 ounces of wine, 12 ounces of beer, or 1.5 ounces of distilled beverage. Although alcohol may raise high-density lipoprotein (HDL) cholesterol levels, it may also increase blood pressure, raise serum triglyceride levels, contribute to weight gain, and cause errors in medication use.

Obese Patients

Most diabetic patients should be encouraged to achieve and maintain a body weight of less than 30% above ideal for their height or a body mass index of less than 30 kg per M^2. Overweight diabetic patients—those with weights exceeding 10% above desirable—also benefit from an exercise and weight-reduction program. Desirable body weight can be estimated quickly as follows: for men, allow 115 pounds for 60 inches of height and 5 pounds for every inch above 60 inches; for women, allow 100 pounds for 60 inches of height and 5 pounds for every inch above 60 inches. When obese Type II patients lose weight, improvements are seen in these parameters: blood glucose levels, glycohemoglobin, blood pressure, and serum cholesterol, LDL cholesterol, triglycerides, and HDL cholesterol levels. Furthermore, weight reduction increases insulin sensitivity and reduces requirements for insulin or oral hypoglycemic agents as well as antihypertensive medications.

Table 3 outlines recommendations for weight-loss programs at different levels of weight excess and obesity. Most obese diabetic patients require medical supervision during weight loss and should not embark on any aggressive weight loss program without careful medical supervision. Patients with body mass indexes (BMIs) < 30 kg per M^2 can safely participate in community programs without medical supervision if they use SMBG and have guidance about adjusting insulin or oral agents. Most patients with BMIs > 30 kg per M^2 require careful medical monitoring, and all patients on very-low-calorie diets must be medically monitored by experienced physicians.

Fundamental Principles. All weight-loss programs should include these three fundamentals:

TABLE 2. **Nutrition Recommendations**

Nutrient	Amount
Carbohydrate	50–60% of calories
Protein	12–15% of calories (0.8 gm/kg)
Fat, total	<30% of calories
Saturated fat	<10% of calories
Monounsaturated fat	12–15% of calories
Polyunsaturated fat	6–8% of calories
Cholesterol	<200 mg/day
Fiber	About 40 gm/day (15–25 gm/ 1000 kcal)
Sodium	<1 gm/1000 kcal

TABLE 3. **Weight Loss Approaches**

BMI (kg/M²)	% Desirable Weight*	Diet Recommendations
<28	110–120	Community program Medical supervision not required
28–30	120–130	High-fiber, weight-reducing diet Meal replacement with food program Minimal medical supervision
30–35	130–160	Very-low-calorie diet with medical supervision High-fiber, weight-reducing diet with minimal medical supervision
35–40	160–180	Very-low-calorie diet with medical supervision
>40	>180	Gastrointestinal surgery should be considered

Abbreviation: BMI = body mass index.

*Values for % desirable weight do not correspond to BMI for all individuals but are given as a further point of reference.

(1) a well-balanced hypocaloric diet, (2) an exercise plan, and (3) careful record keeping of all food intake and exercise. Frequent follow-up is, of course, essential. The diet can be a very-low-calorie diet with adequate protein, vitamins, and minerals or a balanced, low-fat weight-reducing diet. The exercise plan should encourage the patient to expend at least 2000 kcal in physical activity per week; this represents walking about 12 to 18 miles per week. Finally, all food should be recorded at the time eaten.

Physical Activity

Regular aerobic exercise, such as walking, decreases risk for coronary heart disease events and enhances insulin sensitivity for persons with Type II diabetes. Sustained increases in physical activity also can lower blood pressure, raise HDL cholesterol levels, assist in weight management, and improve patients' sense of well-being. Lower insulin or oral agent requirements and decreased medication costs are important by-products of a regular exercise program.

Assessing Risks. Although there are general health benefits and specific diabetes management benefits from exercise, there also are distinct risks. Walking is an exercise that is safe and can be done by virtually everyone who is ambulatory. More vigorous exercise—such as jogging, running, or stair climbing—has these risks: increased likelihood of sudden death while exercising, aggravation of poorly controlled hypertension, hypoglycemia, hyperglycemia, and ketonemia.

Before starting a vigorous program, patients over the age of 35 should undergo an evaluation for hypertension and neuropathy and have an exercise-stress electrocardiogram. Persons with suboptimal blood pressure control may need ambulatory blood pressure monitoring. All patients should monitor their heart rate, which should not exceed 70% of the target heart rate (220 beats per minute minus age).

Glycemic control also affects exercise guidelines. Persons treated with diet alone and most persons taking oral agents can exercise without fear of hypoglycemia or untoward hyperglycemia. Insulin-treated patients need to recognize that vigorous exercise is best undertaken when the blood glucose ranges from 100 to 300 mg per dL because exercise can precipitate hypoglycemia or worsen hyperglycemia. All persons with diabetes should follow these guidelines: (1) use proper footwear; (2) avoid extremes of temperature; (3) inspect feet daily after exercise; and (4) avoid exercise during periods of poor metabolic control. Despite the risks, most diabetic patients gain distinct benefits from a regular walking program.

Oral Hypoglycemic Agents

Diet, exercise, and weight management should be pushed to the maximum before a patient starts taking pharmacologic agents. When fasting plasma glucose values consistently exceed 140 mg per dL, oral agents are usually introduced as the next step. Only sulfonylureas are available in the United States, but biguanide agents such as metformin are used successfully in other countries.

The sulfonylurea agents are safe and effective. The mechanism of action of these agents is complex: they act primarily by stimulating release of insulin from the pancreas, but they may also enhance sensitivity of the liver and peripheral tissues to insulin action. Contraindications to use of sulfonylurea agents include pregnancy or lactation and allergy to sulfonylureas. These agents may not be effective during periods of severe stress.

Some characteristics of the sulfonylurea agents currently available in the United States are compared in Table 4. The first-generation agents (acetohexamide, chlorpropamide, tolazamide, and tolbutamide) are less expensive and are available as generic drugs. Although the first-generation agents are as effective as the second-generation agents, the first-generation agents produce more side effects. Hyponatremia and the alcohol-flushing syndrome do not occur with the second-generation agents, and severe hypoglycemia is much less common with the second-generation agents. The most common side effects with the sulfonylurea agents are gastrointestinal symptoms and skin rashes; rare side effects are hematologic disorders and hepatotoxicity. Results of one study

TABLE 4. **Oral Hypoglycemic Agents**

Generic Name	Brand Name	Dose Range (mg/day)	Daily Frequency
Second-Generation			
Glipizide	Glucotrol	2.5–40	1–2
Glyburide	DiaBeta, Micronase	1.25–20	1–2
First-Generation			
Acetohexamide	Dymelor	250–1500	1–2
Chlorpropamide	Diabinese	100–500	1
Tolazamide	Tolinase	100–1000	1–2
Tolbutamide	Orinase	500–3000	2–3

suggested that oral hypoglycemic agents might increase risk for myocardial infarctions; this suggestion, however, has not been supported by further studies.

Glyburide (Micronase, DiaBeta) and glipizide (Glucatrol) are the most commonly used sulfonylurea agents in the United States; these two agents are very similar. The usual starting dose is 2.5 mg of glyburide or 5.0 mg of glipizide before breakfast. For elderly patients, the starting dose is 1.25 mg of glyburide or 2.5 mg of glipizide before breakfast. The dose is increased every 1 to 2 weeks until glycemic control is achieved or the maximal dose is reached. Usually when the prebreakfast dose exceeds 10 mg, the dose is divided, and one-third to one-half the daily dose is given before the evening meal.

In some patients reactive hypoglycemia develops with the sulfonylureas. When the fasting blood glucose levels are satisfactory, the timing of doses can be adjusted. Some newly diagnosed diabetic patients require sulfonylurea agents for only a few weeks and subsequently can be managed with diet and exercise.

Diabetic patients should be reminded that sulfonylurea agents do not replace diet, exercise, and weight management. These behaviors should be strongly reinforced when oral agents are initiated and at each visit to the physician. Diabetic patients commonly gain weight with oral agents. Two or three pounds of weight gain is acceptable and may be related to better metabolic control. However, a weight gain of more that 5 pounds should be treated by intensive counseling on nutrition and exercise.

Insulin

Usually insulin therapy is reserved for patients who are unable to maintain acceptable glycemic control with diet, exercise, weight management, and oral hypoglycemic agents. Insulin therapy is very effective, restores satisfactory glycemia and well-being, and produces fewer side effects in Type II diabetes than in Type I diabetes. Table 5 summarizes some of the characteristics of commonly used insulins.

In the authors' practice, most Type II diabetic patients are taking sulfonylurea agents when insulin therapy is initiated. Usually they are maintained on the same dose of sulfonylurea agent, and insulin therapy is initiated before the evening meal or at bedtime.

Before insulin therapy is started, techniques of SMBG are reviewed and the patient's glucose meter is checked. SMBG has a critical role in adjusting insulin doses and usually is performed twice daily, before breakfast and supper. Because Type II diabetes is characterized by excessive glucose production by the liver, the elevation in the fasting level of plasma glucose results largely from nocturnal hepatic glucose output. Thus administration of insulin in the evening has theoretical and practical advantages.

TABLE 5. **Insulin Characteristics**

Preparation	Onset (min)	Peak (h)	Duration (h)
Short-Acting			
Regular	15–30	2–5	6–8
Intermediate-Acting			
Isophane (NPH)	1–2	4–12	18–22
Insulin zinc (Lente)	1–3	7–15	18–22
Long-Acting			
Insulin zinc (Ultralente) (human)	3–4	6–16	24–28
Insulin zinc (Ultralente) (beef)	4	10–30	30–36

All values are for human recombinant DNA insulin except as indicated for Ultralente. Representative values are given.

There are many ways of initiating insulin therapy, but all must be tailored to the individual. Isophane (NPH), 10 to 15 units (about 0.2 units per kg), can be started before supper or bedtime. This dose is increased by 5 units every 5 to 10 days if the glucose level measured by SMBG before breakfast remains above 150 mg per dL. If more than 30 units is required, the dose is split and half is given before breakfast and half before supper. When 30 units or more is required twice daily, a mixture of NPH insulin and regular insulin is started. Often the premixed combination of NPH and regular insulin such as 70/30 insulin (providing 70% NPH and 30% regular insulin) is used.

Insulin therapy is fine-tuned on the basis of SMBG values. Most Type II diabetic patients can achieve good to excellent glycemic control by using two injections of a mixture of NPH and regular insulin. For fine-tuning, patients need to measure blood glucose four times daily (before meals and at bedtime). The insulin is adjusted as follows: the prebreakfast regular insulin dose is increased or decreased to regulate the prelunch level of blood glucose; the prebreakfast NPH dose is adjusted to regulate the presupper level of blood glucose; the presupper regular insulin dose is adjusted to regulate the bedtime level of blood glucose; the presupper regular insulin dose is adjusted to regulate the bedtime level of blood glucose; and the presupper NPH dose is adjusted to regulate the prebreakfast level of blood glucose.

After the insulin regimen is fine-tuned, most patients can be managed with twice daily blood glucose measurements, taken before breakfast and supper. If required, regular insulin doses at these times can be increased or decreased by 2 units to 6 units on the basis of blood glucose results or anticipated activity.

Combination Therapy

The use of insulin in combination with sulfonylurea agents is still controversial. Adding insulin at bedtime to a sulfonylurea regimen appears to decrease fasting plasma glucose values without promoting the degree of weight gain seen when good glycemic control is achieved with insulin alone. Whether insulin is used alone or in combination with sulfonylurea agents, patients must be counseled to maintain their diet and exercise program to avoid weight gain. After insulin therapy is initiated, the dose of sulfonylurea agent can be reduced to half the maximum (glipizide, 10 mg twice daily, or glyburide, 5 mg twice daily).

CARDIOVASCULAR RISK FACTOR MANAGEMENT

Cardiovascular disease is twice as common in diabetic men and four times as common in diabetic women as in nondiabetic men and women. Unmodifiable risk factors, including gender and family history, are similar for diabetic and nondiabetic subjects. Major risk factors such as hypercholesterolemia, hypertension, cigarette smoking, obesity, physical inactivity, and poor stress management appear to be equipotent in diabetic and nondiabetic persons. Hypertriglyceridemia, a common finding in Type II diabetes, appears to be a stronger predictor of risk in diabetic than in nondiabetic persons. A low HDL cholesterol value (below 35 mg/dL) is an important risk factor in diabetic and nondiabetic persons but is more prevalent among Type II diabetic patients.

Unique risk factors for diabetic patients are hyperinsulinemia, hyperglycemia, sticky platelets, and an increased susceptibility to oxidation of LDL. Because of the enhanced susceptibility to atherosclerotic disease, risk factors such as hypertension, dyslipidemia, and cigarette smoking must be treated aggressively. Diabetic patients who smoke should be reminded at each office visit that cigarette smoking is especially risky in diabetes. They should be referred to effective smoking cessation programs; Nicorette gum or patches should be prescribed as indicated. Each risk factor should be identified and pursued aggressively.

Hyperlipidemia

Three major lipid problems—increased LDL cholesterol levels, decreased HDL cholesterol levels, and increased triglyceride levels—are seen more frequently in diabetic than in nondiabetic persons. Diabetic persons have additional abnormalities of lipoproteins that are not measured by conventional laboratory testing. Consequently, the dyslipidemias observed with conventional lipid profiles should be aggressively treated with the goal of normalization of levels of serum lipids and lipoproteins.

Treatment of High LDL Cholesterol

A high percentage of diabetic patients have LDL cholesterol values above desirable levels of 130 mg/dL. Intensive diet and medication, if required, should be used to achieve desirable values. A practical stepped approach is to intensify the diabetes diet, add psyllium, and then add pharmacologic agents. Enhancing the diabetes diet, already high in fiber and low in fat and cholesterol, with soluble fiber is the first step. A high-fiber, low-fat diet, including generous amounts of soluble fiber from oat and bean products, effectively lowers LDL cholesterol levels by 10 to 20% in many patients.

Addition of psyllium supplements to the diet is the second step. Starting with one dose of 3.4 grams of psyllium (Sugar-Free Metamucil) and increasing to two doses daily (one dose in liquid twice daily) often decreases the LDL cholesterol level another 5 to 15%. These two steps can decrease LDL cholesterol level from 160 to 190 mg per dL to below 130 mg per dL.

When initial LDL cholesterol values exceed 190 mg per dL, pharmacologic treatment usually is required. If diet and psyllium do not lower the LDL cholesterol level into desirable ranges, addition of a bile acid binder is the third step. Usually one dose of colestipol (Colestid), 5 grams, or cholestyramine (Questran), 4 grams, is mixed with the psyllium and taken twice daily. After 4 to 6 weeks, the dosage can be doubled to two doses twice daily mixed with psyllium and liquid. This addition usually decreases LDL cholesterol levels another 10% to 20%.

When serum triglyceride levels exceed 250 mg per dL, bile acid–binding agents may further increase triglyceride levels. If use of bile acid binders increases triglyceride levels, these agents should be discontinued; 3-hydroxy-3-methylglutaryl coenzyme A (HMG-CoA) reductase inhibitors can be used. Some physicians use nicotinic acid for these derangements, but others believe that nicotinic acid is contraindicated in diabetes.

The fourth step is use of HMG-CoA reductase inhibitors. Usually one dose (e.g., lovastatin [Mevacor], 20 mg, or simvastatin [Zocor], 10 mg) is added to the evening meal or given at bedtime (e.g., pravastatin [Pravachol], 20 mg). Often HMG-CoA reductase inhibitors are added to the regimen of diet, psyllium, and bile acid binders. This addition decreases LDL cholesterol levels another 20%. When initial LDL cholesterol values exceed 200 mg per dL, the HMG-CoA reductase inhibitor dose may have to be doubled; occasional patients need maximal doses to reduce LDL cholesterol levels by more than 40%.

When patients take an array of drugs for hypertension or symptomatic coronary heart disease, the bile acid–binder step can be skipped to avoid interference with drug absorption. Other considerations in managing high LDL cholesterol values include the addition of probucol or antioxidants. Because oxidation of LDL is proposed as a major mechanism in atherosclerosis development, the use of probucol or antioxidant vitamins has theoretical rationale. Although the benefits are not established, the authors recommend 15 mg daily of beta carotene, 500 mg of vitamin C twice daily, and 400 mg of vitamin E daily, as antioxidant adjuncts, for high-risk patients.

Treatment of Low HDL Cholesterol

Type II diabetic patients commonly have low HDL cholesterol levels, and values below 35 mg/dL increase risk for coronary heart disease. Cigarette smoking decreases HDL cholesterol levels and should be aggressively discouraged. Physical activity is the most effective way to raise HDL cholesterol levels. Levels of physical activity should exceed 12 miles of walking per week, with a goal of 20 miles or more of walking per week. Physical activity must be maintained for 3 to 6 months in order to observe the benefits. Oat bran intake raises HDL cholesterol levels slightly. Moderate intake of alcohol also can raise HDL cholesterol levels somewhat; higher alcohol intake (more than 10 drinks per week) may precipitate or worsen hypertension.

Certain pharmacologic agents, notably HMG-CoA reductase inhibitors and gemfibrozil (Lopid), increase HDL cholesterol. Results of clinical trials are not available to support introducing these agents simply for low HDL cholesterol levels. The HMG-CoA reductase inhibitors are indicated if the LDL cholesterol level is elevated, and gemfibrozil is indicated when fasting levels of serum triglycerides exceed 500 mg per dL. Lifestyle measures, including diet, exercise, and nonsmoking, are the mainstay in raising HDL cholesterol levels.

Treatment of Hypertriglyceridemia

Elevated levels of serum triglycerides are part of the dyslipidemia of Type II diabetes. Almost always, high triglyceride levels are related to excessive fat intake, and dietary measures are the primary treatment. Ideal fasting serum triglyceride levels are less than 150 mg per dL; desirable levels are less than 250 mg per dL; and levels above 500 mg per dL require pharmacologic treatment if diet is not effective.

The first step in management of elevated triglyceride levels is nutritional. The diabetes diet should be reinforced with emphasis on low-fat and high-fiber intake. Whereas soluble fibers decrease levels of LDL cholesterol, a combination of soluble and insoluble fibers from wheat bran, whole-grain cereals, fruits, and vegetables lower levels of triglycerides. Weight loss and regular exercise also decrease triglyceride levels. For about 20% of patients, regular intake of alcohol worsens hypertriglyceridemia. They should avoid alcohol for 5 to 7 days to see whether triglyceride levels are lower with abstinence.

Pharmacologic therapy is indicated if fasting levels of triglycerides are consistently above 500 mg per dL on a therapeutic diet. Gemfibrozil, 600 mg twice daily, is the agent of choice. Of course, diet and exercise remain important. As mentioned earlier, some experts recommend nicotinic acid for hypertriglyceridemia, but others believe that this agent should be avoided in diabetes. Fish oil capsules, 2 to 4 grams per day, assist in lowering triglyceride levels in some patients but may worsen glycemic control in patients treated with diet or sulfonylurea agents. Pharmacologic agents play only an adjunctive role in management of significant hypertriglyceridemia because adherence to a low-fat, high-fiber diet is essential for achieving desirable levels of serum triglycerides.

Hypertension

Hypertension is more prevalent among Type II diabetic patients than among nondiabetic persons and accelerates development of retinopathy and nephropathy. Consequently, blood pressure should be carefully monitored in diabetic patients, and mild hypertension should be aggressively treated in order to normalize blood pressure. Nonpharmacologic measures—decreased sodium intake, weight loss, regular exercise, and increased potassium intake—should be attempted before drugs are introduced. The goals of treatment for diabetic individuals just released by the Joint National Committee (JNC V) are to maintain values below 130 mmHg systolic and 85 mmHg diastolic.

Angiotensin-converting enzyme (ACE) inhibitors are emerging as the agents of choice for initial therapy of hypertension for many diabetic patients. These agents are effective, have renal-protective effects, and do not adversely affect glucose or lipid metabolism. The ACE inhibitors are the only agents proved to slow the progression of proteinuria for patients with diabetic nephropathy. Other good agents include calcium-channel blockers and peripheral alpha^1 blockers. Diuretics and beta blockers are not first-line agents because they may worsen hyperglycemia and hyperlipidemia; however, these agents are less expensive than newer agents and are documented to reduce complications of hypertension.

COMPLICATIONS

Hypoglycemia

Hypoglycemia is much less common among insulin-treated Type II diabetic patients than among Type I patients. In Type II diabetes, hypoglycemia is milder and more self-limited; patients usually retain the ability to recognize hypoglycemic episodes. For these reasons, hypoglycemia is not a major problem for most Type II patients. When hypoglycemia does occur, it should be documented by self-measurement of blood glucose levels and followed by intake of 10 to 15 grams of rapidly absorbable carbohydrate. Diabetic patients treated with insulin should carry some form of carbohydrate with them; good choices include four to six Lifesavers, a small box of raisins, 4 to 6 ounces of juice, and 6 ounces of

cola or soda (not diet or sugar-free). The blood glucose level should be rechecked in 15 minutes and more carbohydrate taken if required.

Retinopathy

Diabetes is a major cause of blindness in the United States and is the leading cause of new blindness in adults. Diabetic patients have a 25-fold higher risk for blindness than do nondiabetic persons. Because diabetic retinopathy is often asymptomatic at its most treatable stages and because early treatment reduces risk for visual loss, regular evaluations are crucial. All Type II diabetic patients should have annual examinations, including a history of visual symptoms, measurement of visual acuity, measurement of intraocular pressure, and thorough vitreous and retinal examination with dilation of the pupils. Patients with macular edema or preproliferative or proliferative retinopathy should be referred to an ophthalmologist specializing in retinal diseases.

Nephropathy

After 20 years of diabetes, diabetic renal disease develops in about 5 to 10% of Type II patients. Prevention of renal disease relates to control of blood pressure, prevention of bladder and kidney infections, and avoidance of nephrotoxic drugs and radiologic dyes. Good to excellent glycemic control may reduce risk for nephropathy, but results of appropriate studies, especially for Type II diabetes, are not available. Initially, all diabetic patients should have serum creatinine measurements and a urinalysis with microscopic examination. Ideally, measurement of 12-hour overnight or 24-hour urine albumin excretion should be made annually. These measurements certainly should be made when hypertension is diagnosed or retinopathy is detected and annually thereafter. Microalbuminuria is present when urine albumin excretion is 30 to 300 mg per 24 hours or 20 to 200 μg per minute over a 12- to 24-hour period. Albuminuria is present when 24-hour urine albumin excretion exceeds 300 mg per 24 hours.

When microalbuminuria is detected, hypertension should be intensively treated to maintain normal blood pressures, dietary protein intake should be reduced, nephrotoxic drugs and radiologic dyes should be avoided, and urinary tract infections should be treated promptly. These aggressive measures are vital because experience with Type I diabetes suggests that by 7 years after onset of albuminuria, half the patients have end-stage renal disease.

Neuropathy

Diabetic neuropathies are among the most common complications of diabetes and afflict more than 60% of persons with diabetes of 25 years' duration. Diabetic neuropathies can be classified as peripheral and autonomic neuropathies. Peripheral neuropathies include symmetrical bilateral neuropathy, mononeuropathy, neuropathic ulcer, and diabetic amyotrophy. The major manifestations of autonomic neuropathies include gastroparesis, diabetic diarrhea, constipation, neurogenic bladder, impaired cardiovascular reflexes, orthostatic hypotension, and sexual dysfunction. Only the symptomatic management of selected neuropathic problems is discussed here.

Acute painful neuropathies are uncommon but very unpleasant occurrences in diabetic patients. Local application of capsaicin (Zostrix) can offer relief. Systemic agents such as amitriptyline or carbamazepine may offer relief. The painful phase of these neuropathies usually subsides within 6 months. Mononeuropathies and diabetic amyotrophy usually resolve spontaneously in 3 to 12 months.

Gastroparesis appears to be more common in Type I than in Type II diabetes and can lead to erratic control with unexpected hyperglycemia or hypoglycemia. Sometimes metoclopramide, 10 mg before meals and at bedtime, provides benefits, but chronic use must be monitored because of the tardic dyskinetic side effects. High-fiber intake or psyllium supplements often benefit patients with constipation or diarrhea. Clonidine, metoclopramide, or loperamide may improve diabetic diarrhea.

Foot Care

Diabetic individuals have a 15-fold higher risk for lower extremity gangrene that necessitates amputations than do nondiabetic individuals. Since an estimated 50% of these amputations are preventable, the physician and the patient should devote appropriate attention to foot care and preventive measures. Foot problems result from peripheral neuropathy, peripheral vascular insufficiency, infections, or combinations of these factors. Prevention of foot problems requires regular foot examinations and education of patients by the health care team and awareness and commonsense measures by the patient.

The physician should annually examine the feet, assess the circulation by palpating peripheral pulses and listening for abdominal and femoral bruits, and perform a neurologic examination, including deep tendon reflex testing and tactile and vibratory sensation measurements. At each visit, a history of neurologic, vascular, or foot problems should be obtained, and the feet should be inspected. Appropriate referrals to podiatrists or for special shoes should be made as indicated.

Diabetic patients have the responsibility for inspecting and washing their feet daily, using lubricating oils or creams as required, cutting toenails properly, not cutting calluses or corns, avoiding extremes of temperature, not walking barefooted, wearing appropriate shoes, inspecting their shoes before putting them on, and seeking medical care for skin lesions. The physician needs to ensure that patients receive appropriate instructions in the office or in collaboration with another specialist.

SPECIAL SITUATIONS

Surgery and Serious Illnesses

With attention to glycemic control and avoidance of hypoglycemia, risk involved in elective surgery for diabetic patients is only slightly higher than for nondiabetic persons. Preoperatively, good glycemic control should be achieved and cardiovascular status assessed. The objectives of management are to maintain good glycemic control and normal fluid and electrolyte balance throughout the procedure. Oral feeding should be resumed as soon as possible. Procedures should be scheduled in the early morning if possible.

For major procedures, insulin coverage is usually desirable. Oral agents can be discontinued on the day of hospitalization and human insulin used. Ideally, blood glucose values should be maintained in the range of 100 to 150 mg per dL; values of 150 to 250 mg per dL are acceptable. An intravenous infusion of 5 or 10% glucose is commonly initiated; an intravenous insulin infusion can be used to maintain the blood glucose levels, determined at the patient's bedside by glucose meter, in the desirable range. Alternatively, the intravenous glucose can be initiated and a moderate dose of NPH insulin given subcutaneously. Subcutaneous regular insulin should not be given in the preoperative or operative periods; intravenous regular insulin can be given to control hyperglycemia. Blood glucose values should be measured every 2 hours during the perioperative period. Subsequently, the blood glucose level should be measured every 6 hours until the patient resumes oral feeding.

During serious illnesses, the same techniques can be used. When diabetes is not difficult to control, a mixture of NPH and regular insulin, such as 70/30 insulin, can be given every 12 hours. For more difficult situations, an intravenous insulin infusion can be used to maintain blood glucose values in the desirable range. In intensive care units, the blood glucose level is measured at the patient's bedside every hour, and chemistry panels (glucose and electrolytes) are measured every 6 to 12 hours. Usually 50 units of regular insulin are added to 500 mL of saline, and this is infused at a rate of 10 to 50 mL per hour (1 to 5 units of insulin per hour) with an intravenous infusion pump. Glucose is given intravenously or through the gastrointestinal tract. Subcutaneous NPH infusion should be reinstituted before the insulin drip is discontinued.

Pregnancy

Each year, approximately 10,000 infants are born in the United States to women with diabetes that was recognized before pregnancy. Because management of diabetes before and during pregnancy are critical for the health of the mother and the outcome for the infant, these people should be managed by teams with expertise in diabetes and pregnancy; this specialized management, however, is not discussed here.

Each year, between 60,000 and 90,000 infants are born in the United States to mothers with gestational diabetes. All pregnant women should be screened for gestational diabetes at approximately 24 to 28 weeks of gestation. Screening may be indicated before 24 weeks if there is a history of any of the following: polydipsia or polyuria, recurrent vaginal or urinary tract infections, glycosuria, hydramnios, previous delivery of large infants, or previous gestational diabetes.

For screening, a 50-gram glucose load is given orally, and the plasma glucose is measured 1 hour later; patients do not have to be fasting for the screening test. If the plasma glucose is 140 mg per dL or higher, a 100-gram oral glucose tolerance test is scheduled.

The oral glucose tolerance test follows 3 days of unrestricted diet and a fast of 8 to 14 hours. The patient should remain seated throughout the procedure and should not smoke. A 100-gram oral glucose load is given, and blood is taken in the fasting state and at 1, 2, and 3 hours. The diagnosis of gestational diabetes is established when two or more of the following criteria are met or exceeded: fasting, 105 mg per dL; 1 hour, 190 mg per dL; 2 hours, 165 mg per dL; and 3 hours, 145 mg per dL.

Women with gestational diabetes should be instructed in a diabetes diet and in SMBG. They need to be seen at 1- to 2-week intervals in the physician's office. If fasting plasma glucose values exceed 105 mg per dL or 2-hour postprandial values exceed 120 mg per dL, human insulin therapy should be started. A program of fetal surveillance may be indicated. The glucose tolerance test should be repeated 6 to 8 weeks post partum to determine whether glucose intolerance is still present.

EDUCATION OF PATIENTS

Patients need to be taught basic information about diabetes and its care. All diabetic persons need to know about the nature of diabetes and its inheritance. They need diet instruction and information about exercise. They must be taught to recognize hypoglycemic symptoms, SMBG, and use and side effects of oral hypoglycemic agents and insulin, as appropriate. With well-established diabetes, patients need to be taught principles of foot care, symptoms of eye disease, and symptoms of cardiovascular disease. The efforts of physicians, office staff, and other health professionals should complement available educational material to ensure that persons with diabetes have the knowledge to self-manage the disease.

DIABETES MELLITUS IN CHILDREN AND ADOLESCENTS

method of
WILLIAM L. CLARKE, M.D.
University of Virginia Health Sciences Center
Charlottesville, Virginia

Diabetes mellitus is the most common endocrine disease of childhood with a prevalence of approximately 1 in 600 U.S. school-age children. Childhood and adolescent diabetes mellitus is almost always insulin dependent (IDDM), and current evidence suggests that it is an autoimmune disease that occurs in genetically susceptible persons. Although a variety of environmental factors, including viruses, toxins, and bovine serum albumin antibodies, have been implicated as triggering agents, none has been identified as specifically responsible for initiating the autoimmune destruction of the islet cells in a majority of cases. Newly diagnosed children often exhibit the human leukocyte antigen (HLA) DR3 and/or DR4 haplotype, serum islet cell antibodies, and insulin antibodies. Recent research suggests that the presence of a non–aspartic acid residue at position 57 of the HLA-DQ beta chain is strongly associated with the development of IDDM.

A seasonal variation is observed with increased incidences in the fall and winter. IDDM occurrence peaks at two ages: 5 to 7 years and during adolescence, when an increase in endogenous insulin production is required to offset the insulin resistance associated with the pubertal increase in growth hormone secretion.

The symptoms of hyperglycemia—polydipsia, polyuria, polyphagia, and weight loss—usually do not occur before significant (approximately 90%) destruction of beta cells. This destruction is rarely rapid, and thus methods for identifying the preclinical stage are being sought. Impaired early insulin responses during intravenous glucose tolerance testing are often present in high-risk persons, as are islet cell and insulin antibodies. Although immunotherapeutic trials have recently been initiated, the therapeutic options for reversing or decelerating the destruction of the islet cells are limited or nonexistent.

The diagnosis of IDDM is usually not difficult. In addition to the clinical findings described earlier, a random plasma glucose level of 200 mg per dL or higher in association with urinary ketones is diagnostic. Rarely is an oral glucose tolerance test (OGTT) necessary for diagnosis. Should an OGTT be performed, 1.75 grams per kg (maximum, 75 grams) of glucose is given, and samples for plasma glucose are obtained at baseline and every 30 minutes for 2 hours. The criteria for diagnosis are a fasting plasma glucose level greater than 140 mg per dL, the 2-hour value greater than 200 mg per dL, and at least one intervening value greater than 200 mg per dL.

TREATMENT

Diabetic Ketoacidosis

Despite an apparent increased awareness among the public and the health care community of the early signs and symptoms of IDDM, the diagnosis often is not considered until diabetic ketoacidosis (DKA) occurs. The diagnosis may be particularly elusive in very young children (less than 2 years of age), for whom the symptoms of IDDM mimic those of other more common pediatric illnesses. DKA, other than at diagnosis, may occur in children who are relatively insulinopenic in the presence of severe physiologic stress (e.g., infection) or whose maintenance insulin dose is insufficient to prevent ketosis.

Children with DKA present with significant dehydration and hyperpnea (often with Kussmaul respirations) and a characteristic acetone odor to the breath. The severity of DKA is related to the degree of dehydration, metabolic derangement, and mental status. Children in mild DKA (less than 5% dehydration and arterial pH $\geq$ 7.25) are usually alert. Those with severe DKA (dehydration of 10% or more, pH < 7.1, and serum bicarbonate level < 10 mEq per liter) may be obtunded. After careful assessment of a child's status, the therapeutic principles to be followed include rehydration, insulin administration, potassium replacement, and correction of acidosis.

Many children with mild DKA can be rehydrated orally with electrolyte-rich beverages such as Gatorade (5.8% glucose, 23.5 mEq per liter of sodium, 2.5 mEq per liter of potassium, 17 mEq per liter of chloride, 6.8 mEq per liter of phosphorus) or Pedialyte (5% glucose, 30 mEq per liter of sodium, 20 mEq per liter of potassium, 30 mEq

per liter of chloride, 28 mEq per liter of citrate). Regular insulin is administered subcutaneously at a dose of 0.25 to 0.5 unit per kg every 4 to 6 hours, and oral potassium supplements (10 to 20 mEq every 6 to 12 hours) are given if the serum potassium level is normal or low.

Treatment of the child with moderate to severe DKA is more complex and requires careful monitoring of metabolic and neurologic status. Therapy is divided into resuscitation and replacement phases (Table 1). Initial resuscitation fluids should be intravenous lactated Ringer's solution at a rate of 10 to 20 mL per kg over the first 1 to 2 hours. Lactated Ringer's solution is preferred over isotonic saline because it provides more free water and potassium and less chloride. The lactate is metabolized to bicarbonate to regenerate base. Initial serum sodium values may be falsely depressed as a result of hyperlipidemia or may correctly reflect the shift of intracellular water to the extracellular space (2.5 mEq per liter lowering of sodium for every 100 mg per dL of glucose over 300 mg per dL). Insulin is administered intravenously at a rate of 0.1 unit per kg per hour after an initial bolus of 0.1 unit per kg. Infusion rates can be adjusted to limit the rate of fall of blood glucose levels to between 50 and 100 mg per dL per hour. Dextrose is added to the intravenous fluids when the blood glucose approaches 300 mg per dL, to permit the continued regeneration of base resulting from insulin administration.

Although most children with DKA have a total body potassium depletion (potassium ions exchange at the cell membrane for hydrogen ions, and the resulting serum potassium is lost in the urine), potassium is usually not administered until a child has urinated and the serum potassium level is less than 4.0 mEq per liter. Bicarbonate is often recommended for a pH of 7.0 or lower or if cardiac instability is observed. A dose of 1 to 2 mEq per kg is given over 1 to 2 hours. The use of bicarbonate in DKA is controversial, however, because it increases the need for potassium, tends to shift the hemoglobin O_2 dissociation curve to the left, and may lead to a paradoxical central

TABLE 1. **Fluid Therapy in Moderate to Severe Diabetic Ketoacidosis**

Resuscitation: 1–2 h
Lactated Ringer's solution: 10–20 mL/kg

Replacement: 2–36 h
½ normal saline with 20–40 mEq/L potassium phosphate
Total fluids should not exceed 4 L/M²/24 h
Dextrose may be added to replacement fluids to maintain plasma
Glucose level between 200 and 300 mg/dL

nervous system acidosis. The latter is thought to be a possible cause of cerebral edema.

After resuscitation therapy, replacement therapy designed to correct water and electrolyte deficits over a total of 36 hours is begun. The initial resuscitation fluids should be included in the replacement of the deficit. The metabolic derangements associated with DKA usually do not appear rapidly. Thus once the child is hemodynamically and neurologically stable and a trend toward correction of the metabolic derangements is observed, the remaining abnormalities need not be corrected rapidly.

Replacement fluids include half-normal saline, which provides sufficient sodium and free water, with added potassium. Potassium (20 to 40 mEq per liter) may be given as either potassium chloride or phosphate. Although there is no evidence that phosphate is preferable to potassium chloride, the reduced chloride load and possible replenishment of red blood cell 2,3-diphosphoglycerate may be advantageous. After the resuscitation phase, if the arterial pH is still less than 7.1, sodium bicarbonate (1 mEq per kg) may be given slowly over 1 to 2 hours. Insulin should be continued until the acidosis is cleared. As stated earlier, it may be necessary to administer dextrose intravenously to permit insulin administration without hypoglycemia.

Once acidosis is corrected and the child is able to eat and drink, subcutaneous regular insulin may be substituted for the intravenous insulin. A dose of 0.2 to 0.4 unit per kg every 4 hours is given 15 to 30 minutes before the intravenous insulin is terminated, because the half-life of intravenous insulin is about 10 minutes. Alternatively, a mixture of intermediate- and short-acting insulins, similar to that calculated for chronic maintenance therapy, may be begun. Potassium supplementation may be needed for several days once acidosis is corrected.

The treatment of DKA is usually gratifying to the physician because the patient is initially gravely ill and within 24 to 36 hours is markedly improved. However, the rate of mortality from DKA remains at 0.5 to 18%. Thus caution must be taken to prevent, recognize, and treat early signs of deterioration. Cerebral edema is the most serious complication of the treatment of DKA. Between 4 and 24 hours after the initiation of therapy and, paradoxically, while metabolic parameters appear to be improving, the child experiences a change in mental status often accompanied by a severe headache. These symptoms may rapidly progress to seizures, coma, and alteration in respiration.

Suspected cerebral edema should be treated immediately with a trial of intravenous mannitol (0.2 to 1.0 mg per kg as a 15% solution over 30 minutes). Mannitol should always be readily available during treatment of DKA. The etiology of cerebral edema is unknown but may be related to rapid administration of hypotonic solutions, rapid fall in blood glucose and/or osmolality, inappropriate antidiuretic hormone secretion, and/or central nervous system acidosis. It is important that all physicians caring for children with DKA be aware of this life-threatening complication of treatment and use caution in the administration of intravenous fluids, the lowering of blood glucose, and the administration of sodium bicarbonate. Fluids should not exceed 4 liters per M^2 per day or 3 times daily maintenance. Blood glucose decline should be limited to 100 mg per dL per hour, and bicarbonate should be given only when necessary and then slowly. Other potential complications include vascular thromboses and acute tubular necrosis. Thus monitoring of the patient must include not only a review of laboratory values but also frequent measurements of blood pressure, heart rate, respiratory rate, intake, and output and the evaluation of mental status.

Chronic Management

The goal of IDDM therapy is to achieve and maintain blood glucose levels as close to those of nondiabetic persons as feasible. IDDM, unlike most other medical disorders, necessitates daily decision making by the patient and/or the patient's family, rather than periodic adjustments by the physician, in order to achieve effective disease management. Thus education of the patient and family is essential. Most educational programs use the health care team (physician, nurse educator, nutritionist, psychologist, social worker) approach, in which each team member is responsible for teaching a portion of the curriculum. Initial education must include survival skills such as insulin administration, meal planning, blood glucose monitoring, and the recognition and treatment of hypo- and hyperglycemia.

Diabetes is a disease affecting every aspect of a child's life: what he or she eats, how he or she plays, how he or she is educated, his or her success in forming interpersonal relationships, and his or her career choices. Effective chronic management of diabetes requires that careful attention be paid to assessing the child's lifestyle, educational level and learning abilities, family and peer support system, and recreational preferences. Once survival skills have been taught and the child is settled into a routine, an individualized educational program should be planned to ensure that technical and problem-solving skills taught to the child are age- and developmentally appropriate and that a reasonable amount of responsibility is shared among the child, parents, and health care team. Staged educational curricula for children are available through the American Diabetes Association.

Insulin

Human insulins are now standard therapy for children with IDDM. Although they have a somewhat faster onset of action and shorter duration than insulins of animal origin, their availability, cost, and low level of antigenicity have made them preferable. Initially, subcutaneous insulin is based on weight and given at an average dose of 0.75 unit per kg per day. Newly diagnosed children who have not been in acidosis often require less insulin (0.5 unit per kg per day or less), whereas adolescents' requirements may exceed 1.0 unit per kg per day. Standard therapy includes a mixture of short- and intermediate-acting (NPH or Lente) insulins given twice daily 20 to 30 minutes before breakfast and the evening meal. The morning dose is usually twice as large as the evening dose, and the short-acting doses are usually half as large as the intermediate-acting doses. Adjustments of no more than 10% are made in a single component every 2 to 3 days until premeal and bedtime blood glucose levels are within the targeted range. This range varies in different treatment centers and different age groups but is generally between 75 and 160 mg per dL before meals and between 100 and 160 mg per dL before bed.

Other insulin administration algorithms are shown in Table 2. Intermediate-acting insulin is sometimes given at bedtime rather than before the evening meal to reduce fasting hyperglycemia without precipitating nocturnal hypoglycemia. Ultralente, an insulin with a long duration of action, given once or twice daily with periodic regular insulin to reduce postprandial excursions, is increasingly popular for children or adolescents whose school and recreational schedules include significant day-to-day variability. Children learn to adjust their regular insulin doses for the intensity of their exercise and the size and content of their meals. In general, the more frequently insulin is administered, the smoother the blood glucose control and the more freedom the child has to vary diet and exercise pattern without precipitating hypo- or hyperglycemia.

Continuous subcutaneous insulin infusion systems (pumps), which are important components of intensive insulin therapy, have not met with great acceptance in children and adolescents because they require a level of disease surveillance and decision making that is uncommon among these patients.

Insulin should be stored in the refrigerator but is stable between 35° and 86° F. Injection sites should be rotated among arms, abdomen, thighs and buttocks, but absorption varies from site to site (fastest in the abdomen, slowest in the thighs). Thus frequent rotation may contribute to significant variability in blood glucose readings. In young children with little subcutaneous fat, insulin is given subcutaneously at a 45-degree angle in order to prevent inadvertent intramuscular administration.

Diet

The greatest contributor to variability in blood glucose levels is unquestionably food intake. It is impossible to achieve near-normal glucose levels without controlling the diet. Meals should be planned, given at approximately the same time daily, and, unless insulin is to be varied daily, should consist of relatively stable amounts of calories and carbohydrates. The American Diabetes Association recommends a meal plan with 55 to 60% of calories from carbohydrates, the majority of these being complex; less than 30% fat, the

TABLE 2. **Insulin Administration Algorithms**

Insulin*	Time of Dose	Comments
Regular: NPH (or Lente) Regular: NPH (or Lente)	Prebreakfast Predinner	Most common algorithm ⅔ total dose in morning
Regular: NPH (or Lente) Regular NPH (or Lente)	Prebreakfast Predinner Bedtime	Used to reduce fasting hyperglycemia without precipitating nocturnal hypoglycemia
Ultralente	Prebreakfast or ½ prebreakfast and ½ predinner	40–50% total daily dose as Ultralente
Regular	Before meals	Timing and dose may vary as a result of activity and meal size

*Average Total Daily Insulin Dose = 0.75 units/kg (preadolescents) and 1.0 units/kg (adolescents).

majority being polyunsaturated; and the remainder from protein. Cholesterol intake should be less than 300 mg per day, and salt should be limited to 2 grams daily. These recommendations are similar to those recommended by the American Heart Association and are reasonable guidelines for all persons.

Most nutritionists use the exchange system to teach patients and families how to plan meals. Other systems for categorizing and calculating intake are equally acceptable as long as they are easily understood by the family. The exchange system categorizes all foods into six groups, which are then assigned to each meal in specific numbers to result in a total caloric intake appropriate for age and activity level. Calorie recommendations for children are estimated to be 1000 calories plus 100 cal per year of age and are adjusted upward or downward according to activity level or stage of puberty. Postmenarchal girls with IDDM often must restrict their food intake to less than 2000 calories per day to prevent unwanted weight gain. Total calories may be distributed between meals and snacks to coincide with the child's usual eating pattern and the times of peak insulin action. Usual meal plans consist of three meals and two to three snacks daily.

Exercise

Exercise is important for achieving and maintaining cardiovascular fitness. Whether exercise has a specific role as a treatment modality in IDDM is not clear. Exercise can transiently lower blood glucose levels in well-insulinized persons. The effect of exercise on glucose reduction is greater when insulin is injected into the area to be exercised. Thus the abdomen is the preferred site of insulin administration for most exercising people. There is also a late glucose-lowering effect of exercise that varies from individual to individual. Exercise should be planned for times when the insulin level is not peaking and when sufficient carbohydrates are available to maintain normoglycemia. Unfortunately, most exercise either is unplanned or is planned without regard to the child's diabetes management plan. Thus children who participate in organized athletics may need to reduce the insulin dose or consume an additional snack before the activity. The amount of adjustment must be based on the intensity, duration, and timing of the exercise.

Exercise also may produce a paradoxical increase in blood glucose levels and associated ketonuria when performed during insulinopenic hyperglycemia. Children with IDDM should not exercise vigorously when their blood glucose level is greater than 240 mg per dL.

Monitoring

Blood glucose monitoring is the only effective method for evaluating glycemia by the patient. A variety of reflectance meters are commercially available and produce clinically accurate results that may be used reliably to adjust insulin doses. Most meters can be used by most children by 8 years of age. Initially, blood glucose monitoring should be performed before each meal and at bedtime so that each component of the insulin dose can be adjusted appropriately. In addition, an occasional 0300h test should be performed to guard against nocturnal hypoglycemia. Once glucose levels have stabilized within the target range on a fixed insulin regime, the frequency of monitoring may be reduced to twice daily. In the author's practice, prebreakfast and predinner tests are recommended on Mondays, Wednesdays, and Fridays; prebreakfast and prebedtime tests, on Tuesdays and Thursdays; and prelunch plus one other test, on Saturdays and Sundays. During periods of growth, illness, travel, exercise, or any change of routine, the frequency should be increased in order to ensure proper insulin adjustment. Blood glucose results should be recorded and reviewed periodically by the child and family and brought to clinic visits for review by the health care team.

Most physicians currently monitor glucose control with periodic determinations of glycosylated hemoglobin concentrations. These values reflect average blood glucose levels over the previous 2 to 3 months. Translating glycosylated hemoglobin values into actual average blood glucose levels may be difficult without knowledge of the range and reproducibility of the locally performed tests. Results from different laboratories are not necessarily comparable. Other glycosylated proteins such as fructosamine and albumin are occasionally determined to evaluate short-term glucose control.

Psychosocial Adjustment

As stated earlier, diabetes is a disease affecting lifestyle, and thus it affects more than just intermediary metabolism. Families of children with IDDM experience significant psychological and financial stress. Initial reactions to the diagnosis include grief, denial, and anger. Acceptance may not occur for some time. Children view their disease from their level of development and often believe that they caused IDDM or that their parents could remove it as a reward for good behavior. Diabetes is used as an excuse for misbehavior and poor school performance. It interferes with the adolescent's establishment of independence, peer relationships, and identity development, and it limits career choices. An awareness of these factors is imperative for assisting the child in becoming an independent adult. The average cost of IDDM to the family of a 10-year-old with no complications, no emergency room visits, and no hospitalizations is $2200 per year in Central Virginia. Thus psychological and social work assessments and support are needed on a periodic and yet routine basis.

COMPLICATIONS

Acute

The most serious acute complication of IDDM is hypoglycemia. Hypoglycemia occurs when too much insulin is present for the amount of blood glucose available. This may occur when the insulin level is peaking, when food is omitted, or after periods of excessive exercise. The signs and symptoms of hypoglycemia are categorized as neurogenic (e.g., shakiness, sweatiness, pounding heart) and neuroglycopenic (blurred vision, difficulty concentrating, incoordination). Severe hypoglycemia is characterized by loss of consciousness and/or by seizures and occurs more frequently during intensive insulin therapy.

Not every person with IDDM has all these symptoms when hypoglycemic. Symptoms are unique and reliable to the individual over time. Children who report absence of symptoms during hypoglycemia must be taught to better recognize their early warning signs. Although glucagon secretion to hypoglycemia may be diminished within 3 to 5 years after diagnosis, epinephrine secretion is rarely impaired in childhood IDDM. Children must carry rapid-acting glucose with them at all times, in the form of either commercially available gels or tablets or sugar-containing foods. All family members, teachers, coaches, and others in positions with responsibility for the child with IDDM should learn to inject glucagon (0.5 to 1.0 mg intramuscularly) in case loss of consciousness occurs. Gel or liquid should never be forced into the mouths of unarousable patients because of the risk of aspiration. Injectable glucagon should restore consciousness within 5 to 10 minutes, after which oral treatment may proceed.

Chronic

The micro- and macrovascular complications associated with IDDM include retinopathy, nephropathy, neuropathy, and peripheral vascular disease, and their onset may occur before adulthood. Results from National Institutes of Health–funded prospective, multicenter control and complications trial have recently shown that intensive control of blood glucose can reduce the onset and progression of retinopathy, nephropathy, and neuropathy.

SPECIAL CASE

Very young children with diabetes (toddlers and younger) present special challenges. These children may be exquisitely sensitive to regular insulin, which makes titrating doses in single units difficult. In addition, it may be difficult to adhere to meal plans when the patient refuses to eat. In such circumstances, insulin is often given after rather than before a meal. Exercise in young children is rarely planned and is of variable intensity. The propensity for young children to react to many illnesses with emesis often complicates management and leads to recurrent DKA. Thus the blood glucose target range is modified for these children, and the author attempts to achieve blood glucose levels between 100 and 200 mg per dL 75% of the time.

FUTURE

Current research is centered on defining persons at high risk for development of IDDM and preventing or reversing beta cell destruction before the onset of clinical symptoms. For those previously diagnosed, insulin analogues currently being synthesized may make it easier to mimic the actions of endogenous insulin with subcutaneous injections, and a variety of insulin delivery devices (artificial beta cells) are being designed. Transplantation of beta cells, whole pancreata, and non–islet cell tissue that is genetically engineered to synthesize and secrete insulin in response to glucose is being investigated. Which of these areas will prove most successful is obviously uncertain. Research concerning the diagnosis and treatment of complications is progressing, as are studies defining the psychosocial impairments associated with IDDM.

DIABETIC KETOACIDOSIS

method of
RODNEY A. LORENZ, M.D.
Vanderbilt University
Nashville, Tennessee

Diabetic ketoacidosis (DKA) is caused by insulin deficiency. Its development is promoted by excess of the counterregulatory hormones glucagon, catecholamines, cortisol, and growth hormone, which act synergistically with insulin deficiency to reduce glucose utilization, increase hepatic glucose production, and increase lipolysis and hepatic ketogenesis. These hormonal disturbances cause hyperglycemia and glycosuria with associated increased urinary water and electrolyte losses, as well as ketosis and acidosis that lead to nausea and vomiting. The end result of these processes is a total body deficit of water and electrolytes, often with water loss in excess of solute (i.e., hyperosmolar dehydration). Central nervous system function is impaired with progressively more severe DKA.

The diagnosis of DKA should be considered, therefore, in patients presenting with dehydration and hyperventilation, with or without coma. Vomiting and abdominal pain are common, as is a history of polyuria, polydipsia, and weight loss, especially in new-onset cases. Confirmation of hyperglycemia and ketonuria by rapid bedside methods strongly suggests DKA. Dehydration, decreased level of consciousness, and hyperglycemia without acidosis or ketosis should suggest the less common condition, hyperosmolar nonketotic coma.

INITIAL EVALUATION

The medical history should focus on symptoms suggesting DKA, as outlined earlier, and on other symptoms that might suggest illnesses causing an insulin-resistant state, common examples of which are infection and myocardial infarction. Patients with known diabetes should be questioned about their usual diabetes care practices and level of compliance for clues to the cause of DKA. It is also useful to determine the patient's response to early symptoms of DKA, such as contact with a physician, blood glucose test results, and administration of extra insulin.

The physical examination should emphasize hemodynamic state, signs of dehydration, respiratory status, characterization of level of consciousness, and a careful search for evidence of infection. Abdominal tenderness and even rigidity may be seen in DKA without other causes.

The initial laboratory evaluation should include measurements of arterial blood gases, complete blood counts, measurements of glucose and electrolytes, and urinalysis. Depending on the patient's age and symptoms, other considerations include urine and blood cultures, electrocardiogram, chest x-ray, and measurements of serum calcium, phosphorus, magnesium, amylase, lipase, and osmolality.

The serum amylase level and white blood cell count are frequently elevated in DKA and return to normal within 2 to 3 days. Elevated levels of acetoacetate, commonly seen in DKA, cause false elevations of creatinine as measured by autoanalyzers.

TREATMENT

Principles of Therapy

The basic principles of therapy are to replace deficits of fluid, electrolytes, and carbohydrate and to reverse the catabolic state with insulin. Grading the severity of DKA on the basis of initial laboratory data helps guide therapy. Suggested grading criteria are given in Table 1. The current trend in therapy of DKA is toward slower

TABLE 1. **Criteria for Grading Severity of Diabetic Ketoacidosis**

Symptoms	Dehydration	pH	HCO₃
Severe	7–10%	<7.1	<8
Moderate	5–7%	7.1–7.25	8–12
Mild	<5%	>7.25	<16

correction of deficits. Once the patient is hemodynamically stable and severe acidosis is corrected, there is little need for rapid correction. The hyperosmolality tends to preserve intravascular volume, blood pressure, and renal function better than would be expected for the degree of dehydration.

Most patients with DKA require hospitalization. If acidosis is mild (pH > 7.25), several hours of outpatient therapy with fluids and subcutaneous regular insulin may be attempted. With more severe acidosis, intravenous or intramuscular insulin is recommended because of fears that subcutaneous insulin will not be reliably absorbed in the presence of volume depletion. Admission to an intensive care unit should be considered for patients with altered mental status; hypotension; arrhythmia; complicating cardiac, respiratory, or renal disease; initial pH of less than 7.1; or initial osmolality greater than 300 mOsm per kg H_2O. Careful monitoring of the patient's clinical and laboratory status is essential. A flow sheet should be used to organize the data, including fluid balances, vital signs, pH, glucose, and electrolytes. Initially, vital signs, the pH, and glucose levels are assessed hourly or more often. Electrolytes are measured every 1 or 2 hours. Once the pH exceeds 7.2, the frequency of monitoring may be gradually decreased. Neurologic status should be assessed frequently because of the uncommon occurrence of cerebral edema. Surgical consultation is appropriate if abdominal pain persists after correction of acidosis.

Insulin

There are many alternative methods for delivering insulin during treatment of DKA; probably any method that delivers a dose of at least 0.1 units per kg per hour to the circulation is acceptable. A constant intravenous insulin infusion offers many advantages: simplicity of dosing, predictable insulin effect, and ease of dose adjustment. A convenient way to achieve a dose of 0.1 unit per kg per hour in a constant infusion is to add 100 units of regular insulin to 100 mL of saline (1 unit per mL). This solution should be piggybacked onto replacement fluids so that each can be adjusted independently. Before the infusion begins, 10 to 20 mL of the insulin-saline mixture is run through the tubing to saturate insulin binding on the plastic; the infusion is then begun at 0.1 mL per kg per hour. An infusion pump should always be used to ensure steady flow rate. A fall in serum glucose of 50 to 100 mg per dL per hour is desirable. Depending on the blood glucose response in 2 to 3 hours, the infusion rate can be adjusted. If the patient has not had a satisfactory response in serum bicarbonate, anion gap, pH, or glucose after the initial 2 to 3 hours, the infusion should be checked for technical errors in mixing or delivery of insulin. If none are found, the infusion solution should be replaced and the infusion rate increased (e.g., doubled).

If a constant infusion is started promptly, an initial bolus (loading) dose is not needed. However, if an infusion pump is not immediately available, treatment may be started with an intravenous bolus injection of 0.1 unit per kg. This dose may be repeated every 20 to 30 minutes until the constant infusion is started.

A number of alternatives to constant intravenous infusion have been reported to be effective. These methods have in common the administration of 0.1 to 0.3 unit per kg as either an intravenous or an intramuscular bolus on an hourly basis.

Fluids

All patients with DKA are dehydrated. The extent of fluid loss can be estimated by physical examination, by the guidelines in Table 1, or by comparing present weight to previously recorded weights. More severe DKA or the presence of hypotension suggests the need for more rapid initial fluid resuscitation. Once blood pressure is acceptable and the pH is greater than 7.0, infusion rates can be adjusted to correct the total fluid deficit in 24 to 48 hours; longer periods are used for greater deficits. The total fluid infusion rate should be calculated to correct the deficit as well as replace ongoing urine output and insensible losses.

The serum sodium concentration is usually low in patients with DKA. First there is generally a total body sodium deficit because of urinary losses. Second, the hyperglycemia exerts an osmotic effect, drawing water into the intravascular space and diluting sodium. The expected decrease in serum sodium is about 1.6 mEq per liter for every 100 mg per dL increase in glucose. Third, if the serum is lipemic, the measured level of serum sodium is falsely low. As hyperglycemia is corrected, the serum sodium level should rise. A failure of serum sodium to rise, or a fall, suggests excessive free water administration and too rapid correction of hyperosmolality.

The requirements of fluid resuscitation outlined earlier are usually met if therapy begins with normal saline at a rate of 10 to 20 mL per kg per hour given over the first 1 to 2 hours. Amounts at the higher end of this range are used in cases with hypotension or severe acidosis. The subsequent rate is calculated from the estimated deficit as detailed earlier; a rate of 3 to 6 mL per kg per hour will usually suffice. After the first 2 to 4 hours, saline can be replaced by 0.5 normal saline. Indications for continued use of normal saline include hypotension, depressed level of consciousness, hyponatremia, decrease in serum osmolality greater than 6 mOsm per hour, or glucose level greater than 600 mg per dL. To avoid consumption of low sodium fluids or continued vomiting, patients should not be allowed to drink until acidosis is corrected.

Fluids should be changed to include 5% glucose when the serum glucose approaches 250 mg per dL. The rate of insulin infusion may also need further adjustment at this time. Intravenous fluids may be reduced to maintenance levels or discontinued when pH exceeds 7.3, the serum bicarbonate level is greater than 18 mEq per liter, and the patient is able to resume oral intake.

In patients with cardiac, pulmonary, or renal disease, central venous pressure or Swan-Ganz monitoring may be needed to guide fluid management.

Acidosis

The metabolic acidosis of DKA is caused predominantly by accumulation of β-hydroxybutyrate, with less of a contribution from acetoacetate, lactate, and free fatty acids. In moderate or severe acidosis, respiratory compensation raises the pH, and the depression of bicarbonate or increase in anion gap may be better indicators of the disturbance in acid-base balance.

The question of whether to correct acidosis by giving buffer to patients with DKA has been controversial. Most authorities agree that patients with mild or moderate acidosis (pH > 7.1) do not require buffer. Insulin and fluid therapy alone can restore the pH to normal because bicarbonate is formed as ketoacids are metabolized. There is usually little change in acidosis in the first hour, but clear improvement should be apparent after 3 to 6 hours. In severely dehydrated patients, the pH may drop slightly before it begins to rise again. Acidosis is usually completely corrected within 24 hours.

Although controlled studies have demonstrated no benefits from use of bicarbonate in DKA, some clinicians advocate its administration in severe DKA (pH < 7.1) because of the negative effects of acidosis on cerebral and cardiac function. Possible adverse effects of bicarbonate itself include hypokalemia, paradoxical nervous system acidosis, and decreased tissue oxygen delivery. If bicarbonate is used, it should therefore be given cautiously in a constant infusion with special attention to monitoring serum potassium levels and mental status. The formula mEq $NaHCO_3$ = (anion gap $\times$ kg)/10 estimates the amount of bicarbonate required to correct half the base deficit. This amount is given in a piggyback manner over 4 hours. When the pH reaches 7.1, the bicarbonate infusion may be stopped.

Potassium

Ketoacidosis is always associated with total body potassium depletion, even though the initial serum potassium level may be normal or elevated. As ketoacids accumulate, hydrogen ions move from extracellular fluid to intracellular fluid, with the concurrent exchange of intracellular potassium for hydrogen ions. Serum potassium is maintained in the normal range by renal excretion. When dehydration is severe and glomerular filtration falls, hyperkalemia may ensue. If severe secondary hyperaldosteronism exists or potassium depletion is profound, as it is in patients with marked polyuria for several weeks before diagnosis, hypokalemia may occur.

Treatment of DKA can be expected to produce a fall in serum potassium levels. Insulin causes a cotransport of glucose and potassium into cells. Unless potassium is given, there is a risk of a rapid fall in serum potassium within hours of starting insulin and fluids. Administration of bicarbonate is a further stimulus for a fall in serum potassium.

As a general rule, therefore, potassium should be withheld until the initial serum potassium level is known. Once insulin therapy has been initiated, the patient is producing urine, and the serum potassium is known to be less than 6.0 mEq per liter, potassium may be added to intravenous fluids in a concentration of 40 mEq per liter. Potassium may be given as the chloride salt or equally divided between chloride and phosphate.

Serum potassium should be assessed hourly for the first 4 to 6 hours of therapy and every 2 to 4 hours thereafter until the pH and glucose level are normal. Serial electrocardiographic monitoring can be useful as a screen for extremes of serum potassium level while laboratory results are awaited. Severe acidosis with an initial potassium level below 4.0 mEq per liter may indicate profound potassium depletion. In such instances, potassium concentrations greater than 40 mEq per liter of replacement fluids may be required in order to achieve and maintain normal serum potassium levels. If serum potassium levels fall below 3.0 mEq per liter, there is significant risk of arrhythmia, cardiac arrest, and respiratory muscle paralysis. Immediate modification of intravenous fluids is indicated in such cases.

Glucose

A large quantity of glucose is lost in the urine during DKA. When the blood glucose level is greater than 500 mg per dL, urine glucose levels may approximate 6% (6 grams per dL). Thus an adult or an adolescent with normal renal function may excrete 20 to 30 grams of glucose per hour. Urinary glucose losses in this situation may be greater than the amount of glucose taken up by insulin-stimulated tissues. As blood glucose decreases toward the renal threshold for glucose, urinary glucose excretion becomes a decreasing fraction of the decline in blood glucose. In that situation, the decline in blood glucose is caused predominantly by insulin-induced suppression of hepatic glucose output and, to a lesser extent, increased tissue glucose uptake.

A desirable target for rate of fall of blood glucose levels is 50 to 100 mg per dL per hour, although the initial rate of fall may be higher as rehydration improves renal blood flow and renal glucose clearance. When the blood glucose level approaches 250 to 300 mg per dL, 5% glucose should be added to intravenous fluids. The insulin dose being given is then adjusted to achieve and maintain a target glucose level of 150 to 200 mg per dL. This is close to the renal glucose threshold and therefore minimizes glycosuria and urine volume while also avoiding hypoglycemia. On occasion, the insulin dose required to correct acidosis may be such that 7.5 to 10% dextrose in replacement fluids may be needed to avoid hypoglycemia.

Phosphate

Initial serum phosphate level is usually normal or elevated and falls with correction of DKA. Because of fears of muscle dysfunction or negative effects on hemoglobin's oxygen affinity, thought to be related to phosphate depletion, some authors believe that phosphate supplementation is an essential element of DKA treatment. However, controlled clinical trials have demonstrated no benefit when phosphate salt was included in fluids. If, in the presence of severe hypophosphatemia (e.g., inorganic phosphorus less than 1.0 mg per dL), the clinician wishes to supplement phosphate, half the potassium added to intravenous fluids may be given as the phosphate salt. If this is done, serum calcium levels must be monitored because the infusion of phosphate sometimes causes a fall in serum calcium levels.

COMPLICATIONS

Hypoglycemia and hypokalemia are complications of DKA that can be prevented by frequent monitoring and careful adherence to the procedures outlined earlier.

The most frightening and potentially devastating complication of DKA is cerebral edema. Subclinical cerebral edema may exist in all patients during correction of DKA; symptomatic edema is, fortunately, rare and occurs almost exclusively in children and even more rarely in young adults. Symptoms of cerebral edema usually occur after a period of clinical and biochemical improvement, often 6 to 12 hours after initiation of therapy. Initial symptoms may include irritability, lack of cooperation with treatment or some other subtle change in mentation, headache, or disorientation. These symptoms may progress to include vomiting; seizures; unexpected changes in pulse, blood pressure, or respirations; or diabetes insipidus. In severe cerebral edema, brainstem herniation may occur, with coma, dilated pupils, cranial nerve palsies, incontinence, and cardiorespiratory arrest. Among patients who reach this state, the rates of permanent neurologic sequelae and mortality are very high.

If cerebral edema is suspected, intravenous mannitol should be given immediately in a dose of 0.5 to 1.0 gram per kg, up to 50 grams. A diagnostic emergency computed tomographic scan of the head should be obtained. If cerebral edema is confirmed, the patient should be moved to an intensive care unit for additional therapy such as intubation, hyperventilation, and high-dose glucocorticoids.

Retrospective review of cases of cerebral edema has not identified specific characteristics of patients or modes of therapy that can be implicated as certain causal factors. The most cogent hypothesis to explain cerebral edema is that it results from fluid shifts into the brain, when plasma osmolality drops more quickly than intracellular osmolality. In accord with this hypothesis, cerebral edema tends to occur in patients with long periods of hyperglycemia, such as newly diagnosed patients. Special care should also be exercised in managing patients whose initial sodium level is normal or high, which indicates more severe hyperosmolality. The more frequent occurrence of clinical cerebral edema in children has led many authorities to slow the correction of fluid deficits in this age group.

Another unpredictable and infrequent but well-described complication of DKA is arterial or venous thrombosis or embolism. These events can simulate some aspects of cerebral edema when intracranial vessels are involved.

TRANSITION TO CHRONIC INSULIN THERAPY

Once the blood pH exceeds 7.3, the risk of vomiting is generally minimal and the patient is ready to resume oral intake. Such intake should be limited to clear liquids for the first few hours and expanded as tolerated. When the patient begins ingesting significant caloric loads, additional insulin is required and may conveniently be given subcutaneously. The insulin infusion should be continued until the first subcutaneous dose is effective—for example, 30 minutes after a dose of regular insulin. In patients with previously established insulin regimens, such as twice-daily mixture of regular and NPH, regular insulin alone can be given on a 4- to 6-hour schedule until either the usual morning or evening dose is due.

In patients with newly diagnosed diabetes, the insulin requirement may vary from 0.25 to 2.0 units per kg per day in the days following recovery from DKA. An initial morning (prebreakfast) dose of 0.25 units per kg of NPH insulin can be given plus added regular as indicated by blood glucose levels. Half of the morning dose of NPH can be given before supper. The blood glucose level is determined before each meal and every 4 to 6 hours during the night, and additional regular insulin is given accordingly. The total amount of insulin required in 24 hours can be summed, and two-thirds that amount can be given the following morning as a mixture of NPH and regular insulin.

PREVENTION

Prevention of DKA in patients with known diabetes depends on adequate management during intercurrent illness, pregnancy, or other stress such as surgery or trauma. Insulin is always required on sick days, even when oral intake is reduced. Blood glucose levels must be tested more frequently than usual, up to every 2 to 3 hours. If the glucose level is high, each urine sample should be tested for ketones. Results are used to guide the composition of oral intake and the dose of insulin. For example, a blood glucose level above 250 to 300 mg per dL indicates a need to supplement the usual insulin dose with extra regular insulin. Moderate or severe ketonuria or vomiting indicates a need for immediate contact with the physician. Repeated episodes of DKA indicate a failure of the diabetes management plan, nonadherence to the treatment regimen, poor technique, or significant psychosocial disturbance. Patients with recurrent DKA should have their diabetes care practices reviewed and should be referred for psychological evaluation.

HYPERURICEMIA AND GOUT

method of
ROBERT A. YOOD, M.D.
Saint Vincent Hospital
Worcester, Massachusetts

Gout is caused by deposition of monosodium urate or uric acid crystals. Clinical manifestations of gout include recurrent attacks of acute arthritis, deposition of tophi, uric acid urolithiasis, and, rarely, renal impairment. Hyperuricemia is the common denominator predisposing to crystal deposition and gout. However, in the majority of patients with hyperuricemia, gout never develops, and many patients with hyperuricemia have arthritis as a result of diseases other than gout. Further confusing the evaluation of patients with arthritis is the finding that the serum uric acid may be normal at the time of an acute gouty attack, thus requiring a search for crystals in synovial fluid for proper diagnosis.

Gout is the most common type of inflammatory arthritis in men over the age of 40. Important risk factors for the development of hyperuricemia and gout include male gender, positive family history for gout, obesity, ethanol ingestion, lead exposure, hypertension, renal failure, and ingestion of certain drugs such as diuretics, low-dose salicylates, and cyclosporine (Sandimmune).

HYPERURICEMIA

Hyperuricemia results from either biosynthetic overproduction or renal underexcretion of uric acid or from a combination of both. Excretion either of more than 600 mg of uric acid in a 24-hour period while the patient ingests a purine-free diet or of about 800 mg while the patient is on a normal diet is considered evidence of overproduction of uric acid in the presence of normal renal function. Such overproduction is demonstrated in about 10 to 15% of patients with gout. Approximately two-thirds of uric acid is excreted by the kidney and one-third is eliminated by the gastrointestinal tract. As many as 90% of patients with primary gout have impaired renal excretion of uric acid. The exact mechanism for this impairment is not clear.

CLINICAL FEATURES OF GOUT

In about 80% of cases, the initial attack of gout is monarticular. The most common first site is the great toe metatarsophalangeal joint (podagra), but other joints or bursae in the lower extremities and occasionally the upper extremities may be the initial sites of gout. Gouty arthritis is usually rapid in onset, awakening the patient at night or first noticed upon arising in the morning, and is associated with erythema, warmth, swelling, and exquisite tenderness to touch. There may be extensive soft tissue erythema and swelling that mimics cellulitis. Low-grade fever is common, especially in cases of polyarticular gout. An untreated attack usually lasts for a few days to several weeks, after which there is a gradual return to normal. Provocative factors for gouty arthritis include trauma, surgery, ethanol, and starvation.

The time between the first and second attacks of gout is highly variable. Some patients never have a second attack, although without treatment most have another gouty attack within 2 years. With multiple recurrences, there are usually shorter intervals between attacks, and polyarticular involvement is more common. Although nearly any joint may be affected by gout, involvement of the spine is rare. Eventually, untreated gout may lead to chronic polyarthritis associated with tophaceous destruction of joints and subcutaneous tophi. The most common sites for tophi include the external ear, the olecranon and prepatellar bursae, the ulnar surface of the forearm, and the Achilles tendon. Chronic polyarticular gout may be misdiagnosed as rheumatoid arthritis, especially if tophi are confused with rheumatoid nodules.

DIAGNOSIS

The diagnosis of gout may be suspected on the basis of the clinical features just described. However, podagra is not always caused by gout, and gout occasionally coexists with other disorders such as infectious arthritis or pseudogout. Thus the diagnosis should be made on the basis of identification of needle-shaped urate crystals in synovial fluid aspirated from an affected joint. These crystals appear bright white against a black background when examined in polarized microscopy and are yellow when parallel to the long axis of a first-order red compensator. Synovial fluid should also be examined for cell count, differential, and culture. The synovial fluid leukocyte count in acute gout is elevated, occasionally over 50,000 per mL.

After an acute episode has resolved, it is usually still possible to aspirate the joint and find evidence of urate crystals. An alternative way of making the diagnosis is to aspirate a tophus and examine this material for crystals. In the absence of a crystal diagnosis, a presumptive diagnosis of gout may be based on hyperuricemia and a response to colchicine within 48 hours. Gouty erosions often have a characteristic appearance on x-ray, with a bony overhanging margin.

TREATMENT

Asymptomatic Hyperuricemia

The great majority of patients with asymptomatic hyperuricemia do not require treatment. Asymptomatic hyperuricemia does not appear to lead to significant renal impairment, and only a minority of patients will ever develop gout or urolithiasis. The likelihood of developing acute gout is dependent on the degree and duration of hyperuricemia, often with an interval of decades between the onset of hyperuricemia and the onset of gout. It makes little sense to treat asymptomatic patients with drugs with potential side effects in order to prevent gout in a few. The only exceptions to this might be patients with very high levels of uric acid (over 13 mg per dL) or patients who excrete large amounts of uric acid in the urine (over 1100 mg per 24 hours). Elimination of the underlying cause of hyperuricemia (e.g., diuretics) when possible makes more sense than adding an antihyperuricemic drug. There is little benefit to modification of diet other than to limit alcohol consumption.

Acute Gout

Treatment of acute gout should begin as soon as possible, as delay in treatment often leads to a prolonged attack. Drugs used in the treatment of acute gout include colchicine, nonsteroidal antiinflammatory drugs (NSAIDs), and corticosteroids. The use of oral colchicine for acute gout is limited because of frequent side effects, especially nausea, vomiting, diarrhea, and abdominal pain. When used for acute gout, 0.5 to 0.6 mg of colchicine is usually given orally every hour until joint symptoms improve or until the onset of toxicity. Intravenous colchicine causes less gastrointestinal toxicity but may cause bone marrow suppression and must be used under strict precautions. Intravenous colchicine should be given in a dose of up to 3 mg (usually 1 to 2 mg), diluted in 20 mL of normal saline, infused slowly over at least 10 minutes. Patients chosen for intravenous colchicine should have no renal or hepatic impairment, and no additional oral or intravenous colchicine should be given for 7 days. Because of these restrictions and the risk of marrow suppression, intravenous colchicine is used infrequently.

Indomethacin (Indocin) is often used for the treatment of acute gout, although probably all the NSAIDs are effective when given in full doses (Table 1). The dosage of indomethacin used is often 50 mg three or four times daily for 2 or 3 days and 25 mg three or four times daily for an additional 4 or 5 days or until total resolution of the attack. NSAIDs are usually well tolerated but may cause substantial toxicity. NSAIDs are associated with a significant increase in risk of gastrointestinal ulcer and bleeding. Renal and hepatic impairment appear to occur in fewer than 1% of patients but may be life-threatening. Other manifestations of toxicity include nausea, diarrhea, headache, rash, and fluid retention. NSAIDs should be used cautiously in patients with a history of ulcer disease, renal failure, or congestive heart failure.

Local injection of corticosteroid such as triamcinolone hexacetonide (Aristospan), 20 mg, into an inflamed joint reliably leads to resolution of gout. This treatment is most helpful in patients with monarthritis of a large joint (which may receive injections reliably) and in patients with resistant attacks in whom coexistent infection has been excluded. Recent studies have suggested that adrenocorticotropic hormone (ACTH) given intramuscularly or subcutaneously is very effective in treating acute gout and may be preferred for patients with absolute or relative contraindications to NSAIDs (e.g., gastrointestinal bleeding, anticoagulant therapy, renal failure, or congestive heart failure) or patients unable to take oral medications. ACTH may be given as a single 40-unit injection and may be repeated up to three times daily for several days if needed. Often only one or two injections are necessary, so ACTH may be convenient for outpatient use. Intramuscular triamcinolone acetonide (Kenalog), 60 mg, may be used for acute gout. A second injection may be necessary if there is only a partial response. Oral prednisone is also effective against acute gout, usually in initial doses of 20 to 30 mg daily and tapering over about 10 days.

Prevention of Recurrent Gout

Because a second attack may not occur for years, it is usually advisable to avoid any prophylactic treatment until after the second or third episode of gout. Recurrent attacks may be suppressed by chronic colchicine or low-dose NSAID therapy or by lowering uric acid levels. A disadvantage of using only colchicine and/or NSAIDs is that although they lessen the incidence of acute attacks, they do not prevent deposition of tophi and joint damage. Colchicine prophylaxis is usually in the dose of 0.6 mg twice daily, but should be given once daily to patients with mild renal impairment and avoided in patients with serum creatinine above 2-3 mg per dL because of possible development of toxicity, including myoneuropathy.

Recurrent episodes of gout, appearance of tophi, x-ray evidence of joint erosion, and urolithiasis are indications for antihyperuricemic therapy. Before therapy is started, all signs of inflammation should be absent (traditionally, the author waits 1 month after the acute attack), and prophylactic treatment with colchicine should be begun. If the patient is unable to tolerate colchicine, low-dose NSAIDs (e.g., indomethacin, 25

TABLE 1. **Some Nonsteroidal Anti-Inflammatory Drugs Useful in Treating Acute Gout**

Drug	Initial Dose	Subsequent Dose
Indomethacin (Indocin)	50 mg tid–qid	25 mg bid–qid
Sulindac (Clinoril)	200 mg bid	150–200 mg bid
Ibuprofen (Motrin)	800 mg tid–qid	400–600 mg tid–qid or 800 mg bid
Naproxen (Naprosyn)	500 mg bid–tid	250–375 mg bid–tid or 500 mg bid
Fenoprofen (Nalfon)	600–800 mg qid	200–600 mg tid
Piroxicam (Feldene)	20 mg qd	20 mg qd
Ketoprofen (Orudis)	50–75 mg tid	50–75 mg bid
Tolmetin (Tolectin)	400–600 mg tid	200–400 mg bid–tid or 600 mg bid
Meclofenamate (Meclomen)	100 mg tid–qid	50 mg bid–tid
Diclofenac (Voltaren)	75 mg tid	50–75 mg bid
Flurbiprofen (Ansaid)	100 mg tid	100 mg bid

mg, once or twice daily) may be used for prophylaxis. Colchicine or NSAID prophylaxis should be continued until the uric acid has been normal and the patient free of attacks for 3 to 6 months. Antihyperuricemic therapy is continued indefinitely. Education of patients is essential, with emphasis on the importance of early recognition and treatment of an acute attack, which may be aborted by only a few doses of an NSAID. Patients already receiving antihyperuricemic therapy at the time of acute gout should continue this therapy along with treatment of the acute attack.

Uric acid levels may be lowered by uricosuric agents, usually with probenecid (Benemid) or, occasionally, sulfinpyrazone (Anturane) or by decreasing uric acid production with allopurinol (Zyloprim). Uricosuric agents are indicated only in patients who are under 60 years of age, have essentially normal renal function (creatinine clearance at least 50 mL per minute and preferably 80 mL per minute), have no history of renal stones, and are not overproducers of uric acid. Accordingly, before probenecid is administered, a 24-hour urine uric acid should be obtained. Probenecid is usually started at 250 mg twice daily and may be given in doses up to 1500 mg* twice daily. Side effects, which are infrequent, include skin rash and gastrointestinal complaints. Sulfinpyrazone is usually started at 50 mg twice daily and gradually increased up to 100 mg three to four times daily.

Allopurinol is indicated in patients with urate overproduction, renal stones, renal impairment, age over 60, or inability to take (or failure to respond to) uricosuric agents. Allopurinol is also effective in patients who underexcrete uric acid, so that if a decision is made to use allopurinol instead of a uricosuric drug, it is not necessary to measure 24-hour urinary output of uric acid. Allopurinol is usually started at 300 mg once daily, although lower doses are necessary in cases of renal failure. Doses of up to 600 mg daily may be

required, but such high doses are not often needed. Although allopurinol is usually well-tolerated, side effects, including gastrointestinal upset, diarrhea, headache, and skin rashes, are more common than with probenecid. Serious side effects include alopecia, fever, lymphadenopathy, marrow suppression, hepatic dysfunction, interstitial nephritis, renal failure, and hypersensitivity vasculitis. Allopurinol should not be used with azathioprine (Imuran) or 6-mercaptopurine (Purinethol) because it interferes with the metabolism of those drugs. Because allopurinol is more expensive than probenecid and has more side effects, it is probably wiser to use probenecid to lower serum uric acid when possible.

The dosage of antihyperuricemic therapy should be modified on the basis of the response after 6 months to 1 year, the goal being a uric acid level below 5 to 6 mg per dL. It is also appropriate to monitor x-rays and clinical evidence of tophi, as it is possible for progressive tissue deposition to occur despite normal urate levels. In these cases, higher doses are needed.

HYPERLIPOPROTEINEMIA

method of
ROBERT S. LEES, M.D.
Harvard University/Massachusetts Institute of Technology
Cambridge, Massachusetts

and

ANN M. LEES, M.D.
Harvard Medical School
Boston, Massachusetts

The concept that atherosclerosis is a disease that cannot be prevented and can be treated only by invasive means has been abundantly disproved. Treatment of risk factors, including smoking, hypertension, and diabetes, in addition to lipid disorders, clearly alters

---

*Exceeds dosage recommended by the manufacturer.

the natural history of atherosclerosis before clinical events occur. Multiple studies since 1980 have shown that treatment of lipid disorders can arrest progression and promote regression of existing atherosclerotic lesions. Except in patients with acute abdominal pain, hyperlipoproteinemia is diagnosed by measuring total plasma cholesterol (TC) and triglycerides (TG) at least twice, 1 to 2 weeks apart, at a reliable clinical laboratory. The lipid and lipoprotein cholesterol values at the 50th percentile for the North American population are shown in Table 1.

Hyperlipoproteinemia is a common major risk factor for coronary heart disease. More rarely, hyperlipoproteinemia, specifically hyperglyceridemia, is a cause of severe abdominal pain, with or without acute pancreatitis. Although these complications are relatively rare, their recognition and prompt treatment can resolve an acute abdominal emergency without unnecessary exploratory surgery. Because the diagnosis is frequently overlooked, treatment of severe hyperglyceridemia is discussed first.

HYPERLIPOPROTEINEMIA AND ABDOMINAL PAIN

Severe hyperglyceridemia (TG level > 3000 mg per dL) is associated with two distinct abdominal pain syndromes. The first is hyperglyceridemic abdominal crisis, a syndrome of recurrent abdominal pain without pancreatitis. It often follows a fatty meal in severely hyperglyceridemic patients and is associated with an initial plasma glyceride level of 6000 mg per dL or more. Pain, nausea, and vomiting may be accompanied by fever and leukocytosis. On physical examination, the abdomen may be diffusely tender, or the tenderness may be localized to the liver or spleen. Percussion reveals these organs to be enlarged, because they are engorged with triglycerides; the pain may be caused by capsular stretching. Whole blood may look like cream of tomato soup and plasma like heavy cream. Blood and urine levels of pancreatic enzymes are consistently normal in this syndrome.

Any patient whose clinical picture meets these criteria should be treated immediately with glucose-free intravenous fluids and cessation of oral intake until plasma TG levels are below 1000 mg per dL and symptoms have abated. If left untreated, the syndrome can occasionally trigger acute pancreatitis, the second cause of severe abdominal pain seen in hyperglyceridemia. Although pancreatitis often occurs in the setting of hyperlipemic abdominal crisis, it also may occur as a primary event in hypertriglyceridemia. In either case, the patient can often tell the exact moment when the deep epigastric and back pain of pancreatitis begins. When that occurs, the treatment is identical to that of pancreatitis caused by any other entity.

HYPERLIPOPROTEINEMIA AND ATHEROSCLEROSIS

High TC is usually an indication of elevated levels of low-density lipoprotein (LDL) or very-low-density lipoprotein (VLDL) but occasionally results from elevations of high-density lipoprotein (HDL) alone. Clinically, LDL is measured as LDL cholesterol (LDL-C) and HDL as HDL cholesterol (HDL-C). Because high HDL is a negative risk factor for coronary heart disease and high LDL is a major positive risk factor, the distinction between the two is important. Thus in addition to TC and TG, HDL should be measured in every patient being evaluated for the risk or presence of atherosclerotic cardiovascular disease. From these measurements, LDL can be calculated by the Friedewald equation,

$$LDL = TC - ([0.2 \times TG] + HDL),$$

which is valid for TG levels less than 400 mg per dL. The problem of clinical laboratory variation in lipid measurements has not yet been solved, and so it is worth finding a reliable laboratory. If necessary, a plasma sample might be sent to a laboratory of known accuracy to establish the diagnosis. Women, as well as men, with adverse lipoprotein profiles should be considered at high risk of developing atherosclerosis.

Nowadays, the term "hyperlipoproteinemia," or "hyperlipidemia," is somewhat of a misnomer because depressed levels of HDL may be the only risk factor in some patients and may be associated with severe atherosclerosis. In other patients, elevated levels of plasma lipoprotein (a) [Lp(a)] may be the only risk factor evident. If no other lipid or nonlipid risk factors are present and Lp(a) measurements cannot be made, a tentative diagnosis of elevated Lp(a) may be made in patients with severe coronary disease, and appropriate treatment may be instituted.

TABLE 1. **50th Percentile Plasma Lipid and Lipoprotein Cholesterol Levels***

Age (Years)	TC	LDL-C	HDL-C	TG	Lp(a)
Males					
20–39	160–195	100–130	≈45	80–110	≈13
40–70	205–215	135–145	45–50	130–110	≈13
Females					
20–49	165–205	100–130	50–60	75–95	≈14
50–70	215–235	135–145	≈60	100–120	≈14

Abbreviations: TC = total plasma cholesterol; LDL-C = low-density lipoprotein cholesterol; HDL-C = high-density lipoprotein cholesterol; TG = triglycerides; Lp(a) = lipoprotein (a).

*Approximate values (mg/dL) for the U.S. population. Where a range is given, the beginning of the range applies to the lower end, and the end of the range to the upper end of the age distribution. Age-related data are not available for Lp(a).

Broad guidelines in no way eliminate the necessity of considering each patient individually. The number and degree of lipoprotein abnormalities, the presence of other risk factors, the presence of symptoms or signs of arteriosclerosis or cholesterol deposition, the family history, and the patient's age must all be taken into account in order to determine the most appropriate treatment program. The first line of defense in treating hyperlipidemia is a qualitatively and quantitatively appropriate diet based on the American Heart Association dietary guidelines, as well as cessation of smoking. It is obligatory to treat other risk factors for arteriosclerosis in hyperlipidemic patients, including hypertension, diabetes, cigarette smoking, obesity, and hypothyroidism, when these are present.

CLASSIFICATION OF LIPID ABNORMALITIES

Although a variety of systems have been developed for classifying the hyperlipoproteinemias, most rest on detailed genetic analysis of two to three generations in the patient's family and thus lack the simplicity and cost effectiveness of the Fredrickson-Lees classification, which is a clinical phenotyping system (Table 2). As a result, many physicians classify the patient's hyperlipoproteinemic phenotype inadequately, which can lead to suboptimal treatment.

In brief, 80 to 90% cases of hyperlipoproteinemia in adults are Type II or Type IV. Type II is defined as a primary elevation of LDL cholesterol and is associated with high risk of atherosclerosis; it can be subdivided into Type IIA (elevated LDL alone) and Type IIB (primarily elevated LDL with moderate TG level elevation). Type IV patients, whose atherosclerotic risk is high, have relatively high TG levels as a result of increases in VLDL and commonly also have decreased levels of HDL; the TC may be moderately elevated, inasmuch as VLDL consists of about 20% cholesterol.

Type I hyperlipidemia is very rare and is found usually shortly after birth or in early childhood. Patients present with severe chylomicronemia (greatly elevated TG levels) because of a genetic deficiency or absence of lipoprotein lipase. This syndrome is easily recognizable by lipoprotein electrophoresis. Type I patients are at high risk for pancreatitis and must be treated immediately with a virtually fat-free diet. Their risk of atherosclerosis is relatively low. A presumptive diagnosis of Type I can be made if a fresh blood sample looks like cream of tomato soup and if blood plasma stored overnight in the refrigerator separates into a thick creamy collar and a clear or almost clear infranate.

Type III (dysbetalipoproteinemic) patients, whose atherosclerotic risk is high, usually present as adults with more or less equal elevations of both TC and TG levels and often typical but subtle skin deposits known as planar xanthomas. The disease is associated with an inherited abnormality in apolipoprotein E. The lipo-

TABLE 2. **Description of Lipid Disorders and Selection of Drugs**

Condition	Relative Incidence	Risk of Atherosclerosis	Findings		Drugs of Choice
			Laboratory	*Physical*	
Type I	Rare	Moderate*	TG + + + +	Eruptive xanthomas; abdominal pain	None (low-fat diet)
Type IIA	Common	Very high	TC +/+ + + +	Arcus corneae; xanthelasmas; tendon xanthomas	HMG-CoA reductase inhibitors; niacin; resins; probucol; [estrogen]† apheresis
Type IIB	Common	Very high	TC +/+ + +; TG +/+ +	Arcus corneae; xanthelasmas; tendon xanthomas	Niacin; HMG-CoA reductase inhibitors; probucol gemfibrozil [estrogen]†
Type III	Uncommon	High	TC + + + TG + + +	Eruptive and tuberous xanthomas	Gemfibrozil; niacin
Type IV	Common	High	TG +/+ + + (TC +/+ +)	Arcus corneae; occasionally xanthelasmas	Niacin; gemfibrozil
Type V	Relatively common	Relatively high*	TG + + + + (TC +/+ +)	Eruptive and tuberous xanthomas	Niacin; gemfibrozil; norethindrone acetate
Isolated low HDL	Uncommon	High	HDL <35 mg/dL	Occasionally arcus corneae	Niacin; estrogen†
Elevated Lp(a)	Relatively common	High	Lp(a) >30 mg/dL	None	Niacin; apheresis

Abbreviations: TG = triglycerides; TC = total plasma cholesterol; HMG-CoA = 3-hydroxy-3-methylglutaryl–coenzyme A; HDL = high-density lipoprotein; Lp(a) = lipoprotein (a).
*High risk of pancreatitis
†For post-menopausal women only. See text for details.

protein electrophoretic pattern is often highly suggestive of the disease. Phenotyping is especially important for identifying Type III patients; the disease is uncommon but generally responds well to an appropriate lipid-lowering drug.

Type V hyperlipoproteinemia, less than common but not rare, is found in adults at high risk for atherosclerosis who have markedly elevated TG levels with moderate elevation in TC. Lipoprotein electrophoresis in these patients shows elevation of both chylomicrons and VLDL. Like Type I patients, Type V patients are often at high risk for pancreatitis.

TREATMENT

The primary drugs now in use for lipid disorders include niacin (Nicolar); the HMG-CoA reductase inhibitors lovastatin (Mevacor), pravastatin (Pravachol), and simvastatin (Zocor); the fibrate gemfibrozil (Lopid); the lipid anti-oxidant probucol (Lorelco); and the bile acid–binding resins cholestyramine (Questran) and colestipol (Colestid). Drugs for each phenotype are listed in order of preference in Table 2. Useful drug combinations are listed in Table 3.

Optimal treatment depends on the recognition that diet is the first line of therapy and that the best drug for high LDL cholesterol alone is not necessarily the best drug for elevations of both LDL and TG levels or an elevation of TG level alone. Furthermore, in some patients, two or even three properly chosen drugs at lower doses may be more effective and produce fewer side effects than a single drug at a higher dose.

Normalizing Plasma LDL

Type II hyperlipoproteinemia is characterized by an increase in plasma LDL. In Type IIA patients, elevated LDL level is the only abnormality. In contrast, Type IIB patients have elevated LDL and elevated TG levels, usually accompanied by low HDL levels. The treatment of these two clinical entities is somewhat different. Management of Type IIA is discussed in this section, whereas Type IIB is covered in the section on normalizing TG levels.

Dietary therapy is obligatory for patients with Type IIA hyperlipoproteinemia. In younger subjects with only mild LDL elevation, it may be sufficient. Caloric restriction to achieve as close to ideal weight as possible should be accompanied by a reduction of dietary cholesterol to 200 mg per day and reduction of saturated fat intake to a minimum, with replacement by monounsaturated fats (olive or peanut oil) and some polyunsaturated fats (corn, safflower, sunflower, or canola oil). Margarines with a high monounsaturated content are desirable. Patients with moderate LDL elevations (140 to 165 mg per dL) may experience as much as 20 to 25% lowering of LDL levels on a good diet; those with very high levels (> 200 mg per dL) may have little change, but their response to drug therapy is blunted or even abolished if they are not on an appropriate diet.

The drug of first choice for mild to moderate LDL elevation is one of the three 3-hydroxy-3-methylglutaryl–coenzyme A (HMG-CoA) reductase inhibitors on the U.S. market: lovastatin (Mevacor), pravastatin (Pravachol) and simvastatin (Zocor). In all patients on reductase inhibitors, one should check not only lipids but also liver function tests and creatine phosphokinase monthly for 3 months, then every 3 months for 6 months and every 4 to 6 months thereafter. In patients with mild to moderate isolated LDL elevation (Type IIA), plasma lipids may be normal-

TABLE 3. **Drug Combinations Useful for Treating Lipid Disorders***

Primary Drug	Secondary Drug(s)	Remarks†
High LDL		
HMG-CoA reductase inhibitors (lovastatin, pravastatin, or simvastatin)	Resin (colestipol or cholestyramine); niacin; probucol	If LDL remains elevated
High TG		
Gemfibrozil	Resin	If LDL is elevated
Gemfibrozil	Niacin	If LDL is elevated or HDL is low
Niacin	Resin	If LDL is elevated
Niacin	Probucol	If LDL is elevated
Niacin	Reductase inhibitors	If LDL is elevated
Niacin	Gemfibrozil	If TG remain elevated
Low HDL		
Niacin	Gemfibrozil	If HDL remains low
Estrogen‡	Niacin	If HDL remains low

Abbreviations: LDL = low-density lipoprotein; HMG-CoA = 3-hydroxy-3-methylglutaryl–coenzyme A; TG = triglycerides; HDL = high-density lipoprotein.

*See text for details, including dosages.

†All drug combinations require careful monitoring for side effects, including follow-up visits, liver and skeletal muscle enzymes.

‡*Only* for post-menopausal women. See text for details.

ized with 10 to 20 mg once daily of any of the three, with virtually no side effects. Patients with higher LDL may require 40 mg of lovastatin twice daily or 20 mg of pravastatin or simvastatin twice daily, or more likely, multidrug therapy (to be described). With such therapy, LDL cholesterol may be lowered up to 40% and TG levels lowered to 10 to 15%. In the authors' experience, there is little change in HDL. All three drugs may cause hepatic and skeletal muscle toxicity, as well as insomnia and weight gain. These side effects are relatively uncommon, are dose related, and occur much more often in patients who require multidrug therapy.

The drug of second choice for Type IIA hyperlipoproteinemia is niacin. The authors prescribe only 500-mg tablets, and therapy progresses as rapidly as tolerated to the optimal dose, usually 3 grams daily in divided dose. (The maximal recommended dose is 4 grams daily, which is used in occasional patients.) In all patients taking niacin, one should check not only lipids but also liver function tests and creatine phosphokinase monthly for 3 months, then every 3 months for 6 months and every 4 to 6 months thereafter. Niacin, the drug in longest use for hypercholesterolemia, has many advantages and many disadvantages. Its advantages include LDL lowering of up to 35%, TG level lowering of up to 75%, and, uniquely among available drugs, HDL raising of up to 100% and Lp(a) lowering of up to 50%. Another unique attribute is its cost of a few pennies a tablet, in contrast to a dollar or more for other drugs. Unfortunately, the list of disadvantages of niacin is almost as long. It is a gastric irritant and may activate long-dormant peptic ulcer or cause gastritis. It can elevate blood uric acid levels and produce gout, elevate blood glucose level and exacerbate diabetes, and cause profound hepatotoxicity with (rarely) jaundice or hypoalbuminemia. It commonly causes cutaneous flushing, dry and even scaly skin, and, in rare instances, acanthosis nigricans. Fortunately, all these side effects are reversible when the drug is stopped. Finally, in atherosclerosis regression trials, niacin has been the most effective agent in promoting stability and regression of coronary lesions. In spite of its drawbacks, many patients tolerate niacin at some dose level, and the authors prescribe it frequently, giving the drug always after meals, the first dose after the evening meal, so that flushing is not troublesome during the workday. With continuous regular use, flushing often disappears. If flushing is bothersome, an aspirin tablet (325 mg) before the meal often reduces or abolishes it.

Resins, including cholestyramine (Questran) and colestipol (Colestid), are the drugs of third choice for patients with Type IIA hyperlipoproteinemia, except for children and adolescents, for whom resins may be the first choice. The dose ranges are 4 to 8 grams once or twice daily for cholestyramine and 5 to 10 grams once or twice daily for colestipol. Their advantages include a virtually complete lack of absorption and the potential systemic toxicity that goes with it (because they act within the intestinal lumen) and a moderate LDL-lowering effect (15 to 25%). Their disadvantages include an unpleasant grittiness and multiple gastrointestinal side effects, including bloating, abdominal pain, sometimes severe constipation, and gastrointestinal bleeding. Because resins may decrease the absorption of other medications, they and other drugs should be taken 2 hours apart, which complicates the daily regimen of patients taking multiple drugs. Nevertheless, for patients who do not want or cannot tolerate absorbable drugs, the resins can produce a valuable LDL-lowering effect. In other patients, they are often useful in multidrug therapy and may strongly potentiate reductase inhibitors and niacin.

At menopause, there are often a rise in plasma LDL and a fall in HDL. When these occur, it is advisable to prescribe estrogen replacement therapy (conjugated equine estrogens [Premarin]), 0.625 mg daily, if there are no contraindications such as presence or strong family history of breast or cervical cancer. Women for whom such therapy is most appropriate include those in whom LDL and HDL levels become clearly abnormal and women with a family history of heart disease in either sex. If the HDL level is normal on estrogen replacement but the LDL level remains high, a small dose of a reductase inhibitor (e.g., pravastatin, 10 mg daily) may bring the LDL into the normal range.

Probucol (Lorelco) is the least frequently used but an occasionally valuable drug for lowering the LDL level. It lowers LDL by 10 to 25% and may potentiate reductase inhibitor therapy in patients who respond to little else. Its toxicity in most patients is low, usually manifesting only as occasional diarrhea or foul-smelling perspiration, but rare idiosyncratic reactions—severe vertigo that is easy to mistake for cerebellar hemorrhage, and potentially life-threatening angioneurotic edema—have been well documented. Probucol has two unusual attributes. First, it is an antioxidant and is thought to inhibit LDL oxidation. Unusual reports of the regression of xanthomas with only marginal LDL reduction have been attributed to this antioxidant effect. Second, probucol lowers plasma HDL levels, often dramatically. The significance of this is unclear. Full assessment of the role of probucol in the therapy of hypercholesterolemia must wait until the completion of randomized trials of the drug's effects on clinical event rates and on the progression of atherosclerosis.

For patients with severe hypercholesterolemia who do not respond to drugs, especially patients with atherosclerotic disease, selective LDL apheresis may be lifesaving. Although no system for this is on the market, at least two are in clinical trials in the United States. These systems work by removing blood from an arm vein, separating red blood cells from plasma on-line, removing the LDL by heparin precipitation or by perfusion through an affinity column, recombining the LDL-depleted plasma with the red blood cells, and reinfusing them into the other arm. The entire process is continuous and takes 2 to 4 hours, depending on the device used. It is well tolerated by almost all patients. A few published and several as yet unpublished studies show striking regression of atherosclerosis in patients treated weekly or biweekly with LDL apheresis. The authors have used selective LDL apheresis and, before that was available, nonselective plasmapheresis, for more than 25 years and believe that their efficacy has not been overstated. Patients with homozygous familial hypercholesterolemia have survived in the authors' clinic on apheresis many years longer than their untreated siblings, with regression of xanthomas and no evidence of progression of coronary disease. Drug-resistant patients with total plasma cholesterol higher than 350 mg per dL or LDL cholesterol higher than 200 mg per dL on maximal drug therapy should be considered for LDL apheresis. Liver transplantation is not appropriate therapy for hypercholesterolemia.

Normalizing Plasma Triglycerides

Certain rules apply to all hyperglyceridemic patients (Types I, IIB, III, IV, and V). First, diet is critical. In Type I, which is rare and should preferably be treated by a specialist in lipid disorders, diet is the only therapy currently available. In Types IIB, III, IV, and V, weight should be reduced to as close to ideal as possible. Second, the maintenance diet should be low in cholesterol and saturated fats. In Type V patients, total fat content should be <25% of calories; in the others, about 30%. Third, LDL cholesterol may increase markedly with treatment and should be monitored as described for Type II. If monotherapy raises LDL to abnormal levels, an LDL-lowering drug, usually niacin, sometimes resin, rarely a reductase inhibitor, should be added. Fourth, treatment is different when glucose intolerance is present. Niacin should be a drug of last resort in diabetic patients. If it is given, patients taking insulin require a dose increase; those not taking insulin will require insulin. Finally, all patients taking fibrates, with or without niacin, need careful attention to the potentially insidious onset of myopathy. Malaise, muscle aches, or difficulty in performing physical tasks should cause suspicion of myopathy; plasma creatine phosphokinase (CPK) and, in equivocal cases, aldolase should be measured. In patients on multidrug therapy, CPK should be measured every 3 to 6 months.

In most clinical situations, high to very high plasma TG levels in patients with Type IIB, III, IV, or V hyperlipoproteinemia are associated with low HDL. In patients with increased TG levels, phenotyping of the plasma lipoprotein pattern is very important. For Type IIB patients, the drug of *first choice* is usually niacin (Nicolar), which should be used according to the guidelines already given for Type IIA. Treatment of Type IIB with HMG-CoA reductase inhibitors is usually insufficient to lower the triglyceride levels to normal or to raise the HDL level to normal. Gemfibrozil (Lopid) alone in Type IIB patients may lower TG levels but raise LDL levels even further. It is sometimes useful in combination with niacin or resin. Resins given alone often markedly exacerbate the hyperglyceridemia and lower HDL levels even further. However, either reductase inhibitors or resin may be combined with a low dose of niacin (1 to 2 grams daily) to normalize the plasma lipoprotein pattern in Type IIB patients. The tempting combination of fibrates (to be discussed) with reductase inhibitors is accompanied by a high risk of myopathy, even frank rhabdomyolysis and secondary myoglobinuria and renal failure, and should be used only as a last resort, with very careful follow-up.

Patients with Type III hyperlipoproteinemia are usually remarkably responsive to fibrates such as gemfibrozil (Lopid) and clofibrate (Atromid-S), although the latter is rarely used now. The usual dose of gemfibrozil is 0.6 gram twice daily. Its advantages include a 40 to 80% decrease in TG levels and a 10 to 40% increase in HDL levels, depending on the initial concentration; the higher the initial TG level, the greater the percentage response to gemfibrozil for both TG and HDL. In Type III patients, the response is almost always good, even at relatively low TG levels. Disadvantages are few and include occasional eructation, abdominal pain or diarrhea or both, and, in rare instances, myopathy.

Patients with the Type IV phenotype may respond well to fibrates but often require niacin alone or in combination with a fibrate at the lowest effective dose of each agent to achieve normal lipid levels and to minimize the risk of myopathy. Those with Type V usually do not respond well to fibrates and require niacin or niacin plus a fibrate. In some Type V patients, the disease is resistant to all other drugs and can be controlled only with androgen or progestin therapy. The only such drug available in the United States at present that is of proven use in treating Type V is norethindrone acetate* (Norlutate). At a dose of 5 mg once a day, it lowers TG, raises HDL, and, in the authors' experience, completely prevents pancreatitis, an otherwise constant threat to seriously hyperglyceridemic Type V patients.

Normalizing Plasma HDL

In about 1% of the population, according to the Framingham Study data, HDL is significantly low in the presence of normal TC and TG levels. In such patients, the risk of atherosclerotic death is high. However, low HDL level alone must be treated differently from the low HDL level associated with elevated TG levels. Patients with elevated TG and low HDL levels generally have a significant increase in HDL when the glycerides are normalized, as described earlier. If HDL does not return entirely to normal in treated hyperglyceridemic patients, adding a small dose of niacin or increasing the niacin dose in those already taking it usually normalizes HDL. In patients with normal TG levels, in contrast, low HDL is much harder to treat, and it may not be possible to normalize it with currently available therapy. Weight reduction to ideal weight and treatment with as high a dose of niacin as necessary to normalize HDL (up to a maximum of 4 grams daily in divided doses) or as high a dose as tolerated is, in the authors' experience, the best approach. In all patients taking niacin, liver function tests and CPK measurements should be performed monthly for 3 months, then every 3 months for 6 months, and every 4 to 6 months thereafter. Isolated low HDL in postmenopausal women may be appropriately treated with estrogen replacement therapy (conjugated equine estrogens [Premarin]), 0.625 mg daily, if there are no contraindications such as presence or strong family history of breast or cervical cancer. If HDL remains low on estrogen therapy, niacin should be added to the regimen.

Normalizing Lp(a)

Lp(a) was identified by K. Berg 30 years ago as a heritable lipoprotein antigen with a strong link to coronary heart disease. It is a complex lipoprotein that contains apolipoprotein B, the protein moiety of LDL, disulfide-bonded to apolipoprotein (a), a molecule that closely mimics the structure of plasminogen. Lp(a) accumulates in the arterial

wall just as LDL does, but in addition to bringing excess cholesterol into the vessel, it inhibits tissue plasminogen activator, the enzyme that converts plasminogen into the active thrombolytic enzyme plasmin. This intramural plasmin inhibition probably increases the atherogenicity of Lp(a) but also seems to markedly increase thrombotic occlusions at sites of plaque formation, particularly in smaller arteries such as the coronary vessels. The result is that patients with high Lp(a), even with normal LDL and HDL, are prone to early, severe, and diffuse atherosclerosis; the risk is exacerbated further if high LDL or low HDL or both are also present.

Lp(a) is polymorphic with widely varying numbers of repeating subunits called "kringles" and is difficult to measure accurately. Nevertheless, immunoassays are increasingly available to clinicians, and in patients with normal lipid levels and coronary disease, with coronary disease that is unusually early or severe in relation to the usual risk factors, or with striking family histories of coronary disease, plasma Lp(a) levels should be measured. Values above 30 mg per dL are clearly abnormal and should probably be treated even in the absence of coronary disease. The authors prescribe niacin (up to 4 grams daily, in divided dose), the only drug known to lower Lp(a) levels, and have seen up to 40% reduction in plasma Lp(a). In patients taking niacin, the authors check liver function tests and CPK monthly for 3 months, then every 3 months for 6 months, and every 4 to 6 months thereafter. The only other effective treatment for high Lp(a) is LDL apheresis. All methods used for selective LDL apheresis, including heparin precipitation, dextran sulfate, and antibody columns, remove Lp(a) along with LDL. The authors strongly recommend LDL apheresis for patients at high risk or with severe atherosclerosis who cannot tolerate or do not respond to niacin. It may be lifesaving.

Multidrug Therapy

It is tempting to increase the dose of a first-line drug when a partial response is achieved but the lipoprotein profile does not return to normal. The temptation should often be resisted because the side effects of lipid-lowering drugs usually increase at high dose faster than the therapeutic effects. The authors usually increase the first drug to the maximal recommended dose; if lipids are not normalized or if significant side effects occur, the dose of the first drug is lowered to half or three quarters of the maximal dose, and a second drug is added. Certain drug combinations are especially helpful; these are listed in Table 3.

---

*This use of Norlutate is not listed in the manufacturer's official directive.

Recent data suggest that the combination of a reductase inhibitor with gemfibrozil, which is very effective in Type IIB patients, may be tolerated if a low dose of one drug is given 12 hours apart from a low dose of the other (e.g., pravastatin, 10 to 20 mg in the morning and gemfibrozil 600 mg in the evening). However, use of this combination requires careful clinical and laboratory monitoring of the patient and is contraindicated in patients with diabetes or renal failure.

OBESITY

method of
F. XAVIER PI-SUNYER, M.D.
Columbia University College of Physicians and Surgeons
New York, New York

The treatment of obesity is difficult and often discouraging because the failure rate is extremely high. The primary emphasis must be on self-control rather than on drugs, and what must be recognized by both patient and physician is that the primary agent for change is the patient rather than the physician. Self-motivation and commitment of the patient are required, and the support, understanding, and knowledge of the physician are helpful.

Because physicians are accustomed to giving pharmacologic agents to treat most diseases that they see, they are often not attuned to the tedious task of slow, difficult weight loss, with its relapses, plateaus, and disappointing statistics. Because of this, other health professionals have become involved in treatment. Many dietitians, psychologists, social workers, and nurses advise and treat patients who want to lose weight and can be very helpful. Nevertheless, a physician should monitor the weight loss program and treat any health problems that may develop.

Obesity is extremely common in the United States, and a physician usually requires nothing more than a quick look to determine the need for weight loss. However, because there is much preoccupation with overweight and because social, psychological, and economic rewards are perceived to be derived from a trim look, patients who are not truly obese may wish to lose weight. This should not be allowed. A general table of weight standards for age and height is published by the Gerontology Research Center of the National Institutes of Aging (Table 1). The percentage of body fat also can be calculated and followed during weight loss by using the sum of four subcutaneous skinfolds (Table 2).

Another guideline that can be used is the body mass index (BMI), calculated by dividing the weight in kilograms by the height in meters squared (kg/m^2). Such guidelines have been recommended by the 1985 National Institutes of Health Consensus Development Conference Statement on the Health Implications of Obesity. The U.S. Department of Agriculture has published recommended dietary guidelines for the BMI in the population (Table 3). Below age 35, a BMI of 20 to 25 is a good weight for most people; a BMI of 25 to 27 may lead to some health problems; and one greater than 27 presents an increasing risk of developing health problems. As persons in the United States become older, they gain some weight. Adding one unit of BMI per decade makes allowance for this (see Table 3).

How the fat is distributed on the body also is important to risk of morbidity. An excessive amount of fat in the trunk (central fat, upper body fat) carries more risk than fat on the lower body (peripheral fat, lower body fat), is a better indicator of the presence of risk factors such as hypertension and hyperlipidemia, and is a better predictor of some diseases, such as coronary heart disease and diabetes.

Obesity aggravates or precipitates a number of other diseases, including diabetes mellitus, hypertension, coronary heart disease, congestive heart failure, thromboembolic disease, restrictive lung disease, pickwickian syndrome, gout, degenerative arthritis, gallbladder disease, infertility, and hyperlipoproteinemia. In cases in which one or more of these conditions is present, more stringent standards of weight seems appropriate, such as those of the 1983 Metropolitan Life Insurance Company weight tables. In any case, the physician must recognize that although the loss of weight is likely to ameliorate any associated conditions, therapy targeted specifically for these disorders may be also necessary.

Obesity develops because energy intake exceeds energy expenditure. Once obesity has been attained, however, there may be a new weight plateau at which intake is equivalent to expenditure and weight is stable. To lose weight, energy intake must be decreased and energy expenditure increased in order to disequilibrate the energy balance equation and create a calorie deficit.

TABLE 1. **Age-Specific Weight-for-Height Tables**

Height (feet–inches)	Weight Range (Pounds) for Men and Women by Age (Years)*				
	25	35	45	55	65
4–10	84–111	92–119	99–127	107–135	115–142
4–11	87–115	95–123	103–131	111–139	119–147
5–0	90–119	98–127	106–135	114–143	123–152
5–1	93–123	101–131	110–140	118–148	127–157
5–2	96–127	105–136	113–144	122–153	131–163
5–3	99–131	108–140	117–149	126–158	135–168
5–4	102–135	112–145	121–154	130–163	140–173
5–5	106–140	115–149	125–159	134–168	144–179
5–6	109–144	119–154	129–164	138–174	148–184
5–7	112–148	122–159	133–169	143–179	153–190
5–8	116–153	126–163	137–174	147–184	158–196
5–9	119–157	130–168	141–179	151–190	162–201
5–10	122–162	134–173	145–184	156–195	167–207
5–11	126–167	137–178	149–190	160–201	172–213
6–0	129–171	141–183	153–195	165–207	177–219
6–1	133–176	145–188	157–200	169–213	182–225
6–2	137–181	149–194	162–206	174–219	187–232
6–3	141–186	153–199	166–212	179–225	192–238
6–4	144–191	157–205	171–218	184–231	197–244

*Values in this table are for height without shoes and weight without clothes. To convert inches to centimeters, multiply by 2.54; to convert pounds to kilograms, multiply by 0.455.

Data from Andres R, Gerontology Research Center, National Institute for Aging, Baltimore, MD.

TABLE 2. **Equivalent Fat Content, As a Percentage of Body Weight, for a Range of Values for the Sum of Four Skinfolds* of Males and Females of Different Ages**

Skinfolds (mm)	Males (Age in Years)				Females (Age in Years)			
	17–29	*30–39*	*40–49*	*50+*	*16–29*	*30–39*	*40–49*	*50+*
15	4.8				10.5			
20	8.1	12.2	12.2	12.6	14.1	17.0	19.8	21.4
25	10.5	14.2	15.0	15.6	16.8	19.4	22.2	24.0
30	12.9	16.2	17.7	18.6	19.5	21.8	24.5	26.6
35	14.7	17.7	19.6	20.8	21.5	23.7	26.4	28.5
40	16.4	19.2	21.4	22.9	23.4	25.5	28.2	30.3
45	17.7	20.4	23.0	24.7	25.0	26.9	29.6	31.9
50	19.0	21.5	24.6	26.5	26.5	28.2	31.0	33.4
55	20.1	22.5	25.9	27.9	27.8	29.4	32.1	34.6
60	21.2	23.5	27.1	29.2	29.1	30.6	33.2	35.7
65	22.2	24.3	28.2	30.4	30.2	31.6	34.1	36.7
70	23.1	25.1	29.3	31.6	31.2	32.5	35.0	37.7
75	24.0	25.9	30.3	32.7	32.2	33.4	35.9	38.7
80	24.8	26.6	31.2	33.8	33.1	34.3	36.7	39.6
85	25.5	27.2	32.1	34.8	34.0	35.1	37.5	40.4
90	26.2	27.8	33.0	35.8	34.8	35.8	38.3	41.2
95	26.9	28.4	33.7	36.6	35.6	36.5	39.0	41.9
100	27.6	29.0	34.4	37.4	36.4	37.2	39.7	42.6
105	28.2	29.6	35.1	38.2	37.1	37.9	40.4	43.3
110	28.8	30.1	35.8	39.0	37.8	38.6	41.0	43.9
115	29.4	30.6	36.4	39.7	38.4	39.1	41.5	44.5
120	30.0	31.1	37.0	40.4	39.0	39.6	42.0	45.1
125	31.0	31.5	37.6	41.1	39.6	40.1	42.5	45.7
130	31.5	31.9	38.2	41.8	40.2	40.6	43.0	46.2
135	32.0	32.3	38.7	42.4	40.8	41.1	43.5	46.7
140	32.5	32.7	39.2	43.0	41.3	41.6	44.0	47.2
145	32.9	33.1	39.7	43.6	41.8	42.1	44.5	47.7
150	33.3	33.5	40.2	44.1	42.3	42.6	45.0	48.2
155	33.7	33.9	40.7	44.6	42.8	43.1	45.4	48.7
160	34.1	34.3	41.2	45.1	43.3	43.6	45.8	49.2
165	34.5	34.6	41.6	45.6	43.7	44.0	46.2	49.6
170	34.9	34.8	42.0	46.1	44.1	44.4	46.6	50.0
175	35.3					44.8	47.0	50.4
180	35.6					45.2	47.4	40.8
185	35.9					45.6	47.8	51.2
190						45.9	48.2	51.6
195						46.2	48.5	52.0
200						46.5	48.8	52.4
205							49.1	52.7
210							49.4	53.0

*Biceps, triceps, subscapular, and suprailiac.

From Durnin JVGA, Womersley J: Body fat assessed from total body density and its estimation from skinfold thickness. Br J Nutr *32*:77, 1974. Reprinted with permission of Cambridge University Press.

The three approaches to weight reduction, in order of importance, are diet, exercise, and drugs.

TREATMENT

Goals of Therapy

It is common for patients beginning a weight-loss program to have faulty and unrealistic belief about how rapidly they can lose weight. It is important to instruct them in this regard in order to prevent disappointment and attrition.

One pound of fat is equivalent to 3500 to 4000 kcal. A caloric deficit of 350 kcal per day causes a 1-pound weight loss in 10 days; if the calorie deficit is 700 calories, it will take 5 days. (It may be a bit faster because, particularly initially, a water diuresis also occurs). A regimen of diet and exercise that creates a deficit of 700 to 1000 kcal per day seems reasonable. Thus a man weighing 220 pounds whose calorie intake to maintain weight is 2800 kcal needs to reduce intake to between 1800 and 2100 kcal. Such a diet should enable him to lose between 1 and 2 pounds per week, assuming that there is no increase in activity. It is clear that if this man's ideal body weight is 160 pounds, it will take him between 30 and 60 weeks to reach this weight. A clear realization at the start of the amount of time of sustained effort required to reach the goal that is set is important for keeping a patient motivated and positively reinforced.

TABLE 3. **Body Mass Index Defining Good Weight for Most People**

Age in Years	Body Mass Index (kg/m²)
19–24	19–24
25–34	20–25
35–44	21–26
45–54	22–27
55–64	23–28
65+	24–29

Diet

The most important component of a weight-loss program is the diet. To lose weight successfully obese persons must lower caloric intake and sustain such a reduced intake for a prolonged period. It is important to develop a diet program within the framework of a patient's current food habits and preferences. This is sometimes impossible when dietary habits are so poor that a radical restructuring must take place. However, better compliance occurs in patients for whom it can be done, because such patients are familiar and comfortable with the foods that they are already eating. Factors such as available cooking facilities, ethnic background, and economic background cannot be ignored. Documentation of food intake (e.g., diet records) may be a good method of tracking dietary pitfalls, patterns, and progress, but physicians must beware of perfect records unaccompanied by weight loss. These should serve as a signal that a patient may not be ready to accept the weight problem or be willing to work seriously on improving it.

When available, resting metabolic rate (RMR) should be measured and used to establish a reasonable caloric restriction. This rate multiplied by 1.4 gives a reasonable approximation of 24-hour energy expenditure. For example, a 120-kg male with a measured RMR of 2500 and a calculated 24-hour expenditure of 3500 kcal may choose to lose 1 kg per week on 1500 kcal per day rather than 1.5 kg per week on 1000 kcal per day because quantity of food takes priority over rate of weight loss. Such decisions should be made jointly by the patient and dietitian and/or physician to help promote long-term compliance. A diet should be adequate nutritionally, and this is possible without supplements only in diets of 1000 to 1200 kcals per day or more. To achieve this, patients must be taught to take certain micronutrient-rich foods that they may not be used to eating. With very hypocaloric diets, the nutrients most likely to be in deficit are iron, folacin, vitamin B_6, and zinc. If levels of calories fall below 1100, vitamin and mineral supplements become necessary and should be prescribed by the physi-

cian; a multivitamin/multimineral tablet once a day is enough. Extra macrominerals (sodium, potassium, calcium) are usually not necessary unless subjects go on very-low-calorie diets (300 to 800 kcal), which are not recommended for long-term use.

During weight loss, the emphasis should be on reduction of adipose (rather than lean) tissue. Although there is some obligate loss of lean body mass, it should be kept to a minimum. Lean body mass can generally be spared during weight loss with a protein intake of 1.0 to 1.5 grams per kg ideal body weight (calculated from Table 1). The dietary sources of protein should be of high biologic value (e.g., egg whites, fish, poultry and lean beef, low-fat dairy products). A vegetarian diet is perfectly acceptable, but the concept of protein complementing must be explained and encouraged. The remainder of calories should come from carbohydrate (preferably high-fiber foods) and fat. Although the macronutrient ratio can vary according to the patient's needs and preferences, it is important to obtain some of the antiketogenic and digestive high-fiber benefits of carbohydrate and to get adequate amounts of fat-soluble vitamins and essential fatty acids from the dietary fat.

In all cases of weight reduction, the emphasis should be on micronutrient-dense food choices and away from empty calorie selections. A brief discussion of basic nutrition should help alert the patient to the most appropriate food choices to maximize the caloric restriction. A patient must be taught that alcohol and sweets are not sources of any essential micronutrients. These therefore should be avoided, especially in the early stages of weight reduction, because they provide little more than excess calories. It should be made clear that although some fats are less atherogenic than others, all fats are high-energy, low-micronutrient foods and should be restricted to less than 30% of the total daily calories. Gram for gram, pure fat has more than double the caloric concentration of carbohydrate or protein (9 calories per gram vs. 4 calories per gram). Because carbohydrate often absorbs water upon cooking, the actual caloric density of hydrated carbohydrate on the plate may be as low as 1 to 2 calories per gram. Thus eliminating high-fat foods from the diet should provide a substantial caloric decrease, even if pure carbohydrate foods are substituted. In general, high-fat spreads, condiments, sauces, and gravies are far more detrimental in a weight-reduction program than are bread, potatoes, pasta, or rice.

Many of the more popular media-touted diets have no scientific basis and simply play upon vulnerable persons' desperation to lose weight. Very often they completely ignore the concept of balanced nutrition by totally eliminating or providing insufficient amounts of a particular macronutrient (e.g., protein, carbohydrate, or fat). In time this can result in a concurrent micronutrient imbalance. Such diets are clearly unsound, and if they are followed for any significant time period, serious health consequences such as electrolyte imbalances, deficiency syndromes, or protein-malnutrition can ensue.

Very-low-calorie diets (300 to 500 kcal per day) are potentially dangerous. Although weight loss can be large on such diets, the results are often short-lived. Statistics suggest that a return to prediet weight after solid foods are resumed is the rule. Unless such diets are undertaken in the context of a complete medically supervised, stepwise program in which the very-low-calorie diet is replaced after a few weeks by a higher-calorie balanced diet and intensive behavior modification program, they accomplish little except for periodic loss of water and electrolytes.

To help the patient adhere to a diet balanced in micronutrients and vitamins, it is wise to introduce the concept of the basic six food groups: (1) meat, fish poultry, beans, eggs, and nuts; (2) milk and milk products; (3) bread, cereals, rice, and pasta; (4) fruits; (5) vegetables; and (6) fats and sweets. By selecting from these groups, adequate nutrients can be obtained as follows: group 1 provides protein, fat niacin, riboflavin, iron, phosphorous, and thiamine; group 2 provides protein, fat, vitamins A and D, magnesium, calcium, phosphorous, and zinc; group 3 provides carbohydrate, protein, thiamine, niacin, vitamin E, iron, phosphorous, magnesium, zinc, and copper; groups 4 and 5 provide carbohydrate, vitamins A and C, iron, and magnesium; and group 6 provides essential fatty acids.

Dieters should be encouraged to select a wide variety of food choices within the basic six food groups to help alleviate lack of compliance caused by boredom or monotony. Number of servings per day from each group vary according to the individual's caloric restriction and macronutrient breakdown. Portion sizes should be explained in terms of common household measures (e.g., cups, ounces) and with the aid of food models.

Behavioral Therapy

The traditional technique of handing a patient a printed description of a 1200- or 1500-kcal diet, complete with specific menus and specific portion sizes, was tried for many years but was generally unsuccessful. Because of inadequate education and support, patients quickly dispensed with it.

As an outgrowth of that failure, behavioral therapy has been increasingly employed. The goal in behavioral therapy is to accomplish two things: decrease food intake and increase physical activity. The behavior of a patient is changed in ways that are possible and in reasonable steps, in concert with a physician or group therapy leader who helps one patient or, preferably, a group of patients.

The first step in such therapy is to describe the behavior to be controlled. This means helping the patients become aware of the amount, time, and circumstances of their eating and their activity (or inactivity) patterns. This increases awareness, which is required before corrective measures can be instituted. The second step is to practice control over stimuli that affect eating behavior. Typical stimuli would be persons or situations that increase stress, anxiety, or hostility. The particular stimuli need to be identified, and the patient needs to make an effort to distance himself or herself from them. The third step is to develop techniques to control the act of eating. These include the places where the patient eats, the speed of eating, the size of mouthfuls, the number of times that eating occurs, and the attention paid to eating. Of great importance, it also includes learning the difference in calorie value and nutrient content of foods. Some therapists have suggested that prompt reinforcement of behaviors that delay or control eating are very helpful. This would mean setting up some reward system (e.g., money, entertainment) as positive reinforcement for improved behavior.

The program is adapted to a patient's goals and skills rather than to a physician's idea of how a patient should behave. This individualization of treatment enhances the chances for success in a motivated person.

The advantage of a behavioral approach is that both patient and therapist (which may include the group) focus on the specific environmental variables that seem to govern a particular person's behavior. As A. Stunkard has suggested, "Central to a behavioral analysis is the search by patient and therapist for solutions to problems which are at the same time both relatively modest and potentially soluble." This simplifies and focuses therapy. It has been the experience in the weight control program at St. Luke's/Roosevelt Hospital Center that conducting behavioral therapy in a group setting is highly efficacious. The group setting leads to inquiry and mutual support and encouragement that are conducive to success.

Another advantage of a behavioral approach is that by giving patients the major responsibility for the weight loss strategy, they can attribute increased power to themselves. This tends to reinforce the treatment, inasmuch as when patients believe that the positive results are attributable to their own efforts, they gain increased confidence and desire to continue.

The final and most important advantage of a behavioral approach is that it allows patients to learn to eat under the natural social and environmental conditions with which they live day to day. Thus the habits learned during weight loss can be continued during the difficult period of weight maintenance. This is not possible in programs of very-low-calorie formula diets, in which the patient is taken off natural foods for a period of time and then is suddenly confronted with returning to regular food and having to modify behavior at that point. The learning then comes too little and too late and most often leads to failure and weight regain. It must be remembered that a behavioral program produces the slowest initial weight loss because calorie reduction is not radical and patients are encouraged to eat a hypocaloric but balanced and sensible diet. Patients must be advised to develop a long-term view. Goal weights should be set and perseverance encouraged. Also of importance is that goal weight will often be higher than normal weight. It is imperative that the patient remain in the treatment program not only until goal weight is achieved but also well into the weight maintenance period.

Exercise

Because exercise expends calories, it is a logical part of any weight loss program. Overweight persons are generally inactive, spending much of their day sitting or lying down. Many of them, particularly the heavier ones, have a real problem walking even short distances and climbing steps and tend to avoid situations that require these activities. By staying as sedentary as they do, they are essentially almost at resting metabolic rate for most of the day. These persons must be taught to first walk, then walk faster, and then run or bicycle or do aerobic dance. An exercise program must start slowly. If an obese person is pushed too rapidly, discomfort and avoidance occur. Careful observation for treatment of skin intertrigo, dependent edema, and foot or joint injuries is mandatory.

It is helpful to educate the patient about how many calories are spent in an individual exercise activity. Most tables of calorie expenditure with given levels of activity have been compiled to reflect total caloric expenditure, not the amount over the basal metabolic rate. As a result, the caloric contribution of exercise must be calculated as the difference between the calories expended per minute during exercise and the calories that a person would have expended just sitting. It is instructive and often disappointing to patients to discover just how much exercise they must do to expend a significant number of calories. For instance, if an overweight woman's basal metabolic rate is 1400 kcal per day, lying down awake she expends 1.1 kcal per minute; sitting, about 1.2 kcal per minute; walking slowly, about 1.9 kcal per minute; and walking a treadmill at 4.0 miles per hour, 7.2 kcal per minute. Thus the difference in caloric expenditure between sitting quietly and walking fast on a treadmill (at 4.0 miles per hour) is 5.0 kcal per minute. In an hour, therefore, the energy expended by walking 4 miles is only 360 calories higher than the subject would have expended just quietly sitting. It is important to emphasize that a very significant and persistent commitment to exercise must be present in order for exercise to have any substantial effect on caloric balance and weight loss.

Drugs

Although drugs have a definite role in weight-loss programs, they are often overused and abused. The important point about drug therapy is that it is never primary but always adjunctive. It should under no circumstances ever be the sole therapy but should always be used in conjunction with diet and exercise. Three principles must be kept in mind by the physician: (1) tolerance occurs to many of the drugs used by many people, so that increasing doses may be necessary with time; (2) only a modest effect on appetite occurs, so that using drugs as sole therapy does not work; and (3) all of the drugs have side effects, and because it is unclear whether any one drug is more effective than another, it seems reasonable to use the drugs that seem to have less potential for side effects, including the side effects of addiction or abuse.

The anorectic drugs have a central mode of action. Aside from mazindol, they share in common a phenethylamine group in their molecules. Amphetamine and its analogues (methamphetamine, phenmetrazine, phendimetrazine, benzphetamine, phenylpropanolamine, chlorphentermine,* clortermine,* diethylpropion, and phentermine) exert anorexia via brain catecholamines. Dopaminergic mechanisms also may be involved. Side effects of these drugs are insomnia, excitement, agitation, headache, tremor, dizziness, dry mouth, impotence, hallucinations, confusion, palpitations, tachycardia, assaultiveness, and panic. Fenfluramine is different in that its action is thought to be mediated via central serotoninergic satiety systems. It is not a stimulant but, in fact, is a sedative. Side effects are drowsiness and diarrhea.

*Not available in the United States.

At present, it is not possible to predict who will or will not have side effects of drug therapy and what those side effects will be. Good therapeutic practice mandates that an appetite suppressant not be prescribed without a careful explanation of potential side effects. Also, it is not possible to predict who may become psychologically or physically dependent on these drugs, although this is rare. Careful monitoring of the patient is necessary.

The aforementioned drugs may be particularly helpful in getting a patient through certain difficult periods or times of weight plateaus. It has been suggested that one or a combination of two drugs may prove satisfactory for the long-term treatment of obesity. More research is required in this regard.

Thyroid preparations, digitalis, and diuretics should not be used for weight loss. Inhibitors of carbohydrate absorption (α-amylase, α-glucosidase, and sucrase inhibitors) have not been successful as weight reduction agents. Interest in possible thermogenic agents is growing, but no satisfactory one is available as yet.

Weight Maintenance

Maintaining weight once loss has been achieved is most difficult. There is a persistent tendency to regain the weight and there is experimental evidence, particularly in animal models, that the metabolic rate is abnormally depressed after weight loss and that lipogenic pathways enhancing the reaccretion of fat may be particularly efficient. Although diet may be liberalized after goal weight has been reached, it must be done gradually with daily weight monitoring. It is likely that a limitation of caloric intake will be required indefinitely. All the lifestyle changes learned during the weight loss period should be continued, including a continuation of the exercise program.

Surgery

Surgery may be indicated in patients who are massively obese and who have tried all other forms of therapy and have failed. Because of the significant rates of morbidity and even mortality from the procedure, however, it is indicated only in patients in whom the obesity itself or an associated condition is life-threatening. The surgery should be performed only in centers with adequate support from anesthesia, pulmonary, cardiac, and metabolic divisions. Lifelong follow-up is essential, and the surgeon must truly be interested in such follow-up. The surgery must be considered experimental, because no wholly adequate operation has yet been developed.

The initial procedure was jejunoileal bypass, but it has been abandoned because its side effects were such that the risk/benefit ratio was unacceptable. Problems included electrolyte and vitamin depletion, hepatic toxicity, renal stones, and polyarthritis. As a result, interest has moved to gastric procedures. In gastric bypass, a small 30- to 60-mL pouch is made in the proximal stomach with a very small outlet into the small intestine, so that only a very small amount of food can be eaten at any one time. In gastroplasty, a staple line partitions the stomach into two segments, which are connected by a narrow outlet. This staple line can be horizontal or vertical. The side effects are less common and less serious than with the intestinal operations. However, this operation is technically more difficult. Also, success rates vary, and there have been quite a few failures. These are generally related to poor operative technique or to a patient's eating around the procedure by frequent ingestion of small meals that include high calorie fluids.

VITAMIN DEFICIENCY

method of
RICHARD S. RIVLIN, M.D.
Memorial Sloan-Kettering Cancer Center
New York, New York

In considering the prevention and treatment of vitamin deficiencies, the physician should be aware of a number of general considerations. First, far advanced vitamin deficiencies are rarely encountered singly; multiple deficiencies are the rule. Deficiencies develop gradually, and by the time the classical manifestations are apparent, the deficiencies are far advanced. Alcohol is a major cause of vitamin deficiency and must always be kept in mind when the patient's clinical status is evaluated. Drugs are also a major cause of vitamin deficiency, particularly among elderly, malnourished persons for whom prolonged and multiple-agent therapy has been prescribed.

When a person follows a poor diet pattern, the deficiencies of the vitamins develop in an ordered manner. Thus water-soluble vitamin stores may be depleted in a matter of weeks, whereas several years of inadequate vitamin B_{12} intake are necessary before there is clinically apparent deficiency of the vitamin.

In the process of correction of vitamin deficiency, the physician must remember that large doses of vitamins are in reality drugs, with a toxic-therapeutic ratio and a potential for causing untoward effects. Thus both prevention and treatment of vitamin deficiency require a knowledge of physiology and nutrition.

THIAMINE DEFICIENCY (BERIBERI)

Overt thiamine deficiency in the United States is usually encountered in the setting of chronic alcohol ingestion. Drinking alcohol throughout the day prevents most of the dietary thiamine from being absorbed. It has been estimated that about one-quarter of alcoholic patients admitted to hospitals in the United States show some evidence of thiamine deficiency. It is likely that alcohol has deleterious effects on thiamine metabolism as well as on absorption. When alcohol abuse is superimposed upon a dietary inadequacy of this vitamin, serious neurologic consequences may result.

In developing countries, beriberi is encountered more frequently than in the U.S., particularly when polished rice is a dietary staple, inasmuch as this food contains very little thiamine. Thiamine deficiency may be encountered under conditions in which the metabolic requirement is increased, as in diabetes, cancer, or prolonged fever, or during pregnancy and lactation. Early features of the deficiency state include anorexia, irritability, weight loss, and weakness. Later there is involvement of two major organ systems in the classical syndrome: (a) the cardiovascular system, with beriberi heart disease, and (b) the central and peripheral nervous systems, with peripheral neuropathy and the Wernicke-Korsakoff syndrome.

Prevention

With a diet containing adequate amounts of thiamine-rich sources such as red meat, whole grains, legumes, and nuts, and with avoidance of milled or polished rice, beriberi should be preventable. Thiamine is unstable at alkaline pH and is also heat-sensitive except under acidic conditions below a pH of 5.

The Food and Nutrition Board of the National Research Council, National Academy of Sciences, has established a recommended dietary allowance (RDA) that ranges from 1.2 to 1.5 mg per day for men, depending on age, and 1.0 to 1.1 mg per day for women, depending on age, with an increase of 0.5 mg during pregnancy and lactation. Such figures are intended to meet the needs of nearly all healthy persons and would need to be higher under conditions of increased metabolic requirements.

Treatment

The physician must keep a high index of suspicion that thiamine deficiency may be present when heart disease and/or neurologic manifestations are prominently displayed in a patient who abuses alcohol. In case of doubt the physician should err on the side of treatment, because little untoward effect would result from thiamine injec-

tion when it is not needed. If thiamine deficiency is likely, prompt administration of 50 to 100 mg intramuscularly or intravenously is indicated. Such large doses should be continued for 3 to 4 days, after which 5 to 10 mg can be given orally or intramuscularly.

As noted earlier, in far advanced beriberi it is overwhelmingly likely that other significant deficiencies in vitamins and minerals coexist and also necessitate vigorous treatment. Alcohol abstinence is obviously crucial, and the diet must be adequate in calories and nutrients.

The peripheral neuropathy, manifested by symptoms of numbness, tingling, and burning in the extremities, may be debilitating and responds poorly to analgesics. It is suggested that the patient be kept active and that physiotherapy be instituted early. Recovery from the neurologic disorder may be quite prolonged.

The cardiovascular symptoms of beriberi often resemble those of hyperthyroidism. Heart failure may develop and necessitates digitalis, diuretics, and other drugs. A brisk response to thiamine may obviate the need for a diuretic. Thiamine alone may result in significant improvement in cardiovascular function, with prompt diuresis in cases of failure, but use of standard cardiac medications is generally required for an optimal response and eventual recovery. The possibility that other forms of heart disease, such as alcoholic cardiomyopathy, may be present must be kept in mind.

RIBOFLAVIN (VITAMIN B$_2$) DEFICIENCY

Deficiency of riboflavin is nearly always encountered in the setting of multiple deficiencies. It is important to remember that in addition to being caused by a poor diet, riboflavin deficiency may result from the effects of hormones, drugs, or diseases that impair the body's use of this vitamin. Phototherapy of newborn infants for bilirubin problems may provoke riboflavin deficiency because the vitamin is light-sensitive. Alcohol may also cause riboflavin deficiency by interfering with digestion and absorption. There are other conditions, such as severe burns, trauma, surgery, and dialysis, in which vitamin B$_2$ deficiency may result. Psychotropic drugs, antimalarial agents, and some cancer chemotherapeutic drugs impair the conversion of riboflavin into its active coenzyme derivatives, the most important of which is flavin adenine dinucleotide.

Early in the course of riboflavin deficiency, the patient may exhibit burning and itching of the eyes and mouth, as well as personality disturbances. Later on, angular stomatitis, seborrheic dermatitis, glossitis, and other epithelial abnormalities are found. Cheilosis and angular stomatitis are no longer believed to be specific for riboflavin deficiency. With further progression of the deficiency state, anemia and corneal neovascularization may develop.

Prevention

Riboflavin deficiency should be preventable if the diet contains an adequate supply of milk and dairy products, meat, and green, leafy vegetables. In the United States dairy products are the most important source for the vitamin, and riboflavin nutritional status generally is correlated quite closely with that for calcium. In developing countries, vegetable sources predominate. The RDAs for riboflavin are 1.7 to 1.8 mg for adult males and 1.2 to 1.3 mg for adult females, with an increase of 0.5 mg during pregnancy and lactation.

Treatment

Riboflavin deficiency can be treated with food sources that are rich in this vitamin, such as milk and dairy products, meat, and green, leafy vegetables. Riboflavin can also be administered as a component of a multivitamin tablet. For rapid treatment of riboflavin-deficient patients, doses in the range of 10 to 15 mg per day are recommended. The poor solubility of riboflavin in aqueous solution limits its use in intravenous administration.

NIACIN DEFICIENCY (PELLAGRA)

Pellagra was once quite common in the United States when corn was a dietary staple. Corn is relatively poor in tryptophan, the essential amino acid that serves as a precursor to niacin. At present, niacin deficiency largely results from prolonged alcohol abuse under conditions in which multivitamin deficits prevail. In rare instances, some degree of niacin deficiency may occur after the use of certain drugs that interfere with niacin metabolism, such as isonicotinic acid hydrazine (INH) or 6-mercaptopurine. In the carcinoid syndrome, dietary tryptophan is diverted from niacin synthesis to that of serotonin, and some patients may exhibit signs of pellagra.

Prevention

Niacin deficiency is preventable by a diet that is high in proteins of animal origin, which have a high tryptophan content. Some vegetable proteins also have tryptophan but in lower amounts. Grain products often contain niacin but of relatively low bioavailability. The RDA for niacin is expressed in terms of niacin equivalents; 60 mg of dietary tryptophan yields about 1 mg of niacin synthesized endogenously. Expressed in this manner as niacin equivalents, the RDAs for niacin are 15 to 19 mg in adult males and 13 to 15 mg in adult females, with an additional 5 mg recommended during pregnancy and lactation.

Treatment

Advanced pellagra is a serious disorder, classically known by the four Ds: diarrhea, dermatitis, dementia, and death. Doses in the form of niacinamide in the range of 50 to 150 mg have been given to ill patients; marked clinical improvement is demonstrable within several days. Once these large doses have been administered, maintenance levels of several times the RDA together with a satisfactory diet should be given to the patient. Other measures involved in supportive care include correction of acid-base imbalance, treatment of the skin disease, and recognition that the neurologic impairment may follow a prolonged course.

Niacin in the form of nicotinic acid in much larger doses (3 to 6 g per day) is a first-line drug for management of an elevated serum cholesterol. Niacinamide, another form of niacin, does not cause the flushing symptoms associated with nicotinic acid, nor does it lower the serum cholesterol.

PYRIDOXINE (VITAMIN B₆) DEFICIENCY

Dietary deficiency of pyridoxine occasionally occurs in the United States but almost never as an isolated entity. It is sometimes observed after prolonged therapy with certain pharmacologic agents, such as isoniazid or cycloserine for tuberculosis, both of which are pyridoxine antagonists. Deficiency of pyridoxine occurs commonly in severe alcoholism in association with deficiencies of the other vitamins, as noted earlier.

Prevention

Deficiency of pyridoxine should be preventable by a diet that contains adequate amounts of meat, wheat, nuts, vegetables (particularly beans), fruits, and cereals. Some amount may be lost during pressure cooking. The bioavailability of pyridoxine from food sources varies widely. The RDAs for vitamin B_6 are 2.0 mg for adult males and 1.6 mg for adult females and is increased another 0.5 mg during pregnancy and lactation.

Treatment

The dietary deficiency of pyridoxine can generally be treated with doses in the range of 2 to 10 mg per day. In more severe cases, particularly those occurring during pregnancy, doses in the range of 10 to 20 mg have generally been administered. In the event that deficiency has resulted from a drug that inhibits vitamin B_6 metabolism, as mentioned earlier, somewhat higher doses may be needed, in some instances up to 50 to 100 mg per day. It is advisable to initiate pyridoxine concomitantly with the drug, a practice that is generally followed with INH treatment for tuberculosis but should be applicable more widely with vitamin B_6 antagonists. With L-dopa, however, vitamin B_6 is not prescribed because it is believed by some authorities to interfere with therapeutic efficacy.

Rare cases of a pyridoxine-dependency syndrome, such as pyridoxine-responsive anemia, have generally been treated with doses in the 300 to 500 mg range. It is important to remember that peripheral neuropathy has been reported as a side effect of vitamin B_6 ingestion when 2 grams or more has been used in treatment. It is possible that lower doses, in the neighborhood of 500 mg, may also cause some degree of peripheral neuropathy.

FOLIC ACID DEFICIENCY

Dietary deficiency of folic acid occurs in people who do not consume adequate amounts of rich sources, such as meat, legumes and other vegetables, and fruits. For people who shop infrequently and obtain out-of-date produce, there is some risk of folate deficiency because food folic acid is sensitive to processing, preparation, and storage. Alcohol intake damages the intestinal mucosa, and prolonged abuse, often of an episodic nature, is associated with folate deficiency. Usually the first indication of folate deficiency is a macrocytic anemia, and megaloblastosis may later become more widespread throughout the gastrointestinal tract. Drugs that interfere with folate metabolism, the classic example of which is methotrexate, also produce manifestations of folic acid deficiency.

Prevention

The current RDAs for folic acid are 200 µg per day in adult males and 180 µg per day in adult females, figures that are considerably lower than the 400 µg previously given for adults, both males and females. It is recommended that during pregnancy and lactation, the allowance be increased to 400 and 280 µg, respectively. During pregnancy, the blood volume is greatly increased and folate reserves may be strained, and for this reason, folate intake should be greatly increased.

A new dimension to the role of folic acid during pregnancy has been added by the finding that neural tube defects (NTDs), such as spina bifida and anencephaly, may be reduced in frequency by daily consumption of 0.4 mg of folic acid. The folic acid must be consumed during the first 4 weeks of pregnancy in order to be effective, a period of time in which most women are likely unaware of being pregnant. With these considerations in mind, the Centers for Disease Control have recently recommended that "all women of childbearing age in the United States who are capable of becoming pregnant should consume 0.4 mg of folic acid per day for the purpose of reducing their risk of having a pregnancy affected with spina bifida or other NTDs (neural tube defects)."

Treatment

Folic acid deficiency can be treated by adhering to a diet rich in folate-containing items, such as liver, yeast, green leafy vegetables, legumes, and fruits. Care must be taken not to destroy the food folates during food preparation and storage.

Therapeutic doses in the range of 1 to 2 mg per day can be administered to correct folate deficiency rapidly. In patients receiving anticonvulsant drugs, larger doses may be required to reverse the megaloblastic anemia that may result. One potential risk in administering excessive amounts of folic acid is that it may interfere with the diagnosis of vitamin B_{12} deficiency. At dose levels in excess of 1 mg per day, folic acid may correct the pernicious anemia caused by deficiency of vitamin B_{12} but may not delay the progression of neurologic deterioration. Thus in cases in which combined vitamin deficiency is suspected, vitamin supplementation should include both B_{12} and folic acid.

Currently, the concept being advanced is that certain tissues may have localized folate deficiency that is associated with the development of preneoplastic lesions. In a double-blind trial users of oral contraceptive agents who had cervical dysplasia showed significant improvement with 10 mg per day of folic acid. If these investigations are confirmed and extended, patients will be treated in the future with folic acid as a component of an overall program of cancer prevention.

VITAMIN B_{12} DEFICIENCY

See discussion of treatment of pernicious anemia in Section 5.

VITAMIN A DEFICIENCY

Deficiency of vitamin A is of crucial importance as a worldwide nutritional problem because it is a major cause of blindness in approximately half a million preschool children each year in the developing countries. In these areas, the diet is composed primarily of such items as rice, wheat, maize, and tubers that contain far from adequate amounts of vitamin A and its precursor, beta-carotene. The World Health Organization and other foundations and groups have made great efforts to plan programs to identify people at risk and to institute appropriate preventive measures on a broad scale.

In contrast, vitamin A deficiency in the United States is identified largely with certain risk groups: the urban poor, elderly persons, particularly those living alone, abusers of alcohol, patients with malabsorption diseases, and other persons on a poor diet. Vitamin A deficiency is generally found in a setting in which there are multiple vitamin and mineral deficiencies. Special attention must be paid to deficiency of zinc, a frequent finding in alcoholism, which interferes with the mobilization of vitamin A from its storage site in the liver. This effect is achieved by blocking the release of holo–retinol-binding protein (RBP) from the liver.

The physician must keep in mind that deficiency of vitamin A in the United States may also develop after the long-term use of several medications. Drug-induced nutritional deficiencies in general, particularly those involving vitamin A, occur most frequently among the elderly because they use medications in the largest number and for the most prolonged duration and may have borderline nutritional status to begin with. Among the drugs that are most relevant to vitamin A status are mineral oil, which dissolves this nutrient; other laxatives that accelerate intestinal transit and may diminish the rate of vitamin A absorption; cholestyramine and colestipol, which bind vitamin A; and, under certain conditions, neomycin and colchicine.

Prevention

Deficiency of vitamin A can be prevented by a diet high in carotenes, which serve as precursors to vitamin A. The carotenes, particularly beta-carotene, are derived from plant sources, the richest of which are palm oil, carrots, sweet potatoes, green leafy vegetables, cantaloupe, and papaya. Vitamin A itself is derived from animal sources, such as dairy products, meat, and fish. The commercial preparations of fish oils are rich, sometimes too rich, sources of preformed vitamin A.

The RDA for vitamin A is expressed in terms of retinol equivalents (RE): 1 RE is equal to 1 μg of retinol or 6 μg of beta-carotene. The RDAs are 1000 RE for males and 800 RE for females. This standard nomenclature is nevertheless rarely found on vitamin bottles on which the former system of international units (IU) is used. Expressed in this manner, the RDAs for vitamin A are 5000 IU for adult males and 4000 IU for adult females.

The nutritional value of dietary sources of vitamin A may be compromised when the food items are subject to oxidation, particularly in the presence of light and heat. Antioxidants, such as vitamin E, prevent the loss of vitamin A activity.

Treatment

Vitamin A deficiency has been treated worldwide with single injections of massive amounts (100,000 to 200,000 IU) repeated at intervals of approximately 6 months to 1 year. Such doses have been effective and are associated with remarkably little toxicity, perhaps because body stores are so depleted at the time of therapy. These doses may, however, produce acute toxic symptoms in well-nourished persons.

Clinical vitamin A deficiency in the United States can be treated with either beta-carotene, if there is normal body conversion to vitamin A, or with vitamin A itself. Daily doses in the range of 25,000 IU of beta-carotene are being consumed by many healthy individuals without apparent toxicity of any kind. The yellowish discoloration of the skin associated with prolonged use of beta-carotene is not harmful and may even provide some protection against damaging effects of ultraviolet light from the sun. Vitamin A, in contrast, is quite toxic when ingested in amounts considerably higher than the RDA, especially for prolonged periods. It is probably advisable not to exceed two to three times the RDA for vitamin A in planning a treatment program. Congenital malformations, a particularly disturbing consequence of vitamin A overdosage, have been reported in women consuming 25,000 to 50,000 IU daily during pregnancy. It is not known with certainty what is the lowest dose of vitamin A that would be completely safe as a supplement for pregnant women. Therefore, it is not a good idea for pregnant women to take supplementary vitamin A unless there are specific indications, such as malabsorption or proven deficiency.

At present, there is widespread interest in other therapeutic applications for vitamin A and its derivatives. Large doses of vitamin A have been found to reduce morbidity and mortality rates among children suffering from severe cases of measles. Certain rare forms of leukemia have been found to respond to derivatives of vitamin

A. The therapeutic potential of this vitamin is being expanded greatly in the chemoprevention of cancer. Vitamin A has been found to inhibit cellular differentiation. The toxicity of large doses of vitamin A and its derivatives places important limits on its feasibility in cancer prevention. Attention has turned to beta-carotene and related agents, which in addition to their role as precursors of vitamin A have strong antioxidant activity.

Diminished prevalence of certain cancers has been found among groups of people whose intake of fruits and vegetables is high; this finding is attributable at least in part to the high content of carotenes in the diet. There is some evidence that a combination of antioxidants (i.e., vitamin E, vitamin C, and beta-carotene) may be more effective in chemoprevention than any agent singly. This area of research is innovative and exciting, but it is still too early to make firm recommendations for treatment of the general public in the United States.

VITAMIN D DEFICIENCY

Vitamin D occurs in two major forms, vitamin D_2 (ergocalciferol), which is produced from plant sterols, and vitamin D_3, which is produced in the skin. Scientists are becoming increasingly aware of the important nutritional role of the skin in manufacturing vitamin D_3 under the influence of solar ultraviolet light.

Vitamin D itself is relatively inert biologically and must be converted into its active metabolites to exert its effects. In the kidneys, vitamin D is converted to 25-hydroxyvitamin D (25-OHD), the most important and active derivative. A less active vitamin D derivative, $24,25(OH)_2D$, is also produced from 25-OHD in the kidney. Also, $1,25(OH)_2D_3$ is a steroid in structure, and in function it has many properties of a steroid hormone. Indeed, vitamin D is considered to have hormonal properties.

There are three major sites of action of vitamin D in regulating calcium metabolism. Its best known action is to increase the absorption of calcium, both dietary and secreted, from the intestinal tract. At low doses of vitamin D, the amount of calcium absorbed is linear to the dose given. The second major site of action is on bone, where, together with parathyroid hormone, osteoclastic bone resorption is stimulated. Under a wide variety of conditions, both physiologic and pathologic, the serum calcium level is maintained within a very narrow range at the expense of the calcium derived from bone. The third major site of action of vitamin D is on the kidney tubule to increase the reabsorption of calcium.

Deficiency of vitamin D occurring in infancy and childhood is manifested as rickets, with severe developmental abnormalities. Vitamin D deficiency occurring during adult life results in the pathogenesis of osteomalacia. In a general way, deficiency of vitamin D can result from inadequate intake from dietary sources; from diminished synthesis in the skin; from intestinal malabsorption, as occurs in a variety of diseases; from accelerated catabolism, as caused by certain drugs; and from defects in the conversion of vitamin D into its active derivatives. In a rare genetic disorder, vitamin D–resistant rickets, Type II, the abnormality appears to reside not in the synthesis of the active derivatives but in target organ resistance to their action.

Prevention

Deficiency of vitamin D can be prevented by an adequate diet, conditions favorable to skin synthesis of the vitamin, or both. Results of studies suggest that exposure of small amounts of skin (i.e., the hands and face), for several minutes to the summer sun is enough to meet the nutritional needs of the body. Thus prolonged exposure of the body to sunlight is not necessary to achieve optimal vitamin D synthesis. The goal of preventing skin cancer by avoiding excessive skin exposure to sunlight and sunburn remains compatible with the goal of exposing enough skin to sunlight to achieve adequate synthesis of vitamin D. By contrast, in northern cities, such as Boston, winter sun appears to be ineffective in promoting vitamin D synthesis in the skin. The ability of the skin to synthesize vitamin D is diminished with aging.

In the United States, where foods, particularly milk, are fortified with vitamin D, sources of calcium and vitamin D generally become consumed together. In children and in some adults, having milk with its 10 μg of cholecalciferol (400 IU) in each quart regularly is a good way to ensure adequate vitamin D intake. With persons exposed to abundant sunlight, dietary sources become less important nutritionally, and it is difficult to set an RDA for vitamin D in such persons. The amount of 10 μg of cholecalciferol has been set as the RDA in males from childhood until the age of 24, after which 5 μg is advised. For females, similar recommendations are made except that all pregnant and lactating women are advised to consume 10 μg of cholecalciferol, regardless of age.

Treatment

The goal in the treatment of vitamin D deficiency is to restore bone structure and function to normal and to correct serum concentrations of calcium if inadequate. Rickets, the form of vitamin D deficiency in infants and children, as well as osteomalacia, the manifestation of vitamin D deficiency in adults, responds to the administration of vitamin D if calcium intake is also adequate. For this reason, the physician must first determine that calcium intake is at the level of 1 to 2 grams per day as elemental calcium, either in the form of food sources rich in calcium or by means of supplementation.

The initial doses of vitamin D to be administered in either rickets or osteomalacia are in the range of 400 to 4000 IU per day. Most authorities recommend 2000 to 4000 IU with supplementary calcium. As a frame of reference, a quart of milk is supplemented with 400 IU of vitamin D. Thus consuming a diet high in milk and dairy products is a good way to treat vitamin D deficiency if continued consistently for an adequate period of time. Probably several months' treatment at these high doses is needed, after which doses in the range of 200 to 400 IU are generally adequate. During the treatment period, it is essential to provide exposure to sunlight and to encourage physical exercise of a weight-bearing nature that will facilitate the normal mechanisms of bone renewal.

In the event that the deficiency is complicated by intestinal malabsorption, larger doses of vitamin D, in the range of 10,000 to 25,000 IU or higher, are required. Water-soluble preparations of vitamin D are available and can be administered parenterally if necessary. More calcium, in the range of 2 to 3 grams per day, is also needed. An important consideration to keep in mind is that in some instances of hypocalcemia associated with malabsorption, the provision of supplementary magnesium renders the hypocalcemia less resistant to treatment with calcium and vitamin D. If severe liver disease is present in association with vitamin D deficiency, larger doses of D are also needed, because, as mentioned earlier, the initial conversion of vitamin D to 25-OHD occurs in the liver. If the patient requires certain drugs that bind bile salts (such as cholestyramine) or that increase vitamin D catabolism (such as phenytoin), large doses of D are required for adequate therapy of the vitamin D deficiency.

Vitamin D deficiency complicated by renal disease is only poorly responsive to treatment with vitamin D, because the $1,25(OH)_2D$ derivative is formed inadequately from precursor in the renal parenchyma. For this reason, $1,25(OH)_2D$ (calcitriol) must be given. Most patients respond quite satisfactorily to doses in the range of 0.5 to 1.0 μg per day. A similar strategy of treatment is required in vitamin D–dependent rickets, Type I, in which there is a selective genetic defect (auto-somal recessive) in the conversion of 25-D to $1,25(OH)_2D$. Much higher doses than these must be tried in the case of vitamin D–dependent rickets, Type II, in which the defect is in the receptor response to $1,25(OH)_2D$. Patients with renal disease complicating the vitamin D deficiency also require other ancillary measures, such as phosphate and protein restriction.

VITAMIN E DEFICIENCY

The most widely accepted role for vitamin E is as an antioxidant, and in this capacity it protects cell membranes from damage by free radicals. It has many other properties as well. Dietary vitamin E deficiency tends to be unusual under ordinary circumstances because sources of E are widely available from the food supply. The recognizable cases of vitamin E deficiency tend to arise in debilitated patients who have had severe and prolonged periods of fat malabsorption.

Inborn errors of vitamin E metabolism have been identified recently. In one disorder, familial isolated vitamin E deficiency, there are severe neurologic abnormalities. Because of a genetically determined defect in incorporation of dietary vitamin E into the lipid transport protein VLDL, vitamin E is cleared rapidly from plasma. In another genetic disorder, abetalipoproteinemia, there is a serious defect in the serum transport of vitamin E. A hallmark of this disease is the finding of an extremely low serum cholesterol level.

Prevention

Deficiency of vitamin E can be avoided by regular consumption of the many sources of this vitamin in the food supply. The richest sources of vitamin E in the U.S. diet are vegetable oils, including corn, cottonseed, safflower, and soybean, and the margarines and other products made from these oils. Green leafy vegetables are also good sources of vitamin E. In evaluating the adequacy of any given dietary regimen, one should keep in mind the fact that losses of the vitamin occur during storage, cooking, and food processing, particularly with exposure to high temperatures and oxygen.

Because vitamin E deficiency occurs as a result of severe intestinal malabsorption, it is essential to identify this condition early and to avoid measures that may intensify the degree of malabsorption. For example, cholestyramine and colestipol, resins used in the treatment of hypercholesterolemia, cause malabsorption of vitamin E and should be used at minimal doses if possible.

The RDAs for vitamin E have been set at 10

alpha–tocopherol equivalents (TEs) per day for males aged 11 years and older and at 8 alpha-TEs per day for females aged 11 years and older. It is recommended that women consume 10 alpha-TEs per day during pregnancy and 11 to 12 alpha-TEs during lactation. The storage capacity of the body for vitamin E is considerable.

Treatment

Vitamin E deficiency can be treated satisfactorily with oral preparations of the vitamin. There is a wide margin of safety in the therapeutic administration of the vitamin. Daily doses of vitamin E in the range of 100 to 800 mg can be given safely to nearly all deficient patients. This dose range can be used appropriately in the patients with vitamin E deficiency diagnosed in association with celiac disease, inflammatory bowel disease, or other chronic and prolonged forms of intestinal malabsorption. In such instances, many nutrient deficiencies are likely to be found in association with that of vitamin E, and they too necessitate treatment.

In the genetic disorders of vitamin E metabolism, such as isolated vitamin E deficiency, higher doses of the vitamin, in the range of 800 to 1000 mg and higher, must be taken.

VITAMIN K DEFICIENCY

Vitamin K occurs naturally as K_1 (phylloquinone) from plant sources and as K_2 (menaquinone), which is synthesized by intestinal bacteria and is also present in some animal sources. The most widely appreciated role of vitamin K is in blood clotting, because four clotting factors depend for their action on vitamin K: prothrombin (Factor II), proconvertin (Factor VII), Christmas factor (Factor IX), and Stuart-Prower factor (Factor X).

More recently, an important role for vitamin K in bone metabolism has been identified. Vitamin K is now recognized as being needed for the synthesis of the bone protein osteocalcin and several other bone proteins. Vitamin K antagonists, the anticoagulant drugs warfarin and dicumarol, also interfere with the synthesis of osteocalcin and may result in significant disturbances of bone metabolism, particularly if used during the first and second trimesters of pregnancy.

Prevention

Vitamin K deficiency from diet is an uncommon occurrence. The best food sources are green leafy vegetables, particularly broccoli, brussels sprouts, turnip greens, and spinach. Some vitamin K is also found in animal sources such as liver, bacon, cheese, and butter, as well as in the beverages coffee and green tea.

As a fat-soluble vitamin, vitamin K requires bile salts for its intestinal absorption. The efficiency of absorption is markedly decreased by mineral oil, fat solvents, and laxatives. Thus these agents should be avoided, or doses sharply reduced, in order to avoid vitamin K malabsorption. Prompt treatment of fat malabsorption in such disorders as sprue and inflammatory bowel disease helps prevent the development of vitamin K deficiency subsequently.

The normal intestinal flora synthesize clinically significant amounts of vitamin K and make a substantial nutritional contribution to vitamin K economy. Treatment with antibiotics, particularly when prolonged, leads to recognizable vitamin K deficiency. Therefore, the deficiency can be prevented by restricting the use of antibiotics to times when they are absolutely necessary and avoiding long-term use. Preparations of yogurt containing live cultures may be useful in recolonizing the intestinal tract and helping to restore vitamin K synthesis to normal levels. Moxalactam functions primarily by inhibiting the function of vitamin K in the liver, not by decreasing the flora.

The RDA for vitamin K is based on data indicating that about 1 μg per kg body weight should be adequate to maintain the blood clotting time within a normal range for adults. This parameter in the last analysis is the most appropriate means of defining normal vitamin K status. On the basis of these calculations, the RDAs are 70 to 80 μg per day for men and 65 μg per day for women. There is no increase in the RDA during pregnancy or lactation.

Treatment

Treatment of vitamin K deficiency can be accomplished by adhering to a diet high in the sources of the vitamin that were noted earlier. It may be necessary to administer the vitamin directly, and it has been shown that doses in the range of 50 to 500 μg of phylloquinone for 12 days restore prothrombin times to normal in experimentally deficient subjects. Doses of vitamin K of 1.5 μg per kg body weight have restored prothrombin status to normal when given intravenously. One milligram per os to newborn infants is now recommended for preventing hemorrhagic disease.

Other measures to be considered include restriction of antibiotic administration and efforts to recolonize the intestinal tract, as noted earlier.

VITAMIN C DEFICIENCY (SCURVY)

Vitamin C is a powerful water-soluble antioxidant, and there is much contemporary interest in this action of the vitamin. Vitamin C is involved in lipid and vitamin metabolism, facilitates the intestinal absorption of nonheme iron, and is involved in collagen metabolism, biosynthesis of neurotransmitters, wound healing, immune function, and many other aspects of normal health. Important physical properties of vitamin C include its sensitivity to prolonged storage and cooking at high temperatures, common occurrences that greatly decrease its biologic potency. As an antioxidant, it is destroyed by oxidation, as in exposure to air.

Prevention

The best dietary sources of vitamin C are citrus fruits and green leafy vegetables, particularly broccoli, green peppers, and cabbage. Tomatoes are also a good source. As noted earlier, care must be taken in proper food preparation and storage.

Vitamin C deficiency is common among the urban poor, who may not be able to afford the fresh fruits and vegetables that constitute important sources. Vitamin C deficiency is also common among the elderly, who may shop infrequently and allow produce to be stored longer than is optimal. Food faddism, particularly the macrobiotic diet, adherents of which regularly subject food to pressure cooking, may result in serious vitamin C deficiency. A "tea and toast" diet is virtually devoid of sources of vitamin C. Scurvy develops in alcoholic patients if their diet is deficient in food items containing vitamin C. Thus much vitamin C deficiency could be prevented by making good dietary sources available to urban poor, elderly persons, and others on a subsistence economy; by ensuring that prolonged storage is avoided; by preventing alcohol abuse; and by teaching proper food habits generally.

The RDA has been established to be 60 mg per day in both adult males and females, up to 70 mg per day during pregnancy, and 90 to 95 mg per day during lactation. These estimates are considered generally to be quite generous as doses as low as 10 mg per day have been successful in treating scurvy.

Treatment

In approaching the treatment of scurvy, it is essential to recognize the nutritional deficiency before it becomes extreme. Early symptoms and signs, such as weakness, lethargy, and general malaise, are nonspecific. Pain in the bones and joints, perifollicular hemorrhages, and petechiae should alert the physician to the strong likelihood of scurvy. Swollen, bleeding gums indicate advanced disease, as does edema, oliguria, and peripheral neuropathy.

As noted, a dose of as little as 10 mg per day can treat scurvy satisfactorily, but it is advisable to begin with larger amounts, in the range of 100 to 200 mg per day. Significant improvement should be noted within several days. A good diet is obviously crucial for recovery and for maintenance of health. Such doses should be safe to administer for weeks to months if necessary to restore health to normal.

Rare inborn errors of metabolism, including osteogenesis imperfecta, tyrosinemia, and Chediak-Higashi syndrome, have in case reports been ameliorated by doses in the range of 50 to 200 mg per day. Further experience is needed in the management of these disorders before guidelines can be definitive. Vitamin C at the level of 0.5 to 2 or 3 grams per day has been used to acidify urine. In smaller amounts (40 to 100 mg), ascorbic acid is recommended in order to increase the intestinal absorption of nonheme iron. Patients on a strict vegetarian diet should be encouraged to consume orange juice with their meals because the 40 to 50 mg contained in a glass of orange juice increases the bioavailability of iron from vegetable sources significantly. However, ascorbic acid decreases absorption of copper. Care must be taken to avoid giving potentially toxic doses of vitamin C, and restricting therapeutic doses to the range of 1 to 2 grams should minimize this possibility.

There is great contemporary interest in the potential use of vitamin C alone or in combination with the other antioxidant vitamins, beta-carotene and vitamin E, in the possible prevention of cancer, heart disease, certain manifestations of aging, and other conditions. This is an active area of research, and further investigations are likely to lead to recommendations for the general public as well as for the management of specific disorders.

VITAMIN K DEFICIENCY

method of
BARRY SKIKNE, M.D.
University of Kansas Medical Center
Kansas City, Kansas

and

MARJORIE L. ZUCKER, M.D.
St. Luke's Hospital
Kansas City, Missouri

Vitamin K is essential for normal functioning of the coagulation pathway. This fat-soluble vitamin is responsible for the synthesis of functional coagulation Factors II (prothrombin), VII, IX, and X, as well as the anticoagulant factors responsible for inhibiting coagulation (proteins C and S). Other vitamin K–dependent factors also exist, the most notable being osteocalcin. This protein is found in bone, cartilage, dentin, and other organs and is thought to play a role in their metabolism. Interference with production of functional osteocalcin may be the cause of the congenital bone defects that occur during fetal growth when warfarin is inadvertently administered during pregnancy.

The vitamin K–dependent coagulant proteins are synthesized in the liver and have molecular weights ranging between 42 and 75 kilodaltons (kDa). To become functional, these proteins undergo vitamin K–dependent post-translational modification in the hepatic microsomes, whereby glutamic acid residues near the N-terminal ends of the individual precursor proteins are converted into γ-carboxyglutamic acid residues. This modification allows calcium to bind to these residues. Calcium binding is necessary for the formation of coagulation factor complexes by allowing attachment of these proteins to exposed phospholipids, especially on platelet membranes at the site of activation of primary coagulation. When γ-carboxylation is impaired as a result of vitamin K deficiency or interference with its function, excess amounts of nonfunctional "des-γ-carboxylated" proteins are secreted into the plasma. These are also known as PIVKAs (proteins induced by vitamin K antagonists).

The γ-carboxylation of glutamic acid residues on vitamin K–dependent precursor proteins is dependent on the continuous recycling of vitamin K. Ingested vitamin K quinone is reduced by hydroquinone reductase to vitamin K hydroquinone. Vitamin K hydroquinone serves as cofactor for the conversion of glutamate to γ-carboxyglutamate on the vitamin K–dependent precursor proteins in the presence of a vitamin K–dependent carboxylase (vitamin K epoxidase). This reaction results in the formation of vitamin K epoxide from vitamin K hydroquinone. The cycle is completed by vitamin K epoxide reductase, which converts vitamin K epoxide back to vitamin K quinone for reuse in the cycle. Vitamin K antagonists such as warfarin work by inhibiting vitamin K epoxide reductase and probably hydroquinone reductase as well. Inhibition of these reductases leads to interruption of the vitamin K cycle and accumulation of increased levels of vitamin K epoxide.

The daily vitamin K requirement is 100 to 200 μg, and hepatic vitamin K stores are sufficient to last only 1 to 3 weeks. The primary source of vitamin K is green leafy vegetables. This plant form of the vitamin, phylloquinone (vitamin K_1), accounts for the major portion of the vitamin normally found in the liver. Another important source of vitamin K is menaquinone (vitamin K_2), synthesized by bacteria residing in the intestine. Vitamin K absorption occurs predominantly in the ileum, and bile salts are required for its solubilization in the gastrointestinal tract. In circumstances in which dietary intake of vitamin K_1 is insufficient, vitamin K_2 synthesized by resident intestinal tract bacteria is usually sufficient to maintain a stable vitamin K status.

CAUSES OF VITAMIN K DEFICIENCY

Newborns may be prone to develop vitamin K deficiency. At birth, only minimal amounts of vitamin K are present in stores because of inadequate transfer of vitamin K across the placenta, absence of colonization of the colon by vitamin K–producing bacteria in the fetus, and possible poor vitamin K status of the mother. Vitamin K status may be further compromised by functional immaturity of the liver, which may impair bile salt production, leading to vitamin K malabsorption. Breast-feeding may also play a role, because human breast milk is a poor source of vitamin K. Vitamin K deficiency in newborns, termed "hemorrhagic disease of the newborn," typically occurs in the first 7 to 10 days of life and manifests as skin or mucosal bleeding, bleeding from venipuncture sites, or bleeding from circumcision. More serious manifestations include intracranial and retroperitoneal bleeding. Less commonly, vitamin K deficiency may occur in the third to eighth week of life, particularly in infants who are exclusively breast-fed and/or did not receive vitamin K prophylaxis at birth. Hereditary deficiency of vitamin K is an uncommon disorder that is usually discovered in newborns or later during infancy or childhood.

Vitamin K deficiency rarely occurs as a result of poor dietary intake of the vitamin alone, inasmuch as only minute amounts of the vitamin are required in relation to the quantity of vitamin K present in food. Vitamin K deficiency may be seen in situations in which vitamin K intake is inadequate and intestinal production of vitamin K by bacteria is impaired. This situation typically occurs in severely ill hospitalized patients who have poor dietary intake and are receiving broad-spectrum antibiotic therapy, which eliminates vitamin K–producing intestinal bacteria. Although vitamin K deficiency secondary to antibiotic use is thought to be caused largely by this latter mechanism, certain antibiotics, such as moxalactam and cefamandole, may interfere with the vitamin K–dependent carboxylation of coagulant factors in the liver, hence also causing vitamin K deficiency.

Vitamin K deficiency can occur in any setting in which the production and secretion of bile acids is impaired or malabsorption is present. Typical disorders of the liver associated with impaired bile acid production and secretion include primary biliary cirrhosis and other disorders associated with intrahepatic cholestasis. Disorders of the biliary tree include sclerosing cholangitis or cholelithiasis with common bile duct obstruction. Disorders of the bowel mucosa include Crohn's disease and sprue, as well as short bowel syndromes.

The accidental, surreptitious, or excessive ingestion of vitamin K antagonists (e.g., warfarin) induces a state resembling vitamin K deficiency. The clinical manifestations and laboratory changes are identical to those seen in true vitamin K deficiency. In patients suspected of surreptitiously ingesting warfarin, serum warfarin levels should be measured to confirm these suspicions. Newer rodenticides such as brodifacoum have long-acting effects and should also be considered. These are not detected by serum warfarin assays, and detecting them requires specific assays that are not widely available. Ingestion of high doses of salicylates may also cause vitamin K antagonism via interference with vitamin K epoxide reductase.

LABORATORY CHANGES

Because Factor VII has the shortest half-life of the vitamin K–dependent coagulation factors, the first laboratory manifestation of vitamin K deficiency is prolongation of the prothrombin time. With more profound deficiency, Factors II, IX, and X also decrease significantly, resulting in prolongation of the activated partial thromboplastin time (APTT). A mixture of equal parts of the patient's plasma and normal plasma corrects a prolonged APTT caused by vitamin K deficiency, which rules out the possibility of an inhibitor. The fibrinogen level and thrombin time are normal. Distinguishing vitamin K deficiency from liver disease requires measurement of the thrombin time and individual clotting factors, including fibrinogen and Factor V in addition to Factors II, VII, IX, and X. In liver disease, the thrombin time may be prolonged, and fibrinogen and Factors II, V, VII, IX, and X may be variably reduced, whereas only Factors II, VII, IX, and X are reduced in vitamin K deficiency. Serum levels of the precursor vitamin K–dependent proteins (des-γ-carboxylated proteins) can be measured but their clinical use is limited. When surreptitious warfarin ingestion is suspected, warfarin levels should be measured.

TREATMENT AND PREVENTION

Vitamin K_1 (AquaMEPHYTON, Konakion) should be prophylactically administered within 1 hour of birth at a dose of 1 mg intramuscularly to prevent hemorrhagic disease of the newborn. If there is a particular contraindication to intramuscular injection, oral vitamin K_1 should be given at a dose of 2 to 5 mg. When infants are exclusively breast-fed or have protracted diarrhea or malabsorptive disorders, repeated prophylactic vitamin K_1 injections or oral doses should be administered on a monthly basis. There is no evidence that maternal vitamin K status has a major influence on the newborn's vitamin K status, and improving maternal vita-

min K levels is unnecessary unless they are thought to be deficient.

In hospitalized patients, especially those receiving antibiotics, those with poor dietary intake, and those receiving parenteral nutrition, vitamin K stores should be maintained by an intramuscular dose of 10 mg of vitamin K_1 weekly. If there is a contraindication to intramuscular injection, the dose can be administered intravenously, or 5 mg can be given orally every 3 to 4 days. A 1-mg dose can be added daily to the infused fluids in patients receiving total parenteral nutrition. In patients with malabsorption syndromes, oral administration of vitamin K should be avoided, although on occasion, sufficient amounts may be absorbed if 5 mg of oral vitamin K is taken daily. If oral administration is inadequate, 5 to 10 mg can be self-administered weekly via the subcutaneous route.

The therapy of vitamin K deficiency depends on the clinical setting and the presence or absence of bleeding, as well as on the severity of bleeding. When life-threatening bleeding (e.g., intracranial or gastrointestinal) is present, it is necessary to rapidly correct the coagulopathy by administering fresh-frozen plasma, 15 mL per kg body weight, along with 10 to 20 mg vitamin K_1 intravenously. Fresh-frozen plasma contains sufficient amounts of vitamin K–dependent clotting factors to temporarily correct the disorder. Vitamin K administration should produce partial correction of the prothrombin time by 12 hours and full correction by 24 to 48 hours. Because of the short half-life of Factor VII, it is important to recheck the prothrombin time and APTT after 6 to 12 hours and repeat fresh-frozen plasma administration if the values have not improved significantly and the patient is still bleeding. There are currently no indications for the use of vitamin K–dependent factor concentrates in vitamin K deficiency.

In patients with less severe bleeding, 5 to 10 mg of vitamin K_1 given intramuscularly or intravenously, or 10 to 20 mg given orally, should be sufficient to correct the deficiency. In general, it is preferable to avoid intramuscular injection when the prothrombin time is sufficiently prolonged to cause excess bleeding. When it is necessary to merely correct a prolonged prothrombin time caused by warfarin, the warfarin should be temporarily discontinued for a few days and 1 to 5 mg of vitamin K administered. Administration of excessive amounts of vitamin K may cause transient refractoriness to warfarin when it is reinstituted. Because of the possibility of allergic or anaphylactic reactions with intravenous vitamin K administration, it is necessary to have means of performing resuscitative measures available.

Vitamin K deficiency caused by ingestion of long-acting rodenticides requires long-term vitamin K replacement. Fresh-frozen plasma should be administered in bleeding patients. Large doses of vitamin K, up to 100 mg to 150 mg orally, may be required initially to overcome the effect of these agents. Vitamin K may have to be administered daily over several months until the prothrombin time, which should be regularly monitored, is fully corrected.

OSTEOPOROSIS

method of
URIEL S. BARZEL, M.D.
Albert Einstein College of Medicine
Bronx, New York

Osteoporosis is a condition of bone, present primarily among the aged, in which there is a propensity to fracture spontaneously or as a result of minimal trauma. In this condition, the external size of the bone is normal, but there is too little bone tissue within this envelope to provide adequate skeletal support for the physical stresses of normal daily life and for commonly encountered minor accidents. Osteoporosis is not clinically apparent until the patient presents with a fracture, inasmuch as there is no specific medical or biological marker that would identify it. Some nonspecific radiologic findings are associated with this condition, and some patients may be suspected of having osteoporosis as the result of incidental observations of skeletal structures during radiologic procedures.

CLINICAL MANIFESTATION

Wrist fracture (Colles' fracture) is the most common presenting condition of osteoporosis, followed in frequency by collapse-fractures of spinal vertebrae and by hip fractures. In extreme cases, patients may sustain rib fractures as a result of leaning against a hard surface: the author has seen osteoporotic patients who had fractured ribs as they were leaning on the side of a bathtub while cleaning the tub.

NATURAL HISTORY

The natural history of osteoporosis is one of recurrent, unpredictable, discrete occurrences of fractures, interspersed with periods of months or years of freedom from clinical symptoms. Osteoporotic hip fractures, however, are associated with a 1-year mortality rate of 25 to 50%.

Bone tissue in osteoporosis is completely normal, both histologically and biochemically. Osteoporotic fractures heal normally: there is formation of callus and development of bony union within a few weeks. Fractures in the dorsal spine may cause round back deformity, especially if there are anterior collapses of upper thoracic vertebrae. Fractures in the lower tho-

racic and lumbar spine result, eventually, in the rib cage coming to rest on the iliac crest, a condition described by the patient as the loss of the waistline. These collapses and fractures bring about a marked reduction in height; osteoporotic patients have been known to lose 6 to 10 inches as a result of multiple fractures. The round back deformity and the loss of vertebral height create a bulging of the anterior abdominal muscles and produce chronic constipation because of inability to develop intra-abdominal pressure for adequate evacuation.

ETIOLOGY

A number of conditions have been linked to the development of osteoporosis (Table 1). A major factor is the failure to attain maximum skeletal density at peak development in early adulthood. To some extent, this may be genetic or familial, and to some extent it may be the result of inadequate calcium intake during the formative years. Furthermore, throughout adult life there is an imbalance in bone turnover, in both men and women, whereby bone resorption exceeds bone formation. This results in a slow and inexorable loss of bone, which may reach a clinically significant level in those who failed to achieve maximal density in early adulthood. There are multiple potential contributory factors to this imbalance: inadequate calcium intake throughout adult life and calcium malabsorption, which is frequently present in the elderly, may be two such factors. Inactivity may play an etiologic role in osteoporosis, as suggested by the fact that experimental inactivity in volunteers and immobility in orthopedic or neurologic patients cause negative calcium balance and osteopenia. Results of recent studies imply an abnormal parathyroid response to hypocalcemia, and some investigators propose that an abnormality of vitamin D metabolism may be a contributory factor in osteoporosis. High protein intake, obligatory urinary calcium loss as a result of high sodium intake, and renal tubular calcium leakage have all been described in osteoporosis and may also contribute to its development.

In women, there is an acceleration of bone resorption and an exaggeration of the imbalance between formation and resorption after the cessation of gonadal function at the time of menopause, whether natural or artificial (e.g., bilateral oophorectomy). Because women reach at maturity a smaller skeletal mass than do

TABLE 1. **Factors Associated with Osteoporosis**

Female sex
Menopause
Fair skin
Low calcium intake
Low body weight
Smoking
Alcoholism
Diabetes mellitus
Anorexia nervosa
Pernicious anemia
Inactivity
Excessive activity with secondary amenorrhea

men, and because men do not normally lose gonadal function, women are much more likely to be afflicted by this disease.

ACHIEVEMENT OF SKELETAL INTEGRITY

The achievement of maximal skeletal development requires adequate intake of vitamin D and calcium, as well as physical exercise. Vitamin D may be endogenously synthesized through the exposure of the skin to the ultraviolet rays of the sun for a few minutes a day. Vitamin D is available exogenously in cod liver oil, in deep sea fish, and, in the United States, in some milk formulations that are fortified with vitamin D. (Skim milk, from which all fat has been removed, does not contain the vitamin, which is fat soluble.) Vitamin D is also widely available in therapeutic vitamin capsules. In teenagers and adults, the amount of vitamin D required is 200 to 400 units per day. Because ingestion of excess vitamin D may result in vitamin D toxicity—hypercalciuria and hypercalcemia—megadoses of this vitamin should be discouraged, except in cases of fat malabsorption and of hypoparathyroidism.

The recommended amount of dietary calcium is 800 to 1000 mg daily in adults and twice as much in teenagers. Both vitamin D and calcium can be obtained in adequate amounts from the ingestion of three to four glasses of nonskim milk daily. Calcium is also easily available in multiple over-the-counter products, generally as calcium carbonate, and can be taken as a supplement if the amount of milk ingested is less than recommended. Maintenance of adequate muscle strength, by the performance of calisthenics for 30 to 60 minutes three times a week, is also useful. Excessive exercise may induce amenorrhea, and it then becomes counterproductive because the cessation of ovarian hormone production in this situation results in a negative calcium balance and a significant decrease in skeletal mass similar to that seen in menopause.

MAINTENANCE OF SKELETAL INTEGRITY AND PREVENTION OF OSTEOPOROSIS

Maintenance of the skeletal integrity, once maximal development has been achieved, requires the continuation of adequate intake of calcium and vitamin D and the maintenance of an exercise program. Furthermore, it is recommended that cigarette smoking and excessive alcohol consumption be avoided because these are linked to the development of osteoporosis as well as to other disabilities.

A most important measure in the prevention of osteoporosis in females is cyclic hormone therapy at the time of menopause. Epidemiologic studies, performed in postmenopausal white women, reveal that estrogen administration reduces the risk of osteoporotic fractures by half. Similar studies reveal that the protective effect of estrogen is independent of so-called risk factors such as low body weight or smoking. Thus if there is

no contraindication for hormone therapy, this therapy should be offered to all menopausal women, because rapid bone loss is a universal phenomenon that occurs in all women when estrogen production ceases.

To be effective in preventing the rapid loss of bone, estrogen replacement therapy should be started immediately after bilateral oophorectomy or as soon as possible, and no later than 5 years, after the onset of natural menopause. Once started, estrogen therapy should be continued for at least 5 or 6 years. The optimal treatment regimen recommended today is cyclic therapy with estrogen and progesterone. The minimal effective oral estrogen dose is 25 μg of ethinyl estradiol (Estinyl, Feminone) or 0.625 mg conjugated estrogens (Premarin) (0.300 mg of conjugated estrogen if coupled with high calcium intake) given for 24 days and medroxyprogesterone (Provera, Amen, Curretab), 5 mg per day for the last 12 days of the cycle. Transdermal estrogen administration, 0.05 or 0.1 mg of estradiol (Estraderm) per day, is an approved and effective alternative to oral estrogen and is administered with oral medroxyprogesterone in the last half of the cycle. This therapy prevents hot flushes, maintains vaginal mucosa, and possibly diminishes the risk of acute myocardial infarction in the postmenopausal woman, but there is continued monthly vaginal bleeding. Estrogen therapy is contraindicated in women with breast cancer, family history of breast cancer, and history of thrombophlebitis or thromboembolic disease.

In certain endocrine conditions such as acromegaly, hyperadrenocorticism, and thyrotoxicosis, as well as excess thyroid hormone replacement, gastrectomy, and liver disease, appropriate medical intervention and treatment may help prevent the development of osteoporosis. To the extent possible, acromegaly, hyperadrenocorticism, and thyrotoxicosis should be corrected or kept under optimal control. If patients are given pharmacologic doses of corticosteroids as long-term therapy, some element of protection of the skeleton can be achieved by the coadministration of pharmacologic doses (50,000 to 100,000 units per week) of vitamin D (calciferol) and an adequate calcium intake. Patients receiving thyroxine replacement therapy should be given this hormone in amounts that would maintain normal serum thyroxine and serum thyroid stimulating hormone (TSH) levels. Suppression of the serum TSH level below the normal range should be avoided (except in cases of thyroid cancer, for which this is the therapeutic goal). In postgastrectomy states, osteomalacia may develop unless adequate vitamin D is regularly given in amounts necessary to overcome a degree of malabsorption that is present in this condition.

TREATMENT OF ESTABLISHED OSTEOPOROSIS

When presented with a case of apparent osteoporosis and a fracture, the author treats the actual fracture and, at the same time, reviews the differential diagnosis (Table 2) and initiates a treatment regimen for whatever underlying condition may be responsible for the development of osteoporosis.

Colles' fracture is treated by casting. Spinal collapse is treated with complete bed rest until the acute pain has substantially diminished (72 hours to 2 weeks), followed by gradual mobilization, first to an inclined chair and later to full upright position and re-ambulation. Pain treatment should avoid narcotics, if possible, because of their tendency to cause constipation. A corset may be used for a few weeks to give the spine some support during the period of recovery. Hip fracture necessitates surgical pinning or hip replacement, followed by early ambulation and aggressive physiotherapy.

Beyond the repair of the acute fracture, the anatomic goal of medical therapy in established osteoporosis is to increase the amount of bone tissue and prevent further fractures. Adequate vitamin intake, adequate calcium ingestion (which in the postmenopausal woman rises to 1500 mg per day), and exercise continue to be prescribed in women who have established osteoporosis but do not, per se, improve their bone mineral status. There is epidemiologic evidence that among subjects who have been taking thiazide diuretics for more than 10 years, the rate of osteoporotic fractures is lower. The use of these preparations in subjects with hypercalciuria is clearly justified, but it is not known whether thiazide therapy or a low-sodium diet leads to a positive skeletal balance.

A large number of pharmacologic agents have been under investigation for their possible positive effect on skeletal metabolism (Table 3). According to the literature dealing with the treatment regimens of this condition and with osteoporosis in general, a few caveats must be

TABLE 2. **Differential Diagnosis of Osteoporosis**

Osteomalacia
Acromegaly
Hyperthyroidism
Hyperparathyroidism
Hyperadrenocorticism
Multiple myeloma
Prolonged heparin therapy
Lipid storage disease
Liver disease
Chronic anemia

TABLE 3. **Treatments for Established Osteoporosis**

Generally Accepted or Approved
High-calcium diet
Alkaline calcium supplements
  (e.g., calcium carbonate, calcium citrate malate, calcium citrate*)
Adequate vitamin D intake
Exercise
Calcitonin
Estrogen (oral and transdermal)

Investigational
Sodium fluoride (enteric-coated)
Anabolic agents: methandrostenolone
Low-dose parathyroid hormone
Vitamin D metabolites:
  1,25-dihydroxyvitamin D (calcitriol)
  1α-hydroxyvitamin D
  24,25-dihydroxyvitamin D
Hydrochlorothiazide
Low sodium intake
Diphosphonate (Etidronate)

*Preferred preparation in hypochlorhydria.

kept in mind: (1) Much of the currently available information on osteoporosis is the result of cross-sectional studies in which people born in different years are compared. Such comparisons clearly may not always be justifiable. Comparisons of maximal skeletal development of subjects born in 1910, for instance, with those born in 1945 may be totally invalid because standards of diet and health were markedly different during the times in which these two cohorts grew up and reached maturity. (2) In many ongoing studies of osteoporosis, investigators use currently available methods of bone densitometry and quantitation of bone mineral at different bone sites as their end points of efficacy of interventional regimes. These provide clearly valuable information about bone at these specific, measurable sites but must be viewed critically until they are proved to have a significant correlation with fracture rates. With these caveats in place, osteoporosis therapy can be examined.

Estrogen and progesterone cycles, with the dosages described earlier for preventive therapy, have been shown to have a beneficial effect even at this stage in the natural history of the disease. Unfortunately, estrogen's side effects are unacceptable to most elderly women with established osteoporosis. For example, in a 1-year study in which 70-year-old normal women were given estrogen/gestagen, 44% left the study before its conclusion, two-thirds of them because of "menstrual troubles." In another study, 13% of women with established osteoporosis who were given estrogen therapy required hysterectomy or dilatation and curettage.

Calcitonin (Calcimar, Miacalcin), an injectable hormone with significant effect in Paget's disease, has been approved for treatment of osteoporosis. Available data show that, administered at a dose of 50 to 100 international units (IU) subcutaneously or intramuscularly daily or every other day, salmon calcitonin does have a salutary effect on bone density, but the studies are too short and contain too few subjects to prove that calcitonin treatment prevents osteoporotic fractures. Sodium fluoride has been the subject of intense investigations for more than 10 years. When used therapeutically, in doses of 35 to 70 mg per day, fluoride has effectively increased bone density in only 60% of osteoporotic subjects, the resultant bone has not been histologically normal, and, most important, fracture prevention has not been demonstrated. Furthermore, fluoride therapy is associated with a high rate of gastric and joint complications (a lower rate of these complications is reported for enteric-coated tablets).

Anabolic agents (e.g., stanozolol [Winstrol], 2 to 6 mg daily, 3 weeks out of 4) have a positive effect on bone economy but are unacceptable to most female patients because of the associated masculinizing side effects and because of their negative effects on lipid metabolism. A theory that very-low-dose parathyroid hormone administered parenterally may result in an improved skeletal density and strength is under investigation. The possibility that vitamin D metabolism is faulty in osteoporotic subjects fuels a number of studies of various metabolites of the vitamin. One study reported a beneficial effect of 1,25-dihydroxyvitamin D in the prevention of fractures, but studies on treatment with vitamin D metabolites are inconclusive, as are those on parathyroid hormone injection therapy.

A new approach to the problem of osteoporosis is based on the recently developed concept of ADFR (activate, depress, free, repeat), also called "coherence therapy." This treatment approach is designed to exploit the physiologic sequential coupling of bone resorption and bone formation in bone turnover. Bone turnover and remodeling can be visualized as beginning with osteoclastic resorption, which is later followed by osteoblastic deposition of bone in the same anatomic locations. The aim of ADFR is to stimulate coherent bone resorption ("activate") and then stop it prematurely ("depress"). Thereafter, bone formation proceeds normally ("free"), and eventually the cycle is repeated ("repeat"). The success of this method hinges on the fact that whereas bone resorption would be interrupted pharmacologically, bone formation would be allowed to proceed, physiologically, unhampered. Interrupting the resorptive phase and not the formative phase would achieve excess formation in relation to resorption

and hence a reversal of the previously negative bone balance.

In practice, good results are obtained with this cycling therapy without the "activation" stage of the sequence. "Depression" is achieved by the use of the diphosphonate etidronate (Didronel). This orally administered agent arrests osteoclastic activity and has been used extensively for a number of years to suppress osteoclastic bone resorption in Paget's disease. It is administered at a dose of 400 mg daily, on an empty stomach, for a period of 2 weeks. Thereafter, patients are provided with adequate calcium and vitamin D, but are otherwise not treated ("free"). The treatment cycle is repeated every 10 to 12 weeks. No abnormality has been found on histologic examinations of bone after 150 weeks of ADFR therapy, and a reduction in the depth of resorption cavities has been demonstrated. Furthermore, preliminary data show that over 4 years, there is continuous increase in bone density in all sites examined, as well as a reduction in fracture activity. If confirmed to be effective, this therapeutic approach may prove to provide a safe and a simple long-term management opportunity in established osteoporosis.

PAGET'S DISEASE OF BONE

method of
ROY D. ALTMAN, M.D.
Miami Veterans Affairs Medical Center
Miami, Florida

Paget's disease of bone can be defined as a condition in which there is accelerated remodeling of isolated areas of the mature skeleton. The bone initially undergoes increased absorption by large and active osteoclasts, followed by osteoblastic deposition of bone that is disorganized, often enlarged, interspersed with areas of fibrosis, and (although often heavily calcified) structurally weak.

Paget's disease is occasionally diagnosed on clinical examination by the findings listed in Table 1. However, most often the diagnosis is made from an elevated serum alkaline phosphatase level and by the typical appearance of Paget's disease on the radiograph. A bone scan can determine the extent of bone involvement. Bone biopsy is rarely needed unless sarcoma in Paget's disease or disease metastatic to the Paget's lesion is suspected.

Paget's disease rarely appears before the age of 40, and although the prevalence of disease is approximately 1% of the population, it is suspected that 80% of patients are without clinical findings or complications.

TREATMENT

Not all patients with Paget's disease require therapy, and therapy should have some clearly

TABLE 1. **Complications of Paget's Disease of Bone**

Symptoms or Finding	Pathologic Anatomy
Bone pain	Unknown, periostitis, "bone angina," osteomalacia
Deformity	Softened bone
Fracture	Advancing osteolytic wedge, structurally weak bone, stress fracture of bowed extremity, compression fracture vertebra
Secondary osteoarthritis	Juxta-articular Paget's disease, change in joint congruity, altered gait dynamics
High-output cardiac state	Extensive skeletal involvement; i.e., over ⅓ of the skeleton, serum alkaline phosphatase > 4× upper normal level
Malignancy	Sarcomatous degeneration of involved bone; metastatic malignant disease to pagetic bone
Dizziness/headache	Unknown, massive skull involvement, platybasia (with occipital headache)
Hearing loss	Eighth nerve compression, otosclerosis, invasion of cochlea by pagetic bone
Change in mental status	Platybasia with compression of fourth ventricle
Paraparesis/paraplegia	Cord compression, "spinal artery steal syndrome"
Back pain	Altered gait dynamics, secondary osteoarthritis, active spinal Paget's disease, spinal stenosis, lateral recess syndrome
Hypercalcemia	Hyperparathyroidism, immobilization
Visual loss	Rupture of angioid streak of fundus, optic nerve entrapment

defined goals. For individual patients with a complication of the disease, a therapeutic program can be constructed.

General Measures

Patients should be advised that Paget's disease is rarely a serious illness. Most often, symptoms are mild and readily suppressed by therapy. In patients with symptomatic disease, a variety of physical, medicinal, and surgical measures are often effective in disease control. Death from Paget's disease is almost limited to the fewer than 1% of patients in whom sarcomatous changes develop within the pagetic lesion.

Mechanical devices such as orthoses often correct symptoms related to bowed lower extremities or pelvic deformity. Heel lifts, or, occasionally, medial wedges suffice. Orthopedic procedures indicated for Paget's disease include osteotomy for tibial or femoral deformity, open or closed reduction for fracture, joint arthroplasty for secondary osteoarthritis, and spinal decompression for cord compression. Fractures or osteotomies may necessitate intramedullary rods for stabilization. Because the fractured bone is often soft and tends to bow, the intramedullary rod is commonly left in place indefinitely for continued stabilization. Fractures most often heal without event; however, occasional nonunions occur. The fracture callus is often pagetic. During orthopedic surgery, pagetic bone may be hard and difficult to cut, or it may be soft and may bleed excessively. Medicinal therapy before orthopedic surgery usually reduces excessive bleeding.

Anti-Inflammatory Drugs

High-dose salicylates have been used for their analgesic and anti-inflammatory properties. In addition, they have been shown to retard collagen production and reduce hydroxyproline excretion in pagetic patients. Suppression of prostaglandin levels by indomethacin and other anti-inflammatory agents is believed to decrease skeletal vascularity and bone resorption. In many patients with Paget's disease, pain is related to secondary osteoarthritis. Symptoms related to osteoarthritis may be partly controlled by the use of anti-inflammatory agents.

Guidelines for Suppressive Therapy

Patients selected for suppressive therapy should meet three criteria: they should have symptoms related to Paget's disease, demonstrate active disease by an elevated serum alkaline phosphatase level, and show radiographic evidence of Paget's disease at the symptomatic site.

The author's indications for therapy are outlined on Table 2. The most clear-cut indication for therapy is pain related to Paget's disease and not caused by another phenomenon such as secondary osteoarthritis.

Caution must be exercised in the therapy of patients with lumbar spine involvement from Paget's disease. Although back pain is a common complaint in patients with Paget's disease, Paget's disease per se is an uncommon cause of symptoms. More often, symptoms are caused by musculoskeletal stresses induced by the deformities from Paget's disease and often associated with an arthritic process resulting from the disease.

Paraparesis or paraplegia related to Paget's disease has often been reversed, at least in part, by medicinal therapy. Many affected patients are poor surgical candidates for decompression. Dramatic improvement in paraparesis or paraplegia is believed to be caused by reversal of a "spinal artery steal" syndrome rather than rapid reduction of bone in the spinal canal.

TABLE 2. **Indications for Medicinal Therapy of Paget's Disease**

Sign or Symptom	Calcitonin	Bisphosphonate
Bone pain caused by Paget's disease	+	+
Spinal Paget's disease with paraparesis/paraplegia	+	+
Preoperative orthopedic surgery	+	+
Immobilization hypercalcemia	+	
Nonunion pagetic fracture		+
Osteolytic wedge of long bone on x-ray	+	?
Skull symptoms—headache, dizziness (not platybasia)	+	+
High-output cardiac failure	+	+
Prevent progression of disease (i.e., not correct existing defect):		
Hearing loss (Paget's disease of the petrous ridge)	+	+
Osteoarthritis (Juxta-articular Paget's disease)	+	+
Deformity (Paget's disease of long bones)	+	+
Asymptomatic increase in serum alkaline phosphatase without complication listed above	−	−

Pagetic bone has sometimes been described by orthopedic surgeons as structurally soft and highly vascular. Pretreatment with one of the suppressive agents appears to decrease the vascularity of the pagetic bone and may limit blood loss during orthopedic surgery. The treated bone is likely to heal more normally.

Immobilization-induced hypercalcemia should be treated specifically with calcitonin.

The author's experience with nonunion fractures has been favorable with etidronate; that is, nonunion pagetic fractures often heal shortly after a short course of high-dose etidronate therapy. The physiologic mechanism is not yet understood.

The long bone osteolytic phase of Paget's disease is usually quite symptomatic, and high-quality x-rays may be required for diagnosis. This complication is not common; it has occurred in about 10% of x-rays in the author's series. Calcitonin consistently induces the radiographic appearance of healing during therapy. However, withdrawal of calcitonin is often followed by rapid progression of disease, implying that therapy should not be discontinued. Etidronate inconsistently induces radiographic "healing" and is sometimes associated with disease progression.

It appears that suppressive therapy can inhibit the progression of disease. In the presence of juxta-articular Paget's disease, suppressive therapy may prevent progression to osteoarthritis. In the presence of long bone Paget's disease, suppressive therapy may prevent bowing. In the presence of pelvic Paget's disease, suppressive therapy may prevent the medial migration of the hips with subsequent difficulty in standing erect. In the presence of skull Paget's disease, and involvement of the petrous ridge in particular, suppressive therapy may prevent hearing loss. However, none of these therapies are expected to correct existing hearing loss, deformity, or osteoarthritis. In the presence of any of these complications, therapy is directed at trying to prevent disease progression.

Activity of disease should be followed by periodic testing of Paget's disease of bone, namely, the serum alkaline phosphatase level and, if possible, 24-hour total peptide hydroxyproline excretion in the urine.

Calcitonin

Calcitonin is a 32–amino acid hormone of the thyroid C cells. It has been demonstrated to lower plasma inorganic calcium concentration by action on bone and kidney. It inhibits osteoclastic bone resorption with loss of the ruffled resorption surface of osteoclasts within 1 hour, having some effect within 15 minutes. This effect is probably mediated by cyclic adenosine monophosphate accumulation in the cell and results in reduction in the number of osteoclasts. Even though there is no deficiency of calcitonin in Paget's disease, calcitonin therapy has been demonstrated to suppress clinical and chemical disease. Antibodies to synthetic salmon calcitonin have been demonstrated in patients receiving this agent, and some patients have neutralizing antibodies. Symptoms may be reduced during synthetic salmon or synthetic human calcitonin therapy by the end of the first month of therapy, sometimes dramatically in the first few weeks. Calcitonins induce a more normal histologic picture, with more lamellar than woven bone.

Although considerable variation occurs, synthetic salmon calcitonin (Calcimar, Miacalcin) reduces the chemical expressions of Paget's disease to about 50% of pretreatment levels with a slight loss of effect after 3 to 6 months. After 18 to 24 months of continuous synthetic salmon calcitonin therapy, chemical exacerbation often occurs. If any calcitonin therapy is discontinued, most patients with Paget's disease experience chemical exacerbation of the Paget's disease within 6 months. Antibodies to synthetic salmon calcitonin can occur without clinical resistance and are not present in all patients with resistance.

There appears to be an analgesic effect of synthetic salmon calcitonin that is separate from its effect on suppressing Paget's disease. This analgesic effect may be related to depletion of calcitonin gene–related peptide and substance P from nerve endings. Synthetic human calcitonin (Cibacalcin) does not lose its suppressive chemical effect in most patients for the duration of therapy. However, the net chemical suppression of synthetic human calcitonin on serum chemistries in Paget's disease is usually somewhat less than might be expected with salmon calcitonin. Chemical relapse and clinical relapse do not necessarily coincide; indeed, most patients have a considerable delay in exacerbation of symptoms after withdrawal of calcitonin.

The usual dose of synthetic salmon calcitonin is 100 Medical Research Council (MRC) Units, 0.5 mL subcutaneously or intramuscularly daily, for the first month. The dose can be decreased or the interval between doses increased, depending on the severity of disease and response to therapy. Even though there is no histologic confirmation of benefit, the chemical profiles can be controlled with as little as 50 IU three times a week in many patients. Salmon calcitonin should be refrigerated. It is supplied as 400 IU per 2-mL vial.

Synthetic human calcitonin is supplied as five 0.5-mg doses per box. Each dose is supplied with desiccated calcitonin and the diluent separated in a syringe. The patient breaks the seal between the diluent and the powder, mixes them, and injects. Like that of synthetic salmon calcitonin, the initial dosage of synthetic human calcitonin is a single dose daily for the first month, followed by increases of the interval between doses, depending on the clinical and chemical response.

The most important adverse reactions to the calcitonins are gastrointestinal symptoms (nausea, vomiting, diarrhea, abdominal pain, or cramps), vascular symptoms (flushing of face, tingling of hands and feet), pain at the injection site, urinary frequency, rash, and occasional angioedema. Most symptoms occur within several minutes of injection and last about 1 hour. Hyperparathyroidism, thought to be secondary to calcitonin therapy, has been reported. Adverse reactions are most common during the initial period of therapy and tend to decrease or disappear with continued administration.

Combined plicamycin (Mithracin) and calcitonin have been proposed for severely affected patients. In patients with uncomplicated Paget's disease, the drug could be discontinued after 2 years of therapy. In the presence of a Paget's disease–induced lytic bone lesion, calcitonin probably should be continued indefinitely.

If resistance to salmon calcitonin is suspected, a calcitonin effect on serum calcium level can be tested. Serum calcium level is determined after an overnight fast. Synthetic salmon calcitonin (100 IU) is injected intramuscularly, and serum calcium level is determined 3 to 6 hours afterward. Breakfast is then allowed. If the calcitonin is effective, a decrease of 0.5 mg per dL or more in serum calcium is seen. A decrease of 0.3 mg per dL or less of serum calcitonin is seen in calcitonin resistance.

Another type of calcitonin (eel calcitonin) is under investigation, as are alternative methods of administration (synthetic salmon calcitonin by nasal spray).

Bisphosphonates

The newer approved suppressive agents for Paget's disease are bisphosphonates. The bisphosphonates, or diphosphonates, are pyrophosphate analogues in which the central oxygen of pyrophosphate is replaced with a carbon and that are resistant to pyrophosphatase activity. Serum alkaline phosphatase contains pyrophosphatase activity. Bisphosphonates inhibit the precipitation of calcium phosphate, block the transformation of amorphous calcium phosphate to hydroxyapatite, and inhibit aggregation of calcium apatite crystals into clusters. In addition, they retard dissolution of calcium crystals, disaggregate apatite crystal clusters, peptidize crystals (transform crystals into a colloidal state), and form polynuclear complexes in the presence of calcium. One bisphosphonate, etidronate disodium, can inhibit both soft and hard tissue calcification and inhibit bone resorption. At very high doses in animals, etidronate disodium (Didronel) was shown to inhibit vitamin D absorption from the gastrointestinal tract—a phenomenon not yet demonstrated in humans. Bisphosphonates have a direct effect on macrophage function. Osteoclasts are macrophage-like cells and are of the same stem cell origin. Pagetic osteoclasts appear to be particularly sensitive to the bisphosphonates.

Short- and long-term clinical and chemical suppression of Paget's disease was demonstrated in several studies in which etidronate disodium was used at doses of 5 mg per kg per day for periods of 6 months. Continuation of therapy beyond 6 months does not provide increased clinical or chemical effectiveness. Higher doses can be used for shorter periods of time but are not usually necessary in the initial course of therapy. Clinical improvement may occur after the first month of therapy but is often not apparent until after 3 to 6 months. Clinical improvement is sometimes not apparent until after therapy has been discontinued. Between 15% and 40% of patients receive prolonged clinical and chemical remission from etidronate disodium. The duration of response may be related to the initial dose of medication but is more likely correlated with the pretreatment levels of hydroxyproline excretion and serum alkaline phosphatase.

In general, the number of retreatments needed can be predicted by the height of the initial chemical values: the higher the initial chemical value, the more likely retreatment will be needed. Retreatment, when instituted at a frequency of less than once yearly, is usually effective. In approximately 15% of patients treated with etidronate disodium, the disease becomes refractory to the drug. In cases in which the disease is refractory to 5 mg per kg per day, patients may respond to higher doses. If etidronate disodium is administered at high dosage, administered for prolonged periods of time, or required more than once a year, there is a risk that the disease will become refractory to the drug, that adverse reactions will develop, or both.

In the United States, there appear to be regional differences in the frequency of adverse reactions, such as bone pain. It is tempting to attribute these differences to climate (e.g., sun exposure affecting vitamin D absorption) or hereditary factors. The usual dose of etidronate disodium for Paget's disease is 5 mg per kg per day or 400 mg daily for patients weighing 40 kg (88 pounds) to 80 kg (176 pounds). The drug is supplied in 200-mg and 400-mg tablets. The entire etidronate disodium dose should be administered at one time, midway between breakfast and lunch (or at bedtime) with either black coffee or water. Etidronate disodium adheres to food and milk or other dairy products, preventing absorption, and must be administered on an empty stomach.

Adverse reactions to etidronate disodium include abdominal cramps and diarrhea, hyperphosphatemia, increasing bone pain, and a possible increase in fractures. Abdominal symptoms often subside by altering dosage or time of drug administration. Hyperphosphatemia appears to be a direct renal effect of etidronate disodium in humans that does not occur in animals. Hyperphosphatemia in humans is not related to changes in parathyroid, vitamin D, calcitonin, or calcium homeostasis.

Several other agents have had varying success and may have use in patients in whom disease is refractory to other approved agents. These other agents include intravenous etidronate disodium and intravenous amino-hydroxypropylidene diphosphonate (APD, pamidronate [Aredia]).

Bisphosphonates have been combined with calcitonin; this program seems to be of particular value in severely affected patients. There is clinical and laboratory evidence that when used sequentially, etidronate disodium should be followed, rather than preceded, by calcitonin.

Plicamycin

The first agent that seemed to effectively attack the progression of Paget's disease was plicamycin (Mithracin). This drug, however, is not approved by the U.S. Food and Drug Administration for use in Paget's disease. Plicamycin is a yellow crystalline antibiotic derived from the microorganism *Streptomyces tanashiensis*. It is an inhibitor of DNA-directed RNA synthesis, probably by binding but not DNA-altering. Intravenous administration of 25 µg per kg daily for 10 days results in clinical and chemical benefit in most patients. Smaller doses (10 to 15 µg per kg daily for 10 days) may give similar results. Prolonged remissions of disease may occur. Clinical response to plicamycin is often dramatic. In patients with resistant disease, combination with other agents may be effective.

Widespread use of plicamycin should be limited. The agent has hepatotoxic, nephrotoxic, hematotoxic, and dermatologic reactions. It often causes hypocalcemia, nausea, and vomiting during administration. Many physicians reserve plicamycin for the most seriously affected patients, especially patients with disease that does not respond or that becomes resistant to alternative therapies.

Other Therapies

Although approved by the U.S. Food and Drug Administration for hypercalcemia of malignant disease, gallium nitrate has been tested for Paget's disease. It may have use in refractory cases by either the subcutaneous or the intravenous route.

PARENTERAL NUTRITION IN ADULTS

method of
MARK J. KORUDA, M.D.
University of North Carolina
Chapel Hill, North Carolina

PREOPERATIVE NUTRITIONAL SUPPORT

It has been more than 50 years since H. Studley's landmark study defining the relationship between preoperative weight loss and adverse operative outcome. The mechanisms whereby malnutrition predisposes patients to complications are quite varied. Efforts have been made toward enhancing the perioperative nutritional status of malnourished patients by using total parenteral nutrition (TPN). The presumption is that by improving the nutritional state of the patient, postoperative outcome will improve.

In the past 15 years, numerous reports evaluating the effectiveness of preoperative TPN have been published. These data show that the use of preoperative TPN reduced postoperative complications in only the severely malnourished. In summary, the use of preoperative TPN should be based on an evaluation of nutritional status and an assessment of the degree of malnutrition. If there is no evidence of severe malnutrition (80% of usual body weight or serum albumin levels less than 3.0 grams per dL), there is little compelling evidence to support the routine use of preoperative parenteral nutrition. However, patients who are severely malnourished probably benefit from nutritional supplementation, although the evidence for this remains inconclusive. Table 1 outlines relative indications and contraindications for the use of TPN in surgical patients.

Parenteral Nutrition Access

In order to avoid phlebitis and thrombosis, it is necessary to infuse hypertonic nutrient solutions into a large-diameter, high-flow vein, typically the superior vena cava and less frequently the inferior vena cava. Access to the superior vena cava for the purpose of intravenous nutrient administration is best accomplished by percutaneous cannulation of the subclavian vein. Alter-

natively, a cannula may be directed into the superior vena cava via the internal or external jugular vein, but the location of the catheter exit site in the neck makes it more difficult to secure the catheter and cover the exit site with a sterile dressing. Thus a long-term catheter with the exit site located in the neck is more susceptible to potential contamination and catheter sepsis than is a catheter exiting from the skin of the upper chest.

The introduction of the multilumen catheter, notably the triple-lumen catheter (TLC), in the mid-1980s responded to the need in the critical care setting to deliver a variety of medications, blood, blood products, and infusions to patients with limited venous access. The administration of parenteral nutrition through these multiport catheters has challenged the traditional practice mandating TPN delivery through an inviolate line in an effort to reduce catheter-related sepsis.

Consensus in the catheter-related infection literature remains an elusive goal. Catheter care protocols should differentiate between the various purposes for catheterization, such as dialysis, parenteral nutrition, and pressure monitoring. *Parenteral nutrition infusion should be performed through a dedicated, inviolate port.* Although varying clinical circumstances dictate different insertion sites, a higher incidence of catheter infection has been observed with (1) peripheral versus central lines, (2) lower limb catheterization versus upper limb, and (3) internal jugular versus subclavian catheterization. Most important, the risks and benefits of ongoing catheterization must be reassessed daily and the catheter promptly removed when no longer indicated.

Nutrient Requirements

In the hospitalized patient, the issue of total nutrient intake, enteral or parenteral, is crucial. Too few calories allow excessive catabolism, whereas too many calories impose added cardiopulmonary stress. In addition, the amounts of carbohydrate, fat, amino acids, and protein required to fulfill nutrient requirements are important.

Five basic steps form the framework of the essentials of nutritional support:

1. Prevent malnutrition.
2. Establish energy goals.
3. Select, establish, and maintain feeding access.
4. Choose and design the optimal formula.
5. Monitor the patient to ensure safe and effective results.

The memory aids—KCALS and FACE MTV—

TABLE 1. **Indications and Contraindications for Perioperative Total Parenteral Nutrition**

Indications
Short-bowel syndrome
High-output enterocutaneous fistula
Prolonged postoperative ileus
NPO status for more than 1 week during medical
 management or preoperative work-up
Severe malnutrition (80% of usual body weight or serum
 albumin levels < 3.0 gm/dL)

Relative Indications
Low-output enterocutaneous fistula
Moderate malnutrition (80–90% of usual body weight or
 serum albumin level 3.0–3.5 gm/dL)

Contraindications
Ability to be fed enterally
Terminal disease with poor prognosis
Adequate nutritional status

Abbreviation: NPO = nil per os (nothing by mouth).

are useful for remembering the components of these basic steps (Table 2).

Energy Requirements

The number of calories that should be prescribed to hospitalized patients who require nutritional support is controversial. Just as inadequate caloric prescription can be detrimental to the patient, excessive caloric administration can produce serious metabolic complications.

Energy requirements can be predicted with reasonable accuracy in normal patients by the Harris-Benedict equations:

Males: kcal/24 hours =
$$66.473 + 13.756 \text{ (body weight in kg)} + 5.0033 \text{ (height in cm)} - 6.755 \text{ (age in years)}$$

Females: kcal/24 hours =
$$655.0955 + 9.5634 \text{ (body weight in kg)} + 1.8498 \text{ (height in cm)} - 4.6756 \text{ (age in years)}$$

These equations calculate the expected *basal* energy expenditure (BEE) in kilocalories per 24 hours. To obtain the actual energy expenditure, various coefficients must then be added to the BEE to account for activity and the level of stress. In early recommendations, it was estimated that injury, sepsis, and burns increased energy requirements by 30%, 60%, and 100%, respectively. However, recent reviews question this concept of hypermetabolism; injury and sepsis have been found to increase the metabolic rate only 15 to

TABLE 3. **Stress Factors**

Condition	Stress Factor*
Uncomplicated, semistarvation	0.8
Well-nourished, unstressed	1.0
Multiple trauma (acute phase)	
Normotensive	1.1–1.5
Hypotensive	0.8–1.0
Multiple trauma (recovery)	1.0–1.2
Sepsis (acute phase)	
Normotensive	1.2–1.7
Hypotensive	0.5
Sepsis (recovery)	1.0
Burn 20–40% BSA	
Before skin grafting	1.5–2.0
After skin grafting	1.0–1.3

Abbreviation: BSA = body surface area.
*Multiply the estimated basal energy expenditure (BEE) by the stress factor to yield an estimated resting energy expenditure (REE).

20% above normal. Whenever possible, it is desirable to measure resting energy expenditure by indirect calorimetry. If indirect calorimetry is unavailable, energy requirements should be satisfactorily met by estimating BEE by the Harris-Benedict formula with the use of premorbid body weight and addition of the appropriate stress factor (Table 3). Even more simply, caloric goals can be approximated by providing a nonprotein calorie load of approximately 30 kcal per kg per day.

Protein Requirements

Activation of the metabolic response to injury produces a rapid mobilization of body nitrogen, a process called "autocannibalism," with resultant large increases in urinary nitrogen excretion that are proportionate to the degree of metabolic stress. The requirement for protein is dependent on a variety of metabolic factors, such as the patient's premorbid nutritional status, the amount of nonprotein energy provided, the degree of hypercatabolism, renal function, liver function, and the amount of excessive nitrogen losses in urine, stool, and drainage.

The protein requirement for nitrogen equilibrium in stable adults is 0.8 gram per kg per day. Nitrogen retention increases with increases in either protein or total energy intake. The higher the nitrogen intake, the less dependent is the balance on energy intake. Exogenously administered nitrogen is not very effective in reducing the rate of catabolism. It can, however, increase the rate of protein synthesis and therefore reduce net protein loss. The administration of substantial amounts of amino acid nitrogen must be tempered by the status of hepatic and renal function, which may reduce tolerance to nitrogen loads. Table 4 outlines guidelines for protein administration under a variety of clinical conditions.

TABLE 2. **KCALS and FACE MTV: Essentials of Nutritional Support**

K:	Keep the patient nourished
C:	Calculate the energy and protein goals
A:	Access
L:	List (or think about) the components of the formula and choose amounts best suited for the patient as follows:
F:	Fluids: Should fluids be restricted?
A:	Amino acids/protein: Are special formulas indicated?
C:	Calories: What are the goals and what is the most appropriate mix of carbohydrate and fat calories?
E:	Electrolytes: Are there special electrolyte considerations?
M:	Miscellaneous: Should heparin, insulin, etc., be added?
T:	Trace elements: Are the standard amounts adequate?
V:	Vitamins: Are standard amounts adequate?
S:	Special monitoring to ensure safe and effective nutritional support

TABLE 4. **Guidelines for Protein Administration**

Condition	Protein (gm/kg/day)*
Renal failure, not on dialysis	0.8
Renal failure, on dialysis	1.0
Renal failure, on peritoneal dialysis	1.2
Malnourished, not metabolically stressed	1.0–1.2
Postoperative, no organ failure	1.2–1.5
Severely catabolic, no renal or organ failure	1.5–2.0

*Based on current dry weight unless patient is >140% of desirable weight, in which case use the mean of actual and desirable weights.

Energy Source: Glucose Versus Fat

In general, glucose and lipids are interchangeable as a source for nonprotein calories. Although the cellular uptake of glucose is increased with increasing infusion rates, glucose oxidation plateaus at a maximal infusion rate of 5 to 7 mg per kg per minute (400 to 500 grams per day for a 70-kg patient) in stressed patients. Higher infusion rates stimulate lipogenesis and not glucose oxidation. In addition, fat oxidation persists in trauma patients despite adequate glucose infusion, and in septic patients, a metabolic preference for fat may exist. These factors therefore emphasize the provision of a mixed substrate (glucose and fat) fuel source for critically ill patients.

Fat emulsions are cleared by either lipoprotein lipase activity or the macrophage. If enzyme clearance is reduced, macrophage clearance seems to compensate. Excessive doses of lipid emulsions (>2 to 3 grams per kg per day) have been associated with impaired reticuloendothelial function and interference with polymorphonucleocyte and monocyte migration, chemotaxis, and antigen-induced blastogenesis.

If triglyceride clearance is adequate, lipid emulsions are generally a safe and effective caloric and essential fatty acid source. It is generally recommended to provide 25 to 30% of nonprotein calories as fat (≤1.0 gram per kg per day), to administer the emulsion continuously over a 24-hour period, and to maintain a triglyceride level of less than 350 mg per dL.

Electrolyte and Vitamin Supplementation

It is difficult to define standard electrolyte requirements for hospitalized patients requiring nutritional support. Factors such as perioperative fluid shifts and drainage from nasogastric tubes, biliary drains, fistulas, and wounds mandate close monitoring of fluid and electrolyte changes and tailoring each patient's requirements accordingly.

Although standard electrolyte mixtures are suitable for most patients receiving parenteral nutrition, it is not uncommon for patients to require a specialized electrolyte prescription. Special consideration of individual electrolytes are as follows:

Sodium. Most TPN patients do well after receiving 30 to 50 mEq of sodium per liter of TPN solution. Ongoing fluid losses from ileostomies, gastric drainage, diarrhea, fistulas, or urine necessitate additional supplementation and careful monitoring. Hepatic, renal, and cardiac failure may be indications for sodium restriction.

Potassium. Supplementation of potassium to patients receiving nutritional support is based, in part, on the amount of carbohydrate calories delivered. Typically, 30 to 40 mEq of potassium are required for every 800 kcals. The coupled glucose/potassium transport system shifts potassium rapidly into cells. A significant fall in serum potassium concentration may result if TPN solutions contain an insufficient amount of this cation.

Chloride/Acetate. As with sodium, 30 to 50 mEq of chloride per TPN liter is sufficient under most circumstances. Amino acid mixtures are typically buffered with significant quantities of acetate to prevent acidosis that results from arginine and lysine metabolism. Acetate, in addition to that present in amino acid solutions, is commonly added. Careful electrolyte monitoring is especially indicated in patients at risk for metabolic alkalosis as a result of drainage losses, because supplemental acetate in the TPN exacerbates this alkalosis.

Phosphorus. As with potassium supplementation, phosphorus dosing is related to the amount of glucose administered. In general, 15 mmol of phosphorus should be added per 800 glucose calories. Insufficient phosphorus supplementation produces hypophosphatemia, usually between 2 to 4 days after TPN is started. Severe hypophosphatemia (<1.0 mg per dL) should be corrected *before* TPN begins.

Calcium and Magnesium. Although the quantity of calcium necessary for adult patients receiving nutritional support is not established, 5 to 10 mEq per liter is typically given. Similarly magnesium intake is also on the order of 5 to 10 mEq per liter of TPN. Renal wasting of magnesium as a result of diuretics, cisplatin, or amphotericin usage frequently produces hypomagnesemia, which necessitates supplementation.

Trace Elements. It is difficult to assess trace element status clinically, and serum levels are not correlated with other measures of deficiency. The typical prescription of trace elements includes zinc, 5.0 mg; copper, 1.0 mg; manganese, 500 μg; chromium, 10 μg; and selenium, 60 μg. Zinc is the only trace element for which extra supplementation is likely to be needed. Zinc

TABLE 5. **Metabolic Complications of Parenteral Nutrition**

Glucose
Hyperglycemia
Hypoglycemia

Amino Acids
Hyperchloremic metabolic acidosis
Azotemia
Hyperammonemia

Fats
Hypertriglyceridemia
Essential fatty acid deficiency
Impaired immune function*

Electrolytes
Hypo-, hypernatremia
Hypo-, hyperkalemia
Hypo-, hypercalcemia
Hypo-, hyperphosphatemia
Hypo-, hypermagnesemia

Miscellaneous
Anemia
Bleeding
Liver-associated enzyme elevations

*Possible complication, not verified.

losses in upper gastrointestinal tract fluid reach 17 mg per liter. Therefore, supplementation of additional zinc, up to 25 mg per day, is indicated in patients with large intestinal fluid losses.

Specific vitamin requirements for critically ill patients have not been determined, and the current dosage of intravenous vitamins is based on diverse information. Current recommendations for therapeutic doses of vitamins stipulate that they not exceed 10 times the recommended daily allowance (RDA). These guidelines may still be somewhat liberal for fat-soluble vitamins, which are stored in body fat and thus may become toxic at high levels of intake.

METABOLIC MONITORING AND COMPLICATIONS

Periodic nutritional assessment is required in order to evaluate the adequacy of the nutritional support. Unfortunately, there is no optimal way of evaluating the adequacy of a patient's nutritional support. Body weight changes over ensuing weeks are useful. However, in the day-to-day management of hospitalized patients, short-term changes in body weight reflect more the variations in fluid status than the direct result of nutritional intervention. Changes in the plasma concentrations of proteins with short half-lives such as transferrin, retinol-binding protein, and transthyretin (prealbumin) are commonly used to test the adequacy of nutritional intervention.

None of these is truly a sensitive or specific indicator of nutritional repletion, inasmuch as each is subject to nonnutritional influences on synthesis and degradation.

Nitrogen balance is considered the most consistent and practical method for estimating the adequacy of nutritional support. A nitrogen balance assessment compares the amount of nitrogen a patient receives (generally 1 gram of nitrogen for every 6.25 grams of protein) with the amount of nitrogen lost (urine, stool, integument, drainage).

A wide variety of metabolic complications may occur during parenteral feeding. These can be minimized by frequent monitoring and appropriate adjustment of nutrients in the infusion. Table 5 summarizes many of the potential metabolic complications that may arise during the administration of TPN.

SPECIAL PROBLEMS AND REQUIREMENTS

High Branched-Chain Amino Acid (BCAA) Solutions

The hormonal response to stress (trauma, burn, sepsis) promotes early, increased proteolysis and hydrolysis of BCAA (leucine, isolucine, valine) in skeletal muscle. This process leads to irreversible combustion of BCAA, which the skeletal muscle oxidizes for energy, making available other amino acids (alanine and glutamine) for gluconeogenesis, enzyme synthesis, wound healing, and immune function. Exogenous administration of BCAA as part of TPN or special enteral diets have been proposed to compensate for the altered protein metabolism and blood amino acid levels in stressed patients with a resultant reduction in skeletal muscle catabolism and an increase in protein synthesis. Solutions containing 40 to 50% of the branched-chain amino acids are now available.

In numerous clinical studies, investigators have examined the effect of BCAA administration to critically ill patients. The results are controversial. Well-done randomized, prospective, and controlled studies have demonstrated that BCAA-enriched formulas improve nitrogen retention, visceral protein status, and glucose homeostasis in moderate to severely stressed patients. There has been no significant demonstrable improvement in morbidity, length of hospital stay, or mortality. Therefore, the use of these products should be restricted to the highly catabolic patient, as documented by markedly negative nitrogen balance, increasing blood urea nitrogen, or intolerance to standard diets.

Acute Renal Failure

Patients with renal failure are unable to excrete the end products of nitrogen metabolism, primarily urea, from the body. Urea is generated from dietary amino acids or protein and from endogenous protein. Urea generation can be modulated in part by nutrient intake: decreasing dietary nitrogen intake decreases urea production, and the provision of calories limits the breakdown of endogenous protein and hence lowers urea generation. In general, the goal in the nutritional management of critically ill patients with renal failure is to optimize energy balance but avoid symptoms of uremia, volume overload, and metabolic complications.

The specialized amino acid formulas for renal failure contain essential amino acids as the nitrogen source. In theory, by supplying only essential amino acids, urea production is decreased by recycling nitrogen into the synthesis of non-essential amino acids. In clinical trials these products have not shown clinical superiority over products containing essential and non-essential amino acids. Although survival and improvement in renal function are not enhanced with the use of these products, dialysis requirements may be reduced. Because of the lack of demonstrable clinical efficacy, coupled with the high cost of these formulas, it is recommended that renal failure formulations be used only during the course of *acute* renal failure during attempts to avoid dialysis or to decrease dialysis requirements.

Hepatic Failure and Hepatic Encephalopathy

Protein intake must be altered in patients with advanced hepatic failure and impending encephalopathy. In general, amino acids given intravenously are better tolerated than the equivalent quantity of enteral protein. These patients have elevated blood levels of the aromatic amino acids and low levels of the BCAA. Possible therapeutic approaches in the nutritional management of these patients are to reduce the quantity of dietary amino acids to 20 to 40 grams per day or to administer special amino acid solutions designed to correct the altered concentrations of blood amino acids. The specialized formulas for hepatic encephalopathy contain high quantities of BCAA and low quantities of the aromatic amino acids and methionine. The prospective randomized studies evaluating the efficacy of intravenous hepatic formulations in patients with hepatic encephalopathy suggest that these diets have a beneficial effect on the resolution of encephalopathy and nutritional status and perhaps even an improvement in survival. It is recommended that these preparations be restricted to those patients who exhibit hepatic encephalopathy and not be used in those with non-encephalopathic manifestations of liver disease.

Pulmonary Insufficiency

Nutrition is an important consideration for critically ill patients with respiratory insufficiency, because the maintenance of nutritional status is associated with enhanced ability to wean patients from ventilatory support. High-carbohydrate diets, either parenteral or enteral, and overfeeding have been shown to increase carbon dioxide production, oxygen consumption, and ventilatory requirements. Glucose infusion rates greater than the maximal oxidation rate of glucose, 5 to 7 mg per kg per minute, result in net glycogen and fat synthesis and rather dramatic increases in carbon dioxide production and respiratory quotient (RQ). In patients with compromised pulmonary function, these sequelae can precipitate respiratory failure or complicate weaning from mechanical ventilation. The complete oxidation of fat produces less carbon dioxide than either glucose or protein on a per calorie basis. Replacing carbohydrate calories with fat calories in enteral or parenteral feeding has resulted in reductions in carbon dioxide production, oxygen consumption, and minute ventilation.

The approach to patients with pulmonary compromise should be on an individual basis. Initially, reassess energy requirements to avoid feeding excessive calories by providing maintenance levels or even reducing calories to provide only 80 to 90% of maintenance. Glucose/carbohydrate dosing should be adjusted to 4 to 5 grams per kg per day to avoid carbohydrate-driven increases in RQ. For patients receiving TPN, providing 60 to 70% of energy requirements as carbohydrate and 30 to 40% as lipid suffices in most instances. In practice, the increment in carbon dioxide production from an RQ of 0.7 (all fat) to RQ of 1.0 (all carbohydrate) is only 25% and not likely to be of major consequence in the patient to be weaned. More important, it is during *overfeeding* when the RQ exceeds 1.0 (net lipogenesis) that substantial increases in carbon dioxide production become clinically important.

PARENTERAL FLUID THERAPY FOR INFANTS AND CHILDREN

method of
HOWARD TRACHTMAN, M.D.
Schneider Children's Hospital
New Hyde Park, New York

Parenteral fluid therapy in pediatric patients is indicated in two distinct clinical situations: (1) unusual circumstances, such as during the postoperative period, when an otherwise healthy child is temporarily unable to ingest a sufficient amount of water and electrolytes to maintain the size and composition of the extracellular fluid (ECF) compartment, or (2) conditions in which an infant or child becomes ill and sustains a clinically significant perturbation in the volume or biochemical composition of the extracellular water. Appropriate parenteral solutions are used to enable rapid and safe correction of these abnormalities in a manner that can be continuously monitored.

PHYSIOLOGY OF BODY FLUID HOMEOSTASIS

Water constitutes approximately 60% of the body weight. This proportion is higher in premature and full-term infants, in whom water accounts for nearly 80% of body weight. Body water content is slightly lower in adolescent girls because of increased body fat. The body water is distributed between the intra- and extracellular compartments in a 2:1 ratio. One-quarter of the ECF compartment, or one-twelfth of the total body water, is in the intravascular space, and the remaining portion constitutes the interstitial compartment.

Biologic membranes are freely permeable to water. Therefore, all of the water compartments share the same osmolality, approximately 280 mOsm per kg of water. The major cation in the ECF is sodium, whereas chloride and bicarbonate make up the bulk of the anions. In the intracellular fluid (ICF) space, potassium is the primary cation, and phosphate and protein are the predominant anions.

In the absence of direct measurements, the plasma osmolality can be calculated from the following formula:

$$P_{Osm} = 2[Na^+] + [glucose(mg/dL)]/18 \\ + [BUN(mg/dL)]/3, \qquad (1)$$

where BUN is blood urea nitrogen.

When a child who requires parenteral fluid therapy is evaluated, it is critical to recognize that there are two completely independent pathophysiologic components to the problem. They must be addressed separately and then integrated into a unified treatment regimen.

The first question that must be asked is whether there is a disturbance in the size of the "effective" ECF volume. This is the term applied to the circulating intravascular portion of the total body water that is perfusing vital organs such as the brain, heart, and kidneys. Regulation of the ECF compartment size is achieved through an integrated array of volume receptors that are present in the low- and high-pressure portions of the cardiovascular system. Efferent output to the kidney, mediated by the sympathetic nervous system and a number of circulating hormones, including plasma renin, aldosterone, and atrial natriuretic peptide, modulate renal sodium and water handling to maintain a stable, effective ECF volume.

The primary determinant of the ECF compartment size is total body sodium balance. Under normal circumstances, urinary sodium output matches dietary sodium intake, and there is no change in ECF volume. Because sodium is confined to the ECF space by a range of membrane transport processes, a negative sodium balance (i.e., sodium output exceeds input) results in ECF contraction. This state is clinically categorized as dehydration or, under severe conditions, hypovolemic shock. The accepted term, "dehydration," is a misnomer because it places inappropriate emphasis on water in the pathogenesis of this condition. A more accurate word would be "denatration" to highlight the importance of the disturbance in sodium balance in the pathogenesis of disturbances of the circulating plasma volume. Positive sodium balance yields ECF expansion, a condition that is clinically manifested by hypertension, congestive heart failure, peripheral edema, or pulmonary vascular congestion.

There is no simple laboratory test that can be relied upon to gauge the ECF volume size. Instead, this is a clinical determination that is made by evaluating symptoms and physical signs such as thirst, weight loss, decreased urine output, altered mental status, tachycardia, poor skin color, reduced turgor, dry mucous membranes, and urine-specific gravity. On occasion, invasive maneuvers, such as the insertion of a central venous catheter to measure right atrial pressure, are required in order to enhance the accuracy of the physical examination. There is no scoring system that facilitates estimation of the extent of dehydration, and this remains a skill that is gained through experience and constant exposure to ill children.

The second question that must be asked before parenteral therapy is initiated is whether there is a concomitant osmal disorder. Regulation of plasma osmolality is achieved by modulation of the vasopressin-responsive urinary concentrating mechanism and stimulation of thirst and water intake. These adaptations are controlled through osmoresponsive neurons in the hypothalamus. Under extreme conditions, maintenance of ECF volume takes precedence over stabilization of plasma osmolality.

A derangement in the plasma osmolality indicates that the normal 2:1 ratio for the distribution of the body water between the intra- and extracellular compartments is disturbed. Hyperosmolal states cause water to move down its concentration gradient from the cell to the ECF space and result in relative or absolute contraction of the intracellular water compartment. Conversely, during hypo-osmolal states, water moves from the intravascular compartment into the cell, leading to relative or absolute expansion of the intracellular space. To determine whether there is an abnormality in plasma osmolality, the physician must measure this value directly. In contrast to volume disturbances that mandate a clinical diagnosis, osmal disorders require laboratory confirmation.

There is no a priori link between volume and osmolar disturbances. Children can have hyponatremia with nearly normal ECF volume (e.g., syndrome of inappropriate antidiuretic hormone [SIADH]), hypovolemia (e.g., diarrheal dehydration, adrenal insufficiency, osmotic diuresis) or volume expansion (e.g., acute renal failure, cirrhosis, congestive heart failure). Full understanding of the independent nature of volume and osmolar disturbances is vital in order to devise rational therapeutic regimens for fluid and electrolyte disorders in infants and children.

The treatment of conditions associated with ECF volume expansion such as acute renal failure or congestive heart failure requires primary attention to the underlying disorder. Parenteral fluid management is an important but secondary component in the care of these patients.

TREATMENT

Maintenance Fluid and Electrolyte Therapy

Whenever an infant or child is unable to ingest fluids orally for more than 8 to 12 hours, the physician is forced to administer intravenous solutions to maintain body fluid homeostasis. This situation may arise in a child who must fast preoperatively, in a child who is recovering from a surgical procedure, or in a patient with an alteration in mental status that interferes with normal drinking and swallowing behavior.

The daily requirement for maintenance water intake is necessitated by two routes of ongoing water loss. First, there are insensible losses of free water through evaporative losses through the skin and respiratory tract. In addition, there is an obligatory urine output that is mandated by the daily solute load. The minimal urinary osmolality determines the lower limit of renal water excretion. Factors such as burns, neuroectodermal diseases, and fever increase the daily water requirement by enhancing dermal losses of water. For example, it is estimated that each elevation in temperature above 38° C increases insensible water loss by 12.5%. Tachypnea that might occur during an episode of pneumonia or diabetic ketoacidosis increases the daily water requirement by promoting evaporative losses of water across the respiratory epithelium. The need for maintenance parenteral fluids arises earlier in smaller infants, who are more prone to ECF volume contraction because of a larger ratio of surface area to body volume.

Three methods are commonly used to calculate the maintenance fluid requirement. The first is based on the recognition that water intake is directly related to caloric expenditure and that this value declines with increasing body size. Therefore, the daily fluid need can be calculated, on the basis of body weight (BW), as the sum of three components:

$$
\begin{aligned}
&100 \text{ mL per kg BW for kg 1 to 10} \\
+\ &50 \text{ mL per kg BW for kg 11 to 20} \\
+\ &20 \text{ mL per kg BW for kg} > 20
\end{aligned} \qquad (2)
$$

In the second method, daily fluid requirement is expressed on the basis of body surface area and found to be equal to 1500 mL/M². Many practitioners use this method because there is concern that the first method, which is based on caloric utilization, overestimates fluid requirements in older larger children.

The third method is to break this quantity down into its constituent parts. Thus

$$
\begin{aligned}
&\text{Daily fluid requirement} \\
&= \text{insensible losses} + \text{urine output} \\
&= 400 \text{ mL/M}^2 + \text{urine output}
\end{aligned} \qquad (3)
$$

Although this technique is the most cumbersome to use in clinical practice, it is the most accurate. Moreover, it is the preferred method in a child with acute renal failure, in which case it is unwise to make assumptions about the level of kidney function. Adjustments in this quantity can be made by accounting for the effects of body temperature or respiratory rate on the insensible fluid requirement.

The average daily sodium and potassium requirements in pediatric patients are 3 and 2 mmol per kg per day, respectively. These quantities of electrolytes should be sufficient to prevent any significant fluctuations in ECF volume or serum electrolyte concentrations. However, it is important to recognize that in low-birth-weight infants, daily sodium requirements may be considerably larger (i.e., 4 to 8 mmol per kg per day), because of immaturity of the renal tubular sodium reabsorptive mechanisms. These infants do not gain weight normally, and hyponatremia, hyperreninemia, and hyperaldosteronism develop until the infants are provided sufficient quantities of salt. During short-term parenteral therapy, there is no need to provide an exogenous source of base, because the intrinsic acid-base regulatory systems are adequate for maintenance of the serum bicarbonate level within the physiologic range. Therefore, under most clinical circumstances, the accompanying anion in parenteral solutions is chloride.

Deficit Fluid and Electrolyte Therapy

General Principles

There are three steps in the clinical evaluation of children with dehydration. The first is a complete assessment of the ECF volume status in children that is based on comprehensive attention to a range of symptoms and signs. The most accurate estimate of ECF volume deficit is based on acute alterations in body weight measured on the same scale, because sudden changes in body weight are mainly the consequence of water loss. However, this situation is rarely encountered in practice. Therefore, evaluation of a child's behavior and appearance on physical examination, vital signs, and urinalysis is mandatory. Skin turgor, or the time it takes for capillary refilling after manual blanching of the skin or nail bed, is an especially useful sign for assessing the adequacy of the ECF volume. No scoring system that is comparable with the Glasgow coma scale for the evaluation of altered mental status has been devised to facilitate rapid appraisal of the extent of dehydration; in fact, because of their subjective nature and interobserver variability, physical signs may be less reliable than laboratory determinations such as BUN and serum bicarbonate concentration.

In the past, dehydration in children was scored as mild, moderate, or severe if the estimated loss of weight was less than 5%, 5 to 10%, or more than 10%, respectively. Clinical evidence of shock is supposedly correlated with a more than 15% loss of body weight. However, recent data indicate that these values overestimate the true extent of dehydration in children. Therefore, beyond the neonatal period, it may be more accurate to assign values of less than 3%, 3 to 6%, and more than 6% to mild, moderate, and severe dehydration in children. Greater precision in defining the extent of dehydration is needed in children with significant renal functional impairment or pulmonary or cardiac disease because they may not tolerate excessive fluid administration or they may experience clinical deterioration of the underlying disease.

In any child in whom there is uncertainty about the adequacy of the ECF volume size and perfusion of vital organs, urgent fluid resuscitation is mandatory in order to reverse these abnormalities. Except in select circumstances, such as patients with hemorrhagic shock after trauma, in whom blood is the optimal parenteral fluid, isotonic crystalloids are the preferred solution. They should be administered rapidly through a large-bore intravenous catheter to restore blood pressure. The dose is 20 mL per kg of body weight, and this fluid volume should be repeated until the earliest signs of clinical improvement in the child, such as increased alertness, better skin color, and increased urine output.

If the child has cardiac or pulmonary disease that may confound the clinical assessment of ECF volume, it may be necessary to insert a central venous or Swan-Ganz catheter to more accurately assess the response to ECF volume repletion. If there is a suspicion that the patient has acute or chronic renal failure, it is advisable to be more cautious in the administration of isotonic boluses of crystalloid solutions until the serum biochemical analyses are completed. Thus a full 20–mL per kg dose should be provided initially; however, it should not be repeated as quickly or as often until the level of kidney function is clarified. The author's practice is to disregard the volume of parenteral fluid given as emergency boluses in the calculation of the final therapeutic fluid regimen. However, in a child with normal renal function, this is simply a matter of style that can be left to the discretion of each practitioner.

After a careful examination of the child, the second step is to ascertain the duration of the illness that caused the child to come to medical attention. Acute disease is illness lasting less than 48 hours and chronic disease is one lasting more than 48 hours. This distinction is important in devising a therapeutic rehydration regimen because it indicates how to partition the isotonic fluid losses between the two body water compartments.

The third step in the initial evaluation of a child with dehydration is to determine whether there is a concomitant osmolal disturbance. ECF volume contraction can occur in the presence of a reduced, normal, or elevated plasma osmolality. As stated earlier, this requires laboratory measurement of the serum osmolality. Both hyperosmolality and hypo-osmolality of the circulating plasma volume are associated with disturbances in mental status and can cause profound neurologic symptoms such as seizures and loss of consciousness. Although infants with hypernatremia have a doughy skin texture, are usually more irritable, and may have a high-pitched cry, it is difficult to discriminate osmolal disturbances on the basis of clinical findings.

Specific Scenarios

Isotonic Dehydration. In order to formulate a therapeutic fluid regimen, the daily maintenance water and electrolyte requirements are calculated first. The quantity of fluid must be administered parenterally each day during the rehydration period, when the child is unable to drink normally. The water deficit is then determined by multiplying the estimated percentage dehydration by the admission weight. This weight is an underestimate of the child's true weight; however, calculations based on the premorbid weight do not materially influence the volume or composition of the parenteral fluid regimen. This volume of water represents the isotonic component of the fluid loss that has resulted in contraction of the ECF and ICF spaces. This loss causes the clinical symptoms that prompt the parents to seek medical attention for their children.

In dehydration illness, both the extracellular and intracellular water are affected. However, the relative contribution of these compartments to the total fluid losses depends on the duration of the antecedent illness. It is presumed that in acute dehydration, 80% of the fluid losses are derived from the ECF and 20% from the ICF compartment. In contrast, if the dehydration evolves over a more prolonged period of time, the water loss is more evenly allocated between the two compartments: namely, 60% for ECF and 40% for ICF.

Once the total isotonic loss has been calculated, the electrolyte composition can be determined. It is assumed that the ECF portion has a sodium concentration equal to 140 mmol per liter and contains negligible amounts of potassium. In contrast, the intracellular water is assumed to have a potassium concentration equal to 140 mmol per liter and to be devoid of sodium. By using these values, the electrolyte composition of the ECF and ICF components of fluid loss can be determined. In the absence of an osmolal disturbance, there is no other component to the fluid deficit.

To illustrate these calculations, if a 10-kg child has acute dehydration estimated to be 5% of body weight, the total isotonic fluid loss is 500 mL (Table 1). Because the process is acute, 80% of this loss, or 400 mL, is derived from the ECF and 20%, or 100 mL, is derived from the ICF. The ECF component contains 56 mmol of sodium (0.4 liter × 140 mmol per liter), whereas the ICF portion contains 14 mmol of potassium (0.1 liter × 140 mmol per liter). These fluid and electrolyte quantities are added to the maintenance requirements to yield a repletion solution. The exact electrolyte composition of the solution is determined by normalizing the contents to 1 liter and selecting the closest available solution that is commercially available. Except in low-birth-weight infants, it is rarely necessary to custom formulate a parenteral fluid by adding precise quantities of sodium, potassium, and chloride to a dextrose solution.

The rate of fluid administration in children with isotonic dehydration is determined by adding the maintenance and deficit fluid volumes and dividing by 24 to obtain an hourly infusion rate. It has been customary to provide enough fluid to make up half of the deficit during the first 8 hours of the therapy and the remainder of the deficit over the subsequent 16 hours. However, if emergency bolus therapy has restored organ perfusion and stabilized the child's vital signs, there is no reason to correct the deficit over a period less than 24 hours.

Hypotonic Dehydration. If a child has hypotonic dehydration (Table 2) as a result of a reduction in the serum sodium concentration, the fluid and electrolyte losses can be divided into two portions: an isotonic component that accounts for the symptomatic contraction of the ECF volume, and an additional net sodium loss. The isotonic fluid volume and electrolyte composition are calculated according to the methods outlined in the previous section. The sodium deficiency is determined according to the following formula:

$$\text{Sodium deficit (in mmol)} = 0.6 \times \text{body weight} \times (135 - P_{Na}) \quad (4)$$

Even though sodium is confined to the ECF compartment, the deficit is determined on the basis of the total body weight (0.6 × body weight) because water freely permeates the membranes between all body compartments.

The composition and volume of the parenteral fluid solution needed to treat children with hypotonic dehydration is determined by adding the maintenance and deficit-repletion fluids and the net sodium loss. In general, the repletion fluid contains approximately 100 mmol per liter of sodium chloride, and a 5% dextrose solution containing two-thirds normal saline is suitable in these circumstances.

There has been recent controversy about the optimal rate of correction of hyponatremic dehydration. If a child with hyponatremia has acute neurologic symptoms, a volume of 3% saline must be infused to rapidly raise the serum sodium concentration by 3 to 5 mmol per liter. This increment is sufficient to reduce cerebral edema and

TABLE 1. **Isotonic Dehydration***

Level	Water (mL)	Sodium (mmol)	Potassium (mmol)
Daily maintenance	1000	30	20
Extracellular fluid (80%)	—	56†	0
Deficit	500‡	—	—
Intracellular fluid (20%)	—	0	14§
Total	1500	86	34

*10-kg child, acute illness, estimated 5% dehydration, serum sodium concentration = 138 mmol/L. Each liter of the replacement solution should contain 57 mmol of sodium chloride (86 ÷ 1.5) and 23 mmol of potassium chloride (34 ÷ 1.5). Therefore, use 5% dextrose containing 1/3 normal saline and 20 mmol/L potassium chloride, and infuse the solution at a rate of 63 mL/h (1500 ÷ 24).

†0.4 L × 140 mmol/L.
‡10 kg × 5%.
§0.1 L × 140 mmol/L.

TABLE 2. **Hypotonic Dehydration***

Level	Water (mL)	Sodium (mmol)	Potassium (mmol)
Daily maintenance	1000	30	20
Extracellular fluid (80%)	—	56†	0
Deficit	500‡	—	—
Intracellular fluid (20%)	—	0	14§
Sodium deficit	—	138‖	—
Total	2500	254	54

*10-kg child, acute illness, estimated 5% dehydration, serum sodium concentration = 112 mmol/L. The total solution contains two times the maintenance requirements because the total deficit is to be corrected over 48 h. Each liter of the replacement solution should contain 100 mmol of sodium chloride (254 ÷ 2.5) and 23 mmol of potassium chloride (54 ÷ 2.5). Therefore, use 5% dextrose containing 2/3 normal saline and 20 mmol/L potassium chloride, and infuse the solution at a rate of 52 mL/h (2500 ÷ 48).

†0.4 L × 140 mmol/L.

‡10 kg × 5%.

§0.1 L × 140 mmol/L.

‖0.6 × 10 kg × (135 − 112).

minimize disturbances in central nervous system function. However, after this critical phase is controlled, it is advisable to correct the fluid and electrolyte deficits slowly over at least 48 hours. During prolonged hyponatremia, there is a reduction in cerebral osmolality as a result of the extrusion of electrolytes and organic osmolytes to minimize brain swelling. Overly rapid correction of hypo-osmolal states causes sudden reversal of the plasma-to-brain osmolality before cerebral cells can reaccumulate these solutes. Guidelines for optimal therapy of chronic hyponatremic dehydration are that the serum sodium concentration not increase by more than 25 mmol per 48 hours and that the serum sodium concentration not exceed 135 mmol per hour after 48 hours. These recommendations are designed to prevent the development of central pontine myelinolysis during the treatment of hypo-osmolal states.

Hypertonic Dehydration. If a child has hypertonic dehydration (Table 3) resulting, for example, from an elevated serum sodium or glucose concentration, the fluid deficit can be divided into an isotonic component that results in symptomatic contraction of the ECF space and a net free water loss. It is assumed that all hyperosmolar dehydration states develop on a chronic basis because the ECF is maintained for a more prolonged period at the expense of the ICF space. The isotonic losses are calculated according to the methods outlined in the section on isotonic dehydration. The free water loss is calculated according to the following formula:

$$\text{Free water loss (in liters)} = 0.6 \times \text{body weight} \times (P_{Na}/140 - 1) \quad (5)$$

The repletion solution is calculated by adding the maintenance, isotonic dehydration, and free water loss components. In general, the therapeutic solution contains 30 to 40 mmol per liter of sodium chloride and has a composition that approximates one-fifth to one-fourth normal saline.

The most important feature in the treatment of hyperosmolar dehydration is to correct the hyperosmolality slowly over a minimum of 48 hours. The hazards of rapid correction of hypernatremic dehydration were first highlighted by Laurence

TABLE 3. **Hypertonic Dehydration***

Level	Water (mL)	Sodium (mmol)	Potassium (mmol)
Daily maintenance	1000	30	20
Extracellular fluid (60%)	—	63†	0
Deficit	750‡	—	—
Intracellular fluid (40%)	—	0	42§
Water deficit	1300‖	—	—
Total	4050	123	82

*10-kg child, acute illness, estimated 7.5% dehydration, serum sodium concentration = 170 mmol/L. The total solution contains two times the maintenance requirements because the total deficit is to be corrected over 48 h. Each liter of the replacement solution should contain 30 mmol of sodium chloride (123 ÷ 4.05) and 20 mmol of potassium chloride (82 ÷ 4.05). Therefore, use 5% dextrose containing 1/5–1/4 normal saline and 20 mmol/L potassium chloride, and infuse the solution at a rate of 84 mL/h (4050 ÷ 48).

†0.45 L × 140 mmol/L.

‡10 kg × 7.5%.

§0.3 L × 140 mmol/L.

‖0.6 × 10 kg × (170/140 − 1).

Finberg in 1959. During hyperosmolal states, brain cells accumulate electrolytes and a number of compatible organic osmolytes to prevent cell shrinkage. The recommendation to correct hyperosmolal dehydration slowly is designed to prevent the occurrence of cerebral edema during the therapeutic phase before dissipation of the osmotically active solutes from brain cells.

At present, modifications in infant formula composition have resulted in a lowered sodium content. These changes were instituted to prevent the development of hypertension in the early childhood years. An unexpected consequence of this change has been a steady decline in the incidence of hypernatremic dehydration. However, the hyperglycemia that is observed in untreated diabetic ketoacidosis also results in a severe hyperosmolal state. The recommendation to correct hypernatremic dehydration slowly applies with equal strength to the treatment of severe hyperglycemia. Therefore, careful monitoring of the serum glucose concentration is mandatory, and provision of a parenteral solution containing 100 to 125 mmol per liter of sodium chloride may help prevent the development of hyponatremia and cerebral edema during the treatment of diabetic ketoacidosis.

Associated Problems. All states of ECF volume contraction can interfere with peripheral perfusion and cause a lactic acidosis. However, there may be adverse effects on intracellular acidification and intermediary metabolism associated with the routine use of parenteral sodium bicarbonate. Therefore, it is advisable that bicarbonate be withheld unless there is severe metabolic acidosis (i.e., pH < 7.10), unless there is evidence of myocardial dysfunction, or if systemic acidosis is interfering with the action of other therapeutic agents (e.g., bronchodilators in children with asthma).

In most cases of dehydration, maintenance plus deficit replenishment yield a solution containing 20 to 30 mmol per liter of potassium chloride. If there is an ongoing osmotic diuresis, larger amounts of potassium may be needed. The maximal amount of potassium that can be safely administered and assimilated by the body is 0.3 to 0.5 mmol per kg per hour. In any child with suspected or proven renal failure, provision of potassium-free parenteral solutions is mandatory. Unfortunately, urine output alone may not be an adequate guide to the level of renal function, and it is important to measure the serum creatinine and BUN levels in these situations.

In children with hypernatremic dehydration, the hyperosmolality interferes with insulin and parathormone release, resulting in hyperglycemia and hypocalcemia, respectively. Each of these derangements necessitates special attention during the treatment of hypernatremic dehydration. In children with diabetic ketoacidosis, the serum sodium concentration is lowered by 1.6 mmol per liter for each 100-mg per dL increment above normal in the serum glucose concentration. Provision of a solution containing 100 to 125 mmol per liter of sodium chloride should be adequate to prevent the development of symptomatic hyponatremia during the treatment of diabetic ketoacidosis.

Finally, initiation of parenteral fluid does not cure the underlying disease. Ongoing losses during the fluid and electrolyte repletion period must always be accounted for.

The Endocrine System

ACROMEGALY

method of
MARY LEE VANCE, M.D.
University of Virginia Health Sciences Center
Charlottesville, Virginia

DIAGNOSIS

Acromegaly, excessive growth hormone (GH) secretion by the anterior pituitary, is caused by a pituitary adenoma in more than 99% of cases. Rare causes include ectopic GH-releasing hormone secretion (bronchial carcinoid, pancreatic tumor) stimulating pituitary GH secretion and one reported case of ectopic GH production by a pancreatic tumor. Because of the insidious nature of clinical symptoms and signs, diagnosis may be delayed for 10 to 20 years. Thus, the majority of patients (>80%) at diagnosis have a macroadenoma (>10 mm), frequently with cavernous sinus or dural invasion. The best screening test is measurement of serum insulin-like growth factor-1 (IGF-1), also known as somatomedin C. IGF-1, produced by the liver and other tissues in response to GH, reflects overall GH secretion. IGF-1 production is increased during puberty and pregnancy and is dependent on adequate nutrition. A single GH measurement is misleading because of the pulsatile nature of GH secretion. The definitive test is measurement of GH after oral glucose administration (75 or 100 grams); the normal GH response is reduction to less than 2 μg per liter. Acromegalics have no change, partial reduction, or a paradoxical increase in GH. After biochemical diagnosis, pituitary imaging is required. The best study is a magnetic resonance imaging scan with gadolinium administration. If magnetic resonance imaging is unavailable, a high-resolution computed tomography study (coronal plane, contrast enhancement) is adequate. Additional pretreatment studies include measurement of thyroid hormone level (thyroxine), cortisol, prolactin, and gonadotropins (luteinizing hormone, follicle-stimulating hormone). If the patient has an abnormally low cortisol level, immediate replacement with either hydrocortisone (20 mg on awakening, 10 mg at 6 P.M.) or prednisone (5 mg on awakening, 2.5 mg at 6 P.M.) is necessary. Glucocorticoid replacement should be started before thyroid hormone replacement because thyroid hormone administration to a patient with adrenal insufficiency can precipitate an adrenal crisis. Gonadal steroid replacement (testosterone or estrogen) is not necessary before treatment of acromegaly but should be given if the patient is hypogonadal after treatment to prevent bone loss in men and women and for the cardioprotective effect of estrogen in women.

TREATMENT

The goals of treatment are to reduce GH secretion to normal, reverse headache and visual abnormalities, and preserve other pituitary function. GH hypersecretion is associated with premature mortality and significant morbidity from cardiomegaly, arthritis, sleep apnea, and increased risk of colon polyps and cancer.

Surgery

The preferred approach is the transsphenoidal route because this allows for tumor visualization, avoids the optic chiasm and optic nerves, permits potentially complete resection, and is associated with less morbidity than is the transcranial approach. As with any type of pituitary tumor, the surgical outcome is dependent on two factors: tumor size and the expertise of the neurosurgeon. The presence of a macroadenoma, with suprasellar extension or dural or cavernous sinus invasion, reduces the probability of a surgical cure. Surgery, however, may produce substantial reduction in tumor size and improvement in visual abnormalities, headache, and other symptoms. Approximately 4 to 6 weeks after surgery, IGF-1 measurement and an oral glucose test should be performed. It is prudent to wait to measure IGF-1 because it is protein bound and requires approximately 4 weeks to be cleared. Postoperative imaging should be carried out no earlier than 3 months after surgery because edema and postsurgical changes cannot be distinguished from residual tumor.

Radiation

Pituitary radiation as a primary therapy is ineffective to reduce either tumor size or GH secretion promptly. Reduction of GH to normal may require 10 to 20 years. Thus, radiotherapy is adjunctive therapy for postoperative residual disease and primary therapy for the few patients who cannot undergo surgery.

Medical Therapies

Oral dopamine agonists, bromocriptine (Parlodel), pergolide (Permax), cabergoline,* and lisuride,* decrease serum GH and symptoms of excessive GH. In only a small number, however, is GH or IGF-1 reduced to normal. The bromocriptine dose for treatment of acromegaly is usually 5 mg three or four times a day, which is a larger dose than is used for treatment of hyperprolactinemia. More recently, acromegaly has been treated with a somatostatin analog. Somatostatin is the specific hypothalamic hormone that inhibits GH release; although this hormone was discovered in the 1970s, the need for continuous intravenous administration precluded its use as a long-term treatment. An 8–amino acid analog, octreotide (Sandostatin), was later developed; this peptide is more suppressive of GH than is native somatostatin and has a biologic half-life of 6 to 8 hours after subcutaneous administration. Octreotide decreases GH and IGF-1 in more than 90% of patients, and suppression to normal occurs in 40 to 45%. Although octreotide is more selective in suppressing GH than other hormones, insulin release is decreased for approximately 3 hours after administration. Additionally, gallbladder contractility is decreased, with 18% of acromegalics developing gallstones or sludge. To minimize these potential adverse effects, it is prudent to administer the drug 3 hours after meals. The usual octreotide dose is 100 μg by subcutaneous injection every 6 or 8 hours; some patients have a better response to 300 μg per 24 hours administered continuously with a portable pump as is used for insulin delivery.

*Not available in the United States.

ADRENOCORTICAL INSUFFICIENCY

method of
JAMES C. MELBY, M.D.
Boston University School of Medicine
Boston, Massachusetts

Adrenocortical insufficiency is a life-threatening disorder caused by reduced production of cortisol. In primary adrenal insufficiency, the production of both cortisol and aldosterone is reduced, but in secondary adrenal insufficiency, aldosterone metabolism is not substantially altered, and aldosterone secretory response to sodium deprivation is maintained. It is important to distinguish between primary and secondary adrenocortical insufficiency because the therapy for these conditions is different in the chronic state.

TABLE 1. Chronic Primary Adrenocortical Insufficiency

Autoimmune atrophy	> 70%
Granulomatous disease	> 20%
Tuberculosis	
North American blastomycosis	
Histoplasmosis	
Sarcoidosis	
Acquired immune deficiency syndrome	> 5%
Amyloidosis, hemochromatosis	
Adrenoleukodystrophy	

PRIMARY ADRENOCORTICAL INSUFFICIENCY

Primary adrenocortical insufficiency results from a deficit of cortisol and aldosterone production by the adrenals owing to one or more destructive processes (Table 1). The majority of patients with primary adrenocortical insufficiency, or Addison's disease, have an autoimmune adrenalitis. Evidence for an autoimmune basis for adrenal atrophy is as noted in Table 2.

Approximately 5% of patients with acquired immune deficiency syndrome (AIDS) studied at the San Francisco General Hospital have clinical and biochemical findings of acute adrenal insufficiency. Fifty percent of all patients with AIDS exhibit hyporesponsiveness to either injected corticotropin-releasing hormone or adrenocorticotropic hormone (ACTH) in terms of cortisol secretory activity. Aldosterone production, however, remains normal in many patients with AIDS. Thus, hyperkalemia is not a prominent manifestation of adrenal insufficiency associated with AIDS. Because ACTH levels may be either elevated or subnormal in patients with AIDS, it has been suggested that AIDS encephalitis, basilar meningitis, or autoimmune hypophysitis might be responsible for the initial alterations in hypothalamic-pituitary-adrenocortical function. Patients with AIDS who present with circulatory failure require high-dose replacement therapy of cortisol and long-term replacement doses after acute prostrating illness subsides. Replacement doses do not enhance the

TABLE 2. Autoimmunity in Addison's Disease

Adrenal antibodies in >60%
Association with histocompatibility antigen—HLA B8 or DU3
Association with other autoimmune endocrinopathies
  Autoimmune polyglandular syndrome
    Type I
      Hypoadrenalism
      Hypoparathyroidism
      Mucocutaneous candidiasis
      Hypogonadism
      Chronic acute hepatitis
      Pernicious anemia
    Type II
      Addison's disease
      Hypothyroidism
      Hashimoto's disease
      Type I diabetes mellitus
      Vitiligo
  Schmidt's syndrome

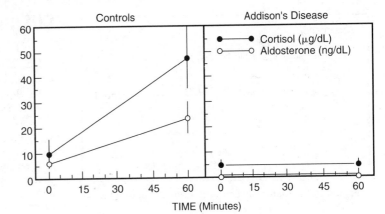

Figure 1. Cortrosyn test.

spread of opportunistic infections. This problem with AIDS could rapidly become one of the most common causes of acute adrenal insufficiency.

SECONDARY ADRENAL INSUFFICIENCY

Secondary adrenal insufficiency may be due to panhypopituitarism or corticotropin deficiency, following exogenous steroid therapy. It is estimated that 8 to 10 million patients are treated with corticosteroids each year. Suppression of the hypothalamic pituitary adrenal system is among the more prominent and potentially hazardous derangements produced by corticosteroids. Some degree of adrenocortical atrophy is apparent in nearly all animal species tested after 10 days of high-dose corticosteroid administration. This atrophy appears to be completely reversible. In a number of studies, feedback inhibition of ACTH and cortisol secretory activity is interfered with for a period of 12 months after a shorter period of 2 weeks of high-dose steroid therapy; stress responses in the pituitary and adrenal glands may be recovered much earlier.

The author has examined the adrenal response to pyrogen stress in relation to the duration and dosage of steroids as well as length of time after cessation of therapy. It was found that the daily doses of less than 20 mg of cortisol or equipotent doses of its synthetic analogues in combination with cessation of corticosteroid therapy for 5 months or more are associated with normal pyrogen stress responsiveness. Thus, acute adrenal insufficiency in these patients is not likely to develop. Similarly, patients receiving alternate-day steroid therapy have little or no attenuation of pyrogen stress response. Most patients receiving 50 mg of cortisol or equipotent doses of synthetic analogues have little response to pyrogen stress 1 month after cessation of steroid therapy regardless of whether therapy had been continued for 1 month or for 8 years. Any patient who has received daily corticosteroid therapy for up to 6 months before arriving in an intensive care unit or an emergency room should receive adrenocortical replacement therapy.

CLINICAL MANIFESTATIONS OF ADRENAL INSUFFICIENCY

Classic manifestations of Addison's disease include pigmentation of the skin, weakness, and postural hy-

potension. Hyperpigmentation results from overproduction of a pigmentary hormone of the anterior pituitary that is secreted in concert with ACTH. Postural hypotension is a result of volume contraction owing to aldosterone deficiency but, more importantly, owing to reduced cardiac output because cortisol is necessary for optimum contractility, and cortisol possesses a positive inotropic effect on the myocardium itself. Serum sodium level is reduced and serum potassium increased in more than 40% of patients with primary adrenocortical insufficiency. In patients who have secondary adrenocortical insufficiency, aldosterone deficiency is not observed, and therefore the serum potassium level is almost never elevated, even though hyponatremia may occur. It should be emphasized that patients with secondary adrenocortical insufficiency *do not* exhibit hyperpigmentation because beta-lipotropin secretion is not increased.

DIAGNOSIS

The laboratory diagnosis of primary adrenocortical insufficiency is as follows. As demonstrated in Table 3 and Figure 1, full evaluation of adrenal function requires measurements of cortisol and aldosterone levels before and after ACTH administration as well as a baseline ACTH value. A saline infusion should be started, and ACTH (250 μg) or cosyntropin (Cortrosyn), the synthetic form of ACTH, is given as an intravenous bolus with a second sample for cortisol and aldosterone obtained at 30, 60, and 120 minutes later. Patients with primary adrenocortical insufficiency exhibit no rise in plasma cortisol and no rise in plasma aldosterone.

The laboratory diagnosis of secondary adrenal insuf-

TABLE 3. **Laboratory Diagnosis of Adrenal Insufficiency**

Plasma cortisol <5 μg/dL (low)
Plasma ACTH >200 pg/mL (high)
Corticotropin stimulation (1–2 h) 250 μg cosyntropin intravenously No rise in plasma cortisol No rise in plasma aldosterone

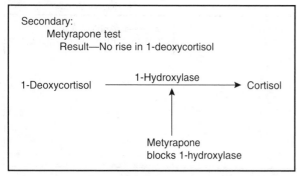

Figure 2. Laboratory diagnosis of secondary adrenal insufficiency.

ficiency rests on the demonstration that metyrapone fails to increase serum levels of 11-deoxycortisol. In patients suspected of having secondary adrenocortical insufficiency, a dose of 750 mg of metyrapone may be given every 4 to 6 hours for 1 day, and plasma levels for 11-deoxycortisol and cortisol are obtained. In general, the 11-deoxycortisol, because of inhibition of 11-hydroxylase, would normally rise more than 10 μg/dL. This test is demonstrated in Figure 2.

TREATMENT

The treatment of primary and secondary adrenocortical insufficiency is identical in the acutely ill. Cortisol as a phosphate or succinate ester is given in a 100-mg bolus intravenously and infused at a rate of 50 mg per hour in an intravenous solution of dextrose and saline. One should not use unobligated water or potassium-containing fluids. Restoration of blood pressure may be apparent within minutes and should be complete after 1 hour in the treatment of acute adrenal insufficiency. Because of the dramatic effects of steroid replacement in these patients, one should adhere to the dictum "when in doubt, treat." Withholding treatment of acute adrenal insufficiency until diagnostic tests have been undertaken is unwarranted when it is suspected because of the potentially lethal consequences of waiting to begin therapy.

Chronic adrenocortical insufficiency requires replacement of cortisol of between 10 and 30 mg daily depending on the patient's response. Perhaps the best single end point for replacement therapy is the presence or absence of postural hypotension. In patients with primary adrenocortical insufficiency, once the amount of glucocorticoid or cortisol has been reduced to 30 mg or less per day, it is necessary to administer between 50 and 100 μg of 9α-fluorocortisol daily to restore normal potassium and sodium metabolism. In patients with secondary adrenal insufficiency, it is not necessary to give mineralocorticoid replacement therapy.

CUSHING'S SYNDROME

method of
PETER J. TRAINER, M.B., and
G. MICHAEL BESSER, M.D., D.Sc.
St. Bartholomew's Hospital
West Smithfield, London, United Kingdom

Cushing's syndrome is the result of prolonged exposure to excessive free circulating glucocorticoids; the first patient was described in 1912, and a group of 12 patients were more fully described in 1932. This brilliant account included all the principal diagnostic features now recognized. The most common cause of Cushing's syndrome is the therapeutic use of glucocorticoids or adrenocorticotropic hormone (ACTH) for the treatment of inflammatory disorders, occasionally without the patient being aware of the glucocorticoids contained in an inhaler or cream. The diagnosis, differential diagnosis, and management of patients with endogenous Cushing's syndrome often constitute one of the most demanding problems of clinical endocrinology.

CLINICAL FEATURES

Excessive exposure to glucocorticoids affects virtually every system of the body. The most common presenting symptoms are weight gain, muscular weakness, lethargy, hirsutism, skin thinning, bruising, and purple striae. Oligomenorrhea and amenorrhea are common in women, with decreased libido and impotence occurring in men. Moderate or severe psychiatric symptoms occur in 65% of patients with Cushing's disease and in 100% of patients with the ectopic ACTH syndrome. Depression is the most frequent feature, whereas frank psychosis is not unusual. Symptoms relating to hypertension, diabetes mellitus, or infection are often encountered. In ACTH-dependent Cushing's syndrome, particularly the ectopic ACTH syndrome, skin pigmentation is common. Local pressure effects owing to a pituitary tumor, such as headaches and visual field loss, are occasionally present at diagnosis. All forms of Cushing's syndrome can be cyclical in activity, and therefore the severity of the signs and symptoms can vary.

A common clinical dilemma is differentiating simple obesity from Cushing's syndrome. A "buffalo" hump is common to both disorders, and pale striae are common in obesity. In the authors' experience, skin thinning, proximal myopathy (reflected by an inability to rise without use of the arms from a squatting position), and purple striae are the most useful features in differentiating obesity from Cushing's syndrome, although purple striae can occur in rapid weight gain of any cause. A short history suggests an adrenal tumor, usually malignant, or a fast-growing source of ectopic ACTH, with pigmentation supporting the latter diagnosis and virilization being in favor of an adrenal tumor.

ETIOLOGY

In the authors' series of 260 patients seen since 1969, pituitary-dependent disease (i.e., Cushing's disease) is four times more common in women than in men, with the most common age for presentation being between 20 and 40 years. More than 90% of cases of ACTH-secreting pituitary adenomas are less than 1 cm in size, i.e., smaller than the normal gland; they are usually basophilic on conventional staining, and on electron microscopy large numbers of neurosecretory granules are seen. These tumors can occasionally grow aggressively into bone and the cavernous sinuses.

Ectopic ACTH excretion has been described in many tumors, the most common being small cell and bronchial lung tumors, with neuroendocrine tumors of the thymus, gastrointestinal tract, and islet cells of the pancreas next in frequency. Rarely ectopic corticotropin-releasing hormone (CRH) secretion is responsible for Cushing's syndrome.

The original classic description of the ectopic ACTH syndrome was of wasting, hyperpigmentation, severe myopathy, hypokalemia, and diabetes mellitus. The vast majority of affected patients have an overt small cell lung tumor. It is now recognized, however, that there is a group of patients with typically slow-growing bronchial carcinoid tumors, all of which are frankly or potentially malignant, and in whom the clinical features are indistinguishable from patients with Cushing's disease. Although some are easily located, many tumors are only a few millimeters in size, and there may be many years between first presentation and identification of the tumor. This is now called the "occult ectopic ACTH syndrome." Both malignant and benign adrenal adenomas can secrete cortisol independent of ACTH and thereby cause Cushing's syndrome. It can be difficult to differentiate between adenomas and carcinomas on histologic grounds unless venous infiltration is present, but most carcinomas are greater than 6 cm in diameter and weigh more than 100 grams. Carcinomas of the adrenal usually secrete more than one class of steroid, typically androgens and occasionally estrogens as well as cortisol.

DIAGNOSIS

The biochemical diagnosis of Cushing's syndrome relies on the demonstration of excess cortisol secretion and desensitization of the normal feedback regulation of the hypothalamic-pituitary-adrenal axis. It is recommended to perform a 48-hour low-dose dexamethasone suppression test in all patients suspected of having Cushing's syndrome. This is performed on an outpatient basis and involves the patient having blood taken for the measurement of cortisol at 9:00 A.M. and thereafter taking 0.5 mg of dexamethasone at 9:00 A.M., 3:00 P.M., 9:00 P.M., and 3:00 A.M. for 48 hours with a second blood sample being taken at 9:00 A.M., i.e., 6 hours after the last dexamethasone tablet. Suppression of serum cortisol to undetectable levels, in the authors' assay, 50 mmol per liter (1.8 µg/100 mL), effectively excludes Cushing's syndrome, although each laboratory should establish its own criteria. The various overnight dexamethasone suppression tests described are unreliable in the diagnosis of Cushing's syndrome, with high false-positive and false-negative rates. They have no advantages over the 48-hour test: both require blood samples before and after dexameth-

asone, and properly instructed patients rarely have difficulty with the timing of medication. Any cause of Cushing's syndrome may show cyclicity in clinical features and steroid secretion, and this may result in inconsistency in results of tests, including false-negative dexamethasone suppression tests. Drugs that induce liver enzymes, such as rifampin, phenytoin, and phenobarbital, can all increase the rate of dexamethasone clearance, resulting in low plasma levels during a dexamethasone test. Failure to appreciate this can result in apparent but false resistance to dexamethasone suppression tests. The glucocorticoid resistance syndrome is another potential cause of lack of suppressibility (i.e., a false-positive result). These patients are typically female and present with hirsutism and menstrual irregularity in the absence of any stigmata of Cushing's syndrome. They have high basal cortisol levels with a circadian rhythm of ACTH and cortisol reset at a higher level and only partial suppression with dexamethasone. The diagnosis can be best confirmed by screening all members of the family because it has autosomal dominant inheritance. The most common reason for a false-positive dexamethasone suppression test is failure to take the tablets correctly.

Only rarely does the measurement of urinary free cortisol (UFC) excretion assist in the diagnosis because the diagnosis is usually clear following a 48-hour low-dose dexamethasone test. Incomplete urine collection can result in false-negative results, and there is no extra information to be gathered from measuring UFC at the same time as plasma cortisol during dexamethasone tests. Patients on drugs, such as metyrapone, that inhibit cortisol secretion have high circulating levels of cortisol precursors, such as 11-deoxycortisol, that cross react in UFC assays, giving spuriously high results.

The insulin tolerance test is occasionally useful in the investigation of suspected Cushing's syndrome, particularly in the differentiation of Cushing's syndrome from depression (see later). In suspected Cushing's syndrome, double the normal dose of insulin is required to induce hypoglycemia (blood glucose <2.2 mmol/L [40 mg/100 mL] plus symptoms): 0.3 units/kg.

CONDITIONS IMITATING CUSHING'S SYNDROME

Depression is both a common symptom of Cushing's syndrome and part of the differential diagnosis. Depression can cause loss of the circadian rhythm of ACTH and cortisol and elevated plasma cortisol levels in association with a failure to suppress in response to a low-dose dexamethasone test. Differentiation between the two conditions in an obese patient may be extremely difficult. Rarely the diagnosis of Cushing's syndrome can be excluded only after depression has been treated, when all the biochemical parameters return to normal. In patients with depression, the cortisol response to hypoglycemia is maintained as opposed to true Cushing's syndrome with secondary depression, in which it is absent.

Alcoholism can produce a clinical and biochemical picture indistinguishable from Cushing's syndrome. ACTH is present in the blood but often at levels rather lower than would be expected from the cortisol levels. The underlying pathogenesis of alcoholic pseudo-Cushing's syndrome is not well understood, and the biochemical abnormalities revert to normal after a few days of abstention from alcohol. This often means that the clinical and biochemical stigmata resolve when the patient is admitted for investigation and can be difficult to distinguish from cyclical Cushing's syndrome.

Obesity is commonly seen in association with diabetes and hypertension; hence, Cushing's syndrome frequently may need to be excluded. Urinary free and plasma cortisol suppress in response to low-dose dexamethasone in obese subjects. The cortisol and ACTH response to CRH is usually attenuated compared with healthy individuals and therefore markedly different from the exaggerated response seen in Cushing's disease (see later).

DIFFERENTIAL DIAGNOSIS OF CUSHING'S SYNDROME

Once Cushing's syndrome has been diagnosed, as already described, investigations should be directed to identifying the precise cause. The 9:00 A.M. plasma ACTH values establish if the cause is ACTH dependent or independent. In the authors' experience, all patients with adrenal tumors have undetectable plasma ACTH values and an obvious adrenal tumor on scanning. The major difficulty is distinguishing between a pituitary and ectopic source of ACTH secretion, a problem necessitating the use of a combination of biochemical and radiologic techniques. No single investigation is infallible, and therefore the diagnosis relies, where possible, on the combined results of several investigations. Cushing's disease is four times more common in women than in men, presenting principally between the ages of 40 and 60 years. Because small cell carcinoma of the lung is more common in men, ectopic ACTH is more common in men. Hence, ACTH-dependent Cushing's syndrome is less likely to be pituitary dependent in a man than in a woman. The classic ectopic ACTH syndrome is clinically distinguishable from Cushing's disease: the principal challenge is differentiating the occult ectopic ACTH secretion from a pituitary source.

The high-dose dexamethasone suppression test is of value in differentiating Cushing's disease from other causes of Cushing's syndrome. Dexamethasone, 2 mg every 6 hours, is given for 48 hours. We perform this on an inpatient basis because the high dose of glucocorticoid can induce psychosis in a Cushing's patient. In Cushing's disease, a fall in cortisol to less than 50% of the basal value is seen in 90% of patients. In all other types of Cushing's syndrome, suppression is not expected; however, uncharacteristic suppression is seen in about 10% of patients with ectopic ACTH syndrome, and lack of suppression is seen in the same proportion of patients with Cushing's disease.

Since 1983, the CRH test has become established as an important tool in the investigation of patients with Cushing's syndrome. Two basal samples are obtained, so that spontaneous pulses of cortisol and ACTH can be identified, before the administration of an intravenous bolus of 100 µg human CRH; thereafter, blood is obtained at 15-minute intervals for 2 hours for measurement of ACTH and cortisol. The ACTH and cortisol responses to CRH are blunted by prior dexamethasone administration, and it is therefore important not to perform a CRH test within 10 days of dexamethasone administration. Typically, patients with pituitary-dependent Cushing's disease show an excessive cortisol and ACTH response to CRH compared with normal individuals, whereas patients with obesity have an attenuated response. The test is therefore of some value in confirming the diagnosis of Cushing's syndrome. Its principal value, however, is in differentiating between a pituitary and ectopic source of ACTH secretion. Only one well-documented case of a patient with the ectopic ACTH syndrome responding to CRH is described, whereas up to 25% of patients with Cushing's disease fail to show a rise in ACTH and cortisol.

In the authors' experience, combining the results of CRH and high-dose dexamethasone suppression tests allows confident discrimination between pituitary and ectopic ACTH secretion. One hundred percent of patients with Cushing's disease have either an exaggerated cortisol response to CRH or show 50% or more suppression to high-dose dexamethasone, whereas no patient with the ectopic ACTH syndrome has shown a similar combination of results.

The metyrapone test was originally described for differentiating pituitary disease from adrenal adenomas, but with the advent of ACTH assays and computed tomography scans, this is no longer a clinical problem. The responses seen in patients with pituitary and ectopic ACTH syndromes overlap markedly, and the test is of no value in differentiating the source of ACTH secretion. The authors have therefore abandoned the metyrapone test.

Plasma potassium is low in 100% of the authors' patients with the ectopic ACTH syndrome but only in 10% of patients with Cushing's disease. It is therefore important to obtain a potassium value before any medication is started. Great care must be taken in the handling of specimens to avoid hemolysis and consequently spuriously normal values, although the bicarbonate may remain high. The discriminatory power of potassium is lost in patients taking diuretics. Diabetes mellitus is more common in the ectopic ACTH syndrome but often occurs also in other causes.

Tumor Markers

Ectopic ACTH secreting tumors commonly co-secrete other peptides, which, in addition to being of value in supporting the existence of an ectopic hormone–secreting tumor, can also be used in localizing the tumor during venous sampling and as a tumor marker to evaluate subsequent therapy. In patients in whom diagnostic difficulty exists, the authors routinely measure β human chorionic gonadotropin, calcitonin, carcinoembryonic antigen, CRH, somatostatin, α-fetoprotein, and growth hormone–releasing hormone.

Computed Tomography and Magnetic Resonance Imaging

Ninety percent of ACTH pituitary adenomas are less than 1 cm in size, and often tumors secreting ACTH cannot be reliably identified on imaging. The latest generation of magnetic resonance imaging scanners is reported to be able to identify pituitary adenomas in up to 80% of patients with Cushing's disease; however, incidental pituitary abnormalities, e.g., functionless tumors and cysts, may be present in up to 25%, and therefore the results of scanning must be interpreted with a knowledge of biochemical findings.

Computed tomography scanning of the chest and abdomen is essential if there is any possibility of an ectopic source of ACTH secretion. Because the primary tumor may be very small, it is necessary to take at least 1-cm contiguous slices through the chest and abdomen using 0.5-cm cuts in regions of concern.

Inferior Petrosal Sinus Sampling

In the last decade, this technique has become established as the most powerful means of discriminating between pituitary and nonpituitary ACTH secretion. Two catheters are inserted into the right femoral vein and guided into each inferior petrosal sinus to sample simultaneously from these veins draining the cavernous sinuses, which receive blood directly from the pituitary. Blood samples for ACTH measurement are obtained before and after 100 μg of CRH is given intravenously.

In the authors' experience, more than 95% of patients with Cushing's disease have a gradient of greater than 2 between the plasma ACTH values obtained from one of the inferior petrosal sinuses and the simultaneous peripheral vein sample. No patient with ectopic ACTH has had a gradient greater than 2. These results are in keeping with the experience of others, some of whom have quoted a specificity and sensitivity of all but 100%. Patients with cyclical Cushing's syndrome must have elevated basal cortisol levels at the time of the procedure because otherwise a false-negative result may be obtained. The ratio regarded as critical depends on the characteristics of the ACTH assay used, and therefore each center must establish its own database. In addition to having a role in establishing the diagnosis, it is also of value in the lateralization of a tumor within the pituitary fossa. In the authors' hands, a gradient of greater than 2 between the two inferior petrosal sinuses correctly lateralizes the tumor in approxiamately 70% of cases. The combined results of pituitary computed tomography or magnetic resonance imaging and petrosal sinus sampling can be of great assistance to the surgeon in planning transsphenoidal selective microadenectomy.

Whole-Body Venous Sampling

In patients suspected of having the ectopic ACTH syndrome, whole-body venous sampling can be of value in confirming and localizing the source of ACTH. A single catheter is introduced, through the right femoral vein, into the superior and inferior vena cava and samples obtained from all the major tributaries. As with inferior petrosal sinus sampling, a peripheral sample is taken simultaneously with the catheter specimens. In addition to measuring plasma ACTH in each sample, any previously identified tumor markers are measured.

Other Investigations

Sputum cytology and bronchoscopy are of value in the occasional patient with suspected ectopic ACTH secretion because the lungs are the most common sites for such tumors. Meta-iodobenzylguanidine (MIBG) and indium-labeled octreotide scanning are of occasional help in identifying the site of ectopic ACTH secretion by carcinoid tumors.

RARE CAUSES OF CUSHING'S SYNDROME

ACTH-dependent adrenal nodules are common in patients with ACTH-dependent adrenal hyperplasia and are usually of no significance because most remain under ACTH control. Rarely Cushing's disease is associated with macronodular adrenal hyperplasia, in which the nodules are autonomous, cortisol levels do not suppress in response to a high-dose dexamethasone suppression test, and no response is seen to CRH. Plasma ACTH levels are usually inappropriately low and intermittently undetectable.

Carney's syndrome is an autosomal dominant condition characterized by mesenchymal tumors, particularly atrial myxomas; spotty skin pigmentation; peripheral nerve tumors; and endocrine disorders. Cushing's syndrome can occur, the results of dexamethasone and CRH tests being the same as in macronodular hyperplasia. The adrenal glands are often normal or small with deeply pigmented nodules.

Very rare cases of ectopic CRH and ACTH-like peptide secreting tumors have been described.

No single test is infallible, and many pitfalls exist in the investigation of Cushing's syndrome. Even after the most meticulous and exhaustive series of investigations, occasionally no clear diagnosis can be established. In such patients, it is reasonable to treat with cortisol-lowering drugs (see later) and to re-investigate after an interval of 3 to 6 months. This situation most commonly arises when the biochemistry points at the occult ectopic ACTH syndrome but no tumor can be identified. Care must be taken to avoid the investigation of cycling patients when the Cushing's syndrome is inactive because otherwise false-negative results arise.

MANAGEMENT

The successful management of Cushing's syndrome depends primarily on establishing the precise cause. Transsphenoidal microadenectomy is accepted as the treatment of choice for Cushing's disease. If a tumor cannot be identified intraoperatively, but preoperative assessment lateralized it, a hemihypophysectomy is performed. In older patients beyond their reproductive years or in patients who are judged unfit to undergo a second operation, particularly if the tumor is not clearly identified preoperatively, the operation of choice is total hypophysectomy. For the reasons outlined subsequently, in all patients with a detectable serum cortisol level after initial surgery, a second hypophysectomy is considered and if thought to be appropriate is performed within 10 days of initial surgery.

All patients undergoing transsphenoidal surgery receive 24 hours of hydrocortisone, 100 mg intramuscularly every 6 hours, the first dose with premedication. If suprasellar extension is present, hydrocortisone is continued for 72 hours. Amoxicillin and flucloxacillin* are likewise begun with the premedication and continued for 5 days or, in the case of a cerebrospinal fluid leak, until it resolves.

To assess the outcome of surgery, serum cortisol is measured at 9:00 A.M. daily for a minimum of 5 days, the first measurement being made at least 12 hours after the last dose of hydrocortisone. In patients with pituitary corticotropin-secreting adenomas, the ACTH-secreting cells in the normal pituitary surrounding the tumor are atrophic, and hence complete excision of the tumor should result in undetectable postoperative cortisol levels, in the authors' assay less than 50 mmol per liter (1.8 μg/100 mL). If serum cortisol is detectable immediately postoperatively, even if subnormal, patients must be regarded as having residual tumor and therefore require consideration for further treatment (see later).

Differences in methodology and definitions of outcome after transsphenoidal surgery make it difficult to compare series, but by the criteria outlined earlier, an experienced pituitary surgeon should render serum cortisol undetectable (i.e., cured) in at least 50% of patients and induce remission in 80 to 90%. Long-term hydrocortisone replacement therapy is often necessary because the hypothalamic-pituitary-adrenal axis can take several years to recover.

Postoperatively, pituitary function must be assessed in detail and followed over the long term. Disturbance of anterior pituitary function is unusual after selective microadenectomy.

In patients with the ectopic ACTH syndrome, clearly curative surgery should be attempted whenever possible. If a bronchial carcinoid is identified, a lobectomy with removal of the regional lymph nodes is indicated because all these tumors should be considered potentially malignant. As with transsphenoidal hypophysectomy, the aim of surgery should be to render serum cortisol undetectable. Failure to do so is indicative of residual tumor. A patient with a bronchial carcinoid and evidence of mediastinal metastases requires postoperative radiotherapy. The authors administer 4000 cGy to the mediastinum in 22 fractions using three fields from a 15-MV linear accelerator.

Unilateral adrenalectomy is the treatment for

both adrenal adenoma and carcinoma even when metastases are present because debulking improves prognosis. All patients with adrenal carcinomas require radiotherapy to the adrenal bed. Bilateral adrenalectomy should cure patients with Cushing's syndrome, although occasionally this is not the case because some gland, particularly around the right adrenal vein, is missed. The place of bilateral adrenalectomy in the treatment of Cushing's disease is, however, greatly limited because with long-term follow-up, approximately 30% of patients develop Nelson's syndrome (high plasma ACTH levels, hyperpigmentation, and an invasive pituitary tumor). To reduce operative morbidity and mortality, plasma cortisol levels must be controlled with drugs, usually metyrapone because of its rapid onset of action (see later). Bilateral adrenalectomy can greatly improve the well-being of a patient with the occult ectopic ACTH syndrome, in whom the tumor cannot be localized and therefore resection is not possible.

Pituitary Radiotherapy

Radiation is administered, from a 6-MV linear accelerator, via a three-field technique (two lateral, one frontal), to a total dose of 4500 cGy in 25 fractions over 35 days. The limitation of radiotherapy is that it can take up to 10 years to be fully effective, and hence patients often require interim medical therapy to control cortisol secretion. Radiotherapy to the pituitary is indicated in patients with pituitary-dependent Cushing's disease who have to have a total adrenalectomy because the condition has not or cannot be cured by hypophysectomy. Radiotherapy usually prevents or at least delays the development of Nelson's syndrome.

Medical Treatment

Drug therapy is effective in controlling cortisol secretion but is not definitive because the effects are fully reversible on stopping treatment. Hence medical therapy is restricted to controlling cortisol secretion; in preparation for surgery; when cortisol levels remain elevated after definitive ablative therapy in acutely unwell, potentially psychotic patients when their condition is life-threatening; and very rarely when detailed investigation has failed to establish the precise cause of the Cushing's syndrome as an interim measure before re-investigation. Medical therapy can be subdivided into drugs acting directly on the adrenal glands and those reducing ACTH secretion. Only drugs acting directly on the adrenal glands are reliably effective. Drug therapy is best moni-

---

*Not available in the United States.

tored by measuring serum cortisol at six points during a single day. The mean should lie in the target range of 150 to 300 nmol per liter (5 to 10 μg/100 mL) because this reflects a normal cortisol production rate.

Ketoconazole* (Nizoral) is the drug of first choice in the treatment of Cushing's syndrome, given in doses between 400 and 1200 mg per day. Ketoconazole inhibits P450-dependent enzymes with effects on cholesterol side-chain cleavage and 11β-hydroxylation. It is of slower onset of action than metyrapone but has the advantage over metyrapone of lowering rather than increasing circulating androgen levels. Hepatotoxicity is a potential problem, and therefore liver function tests, including gamma-glutamyltransferase, should be performed at regular intervals, at least weekly initially.

Metyrapone acts to lower serum cortisol levels by inhibiting the final step in cortisol synthesis: 11β-hydroxylation. Doses of between 1 and 4 grams are usually required, taken in divided doses with food. Metyrapone is fast acting; significant lowering of serum cortisol is seen within 2 hours. In Cushing's disease, despite a rise in ACTH, and in the ectopic ACTH syndrome, it is effective over the long term. Treatment must be carefully monitored to avoid hypoadrenalism. Patients on metyrapone therapy have high circulating levels of 11-deoxycortisol, which cross reacts in some commercial cortisol assays, resulting in misleadingly high results. The major limitation of metyrapone is the rise in circulating androgens and consequent hirsutism in a proportion of women.

Ortho,para,dichlorodiphenyl dichloroethane (o,p′DDD)† is a cytotoxic agent acting on the P450 cytochrome to inhibit cortisol synthesis. It was developed from the insecticide DDT, which was noted to cause hypoadrenalism in dogs. Large doses, up to 10 grams per day, have been used in the treatment of adrenal carcinoma but are associated with unpleasant side effects, such as nausea, vomiting, neuropathy, and ataxia. Used in doses of 2 to 4 grams, however, it is effective in controlling serum cortisol in patients with ACTH-dependent Cushing's syndrome with few if any side effects. It is of slow onset of action, taking 6 to 8 weeks to have full effect, and one must therefore resist the temptation to increase the dose too frequently. The authors generally initiate o,p′DDD therapy in combination with metyrapone and then gradually withdraw the metyrapone and use o,p′DDD as a single agent over the long term.

*Not available in the United States.
†This use of o,p′DDD is not listed in the manufacturer's official directive.

Low-dose o,p′DDD is well tolerated, but its use is limited by acquired hypercholesterolemia. Total and low-density lipoprotein cholesterol has risen in all patients on o,p′DDD. For this reason, despite its effectiveness, we now rarely use o,p′DDD. Preliminary evidence suggests that the hypercholesterolemia of o,p′DDD can be reversed by a hydroxymethylglutaryl coenzyme A reductase inhibitor, such as simvastatin (Zocor). It is also noteworthy that ketoconazole is a potent lowerer of circulating cholesterol levels, and it may be that these drugs act synergistically. Owing to changes in binding proteins, total plasma thyroxine levels fall in patients receiving o,p′DDD, but free hormone levels remain unaltered, and the patient remains euthyroid. A rise in hepatic alkaline phosphatase is normal on starting therapy, and serum urate usually falls owing to increased renal clearance.

In the authors' experience, no other drugs are consistently effective in lowering cortisol secretion. Occasionally a patient shows a dramatic response to bromocriptine* (Parlodel), but such patients are the exception. Cyproheptadine* (Periactin), sodium valproate,* and trilostane* (Modrastane) are rarely effective.

*This use of bromocriptine, cyproheptadine, sodium valproate, and trilostane is not listed in the manufacturer's official directive.

DIABETES INSIPIDUS

method of
JOSEPH G. VERBALIS, M.D., and
ARTHUR GREENBERG, M.D.
University of Pittsburgh School of Medicine
Pittsburgh, Pennsylvania

In diabetes insipidus, diminished plasma arginine vasopressin (AVP) levels cause abnormal urinary losses of solute-free water, with resultant polyuria and polydipsia, and lead to hypertonicity and hypernatremia in some cases. Central diabetes insipidus is characterized by an impairment in pituitary AVP secretion in response to plasma hypertonicity. Release of AVP is subnormal in the partial form of central diabetes insipidus and absent in the complete form. In nephrogenic diabetes insipidus, AVP secretion is normal, but renal sensitivity to its hydro-osmotic effect is impaired or absent.

Central diabetes insipidus is caused by acquired or congenital anatomic lesions that disrupt the hypothalamic–posterior pituitary axis, including pituitary surgery, tumors, trauma, hemorrhage, thrombosis, infarction, or granulomatous disease. Severe nephrogenic diabetes insipidus is most commonly hereditary and congenital, but relief of chronic urinary obstruction or therapy with lithium or other drugs may cause an acquired form severe enough to warrant specific treatment. Short-lived nephrogenic diabetes insipidus from hypokalemia or hypercalcemia responds to correction of the underlying disorder. Other causes of polyuria include primary polydipsia and solute diuresis from glycosuria, mannitol, or diuretic therapy and resolving acute renal failure. Solute diuresis can be excluded by demonstrating that the urine osmolality is below 150 mOsm per kg of H_2O or that the specific gravity is below 1.005. A formal water deprivation test is dangerous and unnecessary if there is significant hypertonicity, but it may be required to diagnose partial diabetes insipidus or for cases in which treatment has already been initiated. The urinary response to exogenous AVP differentiates central from nephrogenic diabetes insipidus in most cases. Plasma AVP levels are confirmatory and are important in equivocal cases, but they are not available on an emergent basis.

TREATMENT

The general goals of treatment are correction of any preexisting water deficits and reduction of the ongoing excessive urinary water losses. The specific therapy required varies with the clinical situation. Awake, ambulatory patients with normal thirst have little body water deficit but benefit greatly from relief of the polyuria and polydipsia that disrupt normal activity. Comatose patients with acute diabetes insipidus after head trauma are unable to drink in response to thirst, and progressive hypertonicity may be life-threatening.

Correction of Water Deficit

The established water deficit may be estimated using the following formula:

$$\text{Water deficit} = 0.6 \times \text{premorbid weight} \times (1 - 140/[Na^+])$$

in which $[Na^+]$ is the serum sodium concentration in milliequivalents per liter. This formula depends on three assumptions: total body water is approximately 60% of weight, no body solute was lost as hypertonicity developed, and the premorbid sodium concentration was 140 mEq per liter.

To reduce the risk of central nervous system damage from protracted exposure to severe hypertonicity, the serum tonicity should be rapidly lowered to the range of 330 mOsm per kg of H_2O. Tonicity may be estimated as twice the serum sodium concentration if there is no hyperglycemia, and measured osmolality may be substituted if azotemia is not present. The brain increases intracellular osmolality by increasing the content of a variety of organic osmolytes as protection against excessive shrinkage during hyper-

tonicity. Because these osmolytes cannot be immediately dissipated, further correction should be spread over 24 to 48 hours to avoid producing cerebral edema during treatment.

The water deficit formula does not take into account ongoing water losses and is only a crude estimate. Frequent serum and urine electrolyte determinations should be made, and the administration rate of oral water or 5% dextrose in water should be adjusted accordingly. For example, the estimated deficit of a 70-kg patient whose serum sodium concentration is 160 mEq per liter is 5.25 liters of water, and administration of water at a rate greater than 200 mL per hour would be required to correct the established deficit over 24 hours. Additional fluid would be needed to keep up with ongoing losses until a definitive response to treatment has occurred.

Pharmacologic Agents

The agents and dosages currently recommended for treatment of diabetes insipidus are listed in Table 1.

Arginine Vasopressin (Pitressin)

AVP is a synthetic form of naturally occurring human vasopressin. Because of the drug's relatively short half-life and propensity to cause acute increases in blood pressure when given intravenously, this route should be avoided. The aqueous solution contains 20 U per mL. This agent is mainly used for acute situations, such as postoperative diabetes insipidus. Repeated dosing is required, and the dose should be titrated to achieve the desired reduction in urine output. AVP is not useful in nephrogenic diabetes insipidus.

Desmopressin Acetate (DDAVP)

One of a number of synthetic congeners of vasopressin, desmopressin (1-deamino-8-D-arginine vasopressin) was developed for therapeutic use because it has a longer half-life than the native form and is devoid of the latter's pressor activity. It is the drug of choice for long-term administration in patients with central diabetes insipidus. The intranasal form is provided as an aqueous solution containing 100 μg per mL in a bottle with a calibrated rhinal tube. The tube is filled to the appropriate graduation line and bent in a U shape. Taking care to retain the fluid within the tube, one end is placed in the mouth and the other approximately 1 cm into the anterior nares. The drug is then puffed into the midportion of the nose deep enough to avoid runoff out the nose but not so far back as to propel the hormone into the throat. Patients require training in how to use

TABLE 1. **Pharmacologic Treatment of Diabetes Insipidus**

Drug	Dose	Onset of Action (h)	Duration of Action (h)	Comments
Arginine vasopressin (AVP; Pitressin)	5–10 U subcutaneously	1–2	2–8	Avoid intravenous use because of risk of acute hypertension
Desmopressin (DDAVP)	50–200 μL (5–20 μg) intranasally	1–2	6–24	Drug of choice for long-term treatment of central diabetes insipidus; higher doses may be helpful in some patients with nephrogenic diabetes insipidus
	1–2 μg intravenously or subcutaneously	1–2	6–24	
Chlorpropamide* (Diabinese)	100–500 mg daily	Delayed	24–48	Potentiates renal effect of AVP; useful in partial central diabetes insipidus
Chlorthalidone* (Hygroton)	50–100 mg daily	2–4	24–48	Reduces renal water clearance; useful in nephrogenic diabetes insipidus; comparable doses of other thiazides are equally effective
Indomethacin* (Indocin)	100–150 mg daily	2–4	6–8	Decreases renal water clearance; useful adjunctive therapy in nephrogenic diabetes insipidus

* Not approved for this use.

the catheter to deliver the prescribed dose reliably. A nasal spray delivering a metered dose of 10 μg in 0.1 mL greatly simplifies dosing, but it has the disadvantage of requiring a fixed dose, which may be more than needed by some patients.

The parenteral form is supplied as a solution containing 4 μg per mL and may be given by intravenous, intramuscular, or subcutaneous routes. The parenteral form is approximately five to ten times more potent than the intranasal preparation, and the recommended dosage is 1 to 2 μg. For both the intranasal and parenteral preparations, increasing the administered dose generally has the effect of prolonging the duration of antidiuresis rather than increasing its magnitude; consequently, altering the dose can be useful to reduce the required frequency of administration.

Chlorpropamide* (Diabinese)

Primarily used as an oral hypoglycemic agent, this sulfonylurea also potentiates the hydro-osmotic effect of AVP in the kidney. It is of no value in nephrogenic diabetes insipidus or in most patients with complete diabetes insipidus, but it can be useful adjunctive therapy in patients with partial central diabetes insipidus. Hypoglycemia may develop, particularly in patients with anterior pituitary insufficiency. Several days of treatment are required before maximal effects are seen.

*This use of chlorpropamide is not listed in the manufacturer's official directive.

Thiazide Diuretics

The natriuretic effect of the thiazide class of diuretics is conferred by their ability to block sodium absorption in the cortical diluting site. Combined with dietary sodium restriction, the drugs cause modest hypovolemia, which stimulates isotonic proximal tubular solute reabsorption and diminishes solute delivery to the more distal diluting site, whose activity has already been partially poisoned. Because these effects markedly diminish renal diluting ability and free water clearance independent of any action of AVP, agents of this class are the mainstay of therapy for nephrogenic diabetes insipidus. Monitoring for hypokalemia is recommended, and supplementation is occasionally required. The dosage of a long-acting thiazide, chlorthalidone (Hygroton), is given in Table 1, but all thiazides are interchangeable. Any drug of the thiazide class may be used with equal potential for benefit, and the physician is advised to use the one with which he or she is most familiar. Care must be exercised in treating patients taking lithium with diuretics because the induced contraction of plasma volume may increase lithium concentrations and worsen potential toxic effects of the therapy.

Nonsteroidal Anti-Inflammatory Agents

Prostaglandins increase renal medullary blood flow and diminish medullary solute reabsorption, effects that modestly decrease the interstitial gradient for water reabsorption. By blocking renal prostaglandin synthesis, nonsteroidal anti-inflammatory drugs can increase non–AVP-mediated water reabsorption and minimal urine osmolality, reducing free water clearance and urine output. Although these agents can be effective in central diabetes insipidus, their main usefulness is as adjunctive therapy in nephrogenic diabetes insipidus, in which more direct antidiuretic therapies are limited. Indomethacin (Indocin), tolmetin (Tolectin), and ibuprofen (Motrin) have been used beneficially. The drugs should be given in three divided doses.

Other Agents

Vasopressin tannate in oil has a 24- to 72-hour duration of action. Because of variable bioavailability, however, it has been supplanted by desmopressin and has recently been withdrawn from production. Clofibrate (Atromid) and carbamazepine (Tegretol) augment release of vasopressin in partial diabetes insipidus, but significant side effects preclude recommending their routine use. Other sulfonylureas share chlorpropamide's effect but are less potent. In particular, the newer generation of oral hypoglycemic agents, such as glipizide (Glucotrol) and glyburide (Micronase), are virtually devoid of any AVP-potentiating effects.

Clinical Situations

Acute Postsurgical or Post-Traumatic Central Diabetes Insipidus

A frequent complication of pituitary surgery or severe head trauma, post-traumatic central diabetes insipidus is usually obvious from the clinical situation. Hypernatremia may develop rapidly, is likely to be severe, and warrants specific therapy with intravenous 5% dextrose in water at a rate estimated from the deficit calculation described previously. Parenteral aqueous vasopressin in a dosage of 5 U subcutaneously or desmopressin in a dosage of 1 to 2 μg intravenously or subcutaneously should be started to reduce urine flow rate and simplify fluid management. Frequent monitoring of urine output and serum electrolytes is required.

After the acute phase, partial or complete resolution of diabetes insipidus often occurs. In some patients, the initial phase of diabetes insipidus is followed by axonal necrosis of vasopressin-secreting neurons with uncontrolled AVP release, potentially leading to water retention and hyponatremia and then to axonal death with cessation of AVP production and recurrent diabetes insipidus; this is the so-called triphasic pattern. AVP requirements may vary at different times. To ensure detection of recovery from diabetes insipidus or a period of inappropriate antidiuresis, the dosage interval for parenteral desmopressin or aqueous vasopressin should be empirically tailored to allow a brief recurrence of polyuria. Postsurgical patients who do not recover need long-term outpatient therapy, usually with desmopressin.

Chronic Central Diabetes Insipidus

Patients with complete central diabetes insipidus should be treated with intranasal desmopressin. Unless the hypothalamic thirst center is also affected by the primary lesion, patients develop thirst when hypertonic. Severe hypertonicity is therefore not a risk in the patient who is alert, ambulatory, and able to drink. Polyuria and polydipsia are inconvenient and disruptive but not life-threatening. Hypotonicity is largely asymptomatic and may be progressive if water intake continues during a period of continuous antidiuresis. Therefore, treatment must be designed to minimize polyuria and polydipsia without an undue risk of hyponatremia from overtreatment. It is best to permit brief, intermittent polyuric episodes, ideally on a daily basis but at least weekly, at the patient's convenience. Treatment must be individualized, usually with an in-hospital trial to determine optimal dosage and interval. This also permits careful education of patients about how to administer the drug intranasally and how to ensure a polyuric phase. Starting at 50 μl, the dose that results in 12 to 24 hours of control should be determined. Most patients require twice-daily dosing, but for some once-daily dosing suffices. Multiple small doses may be preferred because of the high cost of desmopressin. Chlorpropamide may lower the required desmopressin dose and produce an additional economy. A patient with partial central diabetes insipidus can be readily managed with desmopressin, but chlorpropamide alone may be sufficient and simpler in some cases.

Nephrogenic Diabetes Insipidus

By definition, patients with nephrogenic diabetes insipidus are resistant to AVP. Useful treatment measures include sodium restriction and thiazides to reduce renal diluting capacity combined with a prostaglandin synthesis inhibitor. Indomethacin, tolmetin, and ibuprofen have been used, although ibuprofen may be less effective than the others. The combination of thiazides and a nonsteroidal anti-inflammatory agent does not increase urinary osmolality above that of plasma, but the lessening of polyuria is nonetheless beneficial to patients. Although desmopressin is usually not effective in nephrogenic diabetes insipidus, some patients have partial responses with increases in urine osmolality after 6 to 10 μg of this agent.

GOITER

method of
HUGO STUDER, M.D.,
PETER KOPP, M.D., and
LARS ASMIS, M.D.

Inselspital, University of Berne
Berne, Switzerland

Idiopathic (nontoxic or simple) goiter is a slowly developing diffuse or nodular enlargement of the thyroid gland that results from the generation of new follicles. It has to be differentiated from other clinical entities with enlargement of the thyroid (Table 1). Initially thyroid function is normal, but with ongoing nodular transformation, development of subclinical or even overt hyperthyroidism is possible.

Goiter growth results from the generation of new follicles, which may vary in shape, size, and iodine metabolism. Function and morphology of follicular cells widely vary among goiters from different individuals, within different follicles of the same goiter, and even among cells of an individual follicle. The proliferating cell cohorts are scattered throughout the gland; hence, goiter growth is a multicentric process. Because some progenies of follicular cells may replicate faster than others, multiple nodules develop with time in the initially diffusely enlarged gland. Although function and growth of some follicular cells are thyroid-stimulating hormone (TSH) dependent, others may replicate and function autonomously, i.e., by intrinsic mechanisms not dependent on TSH. Therefore, insidiously developing thyrotoxicosis is a familiar corollary of growing nodular goiters owing to excess hormone production by the enlarging mass of autonomously functioning follicles. Apart from follicles with a high iodine turnover, a goiter invariably contains follicles with poor or no iodine metabolism, explaining the scintigraphic finding of "hot" and "cold" nodules.

Although much knowledge about the network of growth-promoting and growth-inhibiting pathways involving overexpression of proto-oncogenes and activation of oncogenes, cytokines, and cellular growth factors as well as their respective receptors has been gathered during the last decade, the precise molecular mechanisms that cause excessive replication of some follicular cells are yet unknown. An individual nodule in a goiter may be polyclonal, i.e., derived from more than one genetically different family, or it may be clonal. Both types of nodules may coexist within the same goiter. The coexistence of both polyclonal and clonal nodules within the same multinodular goiter suggests that some follicular cells with a constitutively high replication rate may evolve into polyclonal nodules. Because replicating cells are prone to a higher incidence of genetic and epigenetic changes, clonal nodules could arise secondarily.

Autonomous replication of any cell cohort either may go on relentlessly, producing rapidly expanding nodules, or may come to a halt for no apparent reason at any moment in the clinical course.

The fundamental process of goitrogenesis is identical regardless of the presence or absence of extrathyroidal growth stimulating agents, such as enhanced TSH levels in endemic goiters or enzyme deficiencies or low levels of growth-enhancing immunoglobulins in a few sporadic goiters. In endemic goiters caused by iodine deficiency, the time sequence of goitrogenesis is accelerated by increased, although barely measurable, TSH levels, but it is not basically altered.

CLINICAL ASSESSMENT

Usually patients with nontoxic goiter present because of a diffuse or multinodular enlargement of the thyroid. Other familiar complaints are difficulty in swallowing, shortness of breath, dysphagia, and hoarseness owing to vocal cord paresis.

The size, structure, and firmness have to be assessed by clinical examination, which should include the palpation of the lymph nodes of the neck. It is essential to evaluate thyroid function by measuring serum TSH and thyroxine. In the case of a TSH level below the normal range, triiodothyronine should also be measured to exclude hyperthyroidism.

Ultrasonography is the "gold standard" to assess the size and structure of a goiter or a thyroid nodule accurately. It is especially helpful in long-term follow-up. The fine-needle aspiration of suspicious nodules controlled by sonography distinguishes nontoxic goiter from neoplastic thyroid enlargement in a high percentage of cases, provided that the smears are evaluated by a skilled cytopathologist.

Isotopic scan studies and radioactive iodine uptake are usually of little help except in the case of intended radioiodine therapy. Reflecting the heterogeneous functional activity of the follicles, the scan usually reveals a patchy uptake. It has to be stressed that scintigraphic studies do not allow reliable discernment of benign from malignant goiters.

TREATMENT

Confronted with a patient bearing a nontoxic goiter, a physician has four therapeutic options:

1. No treatment, but follow-up at regular intervals.
2. Treatment with thyroxine or iodine.
3. Surgical procedures.
4. Radioiodine treatment.

TABLE 1. **Causes of Goiter**

Idiopathic
Iodine deficiency
Goitrogens
Autoimmune thyroid disease
    Graves' disease
    Hashimoto's thyroiditis
Subacute thyroiditis
Neoplastic
    Primary tumor of the thyroid
    Metastasis
Congenital enzyme deficiencies
Thyroid enlargement in pregnancy
Acromegaly

Guidelines for Decision Making

The first step in devising a therapeutic strategy is the unequivocal establishment of euthyroidism because even borderline hyperthyroidism definitely rules out thyroxine treatment. It is important to remember that autonomous growth and autonomous function are entirely independent features of newly generated goiter follicles. Almost every goiter contains follicles with widely differing functional capacity, some of which have high autonomous function. Therefore, insidiously developing hyperthyroidism is a frequently overlooked complication of slowly growing nodular goiter.

The two most important parameters aiding the clinician in making an optimal choice among the four therapeutic options are the careful evaluation of the recent clinical course of the goiter and the patient's age. Indeed, if there is clear evidence of recent growth, active treatment is indicated in all patients, whereas a "wait-and-see" attitude is the method of choice in a middle-aged patient whose nodular goiter was detected by chance during physical examination and appears to remain stable at successive follow-ups. A frequent clinical course in patients older than 30 to 40 years is cessation of active growth of a goiter or of an individual nodule within a goiter.

An active therapeutic approach toward any growing goiter nodule is indicated not only for fear of missing a malignant tumor, but also because this type of nodule remains a problem for an unknown length of time. It requires careful follow-up and possibly lifelong treatment, unless it is surgically removed. This is all the more true the younger the patient is. Because this statement applies to all types of growing nodules regardless of their scintigraphic appearance, routine use of scintigraphy is of little help in decision making, as mentioned earlier. The overall prevalence of malignant tumors in growing nodules is not higher than 15%, probably even much lower in unselected cases. If fine-needle biopsy is positive, malignant growth is certain, but it can never be excluded by a negative result of the cytologic smear.

Thyroxine treatment of euthyroid diffuse and nodular goiters in daily doses of 100 to 150 μg is advocated by many clinicians. This is true for apparently single nodules (most often proved to be multinodular on histologic sections) as well as for multinodular goiters. The correct dose of thyroxine should be aimed at keeping TSH in the lowest normal range while strictly avoiding even borderline hyperthyroidism because of the possible side effects of subclinical hyperthyroidism. There are, however, severe limitations to this form of treatment. Its basic principle is the suppression of TSH, one of the potent growth factors of the thyroid gland. Thyroxine treatment is highly successful in suppressing growth and reducing the volume of endemic goiters caused by iodine deficiency. Nonendemic goiters, however, grow more like benign tumors, in which TSH is only one of the many factors involved in goiter growth. For that reason, these goiters—or individual nodules within such a goiter—grow autonomously, i.e., partly or totally independent of the presence of TSH. Therefore, thyroxine treatment cannot be expected to be effective in sporadic goiter treatment. It may slow down nodular growth and reduce the volume of a goiter but rarely by more than about 30%. This is an insufficient result, particularly in children and young adults, in whom nothing short of the disappearance of thyroid nodules is an acceptable outcome. Furthermore, one cannot be sure that volume reduction involves the entire gland or whether it results merely from morphologic changes localized in other areas, while the truly growing region remains unaffected. Another shortcoming of thyroxine treatment is the frequent necessity to administer the hormone indefinitely after achieving initial success; otherwise the goiter resumes growth within weeks of stopping treatment. Some authors advocate iodine treatment of nodular goiters. There is no evidence, however, that iodine alone is superior to thyroxine treatment. Furthermore, iodide is also delivered by thyroxine because iodine accounts for 65% of its molecular weight.

Thyroxine treatment may be administered in patients with a cytologically benign nodular goiter if the therapeutic effect is regularly monitored by ultrasonography, if euthyroidism can be maintained constantly, and if the long-term compliance of the patient is assured. In the authors' experience, these requirements are seldom met. Younger patients should therefore be referred directly to a surgical treatment. This approach is mandatory if a goiter or any nodule within a nodular goiter continues to grow or resumes growth during thyroxine administration. The surgeon should remove all macroscopically altered tissue following thorough inspection of both thyroid lobes. Histologically small foci of proliferating follicles are often found even within macroscopically normal-appearing tissue.

Radioiodine treatment with iodine-131 is an excellent method to deal with hyperthyroidism in hyperfunctioning large goiters of elderly, frail patients considered to present a high surgical risk. If radioiodine is a therapeutic option, a previous iodine scan is mandatory to localize cold areas not accessible to the isotope because radioiodine destroys only functioning follicles and does not affect follicles with poor iodine uptake. Because growth and function are independent characteristics of a goiter follicle, excessive hormone production can be reliably reduced by radioiodine treatment, while growth may continue. The degree of reduction in goiter volume obtained by therapeutic doses of radioiodine is widely variable and cannot be predicted in an individual patient.

HYPERPARATHYROIDISM AND HYPOPARATHYROIDISM

method of
LINDA BAKER LESTER, M.D., and
MICHAEL R. McCLUNG, M.D.
Providence Medical Center
Portland, Oregon

CALCIUM METABOLISM

Calcium is essential for normal cellular function. Total serum calcium levels are affected by changes in serum protein and are routinely measured on multichemistry panels. Ionized calcium is the biologically active fraction of total calcium. It is maintained within a narrow range, 1.1 to 1.3 mM per liter, despite large swings in calcium absorption during the day. Calcium regulation is obtained by coordination of three major calciotropic hormones: calcitonin, parathyroid hormone (PTH), and 1,25-dihydroxycholecalciferol (calcitriol).

Calcitonin has its major effect at the bone to decrease bone resorption and thus decrease calcium release. The role of calcitonin in normal calcium homeostasis is minimal. Calcitriol, the active metabolite of vitamin D, exerts its major effect on calcium metabolism by stimulating intestinal calcium absorption. It also increases renal tubular reabsorption of calcium and in high doses can increase bone resorption. The synthesis of calcitriol is dependent on PTH, making PTH the major regulator of serum calcium levels.

Parathyroid Hormone

PTH is a single polypeptide chain of 84 amino acids that is secreted from the parathyroid gland. PTH secretion is predominantly regulated by negative feedback control of extracellular ionized calcium. Hypomagnesemia and elevated calcitriol levels can suppress PTH secretion.

PTH has several sites of action in the regulation of calcium balance. It increases bone resorption by increasing osteoclast number and activity. It decreases renal calcium losses by increasing tubular reabsorption of calcium. PTH indirectly increases calcium absorption by stimulating the conversion of 25-hydroxyvitamin D to calcitriol in the kidney. The net effect of PTH action is to increase serum calcium levels.

Measuring Parathyroid Hormone

Several radioimmunoassays are available for the measurement of PTH. Most of the circulating immunoreactive PTH is in biologically inactive mid-region or carboxy terminal fragments. Earlier assays for PTH detected these fragments. These fragments can be secreted in disorders other than primary hyperparathyroidism (HPT) and can accumulate in patients with impaired renal function. There is, therefore, significant overlap with these assays of PTH values found in patients with primary HPT and other disorders, such as hypercalcemia of malignancy. More recently, assays that measure the intact, biologically active molecule rather than inactive fragments have been developed. These assays are a more accurate reflection of PTH secretion and can distinguish between the major causes of hypercalcemia. The measurement of intact PTH has become the assay of choice in evaluating parathyroid function.

PRIMARY HYPERPARATHYROIDISM

Primary HPT is defined as hypercalcemia secondary to excess PTH production. The incidence of primary HPT is between 1 in 500 to 1 in 1000 people. This makes it the third most common endocrine disorder behind diabetes mellitus and thyroid disease. The number of diagnoses has recently increased. This is not due to a true increase in the incidence of the disease but is a reflection of the increased diagnosis of asymptomatic HPT based on screening for hypercalcemia.

The excess PTH is secreted from a benign, solitary adenoma in 85 to 90% of cases. In 10 to 15% of cases, PTH is secreted from hyperplastic glands. When multiglandular disease is present, it is usually associated with either Type I or Type II multiple endocrine neoplasia (MEN) syndromes. Rarely in fewer than 1% of cases, a parathyroid carcinoma is the cause of primary HPT.

The cause of primary HPT is unknown, but a gene defect is likely. Parathyroid adenomas are frequently clonal in origin, suggesting a defect in the gene controlling the regulation of PTH. Gene rearrangements have also been found in patients with primary HPT. Other possible risk factors for the development of primary HPT include a history of neck irradiation as a child or use of the drug lithium.

Hypercalcemia develops in patients with primary HPT because of a loss of the normal feedback control. PTH secretion in patients with adenomas is excessive for the given level of serum calcium secondary to the loss of feedback inhibition by serum calcium. With hyperplasia, the feedback control is normal for the individual cell but the increased number of cells causes oversecretion and hypercalcemia.

Clinical Presentation

Until the 1970s, patients with HPT usually presented with one of the complications of this disease, the most common being nephrocalcinosis. Bone disease was also common, and in primary HPT it is called osteitis fibrosa cystica. This results from increased subperiosteal bone resorption typically in the skull, distal phalanges, or clavicles. These changes can be seen as "salt and pepper" erosions on plain radiographs. Other bone changes include brown tumors and cysts. These bony changes can cause severe pain and deformity. Generalized bone loss or osteopenia can also be a feature of primary HPT. Many patients present with a combination of renal and skeletal disease. Other manifestations of primary HPT are less common but include diffuse neuromuscular weakness, depression, and abdominal pain. Hypertension was thought to be related to HPT, but this is now thought to be a coincidental association and not a causative one.

In the 1970s, automated chemistry evaluations became commonplace. This allowed the diagnosis of primary HPT in an early asymptomatic phase when hypercalcemia is the only manifestation. Since then, the majority of patients are diagnosed in the asymptomatic or minimally symptomatic phases.

Occasionally patients present with severe hypercalcemia from HPT. Serum calcium is markedly elevated, and symptoms may include nausea, vomiting, lethargy, seizures, or coma. This can be life-threatening and requires emergent therapy for acute hypercalcemia. There are no distinguishing clinical signs to separate hypercalcemia of HPT from other causes of hypercalcemia.

Diagnosis

The diagnosis of primary HPT is made by biochemical means and is correlated to the clinical presentation. An elevated ionized or corrected total serum calcium and an elevated intact PTH level are the hallmarks. In the setting of hypercalcemia, intact PTH levels above normal denote HPT. Other associated findings include hypercalciuria (>300 mg calcium in 24 hours) and hypophosphatemia. If hypercalcemia is present but the intact PTH level is suppressed, another cause for the hypercalcemia should be sought, such as a malignancy or granulomatous disease.

Treatment

Surgery

Surgical removal of the abnormal parathyroid gland has been the mainstay of therapy for primary HPT. Parathyroidectomy is successful (>95% of patients are cured) and has a low rate of complications when performed by an experienced surgeon. Surgery is recommended in any case of symptomatic HPT and should be considered in asymptomatic patients (see comment later on nonoperative management). Localization procedures are not routinely recommended before surgery. Choosing a skilled, experienced parathyroid surgeon is the single most important preoperative consideration.

The surgery is performed under general anesthesia. A curvilinear incision is made in the lower neck. The thyroid lobes, recurrent laryngeal nerves, and all four parathyroid glands are identified. In most patients with primary HPT, a single adenoma is found. The most likely location of an adenoma is among the lower parathyroid glands behind the thyroid gland. Occasionally the adenoma may be in an ectopic site, such as in the superior mediastinum, behind the esophagus, up the carotid sheath, or intrathyroidal. If an abnormal parathyroid gland cannot be identified at the time of surgery, the incision should be closed and localization procedures done after the diagnosis of primary HPT is re-confirmed. Localization techniques include computed tomography or magnetic resonance imaging scanning of the neck and superior mediastinum, thallium-technetium scanning, and high-resolution ultrasonography of the neck. Forty to 60% of abnormal parathyroid glands not found at surgery are identified by these techniques. If further evaluation is necessary, selective thyroid arteriography and selective venous sampling for PTH can localize the abnormality in 70 to 85% of cases. These should be performed by skilled angiographers only. Once the abnormality is localized, the patient should be taken back for re-exploration.

In about 10% of patients, all four glands are involved and hyperplastic. The majority of abnormal glands should be removed at the time of surgery to decrease the chance of recurrence. Removal of 3½ glands is recommended in most cases. Total parathyroidectomy and autotransplantation of a small portion of parathyroid tissue into the sternocleidomastoid muscle or muscle pockets in the forearm are recommended for patients with HPT and MEN syndromes.

Complications of Surgery

The complication rate for parathyroidectomy of a single adenoma is quite low when done by a skilled surgeon. Mortality rates are usually low (<1%). Complications that can occur are hypoparathyroidism from damage or removal of all the glands and recurrent laryngeal nerve injury leading to temporary or permanent vocal cord paralysis. These occur in approximately 5% of cases. The extensive exploration with parathyroid hyperplasia or the need for a repeat neck exploration increases the risk of complications.

Postoperative Management

Serum calcium levels should be followed every 6 to 8 hours for the first day and at least daily until hospital discharge. Transient hypocalcemia is frequent, with the nadir in calcium levels occurring on postoperative day 2 to 3. This fall in serum calcium is due to increased bone uptake of calcium (hungry bone syndrome) and sluggish recovery of the previously suppressed normal parathyroid gland. Hungry bone syndrome can be distinguished from postsurgical hypoparathyroidism by the presence of normal to high PTH levels and normal or low serum phophate levels. Management of hypocalcemia is discussed in the following section.

After surgery, patients should be monitored for resolution of primary HPT and for possible complications of surgery. Serum calcium and urinary calcium excretion should be checked several weeks postoperatively to document resolution of hypercalcemia and hypercalciuria. If these values are normal, we recommend continuing a high calcium intake for at least 1 year after surgery in all patients to provide adequate calcium for healing of hyperparathyroid bone disease.

Medical Therapy

There is no adequate medical therapy for primary HPT. Agents that suppress PTH-mediated bone turnover, however, may be useful adjuncts to therapy. Conjugated equine estrogen (Premarin) in doses of 1.25 to 2.5 mg daily may decrease bone resorption and serum calcium levels. This therapy is not recommended as a substitute for parathyroidectomy in patients with severe HPT. In patients with mild or moderate disease, estrogen therapy may stabilize the disease and prevent the need for surgery. These patients require careful interval monitoring.

Other therapies that have been tried include bisphosphonates and calcitonin. Both oral etidronate (Didronel) and salmon calcitonin were found not to be effective either in controlling bone turnover or in lowering serum calcium levels. Recently more potent bisphosphonates, such as pamidronate (Aredia), have been shown to decrease serum calcium transiently in patients with primary HPT. There is no information on long-term therapy, and therefore this should be considered only for short-term correction of hypercalcemia while awaiting surgery or in patients who refuse surgery.

Nonoperative Management

Although the natural history of mild HPT is not completely understood, most patients seem to have a stable course. Monitoring of asymptomatic patients with mild to moderate HPT without sur-

gical treatment has been proposed. Determining if a patient is a surgical candidate is the initial step. Criteria for parathyroidectomy are listed in Table 1. Guidelines for monitoring asymptomatic patients have been developed by a National Institutes of Health (NIH) Consensus Conference. These patients should have serum calcium and urine calcium levels, creatinine clearance, and blood pressure measured every 6 months. Bone densitometry measurements should be assessed yearly to determine rates of bone loss. If the hypercalcemia worsens, if they develop symptoms attributable to hypercalcemia, or if bone loss or other end-organ effects are seen, patients should be considered for surgery.

Patients being followed with mild HPT should be educated to avoid dehydration. There are no current recommendations on calcium intake. Calcium intakes between 500 and 1000 mg daily are recommended.

Pregnancy and Hyperparathyroidism

It is unusual for a patient to present with HPT during pregnancy. These patients are identified when they present with symptoms related to HPT or in conjunction with the evaluation of a neonate with tetany. Nephrolithiasis is the most common presenting symptom during pregnancy. The development of renal stones should prompt evaluation for HPT.

The proportion of patients diagnosed with HPT who are symptomatic is higher during pregnancy compared with nonpregnant patients. This probably reflects the lack of routine screening of serum calcium levels during pregnancy rather than an increased severity of the disease. Intact PTH levels are not altered by pregnancy, and therefore diagnosis of HPT during pregnancy is identical to that in nonpregnant patients. Treatment is also similar. Hormonal therapy and bisphosphonates, however, are contraindicated. Parathyroidectomy is recommended in symptomatic patients and can usually be performed safely during the second trimester. Many patients with mild disease can be followed through their

TABLE 1. **Indications for Parathyroidectomy**

Serum calcium >1.0 mg/dL above normal (11.4–12.0 mg/dL)
History of a life-threatening episode of hypercalcemia
Kidney stones by abdominal x-ray
24-h urine calcium excretion >400 mg
Bone mass 2 standard deviations below normal
Patient age <50 years
Coexisting illness that complicates management
Patient preference for surgery
Creatinine clearance <70% of normal
An unreliable patient for follow-up
Any worsening of status during nonoperative management

pregnancy without need for surgery and undue risk to the patient or infant.

SECONDARY HYPERPARATHYROIDISM

Serum calcium levels and PTH secretion are related by a classic negative feedback system as described earlier. A reduction in serum calcium leads to an appropriate increase in PTH synthesis and secretion. This increase in PTH in response to hypocalcemia is termed secondary HPT. Serum PTH levels in secondary HPT can exceed those seen in primary HPT and are associated with parathyroid hyperplasia. If prolonged, the effect of elevated PTH secretion can result in hyperparathyroid bone disease with osteopenia and osteitis fibrosis cystica.

The major cause of secondary HPT in the United States today is renal failure. Progressive renal failure leads to an impairment in phosphate clearance and a decreased renal mass that subsequently reduces renal 25-hydroxyvitamin D 1-hydroxylase activity. The resulting fall in calcitriol levels causes decreased intestinal calcium absorption, a slight fall in serum calcium, and secondary HPT. Biochemical evidence of secondary HPT may be observed as renal clearance falls below 30 to 40 mL per minute, before the onset of dialysis.

Other causes of secondary HPT include intestinal calcium malabsorption owing to vitamin D deficiency or intestinal diseases, such as celiac disease. With mild to moderate vitamin D deficiency, frank osteomalacia may not occur, whereas secondary HPT may occur early. Hyperparathyroid bone disease is the initial form of skeletal dysfunction in patients with vitamin D deficiency as assessed by histomorphometry. A renal calcium leak with hypercalciuria can produce a significantly negative calcium balance and secondary HPT, especially if combined with a low dietary calcium intake. Renal hypercalciuria may occur as an isolated finding or in conjunction with more generalized abnormalities of proximal tubular function, such as Fanconi's syndrome.

Clinical Presentation

The symptoms of secondary HPT are usually nonspecific and frequently occur much later than the biochemical or radiographic abnormalities. Hypocalcemia is unusual in patients with secondary HPT because serum calcium levels are maintained at the expense of the skeletal calcium stores. Only after prolonged derangement in calcium metabolism is skeletal calcium depleted to the extent that serum calcium levels cannot be supported. At that point, symptoms of hypocal-

cemia occur. Bone pain owing to osteitis fibrosa cystica or osteomalacia may occur in patients with intestinal calcium malabsorption or chronic renal failure. Diffuse skeletal pain that is worse with weight bearing or changes in posture can be a manifestation of this. The hips, lower back, and legs are the most frequently involved areas. Neuromuscular dysfunction similar to that seen in primary HPT may occur and may be accentuated by the effects of vitamin D deficiency. Weakness of the proximal limb musculature is most common and can lead to difficulty climbing stairs and decreased stamina.

Ectopic calcium deposition may occur, especially in patients with chronic renal failure and hyperphosphatemia. This results in pruritus, acute arthritic syndromes, and ischemic necrosis of soft tissues owing to vascular calcification.

Diagnosis

The diagnosis of secondary HPT is confirmed by the demonstration of elevated intact PTH levels in the setting of normal or low serum calcium concentrations. This biochemical profile is also seen in patients with pseudohypoparathyroidism (see discussion of pseudohypoparathyroidism). In patients with renal failure, phosphate levels are elevated along with a low calcitriol level. In patients without renal failure, hypophosphatemia is often present as a manifestation of the renal effect of PTH. Serum alkaline phosphatase is usually elevated, reflecting the PTH-mediated increase in skeletal remodeling.

Treatment

The basis for treatment of secondary HPT is correction of the underlying disorders that led to increased PTH secretion. Specifically this means correction of hypocalcemia. Treatment of secondary HPT associated with chronic renal failure is complex. Initially control of hyperphosphatemia with a low phosphate diet and nonaluminum phosphate binding agents, such as calcium carbonate or calcium citrate, is recommended. Beginning therapy when the patient's glomerular filtration rate is less than 30 to 40 mL per minute is recommended. The authors start with calcium carbonate in a dose of 2 to 3 grams per day and may increase the dose to 8 to 10 grams per day. As renal function deteriorates to clearance rates of less than 20 mL per minute, oral calcitriol (Rocaltrol) therapy in doses of 0.5 to 3.0 μg per day or dihydrotachysterol in doses of 1 to 2 mg per day should be added. For patients with renal failure on dialysis, intravenous calcitriol (Calcijex) is effective. Intravenous calcitriol is usually administered in a dose of 1 μg at the end of a dialysis run once to three times weekly. The goal of therapy is to improve calcium absorption and thus normalize PTH secretion. The effect of therapy can be monitored with repeated measurements of serum intact PTH and serum calcium levels. Great care must be taken in treating patients with calcitriol because it bypasses the regulating steps in vitamin D metabolism. Hypercalcemia may occur, which, in conjunction with hyperphosphatemia, may accelerate the extracellular deposition of calcium.

Treatment of other causes of secondary HPT is dependent on the underlying pathogenesis. Vitamin D deficiency in patients with disorders of intestinal malabsorption is usually corrected by oral ergocalciferol therapy in doses ranging from 1.25 mg (50,000 units) weekly to 5 mg (200,000 units) daily, depending on the severity of the malabsorption. Calcidiol and calcitriol may also be used. They are much more expensive than ergocalciferol (Table 2) but may be absorbed more readily in patients with moderately severe malabsorptive problems. Total daily calcium intake should also be maintained in the range of 1 to 2 grams daily with diet or calcium supplements.

Thiazide diuretics are appropriate treatment for patients with secondary HPT caused by renal calcium wasting. Hydrochlorothiazide, 25 mg twice a day, and chlorthalidone, 25 to 50 mg daily, are effective in reducing renal calcium loss, increasing serum calcium, and suppressing PTH secretion.

HYPOPARATHYROIDISM

Hypoparathyroidism can be divided into two main categories: insufficient amount of PTH (true hypoparathyroidism) or inadequate activity or function of PTH (pseudohypoparathyroidism). The most common cause of true hypoparathyroidism is postsurgical and usually follows extensive thyroid or repeat neck surgeries. The incidence is dependent on the extent of surgery and the skill of the surgeon. It is uncommon following simple thyroid lobectomy but occurs with an incidence of 3 to 5% following total thyroidectomy. Postsurgi-

cal hypoparathyroidism can be temporary, resolving in several weeks, or permanent. Idiopathic hypoparathyroidism is a rare disorder associated with absent or decreased PTH secretion from hypoplastic or damaged glands. One form, DiGeorge's syndrome, occurs as a result of congenital abnormalities in the third and fourth branchial pouches. These patients present in early childhood with infections and abnormalities of cellular immunity. Other patients develop hypoparathyroidism as a part of a polyglandular autoimmune syndrome that includes diabetes mellitus, autoimmune thyroid disease, Addison's disease, pernicious anemia, and candidiasis. Infiltrative disorders (hemochromatosis or amyloidosis) or destructive lesions (metastatic carcinoma) can rarely cause hypoparathyroidism.

Clinical Presentation

Clinical signs and symptoms of hypoparathyroidism are caused by decreased levels of circulating ionized calcium. The magnitude of the symptoms is dependent on the degree of hypocalcemia as well as the rapidity of change, acid-base status, and age at onset. Acute hypocalcemia can present with paresthesias, muscle spasms (carpopedal spasm), tetany, seizures, or even death. Cardiac arrhythmias may occur and are associated with a prolongation of the QT interval.

Chronic hypocalcemia can be associated with dental abnormalities (pitting or delayed eruptions) or subcutaneous calcification. Basal ganglion calcifications and the consequent extrapyramidal syndromes have been associated with chronic hypoparathyroidism. Lenticular cataracts are the most common structural complication of chronic hypocalcemia.

Diagnosis

Hypoparathyroidism is associated with inappropriately low intact PTH levels in the setting of low total and ionized calcium concentration. Hyperphosphatemia is generally present and, in the absence of renal failure, is strongly supportive of hypoparathyroidism. Hypomagnesemia

TABLE 2. **Characteristics of Vitamin D and Metabolites**

Characteristics	Calciferol	Calcifediol	Calcitriol	Dihydro-tachysterol
Need for 1-hydroxylation (kidney function)	+	+	−	−
Need for 25-hydroxylation (liver function)	+	−	−	+
Onset of maximum effect (weeks)	4–12	2–4	0.5–1	1–4
Approximate daily dose (μg)	1000–3000	75–225	0.50–3.00	1000–2000
Frequency of monitoring when initiating therapy	6–8 weeks	2–3 weeks	0.5–1 week	1–2 weeks
Cost per average daily dose	$0.05	$3.40	$1.60	$1.00

may cause hypocalcemia by impairing PTH secretion and action. Consequently hypomagnesemia must be excluded before diagnosis of hypoparathyroidism can be confirmed.

Treatment

Acute Postsurgical Hypocalcemia

Acute hypocalcemia caused by hypoparathyroidism usually occurs after neck surgery. In this setting, serum calcium should be raised quickly to normal levels. If severe symptoms are present (e.g., tetany, laryngospasm, electrocardiogram changes, or seizures), this is best accomplished with intravenous calcium infusion. Calcium chloride and calcium gluconate are the calcium salts commonly used for intravenous injection. Ten-milliliter ampules contain a 10% solution of the salts and provide 272 mg of elemental calcium for calcium chloride and 90 mg of calcium for calcium gluconate. Calcium gluconate is the preferred form because it is less irritating to veins. For rapid correction of hypocalcemia, one or two ampules of calcium gluconate can be given by a slow intravenous push, not to exceed 10 mL in 1 minute. Continuous intravenous infusion of calcium can then be given until oral therapy can be instituted. Five ampules of calcium gluconate (450 mg of calcium) are added to 500 mL of 5% dextrose in water. This is administered by continuous infusion at a rate of 300 to 600 mg of calcium daily. For patients who develop mild hypocalcemia in an early postoperative period, rapid correction of serum calcium is not needed.

When the patient is able to take oral medications, calcium and vitamin D supplementation should begin. Oral therapy is begun with 5 to 10 grams of calcium carbonate (2 to 4 grams of elemental calcium) daily and 0.5 µg per day of calcitriol (Rocaltrol). The authors attempt to keep the serum calcium level in the range of 8 to 9 mg per dL. Resolution of hypoparathyroidism is determined by normal serum phosphate, calcium, and PTH levels. If the hypoparathyroidism does not resolve within 2 months of surgery, long-term therapy for hypoparathyroidism should be started.

Chronic Hypoparathyroidism

Patients with chronic hypoparathyroidism rarely present with symptoms of severe hypocalcemia requiring acute therapy. Usually these patients present with abnormal laboratory tests and mild to moderate neuromuscular symptoms. After the diagnosis is confirmed, therapy is begun with oral calcium supplements and vitamin D. The objective of therapy is to increase calcium levels to the lower part of the normal range (8.5 to 9.0 mg per dL), thereby alleviating symptoms and complications of hypocalcemia without substantially increasing the risk of nephrocalcinosis or ectopic calcification.

Calcium intake should be maintained at 2000 to 4000 mg daily. Often this cannot be accomplished with dietary means alone but requires a calcium supplement. The common supplements are listed in Table 3. Calcium carbonate is used most commonly. It is a more efficient source of calcium than is calcium lactate or calcium gluconate and is much less expensive than calcium citrate. Calcium carbonate is also a weak phosphate binder and may be helpful in controlling the serum phosphate levels. Some patients develop gastrointestinal distress from increased gas production with calcium carbonate. These symptoms can be lessened by switching to another calcium salt.

Serum calcium concentrations in patients with hypoparathyroidism are dependent on calcium intake and absorption because they lack the normal feedback regulatory system. It is important that calcium intake be consistent from day to day. Calcium supplements should be taken throughout the day in several small doses. The authors usually give 20% of the daily calcium dose with each of three meals. The additional 40% of the dose is given at bedtime because the interval between bedtime and breakfast is the longest.

Vitamin D supplementation is also required to sustain serum calcium levels. Ergocalciferol (vitamin D_2) is the common form of vitamin D supplementation. The onset of action is slower than other forms of vitamin D (see Table 2), but it is the least expensive. In patients with mild hypoparathyroidism (serum calcium levels 7.5 to 8.5 mg per dL), 1.25 mg of ergocalciferol three times weekly is an appropriate starting dose. For patients with more severe disease, doses of 1.25 to 5 mg daily may be required. Rarely serum calcium concentrations cannot be normalized with calcium and ergocalciferol. In these patients and those with renal insufficiency, calcitriol (Rocaltrol) therapy must be used in doses of 0.5 to 3.0 µg daily. Calcitriol bypasses renal and hepatic hydroxylation. It has a more rapid onset of action and shorter half-life than does ergocalciferol. Monitoring must be done more frequently with calcitriol treatment given its short half-life and rapidity of change in serum calcium levels.

Some patients have hypercalciuria (urine calcium excretion >300 mg a day) while on therapy to normalize serum calcium levels. They may be at greater risk of nephrocalcinosis and irreversible renal damage. Addition of thiazide diuretics can decrease the hypercalciuria while improving or stabilizing serum calcium levels. Hydrochlorothiazide, 25 mg twice daily, and chlorthalidone,

TABLE 3. **Characteristics of Common Calcium Supplements**

Common Brand Name	Type of Calcium	No. of Tablets = 1000 mg	Side Effects	Cost for 1000 mg
Tums	Calcium carbonate	5	GI distress	$0.20
OsCal	Calcium carbonate	2	GI distress	$0.24
CitraCal	Calcium citrate	5		$0.37
Rugby Calcium Tablets	Calcium gluconate and lactate	22		$1.90

Abbreviation: GI = gastrointestinal.

25 to 50 mg once daily, are usually used. Thiazide administration decreases the dose requirement for vitamin D in many patients. The authors reserve thiazide therapy for those patients not optimally controlled on calcium and vitamin D therapy.

Pregnancy

Treatment of the uncommon patient who has hypoparathyroidism and becomes pregnant is challenging. Overtreatment with calcium and vitamin D can result in increased ionized calcium levels in both the mother and the fetus. This can suppress fetal parathyroid gland development and lead to transient or permanent hypocalcemia from hypoparathyroidism. Undertreatment of the mother results in maternal and fetal hypocalcemia and subsequent hyperplasia of the fetal parathyroid glands. Close monitoring of maternal serum calcium levels during pregnancy can help avoid these problems. Serum calcium levels should be maintained between 8.5 and 9.5 mg per dL. This can be done by maintaining the prepartum dose of vitamin D and altering calcium intakes. In the first two trimeseters, elemental calcium intakes often need to be increased by 500 to 1000 mg daily over their standard intake. During the third trimester, when placental calcitriol synthesis increases, calcium intakes are reduced to 500 to 1000 mg daily less than their prepartum intakes. The responses to changes in therapy are measured monthly by checking serum calcium levels.

Other Therapies

Autotransplantation of parathyroid tissue is recommended in patients undergoing extensive or repeat neck explorations. This helps prevent postoperative hypoparathyroidism in those patients. The tissue is usually transplanted to the sternocleidomastoid muscle or into muscle pockets in the forearm, making future removal relatively easy. Transplantation of cryopreserved parathyroid tissue can also be performed, but the success rate is only 60% compared with 90% with fresh autotransplanted tissue.

PTH may soon be available for use in treatment of hypoparathyroid patients. It is currently available only as an injection, but other forms may become available. The role for PTH in the management of patients with hypoparathyroidism is limited because most patients are easily treated with oral calcium and vitamin D supplementation.

Monitoring Therapy

Careful monitoring is necessary to prevent the complications of therapy, specifically hypercalcemia and hypercalciuria. During the initiation of therapy, serum calcium levels are checked every 4 to 8 weeks. More frequent monitoring is necessary with patients receiving shorter acting vitamin D metabolites (see Table 2). After serum calcium levels are in the desired range, measurement of urinary calcium excretion becomes important. If values exceed 400 mg daily, adjustment of oral calcium intake or the addition of thiazide therapy is indicated.

If hypercalcemia develops during therapy, the dose of vitamin D or its metabolite should be decreased. With long-acting vitamin D, ergocalciferol, calcium supplementation may need to be held while the level of vitamin D in the body slowly decreases. Patients taking shorter acting vitamin D metabolites can be changed to a lower dose and experience a more rapid resolution of the hypercalcemia. Vitamin D toxicity should be avoided because it can precipitate renal insufficiency.

After patients are stabilized on a replacement regimen, their serum and urine calcium levels are checked every 6 to 12 months. Patients need to be educated to avoid volume depletion and to seek medical attention if they experience nausea, vomiting, or diarrhea. Changes in medications should prompt a repeat evaluation of calcium metabolism. Use of thiazide diuretics increases serum calcium, whereas loop diuretics can decrease it. Glucocorticoids can blunt the effect of vitamin D and lead to lower serum calcium levels. Anticonvulsants, cholesterol-binding resins, excess thyroid hormone, and some antibiotics (especially rifampin) increase the degradation of vitamin D and increase vitamin D requirements. Renal function must also be assessed annually. If deterioration in renal function is noted, careful re-evaluation of therapy for hypoparathyroidism is necessary.

Pseudohypoparathyroidism

Pseudohypoparathyroidism refers to a group of disorders characterized by end-organ resistance to PTH. Patients present with hypocalcemia and hyperphosphatemia. In contrast to patients with true hypoparathyroidism, serum PTH levels are elevated. The diagnosis of pseudohypoparathyroidism must be distinguished from disorders of vitamin D metabolism. Both are associated with hypocalcemia and elevated PTH levels. Patients with pseudohypoparathyroidism also have hyperphosphatemia. The treatment of pseudohypoparathyroidism is the same as that of true hypoparathyroidism.

PRIMARY ALDOSTERONISM

method of
SAMI T. AZAR, M.D.
American University of Beirut
Beirut, Lebanon

and

JAMES C. MELBY, M.D.
Boston University School of Medicine
Boston, Massachusetts

Primary aldosteronism is a disorder in which chronic aldosterone excess exists independently or semi-independently of the renin angiotensin system. Aldosterone overproduction results in hypertension, potassium and magnesium depletion, and suppression of plasma renin activity. Estimates of the incidence of primary aldosteronism in the hypertensive population of the United States vary from 0.05% to as high as 2%. The most common adrenal lesion responsible for primary aldosteronism is a solitary adrenocortical adenoma (aldosterone-producing adenoma [APA]) and is responsible for 55 to 60% of cases. Bilateral micronodular or macronodular hyperplasia, also called idiopathic hyperaldosteronism (IHA), accounts for the bulk of the remainder of the cases. Hypersecretion of aldosterone is semiautonomous in most patients with primary aldosteronism with the exceptions of patients with glucocorticoid-suppressible aldosteronism (GSA) and patients with "renin-responsive APA," who are responsive to angiotensin II. A rare subset of patients with primary aldosteronism was recently described, and it consists of patients with primary adrenocortical hyperplasia (PAH), which is unilateral and biochemically behaves similar to APA. Various causes of primary hyperaldosteronism are listed in Table 1.

SCREENING

Screening for primary aldosteronism is usually triggered by finding spontaneous hypokalemia and easily provokable hypokalemia in a hypertensive patient. The

TABLE 1. Causes of Primary Hyperaldosteronism

Aldosterone-Producing Adenoma (APA)
Autonomous
Renin-responsive APA
Adrenocortical Hyperplasia
Idiopathic hyperaldosteronism
Glucocorticoid-suppressible aldosteronism
Primary adrenocortical hyperplasia
Aldosterone-Producing Adrenal Cancer
Ectopic: Ovarian Arrhenoblastoma

hypertension of primary aldosteronism is indistinguishable from that of other disorders. Spontaneous hypokalemia is observed in 80 to 90% of patients with primary aldosteronism, and easily provokable hypokalemia occurs in the remainder. "Easily provokable hypokalemia" refers to hypokalemia induced by the administration of large amounts of sodium chloride for a period of 3 to 5 days. More than 50% of hypertensive patients with spontaneous hypokalemia have primary aldosteronism. In many instances, hypokalemia is the result of treatment with diuretic intake. Thus, if a patient who is taking potassium-wasting diuretics is suspected to have hypokalemia secondary to hyperaldosteronism, the diuretics need to be discontinued for 10 to 14 days and the serum potassium concentration remeasured. A substantial proportion of patients with spontaneous hypokalemia have no symptoms, but marked hypokalemia may be associated with cramps, weakness, polyuria, polydipsia, nocturia, or palpitation. Abnormal glucose tolerance is demonstrable in more than half of the patients and non–insulin dependent diabetes mellitus can be precipitated in patients with genetic susceptibility.

DIAGNOSIS

To establish the diagnosis of primary aldosteronism, diuretic administration should be discontinued for at least 4 weeks, and spironolactone should be withheld for 6 weeks. Antihypertensive sympathetic inhibitors should also be discontinued 1 week before the patient is studied.

The easiest way to evaluate suspected primary aldosteronism is to admit the patient to the hospital. During the week before admission, the patient is allowed unrestricted sodium intake. During the hospitalization, the patient is given a diet containing more than 120 mEq of sodium daily. During the first day of hospitalization, potassium deficit is replaced, and the patient is kept recumbent overnight. The following morning supine (8 A.M.) and 4-hour upright (noon) plasma aldosterone, plasma renin activity, and 18-OH-corticosterone levels are measured; 24-hour urine collection (8 A.M.) for aldosterone and tetrahydroaldosterone is started and then completed on the third day (8 A.M.).

All forms of primary aldosteronism can be diagnosed by the demonstration of inappropriately elevated blood aldosterone concentration, 24-hour urinary aldosterone metabolite (tetrahydroaldosterone) excretion in the presence of suppressed plasma renin activity, or both. The tests are diagnostic with the patient both recumbent and erect. Once the diagnosis of primary aldosteronism is established, the adrenal lesion must be identified and localized.

To distinguish between unilateral and bilateral adrenal disease, and to localize unilateral APA, one can use a variety of tests. Table 2 lists these tests and their approximate accuracy. The authors advocate adrenal computed tomography (CT) scanning or magnetic resonance imaging (MRI) as first-line diagnostic tests for the detection of APA. APA, however, generally measures less than 2 cm in greatest diameter; such lesions are often difficult to visualize by CT and MRI scanning.

Measurements of plasma aldosterone levels at 8 A.M. in the supine position and after 4 hours in upright posture at noon can differentiate APA from IHA in 90% of patients. In patients with APA, plasma aldosterone levels at noon are significantly lower than those at 8 A.M. In comparison, patients with IHA exhibit a rise in plasma aldosterone concentration. 18-Hydroxycorticosterone levels are in excess of 100 μg/dL in APA and less in patients with IHA.

Adrenal imaging with iodocholesterol (^{131}I-6β-iodmethyl-19-nor-cholesterol) (NP-59) gives a functional assessment of this disorder and accurately localized APA in more than 90% of patients. Adrenal scanning is usually performed, after dexamethasone pretreatment to reduce nonadenomatous uptake of isotope. Asymmetrical localization is consistent with APA, and no lateralization is observed in IHA.

Bilateral adrenal venous sampling of aldosterone is the most accurate test in the differential diagnosis of primary aldosteronism. The accuracy of comparative adrenal venous aldosterone levels in confirming either APA or IHA exceeds 90%. Normal adrenal venous aldosterone concentration is between 100 and 400 ng/dL. In APA, the ipsilateral adrenal venous aldosterone concentration is between 1000 and 10,000 ng/dL; more importantly, the ratio of ipsilateral to contralateral aldosterone concentration is usually greater than 10:1. The accuracy of catheter placement can be best evaluated by obtaining simultaneous adrenocorticotropic hormone (ACTH)–stimulated, selective adrenal venous cortisol levels. An aldosterone ratio greater than 10:1 in the presence of a symmetrical ACTH-induced corti-

sol response is diagnostic of an APA. An algorithm for determining the cause of primary aldosteronism is shown in Figure 1.

Patients with "renin-responsive-APAs" behave as though they have idiopathic aldosteronism (IHA), in that, with the erect posture studies, the aldosterone levels rise rather than fall. Furthermore, there are slight increments in plasma renin activity in this condition. As such, the postural aldosterone response cannot be relied on in all cases to distinguish APA (the renin-responsive variety) from IHA.

Patients with "primary adrenal glomerulosa hyperplasia" (PAH) exhibit the features of APA in terms of postural response and 18-hydroxycorticosterone excess.

GSA is characterized by sustained activation of aldosterone secretion and by absence of or reduced aldosterone secretion by angiotensin II. If this disease entity is suspected in a patient with a family history of primary aldosteronism, serum 18-Oxo-cortisol and 18-hydroxycortisol should be measured because they are reported to be increased. These patients do not exhibit a postural response in terms of aldosterone secretory activity. Confirmation of this diagnosis is obtained by demonstration of dexamethasone suppressibility of hypertension.

TREATMENT

The standard treatment of APA, "renin-responsive APA," and PAH is surgical, whereas that of IHA and GSA is medical.

Aldosterone-Producing Adenoma

The treatment for patients with APA (or "renin-responsive APA" and PAH) is surgical removal of the adenoma and the ipsilateral adrenal gland. Poor surgical candidates may be treated medically (see IHA therapy). A posterior surgical approach is associated with few complications and is now the procedure of choice.

Preoperatively patients should be treated with a low-sodium diet, potassium-sparing diuretics, and possibly an antihypertensive agent to control the hypokalemia and hypertension. Few patients may develop hypoaldosteronism after the surgery owing to inadequate function of the contralateral adrenal. During the following 3 to 6 months, awaiting full recovery of the adrenal gland, the patient should be monitored carefully for symptoms and signs of hypovolemia. 9-α-Fluorohydrocortisone* should not be given because it can further suppress and delay the recovery of the adrenal glomerulosa.

Approximately 95% of patients with APA who undergo adrenalectomy become normotensive and normokalemic in the first 3 to 6 months after surgery. Over the next 2 to 3 years, however, ap-

TABLE 2. **Distinction of Aldosterone-Producing Adenoma and Primary Adrenocortical Hyperplasia from Idiopathic Hyperaldosteronism**

	Accuracy (%)
Adrenal CT and MRI scans	75
Posture study	
Aldosterone rise in IHA	} 85
Anomalous aldosterone fall in APA and PAH	
18-OH-corticosterone >100 μg/dL in APA and PAH	80
Adrenal iodoscintigraphy	70
Adrenal venous aldosterone sampling	95

Abbreviations: CT = computed tomography; MRI = magnetic resonance imaging; IHA = idiopathic hyperaldosteronism; APA = aldosterone-producing adenoma; PAH = primary adrenocortical hyperplasia.

*Not available in the United States.

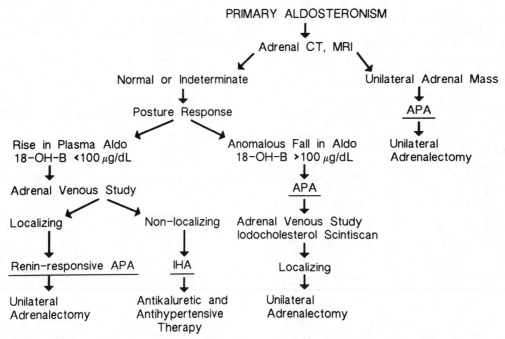

Figure 1. Algorithm for determining the cause of primary aldosteronism. *Abbreviations*: CT = computed tomography; MRI = magnetic resonance imaging; APA = aldosterone-producing adenoma; IHA = idiopathic hyperaldosteronism; Aldo = aldosterone; 18-OH-B = hydroxycorticosterone.

proximately 20 to 25% re-develop hypertension, which is easier to control and is not associated with hypokalemia.

Idiopathic Hyperaldosteronism

To conserve potassium and to lower the blood pressure, patients should be placed on a less than 100-mEq sodium diet. The low-salt diet provides less sodium for exchange with potassium in the distal renal tubule, and mild volume contraction secondary to a low-sodium diet may lead to a decrease in blood pressure. Compliance with a low-sodium diet can be monitored by obtaining a 12-hour urine sample for sodium and creatinine.

Treatment with a potassium-sparing diuretic should be initiated after the diagnostic work-up is completed. Amiloride and spironolactone are considered first-line agents.

Amiloride (Midamor), a non–aldosterone antagonist potassium-sparing diuretic, acts on the distal tubules to block sodium channels in a mineralocorticoid-independent manner. Thus, sodium and chloride excretion increases, whereas potassium excretion decreases. It is available only as 5-mg tablets. The initial dose is 10 mg a day and may be increased at 5-mg intervals up to 40 mg daily. Concurrent potassium supplementation should be avoided because amiloride can increase potassium level, and potassium supplementation may potentially cause hyperkalemia. Gastroin-

testinal disturbances, headaches, mild increase in blood urea nitrogen and uric acid levels, and rarely impotence are among the few side effects of amiloride.

Spironolactone (Aldactone), a competitive antagonist for the mineralocorticoid receptor, is available as 25-, 50-, and 100-mg tablets. The initial dose is 50 mg daily, and it can be increased in increments of 100 mg at 1- or 2-week intervals up to 300 to 400 mg a day. Hypokalemia may respond promptly, but hypertension may take 1 to 2 months to be controlled. The majority of patients become normotensive and normokalemic with spironolactone therapy. The blood pressure and serum potassium level should be monitored closely, and the dose should be titrated based on the potassium level and the blood pressure response. After several months of therapy, spironolactone dose may be reduced to as low as 50 to 100 mg daily. Concurrent potassium supplementation should be avoided because spironolactone alone can increase potassium level by 1.5 to 2 mEq, and potassium supplementation may cause hyperkalemia. Fewer than 20% of patients develop side effects with spironolactone. It decreases testosterone biosynthesis and blocks androgen action, producing menstrual irregularities in women and decreased libido, impotence, and gynecomastia in men. This suggests that this drug may not be considered as a first-line agent in men. Gastrointestinal disturbances can occur with spironolactone treatment and can be minimized if the drug is taken with meals. Drug interaction should be monitored because spironolactone may increase digoxin half-life, and salicylates may interfere with tubular secretion of one active spironolactone metabolite.

Triamterene (Dyrenium), independently of aldosterone, directly affects tubular transport and inhibits potassium excretion. A combination of triamterene and hydrochlorothiazide (Dyazide) has been tried but is much less effective than amiloride or spironolactone in reversing potassium depletion.

For resistant hypokalemia, rather than potassium supplementation, a combination of amiloride and spironolactone may restore the potassium balance. Because spironolactone and amiloride exert their effects by different mechanisms, one should expect synergistic effect on serum potassium. Only a few patients, however, require this regimen to control hypertension, and if the blood pressure is not controlled with one potassium-sparing diuretic, the patient may have renal damage secondary to the long-standing hypertension. If the hypertension secondary to IHA is inadequately controlled with a potassium-sparing agent alone, angiotensin-converting enzyme inhibitors, calcium channel blockers, or thiazide diuretics may be effective if added to the therapeutic regimen. In these patients, converting enzyme inhibitors, such as captopril (Capoten), enalapril (Vasotec), lisinopril (Prinivil, Zestril), and fosinopril (Monopril), are good first choices. They decrease aldosterone secretion and improve blood pressure and potassium level. Calcium channel blockers decrease aldosterone levels in isolated glomerulosa cells and have been used with varying success in treating primary aldosteronism.

Because of the hypothesis that aldosterone production is under tonic dopaminergic inhibition and that there may exist a pituitary aldosterone-stimulating hormone under serotoninergic stimulation, bromocriptine (Parlodel), a dopamine agonist, and cyproheptadine (Periactin), an antiserotoninergic agent, were tested and found to be ineffective in treating primary aldosteronism. Potential new drugs that exploit the ability of atrial natriuretic factor to inhibit aldosterone secretion may prove useful in the future.

For unknown reasons, bilateral adrenalectomy, despite correcting the biochemical abnormalities in patients with bilateral adrenal hyperplasia, is generally ineffective in reversing hypertension, with fewer than 15% of patients becoming normotensive after surgery. In almost every instance, blood pressure falls but not enough to eliminate the need for antihypertensive therapy. In addition, these patients face the problem of adrenal insufficiency. For such little benefit, the need for permanent cortisol and fludrocortisone replacement therapy seems hardly worth it.

Glucocorticoid-Suppressible Aldosteronism

Long-term treatment with physiologic doses of glucocorticoid corrects the hypertension and hyopkalemia of GSA. Rarely large doses of glucocorticoids are required. To avoid the complications associated with long-term steroid administration, GSA may need to be treated in the same way as IHA.

HYPOPITUITARISM

method of
ROBERT J. ANDERSON, M.D.
Creighton University School of Medicine
Omaha, Nebraska

Hypopituitarism implies the loss of one or more of the clinically important pituitary hormones. These include growth hormone (GH), adrenocorticotropic hormone (ACTH), thyroid-stimulating hormone (TSH), follicle-stimulating hormone (FSH), luteinizing hormone (LH), prolactin, and antidiuretic hormone (ADH). The clinical picture of hypopituitarism is often one of a gradual cumulative loss of hormones with increasing debility, but the presentation can be widely variable. A man may have the inexorable onset of fatigue, weakness, decreased libido, impotence, and finally pressure symptoms of headache and visual disturbance associated with an expanding pituitary tumor. Soft, pale, waxy skin with fine facial wrinkles and female body habitus may suggest the diagnosis. Progression may be rapid and dramatic in pituitary apoplexy. Isolated loss of a hormone occurs less frequently. If it is found, care should be exercised to avoid missing progression to a multihormone deficiency. In the setting of large functioning tumors, such as GH-secreting or glycoprotein-secreting adenomas, other pituitary hormone deficiencies should be sought. Common causes of hypopituitarism are pituitary adenoma, craniopharyngioma, traumatic injury, pituitary surgery, irradiation, ischemic necrosis, infiltrative disease, and autoimmune disease (Table 1). Loss of posterior pituitary ADH is not as frequent and suggests pituitary stalk or hypothalamic disease (see the article "Diabetes Insipidus").

There are several guidelines for treatment of hypopituitarism. Hormone deficiency should be documented by baseline testing and further stimulation testing if necessary. The clinical picture is usually one of an endocrine target gland deficiency (for example, low thyroxine) without the corresponding increase in pituitary hormone (a "normal" or low TSH). Except for GH and ADH, hormone replacement is with the target hormones (such as L-thyroxine) because they are less expensive, they can be given orally rather than parenterally, and they are not immunogenic. Finally, even

TABLE 1. **Causes of Hypopituitarism**

Tumors
  Pituitary adenomas—functioning plus nonfunctioning
  Craniopharyngioma
Pituitary Surgery
Traumatic Injury
Infarction/Vascular
  Ischemic necrosis
  Sheehan's syndrome (postpartum pituitary necrosis),
    diabetes mellitus, sickle cell disease
  Pituitary apoplexy—necrosis of tumor
Radiation of Pituitary
  Usually gradual and progressive
Infiltrative and Infectious Diseases
  Sarcoidosis
  Hemochromatosis
  Meningitis
  Tuberculosis
Autoimmune
  Lymphocytic hypophysitis
Idiopathic
Iatrogenic
  Discontinuation of exogenous glucocorticoid treatment or
    inadequate glucocorticoid coverage during stress in
    patients on long-term or intermittent glucocorticoids by
    any route

though the replacement schedules are frequently the same as treatments for primary endocrine deficiencies, follow-up monitoring is not as ideal because the feedback response of the pituitary is lost. Specific treatments are detailed in this article.

GROWTH HORMONE

Diagnosis

GH deficiency in the adult patient only is discussed. The author's practice is to document GH deficiency by demonstrating failure to respond to two separate stimulation tests, such as insulin hypoglycemia (contraindicated in patients with coronary artery disease, seizure disorders, or cerebrovascular insufficiency), L-dopa, or clonidine. Recently hypothalamic GH-releasing hormone (GHRH) sermorelin acetate (Geref) has become available. GHRH is given intravenously and allows a less stressful method for detection of GH response. Insulin-like growth factor-I (IGF-I) (somatomedin-C) provides an averaged indication of GH presence and is a helpful ancillary test. It is important to differentiate a decline in GH secretion signaled by low IGF-I levels in the aging patient from a true GH deficiency.

Treatment

Current practice is not to replace GH in GH-deficient adults. Fascinating recent studies call this approach into question both in pituitary GH-deficient adults and in aging adults with low IGF-I levels owing to decreased GH secretion. Hypo-

pituitary patients experience premature mortality due to cardiovascular disease. Metabolic sequelae associated with the lack of GH may contribute. Subjects treated with GH have an improved sense of well-being and quality of life, increased muscle strength, decreased body fat, increased lean body mass, and a slight increase in spinal bone density. Because of the expense of the recombinant GH preparations and uncertainty about the proper dosage schedule, the use of GH is not yet approved. Treatment of GH-deficient hypopituitary adults and older adults with low IGF-I levels without hypopituitarism is under investigation. Benefits and treatment protocols must be defined clearly because of the adverse effects of decreased glucose tolerance, acromegaly, and cardiovascular complications that occur with excessive doses of GH.

ADRENOCORTICOTROPIC HORMONE

Diagnosis

The diagnosis of secondary adrenal insufficiency is important because this condition is life-threatening. General malaise, fatigue, hypotension, and lack of skin pigmentation are suggestive findings. A careful history is useful to detect exogenous glucocorticoid administration and subsequent interruption of treatment. Exogenous glucocorticoid suppression of the hypothalamic-pituitary-adrenal axis is the most common cause of secondary adrenal insufficiency. The usual findings in secondary hypoadrenalism are a low or "normal" ACTH level (0 to 50 pg/mL) in association with a serum cortisol level of less than 10 µg/dL in the morning or during severe stress. The patient may present in an acute crisis with cardiovascular collapse. A serum cortisol level of less than 20 µg/dL in this situation is highly suggestive. To evaluate any patient suspected of secondary adrenal insufficiency, a rapid adrenocortical screen with the synthetic ACTH cosyntropin (Cortrosyn) usually shows a less than adequate response (cortisol <20 µg/dL at 30 minutes). A normal response does not exclude secondary (pituitary) adrenal insufficiency. The use of insulin-induced hypoglycemia or metyrapone testing to demonstrate lack of cortisol response associated with low ACTH is often not necessary. If the patient has already been treated with glucocorticoids and the clinical picture is not clear, the use of a 1- to 3-day intravenous ACTH infusion documents the presence of adrenal function.

Treatment

The major goal in treatment is to restore normalcy by attempting to reproduce the diurnal rhythm of cortisol production with a glucocorticoid preparation, not ACTH. The author prefers cortisone acetate, 25 mg in the morning and 12.5 mg in the late afternoon, or prednisone, 5 mg in the morning and 2.5 mg in the late afternoon. Hydrocortisone at a dose of 20 mg in the morning and 10 mg in the late afternoon can also be used. The author avoids longer acting preparations, such as dexamethasone, because of the higher occurrence of exogenous Cushing's syndrome and lack of mineralocorticoid effect. A mineralocorticoid preparation is not required in most cases because the renin-angiotensin system should be intact. How do we know how much is enough? There are no precise laboratory means for following this. The best route is to follow the blood pressure, serum electrolytes, and clinical examination and history. The peripheral tissue response is helpful. Occasional patients become cushingoid on the estimated doses and require a smaller, twice-per-day dose or a once-per-day dose. In some situations, the afternoon dose has to be given earlier or later in the day to allow the patient to function as normally as possible.

The glucocorticoids may unmask underlying mild diabetes insipidus in some patients. The author makes certain that the patient understands the need to increase the dose during sick days. Each patient receives a detailed sheet that lists how to adjust the medicine. The patient should double the dose during the 1 to 3 days of a moderate illness such as the "flu" with a low-grade fever (≤100°F) and triple the dose if fever (>100°F) is present. Patients are given prefilled syringes with injectable dexamethasone (Decadron phosphate, 4 mg per mL in 2.5-mL disposable syringe) to use if they are vomiting and cannot get to medical care quickly. Patients administer one half the dose intramuscularly (5 mg) and repeat if necessary every 8 to 12 hours before arriving at the hospital. Patients must get a medical information bracelet or necklace that details their need for cortisol (Medic Alert Foundation International, P.O. Box 1009, Turlock, California 95381-1009; telephone 1-800-344-3226).

Glucocorticoid coverage for surgery and stressful procedures is essentially the same for primary and secondary adrenal insufficiency. The author gives a depot of 100 mg hydrocortisone sodium succinate (Solu-Cortef) intramuscularly on call to surgery and then 50 to 100 mg hydrocortisone intravenously every 6 hours (starting in surgery) the first 24 hours. The dose is decreased by 50% each day as indicated by patient progress until the oral glucocorticoid can be resumed. A preparation of prednisolone (Hydeltrasol) can be used. Prednisolone, 40 mg intramuscularly, is given on call, then 20 to 40 mg every 8 hours is given intravenously for the first 24 hours. The dose is

tapered to 50% of the previous day's dose as tolerated and given every 8 to 12 hours until oral glucocorticoids can be used. Treatment of acute adrenal insufficiency requires intravenous glucocorticoid (Solu-Cortef), 50 to 100 mg every 6 hours; dextrose and saline intravenous fluids; and aggressive review to define the precipitating event (see the article "Adrenocortical Insufficiency").

THYROID-STIMULATING HORMONE

Diagnosis

Patients are clinically hypothyroid but often not as severely myxedematous as patients with primary hypothyroidism. Clinical hypothyroidism with the finding of a low free or total thyroxine (T_4) and a low or "normal" TSH gives the diagnosis of secondary (central) hypothyroidism (for our purposes, this includes hypothalamic hypothyroidism). An absent or blunted response of TSH to intravenous thyrotropin-releasing hormone (TRH) (protirelin [Relefact]) is of limited usefulness because it occurs in only 21% of patients with central hypothyroidism.

Treatment

The great advances that have occurred in titrating thyroid hormone replacement doses with more sensitive TSH assays are lost in hypopituitary patients. In replacement therapy of primary hypothyroidism, our goal is to keep the TSH within the normal range. With this measurement lost in hypopituitary patients, it is best to follow the free T_4 and maintain it within the normal range. The author uses synthetic L-thyroxine (Synthroid, Levothroid, Levoxine) for replacement. Triiodothyronine (Cytomel) is not desirable for long-term replacement because of its short half-life.

A general estimate for thyroxine replacement is 1.6 to 1.8 µg per kg per day. The target final dose is 100 to 125 µg per day in individuals younger than 60 years of age and 75 to 100 µg per day in individuals older than age 60. Variations in requirements occur, and individualization of the dose is necessary. In patients younger than 60 years of age in good health with a short duration of hypothyroidism, the author usually starts at 50 to 75 µg per day and increases by 25-µg increments every 6 to 8 weeks to normalize the free T_4 level. Younger patients may be given the full estimated daily dose without adverse effects. In patients older than age 60, patients with prolonged hypothyroidism (longer than 6 months), and patients with known ischemic heart disease, the author starts with 25 µg per day to avoid aggravation of cardiac disease. The author increases the dose by 25 μg in 4 weeks if there are no adverse symptoms and then increases by 25-μg increments every 6 to 8 weeks until the free T_4 level is normal. The patient is then followed every 6 to 12 months to maintain a normal level. Chronic overreplacement should be avoided to prevent potential accelerated bone loss.

If the thyroid status is not clear from free T_4 measurements, the thyroid hormone–sensitive proteins angiotensin-converting enzyme (ACE) and sex hormone–binding globulin (SHBG) may provide an indirect peripheral measure of T_4 effect. Both increase with elevated thyroid hormone levels. Care is taken to replace cortisol beforehand or concomitantly to avoid precipitating an adrenal crisis with increased metabolic demands of thyroid hormone replacement.

GONADOTROPINS

Diagnosis

Because both LH and FSH are secreted from the gonadotrope, these glycoproteins are usually lost in tandem. The classic presentation in the adult is hypogonadotropic hypogonadism with low or "normal" LH and FSH and low gonadal steroid levels (testosterone in men, estradiol in women). Both men and women experience loss of libido, decline in secondary sex characteristics, and decreased bone density. Women are amenorrheic. Men are impotent. In true deficiency states, there are minimal or absent responses of LH and FSH to multiple intravenous doses of gonadotropin-releasing hormone (GnRH) (gonadorelin [Factrel]). In men and in postmenopausal women, the loss of LH and FSH may be sequential after the loss of GH and may be clinically silent until a pituitary adenoma expands to cause symptomatic defects and compression.

Treatment

Women

Replacement therapy with the gonadal steroid is required in premenopausal women. Premenopausal women with a uterus are given a full schedule to allow menstruation. The author uses oral conjugated estrogens (Premarin) at 0.625 to 1.25 mg per day on days 1 to 25 with medroxyprogesterone (Provera, Amen, Cycrin), 5 to 10 mg per day, added from days 16 to 25. Five to 6 days are allowed for menses. Alternative treatments include oral ethinyl estradiol (Estinyl), 5 to 20 μg per day; oral estradiol (Estrace), 1 to 2 mg per day; or a transdermal system (Estraderm), 0.05- to 0.1-mg patches two times each week on days 1 to 25, in conjunction with medroxyprogesterone

as noted on days 16 to 25. Pregnancy can be attained after induction of ovulation with human menopausal gonadotropins (menotropins [Pergonal]) followed by human chorionic gonadotropin. The procedure is beyond the scope of this article. The addition of small doses of intramuscular testosterone (enanthate or cypionate, 25 to 50 mg each month) can be considered if libido remains decreased as a result of loss of adrenal androgen production stimulated by ACTH. Side effects of acne, hirsutism, and virilization should be avoided. In hypopituitary postmenopausal women, the same considerations apply to the decision for gonadal steroid replacement as apply in a postmenopausal woman with normal pituitary function. The goal is to use hormone treatment to avoid progressive bone loss and osteoporosis without causing side effects.

Men

Replacement therapy is given to men to attempt to normalize sexual function, to maintain secondary sex characteristics, and to prevent bone resorption. It is important to tell the patient that treatment leads to progressive testicular atrophy if the hypopituitarism has not caused it already. In addition, it should be pointed out that fertility is usually lost. Treatment with pulsatile GnRH (if the defect is hypothalamic) or with human chorionic gonadotropin can be attempted to recover fertility. The usual therapy is long-term testosterone replacement. The dose and frequency of testosterone are based primarily on the patient's evaluation of improved strength, energy, libido, and sexual function. The author avoids oral methyltestosterone preparations (Virilan, Android, Metandren, Testred) because of the potential for hepatotoxicity presenting as cholestatic hepatitis, jaundice, or peliosis hepatis. The author prefers testosterone enanthate (Delatestryl) or testosterone cypionate (DEPO-Testosterone) intramuscularly every 2 weeks. This interval avoids the wide fluctuations in levels that can occur with 3- to 4-week intervals. A family member or the patient can give the injections to avoid additional cost. The author starts with 50 to 100 mg for the severely hypogonadal individual and 100 to 200 mg every 2 weeks for most other patients. The dose is individualized and may be adjusted to 300 mg based on response. Monitoring of testosterone replacement is not ideal because no appropriate LH or FSH levels are available to allow an estimate of feedback response. If testosterone levels are measured, they are done at 6 to 9 days after injection for an estimate of the peak value and at 2 weeks to determine the nadir. The goal is to keep the fluctuations of testosterone within the normal range. Problems with acceler-

TABLE 2. **Treatment of Hypopituitarism**

Hormone Lost	Treatment		Monitor
Growth hormone	Investigational in adults		Insulin-like growth factor-I Body composition
Adrenocorticotropic hormone	Cortisone acetate *or* Prednisone *or* Hydrocortisone	25 mg orally, A.M. 12.5 mg orally, P.M. 5.0 mg orally, A.M. 2.5 mg orally, P.M. 20 mg orally, A.M. 10 mg orally, P.M.	Sense of well-being, strength Avoid cushingoid changes Blood pressure, electrolytes

Thyroid-stimulating hormone	L-thyroxine	1.6–1.8 µg/kg/day
		Target dose by age:
		  <60: 100–125 µg/day
		  >60: 75–100 µg/day (may be
		    lower as age increases
			Free thyroxine
			Thyroxine-sensitive proteins
			  (ACE, SHBG) if needed
			Avoid hyperthyroid and
			  hypothyroid signs and
			  symptoms

Luteinizing hormone, follicle-stimulating hormone	*Women*—estrogens day 1–25 *or* *or* *or* *and*	Conjugated, 0.625–1.25 mg/day Estinyl estradiol, 5–20 µg/day Estradiol, 1–2 mg/day Estrogen patch, 0.05–0.1 mg 2 times/week	Menstrual cycle Libido Estrogen-sensitive tissue

	medroxyprogesterone
	    day 16–25
	Men—Intramuscular
	  testosterone ester
		5–10 mg/day
		100–200 mg every 2 weeks
			Libido
			Sexual function
			Testosterone levels in some
			  cases

Prolactin	None		Lactation

Antidiuretic hormone	DDAVP	Intranasal or subcutaneous (see
		  "Diabetes Insipidus" article)
			Thirst
			Intake and output
			Weight
			Serum sodium, urine
			  osmolality

Abbreviations: ACE = angiotensin-converting enzyme; SHBG = sex hormone–binding globulin; DDAVP = 1-deamino-(8-D-arginine)-vasopressin.

ation of benign prostatic hypertrophy, aggression, hepatotoxicity, peliosis hepatis, or polycythemia are uncommon in the author's experience with carefully monitored intramuscular replacement doses. Patients should be warned about the possible occurrence of acne, oily skin, and breast tenderness. Both scrotal and nonscrotal testosterone patches eventually may provide the best treatment when they are available. They are more convenient and provide less erratic levels of testosterone.

PROLACTIN

A well-known clinical situation in which prolactin is lost is postpartum pituitary necrosis and resultant failure of lactation (Sheehan's syndrome). Gradual progression to multihormone deficiency usually ensues. Any woman with hypopituitarism can have failure of prolactin production if pregnancy is attained. Hypoprolactinemia occurs in men, but it is detected less often. The diagnosis is made by documenting a low baseline prolactin level in the absence of any suppressing agent and the lack of prolactin response to TRH.

There is no clear clinical syndrome known in men without prolactin. The hormone may have an effect on sexual behavior, but the effect is not completely clear. Prolactin is not replaced.

ANTIDIURETIC HORMONE

Replacement of ADH is usually required to maintain normal water balance. The vasopressin analogue desmopressin (DDAVP) is used most frequently. Details are given in the article "Diabetes Insipidus."

GENERAL TREATMENT CONSIDERATIONS

Documentation of pituitary hormone loss is essential before treatment. Combined stimulation tests (TRH, GHRH, and GnRH) can be done to increase diagnostic efficiency. Glucocorticoids must be replaced first to avoid life-threatening deterioration. Cortisol is given before or with thyroid hormone to avoid precipitation of a hypoadrenal crisis. Gonadal steroids can be replaced as required. The possibilities for GH treatment will be clarified in the future. Patients can live well with total replacement, but they will be inconvenienced. A patient with panhypopituitarism may need cortisone, L-thyroxine, gonadal steroids, and desmopressin (Table 2). The dose of cortisol must be adjusted during illness. The ability to fine tune the treatment to the best levels for each individual is lacking because the feedback centers are lost. Research into sensitive tissue indicators of adequate replacement will enhance our treatment of this important group of patients.

HYPERPROLACTINEMIA

method of
ANDREW G. FRANTZ, M.D.
Columbia University College of Physicians and Surgeons
New York, New York

Hyperprolactinemia is generally recognized because of presenting symptoms such as amenorrhea, infertility, galactorrhea, or diminished libido or potency or some other condition suggestive of pituitary disease. It is frequently associated with pituitary tumors but may also have a variety of other causes (Table 1).

A complete discussion of the differential diagnosis of hyperprolactinemia is beyond the scope of this article and may be found elsewhere. Nevertheless, it is important to note that in the absence of pregnancy, a serum prolactin level of greater than 300 ng per mL is always, in the author's experience, associated with a pituitary tumor, and levels of 100 ng per mL or more are strongly suggestive of tumor. Most of the conditions listed in Table 1 are associated with relatively modest elevations of serum prolactin. Unless however, there is prompt normalization of the prolactin on withdrawal of a suspected drug or correction of the underlying disorder, such as primary hypothyroidism, however, pituitary radiography by computed tomography (CT) or magnetic resonance imaging (MRI) is indicated to rule out tumor. Occasionally no cause is found despite careful pituitary radiographic examination, and the hyperprolactinemia is labeled idiopathic. In such cases, the suspicion always exists that a small pituitary tumor may in fact be present but for some reason cannot be visualized.

Hyperprolactinemia by itself does not necessarily demand treatment because apart from its effect on gonadal function and a tendency to predispose the patient to osteopenia, there is no evidence at present that long-continued hyperprolactinemia is deleterious. The decision to treat is usually made with one of the following three aims in mind, listed in order of increasing clinical importance.

Cessation of Galactorrhea. Galactorrhea often, but not always, accompanies hyperprolactinemia. When it does, it can usually be stopped or greatly diminished by lowering the serum prolactin concentration. In many cases, however, the galactorrhea is relatively

TABLE 1. **Causes of Hyperprolactinemia**

Physiologic
Sleep
Pregnancy
Nursing
Sexual intercourse with orgasm (stress)

Pharmacologic
Estrogens
Neuroleptic agents
　Phenothiazines
　Butyrophenones
　Sulpiride*
　Pimozide
Non-neuroleptic psychoactive agents
　Clorgyline*
　Pargyline
Antihypertensives
　Alpha-methyldopa
　Reserpine
　Verapamil
Other antidopaminergic agents
　Metoclopramide
　Domperidone*
Histamine H_2-receptor antagonists
　Cimetidine
Opiates
　Morphine
　Methadone
　Pentazocine
　Heroin
Other agents
　Hypoglycemia
　Thyrotropin-releasing hormone
　Arginine

Pathologic
Prolactinoma
Acromegaly
Cushing's disease
Other neurologic conditions
　Craniopharyngioma
　Sarcoidosis
　Granulomas
　Pituitary stalk section
　Head trauma
　Empty sella syndrome
　Epileptic seizures
　Electroconvulsive seizures
Non-neurologic conditions
　Hypothyroidism (primary)
　Addison's disease
　Renal disease
　Chronic alcoholism
　Liver disease
　Chest wall injury, including mastectomy
　Polycystic ovary syndrome

*Not available in the United States.

mild. Treatment with a prolactin-lowering drug, such as bromocriptine, may not be deemed worthwhile in such cases, both because of possible side effects (see later) and because long-term treatment is likely to be necessary, with resumption of the galactorrhea whenever the drug is withdrawn.

Avoidance of Premature Osteoporosis. Hyperprolactinemia in premenopausal women has been associated with a tendency toward generalized osteopenia.

The mechanisms are not altogether clear but probably have to do with diminished estrogen secretion. It is reasonable to suppose that restoration of normal cyclic ovarian function with an increase in overall mean estrogen secretion will diminish the rate of bone loss in such patients, but compelling clinical studies to support such a conclusion are not as yet available. At present, the decision to treat or not with the aim of slowing the progression of osteoporosis must be made on an individual basis; among the factors to be taken into account are the degree of osteopenia, the age of the patient, and the time before likely menopause.

Restoration of Fertility. Hyperprolactinemia of sufficient degree is almost always associated with amenorrhea and infertility. The mechanisms may be multiple but probably involve an abnormality in the tonic or cyclic release of gonadotropin-releasing hormone. Lowering of serum prolactin level close to or within the normal range usually restores ovulatory menses and fertility. Men with prolactin-secreting tumors may experience hypogonadism, impotence, and infertility. Reduction of serum prolactin may cure the infertility, although the success rate among men is somewhat lower than among women. The use of bromocriptine to treat infertility in women with pituitary tumors is discussed in the next section.

TREATMENT

Hyperprolactinemia is found in more than 50% of all patients with pituitary tumors, making the measurement of serum prolactin useful for diagnosis as well as for evaluating the effects of therapy. In most cases, the hyperprolactinemia is due to true hypersecretion by the tumor itself, but in a minority of cases the hypersecretion may result from a nonsecretory tumor (including lesions such as craniopharyngioma) that produces hyperprolactinemia by pressure on the pituitary stalk and interference with the normal flow of prolactin-inhibiting factor (thought to be the same as dopamine) from the hypothalamus to the pituitary. Lesions in this latter category usually produce relatively modest elevations of serum prolactin. When the serum prolactin is above 250 to 300 ng per mL, a true prolactin-secreting tumor is almost always present.

For practical purposes, pituitary tumors are usually classified radiologically into microadenomas (1 cm or less in diameter) and macroadenomas (any larger tumor). Suprasellar extension is also an important consideration because it carries the risk of visual field defects owing to involvement of the optic chiasm. Four methods of dealing with tumors associated with hyperprolactinemia are currently available: (1) observation without treatment; (2) surgery; (3) radiotherapy; and (4) prolactin-lowering drugs, specifically bromocriptine.

Observation Without Treatment

As noted, hyperprolactinemia itself does not necessarily require treatment. If infertility and the other factors discussed previously are not important considerations and if the lesion on MRI or CT is a microadenoma, watchful waiting may well be the best course. Although the number of reports dealing with the long-term natural history of untreated pituitary tumors is not large, those that are available strongly suggest that most microadenomas never progress to macroadenomas. In some cases, the hyperprolactinemia may spontaneously subside over a period of months to years. Under these circumstances, the best course may be to follow the serum prolactin concentration at 6-month to yearly intervals and to perform MRI or CT scanning somewhat less frequently (i.e., at intervals of 1 to 2 years initially) and then less often if there is no change.

Surgery

Most prolactinomas can be successfully approached by the transsphenoidal route, which carries low morbidity and mortality. Transfrontal removal is usually reserved for tumors with significant suprasellar extension and involvement of the optic chiasm. Experienced neurosurgeons achieve normalization of serum prolactin in most patients with microadenomas and in those whose initial serum prolactin level is less than 200 to 250 ng per mL. With larger tumors and higher serum prolactin concentration, the cure rate is appreciably less than 50%. For the largest tumors, complete surgical removal is generally not possible.

With the revival of interest in transsphenoidal pituitary surgery in the early 1970s, spurred by improved techniques, many endocrinologists considered surgery the treatment of choice for prolactinomas. Since then, two factors have combined to limit enthusiasm for surgical therapy. One is a higher than expected incidence of long-term recurrence in patients originally considered cured. This has ranged from 17 to 91%; recurrence has most often involved hyperprolactinemia only and not re-expansion of the tumor. The second factor is the success of drug therapy, particularly bromocriptine, in shrinking prolactinomas as well as in lowering serum prolactin. With the recognition that most microadenomas do not progress to macroadenomas, surgery is used less often, because for small tumors it seems unnecessary and for large ones it is not curative. Nevertheless, there remains a window of size, ranging from the larger microadenomas to the smaller macroadenomas, in which good results can be anticipated after surgery, with avoidance of long-term drug treatment. A particular use of surgery appears to be the treatment of macroadenomas in women who wish to become pregnant. The physiologic enlargement of the pituitary that occurs during pregnancy also takes place in patients with pituitary tumors. Such patients are therefore particularly at risk for visual field compromise during gestation. Even if total removal cannot be accomplished, some debulking of the tumor is considered desirable before attempts at conception.

Radiotherapy

Radiotherapy, usually in the form of 4000 to 5000 rad delivered through multiple ports, is effective in shrinking most prolactinomas. It is also followed, in most cases, by a slow progressive fall of serum prolactin that may continue for years. Before the reintroduction of transsphenoidal surgery and the development of prolactin-lowering drugs, radiotherapy was the treatment of choice for pituitary tumors. It is now used much less, both because of the slowness in the fall of serum prolactin and because of the comparatively high incidence of eventual hypopituitarism. There is also a slight risk of other complications, including lethargy, disturbance of memory, ocular palsies, blindness, and the development of sarcoma in the path of radiation. At present, radiotherapy is reserved for larger tumors for which surgery is not feasible or has been unsuccessful and that have not shown satisfactory shrinkage with bromocriptine.

Bromocriptine and Other Prolactin-Lowering Drugs

Certain ergot derivatives, of which bromocriptine (Parlodel) was the first to be developed and is the most widely used, act as long-acting dopamine agonists and inhibit the secretion of prolactin. They are effective in reducing hyperprolactinemia whether due to tumor or some other cause. Most often, the serum prolactin level can be brought into the normal range or close enough to it to permit the restoration of ovulatory menses. A small proportion of pituitary tumors show little or no response to bromocriptine. In the typical case, serum prolactin falls rapidly (within an hour or two) and remains low as long as the drug is maintained. There is no tendency for escape, even after many months or years of treatment. Withdrawal of the drug almost always results in prompt recurrence of the hyperprolactinemia, although after long treatment the serum prolactin concentration may not always rise to its former height. Besides lowering serum prolactin, ergot derivatives also shrink the majority (75% or more) of prolactin-secreting tumors. Shrinkage may begin within hours of starting the drug and is usually evident, if it is going to occur, within 2 to 4 weeks. Some tumors, particularly large ones associated with severe hyperprolactinemia, may go on shrinking for months or years with continued treatment. Some degree of tumor re-expansion may occur when treatment is stopped; it may occur rapidly after relatively brief therapy if the initial shrinkage has been rapid but tends to occur much more slowly after long-continued treatment. The degree of serum prolactin reduction is not a reliable index of the degree of tumor shrinkage. Major reduction in serum prolactin may occur with little or no change in tumor size, although failure to decline significantly usually means that tumor shrinkage will not occur.

Nausea is the most common side effect of bromocriptine, occurring in at least a third of patients but usually wearing off with continued treatment. It is sufficient to force discontinuation of the drug in 10 to 15% of patients. Postural hypotension may occur after the first or second dose of bromocriptine but rarely thereafter. Other side effects include nasal stuffiness, constipation, and, more rarely, digital vasospasm, cardiac arrhythmias, and psychosis. Bromocriptine antagonizes neuroleptic agents, such as phenothiazines and butyrophenones, and is contraindicated in patients who require those drugs.

To minimize side effects, bromocriptine is usually begun at a small dose and then increased. A typical regimen is 1.25 mg (one-half tablet) at bedtime accompanied by food. After a day or two, this is increased to 1.25 mg twice a day and then gradually to a maintenance level by increasing the dose at 3- to 7-day intervals. To minimize nausea, all doses are usually taken with food. The maintenance dose for most patients is 7.5 mg per day (2.5 mg three times a day) and ranges between 5 and 15 mg per day. Serum prolactin should be measured between 2 and 6 hours after the last dose because suppression may begin to wane after 8 hours. The only other prolactin-lowering drug available in the United States is pergolide (Permax). Its actions and side effects are similar to those of bromocriptine, but its longer duration of action permits once-a-day rather than three times a day dosage in most patients. It is roughly 100 times as potent as bromocriptine on a weight basis, 0.1 mg of pergolide being approximately equal to 5 to 10 mg of bromocriptine. Although currently approved only for the treatment of Parkinson's disease in the United States, pergolide has undergone extensive clinical trials, both in the United States and in Europe, for the treatment of prolactinomas, with a success rate approximately equal to that of bromocriptine. Occasionally one of these two drugs may prove superior to the other in a given patient because of greater reduction of serum prolactin or lesser side effects at a therapeutically effective dose.

The decision to use bromocriptine or surgery as first-line therapy for prolactinomas that seem amenable to surgical resection is still somewhat controversial. In favor of bromocriptine is its simplicity and low risk. Against it is the need for indefinitely continued treatment and the possibility—increasingly remote as time goes on—of the late development of hitherto unanticipated side effects. In favor of surgery is the possibility of obtaining definitive cure, although this is clouded by the reports of late recurrences of hyperprolactinemia in some patients. The availability of an experienced neurosurgeon is essential. The wishes of the patient are an important factor in the decision. Even when surgery is favored, it has frequently been preceded, in the last few years, by a several-week course of bromocriptine to shrink the tumor and facilitate total surgical removal. Whether such preliminary drug treatment improves the overall surgical cure rate is not yet clear.

Pregnancy and Prolactinomas

A final point concerns the treatment of patients with prolactinomas who wish to become pregnant. If the lesion is a microadenoma, current practice is to use bromocriptine to treat the hyperprolactinemia and restore ovulatory menses. As soon as conception is known to have occurred, bromocriptine is withdrawn, and the pregnancy is allowed to proceed. Complications owing to tumor expansion are infrequent in such patients and usually do not require specific therapy. With macroadenomas, there is a somewhat greater risk of complications if bromocriptine is used alone, and consequently many physicians recommend preliminary surgery to reduce tumor size and, it is hoped, cure the hyperprolactinemia and restore menses. If the latter goal is not accomplished, bromocriptine is used as in patients with microadenomas. If complications owing to tumor expansion, particularly progressive reduction of visual fields, do occur during pregnancy, they are usually best dealt with by resuming treatment with bromocriptine.* To date, there is no evidence that bromocriptine treatment, even when maintained throughout gestation, has any deleterious effects on the fetus or on the outcome of pregnancy.

---

*This use of bromocriptine during pregnancy is not listed in the manufacturer's official directive.

HYPOTHYROIDISM

method of
JAMES A. MAGNER, M.D.
East Carolina University School of Medicine
Greenville, North Carolina

PRIMARY HYPOTHYROIDISM

More than 90% of the time, a patient found to have hypothyroidism is afflicted with primary thyroid disease. Hashimoto's (chronic lymphocytic) thyroiditis is the most common cause of hypothyroidism in North America (Table 1). Women are more commonly affected, and the typical natural history reflects a gradual loss of thyroid function over several years, with a gradual elevation of the serum thyroid-stimulating hormone (TSH) level. Rarely immune damage to the thyroid early in the disease may cause brief thyrotoxicosis, so-called Hashi-toxicosis. Nearly all patients have slow progression of this painless disease, so most authorities advise initiation of thyroid hormone replacement early in the course. Of note, serum thyroxine (T_4) levels may remain within the broad range of normal even when the patient has true mild hypothyroidism with mild serum TSH elevation. Most patients have a small goiter. Antimicrosomal (antiperoxidase) antibodies are present in sera of 90% of middle-aged patients but may be negative in young patients. Antithyroglobulin antibodies often become positive only a few years after antimicrosomal antibodies have been positive and presumably represent a response to antigens leaking from the damaged thyroid.

Another common cause of hypothyroidism is prior treatment of hyperthyroidism by thyroid surgery or radioiodine ablation. Elderly patients unable to give good historical information should always have a careful neck inspection to look for a faded surgical scar. Commonly used drugs may also cause hypothyroidism. Lithium interferes with the biosynthesis and release of thyroid hormone and may cause elevated serum TSH levels in patients a few weeks after initiation of therapy. Iodine blocks release of thyroid hormone and inhibits organification of iodide to thyroglobulin. Patients who take "health tonics" or eat kelp may be receiving too much iodine. Amiodarone (Cordarone) is a commonly used antiarrhythmic drug that is fat soluble and remains in the body for many weeks after discontinuation. The drug is rich in iodine, which more commonly induces hypothyroidism than hyperthyroidism in North America. It is prudent to obtain baseline thyroid function tests (including T_4 and triiodothyronine [T_3] by radioimmunoassay and TSH) before initiating amiodarone therapy because interpretation of these tests while taking the drug may prove difficult. For example, a mild elevation of TSH may be seen in patients who are still judged clinically to be euthyroid, and because most have underlying heart disease, thyroid hormone is not prescribed for TSH values less than 10 μU per mL. Iodine-containing expectorants and long-term povidone-iodine (Betadine) use (especially on mucous membranes) may cause hypothyroidism, especially in patients with Hashimoto's thyroiditis. The antithyroid drugs propylthiouracil, methimazole

TABLE 1. **Causes of Hypothyroidism**

Goitrous Hypothyroidism
Hashimoto's (chronic lymphocytic) thyroiditis
Inhibition of thyroid function by antithyroid drugs
  (propylthiouracil, methimazole, perchlorate), lithium,
  iodide excess in autoimmune thyroid disease (amiodarone,
  SSKI, povidone-iodine)
Congenital dyshormonogenesis (produces goiter but rarely
  hypothyroidism)
Endemic goiter (iodine) deficiency (rare in North America)
Infiltrative diseases (rare): amyloidosis, cystinosis, leukemia,
  lymphoma
Peripheral resistance to thyroid hormone

Nongoitrous Hypothyroidism
Radioiodine for hyperthyroidism
Surgical hypothyroidism
Atrophic variant of Hashimoto's thyroiditis
TSH-receptor blocking autoantibodies
External radiation therapy to neck
Pituitary and hypothalamic hypothyroidism

Transient Hypothyroidism
Subacute (granulomatous) thyroiditis
Painless (lymphocytic) thyroiditis
Postpartum thyroiditis

Abbreviations: SSKI = saturated solution of potassium iodide; TSH
= thyroid-stimulating hormone.
From Ross DS: Hypothyroidism. *In* Rakel RE (ed): Conn's Current
Therapy 1992. Philadelphia, WB Saunders Co, 1992.

(Tapazole), and potassium perchlorate (Perchloracap) may cause hypothyroidism.

Temporary thyroid dysfunction lasting a few weeks or months may be caused by several disorders. A viral respiratory infection may damage the thyroid, causing release of stored thyroid hormones and suppression of both serum TSH levels and the 24-hour radioiodine uptake. This subacute (de Quervain's, granulomatous) thyroiditis may present with a tender thyroid gland, often treated with aspirin or prednisone. A 1- to 2-month hyperthyroid phase (sometimes requiring beta-blocking drugs but not treated with antithyroid drugs) may be followed by 1 to 6 months of hypothyroidism that may require thyroid hormone replacement. L-Thyroxine should be stopped at 6 months and serum TSH rechecked 1 month later because long-term hypothyroidism occurs rarely. Painless (lymphocytic) thyroiditis is a clinical entity with an immune system–triggered hyperthyroid phase of a few weeks that may be followed by a few weeks of hypothyroidism. A few patients develop permanent hypothyroidism. The typical hyperthyroidism-hypothyroidism sequence may occur in 5% of postpartum women and tends to recur after other pregnancies. The presence of antimicrosomal antibodies may predict women at risk for postpartum thyroiditis. The syndrome, possibly responsible for many cases of postpartum depression, may occur in up to 20% of women with Type I diabetes mellitus.

Iodine deficiency, once common in the central farmlands of North America, has been eliminated by use of iodized salt and bread. Uncommon causes of hypothyroidism include congenital hypothyroidism, external neck radiotherapy, amyloidosis, and peripheral resistance to thyroid hormone. A recently recognized cause of hypothyroidism is cancer therapy with interleukin-2, interferon-alpha, or granulocyte macrophage–colony stimulating factor.

SECONDARY AND CENTRAL HYPOTHYROIDISM

Fewer than 6% of cases of hypothyroidism are due to secondary or central causes, making the serum TSH level a generally reliable screening tool in most patients with symptoms and signs of hypothyroidism. A deficiency of pituitary TSH secretion may be difficult to distinguish clinically from hypothalamic dysfunction. Biochemical and clinical hypothyroidism is present in both cases with low, normal, or only mildly elevated serum TSH levels. Causes include pituitary or hypothalamic tumors, metastatic lesions, and infiltrating diseases, such as sarcoidosis and histiocytosis X. Rarely head trauma, cranial irradiation, or Sheehan's syndrome may cause TSH deficiency. Congenital TSH deficiency may result from genetic mutations in the TSH-beta subunit gene.

DIAGNOSIS

Patients with hypothyroidism may present with fatigue, constipation, subjective sense of feeling too cool compared with family members, weight gain, edema, muscle cramps or weakness, goiter, and carpal tunnel syndrome. More severe cases may be associated with deep voice, loss of the lateral eyebrows, carotenemia, congestive heart failure, marked bradycardia, ascites, pericardial or pleural effusions, abnormal cognitive function, hyponatremia, anemia, hypercholesterolemia, hyperprolactinemia, hypoventilation, sleep apnea, hypothermia, and coma. Unusual manifestations of hypothyroidism include pituitary enlargement with visual field abnormality, intestinal pseudo-obstruction, bacterial overgrowth with diarrhea, Raynaud's phenomenon, seizures, reticular erythematous mucinosis, acral papulokeratotic lesions, precocious puberty, acquired hemolytic anemia, acquired von Willebrand's disease, acute exertional rhabdomyolysis, cholesterol pericarditis, taste disorders, and psychosis. Hypothyroidism may be more common in persons with primary hypoadrenalism, vitiligo, early ovarian failure, trisomy 4p, and horseshoe kidney.

Although a low serum T_4 level occurs in most patients with hypothyroidism, one must recognize that the normal range for T_4 is broad (generally 4 to 11 μg per dL). If a particular normal individual is frequently retested, the serum total T_4 level is not 4 μg per dL on Monday and 10 μg per dL on Friday but instead varies within 1 or 2 μg per dL. Thus a person may normally have a total T_4 level of 9 μg per dL but after thyroidectomy may have symptoms of hypothyroidism and an elevated TSH level when the total T_4 level is 6 µg per dL, which is still within the broad range of normal for the population (and there is no asterisk on the computer printout). Serum T_4 levels may also remain within the broad normal range in hypothyroid patients with serum protein binding abnormalities, as with estrogen use or chronic hepatitis. Falsely low serum T_4 levels may occur in euthyroid patients with reduced concentrations of thyroxine-binding globulin (TBG), which may be congenital or acquired after treatment with glucocorticoids, androgens, fenclofenac,* asparaginase (Elspar), danazol (Danocrine), and colestipol (Colestid)-niacin. Urine protein loss lowers TBG in the nephrotic syndrome. Phenylbutazone (Butazolidin), phenytoin (Dilantin), salicylates, and high doses of furosemide (Lasix) may displace T_4 from serum binding proteins, lowering serum T_4 levels. Treatment with liothyronine (T_3 or Cytomel) may create frank hyperthyroidism with low T_4 levels.

Thus the serum T_4 level should not be relied on to define the patient's thyroid status (Table 2). Assay of serum TSH is preferred and is elevated in primary hypothyroidism. A caveat is that a few elderly hypothyroid patients may exhibit minimal TSH elevation. The serum TSH is misleading in patients with pituitary or hypothalamic hypothyroidism. The serum TSH may remain suppressed for several days or weeks after hypothyroidism develops in Graves' disease patients treated with radioiodine or drugs, a rare instance of a nonequilibrium state in which the total T_4 or free T_4 level may more accurately reflect the true state of the patient.

---

*Not available in the United States.

TABLE 2. **Causes of Misdiagnosis of Hypothyroidism**

Low Serum T_4
Reduced serum thyroxine-binding globulin
  Genetic factors, androgens, glucocorticoids, danazol, asparaginase, colestipol-niacin, nonthyroidal illness, protein loss by gut, nephrotic syndrome
Displacement of T_4 from binding proteins
  Phenytoin, high-dose salicylates, furosemide in renal failure, fenclofenac,* phenylbutazone, nonthyroidal illness
Liothyronine

Elevated Serum TSH
Recovery phase of nonthyroidal illness
Artifact caused by interfering antimouse IgG antibodies (rare)

---

*Not available in the United States.
  Abbreviations: T_4 = thyroxine; TSH = thyroid-stimulating hormone.
  From Ross DS: Hypothyroidism. *In* Rakel RE (ed): Conn's Current Therapy 1992. Philadelphia, WB Saunders Co, 1992.

Nonthyroidal Illness

Seriously ill patients may exhibit marked declines in serum T_3 levels within a day or two. Serum T_4 levels also generally fall but may be transiently elevated. The serum TSH level is the best guide to the true thyroid status of such patients. Dopamine infusions and high-dose glucocorticoids may lower TSH levels in patients with true primary hypothyroidism. Recovering patients may exhibit a transient rebound of serum TSH values to elevated levels. Most seriously ill patients with TSH levels less than 15 µU per mL require no thyroid hormone replacement.

TREATMENT

Most authorities now agree that synthetic levothyroxine (T_4, Synthroid, Levothroid, Levoxine, Levo-T) is the proper replacement therapy for hypothyroidism (Table 3). Liothyronine (T_3) should not be used routinely because of its short half-life and widely fluctuating serum levels, which theoretically expose cardiac and other tissues to short periods of hyperthyroidism and hypothyroidism. Because of its binding to serum proteins, T_4 has a long serum half-life of about 7 days, and serum levels are stable with once-daily dosing.

Although a few patients may be allergic to the dye used in the yellow 100-µg or green 300-µg tablets, there are few side effects to T_4 therapy. The 50-µg tablet has no dye and may be prescribed for sensitive patients. Although over-the-counter cold remedies caution consumers with thyroid disease, this warning is intended for hyperthyroid patients and is not relevant for euthyroid patients on long-term thyroid hormone therapy.

Thyroid Hormone Preparations

Levothyroxine is available in several generic and proprietary formulations (see Table 3). Tablets at small increments of dosage are available that facilitate the fine titration of thyroid status using serum TSH levels. Because the bioavailability of T_4 may differ between preparations, patients titrated on one brand should not change brands with every prescription refill. Currently the price of brand-name levothyroxine differs little from that of generic formulations, so most authorities avoid prescribing generic levothyroxine, which may have less stringent quality control.

Although liothyronine is not recommended for routine long-term replacement therapy, its short half-life is useful in minimizing hypothyroidism in thyroid cancer patients undergoing whole body scans. Recently it has become available in an in-

TABLE 3. **Thyroid Hormone Preparations**

Generic Name	Brand Names	Approximate Equivalent Dose	Preparations
Levothyroxine	Synthroid Levothroid Levoxine Levo-T	100 µg	24, 50, 75, 88, 100, 112, 125, 150, 175, 200, 300 µg tablets
Liothyronine	Cytomel Triostat	25 µg	5, 25, 50 µg tablets 1 mL vials with 10 µg/mL
Liotrix	Thyrolar Euthroid	1 U	1 unit = T_4 50 µg/T_3 12.5 µg 1 unit = T_4 60 µg/T_3 15 µg ¼, ½, 1, 2, 3 U tablets
Thyroid USP (pork or beef)	Armour Thyroid S-P-T, Thyrar	60–65 mg	65 mg = T_4 38 µg/T_3 9 µg 15, 30, 60, 65, 90, 120, 130, 180, 240, 300 mg tablets
	Thyroid Strong	40 mg	Contains more hormone than thyroid USP 32.5, 65, 130, 195 mg tablets
Thyroglobulin (pork)	Proloid	65 mg	65 mg = T_4 36 µg/T_3 12 µg, 32, 65, 100, 130, 200 mg tablets

Abbreviations: T_4 = thyroxine; T_3 = triiodothyronine.
From Ross DS: Hypothyroidism. *In* Rakel RE (ed): Conn's Current Therapy 1992. Philadelphia, WB Saunders Co, 1992.

travenous form, but its use in myxedema coma remains controversial.

Combinations of T_4 and T_3 (Liotrix) are not recommended because transient hyperthyroidism could precipitate angina or arrhythmias. Thyroid extract or thyroglobulin formulations made from hog or beef thyroid glands also contain both T_4 and T_3, and bioavailability may vary. Rarely a patient may develop allergy to proteins in these preparations. Elderly patients who have been maintained on such preparations for years may resist switching to more modern preparations and may safely be followed on the older preparations if it is recognized that serum T_4 levels may remain in the low-normal range because some of the hormone activity is being provided as T_3. Also, because of reduced bioavailability of a thyroid extract in a particular patient, it may be dangerous to switch from a thyroid extract to the apparently equivalent amount of synthetic hormone using a table of equivalent dose as guidance. A patient on 180 mg thyroid extract daily, for example, should not thoughtlessly be converted to 300 µg of levothyroxine; it would be better to replace the thyroid extract with 100 µg of levothyroxine and recheck the serum TSH level in 4 weeks before raising the dose incrementally.

Initial Therapy

Therapy for hypothyroidism would be straightforward if it were not for coronary artery disease, adrenal insufficiency, or other disorders that may coexist in the patient. Table 4 lists some general rules regarding the initial therapy of hypothyroidism. The clinical assessment of individual patients, however, must take precedence over arbitrary guidelines. Because thyroid hormone increases oxygen consumption by the heart, coronary artery disease symptoms may be precipitated or worsened by therapy. Patients with heart disease, risk factors for heart disease, or long-standing hypothyroidism should be started on a relatively small daily dose of levothyroxine, such as 25 or 50 µg. Split daily doses are not useful because of levothyroxine's long half-life. The dosage may be gradually increased at 1- or 2-month intervals.

In the absence of heart disease, younger patients should be started initially on a nearly full replacement dose of levothyroxine, such as 100 µg daily, to avoid prolonging their symptoms of hypothyroidism. After 6 to 8 weeks, the serum TSH may be checked and the dose adjusted. Onset of hypothyroidism in thyrotoxic patients shortly after radioiodine or thyroid surgery ought to be avoidable by careful follow-up, but should this occur, such patients usually easily tolerate a full dose of levothyroxine as initial therapy.

Some symptoms of hypothyroidism, such as muscle weakness and neuropathies, may persist for many weeks after serum hormone concentrations are rectified. Patients should be so informed, and physicians should be patient and avoid unnecessary diagnostic adventures.

Subclinical Hypothyroidism

Because of the broad normal range for serum T_4 concentrations for the population, an individual may have a normal serum T_4 level and no symptoms but have a mildly elevated TSH level (5 to 15 µU per mL). Such patients have subclinical hypothyroidism, which often results from

TABLE 4. **Guidelines for Initial Levothyroxine Therapy in Adults**

Extremely Cautious
25 μg or less daily for first 4 weeks, then increase by
  increments of 25 μg or less every 4–6 weeks if tolerated
Patients with angina and arrhythmias
Elderly patients
Older patients (>45–50 years) with multiple risk factors
  for coronary heart disease
Older patients with severe or long-standing
  hypothyroidism

Cautious
50 μg daily for first 4 weeks, then increase by increments of
  25–50 μg every 4–6 weeks if tolerated
Older patients (>45–50 years)
Younger patients with multiple risk factors for coronary
  artery disease
Younger patients with severe or long-standing
  hypothyroidism

Routine: Subreplacement Dose
75–100 μg daily for first 4–6 weeks, then increase by
  increments of 25–50 μg every 4–6 weeks if tolerated
Most healthy patients younger than 45–50 years

Rapid: Full Estimated Replacement Dose
Healthy young patients with mild hypothyroidism
Most patients when hypothyroidism occurs shortly after
  surgery or radioiodine treatment of hyperthyroidism,
  unless known cardiac disease is present

From Ross DS: Hypothyroidism. *In* Rakel RE (ed): Conn's Current Therapy 1992. Philadelphia, WB Saunders Co, 1992.

early Hashimoto's disease but can be due to other causes. Thyroiditis, for example, may be asymptomatic and resolve completely. Controversy still exists over whether subclinical hypothyroidism requires treatment. Several randomized prospective trials found little change in serum cholesterol values, although a few treated patients had improved systolic time intervals. Despite their initial asymptomatic state, some patients felt subjectively improved after therapy. Because of the differing natural histories of diseases that may cause subclinical hypothyroidism, many authorities suggest following such patients without therapy and remeasuring the serum TSH after a few weeks. Persistent elevation of TSH may then prompt initiation of thyroid hormone replacement, although elderly patients with cardiac disease may be followed for an additional period. Patients with antimicrosomal antibody titers of 1:1600 or greater have an 80% probability of developing clinical hypothyroidism within 5 years, and early treatment may avoid development of symptoms.

Coexistent Adrenal Insufficiency

A few patients with primary hypothyroidism have autoimmune polyglandular failure and potentially may have adrenal insufficiency, pernicious anemia, hypoparathyroidism, diabetes mellitus, ovarian failure, or rheumatologic diseases. Hypothyroidism may mask adrenal insufficiency, and adrenal crisis may be precipitated by thyroid hormone replacement. Although the possibility of coexistent adrenal insufficiency should be considered in every patient with primary hypothyroidism, it is seldom necessary to exclude this definitively using biochemical testing, such as a stimulation test. This test should be performed, however, in all patients with secondary (pituitary or hypothalamic) hypothyroidism before initiating thyroid hormone therapy.

Monitoring Therapy

Although the average replacement dose of levothyroxine in adults is about 112 μg daily, few patients are precisely "average." Most patients require doses of 100 to 150 μg daily, although elderly patients require less. The precise dose for each patient with primary hypothyroidism may be determined by careful instruction to take the levothyroxine reliably for 6 to 8 weeks (a critical step) and then measuring a TSH value in a sensitive assay. If TSH is outside the normal range (0.5 to 5 μU per mL in most laboratories), a slight dosage change can be instituted for 6 to 8 weeks followed by another TSH measurement. Thereafter many patients remain on the same dose of medication for years, as assessed by annual TSH determination. Data that a given person may have seasonal fluctuations in thyroid hormone requirements remain controversial. Special circumstances, such as pregnancy, are discussed later. Serum T_4 concentrations in patients taking levothyroxine may be slightly higher than the normal range when the TSH measurement is normal and should be no cause for concern.

One cannot rely on the TSH measurement to monitor patients on thyroid hormone therapy who have pituitary or hypothalamic hypothyroidism. One must depend on free T_4 measurements and the clinical status of the patient.

Overtreatment

Because of the broad normal range for serum T_4 levels, one patient with a T_4 level of 10 μg per dL may have a normal TSH level of 2 μU per mL, whereas another patient with a T_4 level of 10 μg per dL may have a suppressed TSH level. Both patients may be asymptomatic. The current view is that the second patient is being slightly overtreated and has subclinical hyperthyroidism. It remains controversial whether such patients are at increased risk over the long term for osteoporosis. Some authors claiming that reduced bone density occurs in such overtreated patients may not have fully allowed for, for instance, a decade of untreated Graves' hyperthyroidism before radioiodine therapy and minimal iatrogenic overtreatment became a factor. Mild overtreatment may induce liver abnormalities, abnormal systolic time intervals, angina, or atrial arrhythmias in some patients, although there is theoretically a small beneficial effect from altered lipid metabolism. Because sensitive TSH testing is now widely available and because dose increments of pills make precise dose titration relatively straightforward, most authorities advise the prudent course of normalizing the TSH level, even if the dangers of mild overtreatment remain uncertain.

Some patients are overtreated intentionally. A patient who had an aggressive thyroid cancer (invasion outside the thyroid or metastases) removed surgically arguably should receive a dose of thyroid hormone that fully suppresses the TSH rather than one that just normalizes the TSH. Some authorities extend the argument and intentionally suppress the TSH in all thyroid cancer patients and even in patients with slowly enlarging benign goiters. Until clinical studies address this issue, the risks and benefits of suppressive therapy should be weighed for each patient, taking into consideration, for example, concomitant risk factors for osteoporosis. Logically the lowest dose of thyroid hormone that accomplishes the desired TSH suppression should be chosen.

SPECIAL TREATMENT SITUATIONS

Hypothyroidism After Radioiodine Therapy

Long-standing hyperthyroidism, as in Graves' disease untreated for many months or years, causes prolonged suppression of TSH. Although serum T_4 levels may fall to hypothyroid levels a few weeks after high doses of radioiodine therapy, in some patients the TSH initially fails to rise. This transient nonequilibrium state may lead to mismanagement by the clinician if only serum TSH levels are monitored. This is an unusual instance when the serum T_4 or free T_4 level is a better indicator of the patient's true metabolic state than is TSH. When serum T_4 falls rapidly to the low normal range in such cases, levothyroxine therapy at 50 or 100 µg per day should be initiated despite the suppressed TSH. Re-evaluation 4 to 6 weeks later then allows titration of the dosage because TSH values may then be more reliable. Efforts should be made to avoid hypothyroidism in Graves' disease patients after radioiodine therapy because some authorities believe

the hypothyroid state may worsen ophthalmopathy.

Pregnancy

The requirement for thyroid hormone increases during pregnancy. Patients who have little functioning thyroid tissue and who have been comfortably maintained over the long term on a constant dose of levothyroxine are found to have an elevated TSH during pregnancy. To prevent mild hypothyroidism, serum TSH levels should be checked once or twice during pregnancy and a slight increase in levothyroxine dose made when indicated. Overtreatment must be avoided, however, because hyperthyroidism may be associated with premature labor. The thyroid status should then be rechecked during the postpartum period because a need for a slight downward adjustment in the dose of levothyroxine would be anticipated.

Emergency Surgery in Hypothyroid Patients

Several published series of hypothyroid patients who underwent major surgical procedures indicate that most did well. Somewhat less anesthesia may be required, serum sodium should be monitored to prevent water intoxication, and the febrile response to postoperative infection may be lessened. Attempts to correct a moderately hypothyroid state rapidly before emergency surgery could induce cardiac arrhythmias, and some studies found no increase in cardiac inotropic status for many days after serum thyroid hormone levels had been normalized, indicating that time for cellular protein synthesis is required. Standard levothyroxine therapy is indicated in most cases of hypothyroidism discovered shortly before or after emergent surgery. Elective surgery should be delayed a few months when possible until a euthyroid state has been attained.

Myxedema Coma

Although myxedema coma is uncommon, recognition and aggressive therapy are necessary. All patients with abnormal mental status should have their necks inspected for a goiter or a scar from prior thyroid surgery. Family members should be questioned about possible prior radioiodine therapy or thyroid disease in the patient. Effective treatment includes adequate ventilation, correction of hypothermia, management of fluid and electrolyte problems, obtaining cultures and initiating therapy for any infections, and glucocorticoid coverage pending assessment of adrenal function. Gradual incremental thyroid hormone replacement is usually recommended in elderly patients without myxedema coma who may have cardiac disease; however, in view of the high mortality associated with myxedema coma, many authorities recommend aggressive thyroid hormone replacement in this disorder. A time-honored regimen includes levothyroxine, 300 to 500 µg as an intravenous loading dose, followed by 50 to 100 µg daily. The oral route of administration is avoided because of fear of reduced bioavailability owing to hypomotility and gut edema. Other authorities favor initial therapy with liothyronine (Cytomel), 20 to 40 µg every 6 to 8 hours, although cardiac arrhythmias may, in theory, be induced. Intravenous liothyronine was formerly specially prepared by pharmacies but has now become available commercially (Triostat).

Transient Hypothyroidism

During the brief hyperthyroid phase of postpartum thyroiditis, subacute thyroiditis, and lymphocytic thyroiditis, patients may be followed on no therapy or treated with beta-blocker drugs (such as atenolol, 50 mg per day). Vigilance must be maintained for the hypothyroid phase that may appear in some patients. When TSH becomes elevated, some authorities prescribe a lower than full replacement dose of levothyroxine (such as 50 or 75 µg per day) and then retest the TSH in 6 to 8 weeks. The therapy is stopped when the TSH normalizes. Alternatively, others favor prescribing a full replacement dose of levothyroxine for 6 months and then stopping therapy. A subsequent TSH value in 4 to 6 weeks confirms euthyroid status off levothyroxine. A minority of patients may require prolonged or lifelong therapy.

Treatment Failures

Nearly all apparent levothyroxine treatment failures are due to noncompliance. Punch-out pill packs may aid the patient's memory. Because of levothyroxine's long half-life, several forgotten doses may be taken all at once. Patients with steatorrhea may truly require higher oral doses. Cholestyramine (Questran) and other resins may interfere with levothyroxine absorption and should be taken at least 4 hours apart from levothyroxine. Loss of T_4 bound to TBG in urine of patients with nephrotic syndrome may rarely require a higher replacement dose of levothyroxine.

Drugs and Hypothyroidism

Hypothyroidism may prolong the effect of sedatives, narcotics, and digoxin and may precipitate clofibrate-induced myopathy. Correction of hypothyroidism may cause bleeding in patients on warfarin because of increased breakdown of vitamin K–dependent clotting factors. Treatment of hypothyroidism may cause more rapid clearance of oral hypoglycemics or insulin such that doses of these drugs may need to be adjusted in diabetics. Phenytoin may increase the metabolism of T_4; the serum TSH level should be used to adjust the dose of levothyroxine.

Congenital Hypothyroidism

Heel-stick screening of all newborns in the United States is now performed. Screening at 3 to 5 days of life seems optimal because this avoids the neonatal surge of TSH, which peaks at 30 minutes after birth and subsides by 48 to 72 hours. Because infants are now discharged quickly, screening is performed at discharge and in most states is based on combined T_4 and TSH screening. Recall rates range from 0.03 to 0.8%. A false-positive rate of one to three normal recalled infants for every congenitally hypothyroid infant is generally seen. Serum testing then identifies the abnormal infant before symptoms or signs are noted. In the United States, the prevalence of congenital hypothyroidism is about 1 in 4000 births and 85% of the time is due to thyroid dysgenesis. Although some authorities suggest that a bone age x-ray, thyroid scan or thyroid ultrasound study and serum thyroglobulin may be indicated, thyroid hormone therapy should not be delayed more than 3 or 4 days. TSH receptor–blocking antibodies may cause transient hypothyroidism in a minority of infants, and antibody measurement can be performed. Newborn screening and early therapy results in normal IQ values in most patients at age 6 to 8.

Long-Standing Therapy but Unclear Diagnosis

Elderly patients who have been on thyroid hormone replacement for many years for uncertain reasons should probably just have their prescriptions refilled; the TSH can be kept in the normal range. Stopping and restarting thyroid therapy in elderly patients can unmask cardiac problems. In a younger patient, a high titer of antimicrosomal antibodies can be reassuring that the long-term therapy was started with good reason. In dubious cases, levothyroxine may be stopped for 6 to 8 weeks; TSH rises transiently as an atrophic gland resumes function in the temporarily hypothyroid patient with a truly intact thyroid. Persistently elevated TSH values signal a need to restart therapy.

HYPERTHYROIDISM

method of
DAVID S. COOPER, M.D.
Sinai Hospital of Baltimore
Baltimore, Maryland

Hyperthyroidism or thyrotoxicosis is a clinical and biochemical state produced when tissues are exposed to excessive circulating quantities of thyroid hormones thyroxine (T_4) and triiodothyronine (T_3). Hyperthyroidism is caused by the uncontrolled secretion or release of thyroid hormone into the bloodstream or by the ingestion of excessive amounts of thyroid hormone. In Graves' disease, the thyroid is stimulated to produce thyroid hormone by thyroid-stimulating autoantibodies, but rarely other factors may stimulate the thyroid and also cause hyperthyroidism—e.g., thyroid-stimulating hormone (TSH) from a pituitary TSH-secreting tumor or human chorionic gonadotropin (hCG) from a choriocarcinoma. Hyperthyroidism may be produced by benign thyroid neoplasia, as in patients with a toxic nodule or toxic multinodular goiter, and it may be produced by thyroid inflammation, with release of thyroid hormone into the bloodstream from damaged follicles in the several forms of thyroiditis. It may also be produced by the ectopic secretion of thyroid hormones by ovarian teratomas (struma ovarii).

It should also be noted that patients may have elevated serum levels of T_4, T_3, or both *without* being hyperthyroid, in situations of increased thyroid hormone binding by thyroid-binding globulin (TBG) or other proteins, in altered peripheral conversion of T_4 to T_3 owing to certain drugs or illness, and in rare patients with congenital peripheral resistance to thyroid hormones. Thus it is of obvious importance first to verify that the patient is hyperthyroid by biochemical means and then to establish the cause of the problem. Graves' disease is, of course, the most frequent cause, regardless of age or sex.

DIAGNOSIS

The laboratory diagnosis of hyperthyroidism is straightforward. Most patients have elevated circulating levels of T_4 and T_3 and an elevated free thyroxine index or directly measured free T_4. In hyperthyroid patients with normal serum T_4 values, serum T_3 should be measured because T_3 toxicosis is seen in 10 to 15% of hyperthyroid patients. In recent years, the development of sensitive assays for TSH has simplified the ability to diagnose milder degrees of hyperthyroidism. It should be apparent that all forms of hyperthyroidism except for the rare pituitary TSH-secreting tumor are associated with low or undetectable serum TSH concentrations. Indeed, a low serum TSH concentration is the sine qua non of hyperthyroidism, and in the absence of severe illness or thyroxine ingestion, this finding should suggest the diagnosis. With the widespread availability of sensitive TSH assays, the thyrotropin-releasing hormone (TRH) test, wherein the TSH response to a bolus of TRH is assessed, has become an obsolete method for diagnosing hyperthyroidism.

The 24-hour radioiodine uptake test is not sensitive or specific for hyperthyroidism because it can be elevated in some patients with hypothyroidism owing to Hashimoto's thyroiditis, and it can be low in hyperthyroid patients with subacute thyroiditis or painless thyroiditis (also called postpartum thyroiditis) and in patients with Graves' disease exposed to iodine-containing compounds. The 24-hour radioiodine uptake test, however, is useful in distinguishing Graves' disease developing in the postpartum period from postpartum thyroiditis and in confirming the diagnosis of subacute thyroiditis.

TREATMENT

Before therapy of hyperthyroidism is undertaken, the precise *cause* of the condition should be ascertained. The vast majority of patients, both young and old, have Graves' disease, although the fraction of patients with toxic multinodular goiter increases with age. Together these two diagnoses account for more than 90% of all cases of hyperthyroidism. It is particularly important to rule out the various forms of thyroiditis as a cause of hyperthyroidism because they spontaneously resolve and require only symptomatic therapy. Fortunately, rapid treatment of hyperthyroidism is rarely necessary, and patients can be managed symptomatically with beta-adrenergic blocking agents until a formal diagnosis can be firmly established.

Because the underlying causes of the immunologic abnormalities in Graves' disease are unknown, treatment centers around direct efforts to lessen thyroid hormone secretion. Although surgery was historically the first form of satisfactory therapy for Graves' disease, it has been replaced by antithyroid drugs and radioiodine as the treatments of choice. Both are effective and safe, and, although neither is perfect, they provide a satisfactory outcome for most patients. The advantage of antithyroid drugs is that they provide the opportunity for the patient to experience a spontaneous remission and thus not require lifelong medication. The disadvantages are that remissions are attained in fewer than 50% of patients and that continuous or repeated courses of drug therapy are usually necessary. Radioiodine is curative but has the disadvantage of causing iatrogenic hypothyroidism in virtually all patients. The management of post-radioiodine hypothyroidism, however, is simpler than managing most patients on long-term antithyroid drug therapy. Therefore, one should not consider radioiodine as a treatment that merely exchanges one thyroid problem for another.

Of course, the major controversy surrounding the use of radioiodine is the possible long-term carcinogenic or mutagenic effects of ionizing radiation. To date, however, despite numerous studies, there are no data that demonstrate that radioiodine therapy for hyperthyroidism is hazardous to the patient, nor has it been shown that it affects subsequent fertility or reproductive outcome when given to women of childbearing age. Thus radioiodine has emerged in the United States as the primary treatment for most women with hyperthyroidism. The use of radioiodine in children and adolescents is more controversial, but it has replaced surgery in most clinics as the second-line therapy, if antithyroid drugs fail owing to drug allergy or poor compliance. Whatever the inclinations and biases of the physician may be, it is important to stress that the participation of the patient in the decision-making process is crucial because all treatments have distinct advantages and disadvantages.

Antithyroid Drug Therapy

If antithyroid drug therapy is selected, one of two thionamide antithyroid drugs is used: propylthiouracil (PTU) or methimazole (Tapazole). Antithyroid drugs are derivatives of thiourea and have as their major property the ability to inhibit thyroid hormone biosynthesis. Thionamides block the utilization of trapped iodide, at a step involving the binding of oxidized iodide to tyrosine residues to form mono- and diiodotyrosine. The coupling of these iodotyrosines to form T_4 and T_3 may also be inhibited by antithyroid drugs. In addition, PTU, but not methimazole, can inhibit T_4 to T_3 conversion in peripheral tissues. A number of studies have suggested, but not proved, that the thionamides have immunosuppressive effects. If so, this might explain why 30 to 50% of patients treated with these drugs undergo a period of remission.

The starting dose of PTU is approximately 300 mg daily, given as two 50-mg tablets every 8 hours. PTU cannot generally be given as a single daily dose, owing to its relatively short duration of action. In contrast, methimazole can be given as a single daily dose. Because it is 10 to 50 times as potent as PTU, starting doses are approximately 5 to 30 mg per day. The time until a euthyroid state is achieved varies, depending on the underlying disease activity, the amount of stored thyroid hormone within the gland, and the dose of antithyroid drug. In general, it takes 4 to 6 weeks for methimazole and 6 to 12 weeks for comparable doses of PTU. For troublesome symptoms, beta-adrenergic blocking drugs are usually given as adjunctive therapy until the thionamides have restored the patient to a euthyroid state. Long-acting beta blockers, such as metoprolol (Lopressor), atenolol (Tenormin), and nadolol (Corgard), and long-acting propranolol (Inderal-LA) are preferable to propranolol (Inderal) itself, which has a short duration of action.

The side effects of antithyroid drugs are somewhat notorious, but they are no different or more frequent than those of most commonly used drugs. Fever, rash, and arthralgias are seen in 1 to 5% of patients; it is sometimes possible to switch to the other drug if a patient develops one of these *minor* side effects. The most dreaded reaction is agranulocytosis, which occurs in about 0.2% of patients. Typically agranulocytosis develops within 90 days of starting thionamide therapy and is heralded by high fever and an infection, usually of the oropharynx. Thus patients should be warned to discontinue their medication if they develop a fever or a sore throat and to call their physician. If agranulocytosis is present, hospitalization and broad-spectrum antibiotic therapy are indicated; fortunately, the white count normalizes within 7 to 10 days in most patients once the medication has been discontinued, and fatalities are extremely rare in the modern era. The administration of granulocyte–colony stimulating factor (G-CSF) may hasten bone marrow recovery. Other *major* side effects, besides agranulocytosis, include toxic hepatitis, vasculitis, and drug-induced lupus erythematosus.

Generally, antithyroid drugs are administered for a period of 1 to 2 years and are then tapered or discontinued to establish whether a remission has occurred. There have been numerous clinical and biochemical markers that have been proposed to assist the clinician in predicting which patients are more likely to achieve a remission with antithyroid drugs. Unfortunately, none have adequate sensitivity or specificity to be of much use in individual patients. In general, remission rates are higher in patients with milder degrees of hyperthyroidism and smaller goiters, who are diagnosed earlier in their illness, and who are treated for longer periods of time with antithyroid agents.

Should a remission be achieved, lifelong follow-up is warranted because most remissions are not permanent. Relapses may be particularly likely to occur in the postpartum period. If a remission is not achieved, the patient is then faced with the choice of a second course of antithyroid drug therapy or radioiodine. It should also be mentioned that some patients who experience remission with antithyroid drug therapy alone eventually develop spontaneous hypothyroidism. The frequency of this phenomenon is approximately 20%.

Radioiodine Therapy

Radioiodine has been in use as a therapy for hyperthyroidism since the 1940s. It is the preferred treatment for most adult patients with Graves' disease, toxic nodules, and toxic multinodular goiter. Radiation damage occurs relatively slowly, which is why it usually takes 2 to 6 months, and sometimes longer, for the full effects to be experienced by the patient. Although the radiation dose delivered to the thyroid gland is high (5000 to 15,000 rad), the radiation dose to the whole body is small in the average patient. In women, it has been estimated that the dose to the ovaries, largely owing to gamma radiation from radioiodine in the urinary bladder, is approximately 0.2 rad per administered mCi of radioiodine. Because a typical radioiodine dose in Graves' disease is 5 to 10 mCi, the ovarian dose would be 1 to 2 rad. This is similar to that which might be obtained after several barium enemas or intravenous pyelograms, well within the range that would be considered safe in terms of reproductive potential. As noted earlier, there is no evidence to support the notion that radioiodine is harmful to women or their offspring.

There are few immediate side effects of radioiodine therapy. Rarely patients complain of anterior neck tenderness 7 to 10 days after therapy, consistent with radiation-induced throiditis, which is managed easily with salicylates. There is a potential for worsening hyperthyroidism soon after radioiodine, secondary to inflammation and release of stored thyroid hormone into the bloodstream. For this reason, elderly patients and patients with cardiac disease are usually pretreated with thionamides before receiving radioiodine; the antithyroid agent blocks the synthesis, but not the release, of thyroid hormone, thereby permitting gradual depletion of glandular thyroid hormonal stores. In general, however, pretreatment with antithyroid agents is not necessary in otherwise healthy young and middle-aged adults, and symptoms can be controlled with beta-adrenergic blocking agents.

The major adverse reaction from radioiodine is iatrogenic hypothyroidism. Indeed, this development is so characteristic that it is considered an inevitable consequence of therapy rather than a side effect. Hypothyroidism develops in at least 50% of patients within the first year after therapy, with a gradual 2 to 3% annual incidence thereafter. Thus, within 10 to 20 years, virtually all patients become hypothyroid. It is therefore mandatory that all radioiodine-treated patients receive lifelong follow-up, with close monitoring of thyroid function, especially the serum TSH level.

For patients with toxic solitary nodules or toxic multinodular goiter, radioiodine is the treatment of choice. This is because these represent benign neoplasms, which never undergo spontaneous remission after a course of antithyroid drug therapy. Because radioiodine is concentrated only in areas within the thyroid that are functioning, the suppressed paranodular areas are spared exposure to the high levels of radiation that are delivered with radioiodine. Therefore hypothyroidism is less of a problem in this setting, although it can occur.

Surgical Therapy

Historically subtotal thyroidectomy is the oldest form of therapy for hyperthyroidism and represented the only form of definitive therapy for many decades. Now with the widespread acceptance of radioiodine, surgery has become a somewhat unusual treatment except in special circumstances: children and adolescents who are allergic to or noncompliant with thionamides, pregnant women who are allergic to thionamides, patients with large goiters, and individuals who prefer definitive therapy but are apprehensive about radioiodine. In the last instance, the decision to operate is based more on emotional factors than on medical science.

Although the mortality rate of subtotal thyroidectomy in recent years is close to zero, recurrent laryngeal nerve damage and hypoparathyroidism continue to occur, albeit rarely. Furthermore, transient hypocalcemia, postoperative bleeding, wound infections, keloids, and unsightly scars develop in a larger proportion of patients.

Immediate hypothyroidism develops in 10 to 60% of patients, with late-onset hypothyroidism developing in an additional 1 to 3% per year. Clearly long-term follow-up is necessary for all patients treated surgically. The development of hypothyroidism depends on a number of factors, including the size of the remnant; the presence of antithyroid antibodies, perhaps reflecting autoimmune destruction of the remnant; and the duration of follow-up. In addition, and perhaps most unfortunately, recurrent hyperthyroidism develops in at least 5% of patients. Recurrences may develop many years after the initial surgery. Radioiodine is the treatment of choice in this situation.

Preparation for subtotal thyroidectomy has undergone an evolution in recent years. Although the use of antithyroid drugs in combination with iodine was standard therapy for several decades, recently preparation with beta-adrenergic blockers with or without potassium iodide has been in vogue. This regimen renders the patient euthyroid faster than would be ordinarily possible if one waited the usual 4 to 12 weeks for thionamides to have their optimal effect. Propranolol (Inderal) or another beta-adrenergic blocking agent is given for several weeks before surgery, in doses sufficient to lower the resting pulse to less than 80 beats per minute (160 to 240 mg per day of propranolol). Patients treated with beta-adrenergic blockers, however, are usually not euthyroid when operated on, even with the addition of iodine to the regimen; because the half-life of thyroxine is 6.9 days, patients may be hyperthyroxinemic postoperatively and require continuing beta-adrenergic blockade. Furthermore, more postoperative problems (e.g., fever and tachycardia) have been observed in patients treated in this manner, especially in patients with severe disease. Therefore unless there is a reason that surgery must be performed quickly, it seems reasonable to prepare the patient in the traditional manner with thionamides until the euthyroid state has been achieved. It is also traditional that potassium iodide, one to three drops of saturated solution of potassium iodide (SSKI) daily, be added to the regimen 10 days before surgery, to decrease blood flow to the gland. If surgery must be performed under emergent conditions, preparation with beta-adrenergic blockers, orally or intravenously, is reasonable. The use of oral cholecystographic agents (see later discussion) should also be considered.

Management of Hyperthyroidism in Pregnancy

Thyrotoxicosis affects approximately 1 in every 500 to 2000 pregnancies. Because radioiodine is contraindicated, antithyroid drugs are the treatment of choice in this situation. Propylthiouracil (PTU) is generally preferred over methimazole (Tapazole) because it crosses the placental barrier poorly and because a minor congenital scalp defect (aplasia cutis) has been associated with methimazole. Methimazole, however, would be an acceptable alternative to PTU, and, in fact, it is the drug of first choice in pregnancy in many parts of the world.

Antithyroid drugs are not teratogenic, but neonatal thyroid function can be affected by transplacental passage. Because fetal wastage and maternal morbidity are significant problems in untreated or inadequately treated thyrotoxicosis, however, the antithyroid drug dosage should be adequate to control the disease, keeping the free thyroxine index in the upper part of the normal or mildly thyrotoxic range. Fortunately, thyrotoxicosis often spontaneously improves in the latter months of pregnancy, permitting the thionamide dose to be lowered or even discontinued. Doses of

PTU below 150 mg per day are rarely associated with fetal thyroid dysfunction. Also, if affected, neonatal thyroid function is usually only mildly depressed, and long-term follow-up of children exposed to thionamides in utero has not shown significant developmental or intellectual deficits. Combined thionamide and thyroxine therapy is not recommended because it does not prevent neonatal hypothyroidism and because it may result in the inadvertent administration of thionamides in doses higher than are really necessary to control the thyrotoxicosis. The clinician should be aware that after delivery, there is often an exacerbation of previously remitted or relatively mild disease. Beta-adrenergic blocking agents can be used early in treatment to alleviate bothersome symptoms and are generally considered to be safe in pregnancy. PTU can be given safely to a nursing mother, although it would be prudent to monitor the baby's thyroid function at periodic intervals.

Thyroid Storm

Thyroid storm is a rare condition characterized by uncompensated thyrotoxicosis, with fever, tachycardia or tachyarrhythmias, and altered mental status. There is almost always a precipitant, usually an infection, surgery, or delivery in a previously untreated or poorly controlled patient. In addition to supportive measures (e.g., intravenous fluids, cooling blankets, mild sedatives), large doses of antithyroid drugs are used to block thyroid hormone synthesis completely. Doses of PTU of 200 to 300 mg every 6 hours are usually recommended; PTU is preferred because of its inhibitory effect on T_4 to T_3 conversion. The drug can be given by nasogastric tube or rectally. In addition to thionamides, iodine is given to block release of thyroid hormone from the gland. Potassium iodide can be given orally as SSKI, five drops three or four times a day. Iodine should be given only after thionamides have been started, to avoid enriching the thyroid gland with iodine and possibly accelerating hormonal synthesis. The use of ipodate sodium (Oragraffin) or iopanoic acid (Telepaque), gallbladder dyes with potent effects on T_4 to T_3 conversion, which also release free iodine into the circulation, is also useful in this setting. Doses of 0.5 to 1.0 gram daily are usually chosen.

Beta-adrenergic blocking agents are a cornerstone of therapy of thyroid storm. Intravenous propranolol (Inderal) (2 to 5 mg every 4 hours or as an infusion at a rate of 5 to 10 mg per hour) or oral propranolol in doses of 160 to 480 mg per 24 hours generally controls tachyarrhythmias and other catecholamine-mediated effects. Esmolol

(Brevibloc) could also be used in this setting, especially if there is a history of pulmonary disease. Stress doses of glucocorticoids are usually recommended in patients with thyroid storm, but the rationale for their use is uncertain. Large doses do inhibit T_4 to T_3 conversion, and steroids may help to stabilize the vascular bed. If conventional therapy fails, thyroid storm can also be managed with plasmapheresis and peritoneal dialysis. Generally, these measures are not necessary.

THYROID CANCER

method of
BARBARA K. KINDER, M.D.
Yale University
New Haven, Connecticut

EVALUATION OF THYROID NEOPLASMS

Because thyroid nodules are extremely common in the general population and thyroid carcinomas relatively rare, means of identifying patients who can be followed nonoperatively are both clinically desirable and cost-effective. The use of thyroid fine-needle aspiration (FNA) cytology is clearly the major advance in thyroidology in recent years. The procedure is simply done, frequently at the first outpatient visit, using a No. 21 gauge needle with immediate preparation of a smeared microscope slide in 95% ethanol for Papanicolaou staining and of a 50% ethanol wash of the residual material in the syringe for cell block. Complications of the procedure are essentially nonexistent, although caution should be exercised in performing the procedure on patients with coagulopathies or who are taking medications associated with clotting abnormalities. The accuracy of FNA is primarily related to the experience of the thyroid cytologist and the adequacy of the specimen, but data from multiple series report sensitivities of 83 to 99% with specificities of 70 to 90%. Cytologic features associated with different thyroid conditions are noted in Table 1. It is important to note that the nuclear features seen in papillary carcinoma on FNA are usually not present on frozen section, so the FNA may be critical for operative decision making. Anaplastic carcinoma and thyroid lymphoma may have similar clinical presentations, which include a rapidly growing, sometimes painful thyroid mass, associated with difficulty swallowing and stridor. In fact, these patients may present as respiratory emergencies, and a prompt decision needs to be made regarding treatment. FNA cytology can reliably differentiate between these entities. The main limitation of FNA is in the differential diagnosis of follicular adenoma and carcinoma.

Since the advent of FNA, the use of imaging modalities has been relegated by the author primarily to the assessment of function of a nodule by radionuclide scanning (warm or hot nodules being less likely to be malignant) and evaluation of the contralateral lobe or of the growth of a nodule over a period of clinical follow-up by ultrasonography. Figure 1 shows an algorithm for the evaluation of thyroid nodules. These are general guidelines: The decision to operate on a patient with a thyroid nodule may be influenced by other clinical factors, such as the age or sex of the patient, the size of the nodule, the presence of clinical symptoms referable to the nodule, and the patient's wishes.

WELL-DIFFERENTIATED THYROID CARCINOMA

The term "well-differentiated thyroid carcinoma" refers to tumors of follicular cell origin that fall into two main groups based on histologic appearance and biologic behavior. The most common and most favorable prognostically are the papillary carcinomas, which have a papillary or frond-like appearance histologically and exhibit characteristic nuclear features, including nuclear grooves and folds and cleared nuclear chromatin ("Orphan Annie" nuclei) on paraffin sections. These neoplasms tend to exhibit intraglandular and extraglandular lymphatic spread, but the presence of lymphatic metastases, in contrast to other cancers, does not generally adversely influence prognosis. Follicular carcinomas do not show the nuclear features of papillary neoplasms but form follicles and exhibit vascular and capsular invasion. Lesions with capsular invasion only have a much more favorable prognosis. Pathologists must take care in the interpretation of follicular neoplasms that have had needle aspirations performed to be sure that "capsular invasion" is not in reality the site of a previous biopsy. Follicular carcinomas are more aggressive than papil-

TABLE 1. **Cytologic Features of Thyroid Conditions**

Cytology	Characteristics
Benign	Bland follicular cells, hemosiderin-laden macrophages, amorphous material
Papillary carcinoma	Nuclear grooves and folds, intranuclear cytoplasmic inclusions, psammoma bodies
Follicular neoplasm	Cellular specimen, paucity of colloid, microfollicular architecture cannot differentiate benign and malignant
Hürthle cell neoplasm	Large cell, abundant granular cytoplasm cannot differentiate benign and malignant
Medullary carcinoma	May mimic papillary or follicular, plasmacytoid features, spindle cells, amyloid
Anaplastic carcinoma	Large pleomorphic cohesive cells, squamoid features, multinucleate cells
Lymphoma	*Large cell:* large, dispersed, monotonous cells *Lymphoplasmacytic:* spectrum from small lymphocytes to plasmacytoid cells

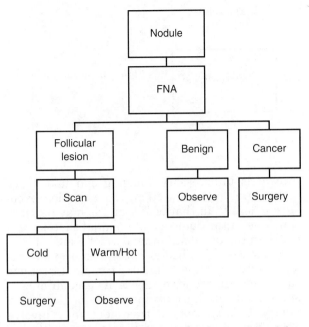

Figure 1. Algorithm for the evaluation of thyroid nodules. FNA = fine needle aspiration.

lary neoplasms and can metastasize hematogenously to lung and bone. Two variants of follicular carcinoma are also recognized: the follicular variant of papillary carcinoma and Hürthle cell carcinoma. The follicular variant of papillary carcinoma does not form papillae but does exhibit the typical nuclear features noted here. This tumor's behavior is biologically similar to that of papillary carcinoma and should be considered under that heading. Hürthle cell neoplasms are oncocytic tumors that, similar to other follicular lesions, are diagnosed as carcinoma when there is evidence of capsular or vascular invasion. Although considered well differentiated, Hürthle cell carcinomas have a significantly worse prognosis than papillary or follicular carcinomas, with a median survival of only 55 months in some series.

Recently a histologically distinctive neoplasm has been described that appears to occupy a clinical niche between well-differentiated and anaplastic carcinomas (Fig. 2). "Insular" or poorly differentiated carcinoma can be identified by the presence of nests or "insulae" of monotonous round cells, sometimes forming follicles. Tumor necrosis is common. The presence of insular carcinoma, even if focal, within an otherwise well-differentiated neoplasm portends a more aggressive course. Thus in a recent series of 25 patients with insular carcinoma, only four patients were alive and free of disease at 5 years.

Treatment

Appropriate treatment of well-differentiated thyroid cancer remains a matter of debate. Proponents of lobectomy and isthmectomy alone point to the usually excellent prognosis of most patients with these tumors and stress the importance of protecting the recurrent laryngeal nerve and parathyroids on the contralateral side. Disadvantages of a unilateral approach include the inability of using radioactive iodine diagnostically or therapeutically and of thyroglobulin as a tumor marker. Most importantly, there are a minority of patients with well-differentiated carcinoma who have more aggressive tumors and whose less favorable clinical course is responsible for the overall recurrence rate for well-differentiated carcinomas of slightly greater than 20% and an overall mortality rate of 10%. Evidence suggests that the clinical course in high-risk patients may be improved by more aggressive initial therapy, such as total or near total thyroidectomy and radioiodine ablation.

Toward that end, a number of clinical scoring systems have been developed to identify prospectively these high-risk patients. The AGES (*A*ge, *G*rade, *E*xtent, *S*ize) and AMES (*A*ge, *M*etastases, *E*xtent, *S*ize, *S*ex), applied by the Mayo and Lahey clinics to their thyroid cancer patients, appear to select those patients at greatest risk of dying of well-differentiated thyroid cancer.

Evaluation of DNA content and ploidy has been useful prognostically in a variety of epithelial neoplasms. There is a general correlation between ploidy and histologic subtype in thyroid tumors, with papillary carcinomas having the lowest percentage and anaplastic tumors the highest percentage of aneuploid tumors. There is some suggestion that aneuploidy may be an independent predictor of mortality in papillary but not in follicular carcinoma, perhaps related to the fact that there is a relatively high incidence of aneuploidy even in benign follicular lesions.

The field of molecular biology may bring additional precision to the assessment of the biologic nature of thyroid cancers. Cytogenetic study of some thyroid tumors has shown rearrangements of chromosome 10 and trisomy 7 that have been associated with a less favorable course in brain tumors. Chromosome 10 is of special interest because the genes for multiple endocrine neoplasia (MEN) Type II and the ret-proto-oncogene have been mapped to the region 10q11-21. Truncation and rearrangement convert this proto-oncogene to an active oncogene that is found in 15 to 20% of papillary (but not follicular, medullary, or anaplastic) thyroid cancers. In addition, *ras* oncogene expression has been shown to be involved in the

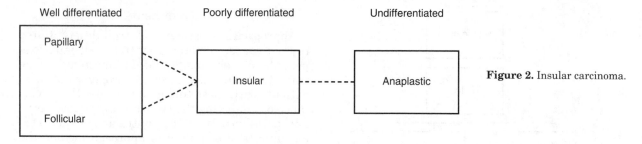

Figure 2. Insular carcinoma.

initiation and progression of thyroid tumors. Correlation of these molecular markers with biologic behavior of thyroid tumors has thus far been inconsistent, so their role in clinical decision making is as yet unclear.

Having arrived at the diagnosis of papillary carcinoma by FNA, the author's approach in most patients, particularly those with clinical features suggesting a less favorable prognosis by the AGES or AMES systems, would be to perform a total lobectomy on the side of the lesion and an intracapsular resection of the contralateral lobe. The author attempts to preserve all parathyroids if this is consistent with gross removal of tumor. The author has had no instances of hypoparathyroidism using this approach. The recurrent and superior (external branch) laryngeal nerves are routinely identified. Nodes in the central compartment are removed, and a functional neck dissection is performed if there are palpable jugular chain nodes.

Postoperative ablation with iodine 131 (^{131}I) is carried out in patients who are judged to be at risk of recurrence. The author prefers to hold thyroid replacement in these patients after surgery for 4 weeks. After assuring an increased thyroid-stimulating hormone (TSH) level, the author scans with 400 mCi of ^{123}I to confirm the presence and determine the amount of residual (usually normal) thyroid tissue. If there is greater than 1 to 2% uptake, the patient is admitted to the hospital for an ablative dose of 100 mCi of ^{131}I. A treatment scan is performed at 1 week as an outpatient procedure to visualize the treated tissue and see whether metastatic uptake is identified. Subsequent scanning and treatment depend on the patient's clinical profile, but treatment of residual or recurrent disease generally requires doses of 150 to 200 mCi with the goal of delivering approximately 20,000 rad to the tumor tissue.

Thyroglobulin levels are measured and in a given patient, when elevated, correlate well with residual and metastatic disease. Recently the use of thallium-201 scintigraphy in the follow-up of patients with differentiated thyroid carcinoma has shown promise. The advantages of this isotope include the fact that thyroid hormone with-

drawal is unnecessary, imaging can take place immediately after injection, the radiation exposure is less than that of ^{131}I, and it may be more sensitive in the detection of residual thyroid cancer than the usual scanning dose of 5 mCi of ^{131}I.

In the case of follicular carcinoma, the diagnosis is often not made until permanent sections can be scrutinized for evidence of vascular or capsular invasion. Capsular invasion alone carries a favorable prognosis, so treatment may involve only TSH suppression and clinical observation. If there is evidence of significant vascular invasion and the patient has other criteria that indicate a more aggressive course, a decision must be made about whether and when to ablate the remaining lobe. Ablation can be accomplished either surgically or with ^{131}I. Radioiodine ablation of a whole lobe is associated with an increased incidence of complications compared with remnant or tumor ablation. These include neck edema syndrome, pain, radiation thyroiditis, and hyperthyroidism. Because reoperation is also an unattractive option, we are inclined to carry out near total thyroidectomy as the primary procedure for large (>4 cm) follicular lesions, particularly in the older or male patient.

Because of its aggressive behavior, Hürthle cell carcinoma should be treated with near total thyroidectomy with ^{131}I ablation. Although these tumors often do not take up radioiodine, some elements of the tumor, including metastatic foci, perhaps more well differentiated, may do so and can be treated.

MEDULLARY CARCINOMA OF THE THYROID

Medullary carcinoma of the thyroid (MCT) arises from the parafollicular or C cells, which are derived from the neural crest and populate the thyroid in mammals during embryologic development. The tumor occurs either sporadically or as part of the MEN II syndrome. In the MEN patients, the process begins as C cell hyperplasia and progresses to carcinoma in situ before becoming frankly invasive carcinoma. C cell hyperplasia can be identified by an inappropriate rise of serum calcitonin following a calcium-pentagastrin infusion, and thus individuals at risk in a kindred can be treated at an early stage of the disease. Because of the variable onset of MCT, screening should begin in infancy for members of the MEN IIB kindreds and in childhood for those in MEN IIA families. Advances in molecular biology now permit presymptomatic identification of gene carriers by screening peripheral blood leukocyte DNA for evidence of markers closely associated with the locus for MEN IIA. The frequency of calcitonin screening can then be individualized based on the patient's predicted genetic risk.

Treatment

Because MCT is multifocal in all patients with MEN II and in a significant percentage of patients with sporadic disease, total thyroidectomy is the procedure of choice. Central lymph nodes should be removed and a modified neck dissection performed if there are palpable jugular chain nodes. Postoperatively calcitonin remains a sensitive tumor marker and may remain elevated in patients who present with bulky disease. Even when biochemical cure is not achieved, many patients do well clinically over years with no foci of tumor clinically identifiable. It is important to realize that MCT can secrete other peptide hormones, notably adrenocorticotropin hormone (ACTH), which may cause clinical symptoms. There is some evidence that the presence of immunohistochemical staining for somatostatin in MCT may be associated with a better prognosis. Radiation therapy may be useful in controlling nonresectable disease. The best results are achieved in kindreds in which patients can be identified and treated early.

ANAPLASTIC CARCINOMA

This aggressive tumor is seen primarily in older patients. The clinical presentation is usually dramatic, with the history of rapid growth of a hard, diffuse neck mass and local symptoms of difficulty swallowing and dyspnea. Diagnosis can be made by FNA as noted earlier.

Treatment

Although the prognosis is dismal, with the majority of patients dying of pulmonary metastases within months, local control should be undertaken with surgery and radiation therapy. In the rare patient who recurs late with local disease alone, re-resection may be indicated. In a single such patient, the author achieved satisfactory local control with a laryngectomy, pharyngectomy, and gastric pullup. Such cases are distinctly unusual.

LYMPHOMA

Thyroid lymphoma is uncommon, representing perhaps 5% of all thyroid malignancies. It is more common in women, and there is a recognized association with Hashimoto's thyroiditis. Clinical presentation may be indistinguishable from that of anaplastic carcinoma. FNA is critical in making this differential diagnosis. Although the diagnosis of large cell lymphoma is usually straightforward, differentiation between lymphoplasmacytoid lymphoma and Hashimoto's thyroiditis may be problematic. In such cases, immunophenotypic evidence of light chain restriction is conclusive evidence of lymphoma because lymphocytes in Hashimoto's thyroiditis should express both types of light chains.

Treatment

Unless the process is clearly confined to the thyroid, lymphoma is not primarily a surgical disease. Multimodality chemotherapy and radiation therapy result in dramatic tumor shrinkage and rapid resolution of airway compromise. Overall 5-year survival is around 70% with the variation in clinical course related to stage and histologic type.

PHEOCHROMOCYTOMA

method of
WILLIAM F. YOUNG, Jr., M.D.
Mayo Medical School
Mayo Clinic and Mayo Foundation
Rochester, Minnesota

Pheochromocytoma is a tumor frequently sought and rarely found. It is associated with spectacular cardiovascular disturbances, and when correctly diagnosed and properly treated, it is curable; when undiagnosed or improperly treated, it can be fatal. Catecholamine-producing tumors that arise from chromaffin cells of the adrenal medulla and sympathetic ganglia are termed "pheochromocytomas" and "paragangliomas." The term "pheochromocytoma," however, has become the generic name for all catecholamine-producing tumors and is used here to refer to both adrenal pheochromocytomas and paragangliomas.

CLINICAL MANIFESTATION

Prevalence estimates for pheochromocytoma vary from 0.01 to 0.1% of the hypertensive population.

These tumors occur equally in men and women, primarily in the third through fifth decades. Patients harboring these tumors may be asymptomatic. Symptoms usually are present, however, and are due to the pharmacologic effects of excess circulating catecholamines. Episodic symptoms include abrupt onset of throbbing headaches, generalized diaphoresis, palpitations, anxiety, chest pain, and abdominal pain. These spells can be extremely variable in their presentation and may be spontaneous or precipitated by postural changes, anxiety, exercise, or maneuvers that increase intra-abdominal pressure. The spell may last 10 to 60 minutes and may occur daily to monthly. The clinical signs include hypertension (paroxysmal in half of the patients and sustained in the other half), orthostatic hypotension, pallor, grade II to IV retinopathy, tremor, and fever. Pheochromocytoma of the urinary bladder is associated with painless hematuria and paroxysmal attacks induced by micturition or bladder distention. Severe, sustained hypertension is the usual presentation in children with pheochromocytoma; in addition, the tumors frequently are extra-adrenal and multiple in this age group.

A "rule of 10" has been quoted for pheochromocytomas: 10% are extra-adrenal, 10% occur in children, 10% are multiple or bilateral, 10% recur after surgical removal, 10% are malignant, and 10% are familial. The familial syndromes include familial pheochromocytoma, multiple endocrine neoplasia (MEN) types IIA (with pheochromocytoma, medullary carcinoma of the thyroid, and primary hyperparathyroidism) and IIB (with pheochromocytoma, medullary carcinoma of the thyroid, mucosal neuromas, thickened corneal nerves, intestinal ganglioneuromatosis, and marfanoid body habitus). Neurofibromatosis (von Recklinghausen's disease) and von Hippel–Lindau syndrome (retinal angiomatosis and cerebellar hemangioblastoma) also are associated with increased incidence of pheochromocytoma. Familial types of pheochromocytoma frequently involve both adrenal glands.

DIAGNOSIS

The diagnostic approach to catecholamine-producing tumors is divided into two series of studies (Fig. 1). First, the diagnosis of a catecholamine-producing tumor must be suspected and then confirmed biochemically by the presence of increased urine or plasma concentrations of catecholamines or their metabolites. Suppression testing with clonidine or provocative testing with glucagon, histamine, or metoclopramide rarely is needed. The differential diagnosis of pheochromocytoma is summarized in Table 1.

The next step is to localize the catecholamine-producing tumor to guide the surgical approach. Computer-assisted adrenal and abdominal imaging (magnetic resonance imaging or computed tomography) is the first localization test. Approximately 90% of these

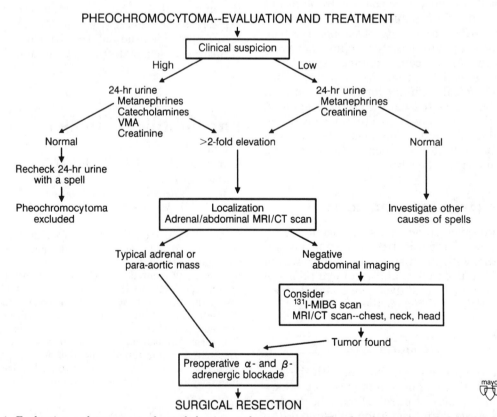

Figure 1. Evaluation and treatment of catecholamine-producing tumors. The details are discussed in the text. VMA = vanillylmandelic acid; CT = computed tomography; MRI = magnetic resonance imaging; ^{131}I-MIBG = ^{131}I-meta-iodobenzylguanidine.

TABLE 1. Differential Diagnosis of Pheochromocytoma Spells

Endocrine
Thyrotoxicosis
Menopausal syndrome
Hypoglycemia
Mastocytosis (systemic or activation disorder)
Hyperadrenergic spells
Renovascular disease
Cardiac
Essential hypertension—labile
Cardiovascular deconditioning
Paroxysmal cardiac arrhythmia
Withdrawal of adrenergic-inhibiting medications (e.g., clonidine)
Monoamine oxidase inhibitor treatment and concomitant ingestion of tyramine or decongestant
Angina
Psychological
Anxiety and panic attacks
Hyperventilation
Sympathomimetic ingestion
Illegal drug ingestion (cocaine, phencyclidine, lysergic acid)
Neurologic
Migraine headache
Diencephalic epilepsy
Fatal familial insomnia
Gold myokymia syndrome

tumors are found in the adrenals, and 98% are in the abdomen. If the abdominal imaging is negative, scintigraphic localization with iodine 131–meta-iodobenzylguanidine (^{131}I-MIBG) is indicated. This radiopharmaceutical accumulates preferentially in catecholamine-producing tumors; however, this procedure is not as sensitive as initially hoped (sensitivity 88%, specificity 99%). Computer-assisted chest, neck, and head imaging and central venous sampling are additional localizing procedures that can be used, although rarely are required. Thorough discussions of the diagnostic investigation of catecholamine-producing tumors are found elsewhere.

The emphasis here is on the therapeutic approach to pheochromocytomas. Hypertension usually is cured by excision of the tumor, and careful preoperative pharmacologic preparation is crucial to successful treatment.

TREATMENT

The treatment of choice for pheochromocytoma is surgical resection. Most of these tumors are benign and can be totally excised. Before the operation, however, the chronic and acute effects of excess circulating catecholamines must be reversed.

Preoperative Management

Combined alpha- and beta-adrenergic blockade is required preoperatively to control blood pressure and to prevent intraoperative hypertensive crises. Alpha-adrenergic blockade should be started at least 10 days preoperatively to allow for expansion of the contracted blood volume. A liberal salt diet is advised during the preoperative period. Once adequate alpha-adrenergic blockade is achieved, beta-adrenergic blockade is initiated (e.g., 3 days preoperatively).

Alpha-Adrenergic Blockade

Phenoxybenzamine (Dibenzyline) is an irreversible long-acting alpha-adrenergic blocking agent (Table 2). Approximately 25% of an oral dose of phenoxybenzamine is absorbed. Phenoxybenzamine is available as 10-mg capsules. The initial dosage is 10 mg orally two times daily; the

TABLE 2. Orally Administered Drugs Used to Treat Patients with Pheochromocytoma

Drug (Trade Name)	Dosage Range (mg/day)*	Side Effects
Alpha-Adrenergic Blocking Agents		
Phenoxybenzamine (Dibenzyline)	20†—100†	Postural hypotension, tachycardia, miosis, nasal congestion, diarrhea, inhibition of ejaculation, fatigue
Prazosin (Minipress)	1–20†	First-dose effect, dizziness, drowsiness, headache, fatigue, palpitations, nausea
Terazosin (Hytrin)	1–20†	First-dose effect, asthenia, blurred vision, dizziness, nasal congestion, nausea, peripheral edema, palpitations, somnolence
Doxazosin (Cardura)	1–20	First-dose effect, orthostasis, peripheral edema, fatigue, somnolence
Combined Alpha- and Beta-Adrenergic Blocking Agent		
Labetalol (Normodyne, Trandate)	200†–1200†	Dizziness, fatigue, nausea, nasal congestion, impotence
Catecholamine Synthesis Inhibitor		
α-Methyl-p-L-tyrosine (Demser)	1000‡–4000‡	Sedation, diarrhea, anxiety, nightmares, crystalluria, galactorrhea, extrapyramidal symptoms

*Given once daily unless otherwise indicated.
†Given as two doses daily.
‡Given in three or four doses daily.

dosage is increased by 10 to 20 mg every 2 days as needed to control the blood pressure and spells. The effects of daily administration are cumulative for nearly a week. The average dose is 20 to 100 mg per day. Side effects include postural hypotension, tachycardia, miosis, nasal congestion, inhibition of ejaculation, diarrhea, and fatigue.

Prazosin (Minipress), terazosin (Hytrin), and doxazosin (Cardura) are selective alpha-adrenergic blocking agents. After oral administration, they are highly bound to plasma proteins. Metabolism occurs primarily in the liver, and the majority of the drug is excreted in the bile and feces. The plasma half-lives of prazosin, terazosin, and doxazosin are approximately 3, 12, and 22 hours. These agents are available as 1-, 2-, 4-, 5-, 8-, and 10-mg tablets/capsules. The initial dose is 1 mg orally at bedtime to avoid the occasional syncope that follows the first dose. The dosage, up to 20 mg orally (in divided doses for prazosin), is then increased every 2 days as needed to control blood pressure. Side effects with prazosin therapy include dizziness, drowsiness, headache, fatigue, palpitations, and nausea. The side effects with terazosin include asthenia, blurred vision, dizziness, nasal congestion, nausea, peripheral edema, palpitations, and somnolence. Because of the more favorable side effect profiles of prazosin, terazosin, and doxazosin, these agents may be preferable to phenoxybenzamine when long-term pharmacologic treatment is indicated (e.g., for metastatic pheochromocytoma).

Phenoxybenzamine is the preferred drug for preoperative preparation because it provides alpha-adrenergic blockade of long duration. Effective alpha-adrenergic blockade permits expansion of blood volume, which usually is severely decreased as a result of excessive adrenergic vasoconstriction.

Beta-Adrenergic Blockade

The beta-adrenergic antagonist should be administered only after alpha-adrenergic blockade is effective because beta-adrenergic blockade alone may result in more severe hypertension owing to the unopposed alpha-adrenergic stimulation. Preoperative beta-adrenergic blockade is indicated to control the tachycardia associated with both the high circulating catecholamine concentrations and the alpha-adrenergic blockade. Caution is indicated if the patient is asthmatic or has congestive heart failure. Chronic catecholamine excess can produce a myocardiopathy, and beta-adrenergic blockade can result in acute pulmonary edema. Noncardioselective beta-adrenergic blockers, such as propranolol (Inderal and Inderal LA) and nadolol (Corgard), or cardioselective beta-adrenergic blockers, such as atenolol (Tenormin) and metoprolol (Lopressor), may be used. (Mechanisms of action, routes of metabolism, dosages, and side effects are discussed elsewhere in this text.) When administration of the beta-adrenergic blocker is begun, the drug should be used cautiously and at a low dose. For example, propranolol is usually started at 10 mg orally twice daily at least 1 week after the initiation of alpha-adrenergic blockade. The dose is then increased as necessary to control the tachycardia.

Labetalol (Normodyne, Trandate) exhibits both selective alpha$_1$-adrenergic and nonselective beta-adrenergic blocking activities in a ratio of approximately 1:3. It is well absorbed after oral administration and is metabolized primarily in the liver; its metabolites are excreted in the urine. Labetalol is available as 100-, 200-, and 300-mg tablets. The dose is 100 mg orally twice a day initially and is increased in increments of 100 mg twice daily every 2 days up to 1200 mg per day if necessary for control of hypertension and spells. Labetalol is contraindicated in patients with nonallergic bronchospasm or congestive heart failure. It has been shown to be an effective agent for the treatment of hypertension associated with catecholamine-producing tumors. Some instances of paradoxical hypertensive responses, however, have been reported, presumably owing to incomplete alpha-adrenergic blockade. Therefore its safety as primary therapy is controversial. Hepatic and cholestatic jaundice have been associated with labetalol therapy on rare occasions. Side effects include dizziness, fatigue, nausea, nasal congestion, and impotence. Its role in the therapy of pheochromocytoma may be in the long-term pharmacologic management of patients with metastatic disease.

Catecholamine Synthesis Inhibitor

Alpha-methyl-L-tyrosine (metyrosine; Demser) inhibits the synthesis of catecholamines by blocking the enzyme tyrosine hydroxylase. It is rapidly absorbed from the gastrointestinal tract, and most of it is excreted in the urine unchanged. Metyrosine is available as 250-mg capsules. The initial dosage is 250 mg orally four times daily. The dosage may be increased by 500 mg per day every 2 days to a maximum of 4 grams per day (1 gram four times per day) as needed for blood pressure control. Side effects include sedation, diarrhea, anxiety, nightmares, crystalluria and urolithiasis, galactorrhea, and extrapyramidal manifestations. Therefore this agent should be used with caution and only when other agents have been ineffective. The extrapyramidal effects of phenothiazines or haloperidol may be potentiated, and their use concomitantly with metyrosine should be avoided. High fluid intake to avoid crystalluria is suggested for any patient taking more than 2 grams daily. Although some centers have used this agent preoperatively, the author has reserved it primarily for those patients who have persistent catecholamine-producing tumors that (for cardiopulmonary reasons) cannot be treated with combined alpha- and beta-adrenergic blockade.

Potential Alternative Agents

Calcium channel antagonists and angiotensin-converting enzyme inhibitors have been reported to control the hypertension associated with pheochromocytoma. Further experience is needed with these agents before any therapeutic recommendations can be made.

Acute Hypertensive Crises

These may occur before or during operation and should be treated with nitroprusside (Nipride) or phentolamine (Regitine) administered intravenously. Phentolamine is a short-acting nonselective alpha-adrenergic blocker. It is available in lyophilized form in vials containing 5 mg. An initial test dose of 1 mg is administered, and, if necessary, this is followed by repeat 5-mg boluses or a continuous infusion. The response to phentolamine is maximal in 2 to 3 minutes after a bolus injection and lasts 10 to 15 minutes. A solution of 100 mg of phentolamine in 500 mL of 5% dextrose and water can be infused at a rate titrated for blood pressure control.

Anesthesia and Surgery

This is a high-risk surgical procedure, and an experienced surgeon and anesthesiologist team are required. The last oral doses of alpha- and beta-adrenergic blockers can be administered early in the morning on the day of operation. Cardiovascular and hemodynamic variables must be monitored closely. Continuous measurement of intra-arterial pressure and heart rhythm is required. In the setting of congestive heart failure or decreased cardiac reserve, monitoring of pulmonary capillary wedge pressure is indicated. Premedication includes minor tranquilizers and barbiturates. Fentanyl and morphine should not be used because of the potential for stimulating catecholamine release from the pheochromocytoma. In addition, parasympathetic nervous system blockade with atropine should be avoided because of associated tachycardia. Induction usually is accomplished with thiopental (Pentothal), and general anesthesia is maintained with a halogenated ether, such as enflurane (Ethrane) or isoflurane (Forane). Hypertensive episodes should be treated with phentolamine (2 to 5 mg intravenously) or nitroprusside (Nipride) intravenous infusion (0.5 to 1.5 µg per kg per minute). Lidocaine (50 to 100 mg intravenously) or esmolol (Brevibloc) (50 to 200 µg per kg per minute intravenously) is used for cardiac arrhythmia.

Because intra-abdominal pheochromocytoma may be multiple and extra-adrenal, an anterior midline abdominal surgical approach is used. If the pheochromocytoma is in the adrenal gland, the entire gland should be removed. If the tumor is malignant, as much tumor as possible should be removed. Because of the bilateral nature of pheochromocytomas (10% in sporadic cases and 50% in familial syndromes), the contralateral adrenal should be palpated and removed if thought to be abnormal. If a bilateral adrenalectomy is planned preoperatively, the patient should receive glucocorticoid stress coverage while awaiting transfer to the operating room. Glucocorticoid coverage should be initiated in the operating room if unexpected bilateral adrenalectomy is necessary. The entire abdomen should be inspected carefully. Ligation of the tumor vasculature and then extirpation are indicated. Paragangliomas of the neck, chest, and urinary bladder require specialized approaches.

Hypotension may occur after surgical resection of the pheochromocytoma and should be treated with fluids and colloids. Postoperative hypotension is less frequent in patients who have had adequate alpha-adrenergic blockade preoperatively. If both adrenal glands had been manipulated, adrenocortical insufficiency should be considered as a potential cause of postoperative hypotension. Hypoglycemia can occur in the immediate postoperative period, and therefore blood glucose levels should be monitored, and the fluid given intravenously should contain 5% dextrose.

Blood pressure usually is normal by the time of dismissal from the hospital. Some patients remain hypertensive for up to 8 weeks postoperatively. Long-standing persistent hypertension does occur and may be related to accidental ligation of a polar renal artery, resetting of baroreceptors, established hemodynamic changes, structural changes of the blood vessels, altered sensitivity of the vessels to pressor substances, renal functional or structural changes, or coincident primary hypertension.

Approximately 2 weeks postoperatively, a 24-hour urine sample should be obtained for measurement of catecholamines and metanephrines. If the levels are normal, the resection of the pheochromocytoma can be considered to have been complete. In major centers, the surgical mortality rate is less than 2%. At the Mayo Clinic, the 30-day perioperative mortality in 110 patients operated between 1980 and 1989 was 0.9%. The survival rate after removal of a benign pheochromocytoma is nearly that of age-matched and sex-matched controls. The 24-hour urinary excretion of catecholamines should be checked annually for at least 5 years as surveillance for recurrence in the adrenal bed, metastatic pheochromocytoma, or delayed appearance of multiple primary tumors.

Malignant Pheochromocytoma (Pheochromoblastoma)

The distinction between benign and malignant catecholamine-producing tumors cannot be made on clinical, biochemical, or histopathologic characteristics. Malignancy is based on finding direct local invasion or disease metastatic to sites that do not have chromaffin tissue, such as lymph nodes, bone, lung, and liver. Metastatic lesions should be resected if possible. Painful skeletal metastatic lesions can be treated with external radiation therapy. In initial studies, local tumor irradiation with ^{131}I-MIBG has proved to be of limited therapeutic value. Further studies with ^{131}I-MIBG may help define a subset of patients with malignant pheochromocytoma who may benefit from this treatment. Although the 5-year survival rate is less than 50%, many of these patients have prolonged survival and minimal morbidity. If the tumor is considered to be aggressive and the quality of life is affected, combination chemotherapy may be considered. A chemotherapy program consisting of cyclophosphamide (Cytoxan, Neosar), vincristine (Oncovin, Vincasar), and dacarbazine (DTIC-Dome) given cyclically every 21 days has proved beneficial but not curative in these patients. Hypertension and spells can be controlled with combined alpha- and beta-adrenergic blockade or inhibition of catecholamine synthesis with metyrosine.

Pheochromocytoma in Pregnancy

Pheochromocytoma in pregnancy can cause the death of both the fetus and the mother. The treatment of hypertensive crises is the same as for nonpregnant patients. Although there is some controversy regarding the most appropriate management, pheochromocytomas should be removed immediately if diagnosed during the first two trimesters of pregnancy. Preoperative preparation is the same as for the nonpregnant patient. If medical therapy is chosen or if the patient is in the third trimester, cesarean section and removal of the pheochromocytoma in the same operation are indicated. Spontaneous labor and delivery should be avoided.

THYROIDITIS

method of
GREGORY P. BECKS, M.D.
University of Western Ontario
London, Ontario, Canada

The thyroiditides encompass a diverse group of thyroid disorders of various causes in which inflammation of the gland is a prominent histologic feature. These may be relatively asymptomatic or self-limited disorders or can be accompanied by long-term abnormalities of thyroid growth (goiter formation, nodularity) or function (hyperthyroidism or hypothyroidism). Therapy is predicated on first making an accurate diagnosis and understanding the natural history or course of the disorder, which may obviate specific therapy in some cases. A useful approach still is to consider thyroiditis as acute, subacute, or chronic.

ACUTE THYROIDITIS

This relatively rare entity is also referred to as suppurative or pyogenic thyroiditis. It is reported to occur most often in women, children, and the elderly. Most often it is caused by an acute bacterial infection of the gland, gram-positive cocci, *Enterobacteriaceae,* or anaerobes. Other causes include infections with fungi, parasites, actinomyces, mycobacteria, and *Pneumocystis carinii,* which can follow a subacute or chronic course. Pathologically the gland is infiltrated by polymorphonuclear leukocytes and lymphocytes with evidence of necrosis and abscess formation. With resolution, fibrosis may develop. Clinical manifestations include localized or diffuse thyroid swelling and inflammatory signs and symptoms, such as pain, tenderness, warmth, and redness. Localized fluctuance suggests abscess formation. Local or systemic features, such as lymphadenopathy, pharyngitis, dysphagia, neck flexion, fever, and sepsis, may also be present. Predisposing factors include underlying nodular thyroid disease; immunosuppressed states; and anatomic aberrations, such as persistence of the thyroglossal duct or a pyriform sinus fistula. Infection can also seed the gland following penetrating trauma or by hematogenous or lymphatic spread from adjacent or contiguous structures. The differential diagnosis includes hemorrhage into a cyst, necrosis in a thyroid nodule or tumor, and painful subacute thyroiditis.

Biochemically there is typically leukocytosis with a left shift. Thyroid function usually remains normal, although hyperthyroxinemia has been reported and is attributed to follicle disruption with release of thyroid hormone. Transient or permanent hypothyroidism may result but is rare. Thyroid antibodies are typically negative.

Thyroid scinitigraphy is not essential for the diagnosis and may be normal but can show hypofunction in involved areas. Ultrasonography demonstrates thyroid enlargement with the appearance of a cystic or complex mass. The diagnosis is confirmed by positive cultures and stains of thyroid fine-needle aspiration biopsy material and is supported by positive blood cultures or pharyngeal swabs. Special stains and cultures may need to be set up if an unusual or atypical infection is suspected.

Abscesses should be surgically drained and appropriate antibiotic therapy administered in the inpatient or outpatient setting, depending on the patient's general condition. Recurrences are rarely seen but should prompt investigation for an anatomic abnormality.

SUBACUTE THYROIDITIS

The two main disorders considered herein, designated as painful and painless subacute thyroiditis, constitute a spectrum of clinical thyroid problems, including 15 to 20% of cases of thyrotoxicosis. Sixty percent of cases of subacute thyroiditis are accounted for by the painful variant, so-called pseudogranulomatous or de Quervain's thyroiditis. This condition most likely represents a stereotypic thyroid inflammatory response to a viral infection, as evidenced by convalescent serologic studies and identification or isolation of viral particles from thyroid tissue. No single virus predominates, but coxsackie and adenovirus, influenza, and mumps have been most commonly identified. There is little evidence for an autoimmune cause; transient changes in thyroid antibody titers, thyroid-stimulating hormone (TSH) receptor antibodies, and thyroid-reactive lymphocytes are considered to be secondary phenomena. An increased risk of developing subacute thyroiditis is associated with human leukocyte antigen (HLA) Bw-35 haplotype in white and Asian populations. Clinically there is a preponderance of cases in women, which may be preceded by an upper respiratory tract infection or a prodrome of malaise, myalgias, and arthralgias. The hallmark is *painful* enlargement of the thyroid gland of variable intensity that may be asymmetrical or migratory, so-called creeping thyroiditis. Patients recognize this as a sore neck or an atypical sore throat. The pain may radiate toward the angle of the jaw, ears, or anterior chest. Accompanying fever is not uncommon, whereas cervical lymphadenopathy is said to be rare.

The histologic picture is one of extensive cellular destruction and desquamation of the thyroid epithelium, which is infiltrated by neutrophils, mononuclear cells, and lymphocytes. Pseudo-giant cells appear owing to masses of colloid surrounded by histiocytes. As a result of a release of thyroid hormone into the circulation, patients may also be mildly to moderately thyrotoxic during the early phase. The differential diagnosis includes early acute thyroiditis, anaplastic thyroid carcinoma or lymphoma, and Graves' disease. Biochemically there is typically an elevated erythrocyte sedimentation rate; normal or elevated leukocyte count; and increased serum thyroxine (T_4), triiodothyronine (T_3), and thyroglobulin levels, while thyrotropin (TSH) is suppressed. During the thyrotoxic phase, which typically lasts 4 to 6 weeks, iodine uptake is low, and the gland may be barely visible on scintigraphy even though there is a readily palpable goiter. The disease course classically includes a subsequent interval of euthyroidism during which time symptoms improve or resolve, followed by a variable period of hypothyroidism over 6 weeks to 3 months, which also resolves spontaneously. Relapses or recurrences are not common, although certainly not unheard of.

Treatment of pain and tenderness in the acute phase includes nonsteroidal anti-inflammatory agents (enteric-coated acetylsalicylic acid, 650 mg orally four times daily) for 7 to 10 days or glucocorticoids (prednisone, 10 mg orally four times daily or equivalent) for 1 to 2 weeks, then tapered to discontinue over a further 2 weeks. Responses may be fairly dramatic with pain relief within 24 hours. Thyrotoxicosis can be treated symptomatically with propranolol (Inderal), 20 to 40 mg four times daily for relief of palpitations, tremor, and agitation or restlessness. The hypothyroid phase may be managed expectantly with biochemical monitoring or, if symptomatic, low-dose levothyroxine (0.05 to 0.1 mg daily) should be prescribed for 3 to 6 months. Only 5% of patients show evidence of biochemical or clinical hypothyroidism in the long term. An increased susceptibility to iodine-induced hypothyroidism has been reported following subacute thyroiditis.

A *painless* variant of subacute thyroiditis is seen approximately 40% of the time. The exact cause of this disorder remains unclear. Present evidence does not favor a viral cause in most cases. Some authorities in the area have suggested an autoimmunity cause, but at present this is not well substantiated. Although the histologic picture is that of a lymphocytic infiltrate, its relationship to chronic autoimmune thyroiditis, including postpartum thyroiditis, is also unclear (see later). There is no specific HLA haplotype identified with this variant. Clinically the disease course is similar to painful subacute thyroiditis, but pain and tenderness in the gland are minimal or absent, with minimal perturbation in the sedimentation rate, no fever, and a modest goiter at most. Thyroid antibody titers tend to be low and may be undetectable. Again thyroid uptake is typically low in association with the thyrotoxic phase. Treatment is entirely expectant or symptomatic: beta blockade for thyrotoxicosis and a course of thyroxine replacement for hypothyroidism.

It should be noted that not all patients pass through all of the typical phases of these disorders. Recovery may proceed directly from the thyrotoxic phase, or this may be so mild as to be overlooked initially, and patients present when they are already entering the euthyroid or hypothyroid phase.

AUTOIMMUNE THYROIDITIS

This is best known as Hashimoto's disease or chronic lymphocytic thyroiditis. Variants include juvenile or adolescent thyroiditis, idiopathic myxedema, postpartum thyroiditis, and possibly some cases of painless or silent thyroiditis (see earlier). Hashimoto's disease is the most common form of thyroiditis, affecting up to 5% of the general population (10% in the elderly), with a definite female predilection. The disorder runs in families, and a genetic predisposition is associated with certain HLA haplotypes in various racial groups, specifically HLA-B8, HLA-DR3 and HLA-DR5 in the white population. It may also be seen in association with other endocrine and nonendocrine autoimmune disorders, including juvenile diabetes mellitus, primary adrenal insufficiency, autoimmune oophoritis, pernicious anemia, rheumatoid arthritis, myasthenia gravis, and inflammatory bowel disease. Autoimmune thyroiditis is also more common with Turner's, Klinefelter's, and Down's syndromes.

As mentioned, various clinical (and biochemical) presentations are recognized. These are often asymptomatic as far as patients are concerned or incidentally discovered by physicians. Most common is goitrous Hashimoto's disease with a diffusely firm, rubbery, or bosselated gland. Pain and tenderness may be encountered but are typically milder than in subacute thyroiditis. Occasionally more or less discrete nodular areas may be present. Regional lymphadenopathy is uncommon. Thyroid antibodies are present in significant or high titers in approximately 80% of individuals. Microsomal or peroxidase antibodies are more common than thyroglobulin antibodies, and titers tend to correlate with disease activity. Although many patients are euthyroid, hypothyroidism is present or develops in 30 to 40% of patients over time. The most sensitive indicator of evolving hypothyroidism is an elevation in serum TSH. Serum T_4 levels are within normal

limits or decreased, whereas serum T_3 levels decline only very late in the course of disease. Patients with Hashimoto's disease are particularly susceptible to iodide-induced, lithium-induced, and amiodarone (Cordarone)-induced hypothyroidism. Pathologically the gland is infiltrated with lymphocytes, sometimes forming germinal centers, with epithelial cell atrophy, eosinophilic changes in parenchymal cells, and variable degrees of fibrosis. A positive diagnosis can be made on fine-needle aspiration biopsy, although this is not routinely required and should be reserved for assessment of nodular areas or goiters that continue to enlarge, when the possibility of neoplasia or lymphoma is to be considered.

An atrophic variant of Hashimoto's thyroiditis is well recognized and may be associated with inhibitory or blocking type antibodies against the TSH receptor. This presents clinically as idiopathic myxedema. Another variant is postpartum thyroiditis, which occurs following 5 to 8% of normal deliveries in the setting of occult autoimmune thyroiditis associated with a transient rebound in immune surveillance following pregnancy. Various cytotoxic mechanisms result in follicle disruption and release of preformed thyroid hormone and thyroglobulin leading typically to biochemical or mild clinical thyrotoxicosis 6 weeks to 3 months postpartum. A goiter may be present, whereas an elevated sedimentation rate, leukocytosis, fever, and pain and tenderness in the gland are typically absent. Low thyroid uptake following radioiodine administration distinguishes this from postpartum relapses of Graves' thyrotoxicosis. Beta-blocker therapy usually suffices for management of thyrotoxic symptoms and can be considered even for nursing mothers. Typically a hypothyroid phase ensues between 6 and 9 months postpartum with spontaneous recovery by 1 year. Patients may be followed expectantly with biochemical monitoring, although thyroxine can be administered for more severe symptoms of hypothyroidism (including depression) and the need for long-term therapy reassessed after 6 to 12 months. Postpartum thyroiditis recurs 25% of the time following subsequent pregnancies and may ultimately culminate in chronic autoimmune thyroiditis.

Hashimoto's thyroiditis may also coexist with Graves' disease. In this case, thyroid function is determined by the balance of thyroid-stimulating antibodies and the functional status of the thyroid follicles. A particularly firm goiter and high titers of thyroid antibodies in an otherwise typical Graves' patient suggests coexistence of the two disorders. It is well documented that Hashimoto's thyroiditis may spontaneously remit, even with recovery from hypothyroidism, and the patient present subsequently with typical Graves' thyrotoxicosis. Graves' disease may culminate in a typical Hashimoto's thyroiditis phase with hypothyroidism.

The author recommends thyroxine therapy in cases of chronic autoimmune thyroiditis if two or more of the following are present; goiter, elevated serum TSH, positive thyroid antibodies, and a documented past or family history of thyroid autoimmunity. Euthyroid patients may be started on a fairly full suppressive dose, 0.1 mg levothyroxine daily, whereas hypothyroid patients are started on 0.025 to 0.05 mg daily and the dose increased at 4- to 6-week intervals based on subsequent TSH levels. The author aims to suppress the TSH level toward the lower limit of normal. A subnormal or undetectable TSH result suggests the possibility of subclinical thyrotoxicosis because most patients remain clinically euthyroid. In some patients, there is concern because of other risk factors for osteoporosis or the presence of coronary artery disease. In this case, a serum free T_4 or free T_3 level should be checked and the thyroxine dose reduced if the level is elevated. In general, average thyroxine requirements are decreased in the elderly and may be increased during pregnancy. Other medications, such as bile acid sequestrants (cholestyramine [Questran] or colestipol [Colestid]), sucralfate (Carafate) and phenytoin (Dilantin), may affect thyroxine absorption and metabolism and necessitate use of higher doses. Thyroxine should be continued more or less indefinitely with a check of the serum TSH level every 1 to 2 years. Goiters or nodules that enlarge despite suppressive or replacement thyroxine therapy should be considered for fine-needle aspiration biopsy or possible thyroid surgery.

INVASIVE FIBROUS THYROIDITIS

Also known as Riedel's thyroiditis or Riedel's struma, this is a rare thyroid disorder of unknown cause typically seen in middle-aged women and is characterized by fibrosis of the thyroid gland and adjacent extrathyroid nerves, blood vessels, and muscles. Associated conditions include salivary and lacrimal gland fibrosis, mediastinal and retroperitoneal fibrosis, and sclerosing cholangitis. There is no conclusive evidence, however, of an autoimmune cause, nor is it readily classified as a collagen vascular disease.

Clinically patients present with painless enlargement of the anterior neck accompanied by a sense of pressure, dysphagia, dyspnea, or hoarseness. A stony hard or woody thyroid is typical with diffuse or asymmetrical involvement. In some cases, the thyroid gland is not enlarged but may be fixed to adjacent structures. Lymphadenopathy and systemic signs and symptoms are unusual. Thyroid function is typically normal, unless the gland is totally obliterated, in which case hypothyroidism may be evident, and thyroid antibodies are negative or present in low titers. Thyroid scintigraphy typically shows hypofunction in involved areas.

Several cases of hypoparathyroidism have been reported in association with Riedel's thyroiditis, but this could be a chance finding. The differential diagnosis includes a fibrous variant of Hashimoto's thyroiditis, painless subacute thyroiditis, and a thyroid adenoma or carcinoma. Histologically there is a bland fibrosis with a minimal inflammatory component, which distinguishes this from the Hashimoto's variant. Arteritis and phlebitis may be seen, and thyroid adenomas are occasionally encountered in the center of fibrotic areas. The diagnosis is confirmed by open surgical biopsy as opposed to fine-needle aspiration biopsy. Surgery may also be indicated to exclude neoplasia as well as for relief of compressive symptoms with resection of the isthmus or occasionally hemithyroidectomy when there is unilateral involvement. Extensive surgery is generally not indicated. Thyroxine therapy is not helpful unless hypothyroidism is evident, and the value of glucocorticoid therapy is unproved. The prognosis is variable in that the disease may remit, stabilize, or progress. Mortality rates of 5 to 10% have been reported related to respiratory obstruction, but this seems excessive given presently available supportive therapy.

MISCELLANEOUS DISORDERS

Focal or patchy thyroiditis may be a histologic feature of a wide variety of other thyroid disorders, not warranting primary consideration or designation as thyroiditis. These include thyroiditis associated with trauma; neoplasms; colloid nodular disease or radiation; and certain drug effects, such as amiodarone administration or hypersensitivity reactions to anticonvulsants and sulfonamides.

Section 9

The Urogenital Tract

BACTERIAL INFECTIONS OF THE URINARY TRACT IN MALES

method of
KEITH N. VAN ARSDALEN, M.D.
Hospital of the University of Pennsylvania
Philadelphia, Pennsylvania

Bacterial infections of the male urinary tract occur in all age groups and may involve all parts of this system from the urethral meatus to the kidneys. With the exception of the first 3 months of life, these infections are much less common in males than in females. In young adults, bacteriuria is 30 times more prevalent in women than in men, but this ratio decreases significantly to approximately 2:1 in the elderly, presumably associated with the development of prostatic enlargement and voiding dysfunction. It has been estimated than fewer than 1% of men between the ages of 50 and 59 years have bacteriuria, with the incidence rising to 3 to 4% by 70 years of age and perhaps to as high as 20% beyond 80 years of age. This figure may be several times higher in hospitalized elderly men.

The ascending route is the most common pathway for bacteria entering the urinary tract, although hematogenous infection may also occur. A zinc salt isolated from prostatic secretions may be an antibacterial factor that, along with the protective length of the male urethra, may normally prevent the retrograde ascent of bacteria into the male urinary tract. Intrinsic bladder defense mechanisms include the hydrokinetic clearance of bacteria through voiding (compromised in patients with outlet obstruction and residual urine), bacterial antiadherence activity of the mucopolysaccharides of the bladder mucosa, and the antimicrobial effects of urine. In the absence of instrumentation, the factors that overwhelm the natural defense mechanisms of the urinary tract are generally unclear.

The pathogenic organisms that usually invade the urinary tract include various serotypes of *Escherichia coli* and, less commonly, other gram-negative rods, including *Klebsiella, Proteus, Enterobacter,* and *Pseudomonas* spp. Gram-positive organisms, such as *Enterococcus* and *Staphylococcus* spp, are occasionally involved. The common sexually transmitted organisms include *Neisseria gonorrhoeae, Chlamydia trachomatis,* and *Ureaplasma urealyticum.* The diagnosis of these organisms and specific sensitivities may be determined by appropriate midstream urine cultures, urethral cultures, or both. Segmental bacterial localization cultures, further investigation of the upper and lower por-

tions of the urinary tract, or both are indicated for the evaluation of recurrent urinary tract infections that imply either bacterial persistence or reinfection. Recurrent infections may be related to urinary tract obstruction, urinary stasis, a foreign body or calculus, or, most commonly, bacterial persistence in the prostate.

URETHRITIS

Urethritis is generally subdivided into gonococcal and nongonococcal. Both forms may be associated with dysuria, itching, and a urethral discharge. The presence of a discharge may be unreliable for diagnosis, however, because one-fourth of men with gonorrhea and two-thirds of men with nongonococcal urethritis (NGU) may not complain of a discharge. Gonococcal urethritis is associated with the gram-negative diplococcus *N. gonorrhoeae.* NGU is diagnosed by demonstrating evidence of urethritis in the absence of gonorrhea. NGU is now approximately twice as common as gonococcal urethritis, with *C. trachomatis* thought to be the most common causative organism followed by *U. urealyticum.* These organisms may coexist with *N. gonorrhoeae* and may account for the development of postgonococcal urethritis if treatment is given only for *N. gonorrhoeae.*

The standard treatment of gonococcal urethritis in men had been with aqueous procaine penicillin G. Owing to the development of resistance to penicillin as the result of the acquisition of a plasmid for penicillinase production, the current Centers for Disease Control (CDC) recommendation for the treatment of gonococcal urethritis is ceftriaxone (Rocephin), 250 mg intramuscularly. Because approximately 30% of men with gonococcal urethritis are simultaneously infected with *C. trachomatis,* which is not sensitive to ceftriaxone, the current recommended treatment for gonococcal urethritis also includes a tetracycline or a tetracycline derivative (doxycycline, 100 mg twice daily) given for 7 days. Alternative therapy for *N. gonorrhoeae* with or without *C. trachomatis* includes ciprofloxacin (Cipro), 500 mg orally once, or ofloxacin (Floxin), 400 mg orally once, followed by doxycycline, 100 mg orally twice daily for 7 days. A third alternative is simply to give ofloxacin, 300 mg orally twice daily for 7 days, but compliance with this longer regimen is essential to assure adequate treatment. As a corollary, in the absence of *N. gonorrhoeae,* NGU may be treated for 7 days with either doxycycline or ofloxacin.

EPIDIDYMO-ORCHITIS

Acute epididymitis generally develops secondary to spread of infection to this area from a primary site in the urethra, prostate, or bladder. Secondary involvement of the testicle in association with acute epididymitis is relatively common. In sexually active men younger than 35 years of age, the most common infecting organisms are those producing urethritis, that is, *N. gonorrhoeae* and *C. trachomatis,* as noted. Although these organisms may also infect older men, the most common organisms in the latter group are the gram-negative rods that are responsible for cystitis and prostatitis.

Treatment of epididymo-orchitis in men with infections suspected to be secondary to sexually transmitted organisms is generally the same as that for the treatment of urethritis, as outlined previously. A tetracycline; a tetracycline derivative; or one of the quinolones, such as ciprofloxacin (Cipro) or ofloxacin (Floxin), should be continued for a minimum of 10 to 14 days, however. Supportive measures include best rest and scrotal elevation. The sexual partner or partners should also be treated. Further evaluation of the genitourinary tract in this setting is usually unrewarding because underlying pathology is rare.

The treatment of epididymo-orchitis secondary to gram-negative bacteriuria begins initially with the administration of broad-spectrum antibiotics. A cephalosporin or a quinolone may be administered orally or intravenously, depending on the clinical setting. A fever higher than 101° F, an elevated white blood cell count, or advancing age usually warrants admission to the hospital and intravenous therapy. The results of the urine culture and sensitivity determine subsequent therapy. Bed rest and scrotal elevation are again important supportive measures. In this setting, the genitourinary tract should be evaluated for underlying pathology. An intravenous urogram may be obtained as soon as the patient is stable, as should an ultrasound-determined residual urine volume. Endoscopy or other instrumentation of the urethra and lower urinary tract should be delayed 4 to 6 weeks after therapy if possible.

PROSTATITIS SYNDROMES

See the article "Prostatitis" later in this section.

CYSTITIS AND PYELONEPHRITIS

Cystitis and pyelonephritis are seen most commonly as ascending infections of the genitourinary tract, particularly from the prostate. In this regard, the most common offending pathogens are the gram-negative rods, although infections caused by gram-positive organisms, such as enterococci and occasionally staphylococci, may also be noted. Acute cystitis without evidence of upper urinary tract infection may initially be treated with oral antibiotics. Commonly used antibiotics that continue to have efficacy include nitrofurantoin (Macrodantin), trimethoprim-sulfamethoxazole double strength (Bactrim DS, Septra DS), or the oral cephalosporins cephalexin (Keflex) and cephradine (Velosef). The newer oral quinolones norfloxacin (Noroxin), ciprofloxacin (Cipro), ofloxacin (Floxin), and lomefloxacin (Maxaquin) are also efficacious and may be particularly useful if there is a known history of chronic bacterial prostatitis. Trimethoprim-sulfamethoxazole may also be useful in this instance.

Therapy for acute pyelonephritis is generally started with gentamicin, 3 to 5 mg per kg per day in three divided intravenous doses, plus ampicillin, 1 gram intravenously every 6 hours. Alternatively, primary intravenous therapy may be given with appropriate third-generation cephalosporin derivatives or penicillin derivatives depending on the culture results and the antibiotic sensitivities. A change may be made to oral therapy after the patient has become afebrile for a minimum of 24 hours. The oral medications noted here may be useful depending on the sensitivities and should be continued for at least 14 days. A complete urologic investigation is warranted in cases of pyelonephritis and cystitis to identify associated genitourinary abnormalities. Lower urinary tract localization cultures are also recommended if there is evidence of recurrent urinary tract infections.

BACTERIAL INFECTIONS OF THE URINARY TRACT IN FEMALES

method of
JOHN A. MATA, M.D.
Louisiana State University Medical Center
Shreveport, Louisiana

Urinary tract infection (UTI) in women is a common problem. Symptoms suggestive of cystitis account for 2 to 5% of primary care visits. Up to 50% of women experience at least one episode of painful voiding (dysuria), half of whom have a culture-proven bacterial

UTI. The prevalence rate of bacteriuria (2 to 10%) increases with age, so it is not uncommon that patients with symptoms of a UTI compose up to 10% of a general practice.

The vast majority of UTIs in women are uncomplicated and usually occur in healthy women. Infections in these individuals respond promptly to treatment. There is a small cohort of patients, however, who have complicating factors (Table 1), who have recurrent or persistent UTIs, or who may have a life-threatening infection.

ETIOLOGY AND DIAGNOSIS

The most common cause of UTI in women is bacterial ascent from the periurethral area by organisms that normally constitute the fecal flora. *Escherichia coli, Staphylococcus* spp, and strains of *Proteus, Klebsiella,* and *Enterobacter* are among the common causative organisms. Bacteriuria (presence of significant 10^2 cfu/mL bacteriuria in an uncontaminated collected urine specimen) is generally preceded by colonization of the periurethral and vaginal mucosa by the infecting organism. The majority of bacteriuric infections occur in the lower tract (cystitis, urethritis), not in the upper tract (pyelonephritis), and in more than 90% of the cases, the infections are uncomplicated but prone to recurrence. Studies of host defenses and bacterial virulence factors suggest that many women burdened with recurrent UTIs are biologically susceptible to bacteriuria, and this is likely a lifelong phenomenon.

The signs and symptoms of UTI in women are characteristic but not specific in that the bladder and urethra respond similarly to a variety of irritative factors. Dysuria, frequency, and urgency are commonly present; however, fever, flank pain, or costovertebral angle tenderness may herald a renal infection in 50% of patients. Patients presenting for the first time with bladder symptoms should be accurately diagnosed before treatment to avoid missing other entities that may mimic a UTI (Table 2). After a history, an abdominal and pelvic examination is helpful to exclude gynecologic conditions. A properly collected, clean-catch midstream or catheterized urine specimen is then analyzed. The new dipstick reagents that test for nitrites and leukocyte esterase are accurate as a screen and are used in addition to a microscopic examination to confirm the presence of bacteriuria and pyuria. A urine culture and sensitivity per se is no longer critical in the majority of women with routine, uncomplicated

TABLE 2. **Differential Diagnosis of Cystitis Symptoms in Women**

Occult pyelonephritis
Sexually transmitted diseases
Vaginitis
Urethral syndrome
Interstitial cystitis
Carcinoma in situ

UTIs but may be prudent on a patient's first visit and in patients suspected to have persistent bacteriuria with organisms such as *Proteus* or an infection that does not seem to be resolving.

MANAGEMENT

Antibiotic Selection

Patients with uncomplicated UTIs respond well to 3-day treatment regimens. This abbreviated course is a good compromise between 1-day therapy and the conventional 7- to 14-day regimens. The relapse rate of 3-day therapy is comparable to longer courses of conventional therapy; such abbreviated therapy is less costly and is associated with fewer drug-induced toxicities. Treatment of symptomatic patients with bacteriuria/pyuria is begun immediately without waiting for culture results (if done). Table 3 summarizes common multiday short-course antibiotics used in 3-day therapy. The various drug classes have their own peculiar side effect profiles, and the physician should be familiar with each of these.

Patients susceptible to *Candida* vaginitis should receive an antibiotic such as nitrofurantoin that is not active on the vaginal flora. More than 90% of women with uncomplicated UTI should be cured with appropriate antimicrobials given in a 3-day course. Some women may benefit from urinary analgesics, such as phenazopyridine (Pyridium), 100 mg orally three times a day, or antispasmodic combinations, such as flavoxate (Urispas), 100 mg orally twice daily. Depending on one's practice, treated patients can call back to report how they are doing or return to the

TABLE 1. **Complicating Factors in Female Urinary Tract Infection**

Diabetes
Stone disease
Chronic catheter
Urethral diverticulum
Immunosuppression
Pregnancy
Neuropathic bladder
Congenital anomalies (reflux)
Urethral stenosis
Urinary tract obstruction

TABLE 3. **Antibiotic Therapy for Female Urinary Tract Infection**

Antimicrobial	3-Day Oral Regimen
Trimethoprim-sulfamethoxazole	160 mg/800 mg bid
Nitrofurantoin (Macrobid)	100 mg bid
Amoxicillin	250–500 mg tid
Cephalexin* (Keflex)	250–500 mg qid
Norfloxacin (Noroxin)	400 mg bid

*Other oral cephalosporins and quinolones with similar effectiveness are available.

office for a confirmatory urine check or culture while off antibiotics.

The greatest risk factors in patients with simple infections include sexual activity, use of diaphragm contraceptives, and a history of an uncomplicated UTI. Plenty of fluids and frequent bladder emptying are helpful. In patients with so-called honeymoon cystitis, pericoital antibiotics, such as trimethoprim-sulfamethoxazole or nitrofurantoin, approximately 2 hours before or after intercourse are effective.

Recurrent Urinary Tract Infections and Prophylactic Antibiotics

In about 20% of women, frequent (two to four per year) reinfections occur after the initial UTI episode. These recurrences are reinfections (not persistence) with new organisms, although it may still be an *E. coli* but of a different serotype. Unfortunately, the majority of women experience another symptomatic UTI within a 2-year period after the initial bout. These again tend to be uncomplicated infections. If these recurrences occur at frequent, closely spaced intervals, such as two or more UTIs in a 6-month period or less, low-dose daily prophylactic therapy or antibiotic self-administration may be indicated.

Prophylactic therapy should have minimal or no adverse effects on the fecal and vaginal flora. Minimal oral dosages at bedtime of trimethoprim, 50 mg; nitrofurantoin, 100 mg; cephalexin, 250 mg; or trimethoprim-sulfamethoxazole (single strength) are useful. Daily treatment reduces reinfections to 5 to 10% of that seen before prophylaxis but does not seem to change an individual patient's propensity to UTIs once prophylactic treatment is discontinued. The typical length of prophylactic therapy is 3 to 6 months. Self-administration of an antibiotic at the first onset of bacteriuria symptoms is a reasonable strategy for motivated patients. Many of the patients on such self-treatment regimens keep urinary dipsticks or dipslide culture tubes available to confirm the presence of pyuria or bacteriuria as they begin a 1- to 3-day short-course treatment regimen. Female patients on chronic prophylaxis, self-treatment, or post-intercourse therapy should all have had previous urine cultures and a good history of previous infections before undertaking one of these therapeutic regimens. It seems that UTI in susceptible women is often a biologic or genetic problem and one in which surgical or mechanical intervention is unlikely to be helpful.

Urinary Tract Infections in Pregnancy

Asymptomatic or symptomatic bacteriuria in pregnant women should be treated when diagnosed during routine prenatal screening. Pregnancy makes bacteriuric women susceptible to acute pyelonephritis and thus may lead to infant morbidity (prematurity). Safe drugs include the penicillins, cephalosporins, and nitrofurantoin. Lower tract infections (cystitis) may be treated by a 3-day antibiotic course. In these patients, it is prudent to check the urine or obtain a culture 2 to 5 days after treatment to make sure one is not dealing with a resistant organism or occult pyelonephritis, which would require culture-specific antibiotics or a longer therapeutic course. Acute pyelonephritis unresponsive to conventional management mandates that one rule out obstruction. Renal ultrasonography early on may be helpful. Because of the hydronephrosis of pregnancy, obstructive uropathy may be difficult to diagnose with certainty, and urologic consultation may be necessary. Sometimes a limited (two to three exposure) intravenous pyelogram is required when the ultrasound study is equivocal and calculi or other causes of obstruction are suspected.

Occult or Acute Pyelonephritis

Pyelonephritis denotes (upper tract) infection in the renal pelvis and parenchyma. Clinicians are alert to this diagnosis in patients with a UTI accompanied by fever or flank pain. A subset of patients also exists who present with only lower tract symptoms who may have occult pyelonephritis and warrant more conventional 7- to 14-day oral therapy. Risk factors for occult pyelonephritis include pregnancy, prolonged symptoms (greater than 1 week), diabetes, and patients with a history of childhood UTI or genitourinary problems (stones, recent instrumentation). Patients with occult pyelonephritis (and many with clinical renal infection) respond well to conventional oral therapy with antibiotics that have good tissue penetration characteristics, such as trimethoprim-sulfamethoxazole, amoxicillin, the quinolones, and some cephalosporins. Ill patients benefit from hospitalization for intravenous fluids and parenteral antibiotics. If a more complicated UTI is suspected, sonographic or radiographic imaging may be warranted. After treatment, a follow-up urinalysis, culture, or both can document a successful treatment outcome.

Complicated Urinary Tract Infections

A small cohort of female patients may have persistent or unresolved bacteriuria secondary to a complicated UTI. A complicated UTI generally occurs in conjunction with any of the following: obstruction (e.g., stones), indwelling urinary

TABLE 4. **Diagnosis in Complicated Urinary Tract Infection**

Upper Tract
Renal/perinephric abscess
Pyonephrosis (infected hydronephrosis)
Acute bacterial nephritis (lobar nephronia)
Xanthogranulomatous pyelonephritis
Emphysematous pyelonephritis

Lower Tract
Cystitis cystica/glandulous
Malakoplakia
Cystitis emphysematosa
Vesicointestinal fistula
Chronic interstitial cystitis

catheter, high postvoid residual urine volumes, anatomic or functional genitourinary abnormalities, renal impairment, and renal transplantation. These patients generally have risk factors (see Table 1) contributing to more serious infections (Table 4). A high index of suspicion is critical for early diagnosis. Management may include intravenous antibiotics, uroradiographic imaging, urologic evaluation, and often adjunctive endourologic or surgical therapy.

Geriatric or neuropathic patients with long-term Foley catheter insertion may present special problems with recurrent UTIs secondary to the foreign body, stones, or *Candida* overgrowth. Asymptomatic or colonized bacteriuria is not treated unless associated with systemic or significant local symptoms or if stone-forming pathogens such as *Proteus* spp are cultured.

Candiduria may be treated with a three-way indwelling urethral catheter using a 5 mg per dL suspension of amphotericin B (50 mg in 1 liter sterile water) at 40 mL per hour or 1 liter per day over 5 to 7 days. Often simply discontinuing long-term antibiotics and removing foreign bodies (catheters), if possible, clear up noninvasive fungal infections of the urinary bladder.

BACTERIAL INFECTIONS OF THE URINARY TRACT IN GIRLS

method of
DAVID B. JOSEPH, M.D.
University of Alabama at Birmingham
Birmingham, Alabama

Prompt evaluation, diagnosis, and treatment of bacterial urinary tract infections (UTIs) in girls is essential to prevent the possibility of renal damage. Significant evidence has shown that even one episode of pyelonephritis can result in renal scarring. Girls under the age of 5 years are at greatest risk to sustain upper urinary tract damage following a UTI. The presenting symptoms in girls who are toilet trained often consists of dysuria, urgency, frequency, and suprapubic discomfort. Other symptoms include hematuria or turbid, malodorous urine. The neonate and infant often present with more subtle findings, such as fever, fussiness, fatigue, poor feeding, and failure to thrive. If a UTI is suspected, the urine must be evaluated.

INCIDENCE AND ETIOLOGY

A conservative estimate from screening programs shows that approximately 1% of girls younger than 1 year of age and 2% of preschool and school-age girls have asymptomatic bacteriuria. A significant number of these children have had a history of diagnosed UTIs or voiding dysfunction. It is estimated that before high school graduation, 5% of girls have had bacteriuria, of which 3% are symptomatic. This likely underestimates the true frequency of symptomatic UTIs in these age groups.

With the possible exception of the neonate, the route of entry for bacteriuria is ascending through the short female urethra. Multiple host defense factors subsequently determine a girl's susceptibility for bacterial colonization. Only 20 to 30% of girls presenting with bacteriuria have an anatomic abnormality, such as vesicoureteral reflux or obstructive uropathy. Many of the remaining children have voiding dysfunction (e.g., bladder instability, incomplete emptying), problems with bowel control (e.g., constipation, perineal soiling), or both.

DIAGNOSIS

Establishing the presence of a UTI requires culture assessment of the urine. It is traditionally accepted that 10^5 cfu per mL defines a UTI when obtained from a midstream clean-voided specimen. Any pure culture in a symptomatic child, however, should be considered positive. Unfortunately, the majority of clean-voided specimens in girls are contaminated even though an effort has been made to clean the perineum. This occurs because of vaginal reflux, which allows for the vaginal flora to be bathed in urine and washed into the collection container. Any questionable specimen should be repeated with a second clean-voided specimen or a catheterized specimen.

A child who is ill and requires hospitalization should have urine obtained for evaluation by either a suprapubic aspirate or catheterized specimen. The suprapubic aspirate can be easily collected using a 21- or 22-gauge needle passed into the bladder one finger breadth above the pubic ramus. Alternatively, a catheterized urine specimen can be obtained. When doing so, it is important not to contaminate the catheter with vaginal flora and to begin the urine collection after the first few milliliters have passed through the catheter, which eliminates bacteria carried into the bladder by the catheter.

Children not yet toilet trained often have a urine specimen collected from a bag. A bag-collected specimen is reliable only if the culture is negative. The potential for paravaginal or perirectal contamination is great, particularly when the bag is left in place longer than 20 minutes. Any bag specimen resulting in a positive culture should be repeated with a second bag specimen or more preferably with a catheterized or suprapubic collection of urine.

EVALUATION

The evaluation of any girl with a suspected UTI begins with a complete history and physical examination. The history details duration of symptoms, previous episodes of UTIs, present voiding habits, and bowel control. Routine physical examination includes height, weight, blood pressure, and temperature. The abdomen is palpated and the spine inspected for occult defects. The perineum, external genitalia, and introitus are assessed for anatomic abnormalities or signs of abuse. A urine specimen is assessed for pH, specific gravity, microscopic evaluation, and culture.

Radiographic imaging is required in all children diagnosed with a UTI. Sonography can be used to evaluate both the upper and the lower urinary tract and is helpful in identifying moderate to high grades of vesicoureteral reflux and most forms of obstructive uropathy. Sonographic imaging of the urinary tract should be undertaken in a timely fashion, particularly in children who appear ill or require hospitalization. Therapy is often directed by the outcome of this examination.

Once the acute inflammatory process has resolved, lower urinary tract evaluation is performed with a voiding cystogram. When the sonographic evaluation is suggestive of vesicoureteral reflux, a conventional (radiographic contrast) study provides appropriate information and anatomic detail. When the previous sonogram is normal, radionuclide cystography is an appropriate means for screening of vesicoureteral reflux. In children who present with the clinical appearance of pyelonephritis, a technetium 99m dimercaptosuccinic acid (DMSA) renal scan may prove helpful in identifying renal scarring and determining the length of therapy. On occasion, an intravenous urogram is required to provide anatomic detail of the urinary tract. Cystoscopy is rarely indicated and should not be performed until initial radiographic imaging has been completed.

TREATMENT

Children who are ill or have symptoms of pyelonephritis must have an accurate urine culture obtained immediately and prompt initiation of broad-spectrum parenteral antibiotics. Adequate coverage is often obtained with the combination of ampicillin and an aminoglycoside or a third-generation cephalosporin. Sensitivity results from the urine culture dictate needed changes. Oral therapy, if sensitive, can begin once the patient's fever has abated. Children who have cystitis but do not appear ill may have treatment deferred until the final urine culture and sensitivity report is available. Full-dose therapy is continued for at least 14 days in cases of suspected pyelonephritis and 7 to 10 days for cases of cystitis. Prophylactic antibiotic therapy should be continued until imaging studies have been completed. Most children tolerate nitrofurantoin macrocrystals, 1 to 2 mg per kg per day, or trimethoprim-sulfamethoxazole suspension, 10 mg per kg per day, for prophylaxis.

Girls with underlying anatomic pathology may require corrective intervention. Children who have either bowel or bladder dysfunction must be placed on a program that includes an appropriate diet and often behavior modification. This program should include a daily bowel movement, timed voiding, and the maintenance of a bowel and bladder diary. Recalcitrant UTIs may require further urologic evaluation and pharmacologic treatment.

CHILDHOOD ENURESIS

method of
WILLIAM FELDMAN, M.D., and
PAUL DICK, M.D.
The Hospital for Sick Children
Toronto, Ontario, Canada

The clinical definition of childhood enuresis (as opposed to the statistical definition) is childhood bladder incontinence that is bothersome to the child and parents. Statistically it is not until age 5 or 6 years that about 90% of children maintain nighttime dryness. Because parents of many 4-year-old boys are not aware that regular bedwetting is common in up to 38% of boys in this age group, knowledge of this normal range may relieve parental anxiety and childhood stress. Girls tend to achieve daytime and nighttime dryness earlier than boys, and persistent nocturnal enuresis is considerably more common in boys. Daytime incontinence is less common than is nocturnal enuresis, and secondary enuresis—a recurrence in children who have been completely dry for months—is also less common.

ETIOLOGY

Several lines of evidence point to the paramount role played by genetics in primary nocturnal enuresis. The concordance rate for enuresis in monozygous twins is double that of dizygous twins. Among children reared and toilet trained by caregivers other than their biologic parents, the most important factor in childhood enuresis was found to be a family history of enuresis. Suggestions that primary nocturnal enuresis is due to altered endogenous vasopressin secretion or to small bladder capacity have not yet been proved. The notion that disturbed nocturnal breathing or snoring from enlarged tonsils can cause enuresis has not been tested by methodologically sound studies.

Most of the medical conditions occasionally associated with enuresis—diabetes, urinary tract infection, disorders of bladder innervation—can be ruled out by history and physical examination. Children with untreated diabetes mellitus or diabetes insipidus always wake up at night to drink and almost always urinate in the toilet, day and night. Children with urinary infection or bladder innervation problems have associated symptoms—frequency, dysuria, or incontinence—both day and night. If the physical examination, including growth, as well as a careful genitourinary examination and anal "wink,"* is normal, few laboratory investigations are required. Urinalysis and culture are rarely helpful but may provide reassurance. Imaging studies of the genitourinary tract are not indicated for the typical patient.

TREATMENT

The child and family should be involved in the therapeutic decision making. The options are as follows:

1. The physician can reassure that there is no medical, psychological, or parenting problem and let time take its course—the enuresis spontaneous remission rate is 15% per year. Motivation using positive reinforcement combined with alleviation of guilt and hostility seems to increase this remission rate.

2. Tricyclic drugs, such as imipramine, are twice as effective as placebo but have a fairly high relapse rate unless tapered slowly. In addition, because accidental or intentional poisoning can be fatal, these drugs should be offered only in safe containers and only to families who are likely to understand the importance of keeping medications away from children. If tricyclics are employed, imipramine or amitriptyline should be used in doses starting at 25 mg at bedtime for 6-year-olds. This dose is often effective even in older children. Adolescents may require as much as 75 mg. If an effective dose has been established without producing somnolence or dry mouth, it should be continued for at least 2 months, then tapered gradually over the next 4 months. Ten-milligram tablets of imipramine may be effective near the end of tapering, whereas no medication may not. Before stopping completely, a trial of alternate-night therapy demonstrating nights without medication to be dry usually signifies a cure.

3. Alarm systems attached to the child's pajamas are effective in up to 70% of children. They have a significant relapse rate but are effective if necessary to be used again.

4. Intranasal desmopressin (DDAVP), an analogue of vasopressin, is effective in short-term trials but is expensive and has a high relapse

rate. DDAVP is used in doses of 20 to 40 μg administered intranasally at bedtime, although some children might be maintained on lower doses. Concerns regarding the rare possibility of hyponatremic complications can be addressed by restricting fluids following the dose of DDAVP until morning.

Because nocturnal enuresis is pathologically benign and ultimately remits spontaneously, treatment options must be extremely safe. DDAVP can be used for settings in which short-term control is important or in which alarms are precluded, such as summer camp. Children who have not responded to motivation and alarm approaches after several months are candidates for a trial of pharmacologic therapy. Other approaches, including hypnosis, other drugs (e.g., diclofenac, anticholinergics), bladder training, and diet, have not been assessed or compared with proven therapies with methodologically sound approaches. Any consideration of novel therapies for childhood nocturnal enuresis must take into account the natural history of remission and the significant response to placebo associated with this condition.

Whichever of the treatment options is chosen, it is important to relieve parental guilt and the child's shame. Enhancement of self-esteem of the parents and child may be as important to the long-term outcome as anything else one does.

URINARY INCONTINENCE

method of
PERRY STARER, M.D.
Mount Sinai School of Medicine
New York, New York

Management of urinary incontinence perplexes and distresses both patient and clinician. Appropriate diagnostic and therapeutic interventions are often overlooked. Instead diapers or catheters are applied, and the problem is concealed. To select the appropriate treatment for an incontinent patient, the cause of the urinary incontinence needs to be determined. Urinary incontinence is the presenting manifestation of a variety of underlying pathologic processes. Incontinence can be classified into the following patterns of presentation: (1) detrusor instability, (2) overflow incontinence, (3) sphincter insufficiency, and (4) functional incontinence. Two or more problems are especially common in elderly patients.

DETRUSOR INSTABILITY

Detrusor instability, which describes the presence of uninhibited detrusor contractions, is a

---

*Stroking the perianal area with a swab or tongue depressor leads to a reflex contraction.

common urodynamic finding among elderly incontinent patients. Involuntary, uninhibited detrusor contractions may be produced either by increased afferent impulses to the central nervous system owing to local disorders in the bladder or urethra (or both) or by a neurologic disorder affecting the inhibitory nervous pathways from cortical and subcortical centers (Table 1). Detrusor instability is the most common cystometric abnormality in patients with voiding problems following a cerebrovascular accident and in patients with Parkinson's disease.

Detrusor instability may be associated with bladder outlet obstruction. Detrusor instability is reversible in the majority of patients undergoing surgery for bladder outlet obstruction. Detrusor instability with poorly sustained contractions has been described. It produces urgency with an inability to empty the bladder completely.

Provocative upright cystometry is helpful in diagnosing involuntary contractions not provoked in the supine position.

Behavioral training with biofeedback should be considered among the first treatments offered to nondemented patients (Table 2). The goals are to train the patient to inhibit detrusor contraction voluntarily and to contract periurethral muscles selectively to prevent urine loss until detrusor inhibition can be achieved. Instead of rushing to the toilet, patients are instructed to contract their sphincter muscles to prevent urine loss and to

TABLE 1. **Diagnosis of Detrusor Instability**

Etiology
Loss of central nervous system inhibition of the detrusor reflex arc (e.g., cerebrovascular accident, demyelinating disease, brain tumor, Parkinson's disease, multiple sclerosis)
Local disorders causing bladder irritation (e.g., urinary infection, bladder tumor)
Bladder outlet obstruction (e.g., benign prostatic hypertrophy)
May occur in elderly patients without neurologic lesions

Symptoms
Urgency, urinary frequency, nocturia
Urinary incontinence while rushing to the toilet
Loss of moderate volumes of urine
Incontinence can occur either day or night
Urine loss may occur in the absence of symptoms of urgency

Physical Examination
May be normal
Neurologic disorders (e.g., hemiparesis, lower extremity spasticity)
Evidence of irritative lesions (e.g., vaginitis)

Postvoiding Residual Urine
Low (unless there is detrusor instability with impaired contractility)

Cystometry
Involuntary bladder contractions

TABLE 2. **Management of Detrusor Instability**

Oxybutynin (Ditropan)
Action: both anticholinergic activity and direct smooth muscle relaxant effect
Dose: 2.5–5 mg PO tid
Side effects: dry mouth, constipation, angle-closure glaucoma, confusion, urinary retention, tachycardia

Propantheline (Pro-Banthine)
Action: antimuscarinic effect plus antinicotinic effect
Dose: 7.5–30 mg PO bid or tid
Side effects: dry mouth, constipation, confusion, urinary retention, tachycardia, orthostatic hypotension, angle-closure glaucoma

Imipramine (Tofranil)
Action: both anticholinergic and alpha-agonist activity
Dose: 10–25 mg PO bid or tid
Side effects: dry mouth, constipation, confusion, urinary retention, orthostatic hypotension, angle-closure glaucoma, sedation, caridac conduction abnormalities

Bladder Training
Patient is taught to resist the sensation of urgency and to increase the interval between voidings

Timed Voiding
Scheduled toileting
Voiding intervals are matched to the patient's usual voiding schedule

wait until urgency subsides before they walk to the toilet.

If present, urinary tract infection should be treated with antibiotics. Patients with involuntary bladder contractions may require additional urologic evaluation to determine the cause of the dysfunction (e.g., inflammation, neoplasm, prostatic hypertrophy).

Pharmacologic management should be considered only after an effort has been made to correct reversible factors contributing to incontinence. Medications should be used in conjunction with a toileting program. Anticholinergic medications have been used in the treatment of detrusor instability to promote urine storage. Oxybutynin chloride has both an anticholinergic effect and a direct spasmolytic effect on the bladder smooth muscle. Oxybutynin chloride at dosages of 2.5 to 5 mg three times per day is safe for use in the elderly. A daily single dose of 5 mg may be given at the time that incontinence is most bothersome. The most common side effect is dryness of the mouth. Imipramine, which has both anticholinergic and alpha-agonist activity, decreases bladder contractility and increases bladder outlet resistance. Medication doses should be low initially, and patients need to be monitored for the development of urinary retention.

The aim of regular toileting is to prevent incontinence by emptying the bladder before reaching the volume at which an involuntary contraction occurs. In contrast to bladder training, the patient is not instructed to delay voiding. Toileting may fail in patients with small bladder capacities (involuntary contractions occurring at volumes less than 150 mL) because toileting more frequently than every 2 hours is difficult.

OVERFLOW INCONTINENCE (URINARY RETENTION)

Urinary retention may occur secondary to bladder outlet obstruction or poor bladder contractions (Table 3). Medications may cause urinary retention. Anticholinergic agents can inhibit bladder contractions. Alpha-adrenergic stimulating agents can increase outlet and urethral pressure. In diabetic patients, urinary retention may occur secondary to autonomic neuropathy. The loss of bladder sensation leads to distention of the bladder, decompensation of the detrusor muscle, and urinary retention. Normal patients may be unable to produce a bladder contraction during cystometric studies even though no abnormality exists. An inability to urinate in front of an audience could be mistaken for bladder dysfunction.

The choice of therapy depends on the cause of retention (Table 4). Surgical treatment may be indicated in the setting of bladder outflow obstruction. Because the symptoms of detrusor instability without infravesical obstruction are similar to the symptoms of prostatism, it is

TABLE 3. **Diagnosis of Overflow Incontinence**

Etiology
Inadequate bladder contractions (e.g., spinal cord lesions, bed rest, calcium channel blockers, anticholinergic medications)
Increased bladder outlet resistance (e.g., benign prostatic hyperplasia, prostate cancer, urethral stricture, uterine prolapse, prolapsing cystocele, fecal impaction, alpha-adrenergic agonist medications)
Impaired bladder sensation (e.g., diabetic neuropathy)

Symptoms
Hesitancy; straining to urinate
Sensation of incomplete bladder emptying; frequent urine loss

Physical Examination
Bladder may be palpable after voiding
Prostate size on rectal examination may be misleading (prostate enlargement can be asymmetrical)
Fecal impaction
Sacral nerve impairment (impaired perineal sensation, absence of anal wink)

Postvoiding Residual Urine
Elevated (>100 mL)
Not elevated if high-pressure bladder contractions overcome outlet resistance

Cystometry
Large bladder volume, poor detrusor contractions may be seen

TABLE 4. **Management of Overflow Incontinence**

Urinary Retention Secondary to Inadequate Bladder Contractions
Intermittent Catheterization
Inserted through the urethra into the bladder every 3–6 h

Credé's Maneuver
Application of manual extrinsic pressure to the bladder

Bethanechol (Urecholine)
Action: cholinergic activity; chronic atonic bladder may not respond
Dose: 50 mg tid
Side effects: sweating, diarrhea, abdominal cramps, bronchospasm, bradycardia
Contraindication: bladder outlet obstruction

Urinary Retention Secondary to Outlet Obstruction
Surgery
Treatment for mechanical obstruction with adequate bladder contractions

Prazosin (Minipress)
Action: alpha-adrenergic blocker
Dose: 1–2 mg PO bid
Side effects: Orthostatic hypotension (initiate dosing in the evening when patient is supine)

important to obtain objective evidence of infravesical obstruction before surgery.

Although bethanechol chloride, a cholinergic agent, is pharmacologically active, it has not been shown to be effective in promoting bladder emptying. Credé's maneuver (the application of steady suprapubic pressure over the full bladder in a caudal direction) is an inefficient method of bladder emptying in a majority of patients. Although prostatectomy is the currently accepted treatment of benign prostatic hyperplasia, the role of pharmacologic therapy is being investigated. The alpha-adrenergic blocker prazosin may have a place in the management of patients with symptoms attributable to bladder outflow obstruction, especially when surgical treatment needs to be delayed. Scheduled toileting may be effective for the diabetic patient with a sensory abnormality that results in infrequent voiding. Intermittent catheterization has a low incidence of symptomatic urinary tract infections and is preferable to an indwelling urethral catheter.

DETRUSOR–URETHRAL SPHINCTER DYSSYNERGIA

Detrusor–external sphincter dyssynergia is the inappropriate contraction or failure of relaxation of the external urethral sphincter during detrusor contractions. This discordant micturition reflex can elevate the residual urine. The normal relationship between the detrusor and the external sphincter is disrupted after spinal cord injury interrupts the pathways connecting the pontine mesencephalic and the sacral micturition centers.

Baclofen, an antispastic drug, decreases external urethral sphincter resistance and reduces residual urine in spinal cord–injured patients.

POST-PROSTATECTOMY INCONTINENCE

Continence after prostatectomy depends on sphincteric efficiency. The cause of incontinence after prostatectomy, however, may be bladder dysfunction (detrusor instability, low bladder wall compliance, or both) rather than sphincteric insufficiency. The preoperative finding of detrusor instability should alert the physician to the possibility of prolonged postoperative symptoms. Persistent postoperative involuntary detrusor contractions are associated with an unfavorable surgical outcome. Comprehensive urodynamic evaluation is essential before treatment can be recommended for incontinence after prostatectomy.

Artificial sphincters have been used for post-prostatectomy incontinence owing to sphincteric insufficiency. The patient must have the manual dexterity to operate the device.

STRESS INCONTINENCE (DECREASE IN BLADDER OUTLET RESISTANCE)

Stress urinary incontinence is the involuntary loss of urine caused by an increase in intra-abdominal pressure but not caused by contraction of the detrusor muscle (Table 5). Before recommending surgical therapy for incontinent women, it is important to determine the cause of their urinary dysfunction. The history should not be relied on solely in determining therapy for incontinence. The presenting symptoms of detrusor in-

TABLE 5. **Diagnosis of Stress Incontinence**

Etiology
Displacement of urethra and bladder neck during exertion
 (e.g., laxity of pelvic muscles)
Urethral sphincter deficiency (e.g., surgical damage, estrogen
 deficiency, alpha-adrenergic antagonists)

Symptoms
Leakage of small amounts of urine with increased abdominal
 pressure
Patients are usually continent of urine at night

Physical Examination
Demonstration of urine loss with coughing (performed with a
 full bladder)
Urine leakage through a correctly positioned urethra
 suggests sphincter deficiency

Postvoiding Residual Urine
Low

Cystometry
Normal

TABLE 6. **Management of Stress Incontinence**

Weight Loss
If overweight

Phenylpropanolamine
Action: alpha-adrenergic agonist
Dose: 25–75 mg PO bid
Side effects: nausea, dry mouth, insomnia, agitation,
 hypertension, cardiac dysrhythmias

Vaginal Pessaries
Designed to reduce pelvic relaxation

Pelvic Muscle Exercises
Increase urethral resistance
Patient must be able to learn the exercises and must
 continue to practice them

Biofeedback
Teaches patient to control sphincter muscle

Estrogen (Intravaginal Cream)
Action: increases urethral resistance in estrogen-deficient
 women; increases alpha-adrenergic sensitivity in urethra
Dose: 0.3–1.25 mg of conjugated estrogen daily
Side effects: endometrial cancer if uterus is intact

Surgery
Urethra and Bladder Displacement
Retropubic suspension
Needle suspension of bladder neck

Urethral Sphincter Deficiency
Sling procedures
Artificial sphincter
Periurethral bulking injection

stability may be confused with anatomic stress incontinence because an increase in intra-abdominal pressure may precipitate an uninhibited detrusor contraction. Although urine loss associated with coughing may be visually demonstrated in patients with stress incontinence, a spontaneous detrusor contraction can occur 5 to 15 seconds after a cough. Because it is difficult to classify the cause of urinary incontinence based on symptoms alone, cystometric studies have been recommended in the evaluation of patients before surgical treatment for stress incontinence. Because detrusor instability may not be detected in the supine position, it is necessary to perform cystometry with postural change and with coughing.

The simple provocative full-bladder stress test is as effective as radiographic or electronic pressure measurement in detecting urethral incompetence producing stress urinary incontinence. The Q-tip test is nonspecific because many postmenopausal patients without stress incontinence have a positive test result. Unless urethral function is compromised, an uncomplicated cystocele is more likely to be associated with urinary retention than with incontinence.

The goal of most operations is to elevate the bladder neck to within the abdominal zone of pressure (Table 6). Urethral sling procedures pass a ribbon of fascia or artificial material beneath the urethra, which elevates and compresses the urethra. In some incontinent women, stress incontinence and detrusor instability may both be present. Both stress incontinence and urgency incontinence may be cured by surgical elevation of the vesical neck.

Although norephedrine, an alpha-adrenoreceptor stimulating agent, produces a significant increase in maximal urethral closure pressure, the therapeutic effect is moderate. Intravaginal estrogen cream increases urethral resistance in estrogen-deficient women. The cream should be applied directly to the urethral orifice. Oral estriol and phenylpropanolamine in combination have been recommended for the treatment of stress urinary incontinence in postmenopausal women.

Pelvic muscle exercise (perivaginal muscle contraction and relaxation) is thought to increase urethral resistance by strengthening the voluntary periurethral and pelvic muscles. It has been recommended that exercises (a 10-second pubococcygeal contraction followed by a 10-second relaxation) be done at least 80 times per day. The primary goal of behavioral training with biofeedback is to enable the patient to contract the periurethral muscles selectively while inhibiting contraction of abdominal muscles. The patient monitors the cystometric tracing or sphincter electromyogram and observes the response of these indicators to attempts to control them. If a vaginal pessary is used, it must be removed and cleaned at least once monthly.

FUNCTIONAL INCONTINENCE

Urinary incontinence can occur in the presence of normal bladder function if the patient is unable to be toileted in an appropriate and timely manner. The patient with normal urodynamic studies may be incontinent owing to functional causes, such as cognitive impairment, immobility, or sedative medications. Improved access to toilet facilities may be achieved through the use of bedside commodes, urinals, and Velcro fasteners instead of zippers. Polyuria (secondary to diabetes, hypercalcemia, congestive heart failure, or diuretic therapy) can overwhelm the urinary storage system.

Detrusor instability alone in an elderly patient may not be sufficient to cause incontinence if the patient is able to alter his or her environment and lifestyle to meet the demands of an unstable bladder. In the setting of an additional stress, however, such as dementia or immobility, incontinence may occur. In this case, the use of an anticholinergic medication may not alleviate incontinence, unless there is also a toileting program to compensate for functional limitations. In stroke patients, the contribution of cognitive impairment and immobility to urinary incontinence needs to be considered as well as interference with the neurologic control of the micturition reflex.

URODYNAMIC STUDIES

Because there is a poor correlation between the presenting symptoms of urinary incontinence and urodynamic abnormalities, patients may require further investigation to determine the cause of the problem and to decide on the treatment. A medical history and physical examination are helpful in predicting urethral incompetence in patients with simple, clear-cut symptoms of exertional or stress incontinence. When the symptoms are urge, mixed (stress and urge), or suggestive of overflow incontinence, cystometry, residual urine measurement, and provocative full-bladder stress testing are needed.

Complex urodynamic tests should be reserved for when symptoms are complex or when treatment has failed. Nonurologic problems (e.g., cognitive dysfunction, immobility, medication effects) that contribute to urinary incontinence should be addressed before considering urodynamic studies.

Although most men with bladder outlet obstruction have a diminished flow rate, uroflowmetry as a single examination cannot distinguish between bladder outlet obstruction and impaired detrusor contractility. The role of the urethral pressure profile in the evaluation of elderly incontinent patients is uncertain. Cystoscopy is indicated in patients with hematuria because of the possibility of bladder stones or carcinoma.

DIAPERS

Although the diaper simplifies nursing care and allows increased mobility and socialization by the patient, it does not cure incontinence. Skin irritation and breakdown may develop if diapers are not changed at appropriate intervals. Before using diapers, an attempt should be made to determine the cause of incontinence and to use the information to choose an effective treatment. In those cases in which specific treatment fails, diapers may be the only alternative.

EPIDIDYMITIS

method of
ALEX F. ALTHAUSEN, M.D.
Harvard Medical School
Boston, Massachusetts

Epididymitis is the most common intrascrotal disease. It occurs at any age but is frequently associated with young adults as a result of urethral inflammation. The symptoms are usually the same regardless of the cause. Pain and tenderness appear first, then swelling. The scrotal skin becomes reddened and often shiny. Fever and malaise are not uncommon as well as a urethral discharge and an accompanying hydrocele.

Acute epididymitis usually resolves within a week to 10 days. A subacute stage, however, may occur in which the epididymis remains swollen and tender for months. Chronic epididymitis presents with recurrent acute attacks and no symptoms between the dormant intervals.

The causes of epididymitis are posterior urethritis, hematogenous infections, trauma, and idiopathic. Posterior urethritis, with retrograde infection down the vas deferens, is the major cause. In the past, the specific organism has been the gonococcus. Now the most common bacteria is *Escherichia coli*. *Chlamydia* and *Mycoplasma* spp are the most common organisms that cause urethritis in the sexually active man. Patients with an active lower urinary tract infection are predisposed to develop epididymitis, again by retrograde vas deferens flow. Bladder outlet obstruction secondary to prostatism or urethral stricture is the most common anatomic abnormality.

Surgical instrumentation of the urethra during cystoscopic procedures and Foley catheter insertion all can set up a urethritis with resultant epididymitis. With the use of prophylactic antibiotics at the time of urethral manipulation, however, the incidence can be greatly diminished.

Hematogenous factors involved in epididymitis and other urologic infections are discussed in the article "Bacterial Infections of the Urinary Tract in Males."

Direct, blunt trauma to the scrotum usually produces an epididymo-orchitis rather than epididymitis alone. If the blow is severe enough, rupture of the intrascrotal tissues can occur, with the onset of exquisite pain, tenderness, and swelling as a result of a rapidly expanding hematoma.

DIAGNOSIS

On physical examination, the patient with acute epididymitis has a scrotal skin that is red, warm, and tense with partial or total obliteration of the rugal folds. The epididymis is tender to the touch, indurated, and enlarged. The globus minor usually becomes involved first. An associated reactive hydrocele may make the testicle difficult to palpate. If an orchitis occurs, there may be no palpable sulcus between the testicle and the epididymis. The spermatic cord is not infrequently involved in the inflammatory process. This not only causes pain in the groin and inguinal canal, but also flank pain. Nausea and vomiting may ensue if the inflammation of the cord (funiculitis) is severe enough. As the epididymis and cord swell, walking may become difficult because of the local as well as the constitutional symptoms.

Digital rectal examination should also be done to ascertain if the prostate, seminal vesicles, or both are tender because this may be the cause as well as the effect of the epididymitis.

The diagnosis of epididymitis is usually evident by history and brief examination of the scrotal contents. The diagnostic problems are to determine the source of inflammation and to rule out testicular neoplasm and acute orchitis. Tuberculosis and mycotic infections are now increasing again as possible causes of epididymoorchitis, especially in the immunodepressed individual.

Any patient in whom the epididymitis does not resolve within 2 weeks of treatment should be evaluated for testicular neoplasm. This is done by careful physical examination combined with scrotal ultrasonography and serum tumor markers (α-fetoprotein and β-human chorionic gonadotropin). If the diagnosis of neoplasm cannot be ruled out by the aforementioned methods, an inguinal, radical, orchiectomy should be considered.

Scrotal ultrasonography is helpful in finding out if the testicle surrounded by the reactive hydrocele is normal. Nuclear medicine flow scans and Doppler flow studies can rule out testicular torsion.

TREATMENT

Urine, urethral, and postmassage prostatic fluid for culture and sensitivities are necessary to determine the treatment-specific antibiotics. Only then can the outcome be more assured for early resolution. The antibiotics should be given for 10 to 14 days. Then the patient needs to be re-examined. If there is little or no resolution of symptoms or decrease in swelling, testicular neoplasm has to be ruled out.

There are, however, many instances in which appropriate cultures are not done because of extenuating circumstances. Broad-spectrum antibiotics, such as the quinolones (which have a high concentration in prostatic and urethral tissues), should be used; ciprofloxacin (Cipro), 500 mg orally twice a day, can be given. If the digital rectal examination of the prostate and seminal vesicles is normal, a 10- to 14-day course of trimethoprim-sulfamethoxazole (Bactrim), double strength, one pill, twice daily suffices. When *Chlamydia* or *Mycoplasma* spp are the suspected agents in sexually transmitted urethritis with subsequent epididymitis, both partners should be treated with tetracycline derivatives: minocycline (Minocin), 100 mg orally twice daily, or doxycycline (Vibramycin), 100 mg orally twice daily. When the patient's dysuria from urethritis is severe enough, phenazopyridine (Pyridium), 100 mg orally four times daily, is beneficial.

Bed rest, scrotal elevation, and ice packs all help to alleviate the local symptoms. Nonsteroidal anti-inflammatory agents, such as indomethacin (Indocin), 25 mg orally three times daily, not only decrease pain, but also the fibrosis or scar tissue in the epididymis and may therefore lessen the chance of recurrence or infertility.

Abscess of the epididymis with local suppuration requires surgical drainage. If a hydrocele develops and becomes painful, aspiration may relieve this for a short time. Definitive treatment, hydrocelectomy, needs to be postponed until the acute inflammation has subsided.

Fortunately, most cases of epididymitis resolve quickly on bed rest, scrotal elevation, antibiotics, and nonsteroidal anti-inflammatory agents. With a chronic, relapsing epididymitis, however, vasostomy or vasectomy should be considered if prolonged use of antibiotics and anti-inflammatory agents does not help.

PRIMARY GLOMERULAR DISEASES

method of
D. C. CATTRAN, M.D.
University of Toronto
Toronto, Ontario, Canada

Primary glomerular diseases refer to a variety of kidney disorders that have in common changes within the glomerulus and often the interstitium of the kidney. These diseases may be associated with clinical features, but often the only features they share are in the urinary sediment, including hematuria, cast formation, and proteinuria, or laboratory abnormalities that indicate impaired renal function. The glomerular injury in the majority of types is believed to be mediated by an immune mechanism, although the specific etiologic diagnosis in almost every case is unknown. This lack of causal factors seriously impairs our ability to understand and classify primary glomerular diseases. Although many different types present with the same features, their natural history and response to therapy is different. The best way to classify these disorders is by histology. Renal tissue can usually be safely and easily obtained via a closed renal biopsy. If following the initial clinical grading into mild, moderate, or severe disease the patient is in the latter two groups, a biopsy should be done so the disease's natural history can be defined and appropriate therapy applied.

CLINICAL PRESENTATIONS

Type 1: Acute Nephritic Syndrome

This syndrome is characterized by a variable degree of either microscopic or macroscopic hematuria, proteinuria that is usually in the 1- to 3-gram-per-day range, and progressive renal functional impairment with a rising serum creatinine, salt and water retention with edema and often hypertension, and occasionally oliguria. The most extreme variant of the acute nephritic syndrome presentation is called rapidly progressive glomerulonephritis. This is an accelerated nephritic picture associated with a doubling of serum creatinine over a period of 2 weeks to 2 months, paralleled by a rapid decline in glomerular filtration rate. Although only 10% of presentations in the primary glomerular disease category are with acute ne-

phritis, it is the most dramatic and urgent group. The most common histologic types presenting in this fashion are diffuse proliferative glomerulonephritis, crescentic glomerulonephritis, membranoproliferative glomerulonephritis, and IgA nephropathy.

Type 2: Nephrotic Syndrome

This syndrome is characterized by edema, severe proteinuria (greater than 3.5 grams per day), and hypoalbuminemia and hypercholesterolemia as revealed by laboratory tests. Twenty percent of patients with the primary glomerulonephropathies present with this picture. The most common associated pathologic types and the age group differences are outlined in Table 1.

Type 3: Asymptomatic Proteinuria/Hematuria

These patients by definition have no clinical findings, and laboratory tests usually reveal normal urea and creatinine values, but their urine sediment usually demonstrates microscopic hematuria with or without casts and proteinuria (trace to 1 gram per liter). This is the mode of presentation in approximately 50% of patients with a primary glomerular disease. The most common histologic correlates are immunoglobulin A (IgA) nephropathy, membranous glomerulopathy, and membranoproliferative glomerulonephritis, but occasionally minimal change disease (MCD) and focal segmental glomerulosclerosis are found.

Type 4: Chronic Nephritis

This category is also largely asymptomatic, although fluid retention with edema, hypertension, or both may be present. Uremic symptoms, such as nausea, vomiting, pruritus, fatigue, and mental slowing, can occur if the renal failure is advanced. In these cases, the urinary sediment findings are often the same as in the asymptomatic group, but instead of normal renal function, these patients commonly have elevated serum creatinine and urea values, reflecting a significant degree of renal failure.

GENERAL THERAPY

Although nonspecific therapy is not discussed with each entity, certain principles can be sum-

TABLE 1. **Idiopathic Nephrotic Syndrome by Type and Percentage**

Histology	Percentage in Children	Percentage in Adults
Minimal change	65	20
Focal segmental glomerulosclerosis	20	20
Membranous	5	40
Membranoproliferative glomerulonephritis	3	5
IgA/IgG nephropathy	2	5
Others	5	10

marized as follows: When edema is a result of a progressive fall in glomerular filtration rate (clinical Types 1 and 4), most patients require, along with sodium restriction in the diet, increasing amounts of the more potent diuretics, such as furosemide (Lasix) and metolazone (Zaroxolyn), to obtain the same net sodium excretion; i.e., with a normal serum creatinine level, 40 mg of furosemide is usually sufficient, but with creatinine values in the 400 to 600 μmol per liter range, up to 120 mg of furosemide twice a day combined with metolazone, 2.5 to 10 mg daily, may be required. Potassium-sparing diuretics should be avoided once the creatinine level is above 300 μmol per liter. This is because the natural history of progressive renal failure is usually associated with increasing difficulty in excreting a potassium load, and thus life-threatening hyperkalemia can be precipitated by drugs that block sodium-potassium exchange.

When edema formation is related to hypoalbuminemia and heavy proteinuria (clinical Type 2), the combination of a loop diuretic, such as furosemide, with an aldosterone antagonist, such as spironolactone (Aldactone), is the most effective form of therapy because the latter blocks the effects of the high aldosterone level that commonly accompanies this syndrome. In both types of edema formation, care should be taken not to overdiurese the patient and cause dehydration because this can produce prerenal azotemia and worsening renal function.

Hypertension is often associated with the glomerulopathies that present with reduced renal function (Types 1 and 4). It is essential that normalization of the blood pressure occurs as soon as possible and that vigilance to ongoing control be maintained. There is little evidence to support one class of antihypertensive agent being better than another, although the newer agents, including calcium channel blockers and angiotensin-converting enzyme (ACE) inhibitors, are in general better tolerated and more potent. Often the blood pressure does become more difficult to control as renal failure worsens, and this type of agent is required. These classes can be used in combination with most diuretic therapies, but remember that hyperkalemia can occur with the ACE inhibitor drugs, especially as renal failure worsens or if the patient is diabetic.

Hyperlipidemia is often found in patients who have either the nephrotic syndrome or significant impairment of renal function (Types 2 and 4). Although preliminary, some data suggest that hypercholesterolemia is an independent risk factor that does accelerate vascular disease in these patients. Dietary therapy should be implemented first, but often this is insufficient treatment. The addition of a competitive inhibitor of hydroxy-methylglutaryl-CoA reductase is effective and should be considered when the cholesterol is above the 80th percentile for an age-matched and sex-matched normal population. Although proper risk-benefit and cost-benefit studies have not yet been completed, our experience indicates these agents are effective and safe if careful monitoring is maintained.

SPECIFIC THERAPY

This section is limited to specific therapy as applied to patients with primary glomerular disease. "Primary" is used to describe glomerulonephritis when the disease process is focused solely in the kidney. The term "secondary" is used when the renal disease is part of a systemic illness. In all histologic types, there are secondary causes that must be considered and ruled out before assuming a primary process. Although a description of all the possible secondary causes is beyond the scope of this article, it is assumed that these causes have been considered before the patient's disease is labeled as primary, and appropriate therapy is initiated.

Minimal Change Glomerulonephritis

Pathology

The glomeruli in MCD by light microscopy are usually entirely normal, immunofluorescence microscopy is negative, and the only abnormality on electron microscopy is diffuse flattening (fusion) of the foot processes of the epithelial cells.

Therapy

Ninety to 100% of children have a complete remission of proteinuria within 8 weeks of starting prednisone treatment at 60 mg/M^2 BSA or 1 to 2 mg per kg per day. Although a high percentage of adults (75 to 80%) also respond to this dose, they may require a more prolonged course, and therefore up to 16 weeks of treatment is recommended before labeling them steroid resistant. An alternate-day steroid regimen with a more rapid reduction in dose has been tried in controlled trials, and although the initial response rate was the same, the relapse rate was twice that of conventional daily treatment. This resulted in a cumulative prednisone dose over 2 years that was higher than in the daily treatment routine, and therefore this approach is not recommended. Despite evidence that spontaneous remissions occur in up to 50% of these patients over a 2- to 3-year period, treatment should not be delayed because of the complications related to the severe proteinuria and subsequent hypoalbuminemia, e.g., thrombosis and spontaneous peritonitis. In the elderly or other risk groups, however, such as those with diabetes mellitus, serious chronic malnutrition, or underlying ulcer disease, in whom the adverse effects of high-dose prednisone are more likely, a shorter course or alternate-day steroids should be considered.

Although this disease type does not progress to renal failure, relapses are common. The decision to treat and for how long becomes more difficult when this occurs. The relapse rates at 1 and 5 years in children are 50% and 80%, and in adults they are 30% and 50%. It is worth noting that the frequency of relapse in children decreases with age, so after children reach puberty, the relapse rate is only 10%.

The relapse group can be further divided into frequently relapsing but steroid-sensitive (SS) and the steroid-dependent (SD) types. The SS patients have periods of complete remission while off all prednisone, and the SD group must be on prednisone continuously to remain protein free. Alkylating agents may induce a complete remission in up to 70% of both these categories, but by 30 months post-treatment, 65% of the SS group versus only 30% of the SD group remain in remission. Both chlorambucil (Leukeran) and cyclophosphamide (Cytoxan) are effective. The experience with cyclophosphamide is greater in North America, and hence it is recommended. The long-term risk of malignancy, gonadal toxicity, or both even in children is minimal as long as the cumulative dose of cyclophosphamide is less than 250 mg per kg, and thus an 8- to 10-week course of 1.5 to 2.5 mg per kg even repeated once is acceptable. The dose should be adjusted to keep the total neutrophil cell count above 1500 per mm^3, and a high fluid intake should be maintained throughout therapy to avoid bladder irritation and gross hematuria. In the elderly patient with MCD, instead of steroid retreatment for the first three to four relapses as is the common practice in children, a short, 8-week course of cyclophosphamide should be considered because complications related to this form of therapy are probably less than those related to an 8- to 10-week course of high-dose oral prednisone.

Focal Segmental Glomerulosclerosis

Pathology

Focal segmental glomerulosclerosis (FSGS) is frequently mistaken for MCD. This is because initially the majority of glomeruli appear unaffected and look normal on light microscopy. The classic sclerotic lesion with or without perisclerotic cellular proliferation is distributed in a focal (i.e., some glomeruli) and segmental (i.e., some parts of an individual glomerulus) fashion.

Therapy

The most common presentation is with a nephrotic syndrome picture associated with a normal creatinine level; however, in contrast to MCD, over the course of 5 to 7 years 50% of the patients progress to renal failure. Hypertension, an increased serum creatinine level, microscopic hematuria, or an active urine sediment may be seen at presentation in FSGS and allow this type to be distinguished from MCD even if the classic pathology is not found on biopsy. Although the percentage of FSGS causing the nephrotic syndrome is lower in adults than in children (see Table 1), in absolute numbers they are equal, and the approach to therapy should be the same in all age groups.

Complete remission during a course of prednisone treatment similar to that used in MCD occurs in 20 to 40% of FSGS patients. There are no specific clinical or histologic features at presentation that can predict this response; therefore a trial of therapy is warranted in all patients. Although the response in adults is less well documented, our own recent study in a nonselected population indicated a similar response rate. A good initial response is also the best predictor of long-term renal survival. Just as in MCD, relapses are to be expected, but they also may respond to repeated steroid courses. The efficacy of alkylating agents in FSGS has not been as well established as in MCD, but a number of open trials have recorded a response rate of up to 20% in steroid-resistant or dependent cases. Therefore a similar 8-week cyclophosphamide trial as in MCD in both adults and children is recommended before assuming they are treatment resistant. The data on the therapeutic benefits of cyclosporine in FSGS is less clear. At present this drug should be viewed as experimental therapy, although it may well turn out to have a role similar to that of the alkylating agents.

Membranous Nephropathy

Pathology

Membranous nephropathy has no significant cellular proliferation or inflammatory changes within the glomeruli on biopsy, but light microscopy does generally reveal thickening of the peripheral capillary walls, and silver staining shows a spike pattern on the epithelial side of the glomerular basement membrane. Immunofluorescence demonstrates the classic uniform granular deposits of IgG and C3 along the peripheral capillary loops, confirming the presence of immune complexes in this area.

Therapy

Most patients present with heavy proteinuria, with 80% in the nephrotic syndrome range. The disease is relatively rare in children, but it is the most common cause of the nephrotic syndrome in adults (see Table 1). The majority of patients at presentation have a benign urine sediment or only microscopic hematuria, have a normal creatinine clearance, and are normotensive. The short-term prognosis is good in this disorder, but by 10 years, approximately 25% are in complete remission, although 20% are in end-stage renal failure, and 55% still have some renal function plus persistent proteinuria. The low percentage with end-stage renal disease combined with an unpredictable spontaneous complete remission rate of 20 to 35% has complicated the evaluation of various drug studies. Initially a short course of high-dose (2 mg per kg) alternate-day prednisone showed an improvement in long-term preservation of glomerular filtration rate, but two recent larger studies have indicated that prednisone is of no benefit in unselected patients with this disorder. An Italian-based study demonstrated, in a randomized controlled trial, better long-term renal function and reduced proteinuria by treatment with pulse methylprednisolone, 1 gram daily for 3 days, then oral prednisone, 0.5 mg per kg per day for 27 days, followed by oral chlorambucil (Leukeran), 0.2 mg per kg for 30 days. This 2-month cycle is then repeated twice, for a total treatment course of 6 months. Significant side effects did occur in 20% of patients on this therapy. Therefore before using this potentially toxic treatment, one should attempt to identify high-risk patients by documenting the persistence of nephrotic-range proteinuria for at least 6 months and perhaps even evidence of a deterioration in renal function as measured by a decreasing creatinine clearance or reciprocal of creatinine. Other therapies, such as long-term pulse or oral cyclophosphamide, or high-dose pulse methylprednisolone alone, have not to date shown an acceptable risk-benefit ratio and need to be studied further before they are recommended. Cyclosporine has recently been shown to be of benefit in progressive cases of membranous nephropathy.

IgA/IgG Nephropathy (Berger's Disease)

Pathology

The disease is characterized by mesangial cell and matrix proliferation on light microscopy associated with mesangial deposition of IgA and commonly IgG complexes by immunofluorescence. Segmental glomerulosclerosis and interstitial fibrosis are both pathologic features that carry a poor prognosis.

Therapy

IgA nephropathy is the most common category of glomerulonephritis found on biopsy in the world; although initially thought to have a benign prognosis, it is now recognized to be one of the top three primary nephropathies that progress to renal failure. Although the classic presentation is with recurrent macroscopic hematuria 2 to 4 days after an upper respiratory infection, more than 75% of cases present with asymptomatic microscopic hematuria, minor proteinuria, or both. A nephrotic syndrome presentation occurs in only 10 to 20% of cases. The pathologic spectrum in IgA nephropathy is broad and paralleled by a variable clinical presentation from microscopic hematuria to rapidly progressive glomerulonephritis. Although the majority of patients have a benign outlook, the presence of proteinuria greater than 1 gram per day, hypertension, or the aforementioned severe pathologic findings are all unfavorable prognostic features. An elevated serum IgA level is seen at some time in 50% of cases, but this is of diagnostic value only and of no prognostic importance.

A variety of treatments, including cytotoxic agents, phenytoin (Dilantin) (which has been shown to lower IgA levels), steroids, and cyclosporine, have been tried, but none has demonstrated a significant benefit. These studies, however, have been small and not directed to the more severely affected group, and therefore although these agents cannot be advocated as effective, they should not be dismissed until proper studies have been performed. Hypertension is a particularly ominous sign in this disorder, and therefore aggressive and meticulous control of blood pressure is advocated in all patients. There is increasing evidence that ACE inhibitor therapy, such as captopril (Capoten), may have a particular benefit in the management of hypertension in IgA patients, and these agents should be considered as primary therapy provided that there are no contraindications.

An interesting but small subgroup of IgA patients presents with the full-blown nephrotic syndrome picture but normal renal function and no interstitial fibrosis or glomerulosclerosis on biopsy. Many of these patients respond as if they had MCD, and an 8- to 10-week course of daily prednisone therapy as in MCD should be tried.

Membranoproliferative Glomerulonephritis

Pathology

There are a number of variants in this category, but their natural history is similar. On light microscopy, they all have a lobular appearance to the glomeruli caused by proliferation of the mesangial cells and associated increase in mesangial matrix. Type 1 membranoproliferative glomerulonephritis (MPGN) is associated with subendothelial immune deposits on electron microscopy, and Type 3 has both subendothelial and subepithelial deposits. Type 2 is generally seen in children and on electron microscopy is associated with a dense deposit, which is not immune complex positive, layered along the basement membrane. This pathology is unique, and this type should probably not be lumped with the rest of the MPGN types.

Therapy

This histologic category presents most commonly with asymptomatic proteinuria (20 to 30%), but acute nephritic (10 to 20%) and nephrotic presentations (10 to 20%) are not uncommon. MPGN is usually the underlying pathology in between 3 and 5% of large biopsy series of primary glomerulonephritis. Type 1 and 3 may be associated with low or normal C3 component of complement, but in Type 2 the level of C3 may be extremely low or even undetectable. Unfortunately, although this is of some aid in the diagnosis of this disorder, the level carries no therapeutic or prognostic significance. Unfavorable prognostic features include persistent (>6 months) nephrotic range proteinuria and persistent elevation of the serum creatinine. Although the overall 5-year renal prognosis in MPGN is good (at > 70%), in those with any of the above features, it falls to 30%. A variety of treatments, including steroids, cytotoxic agents, anticoagulants, and antiplatelet agents, alone and in various combinations, have been tried without proof of benefit. In one controlled trial, a combination of 325 mg daily of acetylsalicylic acid (aspirin) plus dipyridamole (Persantine), 75 mg three times daily, resulted in better long-term preservation of renal function than in the placebo-treated group. This combination may be tried, but the general clinical experience with this routine has not paralleled the controlled trial results.

Diffuse Proliferative Glomerulonephritis

Pathology

Light microscopy reveals a diffuse hypercellularity secondary to endothelial cell proliferation within the glomeruli. There may also be an exudative component, with polymorphonuclear leukocytes noted within the glomerular tufts. In severe cases, epithelial hypercellularity and crescent formations may occur. Large, irregular-sized immune deposits of IgG and complement are seen along the capillary walls on immunofluorescence microscopy.

Therapy

This pattern is classically associated with a poststreptococcal infection, but in many cases an inciting agent cannot be identified. These patients most commonly present with microscopic hematuria, proteinuria, hypertension, and deteriorating renal function, i.e., an acute nephritic syndrome picture. A great majority of children and adults with this disorder experience spontaneous improvement within 2 to 8 weeks. Although there is some concern that mild abnormalities of renal function may persist and lead to chronic renal failure in 15 to 20 years, the great majority heal completely. Treatment is aimed primarily at managing the acute circulatory complications that can occasionally be life-threatening. Treatment may include diuretics, antihypertensive medications, and a salt-restricted diet. Dialysis support may occasionally be required. The rare exception to this excellent prognosis is the patient with diffuse crescent formation. When this occurs, the therapeutic approach changes to that outlined next in the section discussing idiopathic crescentic glomerulonephritis.

Crescentic Glomerulonephritis

Pathology

This type is defined by the presence of proliferating cells within Bowman's space. In their most active phase, the crescents are cellular, but in time they change to fibrocellular and then acellular, with associated glomerular collapse and sclerosis. Immunofluorescence often shows fibrin-related products within the crescent. In the idiopathic crescentic group, glomerular granular capillary wall deposits are seen in 55%, linear deposits in 10%, and no deposits (pauci-immune) in 35% when the tissue is tested against specific immune probes.

Therapy

The great majority (65%) of patients with this type of primary glomerulonephritis present with an acute nephritis picture, but chronic nephritis (25%) and a nephrotic presentation (10%) may occur. In the elderly, congestive cardiac failure is not an uncommon mode of presentation owing to the rapid salt and water retention as glomerular filtration rate declines. The primary renal process can be missed in these patients if the urine is not examined. Unfavorable prognostic features include crescents in more than 75% of the glomeruli, especially if they are acellular; an initial serum creatinine level greater than 600 μmol per liter; and oliguria. Although this is a relatively rare histologic type and represents fewer than 4% of the total cases in large biopsy series, the natural history is poor, as indicated by only a 40% 1-year renal survival when more than 75% of glomeruli have crescents; therefore aggressive therapy is warranted. Pulse methylprednisolone, 5 to 10 mg per kg, given on alternate days for three doses followed by high-dose, alternate-day oral prednisone, 2 mg per kg, for 2 to 3 months has improved the 1-year renal survival from 40 to 70%. The addition of cytotoxic agents, such as pulse cyclophosphamide at 500 mg per M^2 on a monthly basis given for 4 to 6 months, appears to have added a significant benefit in the immune complex and pauci-immune (vasculitic) variants. These frequently have a positive serum test for anti-neutrophilic cytoplasmic antibody (ANCA). The further addition of up to 10 4-liter plasma exchanges in the first 16 days after diagnosis has been advocated in patients who have linear staining and associated circulating antiglomerular basement membrane antibody. Crescentic glomerulonephritis is not uncommon in the elderly, and when the patient is older than 60 years at presentation and other factors, such as infection or other serious concomitant diseases, are present, the aggressiveness of therapy should be tempered by the potential increase in morbidity and mortality in these high-risk patients.

PYELONEPHRITIS

method of
JAMES A. ROBERTS, M.D.
Tulane University School of Medicine
New Orleans, Louisiana

Acute pyelonephritis is a disorder due to bacterial infection of the kidney most often as a result of *Escherichia coli*. A parenchymal infection, it classically is most frequently associated with fever, chills, pain in the flank (with or without radiation to the groin), myalgia, and prostration. There are often associated gastrointestinal symptoms, mainly secondary to paralytic ileus, and fewer than 50% of patients have lower tract urinary symptoms. These classic symptoms, however, are not always found. Indeed, in neonates, the most common symptom is failure to thrive.

Neonatal urinary tract infections have a serious prognosis and are frequently associated with acute pyelonephritis in both males and females. If an abdominal mass is palpated, ultrasonography, intravenous pyelogram, or renal radionuclide studies should be done. The same is true if there is abnormal renal function noted by serum creatinine. All symptomatic infants should be evaluated radiologically, and all boys should be evaluated regardless of age. Ultrasonography and cystogram tend to be the universally approved diagnostic studies.

Acute pyelonephritis in children older than age 1 month is more frequently associated with fever. Therefore during this period, fever remains a danger sign for renal infection, although the diagnosis is made only if urinalysis and culture are done. School-age girls continue to have urinary tract infections but less frequently pyelonephritis.

Acute pyelonephritis in young women is associated with the classic severe symptoms of fever, chills, and often prostration. Flank pain is marked with or without radiation to the groin. The differential diagnosis must include pelvic inflammatory disease, acute cholecystitis, acute appendicitis, perforated viscus, herpes zoster, and lower lobe pneumonia; thus catheterized urine for urinalysis and culture is important. The patient has severe costovertebral angle tenderness and often abdominal tenderness.

E. coli is a less common cause of acute pyelonephritis in the elderly but still causes approximately 60% of the cases. This is probably because of the increased incidence of instrumentation and catheterization in these patients leading to nosocomial infections with organisms such as *Proteus, Klebsiella, Serratia,* or *Pseudomonas* spp. In more than 20%, the predominant symptoms are not genitourinary but instead gastrointestinal or pulmonary symptoms. Radiologic evaluation should be done early, looking for obstructive disorders, such as stone, that lead to continuing sepsis.

THERAPY

Acute pyelonephritis in either the infant or the elderly should be treated as if sepsis were already occurring because it occurs at such a high incidence in these groups. Those adult patients with symptoms and signs of sepsis, such as chills and fever, prostration, and unstable blood pressure, obviously should also be treated the same way. All these patients should soon after admission to the hospital be evaluated radiologically for the possibility of ureteral obstruction because in this case surgical therapy to relieve the obstruction is needed in addition to antibacterial therapy. While awaiting the results of urine culture and sensitivity, standard therapy in adults involves treatment with either a parenteral fluoroquinolone (Cipro, Floxin) in adults allergic to penicillin or a combination of an aminoglycoside (Garamycin) plus a synthetic penicillin, such as piperacillin (Pipracil). (See Tables 1 and 2 for dosage.) The author prefers aztreonam (Azactam) plus ticarcillin (Ticar) for parenteral therapy to prevent the nephrotoxicity of aminoglycosides. A first-generation cephalosporin, such as cefazolin (Ancef), is suggested as initial therapy in the infant or child. Once the results of antibiotic sensitivities are obtained, therapy may be varied. These patients, however, should stay on parenteral therapy until afebrile for at least 24 hours. At this point, oral

TABLE 1. **Antibacterial Dosage for Adults**

Drug	Oral	Intravenous
Amoxicillin (Amoxil)	500 mg q 8 h	
Aztreonam (Azactam)		1000 mg q 12 h
Cefazolin (Ancef)		500 mg q 8 h
Ceftazidime (Fortaz)		1000 mg q 12 h
Ceftazidime (Taxicef)		1000 mg q 12 h
Ciprofloxacin (Cipro)	250 mg bid	400 mg q 12 h
Gentamicin (Garamycin)		1 mg/kg q 8 h
Lomefloxacin (Maxaquin)	400 mg/day	
Norfloxacin (Noroxin)	400 mg bid	
Piperacillin (Pipracil)		70 mg/kg q 8 h
Ofloxacin (Floxin)	300 mg bid	400 mg q 12 h
Ticarcillin (Ticar)		3 gm q 6 h
Ticarcillin–potassium clavulanate (Timentin)		3.1 gm q 6 h
Trimethoprim-sulfamethoxazole (Bactrim DS)	bid	
Trimethoprim-sulfamethoxazole (Bactrim) IV		5 mg/kg as trimethoprim
Trimethoprim-sulfamethoxazole (Septra DS)	bid	

therapy should be begun. The author's first choice if the organism is sensitive is the combination of sulfamethoxazole-trimethoprim (Bactrim, Septra) or a fluoroquinolone (Noroxin, Cipro, Floxin, Maxaquin) with full treatment, parenteral and oral, for 14 days. In young women not showing marked toxicity, outpatient therapy with sulfamethoxazole-trimethoprim (Bactrim, Septra) or a fluoroquinolone may well be advisable if careful follow-up is possible.

Pyelonephritis secondary to *Proteus* spp must also be treated long term and often also needs surgical therapy because pyelonephritis from *Proteus mirabilis* is almost always secondary to stone. Infection with *Pseudomonas* or *Serratia* spp follows instrumentation or catheterization. Should pyelonephritis ensue, therapy is difficult and requires some combination of an aminoglycoside (Garamycin, Tobramycin) or aztreonam (Azactam) and one of the newer synthetic penicil-

lins, such as piperacillin (Pipracil), or a combination of ticarcillin with clavulanate (Timentin) or one of the third-generation cephalosporins, such as ceftazidime (Tazicef, Fortaz).

Treatment of acute pyelonephritis of pregnancy, which usually occurs in the third trimester, is limited by possible fetal effects of some antibacterials. Thus therapy with penicillins (Amoxil, Ticar, Pipracil) or cephalosporins (Ancef) is preferred. Although asymptomatic bacteriuria (100,000 cfu) is usually not treated, that found with pregnancy and diabetes should be because of the high incidence of acute pyelonephritis that may ensue if it is not.

GENITOURINARY TRAUMA

method of
SATISH R. C. VELAGAPUDI, M.D.
State University of New York at Buffalo
Buffalo, New York

and

GREGORY A. BRODERICK, M.D.
Hospital of the University of Pennsylvania
Philadelphia, Pennsylvania

Trauma is the leading cause of death for males between ages 1 and 40 years. After stabilization of life-threatening injuries, complete evaluation of the genitourinary system includes history to establish the mechanism of injury and physical examination before any radiologic evaluation. Radiologic evaluation then should proceed in a caudad to cephalad direction (urethrogram, cystogram, intravenous pyelogram, or computed tomography [CT]).

RENAL INJURIES

The kidney is the most commonly injured organ in the urogenital system. Despite the relatively protected anatomic positions of the kidneys, blunt or penetrating abdominal and thoracic trauma should always raise the suspicion of renal injury. Historically renal injuries are classified according to primary mechanism of injury: Blunt trauma accounts for 80 to 90% of reported renal injuries, whereas penetrating trauma accounts for 10 to 20%. With the advent of semiautomatic weapons and increases in urban violence, the incidence of penetrating abdominal trauma is rising.

Hematuria is the most specific indicator of renal trauma. Significant hematuria has been defined as five red blood cells per high-powered field. Unfortunately, the degree of hematuria does not correlate with the severity of renal injury. In large trauma centers, the dipstick urinalysis method has proved as efficacious as microscopic urinalysis in identifying hematuria.

The clinical signs of blunt renal trauma include contusions, seatbelt marks, lower rib fractures, and frac-

TABLE 2. **Antibacterial Dosage for Children**

Drug	Oral	Intravenous
Amoxicillin (Amoxil)	15 mg/kg q 8 h	
Cefazolin (Ancef)		20 mg/kg q 8 h
Gentamicin (Garamycin)		2 mg/kg q 8 h
Ticarcillin (Ticar)		50 mg/kg q 6 h
Trimethoprim-sulfamethoxazole (Bactrim)	4 mg/kg as trimethoprim q 12 h	
Trimethoprim-sulfamethoxazole (Bactrim) IV (over 2 months of age)		3 mg/kg q 8 h

tures of vertebral bodies and processes. Large retrospective series have clearly shown that the absolute indicators for renal radiographic imaging are gross hematuria or microscopic hematuria associated with shock (systolic blood pressure $\leq$ 90 mmHg). In adults with blunt trauma, stable blood pressures, and microscopic hematuria, the likelihood of major renal injury is less than 1%. In the adult patient with blunt abdominal trauma, no clinical signs of renal trauma, stable blood pressures, and microscopic hematuria, emergency radiographic imaging is not mandated. Unfortunately, in the pediatric patient with microhematuria (>5 red blood cells per high-powered field) and blunt trauma, there is a significant incidence of major renal injury.

After the need for radiologic evaluation has been established, despite normal blood pressures, radiographic imaging should be performed. Selecting the appropriate studies requires coordination with the trauma team and an assessment of the patient's clinical stability. If associated abdominal injuries are suspected, CT scanning is the study of choice. If only renal injuries are suspected, an intravenous pyelogram with nephrotomography may be adequate.

The Organ Injury Scaling Committee of the American Association for the Surgery of Trauma has established a renal injury scale: Grades I and II are minor; Grades III, IV, and V are major. Minor injuries include microscopic or gross hematuria typically associated with renal contusion with contained subcapsular hematoma without parenchymal laceration. Grade II injuries include nonexpanding, perirenal hematoma, or cortical laceration less than 1 cm deep without urinary extravasation. Grade III injuries have parenchymal laceration extending greater than 1 cm into the cortex without urinary extravasation. Grade IV injuries are characterized by parenchymal laceration extending through the corticomedullary junction and into the collecting system with urinary extravasation and laceration or thrombosis of a segmental vessel. Grade V injuries refer to shattered kidneys or avulsion of the main renal artery or vein or thrombosis of the main renal artery.

MANAGEMENT

Minor renal injuries from blunt trauma account for 85% of cases, including contusions, subcapsular hematomas, and minor renal lacerations. These patients are best managed with bed rest, hydration, serial hemoglobin counts, and frequent monitoring of vital signs. Patients with Grade IV and V injuries in general require emergent surgical exploration. Hemodynamic instability secondary to renal bleeding or an expanding pulsatile retroperitoneal hematoma discovered during laparotomy for associated injuries mandates renal exploration.

Relative indications for renal exploration include nonviable tissue associated with a major laceration, urinary extravasation, renal artery thrombosis, and expanding retroperitoneal he-

matoma. In this last-mentioned situation, a two-shot pyelogram is extremely important in that it confirms the presence of two renal units and demonstrates gross urinary extravasation or, by the absence of nephrogram on the affected side, suggests renal vascular injury. Radiographic contrast material is typically administered as a bolus of 2 mL per kg (maximum 150 mL); renal imaging is not possible during profound systemic hypotension. Recent clinical series of blunt trauma have specifically evaluated protocols for nonoperative management of minor and major renal lacerations by serial CT scanning and close clinical monitoring of hemoglobins and blood pressure. These series have clearly highlighted that CT is the most specific modality for staging renal injury. CT scanning is more sensitive than the intravenous pyelogram for detecting urinary extravasation, parenchymal disruption, and segmental infarction.

When the need for exploration has been determined, the preferred approach is a midline transabdominal incision. The midline approach allows simultaneous intra-abdominal exploration and retroperitoneal access. Early vascular control reduces renal loss. The posterior peritoneum is opened at the midline overlying the aorta; if the aorta is not palpable secondary to massive retroperitoneal hematoma, the incision is made medial to the inferior epigastric vein. Dissection is carried upward toward the ligament of Treitz, identifying the left renal vein typically crossing anteriorly over the aorta. Once vascular control has been effected, the colon may be reflected medially, and the underlying hematoma can be safely opened. After debridement of devitalized tissue, collecting system injuries are repaired.

Penetrating Injury

Penetrating abdominal injuries from stab or gunshot wounds are associated with significant renal injury in 8% of cases. There are no reliable clinical signs of major renal injury secondary to penetrating trauma. The initial urinalysis may be normal in one third of patients with significant renal injury after stab or gunshot wounds; there is an especially high risk of renal pedicle injury. All patients with any degree of hematuria who have suffered penetrating injury to the abdomen, flank, or lower back merit radiographic investigation. These patients often have primary surgical staging. Again, in these situations, the intraoperative intravenous pyelogram is performed to establish the presence and function of the contralateral renal unit (solitary kidney occurs in 1 in 1500 cases). Stab wounds to the back or flank can be managed conservatively in the hemodynamically stable patient who has been properly staged with radiographic imaging; this is best done with CT.

Renal Pedicle Injury

Renal vascular injuries are predominantly due to rapid decelerations. Blunt trauma with vascular injury involves the renal artery in 70% of cases, the vein in 20% of cases, and both vessels in 10% of cases. The severity of these deceleration injuries, primarily caused by falls from heights in excess of three stories, is underscored by the fact that 5% of renal pedicle injuries are associated with bilateral renal trauma. Early diagnosis and vascular reconstruction are the only hope for preserving renal function. The majority of renovascular injuries result from penetrating trauma, with patients presenting in shock with at least two other associated abdominal injuries.

Complications of Renal Trauma

The most common immediate postoperative complications of emergency renal explorations include delayed bleeding, urinoma formation, and perinephric abscess. Long-term complications include arteriovenous fistula, renal obstruction, hypertension, and renal atrophy. Renal failure is rare except in the case of repair of a solitary unit. Follow-up of the typical trauma patient has been difficult, but persistent hypertension after renal injury is reported in 5% of cases. The mechanism is presumably elevation of renin/angiotensin from segmental renal ischemia. Arteriovenous fistulas result after penetrating renal injury and have been noted after percutaneous renal biopsies, but surprisingly few have been described as a result of percutaneous nephrostolithotomies.

Ureteral Injuries

Ureteral injuries usually occur as a result of iatrogenic or penetrating abdominal trauma. With the exception of hyperextension/flexion injuries in children, which may result in disruption of the ureteropelvic junction, blunt trauma is rarely responsible for ureteral injury. Ureteral injuries may be classified descriptively. These include avulsion, laceration, crush injury, ligation, devascularization, electrocautery burns, and perforation. The number of ureteral injuries that the practicing urologist encounters secondary to operative damage far exceeds that as a result of spontaneous trauma. Iatrogenic ureteral injuries may be the result of gynecologic operation or oncologic general surgical procedures and commonly occur as a result of urologic endoscopic pro-

cedures. Ureteral injuries may not be accompanied by significant hemorrhage and produce few early signs or symptoms. In one third of reported penetrating ureteral traumas, there is a normal urinalysis. Diagnosis is often made by follow-up intravenous pyelography or CT. Clinical findings can vary, ranging from the development of abdominal ascites owing to urinoma, hydronephrosis, extravasation, and development of perirenal abscess to nonvisualization of a renal unit years after ureteral obstruction. Because of the known tissue devitalizing effect of high-velocity projectiles (blast effect), follow-up intravenous pyelogram performed 5 to 7 days after negative intraoperative two-shot intravenous pyelogram or retroperitoneal exploration may reveal urinary extravasation that did not occur at the time of initial injury.

Treatment of ureteral injuries depends on the anatomic level of trauma, the type of ureteral damage sustained, and the presence of associated bowel injuries. Partial laceration can be managed with internal ureteral stenting with or without retroperitoneal exploration and primary ureteral closure. This is the obvious primary method of managing small ureteral perforations resulting from endoscopic surgery. The options for managing distal ureteral injuries include ureteroneocystostomy with bladder hitch and creation of Boari's flap. Surgical options for more proximal ureteral injuries include ureteroureterostomy, transureteroureterostomy, interposition of small bowel segments, and renal autotransplantation. Not only is the site of ureteral injury important but also the timing for intervention is often a critical management decision. Delayed versus early operative repair should be dictated by the clinical situation. Penetrating trauma resulting in isolated ureteral injury can expeditiously be managed with a minimum of morbidity; this is not the situation when the clinical setting is one of widespread fecal contamination as well. Often trauma or iatrogenic ureteral injury merit the assistance of a skilled genitourinary interventional radiologist.

Bladder Injuries

Bladder injuries result from blunt, penetrating trauma or iatrogenic manipulation. Blunt trauma accounts for the majority of bladder injuries, but most often there is an association with severe pelvic trauma following motor vehicle accidents, falls, and industrial crush injuries. Penetrating injuries to the bladder are less common and represent 25% of cases in large trauma series. Iatrogenic injuries result after endoscopic procedures and open pelvic surgical procedures. Eighty to

90% of bladder trauma is associated with pelvic fracture. From an orthopedic perspective, only a small percentage of pelvic fractures are actually associated with bladder injuries (10 to 16%). Bladder trauma is directly correlated with the severity of pelvic trauma and has been highly associated with forces that disrupt the pelvic ring in an anterior-posterior direction; these fractures are typically described as open book or Malgaigne. Mortality rates are high (22%), not because of the genitourinary trauma but because of associated injuries with extensive pelvic trauma and late complications owing to fluid resuscitation and sepsis.

Bladder ruptures are classified as contusions, interstitial ruptures, intraperitoneal ruptures, and extraperitoneal ruptures. Gross or microscopic hematuria is present in the majority of cases. Extraperitoneal rupture is twice as likely as intraperitoneal rupture, and combined disruption is noted in 12% of cases. Associated renal injuries occur in 2% of cases and urethral injury in 10%. Approximately 50% of patients with gross hematuria in the setting of pelvic fracture have a significant bladder or urethral injury. In cases of delayed or spontaneous intraperitoneal rupture of native bladders or surgically constructed neobladders, azotemia, hyperchloremic metabolic acidosis, and alterations in serum, sodium, and potassium have been noted. These metabolic alterations are secondary to absorption of solutes from the urine. Bladder rupture without associated pelvic fracture is typically due to a kick to the abdomen or sports injury in the presence of a full bladder. Recent reports have cited spontaneous bladder ruptures in children with neobladders as well as augmentation cystoplasties, with recurrent catheter trauma or overdistention being the presumed mechanisms.

Abdominal plain films most efficiently characterize the extent of pelvic trauma for the urologist. An intravenous pyelogram establishes whether there is associated ureteral injury; this is rarely the case with bladder injury. Cystography with postdrainage films is the procedure of choice to evaluate bladder injury. Adequate bladder filling must be obtained with 300 to 400 mL of contrast material; similarly, extravasation below the peritoneal reflection may be unapparent until postdrainage films are reviewed. At least 20% of bladder ruptures are missed on intravenous pyelograms alone. Thirteen percent of bladder ruptures are diagnosed on cystography as a result of postdrainage films alone. Intraperitoneal ruptures are characterized by filling of the paracolic gutters with contrast outlining bowel loops. Extraperitoneal ruptures typically reveal a starburst pattern over the pelvis and diffuse retention of contrast in the pelvis below the acetabular line on postdrainage films. The teardrop bladder is a sign of pelvic hematoma; extravasation below the genitourinary diaphragm may occur in posterior urethral injuries with urine restricted by Colles' and Scarpa's fasciae superficially.

Penetrating bladder injuries should be surgically explored and repaired and an assessment made of intraperitoneal trauma. For intraperitoneal bladder rupture, a transperitoneal approach with closure of the bladder in multiple layers and suprapubic tube drainage is preferred. Small extraperitoneal bladder ruptures can be managed with large-bore catheter drainage and follow-up cystography in 10 days.

Urethral Injuries in Males

Urethral injuries in males are divided into posterior and anterior. Posterior urethral injuries consist of prostatic urethra and membranous portions of the urethra. The anterior urethra consists of the bulbar and pendulous urethras.

Posterior Urethral Injuries

Injuries to the posterior urethra most often result from blunt trauma associated with pelvic fractures. Ninety-five percent of posterior urethral disruptions are associated with pelvic fractures typically involving the pubic rami or diastasis of the symphysis pubis. Ten to 25% of posterior urethral injuries may be associated with bladder rupture; bladder rupture should be suspected if after fluid resuscitation the bladder is not palpable.

The posterior urethra is fixed in place by the urogenital diaphragm and the puboprostatic ligaments. The urethra is typically sheared off proximal to or at the level of the urogenital diaphragm. Blunt posterior urethra trauma may be subclassified into three types: In Type I, the urethra is stretched but not ruptured; in Type II, the prostatomembranous portion of the urethra is ruptured, but the urogenital diaphragm remains intact; and in Type III, both the prostatomembranous portion of the urethra and the urogenital diaphragm are disrupted. Type III is the most common presentation and permits extravasation of urine and contrast above and below the genitourinary diaphragm. The presence of a severe pelvic fracture with evidence of trauma to the pubic rami, blood at the urethral meatus, or the inability to void suggests posterior urethral injury. Blood at the meatus is the most important clinical sign of urethral trauma. All patients should undergo digital rectal examination, as the displaced or "floating" prostate may suggest posterior urethral trauma. Retrograde urethrogram is the study of choice. After fluid resuscitation, the bladder distends and may become palpable on clinical examination; injury through the bladder neck precludes bladder distention.

Traditionally posterior urethral disruptions have been managed by suprapubic cystotomy and delayed urethral repair. If intraperitoneal exploration is to be performed to evaluate or manage associated injuries, a suprapubic tube should be placed at that time. Clear bladder urine suggests no associated bladder injury; still open suprapubic tube placement with bladder inspection is preferred to punch cystotomy. Care should be taken to stay exactly in the midline to open the bladder near its dome and avoid inadvertent opening of the pelvic hematoma. Mortality principally related to severe pelvic trauma is significant and related to hemorrhage. Inadvertent opening of the pelvic hematoma at the time of suprapubic cystotomy may result in brisk and uncontrolled exsanguination. Recently immediate alignment over a Foley catheter placed via cystotomy has been advocated. An intermediate approach has also been taken at some trauma centers, delaying repair for a period of several weeks with suprapubic drainage and then performing definitive urethral repair transperineally with evacuation of the organizing pelvic hematoma. The traditional approach of immediate suprapubic cystotomy and delayed urethral repair at 3 to 6 months has been associated with the least morbidity due to infection of pelvic hematoma, immediate bleeding, and impotence. The incidence of impotence in primary repair is reported at 30 to 80% compared with 10 to 15% for delayed urethral repair. Again in this situation, the urologist should coordinate efforts with both the trauma and the orthopedic teams because opening of the pelvic hematoma can be hemodynamically disastrous, and delayed posterior urethral reconstruction can be complicated by the presence of orthopedic plating across the symphysis. Permanent incontinence is reported in fewer than 5% of series advocating delayed repair.

Anterior Urethral Injuries

Anterior urethral injuries are less frequent and typically less morbid than posterior urethral injuries. They often occur as isolated events, and thus management decisions are directed primarily by urologic concerns. The most common cause of anterior urethral injury is a straddle mechanism with a blow to the perineum, crushing the bulbar urethra upward against the inferior arch of the symphysis pubis. Penetrating trauma from gunshots or stab wounds may injure the anterior urethra and simultaneously the corpora cavernosa. There is typically no disruption of the corporeal bodies in simple straddle injuries.

Patients present with gross blood at the urethral meatus, gross hematuria, or inability to void. Retrograde urethrography is the first study of choice. Complete disruption of the anterior urethra is best managed with suprapubic cystotomy placed percutaneously with or without the assistance of ultrasound guidance and with delayed urethral repair following resolution of pelvic hematoma. Blind stenting of anterior urethral injuries risks conversion of a partial laceration into a complete laceration. Delayed reconstruction after resolution of perineal hematomas is the standard of care for complete urethral transections. The perineal hematoma is related to trauma to surrounding tissue unless Buck's fascia has been disrupted, allowing blood from the corpora spongiosum and urine to dissect freely below Colles' and Scarpa's fasciae. Immediate surgical repair is advocated for urethral stab wounds and delayed repair with minimal debridement of the spongiosum for gunshot wounds.

Female Urethral Injuries

The majority of female urethral injuries result after traumatic vaginal delivery. This form of injury is increasingly rare. Blunt abdominal trauma, pelvic fracture, and associated urethral injury in the female are also rare. Urethral tears associated with vaginal injury and pelvic fracture can occur after a combination of forces, such as deceleration/straddle injuries during high speed motor vehicle or motorcycle accidents. Treatment guidelines in this patient group are less clear because this is a rare injury. Attempts at urethral stenting with a Foley catheter are much less likely to result in inadvertent injury in the female patient with pelvic trauma as opposed to the male. Open pelvic fractures with associated injury of the vagina or rectum merit an open operative approach during which a suprapubic catheter is easily inserted.

Injuries to the Male External Genitalia

The penis, the testes, and the scrotum can be injured by a variety of mechanisms involving blunt, penetrating, and lacerating forces. The goal of initial interventions is to control hemorrhage and preserve vital tissues of sexual and reproductive function.

Penis

The most common mechanism of penile injury is blunt injury sustained during sexual intercourse. The penile fracture results from rupture of the tunica albuginea typically through one of the corpora cavernosa. Rarely does injury involve the corpora spongiosum. Radiographic imaging is not required for diagnosis. The clinical presentation is diagnostic: The patient complains of acute penile pain associated with a popping or cracking sound during coitus. A large hematoma develops as the erection abruptly decompresses; the hematoma deviates the penile shaft away from the site of injury. So long as Buck's fascia is intact, the hematoma remains confined to the penile shaft. Operative repair is the management of first choice; early series of conservative treatment had high complication rates (40%) and prolonged hospital stays. Surgical management consists of evacuation of hematoma and closure of the defect in the tunica albuginea with heavier absorbable sutures. A degloving circumcision is typically adequate and allows exposure to both corpora cavernosa; the injuries are typically distal to the suspensory ligament. Coitus should be avoided for 4 to 6 weeks.

Lacerating or avulsing injuries to the penis are a result of motor vehicle, industrial, or self-inflicted trauma. The majority of penetrating penile injuries are gunshot wounds. A high degree of suspicion for concomitant urethral injury should prompt retrograde urethrography if blood is seen at the meatus. Surgical exploration remains the best way to stage these injuries, and although cavernosography, ultrasonography, and surface coil magnetic resonance imaging would be excellent ways to identify missed injuries, they have little role in the acute trauma setting. Closure of the tunica with minimal debridement of corporal smooth muscle may preserve sexual function. Excess debridement of corporal tissue increases the likelihood of impotence; the corpora cavernosa and spongiosa are highly vascularized, and rubbing away clot on their surfaces usually reveals brisk bleeding and viable tissue. Penile amputation is a rare injury; successful reanastomosis depends on receiving a distal fragment that has been preserved in the trauma field. Reconstruction has as the primary goal re-establishing urethral continuity and anastomosing the corporal bodies. Ligation of the ends of the corporal arteries is recommended with microvascular repair of the dorsal neurovascular bundles with 10–0 nylon restoring inflow and outflow to the glans.

Scrotum and Testes

The scrotum is typically injured by gunshot or motor vehicle or motorcycle accident. Physical examination made early by the urologist is essential because large hematomas form within the scrotal layers. High-resolution near field sonography has come to play a major role in evaluating nontraumatic scrotal and testicular pathology

and should be employed if scrotal contents are not palpable. Hematoma of the skin and dartos layer may be managed conservatively. Open lacerations or gunshot wounds should be debrided, irrigated, and drained. Primary closure can be performed with absorbable suture; there is a distinct difference in managing wound contamination from gunshot or laceration and overt soft infections, such as Fournier's gangrene, in which resection to viable tissue and the open wound management with wet to dry dressings, follow-up quantitative cultures, scrotal regeneration, and delayed closure are the treatments of choice.

Approximately one-half of testicular injuries are due to blunt trauma. Typically overlying hemorrhage and the patient's discomfort preclude adequate physical examination. Scrotal ultrasound scan with color Doppler not only delineates anatomy of testicular and epididymal injury, but also demonstrates symmetry or asymmetry of blood flow within the testes. This new ultrasound technology, which permits real-time assessment of vascular integrity, is equally effective in helping to differentiate acute testicular torsion from early epididymitis.

Testicular ruptures should be explored with debridement of extruded tubules and closure of the tunica with absorbable sutures. Exploration for hematoma of the cord may only compromise testicular blood flow. Experimental evidence suggests that the likelihood of sperm antibody production occurs when the blood testis barrier has been interrupted. Therefore the generation of sperm antibodies and potential for future infertility are a function of the patient's pathology and should not inhibit exploration and closure of the testes whether injury is due to blunt rupture or a penetrating projectile. As in the management of corpora cavernosa rupture in the penis, closure of the fractured testicle is associated with a lower complication rate and reduced hospitalization than those associated with conservative management.

BENIGN PROSTATIC HYPERPLASIA

method of
PAUL O. MADSEN, M.D., PH.D.,
CHRISTOPH SPARWASSER, M.D., and
PETER DRESCHER, M.D.
University of Wisconsin, School of Medicine
Madison, Wisconsin

Benign prostatic hyperplasia (BPH) with associated symptoms of infravesical obstruction is present to some extent in approximately 75% of elderly men. Symptoms of prostatism lead about 30% of all men to undergo some sort of prostatic surgery. In 1989, more than

400,000 prostate operations were performed in the United States, at a estimated cost of $3 billion.

Although BPH is so frequent, its precise cause is still unknown. Age and hormonal status are involved in the development of BPH, and BPH primarily develops within the periurethral prostatic stroma. With increasing growth, the micturition gets afflicted, and longstanding untreated BPH can lead to severe upper urinary tract obstruction possibly followed by secondary infection and renal failure.

SYMPTOMS

Symptoms are described as obstructive or irritative in nature. Obstructive symptoms are attributed to the mechanical obstruction of the prostatic urethra by the hyperplastic tissue and include

Hesitancy.
Weakening of urinary stream.
Intermittent urinary stream.
Feeling of residual urine (incomplete bladder emptying).
Urinary retention.
Postmicturition urinary dribbling.

Irritative symptoms are attributed to involuntary contractions of the vesical detrusor muscle (detrusor instability) and are associated with obstruction in approximately 50% of patients with prostatism. These symptoms include

Nocturia.
Frequency.
Urgency.
Urge incontinence.
Dysuria.

In 25% of cases, these classic symptoms of prostatism can be caused by other diseases, which must be included in differential diagnostic considerations. Irritative symptoms can be caused by urinary tract infection, chronic or interstitial cystitis, cancer of the bladder or prostate, bladder stones, or a great number of neurogenic disorders with associated detrusor hyperreflexia (Parkinson's disease, multiple sclerosis, upper motor neuron lesions). The differential diagnosis of obstructive symptoms includes cancer of the prostate, urethral stricture, or functional obstruction at the level of the bladder neck or external sphincter. Also, neurogenic diseases must be considered.

In the latter group especially, hyposensitivity and consecutive overdistention of the bladder owing to diabetic neuropathy must be kept in mind. Prolapse of a lumbar disk as well as major pelvic surgery can damage the spinal reflex arc of micturition (sacral segments S2-4) and lead to an impaired or even missing detrusor contractility resulting in urinary retention.

DIAGNOSIS

A thorough history is indispensable, including concomitant medical and neurologic diseases, which could mimic symptoms of prostatic hyperplasia. To quantify and to reproduce individual symptoms, various symptom scores have been developed (Boyarsky Score, AUA Score, Madsen and Iversen Score) (Table 1). These scores are helpful in evaluating the results of various therapies. A listing of the actual medications should always complete the initial history because many drugs can affect micturition (e.g., anticholinergics, cholinergic and adrenergic drugs, alpha blockers, tricyclic antidepressants).

The rectal examination assesses size, shape, tenderness, and consistency of the prostate. Palpable nodules or areas of "hardness" should be considered to be prostate cancer until proved otherwise by biopsy. Rectal examination is not helpful in planning further therapy. The size of the prostate is often overestimated or underestimated, and there is no correlation between the size of the prostate and the symptoms. A short neurologic examination of perinanal sensation, anal sphincter tone, and bulbocavernous reflex should follow.

Ultrasound imaging in BPH can help determine the size of the prostate and may be done transabdominally or transrectally. The kidneys can be visualized for signs of obstruction, and residual urine in the bladder can be measured. The latter may be repeated several times because intraindividual variations are high. In routine cases of BPH, ultrasonography of the upper urinary tract may substitute for intravenous pyelography (IVP). Findings such as microscopic hematuria or abnormal urinary cytologic reports or abnormal sonography, however, still are indications for IVP. Cystourethroscopy should be performed before surgery only if information is wanted about the feasibility of performing transurethral versus open prostatic surgery and in case of suspicion of urethral or vesical abnormalities. Measurement of the urinary flow rate is a noninvasive, simple method with a high sensitivity and specifity to detect abnormal micturition patterns. For accurate results, the voided volume should exceed 150 mL. The urinary flow rate, however, cannot distinguish infravesical obstruction from insufficient bladder contractility because both conditions can show identical flow curves. Only simultaneous measurement of the urinary flow rate and intravesical pressure during micturition by multichannel videocysturethrography can establish a diagnosis. A diminished flow in the presence of an adequate detrusor contraction confirms the diagnosis of urethral obstruction. Patients with BPH and maximum urinary flow rates below 10 mL per second profit the most from prostatic surgery.

Extensive urodynamic evaluation should be applied in equivocal conditions, to young patients with prostatism, and to patients with BPH and associated neurogenic diseases or with excessive bladder capacity.

Urinalysis excludes urinary tract infection; the presence of microscopic hematuria requires further workup. Serum electrolytes and creatinine inform about renal function. In 25 to 86% of all patients with BPH, elevated levels of prostate specific antigen (PSA) can be found that demonstrates only a rough correlation between the size of the hyperplastic tissue and the PSA level. In 10% of all transurethral resections for BPH, an incidental carcinoma of the prostate is histologically proved. Thus in cases of a suspicious rectal examination or hypoechoic zones on the transrectal ultrasonography, PSA should be measured.

TABLE 1. **Madsen and Iversen Symptom Score Sheet**

Symptom	0	1	2	3	4
Obstructive					
Stream	Normal	Variable		Weak	Dribbling
Voiding	Normal		Abdominal strain or Credé		
Hesitancy	None			Yes	
Intermittency	None			Yes	
Empty bladder	Don't know or complete	Variable	Incomplete	Single retention	Repeated retention
Incontinence	None		Yes, including terminal dribbling		
Irritative					
Urge	None	Mild	Moderate	Severe (incontinence)	
Nocturia	0–1	2	3–4	>4	
Diuria	q >3 h	q 2–3 h	q <1 h		
Total Score					

TREATMENT

The treatment of BPH is rapidly changing, with many new modalities being tested in clinical trials (Table 2). Surgery remains the principal treatment choice; however, there is a great interest in less or minimal invasive forms of therapy.

Transurethral Resection of the Prostate

Transurethral resection of the prostate (TURP) is usually performed under regional (spinal or peridural) anesthesia. A resectoscope is introduced through the urethra, and large chips of the prostate are removed by electrocautery. Thus the bladder outlet obstruction is relieved; however, the entire prostate is usually not removed. The resection time should not exceed 1 to 1½ hours to avoid a TURP syndrome. This potentially life-threatening complication is caused by intraoperative absorption of large volumes of irrigant fluids by the veins of the prostatic plexus and leads to severe hypervolemia and hyponatremia with consecutive cerebral and cardiac symptoms. To minimize the risk of a TURP syndrome, the use of a suprapubic trocar, leading to lower pressure conditions in the bladder, has been recommended. Postoperatively a catheter is left indwelling for 2 or 3 days.

Improvements in surgical instruments and perioperative care have decreased the mortality rate of TURP substantially to less than 1%. Some concern still exists about increased delayed mortality compared with open surgery, although this is unsubstantiated. Morbidity of TURP includes urinary incontinence owing to damage of the external sphincter in approximately 1%, retrograde ejaculation in up to 80%, and erectile failure in 5 to 10% of patients. Urethral strictures, which are located mainly at the bladder neck and the bulbous urethra, occur in about 10% of patients postoperatively.

In general, TURP is a safe procedure with high efficacy and represents the "gold standard" in treatment of BPH. More than 80% of patients experience subjective improvement, and improvement of urinary flow rate is significant. Nevertheless, about 15% of patients report no benefit 1 year after surgery. The uncertainty about which patient group might or might not benefit from TURP has promoted the search for less invasive alternatives, and many patients prefer a less effective treatment if it also entails less risk.

Transurethral Incision of the Prostate

Transurethral incision of the prostate (TUIP) is a widely accepted method for treating infravesical obstruction caused by BPH of a weight of about 20 grams. The incision is performed unilaterally or bilaterally through the bladder neck and extended to the prostatic apex and deepened down to the prostatic capsule. The efficacy of

TABLE 2. **Treatment Options in Benign Prostatic Hyperplasia**

Transurethral resection of prostate
Transurethral incision of prostate
Open surgery
Transurethral laser-induced prostatectomy
Hyperthermia of the prostate
   Transrectally
   Transurethrally
Transurethral balloon dilatation of the prostate
Prostatic stents and coils
Pharmacotherapy
   Androgen suppression
   Alpha$_1$ blockade
   Aromatase inhibition
   Phytotherapy

TUIP comes close to the results of TURP, and side effects are significantly decreased. Operating time, blood loss, length of catheterization and hospital stay, and incidence of retrograde ejaculation are reduced significantly. Thus for sexually active patients with a small, not infected but obstructive prostate, TUIP represents a true alternative to TURP.

Open Surgery

In cases of a large-volume BPH with a resection time greater than 1½ hours, open surgery is still the method of choice. The operation is performed through a lower abdominal incision, and the prostatic adenoma is enucleated through a retropubic or suprapubic adenomectomy by leaving the prostatic capsule untouched. Transurethral or suprapubic catheters are left in place for 5 to 7 days.

The complications of open surgery are similar to those described for TURP; hospital stay is usually prolonged. Nevertheless, in large prostates, open surgery is an effective, safe treatment.

Transurethral Ultrasound-Guided, Laser-Induced Prostatectomy

The neodymium:yttrium-aluminium-garnet (Nd:YAG) laser is a powerful energy source that has been found to be effective in treatment of superficial bladder cancer. For treatment of BPH, a special device has been developed, consisting of a Nd:YAG laser positioned within an ultrasound transducer. About 20 to 40 watts of laser energy appears to be effective to achieve the desired coagulation necrosis. Only a few patients have been treated with transurethral ultrasound-guided, laser-induced prostatectomy (TULIP) so far, but potential advantages are short hospitalization, rapid treatment time, easy technique, no need for irrigation fluid, and no blood loss. Larger prostates may require more passes of TULIP (8 to 10), and often postoperative urinary retention due to the edema from the necrosis is seen. The results are still preliminary, and long-term results are needed.

Hyperthermia

Microwave hyperthermia appears to bring at least temporary, symptomatic relief to approximately two-thirds of patients. Application of the heat (to temperatures of 42° to 45°C) can be performed transurethrally (transurethral microwave therapy [TUMT]) or transrectally. TUMT seems to be more efficient. Urinary retention owing to prostatic edema is reported to be the only compli-

cation of an otherwise safe method, but also here long-term results of randomized studies are not available. Preliminary data show that more than 50% of patients experience improvement in voiding symptoms, but objective improvement of urinary flow rate still is controversial.

Transurethral Balloon Dilatation of the Prostate

According to some investigators, transurethral balloon dilatation of the prostate (TUDP) seems to be indicated in patients with small prostates, a nonobstructive middle lobe, and good bladder function. TUDP is a simple and safe method with only minimal side effects, but the efficacy varies significantly among different studies, and the long-term results remain uncertain. Patients at high operative risk may temporarily benefit from this minimally invasive procedure.

Prostatic Stents and Coils

Intraprostatic stents or coils are being chosen more frequently as alternatives to permanent catheterization for relief of outflow obstruction in nonoperable patients. The insertion of a temporary or permanent indwelling device, which expands in the prostatic urethra, can be performed as an outpatient procedure. Bacteriuria and irritative symptoms may develop. Ongoing studies will further elucidate the role of these devices.

Pharmacologic Treatment

Enlargement of the prostate in BPH is due to an increase in fibromuscular tissue and the hyperplastic growth of the glandular component. Thus pharmacotherapy has been directed toward relaxation of the prostatic smooth muscle fibers through inhibition of alpha-adrenergic receptors and toward regression of the hyperplastic tissue by hormonal manipulation.

Androgen Suppression

The growth of BPH depends on the presence of the androgenic hormone testosterone and its derivative dehydrotestosterone (via conversion by the enzyme 5 alpha-reductase). The strategy of antiandrogenic therapy in BPH is to interfere with dihydrotestosterone production. Many antiandrogenic drugs have been tried in BPH, but clinical results have been disappointing, or serious side effects, such as loss of libido, impotence, or hepatotoxicity, occurred. At present, the most promising antiandrogenic therapy of BPH is with the 5-alpha reductase inhibitor finasteride. Finasteride (Proscar), 5 mg per day, results in an approximate 20% reduction in prostatic size and a modest improvement of the urinary flow rate and symptom score and has a low rate of adverse effects, mainly a decrease in libido or erectile impotence. Finasteride significantly decreases the serum PSA level, and detection of cancer of the prostate can become more difficult. Finasteride treatment should be considered in patients with moderate symptoms of prostatism. If the patient improves and does not experience side effects, continuation of therapy under careful urologic control is appropriate.

Alpha-Adrenergic Receptor Inhibition (Alpha Blockade)

The tone of prostatic smooth muscle is mediated by the alpha$_1$ adrenoreceptor. Inhibition of alpha$_1$-receptor stimulation through selective or nonselective antagonists relaxes the smooth muscle, resulting in diminution of urethral resistance, improvement of uroflow, and improvement of symptoms. Randomized clinical trials have demonstrated short-term efficacy of selective alpha$_1$ blockade. Selective alpha$_1$ blocking drugs, such as terazosin (Hytrin) and prazosin (Minipress) represent an option for patients with moderate symptoms. The long-term efficacy remains to be established.

PROSTATITIS

method of
RODNEY U. ANDERSON, M.D.
Stanford University School of Medicine
Stanford, California

The medical diagnosis of prostatitis includes a constellation of clinical findings, few of which demonstrate an offending pathogenic microorganism and many of which show little evidence of gland inflammation. The clinician is confronted with unsophisticated diagnostic tools and questionable therapeutic efficacy, leaving him or her to offer only symptomatic treatment and supportive consolation.

Despite this pessimistic assessment of a common disorder in the male, there are specific diagnostic and management decisions that need to be made. The fundamental questions are: (1) Are bacteria involved and (2) is there significant inflammation occurring within the prostate tissue? If the answer is no to both of these questions, one is dealing with a syndrome that has been variously labeled prostatosis, prostatodynia, pelvic myalgia, or pelviperineal pain. The multiple descriptions affirm our lack of knowledge concerning cause, much less treatment.

Histologic findings of prostatitis may be classified as bacterial or nonbacterial and should be accurately diagnosed to facilitate appropriate management and counseling of the patient.

BACTERIAL PROSTATITIS
Acute Bacterial Prostatitis

This unusual problem may occur in both younger and older men and is typically characterized by fever, chills, perineal and suprapubic discomfort, dysuria, and inhibited urinary voiding. The urine examination reveals pus cells and bacterial rods. Digital examination of the prostate is painful, and the gland is swollen and boggy in texture; it may occasionally harbor an abscess. The gland should never be massaged in this condition, however, for fear of disseminating bacteria into the bloodstream and inciting fulminant gram-negative sepsis. If there is enough swelling to inhibit urine flow to any significant degree, particularly in the elderly man, the author advocates placing a temporary small-bore suprapubic catheter for drainage after injection of a first dose of an empirical broad-spectrum parenteral antibiotic, such as ampicillin plus aminoglycoside. These patients can usually be hospitalized pending the outcome of peripheral white blood cell count, blood cultures, identification of the pathogen to switch to oral antibiotics, and clinical response to treatment.

It is important to treat acute prostatitis aggressively and for enough days to ensure elimination of the bacteria from the gland. Drugs that may be taken orally and reach adequate bactericidal concentrations in the prostatic tissue include trimethoprim-sulfamethoxazole (Septra, Bactrim), carbenicillin indanyl sodium (Geocillin), norfloxacin (Noroxin), ciprofloxacin (Cipro), and lomefloxacin (Maxaquin). No one knows the precise period of time one should continue oral antibiotic agents following acute prostatitis, but most clinicians agree that 4 weeks is adequate. After completing treatment, and when the patient is asymptomatic, it is good practice to confirm that no chronic bacterial colonization of the prostate has occurred by performing a lower urinary tract localization study (see later).

Chronic Bacterial Prostatitis

The hallmark of this diagnosis is recurrent urinary tract infection, usually with the same organism. These men are typically asymptomatic, and the urine is clear between episodes; the acute relapses are less impressive than the classic acute prostatitis. In older men, the bacteriuria may even be asymptomatic. A report from Paris suggests that approximately 8 to 10% of human immunodeficiency virus–infected men have bacterial prostatitis; many of these patients also have an associated prostatic abscess diagnosed by ultrasonography.

One approach to prove colonization of the prostate by pathogenic bacteria consists of using nitrofurantoin (Macrodantin) as a urinary tract–sterilizing antimicrobial agent and then performing segmented urine cultures with prostate massage. Collecting and culturing urine and expressed prostatic secretion (EPS) require diligence on the part of the treating physician and attention to detail by the clinical laboratory. The first specimen obtained is the urethral washout, using the patient's first 5 to 10 mL of voided urine. The foreskin should be retracted to prevent skin flora contamination. The second specimen is midstream urine (30 to 50 mL), and one should tell the patient always to retain a little urine in reserve for a final urethral washout specimen following prostate massage. The third specimen is the prostatic fluid obtained by patiently massaging from lateral to midline in each lobe of the gland and expressing a drop or two of fluid down the urethra with compression of the bulbar urethra. A sterile test tube can be used to collect these precious drops of fluid. The patient then collects a fourth specimen as a final urethral washout of 5 to 10 mL. Each of these specimens is cultured, and colony counts of identified bacteria are obtained. The laboratory personnel must be willing and able to report absolute colony counts, even when these are less than 1000 cfu per mL. The author advocates streaking at least 0.1 mL on the agar plate to accommodate the lower counts. If the culture shows a 10-fold difference in growth of the same organism between the urethral washout specimen and the postmassage specimen or EPS, the prostate is considered the source of infection. The organism must be identical to the positive urine culture obtained before sterilizing the urine.

Cytologic analysis should simultaneously be performed to establish the presence of inflammation within the urethra, bladder, or prostate. A drop of sediment stain, such as Sternheimer-Malbin, helps differentiate leukocytes from lecithin granules or spermatids. The author prefers to quantify the count in a hemacytometer as white blood cells per mm^3 (normal up to 1000 in EPS), but most urologists accept greater than 10 per high-power field as indicative of inflammation. Oval fat bodies (macrophages) in the prostatic fluid also suggest chronic inflammation. More than 15 leukocytes per high-power field in the urethral washout and more than 5 in the midstream urine are considered indicative of inflammation. This analysis of the leukocyte pattern, along with assessment of bacterial identification and colony count, should allow the clinician to determine whether chronic bacterial prostatitis exists.

Therapeutic management of chronic bacterial prostatitis poses a challenge. Diffusion of drug into the prostatic tissue is limited, and only those agents mentioned earlier qualify for the job. Erythromycin (E-Mycin) and clindamycin (Cleocin) also penetrate well but are seldom the drugs of choice. If one uses the criteria of cure to include the patient's being symptom free and bacteria free for a minimum of 6 months after completion of oral therapy, the success rate is often only 30 to 40%. Ciprofloxacin has been reported to yield cure rates in the range of 75% at 3-month follow-up. The mean duration of treatment is approximately 2 months. Other, more aggressive treatment regimens include parenteral therapy with aminoglycosides for 7 to 10 days, direct injection of antibiotics into the gland tissue through ultrasound guidance, and extensive removal of prostate tissue through transurethral resection or even total prostatectomy. The transurethral resection may be specifically indicated if there are multiple calculi within the gland acting as infection stones. When specific therapy fails to eradicate the offending organism, one is left with chronic prophylaxis of bacteriuria using low-dose oral antibiotics. The author's preference is 100 mg of nitrofurantoin (Macrodantin) or trimethoprim-sulfamethoxazole (Septra, Bactrim), 80 mg of trimethoprim with 400 mg of sulfamethoxazole, taken each night if the organism is sensitive to these.

NONBACTERIAL PROSTATITIS

The diagnosis of nonbacterial prostatitis implies objective evidence of prostatic inflammation but no documentation of a microorganism as the inciting agent. The patient has symptoms but no laboratory evidence of a causative microorganism—a frustrating dilemma. It is true that some virulent pathogens fail to grow on routine culture media. Considerable effort has been given, for example, to document that *Chlamydia trachomatis* is an offending organism in these cases. This is a gram-negative bacterium with only intracellular growth. This organism as well as *Ureaplasma urealyticum* may be found as urethral commensals, adding confusion to the localization. Similarly, many patients with inflamed prostates and no bacteria have a history of sexually transmitted diseases. Although no prostatic fluid antibodies to either organism can be found in these patients, they do have elevated IgA and IgG levels that may represent some yet unproved inflammatory agent or autoimmune phenomenon to a preceding infection. Prostatic fluid antibodies to either organism have not been documented. In a study of 50 consecutive men diagnosed with nonbacterial prostatitis, only one had a positive finding of

Chlamydia in EPS, and although 44 out of 50 had inflammation on transperineal biopsy, none had *Chlamydia* cultured from the tissue. Nevertheless, other clinicians have been able to demonstrate 8 to 10% of symptomatic men with *Chlamydia* localized to the prostate and clear the organism and symptoms with 3 to 4 weeks of trimethoprim-sulfamethoxazole or tetracycline (Sumycin). In any case, it is probably prudent to look for significant colonization of possible pathogens only when the patient has been completely off all antimicrobial agents for at least 30 days. Until there is further evidence to the contrary, a clinical trial of 2 weeks of tetracycline, doxycycline (Vibramycin), or erythromycin is warranted.

It has been suggested that refluxing urine is an inflammatory agent, causing formation of calculi and perpetuation of the irritated prostate. Outflow obstruction in the form of external sphincter spasm or urethral stricture as well as internal sphincter dyssynergia may play a role. Because of this, the author establishes a working diagnosis of nonbacterial prostatitis with at least two documented localizations of inflammation without bacteria and then studies patients with complex urodynamic and selected endoscopic examinations. In some patients, a transrectal ultrasound examination of the prostate and seminal vesicles is warranted. Criteria are being developed to describe the ultrasound appearance of chronic prostatitis, and a transrectal biopsy confirms the inflammatory process in the stromal tissue. The author continues to look for dilated seminal vesicles as a cause of discomfort as well.

If the presence of urinary outflow obstruction is established—usually a form of internal sphincter dyssynergia—a trial of alpha-adrenergic blocking agents can be initiated. The author urges patients to use hot sitz baths (100° F) and occasionally gives agents such as diazepam (Valium) or tricyclic antidepressants to an obviously stressed and anxious patient. The author urges avoidance of common substances known to irritate the membranes of the genitourinary tract: tobacco, caffeine, chocolate, alcohol, spices, and so forth. At the same time, the author recommends moderation in sexual ejaculation—neither too often nor too seldom.

Adding to the confusion about cause in this malady is a report that in rats spontaneous nonbacterial prostatitis seems to be genetically predetermined, age related, and influenced by hormones; estrogen worsens the condition, and testosterone is helpful. Human studies are needed to clarify any hormonal aspects in men.

PROSTATODYNIA OR PELVIPERINEAL PAIN SYNDROME

This wastebasket medical diagnosis is an admission of failure in medical science. Patients are lumped into this category when they have pain in or near the prostate and no shred of evidence of either microorganisms or an inflammatory condition. The patient describes, usually in excruciating detail, aching, pulling, coldness, itching, orchialgia, subpubic and suprapubic discomfort, rectal discomfort, dysuria, postejaculatory pain, and urethral burning. These individuals often have high stress and anxiety levels with a propensity to somatic awareness. In the author's experience, many of these pelviperineal pain conditions occur as a result of lifestyle: long-distance running, long-distance driving or airflight, weight lifting, biking, and so forth. It is also coincidental how many of these individuals have a history of back injury or complaints of chronic low-back aching. In a few instances, magnetic resonance imaging of the lumbosacral nerve roots can be performed to seek any nerve root compression. If there is also good evidence of urinary dysfunction, the author proceeds with urodynamic testing. Physiologic evidence of sympathetic outflow smooth muscle spasm may be uncovered.

One disease process that may be uncovered in pelviperineal pain and associated urge and frequency complaints is interstitial cystitis; although a rare entity in men, it should be kept in mind when dealing with a complaint of painful prostate. Of course, prostate cancer and bladder carcinoma in situ as well as anal and rectal problems need to be ruled out.

There is a tendency for the physician to judge patients in whom there are no abnormal findings as having a psychosomatic disorder. Accordingly, the best treatment may be psychotherapy but given by a wise and caring physician who has assured himself or herself and the patient that no serious medical illness exists. Otherwise, the patient gives up on the physician in frustration and begins the process all over again with some other practitioner, often in another city.

ACUTE RENAL FAILURE

method of
HEATHER T. SPONSEL, M.D., and
ROBERT J. ANDERSON, M.D.
University of Colorado Health Sciences Center
Denver, Colorado

Acute renal failure (ARF) is the sudden development of renal insufficiency that results in retention of nitrogenous waste in the body. About 5% of all patients admitted to a general medical-surgical hospital and 10 to 20% of intensive care unit patients develop ARF. Moreover, the development of ARF increases mortality by sixfold to eightfold. ARF is one of the few causes of marked organ failure that is potentially completely reversible. The high frequency of occurrence, substantial morbidity and mortality, and potential reversibility of ARF demand a logical diagnostic and therapeutic approach by the clinician.

PRESENTING MANIFESTATIONS

ARF usually comes to the attention of the clinician by finding an increasing blood urea nitrogen (BUN) or serum creatinine (or both) concentration. These nitrogenous waste substances are readily filtered by the kidney and eliminated into the urine. In the absence of glomerular filtration, the BUN usually increases by about 10 to 20 mg per dL per day. Blood urea nitrogen is synthesized in the liver, and this synthesis depends on protein load. Also, filtered urea nitrogen can be reabsorbed by the renal tubules, especially in states of low urine flow. Thus protein loading (e.g., high-protein diet, gastrointestinal bleeding, catabolic state) and low urine flow states (e.g., volume depletion, severe heart failure, obstructive uropathy) can elevate the BUN in the absence of a markedly reduced glomerular filtration rate (GFR). Creatinine is derived from nonenzymatic hydrolysis of creatine that is usually released at a constant rate from skeletal muscle. In the absence of glomerular filtration, serum creatinine increases by 1 to 2 mg per dL per day. If the supply of creatine into the bloodstream is suddenly increased by skeletal muscle injury, a striking elevation of serum creatinine may occur. Also, a small amount of creatinine may be secreted into the urine by renal tubules. Some drugs, such as trimethoprim and cimetidine, may interfere with this tubular secretion, thereby slightly increasing serum creatinine concentration.

A second way in which ARF comes to the attention of the clinician is by a decrease in urine flow. Oliguria (often arbitrarily defined as less than 30 mL per hour or 700 mL per day) almost always indicates the presence of renal failure. Although oliguria is often considered a cardinal feature of ARF, it is important to emphasize that the majority of cases of ARF encountered in the contemporary practice of medicine are nonoliguric. Thus an adequate urine output is not a reliable indicator of normal renal function.

A third way in which ARF rarely comes to the attention of the clinician is by detection of one of the biochemical or clinical consequences of the loss of renal excretory function. Thus, occasionally the development of hyperkalemia, hypocalcemia, hyperphosphatemia, metabolic acidosis, hyperuricemia, anemia, or encephalopathy is the initial manifestation of ARF.

CAUSES

The process of urine formation begins with ultrafiltration of the blood delivered to the kidney; proceeds through intrarenal processing of the ultrafiltrate by tubular reabsorption and secretion; and ends by elimination of the formed urine through the ureters, bladder, and urethra. It follows that ARF is the final common pathway for a number of disease processes acting at these different sites. The initial step when confronted with a patient with ARF is to determine if the renal failure is prerenal (decreased renal perfusion),

postrenal (obstruction to urine flow), or renal (disorders of renal vasculature, glomeruli, interstitium, or tubules) in origin. The major causes of ARF are listed in Table 1.

Prerenal azotemia owing to extracellular fluid volume loss (e.g., burns, diarrhea, diuresis), extracellular fluid volume sequestration (e.g., pancreatitis, peritonitis, sepsis), or a markedly reduced cardiac output (e.g., cardiogenic shock) is the most common cause of ARF, constituting about 50 to 70% of all cases. Moreover, this form of ARF, if treated early, is readily reversible. If left untreated, renal ischemia with acute tubular necrosis (ATN) may result. In prerenal azotemia, the combination of reduced renal perfusion pressure and afferent arteriolar constriction lower glomerular capillary hydrostatic pressure and the process of formation of glomerular ultrafiltrate. This reduced filtration is usually coupled with enhanced renal tubular salt and water reabsorption as the kidney attempts to restore its perfusion toward normal. The combined lowering of GFR and increased tubular reabsorption nearly always leads to an oliguric state.

Two classes of pharmacologic agents, nonsteroidal anti-inflammatory drugs (NSAIDs) and angiotensin-converting enzyme inhibitors (ACEIs), can also induce a form of prerenal azotemia. In the case of NSAIDs, the inhibition of cyclooxygenase leads to a depletion of renal vasodilatory eicosanoids. In the presence of abundant renal vasoconstrictor influence (i.e., norepinephrine, angiotensin II, enhanced renal adrenergic tone), as occurs in edematous disorders, volume depletion, or hypotensive states, severe afferent arteriolar renal vasoconstriction can occur with reduced glomerular

TABLE 1. **Causes of Acute Renal Failure**

Prerenal
Extracellular fluid volume depletion (burns, diarrhea, gastrointestinal hemorrhage, diuresis)
Extracellular fluid volume sequestration (pancreatitis, crush injury, early sepsis)
Impaired cardiac output (severe heart failure, cardiogenic shock)

Postrenal
Extrarenal Obstruction
Bladder outlet obstruction (prostatic disease, urethral occlusion)
Ureteric blockade (tumor, fibrosis, ligature, tissue, pus, stone)

Intrarenal Obstruction
Crystal deposition (uric acid, methotrexate, calcium oxalate, acyclovir)
Protein deposition (plasma cell dyscrasia)

Renal Causes
Renal vascular disorders
　Large vessels (thrombosis, emboli)
　Small vessels (vasculitis, thrombocytopenic purpura, hemolytic-uremic syndrome, malignant hypertension)
Acute glomerulonephritis
Acute interstitial nephritis (drug allergy, hypercalcemia)
Acute tubular necrosis
　Renal ischemia
　Nephrotoxins
　Pigment-induced

capillary filtration pressure and ARF. In the case of ACEIs, the reduction of angiotensin II leads to lowering of renal perfusion pressure and dilation of the efferent arteriole. Together this lowers glomerular capillary filtration pressure and causes ARF. Fortunately, the ARF that can accompany NSAIDs and ACEIs is usually reversible if the offending agent is stopped.

Postrenal azotemia is a less common cause of ARF, making up 1 to 10% of all cases. Postrenal azotemia is almost always treatable. The most frequent cause of extrarenal obstructive uropathy in men is bladder outlet obstruction from prostatic disease. Occasionally extensive prostatic or bladder cancer can occlude the ureteric orifices. Obstruction to urine flow above the level of the bladder is a less common cause of ARF because both ureters must be occluded. An extensive disease process, however, such as retroperitoneal fibrosis or widespread pelvic cancer, can occlude both ureters. In the absence of one kidney or if one kidney is severely diseased, unilateral ureteric obstruction (stone, pus, clot, tissue, ligature) can cause ARF. Obstruction to urine flow can also occur within the kidneys when the distal tubules become occluded with crystals (uric acid, calcium oxalate, acyclovir [zovirax], methotrexate) or with proteinaceous material (myeloma).

Once prerenal and postrenal causes of ARF have been considered, it is appropriate to focus attention on the kidney. When approaching renal causes of ARF, it is helpful to think in terms of the anatomic compartments of the kidney. Disorders of the renal vasculature, such as thrombotic occlusion, emboli, malignant hypertension, thrombotic thrombocytopenic purpura (TTP), hemolytic-uremic syndrome (HUS), and vasculitis, can all cause ARF. Also, acute glomerulonephritis can result in ARF. Acute inflammation of the renal interstitium, as usually results from allergic drug reactions, also produces ARF. Together these vascular, glomerular, and interstitial disorders are relatively uncommon, constituting about 5 to 10% of all cases of ARF. These disorders, however, are often amenable to specific therapy.

The most common renal cause of ARF is tubular injury, often referred to as acute tubular necrosis (ATN). There are essentially three major predisposing factors to ATN, including renal ischemia (prolonged prerenal azotemia), nephrotoxins, and pigmenturia. Prolonged renal hypoperfusion is the most common setting of ATN. There is great variability in the severity and duration of insults that can produce ischemic ATN. About 20 to 40% of all cases of ATN can be attributed to nephrotoxins. Several agents, including antimicrobials (aminoglycosides, amphotericin B, pentamidine), radiographic contrast material, and heavy metals (cisplatin), can all produce ATN. Aminoglycoside-associated ATN usually occurs after 5 to 7 days' exposure to the drug. In some clinical cases and in experimental studies, however, brief (1 to 3 days) exposure to aminoglycosides in patients with underlying renal ischemia may be sufficient to induce ARF. Aminoglycoside-induced ATN is usually nonoliguric, with a mean rise in serum creatinine of 1 to 3 mg per dL.

Exposure to radiographic contrast agents is another acknowledged cause of ATN. Well-documented risk factors include underlying diabetic nephropathy, presence of renal ischemia, high dose of contrast material, and multiple myeloma. Nonionic (low osmolality) contrast agents are less frequently associated with ARF but can still induce ATN. ATN that occurs following contrast exposure may be either oliguric or nonoliguric in nature.

Pigmenturia (either hemoglobinuria from intravascular hemolysis or myoglobinuria from muscle injury) is often associated with ATN. Traumatic injury (i.e., crush injury) is a well-known setting of rhabdomyolysis and ATN. Rhabdomyolysis, however, is also seen in the setting of cocaine use, seizures, heat stroke, alcoholism, strenuous exercise, infections, drug overdose, and a variety of metabolic disturbances. The diagnosis of rhabdomyolysis is often suggested by a disproportionate rate of rise in serum creatinine (>2 mg per dL per day) as well as rapid increases in the serum concentration of substances contained within cells (potassium, lactate dehydrogenase, phosphorus, and uric acid precursors). The triad of elevated serum creatine kinase (skeletal muscle fraction), dipstick (+ for hemoglobin) urine in the absence of hematuria, and the presence of pigmented granular casts on urinalysis is virtually diagnostic of rhabdomyolysis.

CLINICAL APPROACH TO PATIENTS WITH ACUTE RENAL FAILURE

Appropriate management of ARF depends on an accurate assessment of the cause. Thus the first step in approaching the patient with ARF is to ascertain if the renal failure is of prerenal, postrenal, or renal origin. Table 2 suggests a diagnostic sequence to follow.

Chart Review, History, and Physical Examination

A history, physical examination, and review of the medical record is the initial step in assessing the patient with ARF. The overall clinical setting, recent events in the patient's illness, use of medications, and possible toxic exposures should be noted. A history of vomiting, blood loss, diarrhea, diuretic use, burns, or symptoms compatible with heart failure suggests potential prerenal azotemia. A history of decreased size and force of the urine stream; bladder, prostate, pelvic, or intra-abdominal cancer; flank or suprapubic pain; or hematuria or pyuria may suggest postrenal azotemia. A history of a systemic disorder, fever, rash, vascular disease, and musculoskeletal complaints is compatible with a renal vascular, glomerular, or interstitial disorder.

Review of the medical records should focus on indices of volume status (serial weights, intake and output, and hemodynamic measurements when available) to help assess if prerenal azotemia is present. A review of the medication list to determine exposure to potential nephrotoxins is necessary. Delineation of the pattern of urine

TABLE 2. **Diagnostic Approach in Acute Renal Failure**

Chart Review
Recent clinical events
Potential nephrotoxin exposure
Assessment of volume status (serial weights, input and
  output, hemodynamic measurements)
Pattern of urine flow

History and Physical Examination
Evidence of extracellular fluid volume depletion
Evidence of impaired cardiac output
Evidence of edematous disorder
Evidence of systemic disease
Evidence of obstructive uropathy
Evidence of vascular disease

Urinalysis (see Table 3)
Microscopic
Spot chemical parameters

Exclusion of Urinary Tract Obstruction if Necessary
Residual volume
Ultrasonography
Retrograde pyelography

Therapeutic Trials
Extracellular fluid volume expansion
Urinary tract drainage
Discontinuation of nephrotoxins
Improved cardiac index

Special Tests
Blood count (platelet count, red blood cell morphology)
Assessment of renal vasculature (isotope scans, angiography)
Immunologic tests if appropriate (ANA, ANCA, anti-GBM
  antibody)
Renal biopsy

output is often helpful. Anuria almost always denotes the presence of obstructive uropathy. Rarely anuria may indicate the presence of cessation of renal blood flow or rapidly progressive glomerulonephritis. Fluctuating urine volumes may indicate obstructive uropathy. Oliguria is nonspecific, occurring with prerenal, postrenal, and renal causes of ARF.

The physical examination should focus on evidence of extracellular fluid loss, such as orthostatic changes in pulse and blood pressure, dry mucous membranes, decreased skin turgor, and dryness of the axillary and groin areas. The presence of a significant (10 to 20%) fall in orthostatic blood pressure with a rise in pulse rate indicates significant intravascular volume depletion. Orthostatic hypotension, however, is not a sensitive indicator of intravascular volume depletion inasmuch as it may be absent with acute loss of small volumes or with chronic depletion of large volumes. Examination for neck vein distention, pulmonary rales, ventricular gallops, and pedal edema may indicate the presence of heart failure. Occasionally a chest x-ray or cardiac index measurement (i.e., gated blood pool scan) (or both) may be needed to help determine the presence or ab-

sence of heart failure. Rarely invasive monitoring (i.e., measurement of left ventricular filling pressure) may be needed to assess intravascular volume and cardiac status accurately. Abdominal palpation to detect flank, suprapubic, or central abdominal masses may be helpful in assessing the presence of obstructive uropathy and an abdominal aortic aneurysm with possible renal vascular compromise. A rectal and pelvic examination should always be done to assess for possible causes of obstructive uropathy. Examination of the skin may detect a rash that is compatible with drug-induced interstitial nephritis, palpable purpura that is compatible with vasculitis, nonpalpable purpura that is compatible with TTP and HUS, and livedo reticularis that is compatible with vascular insufficiency and renal atheroembolic disease.

Urinalysis and Spot Urine Chemical Analysis

Examination of the urine sediment is of great value in determining the cause of ARF (Table 3). A normal urine sediment suggests the presence of either a prerenal or postrenal cause of ARF. A urinary sediment containing abundant cells, casts, or protein suggests a renal cause of ARF. Specifically the presence of pigmented granular casts or renal epithelial cell casts suggests ATN. The presence of white blood cell casts or eosinophil casts (using Hansel's stain of the urinary sediment) suggests acute interstitial nephritis. The presence of red blood cell casts and heavy proteinuria suggests glomerulonephritis or vasculitis. A dipstick positive urine in the absence of red blood cells suggests the presence of either hemoglobinuria or myoglobinuria.

Analysis of electrolyte composition of the urine may be helpful in differentiating between prerenal and some renal forms of ARF. In prerenal azotemia, the tubules avidly reabsorb sodium in an effort to restore extracellular fluid volume and renal perfusion toward normal. Thus a spot urine sodium concentration is usually less than 30 mEq per liter, and the fractional excretion of sodium (U/P Na ÷ U/P creatinine × 100)* is less than 1%. By contrast, in ATN, the damaged tubules fail to reabsorb sodium normally with a resultant spot urine sodium greater than 50 mEq per liter and a fractional excretion of sodium greater than 1%. It is noteworthy that urinary chemical indices may not be valid after diuretic therapy or in the presence of either glycosuria or bicarbonaturia. Urinary chemical indices are not of value in

*Urine (U) to plasma (P) ratio of sodium concentration divided by the urine (U) to plasma (P) ratio of creatinine concentration multiplied by 100.

TABLE 3. **Urine Findings in Acute Renal Failure**

Condition	Urine Sediment	UNa/FENa
Prerenal Azotemia	Normal or nearly normal (hyaline casts and rare granular casts)	<30 mEq/L/<1.0%
Postrenal Azotemia	Can be normal or can have hematuria, pyuria, and crystals	Not helpful (early can resemble prerenal; late resembles ATN)
Renal Azotemia		
Vascular disorders	Often has RBC	Not helpful (can resemble prerenal)
Glomerulonephritis	RBC, WBC, and granular casts; abundant proteinuria	Not helpful (can resemble prerenal)
Interstitial nephritis	Pyuria, WBC casts, eosinophils, and eosinophilic casts	Not helpful (resembles ATN)
Tubular necrosis	Pigmented granular casts, renal tubular epithelial cells, and granular casts	>30 mEq/L>1%

Abbreviations: UNa = urine sodium concentration; FENa = fractional excretion of sodium; ATN = acute tubular necrosis; RBC = red blood cell; WBC = white blood cell.

determining the presence or absence of obstructive uropathy.

Exclusion of Urinary Tract Obstruction

In patients in whom the cause of ARF remains unclear or in whom the history or physical examination suggests the possibility of obstructive uropathy, further testing is indicated. The first test should be a bladder catheterization for residual volume. A residual volume of more than 100 mL suggests possible bladder outlet obstruction and the need for bladder catheter drainage. If bladder outlet obstruction is not present, occasionally noninvasive testing to examine for ureteric occlusion is indicated. This is most often done by ultrasonography. Rarely the presence of extensive retroperitoneal disease may give a false-negative ultrasonography result (so-called nondilated obstructive uropathy). Computed tomography scanning or magnetic resonance imaging may be helpful to delineate the presence or absence and extent of retroperitoneal disease and ureteral occlusion. In some cases, retrograde pyelography may be needed to exclude ureteric obstruction definitively. Rarely a trial of percutaneous nephrostomy drainage is used when minimally dilated or nondilated obstructive uropathy is suspected.

Other Diagnostic Tests

Sometimes the cause of ARF remains unknown despite careful record review, patient examination, review of standard laboratory data and hemogram, urinalyses, and exclusion of obstructive uropathy. In such cases, a cautious trial of extracellular fluid volume expansion may be indicated if volume-depleted prerenal azotemia is possible. If impaired cardiac output is suspected, a trial of maneuvers that decrease preload and afterload and that increase cardiac contractility may be considered. Careful follow-up of renal function after cessation of all potential nephrotoxins may be worthwhile. In the case of ARF induced by NSAIDs and ACEIs, renal function usually rapidly returns toward normal. If the cause of ARF still remains unknown, a percutaneous renal biopsy should be considered. This procedure may reveal the presence of acute glomerulonephritis or interstitial nephritis that could respond to corticosteroid or other therapy.

MANAGEMENT OF ACUTE TUBULAR NECROSIS

Prevention

In view of the high morbidity and mortality of ATN, maximal attention should be focused on prevention. Prompt, adequate replacement and maintenance of extracellular fluid volume in settings of serious trauma, burns, and extensive surgery may prevent ischemic ATN. In medical settings, aggressive treatment of septic and cardiogenic shock may lower the frequency of ATN. Twenty-five to 30% of medical cases of ARF involve use of nephrotoxic drugs and other therapeutic agents. Thus limitation of use of nephrotoxic drugs and other therapeutic drugs in high-risk groups, modification of dosage, and careful monitoring of renal function are mandatory.

Retrospective studies and clinical experience suggest that maintenance of adequate extracellular fluid volume and renal perfusion with a concomitant relatively high urinary flow rate (>100 mL per hour) may prevent or attenuate ARF in selected high-risk settings (Table 4). In many cases, particularly in elderly patients or patients with underlying cardiac disease, diuretic agents must be administered along with volume expanders to prevent a fluid overload state. In such

TABLE 4. **Clinical Settings in Which Volume Expansion and Solute Diuresis May Be Helpful in Preventing Acute Renal Failure**

Pigmenturia (hemoglobinuria and myoglobinuria)
Crystalluria (uric acid, methotrexate, and acyclovir)
Nephrotoxins (radiographic contrast agents, *cis*platin, amphotericin B)
Major cardiac and vascular surgery
Significant trauma

cases, either a loop diuretic (e.g., furosemide, 20 to 40 mg every 4 to 6 hours) or mannitol (12.5 to 25.0 grams every 4 to 6 hours) may be needed. In general, once the patient is euvolemic, infusion of half-normal saline with 20 to 40 mEq per liter of potassium to match urine output maintains euvolemia. Careful clinical and biochemical monitoring, however, is necessary to prevent volume overload and laboratory complications of forced diuresis, such as hypokalemia, hypomagnesemia, and metabolic alkalosis. In the case of pigmenturia, diuresis should be continued until pigmenturia clears (i.e., urine is no longer dipstick positive for blood). Although experimental data suggest that calcium channel blockers and vasodilators, such as atrial natriuretic peptide, can prevent some forms of ARF, clear clinical indications for use of these agents are not yet available.

Management of the Maintenance Phase

Once reversible prerenal and postrenal forms of ARF as well as renal vascular, glomerular, and interstitial disorders have been excluded, the therapeutic approach outlined in Table 5 should be considered. In these circumstances, consultation with a nephrologist is often helpful. The first consideration is to make sure the patient is euvolemic and cardiac output is optimized. This ensures adequate renal perfusion and blood flow to other vital organs. If the patient remains oliguric despite correction of prerenal factors and exclusion of other treatable causes of ARF, it has be-

TABLE 5. **General Therapeutic Approach in Acute Renal Failure**

Correct prerenal factors and maintain euvolemic state
Attempt to establish a urine output if patient remains oliguric despite correction of prerenal factors and exclusion of obstructive uropathy
Provide adequate (35–40 kcal/day) nutrition
Carefully monitor all drug therapy
Monitor for clinical and biochemical complications (see Table 6)
Reduce risk for infection (remove invasive lines and bladder catheter as quickly as feasible, and institute prophylactic maneuvers to avoid aspiration of gastric contents)
Use extracorporeal therapy when appropriate

come common clinical practice to administer either a potent diuretic agent (e.g., furosemide or bumetanide) or a putative renal vasodilator (e.g., dopamine at <2 to 3 μg per kg per minute) in an attempt to establish adequate urine output. Although definitive proof that diuretics and vasodilators (alone or together) can convert oliguric to nonoliguric ATN and lessen mortality is lacking, nonoliguric forms of ATN are easier to manage clinically. Therefore we usually attempt a trial of furosemide as an intravenous bolus (1 to 5 mg per kg over 30 minutes). Others believe that a continuous intravenous infusion of furosemide (1 mg per kg per hour) is more efficacious. If diuresis does not occur, repetitive high doses of diuretics should not be given, and a trial of dopamine can be considered.

Because most drugs are eliminated, at least in part, by the kidney, careful monitoring of the medication list and, when appropriate, modification of either dosage or dosing interval is necessary in ARF to avoid adverse medication-induced effects. The patient with ARF is at high risk for the development of numerous clinical and biochemical complications of ARF (Table 6). This dictates at least a once-daily careful physical examination. The frequency with which a complete blood count, electrolytes, and serum creatinine and calcium and phosphorus concentrations need to be determined depends on the clinical setting. The frequency of development of clinical and biochemical complications is lowest in nonoliguric patients with mild ARF (peak serum creatinine <3.0 mg per dL) and highest in oliguric, catabolic patients. In general, serum creatinine and electrolytes should be monitored at least daily as long as the creatinine concentration is rising or the patient remains oliguric.

TABLE 6. **Complications of Acute Renal Failure**

Biochemical/Hematologic
Blood urea nitrogen increases (10–20 mg/dL/day)
Creatinine increases (1–2 mg/dL/day)
Potassium increases (0.3–0.5 mEq/L/day)
Bicarbonate decreases (1–2 mEq/L/day)
Calcium decreases
Phosphorus increases
Magnesium increases
Anemia develops
Platelet dysfunction develops

Clinical
Neuropsychiatric (confusion, disorientation, agitation, asterixis, seizures)
Cardiovascular (arrhythmias, pericarditis, hypertension, congestive heart failure)
Gastrointestinal (anorexia, nausea, vomiting, hemorrhage)
Pulmonary (infection, fluid overload)
Infections (lung, intravenous sites, catheters, wounds)

Dietary and Fluid Intake

Once the patient is euvolemic, fluid intake should be restricted to equal urinary and other (i.e., nasogastric) measured losses, allowing 300 to 500 mL per day for insensible losses. Intake of sodium and potassium needs to be carefully monitored, especially in oliguric patients, in whom loss of these substances into the urine is minimal. Generally nonoliguric patients with mild ARF require only modest restriction of sodium and potassium intake, whereas the oliguric patient requires more marked restriction.

Maintenance of adequate nutrition is important in ARF. The goal of nutritional therapy is to achieve positive nitrogen balance without aggravating the signs and symptoms of uremia. Whenever possible, the enteral route should be used. Generally 30 to 50 cal per kg per day is needed. In severely ill catabolic patients, the amount of protein (1.0 to 2.0 mg per kg per day) and calories needed to achieve positive balance is large and requires the parenteral route. Sometimes, especially in catabolic, oliguric patients, the fluid volume required for maintenance of adequate nutrition mandates extracorporeal therapy with ultrafiltration to prevent fluid overload.

Extracorporeal Therapy

Extracorporeal therapy to remove substances normally eliminated by the kidney is rarely required in nonoliguric patients. In oliguric, catabolic patients, dialytic therapy should be instituted if the patient has uremic symptoms; if volume overload is present; or if severe electrolyte disturbances, especially hyperkalemia, are present. Also, many nephrologists institute empirical dialysis to keep the BUN and serum creatinine less than 125 and 10 mg per dL, respectively. Periodic dialysis often simplifies fluid management and provides reduced symptoms.

The method of dialysis employed depends on the expertise and availability of the center at which the patient is hospitalized, the patient's condition, and the indications for dialysis. Most centers routinely use conventional, periodic 3- to 6-hour intermittent hemodialysis. This requires vascular access (often obtained by subclavian or femoral vein cannulation), a stable blood pressure of at least 90 to 100 mmHg, and usually concomitant heparinization. The frequency of the procedure is dictated by blood chemistry, volume status, symptoms, and efficacy of the procedure. Hemodynamic instability with hypotension is the major complication of hemodialysis. Occasionally, especially in noncatabolic patients, peritoneal dialysis, which does not require heparin therapy, can be used.

Recently continuous extracorporeal modalities of blood cleansing therapy have been used increasingly. These procedures have the advantage of providing continuous removal of fluid and solute. These procedures are generally well tolerated and do not induce a large degree of hemodynamic instability. Three of these modalities include continuous arteriovenous hemofiltration (CAVH), continuous arteriovenous hemodialysis (CAVHD), and continuous venovenous hemodialysis (CVVHD). These procedures require either arterial (CAVH and CAVHD) or venous (CVVHD) access and heparinization. In CAVH, the patient's arteriovenous blood pressure gradient results in the convective loss of large volumes of fluid across the highly permeable membrane of the filter. Thus this modality is optimally used when significant volume removal is required (i.e., patients with mild renal failure who require large volumes of parenteral fluid for nutrition). If solute and nitrogenous waste removal is also needed, dialysate fluid can be run through the apparatus, adding diffusive removal of urea nitrogen, creatinine, and potassium to volume removal. This can be done either using the patient's own blood pressure as the driving force (CAVHD) or with venous lines using a blood pump (CVVHD).

PROGNOSIS

Several factors, including health of the patient (severity and reversibility of underlying diseases; Apache II score), severity of the renal failure (urine output, magnitude of rise in serum creatinine, need for dialysis), and number and type of complications from ARF, play determinant roles in ARF outcome. Nonoliguric ATN with only modest (i.e., <2 mg per dL) increases in serum creatinine are generally associated with relatively low mortality (<5 to 20%). By contrast, oliguric ATN that requires dialytic therapy is often associated with greater than 50% mortality, especially if it occurs either in the setting of severe underlying disease or an Apache score greater than 25. In the setting of multiple organ failure, the mortality rate of ATN increases by about 20 to 30% for each organ system that fails.

CHRONIC RENAL FAILURE

method of
BIFF F. PALMER, M.D.
University of Texas Southwestern Medical School
Dallas, Texas

"Chronic renal failure" refers to an irreversible form of renal injury that in nearly every case progresses to end-stage renal disease. Initially, adaptive mechanisms develop in virtually every organ system in the body, which render the typical patient asymptomatic until 70 to 80% of glomerular function is lost. Ultimately, however, the failure of renal excretory function and derangements of metabolic and endocrine function normally maintained by the kidney begin to manifest themselves as the uremic syndrome. The most common symptoms of uremia are referable to the gastrointestinal system (nausea, vomiting, anorexia), the cardiovascular system (hypertension, edema, congestive heart failure), the nervous system (neuropathy, asterixes), and the hematopoietic system (anemia). With the onset of the uremic syndrome, some form of renal replacement therapy must be initiated in order for the patient to survive.

MONITORING THE PROGRESSION OF CHRONIC RENAL FAILURE

During the course of chronic renal failure, the development of signs and symptoms depend on the magnitude of the reduction in renal mass as well as the rapidity with which renal function is lost. Knowledge of the level of renal function at any given time enables the physician to anticipate changes in symptoms, physical findings, and laboratory values so that preventive interventions can be initiated and ultimately the patient can be prepared for renal replacement therapy.

Measurement of the serum creatinine level is the most common way to monitor renal function in a patient with chronic renal failure. The major limitation in the use of this test is its insensitivity in detecting renal function loss until the glomerular filtration rate has declined by more than 50%. The failure of the serum creatinine level to accurately reflect the degree of renal impairment is particularly evident in patients with decreased muscle mass. In this regard, elderly or malnourished patients with advanced chronic renal insufficiency may exhibit only a moderate rise in the serum creatinine despite profound decreases in the glomerular filtration rate.

Measurement of the creatinine clearance level with a 24-hour urine collection is a more accurate way of following renal function. At normal levels of renal function, only a small percentage of creatinine appears in the urine by tubular secretion, whereas the bulk of creatinine is filtered by the glomerulus. As a result, creatinine clearance accurately reflects the glomerular filtration rate. With advancing renal insufficiency, however, the percentage of creatinine that reaches the final urine by tubular secretion increases. In consequence, the creatinine clearance level tends to be an overestimate of the glomerular filtration rate with advancing renal insufficiency.

The most accurate way of following renal function is to directly measure the glomerular filtration rate by measuring the clearance of a compound that is freely filtered by the glomerulus but is neither secreted nor reabsorbed by the tubule. Radiolabeled iothalamate sodium (Glofil) is such a substance that is commercially available for this purpose.

CAUSES OF ACCELERATED LOSS OF RENAL FUNCTION

During the initial evaluation of patients with chronic renal failure, it is important not only to identify the underlying renal disease but also to search assiduously for potentially reversible causes of lost renal function (Table 1). "Prerenal causes" of loss of renal function refer to a decrease in the effective circulatory volume. Excessive dietary salt restriction or overzealous use of diuretics are common causes of volume depletion in these patients. Treatment may consist simply of a short-term discontinuation of diuretic therapy and liberalization of oral salt intake. In patients who are symptomatic, intravenous normal saline may be required but should be given only under careful supervision in order to prevent the acute development of volume overload. A decrease in cardiac output caused by congestive heart failure or pericardial disease can similarly lead to a decrease in effective circulatory volume and result in the development of prerenal azotemia.

Obstruction of the urinary tract represents an important postrenal factor that can result in the reversible loss of additional renal function. Noninvasive methods such as ultrasonography should be used to rule out obstruction of the urinary tract both in the initial evaluation of patients with chronic renal failure and whenever renal function declines at an accelerated rate.

Hypertension

Uncontrolled hypertension is an important cause of accelerated loss of renal function. In addition, uncontrolled hypertension contributes to the progression of atherosclerotic disease and thus has an impact on the overall survival of patients both before and after renal replacement therapy is initiated. As a result, aggressive control of hypertension is an important goal in the management of patients with chronic renal failure.

The goal of management is to lower the blood pressure to normal (<145/90 mmHg). In patients with diabetic nephropathy, further benefit may be achieved by lowering the diastolic pressure to below 80 mmHg. In some patients (particularly those with accelerated hypertension), rapid lowering of the blood pressure may be associated with a transient decline in renal function resulting from the inability of the renal vasculature to autoregulate in a normal manner. Over the long term,

TABLE 1. **Common Reversible Factors in Chronic Renal Failure**

True or Effective Volume Depletion
Excessive diuretic use or salt restriction
Diarrhea, vomiting
Congestive heart failure, pericardial disease
Obstruction of the Urinary Tract
Uncontrolled Hypertension
Nephrotoxins
Aminoglycoside antibiotics, amphotericin B
Nonsteroidal anti-inflammatory agents
Radiocontrast agents
Drug-Induced Interstitial Nephritis

however, a sustained improvement in renal function occurs as long as blood pressure remains controlled. In order to minimize any short-term deterioration in renal function, blood pressure should be lowered in a gradual manner.

The development of hypertension during the course of chronic renal failure is a consequence of an expanding extracellular fluid volume in more than 80% of patients. Initial therapy should be directed toward the restoration of euvolemia and therefore consists of restricting dietary sodium and administration of diuretics. A diet of no added salt (6 to 8 grams of sodium chloride per day) is generally well tolerated and represents a reasonable first step. If diuretics are required, loop diuretics, such as furosemide (Lasix) or bumetanide (Bumex), are the preferred agents. Thiazide diuretics are ineffective at glomerular filtration rates of less than 30 mL per minute. Potassium-sparing diuretics such as spironolactone (Aldactone), triamterene (Dyrenium), and amiloride (Midamor) should be avoided because of the risk of hyperkalemia. Once diuretic therapy is initiated, the patient's volume status must be carefully monitored in order to avoid volume depletion.

Once the patient has been rendered euvolemic, persistent hypertension necessitates an additional agent. Angiotensin-converting enzyme inhibitors not only provide good blood pressure control but also are effective in reducing proteinuria in patients with proteinuria. In addition, these agents have been shown to slow the rate of decline in renal function, particularly in patients with chronic renal failure caused by type 1 diabetes mellitus. Converting enzyme inhibitors must be used with caution in chronic renal failure, however, because they can cause significant increases in the serum potassium concentration in some patients. In addition, in patients with extensive vascular disease with bilateral renal artery stenosis, acute deterioration in renal function can develop when these agents are administered. Calcium channel blockers are effective in controlling blood pressure and are generally well tolerated in patients with chronic renal failure.

Drugs and Toxins

Patients with chronic renal failure are more susceptible to the nephrotoxic effects of therapeutic agents such as aminoglycoside antibiotics, amphotericin B (Fungizone), and nonsteroidal anti-inflamatory agents. It is particularly important to inquire whether a patient is ingesting nonsteroidal anti-inflamatory agents because these drugs are now available on an over-the-counter basis. Drug-induced interstitial nephritis can also result in a reversible form of renal failure. The drugs most commonly associated with the development of interstitial nephritis are the sulfa-containing and beta-lactam antibiotics, xanthine oxidase inhibitors, and sulfa-containing diuretics.

Exposure to radiocontrast agents is associated with enhanced renal toxicity in the setting of chronic renal failure. If a diagnostic test that requires radiocontrast is indicated, a number of precautions can be taken to minimize renal toxicity. Foremost among these is ensuring that the patient's volume status is replete and

that urine flow is brisk. Both states can be accomplished by the intravenous infusion of normal saline at a rate of 150 mL per hour, beginning 4 hours before the procedure and continuing the infusion an additional 4 hours after the dye has been given. Patients need to be monitored closely in order to avoid volume overload, especially those with a history of congestive heart failure.

MANAGEMENT OF METABOLIC DERANGEMENTS

Sodium and Water Balance

As renal mass becomes progressively reduced, the fractional excretion of salt and water increases in the remaining nephrons. This obligatory solute diuresis per remaining nephron results in a relatively fixed amount of salt and water excretion. Under these constraints, patients with chronic renal failure have limits of renal salt and water excretion that are quite narrow in comparison with those of normal subjects.

The optimal salt intake differs from patient to patient and, once prescribed, must be constantly monitored because requirements vary as renal function changes. The goal should be a salt intake that results in a constant weight in which the patient is normotensive and only trace edema is present. A diet of no added salt (6 to 8 grams of sodium chloride per day) is a useful starting point. If a patient's weight begins to decrease over a period of several days and the patient becomes more azotemic, a higher salt intake is required. In addition, during intercurrent illness, supplemental salt can be given in the form of bullion cubes if a deficit in extracellular fluid volume develops. If, in contrast, the patient's weight increases over time and the increase is accompanied by increasing edema and worsening hypertension, further salt restriction is indicated. Once the glomerular filtration rate falls to less than 20 mL per minute, even salt-restricted diets may exceed the excretory capacity of the kidney, and diuretic therapy must be used in order to prevent progressive expansion of the extracellular fluid volume.

The ability to maximally concentrate or dilute the urine becomes progressively impaired as renal function declines. As a result, patients with chronic renal failure are at risk for the development of positive water balance and resultant hyponatremia, as well as negative water balance and hypernatremia. In general, fluid intake should be equal to urine output plus an additional 1000 to 1500 mL per day to account for insensible losses. The treatment of hyponatremia depends on the existing extracellular fluid balance. In volume-overloaded patients, further water restriction is indicated. In hypovolemic patients, water restriction with judicious administration of salt and withdrawing of diuretic therapy is the appropriate management.

Potassium

Potassium balance is generally maintained within normal limits until the glomerular filtration rate falls to less than 10 mL per minute. This balance is achieved by an enhanced potassium excretion rate per remaining nephron as well as increased extrarenal potassium excretion primarily via the colon. The initial approach to treatment of hyperkalemia is the institution of a low-potassium diet (50 to 70 mEq per day). Should hyperkalemia persist, administration of a loop diuretic is a reasonable second step, especially if the patient has demonstrable edema or is hypertensive. Loop diuretics enhance distal sodium delivery and thus serve to enhance potassium secretion by the distal tubule. If the patient is acidotic, sodium bicarbonate administration is an effective way of lowering the serum potassium. This agent also enhances distal sodium delivery and therefore augments potassium secretion from the distal tubule. In addition, the resulting alkalinization causes a shift of potassium into cells.

Some patients continue to remain hyperkalemic despite the therapy just described. In these patients, administration of a potassium-binding resin such as sodium polystyrene sulfonate (Kayexalate) may have to be given on a daily or every-other-day basis. This agent should be given with a bowel cathartic such as sorbitol so as to avoid constipation. Constipation can actually worsen hyperkalemia because potassium secretion by the colon is substantial in patients with advanced renal insufficiency. Magnesium-containing cathartics should be avoided because of the risk of inducing hypermagnesemia in the setting of renal insufficiency.

Acidosis

Under normal conditions, the kidneys are responsible for regenerating consumed bicarbonate, which results from the buffering of daily net acid production. As renal insufficiency progresses, patients typically become acidotic. Initially the acidosis is of the nonanion gap type, but as renal insufficiency becomes far advanced, an anion gap acidosis supervenes. If left untreated, acidosis contributes to bone resorption, may contribute to protein catabolism, and can result in malaise and dyspnea.

Alkali therapy can be given as sodium bicarbonate tablets. Each tablet is 650 mg and contributes 8 mEq of bicarbonate. A useful starting dose is to administer one tablet three times a day and titrate upward in order to maintain the serum bicarbonate level at more than 20 mEq per liter. Alternatively, a sodium citrate solution (Bicitra) can be given; this contributes 1 mEq of bicarbonate per mL of solution. Citrate-containing alkali should not be administered to patients receiving aluminum-containing phosphate binders, because citrate is known to enhance the gastrointestinal absorption of aluminum. Alkali therapy contains a substantial sodium load, and therefore the patient needs to be monitored closely for the development of volume overload.

Calcium and Phosphorus

Disturbances in calcium and phosphate metabolism regularly accompany chronic renal failure and contribute to many of the manifestations of uremia. As the glomerular filtration rate declines, the serum phosphate level begins to increase and causes a reciprocal fall in the serum calcium concentration. In response, parathyroid hormone is stimulated and results in increased phosphate excretion per remaining nephron so that calcium and phosphorus levels return toward normal levels. As renal function continues to decline, calcium and phosphorus levels remain within normal levels but at the expense of an ever-increasing level of parathyroid hormone. Ultimately, enough renal mass is lost such that the hyperphosphaturia per nephron is insufficient to prevent phosphate retention, and hyperphosphatemia becomes sustained.

As renal mass declines, the circulating level of 1,25-dihydroxyvitamin D also begins to fall. Lack of 1,25-dihydroxyvitamin D contributes to the development of hypocalcemia because this hormone normally serves to increase calcium absorption from the gastrointestinal tract and enhances the ability of parathyroid hormone to mobilize calcium from bone. Decreased absorption of calcium from the intestine is further compounded by the low calcium content in the diet of patients with chronic renal failure. Low levels of vitamin D also contribute to the development of secondary hyperparathyroidism because this hormone normally exerts a direct inhibitory effect on the release of parathyroid hormone from the parathyroid gland. Finally, during the course of advancing renal insufficiency, the set point at which calcium suppresses parathyroid hormone release becomes elevated, leading to further elevations in the level of parathyroid hormone.

The primary goal in the management of patients with chronic renal failure is to maintain the serum phosphorus level within normal limits. Initially, the patient should be placed on a phosphate-restricted diet (800 to 1000 mg per day). Dietary sources particularly rich in phosphate include eggs; dairy products such as cream, milk, and cheese; and meat products. Although a few patients may be able to maintain the serum phosphate within normal limits on a restricted diet alone, most patients require a phosphate binder in order to increase fecal excretion of phosphate.

Oral phosphate binders are available as either aluminum or calcium salts. The decision as to which class of binder to administer should rest on the starting phosphate level and the calcium phosphorus product. In patients with a serum phosphorus level of greater than 6 mg per dL or a calcium phosphorus product of greater than 60, the aluminum-containing binders are the appropriate choice. The use of calcium-containing binders in the setting of a high product results in the development of metastatic calcification and therefore should be avoided. The aluminum-containing compounds are considered the most potent phosphate binders and are available as aluminum hydroxide (Amphojel) and aluminum carbonate (Basaljel). As soon as the serum phosphate level is reduced to less than 6 mg per dL and the calcium phosphorus product is less than 60, the aluminum-containing binders should be discontinued so as to avoid the long-term consequences of aluminum toxicity. At this point, the calcium-containing phosphate binders are the preferred agents.

The calcium-containing phosphate binders are available as the calcium salts of carbonate, acetate, and citrate. Recent evidence suggests that calcium acetate (PhosLo) is the most potent phosphate binder within this class. In order to be most effective, all the phosphate binders should be given with meals. The effectiveness can be further enhanced by varying the dose of the binder in proportion to the phosphate content of each meal.

As previously discussed, negative calcium balance tends to develop in patients with advancing renal insufficiency, because of decreased gastrointestinal absorption of calcium and decreased calcium content in the diet. To remain in calcium balance, most patients with chronic renal failure require 1000 to 1500 mg per day of elemental calcium. This is difficult to achieve with diet because many foods that have a high calcium content also have a high phosphorus content and therefore are restricted. In order to overcome this problem, supplemental calcium must be administered and can be given as calcium carbonate or calcium acetate. When given for this indication, calcium should be given between meals. Again, calcium should not be given until the serum phosphate level is normalized, in order to prevent calcium phosphate deposition in the tissues.

In some patients, the serum calcium level remains low despite normalization of the serum phosphate and supplemental oral elemental calcium. In these patients, oral 1,25-dihydroxyvitamin D (Rocaltrol) can be given starting at a dose of 0.25 µg per day in order to increase absorption of calcium from the gastrointestinal tract. Careful monitoring of the patient is required in order to avoid hypercalcemia. The serum phosphorus must also be closely followed as 1,25-dihydroxyvitamin D increases phosphate absorption and therefore could lead to metastatic calcification if the calcium phosphorus product becomes elevated.

Hematologic Abnormalities

Patients with renal insufficiency almost uniformly acquire a normocytic, normochromic anemia that tends to worsen in parallel with advancing azotemia. The etiology of anemia in chronic renal failure is primarily decreased biosynthesis of erythropoietin from the kidney. The use of recombinant human erythropoietin or epoetin alfa (Epogen), now offers the most definitive treatment of the anemia of chronic renal disease. In addition to freeing the patient from repetitive exposure to blood-borne pathogens, iron overload, and sensitization, the use of erythropoietin has been demonstrated to improve cardiovascular and cognitive function and to improve the overall quality of life of patients with chronic renal failure. Although transfusions are clearly indicated for the treatment of acute hemorrhage and cardiovascular instability, this form of therapy should no longer be considered routine in the management of anemia in patients undergoing peritoneal or hemodialysis.

Erythropoietin is administered parentally in doses of 50 to 150 units per kg three times per week to patients on maintenance hemodialysis. Patients receiving peritoneal dialysis and patients not yet on renal replacement therapy can be given erythropoietin subcutaneously three times per week. The target hematocrit should be based on the clinical characteristics of the individual patient. In young patients with no evidence of cardiovascular disease, a target hematocrit of 30 should provide relief of symptoms attributable to anemia. In contrast, older patients with widespread peripheral vascular disease or known coronary artery disease should derive additional benefit from a hematocrit that is closer to normal.

Failure to respond to erythropoietin therapy is most commonly attributable to the presence of iron deficiency. A transferrin saturation of less than 20% or a serum ferritin level of less than 50 μg per liter indicates inadequate iron stores and necessitates prospective iron supplementation, usually given as ferrous sulfate (Feosol), 325 mg twice or three times per day. During the course of therapy, the transferrin saturation and the serum ferritin level should be monitored frequently so as to ensure that iron deficiency does not develop. Other causes of a suboptimal response include the presence of an underlying inflammatory illness, aluminum intoxication, and the presence of hyperparathyroidism.

In patients with advanced chronic renal failure, a qualitative defect in platelet function typically develops. In patients at risk for bleeding complications, three forms of therapy have been shown to be effective in lowering the prolonged bleeding time caused by uremia. First, desmopressin (DDAVP) can be administered intravenously at a dose of 0.3 μg per kg in 50 mL of normal saline infused over 30 minutes. Alternatively, cryoprecipitate (ten bags) can be infused intravenously over 30 minutes. Finally, conjugated estrogens, at a dose of 0.6* mg/kg given intravenously daily for 5 consecutive days, have also been shown to be effective.

Protein Intake

Before the widespread availability of the various forms of renal replacement therapy, rigid control of dietary protein intake was the dominant feature in the management of chronic renal failure. Oftentimes, such strict limitations in protein intake occurred at the expense of severe muscle wasting and other evidence of malnutrition. In view of the readily accessible nature of renal replacement therapy today, dietary management should now be designed in such a way that the onset of the uremic syndrome is delayed and ameliorated, but the patient is nevertheless provided with adequate energy and protein to maintain good nutritional status. With regard to the formulation of nutritional therapy, protein restriction has been demonstrated to slow the progressive nature of renal function loss.

Once the glomerular filtration rate falls below 70 mL per minute, a protein intake of 0.6 to 0.7 grams per kg should be instituted (Table 2). Approximately half of that protein should be of high biologic value, which provides the necessary proportion of essential amino acids. The remainder of the protein can be of lesser quality, usually consisting of grains and vegetables, which tend to enhance the palatability of the diet. In order to ensure neutral or positive nitrogen balance, en-

*This use of conjugated estrogens is not listed in the manufacturer's official directive.

TABLE 2. **Dietary Recommendations for Patients with Chronic Renal Failure and End-Stage Renal Disease**

Substance	Chronic Renal Failure	Hemodialysis and Peritoneal Dialysis
Protein (gm/kg/day)	0.6–0.8	1.2–1.4*
Calories (kcal/kg/day)	35	38
Sodium (gm/day)	6–8	4–6
Potassium (mEq/day)	50–70	50–70
Phosphorus (mg/day)	800	800–1000
Calcium (mg/day)	1200	1500†

*Patients on peritoneal dialysis require at least 1.4 gm/kg due to protein losses across the peritoneal membrane.
†Dietary intake must be supplemented to achieve these levels.

ergy requirements should approximate 35 kcal per kg.

Once hemodialysis is initiated, the protein and energy content of the diet must be augmented. The hemodialysis procedure is catabolic, and there are substantial losses of nutrients into the dialysate. As a result, protein intake should be increased to 1.2 grams per kg per day, and caloric intake should increase to 38 kcal per kg. In patients on peritoneal dialysis, protein intake should be increased to 1.4 grams per kg per day to account for the 6 to 8 grams of protein normally lost across the peritoneal membrane. Again, approximately half of this protein should be of high biologic value.

RENAL REPLACEMENT THERAPY

A number of acute indications warrant the immediate initiation of hemodialysis (Table 3). In the absence of one of these acute conditions, the timing of initiation is somewhat subjective. The

TABLE 3. **Indications for Initiation of Hemodialysis**

Acute Indications
Hyperkalemia unresponsive to conservative management
Uremic pericarditis
Uremic neuropathy
Intractable acidosis
Volume overload unresponsive to diuretic therapy

Chronic Indications
Symptomatic azotemia (decreased appetite, nausea, and vomiting such that nutritional intake is interfered with; declining BUN/creatinine ratio)
Iothalamate sodium (Glofil) clearance <7 mL/min

Abbreviation: BUN = blood urea nitrogen.

symptoms that prompt strong consideration to begin dialysis include a history of decreasing appetite, increasing fatigue, a disturbance in sleep-wake cycles, a metallic taste to food, and the onset of nausea and vomiting. A decline in the ratio of blood urea nitrogen (BUN) to creatinine is an objective sign that suggests that a patient is no longer eating adequately. The longer that initiation of dialysis is delayed, the greater the likelihood that negative nitrogen balance and progressive malnutrition will develop. Procrastination until an acute indication develops may delay the start of therapy 1 to 2 months but is often at the expense of increased patient morbidity.

Dialysis

Dialysis allows for the removal of unwanted solutes on the basis of the diffusion of these solutes across a semipermeable membrane driven by a concentration gradient. Fluid removal, or ultrafiltration, is achieved by the creation of a transmembrane pressure gradient across the dialysis membrane. Provision of dialysis requires reliable and repeated access to the patient's circulation. Creation of an arteriovenous fistula is the preferred vascular access because it is associated with the greatest longevity and the least amount of infectious complications. In elderly patients and patients with extensive vascular disease, vessels may be inadequate for creation of an arteriovenous fistula, and placement of a prosthetic graft may be required. In either case, vascular access should be established when the glomerular filtration rate falls to 10 to 15 mL per minute so as to allow adequate time for the access to fully mature.

Peritoneal Dialysis

Like hemodialysis, solute and fluid removal are achieved by diffusion and ultrafiltration. Solutes diffuse down their concentration gradient across the peritoneal membrane into the dialysate, which is then drained and discarded. Ultrafiltration is achieved by the creation of an osmotic pressure gradient caused by the high glucose concentration in the dialysate.

Peritoneal dialysis is preferred over hemodialysis for patients with cardiovascular instability, patients in whom vascular access cannot be established or maintained, patients who live in areas not readily accessible to dialysis centers, and patients who prefer home dialysis. Conditions that render peritoneal dialysis less feasible include reduced peritoneal surface secondary to adhesions or recurrent peritonitis, the presence of an ostomy, recent abdominal surgery, and

blindness. The most significant complication of peritoneal dialysis is the development of peritonitis and infection of the catheter site.

Continuous ambulatory peritoneal dialysis is typically achieved by the instillation of 2 liters of fluid into the peritoneal cavity, where the fluid is allowed to dwell for 4 to 8 hours while the patient continues his or her daily activities. The fluid is then discarded and the cycle is repeated, usually four to five times per day. In continuous cyclic peritoneal dialysis, an automated cycler is used to provide exchanges of usually 8 liters of dialysis solution while the patient is asleep. One 2-liter exchange dwells in the peritoneal cavity during the remainder of the day.

Transplantation

Renal transplantation has continued to enjoy considerable success as a result of improved donor-recipient selection, immunosuppressive regimens, and methods of treating allograft rejection. Donor transplants from living relatives have the longest graft survival. With the introduction of cyclosporine (Sandimmune), the short-term graft survival of cadaver renal transplants has dramatically improved; the 1-year graft survival rate approaches 88%. In contrast, the long-term survival of cadaver allografts has remained relatively fixed at 7.5 years. The most common cause of late allograft failure is chronic rejection. A patient should be referred for transplantation only if it is determined that the transplantation procedure itself or subsequent immunosuppressive drugs will not confer an excessive risk to that patient. Patients with extensive underlying coronary artery disease, those with underlying chronic infections, and those noncompliant with therapy or prone to drug abuse may be better served by remaining on some other form of renal replacement therapy.

GENITOURINARY TUMORS

method of
IAN M. THOMPSON, M.D., and
JULIUS L. TEAGUE, M.D.
Brooke Army Medical Center
San Antonio, Texas

CARCINOMA OF THE BLADDER

Carcinoma of the urinary bladder is the second most common tumor of the genitourinary tract; approxi-

The opinions or assertions contained herein are those of the authors and do not necessarily reflect those of the U.S. Department of the Army or Department of Defense.

mately 52,300 new cases are diagnosed annually. It is more commonly seen in males than in females, and the risk rises virtually exponentially with age. The reason for this phenomenon is the cumulative effect of various carcinogens on the uroepithelium, the most common of which are cigarette smoke metabolites. A variety of carcinogens have been identified in the urine of cigarette smokers, and these agents are thought to cause 50% of all bladder tumors in men and 31% in women. The process of initiation→promotion→premalignant change→frank cancer may take more than 20 years to occur. Other agents that have been implicated in the development of bladder cancer are a variety of industrial chemicals, including β-naphthylamine and benzene. Of interest, the rate of mortality from bladder cancer has decreased significantly over the past two decades from 4.2 per 100,000 of the general population in 1973 to 3.3 per 100,000 in 1989. The reason for this decrease is unclear, but improvement in treatment and a decreasing rate of invasive disease have been postulated as the causes for this trend.

Most tumors of the bladder are classified as transitional cell carcinomas because they involve the transitional epithelium of the bladder wall. Nevertheless, because of the embryologic origin of these cells, squamous cell carcinoma and adenocarcinoma are occasionally diagnosed. Because most of these tumors grow in a papillary, exophytic manner, the frequent necrosis and sloughing of papillary fronds with transient hematuria are often the events that lead the patient to seek medical care. Other presenting symptoms can include suprapubic pain, obstructive symptoms, ureteral colic, or weight loss or anorexia associated with metastatic disease. The irritative symptoms frequently associated with transitional cell carcinoma often lead to a misdiagnosis of urinary tract infection.

The diagnosis of bladder cancer is suspected by the recognition of a filling defect in the bladder on intravenous pyelogram or a serendipitous finding on ultrasonogram or computerized tomography (CT). However, the most efficient method of diagnosis is cystoscopy with direct visualization of the bladder epithelium. When a bladder tumor is identified, definitive therapy as well as local staging is accomplished by transurethral resection of the bladder tumor (TURBT). At the time of TURBT, examination under anesthesia (EUA) aids in determining the extent of disease. The TNM staging system is displayed in Table 1.

At a minimum, clinical staging must include TURBT pathologic findings as well as EUA. Because of the small but measurable risk of development of upper urinary tract tumors in 2.3% of patients, an IVP is also recommended.

The initial impression of local stage guides the choice of further staging examinations (e.g., for superficial tumors, further staging is of low yield). For advanced tumors (T2+), CT scan of the pelvis and chest x-ray are recommended. Bone scans or liver scans are obtained only if abnormalities of alkaline phosphatase or liver function tests, respectively, are detected.

The vast majority of bladder tumors manifest with early-stage disease (T1 or lower). For these tumors, complete TURBT is usually curative. However, because of the exposure of the entire bladder urothelium to carcinogenic agents, there is a 70% risk that subse-

TABLE 1. TNM Staging System for Bladder Cancer

Stage	Description
Ta	Noninvasive papillary carcinoma
TIS	Carcinoma in situ: flat tumor
T1	Tumor invades subepithelial connective tissue
T2	Tumor invades inner half of superficial muscle
T3a	Tumor invades deep muscle
T3b	Tumor invades perivesical fat
T4a	Tumor invades prostate, uterus, or vagina
T4b	Tumor invades pelvic or abdominal wall
N1	Metastasis to single node, ≤2 cm in greatest diameter
N2	Metastasis to single node, between 2 and 5 cm in greatest diameter
N3	Metastasis to node, >5 cm in greatest diameter

quent tumors will develop. For this reason, *lifelong* follow-up with surveillance cystoscopy is required. Two adverse sequelae in these patients can occur: (1) tumor recurrence and (2) tumor stage progression. The first of these events necessitates additional TURBT; the second may necessitate more morbid therapy (e.g., radical cystectomy) and places the patient at a significantly increased risk of mortality from the disease. To prevent both recurrence and (possibly) progression, high-risk patients may benefit from prophylactic intravesical chemotherapy. Candidates for such adjuvant therapy include those with multiple tumors at diagnosis, carcinoma in situ, or multiple recurrences. Intravesical agents that have been used include doxorubicin (Adriamycin), mitomycin C, thiotepa, and bacille Calmette-Guérin (BCG). Of these, BCG is the most effective in reducing disease recurrence. Results of a recently completed randomized trial also suggest that after 6 weekly instillations, monthly maintenance therapy may further reduce the risk of recurrence.

In patients with higher stage disease (T2+), TURBT usually cannot eradicate disease. Although partial cystectomy is an option for selected patients, the risk of recurrence and the difficulty with obtaining negative surgical margins in many patients makes this treatment appropriate in only a small fraction of cases. For these reasons, the most commonly employed treatment for T2+ disease is radical cystectomy. In males, this extirpative procedure involves removal of the bladder, prostate, seminal vesicles, and, for selected patients, the urethra. In females, the bladder, urethra, and anterior two-thirds of the vagina are removed. In both sexes, pelvic lymphadenectomy is performed. Urinary diversion historically has been performed with the use of an ileal conduit requiring the use of a collecting appliance. Over the past 10 to 20 years, methods of continent diversion to the skin or to the urethra (usually in males), have been developed. Although these techniques require more technical expertise and time to perform, as well as being associated with a higher complication/reoperation rate, they have provided a significant improvement in quality of life for many patients.

Of the patients with advanced (T2+) transitional cell carcinoma, more than 25% die of the disease within

5 years despite aggressive surgical therapy, and the local recurrence rate is 8%. With the advent of effective multiagent chemotherapy (most notably, methotrexate, vinblastine, adriamycin, and cisplatin [MVAC]), a number of centers have reported the use of several cycles of chemotherapy before cystectomy: so-called neoadjuvant therapy. Of patients proceeding to cystectomy following neoadjuvant MVAC, between 20% and 40% have been found to be free of disease in the cystectomy specimen, although metastatic disease has subsequently developed in some. Unfortunately, for some patients, neoadjuvant therapy may delay definitive cystectomy, and the opportunity for cure may be missed. Because this is one of the most urgent questions in urologic oncology, a National Cancer Institute–sponsored randomized study in which neoadjuvant MVAC followed by cystectomy is compared with cystectomy alone is currently accruing patients. Closure of the study is expected in 1996, and results are to be reported thereafter. Patients in whom advanced disease is diagnosed or metastatic disease develops during follow-up can occasionally be treated successfully with MVAC.

Follow-up for patients with superficial bladder tumors includes cytoscopy and bladder wash cytologic studies every 3 months for 2 years, then every 6 months for 3 years, and annually thereafter. A recurrent tumor means starting follow-up over again at every-3-month examinations. Patients who undergo cystectomy should be followed with pelvic CT scans every 6 months for 2 years and annually thereafter. If urethrectomy is not performed, a urethral washing for cytologic examination must be obtained at each visit to rule out urethral recurrence. With proper follow-up and with intravesical therapy when necessary, long-term disease-specific survival for superficial disease is excellent. Long-term disease-free survival for CIS and T1 tumors is somewhat less, generally in the range of 40 to 50%. After radical cystectomy for T2 disease, 5-year survival rates of 50 to 90% can be expected, in comparison with 6 to 60% for T3a and T3b disease. Untreated metastatic disease is almost uniformly fatal within 2 years.

CARCINOMA OF THE PROSTATE

Prostate cancer represents the most common tumor among men in the United States: approximately 165,000 new cases were diagnosed in 1993, and more than 35,000 patients died that year. The most significant determinant of risk for clinical disease is age; disease prevalence increases almost exponentially after age 50. The true prevalence of the disease is unknown, but estimates can be obtained from autopsy series or from series of patients undergoing radical cystectomy for bladder cancer. These series suggest that the risk of disease is more than 30% in men after age 50 and may be as high as 80% in men in their ninth decade of life. Results of recent studies have suggested that this occult disease can occur in as many as 30% of men between the ages of 40 and 50. Clinically evident disease can be expected in between 6 and 8% of men during their lifetime, and about 2% of all deaths in the U.S. male population are caused by prostate cancer.

Patients at the highest risk from the disease are African-Americans and those patients with one or more first-degree relatives (father, brothers) with a history of prostate cancer.

The diagnosis of prostate cancer in 1993 is usually a serendipitous finding. Signs and symptoms of the disease are usually encountered only at an advanced stage; anorexia, bone pain, neurologic deficits, obstructive voiding symptoms, and weight loss are findings characteristic of metastatic disease. Symptoms frequently leading to a diagnosis of prostate cancer are obstructive voiding symptoms, but these symptoms may merely prompt digital rectal examination (DRE), which identifies an otherwise silent nodule resulting from prostate cancer.

With the current emphasis on early detection of prostate cancer, three diagnostic tests are in vogue: DRE, prostate-specific antigen (PSA), and transrectal ultrasonography (TRUS). The latter is generally not recommended for use in a screening algorithm because (1) prostate cancer does not have a pathognomonic echo pattern, (2) the value of TRUS in addition to DRE and PSA is minimal, and (3) the cost of TRUS is considerably higher than that of either DRE or PSA.

The detection of induration or a nodule on DRE is found to be secondary to prostate cancer in 25 to 50% of patients. Although disease in most asymptomatic patients that is diagnosed with DRE is found to be clinically localized, disease in 30 to 70% of patients is pathologically upstaged. PSA is a protein found in significant quantities in the prostate, and serum levels are directly related to the risk of prostate cancer. Elevated levels are also seen in patients with benign prostatic hyperplasia (BPH), prostatitis, and prostatic infarct. In general, the highest levels are seen in patients with prostate cancer but significant overlap exists with BPH because of its virtual endemic prevalence. According to a monoclonal assay with an upper limit of normal of 4 ng/mL, the risks of prostate cancer are 25% in patients with levels of PSA between 4 and 10 ng/mL and 50% in those with levels over 10 ng/mL.

The role of early diagnosis and screening for prostate cancer at this time is unknown, primarily because of the extremely high prevalence of the disease and its unknown natural history. As a result of questions regarding whether screening is effective, the National Cancer Institute is currently beginning a trial in which patients are randomly subjected to annual screening with DRE and PSA or to follow-up alone; the ultimate end point is a reduction in the rate of mortality from prostate cancer.

Prostate cancer is most frequently diagnosed through needle biopsy although unsuspected disease is found at transurethral resection of the prostate (TURP) in as many as 10% of all patients. Virtually 100% of cases are adenocarcinomas. After a histologic diagnosis has been established, staging is performed (Table 2). At a minimum, staging should include prostatic acid phosphatase (PAP) and bone scan in all patients. PAP is useful because an elevated enzymatic value is virtually always indicative of metastatic disease. PSA has been suggested to be useful because low values (e.g., <20 ng/mL) are almost never associated with bony metastases (and therefore in patients

TABLE 2. **TNM Staging System for Prostate Cancer**

Stage	Description
T1a	Incidentally detected tumor, ≤5% of resected tissue
T1b	Incidentally detected tumor, >5% of resected tissue
T1c	Impalpable tumor, detected by needle biopsy (usually because of elevated prostate-specific antigen level)
T2a	Tumor confined to prostate, <50% of lobe involved
T2b	Tumor confined to prostate, >50% of lobe involved but not both lobes
T2c	Tumor confined to prostate, involves both lobes
T3a	Unilateral extension through prostate capsule
T3b	Bilateral extension through prostate capsule
T3c	Tumor invades seminal vesicle(s)
T4a	Tumor invades bladder neck, external sphincter, or rectum
T4b	Tumor invades levator muscles and/or fixed to pelvic wall
N1	Metastasis to lymph node, ≤2 cm in greatest diameter
N2	Metastasis to lymph node, >2 cm but ≤5 cm in greatest diameter
N3	Metastasis to lymph node(s), >5 cm in greatest diameter

with values of <20 ng/mL, bone scans might be omitted). It must be emphasized that DRE, when performed by an experienced urologist, is extremely useful in assessing the presence of local extraprostatic disease.

Multiple treatment options exist for localized prostate cancer. Studies of the natural history of untreated stages A and B disease attest to the slow progression of these lesions with disease-specific survival rates in excess of 85% at 10 years. For this reason, a "watch and wait" policy for older patients and those with significant other comorbid conditions is a reasonable option. For younger patients with a long life expectancy (≥10 years), treatment for cure can be accomplished with radical prostatectomy, radiotherapy, or interstitial radiotherapy (brachytherapy). Brachytherapy has been used longest with iodine 125. Local control rates with this method have been disappointing—significantly lower than those achieved with external beam radiotherapy. Newer methods of implantation and newer isotopes are being investigated, but it must be stressed that 10- and 15-year statistics are necessary for the evaluation of treatment for prostate cancer and that such data are unavailable for these newer techniques. Radical prostatectomy is one of the oldest methods of treatment and many series have reported excellent 10-, 15-, and 20-year survival rates. Recent innovations have led to reduced rates of morbidity after surgery with virtually 100% continence, less than 1% perioperative mortality, and few patients requiring postoperative homologous blood transfusion. Problems with radical prostatectomy include the high rate of pathologic upstaging (positive surgical margins or seminal vesicle invasion): between 30% and 50% of patients. In addition, measurable PSA (serologic failure) develops in 20 to 40% of patients after radical prostatectomy. A reduction in these rates may be achieved with more intense screening of patients and earlier

diagnosis. External-beam radiation therapy (XRT) has undergone many refinements and has produced excellent disease-specific survival rates among patients with localized disease. Approximately 70 Gy (about 35 treatments over 7 weeks) are administered, and serious complications are quite uncommon. The long-term efficacy of this treatment has been questioned because of the evidence of residual disease in prostate biopsy specimens 2 or more years after treatment and the fact that patients with persistent disease in biopsy specimens seem to have a poorer prognosis.

The optimal treatment of locally advanced disease is unknown, but the most commonly employed current treatments include hormonal therapy, TURP for symptoms, and XRT. There is little evidence that any one treatment has greater efficacy. The cornerstone of treatment for metastatic disease is hormonal therapy, which is predicated on a reduction in androgens available to prostate cancer cells. This treatment is not curative, and disease relapse is the rule, probably as a result of populations of tumor cells that are androgen independent. There are multiple methods by which hormonal treatment can be achieved. Table 3 is a partial listing that includes benefits and risks of each.

Monotherapy, when chosen, usually consists of orchiectomy, estrogens, or luteinizing hormone–releasing hormone (LHRH)–agonist therapy. For many patients, orchiectomy is the simplest form of therapy, and compliance is not an issue. Estrogen therapy has generally been abandoned in the United States because of the significantly increased risk of cardiovascular mortality. LHRH-agonist therapy may be more acceptable to many patients, but if it is chosen, some form of block-

TABLE 3. **Options for Hormonal Treatment of Prostate Cancer**

Treatment	Advantage	Disadvantage
Bilateral orchiectomy	Inexpensive 100% compliance Minimal morbidity	Hot flashes Psychological effect Decreased libido/ erections
Estrogens (oral)	Inexpensive	High risk of cardiovascular/ thromboembolic complications Gynecomastia Hot flashes Decreased libido/ erections
Luteinizing hormone–releasing hormone agonists	Convenient (q month dosing)	Very expensive Flare phenomenon Decreased libido/ erections
Antiandrogens	Maintenance of potency	Very expensive Elevated testosterone
Combined androgen blockade	Possibly improved survival	Extremely expensive Combines complications of antiandrogen and either LHRH agonist or orchiectomy

ade of the initial rise in serum testosterone must be administered for 1 to 2 months. (This is usually accomplished with an antiandrogen.) The relative efficacy of an antiandrogen alone is unknown, but such a regimen is usually not chosen because of the rise in testosterone that occurs with treatment. A number of authors have espoused the advantages of combined androgen blockade, in which residual circulating androgens of adrenal origin are "blocked" with the addition of an antiandrogen. An initial National Cancer Institute–sponsored trial demonstrated a modest increase in median survival in patients treated with LHRH-agonist and flutamide (Eulexin), an antiandrogen, as opposed to LHRH-agonist alone. Because of concerns that this difference may be attributable only to the initial flare in with LHRH-agonist–treated patients, a subsequent study in which orchiectomy plus flutamide was compared with orchiectomy alone was initiated. Accrual to this study was expected to be complete during the summer of 1993, and results of that study will probably set the standard for management of patients for years to come.

Despite these advances, the prognosis of patients with metastatic disease is poor; the median length of survival is 2 years. After a patient exhibits hormonal-refractory disease, death usually occurs within 1 year. Chemotherapy or other second-line treatment is generally ineffective and is not recommended unless conducted in an investigational program.

TUMORS OF THE KIDNEY

The frequency of diagnosed renal tumors increased slightly over the past decade; approximately 27,200 cases were diagnosed in 1993. The male: female ratio is approximately 2:1, and the incidence of disease increases dramatically with age. The majority of renal tumors in adults are adenocarcinomas arising from the renal parenchyma, but approximately 8% arise from the transitional epithelium of the collecting system and are therefore transitional cell carcinomas. The prognoses and treatments of these two entities are distinctly different, and a preoperative diagnosis is of significant importance. Factors predisposing to the development of renal cell carcinoma are poorly understood, but several agents, including cigarette smoking and phenacetin ingestion, have been linked to the development of transitional cell carcinoma.

Symptoms that may lead to the diagnosis of renal tumors include hematuria, flank pain, flank mass, and weight loss. Renal tumors are notorious for manifesting with a bizarre constellation of symptoms that taxes the diagnostic acumen of clinicians. With increasing frequency these tumors are diagnosed serendipitously because of their appearance on an imaging study performed for other reasons (e.g., right upper quadrant ultrasonography for cholelithiasis). It has been demonstrated that tumors diagnosed in this manner are of a lower stage and carry a better prognosis than do tumors detected through other means.

The preoperative diagnosis of renal tumors virtually always remains uncertain until confirmed surgically. Radiographic characteristics of renal cell carcinoma and transitional cell carcinoma of the kidney on various studies are demonstrated in Table 4.

With intelligently selected imaging studies, the majority of renal tumors can be properly classified. In the presence of a solid mass, the likelihood of a malignant neoplasm exceeds 95%. For this reason, in the majority of such cases, a preliminary biopsy (e.g., needle biopsy) is unnecessary. The most frequently entertained differential diagnosis is that of a complex renal mass, one that does not meet all the accepted criteria of a simple cyst. It can be extremely difficult to establish this diagnosis, and the collaboration of experienced urologists and radiologists is often required in order to establish the best method of diagnosis and treatment. Ancillary testing can include needle aspiration, magnetic resonance imaging, and arteriography. In cases raising suspicions of transitional cell carcinoma, ureteroscopy with cytologic evaluation or ureteroscopic biopsy may prove useful. Renal cell carcinoma can invade the renal vein in the form of a thrombus that can propagate into the inferior vena cava and up to the right atrium.

The staging system for renal tumors is shown in Table 5. Poor local prognostic factors include nodal disease, positive surgical margins, and invasion beyond the renal capsule. In general, a renal vein thrombus, unless invading the caval wall, does not confer a poorer prognosis on the local tumor stage. Because renal cell carcinoma has a distinct affinity for pulmonary (and occasionally bone) metastases, the minimal staging studies required include abdominal CT, chest x-ray, liver function tests, and alkaline phosphatase measurement. If the last level is elevated, a bone scan is required. In the authors' experience, with the exception of small, peripheral lesions, renal ultrasonography is the preferred initial study for ruling out the possibility of a caval tumor thrombus.

TABLE 4. **Radiographic Findings with Renal Tumors**

Study	Renal Cell Carcinoma	Transitional Cell Carcinoma
Intravenous pyelogram	Mass effect Calyces splayed about mass Peripheral mass Nonfunction	Filling defect in collecting system Obstruction of segment of collecting system Central mass
Ultrasonography	Peripheral mass Possible thrombus in renal vein or inferior vena cava	Central mass If large, involves hilum Thrombus extremely rare
Computed tomography	Peripheral mass HU >10 Frequently enhances with contrast Possible lymph node involvement Possible thrombus	Central mass Invades hilum Possible lymph node involvement
Retrograde pyelogram	Splayed calyces	Filling defect

TABLE 5. **TNM Staging System for Tumors of the Kidney**

Stage	Description
T1	Tumor ≤2.5 cm in greatest diameter, limited to kidney
T2	Tumor >2.5 cm in greatest diameter, limited to the kidney
T3a	Tumor invades adrenal gland or perinephric tissues but not beyond Gerota's fascia
T3b	Tumor grossly extends into renal vein(s) or inferior vena cava below diaphragm
T3c	Tumor grossly extends into vena cava above diaphragm
T4	Tumor invades beyond Gerota's fascia
N1	Metastasis to lymph node, ≤2 cm in greatest diameter
N2	Metastasis to lymph node, >2 cm but <5 cm in greatest diameter
N3	Metastasis to lymph node, >5 cm in greatest diameter

Because nonsurgical treatment of both renal cell carcinoma and transitional cell carcinoma is largely ineffective, the treatment of choice is extirpative surgery. In the presence of a normal contralateral renal unit, transitional cell carcinoma is best treated with nephroureterectomy. Like transitional cell carcinoma of the urinary bladder, renal transitional cell carcinoma can be considered a "field change" phenomenon, and nephrectomy alone without removal of the ureteral stump leaves the patient at a high risk of recurrent disease. In patients with solitary kidneys or compromised renal function and with superficial tumors accessible to endoscopic management, it is possible to achieve local control with a combination of fulguration, laser therapy, and resection. In such cases, surveillance is required, much as for transitional cell carcinoma of the urinary bladder.

The gold standard for the management of renal cell carcinoma is radical nephrectomy. In this procedure, early vascular control is obtained to reduce the likelihood of tumor dissemination during renal mobilization, and the kidney is removed, leaving Gerota's fascia and the perinephric fat intact. If a renal vein or caval thrombus is present, the surgical management plan is altered (often radically, to include profound hypothermia and circulatory arrest) to allow vascular control with thrombus removal.

Adjuvant therapy after surgical removal of the kidney for transitional cell or renal cell carcinoma is of questionable value. Possible adjuvant agents include MVAC or interferon, respectively, but neither has established efficacy in this setting. Patients who have been treated for renal transitional cell carcinoma must be observed in a manner similar to that of patients with transitional cell carcinoma of the bladder, with periodic cystoscopy and imaging of the contralateral collecting system and ureter. In as many as 75% of these patients, bladder tumors subsequently develop. Similarly, patients who have undergone nephrectomy for renal cell carcinoma must undergo periodic follow-up for evidence of recurrence. Because recurrences are most likely in the abdomen or lungs, follow-up should include periodic abdominal CT and chest x-ray. (Nihilists could argue that follow-up is unnecessary because therapy at relapse is generally ineffective.) The 5-year survival rate for patients with pathologically localized disease is 85% for renal cell carcinoma and tumors of the renal pelvis, in comparison with 9% for metastatic disease.

Unfortunately, the success rate for the treatment of metastatic transitional cell or renal cell carcinoma is extremely poor. Transitional cell carcinoma is probably best treated with MVAC, but only anecdotal reports of its efficacy are available. An impressively long list of agents have been used for metastatic renal cell carcinoma, but responses are rare, and few anecdotes of long-term disease-free survival have been reported. The opinion of many authorities is that should treatment be employed for advanced disease, the patient is best served by participating in an investigational protocol. The National Cancer Institute currently sponsors a myriad of such studies at a large number of U.S. institutions.

CANCER OF THE TESTIS

Tumors of the testis are uncommon neoplasms; only 6,600 new cases are diagnosed annually in the United States. The age-adjusted incidence rate is 4.8 per 100,000 for all races. Despite this small number, the diagnosis of testis cancer is of extreme importance because it strikes men at a young age and because it is almost uniformly curable. Testis tumors are most commonly diagnosed between the ages of 20 and 35, although they can be found in neonates and in nonagenarians. The risk of developing this disease increases significantly in men with a history of cryptorchidism; this group constitutes 10% of all patients with this disease. For reasons that are unclear, testis tumors are distinctly uncommon in African Americans.

The manifestations of testicular tumors are extremely variable. Ideally, all tumors should be diagnosed by patients during weekly testicular self-examination. Unfortunately, most tumors are painless, and many patients postpone seeking treatment out of embarrassment or fear. In addition, many testicular tumors are initially misdiagnosed as trauma or epididymitis by health care providers, which further delays definitive treatment. The suspicion of a testicular tumor should begin with the finding on physical examination of a solid mass interrupting the normal contour of the tunic surrounding the testis. In uncertain cases, high-resolution testicular ultrasonography can be very helpful. With a working diagnosis of testicular carcinoma, radical (inguinal) orchiectomy is indicated. In unusual circumstances when the diagnosis is uncertain, inguinal exploration, testis biopsy, and frozen section interpretation can aid with management plans.

Testicular tumors can be histologically segregated into two groups: seminomas and nonseminomas. The latter contains multiple types of germ cell tumors. Radical orchiectomy specimens provide pathologists with tissue to appropriately categorize the tumor into one or the other category as well as to provide local tumor staging (T stage). In general, testis tumors metastasize by first gaining access into the lymphatic channels of the testis and adnexa and subsequently traveling along lymphatic channels to the "landing zone" lymph nodes of the retroperitoneum. These nodal regions correspond to the source of vascular supply to the testis: the pre- and periaortic lymph nodes on the left and the precaval and interaortocaval nodes on the right. From there, spread via the thoracic duct and subsequent hematogenous spread to the lungs is the most frequent subsequent route of metastasis.

Diagnosis of testicular tumors is generally obtained from radical inguinal orchiectomy. With the finding of a solid, nonpainful mass in the testis, inguinal orchiectomy is indicated. (Confirmation may be made in some cases with the use of testicular sonography, but this examination is usually redundant in patients with a solid mass.) Needle aspiration or biopsy is contraindicated because spillage of tumor cells can radically alter the patterns of metastasis. If the etiology of a mass is uncertain, open surgical testicular biopsy with vascular control and frozen section evaluation is indicated.

The staging system for testicular tumors is shown in Table 6. The staging system is logically based on the orderly progression from disease limited to the testis to spread to the retroperitoneum to metastatic disease in the lung. Staging studies essential for the evaluation of the patient with testis cancer include x-ray (or CT) of the chest and CT of the abdomen. Serologic studies, including measurements of alpha-fetoprotein, human chorionic gonadotropin–beta (hCG-beta), and lactate dehydrogenase, are essential for staging the disease as well as for follow-up. Although seminomas can be associated with elevations in hCG-beta and lactate dehydrogenase levels, an elevation in alpha-fetoprotein level is pathognomonic of nonseminomatous disease.

Treatment for malignant neoplasms of the testis is based on both stage and histologic findings. Generally employed treatment of testis cancer is displayed in Table 7.

Seminoma is significantly more radiation sensitive than are nonseminomatous tumors. As a result, for disease that appears to be localized to the testis or with nonbulky retroperitoneal spread, radiation therapy to the retroperitoneum is employed for seminoma. For more bulky disease, cisplatin-based chemotherapy is employed for therapy. The best form of therapy for residual radiographically detectable masses after chemotherapy for seminoma remains uncertain. Although resection of residual disease offers both a chance for cure and histologic confirmation, the scirrhous nature

of seminoma after chemotherapy makes surgical resection extraordinarily difficult. As a result, many institutions prefer to treat these masses with radiotherapy or observation.

Nonseminomatous germ cell tumors spread in a similar fashion but are less radiosensitive. Because, with current radiographic staging, 75% of patients with clinically stage A disease are cured with orchiectomy alone and because of the availability of chemotherapy with excellent response rates, observation has been offered for patients with stage A disease at a number of centers. Although rates of survival are similar to those for immediate retroperitoneal lymph node dissection (RPLND), the meticulous follow-up required for these patients makes the replication of these results unlikely in the general population of patients. It is for this reason that RPLND remains the standard treatment for patients with stages A and B1 disease. The principal complication of RPLND is the lack of seminal emission; this can be mitigated by nerve-sparing approaches or by semen banking preoperatively. For patients with stage B2 or C disease, chemotherapy with resection of residual masses is appropriate because as many as 60% of residual masses contain either persistent carcinoma or teratoma. (Although teratoma generally does not metastasize, local growth and impingement upon local structures can cause significant morbidity.)

TABLE 7. **Management of Testis Cancer, By Stage**

Stage	Seminoma	Non-seminoma
T1–T4, N0	Radiation therapy to the retroperitoneum	Observation RPLND
T1–T4, N1–N2	Radiation therapy to the retroperitoneum	RPLND ± chemotherapy
T1–T4, N3	Chemotherapy with radiation therapy as needed	Chemotherapy with adjuvant RPLND
Distant metastases	Chemotherapy	Chemotherapy with resection of residual tumor as necessary

Abbreviation: RPLND = retroperitoneal lymph node dissection.

TABLE 6. **TNM Staging System for Testis Cancer**

Stage	Description
TIS	Intratubular tumor: preinvasive cancer
T1	Tumor limited to testis, including rete testis
T2	Tumor invades beyond tunica albuginea or into epididymis
T3	Tumor invades spermatic cord
T4	Tumor invades scrotum
N1	Metastasis to node, ≤2 cm in greatest dimension
N2	Metastasis to node, >2 cm but <5 cm in greatest diameter
N3	Metastasis to node, >5 cm in greatest diameter

GENITOURINARY MALIGNANCIES OF CHILDHOOD

Three of the five most common solid malignancies in childhood can originate in the genitourinary tract. Fortunately, the overall incidence of solid malignancies among children is low so that the absolute number of children affected annually with these tumors (neuroblastoma, Wilms' tumor, rhabdomyosarcoma) is small. Testicular tumors are uncommon in childhood but are mentioned because of the importance of early diagnosis in successful intervention.

Neuroblastoma

Neuroblastoma is the second most common solid tumor in children. The incidence varies with race and is reported as 9.6 per million in white children and 7.0 per million in black children. Neuroblastoma generally manifests early in childhood; half of affected children are less than 2 years old at the time of diagnosis. Because these tumors are of neural crest origin, they can develop anywhere from the head to the pelvis along the sympathetic chain. More than half are located in the abdomen, and two-thirds of these arise from the adrenal gland.

Diagnosis

The child with neuroblastoma often appears sickly and has a history of weight loss, anorexia, and malaise. On physical examination, a firm, fixed, irregular abdominal mass that extends across the midline is routinely seen. In infants, the most common metastatic site is the liver, and with extensive involvement, it may be palpably enlarged. Bone metastases are more commonly seen in older children. Metastatic disease can also be found periorbitally with resulting proptosis.

If an abdominal mass is present, the best initial study is abdominal ultrasonography. This study distinguishes between solid and cystic masses and can greatly aid in the differential diagnosis of any abdominal mass. Ultrasonography can also evaluate the liver for metastatic disease, determine the patency of the major abdominal vessels, and ascertain the presence of hydronephrosis or renal involvement. Intravenous pyelography generally shows a mass with stippled calcification throughout and distortion of the renal axis. The renal calyces are not deformed as they are with Wilms' tumor.

Radiologic evaluation should also include CT scan to further delineate the tumor and bone scan, skeletal survey, and chest films to look for metastatic disease. Nuclear medicine studies with iodine ^{131}I-meta-iodobenzylguanidine can be used to localize metastatic disease. Bone marrow aspirate is positive in 70% of neuroblastoma patients and should be performed routinely.

The vast majority of neuroblastomas are metabolically active and produce significant amounts of catecholamines. The measurement of the breakdown products of the catecholamines vanillylmandelic acid and homovanillic acid in the urine provides the best diagnostic test for neuroblastoma. Ninety-five percent of patients with neuroblastoma exhibit an elevation in urine vanillylmandelic acid, homovanillic acid, or both. Twenty-four-hour urine collections are classically used for this determination, but tests are available for spot urine samples as well.

Accurate staging is critical for prognosis and is based on the results of clinical and pathologic data (Table 8). Among patients with stages I and II disease, the survival rate is 80%, whereas with stage III it is 37% and with stage IV, only 7%. Stage IV-S is unusual in that survival among these patients is comparable with that among patients with stages I and II disease.

The age of the patient, the serum ferritin level, and the Shimada index are also important prognostic indicators. Age is inversely related to survival; the survival rate is 74% among patients less than 1 year old, whereas it is 12% among patients older than 2. Ferritin, a serum protein, is excreted by neuroblastoma. Normal serum levels of ferritin imply a less active tumor and are associated with a better prognosis, especially in stage III disease. The Shimada index uses histopathologic data and combines the number of mitotic cells per high-power field, the tumor stroma, the immature cell distribution, and the age of the patient. These factors can accurately distinguish patients with tumors that carry favorable or unfavorable prognoses.

Treatment

Treatment for patients with favorable tumor parameters is surgical excision of the mass possibly followed by chemotherapy or radiation. Regardless of the treatment plan, patients with favorable prognostic factors generally do well. The main goal in this group of patients is to minimize treatment morbidity. Patients with unfavorable prognoses tend to do poorly regardless of treatment. Surgery plays a much smaller role in these patients. If the diagnosis is not in doubt and tissue confirmation is not needed, initial surgery can be avoided. Treatment can begin with aggressive chemotherapy and radiation followed by surgical excision of remaining tumor if appropriate.

Wilms' Tumor

Wilms' tumor (nephroblastoma) is the fifth most common malignancy of childhood; the over-

TABLE 8. **Staging System for Neuroblastoma**

Stage I	Tumor limited to organ or site of origin
Stage II	Tumor extending in continuity beyond organ of origin but not across midline
Stage III	Tumor extending in continuity across midline
Stage IV	Distant metastases to bone, bone marrow, lung, liver, skin, soft tissue, distant lymph nodes
Stage IV-S	Disease that would otherwise be stage I or II with spread of tumor to liver, skin, or marrow only

all incidence is 7 per million. There is little difference between numbers of males and females affected. With an average age at presentation of 3.5 years, patients with Wilms' tumor tend to be older than patients with neuroblastoma. These tumors may arise from rests of metanephric blastema within the kidney, especially in patients with multifocal and bilateral disease. An abnormality in chromosome 11 has been identified in many patients with Wilms' tumor.

There is a definite association of Wilms' tumor with certain clinical syndromes and anomalies. The most striking are hemihypertrophy, sporadic aniridia, and Beckwith-Wiedemann syndrome. The incidence of Wilms' tumor in patients with any of these conditions is significantly elevated, and routine imaging of the kidneys, generally with ultrasonography, is recommended until these patients are at least 7 years old.

Diagnosis

The patient with Wilms' tumor usually manifests with an asymptomatic abdominal mass. Unlike patients with neuroblastoma, these children generally appear healthy. The mass is usually smooth and does not extend across the midline. Imaging studies begin with abdominal ultrasonography. This study can reveal the solid nature of the mass and often determines the patency of the renal vessels and inferior vena cava. Intravenous pyelogram classically shows the widely splayed and attenuated calyces characteristic of an intrarenal mass. CT of the abdomen and chest is helpful in the search for metastatic disease. Magnetic resonance imaging may provide information equal to that of the CT scan without radiation, but this is as yet unproved. Bone scan and bone marrow aspirate are generally not necessary. Percutaneous biopsy is not routinely performed. The determination of an accurate tissue diagnosis rests on the results of surgical exploration.

Treatment

The therapy of Wilms' tumor has undergone great advances in recent years largely as a result of the efforts of the National Wilms' Tumor Study group. Three of these studies have been completed, and a fourth is in progress. Much has been learned in regard to the efficacy of chemotherapy, the need for radiation, and the importance of tumor histology for prognosis and therapy. In the case of unilateral disease, treatment begins with a complete surgical exploration. The contralateral kidney is first completely mobilized and examined to ensure that there is no evidence of bilateral disease. If the tumor is resectable and there is no evidence of metastatic disease, a radi-

TABLE 9. Staging of Wilms' Tumor

Stage I	Tumor limited to kidney, completely excised, no capsular rupture, no residual tumor
Stage II	Tumor extends beyond kidney, but is completely excised; biopsy or local spillage
Stage III	Residual nonhematogenous tumor confined to abdomen, lymph node involvement; tumor extends beyond margins of resection
Stage IV	Spread beyond stage III (lung, brain, bone, liver)
Stage V	Bilateral renal disease at diagnosis

cal nephrectomy is performed. If the size of the tumor precludes resection or if there is evidence of bilateral or metastatic disease, multiple biopsy specimens are taken and adjuvant therapy is instituted.

Adjuvant therapy is based on the stage of the disease as determined by radiographic studies and surgical exploration as well as the histologic features of the tumor (Table 9). Chemotherapy with doxorubicin (Adriamycin), vincristine, and bleomycin (Blenoxane) is the cornerstone of treatment in advanced-stage disease. Current protocols focus on reducing the morbidity of treatment while maintaining the high cure rates achieved by previous treatment regimens. The exception to this approach is in patients with unfavorable histologic findings in whom aggressive therapy is still mandatory. Second-look surgery may be feasible after chemotherapy in order to remove any residual masses. Radiotherapy is reserved for cases in which local tumor spread is demonstrated.

Cure rates in Wilms' tumor are directly related to the stage and histologic features of the disease (Table 10). Overall, histologic features play a more important role in prognosis than does any other variable.

Rhabdomyosarcoma

Rhabdomyosarcoma is the third most common solid tumor in children. It arises from the same embryonal cells as striated muscle and can occur anywhere in the body. The incidence of genitourinary rhabdomyosarcoma is 0.5 to 0.7 case per 1 million children less than 15 years old. There is a

TABLE 10. Cure Rates in Wilms' Tumor

Histologic Findings	Stage	% Relapse Free at 4 Years
Favorable	I	90%
Favorable	II	87%
Favorable	III	80%
Favorable	IV	75%
Unfavorable	I–III	65%
Unfavorable	IV	55%

TABLE 11. **Staging System for Rhabdomyosarcoma**

Stage	Description
I	Localized disease, completely resected, confined to organ of origin
II	Total resection with evidence of regional spread
III	Incomplete resection with residual disease
IV	Distant metastases

slight male predominance. Fifteen to twenty percent of all rhabdomyosarcomas occur in the genitourinary tract. Rhabdomyosarcoma has been associated with congenital disorders such as neurofibromatosis and fetal alcohol syndrome.

Diagnosis

The presenting signs and symptoms of genitourinary rhabdomyosarcoma are determined by the organ of origin. Bladder rhabdomyosarcoma can infiltrate the trigone and cause bladder outlet obstruction with resulting infection or hydronephrosis. Tumor tissue fragments may be passed in the urine, and there may be hematuria. Rhabdomyosarcoma can also arise from the prostate and cause symptoms similar to those of bladder rhabdomyosarcoma. Prostate rhabdomyosarcoma may cause constipation by extensive local infiltration of the rectal wall and is generally palpable on rectal examination. Rhabdomyosarcoma of the female genital tract manifests as a vaginal mass or bloody vaginal discharge.

Radiographic evaluation begins with ultrasonography. A mass may be seen displacing the bladder or causing uterine enlargement. Ultrasonography is also helpful in determining whether there is hydronephrosis. A voiding cystourethrogram can demonstrate bladder displacement and involvement. CT scan and magnetic resonance imaging further delineate pelvic masses and allow for complete clinical staging.

Final diagnosis rests on the microscopic examination of adequate tissue samples. With tumors of the lower genitourinary tract, this is usually done through endoscopic biopsy of the lesion. Needle biopsy can be performed as well. Uterine tumors are best diagnosed by dilatation and curettage.

Treatment

Treatment of genitourinary (pelvic) rhabdomyosarcoma has undergone extensive change since the initiation of the Intergroup Rhabdomyosarcoma Study in 1972. Initially, the cornerstone of therapy was surgical excision of the mass, which often required anterior pelvic exenteration and urinary diversion. This was then followed by radiation therapy. This approach was associated with significant morbidity and cure rates of only 40 to 70%. Three study protocols have been completed, and a fourth is in progress.

The development of effective chemotherapy regimens has greatly enhanced cure rates and decreased long-term morbidity. Treatment now begins with surgical biopsy as outlined earlier, followed by chemotherapy. The chemotherapy regimen used is based on the stage of the disease (Table 11). Radiation therapy may also be used in advanced-stage disease. Overall survival rates are related to clinical stage; 77% of patients achieve long-term survival. Current treatment plans not only result in improved survival but also greatly decrease the morbidity of treatment. In the majority of patients, the bladder is preserved, and exenteration is generally needed only for recurrent disease.

Testicular Tumors

Testicular tumors in children account for 1 to 2% of pediatric solid tumors. In contrast to adult patients, in whom germ cell tumors predominate, the most common testicular neoplasm in young pediatric patients is the yolk sac tumor (Table 12).

Diagnosis

Testicular tumors most commonly manifest as painless scrotal masses. Differential diagnosis in the child with a scrotal mass should include testicular torsion, epididymitis, incarcerated inguinal hernia, and hydrocele. In the case of a testicular tumor, the testis is very firm and is usually globally enlarged. The spermatic cord is generally not involved, and unlike a hydrocele, the mass does not transilluminate. Functional tumors such as those of Leydig cell origin may manifest with precocious puberty or gynecomastia. Scrotal ultrasonography with Doppler imaging of the spermatic vessels and nuclear testicular scanning can be helpful in establishing the accurate diagnosis. If tumor is suspected, serum markers such as alpha-fetoprotein and hCG-beta should be obtained before any therapy.

TABLE 12. **Distribution of Testis Tumors in Childhood**

Pathologic Findings	Percentage of Cases
Yolk sac tumor	63%
Teratoma	15%
Gonadal stromal tumor	5%
Leydig cell tumor	1%
Sertoli cell tumor	1%
Other tumors	15%

Treatment

Treatment begins with surgical exploration and radical orchiectomy to obtain an accurate tissue diagnosis. Percutaneous biopsy of the testis should be avoided. If the tumor is of the yolk sac variety, orchiectomy is usually curative. CT of the abdomen should be obtained to rule out metastatic disease, but retroperitoneal masses are rare. If tumor markers and CT are normal, the patient does not require further therapy and can be observed with frequent repeat markers, physical examination, chest x-ray, and abdominal ultrasonography or CT. Follow-up should be continued for at least 2 years. If there is evidence of metastatic disease, aggressive treatment with chemotherapy and possible retroperitoneal lymph node dissection are indicated.

Pediatric patients with seminoma are managed in the same way as adults. Treatment may involve retroperitoneal exploration, chemotherapy, and radiotherapy as has been discussed previously.

URETHRAL STRICTURE

method of
GEORGE D. WEBSTER, M.B., and
SCOTT A. MacDIARMID, M.D.
Duke University Medical Center
Durham, North Carolina

A stricture is a narrowing of the urethra as a result of scar tissue. Some urethral strictures are congenital, but the majority are acquired, secondary to either trauma or inflammation. Trauma may be blunt, penetrating, or from transurethral instrumentation. The majority of inflammatory strictures are caused by sexually transmitted diseases. The true incidence of this disease is unknown but is probably decreasing as a result of both the lower incidence and better treatment of gonoccocal urethritis and the increasing usage of seat belts. Common symptoms include a weakened urinary stream, frequency, and dysuria; less common symptoms include hematuria. Severe cases may result in urinary retention. Poor bladder emptying commonly leads to urinary tract infections, some of which are refractory to antibiotics. In rare cases, an infected stricture can progress to a periurethral abscess, a urethrocutaneous fistula, and renal failure. Irregular strictures in elderly men that are excessively friable and become increasingly resistant to conservative management may represent urethral carcinoma. The diagnosis and local extent of the stricture is made in most cases by a retrograde urethrogram and cystoscopy, but a voiding cystourethrogram may also be required. Patients with strictures associated with findings of bladder obstruction should undergo intravenous pyelography to assess the upper urinary tract, and all patients require urinalysis, urine culture, and serum chemistry studies.

TREATMENT

Factors that determine the management of a stricture include location, etiology, proximity to the sphincter mechanisms, the presence of adverse local factors (fistulae, false passages, etc.), and the degree of obstruction. Urinary retention should be acutely managed with a percutaneous suprapubic tube, followed by disease documentation through the aforementioned techniques. Blind dilatation before identifying the stricture characteristics may lead to further compromise of the urethra and is discouraged.

The management of urethral stricture disease is divided into two broad categories: (1) nonsurgical management (urethral dilatation or direct-vision internal urethrotomy) and (2) open surgical urethroplasty. For centuries, nonsurgical techniques have been the therapeutic mainstay, but unfortunately they have been more palliative than curative; this emphasizes the need for surgical management in many patients.

Urethral Dilatation

The majority of patients are best managed, at least initially, by either urethral dilatation or direct-vision internal urethrotomy. In general, urethral dilatation is successful only for strictures associated with minimal spongiofibrosis, and it can be easily performed under instillational anesthesia. With a well-lubricated van Buren sound, the scar tissue should be progressively dilated on a weekly basis until a caliber of 24 French is achieved. Small-caliber sounds (< 18 Fr) indicate traumatic sharp tips and should be avoided. Filiform bougies and followers are an excellent alternative tool, especially when sounds cannot be negotiated through the stricture. They have the advantage of being able to be inserted under direct cystoscopic vision, making dilatation of narrow, tortuous strictures much safer. Traumatic dilatation should be avoided because it results in urethral tearing with subsequent urine extravasation and worsening of the spongiofibrosis. Liberal usage of antibiotics to treat associated urinary tract infections and to prevent dilatation-induced sepsis is highly recommended. Intermittent home self-dilatation with a well-lubricated catheter is an excellent alternative for managing rapidly recurring stricture disease in patients who refuse or are not appropriate candidates for open urethroplasty.

Direct-Vision Internal Urethrotomy

Direct-vision internal urethrotomy is most highly successful when used to treat short strictures with minimal spongiofibrosis and in the bulbar urethra; short-term success rates approach 85%. The scar should be incised at full thickness and at the 12 o'clock position to avoid the urethral vasculature. Success requires that the incised cleft re-epithelialize in the opened position, but unfortunately this cannot be guaranteed, even by prolonged catheterization. The majority of catheters are removed within 1 to 7 days, depending on the density of the stricture, the depth of incision, and the amount of urethral bleeding. Instillational anesthesia is appropriate in many cases, but more aggressive incision of dense strictures with higher risk of significant bleeding should be performed under regional or general anesthesia, and all cases should be covered with antibiotics. Repetitive urethrotomies should be discouraged because they can advance the peripheral and longitudinal extent of scarring and make subsequent urethroplasty more difficult.

Open Surgical Urethroplasty

In a number of circumstances, nonsurgical therapy is inappropriate, and the strictures are best managed by open urethroplasty (Table 1). No single repair is appropriate for the management of all urethral stricture disease, and proper selection is dictated by the site, etiology, length, and multiplicity of the stricture; by the presence of adverse local factors; and by the surgeon's experience and personal bias. Repairs are best classified as anastomotic or substitution procedures. Anastomotic repairs rely on the excision of the scar and reanastomosis of healthy urethral margins. Substitution operations are performed in one or two stages and entail the use of either grafts or flaps of penile or other non–hair-bearing skin to reconstruct the urethra.

Anastomotic Repairs

Anastomotic repairs are used preferably in two unique situations. Short post-traumatic strictures of the bulbar urethra, which classically fol-low a straddle injury, generally have minimal spongiofibrosis and are optimally managed by anastomotic repair. Obliterative distraction defects of the membranous urethra after pelvic fracture are also best treated by an elaborate "progressive" anastomotic repair through a perineal approach.

Substitution Repairs

Inflammatory strictures and those that recur after previous failed nonoperative and operative repairs are usually long with adjacent spongiofibrosis and are best managed by substitution techniques in one or two stages, depending on their length and complexity. In the majority of cases, the graft or flap is used as a one-stage operation to augment the size of the urethral lumen at the site of the stricture incision, although if scarring is excessive, full circumference replacement of a portion of the urethra may be necessary. Two-stage repairs are used primarily for long strictures or for those associated with adverse local factors that might militate against flap or graft survival. The urethra is marsupialized to the surrounding skin in the first stage and reconstructed 4 to 6 months later in the second stage by retubularization.

RENAL CALCULI

method of
JOHN R. BURNS, M.D.
University of Alabama at Birmingham
Birmingham, Alabama

Urolithiasis is a chronic disease. Of patients who have a urinary stone, 50% have a recurrent stone within 10 years. Long-term follow-up of urinary stone formers is necessary to assess both the effectiveness of treatment and a patient's compliance with treatment. Proper management of a recurrent stone former involves a long-term commitment by both patient and physician.

New surgical therapies for urolithiasis include extracorporeal shock wave lithotripsy (ESWL), percutaneous nephrolithotomy, and ureteroscopy. Although these therapies are widely available and cause minimal morbidity, they are useful only for removing existing stones and have no effect on the rate of recurrence. In the rush to employ new technologies, many physicians have forgotten the benefits of medical therapy in treating urolithiasis. Because the cost of a single ESWL treatment may be $10,000, the surgical management of the disease is extremely expensive. In contrast, the cost of medical therapy, including office visits, is usually less than $1,000 per year.

In the United States, sterile calcium (calcium oxalate

TABLE 1. **Indications for Open Urethroplasty**

Nonsurgical therapy required >2×/year
Recurrent strictures in children
Local adverse factors (fistuli, etc.)
Dense spongiofibrosis
Prior sepsis with nonsurgical therapy
Obliterative strictures

and calcium phosphate) calculi account for approximately 80% of urinary calculi. Other commonly encountered calculi are struvite (magnesium ammonium phosphate, infected phosphate), uric acid, and cystine. Although the management of the different calculi varies in many respects, the need for adequate hydration and for modification of dietary habits is common to patients with stones of all types.

DIAGNOSTIC CONSIDERATIONS

All patients with recurrent urolithiasis should undergo full investigation. What constitutes full evaluation is controversial, and the author's approach is included in the discussion of each stone type. Patients with cystine, uric acid, and infected phosphate calculi should be evaluated completely. The extent of evaluation of a patient with an initial episode of sterile calcium lithiasis depends on age, sex, and race. Children require complete investigation. Because "idiopathic" stone disease is uncommon in blacks, the etiology should be determined. For a white adult with a first sterile calcium stone, laboratory evaluation consisting of stone analysis, measurement of SMA 18, and determination of urinary acidification is adequate.

In the initial visit to the author's stone clinic, a patient is instructed to bring a 24-hour urine collection (without preservative) and a diet record. The diet record includes the amounts of all foods, liquids, and medications consumed each day over a 1-week period. If the patient's urine in clinic has a pH higher than 5.5., the patient is instructed to record the pH, measured with nitrazine paper, of the first two specimens of voided urine each day for 1 week. The ability to acidify urine to a pH of 5.5 or below effectively eliminates the possibility of renal tubular acidosis. Any stone previously passed is sent to a specialized laboratory for analysis.

TREATMENT

General Therapy

Regardless of stone type, increasing the fluid intake is the most effective method of preventing stone recurrence. Rather than prescribing consumption of a fixed amount of fluid (such as 1 gallon per day), it is more effective to focus on urine output. Although a daily urine output of 3 to 4 liters is ideal, most patients cannot achieve this output. The average person has a daily urine output of approximately 1 liter. If a patient can maintain a daily output of 2 liters, the chance of stone recurrence decreases by 66%; a daily output of 3 liters diminishes the chance of recurrence by 90%. Patients are instructed to distribute their fluid intake throughout the day. Risk is maximal in the 2 to 3 hours after a meal and during sleep, so it is necessary to stay well hydrated during these periods. Fluid intake during the evening is sufficient if a patient is required to awaken once to urinate during sleeping hours.

Most large studies dealing with treatment for urolithiasis have demonstrated a placebo effect of 50% or greater. The placebo effect probably occurs as a result of changes in diet and hydration. Patients are instructed as to proper diet on the basis of stone analysis, and the beneficial effects of hydration are stressed.

Cystine Calculi. Patients should submit a 24-hour urine collection for quantitative cystine analysis. Urine of all consanguineous relatives should be screened for cystine with a sodium nitroprusside test.

The mainstay of therapy in these patients is hydration. The solubility of urinary cystine is 300 mg in 1 liter of urine at a pH of 5.5. A patient who excretes 450 mg of cystine each day could therefore be managed by maintaining a daily urine output of 2 liters spaced evenly throughout the day. Solubility increases above a pH of 7.5; however, it is difficult for patients to maintain this degree of alkalinization.

In patients with markedly increased cystine excretion (>1 gram per day), D-penicillamine (Cuprimine), 250 to 500 mg four times daily, is often necessary. The usefulness of penicillamine is, however, often limited by its toxicity. Common adverse effects include rashes, arthralgia, fever, and proteinuria. An alternative therapy with fewer reported adverse effects is α-mercaptopropionylglycine (tiopronin [Thiola]).

Uric Acid Calculi. A 24-hour urine sample for uric acid excretion should be obtained. Serum calcium levels should be determined in order to rule out hyperparathyroidism, because uric acid urolithiasis and calcium urolithiasis may coexist. Initial therapy for uric acid stone formers includes limitation of protein to 56 grams per day and an increase in fluid intake.

Uric acid calculi form either from excessive excretion of uric acid or from a persistently acidic urine. In a patient with high uric acid excretion (>750 mg per day) that persists after protein intake is limited, allopurinol can be added in a single daily dose of 300 mg. In patients with normal uric acid excretion and persistently acidic urine, alkalinization therapy is effective. The vast majority of uric acid calculi can be dissolved with intensive alkali therapy. Surgical therapy for uric acid calculi should be considered only after alkalinization therapy fails. Sufficient alkali is administered to achieve a constant urinary pH of 6.7 to 7.0. Either sodium bicarbonate or potassium citrate is taken at 6-hour intervals. After stone dissolution is complete, recurrent calculi can often be prevented with a single daily dose of alkali.

Infected Phosphate Calculi. Infected phosphate calculi are composed of a mixture of struvite—$Mg(NH_4)(PO_4) \cdot 6H_2O$—and carbonate-apatite—$Ca_{10}(PO_4)_6(CO_3)(H_2O)$. These calculi form only after the introduction of a urease-positive bacterial urinary infection, most often with *Proteus* spp. Patients with neurogenic bladder or foreign bodies in contact with the urinary stream are at high risk for this type of calculi.

The initial management of infected phosphate calculi should be surgical, because infection cannot be adequately controlled until the kidney is free of stones. Surgery can consist of open lithotomy, percutaneous nephrolithotomy, or ESWL, depending on stone size and configuration. Oral antibiotics are given for 1 week before surgery and for at least 2 to 3 weeks after surgery.

Before surgery, serum calcium levels should be measured. In many menopausal women with infected phosphate calculi, hyperparathyroidism is an underlying disease, and infection is superimposed on metabolic calculi. If hyperparathyroidism is documented, it should be corrected before surgical treatment of the calculi.

The key to preventing recurrent infected phosphate calculi is to recognize and promptly treat any new infection. Long-term low-dose antibiotic therapy (penicillin or ampicillin, 250 mg once a day) is often effective in preventing recurrent infection. Patients should avoid magnesium-containing medications such as milk of magnesia, Maalox, and Mylanta.

If these measures are unsuccessful, administration of acetohydroxamic acid (Lithostat) can be considered. Acetohydroxamic acid inhibits the action of bacterial urease. Unfortunately, it can be associated with a number of serious adverse effects, which limits its usefulness.

Sterile Calcium Calculi. Possible metabolic causes of calcium urolithiasis should first be eliminated. Primary hyperparathyroidism, renal tubular acidosis, and medullary sponge kidney disease account for over 90% of metabolic sterile calcium calculi. Primary hyperparathyroidism can usually be ruled out with a determination of fasting serum calcium levels. If the calcium concentration is greater than 10.2 mg per dL, a parathyroid hormone level should be checked.

Renal tubular acidosis accounts for fewer than 1% of stone formers in most series. The diagnosis is suspected if a patient cannot acidify a morning urine to a pH of 5.5 or less. Treatment consists of administration of absorbable alkali, with 100 to 150 mEq per day of cation taken in four equally divided doses. Alkali is usually given as potassium citrate tablets with the dose titrated until the systemic acidosis is corrected and until urinary citrate excretion has been maximized.

Patients with medullary sponge kidney disease are managed with hydration, dietary modification, and control of infection. Hydrochlorothiazide (25 mg every 12 hours) can be added if these measures fail.

After metabolic causes of calcium urolithiasis are ruled out, what is left is a large group of "idiopathic stone formers." With the use of an extensive outpatient evaluation, this group of patients can be subdivided into various categories, including those with absorptive hypercalciuria, renal leak hypercalciuria, hyperuricosuric calcium oxalate urolithiasis, hypocitraturia, and enteric hyperoxaluria. Although some authorities still recommend this type of evaluation, most experts believe that such a detailed classification is not useful. The author's current evaluation for recurrent stone formers consists of a measurement of fasting SMA 18 and a 24-hour urine sample for volume and levels of creatinine, calcium, oxalate, uric acid, citrate, and magnesium. The urine is collected while the patient is on an unrestricted diet.

For a recurrent sterile calcium stone former with low urinary output and a highly lithogenic diet, medication is initially withheld. The patient is given a several-month trial period in which to adhere to a low-calcium, low-oxalate diet and to increase fluid intake. A 24-hour urine collection is obtained after 2 to 3 months. Urine volume and the concentrations of the offending stone salts (calcium, oxalate, and uric acid) are measured. If these characteristics do not show improvement or if the patient forms a recurrent calculus during this time period, medical therapy is started.

Medical Therapy

Thiazides. Hydrochlorothiazide is effective in treatment for sterile calcium stones. It is most effective in patients with hypercalciuria (>250 mg per 24 hours). It is, however, also effective in patients with normal urinary calcium levels and should be considered in any patient with sterile calcium stones who does not respond to diet modification and increased hydration. Hydrochlorothiazide acts primarily by decreasing urinary calcium. The mean reduction is 150 mg per day. The decrease in urinary calcium is maximal within 1 to 2 weeks.

The major adverse effects of thiazides are hypokalemia, hyperglycemia, and hyperuricemia. Potassium supplements are required in approximately 50% of patients and are usually administered as potassium citrate tablets. Administration of potassium prevents the common adverse effects of lassitude, dizziness, and muscle weakness. Side effects of thiazide therapy occur in 30 to 35% of patients, usually early in the course of treatment. To reduce the incidence of side effects, patients should start with 25 mg per day for several weeks until the maintenance dosage of 25 mg twice a day is reached.

Phosphates. Treatment with orthophosphates increases the urinary excretion of pyrophosphate, a known inhibitor of calcium phosphate and calcium oxalate crystallization. The urinary calcium level also decreases; the effect is most pronounced in patients with hypercalciuria.

Orthophosphates are available as acidic, neutral, or alkaline preparations; most patients are treated with a neutral preparation. The minimal effective dose for men is 1500 mg or more of phosphorus given in divided doses at 8-hour intervals. A slightly smaller dose, 1250 mg, may be effective in women.

The major side effect of orthophosphate therapy is diarrhea and occurs to some extent in all patients. Orthophosphate therapy is currently used in a very small percentage of patients with calcium urolithiasis.

Potassium Citrate. Hypocitraturia is commonly encountered in patients with renal tubular acidosis and in those with chronic diarrhea. Hypocitraturia can also occur in conjunction with other abnormalities such as hypercalciuria and hyperuricosuria. Potassium citrate tablets are commonly administered to patients with hypocitraturia. By providing an alkali load, potassium citrate raises urinary pH, thereby increasing the excretion of urinary citrate, a known inhibitor of calcium oxalate and calcium phosphate crystallization. In patients with hypocitraturia (<320 mg per day), potassium citrate is given at a starting dose of 20 mEq orally three times daily. The dose is titrated until normal urinary citrate excretion is restored. A combination of hydrochlorothiazide and potassium citrate is effective in the vast majority of patients with sterile calcium stones.

Allopurinol. The use of allopurinol (300 mg once daily) in the treatment of sterile calcium calculi is controversial. Some series show that in calcium oxalate stone formers with hyperuricosuria, allopurinol markedly reduces the incidence of stone recurrence. The rationale for this beneficial effect is unclear.

In most calcium oxalate stone formers, hyperuricosuria is caused by excessive purine ingestion. A reduction in animal meat protein to 6 to 8 ounces per day usually reduces uric acid excretion to an acceptable level. Because of the potential adverse effects of allopurinol, it is reserved for patients who form mixed calcium oxalate-uric acid calculi that cannot be controlled by dietary or other conservative measures.

Surgical Therapy

The surgical treatment of urinary calculi has changed dramatically over the past 10 years. Whereas open surgical lithotomy was previously the only available treatment, only a very small percentage of calculi are currently treated with open surgery. With the wide assortment of treatment modalities currently available, the clinician is now faced with the decision of which noninvasive therapy to choose.

More than 90% of renal calculi are best managed with ESWL. Lithotripsy can be used for calculi in the renal pelvis, calyces, and ureter. ESWL is the preferred treatment for renal calculi less than 2 cm in diameter, assuming normal renal anatomy. Although calculi more than 2 cm in diameter can be fragmented with ESWL, fragmentation is often incomplete, resulting in excessive complications and the need for repeated ESWL. The decision to treat large renal calculi (>2 cm in diameter) with ESWL is often based on the density of the calculus on a plain radiograph because calculi of low density are easily fragmented with ESWL.

Infection-induced calculi are often branched in configuration. Branched calculi form a cast of the collecting system, filling the renal pelvis and one or all of the calyces. Before the development of minimally invasive surgical therapies, branched calculi were treated with open surgical lithotomy. The current treatment of these calculi is controversial. Large branched calculi are usually treated with a combination of techniques. The calculus is first debulked with a percutaneous nephrolithotomy; a portion of the calculus is left untreated. The residual calculus is then treated with ESWL. After 1 to 2 weeks for fragments to pass, the collecting system is visualized through the original nephrostomy tract, and any remaining fragments are removed. An alternative to repeated nephroscopy is irrigation of the collecting system with hemiacidrin (Renacidin), an acidic irrigating solution. Hemiacidrin solution acts by markedly increasing the solubility of struvite and carbonate-apatite, promoting dissolution of stones.

When a branched calculus fills the entire collecting system, an open surgical approach is nonetheless justified. The surgical procedure, termed an "anatrophic nephrolithotomy," involves instituting renal hypothermia, clamping the renal artery, and then splitting the kidney along an avascular plane. The calculus is removed, and intraoperative radiographs are obtained to ensure a stone-free result. Although this procedure is extremely effective, most patients are reluctant to have open surgery and instead opt for a less invasive, albeit less effective, procedure.

Ureteral calculi can also be treated in a variety of ways. Before ESWL and ureteroscopy, most ureteral calculi were managed with watchful waiting. Surgery was indicated for patients with severe, unremitting pain, superimposed infection, or a failure of the stone to progress down the ureter. Patients were often treated conservatively for several months before surgery was indicated.

A patient with a symptomatic ureteral calculus is now often treated soon after the diagnosis is established. ESWL is the preferred treatment for calculi in the proximal two-thirds of the ureter. For calculi in the distal third of the ureter, either ureteroscopy or ESWL is used. Although ureteroscopy is more effective than ESWL for distal calculi, ureteroscopy has a higher complication rate, especially when performed only occasionally by a practitioner. The role of watchful waiting, however, should not be forgotten, because more than 90% of calculi less than 4 mm in diameter pass spontaneously if sufficient time is allowed.

SUMMARY

It is estimated that urinary calculi eventually form in as many as 12% of the population of the United States. A stone former has a 50% chance of stone recurrence within 10 years. Sterile calcium calculi account for 80% of urinary calculi. A patient with a urinary calculus should be evaluated in order to discover any correctable metabolic abnormality.

The mainstay of therapy for patients with sterile calcium stones is diet and adequate hydration. Approximately 70% of stone formers can be effectively managed in this manner. If calculi continue to recur despite these measures, patients should be offered medical therapy.

New treatment modalities have markedly decreased the morbidity of urinary stone disease. Open surgical lithotomy is now seldom necessary. Despite the ease of treating patients with "surgical" stone disease, clinicians and patients should be reminded that the optimal treatment is still the prevention of recurrent urinary calculi.

The Sexually Transmitted Diseases

CHANCROID

method of
DAVID H. MARTIN, M.D.
Louisiana State University Medical Center
New Orleans, Louisiana

Chancroid, caused by the gram negative bacillus *Haemophilus ducreyi*, may be the most prevalent cause of genital ulcer disease worldwide. In the United States, the disease had nearly disappeared by the 1970s. However, beginning in the early 1980s, isolated outbreaks began to appear once again. Initially the disease occurred primarily among migrant workers and was associated with door-to-door prostitution, but by the mid-1980s the disease established itself endemically in a number of urban centers such as Dallas, the New York–Philadelphia metroplex, and Miami. In 1987, 5,047 cases were reported to the Centers for Disease Control in Atlanta, Georgia. Although the number of reported cases has gradually declined since then, chancroid has established itself in even more locations, primarily in the southeastern United States.

The major public health problem associated with chancroid is that African studies have shown it to be an important cofactor for the heterosexual transmission of the human immunodeficiency virus (HIV). In the United States, chancroid is linked to the sexual behavior associated with crack cocaine abuse. The combination of high risk for both chancroid and HIV infection among cocaine abusers creates the potential for a disastrous rise in the incidence of acquired immune deficiency syndrome (AIDS) in this population.

Chancroid classically manifests as multiple, painful ulcers that have purulent bases and ragged, undermined borders. Because lesions are usually not indurated, they are often referred to in the older literature as "soft chancres." In 50 to 60% of men with chancroid, inguinal lymphadenopathy, which is usually unilateral, develops. In a small proportion of cases, the inguinal node masses, or buboes, become fluctuant and may rupture, resulting in a draining abscess. Despite the distinctive features of classical chancroid, it is clear that there is considerable overlap between this disease, syphilis, and genital herpes, making accurate clinical diagnosis very difficult.

For reasons that are not clear, the ratio of male to female chancroid cases ranges from 3:1 to 25:1. In part, this may be because internal lesions in women often go unnoticed, as is the case in primary syphilis. However, the male-to-female ratio for chancroid cases is higher than that for primary syphilis, which suggests that there are other reasons for this phenomenon.

Laboratory confirmation of the diagnosis of chancroid is difficult because *H. ducreyi* has special in vitro growth requirements. Most clinical laboratories cannot successfully cultivate this slow-growing organism, especially from ulcers in which overgrowth of contaminating skin flora is a major problem. In most practice settings, the diagnosis is usually made by ruling out syphilis and herpes simplex virus infection. Unfortunately, this approach is often not helpful in guiding therapy, especially when dark-field microscopy is not available. Therefore, by necessity, treatment is empirical and should be guided by knowledge of the incidence of chancroid in a given geographic area. A useful clue to the presence of the disease is the observation of "treatment failures" among patients with primary syphilis caused by *Treponema pallidum* and *H. ducreyi* co-infection, as well as among patients with chancroid misdiagnosed as syphilis. Another clue is an increased incidence of patients presenting to local acute care facilities for the treatment of painful inguinal buboes.

TREATMENT

Although increasing resistance to some of the older drugs used to treat this disease has been observed over the past 10 years, there remain a number of drugs, both old and new, that have good activity against *H. ducreyi*. Ceftriaxone (Rocephin), in a single 250-mg intramuscular dose, is effective for both ulcers and buboes. The only drawbacks to this approach are the inconvenience of intramuscular administration and the relatively high cost of the drug.

As with ceftriaxone, there has been no evidence of development of erythromycin resistance among *H. ducreyi* strains worldwide. Erythromycin, 500 mg orally four times daily for 7 days, is the standard therapy. Results of one recent study suggest that as little as 500 mg three times a day for 5 days also may be effective.

Sulfonamide resistance among *H. ducreyi* strains has steadily increased worldwide; more recently, trimethoprim resistance has become a problem in both Thailand and Africa. At one time, a single high dose of trimethoprim-sulfamethoxazole was widely used for chancroid. Although increased failure rates were first reported with single-dose therapy, failures have been noted recently in the Far East and Africa with the multiple-dose regimens as well. Recent in vivo and in vitro experience with trimethoprim-sulfamethoxazole in the United States is limited; therefore, this drug probably should not be used any longer, in view of the availability of effective alternatives.

A number of the newly developed broad-spectrum oral antibiotics have promise for the therapy of chancroid. Among the quinolones available in the United States, ciprofloxacin (Cipro) has been studied most extensively; it appears to be effective in a single 500-mg dose, although 500 mg twice daily for 3 days is the currently recommended dose. Fleroxacin, a new quinolone not currently available in the United States, also has been found to cure most cases when given as a single dose. Almost all *H. ducreyi* strains produce beta-lactamase and therefore are resistant to ampicillin alone, but ampicillin–clavulanate potassium (Augmentin), 500/125 mg three times daily by mouth for 7 days, is effective. Finally, recent studies have shown that cure rates for the new macrolide azithromycin (Zithromax), given as a single 1-gram oral dose, are equal to those for intramuscular ceftriaxone.

Studies from Africa suggest that HIV-infected persons with chancroid are more difficult to treat. Failure rates of 20 to 50% have been reported among these patients after treatment with single doses of a number of the drugs discussed earlier. Thus patients with chancroid who are known to be HIV-infected should be treated with one of the multiple-dose regimens and should be monitored closely for evidence of an appropriate therapeutic response.

In view of the difficulty in clinically distinguishing syphilis and chancroid and the fact that the two diseases may coexist in 10 to 20% of cases, patients suspected of having chancroid who have not had a negative dark-field examination result should also be treated for primary syphilis unless adequate follow-up can be ensured. It is important that all recent sexual contacts of patients suspected of having chancroid be treated as well.

Fluctuant buboes should be drained in order to prevent rupture. Insertion of an 18-gauge needle into the center of the lesion through normal skin at the margin of inflammation is the simplest approach. Some of these patients may require one or more reaspirations. Large-node masses may become fluctuant after treatment with effective antibiotics. This development should not be taken as evidence of treatment failure, because the pus aspirated from these lesions is usually sterile.

GONORRHEA

method of
RODNEY A. MICHAEL, M.D.
Uniformed Services University of the Health Sciences
Bethesda, Maryland

and

RONALD H. COOPER, M.D.*
Madigan Army Medical Center
Tacoma, Washington

The 1970s and 1980s saw the emergence and spread of penicillin- and tetracycline-resistant *Neisseria gonorrhoeae*. Coincidentally, the 1980s also witnessed the development of antimicrobial agents with markedly improved activity, including reliable activity against multiresistant strains. The current mainstay of therapy for uncomplicated gonococcal infection is single-dose, intramuscular ceftriaxone (Rocephin). However, the development of potent new oral agents, including the oral third-generation cephalosporin cefixime (Suprax) and the fluoroquinolones ciprofloxacin (Cipro) and ofloxacin (Floxin), promises highly effective, single-dose therapy of uncomplicated gonococcal infections. The new macrolide antibiotics, azithromycin (Zithromax) and clarithromycin (Biaxin), offer additional alternatives.

The spectrum of illness caused by *N. gonorrhoeae* ranges from uncomplicated urethritis to deep tissue infection complicated by multiple other pathogens. With the possible exception of male urethritis, the clinical diagnosis of gonococcal infection (including positive Gram's stains) should be confirmed with cultures. However, treatment should be initiated empirically while the results of cultures or other diagnostic tests are pending.

After a course of therapy, cultures should be performed if feasible, especially if symptoms persist, if a complicated infection is being treated, or if alternative therapeutic regimens are used. All patients presenting with gonococcal infection or other sexually transmitted diseases (STD) should be routinely tested for syphilis and routinely offered testing for human immunodeficiency virus (HIV) infection. A patient receiving treatment with antibiotics other than a penicillin or cephalosporin should be retested for syphilis 6 to 12 weeks after the initial evaluation.

As many as 45% of patients presenting with gonococcal genital infection have concomitant infection with *Chlamydia trachomatis*. Because current diagnostic tests for chlamydial infections do not permit a timely or reliable diagnosis, patients should be treated presumptively for that organism. Sexual partners of infected patients should be evaluated, undergo culture,

---

*The views of the authors do not necessarily reflect the position of the Department of the Army or the Department of Defense.

and be treated presumptively for gonococcal and chlamydial infection, regardless of their symptom status.

TREATMENT OF ADULTS

Uncomplicated Genital, Rectal, or Pharyngeal Infection

The current recommendation of the United States Public Health Service (USPHS) for uncomplicated genital, rectal, or pharyngeal gonococcal infection is 250 mg of intramuscular ceftriaxone in a single dose, followed by 100 mg of doxycycline (Vibramycin) taken orally two times daily for 7 days. Clinical trials have demonstrated equivalent efficacy with oral cefixime, administered as single doses of 400 or 800 mg. The cost of a 400-mg dose of cefixime is somewhat less than that of a 250-mg dose of ceftriaxone given intramuscularly. The 400-mg dose of cefixime has fewer gastrointestinal effects than the 800-mg dose, with essentially equivalent efficacy. The authors have used a single-dose regimen of 400 mg of cefixime in their STD clinic since 1991 with excellent results.

Patients with immediate hypersensitivity reactions to penicillin and cephalosporin antibiotics can be treated with several other regimens, but there are some caveats. Spectinomycin (Trobicin) is highly effective for gonococcal urethritis and proctitis but not for pharyngeal infection. It does not eradicate incubating syphilis. Ciprofloxacin or ofloxacin may be considered for infection at all sites, but there is less experience with these agents, and they are not effective against incubating syphilis. Quinolones are contraindicated in adolescents younger than 16 years of age and in pregnant or nursing women.

Ampicillin (Amcill), 3.5 grams, or amoxicillin (Amoxil), 3.0 grams, combined with 1 gram of probenecid (Benemid) should be considered as therapy only if a patient is known to be infected with a strain of *N. gonorrhoeae* susceptible to penicillin.

Pelvic Inflammatory Disease

Pelvic inflammatory disease (PID) may involve any part of the upper genital tract in women. The microbiology of PID is complex and should be presumed to include *N. gonorrhoeae*, *C. trachomatis*, enteric gram-negative bacilli, streptococci, and anaerobes, including *Bacteroides fragilis*. Patients with first-time episodes of PID are more frequently infected with *N. gonorrhoeae* and *C. trachomatis*. Patients with prior episodes of PID present more frequently with mixed infections. The diagnosis of PID may be difficult, and its manifestation may be indistinguishable from those of other serious intra-abdominal conditions, such as appendicitis, ectopic pregnancy, and abscess. In some cases, laparoscopy or culdocentesis may be necessary for diagnosis.

Hospitalization and intravenous therapy offer optimal treatment for most patients presumed to have PID. This treatment facilitates evaluation and helps ensure the clinical stability of patients. If appendicitis, ectopic pregnancy, or pelvic abscess cannot be ruled out, hospitalization is mandatory. Other strong indications for inpatient management include significant systemic toxicity, nausea and vomiting, failure of outpatient therapy, pregnancy, or inability to comply with outpatient management.

Precise bacteriologic diagnosis is usually not available without invasive sampling. Empirical treatment of PID should include coverage for the general classes of organisms mentioned earlier. Current USPHS recommendations for treatment are shown in Table 1, regimens 9 and 10. If infection with *N. gonorrhoeae* or *C. trachomatis* is more likely, regimen 9, which includes cefotetan (Cefotan), is preferred. According to documented antimicrobial susceptibility data, a regimen consisting of parenteral ceftriaxone, oral or parenteral metronidazole (Flagyl), and oral or parenteral doxycycline (Table 1, regimen 11) should have equivalent efficacy and the advantage of greater convenience of administration. The authors have used this regimen with clinical success. Regardless of the chosen regimen, intrauterine devices must be removed. The outpatient management of PID requires close follow-up care and early admission in the event of treatment failure.

Disseminated Gonococcal Infection

Gonococcal arthritis-dermatitis syndrome is the most common clinical manifestation of disseminated gonococcal infection (DGI) and consists of tenosynovitis, arthritis, and a pustular or papular rash in a young, sexually active patient. Cultures of all involved sites are frequently negative, and therapy often must be administered presumptively, on the basis of clinical presentation alone. Patients should be treated with parenteral ceftriaxone for at least 3 days, followed by oral cefixime to complete 7 days of therapy. Patients allergic to the cephalosporin antibiotics may be treated alternatively with intramuscular spectinomycin for 72 hours, followed by an oral quinolone to complete 7 days of therapy.

Meningitis and endocarditis may complicate bacteremic gonococcal infection. Although treatment regimens have not been well established, 2 grams of parenteral ceftriaxone twice daily for 10 to 14 days for meningitis, and 1 to 2 grams twice daily for 4 weeks for endocarditis, should result in a high degree of success.

TABLE 1. **Treatment of Adult Gonococcal Infections**

Syndrome or Site of Infection	First Choice	Alternate
Uncomplicated	1 or 2	5 or 6
Urethritis	plus 12	plus 12
Cervicitis		
Proctitis		
Pharyngitis	1 or 2	6
Epididymitis	1 or 2	5 or 6
	plus 13	plus 13
Conjunctivitis (not septic)	3	7
Disseminated gonococcal infection (no meningitis or endocarditis)	4 plus 12	8 plus 12
Pelvic inflammatory disease		
Hospitalized	9, 10, or 11	
Outpatient	1 plus 13	5, 6, or 14 plus 13

Regimens
1. Ceftriaxone, 250 mg IM, one time.
2. Cefixime, 400 mg PO, one time.
3. Ceftriaxone, 1 gm IM, one time.
4. Ceftriaxone, 1 gm IV daily for at least 72 hours, then cefixime, 400 mg PO, once daily to complete 7 days of therapy.
5. Spectinomycin, 2 gm IM, one time.
6. Ciprofloxacin, 500 mg PO, one time or ofloxacin, 400 mg PO, one time.
7. Ciprofloxacin, 750 mg PO, one time.
8. Spectinomycin, 2 gm IM every 12 hours for at least 72 hours, then ciprofloxacin, 500 mg PO, daily or ofloxacin, 400 mg PO, daily to complete 10 days of therapy.
9. Cefotetan, 2 gm IV every 12 hours, plus doxycycline, 100 mg PO bid or IV for at least 4 days and until the patient is clinically improved for at least 48 hours; then continue doxycycline, 100 mg PO bid to complete 14 days of therapy.
10. Clindamycin, 900 mg IV every 8 hours and gentamicin, 2 mg per kg IV once followed by 1.5 mg per kg every 8 hours for at least 4 days and until the patient is clinically improved for at least 48 hours; then continue doxycycline, 100 mg PO bid to complete 14 days of therapy.
11. Ceftriaxone, 1 gm IV daily plus metronidazole, 500 mg PO or IV every 12 hours plus doxycycline, 100 mg PO bid or IV every 12 hours for at least 4 days and until the patient is clinically improved for at least 48 hours; then continue doxycycline, 100 mg PO bid to complete 14 days of therapy.
12. Doxycycline, 100 mg PO, twice daily for 7 days.
13. Doxycycline, 100 mg PO, twice daily for 14 days.
14. Cefixime, 800 mg PO, one time.
Abbreviations: IM = intramuscularly; PO = per os (orally); IV = intravenously.

Infections at Other Sites

Epididymitis is most frequently caused by *C. trachomatis* but may also be caused by *N. gonorrhoeae*. Most patients can be treated successfully with antibiotics as outlined for uncomplicated gonococcal infection, except that doxycycline therapy for *C. trachomatis* should be extended to 14 days. Nonsteroidal anti-inflammatory drugs (e.g., ibuprofen [Motrin]) and scrotal support are adjuncts to successful management of acute epididymitis.

Conjunctivitis is an unusual infection in adults. Rapid initiation of parenteral antibiotic therapy (not topical) is necessary for successful management. In the absence of septicemia, treat-

ment with a single dose of ceftriaxone is sufficient. Patients with septicemia and ophthalmic infection should be hospitalized and treated for 5 to 7 days with 1 gram of ceftriaxone given intravenously daily. All patients with gonococcal eye infections should undergo ophthalmologic evaluation and careful slit-lamp examinations to detect possible complications.

Gonorrhea in Pregnancy

The clinical manifestations of gonorrhea are not significantly different during pregnancy. However, the presence of active gonococcal infection during pregnancy may result in obstetric complications, underscoring the importance of prompt recognition and treatment. Treatment for gonorrhea during pregnancy is identical to that used for nonpregnant adults, except that ciprofloxacin should be avoided and chlamydial infection should be treated with erythromycin (base or stearate, 500 mg orally four times daily, or ethylsuccinate, 800 mg orally four times daily for 7 days) instead of doxycycline. One gram of azithromycin (Zithromax) orally as a single dose is safe and effective therapy for chlamydial infection during pregnancy and can be used in patients intolerant of erythromycin.

TREATMENT OF CHILDREN AND INFANTS

Gonococcal infection of children is relatively rare, and treatment regimens have not been as well studied or established as for adults. Consultation with a pediatric infectious disease specialist is recommended when questions arise. These treatment regimens represent current USPHS guidelines.

Children who weigh 45 kg or more should be treated with adult regimens, as previously outlined. Children who weigh less than 45 kg with uncomplicated genital, rectal, or pharyngeal infection should receive 125 mg of ceftriaxone intramuscularly one time. Although not studied in children, oral cefixime (400 mg one time) should provide equal efficacy. Children 8 years of age or older should receive 100 mg of doxycycline orally two times daily for 7 days. All children with gonococcal infection should be considered victims of child abuse and evaluated for that possibility. Concomitant infection with syphilis, HIV, and *C. trachomatis* should be considered and ruled out during the initial evaluation.

Neonates born to mothers with gonococcal infection are at risk for ophthalmic and disseminated infection. In the absence of clinically obvious neonatal infection, presumptive treatment should be given. The USPHS currently recommends 125 mg of ceftriaxone given intramuscularly in a single dose. However, there is a theoretical risk associated with the use of ceftriaxone in neonates, especially if they also have hyperbilirubinemia, and its use is relatively contraindicated in this setting. Many experts instead choose to treat with 50 to 100 mg of cefotaxime (Claforan) per kg of body weight, given intramuscularly in a single dose.

Neonates clinically infected with *N. gonorrhoeae* (e.g., DGI, ophthalmic infection) should be hospitalized and receive treatment with 25 mg of cefotaxime per kg of body weight, given parenterally every 12 hours for 7 days.

Infants older than 2 weeks of age with clinical gonococcal infection should be hospitalized and may be treated with 25 mg of cefotaxime per kg two times daily or 50 mg of ceftriaxone per kg once daily; both drugs are given parenterally. Treatment should be prolonged if meningitis or endocarditis complicates the infectious process.

NONGONOCOCCAL URETHRITIS IN MEN

method of
JOHN A. MATA, M.D.
Louisiana State University Medical Center
Shreveport, Louisiana

Nongonococcal urethritis (NGU), formerly called "nonspecific urethritis," is the most common sexually transmitted disease (STD) in men in North America. NGU is a syndrome with several causes (Table 1). *Chlamydia trachomatis* is the most common sexually transmitted pathogen and causes 30 to 50% of the cases of NGU in heterosexual men. Homosexual men are more likely to have gonococcal urethritis. *Ureaplasma urealyticum* is the cause of NGU in 20 to 40% of males. Other etiologic agents are possible, but in 20 to 30%, the precise cause of NGU is unknown. NGU is diagnosed only after gonococcal urethritis has been

TABLE 1. **Etiology of Nongonococcal Urethritis in Men**

Chlamydia trachomatis	30–50%
Ureaplasma urealyticum	30–40%
Unknown	20–30%
Trichomonas vaginalis	1–3%
Herpes simplex	1–2%
Cytomegalovirus	<1%
Adenovirus	<1%
Yeast	<1%
Gardnerella vaginalis	Rare
Staphylococcus saprophyticus	Rare
Others	Rare

ruled out, and it classically responds promptly to antibiotic therapy. Also, as in most STDs, concurrent treatment of the patient's sexual partner is mandatory.

DIAGNOSIS

The incubation period of NGU (1 to 2 weeks) is longer than that of gonococcal urethritis. Signs and symptoms include urethral discharge, urethral itching, and dysuria. The urethral discharge is mild to moderate in quantity and whitish or clear, but occasionally it is thick and purulent. Urethral inflammation is confirmed by the presence of four or more white blood cells per field on oil-immersion magnification on Gram's stain smear of an endourethral swab. This should confirm urethritis and rule out *Neisseria gonorrhoeae*.

Chlamydia trachomatis is an obligate intracellular parasitic bacterium and is best cultured with an endourethral swab from an area 2 to 3 cm inside the urethral meatus. Chlamydia-positive and chlamydia-negative NGU cannot be differentiated clinically. Because cultures require 2 to 3 days for initial results and are not widely available, other, more rapid (although less sensitive) techniques exist to document chlamydial infections. Solid-phase enzyme immunoassay (Chlamydiazyne) and monoclonal antibodies with fluorescent labels (Microtrak Assay) can be used to identify chlamydial antigens in exudates. Polymerase chain reaction technology is also being applied for *C. trachomatis* detection. It is important to know what tests are available locally in order to detect this common and potentially dangerous pathogen. For practical purposes, the history and clinical findings of urethritis, without intracellular gram-negative diplococci on Gram's stain, is evidence enough to warrant initiation of treatment.

TREATMENT

The recommended regimen for uncomplicated urethral *C. trachomatis* infections is doxycycline, 100 mg orally two times a day for 7 days, or tetracycline, 500 mg orally four times a day for 7 days. It is essential to treat persons in sexual contact with known patients. Alternative regimens include erythromycin base, 250 mg orally four times a day for 7 days, or erythromycin ethylsuccinate, 400 mg orally four times a day for 7 days. If erythromycin is not tolerated, sulfisoxazole, 500 mg orally four times a day for 10 days, may be effective. Follow-up test for cure evaluation is unnecessary in routine cases when treatment has been completed.

A recent controlled trial of a single dose of azithromycin (Zithromax) for the treatment of chlamydial urethritis has been shown to be as effective as a 7-day course of doxycycline. This may have important implications in the treatment of groups at risk for noncompliance with the medication regimen.

Management of recurrent or persistent NGU symptoms requires a focused approach to detecting a specific cause. For example, if *Trichomonas vaginalis* is the etiologic agent, metronidazole (Flagyl), 250 mg orally three times a day for 7 days is effective. Potassium hydroxide smears for possible fungi are important in the etiologic search. Herpes simplex infection should also be considered. Tetracycline-resistant *Ureaplasma urealyticum* is also a cause of persistent NGU. These resistant strains are responsive to erythromycin. Recurrence caused by reinfection can be prevented if the patient's sexual partner is also treated.

NGU symptoms sometimes persist after multiple courses of antibiotics. These difficult cases should be referred to a STD specialist or urologist. Uroflowmetry and cystoscopy are sometimes necessary to rule out urethral stricture disease, foreign bodies, or intra-urethral condyloma. Concurrent examination of the sexual partner is helpful in recurrent reinfection. In summary, *C. trachomatis* is a potentially serious pathogen and is considered the causative agent in NGU until proved otherwise. The patient and all sexual partners should be treated promptly and effectively.

GRANULOMA INGUINALE
(Donovanosis)

method of
J. ERIC BAUWENS, M.D.
Harborview Medical Center
Seattle, Washington

Granuloma inguinale is a chronic, progressive, ulcerative disease that is probably transmitted sexually. The causative agent, *Calymmatobacterium granulomatis,* is a gram-negative, obligate intracellular organism. The disease is a common cause of genital ulcers in South Africa and southeast India, but it is rare in the United States and Europe. It also occurs in small endemic regions of Asia, Australia, New Guinea, South America, and the Caribbean.

After an incubation period of 3 to 40 days, the infection first manifests as a pruritic papule, located most commonly on the labia or distal penis. Lesions characteristically evolve into beefy-red, heaped-up, painless ulcers that bleed easily. Multiple ulcers may coalesce as they spread to surrounding tissue. Lymphadenopathy or systemic symptoms are uncommon.

The differential diagnosis includes syphilis, ulcerated genital warts, squamous cell carcinoma, chancroid, lymphogranuloma venereum, and cutaneous amebiasis. Verrucous forms, particularly in the perianal area, can be confused with condyloma latum of secondary syphilis. Wright's or Giemsa staining of direct smears or biopsies identifies Donovan bodies (i.e., multiple, bipolar-staining bacilli within histiocytes) in

60 to 80% of patients with granuloma inguinale and confirms the diagnosis. No culture or reliable serologic testing is available for routine diagnosis.

TREATMENT

Antibiotic therapy should be individualized. Tetracycline (Panmycin), in a dose of 500 mg taken orally four times daily, or double-strength co-trimoxazole (Bactrim), consisting of 160 mg of trimethoprim and 800 mg of sulfamethoxazole and taken as 1 tablet (or 2 single-strength tablets) twice daily, should be administered until the lesion is completely healed. Treatment alternatives include norfloxacin (Noroxin), chloramphenicol (Chloromycetin), and gentamicin (Garamycin). Pregnant women can be treated with 500 mg of erythromycin, taken orally four times daily.

Sequelae of granuloma inguinale include lymphedema, strictures, and fistulas, which may be ameliorated by reconstructive surgery. Antibiotic therapy should be administered before surgical treatment to prevent spread of active infection.

Patients with granuloma inguinale should be screened for other sexually transmitted diseases, and contacts should be traced. Treatment of lesion-free sexual contacts is not recommended.

LYMPHOGRANULOMA VENEREUM
(LGV)

method of
J. ERIC BAUWENS, M.D.
Harborview Medical Center
Seattle, Washington

Lymphogranuloma venereum (LGV) is a sexually transmitted disease caused by *Chlamydia trachomatis* serovars L1, L2, or L3. This chronic, invasive infection is endemic in parts of Asia, Africa, India, South America, and the Caribbean. The disease is uncommon in the United States and other developed countries in temperate climates.

The infection typically begins as an inconspicuous genital papule or ulcer. Regional lymphadenitis, fever, and constitutional symptoms occur 2 to 4 weeks later. Inguinal lymphadenopathy is the most common secondary manifestation of LGV. The "groove sign," prominent femoral and inguinal lymphadenopathy separated by Poupart's ligament, strongly suggests LGV. Progressive lymphadenitis with suppuration and lymphedema occur in some untreated patients. Depending on the location of progressive infection, fistulas, ulcers, strictures, and scarring can occur.

In the United States, the most frequent manifestation of LGV is acute proctocolitis in gay men, generally manifested by rectal pain, bleeding, mucopurulent discharge, and tenesmus. The clinical and histologic appearance of granulomatous inflammation may mimic inflammatory bowel disease. Inguinal lymphoadenopathy is usually absent in patients with proctocolitis.

The diagnosis of LGV is suggested by a compatible epidemiologic and clinical presentation and is confirmed by serologic testing or culture. A chlamydial complement fixation titer of 1:64 or greater or the isolation of *C. trachomatis* from a genital ulcer or lymph node aspirate confirms the diagnosis of LGV. Rectal cultures for *C. trachomatis* can also be performed, but because non-LGV serotypes of *C. trachomatis* can also cause proctocolitis, a positive rectal culture is not diagnostic of LGV.

TREATMENT

Tetracycline (Panmycin) in a dose of 500 mg taken orally four times daily or 100 mg of doxycycline (Vibramycin) taken orally twice daily is the primary treatment for LGV. Proctocolitis or lymphadenitis should be treated for a minimum of 14 days. An alternative is 500 mg of erythromycin taken orally four times daily.

Patients with extensive lymphadenitis may require aspiration of buboes to prevent rupture. Reconstructive surgical treatment may benefit patients with strictures and fistulas. A patient should receive antibiotic therapy for several weeks before surgery.

Patients with LGV should be screened for other sexually transmitted diseases. Sexual contacts should be examined and supply culture specimens and should receive tetracycline, doxycycline, or erythromycin for 7 days.

SYPHILIS

method of
JUSTIN D. RADOLF, M.D.
University of Texas Southwestern Medical Center
Dallas, Texas

After alarming increases throughout the latter part of the 1980s, incidence rates for new cases of syphilis have declined significantly in the 1990s. Despite this trend, the management of syphilis, particularly early infection, is for several reasons hotly debated. First, it has long been recognized that spirochetemia and central nervous system invasion by *Treponema pallidum* occur very early in acquired syphilis, usually long before the onset of neurologic symptoms. Second, a substantial proportion of patients with early syphilis have concomitant human immunodeficiency virus (HIV) infection. Third, numerous case reports have documented that such patients appear to be at increased risk for relapse with neurologic or ophthalmologic complications that follow the administration of treatment regimens employing intramuscular penicillin G benzathine. Although authorities generally agree about the management of syphilis in patients without HIV infection, no consensus exists with regard to patients with concomitant HIV disease. The treatment guidelines presented here are based largely on those endorsed by the Centers for Disease Control.

TREATMENT

Principles

For the treatment of all stages of syphilis (Table 1), penicillin is the drug of choice. This statement is based on the exquisite sensitivity of *T. pallidum* to this agent in both in vitro and animal studies and on the drug's outstanding clinical track record. Debates over the use of penicillin for the treatment of syphilis center on the appropriate dosages of the antibiotic and the duration of therapy, not on the drug's efficacy. There is no evidence that the sensitivity of *T. pallidum* to penicillin or similar agents, such as ampicillin and amoxicillin, has diminished since the introduction of penicillin.

Studies in the rabbit model, and subsequently in patients, confirmed that prolonged treponemicidal levels of penicillin (0.03 IU per mL or 0.018 µg/per mL) are needed in order to eradicate the syphilis spirochete. For this reason, all treatment schedules maintain therapeutic penicillin levels for extended periods. Invasion of the central nervous system by *T. pallidum* occurs frequently in early syphilis even in the absence of neurologic complications. Regimens employing penicillin G benzathine for early syphilis fail to achieve treponemicidal antimicrobial levels within the cerebrospinal fluid (CSF), and yet the vast majority of patients with early syphilis who receive such regimens do not experience neurologic relapse. It has been conjectured, therefore, that the host immune response acts in concert with the small amount of antibiotic that penetrates the blood-brain barrier to eradicate *T. pallidum* from the central nervous system of patients with early syphilis treated with intramuscular penicillin G benzathine.

Tetracycline, erythromycin, and chloramphenicol, agents long used in penicillin-allergic patients, appear to be less efficacious both in vitro and in vivo; there also is much less clinical experience with these agents. Several newer beta-lactam drugs, particularly ceftriaxone (Rocephin), have excellent in vitro activity against *T. pallidum,* and the limited clinical experience with these agents is promising. However, optimal treatment schedules for these agents have not been determined, and they should not be considered first-line drugs until they have been compared with penicillin in large prospective clinical trials. Quinolones and trimethoprim-sulfameth-

TABLE 1. **Therapeutic Guidelines for Syphilis**[1]

Stage of Infection	Regimens for Non–Penicillin-Allergic Patients	Alternative Regimens for Penicillin-Allergic Patients[2]
Early Syphilis HIV-negative	Penicillin G benzathine, 2.4 million U IM as a single dose	Doxycycline, 100 mg PO bid × 14 days or Tetracycline, 500 mg PO qid × 14 days
HIV-positive with >400 CD4[+] cells/mm[3] or <400 CD4[+] cells *and* normal CSF[3]	Penicillin G benzathine, 7.2 million U (2.4 million million U/week IM × 3 weeks)	Doxycycline, 100 mg PO bid × 28 days or Tetracycline, 500 mg PO qid × 28 days
HIV-positive with <400 CD4[+] cells/mm[3] and significant CSF abnormalities[3]	Same as for neurosyphilis	Penicillin densensitization or Consider alternative regimens[4]
Late Latent or Syphilis of Unknown Duration[5]	Penicillin G benzathine, 2.4 million U IM × 3 consecutive weeks (7.2 million U total)	Doxycycline, 100 mg PO bid × 28 days or Tetracycline, 500 mg PO qid × 28 days
Tertiary Syphilis Cardiovascular or benign tertiary (gummatous)[5]	Penicillin G benzathine, 2.4 million U IM × 3 consecutive weeks	Doxycycline, 100 mg PO bid × 28 days or Tetracycline, 500 mg PO qid × 28 days
Neurosyphilis (symptomatic and asymptomatic)	Aqueous crystalline penicillin G, 12–24 million U/day × 10 to 14 days or Aqueous procaine penicillin G, 2.4 million U/day IM × 10 days, plus probenecid, 500 mg PO qid × 10 days	Penicillin desensitization (see text)[6]
Syphilis in Pregnancy	Treat according to stage	Penicillin desensitization (see text)[7]
Congenital Syphilis[8]	Aqueous penicillin G procaine, 50,000 U/kg/day IM × 10–14 days or Aqueous crystalline penicillin G, 50,000 U/kg IV, in 2 or 3 divided doses per day × 10–14 days or Penicillin G benzathine, 50,000 U/kg IM in a single dose[9]	

[1]Prospective, randomized studies of therapeutic regimens have never been performed; recommendations are extrapolated from clinical literature.

[2]Clinical data for evaluation of all syphilis regimens not employing penicillin are extremely limited.

[3]Recommendations for HIV-positive patients with early syphilis are the author's.

[4]Ceftriaxone, 1–2 gm/day IM × 10–14 days, or doxycycline, 200 mg/day PO bid × 28 days.

[5]To rule out asymptomatic neurosyphilis, CSF examination is advised for patients with syphilis of unknown duration, latent syphilis, and tertiary syphilis without neurologic signs (see text).

[6]In patients with neurosyphilis and a history of penicillin allergy, penicillin hypersensitivity should be confirmed by skin testing. If skin tests are reactive, desensitization should be performed (see text).

[7]Use of erythromycin for penicillin-allergic pregnant patients has resulted in an unacceptably high failure rate in neonates. Such patients should be skin tested to confirm penicillin hypersensitivity, and if they are reactive, densensitization should be performed (see text).

[8]Recommended doses are for neonates.

[9]Used *only* for infants without evidence of active disease, with normal CSF, and with nontreponemal test titers less than or equal to maternal values.

Abbreviations: HIV = human immunodeficiency virus; IM = intramuscularly; PO = per os (orally); CSF = cerebrospinal fluid; IV = intravenously.

Based on Centers for Disease Control treatment guidelines for sexually transmitted disease. MMWR *38*(suppl):5, 1989. Modified with permission from Table 291–2 in Radolf JD, and Isaacs RD: Syphilis. *In* Kelley WN (ed): Textbook of Internal Medicine, 2nd ed. Philadelphia, JB Lippincott, 1990.

oxazole, antimicrobials commonly used for the treatment of other bacterial genitourinary infections, have poor in vitro activity against *T. pallidum* and should never be relied upon for the treatment of active or incubating syphilis. Although the new macrolide azithromycin (Zithromax) has excellent in vitro activity against *T. pallidum* and compared favorably with penicillin G benzathine in the rabbit syphilis model, clinical experience with it is extremely limited.

Early Syphilis in HIV-Seronegative Patients

Early syphilis is the period of maximal infectiousness and includes incubating, primary, secondary, and early latent (usually defined as the first year of infection) disease. Intramuscular administration of 2.4 million U of penicillin G benzathine (1.2 million U in each buttock) achieves cure rates well in excess of 95%. Penicillin-allergic patients with early syphilis should receive tetracycline, 500 mg orally four times per day, or doxycycline, 100 mg orally twice a day, for a total of 14 days.

Post-Treatment Follow-Up

After the clinical manifestations of early syphilis dissipate (usually within several weeks of therapy), it is essential that quantitative nontreponemal tests be conducted to document that a cure has been achieved. It was formerly held that titers in nontreponemal tests fell fourfold and eightfold 3 months and 6 months, respectively, after therapy of early syphilis and that they became nonreactive within 2 years. However, more recent data indicate that smaller declines in nontreponemal test titers within the first year of therapy are acceptable and that failure of these tests to become nonreactive (i.e., to serorevert) does not necessarily indicate treatment failure, particularly if antibody titers reach low, stable titers.

Early Syphilis in HIV-Infected Patients

A number of case reports have documented neurologic relapse or ophthalmologic relapse or both after the administration of recommended doses of penicillin G benzathine to HIV-infected patients with early syphilis. Nevertheless, the magnitude of the increased risk for treatment failure and the level of immunosuppression at which such increased risk becomes manifest are unknown. HIV-infected patients with CD4$^+$ counts greater than 400 per mm^3 should receive the same treatment as HIV-seronegative patients, along with close follow-up to identify possible treatment failure that necessitates more intensive antibiotic therapy. Although treatment failure and the development of neurosyphilis have not been correlated with depression of the absolute CD4$^+$ count below specific levels, lumbar puncture is advisable for HIV-positive patients with CD4$^+$ counts lower than 400 per mm^3, regardless of whether neurologic symptoms are pres-

ent. High-dose intravenous penicillin (3 to 4 million U intravenously every 4 hours) should be administered for 10 days if significant cerebrospinal fluid abnormalities that cannot be attributed to other causes (HIV infection alone often causes minor cerebrospinal fluid abnormalities) are present. Otherwise, 7.2 million U of penicillin G benzathine (2.4 million U weekly for 3 consecutive weeks) should be administered intramuscularly. Currently, few data are available with regard to the course of nontreponemal tests in HIV-infected syphilis patients after therapy with penicillin G benzathine. All such patients should be monitored extremely closely to identify possible treatment failure; lumbar puncture is indicated under such circumstances.

Late Syphilis

Late Latent Gummatous and Cardiovascular Syphilis

Late syphilis includes all syphilis infections lasting 1 year or longer. Patients with syphilis of undetermined duration (i.e., asymptomatic persons without a history of recent manifestations of early syphilis and without documented nonreactive syphilis serologic findings in the year before presentation) are considered to have late syphilis. Ideally, all late syphilis patients should undergo lumbar puncture to rule out asymptomatic neurosyphilis before receiving therapy. The highest priority for lumbar puncture should be accorded to patients with nontreponemal test titers of 1:32 or higher and to patients who are HIV-seropositive. Patients with abnormal CSF parameters unattributable to other causes should be treated for asymptomatic neurosyphilis. In the absence of other CSF abnormalities, treponemal tests reactive in the CSF should not be considered evidence for neurosyphilis. Once asymptomatic neurosyphilis has been ruled out, treatment of late syphilis consists of 7.2 million U of penicillin G benzathine (2.4 million U per week intramuscularly for 3 weeks). Penicillin-allergic patients should receive either tetracycline, 500 mg orally four times per day, or doxycycline, 100 mg orally twice a day, for 28 days. In patients with late syphilis, low nontreponemal test titers frequently fail to decrease significantly after therapy. Such patients are considered "serofast" and do not require retreatment.

Neurosyphilis

All patients with neurologic abnormalities attributable to syphilis should be treated for neurosyphilis *regardless* of stage or HIV status. Otic or ophthalmologic involvement, particularly posterior uveitis or optic neuritis, also should be managed as neurosyphilis. The antibiotic regimen that can best be relied upon to cure neuro-syphilis (symptomatic or asymptomatic) is aqueous crystalline penicillin G, 3 to 4 million U given every 4 hours for 10 to 14 days. An alternative outpatient regimen consists of 2.4 million U of penicillin G procaine intramuscularly for 10 to 14 days along with probenecid, 500 mg orally four times per day. It is no longer considered necessary to follow either regimen with intramuscular penicillin G benzathine. In view of the paucity of data supporting the use of agents other than penicillin for the treatment of neurosyphilis, a history of penicillin allergy should be confirmed by skin testing, followed, if necessary, by desensitization.

Patients treated for neurosyphilis should be monitored for a minimum of 2 years after therapy. Pleocytosis is the most reliable indicator of disease activity; the number of cells should improve significantly within 6 months after therapy and normalize within 1 year. Failure to do so indicates the need for retreatment. An elevated cerebrospinal fluid protein level and/or a reactive Venereal Disease Research Laboratories test of the CSF (CSF-VDRL) may take years to normalize even in adequately treated cases.

Syphilis During Pregnancy

Treatment schedules for pregnant women with syphilis are the same as those for nonpregnant women, with the exception that doxycycline should never be given to pregnant women. Because a number of treatment failures have been reported in infants born to penicillin-allergic women treated with erythromycin, penicillin allergy should be confirmed by skin testing, and patients should, if necessary, be desensitized for penicillin therapy. Ultrasonography should be performed on all women in the third trimester with untreated syphilis in order to assess the condition of the fetus. If evidence of fetal infection is found, the woman should be hospitalized and managed in consultation with an obstetrician.

Pregnant women treated in the last trimester of pregnancy are at increased risk of premature labor resulting from precipitation of a Jarisch-Herxheimer reaction (see later discussion). Patients should be advised to seek medical attention if contractions or any change in fetal movements occur after treatment.

Congenital Syphilis

All infants born to women with untreated syphilis are at risk for congenital syphilis. Infants should be treated with aqueous crystalline penicillin G, 50,000 units per kg per day intravenously every 8 to 12 hours for at least 10 days if there is any evidence of active disease or if one or more of the following are present: (1) reactive CSF-VDRL, (2) pleocytosis and/or elevated CSF protein levels, (3) quantitative nontreponemal serologic test titer fourfold or more greater than the mother's, and (4) positive IgM test for *T. palli-dum*–specific antibodies. Asymptomatic infants with nontreponemal test titers less than or equal to maternal titers and normal CSF parameters may receive penicillin G benzathine, 50,000 U per kg intramuscularly in a single dose.

Jarisch-Herxheimer Reaction

Within several hours of therapy, a substantial proportion of patients with early syphilis may experience constitutional symptoms (headache, fever, myalgia), mild hypotension, and worsening of specific syphilis manifestations. This phenomenon, the Jarisch-Herxheimer reaction, should be treated with salicylates (acetaminophen in pregnant women) or, in severe cases, with prednisone. A localized Jarisch-Herxheimer reaction also may manifest as transient worsening of neurologic, otic, or ophthalmologic symptoms soon after therapy and should be treated with prednisone. Patients should be warned of the possibility of the Jarisch-Herxheimer reaction before therapy and instructed with regard to self-medication and the need for contacting the physician.

Diseases of Allergy

ANAPHYLAXIS AND SERUM SICKNESS

method of
REBECCA B. RABY, M.D., and
MICHAEL S. BLAISS, M.D.
University of Tennessee, Memphis
Memphis, Tennessee

Anaphylaxis is a potentially fatal, acute systemic reaction resulting from the release of potent chemical mediators from tissue mast cells and peripheral blood basophils. It is estimated to occur in one of every 2700 hospitalized patients. Classical anaphylaxis is an immunologic reaction involving IgE in the release of chemical mediators. Anaphylactoid reactions have the same clinical manifestations as classic anaphylaxis but are not caused by the IgE-mediated release of chemical mediators from mast cells and basophils. Clinical symptoms of anaphylaxis can range from mild cutaneous manifestations such as generalized erythema, urticaria, and angioedema to life-threatening hypotension and cardiac arrhythmias. The most common causes are drugs, food and food additives, insect stings, and physical factors, such as exercise. In rare cases of anaphylaxis, an etiologic agent is never identified.

Serum sickness, as opposed to anaphylaxis, is an immune reaction involving IgG, IgM, or both circulating immune complexes to foreign antigens. Clinical symptoms classically occur 6 to 21 days after exposure to the antigen. Symptoms commonly seen in serum sickness are urticaria, fever, lymphadenopathy, and joint pain. True serum sickness is an infrequent event in humans today.

PATHOPHYSIOLOGY

Classical anaphylaxis is an IgE-mediated reaction to a foreign antigen, whether it is a protein, a polysaccharide, or a hapten. In susceptible persons, initial exposure to an antigen results in the production of specific IgE antibodies to that antigen. These antibodies bind to IgE receptors on the surface of mast cells and basophils. On re-exposure, the antigen can bind and cross-link the IgE antibodies on these cells. This leads to changes in the cell membrane with degranulation and release of chemical mediators, which include histamine, leukotrienes, prostaglandins, kallikrein, platelet activating factor, and eosinophil and neutrophil chemotactic factors. These mediators produce the clinical symptoms of anaphylaxis by causing vasodilation, increased vascular permeability, and smooth muscle contraction.

Several mechanisms can lead to anaphylactoid reactions. One is the activation of the complement system, resulting in the formation of anaphylatoxins C3a and C5a. These proteins can directly trigger mast cell and basophil degranulation, releasing the same potent mediators. Blood products can induce this type of reaction. Another mechanism is the direct action of certain agents, such as hyperosmolar radiocontrast media and opiates, on mast cells and basophils with the release of mediators. This mechanism is independent of IgE and complement. Anaphylactoid reactions can also occur in situations in which the mechanism is not clearly understood; these reactions include systemic reactions initiated by exercise, aspirin, nonsteroidal anti-inflammatory drugs, and synthetic steroid hormones. Idiopathic anaphylaxis is a rare syndrome for which no triggering agent can be identified.

SIGNS AND SYMPTOMS

Anaphylaxis manifests with a spectrum of symptoms ranging from mild to fatal within minutes. The overwhelming majority of reactions occur within 1 hour of exposure to the inciting agent. In some persons, the onset of the symptoms may be delayed for several hours. The most commonly affected organ systems are the skin, gastrointestinal tract, respiratory tract, and cardiovascular system. The severity of an individual's response is dependent on rate, amount, and site of mediator release as well as any personal risk factors such as asthma, underlying cardiac disease, and use of beta-blockers.

Skin manifestations are most commonly the first indications of anaphylaxis. These may include erythema, pruritus, urticaria, and angioedema. Swelling of the lips or tongue can impair ventilation, and swelling of the larynx, epiglottis, and surrounding tissue can cause upper airway obstruction with resultant stridor or suffocation. Gastrointestinal manifestations of anaphylaxis include nausea, vomiting, cramping abdominal pain, and diarrhea, which is often bloody. Respiratory symptoms include dyspnea, tachypnea, and wheezing. Hypotension and cardiac arrhythmias and arrest can also occur (Table 1).

When the aforementioned signs or symptoms of anaphylaxis occur within minutes of exposure to a known causative agent, it is usually not difficult to make the diagnosis of anaphylaxis. However, if the precipitating event is not known, the diagnosis could be confused with many other medical emergencies that clinically mimic anaphylaxis (Table 2). The condition most fre-

TABLE 1. Clinical Manifestations of Anaphylaxis

System/Structure	Symptoms
Skin	Erythema, general pruritus, urticaria, angioedema
Eye	Pruritus, conjunctival injection, lacrimation
Nose	Pruritus, congestion, sneezing, clear rhinorrhea
Upper airways	Sensation of narrowing airways, hoarseness, stridor, oropharyngeal or laryngeal edema, cough, complete obstruction
Lower airways	Dyspnea, tachypnea, use of accessory muscles, cyanosis, wheezing, respiratory arrest
Cardiovascular	Tachycardia, hypotension, arrhythmias, cardiac arrest
Gastrointestinal	Nausea, vomiting, cramping abdominal pain, diarrhea (often bloody)
Neurologic	Dizziness, weakness, syncope, seizures
Miscellaneous	Uterine contractions, intravascular coagulation, fibrinolysis

TABLE 2. Differential Diagnosis of Anaphylaxis

Vasovagal response
Primary cardiac event
Globus hystericus
Scombroid poisoning
Hyperventilation
Hereditary angioneurotic edema
Carcinoid
Systemic mastocytosis
Cold urticaria
Foreign body in trachea
Stroke
Medication overdose
Pheochromocytoma

quently mistaken for anaphylaxis is a vasovagal episode. Vasovagal episodes are usually preceded by a stressful or frightening event and are characterized by sweating, pallor, hypotension, and bradycardia. These attacks can usually be distinguished from anaphylaxis by the lack of pruritus, urticaria, and bronchospasm. The distinction between anaphylaxis and a primary cardiac event may be difficult, especially if the event is preceded by what seems to be an anaphylaxis-inducing exposure (i.e., insect sting, drug or food ingestion, etc.).

A complete cardiac evaluation and allergic work-up may be indicated. Table 3 lists criteria that may help make a diagnosis of anaphylaxis in people in whom the diagnosis may not be readily apparent. Measurement of serum levels of mast cell tryptase may help confirm an anaphylactic reaction. Unlike plasma histamine level, which usually declines within 30 minutes of an anaphylactic reaction, mast cell tryptase level peaks 60 to 90 minutes after anaphylaxis and has an approximately 3-hour half-clearance time.

CAUSATIVE AGENTS

There are hundreds of agents that can cause anaphylactic reactions (Table 4). The most common offenders are drugs, insect stings, and food substances. Penicillin remains one of the major medications that cause anaphylaxis. Deaths are more common when it is administered parenterally than orally. Of the people who have died from penicillin anaphylaxis, 75% had no history of previous reaction to penicillin. After injection (or ingestion), penicillin is metabolized into major and minor components or determinants. The minor determinant, which constitutes only 5% of the metabolites, is believed to be responsible for anaphylaxis in most persons sensitive to penicillin. Skin testing by a trained allergist with these me-

tabolites can be used to determine the potential of a serious reaction in patients with a history of penicillin allergy. It is estimated that about 2 to 7% of patients allergic to penicillin (history and skin test positive) are allergic to cephalosporins and therefore should not receive them.

Foods are another common cause of anaphylaxis. Legumes (peanuts, peas, soybeans, and beans), nuts, fish, shellfish, cow's milk, and eggs are the most common food allergens. Most anaphylactic reactions resulting from insect sting or bite are caused by an insect in the order Hymenoptera, which includes fire ants, hornets, yellow jackets, wasps, and honey bees. All patients with anaphylaxis caused by one of these insects should undergo venom skin testing by a trained allergist in order to document sensitivity. Of interest also is the contribution of physical factors to anaphylactic or anaphylactoid reactions. Many of these are not well understood, but exercise, cold, heat, and sunlight have all been implicated as causative agents.

Rubber (latex) products have recently been in-

TABLE 3. Diagnosis of Anaphylaxis*

At least one of the following must be present: acute hypotension, bronchial obstruction, or upper airway obstruction (cardiac or respiratory arrest)
Presence of distinctive allergic symptoms and signs in other systems
Recent exposure to agents or activities known to be capable of inducing anaphylaxis
Evidence of IgE to an agent encountered just before onset of anaphylaxis
Absence of conditions that can mimic anaphylaxis
Elevated serum levels of mast cell tryptase
Elevated levels of other molecules associated wtih mast cell secretion: plasma and urinary histamine and metabolites, serum high–molecular-weight neutrophil chemotactic factor, and urinary PGD_2 metabolites

*Effective therapy of acute anaphylaxis requires accurate diagnosis based upon clinical criteria.
Abbreviation: PGD_2 = prostaglandin D_2.
From Sullivan TJ: Systemic anaphylaxis. *In* Lichtenstein LM, and Fauci AS (eds): Current Therapy in Allergy, Immunology, and Rheumatology–2. Philadelphia, BC Decker, 1988.

TABLE 4. **Common Causes of Anaphylaxis**

Penicillin and derivatives
Cephalosporins
Tetracycline
Allergy extracts
Human seminal plasma
Streptokinase
L-asparaginase
Insulin
Opiates
Aspirin
Nonsteroidal anti-inflammatory agents
Radiocontrast media
Blood products
Milk
Eggs
Legumes
Nuts
Shellfish
Fish
Stinging insects
Cold
Exercise
Heat
Rubber (latex)

volved in more and more anaphylactic reactions. Many reports have documented anaphylaxis during surgical and radiologic procedures that was caused by latex objects such as gloves and catheters. Three groups appear to be at high risk for anaphylaxis to latex: medical personnel, people with a history of pruritus from exposure to latex objects, and patients with spina bifida. In these patients, latex sensitization develops because of multiple surgical procedures. Skin testing is available in some medical centers to confirm the diagnosis.

TREATMENT

Because acute anaphylaxis can be a life-threatening event, assessment and management must begin without delay (Table 5). This requires rapid evaluation of recent events, assessment of the severity of the clinical manifestations, rate of progression of symptoms, and a medical history, including known allergies, present medications, and underlying health problems. Simultaneously, the "ABCs" of emergency management should be implemented: Is the patient's *a*irway patent or obstructed? Is it in potential danger of becoming obstructed in the near future? Is the patient ventilating (i.e., *b*reathing)? If so, the patient should immediately be given high-flow oxygen and placed in a recumbent position with feet elevated above the heart (Trendelenburg's position). Is the patient's *c*irculatory system compromised?

After initial rapid assessment, epinephrine should be administered. Many deaths from anaphylaxis could have been prevented if epineph-

rine was given at the first sign of symptoms. The recommended dose of epinephrine 1:1000 is 0.01 mL per kg, up to 0.30 mL administered subcutaneously, to be repeated every 15 minutes if indicated. If the inciting event was an injection (i.e., insect sting, drug injection), a tourniquet should be placed proximal to the site of injury. Epinephrine can be given subcutaneously near the injection site to help retard systemic absorption of the offending agent.

Although not effective in the acute management of anaphylaxis, H_1 antihistamines, H_2 antihistamines, and corticosteroids are commonly administered. H_1 antihistamines, such as diphenhydramine (Benadryl), 1 to 2 mg per kg intravenously or intramuscularly up to 50 mg every 4 to 6 hours, help control the pruritus and skin manifestations. The use of H_2 antihistamines, such as ranitidine (Zantac), in conjunction with H_1 antihistamines may be beneficial in treating hypotension. Corticosteroids, such as hydrocortisone, 5 to 10 mg per kg intravenously up to 500 mg every 4 to 6 hours, may prevent a protracted course of anaphylaxis and decrease the magnitude of late sequelae.

After these initial steps, the patient's response should be reassessed in order to determine the next course of therapy. Should the patient be hy-

TABLE 5. **Management of Anaphylaxis**

1. Place patient in recumbent position with feet elevated
2. Secure and maintain airway, administer oxygen at 4–6 L/min
3. Epinephrine 1:1000, 0.01 mL/kg up to 0.30 mL SC; repeat every 15 minutes if necessary
4. Tourniquet above injection site and infiltrate site with additional epinephrine 1:1000, 0.01 mL/kg 0.10 to 0.20 mL SC
5. Administer diphenhydramine, 1–2 mg/kg IM or IV up to 50 mg every 4–6 h
6. Administer corticosteroids such as hydrocortisone, 5–10 mg/kg up to 500 mg IV every 4–6 h
7. Administer ranitidine, 12.5 mg to 50 mg IV every 6–8 h
8. Monitor vital signs frequently
9. If patient is hypotensive after epinephrine therapy, administer IV normal saline or colloids to replace intravascular fluid loss
10. If hypotension persists, administer norepinephrine bitartrate, 2–8 μg/min, or dopamine, 2–10 μg/kg/min, to maintain blood pressure
11. If hypotension is caused by beta-blockage, administer glucagon, 1–5 mg IV over 1 min, and begin continuous infusion 1–5 mg/h
12. Administer specific antiarrhythmic agents if indicated
13. For persistent bronchospasm, administer aminophylline, 6 mg/kg IV over 20 minutes, then continuous IV aminophylline drip at 0.9 mg/kg/h; monitor theophylline level; aerosolized beta$_2$-agonist as needed
14. Keep patient in observation for at least 6 to 8 h in case of a protracted course

Abbreviations: SC = subcutaneously; IM = intramuscularly; IV = intravenously.

potensive after subcutaneous epinephrine administration, treatment with volume expanders is indicated. The hypotension is a result of intravascular volume depletion secondary to increased capillary permeability as well as to vasodilation and decreased arteriolar tone. Normal saline or colloid may be used and administered at a rapid rate (in adults, as fast as 100 mL per minute). The patient's response, urine output, cardiovascular status, and age should be used as guidelines for the total amount of fluid to be given. Usually, a total of 3 liters can be given rapidly to an adult without ill effect. If hypotension persists, norepinephrine bitartrate, 2 to 8 µg per minute, or dopamine, 2 to 10 µg per kg per minute, should be administered to maintain blood pressure. The rate of infusion should be adjusted to maintain a systolic blood pressure of at least 80 to 100 mmHg.

Cardiac arrhythmias resulting from a combination of the chemical mediators, from hypoxia, from hypotension, and from the epinephrine itself can lead to cardiogenic shock. This condition necessitates the use of specific antiarrhythmic agents. Resistance to epinephrine may be seen in patients with a history of cardiac disease and on beta-blocking agents. In these situations, the use of glucagon, 1 to 5 mg intravenously over 1 minute and administered in a continuous drip, can partially overcome this resistance. Bronchospastic symptoms can be managed in a similar manner as those of status asthmaticus, with the use of beta-agonist aerosols and intravenous aminophylline therapy. Patients with severe anaphylaxis should be observed for at least 6 to 8 hours because of the possibility of a protracted course.

PREVENTION

Prevention of recurrence of anaphylaxis is aimed at identifying the etiologic agent and education of patients. Once the causative agent is identified, the treatment of choice is avoidance especially in food, drug, and latex allergy. If avoidance is not possible, however, other measures of prevention are available. In patients with a history of anaphylaxis in response to radiocontrast media, a premedication protocol is available (Table 6). Venom immunotherapy should be offered to all patients with documented Hymenoptera anaphylaxis. It has been shown to be effective in the prevention of anaphylaxis in more than 95% of treated patients. In patients with a positive history and positive skin test responses to penicillin to whom penicillin or one of its derivatives must be administered, desensitization protocols are available.

All patients with a history of anaphylaxis

TABLE 6. **Premedication for Radiocontrast Media Reactions**

1. Prednisone, 50 mg orally, 13, 7, and 1 h before the procedure
2. Diphenhydramine, 50 mg intramuscularly, 1 h before the procedure
3. Ephedrine, 25 mg orally, 1 hour before the procedure, unless the patient has underlying cardiovascular disease

should wear a medical identification bracelet (Medic-Alert) to inform medical personnel of their known allergies. They should be equipped with and educated in the use of self-administered epinephrine such as EpiPen and Ana-Kit/Ana-Guard. If exposure to the anaphylactic agent occurs, patients should immediately use the epinephrine and promptly go to a medical facility for evaluation.

SERUM SICKNESS

Serum sickness is a syndrome involving IgG, IgM, or both circulating immune complexes that was first described with the use of foreign antiserums. Today, the most common causes are medications (Table 7). The disease is usually milder in children and more severe in adults. As described in animal models, after a latent period of a few days when antigen is present in excess, antibodies (IgG or IgM) that interact with the antigen are made, forming soluble circulating immune complexes. These complexes, if not removed from the circulation, are capable of migrating into vascular walls, where they may fix and activate complement. Monocytes and macrophages may be chemically attracted to these areas and contribute to tissue destruction as well. The resulting inflammation can lead to the vasculitis. Signs and symptoms of serum sickness are shown in Table 8. Cutaneous eruptions are seen in more than 90% of all patients and include urticaria, maculopapular or purpuric lesions, and erythema multiforme. A characteristic band of erythema on the plantar and palmar junctions of the feet and hands has been described. Nearly all

TABLE 7. **Common Causes of Serum Sickness**

Penicillin and derivatives
Cephalosporins
Sulfonamides
Hydantoins
Blood products
Phenylbutazone
Naproxen (Naproxyn)
Thiazides
Propranolol
Metronidazole

TABLE 8. **Symptoms of Serum Sickness**

Symptoms	Frequency (%)
Fever, malaise	100
Cutaneous eruptions	90
Arthralgia	50–75
Myalgia	25–50
Lymphadenopathy	10–20
Glomerulonephritis	Rare

From Younger RE: Anaphylaxis and serum sickness. *In* Rakel RE (ed): Conn's Current Therapy. Philadelphia, WB Saunders, 1992, pp 681–84.

patients have a mild fever, although it is higher in the more severe cases. Most have peripheral edema and arthritis or arthralgia. In the most severe cases, glomerulonephritis, peripheral neuritis, and, rarely, Guillain-Barré syndrome may be present. Symptoms usually occur 7 to 21 days after exposure to the agent. In previously sensitized patients, the symptoms may occur as soon as 24 hours after re-exposure. Most serum sickness–type reactions are considered mild and resolve spontaneously within 2 to 3 weeks.

If the patient is still receiving the offending antigen when serum sickness occurs, it should be discontinued immediately. Treatment is generally directed at symptomatic relief. Antihistamines relieve the pruritus, and nonsteroidal anti-inflammatory agents relieve the fever and arthralgias. If symptoms persist or worsen despite these measures, it may be necessary to administer corticosteroids. Prednisone, 1 to 2 mg per kg per day (maximal dose: 60 mg), tapering over 5 to 7 days and followed by a smaller daily morning dose for 1 week, usually provides good results. Shorter courses of corticosteroids may not be effective.

There is no definitive laboratory test for diagnosis of serum sickness. It is usually based on the history and clinical presentation. However, the erythrocyte sedimentation rate is usually mildly elevated, and there may be peripheral eosinophilia with leukocytosis or leukopenia, proteinuria, hematuria, decreased complement levels (CH50, C3, C4), and electrocardiographic changes. Circulating immune complexes may also be detected in some patients by using C1q binding assays or Raji cell immunoassays. Because serum sickness is a clinical syndrome with many similarities to other inflammatory diseases, re-evaluation of the diagnosis is indicated if the symptoms persist for longer than 3 weeks. In adults, other vasculitides are often confused with serum sickness, as is juvenile rheumatoid arthritis in children.

ASTHMA IN ADOLESCENTS AND ADULTS

method of
DAVID A. KHAN, M.D., and
JAMES T. C. LI, M.D., Ph.D.
Mayo Clinic and Foundation
Rochester, Minnesota

Within the past few years there has been a rise in asthma-related mortality. From 1980 to 1987, the number of deaths due to asthma increased 31%. There has been an upward trend in asthma-related mortality for all age groups over 4 years old (highest in the >65-year-old age group), and the death rate among blacks is almost three times that of whites. The preeminent factor associated with a favorable impact on asthma mortality is proper management, including effective maintenance of stable asthma and prompt treatment of asthma exacerbations with anti-inflammatory therapy.

Asthma has been defined as a chronic airway disorder characterized by variable obstruction, eosinophilic inflammation, and hyperresponsiveness of the airways. The prevalence of asthma among adolescents and adults is approximately 4 to 9%; at younger ages, more males are affected, and the incidence among females increases after menopause.

PATHOPHYSIOLOGY

The pathologic features of asthma have been known since the nineteenth century, although the knowledge of the inflammatory nature of asthma has only recently made an impact on its management. Initial pathologic evaluations were limited to autopsy specimens from cases of fatal asthma, which demonstrated mucus plugging, desquamated epithelium, mucosal edema, smooth muscle and glandular hypertrophy, basement membrane thickening, and inflammatory infiltrates with a predominance of eosinophils.

Bronchoalveolar Lavage and Bronchial Biopsy

Within the past decade, the technique of bronchoscopy with bronchoalveolar lavage (BAL) has been used to study the pathology of asthma in vivo. BAL studies have shown an inflammatory influx of eosinophils, mast cells, T lymphocytes, and, to a lesser extent, neutrophils. A potpourri of cellular mediators has also been detected in BAL fluid. Bronchial biopsy specimens from asthmatic patients show an inflammatory infiltrate consisting of eosinophils, T cells, and macrophages, similar to airway specimens obtained from patients with fatal asthma.

The sputum from asthmatic patients shows eosinophils along with the granule proteins, major basic protein (MBP), eosinophil-derived neurotoxin (EDN), and eosinophil cationic protein (ECP). MBP is toxic to respiratory epithelium, producing many changes similar to those found in specimens of fatal asthma. The total eosinophil count in peripheral blood is often elevated in asthmatic patients and can aid in diagnosis and therapy.

Late-Phase Reactions

When a patient with allergic asthma is challenged with an allergenic aerosol, early-phase bronchoconstriction occurs within minutes of exposure to antigen. Beta-adrenergic agonists and cromolyn sodium are effective at blocking this early-phase reaction. The late-phase reaction typically occurs 4 to 6 hours later and is characterized by a cellular influx of eosinophils, which can release toxic granule proteins (such as MBP), T cells capable of releasing cytokines, and macrophages, basophils, and neutrophils. Aerosol corticosteroids and cromolyn sodium are effective in attenuating this late-phase reaction. The pathologic similarities between the late-phase reaction and chronic asthma has led to the theory of allergic asthma as a perpetual late-phase reaction.

Airway Hyperresponsiveness

One of the hallmarks of asthma is bronchial hyperresponsiveness. The hyperresponsive airway constricts after exposure to respiratory irritants, cold air, exercise, and the pharmacologic agents methacholine and histamine. This is the basis of the methacholine challenge. The degree of airway hyperresponsiveness is correlated with the severity of asthma and may be caused by physical inflammation of the airway, epithelial injury, or disorders in neural regulation such as beta-adrenergic dysfunction, increased parasympathetic response, or release of neuropeptides such as calcitonin related gene product (CRGP) or substance P from nonadrenergic-noncholinergic nerves. Bronchial hyperresponsiveness is augmented by allergic reactions and viral infections. These viruses may also have a role in the pathogenesis of asthma by causing epithelial damage directly, enhancing mediator release, or initiating production of specific IgE. Diurnal variation of forced expiratory volumes and flow rates in nocturnal asthma is another example of increased airway hyperresponsiveness.

Pulmonary Function

Alterations in pulmonary function in asthma include increased airway resistance, decreased forced expiratory volumes and flow rates, hyperinflation (as demonstrated by an elevated residual volume and occasionally an elevated diffusion capacity), and ventilation/perfusion abnormalities. Metabolic changes that may be present include reduced arterial oxygen tension and respiratory alkalosis. Pulsus paradoxus and electrocardiographic changes of sinus tachycardia, right axis deviation, P-pulmonale, and right ventricular strain may also occur with more severe asthma.

DIAGNOSIS

History

History is the most important component of the diagnosis of asthma and is crucial for determining prognosis and management (Table 1). Symptoms include nocturnal exacerbations, episodic or chronic symptoms, and triggering factors. Symptoms of conjunctivitis, rhinitis, and skin rash may be caused by coexisting diseases such as allergic rhinoconjunctivitis, nasal polyposis, sinusitis, and eczema. Special historical features of adolescent patients include the amount of school missed, medication compliance, self-esteem, and ability to participate in physical education class and other activities. Occupational asthma is an important type of asthma that is often unrecognized (Table 2). The clinician must take a careful occupational history and intervene promptly if occupational asthma is present.

Physical Examination

The physical examination is less helpful than the history both in diagnosis and in management. The chest examination may be normal or may reveal hyperinflation, prolonged expiration, wheezing, or diminished breath sounds. Correlation between physical findings and severity of asthma is poor. The nose

TABLE 1. **Components of Asthma History**

Symptoms
Wheeze
Dyspnea
Chest tightness
Cough
Nighttime awakening
Sputum production

Triggers
Exercise
Activity
Cold air
Respiratory infections
Seasonal change
Environmental irritants
    Work
    Hobbies
    Home
    Bedroom
    Pets
    Cigarette smoke
Animals
Aspirin

Severity
Emergency room visits
Hospitalizations
Work absenteeism
Asthma medication use
Sleep habits
Frequency of symptoms
Exercise capacity

Compliance
Perception of severity
Lifestyle
Psychosocial factors

Family History
Asthma
Allergic rhinitis
Eczema
Pulmonary disorders

TABLE 2. **Causes of Occupational Asthma**

Allergen	Example	Occupation or Industry
Animal proteins	Cat, mouse, guinea pig	Laboratory workers, veterinarians
Plant proteins	Flour	Bakers, food workers, dockworkers
Vegetable gums	Acacia	Printers
Acid anhydrides	Trimellitic (TMA)	Plastic, epoxy resin
Metallic salts	Platinum chloride	Nickel, platinum, chromium, vanadium workers
Diisocyanates	Toluene diisocyanate (TDI)	Auto, paint, plastics, polyurethane foam workers
Antibiotics	Penicillin	Pharmaceutical
Fluxes	Colophony	Solderers, welders
Persulfate salts	Hair bleach	Beauticians
Ethylenediamine	Hair dye	Beauticians
Extract of henna	Hair dye	Beauticians
Wood dusts	Western red cedar	Woodworkers

should be examined for mucosal edema and polyps, and the skin should be examined for eczema.

Laboratory Studies

Pulmonary Function Tests. Pulmonary function testing is useful for diagnosis and crucial in management of asthma. A peak flow meter can be helpful if it demonstrates decreased flow rates that are reversible with treatment or variable over time. However, peak flow rates are effort-dependent and often can be normal despite significant obstruction. Airway obstruction in asthma results in a decreased forced expiratory volume in 1 second (FEV_1), normal or proportionately reduced vital capacity, and a reduced ratio of FEV_1 to forced vital capacity [FVC]). Measurement of FEV_1 by spirometry is the most useful test for asthma. Repeated measurements of FEV_1 over time or after treatment helps establish the variable obstruction in asthma and provides a good estimate of severity. Plethysmography measures residual volume, which is often increased in asthma. The diffusion capacity is normal or sometimes elevated in asthmatic patients and therefore can help differentiate asthma from other obstructive lung diseases. The authors obtain plethysmography with a diffusion capacity in cases in which the diagnosis of asthma is not certain or if treatment is unsuccessful.

A key to diagnosing asthma is the demonstration of reversible airway obstruction. This reversibility can be revealed by measuring the response to a bronchodilator or the response to anti-inflammatory therapy. Patients with airway obstruction unresponsive to bronchodilator (<10% change in FEV_1) may require a course of oral steroids (e.g., prednisone, 40 mg per day for 7 to 14 days) and repeated spirometry to document reversibility. This diagnostic trial of systemic steroids can aid in differentiating asthma from irreversible obstructive lung disease.

Patients with mild asthma may not demonstrate obstruction on spirometry, and bronchoprovocation methods may contribute to the diagnosis of asthma. The most common bronchoprovocation techniques are the methacholine, histamine, and exercise challenge tests. The most widely used is the methacholine (Mecholyl) challenge. This is considered positive if the FEV_1 drops by 20% after challenge. The authors administer up to five breaths of nebulized methacholine at 25 mg per mL. These tests are used for patients with normal spirometry results, with an atypical history of asthma, with chronic cough, or with exertional dyspnea. The sensitivity of the test approaches 100% in symptomatic asthmatic patients. However, nonasthmatic patients with allergic rhinitis, a viral infection, chronic obstructive lung disease (COLD), bronchiectasis, and cystic fibrosis can demonstrate positive results of challenges.

Allergy Testing. Asthmatic patients who provide a history suggestive of an allergic trigger may benefit from allergy testing. However, the allergic component of asthma is sometimes difficult to elucidate by history alone. For example, patients allergic to dust mites usually have perennial symptoms, which can be clinically indistinguishable from nonallergic asthma.

There are basically two types of allergy tests available: skin tests and in vitro tests (the radioallergosorbent test [RAST]). Skin test methods have the advantage of immediate results, lower cost, and improved sensitivity in comparison with RAST. The in vitro assays measure specific IgE to specific antigens in serum. Test results are usually not available for a few days and are more costly. In vitro assays may be indicated in patients with dermographism or atopic dermatitis or who may be taking long-acting antihistamines such as astemizole (Hismanal).

Significant aeroallergens in asthma include tree, grass, and weed pollens; outdoor and indoor molds; insect or arthropod emanations (cockroach and dust mites); and dander of animals such as dogs and cats. Food allergy almost never plays a role in chronic asthma and therefore should not be part of routine allergy testing in asthmatic patients.

Other Tests. Asthmatics may have elevated numbers of eosinophils in sputum and blood. The total IgE level can be elevated in patients with allergic asthma, patients with allergic bronchopulmonary aspergillosis, and smokers. Chest x-rays are usually normal but may demonstrate hyperinflation or complications of asthma such as pneumothorax, pneumomediastinum, atelectasis, pneumonia, or allergic bronchopulmonary aspergillosis. Arterial blood gases are not helpful in diagnosing asthma but can be helpful in assessing respiratory failure.

TABLE 3. **Differential Diagnosis**

Differential Diagnosis of Wheezing
Chronic obstructive lung disease
Extrathoracic obstruction
Vocal cord dysfunction
Congestive heart failure
Sarcoidosis
Pulmonary embolism
Hyperventilation syndrome

Diseases Complicating Asthma
Nasal polyposis
Sinusitis
Gastroesophageal reflux
Hyperthyroidism
Allergic bronchopulmonary aspergillosis
Churg-Strauss vasculitis
Obstructive sleep apnea

Differential Diagnosis

Guided by a careful history and appropriate testing (including spirometry), clinicians can usually make the diagnosis of asthma without difficulty. The differential diagnosis of asthma includes a variety of cardiopulmonary and upper airway disorders (Table 3). COLD may be distinguished by a smoking history, evidence of irreversible obstruction despite treatment, and a diminished diffusion capacity. Some patients may have a component of both asthma and COLD. Extrathoracic obstruction should be considered in patients with inspiratory wheezing or stridor. Paradoxical vocal cord dysfunction is a condition often seen in younger women and in medical personnel who have inspiratory difficulty. The diagnosis is made by laryngoscopy during an attack, in which paradoxical apposition of the cords is shown during inspiration, or by spirometry, including an inspiratory flow-loop. Diseases that may complicate asthma (Table 3) should be suspected when a patient's therapeutic goals are not being achieved.

TREATMENT

Goals of Therapy

The key to success in managing asthma is establishing therapeutic goals that guide all management decisions. Achievement of these goals determines the extent and the type of treatment. The National Heart and Lung Institute convened an expert panel that issued guidelines on the management of asthma (Table 4).

TABLE 4. **Goals of Therapy**

Maintain normal activity levels (including exercise)
Maintain (near) "normal" pulmonary function rates
Prevent chronic and troublesome symptoms (e.g., coughing or breathlessness in the night, in the early morning, or after exertion)
Prevent recurrent exacerbations of asthma
Avoid adverse effects from asthma medications

From the National Asthma Education Program Expert Panel Report—1991.

Education of Patients

Several studies have demonstrated the effectiveness of proper education of patients in reducing the morbidity in asthma; however, among the various management tools, it is perhaps the least used. Education of asthmatic patients is multifaceted and includes forming a partnership between the physician and the patient to provide the patient with an active role in management; outlining specific goals; and stressing the need for long-term follow-up because of the nature of the chronic disease. The patient should understand the nature of asthma, warning signs and symptoms, and the significant triggers. The patient should practice avoidance measures when appropriate, monitor peak expiratory flow rates at home, and avoid overuse of medications. Instructions should be both written and verbal for maintenance therapy and should include a detailed and specific action plan for asthma exacerbations. Patients should be aware of early signs of asthma exacerbation such as decreased peak expiratory flow rates and nocturnal symptoms and be cognizant of the necessity of early treatment. The action plan should include specific therapy for exacerbations (such as increase in self-medication and emergency telephone numbers to call) as well as indications for emergency care (such as difficulty walking or talking, peak flow of <50% of normal, retractions, and absence of response to medications).

Because 25 to 50% of asthmatic patients use inhalers improperly, learning correct inhaler technique is another important educational objective. In order to enhance compliance, the physician must review the indications for and the acute and long-term side effects of preventative medications. Other compliance issues include cost, complicated medicine schedules, and steroid phobia. Medical care availability and cost, underestimation of the severity of asthma, the stigma of illness, and cultural factors may also contribute to poor outcomes. Adolescents have additional compliance issues, including the administration of medications at school (and consequent disruption of class schedules), being perceived as different from their peers, and parental conflicts.

Measurements of Lung Function

Several studies have demonstrated that subjective assessment of lung function both by patients and by physicians are poorly correlated with measured pulmonary function. Moreover, underestimation of asthma severity is linked to increased rates of morbidity and mortality. For these reasons, an objective measurement of pulmonary function with either spirometry or a peak flow meter is mandatory for the proper management of asthma. It is analogous to using a sphygmomanometer for monitoring hypertension or blood glucose in diabetes. Spirometry is useful during the initial assessment and thereafter can be repeated, depending on the severity and response to treatment.

Environmental Control Measures

Environmental control is the cornerstone of allergy therapy, and its proper use can help achieve the goals of therapy with fewer medications. Patients allergic to outdoor molds and pollens can decrease their allergen exposure by limiting outdoor activity during relevant seasons and staying in an air-conditioned environment.

Dust mites are a significant allergen for many asthmatic patients. The allergen is found in the feces and body parts of these humidity-dependent microorganisms and is abundant in pillows, mattresses, carpets, and upholstered furniture. Vacuuming does little to remove the allergen. Effective control measures include encasing pillows and mattresses with plastic, washing bedding in water warmer than 130° F, reducing humidity to less than 50%, and, if possible, removal of carpeting, especially in the bedroom. Dehumidifiers should be cleaned to prevent the growth of indoor molds.

Other indoor allergens include cockroaches and pets. In addition to allergens, strong odors and sprays and indoor pollutants such as smoke from cigarettes, wood stoves, and fireplaces should be avoided. Outdoor pollutants such as ozone and sulfur dioxide can adversely affect asthmatic patients, and exposure should be minimized.

Drug-Induced Asthma

Beta-blockers (even topical eye drops) should be avoided. Aspirin and nonsteroidal anti-inflammatory drugs can provoke profound asthma exacerbations in the 4 to 20% of asthmatic patients who are sensitive to these agents. Asthmatic patients are at increased risk of anaphylactoid reactions from radiocontrast material. Angiotensin-converting enzyme inhibitors are not contraindicated, but patients taking them should be monitored for the development of a drug-induced cough. Sulfites, food additives often found in salad bar items, potatoes, beer, and wine, trigger an exacerbation in 4% of asthmatic patients.

Pharmacotherapy

Anti-Inflammatory Agents

In view of the inflammatory nature of asthma, there has been a general trend toward the greater use of anti-inflammatory agents. This therapy is underused in many asthmatic patients despite proof of safety and efficacy.

CORTICOSTEROIDS

Corticosteroids are the most effective anti-inflammatory agents available for the treatment of asthma. Several mechanisms have been proposed to explain the actions of corticosteroids, including interference with arachidonic acid metabolism, prevention of activation and directed migration of inflammatory cells, inhibition of cytokine production, and increased responsiveness of beta receptors of airway smooth muscle. Corticosteroids can be administered by inhalation, orally, or parenterally. All of these routes are useful in specific facets of the treatment of asthma.

Inhaled corticosteroids such as beclomethasone (Vanceril, Beclovent), triamcinolone (Azmacort), and flunisolide (Aerobid) are very effective in treating the inflammatory component of asthma. The response to these medications is dose-dependent, and evidence of improvement usually takes a few weeks. Adverse effects are mainly a result of local deposition causing thrush, dysphonia, and occasional coughing, all of which can be greatly reduced with a spacer and rinsing the mouth after use. Systemic effects of inhaled steroids are very infrequent at the approved dosages, although growth retardation in children has been reported.

Oral corticosteroids are extremely effective for acute exacerbations and have been shown to decrease the number of hospitalizations, the number of emergency room visits, and the morbidity associated with asthma. The onset of action, usually within 3 to 12 hours, is much more rapid than that of inhaled corticosteroids. Acute adverse effects are transient and include weight gain, increased appetite, mood alteration, hyperglycemia, and hypokalemia. The authors prefer oral steroid preparations to intramuscular glucocorticoids for acute exacerbations because the dose and schedule can be more precisely controlled. Intravenous steroids are indicated in the hospital setting.

Chronic therapy with oral steroids is also quite efficacious, but adverse effects such as osteoporosis, hypertension, myopathy, Cushing's syndrome, cataracts, and adrenal suppression make this form of therapy too toxic for all but the most refractory cases of asthma. An adequate trial of inhaled steroids should always be initiated before a patient is committed to chronic oral steroids and its associated problems.

CROMOLYN SODIUM

Cromolyn sodium (Intal) is a nonsteroidal anti-inflammatory drug whose mechanism of action is not fully understood. Cromolyn sodium blocks both early- and late-phase allergen-induced bronchoconstriction. A 4 to 6 week trial is sufficient for determining efficacy. It is unclear whether there is any advantage to using cromolyn sodium in combination with inhaled steroids, and in the authors' experience, it is rarely beneficial in severe asthma. The adverse effects of this drug are limited to occasional coughing upon inhalation of the powder formulation.

NEDOCROMIL SODIUM

Nedocromil sodium (Tilade) is a pyranoquinolone derivative that has recently become available in the United States. Its actions are similar to those of cromolyn sodium, but it may be more potent. Nedocromil sodium has been shown to reduce nonspecific airway reactivity in atopic and nonatopic patients and has no significant adverse effects.

Bronchodilators

BETA-ADRENERGIC AGONISTS

Beta-adrenergic agents are classified according to their degree of selectivity for beta$_1$ and beta$_2$ receptors. Beta$_2$ selective agents include albuterol (Ventolin, Proventil), pirbuterol (Maxair), bitolterol (Tornalate), and terbutaline (Brethaire, Brethine). Nonselective beta-adrenergic agonists include ephedrine, isoetharine (Bronkosol, Bronkometer), epinephrine (Primatene), isoproterenol (Isuprel), and metaproterenol (Alupent). The beta$_2$ selective agonists are the medications most widely used for asthma. These agents relax airway smooth muscle and modulate mediator release from mast cells and basophils. Their duration of action after inhalation is 4 to 6 hours, although new 12-hour agents such as salmeterol may soon become available in the United States.

Beta$_2$ agonists can be administered orally, in an inhaled form via a metered dose inhaler (MDI) or powder inhaler, or as an aerosolized liquid. The MDI or powder inhaler is preferred for chronic use because inhaled beta agonists provide greater bronchodilation than do oral preparations and fewer side effects such as tremor, anxiety, and hypokalemia than do nebulized aerosols. Beta$_2$ agonists are the initial treatment of choice for acute exacerbations of asthma and in the prevention of exercise induced asthma.

Recently, a controversy has arisen over the regular use of beta$_2$ agonists and their association with worsening control and increased morbidity of asthma. This data has been extended to include several classes of beta$_2$ agonists as well as other bronchodilators such as theophylline and ipratropium bromide. Because this area remains a topic for debate, the authors recommend that for chronic asthma, beta$_2$ agonists be used only as needed, instead of on a scheduled routine, preferably fewer than four times daily.

METHYLXANTHINES

Theophylline and aminophylline have been used extensively in the treatment of asthma. Their mechanism of action is unknown, although some studies have shown extrapulmonary and anti-inflammatory effects. In vitro, theophylline inhibits phosphodiesterase, but the concentration at which this occurs is not likely to be reached in vivo. A recent multicenter asthma treatment study comparing theophylline with inhaled beclomethasone demonstrated overall superiority of beclomethasone, but not by a wide margin. For nocturnal asthma, the authors recommend sustained-release theophylline (Uniphyl, 400 to 800 mg) or sustained-release albuterol (Proventil Repetabs, 4 mg) every evening.

The major drawback to these drugs is their narrow therapeutic range and significant potential for toxicity. Drug levels of 5 to 15 µg per mL are usually adequate, and yet toxicity can occur even in this range. Several factors can affect theophylline metabolism, including febrile illness, hepatic disease, congestive heart failure, pregnancy, and other drugs such as cimetidine, erythromycin, and quinolones. The signs and symptoms of toxicity include nausea, vomiting, and tachycardia and can progress to seizures and arrhythmias. A recent study of school-aged children and adolescents demonstrated no difference in academic achievement between theophylline-treated children and sibling controls.

ANTICHOLINERGIC AGENTS

Ipratropium bromide (Atrovent) has gained popularity over other anticholinergic agents because of its lack of systemic effects. It is thought to act by blocking postganglionic efferent vagal pathways, thus reducing intrinsic vagal tone, and has been shown to block reflex bronchoconstriction to irritants. Ipratropium bromide has a slower onset and is a weaker bronchodilator than beta$_2$ agonists but may be helpful for patients unable to tolerate beta$_2$ agonist–associated tremor. Unfortunately, not all asthmatic patients respond to ipratropium bromide, and its use in treating asthma is currently not approved by the U.S. Food and Drug Administration.

Spacer Devices

Spacer devices come in a variety of shapes and sizes but are all very similar conceptually. These devices are simply chambers placed over the opening of an MDI to physically distance the device from the oropharynx, allowing improved drug delivery to the airways as well as reducing oropharyngeal deposition and hence local side effects. In view of these characteristics, their use is especially beneficial for the delivery of inhaled corticosteroids, and they should be used in all patients who require these agents. In addition, spacers are useful aids to patients with difficulty coordinating inhalation with hand actuation of an MDI. Because these spacers are somewhat cumbersome and do not fit easily into one's pocket, administering inhaled corticosteroids twice daily while the patient is home improves compliance. This is especially important among adolescents who are reluctant to use inhalers in front of their peers, especially if the inhalers are attached to a bulky spacer device.

Immunotherapy

Immunotherapy (also known as desensitization or hyposensitization) for asthma has been shown to be effective in double-blind placebo-controlled studies for grass pollen, cat, dust mite, *Alternaria* (an outdoor mold), and ragweed. Asthmatic patients in whom allergy plays a significant role and who demonstrate positive reactions in allergy skin tests or RAST to relevant allergens are candidates for immunotherapy. Immunotherapy should be avoided in patients with severe asthma (FEV_1 < 70%), patients without allergic disease, and patients with significant coronary artery disease. Immunotherapy injections should be administered in an office equipped for treating life-threatening reactions. Once a monthly maintenance dose is achieved, immunotherapy should be continued for 3 to 5 years and then reassessed. If, however, there has been no improvement after 1 year, further therapy is unlikely to be beneficial. In addition to local reactions consisting of mild swelling and pruritus, immunotherapy carries a risk of systemic reactions (which are usually mild). From 1945 to 1984, 30 fatalities from immunotherapy were reported in a retrospective national survey of allergists. In view of the estimated 7 to 10 million injections administered per year, this mortality figure is quite low. Immunotherapy with sublingual drops and bacterial, food, and *Candida* extracts are all unproven forms of therapy and should be avoided.

Maintenance Therapy

Pharmacotherapy in asthma is tailored to the individual, and because asthma is a fluctuant disease, therapy must be equally flexible. Treatment guidelines are summarized in Table 5. In general, mildly asthmatic patients with episodic symp-toms require treatment only as needed, usually an inhaled beta$_2$ agonist. When symptoms are more persistent and especially if spirometry is abnormal, daily inhaled anti-inflammatory agents are indicated. A trial of cromolyn sodium may be worthwhile, especially in younger patients, before inhaled glucocorticoids (which may affect growth) are initiated.

Although animal studies have shown that inhaled corticosteroids vary somewhat in their degree of topical (i.e., bronchial) and systemic potency, they are all effective agents. Choosing one type of inhaled corticosteroid over another is usually not as critical as titrating the dose. The authors recommend that patients administer their inhaled medications one puff at a time without waiting between inhalations.

As the severity of asthma increases, so does the need for higher doses of inhaled corticosteroids. Often a short burst of oral steroids is required in order to gain immediate control of the inflammation. This also provides an opportunity to measure pulmonary function at its peak and to determine the extent of reversibility. It is crucial to keep the goals of therapy in mind. This requires repeated objective pulmonary function measurements as dictated by the patient's response to therapy. Once these goals are met, medication can be gradually tapered to the lowest amount that maintains control. During return visits, physicians should review inhaler technique, peak flow records, medications, environmental control, and overall compliance.

Several studies have identified characteristics of patients that are associated with increased asthma mortality (Table 6). These asthmatic patients require more intensive management, careful monitoring, and special attention to education.

If the goals of therapy are not strictly met despite treatment, referral of the patient to an asthma specialist is strongly recommended. Consultation by an allergist should be considered in any patient in whom the question of an allergic component of their asthma exists. Steroid-dependent asthmatic patients should always be under the additional care of a specialist.

Exacerbation Management

Home Management

Part of the education process includes providing an action plan specifically outlining management of asthma exacerbations (see the Education of Patients section). The action plan should stress prompt treatment, early use of oral steroids for exacerbations, and monitoring response to therapy with a peak flowmeter. Individual patients

TABLE 5. **Asthma Maintenance Pharmacotherapy**

Mild	Moderate	Severe
Criteria		
Episodic symptoms	Symptoms almost daily	Continuous symptoms
Normal spirometry	Abnormal spirometry	FEV_1 <60%
	Uses β_2-agonist inhaler almost daily	Exacerbations despite treatment
Initial Therapy		
β_2-agonist inhaler prn, 2 puffs 3 times daily (or fewer) and 30 min before exposure to triggers	β_2-agonist, 2 puffs tid-qid prn	β_2-agonist inhaler, tid-qid prn
	Beclomethasone, 4 puffs bid, or triamcinolone, 4 puffs bid, or flunisolide, 2 puffs bid, or cromolyn sodium, 2 puffs qid, or theophylline, bid	Oral prednisone, 20 mg bid × 1–2 weeks, then taper × 2–3 weeks
		Beclomethasone or triamcinolone, 8–10 puffs bid, or flunisolide, 4 puffs bid
		Theophylline at therapeutic levels
Further Therapy		
Cromolyn sodium, 2 puffs before exposure to triggers	Beclomethasone, 5–8 puffs bid, or triamcinolone, 5–8 puffs bid, or flunisolide, 3–4 puffs bid	High-dose inhaled corticosteroids (e.g., 20–30 puffs/day)
	Consider adding theophylline	Consider ipratropium bromide qid
	Consider prednisone burst, 20 mg bid × 1 week, then taper 1–2 weeks	Daily or alternate-day prednisone as a last resort

Abbreviations: FEV_1 = 1-s forced expiratory volume.

may benefit from home use of oral steroid tablets, nebulizers, and injectable epinephrine.

Emergency Room Care

An often underused and yet critical tool for the assessment and management of asthma in the emergency room is the use of spirometry or peak flow devices. All asthmatic patients require objective measurements of airway flow before and after therapy to assess response to treatment. A focused history is crucial for management decisions. The severity, time of onset, allergic exposure, medication use (especially corticosteroids), and history of prior hospitalization or intensive care unit care are all important components of the history. Physical examination should be directed toward vital signs, chest auscultation, and observation of the use of accessory muscles of respiration and diaphoresis. It is imperative to realize that a silent chest may represent severe airway obstruction.

Therapeutic guidelines are listed in Figure 1. The majority of asthmatic patients can be managed successfully in the emergency room without any laboratory studies other than spirometry. Chest radiographs should be obtained if a complicating pulmonary process is suspected. A complete blood count may be helpful in patients who

TABLE 6. **Risk Factors For Fatal Asthma**

Prior intubation
Previous life-threatening attack
Hospitalization or emergency room visit within past year
Noncompliance with treatment
Psychiatric/psychosocial problems
Recent taper of systemic steroids

are febrile or producing purulent sputum. Theophylline levels should be obtained in patients taking this drug. Arterial blood gases should be measured in severe exacerbations when the patient is too breathless to speak, exhibits hypoventilation or cyanosis, generates peak expiratory flow rates or an FEV_1 30% less than predicted after initial treatment, or is a candidate for hospital admission.

The decision regarding which asthmatic patients can be safely discharged may be difficult in patients with moderately severe asthma exacerbations. High-risk patients (Table 6), those with inadequate access to care at home or inadequate transportation back to the emergency room, and those with prolonged symptoms before they sought care should be considered for hospitalization. Asthmatic patients who demonstrate sustained improvement 1 hour after a beta$_2$ agonist treatment may be considered for discharge. Discharge planning should include continued aerosol beta$_2$ agonist therapy, oral steroids in most cases, a review of proper inhaler technique, an action plan, and follow-up within 1 to 3 days.

Hospital Management

Therapy for hospitalized asthmatic patients is an extension of therapy initiated in the emergency room. Aerosol beta$_2$ agonists should be continued at the same frequency and then tapered as tolerated to every 4 hours. Recent literature suggests that MDIs are an effective alternative to nebulizer therapy; however, MDI technique and delivery may be compromised during a severe asthma attack. Corticosteroids should be administered intravenously in an initial dose comparable with methylprednisolone (Solu-Medrol),

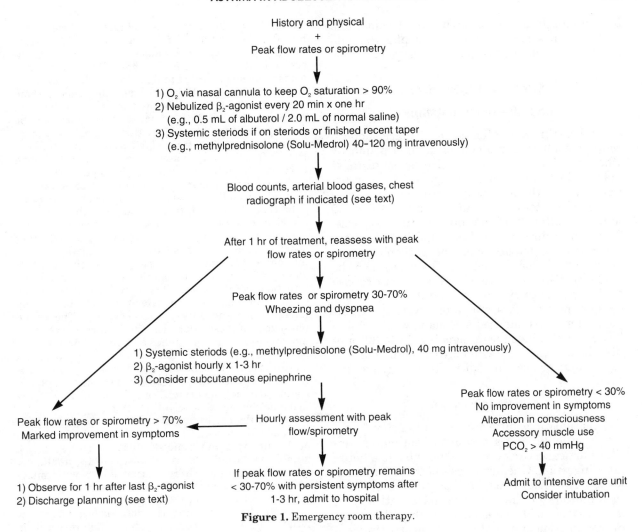

Figure 1. Emergency room therapy.

40 mg every 6 hours, although results of some studies suggest that oral steroids may be as efficacious. Aminophylline currently is not recommended for short-term use in the emergency room but may be helpful for some hospitalized asthmatic patients. Theophylline can be administered orally if the patient is not vomiting or intravenously with a loading dose of 6 mg per kg over 20 minutes (if the patient is not already taking theophylline) and a maintenance drip of 0.5 mg per kg per hour. The first aminophylline level should be obtained 6 hours after the maintenance infusion begins, and the dose should be adjusted to maintain a level of 5 to 15 µg per mL. Supplemental oxygen should be continued as long as required in order to keep the oxygen saturation higher than 90%. Routine use of antibiotics is not recommended because the majority of infection-induced attacks are caused by viruses. Mucolytics and sedatives may be harmful and have no added

benefit. Ipratropium bromide probably adds no additional benefit to beta$_2$ agonist therapy but may be useful for individual patients.

Continued objective monitoring of pulmonary function is required in order to assess the response to therapy and guide further management decisions. This can be achieved by measuring peak expiratory flow rates three times a day and spirometry daily.

Discharge preparations begin with converting to oral medications and ensuring that the patient is clinically stable while receiving inhaler therapy and demonstrating proper technique. There are no well-defined clinical criteria for discharge, but premature discharge can result in recurrent exacerbations, sometimes fatal. Patients should be minimally symptomatic without wheezes, not be awakening to use medications at night, and have a peak expiratory flow rate or FEV$_1$ of more than 70%. Steroid tapering should be determined by the length of stay, prior use of steroids, and prehospitalization severity. Action plans should be reviewed and follow-up care arranged.

SPECIAL PROBLEMS

Exercise-Induced Asthma

Some asthmatic patients, particularly adolescents, may have symptoms of asthma primarily when provoked by exercise. However, exercise may be just one of many triggers for other patients with asthma. Airway narrowing peaks 5 to 10 minutes after exercise and usually resolves 30 minutes after termination of the exercise. Changes in airway osmolality and heat loss are thought to be important in the pathophysiology of exercise-induced asthma. Diagnosis can be made by history and confirmed with an exercise challenge, measuring peak expiratory flow rates or spirometry before and after exercise. Treatment of exercise-induced asthma is with prophylactic use of inhaled $beta_2$ agonists 15 to 30 minutes before exercise. Cromolyn sodium may be substituted or used in addition to a $beta_2$ agonist.

Aspirin Idiosyncrasy

Sensitivity to aspirin occurs in 4 to 20% of asthmatic patients, and symptoms of asthma, rhinitis, or urticaria can develop 30 minutes to 4 hours after ingestion. One hypothesis of the mechanism for aspirin idiosyncrasy is thought to be related to inhibition of the cyclooxygenase pathway in arachidonic acid metabolism with subsequent overproduction of potent bronchoconstricting leukotrienes. Patients with the triad of asthma, nasal polyps, and aspirin sensitivity tend to have more severe asthma, often becoming steroid dependent. It is important to recognize that most nonsteroidal anti-inflammatory drugs can cause reactions in aspirin-sensitive patients and that aspirin idiosyncrasy can develop de novo after years of asymptomatic exposure.

ASTHMA IN CHILDREN

method of
GERALD B. KOLSKI, M.D., Ph.D., and
NICHOLAS A. ORFAN, M.D.
Mary Imogene Bassett Hospital
Cooperstown, New York

Asthma is one of the leading causes of morbidity in infants and children. It is associated with staggering health costs: It is estimated that the direct cost in 1990 dollars in health expenditure for asthma was approxi-

mately $3.4 billion, and the indirect costs were estimated to be another $2.5 billion dollars. These costs are likely to increase because of the continuing increase in the prevalence of asthma. Despite the large sums of money invested in direct and indirect costs for asthma treatment, the rate of mortality from asthma continues to rise. Not only the trends in cost but also morbidity and mortality from asthma prompted the development of guidelines for the diagnosis and management of asthma from the National Institutes of Health (NIH), U.S. Department of Health and Human Services, which became available in August 1991.

The pathophysiology of asthma has become far better understood in the last decade. The current working definition of asthma is a lung disease with the following characteristics: (1) airway obstruction that is reversible (but not completely so in some patients) either spontaneously or with treatment, (2) airway inflammation, and (3) increased airway responsiveness to a variety of stimuli. This definition focuses on the obstruction and its reversibility as well as what has become more apparent in recent years: the airway inflammation and airway responsiveness. The pathophysiology of these alterations in the airway is coming under closer scrutiny. Studies of bronchial provocation, as well as bronchial alveolar lavage, have provided a more dynamic look at the airways of asthmatic patients. Previous work has always focused on autopsy specimens and did not give an understanding of the dynamic changes that occur in asthma.

Most of the experimental studies of the pathophysiology of asthma have focused on the bronchial response of the airway to antigenic stimulation. This antigenic stimulation usually leads to mast cell degranulation. Mast cell degranulation is associated both with immediate release of preformed mediators from granules and with release of secondary mediators. Primary mediators include histamine, chemotactic factors, proteolytic enzymes, and heparin. The initial response is characterized by significant smooth muscle bronchoconstriction and the recruitment of other inflammatory cells, including neutrophils, eosinophils, and mononuclear cells, to the airway. In bronchial alveolar lavage specimens, accumulation of basophils, lymphocytes, and monocyte macrophages has been seen later (4 to 8 hours) in the airway. Lavage of the airways has demonstrated the release of cytokines, as well as of vasoactive factors and arachidonic acid metabolites.

Activation of epithelial and endothelial cells does appear to occur, thereby enhancing inflammatory responses. Release of interleukins-3 to -6, tumor necrosis factor, and interferon-gamma has been demonstrated in the inflammatory response. Release of interleukins-4 and -5 can up regulate IGE production as well as mast cell growth. Interestingly, not all these factors are seen with every challenge. An immediate reaction can be discerned from a late-phase reaction during an antigen challenge. The early-phase bronchoconstriction in asthma is thought to be caused by the primary mediators, whereas the secondary, or late-phase, reaction appears to be caused by recruited inflammatory cells. It appears that this late-phase reaction is the one that causes significant airway damage and leads to increased airway reactivity.

Bronchial hyperresponsiveness is the classic hallmark of asthma. It has been shown that airway hyperresponsiveness can be modulated by a number of factors. Seasonal allergies clearly may render the airway more responsive to other stimuli such as infectious agents, exercise, and irritants. The interplay of various stimuli that affects airway responsiveness mediates episodes of asthma and guides management of individual patients at various times. The recent NIH guidelines as well as expert panels have clearly altered the focus from treating the bronchospasm to treating the inflammatory component of the asthma. Treatment of the inflammatory component is the only way that the physician-patient team can reduce hyperresponsiveness. None of the current medications for treatment of bronchospasm have been shown to significantly alter airway responsiveness.

The diagnosis of asthma is often more difficult in infants and young children than in adults. Some of the mechanisms to evaluate airway dynamics in adults are obviously not applicable in young infants and preschool children. Pulmonary function testing, in which an effort is made to assess airway obstruction and its response to bronchodilators, is dependent on the cooperation, knowledge, and compliance of the patient. In older children and adolescents, the most common measurable parameters used in supporting the diagnosis of asthma include forced vital capacity (FVC), the forced expiratory volume in 1 second (FEV_1) the midexhalation forced expiratory flow (FEF_{25-75}), and their response to bronchodilators. A 15% increase in FEV_1 from baseline and a 20% increase in FEF_{25-75} from baseline after bronchodilation therapy (albuterol, 2.5 mg per nebulizer puff) are believed to be diagnostic of asthma. If there is no evidence of obstruction in baseline pulmonary functions, bronchial provocation challenge may be indicated in order to confirm the diagnosis. Bronchial provocation with methacholine or histamine or, if this is not possible, exercise challenge or hyperventilation of cold air can be used to promote bronchoconstriction. There is a strong correlation between the findings obtained through these various methods. Bronchial provocation should be performed only by clinicians well versed in this technique because there is a risk of inducing severe bronchospasm.

If the child is too young or if provocation tests cannot be performed, there are other ways of assessing whether significant asthmatic episodes are occurring. In infants, a therapeutic response to bronchodilators with improvement in respiratory function, oxygenation, work of breathing, and coughing indicates reversible bronchospasm. Recurrent episodes of wheezing and response to bronchodilators can obviously confirm the diagnosis.

Hyperinflation on chest x-ray is suggestive of small airway disease and mucus plugging. In infants, this is consistent with bronchiolitis or asthma. The onset of wheezing during infancy should suggest some congenital anomaly such as bronchomalacia or impingement on the airway by webs or vascular rings. In children with recurrent pulmonary infections, cystic fibrosis must be ruled out. Asymmetric breath sounds or wheezing should raise suspicion of aspiration of a foreign body. Aspiration of a foreign body may be associated with a gagging or coughing episode prior to the onset of wheezing.

In most children with asthma, certain factors trigger the episodes of obstruction. These triggering factors play an important role in how a child's symptoms are managed. The most frequent triggers for asthma are allergies, infections, exercise, irritants, weather changes, and medications. A stepwise approach for treating children with asthma includes avoidance measures or environmental control, medications and immunotherapy.

Recent reports from England show that early exposure to dust mites during infancy is a predisposing factor for the development of asthma. The level of environmental dust mite antigen was shown to be correlated with the development of asthma. In urban populations, exposure to potent allergens such as cockroach and dust mite antigens may be a major factor in childhood asthma. Animal exposure in suburban as well as urban populations is often associated with the development of asthma. In order to evaluate whether these factors play a role in a child's asthma, specific allergy testing is often necessary. Specific testing is most efficiently, inexpensively, and accurately accomplished through skin testing methods. Allergies in children develop with exposure to allergen. Infants are most commonly allergic to perennial allergens or foods. There is no other time in life when exposure to potential allergens is more repetitive than during the introduction of foods and formulas. As children grow older and begin to be exposed to pollens and the outdoor environment, allergies to these substances may develop. The clinician must be aware of a broadening environment during infancy as well as early childhood. Children may spend time at day care centers, and babysitters and these environments need to be included in any evaluation in order to determine which etiologic factors are exacerbating asthma in a child.

The most effective way to reduce allergen exposure is to focus on the area in which an infant or a child spends the most time. The factors that affect dust mite exposure most dramatically are the moisture, or humidity content, of the environment and the presence of humans. Dust mites need moisture and human dander in order to multiply. In addition to promoting dust mite growth, moisture is also a factor in increasing mold growth and, consequently, mold exposure. Molds and dust mites are common exacerbating allergens in children with asthma. The presence of these allergens is often enhanced by the use of vaporizers in children's bedrooms for acute upper respiratory tract infections. Vaporizers are started during colds but, unfortunately, are often continued when children continue to have symptoms that may be allergy related.

The most effective way to manage dust mite and mold growth is to control humidity at levels below 50% and to eliminate any mold that is present by using half-strength bleach or Lysol. In recent years, a number of allergy solutions and acaricides (mite killers) have been developed to decrease the content of dust mites in the environment and limit their regrowth. If allergy to animals is a significant problem, pets can be either removed from the environment or washed once per week to reduce dander shedding. Alternatively, dander allergenicity can be reduced by using special sprays on furniture and rugs to denature the allergenic protein. In almost all circumstances, pets should be banned from the children's environments or limited to areas where the children spend very little time. If a child comes in contact with the animals, he or she should wash thoroughly and should especially avoid the animals when he or she is wearing pajamas.

In addition to the perennial allergens just discussed, cigarette smoke has been shown to be potent factor in increasing respiratory problems in children. Passive smoke from maternal smoking has been associated with a two- to three-fold increase in number of respiratory illnesses as well as asthma problems. Cigarette smoke is an irritant that not only promotes bronchospasm but also increases mucus production as well as decreases mucociliary clearance, thus predisposing to infection.

In trying to decide which medications may be necessary to treat asthmatic children, it is important to focus on three factors: (1) the severity of the illness, (2) the frequency of the asthmatic episodes, and (3) the effect of the treatment on function in school or home. International investigations of asthma have focused on trying to treat the symptoms in the most effective manner without predisposing patients to secondary consequences of toxicity or increased morbidity.

PHARMACOLOGIC MANAGEMENT

Cromolyn Sodium

Cromolyn sodium (Intal), or disodium cromoglycate, is an effective first-line treatment of asthma. It focuses on the inflammatory component of the asthmatic process and acts as a mast cell stabilizer. It appears to have the effect of preventing both the early- and late-phase reactions in bronchial provocation tests. It is well tolerated and available in a number of preparations for use as an inhalant. It is the only pharmacologic agent without any long-term side effects or any significant association with morbidity or mortality.

Cromolyn sodium can be used prophylactically approximately 5 to 10 minutes before exercise or allergy exposure. It can also be used chronically to decrease airway hyperresponsiveness by use three or four times per day in inhaled form either as a metered-dose inhaler powder or as a nebulized preparation. The inhaled powder does contain lactose, and so it can cause problems in lactose-intolerant people. It also can cause a significant irritant cough in some patients. Because it is a preventive medicine, compliance is often a problem. Patients do not experience any immediate benefit from its use, and irregular use results in inadequate therapeutic benefit.

Cromolyn sodium is effective in children, especially in those with significant atopy. It has been used in infants, toddlers, and adolescents without side effects. When delivered in a metered-dose inhaler, it can be used with a spacer to increase delivery to the lung. The normal dose is two inhalations given three or four times per day. As a preparation for nebulization, it is available in (unit dose) glass ampules to be used either by itself or with bronchodilators. Because cromolyn sodium for nebulization is made with distilled water, some patients experience an immediate decrease in pulmonary function (bronchoconstriction) if cromolyn sodium is used alone.

Corticosteroids

With the recognition that asthma has a significant inflammatory component, corticosteroids have become widely used as potent anti-inflammatory agents. In addition to an anti-inflammatory effect, they appear to restore beta$_2$-adrenergic responsiveness. They are effective in inhibiting release of arachidonic acid and production of secondary mediators. In most studies, they have an effect on the late-phase allergic reaction but not on the early-phase reaction. Numerous topical formulations are available in the United States, including beclomethasone (Vanceril, Beclovent), flunisolide (Aerobid), and triamcinolone (Azmacort). These agents, when used in prescribed doses, are usually not associated with significant adrenal suppression. However, if given in higher doses, they can cause significant adrenal suppression and have been associated with the development of cataracts. They have been shown to have a significant effect on airway responsiveness and, along with cromolyn sodium, are the only agents that appear to decrease airway responsiveness.

The different preparations have different dosing recommendations, but for the most part, two inhalations from two to four times per day are required. If adequate control of asthma cannot be maintained with inhaled corticosteroids or cromolyn sodium, oral corticosteroids may be necessary. At present, these medications can be given in the form of oral prednisone, oral prednisolone, or oral methylprednisolone. A short course of oral steroids can be administered, beginning with approximately 2 mg per kg per day and then tapering over 7 to 10 days. If a patient continues to experience relapse on short courses of steroids, chronic alternate-day corticosteroids may be needed. These should be given at the lowest possible dose that maintains control of the asthma. Oral corticosteroids are available in tablets as well as in liquid preparations, and the dosing guidelines just outlined should be followed according to the known concentration of steroid in each preparation. In children, because of the effects on growth as well as hormonal function, it is important to find the lowest effective dose of inhaled or oral corticosteroids. In order to maximize the benefits of inhaled corticosteroids, a spacer, which allows better delivery to the lung, should be used. In infants, an aerochamber with a face mask is available. The parents should be cautioned that rinsing the mouth after using inhaled corticosteroids is important in that it reduces the incidence of oral thrush.

Beta-Adrenergic Agonists

The beta-adrenergic agonists have been the focus of major discussions in the past few years. These drugs are potent bronchodilators, and the newer agents have longer durations of action. With the development of more selective beta$_2$ agents, there has been considerable impetus to use these as the primary agents in the treatment of asthma. Because the relatively short-acting isoproterenol and isoetharine have less selectivity, most pulmonologists and allergists have preferred the more selective beta$_2$ agents metaproterenol (Alupent, Metaprel), albuterol (Ventolin, Proventil), terbutaline (Brethine), and pirbuterol (Maxair). Although these agents have been shown to be fairly effective in reversing bronchospasm, no studies have shown them to be potent anti-inflammatory agents. Because these agents are not anti-inflammatory agents, they appear to be unable to reduce airway responsiveness and should not be used regularly for a prolonged period of time without some anti-inflammatory preparation (either corticosteroids or cromolyn sodium). They are the most effective agents for reversing immediate bronchospasm and can be delivered orally as well as by inhalation.

The inhalation route allows the administration of these agents via nebulizer or metered-dose inhaler. The use of inhaled preparations minimizes the side effects that are often seen with the oral preparations. The oral preparations are frequently associated with significant tremor, nervousness, and palpitations, as well as occasional gastrointestinal upset. The oral beta agonists are often used in infants and small children, in whom the use of inhalers or nebulizers is difficult or ineffective. Overuse of these agents has been associated with increased rates of mortality from asthma. Results of recent studies indicate that the use of more than one canister per month is associated with a two- to fivefold increase in the rate of mortality from some of these agents. If used in a metered-dose inhaler, they should be used with a spacer to maximize benefit and minimize side effects. If they are to be used with a nebulizer, they should be mixed with normal saline or cromolyn sodium. A number of air compressors are available for nebulization. Suggested dosing for beta agonist preparations is shown in Table 1. In older children, oral slow-release pills are available. However, like the liquid preparations, they should be used in the manner outlined earlier.

Use of systemic adrenaline or epinephrine may be accomplished by prescribing epinephrine preparations (EpiPen, Ana-Kit). These are recommended for patients who respond with anaphylaxis to insect stings or to other agents such as foods, but they are not recommended for use in the chronic management of asthma. In rare situations, home administration of epinephrine is necessary.

Theophylline

Since 1990, the methyxanthines have fallen into disrepute. This has been the result primarily of actions by clinical lawyers' associations and numerous successful civil suits against physicians and hospitals for theophylline toxicity. Despite these developments, there is still considerable evidence that these preparations benefit children with asthma. Like the beta-adrenergic agents, the theophylline preparations do not have a marked anti-inflammatory role and appear to be effective primarily as bronchodilators. Because of the slow-release characteristics of numerous preparations, these medications offer the advantage of long duration of action. This may obviate the need for inhalation devices and the cooperation and coordination of the patient that are required for inhaling medications properly.

A number of studies have called into question the effects on behavior that have previously been attributed to theophylline, especially in terms of school performance. Certain patients appear to be stimulated by, and have some tremor as well as nausea and vomiting with, these preparations. In order to minimize these side effects, lower doses than were historically prescribed may be used. The therapeutic index is fairly narrow, and frequently theophylline is effective at doses achieving serum levels as low as 5 to 10 μg per mL. Most serious toxic reactions to theophylline, such as seizures, arrhythmias, and death, occur at serum levels above 30 μg per mL; however, even at lower serum levels, theophylline seems to reduce the seizure threshold. The availability of the longer acting beta$_2$ agonists as well as the emphasis on anti-inflammatory therapy for asthma has recently discouraged use of theophylline as first-line therapy. It is possible, however, that the increased mortality rate noted with chronic beta agonist use may prompt a resumption of the cautious use of theophylline. Table 2 shows some guidelines for theophylline dosing. The goal, however, is to maintain theophylline serum levels in the range of 5 to 15 μg per mL.

TABLE 1. **Dosages for Therapy in Childhood Asthma**

Beta$_2$ Agonists

Inhaled

Examples: Albuterol, metaproterenol, bitolterol, terbutaline, pirbuterol

MODE OF ADMINISTRATION

MDI	2 puffs q 4–6 h
Dry powder inhaler	1 capsule q 4–6 h
Nebulizer solution*	Albuterol, 5 mg/mL; 0.1–0.15 mg/kg in 2 mL of saline q 4–6 hours; maximum, 5.0 mg
	Metaproterenol 50 mg/mL; 0.25–0.50mg/kg in 2 mL of saline q 4–6 h; maximum, 15.0 mg

Oral

LIQUIDS

Albuterol	0.1–0.15 mg/kg q 4–6 h
Metaproterenol	0.3–0.5 mg/kg q 4–6 h

TABLETS

Albuterol	2- or 4-mg tablet, q 4–6 h
	4-mg sustained-release tablet q 12 h
Metaproterenol	10- or 20-mg tablet q 4–6 h
Terbutaline	2.5- or 5.0-mg tablet q 4–6 h

Cromolyn Sodium

MDI	1 mg/puff; 2 puffs bid-qid
Dry powder inhaler	20 mg/capsule; 1 capsule bid-qid
Nebulizer solution	20 mg/2 mL ampule; 1 ampule bid-qid

Theophylline

Liquid
Tablets, capsules
Sustained-release tablets, capsules
Dosage to achieve serum concentration of 5–15 μg/mL

Corticosteroids

Inhaled†

Beclomethasone	42 μg/puff 2–4 puffs bid-qid
Triamcinolone	100 μg/puff 2–4 puffs bid-qid
Flunisolide	250 μg/puff 2–4 puffs bid

Oral‡

LIQUIDS

Prednisone	5 mg/5 mL
Prednisolone	5 mg/5 mL
	15 mg/5 mL

TABLETS

Prednisone	1, 2.5, 5, 10, 20, 25, 50 mg
Prednisolone	5 mg
Methylprednisolone	2, 4, 8, 16, 24, 32 mg

*Premixed solutions are available. It is suggested that the per kg dosage recommendations be followed.

†Consider use of spacer devices to minimize local adverse effects.

‡For acute exacerbations, doses of 1–2 mg/kg in single or divided doses are used initially and are then modified. Reassess in 3 days, as only a short burst may be needed. There is no need to taper a short (3- to 5-day) course of therapy. If therapy extends beyond this period, it may be appropriate to taper the dosage. For chronic dosage, the lowest possible alternate-day morning dosage should be established.

Abbreviation: MDI = metered-dose inhaler.

From National Institutes of Health, U.S. Department of Health and Human Services: Executive Summary: Guidelines for the Diagnosis and Management of Asthma. Washington, DC, U.S. Government Printing Office, 1991.

Other Preparations

Anticholinergics. Anticholinergic agents such as ipratropium bromide (Atrovent) have been available in the United States since the late 1980s. These agents appear to have some bronchodilator capability as well as the ability to decrease mucus production. They have been fairly effective in adults, especially those with chronic bronchitis, and appear to have the most potent effects on large airways. They may be therapeutically additive with the beta agonists and may have an effect on irritant-induced asthma. Ipratropium bromide is available only in a metered-dose inhaler and is not approved for use in children.

Antihistamines. The Academy of Allergy and Immunology and most practicing physicians have found that antihistamines (despite the labels from most pharmaceutical companies) do not exacerbate asthma and may be used in patients with severe allergic as well as asthmatic symptoms. They are most effective in situations in which significant allergic rhinitis causes difficulty with nasal breathing and effective control of upper airway disease is required. H$_1$ antihistamines are available in numerous preparations. Clinicians should note that none of the new long acting, nonsedating antihistamines (terfenadine [Seldane], astemizole [Hismanal]) are approved for use in children, and they must be used with caution because they have been linked to significant cardiac arrhythmias in overdose and drug-interaction situations.

OVERALL MANAGEMENT OF ASTHMA IN CHILDREN

Children who have relatively mild asthma with only intermittent wheezing and no significant alterations in pulmonary status at baseline can be treated with inhaled beta agonists. Children less than 5 years of age may receive doses either with a nebulizer or with a metered-dose inhaler and a face mask. If neither of these are possible, oral beta agonist syrups are available. If the asthma symptoms necessitate treatment several times a day or frequently in a given week, some effort should be made to use cromolyn sodium or corticosteroids as anti-inflammatory agents. The NIH guidelines for drug therapy are presented in Table 1.

The charts shown in Figures 1 and 2 outline the management of children with chronic moderate or severe asthma. It is important to understand both the treatment of bronchospasm and the treatment of airway inflammation. The goal should always be to minimize the use of the beta agonists for chronic therapy by controlling airway

TABLE 2. **Dosages of Drugs in Acute Exacerbations of Asthma in Children**

Drug	Available Form	Dosage	Comment
Inhaled Beta₂ Agonist			
Albuterol			
Metered-dose inhaler	90 μg/puff	2 inhalations every 5 min for total of 12 puffs, with monitoring of PEFR or FEV$_1$ to document response	If not improved, switch to nebulizer; if improved, decrease to 4 puffs every h
Nebulizer solution	0.5% (5 mg/mL)	0.1–0.15 mg/kg/dose up to 5 mg every 20 min for 1–2 h (minimum dose, 1.25 mg/dose) 0.5 mg/kg/h by continuous nebulization (maximum, 15 mg/hour)	If improved, decrease to 1–2 h; if not improved, use by continuous inhalation
Metaproterenol			
Metered-dose inhaler	650 μg/puff	2 inhalations	Frequent high-dose administration has not been evaluated. Metaproterenol is not interchangeable with beta₂ agonists albuterol and terbutaline
Nebulizer solution	5% (50 mg/mL)	0.1–0.3 mL (5–15 mg); do not exceed 15 mg	
	0.6% unit dose vial of 2.5 mL (15 mg)	As above 5–15 mg; do not exceed 15 mg	
Terbutaline			
Metered-dose inhaler	200 μg/puff	2 inhalations every 5 min for a total of 12 puffs	
Injectable solution used in nebulizer	0.1% (1 mg/1 mL) solution in 0.9% NaCl solution for injection Not FDA approved for inhalation		Not recommended as not available as nebulizer solution; offers no advantage over albuterol, which is available as nebulizer solution
Systemic Beta Agonist			
Epinephrine HCl	1:1000 (1 mg/mL)	0.01 mg/kg up to 0.3 mg subcutaneously every 20 min for 3 doses	Inhaled beta₂ agonist preferred
Terbutaline	(0.1%) 1 mg/mL solution for injection in 0.9% NaCl	Subcutaneous 0.01 mg/kg up to 0.3 mg every 2–6 h as needed; intravenous 10 μg/kg over 10 min loading dose; maintenance: 0.4 μg/kg/min; increase as necessary by 0.2 μg/kg/min and expect to use 3–6 μg/kg/min	Inhaled beta₂ agonist preferred
Methylxanthines			

Theophylline	Aminophylline (80% anhydrous theophylline)	Loading dose:* If theophylline concentration known: every 1 mg/kg of aminophylline gives 2 μg/mL increase in concentration
		Loading dose:* If theophylline concentration is unknown: 6 mg/kg aminophylline (no previous theophylline); 3 mg/kg aminophylline (previous theophylline)
		Constant Infusion Rates:* Infusion rates to obtain a mean steady-state concentration of 15 μg/mL, by age:
		  1–6 months
		  6 months–1 year
		  1–9 years
		  10–16 years
			
			0.5 mg/kg/h aminophylline
			1.0 mg/kg/h aminophylline
			1.5 mg/kg/h aminophylline
			1.2 mg/kg/h aminophylline

Corticosteroids			
Outpatients	Oral prednisone, prednisolone, or methylprednisolone	1–2 mg/kg/day in single or divided doses	Reassess at 3 days as only a short burst may be needed; no need to taper dose
Emergency Department or hospitalized patients	Methylprednisolone IV or PO	1–2 mg/kg/dose every 6 h for 24 h then 1–2 mg/kg/day in divided doses q 8–12 h	Length depends on response; may only need a few days

*Check serum concentration at approximately 1, 12, and 24 h after starting the infusion.

Abbreviations: PEFR = peak expiratory flow rate; FEV$_1$ = forced expiratory volume in 1 second; IV = intravenous; PO = per os (orally).

From National Institutes of Health, U.S. Department of Health and Human Services: Executive Summary: Guidelines for the Diagnosis and Management of Asthma. Washington, DC, U.S. Government Printing Office, 1991.

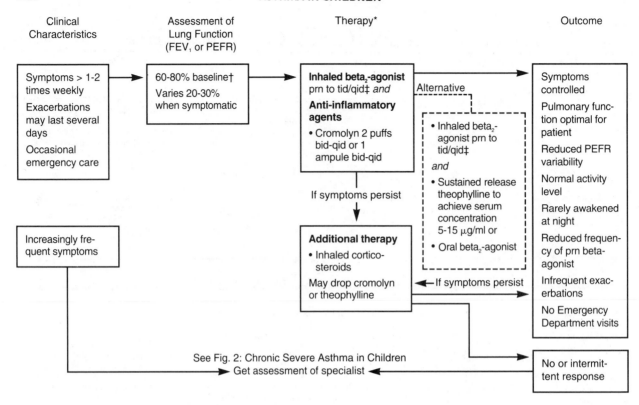

*All therapy must include patient education about prevention (including environmental control where appropriate) as well as control of symptoms.

†PEFR % baseline refers to the norm for the individual, established by the clinician. This may be % predicted based on standardized norms or % patient's personal best.

‡If exceed 3-4 doses a day, consider additional therapy other than inhaled beta₂-agonist.

Figure 1. Management of asthma in children: chronic moderate asthma. *Abbreviations:* FEV_1 = forced expiratory volume in 1 second; PEFR = peak expiratory flow rate. (From National Institutes of Health, U.S. Department of Health and Human Services: Executive Summary: Guidelines for the Diagnosis and Management of Asthma. Washington, DC, U.S. Government Printing Office, 1991.)

inflammation. Peak flowmeters should be available in most primary care physicians' offices so that they can assess the degree of airway obstruction in older children and adolescents. The clinical examination often does not show evidence of wheezing even when significant obstruction is evident on peak flow or pulmonary function testing. In these situations, many patients have significant nocturnal (or exercise-provoked) symptoms. If inhaled steroids and cromolyn sodium are not effective, oral theophylline and oral corticosteroids may be necessary in order to help control symptoms. The goal of therapy should always be to normalize a patient's lifestyle and allow for restful sleep and participation in sports activities.

In acute exacerbations of asthma, it is important to measure a patient's respiratory parameters in order to assess asthma severity. Severity can be estimated by observing the patient's color, use of accessory muscles, inspiration and expiration on auscultation, and central nervous system status. These clinical indicators should be used

in conjunction with measures of oxygenation such as pulse oximetry, as well as lung function as measured by peak flows. After severity is assessed, management in the hospital setting or emergency room should start with oxygen. Enough oxygen should be given to keep an arterial oxygen saturation greater than 95%. The guidelines for asthma therapy given in the accompanying charts shown in Figures 3 and 4 were developed by an NIH task force.

In the acute situation, nebulized beta agonists have been given on a continuous basis or as often as every 20 minutes. Caution must be used because of the hypokalemia that accompanies beta agonist use and overuse. Cardiac monitoring should be available if more frequent beta agonist use is anticipated. Dosing for acute asthma is shown in Table 2. Most emergency room studies have shown that use of corticosteroids in the emergency room decreases the likelihood that asthmatic patients who are discharged from the emergency room will return. If a patient is to be

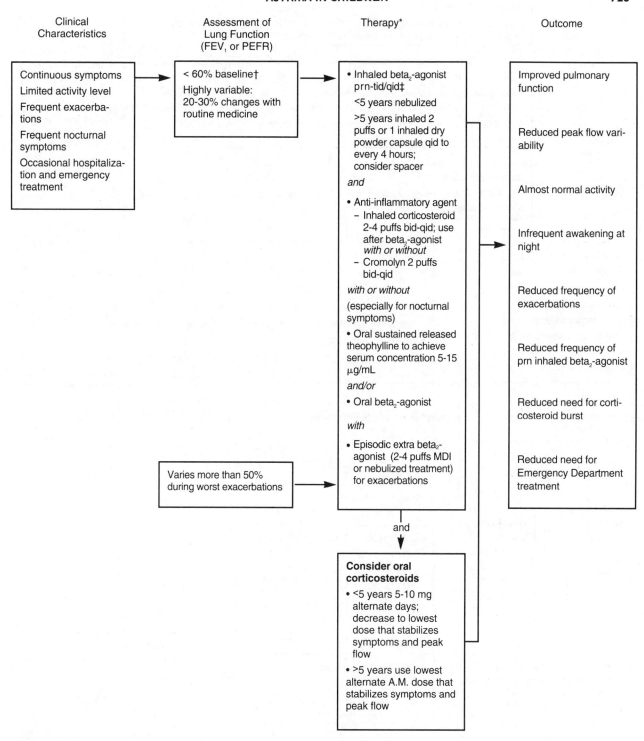

| Clinical Characteristics | Assessment of Lung Function (FEV₁ or PEFR) | Therapy* | Outcome |

Clinical Characteristics:
- Continuous symptoms
- Limited activity level
- Frequent exacerbations
- Frequent nocturnal symptoms
- Occasional hospitalization and emergency treatment

Assessment of Lung Function (FEV₁ or PEFR):
- < 60% baseline†
- Highly variable: 20-30% changes with routine medicine

- Varies more than 50% during worst exacerbations

Therapy*:
- Inhaled beta₂-agonist prn-tid/qid‡
  - <5 years nebulized
  - >5 years inhaled 2 puffs or 1 inhaled dry powder capsule qid to every 4 hours; consider spacer

  and

- Anti-inflammatory agent
  - Inhaled corticosteroid 2-4 puffs bid-qid; use after beta₂-agonist *with or without*
  - Cromolyn 2 puffs bid-qid

  with or without

  (especially for nocturnal symptoms)

- Oral sustained released theophylline to achieve serum concentration 5-15 μg/mL

  and/or

- Oral beta₂-agonist

  with

- Episodic extra beta₂-agonist (2-4 puffs MDI or nebulized treatment) for exacerbations

and

Consider oral corticosteroids
- <5 years 5-10 mg alternate days; decrease to lowest dose that stabilizes symptoms and peak flow
- >5 years use lowest alternate A.M. dose that stabilizes symptoms and peak flow

Outcome:
- Improved pulmonary function
- Reduced peak flow variability
- Almost normal activity
- Infrequent awakening at night
- Reduced frequency of exacerbations
- Reduced frequency of prn inhaled beta₂-agonist
- Reduced need for corticosteroid burst
- Reduced need for Emergency Department treatment

NOTE: Individuals with severe asthma should be evaluated by an asthma specialist.

*All therapy must include patient education about prevention (including environmental control where appropriate) as well as control of symptoms.

†PEFR % baseline refers to the norm for the individual, established by the clinician. This may be % predicted of standardized norms or % patient's personal best.

‡If exceed 3-4 doses a day, consider additional therapy other than inhaled beta₂-agonist.

Figure 2. Management of asthma in children: chronic severe asthma. *Abbreviations:* FEV₁ = forced expiratory volume in 1 second; PEFR = peak expiratory flow rate; MDI = metered-dose inhaler. (From National Institutes of Health, U.S. Department of Health and Human Services: Executive Summary: Guidelines for the Diagnosis and Management of Asthma. Washington, DC, U.S. Government Printing Office, 1991.)

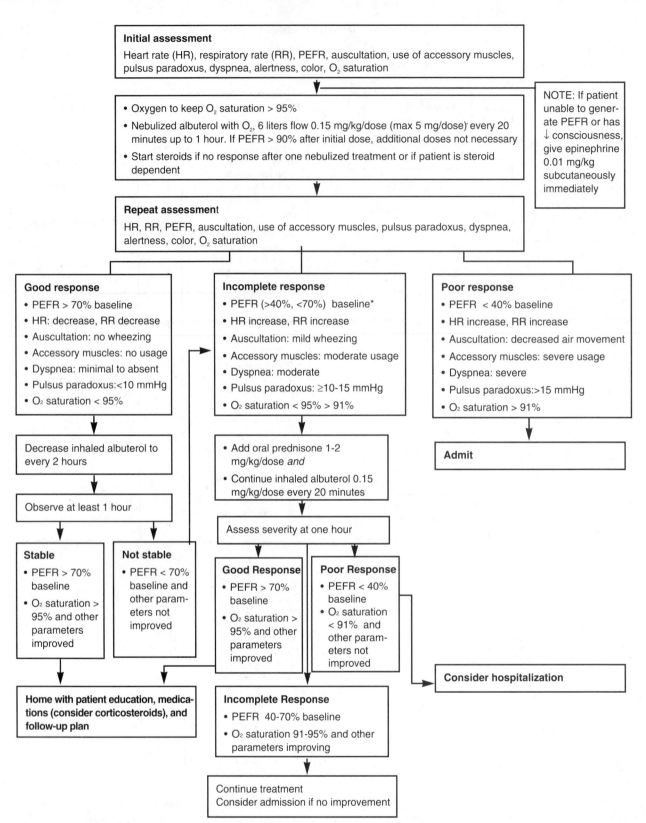

Initial assessment

Heart rate (HR), respiratory rate (RR), PEFR, auscultation, use of accessory muscles, pulsus paradoxus, dyspnea, alertness, color, O_2 saturation

- Oxygen to keep O_2 saturation > 95%
- Nebulized albuterol with O_2, 6 liters flow 0.15 mg/kg/dose (max 5 mg/dose) every 20 minutes up to 1 hour. If PEFR > 90% after initial dose, additional doses not necessary
- Start steroids if no response after one nebulized treatment or if patient is steroid dependent

NOTE: If patient unable to generate PEFR or has ↓ consciousness, give epinephrine 0.01 mg/kg subcutaneously immediately

Repeat assessment

HR, RR, PEFR, auscultation, use of accessory muscles, pulsus paradoxus, dyspnea, alertness, color, O_2 saturation

Good response
- PEFR > 70% baseline
- HR: decrease, RR decrease
- Auscultation: no wheezing
- Accessory muscles: no usage
- Dyspnea: minimal to absent
- Pulsus paradoxus:<10 mmHg
- O_2 saturation < 95%

Incomplete response
- PEFR (>40%, <70%) baseline*
- HR increase, RR increase
- Auscultation: mild wheezing
- Accessory muscles: moderate usage
- Dyspnea: moderate
- Pulsus paradoxus: ≥10-15 mmHg
- O_2 saturation < 95% > 91%

Poor response
- PEFR < 40% baseline
- HR increase, RR increase
- Auscultation: decreased air movement
- Accessory muscles: severe usage
- Dyspnea: severe
- Pulsus paradoxus:>15 mmHg
- O_2 saturation > 91%

Decrease inhaled albuterol to every 2 hours

- Add oral prednisone 1-2 mg/kg/dose *and*
- Continue inhaled albuterol 0.15 mg/kg/dose every 20 minutes

Admit

Observe at least 1 hour

Assess severity at one hour

Stable
- PEFR > 70% baseline
- O_2 saturation > 95% and other parameters improved

Not stable
- PEFR < 70% baseline and other parameters not improved

Good Response
- PEFR > 70% baseline
- O_2 saturation > 95% and other parameters improved

Poor Response
- PEFR < 40% baseline
- O_2 saturation < 91% and other parameters not improved

Consider hospitalization

Home with patient education, medications (consider corticosteroids), and follow-up plan

Incomplete Response
- PEFR 40-70% baseline
- O_2 saturation 91-95% and other parameters improving

Continue treatment
Consider admission if no improvement

NOTE: Therapies are often available in a physician's office. However, most acutely severe exacerbations of asthma require a complete course of therapy in an Emergency Department.

*PEFR % baseline refers to the norm for the individual, established by the clinician. This may be % predicted based on standardized norms or the patient's personal best.

Figure 3. Acute exacerbations of asthma in children: Emergency Department management. *Abbreviation:* PEFR = peak expiratory flow rate. (From National Institutes of Health, U.S. Department of Health and Human Services: Executive Summary: Guidelines for the Diagnosis and Management of Asthma. Washington, DC, U.S. Government Printing Office, 1991.)

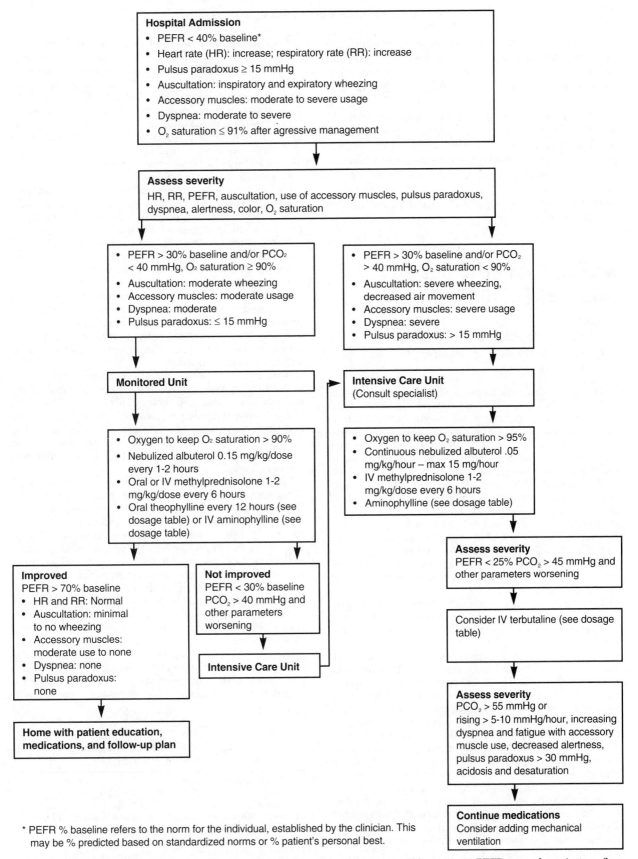

Figure 4. Acute exacerbations of asthma in children: hospital management. *Abbreviations:* PEFR = peak expiratory flow rate; IV = intravenous. (From National Institutes of Health, U.S. Department of Health and Human Services: Executive Summary: Guidelines for the Diagnosis and Management of Asthma. Washington, DC, U.S. Government Printing Office, 1991.)

admitted to the hospital because of an inadequate response to medication in the emergency room, the use of the beta agonists should be accompanied by use of theophylline and intravenous corticosteroids at appropriate doses (see Table 2). If despite maximal therapy the patient continues to deteriorate (i.e., carbon dioxide tension > 45 mmHg and rising, dyspnea increasing, pulsus paradoxus > 30 mmHg), mechanical ventilation may be necessary. Mechanical ventilation should be undertaken only at an institution familiar with the ventilatory patterns needed for appropriate treatment.

ALLERGIC RHINITIS DUE TO INHALANT FACTORS

method of
GAIL G. SHAPIRO, M.D.
University of Washington School of Medicine
Seattle, Washington

Allergic rhinitis is a common disorder; the incidence is 10 to 12% in the U.S. population. It is the most common cause of chronic nasal congestion in children. Its major features are nasal mucosal edema and mucus hypersecretion secondary to an immunologic reaction between environmental antigens and nasal mucosal mast cells and basophils. Although all people have such mucosal cells, only allergic persons have cell-bound IgE that specifically interacts with antigens (allergens) so as to set off an inflammatory event. The conjugation of cell-bound IgE and allergen molecules results in the release of chemical mediators that are capable of causing vasodilation, increased mucosal permeability, increased mucus production, influx of inflammatory cells, and increased sensitivity to subsequent allergen exposure.

This nasal allergic reaction may result in isolated immediate mast cell mediator release. In this case, mediators such as histamine, prostaglandin D_2, N-α-tosyl-L-arginine methyl ester (TAME), and kinins produce direct and reflex-mediated changes in nasal vascular permeability and mucus secretion that are relatively short-lived. In other cases, this early-phase reaction is followed hours later by a late-phase reaction. It is thought that chemotactic mediators from the early event stimulate inflammatory cell influx (e.g., eosinophils, neutrophils) into the nasal membranes. These inflammatory cells play a role in the late phase reaction. Also, basophils, which are present in the stimulated respiratory epithelium, play a major role by secreting more histamine, TAME, and kinins.

Consequently, an allergen exposure creates a disorder that greatly outlives the duration of the exposure. Even days after a significant exposure, inflammatory changes may still be noticeable in the nasal airway.

DIAGNOSIS

Although allergic rhinitis is an extremely common cause of chronic rhinitis, other problems should be considered during evaluation of patients with chronic nasal obstruction (Table 1). Structural anomalies certainly distort airway patency (e.g., severe nasal septal deviation and nasal polyps). Nasal polyps generally emanate from the sinus cavities into the nasal vault. They occur in nonallergic as well as allergic persons. Unlike swollen nasal mucosa, which is pink, polyps are grayish, gelatinous projections that droop down from the upper nasal vault and may appear as shiny globules or as large fingerlike projections.

Hypertrophic, erythematous nasal mucosa may develop secondary to overuse of topical vasoconstrictor nose sprays; this condition is known as rhinitis medicamentosa. Similar-appearing mucosa with purulent nasal secretions suggests infectious rhinosinusitis.

Nasal edema with clear, thin secretions may represent vasomotor rhinitis. This condition is seen more often in adults than in children. Sufferers typically have chronic congestion and rhinorrhea that are exacerbated by temperature changes, pollution, irritating fumes, and tobacco smoke. These irritants appear to provoke symptoms on an autonomic rather than an immunologic basis. Some patients with vasomotor rhinitis complain of copious thin, watery nasal secretions without much congestion.

A condition known as nonallergic eosinophilic rhinitis mimics allergic rhinitis remarkably. Patients complain of congestion and watery rhinorrhea. The nasal mucosa appears pale and edematous, and secretions are thick and clear. Microscopic examination of the secretions reveals mainly eosinophils. In spite of these findings, results of skin testing to common allergens are negative.

The usual features of allergic rhinitis are nasal congestion, rhinorrhea, sneezing, and nasal itching. Some patients complain of constantly feeling as if they have a cold. Some experience itching of the palate or ear as a result of common fifth cranial nerve innervation of the nose and ear canal. Youngsters may habitually rub their noses or make strange facial gestures to overcome nasal pruritus. Dark periorbital circles have been called "allergic shiners."

Allergic rhinitis may be an etiologic factor for chronic or recurrent acute sinusitis as well as for eustachian tube dysfunction and middle ear problems, including infections, effusions, and conductive hearing loss. Allergic rhinitis may be episodic or continual, depending on the spectrum of allergens affecting a patient. When the predominant allergens are pollens, symptoms are confined to pollinating seasons, usually spring and

TABLE 1. **Differential Diagnosis of Allergic Rhinitis**

Infectious rhinosinusitis
  Viral
  Bacterial
Chronic inflammatory sinusitis with or without nasal polyps
Non–allergic rhinitis with eosinophilia
Vasomotor rhinitis
Rhinitis medicamentosa
Structural problems
  Septal deformity
  Tumor

summer. Of course, warmer regions have pollen year round. In general, trees are pollinated in early spring, followed by grasses and then weeds in summer. Ragweed season, the major problem time in the eastern and midwestern United States, extends from August until the first frost, usually in mid-October.

Usually, people with year-round (perennial) allergic rhinitis have sensitivity to dust, mold, or animal dander and may also react to pollen. Aggravating allergens exist in the work place or at a babysitter's home. In taking an environmental history, these factors must be explored (Table 2).

Recent investigations have identified late-phase allergic reactivity after allergen exposure in some persons. These patients have the anticipated release of allergic mediators within minutes of allergen exposure. Then several hours later, they again experience release of mediators and allergic symptoms. In some cases in which recurrent or chronic allergen exposure occurs, there may be a continuum of symptoms as immediate- and late-phase reactions alternate and actually blend together. The late-phase reaction obviously contributes to difficulties in assigning cause and effect to allergic reactions.

Physical Examination

The physician should be aware of previously mentioned clues: nose rubbing, dark circles around the eyes, sneezing, and rhinorrhea. Allergic conjunctivitis may be a concomitant finding that is apparent as injection or edema of the bulbar conjunctiva, sometimes so severe as to produce a gelatinous appearance. The hard palate may show petechiae; these result from negative pressure exerted by the tongue as the patient attempts to scratch the itchy palate, usually producing unique clucking noises in the process.

The typical appearance of the allergic nasal vault is swollen, pale pink mucosa overlying the turbinates along with thin, colorless secretions. This prototype appearance, however, is frequently replaced by a less classic one. The nasal vault may look normal; the mucosa may be erythematous; secretions may be turbid. These deviations may occur because at the time of the examination, the patient is asymptomatic, has an upper respiratory infection, or has a distinctive individual pattern of disease.

Diagnostic Aids

The microscopic evaluation of nasal secretions provides information valuable for making a diagnosis. The patient blows his or her nose into plastic wrap; alternatively, a swab or brush can be used to obtain the specimen. The secretions are wiped onto a glass slide, which is then heat-fixed and stained with Hansel's stain (Table 3). The presence of more than 5 to 10% eosinophils per field suggests allergic rhinitis. However, the less common problems, nonallergic rhinitis with eosinophilia and nasal polyposis (with or without concomitant allergic rhinitis), cannot be discounted. A prevalence of neutrophils suggests infectious rhinitis, most likely related to a viral syndrome if acute or to bacterial rhinosinusitis if more longstanding. If there are watery secretions that yield few cells, vasomotor rhinitis is quite likely, although it is possible that the patient has allergic rhinitis but is currently asymptomatic.

TABLE 2. **Environmental Considerations in Allergic Rhinitis**

Examples of Factors Meriting Consideration	Reasons for Determining
Home Construction	
Heating system	
Radiator	
Forced air	Possibility for central filtering of forced air systems
Wood	Pollutants from wood stoves
Baseboard	Poor air circulation and mold growth from noncirculating baseboard heat
Humidity	More humid, greater likelihood of dust mite and mold
Cleaning Regimen	
Ownership of vacuum cleaner, frequency of dusting and vacuuming, frequency of cleaning drapery and carpet	May influence dust mite population in the home
Household Contents	
Age of carpeting, age of furnishings, quantity of overstuffed articles	The older, the more likely as sources of dust mites
Pets	Source of animal allergies
Bedroom	
Carpeting, window coverings, mattresses	Dust mites likely in carpets, overstuffed mattresses, and furniture
Bedding materials, stuffed toys	Feathers in bedding attract dust mites and are allergens themselves
Ambient Air Quality	
Exposure to tobacco smoke	Pollutants and irritants
Exposure to wood stove	Pollutants and irritants

Allergy skin testing plays an important role in distinguishing the several diagnostic possibilities. Extracts of common aeroallergens are applied to the epidermis in such a way as to reproduce the interaction of environmental allergen and mast cell–bound IgE that occurs in the nose. Initial testing is usually epicutaneous (e.g., prick, puncture, or scratch). A drop of an extract of each allergen in question is applied to the skin of the back or flexor surface of the forearms, and then a needle is used to pierce the skin superficially, enough to bring antigen and mediator-containing cells into contact. Within 15 to 20 minutes, a wheal and flare appear if significant amounts of histamine are released. There is a strong correlation between positive epicutaneous skin test responses to inhaled allergens and clinical symptoms on exposure. Because this testing is not always adequately sensitive, intradermal skin testing may be needed. A small quantity of allergen is directly injected into the epidermis of the dorsal surface of the upper arm. Again, a wheal and flare reaction occurring with 15 to 20 minutes of exposure indicates IgE reaction against the allergen. The correlation of intradermal test positivity and actual symptoms from exposure to a particular allergen is less commanding than for epicutaneous test reactions.

An alternative approach to diagnosis is in vitro measurement of allergen-specific IgE. The patient's serum is incubated with an inert carrier material coated with allergen. Serum IgE to specific allergen reacts with the allergen-carrier complex to form an IgE–allergen-carrier complex that can be radiolabeled and then quantitated. The prototype of this method of testing is the radioallergosorbent test (RAST). In general, such in vitro methods are more costly and less sensitive than skin testing and are rarely preferable. The measurement of total serum IgE has limited value in the diagnosis of allergic rhinitis. Because it is elevated in only about 45% of cases, it is helpful when positive but not when negative.

The decision to conduct skin tests or to treat allergic rhinitis empirically depends on the chronicity and severity of the problem. In some situations, brief courses of antihistamines or decongestants provide satisfactory relief, and no in-depth evaluation need be done.

TREATMENT

Avoidance

The common allergens provoking allergic rhinitis are house dust mites, molds, animal proteins, and pollens. Insect antigens (especially

TABLE 3. Technique of Staining Nasal Secretions

1. Transfer specimen to glass slide, dry, and fix with heat
2. Stain for 30 s with Hansel's stain (1:500 eosin and 1:200 methylene blue in alcohol)
3. Add distilled water for 30 s to take up stain
4. Wash with water
5. Decolorize with methanol or 95% ethyl alcohol (do not over-decolorize)
6. Dry and examine under oil immersion

TABLE 4. Environmental Control Suggestions

Exposure	Intervention
Airborne irritants	Avoid tobacco smoke, wood stoves, noxious fumes; consider problem of off-gassing from pressboard products (e.g., new cabinets)
Dust mites	Remove carpet if possible, use acaricides if not:
	Tannic acid solution 3%:* spray on carpets and stuffed furniture every month (denatures mite and pet antigen, but does not kill mites)
	Benzylbenzoate: spread on carpets every 2–3 months (denatures antigen and kills mites with repeated use)
	Place plastic zippered cover on mattress and box spring cover
	Wash pillow, blankets, and sheets in hot water weekly
Mold	Decrease humidity in home to <50% relative humidity
	Apply bleach-containing cleaners to visible mildew

*Available from Allergy Control Products, 96 Danbury Road, Ridgefield, CT 06877.

from cockroaches) are important in certain parts of the United States. The most effective therapy is avoidance of the inciting allergens (Table 4). In the case of animal exposures, this may represent severe sacrifice: the emotional attachment to pets must be weighted against the degree of disease involvement and relief through other modalities.

House dust mites are ubiquitous microscopic creatures that live off human skin scales. They thrive in climates with high relative humidity, and they avoid ambient daylight. They are therefore abundant in stuffed furniture, mattresses, and carpets, where they leave fecal particles that are more antigenic than the mites themselves.

Dust mites do not survive extremes of boiling and freezing and do not proliferate in dry relative humidity. Their effects may be minimized by such measures as decreasing moisture, removing carpets, and encasing mattresses in nonporous plasticized covers. Hot-water washing of bedding, including pillows and blankets, on a weekly to biweekly basis appears to be helpful (temperature >130° F). Placing unwashable stuffed toys in a hot dryer or a freezer may be helpful, although few firm data exist to validate these measures. Acaricides (dust mite killers) are in the developmental stages but are receiving considerable attention. Benzyl benzoate powder* for application to carpets on an every-6-month basis

*Acarosan available from Fisons Corporation, P.O. Box 1766, Rochester, New York 14603.

is commercially available. Evaluations of its effectiveness are conflicting. It is likely that it must be applied and then left in place for at least 12 hours rather than the shorter time recommended with the product instructions and that it needs to be used more often than the advertised every 6 months. Tannic acid solution (3%)* is also available commercially for application to carpets and upholstery. Although it does not kill mites, tannic acid appears to denature mite and pet antigens, rendering them nonimmunogenic. It probably should be used every month rather than the advertised every 2 to 3 months.

Mold avoidance also involves measures to decrease household humidity. Heating and cooling systems should be checked to eliminate mold reservoirs. A layer of heavy plastic (Visqueen) in the crawl space of a home decreases moisture problems and mold. At times, a dehumidifier may be necessary. An application of liquid laundry bleach removes mold growth on window frames and bathroom tiles.

Pollen avoidance is extremely difficult because these allergens are so widespread at certain times of year. Keeping doors and windows closed and using air conditioning will effectively filter most pollen from the home. These measures are ineffective, however, for people with an outdoors-oriented lifestyle. Similarly, it is impractical in parts of the country in which air conditioning is unnecessary for temperature control. High-efficiency filters (electrostatic precipitators, high-efficiency particulate air [HEPA] filters) remove particulate matter, including pollens, mold spores, and mites. They, too, are most effective if doors and windows are kept closed. The correlation between their use and control of rhinitis symptoms is unclear.

Although environmental control is the theoretical ideal for managing allergic rhinitis, it is difficult to institute and to sustain. The impressive improvement seen in many instances in which these preventative measures have been accomplished encourages patients to continue with these recommendations. Nevertheless, complicated lifestyles involving such confounding factors as rental homes, work environment, dual-parent—and therefore dual-household—custody of children, and day care settings are important factors that force the use of other approaches.

Pharmacologic Intervention

Antihistamines are first-line therapy for allergic rhinitis. They competitively inhibit the al-

lergic mediator histamine at its receptor sites. Although there are both H_1 and H_2 receptors in the tissues of the upper airway, H_1 receptors are most relevant to allergic rhinitis. Antihistamines block both the vasodilation that results from stimulation of the blood vessels by H_1 receptor–histamine interaction and the mucous gland hypersecretion and sneezing that result from reflex initiation caused by the stimulation of H_1 receptors on sensory nerves by histamine. In terms of symptomatic benefit, antihistamines are most effective for diminishing nasal itch and hypersecretion but do not effectively decrease mucous membrane swelling.

Antihistamines are classified on the basis of chemical structure; some newer agents are considered "miscellaneous" because they do not fall into the established six categories (Table 5). Familiarity with a representative drug from each of several classes enables clinicians to alternate among these classes, which is necessary because tachyphylaxis or adverse side effects often make alternative choices necessary. Terfenadine (Seldane) and astemizole (Hismanal) were the first antihistamines approved by the U.S. Food and Drug Administration (FDA) that do not cross the blood-brain barrier. They do not usually cause drowsiness. Terfenadine is FDA-approved in the United States for children over 12 years of age, but it is available in a liquid form in other parts of the world and has been used successfully in younger children. Its potency is similar to that of chlorpheniramine, but it is much more expensive. Although terfenadine is available in Canada and elsewhere as an over-the-counter product, recent reports of QT interval prolongation and arrhythmias, including *torsades de pointes* in patients receiving terfenadine, make the adoption of over-the-counter status in the United States unlikely at this time. These adverse effects appear to be related to increased serum concentration of terfenadine as a result of excessive dosages (>1 tablet twice a day) and to impaired metabolism in the liver, as in patients with known hepatic dysfunction and in those receiving concomitant macrolide antibiotics (e.g., erythromycin or ketoconazole [Nizoral]).

Astemizole differs from terfenadine in having a much slower onset and much longer duration of action. To overcome this, it was in the past sometimes given in a dosage of 30 mg daily for several days to accomplish a loading affect, after which 10 mg daily, the customary dose, was continued. As with terfenadine, high doses of astemizole seem to be arrhythmogenic, and this loading practice is not now recommended. Consequently, patients must be counseled to wait up to 2 weeks before deciding whether it is effective for them. The activity of astemizole is so prolonged that it

*Allergy Control Solution available from Allergy Control Products, Inc., 96 Danbury Road, Ridgefield, Connecticut 06877.

TABLE 5. **Classification of Commonly Used Antihistamines**

Class and Examples	Trade Names	Usual Adult Dosage	Central Nervous System Sedation	Antihistaminic Activity	Anticholinergic Activity
Ethanolamines					
Diphenydramine	Benadryl	25–50 mg q 6 h	Marked	Moderate	Marked
Clemastine*	Tavist	1.34–2.68 mg bid, tid	Marked	Moderate	Marked
Dimenhydrinate	Dramamine	50–100 mg q 4–6 h	Marked	Moderate	Marked
Ethylenediamines					
Tripelennamine	PBZ	25–50 mg q 4–6 h	Relatively mild	Mild to moderate	Mild if any
Pyrilamine*	Nisaval	25 mg q 12 h	Relatively mild	Mild to moderate	Mild if any
Alkylamine					
Chlorpheniramine	Chlor-Trimeton	4 mg q 4–6 h	Mild	Marked	Moderate
Brompheniramine	Dimetane	4 mg q 4–6 h	Mild	Marked	Moderate
Triprolidine	Actidil	2.5 mg q 6 h	Mild	Marked	Moderate
Piperidines					
Azatadine*	Optimine	1–2 mg q 12 h	Mild to moderate	Moderate	Moderate
Cyproheptadine*	Periactin	4 mg q 6–8 h	Mild to moderate	Moderate	Moderate
Phenothiazines					
Promethazine*	Phenergan	12.5–50 mg q 4–6 h	Marked	Marked	Marked
Trimeprazine*	Temaril	2.5 mg q 6 h	Marked	Marked	Marked
Piperazines					
Hydroxyzine*	Atarax, Vistaril	10–50 mg q 6 h	Mild	Moderate	Mild
Cyclizine	Marezine	50 mg q 4–6 h	Mild	Mild	Mild
Meclizine*	Antivert	25–100 mg/day in divided doses	Mild	Mild	Mild
Others (Second-Generation Antihistamines)					
Terfenadine*	Seldane	60 mg bid	Essentially none	Moderate to marked	None to very little
Astemizole*	Hismanal	10 mg qd	Essentially none	Moderate to marked	None to very little
Loratadine	Claritin	10 mg qd	Essentially none	Moderate to marked	None to very little

*Prescription needed (others are over the counter or nonprescription drugs).

must be discontinued a month or more before allergy skin tests in order to avoid histamine-induced wheal suppression. Most other antihistamines must be discontinued for only 24 to 48 hours. The long half-life of astemizole is a consideration in the treatment of women who may become pregnant because this drug, which is not recommended during pregnancy, cannot be readily removed from the system.

Recently, a third non-sedating antihistamine, loratadine (Claritin), has been approved. It is formulated as a 10-mg tablet for once daily dosing. It appears to have a fairly rapid onset of action with activity noted in about 30 minutes and lasting for 24 hours. At this time, drug interactions and arrhythmias have not been a problem.

The oral decongestants phenylpropanolamine, phenylephrine, and pseudoephedrine are alpha-adrenergic agents capable of producing vasoconstriction of nasal mucous membranes that is adequate for reducing edema. They work well in conjunction with antihistamines. Currently, a large number of combination products contain antihistamine and decongestant in one preparation. Although this increases convenience and patients' compliance with medication regimens, it prevents individualized dosage adjustments. However, because little is currently known about dose-response relationships and kinetics of most of these preparations, these fixed combinations remain practical and popular. A particularly popular combination drug is terfenadine, 60 mg, with time-release pseudoephedrine, 120 mg (Seldane D).

Topical decongestants are poor choices for treating chronic rhinitis. With repeated use, they tend to cause decongestion for less sustained periods of time, which leads both to overuse and to rebound vasodilation with increased congestion. This iatrogenic congestion is known as rhinitis medicamentosa.

Cromolyn sodium, long used for asthma therapy, is an alternative to antihistamines as primary therapy for treatment of allergic rhinitis. A 4% solution of cromolyn sodium (Nasalcrom) is used as a nasal spray and may act by preventing release of allergic mediators. The usual dosage is one spray per nostril three to six times daily; each spray delivers 5.2 mg of cromolyn sodium. Cromolyn sodium is effective only as a prophylactic agent, and for best results, it must be used regularly rather than only after symptoms occur. Adverse effects are uncommon and benign and include transient sneezing, nasal stinging, and headache, which remit when the drug is discontinued.

Nasal administration of corticosteroids is an extremely effective therapy for allergic rhinitis. It is usually used for brief intervals when the previously mentioned agents are inadequate. Corticosteroids appear to diminish histamine release and to alter the pathways that lead to the production of mediators from arachidonic acid. Until recently, available corticosteroid nasal sprays were systemically absorbed to a significant degree. Intranasal beclomethasone (Beconase, Vancenase), flunisolide (Nasalide), and triamcinolone (Nasacort) are highly active topically and are very poorly absorbed from the mucosa. The portion that is swallowed and absorbed from the gastrointestinal tract is rapidly metabolized to an inactive form. These new preparations have greatly improved the safety of long-term topical corticosteroid therapy. They are generally used for several weeks during rhinitis exacerbations, although longer treatment periods may be needed during pollen seasons and for especially severe, chronic, perennial rhinitis. Often concomitant therapy with antihistamines and decongestants is continued during this period. The customary dosage is two puffs per nostril two to four times daily, although a once-a-day preparation is available (Nasacort). Most complaints concern nasal stinging and nosebleeds, which remit when use of the drug is discontinued. Perforation of the nasal septum has also been reported but is extremely uncommon.

Systemic corticosteroid therapy is rarely needed for allergic rhinitis. In patients who have severe involvement that appears to be refractory to other therapy, a short course of oral, short-acting steroid (e.g., prednisone) is helpful. Long-term use puts patients at risk of numerous steroid-induced adverse effects, which may well be more worrisome than the initial rhinitis complaints. Intramuscular steroid injection has produced unsightly keloid formation and subcutaneous fat atrophy, which have been the bases for malpractice suits. Injection of steroids into the turbinates has been linked to blindness as a result of intra-arterial embolization of the mixture.

Reasonable certainty about the etiology of rhinitis dramatically enhances success with medical management. A patient with vasomotor rhinitis does not benefit from nasal steroids or cromolyn sodium. Decongestants as well as antihistamines (with their atropine-like drying effect) are most useful. For nonallergic rhinitis with eosinophilia, antihistamines and decongestants may be of some benefit, but topical nasal steroids produce the best results. Nasal polyposis may necessitate a short course of relatively high-dose daily steroid therapy (40 to 60 mg of prednisone each morning for 1 week in an adult), followed by chronic use of a topical nasal steroid. Chronic infectious rhinitis, as with sinusitis, necessitates appropriate antimicrobial therapy in addition to decongestants. Rhinitis medicamentosa necessitates discontinuation of the initiating agent. The use of a topical nasal steroid spray aids in weaning the patient from the topical decongestant.

Immunotherapy

Immunotherapy, also known as desensitization or hyposensitization, is the injection of allergens to which an individual is immunologically sensitive for the purpose of building tolerance to those allergens. Many studies attest to its usefulness, provided that appropriate patients are selected and appropriate allergenic extract and dosing are used. Immunotherapy is usually reserved for allergic patients who continue to have recalcitrant disease after optimal avoidance measures and pharmacologic intervention have been conducted. Many of these patients suffer from sensitivity to pollens that are present much of the year and thus reduce the impact of environmental control measures. Immunotherapy is ordinarily limited to such patients because it is a costly investment of time and money. In view of this, it should be recognized that the chronic use of such medications as nonsedating antihistamines and nasal steroids is a very expensive proposition. The reasonable chance of minimizing such cost with immunotherapy sometimes makes this injection therapy a cost-effective intervention.

Usually patients receive injections once to twice weekly for several months and eventually reach a monthly regimen, which is continued for several years. After this, the majority of patients who have experienced symptomatic benefit continue to do so because of maintained immunologic tolerance to the specific allergens against which they were immunized.

Before immunotherapy is initiated, a patient's sensitivity to allergens should be confirmed by skin testing. Only clinically significant allergens with such skin test verification should be added to the treatment mixture. Therapy is usually confined to house dust, mite, pollen, and certain mold allergens. Evidence for efficacy with mold antigens is limited. Standardized cat antigen for immunotherapy has become commercially available.

Immunotherapy is usually initiated at a concentration one order of magnitude less than that which produces a 5-mm wheal on skin-prick testing. The initial concentration is frequently 1:100,000. Patients receive 0.05 mL of the solution, and subsequent injections once to twice weekly increase to 0.5 mg. Patients then begin receiving injections with the 1:10,000 concentration and progress as before, eventually reaching the 1:1000 and finally the 1:100 concentrations. Then a maintenance dosage (usually 0.2 or 0.3 mL) is selected and given every 2 to 4 weeks. There are many variations of this schedule, but all follow the principle of gradual progression from a diluted to a concentrated antigen mixture.

Benefits of immunotherapy are often achieved in the first year. Most patients receive such therapy for 3 to 5 years. After this time, many of those who have responded seem to retain symptomatic benefit even when immunotherapy is discontinued. Responsiveness is thought to be related to production of IgE-blocking antibodies, down-regulation of IgE production, and decreased releasability by mediator-containing cells (i.e., mast cells and basophils).

Physicians who administer immunotherapy must be prepared to treat anaphylaxis. Patients are most at risk as they progress to higher antigen doses. Nevertheless, anaphylaxis can occur at any time. Life-threatening anaphylaxis occurs most commonly immediately after the injection. For this reason, patients should remain in the clinic for 30 minutes after their injection so that they can be observed for possible systemic complications. Quite commonly, patients experience local reactions at the injection site. If a large immediate- or late-phase local reaction occurs, the immunotherapeutic dosage should be decreased and then increased slowly if reactions diminish.

Approach to Treating the Patient

To apply these therapeutic modalities most effectively, assessment and intervention should proceed in a stepwise manner. Many patients re-

TABLE 6. **Approach to Allergic Rhinitis**

Consider differential diagnosis entities, including allergic rhinitis with secondary sinusitis, which necessitates antimicrobial therapy in addition to allergic rhinitis therapy. If allergic rhinitis is most likely, follow a program based on duration and severity of symptoms.

Recent Onset of Symptoms (e.g., Nasal Congestion, Sneezing)
Oral antihistamines ± oral decongestant
         or
Nasal cromolyn

Persistent Symptoms for Several Months
Allergy history, pertinent skin testing
Institute appropriate avoidance measures
Oral antihistamines and oral decongestant
Nasal corticosteroids

Continuation of Symptoms
Increase environmental efforts
Alternative oral antihistamine and decongestant
Increase dose of nasal corticosteroid
Consider immunotherapy

spond to the first antihistamine that is prescribed; other patients fail to do so or may encounter adverse effects. If a patient requires chronic use of antihistamines and decongestants and is still symptomatic, nasal steroids are a helpful addition. If the patient requires several agents for significant lengths of time, careful attention must be paid to environmental factors that may be precipitating the difficulties. Allergy testing may be helpful at this juncture. The schema in Table 6 represents a stepwise approach to treating patients with allergic rhinitis.

ALLERGIC REACTIONS TO DRUGS

method of
KATHY R. SONENTHAL, M.D.
Cook County Hospital
Chicago, Illinois

and

LESLIE C. GRAMMER, M.D.
Northwestern University Medical School
Chicago, Illinois

An adverse drug reaction is any untoward and accidental response that occurs after a drug is given appropriately for therapeutic, diagnostic, or prophylactic purposes. Between 15% and 30% of patients on medical services experience adverse drug reactions. Allergic reactions to drugs are adverse reactions in which an immunologic mechanism has been demonstrated or is presumed.

There are several risk factors for drug allergy. Sensitization to a drug is more likely to occur after higher doses and longer durations of exposure. Immune responses to drugs often occur in patients with specific human lymphocyte antigen (HLA) phenotypes and with certain drug metabolism susceptibilities. Topical application of a drug is associated more with increased incidence of sensitization than is parenteral administration, which is more sensitizing than oral administration. Allergic drug reactions occur less frequently in children. Patients who have histories of multiple-drug sensitivities tend to have reactions to unrelated drugs. Clinical expression of drug allergies is also influenced by concurrent medical therapy and illnesses. Many physicians think that patients who are atopic are at no greater risk of having a drug allergy than are nonatopic patients.

Allergic reactions to drugs are caused by specific interactions between the drugs or their metabolites with elements of the immune system. Most drugs are low-molecular-weight molecules, so the drug or reactive drug metabolites must combine with tissue, plasma proteins, or cells to form drug-protein or drug metabolite-protein complexes. These complexes must have multiple antigenic combining sites to stimulate a drug-specific immune response and to provoke an allergic reaction. After initial exposure to the drug, a latent period ensues before the onset of a hypersensitivity reaction. This latent period, which lasts approximately 10 to 20 days, is when the drug/drug-metabolite complexes stimulate the production of many immune effector cells and antibodies, causing allergic sensitization. After re-exposure to the drug, the latent period may be very short.

The drugs most frequently implicated in allergic drug reactions include penicillins, cephalosporins, aspirin and other nonsteroidal anti-inflammatory drugs, sulfonamides, iodinated contrast media, anticonvulsants, organ extracts (including insulin), antisera and vaccines, allopurinol (Zyloprim), erythromycin (E-Mycin), antihypertensive agents (e.g., methyldopa [Aldomet], hydralazine [Apresoline]), antituberculous drugs, antimalarials, antiarrhythmic agents (e.g., procainamide [Pronestyl], quinidine [Quinaglute]), enzymes (e.g., chymopapain, streptokinase), biologic modifiers (e.g., interleukin-1), and blood products.

MECHANISMS OF ALLERGIC DRUG REACTIONS

Drug reactions can theoretically fit into one or more of the Coombs and Gell classification of hypersensitivity reactions. Type I, or immediate, hypersensitivity is mediated by IgE antibody. Antigens cross-link the IgE that is attached to the surface of mast cells, which results in mediator release. Clinical findings include anaphylaxis, urticaria, angioedema, and bronchospasm. Type II, or cytotoxic, hypersensitivity is mediated by IgG and IgM. Complement may or may not be involved in these reactions. Clinical findings include immune hemolytic anemia, thrombocytopenia, and leukopenia. Type III hypersensitivity, or Arthus reactions, are mediated by antigen-antibody complexes and complement activation. Immune complexes are deposited in tissues. Clinical findings include serum sickness–type disease. Type IV, or cell-mediated, hypersensitivity reactions are mediated by sensitized T lymphocytes. These are delayed reactions. Clinical findings include contact dermatitis.

Immunologic drug reactions of uncertain or mixed pathophysiology have been described. Skin eruptions are the most prevalent form of adverse drug reactions. There are many cutaneous manifestations, including maculopapular, erythematous rashes, eczema, erythema multiforme, photosensitivity reactions, vesiculobullous eruptions, exfoliative dermatitis, and fixed drug eruptions. Some reactions, including Stevens-Johnson syndrome and toxic epidermal necrolysis, involve both the skin and mucous membranes. The exact mechanism of these reactions is not understood.

Another adverse drug reaction is fever, which can occur alone or in association with dermatitis, vasculitis, or immune complex reactions. A drug fever usually begins 1 week to 10 days after initiation of the drug. Fever may be induced by reactions that release endogenous pyrogens from neutrophils.

Several pulmonary hypersensitivity reactions, including alveolar or interstitial pneumonitis, pulmonary edema, and fibrosis, are secondary to drugs and thought to be immune mediated. Sometimes, eosinophilic pneumonitis can be seen. Immunologic reactions to drugs are also associated with other organ systems. Hepatic hypersensitivity reactions have caused cholestatic or hepatocellular changes. Drugs have been implicated in renal hypersensitivity reactions, including some cases of interstitial nephritis, and generalized lymphadenopathy has been associated with certain drugs.

Pseudoallergic drug reactions behave as if driven by an immune mechanism, but no such mechanism exists. For example, a drug can lead to nonspecific release of mediators, directly resulting in an anaphylactoid reaction. This type of reaction can be seen with the administration of iodinated radiocontrast media (RCM), opiates, and some intravenous anesthetics.

DIAGNOSIS

The diagnosis of a drug allergy is usually based on a detailed history and physical examination. The history should include the time course, manifestations, and treatment of the reactions. It should also be determined whether the patient continued to receive the drug after the onset of the reaction and what the outcome was. It is often difficult to identify the exact drug, because hospitalized adult patients receive an average of 10 drugs during a stay, and outpatient adults receive an average of two regular medications.

In vitro tests used to diagnose drug allergies are not very helpful. The radioallergosorbent test (RAST) is the most commonly used in vitro test for IgE-mediated reactions. This radioimmunoassay detects circulating allergen-specific immunoglobulins, but it often fails to detect circulating antibodies. Another drawback is the very limited knowledge of the drug metabolites that act as antigens.

In vivo testing is the preferred method for diagnosing a drug allergy. This is accomplished by skin testing or careful readministration of the drug, which should be done by physicians who know the testing protocols, risks, and complications of challenging a patient with a potentially allergenic drug.

Skin testing with drugs that are complete antigens and with haptens that are well characterized is the most rapid, useful, and sensitive method of demonstrating IgE antibody, but skin tests cannot assess the risk of other types of allergic reactions, including drug fevers and rashes. Skin testing is limited by the lack of knowledge of all of the relevant metabolites that may cause reactions. It is applicable for high-molecular-weight proteins (e.g., insulin) and for certain haptens, such as the major (produced in large quantities) and minor (produced in small quantities) determinants of penicillin. Skin testing with low-molecular-weight chemicals often produces an irritant reaction that may incorrectly be interpreted as IgE mediated. Skin testing for penicillin is itself often limited by the unavailability of minor determinant reagents that are responsible for many of the allergic reactions. In performing skin tests only with the major determinant, penicilloyl-polylysine (Pre-Pen), approximately 90% of the patients at risk for acute allergic reactions to penicillin therapy are detected.

If skin testing is unavailable, if a drug is essential,

and if no substitutes are available, test dosing should be performed by an experienced physician under controlled and monitored conditions with emergency treatment available. With test dosing, the drug is given by the recommended route and incrementally increased until a minimal drug reaction occurs or a therapeutic dose is achieved. Beginning dilutions can range from 1:1,000,000 to 1:1000 of the final dose, depending on the previous reaction, the experience of the physician, and the drug. Concentrations are usually increased by a factor of 10 until full strength is reached. The rationale behind this procedure is that in an allergic person, there is a dose of drug so low that no adverse reaction occurs and if an allergic reaction does occur, it manifests at a minimal dose with a minimal reaction that can be easily treated.

Skin testing and test dosing can identify immediate reactions, but they do not rule out late immunologic reactions, some of which may be severe (e.g., Stevens-Johnson syndrome).

TREATMENT

The basic treatment for drug allergy is to avoid the drug to which there is a suspected allergy. In most cases, an alternative pharmacologic agent can be found.

After a patient has a reaction to a drug, certain precautions can decrease morbidity and mortality risks. These precautions include the early diagnosis of a drug-related reaction, immediately stopping the drug that is the suspected allergen, and immediately initiating therapy. If a patient is on multiple medications, the drug most likely to cause the reaction should be immediately stopped, and any other essential medications should be switched to non-cross-reacting agents. Agents least likely to have caused the reaction may be cautiously introduced at a later time if there is a definite indication. Symptomatic and supportive care should be initiated after the reaction occurs and should continue until the reaction abates. Anaphylaxis should be treated with epinephrine, antihistamines, corticosteroids, vasopressors, and other resuscitative measures as required. Serum sickness may be treated with antihistamines and corticosteroids. There is controversy about the treatment of Stevens-Johnson syndrome, but the authors believe it should be treated with corticosteroids, at least 1 mg per kg per day of prednisone (Deltasone) or its intravenous equivalent.

Drug Desensitization

The administration of a drug to a patient in whom a drug allergy has been established, who needs that drug for clearly defined medical reasons, and for whom no alternative drug is available can be achieved by drug desensitization. This should not be confused with test dosing. Desensitization is a very hazardous procedure, and it is potentially life-threatening. It should be done by a specialist in a controlled setting, such as an intensive care unit, with emergency therapy available. Drug desensitization involves exposing the patient to increasing concentrations of antigens according to a specific protocol. The initial dose used and the route of administration and rapidity of incremental increases in the dose depends on the drug, the urgency of drug therapy, and the prior reaction. Desensitization is useful for IgE-mediated reactions only during the treatment course for which it is attempted; it does not reduce the future risk of reactions to that drug.

Drug Sensitivities

Beta-Lactams. Penicillin and its derivatives cause almost every form of allergic drug reaction. Penicillin is the most common cause of anaphylaxis from drugs, with a frequency of approximately 1%. IgE antibodies against penicillin decrease over time, and in approximately 50% of patients, skin test results are negative 5 years after an allergic reaction, and in 75 to 80% skin test results are negative 10 or more years after a reaction, which is why skin testing for the major and minor determinants of penicillin is important. Patients who are allergic to penicillin according to history and skin tests should be considered allergic to all semisynthetic penicillins. There is some cross-reactivity in allergenicity to penicillins and cephalosporins, and the risk of a reaction to a cephalosporin in a penicillin-allergic patient has been estimated at 5 to 16%, but it may be as low as 2%.

Radiocontrast Media. RCM is commonly used in diagnostic radiology. Approximately 1.7% of patients experience anaphylactoid reactions to RCM. The true mechanism of this reaction is unknown. Low-osmolality RCM agents seem to decrease the risk of anaphylactoid reactions. This reaction is not IgE mediated, and there are no tests that can be done to predict the risk. Many pretreatment regimens can be used to reduce the risk of a reaction, but a reaction, even a life-threatening one, may still occur. One pretreatment regimen involves the use of 50 mg of prednisone taken orally 13 hours before, 7 hours before, and 1 hour before the procedure; 50 mg of diphenhydramine (Benadryl) taken orally 1 hour before the procedure; and 25 mg of ephedrine taken orally 1 hour before the procedure if not contraindicated.

Aspirin. There are many adverse reactions to aspirin, and there are also allergic-like reactions. There are patients who have nasal polyps and corticosteroid-dependent asthma in whom aspirin or other nonsteroidal anti-inflammatory agents (NSAIDs) trigger severe bronchospasm. Many patients with asthma without a history of aspirin intolerance have been reported to have substantially decreased expiratory flow rates after aspirin ingestion. One theory about the pathogenesis of aspirin intolerance is that aspirin and related drugs block the cyclooxygenase pathway for prostaglandin synthesis and therefore shunt the metabolites of arachidonic acid to the lipoxygenase pathway, which increases the production of leukotrienes. Leukotrienes may mediate the asthmatic response. The treatment of aspirin sensitivity is avoidance, although desensitization protocols may be employed in specific situations. In some patients, urticaria and angioedema develop with aspirin or other NSAIDs.

Insulin. Patients experience reactions to all types of insulin, although human insulin is usually less allergenic than porcine insulin, which is less allergenic than bovine insulin. In about half of all diabetics, some sort of local reaction develops at the site of insulin therapy. Most of these reactions resolve spontaneously with continued insulin therapy and do not necessitate treatment or necessitate only antihistamines. Systemic allergic reactions to insulin are less common, with an incidence of 0.1 to 0.2%. Most of these patients have a positive IgE-mediated skin reaction to insulin. If the evaluation occurs less than 48 hours after the reaction, the insulin dose can be decreased to one-third and then gradually increased until a therapeutic level has been obtained. If the evaluation occurs more than 48 hours after the last insulin injection, desensitization is necessary.

One form of immunologic insulin resistance is associated with high levels of circulating antibodies (mostly IgG) to insulin. It usually subsides after a few months, but cortico-steroid therapy may decrease insulin requirements.

ALLERGIC REACTIONS TO INSECT STINGS

method of
DAVID F. GRAFT, M.D.
Park Nicollet Medical Center
Minneapolis, Minnesota

Systemic allergic reactions resulting from the stings of insects of the order Hymenoptera (honeybees, yellow jackets, hornets, wasps, and imported fire ants) affect 1% of the U.S. population and may be mild, with only cutaneous symptoms (pruritus, urticaria, angioedema), or severe, with potentially life-threatening symptoms (laryngeal edema, bronchospasm, hypotension). Approximately 50 deaths per year are attributed to insect stings in the United States. Only one or two occur in children; the number of deaths increases gradually with age, reaching 10 deaths per year for persons aged 40 to 49, 50 to 59, and 60 to 69 years. The true incidence of insect sting–related fatalities may be even higher because sudden deaths on the golf course or at poolside may be ascribed mistakenly to heart attacks or strokes. The results of the morbidity of insect sting hypersensitivity include alterations in lifestyles, work patterns, and leisure activities to avoid future stings. A large local reaction occurs in 10% of people and consists of swelling greater than 5 cm in diameter that persists for longer than 24 hours.

ACUTE MANAGEMENT

Patients with anaphylaxis require careful observation. A subcutaneous injection of epinephrine (1:1000) at a dose of 0.3 to 0.5 mL (in children, 0.01 mL per kg; maximum, 0.3 mL) is the cornerstone of management and often is sufficient to terminate a reaction. This may be repeated in 10 to 15 minutes if necessary. An oral antihistamine such as diphenhydramine hydrochloride (Benadryl), 12.5 to 50 mg, is also usually given. It may lessen urticaria or other cutaneous symptoms, but in more serious or progressive reactions, its use should not delay the administration of epinephrine. Diphenhydramine (Benadryl) may also be administered parenterally (50 mg in adults; 5 mg per kg per 24 hours in children) for more serious reactions.

Inhaled sympathomimetic agents such as isoproterenol or albuterol may decrease bronchoconstriction but do not address other systemic manifestations such as shock. Aminophylline may be helpful if bronchoconstriction persists after administration of epinephrine. Severe reactions often necessitate treatment with oxygen, H_2 antihistamines such as cimetidine (Tagamet), volume expanders, and pressor agents. Corticosteroids such as prednisone (0.5 to 1 mg per kg per 24 hours) are commonly used, but their delayed onset of action (4 to 6 hours) limits their effectiveness in the early stages of treatment. Intubation or tracheostomy is indicated for severe upper airway edema that does not respond to therapy. Allergic reactions are generally more severe in patients who take beta-blocking drugs. Furthermore, reactions in these patients may be more difficult to treat because beta blockers impede the response to epinephrine and other sympathomimetic medications. Glucagon, 2 to 5 units given over 2 minutes intravenously, may be helpful in this clinical situation.

Systemic reactions commencing more than several hours after a sting are usually manifested in only mild symptoms. Most are easily managed with oral antihistamines and observation. On occasion, anaphylaxis may be prolonged or biphasic. Close observation and continued treatment are essential in these situations. The administration of corticosteroids as early in treatment as feasible may help to diminish later symptoms.

Treatment recommendations for large local reactions include application of ice packs to and elevation of the affected limb and antihistamines. A short course of prednisone (0.5 to 1 mg per kg per day for 5 days), especially if initiated immediately after the sting, may be the best treatment for massive local reactions.

DECREASING FUTURE REACTIONS

Preventing Stings

Future stings can be avoided by taking common sense precautions to significantly reduce exposure. Because many stings in children occur when they step on a bee, shoes should always be worn outside. Hives and nests around the home should be exterminated. Good sanitation should be practiced because garbage and outdoor food, especially canned drinks, attract yellow jackets. Perfumes and dark and floral-patterned clothing should be avoided.

Emergency Epinephrine

To encourage prompt treatment, epinephrine is available in emergency kits for self-administration (Table 1). These are used by insect sting–allergic people immediately after the sting in order to "buy time" to get to a medical facility. The Ana-Kit contains a preloaded syringe that can deliver two 0.3-mL doses of epinephrine. Incre-

TABLE 1. **Epinephrine Injection Kits for Emergency Self-treatment of Systemic Reactions to Insect Stings**

Injection Kit	Dosage
EpiPen*	Delivers 0.3 mL 1:1000 (0.3 mg of epinephrine)
EpiPen Jr.*	Delivers 0.3 mL 1:2000 (0.15 mg of epinephrine)
Ana-Kit†	Delivers two doses of 0.3 mL 1:1000 (total, 0.6 mg of epinephrine)

*The EpiPen and EpiPen Jr. are spring-loaded automatic injectors and are distributed by Center Laboratories, Port Washington, New York.

†Ana-Kit is capable of delivering fractional doses and is distributed by Hollister-Stier Laboratories, Spokane, Washington.

From Graft DF: Insect strings. In Gellis SS, and Kagan BM (eds): Current Pediatric Therapy. Philadelphia, WB Saunders, 1990.

mental doses may also be given. The physician who prescribes this kit must provide thorough instruction and must be confident that the patient can perform the injection procedure. These kits can be confusing to nonmedical personnel, and some patients have a tremendous fear of needles. A practice self-injection with saline resolves this issue. The EpiPen (0.3 mg of epinephrine) and EpiPen Jr. (0.15 mg of epinephrine) offer a concealed needle and a pressure-sensitive spring-loaded injection device that make them suitable for patients and families who are uncomfortable with the injection process. Medihaler-Epi (10 to 30 inhalations; 1.6 to 4.8 mg of epinephrine), may also be used to achieve therapeutic levels of epinephrine in plasma and may be especially helpful for laryngeal edema and bronchospasm. Patients who are receiving maintenance injections of venom immunotherapy are advised that emergency self-treatment will probably not be required; however, they should have the kit available if they are far from medical facilities. The wearing of a Medic-Alert bracelet is also advised.

Venom Immunotherapy

The clinical history is the key to determining the need for venom immunotherapy (Table 2). A careful history discloses the type, degree, and time course of symptoms and often reveals the culprit insect. A patient who has experienced a sting-induced systemic reaction should be referred to an allergist, who will perform skin tests with dilute solutions of honeybee, yellow jacket, yellow hornet, white-faced hornet, and Polistes wasp venoms. Radioallergosorbent testing (RAST) cannot replace venom skin testing but may provide additional information. Whole-body extract materials were used before 1979 to diagnose and treat insect allergy, but they were shown to be ineffective, and venoms supplanted their use. However, to date, fire ant venom has only been available in small research quantities; fortunately, the fire ant whole-body extract material seems more potent than those previously available for the other Hymenoptera species and has been successfully used for skin testing and treatment. If the reaction was severe (potentially life-threatening symptoms of bronchospasm, laryngeal edema, shock) and the venom test result is positive, immunotherapy with the appropriate venom or venoms is commenced. Because the recurrence rate in children with a history of milder cutaneous reactions is only 10%, venom treatment is not required. Patients with large local reactions or negative skin test results also are not candidates for venom therapy.

TABLE 2. **Selection of Patients for Venom Immunotherapy**

Sting Reaction	Skin Test/RAST	Venom Immunotherapy
1. Systemic, non–life-threatening (child): immediate, generalized, confined to skin (urticaria, angioedema, erythema, pruritus)	+ or −	No
2. Systemic, life-threatening (child): immediate, generalized, may involve cutaneous symptoms but also has respiratory (laryngeal edema or bronchospasm) or cardiovascular symptoms (hypotension/shock)	+	Yes
3. Systemic (adult)	+	Yes
4. Systemic	−	No
5. Large local (>2 inches [5 cm] in diameter; >24 hours)	+ or −	No
6. Normal (<2 inches [5 cm] in diameter; <24 hours)	+ or −	No

Abbreviation: RAST = radioallergosorbent test.
From Graft DF: Insect stings. *In* Gellis SS, and Kagan BM (eds): Current Pediatric Therapy. Philadelphia, WB Saunders, 1990.

Increasing amounts of venom are given weekly for several months until the 100 µg dose (equivalent of two stings) is reached. Maintenance injections are given every 4 weeks during the first year of treatment, and then the interval can be extended to 6 weeks. Venom therapy is highly effective, protecting 97% of patients from reactions to challenge stings administered in-hospital (the risk of an allergic reaction for untreated insect sting–allergic persons is probably about 60%). The disadvantages of venom treatment include cost and systemic and local reactions to injections. No long-term side effects have been reported. In about 25% of patients, negative skin test results develop after 3 to 5 years of treatment, and these patients may be able to discontinue therapy. Furthermore, 5 years' worth of venom injections is probably sufficient for the majority of patients; patients who have very severe reactions constitute the major exceptions.

Section 12

Diseases of the Skin

ACNE VULGARIS AND ROSACEA

method of
DONALD P. LOOKINGBILL, M.D.
*Pennsylvania State University—College of
Medicine*
Hershey, Pennsylvania

Acne affects most teenagers and many patients in their twenties and thirties. The pathogenesis involves androgen stimulation of sebum production; keratinous obstruction of the sebaceous follicle outlet, leading to accumulation of keratin and sebum with the formation of open and closed comedones (i.e., blackheads and whiteheads); and bacterial *(Propionibacterium acnes)* colonization of the trapped sebum, inciting an inflammatory reaction that produces inflammatory papules, pustules, nodules, and cysts. Most therapeutic measures are directed toward diminishing outlet obstruction and inflammatory reactions.

TREATMENT OF ACNE

Most of my acne patients are treated with a combination of topical and systemic agents, specifically topical tretinoin (Retin-A), and topical benzoyl peroxide in combination with an oral antibiotic. I instruct patients to apply their topical preparations to the entire area affected by acne (e.g., the entire face), rather than to isolated spots. At the initial visit, I discuss the importance of diet, washing, and not picking the lesions. Because there is no evidence to implicate specific foods in the pathogenesis of acne, I do not recommend any dietary restrictions, except for suggesting a nutritious well-balanced diet. Acne cannot be washed away, but twice-daily facial cleansing is recommended. Specific acne cleansers are not necessary. Most acne patients pick at their lesions, which increases the chances for scarring. I vigorously discourage this practice. Patients must understand that results from therapy require time. I usually schedule the first follow-up visit in 2 months and, thereafter, see patients at 2- to 4-month intervals.

Topical Therapy

Three types of useful topical agents are tretinoin, benzoyl peroxide, and topical antibiotics.

Topical Tretinoin. Tretinoin acts primarily on the abnormal follicular keratinization and is the most effective topical agent in the treatment of comedones. It can be used as monotherapy for the uncommon patient with pure comedonal acne. Tretinoin is available in three different vehicles and a variety of concentrations. The mildest preparations are the 0.025% and 0.05% creams and the 0.01% gel. Intermediate-strength preparations are the 0.1% cream and 0.025% gel. The strongest preparation is a 0.05% solution.

At their first visit, patients are started on the least irritating preparations, which are applied at bedtime. If the skin is dry, the cream vehicle is selected; if it is oily, the gel is preferred. Even with the mildest formulations, irritation may occur, and the patients should be warned. With continued use, the skin usually becomes accustomed to the irritant effects of tretinoin, and if the desired therapeutic effect is not achieved, the concentrations of the tretinoin can be advanced at future visits.

Although tretinoin does not photosensitize, it does irritate the skin, and sunlight may add to this irritation. Use of a sunscreen is advised at times of sun exposure. Because tretinoin is expensive, its use is usually confined to the face.

Benzoyl Peroxide. Benzoyl peroxide affects follicular keratinization and the *Propionibacterium acnes* bacteria. It can be used as a single agent for patients with mild acne. There are many benzoyl peroxide preparations on the market. Some are over-the-counter products, and others require a prescription. Preparations are available in concentrations of 2.5%, 5%, and 10%. Most are gels, some of which are less drying than others. For example, Desquam-E (E for emollient) Gel was developed to be less drying than Desquam-X, and Persa-Gel-W (W for water) and Benzac-W gel are less drying than their parent formulations. Therapy is initiated with the lower concentrations and applied in the morning to the entire facial area. In patients with acne of the upper trunk, benzoyl peroxide may also be used at night on these areas.

Like tretinoin, benzoyl peroxide may cause irritation of the skin, but this effect usually becomes less troublesome with continued use. A patient may rarely develop an allergic reaction to benzoyl peroxide. The severe reaction lasts for many days after discontinuing the drug, unlike the usual time of 1 or 2 days for simple irritation. If allergy occurs, the patient should never again use benzoyl peroxide preparations. All patients should be advised that benzoyl peroxide bleaches bedding and articles of clothing that come in contact with it.

Topical Antibiotics. Topical antibiotics exert their effect on the *Propionibacterium acnes* bacteria. The two major drugs in use are erythromycin (ATS, EryDerm, Erycette, Staticin, T-stat), which is available in gels, solutions, saturated swabs, and ointment formulations, and clindamycin (Cleocin-T), available in a gel, solution, and lotion. We use these agents primarily in patients with mild to moderately severe inflammatory acne who fail to respond to tretinoin or benzoyl peroxide or are unduly irritated by those agents.

Topical Combinations. A combination of 5% benzoyl peroxide and 3% erythromycin in a topical gel (Benzamycin) is somewhat superior to either of the agents used singly. It must be kept refrigerated and is moderately expensive.

Acne Washes. Acne washes are convenient for treating large areas of acne, particularly the chest and back. The two agents that I employ are benzoyl peroxide washes (Desquam-X 10 Wash) and chlorhexidine (Hibiclens). Both agents are effective against the *Propionibacterium acnes* organism, but chlorhexidine is much less expensive.

Systemic Therapy

Systemic Antibiotics. Antibiotics act on the bacteria involved in acne. They may also have an anti-inflammatory effect. Typically, I start patients on twice-daily therapy for the first 2 months. If the acne is well controlled at that point, the antibiotics are tapered over the next several months while maintaining topical therapy. Some patients require long-term antibiotic therapy, and bacterial resistance to a specific antibiotic can develop. Changing to an alternative drug is often useful.

Tetracycline is the antibiotic most frequently employed. It is inexpensive and usually well tolerated. For most patients, the usual starting dose is 500 mg twice daily. Patients should be instructed to take the medication on an empty stomach, because food (particularly dairy products) interferes with its absorption. Side effects from tetracycline are uncommon. Vaginal candidiasis may develop in women, particularly those on birth control pills. Tetracycline has also been implicated as reducing the efficacy of birth con-

trol pills, but this has not been proven. However, if a physician or patient is concerned about this possible interaction, erythromycin is a safe alternative. Photosensitivity rarely occurs during tetracycline use. It more frequently occurs with doxycycline (Vibramycin).

Erythromycin is the second most frequently employed antibiotic. It is somewhat more expensive than tetracycline but still moderately priced. The standard starting dose is 500 mg twice daily or its equivalent. Gastrointestinal side effects are more frequent than with tetracycline, but if this is a problem, many erythromycin preparations can be taken with meals, because food interferes much less with their absorption than with the absorption of tetracycline.

If tetracycline and erythromycin fail, alternative antibiotics can be considered. Doxycycline and minocycline (Minocin), 100 to 200 mg daily, may be somewhat more effective than tetracycline, but doxycycline occasionally causes photosensitivity and minocycline is very expensive. Trimethoprim-sulfamethoxazole (Bactrim) is efficacious, but side effects are of concern, including rashes and rare cases of agranulocytosis. Clindamycin (Cleocin) had been more commonly used in the treatment of acne, before cases of pseudomembranous colitis were reported from its use.

Retinoids. The development of 13-*cis*-retinoic acid (Accutane) revolutionized the treatment of severe, therapy-resistant acne. This agent profoundly shrinks sebaceous glands and reduces follicular hyperkeratinization. Other therapies primarily control the acne process until the patient "outgrows it," but Accutane induces long-term (sometimes indefinite) remissions in many patients. Its use is restricted to nodulocystic acne, severe papulopostular acne, scarring acne, and debilitating acne in patients who have not responded to the treatment modalities previously discussed. The drug is prescribed in a dose of 1 mg per kg daily for 20 weeks. During the first month, some patients notice a flare of their disease. This reaction can sometimes be obviated by employing the drug at half dosage for the first month and advancing to the full dose after that.

Side effects are numerous. Of most concern is the teratogenic effects of this and all other retinoids. Therefore, it must be used with great caution in women of childbearing age. The manufacturer of the drug provides an informational kit that includes consent forms for women contemplating this therapy. Women must be employing effective birth control measures, and a pregnancy test must be performed before initiating therapy and at monthly intervals thereafter. It is critical that physicians and patients who use Accutane be fully aware of its teratogenic risk and follow carefully the guidelines outlined for its use in women.

Other side effects are associated with the use of Accutane. Frequent side effects include chapped lips, red and dry skin, dry eyes (therefore, contact lenses should not be used), and dryness of the nose sometimes accompanied by nosebleeds. Less frequently, patients may develop severe headaches due to pseudotumor cerebri, muscle or joint aching, fatigue, hair loss, and a multitude of other reactions. Because retinoids can increase plasma lipids, blood levels should be monitored. Mild bony exostoses of cervical vertebrae have been detected radiographically in some patients.

Accutane is taken for 20 weeks; after a 20-week course of Accutane, most patients are clear of acne, and many remain so for an indefinite period. Those who relapse do so slowly over the course of many months to years. Relapses are usually milder than the initial condition and can usually be managed with standard therapy. Accutane is quite expensive.

Hormonal Therapy. Because androgens stimulate sebum production, antiandrogen therapy has been employed in acne, but it is reserved mainly for women with androgen excess in whom standard therapy has failed. Women may be suspected of androgen excess if their acne is resistant to therapy or if they have accompanying hirsutism or irregular menses. In such women, I order a free and total testosterone to screen for ovarian hypersecretion and a serum dehydroepiandrosterone sulfate level for adrenal androgen excess. For mild increases in testosterone, estrogen therapy (i.e., birth control pills) may be used, but because the progestin in some birth control pills can have androgenic activity, an unopposed estrogen product should be selected, for example, Demulen. Mild elevations of the adrenal androgen dehydroepiandrosterone sulfate can be treated with a low-dose corticosteroid (e.g., 2.5 mg of prednisone) taken at bedtime.

Antiandrogens have occasionally been employed for treating acne. Cyproterone acetate is available in Europe but not in the United States. In the United States, spironolactone (Aldactone), has been used for this purpose in a daily dosage of 100 to 200 mg.* This agent can improve acne, but women must employ birth control measures (preferably birth control pills) simultaneously because of the theoretical risk of feminizing a developing male fetus by exposure to spironolactone. Other side effects of spironolactone include breast tenderness and break-through bleeding.

---

*This use of spironolactone is not listed in the manufacturer's official directive.

Accutane and hormonal therapy are not first-line choices for the treatment of acne. Most patients respond quite satisfactorily to topical agents and systemic antibiotics.

TREATMENT OF ROSACEA

Rosacea is an acneiform condition that affects middle-aged patients. It is characterized by papules and pustules occurring on a background of erythema and telangiectasia of facial skin. The process tends to affect mainly the middle third of the face, from forehead to chin. Comedones are not typically present. Some patients with rosacea develop the thickened skin and enlarged sebaceous glands of rhinophyma.

Topical Therapy

Tretinoin and benzoyl peroxide preparations aggravate the erythema and are usually not employed. Topical antibiotics can be helpful. Topical metronidazole (MetroGel) applied twice daily is the most effective topical therapy for rosacea. It is applied for several months and then tapered. Recurrences are common and re-treatment can be safely instituted.

Systemic Therapy

As in acne vulgaris, systemic antibiotics are effective in treating rosacea. Lower dosages can often be employed; for example, tetracycline or erythromycin in a dose of 250 mg twice daily. After the first month, the dosage can often be lowered and the drug ultimately discontinued. Recurrences are common, and repeated courses of antibiotics may be needed. Antibiotics are also helpful in treating the blepharitis and keratitis that are occasionally associated with rosacea.

Rosacea that fails to respond to the above measures may be treated with low-dose (0.5 mg per kg) Accutane for a 20-week course. Results are usually good, but recurrences are common.

Surgical Therapy

Medical treatment has a limited effect on erythema and no impact on telangiectasia. If desired, telangiectasias can be treated with electrosurgery or laser therapy. Rhinophyma may be treated with curettage, dermabrasion, or laser therapy.

HAIR DISORDERS

method of
JAMES D. STROUD, M.D.
Wayne State University
Detroit, Michigan

In adults, four types of hair loss account for 90% of all diagnoses made in hair-loss patients. The "big four" are (1) androgenetic alopecia (common baldness), (2) traction/chemical alopecia, (3) alopecia areata, and (4) telogen effluvium.

In children, tinea capitis and trichotillomania are additional important diagnostic considerations. Making the correct diagnosis will allow the physician to effectively manage the vast majority of patients who present with hair loss.

ANDROGENETIC ALOPECIA (COMMON BALDNESS)

Androgenetic alopecia is inherited as an autosomal dominant trait with variable expression. It is caused by the action of androgens on genetically predisposed hair follicles. In men, balding occurs over the vertex and occipital scalp, while in women the hair is diffusely thin.

The ideal medical treatment for androgenetic alopecia is not yet available. Two percent minoxidil topical solution (Rogaine) may help retard further progression of hair loss, but in my experience it is only minimally effective in regrowing cosmetically acceptable new hair. Spironolactone (Aldactone)* can be used in women with androgen excess in doses ranging from 50 to 200 mg per day. Estrogen-dominant birth control pills in young women and oral estrogen in menopausal women may be helpful. Hair transplantation combined with scalp reduction techniques offer a more permanent solution and can be performed in both men and women.

TRACTION/CHEMICAL ALOPECIA

Traction alopecia is common in my practice, particularly in black girls and women. Hair styles that apply tension to the hair for long periods cause alopecia. Most cases, especially in children, are reversible. If the traction is maintained for years, however, as is the usual case, the alopecia may be permanent. Prolonged traction on hair produces fibrosis of the hair root and irreversible alopecia.

Traction alopecia is characterized clinically by noninflammatory linear areas of hair loss at the margins of the hairline, along the part line, or scattered throughout the scalp depending on the type of hair styling procedures used. Hot comb alopecia occurs most commonly around the periphery of the scalp.

Frequently, patients who use damaging hair styling procedures will try permanent waving as a method of styling their hair. This also may result in hair breakage if it is done improperly, if too much tension is applied during waving, if the solution is left on too long, or if it is too strong.

Affected patients should avoid the use of tight ponytails, braids, cornrowing, and nightly rollers and curlers. Patients should be advised to stop all hair straightening procedures and to avoid all other tension-producing trauma. A "natural" hair style is best for these patients. Occasionally, patients may try one of the milder bisulfite home permanents, which are said to be less damaging to the hair.

ALOPECIA AREATA

Alopecia areata is characterized by the sudden onset of asymptomatic, noninflammatory round bald patches located on any hair-bearing part of the body, but most commonly on the scalp. The cause of alopecia areata is unknown, but current theory presumes an altered immune state.

Patients with alopecia areata need encouragement and psychological support. There are many recommended treatments, none of which are uniformly successful, and there is no convincing evidence that any treatment alters the natural history of alopecia areata. In children, first-time treatment is with topical anthralin* cream (0.1, 0.25, 0.50, 1.0%) applied for 20 minutes and washed off. The duration of application and potency of medication can be slowly increased as tolerated. Potent topical steroids can be tried for 6 to 12 weeks. Super-high potency topical steroids can be used for a maximum of 2 weeks, followed by a rest period before reapplication. The most effective treatment for localized areas of alopecia is intralesional corticosteroids. Triamcinolone acetonide suspension, 3 mg per ml is injected by using a 30-gauge, .05-inch long needle. The drug should be injected into the mid to deep dermis, avoiding the subcutaneous tissue. A maximum of 10 mg is injected per visit and each site is injected no more than once a month. It is a good idea to "map" on the chart areas that have been injected to avoid injecting into the same area. Systemic steroids should be used with caution.

TELOGEN EFFLUVIUM

Telogen effluvium is excessive loss of normal club hairs from normal telogen (resting) follicles.

---

*This use of spironolactone is not listed in the manufacturer's official directive.

*This use of anthralin is not listed in the manufacturer's official directive.

The growing hair follicle responds to stress by regressing to the resting telogen stage.

Telogen effluvium is provoked by a host of different stimuli, including high fever, childbirth, severe illness, surgery, hypothyroidism, crash diets, and medications. The excessive scalp hair loss occurs 1 to 4 months after the stressful event. The amount of hair shed daily is in excess of 100 hairs per day and may last for months.

Treatment is primarily by recognition of the precipitating stressful event. The hair will normally regrow fully within 1 year. Treatment of underlying disease states and withdrawal of drugs are sometimes indicated.

TINEA CAPITIS

Every child with scalp hair loss should be considered to have tinea capitis until a negative KOH and fungal culture prove otherwise. The clinical appearance of tinea capitis may vary from a few patches of noninflammatory alopecia to a severe inflammatory process.

Treatment is with oral griseofulvin for 6 to 8 weeks. Supplemental therapy with selenium sulfide (Selsun) shampoo and topical antifungal creams is useful.

TRICHOTILLOMANIA

Trichotillomania is the compulsion to pull out one's own hair. Clinical diagnosis is often difficult and confusion with other hair loss disorders is frequent. A scalp biopsy is very helpful in making the diagnosis.

Most cases resolve spontaneously. Confrontation of the patient may result in improvement. Behavioral modification and psychotherapy are indicated in more severe cases.

CANCER OF THE SKIN

method of
ROBERT E. CLARK, M.D., Ph.D.
Duke University Medical Center
Durham, North Carolina

Cancer of the skin is the most common cancer diagnosed in humans: one in three cancers is a skin cancer. The frequent occurrence of skin cancer in sun-exposed areas facilitates early diagnosis and treatment. Individuals with a previous history of skin cancer, family history of skin cancer, or evidence of chronic solar damage should be examined for these malignancies.

EPIDEMIOLOGY AND ETIOLOGY

Skin cancer commonly affects individuals of the white race. Overall, one in six whites will develop skin cancer in their lifetime. Individuals at highest risk have a fair complexion, sunburn easily, and have blond or red hair and blue eyes.

Behavioral patterns of sun exposure over the past 50 years have contributed to the rising incidence of skin cancer in the white population of the United States. Approximately 80% of the ultraviolet radiation damage to the skin occurs by the age of 20 years. An additional 30 to 40 years is required for transformation of this damage into a frank malignancy. Therefore, prophylactic measures in the early years of life is important in preventing skin cancer, photodamage, and premature photoaging.

The three most common types of skin cancer are basal cell carcinoma (80%), squamous cell carcinoma (12%), and malignant melanoma (4.5%). More than 550,000 new cases of basal cell carcinoma are diagnosed each year in the United States. Approximately 80% of basal cell carcinomas occur in sun-exposed areas of the head and neck and dorsum of the hands. One-third of basal cell carcinomas occur on the nose, and 90% are related to a past history of solar damage to the skin. These tumors originate from the basal cell layer of the epidermis.

Squamous cell carcinoma is the second most common skin cancer. Approximately 130,000 new cases will be diagnosed this year. Squamous cell carcinoma predominantly arises in solar-damaged skin. The increased incidence of metastasis of squamous cell carcinoma necessitates concern for adequate removal of this tumor. Approximately 25% of all deaths due to skin cancer result from squamous cell carcinoma. Squamous cell carcinoma arising on the lower lip, burn scars, chronic osteomyelitis sinus tracts, or leg ulcers have a high incidence (15% to 30%) of metastasis. Fifty to 75% of individuals with metastatic squamous cell carcinoma will die of their disease.

The cell of origin for squamous cell carcinoma is the epidermal keratinocyte. Ultraviolet radiation damage from the sun is the primary etiologic agent for squamous cell carcinoma. This tumor is also induced by ingestion of arsenic in medications or contaminated water. Additional etiologic agents include x-rays, immunosuppressive states, human papilloma viruses, and exposure to chemical carcinogens as found in shale oil derivatives.

Malignant melanoma is the most dangerous type of skin cancer. Thirty-two thousand new cases of invasive malignant melanoma will be diagnosed this year with an additional 6300 cases of malignant melanoma in situ. Seventy-five percent of all skin cancer deaths are due to metastatic malignant melanoma.

Malignant melanoma develops from pigment-forming cells in the skin. Ten percent of all malignant melanomas occur in families with a familial predisposition to developing this tumor; however, most cases are spontaneous in origin. The back is the most common location for malignant melanoma in men, while the lower extremity is more commonly affected in women. The incidence of malignant melanoma has increased by 1500% since 1935. The current lifetime risk for developing malignant melanoma for an individual born at this time is 1 in 105. At current rates of increase, this is projected to be a 1 in 75 risk for individuals born in the year 2000.

Intermittent high doses of ultraviolet B light are thought to contribute to the increasing incidence of malignant melanoma. Therefore, behavioral patterns of sun-exposure dramatically affect the incidence of this disease. In blacks malignant melanoma involves more frequently the palms, soles, and subungual regions.

CLINICAL MANIFESTATIONS

Basal cell carcinoma commonly presents as a flesh-colored, pearly, or waxy papule. Eighty percent of lesions occur in sun-exposed areas and most involve the head and neck region. The nose is the most common location. A nonhealing sore or recurrent bleeding is a cardinal sign of this tumor. Basal cell carcinomas that are recurrent, infiltrative, or morpheaform often present as hypopigmented skin plaques. These varieties of basal cell carcinomas typically have indistinct clinical margins and high rates of recurrence following excisional surgery, electrodesiccation and curettage, or cryosurgery. Superficial basal cell carcinomas commonly occur on the trunk and may present as an erythematous scaling eruption.

Squamous cell carcinoma typically presents as an erythematous or flesh-colored nodule with ulceration and a keratin-filled crater. These tumors most often arise in skin with chronic solar damage but can also involve the mucous membranes. Nonhealing leg ulcers, chronic osteomyelitis sinus tracts, and skin lesions arising in burn scars should be biopsied to rule out an underlying squamous cell carcinoma. Regional metastases from squamous cell carcinoma arising in sun-damaged skin occur in 5% of cases. The incidence of metastases from the lip and tumor arising in nonhealing wounds varies from 18% to 30%.

Malignant melanoma commonly presents as a brown or black pigmented skin lesion. The tumor typically has a mixture of colors including black, brown, red, or blue. The borders are irregular and notched with overall asymmetry of the lesion. The diameter is typically greater than 6 mm. The deeper the tissue invasion from melanoma, the greater the incidence of metastasis and death from this disease. Early diagnosis and excision can be lifesaving.

TREATMENT

Because treatment recommendations for skin cancers are based on the type of tumor, accurate histologic diagnosis is necessary. Biopsy of basal cell carcinoma and squamous cell carcinoma can be performed by shave biopsy, punch biopsy, incisional, or excisional biopsy. Malignant melanoma should be biopsied by excision, if the tumor is small, or by punch biopsy or incisional biopsy if larger.

Malignant melanoma is treated by excision with margins dependent upon the depth of tumor invasion into the skin. Due to the potential for metastatic disease and death from this tumor, it is recommended that excisional treatment be done by a dermatologic surgeon or surgical oncologist.

The following modalities can be utilized for treatment of basal cell carcinoma or squamous cell carcinoma.

Excisional Surgery. Conventional excisional surgery is the most common method for treatment of basal cell carcinoma and squamous cell carcinoma. Histologic examination of the tissue margins is utilized to determine the radial and vertical extension of the tumor. This tissue processing technique is limited by the fact that 1% or less of the tissue margins are examined by the pathologist; hence, conventional excisional surgery results in a 5-year cure rate of approximately 80%. However, this cure rate drops rapidly for tumors 2 cm or more in diameter. Typically, a 3-mm to 5-mm margin of clinically normal appearing tissue is excised.

Electrodesiccation and Curettage. Electrodesiccation and curettage is a commonly used method of treating small ($\leq$1 cm) basal cell carcinomas and squamous cell carcinomas. Typically, the tumor should be located in a cosmetically insignificant area as the wound heals by second intention. The procedure is performed by curetting the tumor from the skin followed by electrodesiccation of the base of the wound. This procedure is repeated twice more, resulting in a shallow ulceration that is then allowed to heal without closure. Five-year cure rates for low-risk tumors treated by this method are approximately 90%. Electrodesiccation and curettage should not be used for recurrent tumors, morpheaform basal cell carcinomas, or tumors located in high-risk areas for recurrence such as around the eyes, ears, nose, and mouth.

Cryosurgery. Cryosurgery using liquid nitrogen for treatment of small basal cell carcinomas and squamous cell carcinomas results in a 5-year cure rate of approximately 90%. Thermocouples can be used for accurate depth of freezing. Wounds resulting from this procedure are allowed to heal by second intention. Hypopigmented scarring is typical and cosmesis should be considered prior to utilization of this modality. Recurrent tumors or tumors with infiltrative patterns should not be treated by this method.

Mohs' Micrographic Surgery. Mohs' micrographic surgery is a technically complex surgical procedure for excising basal cell carcinomas and squamous cell carcinomas of any subtype. This specialized technique facilitates complete removal of the tumor by examining virtually 100% of all tissue margins and thus minimizes the removal of uninvolved normal adjacent skin. This surgical modality allows for careful microscopic control and removal of tumor and has a 5-year cure rate of 97 to 99% for basal cell carcinoma and 90 to 95% for squamous cell carcinoma. This surgical technique is especially advantageous in areas of cosmetic importance in the head and neck. Mohs' micrographic surgery is indicated for treatment of recurrent tumors or tumors in the periocular, perinasal, perioral, or periauricular regions. Tumors with aggressive histologic features such as morpheaform basal cell carcinoma are best treated by this method.

Radiation Therapy. Radiation therapy for skin cancers is typically reserved for individuals who are unable or unwilling to undergo surgical procedures. X-ray therapy results in a 5-year cure rate of approximately 90% for small basal and squamous cell carcinomas. Initial cosmetic results are acceptable; however, chronic radiation damage results in cosmetically disfiguring yellow, depressed scars with time. The radiation is delivered in fractionated doses distributed over 2 to 6 weeks on a 5-day per week delivery schedule. This treatment method is not recommended for individuals who have an anticipated life expectancy of 10 years or greater.

Experimental Therapies. A variety of nonsurgical treatments for cutaneous malignancies have been introduced. Interferon-alpha-2b is effective in the treatment of small superficial basal cell carcinomas when injected intralesionally at a dose of 3 million units, three times weekly for 3 weeks. Histologic cure rates range from 50% or higher 1 year after treatment. This method is unlikely to replace surgical procedures but may be effective for selected individuals.

Isotretinoin (Accutane) and etretinate (Tegison) are synthetic retinoids that are effective preventative agents for patients who are predisposed to the development of multiple basal cell and squamous cell carcinomas. Immunosuppressed individuals with multiple squamous cell carcinomas can be maintained on retinoids to reduce the rate of transformation of premalignant skin lesions to frank malignancy. Also, patients with the nevoid basal cell carcinoma syndrome have been maintained on synthetic retinoids with reduction in the rate of development of basal cell carcinomas.

Intralesional chemotherapy agents such as 5-fluorouracil and methotrexate have been used to treat superficial skin cancers with only moderate success.

Photodynamic therapy is a newly developing field of treatment for cutaneous malignancies. This technique involves intravenous or topical administration of porphyrin derivatives. Selective uptake of the porphyrin derivative by the tumor followed by activation with a laser destroys the tumor cells. Initial studies have demonstrated high rates of recurrence for this treatment modality, and further study is necessary before this technique can be recommended for treatment of cutaneous malignancies.

PREVENTION

Solar exposure during the first 20 years of life is typically responsible for the sun-induced damage to the skin that evolves into cutaneous malignancies. Proper education of grandparents, parents, and children is important in reducing the rising incidence of skin cancer. Sun-protective measures are instrumental in minimizing solar damage. The peak hours for ultraviolet exposure are from 10:00 A.M. to 3:00 P.M. It is recommended that patients minimize sun exposure during these time periods and utilize sunscreens with an SPF of 15 or greater. Clothing with a tight weave pattern along with hats serve a protective function. Patients should be advised to avoid behavior that results in overexposure to solar radiation. Development of new and better sunscreens will help to reduce the rates of skin cancer.

PROGNOSIS

Routine skin examination by the patient and regular visits to the physician are helpful in early diagnosis of skin cancer. Suspicious lesions require histologic diagnosis. Early treatment is essential to a favorable outcome.

PAPULOSQUAMOUS DISEASES

method of
CRAIG A. ELMETS, M.D.
Case Western Reserve University
Cleveland, Ohio

The papulosquamous diseases are a heterogeneous group of cutaneous disorders whose common clinical feature is the presence of erythematous papules or plaques surrounded by variable degrees of scale. Because the basis for their classification together is a physical finding rather than a specific etiologic agent, the treatment for each condition is, for the most part, unique to each pathologic entity. A list of papulosquamous disorders is presented in Table 1. Although lupus erythematosus and secondary syphilis are considered to be papulosquamous disorders, they fit into other classification schemes as well. Their treatment is presented elsewhere in this book. Eczematous processes and superficial dermatophyte infections, classified separately by dermatologists, and some forms of cutaneous T cell lymphoma may also display clinical features that, at times, appear to be papulosquamous in nature.

TABLE 1. **Papulosquamous Diseases**

Psoriasis
Reiter's syndrome
Seborrheic dermatitis
Parapsoriasis
Lichen planus
Lichen nitidus
Lichen striatus
Pityriasis rosea
Secondary syphilis
Lupus erythematosus

May Simulate Papulosquamous Diseases
Viral exanthems
Cutaneous T cell lymphoma
Eczema
Dermatophyte infections
Tinea versicolor

PSORIASIS

Psoriasis is an inflammatory disease of epidermal hyperproliferation that affects over three million individuals in the United States. It is characterized by the development of widespread well-circumscribed "ham-red" erythematous plaques with a thick whitish scale. With the exception of an inflammatory arthritis that develops in approximately 6% of patients, the disease is restricted to the skin. Sites of predilection include the extensor surfaces of the elbows and knees, the intergluteal cleft, the nails, and the scalp, although almost any area of the skin may be involved. The plaques are unsightly and pruritic, and the disease is associated with considerable emotional distress. The course of the disease, which can begin at any age, is chronic and is characterized by exacerbations and remissions.

The treatment of psoriasis depends to a large extent on the severity of the disease and the patient's response to prior therapeutic maneuvers. In general, the disease is managed with topical medications first; ultraviolet light phototherapy is added if topical agents alone fail; systemic therapeutic agents are reserved for severe or resistant cases.

Topical Agents

Topical Corticosteroids. Topical corticosteroids are the most common topical preparations employed for psoriasis. For nonintertriginous, non–hair-bearing areas of skin, therapy should be initiated with a midpotency topical steroid such as 0.1% triamcinolone (Kenalog, Aristocort) cream or ointment applied two to three times daily. Should this fail, more potent topical steroids such as fluocinonide 0.05% (Lidex) or desoximetasone 0.25% (Topicort) are often employed and are applied on a twice-a-day basis. Ultrapo-

tent topical steroids such as clobetasol (Temovate) or betamethasone dipropionate 0.05% (Diprolene) are quite effective in psoriasis, but are known to cause atrophy of the skin when used for extended periods of time. They should be reserved for cases in which less potent preparations are ineffective. When they are employed, they should be applied to localized areas of skin for a limited period of time (e.g. daily for 2 weeks).

Most topical steroids are available in ointment and cream formulations. Creams are cosmetically more acceptable, but for a given corticosteroid preparation, the ointment is more potent. In addition, ointments are more effective at loosening and removing psoriatic scales.

One can achieve increased penetration into the skin and enhanced therapeutic efficacy by applying topical steroids under an occlusive dressing for 1 to 8 hours. This strategy is commonly employed to treat more resistant areas of psoriasis. For small areas of skin, commercially available patches (Actiderm Dermatological Patch) have been designed specifically for this purpose, although plastic wrap works as well. Occlusion of large areas of skin can be achieved with vinyl occlusion suits. Occlusion should not be utilized for extended periods of time because of the enhanced potential for local and systemic complications of corticosteroid therapy.

For psoriasis involving the face and intertriginous areas, only low-potency topical steroid creams (2½% hydrocortisone, alclometasone dipropionate [Aclovate], desonide [DesOwen]) should be applied to reduce the risk of local adverse side effects, including telangiectasias and striae. For scalp psoriasis, the addition of topical corticosteroid solutions (0.1% triamcinolone [Kenalog], fluocinolone [Synalar] or fluocinonide 0.05% [Lidex]) can be applied on a twice daily basis as an adjunct to tar shampoos, which remain the first line of therapy for psoriasis in that area.

Once the psoriasis is controlled to the patient's satisfaction, it is important to attempt to reduce either the potency or the frequency of the applied topical steroid to the minimum amount and frequency required to maintain control of the disease. One disadvantage to the exclusive use of topical steroids in psoriasis is that if they are withdrawn too rapidly, a rebound in the severity of disease is often observed. Thus, a slow taper of medications is advisable.

Tars. Crude coal tar and related compounds have been used for many years in the management of psoriasis. Tars typically require longer periods of time than topical steroids to induce a response and are cosmetically less acceptable. However, they have relatively few side effects, and unlike steroids, they do not produce a rebound phenomenon when they are withdrawn. Tar formulations are available as ointments (5% liquid Carbonis Detergens in hydrophilic ointment), gels (Estar gel), bath oils (Balnetar bath) and shampoos (Ionil-T, T-gel). Tar shampoos are the first line of therapy for scalp psoriasis. They are often combined with ultraviolet B phototherapy (see below).

Other Topical Preparations. Anthralin in a 0.1 to 1.0% formulation (Anthra-Derm, Dithrocreme) applied for 30 minutes to 2 hours per day and then removed with soap and water or mineral oil is another topical medication used for psoriasis. Although it is quite effective, the treatment is messy and stains both clothing and the treated skin sites. These undesirable side effects reduce patient compliance.

Salicylic acid (Keralyt Gel) is a potent keratolytic agent that is often added to other forms of therapy when psoriatic plaques are covered by a thick scale. Loosening and removal of such scale with the salicylic acid facilitates penetration of other forms of topical therapy.

Ultraviolet Phototherapy

Ultraviolet B phototherapy: Ultraviolet B (UVB) phototherapy is usually administered three times weekly in a UVB light box beginning at two-thirds the dose necessary to cause a mild erythema reaction. The UVB dose is increased by 10 to 15% with each treatment. The major acute adverse reaction to this form of therapy is production of a sunburn reaction, which can cause exacerbation of the psoriasis, since psoriasis is known to spread to areas of epidermal injury.

A synergistic therapeutic effect can be achieved in psoriasis by combining UVB light with topical application of tar. The tar, either as 5% liquid Carbonis Detergens in hydrophilic ointment, Estar gel, or Balnetar bath, is applied 30 minutes to 2 hours before the UVB treatment.

PUVA. Psoralen plus ultraviolet A (UVA) radiation, also known as PUVA, combines the oral administration of the photosensitizing compound 8-methoxypsoralen (methoxsalen) with total body exposure to high-intensity ultraviolet A radiation. Methoxsalen (Oxsoralen-Ultra) is usually started at a dose of 0.5 mg per kg, which is given 1½ hours before treatment in a UVA light box. The UVA dose administered is usually two-thirds of the dose necessary to produce a mild erythema and is increased by 10 to 15% thereafter. Patients are started on three treatments per week. Patients should be evaluated for clinical or serologic evidence of lupus erythematosus, cataracts, or skin cancer prior to initiation of PUVA therapy and periodically thereafter, since each of these diseases is a contraindication to therapy. Moreover, since squamous cell carcinoma of the scrotum and formation of cataracts are known side effects of this form of therapy, patients should be instructed to wear an athletic supporter and eye goggles while receiving the UVA treatment and should use glasses that filter UVA radiation for 24 hours after taking the 8-methoxypsoralen.

Systemic Agents

Because of their potential for serious side effects, systemic agents should be reserved for those patients whose psoriasis is extensive or who have not responded to more conservative therapy. The drugs should be administered only by experienced physicians familiar with their use in psoriatic patients.

Methotrexate is given orally in doses of 15 to 25 mg per week. The total dose is generally divided into thirds and is given at 12-hour intervals over 36 hours. Because of the potential of methotrexate to produce hepatic fibrosis and cirrhosis when administered on a chronic basis, pretreatment and yearly liver biopsies should be performed. Hematologic and hepatic function should be monitored frequently with blood tests.

The aromatic retinoid etretinate (Tegison) is administered in doses ranging from 0.75 to 1.0 mg/kg daily and is often combined with PUVA therapy. This vitamin A analog has many adverse side effects including hepatotoxicity, pseudotumor cerebri, hypertriglyceridemia, hyperostoses, xerosis, cheilitis, and alopecia. Etretinate is also a well-recognized teratogen. Women of childbearing age should not, in general, use this medication for psoriasis.

The immunosuppressive medication cyclosporine* (Sandimmune), in doses ranging from 3 to 5 mg per kg per day, has recently been discovered to be a potent antipsoriatic agent. The major side effects of this immunosuppressive medication include hypertension, nephrotoxicity, hyperkalemia, gastrointestinal disorders, myalgias, and fatigue. Its long-term side effects remain to be determined.

Oral steroids, while effective, should not be used for psoriasis, except under life-threatening conditions because of the potential for a severe flare or for the emergence of a pustular variant of the disease when the steroids are withdrawn.

SEBORRHEIC DERMATITIS

Seborrheic dermatitis is a very common clinical problem. Patients complain of scaling, itching

---

*This use of Sandimmune is not listed in the manufacturer's official directive.

and sometimes erythema in the scalp, eyebrows, central area of the face, ear canals, presternal area of the chest, and intertriginous areas. Seborrheic dermatitis involving the scalp can be easily managed solely by shampoos. Among the variety available are tar shampoos (T/Gel, Ionil T), pyrithione zinc (Zincon), selenium sulfide (Selsun Gold), and ketoconazole (Nizoral). At least one of these should be included in any therapeutic regimen on an every day or every other day basis. Topical steroid solutions (0.1% triamcinolone, [Kenalog] fluocinolone 0.025% [Synalar], fluocinonide 0.05% [Lidex]), applied once or twice a day, are often added to the regimen for the erythema and pruritus. Overnight occlusion with a shower cap nightly for 1 to 2 weeks increases the efficacy of the topical steroids. When involved areas of the scalp are covered by a thick scale, it is advisable to first remove the scale with a keratolytic agent (P&S Liquid) to allow for greater penetration of the other therapeutic agents employed. This medication is applied overnight under a shower cap. The scalp is shampooed the next morning and topical corticosteroids are administered at that time.

Involvement of areas of the body other than the scalp are generally managed by topical steroid preparations. Low-potency creams (1 to 2½% hydrocortisone, desonide [DesOwen], alclometasone diproprionate [Aclovate]) are used for the face, ear canals and intertriginous areas. Medium potency topical steroid creams (0.1% triamcinolone) are recommended for other areas of involvement. Because of recent evidence that an overgrowth of the yeast *Pityrosporum ovale* is involved in the pathogenesis of seborrheic dermatitis, topical ketoconazole cream is an additional therapeutic option.

LICHEN PLANUS

Lichen planus is an inflammatory skin disease that is characterized by the abrupt onset of exceptionally pruritic polygonal flat-topped violaceous papules. Characteristic areas of involvement include the flexor surfaces of the wrists, dorsal surfaces of the hands, glans penis, and anterior aspects of the lower legs. Involvement of the mucous membranes occurs in about 50% of cases and in that location the lesions are often detected as lacy white patches. In many cases, the disease lasts for variable lengths of time, (6 to 18 months) and then resolves spontaneously. However, some individuals develop a chronic form that can last for decades.

Although for most cases no etiology can be found, a number of drugs and chemicals have been found to cause a lichen planus–like eruption

TABLE 2. **Drugs that Cause a Lichen Planus–Like Eruption**

Gold
Quinidine
Quinacrine
Chloroquine
Phenothiazine derivatives
Thiazides
Captopril
Naproxen
Streptomycin
Para-aminosalicylic acid

(Table 2). Thus, a careful history to identify exposure to such agents is mandatory because their removal can be curative. For the majority of individuals, some type of topical or systemic therapy is required. Cure of the disease can be achieved in some patients by a short course of oral prednisone (40 mg per day for 2 weeks and then tapering for an additional 2 to 4 weeks). In patients with mild disease or in patients who do not respond to oral steroids, application of a potent topical steroid (fluocinonide 0.05%) is beneficial. Oral antipruritic agents such as hydroxyzine (Atarax) at a dose of 25 mg every 4 to 6 hours can be given to control any associated pruritus. In patients with extensive disease who have not responded to other forms of therapy, treatment with PUVA may be required. In most instances, treatment of oral lesions is unnecessary.

PITYRIASIS ROSEA

Pityriasis rosea is a disease of unknown etiology that typically affects children and young adults. The disease often begins with a "herald patch," a round or oval erythematous slightly elevated plaque with scale measuring 2 to 5 cm in diameter. Over the next several days, crops of asymptomatic to moderately pruritic plaques with a collarette of scale appear over the trunk, upper arms, and upper legs. These have the same clinical appearance as the herald patch but are smaller in size. The lesions tend to be distributed along the skin lines, in what is termed a Christmas tree distribution. The eruption typically lasts for 2 to 6 weeks and then resolves spontaneously.

In most patients, reassurance is all that is necessary. Oral (hydroxyzine) or topical (Sarna) antipruritic agents or 0.1% triamcinolone cream can be given when the pruritus is severe enough to require treatment or when the appearance of the lesions is a cosmetic problem.

PARAPSORIASIS

Parapsoriasis refers to an ill-defined group of cutaneous disorders that are often classified into acute and chronic forms. Acute parapsoriasis manifests as vesiculopapules over extensive areas of the body and may be confused with varicella. It bears little resemblance to other papulosquamous diseases and its management should be undertaken only by a physician experienced in the care of these patients.

Chronic parapsoriasis is characterized by salmon red plaques of variable size and may have a clinical appearance similar to that of psoriasis or nummular dermatitis. Although the diagnosis is largely made by exclusion, it is one that is important to establish, since some patients, particularly those in whom large plaques (>5 cm) predominate, are at risk for progression to cutaneous T cell lymphoma.

Therapeutic options in chronic parapsoriasis are limited. Although topical corticosteroids and emollients are often employed, they do little to influence the course of the disease. Phototherapy with UVB or with PUVA have also been employed with variable results.

CONNECTIVE TISSUE DISEASES

method of
LESTER D. MILLER, M.D.
Dominican Santa Cruz Hospital
Santa Cruz, California

SYSTEMIC LUPUS ERYTHEMATOSUS

Systemic lupus erythematosus (SLE) is a complex multisystem disease in which aberrant immune regulation results in the production of numerous autoantibodies reacting with nuclear and cytoplasmic cellular components. Antigen-antibody circulating immune complexes are produced, which are deposited in blood vessel walls of diverse organ systems (e.g., the kidney, resulting in glomerulonephritis). Table 1, adapted from the 1982 American Rheumatism Association criteria for the diagnosis of SLE, illustrates the multidimensional aspects of the disease. The criteria were developed primarily for selecting patients with SLE for large clinical studies. However, there is utility in applying them to individual cases of SLE. The presence of 4 of the 11 ARA criteria makes the diagnosis of SLE likely. Diagnosis of an individual case can be difficult if a patient has borderline clinical signs or symptoms and weakly reactive autoantibody studies. Table 2 illustrates common antibodies associated with SLE and other connective tissue diseases. Antibodies to double-stranded native DNA (anti-dsDNA) and anti-Sm antibodies have a high degree of specificity for SLE, and this is especially

TABLE 1. **Criteria for the Diagnosis of Systemic Lupus Erythematosus**

Malar rash
Discoid rash
Photosensitivity to sunlight
Oral ulcerations
Nonerosive polyarthritis
Serositis: pleuritis, pericarditis
Proteinuria >500 mg per day, cellular casts
Neurologic: seizures, psychosis
Hematologic: Leukopenia, hemolytic anemia, lymphopenia, thrombocytopenia
Immunologic: Anti-dsDNA or anti-Sm antibodies
Positive antinuclear antibody (in the absence of drugs known to induce SLE)

Adapted from the 1982 American Rheumatism Association Criteria for the Diagnosis of Systemic Lupus Erythematosus. Tan EM, Cohen AS, Fries JF, et al: The 1982 Revised Criteria for the Classification of SLE. Arthritis Rheum 25:1271, 1982.

true when these antibodies are present in conjunction with low serum complement levels.

There is now a considerable body of scientific evidence that patients have a genetic predisposition to SLE. When testing for genetic markers is readily available in commercial laboratories it will allow for better disease classification and prognostication.

SLE is predominantly a disease of young and middle-aged women between the ages of 15 and 50. The female-to-male ratio is 8 or 9:1. Cumulative survival rates in SLE range between 88 and 97% at 5 years and between 71 and 90% at 10 years. About 10% of a patient's close relatives may have SLE or a related connective tissue disease.

Drug-Induced Disease

It is vital to ask patients about prior and current prescribed medications, as drug-induced

TABLE 2. **Antinuclear Antibody Associations with Connective Tissue Diseases**

Antibody	Disease
Anti-ds DNA	SLE
Anti-Sm	SLE
Anti-centromere	CREST variant of scleroderma
Anti-topoisomerase I (SCL-70)	Diffuse scleroderma
Anti-U1RNP (RNP)	Overlap syndromes (MCTD)
Anti-Ro (SSA)	Sjögren's syndrome; subacute cutaneous lupus erythematosus
Anti-La (SSB)	Sjögren's syndrome
Anti-histone	Drug-induced SLE
Peripheral or rim pattern ANA	SLE
Speckled pattern ANA	Overlap (MCTD), SLE, scleroderma
Nucleolar pattern ANA	Scleroderma

Abbreviations: SLE = Systemic lupus erythematosus; ANA = antinuclear antibody; MCTD = mixed connective tissue disease.

SLE is common. Some of the leading inducing agents are procainamide (Pronestyl), hydralazine (Apresoline), isoniazid (INH), and chlorpromazine (Thorazine). In addition, a host of other medications have been reported to induce SLE. Most patients with drug-induced disease *do not* develop renal or central nervous system complications. By definition, all patients with drug-induced SLE have positive antinuclear antibodies. The presence of antihistone antibodies, however, is more specific evidence of this condition. Treatment involves withdrawal of the offending agent. However, in some cases SLE symptoms can persist for months and require interim therapy with corticosteroids.

Treatment

Skin Manifestations

Skin manifestations of SLE are broad, ranging from the classic butterfly malar rash to cutaneous vasculitic lesions. Photosensitivity is present in 10 to 60% of patients. Sunscreens with high sun protection factors are helpful for some patients, but it is best to avoid prolonged exposure to ultraviolet rays altogether.

Discoid lupus erythematosus (DLE) can occur alone or in conjunction with SLE. Discoid lesions often occur on the scalp, face, and neck and can be disfiguring in certain cases. The lesions are often well-circumscribed erythematous plaques with scaling and follicular plugging. As discoid lesions progress, there is often atrophic scarring and associated depigmentation.

Subacute Cutaneous Lupus (SCL) affects a unique subset of patients who present with a more diffuse rash consisting of scaly and erythematous macules and papules. The rash can be extensive, covering the face, trunk, and extremities. It some cases the lesions have prominent erythematous annular borders. SCL eruptions sometimes resemble psoriasis. There is a strong association between SCL and anti-Ro (SSA) antibodies (Table 2), which are present in up to 80% of these patients.

Treatment of sparsely distributed discoid lesions consists of topical steroids. While it is always preferable to use hydrocortisone on the face, it is often not potent enough, and a thin film of halogenated steroids such as fluocinonide 0.05% (Lidex) or betamethasone dipropionate 0.05% (Diprolene) can be applied once or twice daily to affected areas. These medications can lead to steroid atrophy of facial skin, as can discoid lupus itself. Occasionally lesions are directly injected with triamcinolone (Kenalog) in a concentration of 2.5 mg per ml. This, however, is best left to an experienced dermatologist.

Hydroxychloroquine (Plaquenil) is also an extremely valuable drug for the treatment of lupus skin conditions. The drug is administered orally in a dosage of 6.5 mg per kg of body weight with a maximum single dosage of 400 mg orally per day. The drug should be reduced in patients with azotemia and in patients over the age of 65 who are likely to have diminished renal function. At these dosage levels, ocular toxicity is very rare. Nonetheless, patients should always be encouraged to have eye examinations every 6 months to exclude retinal damage. In certain situations, chloroquine phosphate (Aralen) at a dose of 250 mg orally per day may have to be substituted for hydroxychloroquine.

When skin disease is severe or widely distributed, systemic steroids are indicated. Dosages of 1 mg per kg to a maximum of 60 mg of prednisone orally per day may be needed initially. This dosage can then be gradually tapered to maintenance levels of 5 to 15 mg per day.

Joint Involvement

The arthritis of SLE is typically a nondeforming polyarthritis involving the small joints of the hands and wrists but can involve virtually any synovial joint. In most cases the appearance mimics that of early-onset rheumatoid arthritis. However, unlike rheumatoid disease, erosive changes on x-ray are rare. Reducible swan-neck deformities of the fingers are frequently seen.

Initial therapy is with aspirin or standard dosages of nonsteroidal anti-inflammatory drugs (NSAIDs) (e.g., naproxen [Naprosyn], 500 mg orally twice daily). Plaquenil is valuable and is used in the same dosages discussed in the section on skin manifestations. In cases in which the synovitis is resistant to conventional therapy, 5 to 10 mg of prednisone orally per day is beneficial and may be needed long term.

Renal Involvement

Renal involvement is potentially one of the most serious complications of SLE. Individuals presenting with proteinuria and an active urinary sediment should receive a thorough serologic evaluation, and renal biopsy should be done in selected cases. Anti–double-stranded DNA (anti-dsDNA), C'3, C'4, CH50 (total hemolytic complement), serum creatinine, blood urea nitrogen (BUN), 24-hour urinary protein, and creatinine clearance should be measured. Patients with active renal disease commonly have elevated titers of anti-dsDNA and low serum complement levels. It cannot be overemphasized that the patient's blood pressure needs to be carefully monitored and aggressively treated to keep the diastolic pressure below 90 mmHg.

Renal biopsy is pursued to assess the severity of kidney involvement and to see if pathologic changes appear reversible. Patients with focal proliferative, diffuse proliferative, and mixed membranoproliferative nephritis often need aggressive treatment. The biopsy is helpful in demonstrating evidence of irreversible glomerular sclerosis or interstitial inflammation, both of which herald a poor outcome and a high likelihood of eventual dialysis. Patients with primarily mesangial disease or pure membranous nephritis have a better prognosis and do not usually require long-term high-dose corticosteroid therapy.

If the laboratory, pathologic, and clinical evaluations indicate active glomerulonephritis, treatment with prednisone, 1 mg per kg per day in a single or divided dose (to a maximum dosage of 60 to 80 mg), should be started. In clinical situations that appear urgent, intravenous pulses of methylprednisolone (Solu-Medrol), 1 gram daily for 3 days, may be of some benefit.

It is the use of intravenous pulses of cyclophosphamide (Cytoxan) in doses of 500 to 750 mg per M^2 of body surface area that has revolutionized the treatment of lupus nephritis. Cyclophosphamide has not only delayed the onset of renal failure, but in many cases, prevented it. Intravenous cyclophosphamide is given monthly for approximately 6 months. If the patient responds satisfactorily, the drug can be given less frequently with pulses every 2 to 3 months. In many cases patients may be able to terminate intravenous cyclophosphamide cytoxan after 1 to 3 years. Mesna (Mesnex), can be infused intravenously to help prevent hemorrhagic cystitis. Cyclophosphamide can also be given orally (1 to 2 mg per kg per day), but results are clearly superior with intravenous administration.

It is important to bear in mind that long-term administration of cyclophosphamide is associated with an increased risk of bladder cancer, ovarian failure, herpes zoster, and other infections. In patients who do not respond to cyclophosphamide, azathioprine (Imuran) has been used in an oral daily dose of 1.0 to 2.5 mg per kg. End-stage renal involvement in SLE is handled in standard fashion with hemodialysis. Some patients may be candidates for renal transplantation depending on their age and health status.

Neurologic Involvement

Nervous system involvement in SLE is wide ranging and can include psychosis, epileptic seizures, chorea, stroke syndromes, cranial nerve involvement, optic neuritis, ophthalmoplegias, peripheral neuropathies, and mononeuritis multiplex. Aseptic meningitis, multiple sclerosis–like syndromes, and transverse myelitis have also been reported.

Nervous system involvement is a perplexing area to manage. The difficulty comes in trying to establish whether the clinical problem is SLE related or due to other causes. Infection must be ruled out when meningitis is present, and this is especially true in patients on cytotoxic therapy. Some cases of aseptic meningitis in SLE patients have been associated with the use of ibuprofen. Psychotic behavior raises the question of whether steroids are the offending agent. In general, steroid psychosis is a rare phenomenon and the problem is often attributable to active SLE, especially when seen in conjunction with objective neurologic events (i.e., neuropathies). There are no specific laboratory tests that can unequivocally define the problem of central nervous system (CNS) lupus. The cerebrospinal fluid (CSF) is often abnormal with a few lymphocytes. The CSF protein may be elevated and the results of electroencephalography, computed tomography scans, and magnetic resonance imaging can be nonspecifically abnormal.

Treatment of CNS lupus often requires prednisone at a dosage of 1 mg per kg (maximum 60–80 mg) orally per day. Higher dosages have been used but as the dose approaches 100 mg of prednisone per day the risk of opportunistic infection increases. When faced with a rapidly deteriorating patient a trial of methylprednisolone pulse therapy, as outlined in the section on the treatment of renal disease, can sometimes be helpful. Intravenous pulses of cyclophosphamide (see Renal Involvement for dosages) can also be tried in severely ill patients. Patients who develop focal or grand mal seizures should be treated with standard anticonvulsants.

Cardiac Involvement

Pericardial disease is extremely common in SLE. Echocardiography has revealed that numerous patients have asymptomatic pericardial effusions. In rare cases, pericardial effusions can be massive and lead to life-threatening tamponade.

Minor effusions can be managed with a trial of indomethacin (Indocin), 75 mg sustained release capsules orally twice daily, or other NSAIDs. Larger, symptomatic effusions should be managed with prednisone in initial dosages from 40 to 60 mg orally per day and tapered accordingly.

Other manifestations of cardiac disease include myocarditis, myocardial infarction, and Libman-Sacks verrucous endocarditis. The latter two may be associated with anticardiolipin antibodies.

Pulmonary Involvement

Pleurisy and small areas of plate-like atelectasis are the most common manifestations of SLE in the lung. However patients may develop interstitial lung disease, pulmonary hemmorrhage, and the rare dreaded complication, acute lupus pneumonitis, which has a 50% fatality rate. Treatment consists of NSAIDs for pleurisy and prednisone for more advanced pulmonary problems (see Cardiac Involvement for dosages). Intravenous cyclophosphamide is added in life-threatening disease.

Hematologic Involvement

Leukopenia (white cell count less than 4000 cells/mm³) is extremely common in SLE but rarely needs to be treated. The anemia of chronic disease with low hemoglobin, hematocrit, and normal indices is the general rule in SLE. Approximately 10% of patients develop autoimmune hemolytic anemia, which is generally responsive to corticosteroid therapy. Thrombocytopenia is present in approximately 15% of patients but is usually not treated unless counts fall below 50,000 platelets per mm³. When platelets fall to dangerously low levels, prednisone is tried in a daily dosage of 1 mg per kg orally (60 to 80 mg maximum daily dose). Counts usually rebound over 2 to 8 weeks, but in nonresponders, the mild androgenic steroid danazol (Danocrine) can be used in dosages ranging from 200 to 800 mg orally per day (average dose 600 mg). Alternatives are intravenous gamma globulin and cytotoxic drugs such as intravenous cyclophosphamide and oral azathioprine (Imuran) in varying dosage regimens that are beyond the scope of this discussion. In severe cases, surgical splenectomy may be indicated.

Antiphospholipid Syndrome

Between 20 and 50% of patients with SLE have detectable antiphospholipid antibodies, making it imperative to test all patients. The most common of these are anticardiolipin antibodies that show a strong association with specific clinical aspects of SLE. Laboratories commonly report three isotypes, anti-IgA, anti-IgM, and anti-IgG. Patients with high-titer anti-IgG cardiolipin antibodies are at the greatest risk of developing one or more of the clinical manifestations of the antiphospholipid syndrome (Table 3).

Some of these same patients may have had a biologic false-positive syphilis serology (positive VDRL or RPR) or a prolonged partial thromboplastin time due to the so-called "lupus anti-coagulant." In some cases patients will not fulfill the diagnostic criteria for SLE (see Table 1) and will be classified as having "primary" antiphospholipid syndrome.

Recommendations for treatment of the antiphospholipid syndrome vary. One "baby" aspirin (81 mg tablet) orally per day is recommended for

TABLE 3. Clinical Manifestations of the Antiphospholipid Syndrome

Thrombocytopenia
Thrombophlebitis
Pulmonary embolism
Recurrent miscarriages
Migraine
Transient ischemic attacks
Stroke
Myocardial infarction
Libman-Sacks cardiac valvular vegetations
Livedo reticularis

patients with high titer anti-IgG cardiolipin antibodies or a prior history of significant vascular events. Major events, such as a stroke, recurrent thrombophlebitis, or pulmonary embolism require initial heparin therapy and possible lifelong treatment with Coumadin. Treatment with prednisone does not appear to affect the titer of anticardiolipin antibodies or protect patients from serious vascular complications. However, in patients who have had recurrent miscarriages, low-dose aspirin with or without prednisone can be tried in an effort to prevent fetal loss. This type of therapy has had only limited success.

Complications of Treatment

While treatment with corticosteroids has enhanced the survival of patients with SLE, it has also been responsible for considerable morbidity and mortality. Corticosteroids contribute to the development of avascular necrosis of bone, especially in the femoral heads, which can lead to premature secondary osteoarthritis and the need for total hip arthroplasty.

Steroids can also accelerate osteoporosis, cataract formation, glaucoma, and glucose intolerance. Furthermore, corticosteroids have been implicated in accelerating atherosclerosis, leading to premature myocardial infarction. Young women with SLE are particularly at risk for this complication. Therefore, monitoring of the patient's dietary intake, blood pressure, and exercise program is imperative.

POLYMYOSITIS AND DERMATOMYOSITIS

Polymyositis and dermatomyositis (PM/DM) belong to a group of uncommon diseases called the idiopathic inflammatory myopathies. Both PM and DM can occur at almost any age with a 2:1 female-to-male ratio. Age-adjusted incidence rates range from 1 to 5 cases per million population per year. There is a bimodal distribution with a peak in childhood below the age of 15 that represents childhood PM/DM and a second peak in adulthood between 45 and 55 years.

PM/DM have many common manifestations, which include symmetric proximal muscle weakness, elevated levels of muscle enzymes in the serum (e.g., creatine kinase, aldolase) characteristic electromyograms with increased insertional activity, polyphasic and fibrillation potentials, and positive sharp waves.

DM is further characterized by an erythematous papular rash over the extensor aspects of the knuckles (Gottron's papules) or elbows and in the V of the neck. Patients frequently have a dusky violaceous rash over the upper eyelids with associated periorbital edema, the so-called heliotrope sign, which occurs in approximately 25% of patients with DM. Digital erythema in the periungual areas and on the fingertips is also common.

Although some cases of PM/DM seem clinically straightforward, it is strongly recommended that a muscle biopsy be performed for confirmation of the diagnosis. If special metabolic stains are available they should also be done. Pathology sections typically show an inflammatory cellular infiltrate with lymphocytes, plasma cells, and polys. There is also evidence of muscle degeneration and phagocytosis.

The clinician should bear in mind that other conditions can mimic PM, such as drug-induced myopathies (e.g., gemfibrozil [Lopid] and lovastatin [Mevacor]). Hypothyroidism, viral myositis, alcoholic myopathy, metabolic myopathies, and inclusion body myositis can all mimic this disease as well.

DM and PM can both be associated with malignancies in older patients, although the primary statistical association is with DM. The literature on this subject is lengthy and there is controversy about the frequency of malignancy in DM (estimates range from 8 to 25% of patients). It is often not productive to search long and hard for a tumor if there are no apparent symptoms at the time of the initial evaluation. However, a standard chest x-ray, mammogram, pelvic examination and ultrasound, and a screen for occult blood in the stool are reasonable for the older patient.

The most serious complications of PM/DM involve the respiratory system. One possible complication is aspiration pneumonia secondary to difficulty in controlling the muscles of deglutition. Failure of respiratory musculature can lead to the need for intensive care and ventilator support. In rare situations the patient can develop progressive pulmonary interstitial fibrosis leading to death. This complication is frequently unresponsive to treatment with corticosteroids or cytotoxic drugs.

Treatment

Treatment of PM/DM requires a trial of corticosteroid therapy despite the fact that adequate controlled trials have not been done. Prednisone dosage is 1 mg per kg with starting doses frequently in the range of 60 mg orally in a single or divided dose. High-dose prednisone is warranted for about 3 months with gradual tapering to lower levels. It is important to recognize that in some cases the creatine kinase (CK) levels never normalize with therapy.

If the patient's muscle tone and strength return, it is not necessary to push steroid dosages higher simply to normalize the CK. On the other hand, if there is a poor clinical response and little restoration of strength, a second-line agent should be added, and methotrexate is the drug of choice in that situation. This drug can be administered orally, intramuscularly, or intravenously and the initial dosage is generally 10 to 15 mg per week orally. This level is maintained, raised, or lowered depending on the patient's clinical response. It is not common for dosages of oral methotrexate to exceed 20 to 25 mg per week. Intravenous weekly dosages can rise to 35 to 50 mg per week in some cases. The drug is monitored with monthly complete blood counts and chemistry panels that include liver function tests. Methotrexate cannot be used in patients with pre-existing liver disease or those who consistently imbibe alcohol. Methotrexate must also be given with caution in patients who have azotemia. If methotrexate fails, azathioprine can be tried in a dosage of 1.5 to 2.0 mg per kg orally daily.

Treatment of an underlying malignancy often ameliorates symptoms of dermatomyositis, even though tumors are not generally curable at this stage of the disease.

SCLERODERMA

Scleroderma, or systemic sclerosis, is a relatively rare connective tissue disease characterized by increased thickening and fibrosis of the skin secondary to deposition of dermal collagen. The skin becomes tethered to the underlying connective tissue. Thickening is found in both proximal and distal areas of the extremities where there is tight fibrotic skin around the fingers. Resorption of the pulp of the digital tips with small distal ulcerations are common, a condition known as sclerodactyly. Raynaud's phenomenon is the most common initial symptom of scleroderma.

Scleroderma is divided into two broad subclasses: limited and diffuse. The limited form of the disease is referred to as the CREST syndrome, which comprises Calcinosis cutis, Raynaud's phenomenon, Esophageal dismotility, Sclerodactyly, and Telangiectasias. The limited form of scleroderma generally carries a more favorable prognosis than the diffuse form. Skin involvement is more rapid and more severe in diffuse scleroderma. Proximal areas such as the upper arms, chest, abdomen, and thighs are frequently involved. As the disease progresses, distal involvement of the hands occurs. Patients with diffuse disease can develop pulmonary interstitial fibrosis, renal involvement, and cardiac problems, and generally have more severe and potentially life-threatening complications than CREST patients.

Scleroderma has its peak incidence between the ages of 45 and 64 with a female-to-male ratio of approximately 3:1. The disease is rare prior to puberty. Currently, no strong genetic markers for the disease have been identified. However, certain autoantibodies are present in scleroderma that have helped to define clinical subgroups of the disease (see Table 2). In the limited form (CREST) there is an increased frequency of anti-centromere antibodies (range between 50 to 96%) while in diffuse scleroderma approximately 30% of patients have antitopoisomerase I (previously anti-Scl 70) antibodies.

Localized Scleroderma

There are localized forms of scleroderma that are not associated with systemic disease. These include scleroderma morphea and linear scleroderma. The linear localized forms can produce disfigurement and limb contractures. The latter has a predilection for children. The patient's sera may have low-titer or nonexistent autoantibodies. There is no effective treatment for localized scleroderma.

Environmental Exposures

Environmental chemicals have been implicated in scleroderma-type syndromes; these include polyvinyl chloride, trichlorethylene, and silica. In addition, there have been reports linking the onset of scleroderma to silicon breast implants, but the evidence is far from conclusive.

Eosinophilia myalgia syndrome, secondary to ingestion of contaminated batches of L-tryptophan, has some scleroderma-like manifestations. Although this nutritional supplement has been withdrawn from the market, this episode should serve as a reminder to clinicians to consider patient exposure to chemicals in the home and work environment.

Treatment

There is no effective therapy for systemic scleroderma, although there are treatments for certain complications of the disease. D-penicillamine (DePen, Cuprimine) has been tried in patients with diffuse scleroderma. The usual starting dose is 250 mg orally per day with incremental increases about every 2 to 3 months to 750 mg or 1000 mg per day.

Some patients may benefit from such a trial with noticable reduction of skin thickness and tightness. Unfortunately D-penicillamine is a toxic drug and side effects requiring discontinuation are common. Frequent monitoring of the blood count, urinalysis, and chemistry profile is necessary.

Numerous other therapies ranging from cytotoxic agents to plasmapheresis have been tried with little or no benefit.

Cutaneous Involvement

No topical therapy has been found to prevent progressive fibrosis of the skin. Over-the-counter emollients are helpful in keeping the skin moist, and they may also lessen the tendency of the skin to crack and become secondarily infected. Digital ischemia from Raynaud's phenomena (see next section) frequently leads to digital tip ulcers. In the limited CREST form of the disease, subcutaneous calcinosis develops around the fingers, elbows, knees, and other pressure points. The calcific deposits often become large, protrude through the skin, and become a nidus for bacterial infection. There is currently no effective medical therapy for calcinosis cutis. Proper skin hygiene and antibiotics are used in tandem for treating local infections.

Raynaud's Phenomenon

Raynaud's phenomenon is found in nearly all patients (98%) with scleroderma In CREST, it frequently precedes the onset of recognizable disease by 5 to 10 years. In diffuse scleroderma, the onset is often coincident with the development of skin thickening. Treatment of Raynaud's phenomenon involves the use of calcium channel blockers. Nifedipine, in an extended-release preparation (Procardia XL), is commonly used in a starting dose of 30 mg daily. This initial dose can be titrated upward to 60 mg or 90 mg daily. Other calcium channel blockers such as diltiazem (Cardizem), in dosages starting at 30 to 60 mg three or four times per day, can also be used. A sustained-release preparation in a single daily dose is another option. Some clinicians find that patients benefit from alpha-adrenergic blockers such as prazosin (Minipress), starting at 1 mg two or three times per day, with careful upward titration. In individuals with digital tip ulcerations a trial of nitroglycerine ointment may be helpful due to its local vasodilatory effect.

Patients should always be advised to avoid prolonged cold exposure and to wear gloves as needed. They should also avoid over-the-counter cold remedies (e.g., nasal sprays) that contain vasoconstrictors.

Pulmonary Involvement

In diffuse scleroderma, patients frequently complain of dyspnea and are subsequently found to have pulmonary fibrosis. The condition is usually progressive and often leads to respiratory failure and death. Early signs of pulmonary fibrosis include abnormal pulmonary function tests, especially the diffusing capacity, and radiographic signs of fibrosis in the lung bases. The latter can seen by CT scan in its early stages; in later stages the standard chest film is adequate to determine the degree of lung involvement. There is no reliable treatment for progressive pulmonary fibrosis although in early stages prednisone has been tried.

Pulmonary hypertension without pulmonary fibrosis can occur in patients with the CREST syndrome. This can be a rapidly fatal complication of the disease and is generally unresponsive to calcium channel blockers. Nonetheless, drugs such as nifedipine (Procardia) and diltiazem (Cardizem) should be tried in full therapeutic dosages.

Renal Involvement

One of the leading causes of death in the past was scleroderma renal crisis with severe hypertension and azotemia. However, the advent of angiotensin-converting enzyme inhibitors such as captopril (Capoten), enalapril (Vasotec), and lisinopril (Prinivil) have enabled us to take a quantum leap in the management of this dreaded problem. Early and agressive treatment with these agents will often abort renal and hypertensive crises and prolong the life of the patient. Unfortunately, not all patients respond to this therapy and their disease may progress to renal failure.

Captopril can be tried first in a dosage of 12.5 mg or 25 mg two or three times per day. Depending on response, it can be titrated upward. Enalapril, starting at 5 mg daily, or lisinopril, starting at 10 mg daily, can also be tried and the dosage adjusted upward as needed. Captopril, with a half-life of 2 to 3 hours, is preferable in crisis situations.

Patients with diffuse scleroderma should learn how to monitor their own blood pressure so that diastolic elevations of 10 mmHg or more can be found and treated promptly.

Gastrointestinal Involvement

Esophageal dysmotility is very common in scleroderma. Propulsion of both solids and liquids is abnormal, and patients may develop chronic erosive esophagitis with reflux and strictures. Treatment includes the use of H_2 blockers such as ranitidine (Zantac), 150 mg twice daily or cimetidine (Tagamet) 400 mg twice daily. The pump inhibitor omeprazole (Prilosec), 20 mg orally per day for up to 60 days, is also effective.

Patients in the late stages of scleroderma often develop hypomotility of the intestines, which can produce abdominal bloating, diarrhea, or obstructive symptoms. Large wide-mouthed diverticuli can be seen in the large intestine on barium enema with markedly prolonged barium transit times. These individuals are prone to malabsorption from stasis in the gut and secondary bacterial overgrowth. This can sometimes be alleviated by broad-spectrum antibiotics such as amoxicillin, 250 mg or 500 mg orally three times daily, or doxycycline, 100 mg orally twice daily, given in alternating monthly cycles.

In CREST patients, primary biliary cirrhosis has been described. Serology for antimitochondrial antibodies should be obtained in these patients.

Articular and Muscular Involvement

Inflammatory synovitis involving the joints is not usually a problem in scleroderma; most joint problems are an outgrowth of the skin disease itself. Early-onset skin disease in scleroderma produces diffuse edema and puffiness of the hands. Low-dose corticosteroids (e.g., prednisone, 5 to 10 mg orally daily) are quite effective for this problem, although long-term administration of steroids should be avoided. The most significant long-term problem is skin tightening, leading to flexion contractures of the fingers and larger joints. Tethering of skin to tendon sheaths produces tendon friction rubs, which are audible with a stethoscope.

Muscular involvement usually takes the form of inflammatory myopathy. Patients can develop a mild, so-called "simple" myopathy in which the creatine kinase is only slightly elevated and there is little overt weakness. A more profound myopathy, indistinguishable from idiopathic polymyositis, also occurs. These patients usually have an "overlap syndrome" with features of two or more connective tissue diseases. In cases in which myositis resembles polymyositis, moderate- to high-dose prednisone (40 to 60 mg orally per day) should be used and tapered in accordance with the clinical response. In resistant cases, methotrexate may have to be used (see section on treatment of PM/DM).

SJÖGREN'S SYNDROME

Sjögren's syndrome, or keratoconjunctivitis sicca, characteristically presents as dryness of the eyes and mucous membranes of the mouth. Biopsy of the minor salivary glands inside the lower lip typically reveals lymphocytic infiltration of the glands. When Sjögren's syndrome occurs alone it is termed primary Sjögren's Syndrome; when it is seen in conjunction with connective tissue diseases such as SLE, polymyositis, scleroderma, or rheumatoid arthritis, it is classified as secondary Sjögren's syndrome. Serologic studies commonly reveal the presence of anti-Ro (SSA) or anti-La (SSB) antibodies (see Table 2). The rheumatoid factor assay is also frequently positive.

Sjögren's patients can present with a diversity of clinical features, including parotid gland enlargement, myositis, nervous system involvement (both central and peripheral), interstitial lung disease, hyperglobulinemic purpura, renal tubular acidosis, and vasculitis. In fewer than 5% of patients, non–Hodgkin's lymphomas or Waldenström's macroglobulinemia may develop. Autoantibodies frequently disappear in patients with these lymphoproliferative diseases.

Treatment of Sjögren's syndrome depends on the patient's symptoms. Artificial tears are helpful in alleviating dryness of the eyes: some popular brands include Liquifilm tears, Tears Plus, Refresh, and Hypotears. Ocular ointments such as Lacri-Lube and Lacrisert can also be used. Extra fluids at mealtime can help dry mouth symptoms, and artifical saliva preparations, such as Salivart and Mouth Cote, are also helpful. Arthralgia and myalgias associated with Sjögren's syndrome may respond to standard NSAIDs (e.g., naproxen [Naprosyn] 500 mg orally twice daily). Hydroxychloroquine (Plaquenil), 200 to 400 mg orally per day, is also beneficial in some cases. When serious problems, such as systemic vasculitis, occur in conjunction with Sjögren's syndrome, corticosteroids or cytotoxic drugs or both are utilized.

OVERLAP SYNDROMES AND MIXED CONNECTIVE TISSUE DISEASE

It is not uncommon for patients to have features of more than one connective tissue disease. Systemic lupus erythematosus, scleroderma, and polymyositis frequently overlap. These individuals often have anti-nuclear antibodies in high titer with a speckled pattern, and markedly elevated anti-RNP antibodies are also present. It was thought at one time that these coexistent disorders constituted a unique subset called mixed connective tissue disease. However, when these patients are followed over time, it is clear that they do not fall neatly into one specific diagnostic group, although scleroderma-like features often predominate. It is probably most appropriate to classify these patients as having an overlap syndrome and to then treat the dominant symptoms as outlined in the earlier sections of this chapter.

CUTANEOUS VASCULITIS

method of
JEFFREY P. CALLEN, M.D.
University of Louisville
Louisville, Kentucky

The term "cutaneous vasculitis" refers to a number of syndromes. Leukocytoclastic vasculitis is a specific histopathologic entity that is observed in many of the conditions within the vasculitic spectrum. In general, involvement of the skin by vasculitis is most frequently manifested by an abnormality of the small vessels, and the clinical correlate is either palpable purpura or urticarial lesions. When larger vessels are involved, the manifestation may be a nodule, livedo reticularis, and/or cutaneous ulceration. Although circulating immune complexes are involved in the pathogenesis of many of the vasculitic syndromes, the exact pathogenetic mechanisms have not been fully elucidated. However, even when the skin is seemingly the only organ involved, vasculitis should be thought of as a systemic process.

Syndromes that can involve the small cutaneous vessels include hypersensitivity vasculitis, Henoch-Schönlein purpura, vasculitis associated with paraproteinemias, vasculitis as part of a collagen vascular disorder, and hypocomplementemic (urticarial) vasculitis. Although some patients with Wegener's granulomatosis or other diseases of the medium-sized vessels may have cutaneous small vessel disease, most will have other manifestations in the skin. Therefore, prior to any pharmacologic therapy, a thorough evaluation for associated disorders and etiologic factors as well as an assessment of the potential for active systemic disease must be carried out.

EVALUATION

Evaluation of the patient with cutaneous vasculitis is useful in determining the etiologic and associated factors and in assessing prognosis. Historical information can reveal the presence of a preceding disorder, medications taken prior to onset, the presence of an infection, and symptoms suggestive of systemic involvement. On physical examination, both the type of cutaneous lesion and the extent of disease are of prognostic importance. Tissue confirmation of vasculitis is almost always necessary and should be performed on an early lesion (<48 hours old) if possible. Immunofluorescence microscopy is helpful when the possibility of Henoch-Schönlein purpura is considered, particularly in adults. A complete laboratory evaluation is also helpful and should include a complete blood count, urinalysis, cryoglobulin determination, protein electrophoresis, hepatitis B surface antigen test, antinuclear antibody test, and possibly an anti-Ro (SS-A) test, tests of renal function, and a chest roentgenogram. The presence of antineutrophil cytoplasmic antibody has been correlated with Wegener's granulomatosis but can also occur in other vasculitic syndromes, such as polyarteritis nodosa and microscopic polyarteritis.

TREATMENT

General Measures

An obvious but often overlooked manuever is the removal or therapy of an associated condition or etiologic factor. Identification and treatment of infection, discontinuation of medicaments or other ingestants, and therapy directed against the production of an abnormal protein are most important. In a recent report from investigators in Italy, five patients were put on an elimination diet, which resulted in control of their disease. With reintroduction of foods and food dyes, they were able to identify the offending agent and continued control was possible. This manuever is perhaps most useful in patients with chronic but non–life-threatening vasculitis. Because lesions are more frequent and more severe on dependent areas and cooler (acral) areas of the body, frequent turning, elevation, and a warm environment are helpful.

Disease-Specific Considerations

The different vasculitic syndromes vary in their prognosis and severity, and thus may not all require the same therapeutic measures. Hypersensitivity vasculitis and Henoch-Schönlein purpura are often self-limited and the patients do not need to be treated aggressively. Polyarteritis nodosa (which more often involves internal organ systems, in particular the kidneys), Wegener's granulomatosis, and systemic necrotizing vasculitis are potentially life-threatening conditions. Many untreated patients will succumb to the disease from renal or central nervous system involvement. Urticarial vasculitis may be a chronic condition with a benign course, or in the presence of hypocomplementemia, may be complicated by chronic obstructive pulmonary disease. The chronic nature of the process necessitates continual suppressive therapy. Vasculitis complicating rheumatoid arthritis, lupus erythematosus, or Sjögren's syndrome varies from benign palpable purpura to severe life-threatening disease, and therapy depends on the severity of the process. In patients with a paraproteinemia, the therapy for the abnormal protein may differ from that needed for the cutaneous vasculitis.

Nonimmunologic Drug Therapy

In patients with urticarial vasculitis or palpable purpura, antihistamines have often been suggested as first-line therapy, based on the observation that injected histamine allows deposition of immune complexes in the vessel walls with eventual vasculitis histopathologically. In patients with palpable purpura, antihistamines have rarely if ever been effective in my practice. However, in patients with urticarial vasculitis, I generally begin therapy with a nonsporific agent such as astemizole (Hismanal) each morning and an H_1 inhibitor in the evening. Furthermore, an agent such as doxepin may have both H_1 and H_2 inhibiting effects and is preferable in some cases.

Various nonsteroidal anti-inflammatory drugs (NSAIDs) have been used in vasculitic syndromes. In particular, patients with urticarial vasculitis may respond to ibuprofen or indomethacin. The therapeutic benefit of NSAIDs comes from their effect on prostaglandins and leukotrienes and, for some, on platelet aggregation. In my experience, NSAIDs have not been particularly effective in urticarial vasculitis as well as in other cutaneous vasculitic syndromes. It is the rare patient who will respond to a NSAID.

Antimalarials such as hydroxychloroquine (Plaquenil) and chloroquine have been used in vasculitis. While they are effective for cutaneous lupus erythematosus, they have not been effective for vasculitis even in my patients with lupus erythematosus.

Diaminodiphenyl sulfone (dapsone, DDS) has received some recent attention. It is effective for dermatitis herpetiformis, a disease characterized by neutrophilic papillitis, and has various effects on leukocytes. It is the treatment of choice for the rare cutaneous vasculitic syndrome of erythema elevatum diutinum. In selected patients, it has been effective in controlling the manifestations of palpable purpura in doses of 100 to 200 mg per day. In general, it is my second choice after colchicine, and thus I may be selecting patients with recalcitrant disease, which might explain the lack of effect I have observed in my patients. Those of my colleagues who employ dapsone therapy before colchicine have observed the same findings with colchicine as I have with dapsone. Thus the choice of whether to begin with colchicine or dapsone is one of style rather than substance.

Colchicine has been reported to be effective for cutaneous vasculitis manifested by palpable purpura or urticarial lesions. Colchicine is an alkaloid derived from a crocus-like plant, *Colchicum autumnale*. Its effects in vasculitis are related to a blockade of disease expression. Colchicine inhibits leukocyte chemotaxis, blocks the release of lysosomal enzymes, inhibits DNA synthesis and cell proliferation, and may inhibit the effects of prostaglandins. Its use in vasculitis is limited to anecdotal reports and a small number of open label studies. Of the 50-plus patients I have treated and observed, colchicine has been effective in about 35, nonevaluable in about 5, and ineffective in the remaining 10. The agent is used in a dose of 0.6 mg given orally twice daily. If tolerated, its effects can be seen within 7 to 14 days, and thus therapy beyond 2 weeks is not likely to be beneficial. In patients with associated arthralgias or arthritis, colchicine has also been of some benefit. Immune complexes are unaffected by the drug, and this leads me to believe that the mechanism of action is a suppression of disease expression. Long-term effective therapy (up to 10 years) without side effects has been achieved in some of my patients, who are regularly monitored with complete blood counts.

Corticosteroids

Systemic corticosteroids are useful in most patients with vasculitis, but because of multiple potential toxic effects their use should be limited to patients with severe disease or those in whom the therapy is expected to be short-term. The absolute indications for systemic corticosteroids include a rapid progressive course, neurologic involvement, renal involvement with loss of function, carditis or coronary vasculitis, and severe pulmonary disease with cavitation or infiltration. Among the relative indications are chronic cutaneous disease unresponsive to other agents, peripheral neuropathy, chronic lung disease, weight loss, and fever.

Corticosteroids should be given in moderate to high daily dosages. I use prednisone at a starting dose of 60 to 80 mg per day in a divided dose. Divided dosage is clinically more effective than a single morning dose, even in equivalent milligram for milligram doses. However, the increased efficacy is accompanied by an increased risk of side effects (see further on). The drug is continued until the signs and symptoms of vasculitis have been controlled, at which point a switch to a single morning dose should be attempted, and the dosage then slowly tapered. Tapering should take place over a period about twice the length of the active treatment phase. If reactivation of the disease occurs, the original dosage should be reinstituted, followed by a slow taper.

Recently, intravenous administration of methylprednisolone in high doses (1 gram per day for 5 days) has been used in patients with acute fulminating vasculitis. This therapy is not without risk: sudden electrolyte shifts, cardiac arrhythmias, and cardiac arrests have been reported. The patient must be carefully monitored throughout therapy. This is a stopgap measure for severe disease, and other means of disease suppression are necessary for long-term control of the vasculitic process.

Corticosteroids, as mentioned, are frequently accompanied by side effects. Careful monitoring for diabetes mellitus, hypertension, peptic ulcer disease, osteoporosis, cataract formation, and glaucoma is important. Also, reactivation of *Mycobacterium tuberculosis* infection can occur, and attempts to identify the at-risk patient should be made at the onset of therapy. It has recently been pointed out that reliable skin testing can be done during the first few days to weeks of therapy with systemic corticosteroids, and thus therapy need not be delayed until results of the skin test are available.

Immunosuppressives

Patients who fail to respond to systemic corticosteroids, who develop steroid-related side effects, or in whom the disease is severe may be treated with an immunosuppressive agent. The agents most often used in vasculitis are alkylating agents, such as cyclophosphamide (Cytoxan) and chlorambucil (Leukeran), antimetabolites such as azathioprine (Imuran), the folate antagonist methotrexate (Rheumatrex), and cyclosporine (Sandimmune). Earlier studies suggested that cyclophosphamide was the therapy of choice in conditions such as severe necrotizing vasculitis and Wegener's granulomatosis, but recent reports indicate that methotrexate may be equally effective in Wegener's granulomatosis. Cyclophosphamide has been used in a daily oral dose of 1 to 2 mg per kg. It is administered in the morning, and the patient is given adequate hydration throughout the day to prevent hemorrhagic cystitis. This agent should not be given during pregnancy. Its beneficial effects are often not seen until 4 to 6 weeks. Recently, cyclophosphamide has been administered in intermittent intravenous pulses; this method avoids some of the potential long-term toxicity, but hemorrhagic cystitis remains a possibility. Chlorambucil is an agent with a presumably similar mechanism of action, but without associated bladder toxicity, but it has been much less well studied. Both cyclophosphamide and chlorambucil have been linked to an increased risk of neoplasia, in particular lymphoreticular malignancies.

Azathioprine has recently been reported to be useful in patients with severe refractory cutaneous vasculitis and in patients with rheumatoid vasculitis. It has also been used in severe necrotizing vasculitis, polyarteritis nodosa, and Wegener's granulomatosis, but it is probably less effective than cyclophosphamide in these conditions. It is administered in a single oral dose of 1 to 2 mg per kg. The primary toxicities are drug-induced fever, pancreatitis, hepatitis, and bone marrow toxicity. The onset of action is also delayed, occurring within 4 to 6 weeks. Long-term toxicity, including the risk of neoplasia, has recently been studied in patients with rheumatoid arthritis, but the risk of subsequent malignancy was no greater in the azathioprine-treated patients than in those with similar disease who were not given azathioprine.

Low-dose weekly methotrexate (7.5 to 15 mg) has been used to treat patients with Wegener's granulomatosis, rheumatoid vasculitis, and cutaneous polyarteritis nodosa. Methotrexate can be administered orally, intramuscularly, or intravenously. Renal function should be carefully assessed prior to initiating therapy, since failure to excrete the methotrexate increases the potential for severe toxicity. Initial monitoring of patients treated with methotrexate should include frequent complete blood counts and liver function tests. Long-term therapy requires periodic liver biopsies to monitor for potential fibrosis and cirrhosis.

Cyclosporine is a relatively new agent developed to prevent transplant rejection. The mechanism of its action is unknown. It is administered in doses of 3 to 8 mg per kg per day, and its side effects are closely linked. Renal toxicity is a limiting factor, and careful monitoring of renal function and blood pressure is necessary. Blood levels (trough) can be obtained, but it is not clear how meaningful they are in terms of toxicity or effect. Clinical experience with cyclosporine in patients with vasculitis is anecdotal.

Plasmapheresis

Plasma exchange can be an adjunct to therapy for severe diseases characterized by circulating immunoreactants, such as vasculitis. A number of exchanges are required and they must be performed in a hospital setting. This therapy can protect patients through a severe flare of disease, although systemic therapy with corticosteroids and/or immunosuppressives is required for long-term control of the disease process.

DISEASES OF THE NAILS
method of
ECKART HANEKE, M.D.
Ferdinand-Sauerbruch Hospital
Wuppertal, Germany

INFECTIONS OF THE NAIL ORGAN
Onychomycoses

Fungal infections of the nails are collectively called "onychomycoses," whereas "tinea unguium" refers to dermatophyte infections that involve the nails. Onychomycoses are the most common nail diseases, accounting for 15 to 40% of all cases. About one-quarter of all dermatomycoses are estimated to be nail infections. Furthermore, they are the most difficult to treat of all fungal skin diseases. The main considerations in the differential diagnosis are onychodystrophies, as seen after trauma or repeated minor damage or in impaired arterial and venous circulation, lymphatic obstruction, peripheral neuropathy, and diabetes, as well as nail psoriasis, Reiter's disease, eczematous dermatitis, lichen planus, and alopecia areata unguium. Onychomycoses are exceptional in children and rare in young adults, but their prevalence increases steadily with age. Whenever one sees a single nail affected, trauma should be considered.

Trichophyton rubrum accounts for about 80 to 85% of all infections, *T. mentagrophytes (interdigitale)* for about 10 to 15%, and *Epidermophyton floccosum* for 2 to 3%. Molds usually infect already damaged nails and hence may be found in association with dermatophytes, but *Hendersonula toruloidea* and *Scytalidium hyalinum* can primarily infect nails. *Candida albicans* and other *Candida* species are mainly found in fingernails. Onychomycoses can take many forms and must be distinguished according to pathogenesis, mode of invasion, and to a certain degree the type of pathogenic fungus.

Distal subungual onychomycosis is by far the most frequent type of infection. It develops from an infection of the hyponychium, which is commonly an extension of tinea pedis or manuum. The fungal infection initially causes a mild inflammation of the nail bed with consequent hyperkeratosis. With the gradual proximal advancement of the infection, the nail bed epithelium takes on an epidermal configuration and produces a horny layer. This allows further fungal invasion and also gives rise to onycholysis, since this keratosis prevents normal nail plate–nail bed adherence. This mechanism of fungal invasion also explains why the nail plate is seldom invaded by the fungus. Gradually, discoloration, subungual hyperkeratosis, onycholysis, and finally plate destruction occur.

Proximal subungual onychomycosis develops from an infection of the proximal nail fold when the fungus invades the cuticle and also grows in the stratum corneum of the eponychium toward the matrix. When the fungus reaches the depth of the nail pocket at the proximal end of the matrix, it is incorporated into the growing nail plate and transported away from the matrix epithelium. This is why the inflammatory changes are relatively mild and why the fungus invades the nail plate at different levels. In immunocompetent patients, it takes a long time for the fungus to travel along the matrix distally to the nail bed. However, this formerly very rare type of onychomycosis is now commonly seen in AIDS patients, in whom it is rapidly progressive.

Superficial white onychomycosis is due to *Trichophyton mentagrophytes* in the vast majority of cases and is seen only on the toenails. Molds are unusual etiologic agents, and *Trichophyton rubrum* has only recently been seen in AIDS patients. Histopathology reveals huge amounts of spores arranged in chains on the surface and in superficial splits of the nail plate. This growth pattern is consistent with the saprophytic form of *T. mentagrophytes.*

Total dystrophic onychomycosis can develop in any of the previously mentioned fungal nail infections, with the exception of superficial white onychomycosis in immunocompetent patients. Chronic mucocutaneous candidiasis, a rare condition characterized by a variety of immune defects, produces a primary total dystrophic onychomycosis, in which there are irregular keratin masses instead of an orderly nail plate. The nail bed and matrix are papillomatous, and there is a chronic inflammatory infiltrate. *T. rubrum* may coexist with *Candida albicans.*

Diagnosis

Since treatment of any fungal nail infection is tedious and time consuming, the diagnosis of onychomycosis must be confirmed by laboratory examinations either to exclude nonfungal diseases or to determine the fungus species and the best therapeutic agent.

In *superficial white onychomycosis,* the surface may be scraped for a potassium hydroxide (KOH) wet mount and mycologic culture. With a sharp scalpel, a slice of the nail plate is cut tangentially and processed for histopathology. Periodic acid–Schiff (PAS), Grocott, or Gridley stains nicely stain the organism and demonstrate their superficial seating.

Distal subungual onychomycosis exhibits a variable amount of subungual keratin harboring most of the fungal organisms. The nail plate should be cut as proximally as possible to expose the advancing border of the infection, where most of the fungi are found. Here the keratin is used for KOH mounts, histopathology, and culture; the trimmed nail plate is not ideal for culture since it contains few fungal elements.

In *proximal (white) subungual onychomycosis,* which is characterized by the sudden appearance of whitish opaque spots in the nail, abundant fungi are found in the nail plate. A punch biopsy of the nail plate can easily be taken from this area. The digit is immersed in warm water for about 5 to 10 minutes to soften the nail plate, which is cautiously punched. Since no anesthesia is used, the patient will let you know if you cut too deeply. The plate is cut, and one piece may be processed for histopathology and the remainder cut into small pieces for culture.

In *total dystrophic onychomycosis,* the nail surface is often heavily colonized with airborne saprophytes. Cleansing with 70% alcohol and scraping away the most superficial keratotic debris may be necessary before taking material for KOH mounts and culture.

KOH mounts are easy to perform. A few drops of 10 or 20% KOH are placed on a glass slide, and scrapings are immersed and finally coverslipped. When the slide is gently heated over an alcohol flame, the keratin is slowly dissolved by the KOH, whereas the fungi remain intact. The latter are seen under the microscope as strongly refractile structures; however, neither determination of fungal species nor differentiation from cloth fibers and other structures such as cell and lipid droplet borders is possible. Different media can be used for culture, but Sabouraud's and Kimmig's agars are both cheap and reliable. So-called dermatophyte or Candida-specific media contain substances that inhibit the growth of many other organisms but also, to a certain degree, some dermatophytes, and "Candida-selective" agar is not really selective. For toenails, two media—one with and one without ActiDione—are recommended to prevent molds from overgrowing dermatophytes. Nevertheless, cultures often remain negative despite unequivocal proof of a nail mycosis.

Treatment

Superficial white onychomycosis is easy to treat as long as the white area does not extend to or under the proximal nail fold. The surface is treated with an antimycotic solution, which is allowed to dry and then covered with antifungal cream. Softening of the nail surface with a 40% urea ointment to allow removal of fungus-containing nail layers and enhance penetration of the antimycotic agents shortens therapy.

All other types of onychomycoses are notoriously recalcitrant, demanding long-term treatment and optimal patient compliance. The therapeutic strategy depends on the clinical type and severity of onychomycosis, the pathogenic fungus, and predisposing factors.

If it does not involve too many nails and more than 60% of the nail area, *distal lateral subungual onychomycosis* can be treated with one of the recently developed topical formulations such as 1% bifonazole–40% urea* ointment (Mycospor Nail Set), amorolfine* nail lacquer, or ciclopirox (Loprox) nail lacquer. The former is applied under occlusive dressing and softens the nail plate considerably so that it can be atraumatically removed to expose the nail bed, which is the site of infection. Treatment is then continued with an antimycotic solution and/or ointment and the atraumatic removal of onycholytic nail and nail bed hyperkeratoses is repeated at intervals until a completely healthy nail has grown out.

Amorolfine* (Loceryl) is a new antifungal with both fungistatic and fungicidal action at very low concentrations. It is incorporated into a film-forming solution that steadily releases the active substance over several days, so it need be applied only twice a week. Its advantage is that the nail plate does not need to be cut away, but it is not recommended when the fungus has reached the matrix. Response rates are nearly 90% in fingernail infections and approach 70% in toenail infections.

Ciclopirox is a fungicidal substance that has the same antimycotic properties as ciclopiroxolamine (Loprox) but is more readily released from the lacquer-forming solution. It is applied once daily and the lacquer remnants are removed once weekly before reapplication of the preparation. Response rates are 90% in fingernail and 70% in toenail mycoses.

The mainstay of onychomycosis therapy is systemic treatment. Griseofulvin has been used for more than 30 years; however, its effectiveness has been limited, with cure rates of approximately 50 to 60% in fingernails and 20% in toenails. Recurrence rates approach 100% in toenails, and long-term if not lifelong prophylaxis is usually advised. The recommended dose is 500 mg micronized, or 330 mg ultramicronized, griseofulvin daily, but after a few months this usually turns out to be insufficient, so that the dose has to be doubled and after a few more months even tripled. Griseofulvin is usually well tolerated; gastrointestinal symptoms and headache are the most common adverse effects. Absorption is increased when taken with a meal rich in fats. Treatment duration is a minimum of 6 to 8

months for fingernails and 12 to 18 months for toenails. It is active only against dermatophytes; mixed as well as nondermatophytic infections do not respond. Griseofulvin is incorporated into the growing nail, but no data are available concerning its penetration into the subungual hyperkeratoses harboring the fungi. It is essential to remove as much of the infected nail plate and nail bed keratoses as possible, preferably by atraumatic avulsion, to shorten therapy and enhance cure rates. The slower the nail grows, the poorer the response rate.

Ketoconazole (Nizoral) is the first oral broad-spectrum azole antimycotic. It is more active than griseofulvin and dramatic results have been achieved in nail infections with chronic mucocutaneous candidiasis. The usual dose is 200 mg once a day with breakfast, but this may be increased to 200 mg twice daily. Treatment continues until a healthy nail has grown out. Hepatotoxic reactions, which on rare occasions have been fatal, limit its use for onychomycosis. This risk appears to be higher in patients who recently received griseofulvin. Doses higher than 200 mg per day can interfere with androgen biosynthesis and cause gynecomastia and even impotence.

Three new orally active antifungal substances have proved effective in onychomycosis. Fluconazole (Diflucan) is an azole antimycotic that is water soluble, well absorbed from the gastrointestinal tract, not metabolized by the liver, and excreted mainly unchanged by the kidneys. Only 11% is protein bound in the serum, and it is rapidly distributed in all body fluids. Promising results were achieved with 150 mg once weekly and with 100 mg per day.

Itraconazole (Sporanox) is another azole antimycotic that has shown promising results in onychomycoses. It is strongly lipophilic but well absorbed from the gastrointestinal tract. It is bound to plasma proteins but rapidly distributed to the skin. Because it binds specifically to fungal cytochrome P450, it does not interfere with human androgen synthesis and is better tolerated than ketoconazole. At a dose of 200 mg a day, a 3-month course for fingernails and a 6-month course for toenails give cure rates of more than 70%, with both clinical and mycologic cures increasing even after withdrawal of the drug. Recurrence rates are much lower than with griseofulvin.

Terbinafine* (Lamisil), an orally effective allylamine derivative, is already in use for onychomycoses in several European countries. It is lipophilic, well absorbed from the gastrointestinal tract, does not interfere with the cytochrome

---

*Not available in the United States.

*Not available in the United States.

P450 system, and is well tolerated. Side effects are mainly gastrointestinal, but loss of taste has been observed in a few cases. The daily dose is 250 mg, and 3 months of treatment are sufficient to cure roughly 90% of fingernail mycoses, but a 6-month course is recommended for toenails. Terbinafine is fungistatic and fungicidal, and both clinical and mycologic cure rates increase after the cessation of therapy at 3 and 6 months, respectively. Recurrence rates are surprisingly low.

Proximal subungual onychomycosis is primarily treated systemically with any of the oral antimycotics. Removal of the diseased nail plate may decrease treatment duration and enhance cure rates.

Total dystrophic onychomycosis can develop from distal or proximal subungual onychomycosis and may be due to dermatophytes or may be primary and caused by *C. albicans*. However, serious secondary infection by bacteria and saprophytic or pathogenic fungi is often present, considerably limiting the use of griseofulvin. Radical removal of infected nail remnants and keratotic debris is necessary in conjunction with systemic treatment. Ketoconazole, itraconazole, or fluconazole is indicated for nail lesions in chronic mucocutaneous candidiasis. Surgical nail avulsion and gentle curettage of the matrix and nail bed may be necessary if conservative treatment fails.

Nail Avulsion

Trauma is one of the most important predisposing factors for fungal nail infections. As the most serious iatrogenic trauma, nail avulsion should be limited to exceptional cases of onychomycoses refractory to consistent combined conservative treatment. Persons requesting nail avulsions usually want a "radical cure" and are not patient and compliant enough to benefit from long-term conservative treatment. Furthermore, avulsion is often mistaken for the therapy itself but in fact is just its start.

Partial nail avulsion is preferable to total avulsion; e.g., when one half of the nail is affected, it is sufficient to remove that portion. The commonly performed distal approach in nail avulsion is more traumatizing than the proximal approach, in which a nail elevator is introduced under the proximal nail fold to free it from the underlying nail plate and then slipped around the nail plate's proximal end under the nail. Moving the elevator gently back and forth frees the plate from the matrix and the nail bed.

Paronychia

Paronychia, the inflammation of the periungual soft tissues, can occur as an acute disease, but more often it is chronic with or without subacute flare-ups. Chronic paronychia is frequently due to *C. albicans* and bacteria, but foreign bodies can mimic *Candida* paronychia. Chronic paronychia leads to thickening of the proximal nail fold with loss of the cuticle and of the eponychium–nail bed attachment so that a probe can be inserted into the nail pocket to obtain material for mycologic and bacteriologic cultures. Predisposing factors are moisture and carbohydrate contacts, and this condition is seen mainly in homemakers, confectioners, bartenders, and fishmongers. Cracks in the cuticle can aid propagation of the condition in the beginning, but it is the chronic thickening of the proximal nail fold that causes the cuticle to completely disappear. Treatment is two-armed: avoiding the most important predisposing factor (i.e., moisture) and applying antimicrobial agents under the proximal nail fold. To avoid moisture the patient is warned not to wash his or her hands more often than three times a day and a hair dryer should be used after the towel. Dishwashing, preparing meals, and household work are done only with cotton gloves under heavy-duty rubber gloves, but even then the cotton gloves have to be changed regularly before they become wet with perspiration. When foreign material is suspected to have penetrated under the proximal nail fold, the fine jet of water from a mouth douche can be used to clean the nail pocket, which is then dried with a fine cotton swab and then a hair dryer. Topical treatment consists of antimycotic solutions, preferably those with antibacterial action (e.g., econazole [Spectazole], fenticonazole* [Lomexin]); these solutions reach the most proximal part of the infection by capillary diffusion. These topicals should be applied several times a day using a very soft nail or hand brush, allowed to dry, and then covered with a cream preparation. If *C. albicans* is repeatedly grown, a 10-day course of 200 to 400 mg ketoconazole or 100 to 200 mg itraconazole is helpful. Corticosteroids are usually not necessary. Very long-standing paronychia may cause the proximal nail fold to become nearly bone hard. This is best treated by excision of a crescent of tissue; healing is more rapid when the excisional margin is beveled according to the natural angle of the nail fold's free edge.

Mycotic onycholysis is treated exactly like chronic mycotic paronychia, except that the onycholytic portion of the nail plate has to be cut every 4 weeks.

---

*Not available in the United States.

Bacterial Infections

Whitlows are the most common bacterial infections of the nail organ. The most superficial type is a particular form of impetigo, mainly staphylococcal, also called *bulla repens* or *bulla rodens*. In contrast to common impetigo, the blister roof is more durable and the blisters can remain intact for 5 to 10 days and slowly enlarge to surround the nail. Treatment consists of complete removal of the blister roof, antiseptic soaks, and antimicrobial or antibiotic impregnated dressings to be changed twice daily, then after 2 or 3 days once daily.

Any whitlow can extend more deeply into the tissue to give rise to a *felon* that connects to the tendon sheath or extends under the nail plate. This should immediately be treated with systemic antibiotics selected according to culture-proven sensitivity or with staphylococcus-proof antibiotics. Any pyogenic infection of the nail matrix lasting longer than 48 hours can cause permanent nail damage, particularly in children. One should cut the nail plate over the subungual lake of pus, drain the pus, use antibacterial baths, initially twice daily, then once daily, and splint the finger and hand.

Viral Infections

Recurrent herpes simplex of the periungual skin is more frequent than commonly believed. However, it is usually not diagnosed and is mistakenly treated by surgeons as a whitlow or felon. A *herpetic whitlow* is due to herpes simplex virus type 1 or 2 and is often seen in medical personnel and dentists. In contrast to labial herpes simplex, it is accompanied by severe pain, lymphangitis, and frequently tender lymphadenitis. Treatment is essentially conservative. Severe symptoms and inability to perform professional activities warrant systemic treatment with oral acyclovir (Zovirax), 200 mg five times daily.

Periungual warts are the most frequent viral infection. Human papillomavirus causes both common and palmar plantar warts. They are easily diagnosed in children; however, several benign tumors and Bowen's disease must be differentiated in adults. Treatment consists of supportive and specific measures.

Warts prefer cool skin, and therefore bathing the hand or foot in very hot water twice a day to improve blood circulation is recommended. Additional trauma from biting, picking, or scratching must be avoided. Especially in children, suggestion therapy may be tried (e.g., gentian violet or eosin painting plus ultraviolet radiation). Specific treatment is preferably conservative. No antiviral

drug is effective against human papillomaviruses, but there is a wide choice of keratolytic and caustic agents, and their selection depends on personal experience and preferences, practicability, possible pain of the procedure, number of warts and their location, and previous treatment. My first choice is saturated monochloroacetic acid which is applied sparingly and allowed to dry. It is then covered with a 40% salicylic acid plaster overlapping the wart by a few millimeters and held in place for a week by simple adhesive tape. This permits the patient to take hot hand or foot baths twice a day without loosening of the tape. Once a week, the tape and salicylic acid plaster are removed after the hot bath, the necrotic superficial portions of the wart are curetted, and the procedure is repeated until the wart is gone. Depending upon the amount of monochloroacetic acid applied, a dull pain may commence a few hours after application and last up to 24 hours. If it is intolerable, the dressing is removed and the digit is soaked in lukewarm or even cool water, and the salicylic acid plaster is reapplied a few hours later. The success rate is greater than 80% with proper patient compliance. Subungual warts first require removal of the nail plate covering the wart; this can be done under local anesthesia, preferably a digital block.

Alternative conservative therapies include concentrated salicylic acid ointments or lacquers, the latter frequently in combination with lactic acid (Duofilm), cantharidine (Cantharone), which produces a blister that tears the wart out from the bottom, or intralesional bleomycin (0.1 μg per ml).

Warts are essentially benign infectious fibroepitheliomas with a natural life span of approximately 5 years. Any operation resulting in scarring or mutilation constitutes therapeutic "overkill." The most frequent surgical procedure is curettage, which is performed under digital block anesthesia. Since bleeding may be considerable, antibiotic tulle gras and thick gauze padding should be applied for 24 hours. Then the hand or foot is soaked so that the gauze floats off of the wound—a painless procedure. Electrodesiccation is not recommended since it can induce scarring or even matrix damage. This is also the reason why electrosurgical wart removal cannot be recommended for periungual and subungual warts. Cryosurgery may be successful if done by an experienced person. However, freezing times must be limited over the proximal nail fold to avoid damage to the matrix. Postcryosurgical edema can cause extreme pain, warranting the administration of nonsteroidal anti-inflammatory agents or aspirin the evening prior to cryosurgery.

Infestations

Scabies mites infect the hyponychium in Norwegian scabies, in severe immunodeficiency such as AIDS, lymphoma, or histiocytosis X, and occasionally in elderly persons. Usually moderate subungual hyperkeratosis develops, which can persist even after otherwise successful treatment and give rise to repeated relapses and small epidemics. Treatment must include all of the skin surface from the neck to the toes, and in the case of sub- and periungual scabies, the scabicide should be applied with a "surgical hand wash" twice a day for at least 3 days.

Tungiasis is caused by the fertilized female sandflea, *Tunga penetrans,* which digs into the plantar skin, particularly under and around the nail. It enters the skin with its abdomen pointing outwards and can mimic a foreign body granuloma. Secondary infection is common. Cautious removal under regional block anesthesia is recommended.

THE NAIL IN DERMATOLOGIC DISEASE

Psoriasis is the skin disease with the highest incidence of nail involvement. Nail lesions are found in about 50% of psoriasis patients when first seen, but there is a greater than 90% chance of developing nail changes over the lifetime. The characteristic pits are due to minute short-term psoriatic lesions of the most proximal portion of the matrix. Salmon patches are psoriasis plaques of the nail bed, which when involving the hyponychium, can cause onycholysis. Severe matrix involvement causes nail destruction.

Treatment of nail psoriasis is difficult. Pits are best left untreated; if they cause cosmetic embarassment, nail varnish or artificial nails can be applied. Psoriasis of the nail bed and hyponychium can be treated with potent corticosteroid solutions that spread under the nail by capillary action. However, secondary bacterial and yeast infections do occur and can act like the Koebner phenomenon in exacerbating subungual psoriasis. To avoid secondary infection, the fingers should be dipped once or twice daily into an antimicrobial solution such as chlorhexidine, hexamidine, or hexachlorophene or even an azole antimycotic solution. Psoriasis of the nail folds responds to anthralin (Dithranol), but most patients find this cosmetically unacceptable since it stains the fingers and nails. The most recent advance in psoriasis therapy, calcipotriol ointment* (Daivonex, Psorcutan), is a very useful, cosmetically acceptable alternative. A nearly 90% improvement has also been achieved with 1% 5-fluorouracil cream (Efudex) applied twice daily to the nail region. Intralesional-subungual injection of triamcinolone acetonide crystal suspension (Kenalog) is the optimal treatment. Under regional anesthesia, about 0.1 ml is injected into the proximal nail fold on either side of the extensor tendon insertion or under the nail bed. Although radiation can bring about dramatic improvement, it is not recommended since patients frequently insist on repeated courses, and they will seek out another radiotherapist when they are refused further x-ray treatments, risking chronic radiodermatitis, nail dystrophy, and cancer.

Any effective systemic treatment for psoriasis is usually also beneficial for the nail lesions; this is true for photochemotherapy with 8-methoxypsoralene and ultraviolet A (PUVA), for cyclosporine, and for retinoids. However, etretinate (Tegison, Tigason*) can be destructive to the nails, although it is the treatment of choice for pustular psoriasis and acrodermatitis continua suppurativa. Its metabolite, acitretin* (Neo-Tegison, Neo-Tigason), has virtually the same spectrum of action as etretinate.

Reiter's disease frequently affects the nail and may not be distinguishable from ungual psoriasis. Treatment is the same as for severe nail psoriasis.

Eczematous dermatitis of the nail apparatus is mainly seen in allergic contact dermatitis, especially in hairdressers, in atopic hand dermatitis, and in immediate-type contact allergy to food allergens. In allergic contact dermatitis, oozing papulovesicles and reddening gradually develop into chronic eczema with thickening of the proximal nail fold, loss of the cuticle and eponychium–nail bed adherence, nail plate deformation with irregular horizontal grooves and ridges, and discoloration. Nail involvement in dyshidrotic atopic dermatitis may look very similar.

The mainstay of treatment in allergic contact dermatitis is strict and consistent avoidance of allergens, moisture, and other irritants. Potent topical steroids to be applied as a solution for involvement of the eponychium and nail bed and as a cream for periungual skin can usually be followed by a moderately potent steroid after a week and finally a weak one. Recurrences occur even with allergen restriction, probably due to nonspecific primary irritation. It is not unusual to have a two-phase eczema with specific sensitization consequent to chronic irritant dermatitis when rubber gloves are worn and the patient develops an allergy to rubber chemicals. Nail involvement in chronic atopic dermatitis is more

---

*Not available in the United States.

*Not available in the United States.

recalcitrant and may occasionally require intralesional steroid injections.

Ungual lichen planus is seen in about 10% of all lichen planus patients or can occur as an isolated nail disease. The proximal matrix and eponychium are most frequently affected, hence the loss of luster and nail sheen, the rough ridging, and the thickening of the proximal nail fold. Extensive matrix involvement can cause pterygium formation. Treatment is usually unrewarding. High-potency steroids are rubbed in twice daily with salicylic acid to enhance penetration. Intralesional steroid injections repeated every month may be necessary in severe cases with pterygium formation or even ulceration. Oral steroids must be given in doses several times greater than the Cushing threshold and thus cannot be recommended. Oral retinoids (etretinate, acitretin) are commonly disappointing as is topical cyclosporine.

Alopecia areata can be accompanied by a spongiotic dermatitis of the matrix and nail bed with consequent dense fine pitting, loss of luster, friability, thickening, and dirty grayish discoloration of the nail plate. Nail shedding does not occur. Treatment is not very successful. High-potency topical steroids may be tried, followed by intralesional steroid injections if topicals do not produce a response. Often the nail lesions run a course similar to the hair loss, with spontaneous remissions and recurrences. In general, the nail lesions are most severe and persistent in universal alopecia areata.

Virtually all *autoimmune bullous dermatoses* such as pemphigus vulgaris, bullous pemphigoid, cicatricial pemphigoid, and epidermolysis bullosa acquisita may occasionally produce nail lesions. Systemic corticosteroids, preferably in combination with immunosuppressants, will clear all lesions. Topical antibiotics are occasionally required to combat secondary bacterial or yeast infections. Nail involvement in Stevens-Johnson and Lyell's syndrome can cause permanent nail loss when nails heal with scarring. Potent topical steroids are indicated to avoid scarring.

SPECIFIC NAIL DISORDERS

Twenty-nail dystrophy is an acquired, idiopathic nail dystrophy in which all the nails become uniformly rough, pitted, or ridged. It develops insidiously in childhood and resolves spontaneously with age. It has inconclusively been associated with lichen planus, alopecia areata, and psoriasis. The best management is thorough explanation and avoidance of all therapeutic attempts.

Brittle nails are frequent in women, but men rarely complain of this condition. Several clinical types have to be differentiated: (1) onychorrhexis, in which a series of fine parallel superficial furrows appears, often with an isolated split extending proximally, (2) breaking of the nail, resulting in a crenellated margin, (3) transverse splitting and breaking of the lateral edge close to the distal margin, which prevents the nail from growing long, and (4) onychoschisis, the horizontal splitting of nail layers at the free margin of the plate. A vast array of causes has been offered; however, except for chronic minor trauma from chronic immersion in water, detergents, organic solvents and mineral oils, alkalis, oxidizing agents, and cosmetic hair and nail procedures, none has been confirmed.

Nails in women appear to be much more susceptible to brittleness than those of men. Treatment includes strict avoidance of any possible cause, particularly moisture. Topical therapy is rarely helpful, although some authors recommend massaging the nail with an emollient; any potential benefit may well be due to the mechanical effect of massage with improvement of peripheral circulation. Soft nails may be hardened by applying a base coat, nail polish, and hard top coat. A variety of different treatments have been advocated, biotin 2.5 mg daily being the most recent one. Other therapies include oral iron; daily doses of evening primrose oil (six capsules, each containing 40 mg of gamma-linoleic acid), pyridoxine (30 mg), or ascorbic acid (2 to 3 grams); low dose vitamin A; and gelatin. However, it takes a minimum of 6 months for fingernails to regrow, so all drugs have to be taken for at least half a year before being evaluated.

Hangnails (agnails) are small triangular tags of hard keratotic epidermis of the proximal nail fold that are painful and can be the portal of entry for bacterial infections. In addition to hereditary susceptibility, hydration and dehydration and dry skin appear to be common precipitating factors. Hangnails should be cut with fine sharp scissors, not torn! Abundant use of bland emollients, under occlusion overnight, is beneficial.

Ingrown toenails are a frequent ailment often limiting physical activity. Five different types have to be differentiated: (1) neonatal form with an incompletely grown-out nail, (2) neonatal-infantile form due to a hypertrophic lateral lip, (3) infantile form due to congenital malalignment of the great toenail, (4) adolescent form, the most frequent type, mainly seen in tall youngsters with a very wide, often overcurved nail and hyperhidrosis of the feet, and (5) adult form due to a thick, inelastic, overcurved nail plate.

The *neonatal ingrown toenail* is due to a distal nail fold and to distally narrowing lateral nail folds. Consistent massage of the nail walls in distal-volar and lateral-volar directions, respectively, will gradually free the nail and allow it to grow out. Recurrences do not occur. No surgery is necessary. The *hypertrophic lateral lip (neonatal-infantile) form* is always treated conservatively with massage of the lateral nail fold to keep it away from the nail plate.

Congenital malalignment of the great toenail is a lateral deviation of the nail that can lead to transverse ridging and waving, partial nail shedding, onycholysis with permanent shrinking of the nail bed, discoloration, permanent onychodystrophy, and ingrown toenail. Any of these signs indicates that surgical realignment of the nail's long axis is necessary. This is best done before age 2. A crescentic wedge of tissue is excised from the tip of the toe under general anesthesia, and the entire nail apparatus is dissected from the bone and swung to achieve a correct longitudinal axis. Healing is generally uneventful.

Ingrown toenails are most frequent in school children and young adolescents. Whatever the precipitating factor, there is a discrepancy between the wide nail plate and the narrow nail bed. It is therefore logical to narrow the nail plate, leaving the nail bed and lateral nail folds intact. The optimal treatment is thus selective lateral matrix horn resection, either by surgical excision or by cautery using liquefied phenol (90% phenol). A digital block is performed at the base of the toe with 2 to 3 ml 2% lidocaine, the ingrown nail plate is cut longitudinally about one-fifth the distance from its margins, both lateral nail strips are avulsed after having been freed from the eponychium and nail bed, and the matrix is completely dried of blood. Under hemostasis, liquified phenol is vigorously rubbed for 2 to 3 minutes into each corner of the matrix. If there is abundant granulation tissue this may be gently cauterized with phenol for a few seconds. Small antibiotic tablets are placed into the wound cavities and a thick padded dressing with abundant antimicrobial ointment is applied for 24 hours. This is changed daily in a warm footbath containing povidone-iodine soap. Provided the cautery was long enough and the phenol had not been inactivated by blood, there will be no recurrences. This method is extremely simple and safe; toxicity from the minute areas treated by phenol has not been observed. Surgical dissection of the matrix horns is an alternative, but it requires considerable surgical skill and experience. However, healing is more rapid after surgical excision than after phenol cautery.

Overcurvature of the nails *(pincer nails)* is hereditary if symmetric and also involving several lesser toes, whereas foot deformities, chronic psoriasis, and digital osteoarthritis commonly cause asymmetric pincer nails. Most cases produce remarkably little symptomatology, but pain can sometimes be excruciating when the lateral nail margin digs deeply into the soft tissue. X-ray films virtually always show a widening of the base of the distal phalanx resulting in a distally increasing inward curving of the nail. Orthonyx treatment with elastic steel nail braces is therefore useless. Treatment is entirely surgical with resection of the lateral matrix horns and longitudinal incision of the nail bed to allow it to be dissected from the underlying bone and spread. Reverse tie-over sutures keep the spread nail bed in place.

TRAUMA

The most frequent sequela to trauma is *hematoma*, which commonly results from a blow of a hammer or a crush injury from a door. Depending on the intensity of trauma, the hematoma may involve part or all of the nail bed and matrix. Small hematomas usually do not require treatment. Hematomas involving less than 50% of the nail field may be cautiously drained by burning a hole into the nail plate with the red-hot end of a paper clip. Hematomas greater than 50% usually involve nail bed and matrix and often also bone fractures. A radiograph should be taken, and meticulous repair by an experienced hand surgeon is mandatory.

Nail habits are not rare and are most commonly seen on thumb nails as a washboard deformity of the median portion of the plate. This is almost always associated with a very large lunula and loss of the cuticle since the patients push the proximal nail fold back to the dead end of the nail pocket. This condition is symmetric when the thumb nail of the opposite hand is used to push back the cuticle, but occurs on only one thumb when the index finger of the same hand is used. It is often mistaken for Heller's median caliniform dystrophy. Onychotillomania (habitual picking, filing, and cutting until virtually all of the nail plate is removed) is a less common habit. Treatment is difficult because most patients will not admit to their habit and insist on a somatic etiology.

TUMORS OF THE NAIL APPARATUS

Many benign and malignant tumors occur under and around the nail. Only the most common and most important tumors are dealt with in this section.

Benign Tumors

Myxoid pseudocyst is a common lesion of the proximal nail fold. About 80 to 90% occur on the fingers. They usually present as an ill-defined, elastic, flesh-colored tumor sparing the midline of the nail. A longitudinal depression in the nail plate results from continuous pressure on the matrix. Any puncture of the pseudocyst will reduce this pressure and cause transverse rims in the depression. Myxoid pseudocysts are degenerative lesions, not true tumors. Repeated needlings and expression, injection of hyaluronidase, sclerosing agents, or steroid crystals are followed by frequent recurrences. Cryosurgery by the experienced operator achieves cure rates of up to 80%.

When complete surgical removal is undertaken, a digital block is performed and 0.1 to 0.2 ml of sterile methylene blue solution is injected into the distal interphalangeal joint via the volar crease. This will stain the stalk from the pseudocyst to the joint and the true extent of the lesion becomes apparent. An incision is made around the tumefaction, and a small transposition flap is incised. The lesion is meticulously dissected and the flap raised. Any extension of the lesion can now be seen due to the methylene blue and should be removed. The stalk is followed and resected and the incision is closed with 6-0 resorbable sutures. The flap is transposed into the primary defect and sutured. The secondary defect is allowed to heal by secondary intention. This treatment yields excellent functional and cosmetic results with a recurrence rate less than 2%.

Periungual fibromas and *fibrokeratomas* are not rare. Their treatment is relatively simple. *Multiple fibromas* in tuberous sclerosis (Koenen tumors) are cut at their base and the wound surface is allowed to epithelialize by secondary intention.

Fibrokeratomas are acquired benign tumors that often arise in the nail pocket, most frequently from the proximal matrix. They have a fibromatous core that must be enucleated down to the bone in order to prevent recurrences. If the fibrokeratoma emerges from within the nail plate, two lateral incisions are made and the proximal nail fold is reflected back. A No. 11 scalpel is inserted between the nail plate surrounding the tumor and the tumor itself and advanced in the natural split down to the bone to dissect the fibrokeratoma from the periosteum. Usually, the matrix defect cannot be sutured but heals uneventfully by secondary intention. The nail deformation, commonly a longitudinal depression, will disappear spontaneously.

Subungual filamentous tumors are common lesions characterized by a longitudinal whitish or reddish line in the nail plate, which is due to a keratotic rim on the undersurface of the nail plate. This can be easily seen in unmanicured nails. The subungual filamentous tumor is probably an extremely thin subungual fibrokeratoma. Treatment is necessary only when it results in a split nail; otherwise it can be pared down painlessly.

Giant cell synovialoma, one of the most common tumors of the hand, can be found in the proximal nail fold area. It usually presents as a multilobulate, firm, subcutaneous tumor that can invade the overlying dermis and interfere with nail growth. It is removed by dissection from the surrounding tissue, along with any involved skin. The defect is covered with a full-thickness skin graft taken from an area of thin skin or a Wolfe-Krause graft.

The *glomus tumor* is the most characteristic subungual tumor. It is associated with radiating pain, which is either spontaneous or evoked by minor trauma or cold. The pain is often relieved by a tourniquet. Clinically, the tumor presents as a bluish-red spot in the nail bed that is extremely tender on probing. Small lesions can be removed after punching or cutting a hole in the nail plate that is about 50% larger than the glomus tumor. The nail bed is then incised longitudinally, and the tumor, which usually looks like a small grayish pea, is dissected from the surrounding tissue. Tumors in a lateral position are removed by an L-shaped incision of the tip of the finger allowing dissection of the nail bed from the bone until the lesion is reached.

Malignant Tumors

Bowen's disease of the nail organ is not rare, although it can mimic common warts, butcher's nodule (tuberculosis cutis verrucosa), chronic paronychia, granulation tissue, and even fibrokeratoma. Rare variants may be pigmented. Its onset is insidious, and it is usually asymptomatic. Human papillomavirus 16, 35, and other types have been detected in a number of ungual Bowen's lesions. Treatment of choice is complete surgical excision with microscopic control of the excision margins. Depending on its size, the resultant defect will require flap or graft closure. Serial and step sections of the surgical specimen are essential to histopathologically rule out invasive squamous cell carcinoma.

Squamous cell carcinoma is a slow-growing, low-grade malignancy that can develop from ungual Bowen's disease or de novo but is also found after trauma, in chronic radiodermatitis, and in osteitis terminalis. Major differential diagnostic considerations are paronychia, ingrown nail, pyogenic granuloma, warts, and amelanotic melanoma. Complete surgical excision is mandatory and should be done by Mohs micrographic surgery.

Melanonychia Striata and Melanoma

The nail apparatus contains melanocytes that are normally nonfunctional. However, both benign and malignant melanocytic lesions can arise in the nail matrix, bed, or periungual tissue. Any lesion of the matrix that continually produces melanin in quantities that can no longer be completely degraded by the keratinocytes will result in a longitudinal brown to black streak. This may be due to a focus of active melanocytes, a lentigo, or a melanocytic nevus, but also to a malignant melanoma. Multiple pigmented bands are seen in dark-skinned people, after PUVA therapy, in adrenal insufficiency, malnutrition, AIDS, or after treatment with zidovudine (Retrovir), antimalarials, or minocycline (Minocin). Any longitudinal band in a fair-complexioned individual is suspicious and should be biopsied; excisional biopsy is usually necessary to make the correct diagnosis. Hutchinson's melanotic whitlow, the spreading of melanin pigmentation to periungual skin, is usually associated with ungual melanoma. Although malignant melanonychia striata is commonly dark brown, subungual melanoma may masquerade as a light-brown band, and 20 to 25% of ungual melanomas are amelanotic, mimicking pyogenic granuloma, granulation tissue, or ingrown nail. Bands wider than 5 to 6 mm are usually malignant, and darkening and widening of a light-brown band in a black or Asian individual is suggestive of melanoma. Bleeding, ulceration, and onychodystrophy are characteristic of ungual melanoma.

A considerable proportion of patients present only after trauma to the nail, and a subungual hematoma or infection may obscure the clinical picture. If this is the case, pigmented material should be scraped from the nail, boiled in a test tube, and tested for blood content. Blood tends to grow out with the nail and usually has a horizontal border proximally. Microbial pigment can be seen on histologic slides as a diffuse brownish staining, whereas melanin is finely granular and stains with an argentaffin reaction.

When confronted with a pigmented nail lesion, one has to consider that overtreatment of a benign alteration may cause unnecessary mutilation but delay in diagnosis and treatment may allow the melanoma to disseminate. An individual approach is therefore proposed: Narrow bands are diagnosed and treated by punching the lesion out after having reflected the proximal nail fold and identified the melanocytic lesion. Lesions in far lateral position are removed using the technique of lateral longitudinal nail biopsy, which will eventually result in a somewhat narrower nail. Wider lesions are either biopsied, or a transversally oriented fusiform excision is performed. Hutchinson's melanotic whitlow is a widespread (in situ) melanoma and requires wide excision of the nail organ as does any early invasive melanoma. Advanced malignant melanoma may require amputation of the digit.

KELOIDS

method of
JOUNI UITTO, M.D., PH.D.
Jefferson Medical College of Thomas Jefferson University
Philadelphia, Pennsylvania

CLINICAL FEATURES

Keloids manifest as hard, elevated fibrous tumors with predilection for sites on the upper back, chest, and ear lobes. Their appearance is associated with trauma, which may be quite mild and go unnoticed by the patient. Young patients are more likely to develop keloids than the elderly. There appears to be a racial predisposition, inasmuch as keloids are more common in blacks and Asians than in whites. Also, in about 10% of the European white patients with keloids, there is a positive family history of similar lesions. Thus, keloids are acquired cutaneous lesions with a clear genetic predisposition.

Hypertrophic scars are clinically similar to keloids, but the distinction between these two types of lesions lies in the fact that hypertrophic scars are confined to the original wound margins, while keloids extend beyond the original site of the trauma.

Histopathology of keloids reveals that they are composed of excess connective tissue, primarily collagen. Recent biochemical and molecular biologic studies have disclosed that the growth and development of keloids is accompanied by enhanced expression of several of the collagen genes. Transforming growth factor-β, a multifunctional cytokine, may play a role in enhancing the collagen accumulation.

TREATMENT

In general, the treatment of keloids is difficult, and often only partially successful. Furthermore, keloids have a particular tendency to recur after surgical excision. The management of keloids consists of intralesional injections of high-potency glucocorticosteroids combined in selected cases with surgical removal of the excess tissue. The surgical removal of tissue can be accomplished by conventional surgery by scalpel, or the bulk of excess tissue can be ablated by a CO_2 laser. Nevertheless, in both cases, the lesions tend to regrow unless the procedure is coupled with intralesional injection of steroids, such as triamcinolone acetonide. This long-acting glucocorticoid decreases collagen synthesis, and when injected without accompanying surgical procedure, it results in gradual softening of the lesions. Triamcinolone acetonide should be diluted with lidocaine to lessen the pain, although initial injections to the hard lesions may be painful nevertheless. Relatively high concentrations (up to 40 mg per ml) of the steroid should be used. The injections can be repeated at 3-week intervals until the desired degree of flattening and softening of the lesion has been achieved.

Application of constant pressure has been suggested for the prevention and treatment of keloids. Although this treatment modality may be somewhat helpful, it requires the application of constant pressure, such as use of custom-fitted Jobst garments, which are often unacceptable to the patient. Recently, topical application of silicon sheets or gels, with or without the accompanying use of pressure, has been advocated. This treatment method appears to ameliorate the clinical symptoms, such as itching, and lead to softening of the lesions, but the mechanism of action and the long-term benefits remain to be elucidated.

Other lasers, besides the CO_2, such as the neodynium:YAG laser, have been suggested to soften keloids through "bioinhibition" of collagen synthesis. This approach is still experimental and its usefulness remains to be tested.

Other experimental approaches for treatment of keloids include pharmacologic inhibitors of collagen biosynthesis. Among them, interferon-γ, an inhibitor of collagen transcription, has been suggested to soften keloids. Similarly, topical application of all-*trans*-retinoic acid has been shown to reduce the size of keloids. However, the reduction has been only modest, and the long-term benefits from these approaches have not been established. Even more experimental is the use of other potential inhibitors of collagen deposition, including β-aminopropionitrile and D-penicillamine, which have been suggested to be helpful in other systemic fibrotic conditions, such as scleroderma.

PREVENTION

The best means of preventing keloids is avoidance of trauma and deferral of elective surgical procedures in patients with known tendency to keloid formation. If surgery is necessary, procedures that increase the length of the scar, such as Z-plasties and W-plasties, should be avoided. All wounds should be closed with small sutures placed close to the edge of the wounds, and the sutures should be removed as early as possible during the wound healing process.

WARTS
(Verruca Vulgaris)

method of
JENNIFER L. VESPER, M.D., and
NEIL A. FENSKE, M.D.
University of South Florida College of Medicine
Tampa, Florida

Human papilloma virus (HPV) infection causes the common wart. HPV is a member of the family Papovaviridae, which are nonenveloped viruses containing circular double-stranded DNA. Papilloma viruses are thought to be highly species specific.

Different HPV types are defined by the degree of DNA hybridization; the DNA of a new virus type cross-hybridizes less than 50% with the DNA of the previously identified types. Of the more than 60 types of HPV identified, types 1,2,4, and 7 manifest clinically as common warts, types 3 and 10 as flat warts, and types 1,2, and 4 as plantar warts. Several HPV types are associated with condylomata acuminata as well as cervical and mucous membrane infection. Of these, types 16, 18, 31, and 33 are known to be a strong risk factor for malignancy. HPV-16 is the type most frequently associated with cervical cancer.

EPIDEMIOLOGY

HPV infection is problematic worldwide. It most frequently affects children and young adults, in whom the incidence may be as high as 10%. Warts are spread from person to person as well as through autoinoculation and less commonly from fomites. If stored in glycerol, the virus can remain infectious for months to years. Although HPV is resistant to freezing or desiccation, infectivity can be blocked by treatment with detergents or temperatures greater than 55° C.

Not all warts are equally contagious. Factors that can affect infectivity include the quantity of virus in the wart (older warts usually have a lower concentration), the location of the wart, and the degree of exposure to the potential host as well as the immunologic status of this host. Patients with impaired cellular immunity have a significantly increased incidence of HPV infection. For example, more than 40% of renal transplant patients receiving immunosuppressive therapy become infected with HPV.

The incubation period for HPV infection can be as short as 4 weeks or as long as several months. All types of squamous epithelia can be infected; the appearance of the wart is affected by both the site of infection and the virus type.

CLINICAL MANIFESTATIONS AND DIFFERENTIAL DIAGNOSIS

Warts that occur on the hands are typically flesh-colored papules that eventually grow into yellowish gray verrucous hyperkeratotic papules. Flat warts, frequently found on the face, neck, and legs (often spread by shaving) are subtle 1- to 4-mm, round to oval, gray or yellowish brown, slightly raised papules. Warts on the plantar surface of the feet tend to grow inward and are often painful. Even though these warts are often considered "deep," like all warts they are confined to the epidermis and simply displace the dermis.

Sometimes corns (clavi) and calluses can be mistaken for plantar warts, but they can be differentiated by paring off the hyperkeratotic surface of the lesion and observing the freshly exposed surface. Verrucae obscure the normal skin lines and have small black dots representing thrombosed capillaries that have grown up the papillary projections of the wart. On the other hand, clavi have a hard translucent central core and frequently overlie the metatarsal heads. Clavi are quite painful until the core is removed by separating it from the normal skin with a #15 surgical blade and lifting it out. Lastly, calluses can be distinguished by the presence of normal skin lines after the roughened surface is pared away.

TREATMENT

The ideal treatment of verruca vulgaris would be one that is easy to perform, inexpensive, rapidly effective (with a low recurrence rate), and gives a cosmetically acceptable outcome. Unfortunately, no therapy fulfills all of these criteria. Instead a systematic approach is recommended.

First, the patient must understand that there are many ways to treat warts that are generally effective but require perseverence for complete resolution. The most simple, least traumatic treatments should be attempted first. These include topical cantharidin, topical keratolytic preparations, and cryosurgery.

Cantharidin (Cantharone), blister beetle extract, works by causing blister formation at the junction between the dermis and the epidermis. This is an excellent therapy for young children who do not tolerate cryosurgery well and for periungual warts. Unfortunately, one of the potential adverse outcomes is dissemination of the HPV to the blister edge where a subsequent ring of small verrucous papules can form.

Keratolytic agents, most commonly salicylic acid and lactic acid preparations, are often very effective but require a diligent patient. Ideally the patient applies the preparation twice a day after removing the dead hyperkeratotic layers by "sanding" the surface away with a pumice stone or an emery board. Penetration of the medication is improved if the lesion is soaked in warm water prior to treatment. Therapy should be continued until there is no interruption of the normal skin lines.

Cryosurgery is considered the first line of therapy by many clinicians. It can be applied by a cotton swab or with a spray canister. If cotton swabs are used, it is important not to reintroduce the swab into the main supply since the virus can remain alive in the liquid nitrogen and subse-quently be transmitted to the next patient. Many clinicians avoid this by pouring a small aliquot into a Styrofoam cup before dipping the swab into the liquid. The liquid nitrogen should be applied so that a small rim of normal-appearing tissue around the lesion also appears white. The area should remain frozen for several seconds depending on the size of the lesion and its location.

Cryosurgery is usually tolerated well. The pain from the procedure lasts about 5 minutes and mild discomfort for a few hours more. Blister formation (often hemorrhagic) frequently occurs within 24 hours after treatment. The blister should be allowed to remain intact unless the pressure is painful. If this is the case, the blister can be drained while leaving the roof intact to act as a natural dressing. As long as progress is being made, cryosurgery can be continued at 2- to 3-week intervals. If progress is slow, treatment can be attempted at weekly intervals before changing to another therapy. Cryosurgery should be avoided if possible in dark-skinned individuals since post-therapy hypopigmentation may occur.

Flat warts present a unique challenge because they are frequently multiple and often affect the face where potentially scarring procedures should be avoided. Retinoic acid cream applied at bedtime in a strength high enough to prompt moderate irritation and fine scaling clears flat warts in 50% of patients after several weeks of therapy. If this alone does not prove to be effective, some suggest light cryosurgery to individual lesions. Application of 5% 5-fluorouracil cream (Efudex), twice a day for 3 to 5 weeks is an alternative, although, as with many of the other therapies, 5-fluorouracil carries a risk of postinflammatory hyperpigmentation.

If individual lesions prove resistant to these therapies, various alternative surgical techniques can be employed. However, recurrences can occur, risk of scar formation is slightly higher, and local anesthesia must be used. Blunt dissection carries a low risk of scarring if the normal skin is not disturbed. The line of cleavage between the lesion and normal skin is delineated with blunt-tipped scissors, and the wart is gently separated from the surrounding skin and lifted out. Some clinicians advocate light curettage or electrodesiccation of the base to help reduce the recurrence rate, but these techniques increase the risk of pigmentary changes and scarring. Another technique is to enucleate the wart with a curet followed by electrodesiccation of the base to destroy the remaining lesion, but one must be careful, since overaggressive therapy can lead to excessive scar formation.

Additional therapies include contact immunotherapy, intralesional bleomycin, and carbon dioxide laser surgery. Contact immunotherapy, although still controversial, utilizes immunogens such as dinitrochlorobenzene (DNCB). The patient is sensitized by applying a small amount of the immunogen on the same extremity as the lesion. Erythema and blistering in the sensitized area indicate an active immune response. The following week, the same immunogen is painted onto the lesion, an allergic response to the sensitizer occurs, and the innocent bystander, the wart, is subsequently destroyed. Serial treatments may be required.

Injection of bleomycin sulfate 0.1% directly into the wart is often successful after two to three treatments. Although very little medication is required, it is quite expensive and the bleomycin is stable for only 60 days even when refrigerated. Bleomycin should be administered by an experienced clinician due to the risk of extensive tissue necrosis.

Carbon dioxide lasers have also been used in the treatment of cutaneous and mucosal verrucous lesions. Most of the studies reporting the efficacy of lasers in the treatment of HPV-induced lesions have focused on genital lesions. The laser is effective in treating clinically visible lesions; however, among its disadvantages are the expense of therapy, risk of fire, scar formation, and airborne contagion in the plume that can introduce the virus into the upper respiratory tract of the patient or personnel.

Large chronic refractory lesions may necessitate biopsy to rule out carcinomatous degeneration.

NEVI

method of
EDWARD M. YOUNG, Jr., M.D.
*Sidell, Erickson, McCleary and Young
Dermatology Surgical and Medical Group
Sherman Oaks, California*

Melanocytic nevi, also called nevocellular nevi or moles, are common benign pigment cell tumors. The term "nevus" ("new growth") has two meanings: usually, it refers to an acquired melanocytic nevus; however, it can also designate a congenital proliferation of various mature skin structures. For example, nevus sebaceus, nevus flammeus, and eccrine nevus refer to congenital proliferations of sebaceous glands, blood vessels, and eccrine sweat glands, respectively.

The medical importance of melanocytic nevi lies in their possible transformation into malignant melanoma. Increased ultraviolet exposure from sunbathing, outdoor recreation, and the thinning of the stratospheric ozone layer are all believed to be at least partly responsible for the epidemic rise in the incidence of malignant melanoma.

CLASSIFICATION

Clinically, melanocytic nevi appear as brown or black macules or patches (flat areas) and as pigmented or flesh-colored papules or nodules (raised growths). Histologically, nevi are classified according to the location of nevomelanocytes (nevus cells) within the skin.

Melanocytes originate from the ectodermal neural crest, then migrate to the basal cell layer of the epidermis. Most nevi appear during childhood and adolescence, then gradually regress during adulthood. Two exceptions to this rule, congenital nevi and dysplastic nevi, evolve differently and have a much higher incidence of malignant transformation.

The three major types of melanocytic nevi are junctional nevi, compound nevi, and intradermal nevi. Histologically, *junctional nevi* demonstrate clusters or nests of nevus cells in the lower epidermis at the junction of the dermis. In contrast, *intradermal nevi* display nests, cords, and strands of nevomelanocytes solely within the dermis. *Compound nevi* exhibit nests of nevus cells both at the demoepidermal junction and within the dermis (Table 1).

Sun exposure influences the development of nevi: most nevi are located on sun-exposed areas, such as the face, but are relatively uncommon in sun-protected areas, such as the axilla. Intense sun exposure also predisposes nevi toward malignant transformation.

Pigmented nevi appear brown or black due to melanin, produced in response to ultraviolet irradiation. Nevus cells at the dermoepidermal junction receive more ultraviolet light and produce more melanin than do nevus cells deep within the dermis. Junctional nevi appear as brown or black macules, whereas intradermal nevi usually appear as flesh-colored, dome-shaped papules. Compound nevi share features of both junctional and intradermal nevi; they usually appear as slightly elevated, light or dark brown papules. Overlap occurs among these three divisions; clinical appearance is not a substitute for histologic diagnosis.

The prevalence of acquired nevi is extremely high. Nearly everyone develops at least one melanocytic nevus during his or her lifetime. Acquired nevi usually appear during childhood, mainly between 2 and 6 years of age; they rarely appear after 40 years of age. A melanocytic nevus begins as a pigmented junctional nevus in childhood, then matures to form a less deeply pigmented compound nevus, and finally regresses into a flesh-colored intradermal nevus in adulthood. In later life, pigmented nevi tend to involute and eventually disappear.

Two important exceptions to this life cycle are congenital and dysplastic nevi, both of which also exhibit a much higher incidence of malignant transformation than do common acquired nevi. Congenital nevi manifest at birth; in contrast, dysplastic nevi appear during adolescence and continue to develop during adulthood. In addition, nevi on the palms, soles, and genitals may appear later in life, usually persisting as junctional nevi. Existing nevi may darken and new nevi may ap-

TABLE 1. **Categories of Acquired Nevocellular Nevi**

Type of Nevus	Common Age at Presentation	Morphology	Color	Histology
Junctional	Infancy, childhood	Flat, symmetrical, oval, regular border, hairless	Brown to black	Nevus cells in lower epidermis at junction of dermis
Compound	Childhood, early adulthood	Slightly elevated, symmetrical, dome shaped or warty, often hairy	Flesh to dark brown	Nevus cells in lower epidermis and upper dermis
Intradermal	Adults	Dome shaped with narrow or broad base, warty, occasionally hairy	Flesh to dark brown	Nevus cells in deep dermis

From Goldminz D: Nevi. *In* Rakel RE (ed): Conn's Current Therapy 1993. Philadelphia, WB Saunders, 1993, p 775.

pear during pregnancy, with hormonal therapy (oral contraceptive use and postmenopausal estrogen replacement therapy), and after intense sun exposure.

SPECIAL TYPES

In addition to the three major nevi described above, special types of melanocytic nevi include congenital nevus, dysplastic nevus, dermal melanocytosis, and Spitz's nevus.

Congenital nevi are present at birth as flat, occasionally hairy, brown or black macules or patches that may become verrucous and nodular with age. They range in size from a few millimeters to several centimeters in diameter. Small congenital nevi (i.e., <1.5 cm in diameter) occur in approximately 1% of newborns, whereas larger congenital nevi occur in 0.2% of newborns. The melanocytes in a congenital nevus penetrate into the deep dermis and subcutaneous fat. The likelihood of malignant transformation within a congenital nevus is high, especially in a large congenital nevus during the first decade of life. For this reason, complete full-thickness excision of congenital nevi is advisable sometime during the first 10 years of life or immediately if the nevus appears to be undergoing malignant transformation.

A *dysplastic nevus* (also called Clark's nevus) is an *atypical* acquired nevus that can also be a precursor to malignant melanoma. Dysplastic nevi clinically demonstrate one or more of the ABCD warning signs of early melanoma (Table 2): *A*symmetry, *B*order irregularity, *C*olor variation, and *D*iameter greater than 6 mm (about the size of a pencil eraser). Dysplastic nevi usually appear after puberty and may number more than 100. On the other hand, common acquired nevi appear earlier and usually number less than 40. Dysplastic nevi are more atypical than common nevi both clinically and histologically.

Dysplastic nevus syndrome (DNS) occurs when patients continue to develop several dysplastic nevi during adolescence and adulthood. Some of these patients may have a personal and/or family history of melanoma, and all are at an increased lifetime risk for developing malignant melanoma. DNS can occur in a familial form, affecting parents, siblings, and/or children of an affected patient, or it can occur sporadically, in the absence of affected relatives, due to an autosomal dominant mutation. The lifetime incidence of malignant melanoma can approach 100% in patients with familial DNS. Therefore, periodic examination of the entire skin, oral mucosa, and intraocular structures is mandatory in order to detect early melanoma. Sun avoidance and sunscreens are essential for these patients.

Dermal melanocytosis refers to deeply pigmented melanocytes within the dermis. Clinically, these lesions appear blue or black due to scattering of visible light, termed the Tyndall effect. Examples of dermal melanocytosis include blue nevus, lumbosacral melanocytosis of infants (also called Mongolian spot), nevus of Ito (involving the shoulder region) and nevus of Ota (involving the periorbital region). A combined nevus consists of a blue nevus below a junctional, compound, or intradermal nevus.

Spitz's spindle cell and epithelioid cell nevus was formerly (and misleadingly) termed benign juvenile melanoma. Fortunately, it is a benign, clinically distinctive compound nevus that typically appears in children as a red or red-brown dome-shaped papule. Histologically, it may resemble malignant melanoma in some aspects. However, the benign clinical course of Spitz's nevus warrants purging the ominous "melanoma" from its name.

DIAGNOSIS AND DIFFERENTIAL DIAGNOSIS

While clinical appearance provides valuable clues to diagnosis, histologic examination is essential for all nevi, including those removed for purely cosmetic reasons. This is because skin cancers in general, and malignant melanoma in particular, are preventable and

TABLE 2. **Danger Signs Suggesting Malignant Transformation**

A	Asymmetry
B	Border changes (irregularity, satellite pigmentation, surrounding erythema, halo)
C	Color variation (darkening, loss of color, spread of color, red, white, blue)
D	Diameter enlargement (larger than 6 mm)
Other	Changes in surface characteristics (scaliness, erosion, oozing, crusting, bleeding, ulceration) Symptoms (pruritus, tenderness, pain)

From Goldminz D: Nevi. *In* Rakel RE (ed): Conn's Current Therapy 1993. Philadelphia, WB Saunders, 1993, p 775.

curable if detected early. Indications for biopsy include the ABCD warning signs of early melanoma (see Table 2) as well as any recent change in a nevus, such as ulceration, irritation, pruritus, bleeding, pain, or tenderness.

Histologic features of benign nevi include well-organized nests, cords, and strands of melanocytes that mature by becoming smaller as they move deeper into the dermis. In contrast, dysplastic nevi exhibit atypical melanocytic hyperplasia, nuclear atypia, or both. *Atypical melanocytic hyperplasia* (AMH) is defined as proliferation and abnormal architectural grouping of melanocytes. AMH can occur as a focal or continuous horizontal (lentiginous) band and as a vertical (Pagetoid) distribution of nevomelanocytes within the epidermis. AMH can be graded from mild to moderate to severe, with severe AMH being equivalent to melanoma in situ. Nuclear atypia consists of enlarged, hyperchromatic nuclei with abundant chromatin, prominent nucleoli, and/or mitotic figures.

The clinical differential diagnosis of pigmented lesions is extensive. The following is merely a partial list of common simulators of melanocytic nevi. Junctional nevus resembles lentigo, lentigo maligna, lentigo maligna melanoma, ephelis (freckle), café au lait macule of neurofibromatosis, and thrombosed hemangioma. Compound nevus mimics dermatofibroma, pigmented basal cell carcinoma, and seborrheic keratosis. Dermal nevus imitates basal cell carcinoma, sebaceous hyperplasia, fibrous papule, and neurofibroma. Blue nevus resembles traumatic tattoo from implanted pencil lead, Kaposi's hemorrhagic sarcoma, and nodular melanoma. Spitz's nevus suggests hemangioma and insect bite. Congenital nevi are distinguished by being present at birth. A dysplastic nevus resembles early malignant melanoma and may be a precursor to it.

The histologic differential diagnosis of melanocytic nevi, especially those with spindle-shaped cells, includes neural tumors (neurofibroma, schwannoma), fibrohistiocytic tumors (dermatofibroma, histiocytoma), spindle cell squamous cell carcinoma, and spindle cell melanoma. The S-100 immunoperoxidase stain is useful to confirm the melanocytic or neural origin of a spindle cell tumor. The Fontana-Masson melanin stain distinguishes melanin-positive nevi from some hemosiderin-positive dermatofibromas.

TREATMENT

Treatment decisions depend upon whether the nevus is undergoing malignant transformation. Therefore, any suspicious nevus, and even clinically benign nevi removed for purely cosmetic reasons, should be submitted for histologic examination in order to exclude malignant melanoma and melanoma in situ.

Histopathologic diagnosis ultimately determines the medically acceptable treatment options for nevi. These range from reassurance and observation for obviously clinically benign nevi to tangential shave excision, incisional wedge or punch biopsy, sequentially staged excisions, and complete full-thickness excision, depending on the diagnosis. However, destructive procedures alone, such as electrocautery, liquid nitrogen cryosurgery, laser vaporization, and chemical treatments (trichloroacetic acid peel and hydroquinone bleaches), should be avoided. Such procedures yield only damaged tissue that cannot be submitted for histopathologic examination. In addition, hydroquinone bleaching agents can confound or delay diagnosis by altering or removing pigment without destroying the atypical melanocytes.

Tangential shave excision involves horizontal removal of the upper dermal and epidermal component of a nevus. The outline of the nevus is first marked with ink for accurate visualization, since even careful subsequent injection of local anesthetic can distort the clinical borders. A No. 15 scalpel blade is used to shave or slice the nevus as level with the surrounding skin as possible. Delicate curettage can be used to smooth any rough edges. Hemostasis is achieved with very light electrocautery, aluminum chloride solution, or, for minimal tissue damage, direct pressure with a gauze pad. The tangential shave technique is especially useful for cosmetic removal of nevi and for biopsy of junctional nevi. Since hair roots are preserved with shallow shave excision, any thick hairs within the nevus are likely to regrow, a cosmetic annoyance. Also, if any nevus cells remain at the base, the nevus can recur and repigment darkly, even if it originally lacked pigment. Complete re-excision is advisable for all clinically atypical recurrent nevi. The histopathology of a clinically benign recurrent nevus may resemble that of malignant melanoma. The pathologist should therefore also review the histology of the original nevus in order to prevent erroneous diagnosis and overtreatment for a malignant melanoma. If the recurrent nevus clinically extends beyond the original borders of the biopsy site, however, it truly may be transforming into melanoma.

Incisional biopsy, including wedge incision and punch biopsy, consists of full-thickness removal down to the subcutaneous fat. Elliptical wedge incision and circular punch biopsy can be used to obtain a sample of the darkest or thickest area of a large nevus. Punch biopsy can also completely remove a small, dark, deep nevus, such as a blue nevus, compound nevus, or combined nevus.

Sequentially staged (partial) incisions allow the gradual removal of a large circular or oval nevus with the shortest possible scar. With a standard elliptical excision, the resulting scar is three times the width of the lesion; however, multiple smaller concentric or adjacent partial elliptical incisions can remove the same lesion with a final scar no longer than the original lesion. This is an important tissue-sparing technique especially for large round or oval nevi, such as some giant congenital nevi. Sequentially staged incisions can also preserve vital anatomic function when a nevus involves the ear, eyelid, nose, mouth, hand, foot, digit, or genitals. The main disadvantage is that multiple surgical procedures are required.

Complete excision with adequate marginal clearance is essential for any lesion suspected to be a malignant melanoma.

MALIGNANT MELANOMA

method of
PHILIP D. SHENEFELT, M.D.
University of South Florida
Tampa, Florida

Malignant melanoma accounts for 3% of all new cancers and about 2% of cancer deaths each year. Roughly 30% start within a pre-existing nevus cell nevus, while 70% arise de novo. Malignant melanoma frequently occurs on intermittently sun-exposed areas such as the back or the calf of the leg. Early removal usually produces a cure, but advanced melanoma commonly metastasizes with a high risk of death. In 1993, the incidence of malignant melanoma in the United States was about 32,000, or 12.8 per 100,000 population. There were about 6800 deaths from malignant melanoma in the United States in 1993; the death rate for men was 3.2 per 100,000 population compared to 2.2 per 100,000 for women. The incidence of malignant melanoma has been increasing rapidly, with a four-fold increase in incidence in the United States from the 1960s to the 1980s. Intermittent strong sun exposure, especially early in life, is believed to be the primary environmental factor related to malignant melanoma. Lifestyle changes and decreased atmospheric ozone have both increased exposure to ultraviolet light, and this is believed to be responsible for the rising incidence of this disease.

Genetics also plays a role. Those with skin type I (always burn, never tan) or II (always burn, sometimes tan) are at greatest risk for malignant melanoma. Those with skin type III (sometimes burn, always tan) are at moderate risk. Persons with skin type IV (never burn, always tan), skin type V (never burn, olive baseline color), or VI (black) generally are at low risk. Individuals with atypical/dysplastic nevi are at higher than average risk for developing malignant melanoma. For patients with sporadic atypical/dysplastic nevi, the risk of malignant melanoma is six times that of the general population, and patients with familial dysplastic nevus syndrome are at even higher risk.

Malignant melanoma occurs in all age groups. In young white adults between the ages of 25 and 29, malignant melanoma is the most frequent kind of cancer. There is no overall gender predilection. Women outnumber men by up to 2:1 in developing malignant melanoma before age 40, but the ratio begins to reverse thereafter, and by age 80 the disease is seen twice as frequently in men.

Risk factors for the development of cutaneous malignant melanoma include Caucasian race, a higher than average number of benign nevus cell nevi, fair complexion, freckling, atypical/dysplastic nevi, and a personal or family history of malignant melanoma.

Because early diagnosis is crucial, it is important that the patient's skin be checked once every few years. Annual total body skin examinations are recommended for fair-skinned patients who sunburn easily. Individuals who have already had skin cancers or precancers and those with atypical nevi should be checked twice a year and should be taught to do skin self-examinations monthly.

DIAGNOSIS

There are four clinical subtypes of malignant melanoma. The most common is *superficial spreading malignant melanoma,* which accounts for about 70% of all melanomas. It usually shows the ABCD signs of *A*symmetry, *B*order irregular, *C*olor variation within the lesion, and *D*iameter larger than a pencil eraser (6 mm). Superficial spreading malignant melanoma has variegated patches of blue, black, or brown pigmentation, often with areas of white and red. The borders are irregular and may be notched. Advanced lesions may ulcerate or form an elevated tumor. It occurs most commonly on intermittently or chronically sun-exposed areas. Melanomas typically enlarge in diameter before invading deeper into the tissue. This provides an opportunity to identify and remove the tumor before it metastasizes.

Nodular malignant melanoma is an elevated dark brown to black or rarely reddish (amelanotic) nodule without peripheral lentiginous spread. Ulceration can occur. It most commonly develops on chronically or intermittently sun-exposed areas. It may develop deep in a congenital nevus as a palpable nodule. Often it has invaded deeply and metastasized prior to recognition, giving it a poor prognosis.

Lentigo maligna melanoma is a thickened darker area in a lentigo maligna, usually located on chronically sun-exposed facial skin in the elderly. Often the lentigo maligna has been present for years prior to the development of the invasive malignant melanoma. The prognosis is usually good provided that the lesion is not too deep.

Acral lentiginous melanoma is a variegated brown to black macule or flat patch with irregular borders located on the palm, or sole, or digit. It can occur in blacks. The spindle-shaped cells usually grow superficially for some time before invading deep. Unfortunately, this form of malignant melanoma is frequently recognized late in its development, leading to a poor prognosis. When located in the nail matrix, the melanoma can produce a wide pigmented band in the nail.

The differential diagnosis of malignant melanoma includes lentigo, seborrheic keratosis, nevus cell nevus, dysplastic nevus, pigmented basal cell carcinoma, and angiokeratoma. Biopsy should be excisional to include the borders and the deep portion. In very large lesions, a preliminary deep punch biopsy can be performed. Microscopic examination shows malignant cells with variable pigmentation in the upper dermis and extending upward within the epidermis. Diagnosis is based on clinical suspicion confirmed by biopsy.

PROGNOSIS

The course and prognosis of malignant melanoma is progressive with rare spontaneous involution. Increased thickness of the melanoma is a bad prognostic sign. Metastatic spread is generally fatal. Early recognition and prompt surgical excision of a malignant melanoma with adequate margins are critical to increasing the patient's chance of long-term survival.

Important prognostic factors for malignant melanoma include depth of invasion, number of mitoses, ulceration, regression, association with a pre-existing nevus, stage of spread, location on the body, sex, and age.

Clark levels and Breslow thickness are indicators of malignant melanoma thickness and propensity to metastasize. Clark level I refers to an in situ lesion at the dermatoepidermal junction, while a Clark level II melanoma has invaded the papillary dermis. Clark level III tumors abut the reticular dermis, and Clark level IV tumors invade the reticular dermis. Clark level V melanomas extend below the dermis. Ten-year survival varies from over 95% for Clark levels I and II to about 40% for Clark levels IV and V.

Breslow thickness is measured from the granular layer of the epidermis to the deepest portion of the tumor. Depth intervals in multiples of 0.75 mm are utilized for prognosis. Lesions with a depth of less than 0.76 mm have a good prognosis. The prognosis becomes progressively worse for depths of 0.76 to 1.50 mm, 1.51 to 2.25 mm, 2.26 to 3.00 mm, and greater than 3.00 mm.

Large numbers of mitoses in the tumor carry a poorer prognosis, as does ulceration. Regression most often occurs in a thinner lesion but may indicate a poorer prognosis. Association with a pre-existing acquired nevocellular nevus indicates a more favorable prognosis, while association with a congenital nevus carries a worse prognosis.

Tumor spread is grouped into Stage I, nonmetastatic local disease, Stage II, regional lymph node involvement, and Stage III, disseminated disease. The prognosis is poor for Stage II and very poor for Stage III. The current 5-year survival rates for malignant melanoma are 91% for Stage I, 54% for Stage II, and 13% for Stage III. Fortunately, 81% of malignant melanomas are at Stage I when diagnosed, while 8% are at Stage II, and only 4% are at Stage III.

Location of malignant melanoma on the forearms and legs carries a better prognosis, while location on the hands, feet, trunk, and head indicates a worse prognosis. Females tend to fare better than males, and young better than old. The 10-year survival is 83% for women versus 73% for men. Pregnancy is not an adverse prognostic factor.

TREATMENT

Treatment of malignant melanoma is excision of the lesion. For lesions thinner than 0.76 mm, a 1-cm margin laterally including underlying fat is considered sufficient. For thicker lesions, a 2- to 3-cm lateral margin is recommended. Locally recurrent malignant melanoma or malignant melanoma in a cosmetically important location may best be treated with conservative excision by the Mohs micrographically controlled technique.

Lymph node dissection is indicated if palpable regional lymph nodes are present. A Clark level of IV or V is also an indication to consider regional lymph node dissection, but this is more controversial.

Treatment for metastatic malignant melanoma continues to be disappointing. Chemotherapy and immunotherapy have been successful in a small percentage of cases. Referral to a regional or national cancer center for participation in clinical trials may be considered.

Any patient who has had a malignant melanoma requires follow-up for at least 10 years. For Clark level I or II, Stage I malignant melanoma, the patient should be seen every 6 months for 2 years, then yearly. A yearly history, physical examination, and chest x-ray are recommended. For Clark level III and beyond or Stage II malignant melanoma, follow-up should be every 3 months for 5 years, then every 6 months.

PREMALIGNANT LESIONS OF THE SKIN

method of
GARY D. MONHEIT, M.D.
University of Alabama Medical Center
Birmingham, Alabama

The clinical term "precancer" is used to describe those skin lesions that have a tendency to develop into skin cancer with time. Included in this category are skin lesions that have a propensity to develop skin cancer, skin lesions that degenerate into skin cancer, and noninvasive epidermal cancers, i.e., carcinoma in situ. It is important to recognize these lesions in their precancerous or nonmalignant stages, since treatment or removal will give a complete cure. Identification of these precancerous conditions allows patients and families to have appropriate counseling for prevention and treatment (Table 1).

The vast majority of skin cancers are the result of cumulative ultraviolet damage. Even small repetitive exposures to ultraviolet light on a continuing basis will result in precancer and eventual skin cancer in susceptible skin. Ultraviolet B irradiation plays the major role in skin carcinogenesis. A history of repeated sunburns is associated with early development of precancerous growths.

Susceptible skin types for preskin cancer are those

TABLE 1. **Premalignant Skin Lesions**

Premalignant Lesion or Condition	Carcinogen or Cause	Resultant Carcinoma
Actinic keratosis	Ultraviolet light, photo types I and II	Squamous cell carcinoma, basal cell carcinoma
Actinic cheilitis	Ultraviolet light, tobacco, heat (thermal damage)	Squamous cell carcinoma
Leukoplakia—mucosal	Tobacco	Squamous cell carcinoma
Bowen's disease	Carcinoma in situ	Squamous cell carcinoma
Arsenical keratosis	Chronic arsenic exposure	Squamous cell carcinoma, basal cell carcinoma
Bowenoid papulosis	Viral oncogenesis, papillomavirus	Questionable squamous cell carcinoma
Giant condyloma	Papillomavirus	Verrucous carcinoma
Chronic plantar verrucae	Papillomavirus	Cunilate carcinoma
Florid oral papillomatosis	Papillomavirus	Squamous cell carcinoma
Radiodermatitis, chronic	Radiation overexposure	Squamous cell carcinoma
Scars or chronic burns	Predisposition to ultraviolet transformation	Squamous cell carcinoma
Erythema ab igne	Chronic heat and thermal injury	Squamous cell carcinoma
Xeroderma pigmentosum	Autosomal dominant genetic deficiency in repair of ultraviolet damage	Squamous cell carcinoma, basal cell carcinoma, melanoma
Basal cell nevus syndrome	Autosomal dominant genodermatosis with palmar pits, bone cysts, and basal cell carcinoma	Basal cell carcinoma
Precancerous skin diseases	Lichen sclerosis et atrophicus, ulcerative lichen planus, discoid lupus erythematosus	Squamous cell carcinoma
Dysplastic nevus	Large number of irregular and larger than normal moles	Malignant melanoma
Lentigo maligna	Ultraviolet exposure, lentigines	Invasive melanoma
Congenital nevus	Birthmarks, nevi, large lesions at greater risk	Malignant melanoma

that have little natural ultraviolet protection. Fitzpatrick's classification of skin types is based on the propensity of the skin to tan (facultative melanogenesis) (Table 2). Skin photo types I, II, and III are most susceptible to sun damage and its cumulative effects. The highest incidence of nonmelanoma skin cancer is in whites who do not tan (skin photo types I and II) and have chronic sun exposure. It is important to recognize these individuals so they can receive appropriate counseling in skin protection and in self-examination to recognize precancer and early skin cancer. Physician recognition of precancerous lesions may prevent the progression to skin cancer in those at greatest risk.

ACTINIC KERATOSES

Actinic keratoses are the most common premalignant skin growths. They appear on sun-exposed areas of individuals with well-advanced ultraviolet damage with associated solar elastosis, lentigines, and collagenosis. Actinic keratoses are also called "solar keratoses," suggesting a link to sun exposure, but they can be caused by artificial sources of ultraviolet radiation such as tanning beds and even chronic x-ray irradiation. In the past, these lesions were seen mainly in people who farmed or worked in other outdoor professions. Today, however, as a result of excessive recreational sun exposure, it is not uncommon to see patients in their late teens and early twenties with actinic keratoses. Sun exposure early in life carries the greatest risk of developing precancerous and cancerous lesions.

Actinic keratoses present as well-circumscribed lesions that tend to be rough and scaly on sun-exposed areas of the skin. They are thickened keratotic plaques on erythematous or pigmented bases. The scaly patches are sharp, recur with peeling, and may bleed. In addition, they are seen on skin that has other signs of chronic irradiation changes, such as telangiectasias, solar elastosis, and lentigines.

The actinic keratosis is a precancerous epidermal growth with a 20% incidence of progression to squamous cell carcinoma. Of equal importance is the number of squamous cell carcinomas found with associated actinic keratoses. In one series, it was noted that 60% of squamous cell carcinomas developed from pre-existing actinic keratoses.

The importance of actinic keratoses is threefold:

1. The presence of these lesions indicates significant ultraviolet damage in an individual at risk of skin cancer. The patient should be followed regularly to detect early skin cancer and encourage self-examination.

TABLE 2. **Fitzpatrick's Classification of Skin Type**

Skin Type	Color	Reaction to Sun
I	Very white or freckled	Always burn
II	White	Usually burn
III	White to olive	Sometimes burn
IV	Brown	Rarely burn
V	Dark brown	Very rarely burn
VI	Black	Never burn

2. Removal of the actinic keratosis will prevent their evolution into skin cancer.

3. Actinic keratoses are preventible with the appropriate use of sunscreens.

These individuals should be instructed to (1) use sunscreens with a sun protective factor (SPF) of 15 or greater; (2) wear protective clothing, broad-brimmed hats, and sunglasses; and (3) avoid sun during the peak hours of 10:00 A.M. to 2:00 P.M.

Treatment consists of conservative destructive modalities (Table 3). These include topical chemotherapy, cryosurgery, electrodestruction, shave excision, chem-exfoliation (chemical peel), and dermabrasion.

ACTINIC CHEILITIS AND LEUKOPLAKIA

The lower lip vermilion commonly develops chronic ultraviolet degeneration that presents as scaly erythematous patches with focal hyperkeratosis. Similar white patches on the mucosa, leukoplakia, are the result of chronic inflammation and irradiation. The most common cause of leukoplakia is nicotine from chewing tobacco, cigarettes, or pipes. Squamous cell carcinoma can result from actinic cheilitis or from leukoplakia. The incidence of metastasis of the resultant squamous cell carcinoma is greater on lip than on skin, and mucous membrane than on lip. Any suspicious area should be biopsied prior to destruction to exclude the diagnosis of evolving squamous cell carcinoma. Methods of treatment include topical chemotherapy, cryosurgery, electrosurgery, and CO_2 laser vaporization.

BOWEN'S DISEASE

Bowen's disease represents squamous cell carcinoma in situ involving the epidermis and epidermal adnexae, including the pilosebaceous apparatus and eccrine ducts. Though there is some evidence that actinic keratoses can evolve into Bowen's disease, which in turn develops into invasive carcinoma, it is more likely that Bowen's disease is a distinctive clinical and histopathologic entity.

Clinically, Bowen's disease presents as eczematous patches or plaques on sun-protected as well as sun-exposed areas of the skin. It may be confused with tinea corporis, seborrheic dermatitis, and other papulosquamoid dermatitis; however, it will continue to enlarge centripetally in the face of treatment for these skin diseases. A biopsy will confirm the diagnosis of Bowen's disease by demonstrating squamous cell carcinoma confined to the epidermis.

Several unusual clinical variants of Bowen's disease have been identified. *Erythroplasia of Queyrat* is a type of squamous cell carcinoma in situ that presents as a velvety red plaque found on the glans penis or foreskin mucosa. It can also involve the vulvar, oral, or anal mucosa and can spread to glabrous skin, such as the penile shaft. Histopathologically, it is indistinguishable from Bowen's disease; however, erythroplasia has a higher propensity for dermal invasion and subsequent metastasis.

Bowenoid papulosis, which presents as discreet hyperpigmented papules in the genital area, is thought to be associated with the human papillomavirus. The genital papules are considered potentially precancerous, based on their histopatho-

TABLE 3. **Treatment of Actinic Keratosis**

Modality	Agent	Advantages	Disadvantages
Topical chemotherapy	5-Fluorouracil	Simple, inexpensive, patient applies to localized areas or individual lesions, can reveal occult growths in areas treated	Morbidity—6 weeks of inflamed lesions, treatment failures frequent
Cryosurgery	Liquid nitrogen	Simple, nonexcisional office procedure, anesthesia not necessary, 3–5 days for healing, effective for most individual keratoses	Discomfort, blisters, can cause hypopigmentation
Electrodesiccation	Cautery or desiccation, CO_2 laser surgery	Effective for thicker keratoses, cutaneous horns, hyperkeratotic keratoses	Hypopigmentation, scarring, requires anesthesia
Chem-exfoliation (chemical peeling)	Trichloracetic acid, phenol, combination agents	Effective as a full-face preventive treatment for advanced photodamage of the skin	Morbidity, healing time 1 week, more complicated procedure technically
Dermabrasion	Dermabrasive surgical tools	Most effective method of removal with least incidence of recurrence	Extensive surgical procedure, 2 weeks' healing
Shave excision	Surgical procedure	Questionable lesions can be confirmed histologically, e.g., hypertrophic actinic keratosis vs. squamous cell carcinoma	Anesthesia necessary, surgery can produce a scar

logic appearance, and should be destroyed by conservative measures. Bowen's disease is also associated with chronic radiation dermatitis, arsenical dermatitis, viral infections (verrucae or condylomas on the skin or mucosa), and trauma (tick bite nodules, vaccination scars, old burn scars, and chronic thermal injury).

As mentioned, Bowen's disease is a form of squamous cell carcinoma in situ, and treatment should include eradication of all the neoplasia. This may be more difficult than removal of actinic keratoses, as Bowen's disease involves the pilosebaceous apparatus. This makes recurrence common with only superficial destruction of the epidermis. Methods of treatment include aggressive topical chemotherapy, deep cryosurgery, radiation therapy, laser and electrosurgical destruction, and surgical excision. In some patients, Mohs micrographic technique is necessary to fully remove the silent extensions of cancer in the epidermis and the pilosebaceous apparatus. One should be more aggressive in treating these lesions because of their high recurrence rates and their ability to invade the dermis and metastasize.

HUMAN PAPILLOMAVIRUS INFECTION

Human papillomavirus (HPV) infection has, in some cases, been associated with squamous cell carcinoma. One example is the association of HPV types 11, 16, and 32 with the transformation of vaginal HPV infection into cervical carcinoma. The giant condyloma acuminatum of Buschke-Lowenstein can degenerate into squamous cell carcinoma. Other HPV growths with the potential for malignant change include oral florid papillomatosis, HPV 16–associated nail fold and nail bed verrucae, and the resistant large plantar wart that evolves into the cunilate carcinoma. These precancerous viral infections should be documented by biopsy and eradicated when possible.

MISCELLANEOUS CONDITIONS

Other skin conditions can develop into precancerous and cancerous lesions. *Chronic radiation exposure,* either therapeutic or accidental, can eventuate in chronic radiation dermatitis, characterized by mottled, atrophic skin with telangiectasias and scattered keratoses. These epidermal lesions may resemble actinic keratoses. These patients can develop Bowen's disease, which can progress to squamous cell carcinoma.

Arsenical keratoses are associated with chronic arsenic ingestion—either therapeutic (Fowler's solution), or accidental (water or insecticide ex-

posure). These scattered keratoses can degenerate into Bowen's disease and squamous cell carcinoma.

Long-standing ulcerated patches of *lichen planus, discoid lupus erythematosus,* and *lichen sclerosus et atrophicus* can develop into Bowen's disease and squamous cell carcinoma. A nonhealing ulcer within a lesion of chronic skin disease can undergo carcinomatous change, and biopsy should be performed.

There are rare genetic disorders that are associated with the development of skin cancer. The lack of protective pigmentation in *albinism* can lead to the rapid progression of precancers and cancerous lesions. *Xeroderma pigmentosum* is due to a defect in DNA repair and results in the early development of squamous cell carcinoma, basal cell carcinoma, and melanoma. This disorder is characterized by premature photoaging of the skin in childhood with actinic keratoses, lentigines, and skin cancer. Avoidance of ultraviolet radiation is necessary to prevent fatal skin cancer.

MELANOMA

Melanoma, the most deadly form of skin cancer, derives from the pigment cell population of the epidermis. By far, the leading environmental cause of melanoma is solar ultraviolet irradiation of both chronic and intermittent duration. Susceptible individuals are those with very fair skin (skin photo types I and II) who have had sunburns in childhood and early life. They are particularly at risk for the development of melanoma 20 years later. Patients with many moles, especially atypical moles, are at greater risk for the development of melanoma. The unusual nevus referred to as *dysplastic, or Clark's nevus* serves as a marker for this melanoma-prone skin type. The Clark's nevus is often large, (greater than 5 mm in diameter), irregularly bordered and colored, and poorly marginated. It may have clinical features similar to melanoma or its own characteristic features. Patients with multiple dysplastic nevi usually have relatives with melanoma and are at increased risk of developing melanoma. They should be examined periodically and educated in self-examination and should limit their ultraviolet exposure. Any nevus that is suspected of being a melanoma or has undergone recent change should be biopsied or excised (see next section).

Of similar concern is the enlarging *actinic freckle* in the older patient. The *Hutchinson's freckle,* or *pre-malignant lentigo maligna,* is a melanoma in situ that will eventuate in invasive malignant melanoma. It usually presents on sun-exposed areas of the face, hands, and arms as a larger than normal actinic lentigo with irregular borders, mottled coloration, and indistinct margination. As with Bowen's disease, this melanoma in situ involves both the epidermis and the pilosebaceous apparatus and thus presents a greater treatment challenge than simple lentigines. Therapy with excision or destruction must eradicate the epidermal component as well as penetrate more deeply into hair follicles.

Whether melanoma results from sun exposure, genetic traits, or a combination of factors, the key to saving the patient is early discovery and treatment. For this reason, the recognition of precancerous skin types and lesions is especially important in the prevention of melanoma. In evaluating patients at risk for melanoma, one should:

1. Obtain a careful family history for melanoma. There is a two to fourfold increase in the risk of melanoma with a positive familial history of melanoma.

2. Question the patient about sun exposure and sunburn for classification into the correct skin photo type.

3. Assess the number and types of moles.

4. Search for dysplastic nevi and melanoma.

BIOPSY

All lesions suspected of being either precancers or cancers should be biopsied. The cutaneous biopsy is a useful diagnostic procedure that can be readily performed with minimal risk to the patient. The type of biopsy selected should give maximal information on the type of skin disease, the level of invasion, and the etiology. For this reason, a shave biopsy may be sufficient to diagnose actinic keratosis or Bowen's disease, but suspicious pigmented lesions should undergo excisional or punch biopsy to assess depth of penetration and tumor thickness.

A new instrument, the dermascope, is being used to evaluate the characteristic features of suspicious nevi and substantiate the need for biopsy. Dermascopy, also called epiluminescent microscopy, is an inexpensive and noninvasive procedure that provides additional clinical information in the evaluation of pigmented skin lesions.

BACTERIAL DISEASES OF THE SKIN

method of
MORTON N. SWARTZ, M.D.
Harvard Medical School
Boston, Massachusetts

IMPETIGO

Impetigo is a superficial, painless infection of the skin, typically on exposed surfaces. It begins as vesicles that rapidly pustulate, rupture, and form golden-yellow crusts. Previously, group A streptococci have been the cause in 90% of cases, and *Staphylococcus aureus* in the remainder. In the past decade, *S. aureus* has been implicated increasingly frequently. When both species are isolated from a lesion, group A streptococci are usually the etiologic agent and staphylococci are secondary invaders.

Impetigo is most common in children and is highly communicable, particularly in families. Principal concerns are appearance, secondary infection, and glomerulonephritis. Penicillin is the treatment of choice, administered either as a single intramuscular injection of benzathine penicillin (300,000 to 900,000 units for children; 1.2 million units for adults) or oral penicillin V (15 to 50 mg per kg per day in four divided doses for 10 days). In the penicillin-allergic patient, erythromycin is a suitable alternative: the dosage for children is 30 to 50 mg per kg per day orally in divided doses four times daily and for adults, 250 to 500 mg orally four times daily. Duration of treatment is 10 days. A topical antibiotic, 2% mupirocin (Bactroban) ointment, applied to lesions can be effective treatment, but it does not have the value of penicillin in eradicating pharyngeal carriage of group A streptococci. Local care (removal of crusts by soaking with soap and water) may be helpful. When *S. aureus* appears to be the primary cause or is a significant secondary invader, some physicians favor the following alternative approaches (which are more expensive): (1) cefadroxil (Duracef) 30 mg per kg per day orally in divided doses every 12 hours for children and 1 gram once daily for adults; (2) cephalexin (Keflex), 500 mg orally twice daily for adults; or (3) amoxicillin-clavulanic acid (Augmentin), 250 mg orally three times daily for adults.

Bullous impetigo, a less common form, occurs chiefly in newborns and younger children and is characterized by flaccid bullae that readily rupture. *S. aureus* strains producing an exfoliative toxin are the etiology. Treatment consists of a penicillinase-resistant penicillin such as dicloxacillin (Dynapen) (25 mg per kg per day orally in four divided doses for children).

ERYSIPELAS

Erysipelas is a distinctive bright red, sharply demarcated, superficial cellulitis of the skin with prominent dermal lymphatic involvement. Fever is a feature. The causative microorganisms are almost always group A beta-hemolytic streptococci (uncommonly group B, C, or G) or rarely *S. aureus*. Penicillin is the drug of choice; the dosage for adults varies from 600,000 units of procaine penicillin intramuscularly twice daily for mild, early cases to 2 million units of aqueous penicillin G intravenously every 4 to 6 hours for more severe, extensive cases. Treatment is continued for 10 days, longer if needed. For adults allergic to penicillin, erythromycin, 500 mg orally four times daily, is an alternative. For more seriously ill penicillin-allergic patients, erythromycin should be given intravenously, or clindamycin (Cleocin), 600 mg intravenously every 8 hours, should be substituted. In the occasional instance in which *S. aureus* is considered a possible cause, and when the patient has serious and extensive involvement, a penicillinase-resistant penicillin such as nafcillin (Unipen), 6 to 10 grams daily intravenously in divided doses every 4 hours, should be employed. If there is reason to suspect a methicillin-resistant *S. aureus* or if the patient is allergic to penicillin, vancomycin (Vancocin), 0.5 gram intravenously every 12 hours, is an alternative.

LYMPHANGITIS

Lymphangitis is an inflammation of lymphatic channels in subcutaneous tissue. Acute lymphangitis is characterized by red linear streaks extending from the initial infection toward regional lymph nodes. Spread of infection is usually rapid and often complicated by bacteremia. Acute lymphangitis is most commonly due to group A streptococci, occasionally to *S. aureus,* and rarely, to *Pasteurella multocida* following a cat bite. Treatment of mildly ill adults should consist initially of aqueous procaine penicillin G (Wycillin), 600,000 units intramuscularly once or twice daily, with supplementary oral penicillin V, 0.5 gram every 6 hours. In more acutely ill patients hospitalization and more intensive penicillin G treatment (0.6 to 2.0 million units intravenously every 4 to 6 hours) is indicated. A penicillinase-resistant penicillin such as nafcillin (Nafcil), 1.0 to 1.5 grams intravenously every 4 hours in adults, or a first-generation cephalosporin such as cefazolin (Kefzol), 1.0 to 1.5 grams intravenously every 6 hours, should be used in treatment of seriously ill patients in whom *S. aureus* is a likely cause. When penicillin allergy or methicillin resistance is a consideration, vancomycin, 0.5 to 1.0 gram intravenously every 12 hours, or clindamycin, 0.6 gram intravenously every 6 to 8 hours, is an alternative. When lymphangitis occurs following a cat bite, initial therapy might include additional coverage for *P. multocida,* such as amoxicillin-clavulanic acid, 250 to 500 mg orally every 8 hours for an adult, or if parenteral therapy is indicated, ampicillin-sulbactam (Unasyn), 1.5 gram intravenously every 6 hours.

Chronic granulomatous lymphangitis consists of multiple subcutaneous nodules extending proximally along the course of thickened regional lymphatics. There is little pain or evidence of systemic reaction. The nodules may be erythematous or exhibit normal skin color. The initial inoculation site may become a chancriform ulcer. Infectious agents causing chronic lymphangitis are principally *Sporothrix schenckii* (sporotrichosis) and *Mycobacterium marinum* (swimming pool granuloma). *Nocardia braziliensis, N. asteroides,* and *M. kansasii* are rare causes of this syndrome. Recurrent episodes of acute lymphangitis and lymphadenitis are a feature of filariasis due to *Wuchereria bancrofti* (or sometimes to *Brugia malayi*), which is endemic to Africa, Southeast Asia, and tropical South America. *S. schenckii* commonly is introduced by minor trauma from a barberry or rose bush or while handling sphagnum moss in gardening. Infection with *M. marinum,* an atypical mycobacterium that grows best at 25 to 32° C, occurs in persons in contact with fish tanks or swimming pools, and such an epidemiologic background usually provides the necessary clues to direct therapy. When such exposures have not occurred (or when a patient has had both types of exposure), a biopsy (with culture) is necessary for selection of antimicrobial therapy. The bacterial causes of nodular lymphangitis are the mycobacterial and nocardial species noted above. The treatment of choice for *M. marinum* infection in adults consists of rifampin* (Rifadin, Rimactane), 600 mg orally daily, plus ethambutol (Myambutol), 15 mg per kg per day for 6 to 12 weeks. Alternative drugs include oral doxycycline (Vibramycin), 100 mg twice daily, or minocycline (Minocin), 100 mg twice daily for 6 to 8 weeks, or oral trimethoprim-sulfamethoxazole 1 DS tablet twice daily. Treatment is continued for a few weeks following clinical resolution. Treatment of nodular lymphangitis due to *Nocardia* consists of trimethoprim-sulfamethoxazole, 1 DS tablet twice daily, or a sulfonamide such as sulfisoxazole (Gantrisin) or sulfadiazine. Minocycline, 100 mg orally twice daily, is an alternative. Nodular lymphangitis due to *M. kansasii* infection is commonly treated with a

---

*This use of rifampin is not listed in the manufacturer's official directive.

combination of INH, rifampin, and ethambutol initially, pending susceptibility testing.

CELLULITIS

Cellulitis is an acute, painful, spreading inflammation of the skin extending to subcutaneous tissues. Predisposing factors include an antecedent abrasion or puncture wound or underlying skin lesion such as tinea pedis that becomes secondarily infected. Sometimes no portal of entry is evident, and rarely, cellulitis may result from bacteremic spread of infection. It is prone to develop (and spread rapidly) in areas of pre-existing edema such as those associated with peripheral venous stasis or congestive failure. The involved area is markedly red, hot, swollen, and tender, but unlike erysipelas, the margins are not sharply demarcated. Systemic manifestations, including fever, chills, and malaise, are evident. Bacterial species most commonly implicated are group A streptococci and *S. aureus*. Other streptococci belonging to group C, G, or B (the latter particularly in neonates or diabetics) are sometimes responsible. Less commonly involved bacteria include *Haemophilus influenzae* type b (lesions involving the face and neck; principally in children below 3 years of age); *Streptococcus pneumoniae* (acquired through the bacteremic route); and *Escherichia coli, Serratia, Proteus*, and anaerobes (the latter four producing cellulitis in the setting of diabetes and foot ulcers or in immunocompromised or granulocytopenic patients). Aspiration and culture of the advancing margin of cellulitis have usually not been helpful in bacteriologic diagnosis; aspirates from the point of maximal inflammation (particularly if early fluctuance is present) or from associated bullae may provide a higher yield.

Treatment of mild, early cellulitis, when there is no initial clue as to etiology or when staphylococcal etiology is suspected, should involve oral therapy with a penicillinase-resistant penicillin (e.g., cloxacillin 0.25 to 0.5 gram every 6 hours) or a cephalosporin (cephalexin 0.5 gram every 6 hours). For patients allergic to penicillin, erythromycin, 0.5 gram every 6 hours, and clindamycin, 300 mg every 6 to 8 hours, are alternatives. For more severe cellulitis, in which either streptococcal or staphylococcal etiologies are likely, treatment with nafcillin, 1.0 to 1.5 grams intravenously every 4 hours, cephapirin (Cefadyl), 1 to 2 grams intravenously every 6 hours, or cefazolin, 1 to 2 grams intravenously every 8 hours, is appropriate. Vancomycin, 1 gram intravenously every 12 hours, and clindamycin, 600 mg intravenously every 8 hours, are alternatives when the patient is allergic to penicillin or when methicillin-resistant *S. aureus* is suspected.

In view of the prevalence of ampicillin-resistance in *H. influenzae* type b (30 to 40%), treatment of presumed *H. influenzae* cellulitis should rely on a third-generation cephalosporin. Such would include intravenous ceftriaxone (Rocephin) (50 to 100 mg per kg daily in divided doses every 12 hours for children; in adults, 1 gram every 12 hours) or intravenous cefotaxime (Claforan) 50 to 180 mg per kg daily in divided doses every 4 to 6 hours for children; in adults, 2 grams every 6 to 8 hours). Ampicillin can be used once the *H. influenzae* strain is identified (often isolated in blood cultures) and can be shown to be ampicillin susceptible. Chloramphenicol is an alternative for use in a highly penicillin (and cephalosporin)-allergic individual.

Initial local care consists of immobilization and elevation of the affected limb to reduce swelling. A foot board is helpful to keep bedclothes off the sensitive skin. Loose sterile dressings can be used to protect areas of denuded epidermis.

Recurrent Cellulitis

Recurrent episodes of cellulitis may occur in patients with chronic lymphedema (due to prior episodes of lymphangitis, erysipelas, or lymphatic obliteration as a consequence of harvesting of saphenous veins for coronary artery bypass grafting). These episodes are presumed due to streptococci (groups A, B, C, G) on the basis of the clinical picture, the few isolates, and response to penicillin. Treatment of acute episodes usually requires high-dose intravenous therapy with penicillin (or nafcillin). The portal of entry for invading bacteria is often a break in the skin in the interdigital web spaces due to tinea pedis. An important element in management and prophylaxis against further recurrences is topical treatment of the interdigital dermatophytosis with miconazole or clotrimazole cream. Elastic stockings (to reduce edema) can help prevent recurrences. If recurrences continue despite such measures, prophylactic antibiotic use is reasonable: penicillin V, 250 to 500 mg orally daily, or in the penicillin-allergic patient, erythromycin, 250 mg daily.

Cellulitis Following Water Exposure

Aeromonas hydrophila can produce a severe, rapidly progressive cellulitis or even myonecrosis, following an abrasion or penetrating trauma in fresh water. The organism is usually susceptible to ciprofloxacin, gentamicin, trimethoprim-sulfamethoxazole, third generation cephalosporins, aztreonam, imipenem, and chloramphenicol and is variably susceptible to tetracyclines.

Cellulitis, with bullous lesions or necrotic ulcers, caused by *Vibrio* spp (e.g., *V. vulnificus*), can result from a traumatic wound sustained in salt water or from lacerations from shellfish. Large hemorrhagic bullae with surrounding cellulitis can occur, as a result of bacteremia, following ingestion of raw shellfish by patients with hepatic cirrhosis or hemochromatosis. Treatment consists of tetracycline, (0.5 gram orally four times daily) or doxycycline, 100 mg orally or intravenously every 12 hours. *V. vulnificus* is also susceptible to gentamicin, chloramphenicol, and cefotaxime.

STREPTOCOCCAL GANGRENE AND NECROTIZING FASCIITIS

Hemolytic streptococcal gangrene (also known as streptococcal necrotizing fasciitis) begins, either at a site of trauma or without any obvious portal of entry, as a localized, painful, swollen, erythematous area. Yellowish to red-black bullae subsequently develop. The lesion progresses to become a sharply demarcated necrotic area resembling a third-degree burn. The primary process extends more widely in the subcutaneous tissues along fascial planes than is evidenced by the extent of the cutaneous gangrene. This type of gangrene is due to beta-hemolytic streptococci (usually group A, occasionally group C or G). Bacteremia is frequent. This life-threatening infection requires prompt diagnosis and treatment. Immediate surgical débridement extending through the deep fascia and beyond the gangrenous and undermined areas is essential. Antimicrobial therapy consists of intravenous aqueous penicillin G, 1 to 2 million units every 4 hours; if *S. aureus* involvement is suspected, nafcillin, 1.5 to 2.0 grams intravenously every 4 to 6 hours, should be used.

Necrotizing fasciitis, other than the form due to group A streptococci, is a mixed infection involving anaerobes (e.g., *Bacteroides, Peptostreptococcus*) as well as one or more facultative species (e.g., *E. coli, Enterobacter, Proteus,* non-group A streptococci). This infection is acute and commonly follows antecedent injury, surgery, perirectal abscess, decubitus ulcer, or intestinal perforation. Necrotizing fasciitis originating in the abdomen (e.g., from occult diverticulitis) may manifest itself in the thigh. The initial appearance of the lesion is much like that of cellulitis, but bullae and skin necrosis soon develop and crepitus is often present. Prompt exploration of the involved area is essential. Ready passage of a hemostat through a plane just superficial to the deep fascia is characteristic. Foul odor is often present. Débridement, with removal of all necrotic fat and fascia, should be extended beyond the area of involvement until normal fascia is reached and the wound left open. A "second look" procedure 24 to 48 hours later is indicated if any uncertainty exists regarding adequacy of the initial débridement.

Preliminary antimicrobial selection is based on knowledge of the usual aerobic and anaerobic species in such a mixed infection. Treatment includes regimens often employed for intra-abdominal infections: (1) combination of ampicillin (1 to 2 grams intravenously every 4 hours) or penicillin G (1 to 2 million units intravenously every 4 hours) and metronidazole (500 mg intravenously every 6 hours) plus an aminoglycoside (such as tobramycin or gentamicin in a dose of 1.5 mg per kg every 8 hours); (2) clindamycin (600 mg intravenously every 6 to 8 hours) plus an aminoglycoside. Modifications in antimicrobials are made based on results of gram-stained smears and cultures.

POSTOPERATIVE WOUND INFECTIONS

Two types of life-threatening infection that occur shortly (6 to 48 hours) after surgery are group A streptococcal cellulitis and gas gangrene. Both are uncommon, but prompt recognition is essential since progression is rapid. Fever and hypotension may be initial manifestations of the former at a time when inflammation about the incision is minor. A small amount of thin exudate containing gram-positive cocci in chains can be expressed from the wound. Treatment involves penicillin G in high doses (1 to 2 million units intravenously every 3 or 4 hours).

Gas gangrene is a rapidly progressive, toxemic, potentially lethal clostridial (usually *C. perfringens*) infection of the skeletal muscle that sometimes follows abdominal surgery, but usually occurs in the setting of a dirty traumatic wound. The involved area is tender, tense with edema, and has a yellowish or bronze discoloration. Crepitus is present but not marked. Tense blebs containing thin grey or dark fluid are present. Gram-stained smear of an aspirate shows many large gram-positive bacilli with blunt ends but few polymorphonuclear leukocytes. Treatment includes immediate excision and débridement of involved muscles and amputation when necessary. Antibiotic therapy consists of penicillin G, 1 to 2 million units intravenously every 2 to 3 hours. A second antibiotic (chloramphenicol, metronidazole) is added when smears of wound exudate show gram-negative bacilli as well.

Most postoperative wound infections become manifest several days later as cellulitis or abscess. *S. aureus* is the common causative organism, but prominent nosocomial pathogens are also considerations. Findings on gram-stained smear and culture provide guides to antimicrobial selection. Surgical measures include drainage of abscesses, removal of sutures, and débridement.

SECONDARY INFECTIONS COMPLICATING SKIN ULCERS

Chronic diabetic foot ulcers and decubitus ulcers are commonly colonized with mixtures of both anaerobic (e.g., *Bacteroides, Peptostreptococcus, Clostridium species*) and aerobic (e.g., *Proteus, Pseudomonas, Enterobacter, Enterococcus,* various streptococci, *S. aureus*) organisms. Cellulitis and subcutaneous abscesses can complicate these processes. Extension to underlying bone can result in chronic osteomyelitis. Evaluation of diabetic and ischemic foot ulcers includes Doppler flow measurement of arterial supply to determine the need for vascular surgery or amputation. Aerobic and anaerobic cultures of deep tissue specimens from wound débridement are of greater value than culture of exudate from the ulcer surface, which contains many contaminating organisms. Initial treatment, prior to receiving results of bacteriologic studies, might consist of a combination of clindamycin and an aminoglycoside (gentamicin or tobramycin), provided that renal function is not compromised. Another combination might include cefoxitin (Mefoxin) or a first-generation cephalosporin, such as cefazolin, plus an aminoglycoside. Other drugs that can be substituted for an aminoglycoside when renal function is likely to be impaired include ciprofloxacin (Cipro), ceftazidime (Fortaz), aztreonam (Azactam), ticarcillin plus clavulanate (Timentin), ampicillin plus sulbactam (Unasyn), or imipenem-cilastatin (Primaxin).

HAIR FOLLICLE INFECTIONS

Folliculitis consists of small erythematous papules, often topped with central pustules, located in hair follicles. A furuncle or a boil is a deep, tender inflammatory nodule that involves an area surrounding a hair follicle. A carbuncle is a larger, deeper, more indurated infection occurring under areas of thickened skin (nape of neck, back, upper lip, thighs). With progression, drainage occurs externally through multiple hair follicles. Factors predisposing to furunculosis or contributing to its severity include obesity, poor skin hygiene, blood dyscrasias, defective neutrophil function, corticosteroid treatment, diabetes mellitus, and preexisting skin lesions (scabies, pediculosis).

Folliculitis

The bacteriology of folliculitis is varied. That accompanying acne is associated with *Propionibacterium acnes. S. aureus* is a common cause, particularly in children. *Pseudomonas aeruginosa* may be the etiology in occasional cases following exposure in a swimming pool or Jacuzzi. Fungi, such as *Candida* and *Malassezia (Pityrosporum),* can occasionally cause folliculitis.

For folliculitis associated with acne or in the bearded areas, topical antibiotic solutions (2% erythromycin or 1% clindamycin [Cleocin T]) applied twice daily may be helpful. Local therapy includes skin cleansing with a topical antiseptic such as chlorhexidine (4%) solution (Hibiclens). Extensive folliculitis responds to systemic treatment with erythromycin, 250 mg orally four times daily, cephalexin, 250 mg orally four times daily or clindamycin, 150 mg orally four times daily. *P. aeruginosa* folliculitis usually clears spontaneously in 4 or 5 days with cessation of exposure to the source of infection.

Furunculosis and Carbuncles

Uncomplicated furuncles are treated with hot compresses several times daily to localize infection and promote drainage. More serious lesions, including those associated with surrounding cellulitis, fever, or carbuncles and those about the midline of the face and in the nares, require systemic antimicrobial therapy. Oral therapy with dicloxacillin, 0.25 to 0.5 gram four times daily, cephalexin, 0.5 gram four times daily, or clindamycin, 0.3 gram four times daily is appropriate initially. For more serious infections, intravenous therapy is necessary: nafcillin, 2 grams every 6 hours, cephapirin (Cefadyl), 2 grams every 6 hours, or if methicillin resistance is likely or the patient is allergic to penicillin, vancomycin (Vancocin), 0.25 to 0.5 gram every 6 hours. Localized, fluctuant lesions should be surgically drained.

Recurrent Furunculosis

Generalized skin care with soap and water (or 4% chlorhexidine antimicrobial soap solution) is important to reduce staphyloccal skin carriage. Underclothing and sheets should be laundered at high temperatures and changed often. Washclothes should be washed thoroughly in hot water after each use and changed frequently. Draining lesions should be covered with sterile dressings to prevent autoinoculation. Dressings should be changed frequently and discarded in a sealed paper bag. In refractory cases measures may be indicated to reduce nasal carriage of *S. aureus:* (1) intranasal application of a 2% mupirocin ointment in a soft paraffin base for 5 to 7 days (or similar application of bacitracin ointment); or (2) oral antimicrobials (e.g., rifampin [Rifadin], 600 mg daily for 10 days) have been effective in eradicating *S. aureus* from nasal carriers for periods of many weeks. However, selection of rifampin-resistant strains does occur. Addition of a second drug (dicloxacillin if the strain is methicillin susceptible; trimethoprim-sulfamethoxazole; ciprofloxacin; minocycline) can reduce emergence of rifampin resistance.

VIRAL DISEASES OF THE SKIN

method of
STEPHEN K. TYRING, M.D., Ph.D.
University of Texas Medical Branch
Galveston, Texas

Whereas many families of viruses produce lesions of the skin, the clinical manifestations of three of these families are usually limited to the skin and mucous membranes. These virus families include: most herpesviruses as well as papillomaviruses and poxviruses. Twelve antiviral drugs have received Food and Drug Administration (FDA) approval thus far, and many are used in the therapy of viral diseases of the skin and mucous membranes. However, treatment of most viral lesions of the skin is mainly symptomatic.

HERPESVIRUSES

Often when the word "herpes" is used, one thinks of "genital herpes" or "cold sores." It is true that both conditions are due to infection with the herpes simplex viruses, but the human herpesvirus family actually comprises seven members, six of which are closely associated with human disease. In fact, the herpesviruses are so common that almost everyone in the United States has been infected and affected by them. These six herpesviruses are (1) herpes simplex virus 1, most often associated with "cold sores"; (2) herpes simplex virus 2, most often associated with genital herpes; (3) varicella zoster virus, the cause of both chickenpox and shingles; (4) Epstein-Barr virus, the cause of infectious mononucleosis; (5) cytomegalovirus, which is associated with certain birth defects and is a frequent cause of eye disease, including blindness, in AIDS patients; and (6) herpes virus 6, the cause of roseola, a usually mild childhood disease. The following discussion focuses on the herpes simplex viruses and the varicella zoster virus.

Herpes Simplex Viruses

In general, herpes simplex viruses (HSV) 1 and 2 are found at different sites in the body, with HSV 1 responsible for at least 90% of "cold sores" and HSV 2 causing at least 90% of genital herpes. The remaining cases of "cold sores" and genital herpes are associated with HSV 2 and HSV 1, respectively. The initial infection with either type of HSV can be the most disabling, with widespread blistering of the body site associated with severe discomfort and a healing time of 3 to 4 weeks (without therapy). Often, however, a person's first symptomatic episode is not a true "primary" infection since the virus may already have been in their body for an extended time period. Recurrences are usually less severe but still bothersome, and lesions usually heal in less than 2 weeks without therapy. The majority of persons who are infected with either HSV 1 or 2 have no symptoms, although the virus can hide in the person's body, specifically in one or more nerves. Likewise, not everyone who has a primary (initial) outbreak of herpes will have a recurrence. Antibodies to HSV 1 and 2 can be found in millions of adults who deny ever having had an outbreak of "cold sores" or genital herpes.

Clinical manifestations of HSV infection usually progress from a prodrome of burning and tingling to erythema, then blisters, then ulcers, then crusts, and finally to healing. What triggers an outbreak of herpes is not always clear, but it often follows some type of emotional or physical stress, which can be intense sunlight exposure for "cold sores" or menstruation for genital herpes in women. Often, however, the triggering event is not known. In persons whose immune systems are impaired, such as with cancer, AIDS, or organ transplant patients, episodes of HSV infection can be chronic in that one recurrence does not completely heal before the next recurrence starts.

Whereas HSV infection in otherwise healthy persons can be very uncomfortable, the effects are usually temporary. In contrast, genital herpes in a pregnant woman can result in birth defects or even infant death. In the past, HSV 2 was thought to be responsible for cervical cancer. However, another virus, the human papillomavirus, is now believed to be primarily responsible for this cancer, although HSV 2 may still act as a "helper virus."

Herpes simplex infection is not restricted to the mouth and genitalia; both HSV 1 and 2 can affect any site on the body. Herpetic infection of the eyes can be severe, resulting in impaired vision or even blindness if not treated. Although very rare, herpes simplex can also infect the brain, producing herpes encephalitis, a potentially fatal condition.

Treatment

The time to healing of herpetic lesions can be markedly shortened by antiviral therapy, and in fact, some episodes can be totally prevented if therapy is initiated early enough during the prodromal phase or if daily suppressive therapy is given to those individuals who have frequent recurrences. Whereas a number of antiherpes drugs are available, such as idoxuridine (Herplex, Stoxil), and vidarabine (Vira A), by far the safest and most effective antiherpes drug is acyclovir (Zovirax), which is available as a cream, a capsule, and an intravenous preparation (Table 1). Both oral and intravenous acyclovir are highly effective, but neither acyclovir nor any other drug has been demonstrated to rid the body of HSV. Acyclovir is very safe, rarely producing any side effects. It is activated by thymidine kinase produced by the virus and therefore works only where it is needed, i.e., in cells infected by HSV. In addition to the fact that it is a treatment and not a cure, the primary drawback to the use of acyclovir is its expense. Five 200-mg capsules a day are recommended to treat a recurrence, and two to four 200-mg capsules per day are recommended for prophylaxis in recurrence-prone individuals.

Vaccines for herpes simplex have been tested but so far have not been effective. Newer vaccines for HSV as well as other antiherpes drugs are currently under investigation.

Varicella Zoster Virus

The varicella zoster virus (VZV) is a unique herpesvirus in that it causes two very different diseases, chickenpox and shingles (also known as herpes zoster). Chickenpox is highly contagious and can be spread via airborne droplets, sneezing or coughing. In children, chickenpox is usually not a severe disease and resolves in 2 to 3 weeks in otherwise healthy hosts. In some adults and in children with impaired immunity, however, chickenpox can be a very serious and potentially fatal disease. Whereas symptomatic treatment is usually sufficient in most children, chickenpox in persons with cancer, AIDS, and other immunodeficient states requires antiviral therapy (e.g., acyclovir).

When the skin lesions of chickenpox heal, the virus remains latent in a cranial nerve ganglion or in the dorsal root of a spinal nerve and can later reappear to produce a completely different disease, shingles (herpes zoster). Shingles affects approximately 20% of persons at some time in their lives. It is more common in persons over 50 years of age, but it can be seen in persons of any age, and it is not uncommon in younger individuals with impaired immunity. The skin lesions of shingles appear first as erythema, then vesicles, then pustules, and finally progress to crusts, which fall off after 3 to 4 weeks. These skin lesions follow the distribution of a single nerve and are therefore seen on only one side of the body, often the trunk, but sometimes on the arm, leg, or face. If the nerves that supply the eye are affected, partial or total loss of vision can result if shingles is not treated.

Although caused by the same virus, shingles is much less contagious than chickenpox. A person who has never had chickenpox can develop this disease following direct contact with the skin lesions of a person with shingles. Shingles, however, cannot be passed from one person to another, since it only develops from a reactivation of latent VZV in the nervous system of a person who has had chickenpox.

TABLE 1. **Treatment of Herpesvirus Infections with Acyclovir***

Herpes Simplex Viruses (HSVs) Treatment		Suppression	Varicella Zoster Virus (VZV) Treatment	
NORMAL HOSTS				
Initial episode: 200 mg PO 5 times/ day × 10 days or 5 mg/kg iv q 8 h × 5 days or 5% ointment topically qid × 7 days†	Recurrent episode: 200 mg PO 5 times/ day × 5 days	400 mg PO bid	Primary varicella (children): 20 mg/kg PO qid × 5 days (maximal dose, 800 mg PO qid) (adults): 800 mg PO 5 times/ day × 7–10 days	Herpes zoster: 800 mg PO 5 times/ day × 7–10 days
IMMUNOCOMPROMISED PATIENTS				
200–400 mg PO 5 times/day × 10 days, or 5 mg/kg iv q 8 h × 7–10 days, ‡ or 5% ointment topically qid × 7 days†		≥ 400 mg PO bid	10 mg/kg iv q 8 h × 7–10 days§	10 mg/kg q 8 h × 7–10 days

*Doses of acyclovir are for adults with normal renal function unless otherwise noted.
†Less effective than the oral or the intravenous route; topical therapy should be used for minor outbreaks.
‡A dose of 250 mg per square meter of body surface area should be given to children under 12 years of age.
§A dose of 500 mg per square meter of body surface area should be given to children under 12 years of age.

Treatment

Acyclovir is FDA approved for the treatment of chickenpox and herpes zoster, but antiviral therapy is not always indicated in otherwise healthy persons with these conditions. When used for therapy of VZV infections, however, the dosage of acyclovir must be significantly higher than for treatment of HSV infections. Specifically, acyclovir, 800 mg orally five times per day for 7 to 10 days, is necessary for therapy of herpes zoster or of chickenpox in adults. If the patient is severely immunocompromised, or otherwise requires intravenous therapy, the recommended dosage is 10 mg of acyclovir per kg body weight three times per day. Acyclovir cream has no proven efficacy in treatment of VZV infections. Systemic acyclovir is clearly indicated for VZV infections in immunocompromised patients, for chickenpox in adults, and for shingles in patients over 50 years of age. It is important to treat VZV infections as early in the course as possible since starting acyclovir after the third day of development of vesicles has questionable benefits.

Because disseminated zoster is rare, the usual reason for treating shingles is prevention of postherpetic neuralgia (PHN). Acyclovir is of only modest benefit in preventing PHN. Prednisone was widely used for prevention of PHN before the availability of acyclovir but is associated with more side effects. One study is currently underway that compares the efficacies of acyclovir or prednisone with those of the drugs in combination. Although PHN is more easily prevented than treated, therapy can be undertaken with analgesics, antidepressants (e.g., amitriptyline), substance P inhibitors (capsaicin [Zostrix]), and nerve blocks. A VZV vaccine is widely used in Japan and Europe but is available in the United States only for prophylaxis in immunocompromised children. FDA approval of the VZV vaccine for general use in healthy children is expected in 1994.

HUMAN PAPILLOMAVIRUSES

A total of 68 human papillomavirus (HPV) types have been identified. Members of the HPV family have not been successfully grown in tissue culture, but HPV types can be distinguished by DNA hybridization. Some HPV types are very common while others are extremely rare. One or more of approximately 18 different papillomaviruses can be found in epidermodysplasia verruciformis, which is a rare condition, but most of these HPV types are not found in other clinical settings. A limited number of these HPV types are associated with a high rate of malignant conversion to squamous cell carcinoma when infected skin is exposed to ultraviolet light (e.g., sunlight). More common HPV infections can be divided into anogenital and nonanogenital types.

Anogenital HPV Infections

These HPV types can be classified as having low malignant potential (e.g., HPV 6 and HPV 11), intermediate malignant potential (e.g., HPV 31, HPV 33, and HPV 35), and high malignant potential (e.g., HPV 16 and HPV 18). Types 6 and 11 are responsible for venereal warts, condylomata acuminata, which is considered the most common viral sexually transmitted disease. These warts can present as verrucous, flat, or pedunculated papules on the skin and mucous membranes. In addition to being a cosmetic problem, they can produce large cauliflower-like lesions that are painful and malodorous, bleed easily, and can block the passage of body fluids. Not only can genital warts make sexual intercourse very difficult, they can actually grow so large during pregnancy that they can interfere with vaginal delivery.

Treatment

Initial therapy for genital warts is usually symptomatic, involving chemotherapeutic and cytodestructive techniques. Chemotherapeutic agents include bichloroacetic acid, trichloroacetic acid, 5-fluorouracil cream, and podofilox (podophyllotoxin) (Condylox). The last-named agent is the active ingredient in the crude resin podophyllin, which was widely used in the past but has toxic potential and lacks reproducible clinical results. The reproducible clinical activity and low toxicity of podofilox have made it the chemotherapeutic agent of choice for many physicians.

Cytodestructive treatment for genital warts includes cryotherapy using such agents as liquid nitrogen. Surgical therapies include simple excision, laser surgery, and electrosurgery.

The only antiviral drug approved for treatment of genital warts is interferon-alpha, which has been demonstrated to eliminate over 70% of genital warts when used intralesionally or subcutaneously (locally). A mild flu-like syndrome is often seen after the first injection of interferon, but almost all patients develop tolerance to side effects by the second or third in a series of injections. Although the recurrence rate of genital warts after clearing with interferon is usually less than that following nonantiviral therapy, the clinical response with interferon therapy is often slower than with other therapies. In very large lesions, interferon may not be effective as monotherapy.

Interferon is most efficacious in combination

with nonantiviral therapy. For example, with smaller genital warts, the patient can self-administer topical podofilox twice daily for 3 days, stop therapy for 4 days, and then repeat the cycle as necessary. During the same period, the patient can simultaneously receive local subcutaneous interferon therapy two or three times per week. Large or numerous genital warts can be surgically removed and the area treated with local subcutaneous interferon to reduce the recurrence rate. Either combination should result in a rapid response due to the nonantiviral therapy and a low recurrence rate due to the interferon treatment.

Nonanogenital HPV Infections

The most common HPV-related lesions outside of the anogenital area include plantar warts (HPV 1), verruca vulgaris (common warts) (HPV 2), and flat warts (HPV 3). Aside from their appearance and their potential for infectivity, most warts are asymptomatic except when located on weight-bearing surfaces. Plantar warts can make standing or walking very uncomfortable.

Treatment

Neither interferon nor any other antiviral drug is approved for treatment of nongenital warts, although a few case reports suggest that interferon may have some efficacy against these warts. Standard therapy for nongenital warts includes salicylic or lactic acids, keratolytic compounds, cantharidin, liquid nitrogen, electrosurgery, and sometimes even laser surgery.

POXVIRUSES

The only poxvirus infection commonly seen today is molluscum contagiosum, in which 4 to 6 mm smooth papules with a central umbilication can be seen as a (usually) nonsexually transmitted disease on any part of the body in children and as a (usually) sexually transmitted disease on the genitalia of adults. A much more aggressive presentation of molluscum contagiosum has become more frequent recently due to the prevalence of acquired immunodeficiency syndrome. Molluscum lesions can cover much of the body surface in AIDS patients. Less common diseases due to poxviruses include orf and milker's nodules, which are occasionally seen on the hands of persons who work with sheep and cattle. Both diseases may be due to the same virus, which produces nodules, tender plaques, or abscesses but no systemic symptoms.

Treatment

Therapy of molluscum contagiosum in nonimmunocompromised patients is usually simple and can involve such procedures as: expressing the molluscum body from an incised papule or use of liquid nitrogen with or without curetting. Since they often have many thousands of molluscum papules, the success of such simple destructive therapies in AIDS patients is very limited. Interferon-alpha therapy is effective in eradicating molluscum contagiosum in nonimmunocompromised patients but has limited usefulness in AIDS patients. Self-administered topical application of podofilox, however, is fairly effective even in AIDS patients. When podofilox is combined with systemic interferon, the clinical effects are often additive to synergistic.

No specific antiviral therapy exists for orf or milker's nodules, but none is needed since both conditions spontaneously resolve in 3 to 4 weeks.

PARASITIC DISEASES OF THE SKIN

method of
NILDE COSTANTE, M.D., and
KEYOUMARS SOLTANI, M.D.
The University of Chicago
Chicago, Illinois

Parasitic diseases of the skin include a wide spectrum of infestations. Some of these parasites are not encountered in the United States (Table 1), except by travelers to endemic areas. Others such as pediculosis, tick bites, and scabies are seen throughout the country. Swimmer's itch and creeping eruption (larva migrans) also exist in certain areas. To a great extent, the clinical manifestations of these skin disorders result from host immunologic responses as well as mechanical irritation.

SCABIES

Scabies is acquired by direct contact with the mite *Sarcoptes scabiei*. After the female mite burrows and lays eggs in the keratinized epithelium for 4 to 6 weeks, larvae migrate to the skin surface and develop into the adult stage within a week.

Pruritus often develops within 3 weeks of the initial infestation, with papules, vesicles, burrows, and secondary pyoderma over the finger webs, toes, axillae, areolae, groin, genitals, buttocks, and waist. In previously uninfected hosts, erythema and itching are initially mild or absent. In reinfested patients, there is no latent period, and skin lesions with intense pruritus appear promptly after infestation due to previous sensi-

TABLE 1. **Major Parasitic Diseases of the Skin**

Skin Disease	Parasite	Treatment
Scabies	*Sarcoptes scabiei*	Permethrin cream, lindane cream or lotion, sulfur cream, malathion lotion, benzyl benzoate lotion or emulsion, crotamiton cream or lotion (see text)
Pediculosis capitis/corporis/pubis	*Pediculus humanus* var. *capitis*/var. *corporis, Phthirus pubis*	Permethrin rinse, cream, or shampoo, lindane shampoo, cream, or lotion, malathion lotion, crotamiton lotion or cream, pyrethrins with piperonyl butoxide (see text)
Amebiasis cutis	*Entamoeba histolytica*	Metronidazole (Flagyl) 750 mg PO q 8 h for 5–10 days; iodoquinol (Yodoxin) 650 gm PO q 8 h for 20 days
Trichomoniasis	*Trichomonas vaginalis*	Metronidazole (Flagyl), 2 gm PO single dose or 250 mg q 8 h for 7 days
Simple cutaneous leishmaniasis	*Leishmania tropica*	Local treatment: cryotherapy; sodium stibogluconate (Pentostam) or meglumine antimonate (Glucantime) intralesionally
Cutaneous leishmaniasis (late ulcerative type/secondarily infected)	*Leishmania tropica*	Systemic: sodium stibogluconate (Pentostam) 20 mg/kg/day IV or IM or rifampicin (Rifampin) 600 mg/day for 10 days
Mucocutaneous leishmaniasis	*Leishmania braziliensis*	Amphotericin B (0.5–1 mg/kg/day in IV infusion)
Cercarial dermatitis	Schistosomes	Topical steroids or antihistaminics
Cysticercosis cutis	*Taenia solium*	Praziquantel 10 mg/kg
Enterobiasis	*Enterobius vermicularis*	Pyrvinium pamoate (Povan)* 5 mg/kg PO single dose
		Mebendazole (Flagyl) 100 mg PO single dose
Elephantiasis tropica loiasis	Filariae	Diethylcarbamazine (Hetrazan)* Surgery
Larva migrans/ground itch	Hookworms	Thiabendazole (Mintezol)
	Ancylostoma braziliens, Necator americanus	Mebendazole (Vermox)
Onchocerciasis	*Onchocerca volvulus*	Ivermectin/diethylcarbamazine

*Not available in the United States.

tization. Young children and elderly patients may have significant involvement of the palms, soles, scalp, and face. In immunocompromised and debilitated patients who lack proper inflammatory responses, the skin may be heavily infested, resulting in the crusted (Norwegian) form of scabies with numerous mites present in the hyperkeratotic lesions and severe nail involvement. Scabies is usually contracted by direct personal contact, but infestation by contact with contaminated towels, linens, and clothing is possible since the female mite can survive 3 days away from the skin. The clinical picture is suggestive of the diagnosis, which can be confirmed by microscopic demonstration of the mite.

Treatment

The entire body must be treated from head to toe, being careful to avoid the eyes, mouth, or other mucosal epithelia. Papules and itching persist for 1 or 2 weeks even after treatment and elimination of the mites due to the persistence of a delayed hypersensitivity reaction. In infants and debilitated patients, the head and face particularly require treatment. Household contacts need to be treated simultaneously. Laundering linens and clothing will effectively eliminate mites.

Permethrin 5% cream (Elimite) applied once overnight is a highly effective scabicide with low toxicity. It is not recommended for pregnant women and infants under 2 months of age. Gamma benzene hexachloride (lindane) lotion or cream (Kwell) although very effective, is not used as frequently as previously. It occasionally displays some neurotoxicity, especially in children. It is applied overnight for two consecutive nights, and treatment can be repeated after 1 week. In small children, the medication should be left on the skin for no more than 2 hours. In pregnant women and infants, 5 to 10% sulfur in petrolatum or a moisturizing cream base is effective and safe, and should be used in several overnight applications and repeated after 1 week. Crotamiton (Eurax) is administered in two overnight applications for 2 consecutive days, washed off 24 hours after the last application, and repeated in 1 week. Eurax is not very effective but it has some antipruritic effects. Malathion 0.5 to 1.0% lotion

(Ovide, Prioderm) and benzyl benzoate 20 to 50% in lotion or emulsion form are valuable alternatives.

Patients must be advised of the persistence of itching for several days or weeks after treatment, which may be helped by topical steroids.

Treatment for Norwegian scabies is the same as for ordinary scabies, although keratolytic agents, daily trimming of nails and scrubbing of subungual areas with lindane is advised.

PEDICULOSIS

Pediculus humanus and *Phthirus pubis* are the two species of lice that infest humans.

Pediculosis Capitis

This infestation is caused by *Pediculus humanus* var. *capitis*. Children are more frequently infested. Head lice are scattered over the scalp, especially at the nape of the neck. There is usually intense pruritus of the scalp, caused by the saliva of the louse and its feces when injected into the skin through the puncture wound. Furunculosis, impetigo, and cervical lymphadenopathy are common complications of pediculosis capitis.

Pediculosis capitis is transmitted by close contact as well as through combs, bed linen, and clothing. The adult louse can survive for 10 days away from the human body, while nits can survive up to 3 weeks. The clinical diagnosis is confirmed by microscopic examination of the lice or nits. White fluorescent specks on the hair and scalp can be seen under Wood's light.

Treatment

Treatment is directed toward the destruction of the lice and ova. Permethrin 1% cream rinse (Nix) is very effective and relatively nontoxic. It is applied for 10 minutes, washed off, and reapplied after a week. Lindane 1% shampoo (Kwell, Scabene) should be left on the scalp for several minutes and rinsed out. Malathion lotion (Prioderm, Ovide) can also be applied for 10 minutes. Crotamiton (Eurax) cream or lotion is less effective than lindane and can be applied for 24 hours followed by shampooing.

Pyrethrin combined with piperonyl butoxide (RID, Pronto shampoo) is an alternative and must be applied for 10 minutes and washed off. Nits should be removed with a fine-tooth comb. For eyelash involvement, petrolatum (Vaseline) can be used twice daily followed by mechanical removal of the nits. More recently a formic acid preparation (Step 2) has been introduced that effectively removes dead nits from the hair shaft.

Pediculosis Corporis

This infestation is caused by *Pediculus humanus* var. *corporis*. Body lice are important vectors of disease, transmitting epidemic typhus, trench fever, and relapsing fever. The lice live at the sites of pressure such as beneath bras or belts or in bedding. They cause intense pruritus and papular urticaria. The infected lesions have an eczematous appearance resembling scabies except for the sparing of the hands and feet and predilection for the upper back. Diagnosis is made by clinical presentation and confirmed by finding the lice or nits in clothing or bedding.

Treatment

Laundering of clothing and bedding is essential. Pruritus is symptomatically treated. The majority of the treatments used for scabies are effective in pediculosis (see Table 1). Treatment of persons in close contact with infected patients is advised.

Pediculosis Pubis

Pediculosis pubis is a sexually transmitted disease caused by *Phthirus pubis*. The infestation can also be transmitted by contact with clothing, bedding, or towels. It is limited to the genital area but may occasionally involve the axillae, eyelashes, beard, and other hairy areas. It causes mild to severe pruritus in the affected areas. The lice can be seen on the skin as yellowish brown specks. Occasionally, nonpruritic hyperpigmented spots, known as maculae cerulae, can be detected on the skin.

Treatment

Most treatments that are effective in scabies also work for pediculosis pubis. Persons in close contact with the patient should be treated.

CERCARIAL DERMATITIS

Many schistosome cercariae that ordinarily infect birds and semiaquatic mammals can penetrate human skin, producing a cutaneous inflammatory response. Fresh-water lakes and some marine beaches may contain cercariae that cause swimmer's itch or marine dermatitis, respectively. Exposure to either type of cercariae will sensitize people to both.

The cycle begins when eggs present in the feces of definitive hosts enter the water, where a mollusc serves as an intermediate host in which the parasites will develop to cercariae that are finally liberated under appropriate conditions to enter the skin of birds or other mammals to complete the cycle. Human beings are inadvertent hosts, and although the cercariae may penetrate their skin they cannot develop further. Immediately after immersion penetration of the larvae through the skin causes local erythema and pruritus followed by delayed onset of pruritic papules and vesicles.

Treatment

Treatment is directed toward symptomatic relief of pruritus with topical steroids or antihistamines.

MYIASIS

Myiasis is caused by invasion of animals or humans by fly larvae. The infestation can be primary (furuncular myiasis) if the larva penetrates the skin or secondary if it invades a pre-existing wound or ulcer. A creeping eruption due to intradermal migration of the larvae is another type of presentation. Myiasis can be obligatory or facultative. Myiasis is caused by many species of flies, but North American furuncular myiasis is commonly caused by larvae of the genus *Cuterebra*. Patients seen in the United States frequently have a history of travel to endemic areas. Furuncular myiasis is characterized by an erythematous papule 2 to 4 mm in diameter that may be tender and may have a central pore. The face, scalp, neck, shoulders, and chest are frequently involved. Lesions contain one or more larvae depending on the fly species.

Treatment

Treatment consists of débridement and removal of the larvae and prevention of secondary bacterial infections. Application of petroleum jelly to the pores will force the larvae to come out for air so they can easily be removed for diagnosis and treatment.

SUPERFICIAL FUNGAL INFECTIONS OF THE SKIN

method of
FREDERIC W. STEARNS, M.D.
St. Francis Hospital
Tulsa, Oklahoma

Superficial fungal infections occur frequently and are responsible for 4% of all visits to dermatologists. Dermatophytes, *Candida* species, and *Pityrosporum orbiculare* are the organisms most commonly involved. Diagnosis requires recognition of the usual clinical picture and typically annular scaling erythema and demonstration of the organism directly in the scales or in selective culture media.

TREATMENT

Topical treatment is either the sole modality or an adjunct to systemic therapy. Notable exceptions are dermatophytes in hair or nails (tinea capitis, onychomycosis), in which topical therapy is ineffective. Currently available topical agents are (1) imidazoles—clotrimazole (Lotrimin), miconazole (Micatin), oxiconazole (Oxistat), econazole (Spectazole), sulconazole (Exelderm), and ketoconazole (Nizoral); (2) polyenes—amphotericin B (Fungizone) and nystatin (Mycostatin) effective only for *Candida;* and (3) naftifine (Naftin) for tinea and ciclopirox (Loprox) for both tinea and *Candida.*

Griseofulvin (Fulvicin, Grisactin, GrisPEG) has been the standard treatment for dermatophytoses for years. It is fungistatic, ineffective against yeasts, and should be taken in full dosage until the infection clears. Absorption improves with milk or food. Side effects include headaches, gastrointestinal distress, and less commonly, alcohol interaction, urticaria, and phototoxicity. Dose-response of warfarin (Coumadin), phenobarbital, and related medications will vary when given with griseofulvin due to hepatic enzyme induction.

Ketoconazole is an oral, fungistatic, imidazole effective for candidiasis, dermatophytoses, and other systemic mycoses. The usual dosage is 200 to 400 mg daily with juice. Hepatotoxicity is idiosyncratic, rare, but hazardous and necessitates monitoring. Androgenic suppression leading to gynecomastia, oligospermia, and impotence resolves after the drug is stopped but can be distressing.

Fluconazole (Diflucan) and itraconazole (Sporanox) are new triazoles that promise to be effective against both dermatophytes and yeasts. Because their initial indications are limited, usage for superficial infections is largely anecdotal. Side effects seem infrequent. Cost is a factor with prolonged treatment. The lipophilic nature of these compounds makes intermittent dosing practicable, and fluconazole is commonly taken once or twice weekly. Drug-drug interactions are common, occurring with digoxin, cyclosporine, phenytoin, rifampin, H_2 antagonists, anticoagulants, isoniazid, and oral hypoglycemic agents, so dosage adjustments may be necessary with concomitant usage. Fluconazole has proven valuable in persistent/resistant/mixed infections, but more information is necessary before guidelines can be given for itraconazole.

TINEA VERSICOLOR

A lipophilic organism, *Pityrosporum orbiculare,* causes discrete and confluent plaques of hyper- and hypopigmented scaling on the trunk and proximal extremities. It is frequently asymptomatic, but it can cause considerable itching when the individual sweats. Because this organism requires oil to grow, topical creams and lotions should be eliminated. The scalp should be treated with the body, since it frequently serves as a reservoir for the organism. Selenium sulfide suspension (2.5%) (Exsel, Selsun) should be applied twice weekly to all involved areas, allowed to dry, left on overnight, then showered off following a shampoo with the suspension. Ketoconazole can be used for severe cases: 400 mg is taken once a week 2 hours before exercise. Fluconazole and itraconazole are probably effective, but treatment regimens have not been formulated. Topical antifungal creams are effective, but the cost and inconvenience of applying them frequently to large body surface areas make them impractical. Older remedies such as sodium thiosulfate solution, propylene glycol in water, and sulfur and salicylic acid (SAS) soap may help prevent recurrences. Relapses are common, and many seem linked to tanning beds. Dyschromia, either hyper- or hypopigmented, resolves slowly after successful treatment.

CANDIDA

The yeast *Candida albicans* invades warm, wet areas of the skin, particularly skin folds (axillae, groin, gluteal cleft, inframammary, digital webs, and under the foreskin), nails (onychia, paronychia), and mucous membranes. Nurses, bartenders, dairy farmers, mothers of young children, and others doing "wet work" frequently have nail infection with *Candida.* Thrush and crural candidiasis are seen following antibiotic therapy and in newborns. Angular cheilitis frequently occurs with dentures. Diabetes, obesity, immunosuppression, and systemic antibiotics all predispose to candidiasis. Occluded areas become beefy red with peripheral scaling and follicular ("satellite") pustules. Demonstration of the organism with a wet prep (hanging drop, KOH, Swartz-Lamkin stain) is diagnostic.

Topical amphotericin B is the most effective agent, but nystatin, imidazoles (e.g., miconazole, econazole), and ciclopirox (Loprox) sometimes work well. Wet compresses with Burow's solution kill yeast and provide symptomatic relief. Older preparations such as gentian violet and Castellani's paint are inexpensive and effective but messy; 5% thymol in chloroform works well under and around nails. Drying the area is important, and a hair dryer is good for hard-to-reach areas like nails, toe webs, and groin folds. Reducing intestinal tract colonization with oral nystatin, 500,000 units twice daily for 2 weeks, prevents "seeding" of involved areas. Troches and pastilles (Clotrimazole [Mycelex], nystatin [Mycostatin]) are convenient for oral involvement, and chlorhexidene (Peridex) helps denture infestation. Fluconazole, 200 mg every other day, is beneficial in resistant cases and may supplant ketoconazole for treatment of chronic mucocutaneous candidiasis.

DERMATOPHYTE INFECTIONS

Dermatophytes invade and inhabit the stratum corneum, the devascularized keratin layer of the epidermis. The clinical picture depends upon the infecting organism, the infected site, and the immune response of the host. The genera *Trichophyton, Microsporum,* and *Epidermophyton* account for most dermatophyte disease. Five species (*T. rubrum, T. tonsurans, T. mentagrophytes, M. canis, E. floccosum*) produce most infections, with *T. verrucosum* common in agricultural regions.

Tinea capitis is usually found in children, presenting either as a diffuse mild scalp scaling, "black dot" ringworm with patchy hair loss and broken hairs, or the boggy, exudative kerion. Tinea barbae and Majocchi's granuloma are deep infections of shaved hairs. KOH preparations of infected hairs show spores and hyphae in the hair shaft (endothrix) or outside it (ectothrix). Only *Microsporum* species fluoresce with Wood's light, and the nonfluorescing *T. tonsurans* is now the most common cause of tinea capitis. When ringworm occurs, household pets and family members, including adults, should be examined. Topical medications will not clear hair infections, but selenium sulfide shampoo (Exsel, Selsun) hastens clearing and decreases contagion. Griseofulvin, 10 to 15 mg per kg per day, given after meals, usually brings about clearing in 6 to 8 weeks. Ketoconazole and fluconazole are also effective for adults; prolonged treatment is necessary. Kerions occasionally require systemic corticosteroids or potassium iodide to prevent febrile hypersensitivity reactions during initial therapy.

Tinea corporis ("jungle rot") and tinea cruris ("jock itch") are characterized by well-marginated plaques of annular scaling and can occur separately or together. *T. rubrum, T. mentagrophytes, M. canis,* and *E. floccosum* commonly produce these conditions. The organisms are admirably suited for their environment, and infections can recur or persist for years. KOH preparations or fungal cultures differentiate these conditions from nummular eczema, neurodermatitis, seborrheic dermatitis, psoriasis, and cutaneous candidiasis. Topical treatment with an imidazole preparation applied daily is usually adequate; treatment of areas adjacent to the visible changes and treatment for 2 weeks after disappearance increase cure rates. Griseofulvin, ketoconazole, or fluconazole may be necessary for widespread disease, especially with infected hairs, and is frequently necessary for immunocompromised patients.

Tinea pedis ("athlete's foot") presents as interdigital scaling and maceration, vesicles on the proximal foot, or diffuse scaling on the sole. It can be a point of entry for bacteria causing lymphangitis or erysipelas, especially in elderly or diabetic patients. *T. rubrum* and *T. mentagrophytes* are the most common organisms. Most imidazoles are effective applied once daily for a prolonged time, usually 3 months or more. Subsequent weekly application or use of Whitfield's ointment can prevent recurrences. Stubborn or resistent cases require griseofulvin, 500 mg twice daily, ketoconazole, 200 to 400 mg daily, or fluconazole, 200 mg twice weekly. Feet are kept dry with Zeasorb powder and avoidance of rubber-soled footgear. Tinea manuum often appears in concert with tinea pedis, presenting as persistent, often unilateral, palmar scaling. It requires systemic antifungals for clearing.

Onychomycosis is the most stubborn dermatophyte infection, trying patients and practitioners alike. Before beginning treatment, positive identification should be made, since a variety of yeasts and occasionally *Pseudomonas* infections can give a similar appearance, and treatment for one may not affect the other. The fungus may colonize distally, showing thickening, discoloration, and debris that lifts the nail plate from its bed, or superficially, showing white scaling areas on top of the nail plate. Occasionally, infection begins proximally and the nail plate will begin to separate at the cuticle. Treatment aims at supressing the fungus as the nail grows out; this takes 4 to 6 months for fingernails and 12 to 24 months for toenails. Griseofulvin, ketoconazole, or fluconazole should be used in full dosages. Fingernails respond better than toenails, where recurrences are common. Toenails follow the "third" rule: 1/3 do well, 1/3 improve but recur, and 1/3 fail to respond. Removing an affected nail and treating the nail bed with an imidazole as the new nail grows increases success, and using 5% thymol in chloroform to dry distal onycholysis helps, but other topical measures waste time, money, and effort. Again, follow-up measures stressing dryness, treating associated hyperhidrosis with aluminum chloride hexahydrate (Drysol) at bedtime, and avoiding trauma to the nail plate help prevent recurrences.

DISEASES OF THE MOUTH

method of
DRORE EISEN, M.D., D.D.S.
Cincinnati, Ohio

BENIGN NEOPLASMS AND DISTURBANCES OF DEVELOPMENT

Torus Palatinus and Torus Mandibularis. These slowly enlarging masses arise either in the midline of the hard palate (torus palatinus) or on the lingual surface of the mandible (torus mandibularis). These benign, bony protuberances are often inherited in a Mendelian dominant pattern. Although they are generally asymptomatic and require no treatment, they occasionally can become traumatized and ulcerated. Furthermore, they are often surgically removed to facilitate the construction of dental prostheses.

Fibroma. These are the most common soft tissue tumors of the oral cavity, occurring most frequently on the buccal mucosa. They appear as smooth, pink papules or nodules and can be either sessile or pedunculated. Although some represent true neoplasms, most probably result from trauma and chronic irritation. Treatment consists of simple surgical resection.

Lipoma. This fatty tumor is a benign, slow-growing neoplasm. It occurs in the oral cavity, most commonly on the buccal mucosa, as a soft, yellow nodule. Excision is both diagnostic and therapeutic.

Hemangioma. This common oral tumor can either be congenital or develop during childhood or, less commonly, later in life. It presents as a flat or raised lesion in shades of blue, red, or purple. Women are affected twice as often as men, and the most common sites of occurrence are the lips and tongue. Congenital lesions often spontaneously involute; however, those that ulcerate, hemorrhage, or interfere with eating and other oral functions require treatment. Hemangiomata can be surgically removed or treated by a variety of methods, including laser surgery, cryosurgery, injection of sclerosing agents, and compression therapy.

Lymphangioma. This benign tumor of the lymphatic vessels is usually present at birth or shortly thereafter. It most commonly occurs on the tongue and can be a cause of macroglossia. While deep lesions appear as nonspecific masses, superficial lesions exhibit the pathognomonic appearance of a nodular, pebbly surface of pink and grey projections. These lesions are often surgically removed; however, because of their infiltrative nature, recurrences are common.

Fordyce's Granules. These ectopic sebaceous glands are most commonly observed on the buccal mucosa and vermilion border. They appear as yellow papules that often coalesce into plaques. Fordyce's granules are benign and are of no clinical significance.

Lip Pits. Unilateral or bilateral congenital pits can be commonly found at the commissures. Rarely, paramedian lip pits are seen on the lower lip on either side of the midline. The latter has been associated with cleft lip or palate and other developmental anomalies. Although lip pits may express the contents of an underlying minor salivary gland, they are benign and need be surgically excised only for aesthetic reasons.

Pleomorphic Adenoma. This slow-growing tumor represents the most common salivary gland neoplasm of the oral cavity. It occurs most commonly on the hard palate as a smooth, submucosal mass that rarely ulcerates. Treatment is by complete surgical resection.

Nevomelanocytic Nevus. Nevi rarely occur in the oral cavity and should be differentiated from other causes of oral pigmentation. The majority occur on the hard palate and gingiva where oral melanomas also most commonly arise. Surgical excision of all intraoral nevi is recommended since differentiation from early oral melanoma cannot be made by clinical findings alone.

Congenital Epulis. These rare tumors occur most often on the anterior alveolar ridge of infants as protuberant, smooth, pink masses that are frequently pedunculated. Recurrences after surgical resection are not common.

Peripheral Ossifying Fibroma. This common tumor affects mainly children and teenagers. Clinically, a sessile or pedunculated nodule arises on the gingiva. The lesions are usually smooth and pink, although they may be ulcerated. Treatment by excision is diagnostic and curative, although recurrences are not uncommon.

Odontogenic Cyst. This group of cysts arises from epithelium derived from the development of the dental apparatus. Most are discovered radiographically as well-circumscribed radiolucencies. Although benign, these can display considerable growth potential, resulting in expansion and destruction of bone. Malignant transformation of the lining epithelium has been reported. Treatment consists of surgical resection; recurrences are uncommon.

Ameloblastoma. These are benign, odontogenic tumors; however, by their growth pattern, they mimic malignancies. Although painless and slow growing, as they enlarge, they can cause loosening of teeth, bone destruction, paresthesias, and disfigurement. More than two-thirds occur in the mandible, and they are diagnosed most commonly between the ages of 30 and 50. These aggressive tumors require complete surgical re-

moval. Radiation therapy has also been employed as therapy.

PREMALIGNANT AND MALIGNANT NEOPLASMS

Oral Melanoma. The dismal prognosis of oral melanoma is partly due to the lack of early recognition by patients and physicians. The majority arise on the palate and maxillary alveolar ridge. Some tumors appear as nodules and grow rapidly, causing pain, bleeding, and loosening of teeth. Many, however, appear as innocent pigmented macules and have a prolonged vertical growth phase before becoming invasive. The presence of unexplained oral pigmentation, especially on the palate, necessitates a biopsy. Oral melanomas often are treated by wide surgical resection and adjuvant chemotherapy and radiotherapy in selected cases.

Squamous Cell Carcinoma. These tumors, which predominantly affect the middle-aged and elderly, account for 90% of all malignancies of the oral cavity. Men are affected twice as often as women. Tobacco and alcohol as well as other carcinogens have been implicated as causative factors. The lower lip and lateral surfaces of the tongue are the most frequent sites of occurrence, but the floor of the mouth, gingiva, buccal mucosa, and soft palate are also frequently involved. Early lesions are often asymptomatic and appear as raised white or red plaques. Ulcerations with rolled, indurated borders and exophytic masses usually represent advanced lesions.

Surgery and radiation therapy, alone or in combination, have been utilized in the treatment of oral squamous cell carcinomas. The prognosis is influenced by the site, size, and spread of the tumor. Metastases from intraoral tumors are common, which accounts for the poor survival rate of these malignancies.

Leukoplakia. Leukoplakia is a keratotic, white plaque that cannot be characterized clinically or pathologically as any other disease. Clinically, these lesions are asymptomatic and are usually discovered during a routine oral examination. They can occur anywhere in the oral cavity, but most frequently seen on the tongue, buccal mucosa, alveolar mucosa, and floor of the mouth. When these lesions are examined histologically, approximately three-fourths will show only benign, keratotic changes; the remaining one-fourth will demonstrate dysplasia, carcinoma in situ, or squamous cell carcinoma.

The causes of leukoplakia are as varied as the histologic appearance of these lesions; most are considered to arise from chronic irritation, such as local trauma from teeth or restorations or from tobacco or alcohol consumption. Biopsy is warranted to differentiate leukoplakia from other specific white oral lesions and to exclude histologic features of dysplasia or carcinoma. Histologically benign lesions often regress, especially when local irritation, such as that from a sharp tooth or filling, is corrected. Scalpel and laser surgery have been employed when premalignant or malignant features are demonstrated. Recently, beta-carotene and vitamin A analogues have been employed in the treatment of selected cases.

Erythroplakia. Like "leukoplakia," "erythroplakia" is a clinical term describing any red patch on the oral mucosa not caused by inflammation. Unlike leukoplakia, however, approximately 90% of these lesions prove to be carcinoma in situ or invasive carcinoma on histologic examination. They are often asymptomatic velvety red plaques that are easily overlooked. A biopsy is mandatory for all persistent red plaques, and surgical resection is indicated if precancerous or cancerous changes are identified.

Kaposi's Sarcoma. This malignant vascular tumor is present in approximately 15 to 25% of patients with acquired immunodeficiency syndrome (AIDS). Although many lesions are asymptomatic and appear as blue-red macules, others may present as nodules, causing local tissue destruction and pain. The great majority of lesions occur on the hard palate, and multiple tumors are common. AIDS patients who have oral lesions often experience a more aggressive clinical course. Scalpel and laser surgery, radiation, and intralesional vinblastine have been used as treatment modalities.

Leukemia. Oral cavity lesions are common in all types of leukemia but are most prevalent in myelocytic (monocytic) leukemias. Gingival hyperplasia with bleeding is frequently noted. Other primary clinical manifestations of leukemia include oral ulcerations, hemorrhagic lesions, and destruction of alveolar bone resulting in loose teeth. These oral symptoms may be the first clinical manifestations of leukemia. Oral lesions usually respond to therapy of the underlying disease. Dental evaluation and requisite treatment prior to chemotherapy are essential in order to eradicate potential sources of infection that could become problematic with reduced autoimmunity.

INJURIES OF THE ORAL CAVITY

Traumatic Ulcers. Traumatic ulcerations of the oral cavity are commonly encountered. Self-inflicted injuries from biting the mucosa, toothbrush injuries, ill-fitting dentures, rough teeth and restorations, accidents and iatrogenic injuries during dental procedures will result in ulcerations that usually can be diagnosed by their clinical features and history. Ulcerations that persist for prolonged periods require biopsy to exclude carcinoma.

Inflammatory Papillary Hyperplasia. This condition is associated with ill-fitting dentures or continuous daily wear of dentures without regular removal. The hard palate exhibits red, edematous papules that often coalesce into plaques. Occasionally the alveolar mucosa may be involved. Various degrees of inflammation may be present, and lesions are often secondarily infected with *Candida*. Having patients remove their dentures nightly or remaking ill-fitting dentures usually results in partial or complete regression of the lesion. Candidiasis should be treated with clotrimazole or nystatin.

Nicotine Stomatitis. This condition occurs in patients who smoke pipes and cigars. The palate typically develops diffuse white papules with small, red, depressed centers. Each papule represents a dilated and partially occluded orifice of minor salivary glands. The lesions usually disappear after the cessation of smoking.

Mucocele. This common lesion results from trauma to a salivary duct, usually incurred by biting the lip. The great majority occurs on the lower lip, but lesions can appear in other locations. Clinically, mucoceles present as blue, translucent masses when superficial, and pink, firm nodules when deep. Aspiration yields a viscous, clear fluid. Surgical excision of the lesion and the adjacent salivary gland acini is the treatment of choice.

Ranula. This retention cyst occurs in the floor of the mouth and arises from sublingual or submandibular glands. Lesions are usually asymptomatic and unilateral. Treatment consists of either excising or unroofing the lesion.

Amalgam Tattoo. This common lesion is caused by the introduction of dental filling material (amalgam) into the oral soft tissue during dental procedures. Bluish-black tattoos appear most commonly on the gingiva and buccal mucosa and are asymptomatic. The diagnosis can usually be established clinically and supported by the dental history. Occasionally a radiograph of the lesion will demonstrate metallic radiopacities. A biopsy should be performed on lesions when the diagnosis is uncertain.

Pyogenic Granuloma. These lesions arise as a response to local trauma or irritation. Clinically, an elevated pedunculated or sessile nodule develops, often rapidly. Lesions are usually red and vascular and ulcerate or bleed frequently. They are treated by surgical excision. When located on the gingiva, it is important to remove local factors such as calculus and plaque from adjacent teeth since these can act as irritants leading to recurrences. The pregnancy tumor is clinically and histologically identical to a pyogenic granuloma. Surgical excision of pregnancy tumors should be postponed until after childbirth, since many will spontaneously regress.

Hairy Tongue. Hypertrophy of the filiform papillae results in a matted layer of elongated papillae on the dorsum of the tongue. Depending upon the cause, the papillae will stain yellow, white, brown, or black and appear as elongated hairs. Common causes include smoking, poor oral hygiene, radiation therapy, foods, and antibiotics resulting in overgrowth of chromogenic organisms. Brushing and scraping the tongue with a toothbrush often causes desquamation of the papillae. Long papillae can be snipped with scissors.

Benign Migratory Glossitis (Geographic Tongue). This common inflammatory condition of the tongue is generally asymptomatic. Red patches with white, elevated borders occur on the dorsal and lateral surfaces of the tongue. As its name implies, the lesions are migratory, returning to a normal appearance before new lesions appear elsewhere. If burning and stinging are present, patients can be treated with a potent topical corticosteroid such as fluocinonide gel or ointment (Lidex) three times daily. Various mouth rinses containing hydrogen peroxide, diphenhydramine and tetracycline may also be beneficial.

Contact Stomatitis. Inflammatory changes in any mucosal surface can occur as an allergic reaction to a variety of causative agents. Pain, swelling, erythema, vesiculation, and erosions are frequently encountered. Common offending agents include toothpastes and mouth rinses, foods, cosmetics, and dental materials. Treatment may require systemic corticosteroids if the allergic reaction results in erosions. Otherwise, potent topical corticosteroids and avoidance of the allergen will result in remission.

Melkersson-Rosenthal Syndrome. This disorder of unknown etiology is characterized by a granulomatous infiltrate of the oral soft tissues. Recurrent episodes of swelling eventually result in an edematous and rubbery tissue most commonly in the lips. The gingiva and buccal mucosa may be affected as well. The swelling can occur alone or as part of a triad with Bell's palsy and fissured (scrotal) tongue. Systemic conditions with identical histologic findings, including Crohn's disease and sarcoid, should be excluded. There is no specific treatment for this condition; however, intralesional and systemic corticosteroids as well as the removal of dental foci of infection have occasionally been of benefit.

Sialolithiasis. Patients with obstructions of a salivary gland often will complain of pain after meals when saliva flow is stimulated. Occlusion of the duct by calcified stones prevents the flow of saliva, producing discomfort. Small stones may be manipulated and removed with a probe, whereas large ones almost always require surgical removal.

Angular Cheilitis. This frequently encountered inflammatory condition manifests as fissuring and exudation at the corners of the mouth. Various causes of excessive salivation and drooling at the corners of the mouth produce a similar clinical pattern. These include overclosure of the bite in edentulous patients, orthodontic braces, and habitual licking of the lips. Candidiasis and *Staphylococcus aureus* infections can also produce angular cheilitis, as can ariboflavinosis. Treatment is directed at eliminating predisposing factors and reducing excessive salivation. Symptomatic relief is achieved by applying combinations of mild topical corticosteroids, antibiotics, and antifungal ointments. Hydrocortisone 2.5% ointment mixed with equal parts of ketoconazole (Nizoral) cream applied twice daily usually results in rapid improvement.

Epulis Fissuratum. This reactive inflammatory response occurs in edentulous patients wearing poorly fitting dentures. Excessive folds of tissue, pink or red in color, arise from the sulci anterior or posterior to the alveolar ridge. Excising the redundant tissue and remaking the dentures prevents recurrences.

INFECTIONS

Herpes. Primary herpetic gingivostomatitis, the primary herpes infection, usually occurs in young children, although teenagers and adults may occasionally be affected. Fever accompanies painful and edematous gingiva with widespread oral ulcerations. Therapy with systemic acyclovir (Zovirax), 200 mg five times daily for 7 days, shortens the duration of the disease.

Following the primary infection, the virus remains dormant until reactivated, recurring most commonly on the lips (recurrent herpes labialis). Prodromal symptoms of burning and pain precede the development of small vesicles, which subsequently rupture and crust over. Spontaneous healing usually occurs in 7 to 14 days. Topical and systemic acyclovir (Zovirax) may shorten the duration of the disease if started during the prodromal phase or shortly thereafter. Recurrent intraoral herpes infection is less common than herpes labialis and manifests as small ulcerations resembling aphthae. The attached gingiva and hard palate are most commonly involved. These lesions may be treated as above; however, they will usually heal spontaneously within 7 days.

Herpangina. This infection, caused by a Coxsackie virus, usually affects children and teenagers. Small vesicles and ulcerations are seen on the soft palate, uvula, and oropharynx. Patients often have accompanying viral symptoms, including fever and malaise, and oral pain creates difficulty in eating and swallowing. The diagnosis is based upon the clinical findings, and healing occurs within 7 to 10 days without any treatment.

Hand, Foot, and Mouth Disease. This disorder, like herpangina, is caused by Coxsackie viruses. Oral lesions are almost always present, most frequently on the hard palate and tongue. Small vesicles and ulcerations often result in significant discomfort. Cutaneous lesions characterized by small vesicles and erythema occur on the hands, feet, and occasionally the buttocks. Topical anesthetics, including lidocaine and diphenhydramine, are palliative until the disease resolves spontaneously in 7 to 14 days.

Candidiasis (Thrush). This opportunistic infection is caused most commonly by *Candida albicans*. Although healthy individuals without any predisposing conditions may be affected, candidiasis occurs mainly when local or systemic alterations allow favorable overgrowth of the yeast organism. Infants, immunocompromised and chronically ill patients, diabetics, and those taking antibiotics, corticosteroids, and chemotherapy for prolonged periods are most predisposed to candidiasis. Clinically, candidiasis can appear in several forms, most commonly as white plaques that can be easily wiped off, revealing a raw, bleeding surface. Other clinical presentations include pseudomembranous white lesions, chronic hyperplastic white lesions, and atrophic red plaques. All forms may be diagnosed by microscopic examination for hyphae or by culture.

In managing patients with candidiasis, identifying and eliminating predisposing or precipitating factors are as important as antifungal therapy. Topical agents, including nystatin oral suspension (Mycostatin), 400,000 to 600,000 units four times daily, and clotrimazole troches (Mycelex), five times daily for 2 weeks, are usually successful. Recurrences are common unless antifungal therapy is continued for several weeks following the disappearance of the oral lesions. Systemic agents, such as ketoconazole (Nizoral), can be prescribed for resistant cases or for those suffering from chronic mucocutaneous candidiasis.

Median Rhomboid Glossitis. This lesion appears as a red patch or nodule on the dorsal surface of the tongue in the midline. There is loss of the filiform papillae within the lesion, causing it to appear smooth and clinically distinct. Although once considered to be a developmental anomaly, it is now felt to represent a local candidal infection. Antifungal therapy often results in complete resolution.

Oral Hairy Leukoplakia. These lesions, which harbor Epstein-Barr virus, occur most commonly on the lateral surfaces of the tongue and may be unilateral or bilateral. Clinically, they are often corrugated, rough plaques that cause no discomfort. The importance of identifying these lesions lies in the fact that almost all patients with this condition are infected with human immunodeficiency virus and will develop AIDS within 2 to 3 years. Treatment includes topical retinoids (Retin-A gel 0.1%), surgery, and systemic acyclovir (Zovirax).

Viral Warts. Oral warts are caused by the human papillomavirus. Condylomata acuminata (venereal warts) occur mainly in the anogenital area but can spread to the oral cavity through oral-genital contact. Verruca vulgaris (common warts) can involve the oral cavity, often in conjunction with cutaneous warts. Treatment of warts consists of excision, cryosurgery, electrodesiccation, or occasionally chemical destruction.

Acute Necrotizing Ulcerative Gingivitis. In some patients with lowered resistance to infections (AIDS) and poor oral hygiene, and infection with oral bacilli and spirochetes results in this ulcerative form of gingivitis. Young adults are most commonly afflicted. Clinically, a grey-white pseudomembrane covers ulcerations that start in the interdental papillae, but diffuse areas of involvement may be found. Patients frequently complain of gingival tenderness and pain, bleeding, fetid odor, and difficulty in eating. Low-grade fevers and lymphadenopathy are also commonly encountered.

In mild cases, an intense oral hygiene program accompanied by hydrogen peroxide rinses and analgesics will effect complete resolution. In more severe cases, systemic antibiotics such as penicillin or erythromycin will cause rapid improvement. Periodontal surgery may be necessary after the disease regresses.

Syphilis. The oral cavity may be the site of involvement in all stages of syphilis. Extragenital chancres in primary syphilis are found most commonly on the lips, accompanied by lymphadenopathy. Painful ulcerations usually resolve within 3 to 4 weeks. The mucous patch characterized by a painless, grayish-white lesion, usually on the tongue, is frequently seen in secondary syphilis, and syphilitic pharyngitis with necrosis is also common during this stage. In the tertiary stage of syphilis, there may be a pathognomonic atrophic glossitis, with loss of the papillae and atrophy of the tongue musculature. Oral gummas involving the palate and tongue are infrequently seen. Patients with congenital syphilis often develop abnormalities of teeth, most commonly Hutchinson's incisors and mulberry molars.

VESICULOEROSIVE ORAL DISEASES

Lichen Planus. This common inflammatory condition of the oral cavity affects 1% of the general population with the peak incidence in the fourth to sixth decades of life. Although the etiology is unknown, lichen planus is felt to be an autoimmune disorder that can involve the skin. The posterior buccal mucosa and tongue are most commonly affected, although any oral site may be involved. White reticulated lesions, papules, and plaques are seen most frequently and, if asymptomatic, do not require treatment. Many patients display red atrophic lesions and erosions that can cause considerable discomfort and morbidity.

Treatment for such patients includes topical, injectable, and systemic corticosteroids and retinoids, but none is universally effective. Triamcinolone acetonide 0.1% (Kenalog in Orabase) or fluocinonide gel (Lidex gel) applied four times daily reduces inflammation and pain. Secondary candidiasis frequently is encountered in oral lichen planus and should be treated appropriately. Patients with malignant transformation of oral lichen planus have been reported, and patients with chronic erosions should be monitored closely for the development of oral squamous cell carcinoma.

Pemphigus Vulgaris. This autoimmune disease, which occurs most commonly in the fifth to sixth decades of life, causes significant morbidity and is potentially fatal. The disease originates in the oral cavity in the majority of patients and subsequently involves the skin in the form of vesicles and blisters. Oral lesions are characterized by blisters that rupture and leave large, painful erosions on the palate, gingiva, tongue, and buccal mucosa. The diagnosis is established by histopathologic and immunopathologic biopsies. Therapy consists of high doses of systemic corticosteroids often combined with various immunosuppressive agents, including azathioprine (Imuran), cyclophosphamide (Cytoxan), and gold therapy. Titers of circulating autoantibodies in serum correlate with the severity of the disease and can be useful in monitoring the response to therapy.

Cicatricial Pemphigoid. This autoimmune disease occurs most commonly in the sixth to seventh decades of life and almost always involves the oral cavity. Patients generally present with desquamation of the gingiva; however, widespread erosions can also be observed. Unlike pemphigus vulgaris, the skin is rarely involved and the disease is not fatal. However, cicatricial pemphigoid can cause great morbidity. Ocular involvement is frequent and can lead to scarring, symblepharon, and loss of vision. The diagnosis is established by histologic and immunofluorescent biopsies. Topical and systemic corticosteroids, dapsone, and other immunosuppressive agents have been utilized in treatment, depending upon the severity of the condition.

Bullous Pemphigoid. Like pemphigus vulgaris and cicatricial pemphigoid, this autoimmune disorder produces vesiculoerosive lesions of the oral cavity, although these are seen in only 30 to 35% of patients. In the usual case, there are only a few superficial erosions; however, extensive ulcerations with desquamation of the gingiva can afflict some patients. Corticosteroids and immunosuppressive agents are used in the treatment of this condition. Recently, a combination of nicotinamide and tetracycline has proved beneficial.

Erythema Multiforme. This vesiculoerosive disease commonly affects the oral cavity. Although in the majority the disease process is self-limited, severe, life-threatening cases occur, and the degree of oral involvement correlates with the severity of the disease. Multiple, painful erosions in the oral cavity make eating and speaking difficult. Hemorrhagic crusting of the lips, when present, is useful in establishing the diagnosis. Although various precipitating factors have been identified, including reactions to infections and drugs, many cases remain idiopathic. Extensive skin involvement is not uncommon, and in the more severe cases, ocular involvement can lead to blindness. Most episodes will spontaneously resolve within 3 to 6 weeks and need only symptomatic care. Recurrent episodes will necessitate a careful search for an underlying cause. Systemic and topical corticosteroids are often used in patients with severe oral involvement.

Recurrent Aphthous Stomatitis (Canker Sores). This is a common disorder of the oral mucosa affecting approximately 20% of the general population. The disease is characterized by the recurrent development of one or several ulcerations on nonkeratinized mucosa. "Minor" aphthous ulcers typically heal spontaneously within 7 to 14 days, whereas "major" aphthous ulcers can take as long as 4 to 6 weeks to resolve, not uncommonly with scarring. Although the episodes are self-limiting, some patients suffer with the continuous development of severe ulcerations. The etiology of recurrent aphthous stomatitis is unknown; however, it is felt to be an immune-mediated disorder. Patients who exhibit recurrent episodes require a careful evaluation to exclude a systemic illness in which recurrent oral ulcerations are a clinical feature. These include inflammatory bowel disease, hematologic diseases, nutritional deficiencies, and connective tissue disorders. Trauma to the oral cavity commonly induces new lesions to form, and premenstrual flare-ups have been reported.

All treatments for recurrent aphthous stomatitis are palliative and none are curative. Symptomatic relief can be achieved with a number of topical agents, including antibiotics, anesthetics, and corticosteroids. Specifically, lidocaine (Xylocaine ointment 5% or viscous), diphenhydramine (Benadryl elixir), dyclonine (Dyclone), and tannic acid preparations (Zilactin) can be applied directly to ulcers for pain relief. Tetracycline or erythromycin elixirs can be used as an oral rinse four times daily to shorten the duration and decrease the pain of the ulcerations. Triamcinolone acetonide (Kenalog in Orabase) can be applied four to six times daily to ulcerations for pain relief. Systemic agents that have been used with varying success include antibiotics, corticosteroids, colchicine, dapsone, acyclovir, and levamisole. Before any therapy is initiated, predisposing factors or underlying illnesses should be identified.

DISORDERS OF THE TEETH AND SURROUNDING STRUCTURES

Dental Caries. Cavities are formed by the demineralization of the inorganic portion and destruction of the organic material of the tooth by microorganisms that inhabit the oral cavity. Dental plaque, consisting of microbial or bacterial plaque with various salivary components, develops on teeth and contributes to the initiation of the carious lesion. The reduction in tooth decay during the past decade is in part due to the addition of fluoride to water supplies and the use of fluoride supplements. The carious portion of the tooth can be removed by dentists, and the remaining defect filled with a restorative material. Without treatment, the process progresses and can lead to tooth destruction and further complications.

Pulp and Periapical Diseases. Pulpitis, an inflammatory condition of the dental connective tissue, is the result of either a large, carious lesion or a traumatic event. Acute episodes result in pain, especially with thermal stimuli, whereas pain may be absent or minimal in chronic pulpitis. The treatment for either is the same and consists of root canal therapy or extraction of the tooth. Pulpitis can spread through the roots of the tooth and into the periapical structures, causing periapical granulomas and apical periodontal cysts, which can be detected by radiographs. The involved tooth often needs to be extracted, and the periapical tissue curetted. If left untreated,

these granulomas and cysts can expand, causing bone resorption, or develop into a periapical abscess. Periapical abscesses can also arise from a traumatic tooth injury. Pain, fever, and lymphadenopathy are not uncommon. If untreated by drainage, the periapical abscess can lead to osteomyelitis, cellulitis, or bacteremia.

Gingivitis. Inflammation of the gingiva can be acute or chronic, the latter being more common and almost universal in older patients. Inflammation beginning in the interdental papillae and spreading to include the gingiva immediately surrounding the teeth is clinically recognized by erythema, tissue enlargement, and loss of normal architecture, including stippling. Local factors (including plaque and calculus formation) and systemic factors (including nutritional disturbances, pregnancy, and diabetes) are known to cause or aggravate gingivitis. Daily brushing and flossing combined with an optimal oral hygiene program will prevent or minimize the severity of this condition.

Periodontitis. This inflammatory condition of the periodontal structures including the alveolar bone and periodontal ligament is preceded by gingivitis and is seen most commonly in adults. With progressive gingivitis, deep, gingival crevices, termed "periodontal pockets," will develop. The gingiva becomes edematous and easily bleeds as the disease advances. Calculus above and below the gingiva is usually clinically evident and contributes to the severity of the disease. Gingival recession, alveolar bone destruction, and tooth loss can occur, depending upon the extent of the disease. Radiographic abnormalities are apparent and are useful in determining the optimal treatment regimen, which includes calculus and plaque control as well as surgical correction in severe cases.

Tooth Anomalies. Hypodontia refers to the congenital absence of one or more teeth, whereas anodontia is the congenital absence of all teeth. Hypodontia is not infrequent and commonly involves the maxillary lateral incisors and the third molars (wisdom teeth). Various syndromes, most notably the ectodermal dysplasias, are associated with hypodontia. Supernumerary teeth (additional teeth within the dental arch) are most often found in the anterior maxilla in the midline. If these teeth are allowed to erupt, they can cause crowding of the existing teeth and resorption of adjacent teeth. Although they can occur as an isolated event, multiple supernumerary teeth have been associated with various syndromes, including cleidocranial dysplasia and Gardner's syndrome.

Abrasion and Erosion of Teeth. Abrasion refers to the destruction of tooth structure by an abnormal mechanical force, most commonly improper toothbrushing. An abrasive dentifrice or excessive brushing can result in a wedge-shaped notch at the crown-root junction. Other less common causes of abrasion are related to various habits, such as placing foreign objects between the teeth (e.g., nails, toothpicks, and pipes), which abrades the anterior teeth.

Erosion is defined as the loss of tooth structure by a chemical process. The etiology of this disorder is unknown in many cases. Patients who expose their teeth to an acid pH, through sucking on acidic candy, regurgitation of the stomach contents, or chronic vomiting as in bulimia are not infrequently found to have tooth erosion. Various patterns of erosion can often lead to identification of the underlying cause.

MISCELLANEOUS DISORDERS OF THE ORAL CAVITY

Nutritional Deficiencies. Vitamin deficiency results in a number of characteristic oral lesions, mainly involving the tongue or lips. A lack of thiamine, nicotinic acid, pyridoxine, or folic acid produces various forms of glossitis. The tongue is usually atrophic, devoid of papillae, swollen, and red. Erosions and pain may also be present. Angular cheilitis may be seen with riboflavin deficiencies accompanied by a reddened and enlarged tongue. Vitamin C deficiency can manifest itself as swollen and bleeding gingiva and, in chronic cases, loosening of teeth. None of these oral changes is pathognomonic; however, replacement of the deficient vitamin usually results in prompt improvement.

Oral Pigmentary Disturbances. A growing list of drugs can cause oral pigmentation. Antimalarial agents and amiodarone cause pigmentation of the palate, while zidovudine (Retrovir) produces a more diffuse oral pigmentation. Heavy metals, such as bismuth, lead, and mercury, result in staining, usually along the gingival margin. A number of systemic disorders also can produce striking intraoral pigmentary changes. The diffuse oral pigmentation in Addison's disease and Peutz-Jeghers syndrome is prominent and aids in establishing the diagnosis. Hemochromatosis, jaundice, ochronosis, and Albright's disease also display varying degrees of intraoral pigmentation.

Glossodynia (Burning Tongue Syndrome). This disorder of unknown etiology is relatively common and most frequently affects menopausal and postmenopausal women. Patients complain of burning and stinging of the tongue and occasionally of other oral structures. Despite the continuous symptomatic discomfort, examination of the oral cavity reveals no abnormality. The etiology of glossodynia is multifactorial, and each patient requires careful evaluation to identify a reversible cause. Drug reactions, metabolic disorders, including vitamin deficiencies and diabetes, infections, and dental disorders are some of the more commonly identified causes. When no pathologic condition is discovered, treatment with low doses of chlordiazepoxide (Librium) or amitriptyline (Elavil) has had some success.

VENOUS (STASIS) ULCERS

method of
HENRY H. ROENIGK, JR., M.D.
Northwestern University Medical School
Chicago, Illinois

Venous (stasis) ulcers, the most common type of leg ulcers, are part of the continuum of skin changes caused by stasis dermatitis. Chronic venous insufficiency produces skin changes that progress from edema, to dermatitis, to ulceration, and finally to infection.

PATHOLOGY AND PATHOGENESIS

The veins of the leg can be classified as deep, superficial, or communicating (perforating). The communicating veins perforate the deep fascial layer and connect the superficial to the deep veins. Each perforating vein has a valve that allows blood to pass in one direction only from the superficial to the deep system.

The venous pressure in the leg is normally low during walking or exercise because compression of the calf muscles forces the blood upward while the vein valves prevent retrograde flow. When extensive thrombophlebitis of the deep veins occurs, however, many valves are destroyed during the healing process and the venous walls are weakened. This incompetence in the deep and perforating veins produces ambulatory venous hypertension. There is excessive loss of fluid from the bloodstream to the extracellular spaces, and congestion and edema eventually develop. These stasis changes are often aggravated by scratching, overtreatment, or sensitization to the many proprietary preparations applied to the leg before the patient seeks professional help.

Stasis ulcer itself is an uncommon complication of varicose veins but is often associated with incompetent perforating veins that lead into the area of the ulcer.

CLINICAL FEATURES

Stasis ulcerations usually occur in the ankle region over the medial malleolus and only rarely on the feet, upper leg, or thigh. Ulcers often develop in areas of indurated cellulitis or dermatitis. There is usually brown pigmentation in the surrounding skin, and the affected leg is often edematous. The ulcers can develop spontaneously or can be secondary to minor trauma, as from bumping or scratching. The size of the ulcer varies greatly, but if neglected, it can extend to involve almost the entire circumference of the leg. The base of the ulcer is usually moist with extensive granulations and is frequently secondarily infected. Ulcers may or may not be painful but are never as painful as ischemic ulcers. The discomfort is often greatly relieved by rest and elevation. After an ulceration has healed, there is a tendency for recurrence in the same area.

DIFFERENTIAL DIAGNOSIS

Ulcers have many causes, including arterial insufficiency, vasculitis, hematologic infections, metabolic disorders, and tumors. However, a history of thrombophlebitis or edema and the presence of varicose or dilated veins, stasis pigmentation, induration, and dermatitis make chronic venous insufficiency the chief suspect in the search for the cause of the ulcer.

Arteriovenous fistulas should be considered in all cases of chronic venous insufficiency. The history of a penetrating injury and the presence of a thrill and bruit may indicate a traumatic arteriovenous fistula.

It is important to differentiate ischemic ulcers caused by arteriosclerosis and stasis ulcers. Ischemic ulcers usually develop more distally on the feet and toes, they are more painful, and some relief is obtained by dependency.

Hypertensive ischemic ulcers are usually found on the lateral or posterior aspect of the lower leg, are very painful, and often are surrounded by a purplish, cyanotic rim of ischemic tissue.

In lymphedema there is diffuse thickening and prominence of the skin and subcutaneous tissue that is not a feature of the edema of chronic venous insufficiency. The edema does not decrease on elevation of the leg in lymphedema.

TREATMENT

Acute Stasis Dermatitis

If weeping acute dermatitis accompanies the stasis ulcer, the leg is best treated by bed rest and wet compresses, which should be changed every 2 to 3 hours. The wet dressings should not be enclosed in a plastic covering, since this will result in maceration of tissues and will prevent the evaporation necessary for healing. The following solutions are suggested for compresses: (1) aluminum acetate (Burows's solution) 0.5%, (2) isotonic saline solution 0.9%, or (3) acetic acid solution 1%. Between compresses, application of a drying anti-inflammatory topical steroid or steroid/antibiotic ointment or cream will help clear the dermatitis.

Subacute Stasis Dermatitis

When the acute phase of the dermatitis has subsided and the patient becomes more ambulatory, recurrence of edema after prolonged stand-

ing must be prevented; if it is not, acute dermatitis may promptly recur. The use of a modified Unna paste boot dressing is ideal in this situation. These flesh-colored roll bandages are impregnated with a paste of zinc oxide, calamine, glycerin, and gelatin. Their use eliminates the need for bed rest or extensive hospital care.

To apply the Unna boot, the leg is first cleansed with lukewarm water or mineral oil to remove any debris or medication residue. Any of the following topical medications can then be applied to the leg: (1) gentian violet 1%, (2) fluocinolone acetonide (Synalar) cream or ointment 0.025% (or any other topical corticosteroid preparation), or (3) topical antibiotics alone, such as ointments containing polymyxin B, bacitracin, and neomycin (Polysporin, Neosporin); erythromycin; or gentamicin sulfate (Garamycin).

The modified Unna boot is applied from an area just proximal to the toes to just below the popliteal space. The foot should be kept at a right angle to minimize chafing. A circular turn is made around the foot, then the bandage is directed obliquely over the heel as would be done in applying an elastic bandage. This is repeated until the calf has been adequately covered. The first layers of the boot should be snug, and the bandage roll should be cut frequently during its application to ensure a flat surface. It should be applied in a "pressure gradient" manner, with the greatest pressure applied at the ankle and lower third of the leg and progressively diminishing pressure over the upper two-thirds of the leg. Care should be taken not to apply the bandage too loosely or too tightly. A double layer of Tubegauze is placed over the Unna boot and secured at the upper and lower limits with tape, which should not be placed directly on the skin. This dressing is usually changed at weekly intervals unless excessive drainage necessitates changing every 3 to 5 days.

Alternatives to the Unna boot include an absorbent dressing (Allevlyn*) that is held in place by a light, white compression liner. During the day when the patient is active, the compression liner is covered by a heavy support stocking with a posterior zipper. The dressing can be removed nightly to allow the leg to be bathed.

Stasis Ulcers

The general principles of management of a stasis ulcer are the same as those for subacute stasis dermatitis. The ulcer is cleansed and gently débrided. If there is considerable secondary infection, an occlusive dressing should not be applied. Bed rest and compresses are recom-

---

*Smith and Nephew Medical, Massillon, Ohio.

mended, as mentioned previously, until the infection subsides. Pyogenic crusts should be removed, and any drainage should be cultured before antibiotic therapy. Topical antibiotic ointments can be applied between the compresses. If cellulitis, lymphangitis, or septicemia is present, intravenous and oral systemic antibiotic therapy is indicated. The choice of antibiotics should be dictated by the culture and sensitivity reports. The Unna boot is used in the manner as outlined for subacute stasis dermatitis.

Débridement

Topical enzymes, antibiotics, and DuoDerm (see next section) are often used to débride leg ulcers and develop healthy granulation tissue. Another excellent method of local débridement is the application of topical viscous lidocaine (Xylocaine) and the use of a small, sharp curet to remove the eschar that adheres to the granulation tissue and inhibits re-epithelialization of the ulcer. Occasionally, forceps and small scissors can be used to cut away thicker eschar that cannot be removed by the curet.

DuoDerm beads débride ulcers by absorbing wound debris. The beads are highly hydrophilic and absorb fluid until saturated, swelling in the process. When placed on a discharging ulcer surface, the beads absorb the exudate, bacteria, and tissue degradation residues from the ulcer surface.

Wound Dressings

It is well accepted that epithelial migration occurs more readily in a moist environment such as that created by occlusive dressings. In the past few years, new dressings have been developed that do more than just cover the wound and keep it clean; some examples are Op-Site, Tegaderm (polyrethan) bioclusive, Vigilon (polyethylene oxdihydrogel with polyethylene film backing, thicker hydrogel films on both sides, and gel in the middle), and DuoDerm (hydrocolloid material surrounded by an inert, hydrophobic polymer that is adhesive). These occlusive or semiocclusive dressings vary in the degree of débridement, cleansing, and wound granulation that speeds the healing process.

Most of these dressings, except DuoDerm and Vigilon, will transport water, and all except DuoDerm will transport oxygen. They all absorb bacteria, except Vigilon, and only DuoDerm is not transparent. All except Vigilon are self-adhesive. Excessive fluid can accumulate under some of these dressings, especially Op-Site. Exacerbation of infection and cellulitis may develop if these dressings are used on an infected leg ulcer. They are best used when all infection is cleared, there is good granulation tissue, and re-epithelialization is sought. These dressings can be used under an Unna boot or elastic bandage but should be changed every 2 to 3 days.

When the edema has receded and the infection has cleared, new granulation tissue will start to appear. Once this tissue fills the ulcer, re-epithelialization will start from the edges and occasionally from islands of granulation tissue in the center of the ulcer. If rapid re-epithelialization is occurring, continued use of wound dressings and the Unna boot will result in complete healing of the ulcer with a combination of scar tissue and new epithelium.

Surgical Management

The final goal in the treatment of leg ulcers is to provide adequate skin coverage. With ulcers that have poor granulation tissue and necrotic or fibrotic tissue at the border that shows no sign of epithelial ingrowth after conservative measures, more aggressive (surgical) approaches must be considered.

When healthy granulation tissue has become established in the ulcer base and the surrounding inflammation has subsided, the patient is ready for pinch grafting if this is the planned surgical procedure. The donor area (usually on the anterior thigh) is prepared by shaving, if necessary, and washing with povidone-iodine soap. Sterile technique should be maintained when working in the donor area, but strict sterile technique is not necessary in the recipient site.

Circular areas of 5 to 10 mm are marked in parallel rows on the upper thigh with gentian violet and then injected intradermally with 1% lidocaine. This serves two purposes: it provides anesthesia and it elevates the skin for easy removal of small epidermal or dermal grafts. Anesthesia can also be produced with a field block, in which case elevations are produced by injection of sterile saline under each circle. A curved needle or the tip of a 30-gauge needle is placed at the center of a circle and used to further tent the skin. A single-edged razor blade or No. 15 scalpel blade is used to cut a split-thickness graft. The depth of the pinch graft should be 1 to 2 mm or to the mid-dermis. Subcutaneous fat taken with the graft interfaces with the "take" and can result in undue scarring in the donor area.

As grafts are removed, they are placed in a Petri dish containing gauze moistened with saline and then transferred for placement on the ulcer. With a 25-gauge needle or forceps, the grafts are placed on the ulcer bed next to, but not touching, each other until the defect is covered. The placement of the pinch grafts can be facilitated by marking them with gentian violet on the epidermal side. After placement of the grafts, the practitioner must allow 1 to 2 mm of clearance at the margins of the ulcer, because epithelium growing in from the edges of the ulcer may prevent the border grafts from taking.

The area is sprayed with Skin Prep, a spray adhesive dressing, or a topical antibiotic is carefully applied over the grafts. A semipermeable membrane, such as Vigilon or OpSite, is then applied on the grafted ulcer with its edges extending approximately 3 cm beyond the margin of the ulcer.

To prevent the grafts from tenting and losing contact with the ulcer base, gauze cut to the approximate size of the ulcer is placed over the ulcer bed. A circular piece of thick gauze slightly larger than the ulcer is placed over the first piece of gauze to protect the grafts and provide pressure on the tissue surrounding the ulcer. An elastic dressing is wrapped around the ulcer directly over the gauze to apply minimal pressure. The patient should be kept on strict bed rest for 72 hours, with limited ambulation after the first 72 hours in a wheelchair with the leg elevated thereafter.

The ulcer is examined through the adhesive membrane at 48 hours and daily thereafter. If fluid collects beneath the membrane, it may be punctured and the fluid drained. If infection develops, the membrane should be removed. However, with an adequate pressure dressing, any fluid that forms tends to drain from under the edges of the membrane. The membrane is removed from the ulcer 7 to 10 days after grafting. Should any of the grafts become dislodged, they are repositioned and the wound dressed again. Once the semipermeable membrane is removed, the wound is dressed by applying a 4×4 inch gauze pad and elastic bandage, which are changed daily. Periods of ambulation may begin a week after grafting; however, elevation of the leg should be continued until healing is complete, usually a matter of 2 to 4 weeks.

When there is adequate granulation tissue in the ulcer bed, an alternative to pinch grafting is the split-thickness skin graft. The technique is similar to that for grafts placed in other areas of the body. The anterior thigh is usually chosen as the donor site.

For ulcers with exposed bone or tendon, fully vascularized full-thickness skin and subcutaneous tissue must be applied. Split-thickness skin grafts do not become revascularized when placed upon exposed bone denuded of its periosteum or on tendon denuded of paratendon. This situation is not common with leg ulcers, but when it does occur, the defect is usually over an exposed tibia. Full-thickness vascularized tissue may be provided by local flaps, cross-leg pedicle flaps, or the application of distant tissue in the form of a free flap transfer revascularized by microvascular technique.

Generalized Eczematization

In patients with severe stasis dermatitis and ulceration, a generalized eczematous eruption may develop. This can often be controlled by topical corticosteroids and antihistamines, such as cyproheptadine (Periactin), 4 mg four times daily. It may be necessary in severe cases to give systemic corticosteroids orally or intramuscularly.

Neurodermatitis

Because of lichenification from "habit scratching," an associated neurodermatitis of the legs may develop. If this occurs, the application of fluocinolone acetonide (Synalar), 0.025%, or other potent topical corticosteroids under plastic food wrap at bedtime may be helpful. Intralesional injection of triamcinolone acetonide (parenteral Kenalog) suspension (10 mg per mL) into localized neurodermatitis may bring more prompt relief of the pruritus.

Chronic Venous Insufficiency

After the acute and subacute stages of dermatitis have subsided and the cellulitis and ulcerations have healed, the treatment of chronic venous insufficiency is not finished. The patient must understand that he or she has a lifelong problem and that continuous supportive measures will be necessary to prevent future complications.

Elastic bandages and proprietary elastic stockings are not satisfactory for most patients. Individually measured, "pressure-gradient" support stockings, such as the Jobst stocking, are preferred. Directions for Jobst stocking measurements are furnished by the company. Measurement should be made only after all edema has subsided or after the patient's legs have been mechanically pumped to make them edema free. Camp stockings, Sigvaris 902 series stockings, and MediStrumpf stockings may also be useful effective.

The patient should put on the supportive stockings before arising and remove them just before retiring. It is usually necessary to purchase new stockings every 3 to 4 months because the stockings will stretch out.

DECUBITUS ULCER

method of
WILLARD D. STECK, M.D.
Cleveland Clinic Foundation
Cleveland, Ohio

Decubitus ulcers are also called pressure sores, pressure ulcers, and bedsores, or as here, simply sores or ulcers. They result from necrosis that begins deep in tissues where skin has been exposed to prolonged pressure. They occur over the bony prominences of the sacrum, heels, trochanters, ischia, scapulae, malleoli, or scalp in patients who lie or sit in unvarying positions or on unyielding surfaces.

Bedsores plague those who, for reasons of age, injury, or disease, have impaired activity, mobility, sensory perception, or nutrition, and whose skin is harmed by friction, shearing forces, or improper water content. The Braden Scale is one of several guides that help to identify patients at risk. (These are described frequently in the journal *Decubitus*).

Recent therapeutic advances have made the caregiver's task easier. Biotechnology has provided an array of treatment aids, some very helpful and others that border on baldfaced quackery. Biologic research probes the molecular mechanisms of ischemic tissue damage, a subject that is complex, poorly understood, and mostly irrelevant to clinical management.

The Agency for Health Care Clinical Practice Guidelines #3* roughly codify techniques for prediction and prevention of pressure ulcers in adults. These will likely become a standard of care, at least for purposes of documentation.

All bedsores probably could be prevented if there were no constraints on moving, feeding, cleansing, or supporting every patient. However, certain neuropathic disorders, surgical operations, or orthopedic requirements may make it impossible or impractical to use adequate preventive measures. Some courts have ruled that a pressure ulcer is prima facie evidence of neglect. Yet, that "neglect" may be justified when prevention and treatment conflict with primary goals of confinement, when scant resources must go to more important work, or when the patient will certainly expire in a few days in any case. Documentation in these situations must be persuasive.

PREVENTION

Examination for and charting of risk factors must be done immediately upon assumption of care and every day until discharge.

1. Search the entire body surface daily for evidence of pressure damage. Pallor, erythema, abrasion, or maceration signal danger.

2. Shift weight at least every 2 hours, provided it does not cause undue pain or conflict with more important goals.

3. Hospital mattresses are stiff, hot, and prone to

---

*AHCR Publications, PO Box 8547, Silver Spring, Md 20907.

cause sweating, irritation, and shearing injury. A light, cotton blanket, folded smoothly and placed between the mattress and sheet may prevent damage. Use foam mattress overlays (e.g., Bioclinic Egg Crate, GeoMatt, Lotus) with higher risk patients. Some may require low airloss beds (e.g., Kinair, Flexicare, Apropos). One air cushion device automatically turns the patient from one side to the other every few minutes (Dr. Volkner's Lamellar Turning Mattress). Such highly effective dynamic weight dispersion devices usually require an order from an institution's Skin Care Team because of their extra cost. Keep the head of the bed low much of the time to avoid sacral area shearing. Heel cushions should be used; a number of good ones are available, from inexpensive (Bioclinic Eggcrate) to moderate (Posey, Lunax Boot, Stryker Air-Shoe), to expensive (L'Nard Multi-Podus). Heel rings or donut pads may do more harm than good.

4. Keep the skin clean and dry with a minimum of irritation. Soap and water, used gently, may be best. One capful of Alpha Keri Bath Oil in 1 quart of tepid H_2O is effective when skin is dry; povidone iodine (Betadine) solution, 30 ml in 500 ml H_2O, is good when skin is too moist, as is plain rubbing alcohol.

5. Clean up excretory soilage at once. If it cannot be kept off the skin, use a protective cream or paste. Ordinary zinc oxide ointment or paste works very well, provided one understands how to remove it. This is done by cleansing with a gauze sponge soaked with mineral oil, rather than by trying to wash it away.

6. Avoid massage over bony prominences to avoid risk of shearing injury.

TREATMENT

1. Continue daily examination, skin care, cleansing, protection, turning, and weight dispersion. The first cutaneous evidence of actual tissue breakdown is persistent erythema. Shea's method of staging is useful for documentation of damage. Skin changes are classified as follows: Stage I, nonblanching erythema that does not disappear within 24 hours after pressure has been relieved; II, a superficial skin lesion such as a blister, fissure, or abrasion; III, a break through the skin exposing subcutaneous tissue and having defined margins; and IV, a lesion that exposes muscle or bone.

2. Treat tissue infection with systemic measures that seem appropriate. Culture usually reveals a variety of opportunistic colonizers that do not necessarily require specific therapy. Most of the modern cleansers and dressing materials tend to inhibit microbial growth.

3. Manage Stage I and II damage with gentle cleansing, relief of pressure by whatever means necessary, and dressings that pad and protect while absorbing exudation. It may be necessary to go from passive to dynamic to weight dispersion aids.

4. Use the new spray cleansers (e.g., Constant-

Clens, Ultra Klenz) for convenience, particularly during dressing changes for deeper sores.

5. Use hydrocolloid dressings to protect skin at risk from soilage, wetness, and the trauma of frequent cleansing. DuoDerm is widely available and represents the current standard. Comfeel Ulcus and Cutinova Hydro are similar. All work well alone on shallow lesions or in conjunction with hydrocolloid paste to fill the space of deeper sores. The edges of these dressings should extend about 1½ inches beyond the ulcer on all sides. The dressings will bulge as they absorb exudate; this should not be confused with an accumulation of pus. Hydrogel dressings (Transorb, Mitraflex) are also absorbent and useful on shallow wounds.

6. Débride Stage III and IV ulcers carefully. Remove frankly necrotic tissue as conservatively as possible. This is not preparation for grafting. Enzymatic débridement may occasionally be useful but is seldom necessary. Yellow fibrin deposition on an ulcer base does no harm.

7. Obliterate dead space and manage the exudate with as few dressing changes as possible. The new calcium alginate materials (Aldosteril, Sorbisan) absorb great quantities of liquid, are hemostatic and bacteriostatic, and can encourage growth of granulation tissue. They need changing only when they become saturated. When the wound becomes more shallow, a hydrocolloid paste and dressing may be used and can be left in place for up to 1 week between changes.

8. In the absence of the hydrocolloids and alginates, one can still use iodoform gauze to pack deep wounds and zinc oxide paste for shallow ones—inexpensive but effective methods. These agents just take a little more time, effort, and skill to use.

9. When all else fails and severe ulceration persists, do not use hyperbaric oxygen; rather, ask for help from the plastic surgeons. Provided the patient is viable and can withstand the rigors of surgery, the rotation of tissues may allow healing. However, such surgery should not be undertaken simply in the hope of easing the burden of care.

10. Do not let good work and careful decision making be overlooked for lack of adequate documentation.

ATOPIC DERMATITIS

method of
ROBERT S. LESTER, M.D.
Sunnybrook Health Science Centre
Toronto, Ontario, Canada

"Atopy" means "strange," and the term was first used in 1923 to describe a human hypersensitive state (asthma and hay fever) characterized by an enhanced capacity to form "reagins" in response to a variety of antigens. In 1933, the term "atopic dermatitis" was coined to refer to an inflammatory skin disease marked by intense pruritus and a tendency to lichenification of the skin. Approximately two-thirds of children with atopic dermatitis have a positive family history for atopic disease, and 50 to 80% of these children will develop other atopic disorders, usually allergic rhinitis or asthma.

Patients with atopic dermatitis demonstrate a variety of immune system abnormalities. They have increased susceptibility to cutaneous dissemination of certain viral infections such as herpes simplex and vaccinia; decreased delayed type hypersensitive response to common microbial antigens; a low incidence of sensitization to contact allergens; decreased lymphocyte response to mitogens and antigens; and defective granulocyte and monocyte chemotaxis. Serum IgE concentrations may be elevated, and most have positive prick skin tests and radioallergosorbent tests (RASTs) to various allergens.

CLINICAL FEATURES
(Table 1)

Some form of atopy occurs in approximately 20% of the population, with the approximate incidence of skin disease being 3 to 5%. The disease usually presents around the age of 3 months, with 60% of cases of atopic dermatitis presenting before the age of 1 year, and almost 85% before the age of 3. The primary symptom of atopic dermatitis is pruritus with its concomitant scratch response. There is controversy as to whether atopic dermatitis represents "a rash that itches" or "an

TABLE 1. **Identifying Characteristics of Atopic Dermatitis**

Major Criteria (Seen in All Patients)
Pruritus
Typical morphology and distribution of lesions
Facial and extensor involvement in infants
Flexural lichenification in older children and adults
Tendency toward chronic or chronically relapsing dermatitis

Common Findings (At Least Two)
Personal or family history of atopic disease (asthma, allergic rhinitis, atopic dermatitis)
Immediate skin test reactivity
White dermatographism and/or delayed blanch to cholinergic agents
Anterior subcapsular cataracts

Associated Findings (At Least Four)
Xerosis/ichthyosis/hyperlinear palms and soles
Pityriasis alba
Keratosis pilaris
Dennie-Morgan infraorbital fold
Elevated serum IgE
Keratoconus
Tendency toward nonspecific hand dermatitis
Tendency toward repeated cutaneous infections

Adapted from Hanifin JM, and Lobitz WC: Newer concepts of atopic dermatitis. Arch Dermatol *113*:663, 1977. Copyright 1977, American Medical Association.

itch that rashes." Atopics have a lower itch threshold and a longer duration of itch. Atopic inflammation begins abruptly with erythema and severe pruritus, and the skin surface is modified by scratching. There does not seem to be a single primary lesion but rather several patterns and types of lesions, including papules, eczematous dermatitis with erythema and scaling, and lichenification or thickening of the skin with accentuation of the normal skin markings.

Although the cutaneous manifestations of the atopic diathesis are varied, they have characteristic age-determined patterns, and atopic dermatitis has been arbitrarily divided into three phases.

Infant Phase (Birth to 2 Years)

Infants typically develop the first signs of inflammation during the third month. The eruption characteristically involves the face and lateral aspects of the lower legs but can occur elsewhere. As the eruption progresses, the infant may become uncomfortable, restless, and agitated during sleep.

Childhood Phase (2 to 12 Years)

The most common and characteristic appearance of this phase is inflammation and lichenification in the flexural areas such as the antecubital fossae, popliteal fossae, neck, wrists, and ankles. In severe cases, the inflammation and pruritus may become incapacitating with disturbance in sleep and inability to perform at school.

Adult Phase (12 Years to Adult)

As in the childhood phase, localized inflammation with lichenification is the most common pattern. Hand dermatitis may be the most characteristic expression of atopic diathesis in adults. Many develop eyelid dermatitis and localized areas of lichenification in the anogenital area.

Associated Features

Dry Skin and Xerosis. Dry skin, or atopic xerosis, is a characteristic feature of atopic dermatitis and is principally independent of eczematous eruptions. Noneczematous, atopic dry skin shows enhanced transepidermal water loss denoting an impaired water permeability barrier function. The water permeability barrier is formed by intercellular lipid lamellae located between the horny cells of the stratum corneum. The lipids are provided via exocytosis in membrane-coating granules. Recent studies suggest that some pathologic extrusion mechanism in membrane-coating granules in atopic dry skin may be responsible, at least partly, for recently detected biochemical alterations of epidermal lipids and for the deficient water permeability barrier. The unsuccessful attempts of the atopic epidermis to recover and compensate for disturbed barrier function may elicit immunologic and inflammatory mediators in the epidermis, leading to clinically visible atopic dermatitis lesions.

Ichthyosis Vulgaris. The dominant form of ichthyosis vulgaris is found in patients with atopic dermatitis and is usually manifested as rectangular, dry scales found predominantly on the extensor aspects of the arms and legs. This condition tends to improve with age.

Keratosis Pilaris. This condition is so common that it is probably physiologic. However, it occurs more commonly in patients with atopic dermatitis and manifests as small (1 to 2 mm), rough, follicular papules or pustules involving mainly the posterolateral aspect of the upper arms and the anterior thighs. Keratosis pilaris can occur at any age, but is most common in young children and peaks during adolescence. There is usually spontaneous improvement.

Pityriasis Alba. This common disorder is characterized by asymptomatic, hypopigmented, finely scaling plaques, usually on the face and lateral upper arms. It tends to appear in young children and usually disappears by early adulthood. Lesions become more obvious during the summer when they fail to tan.

Hyperlinear Palmar Creases. Atopic patients frequently demonstrate an accentuation of the major skin creases of the palms. This may be present in infancy but becomes more prominent as age and severity of skin inflammation increase.

Atopic Pleats. The appearance of an extra line on the lower eyelid (Dennie-Morgan infraorbital fold) has been considered a distinguishing feature of the patient with atopic dermatitis. However, this extra line is an unreliable sign of the atopic state.

Cataracts and Keratoconus. Anterior subcapsular cataracts occur in up to 13% of patients with atopic dermatitis, mainly young adults. They are usually asymptomatic and tend to accelerate with an acute exacerbation of the disease. Keratoconus has been reported in 3% of patients with atopic dermatitis and occurs independently of the cataracts.

Exacerbating Factors

Many factors promote dryness or increase the desire to scratch, both of which worsen atopic dermatitis. Understanding and controlling these aggravating factors are essential to the successful management of atopic dermatitis.

Temperature Change. Patients with atopic dermatitis cannot tolerate sudden changes in temperature. Sweating induces itching, particularly in the flexural areas, to a greater extent than in the normal individual. In addition, a sudden lowering of body temperature, as occurs when leaving a warm shower, for example, can promote itching.

Decreased Humidity. Atopic xerosis is associated with increased transepidermal water loss, which indirectly reflects a defective water permeability barrier. Since cold air cannot support much humidity, atopic xerosis becomes worse during winter months. Dry skin is less supple, more fragile, and more easily irritated. Excessive washing of the skin removes water-binding lipids and exacerbates the problems induced by decreased humidity.

Primary Irritants. Wool, household and industrial chemicals, cosmetics, and some soaps and detergents can promote irritation and inflammation of the skin of atopics, often interpreted as an allergic reaction. However, although allergic contact dermatitis can occur in patients with atopic dermatitis, it is much less frequent than in normal individuals.

Allergens. There are significant data suggesting that food allergens and aeroallergens can exacerbate skin disease in a significant subset of patients with atopic dermatitis. Egg, peanuts, milk, soy, wheat, and fish account for over 90% of food allergens that exacerbate atopic dermatitis. House dust mites, animal dander, and pollen have been implicated in the exacerbation of atopic dermatitis, but there have been few controlled trials investigating the role of aeroallergens in the pathogenesis of atopic dermatitis. (The role of allergens is discussed further at the end of this article.)

Emotional Stress. Stress can have a profound effect on the course of atopic dermatitis. This is often aggravated by the anger, anxiety, and frustration associated with chronic disease. It is important to emphasize that atopic dermatitis is not caused by nerves but is an inherited disease aggravated in a nonspecific way by emotional stress.

Infections. Superficial bacterial, fungal, or viral infections commonly occur in patients with moderate to severe atopic dermatitis. *Staphylococcus aureus* is the common agent causing bacterial infections of the skin and may be recovered from approximately 70% of patients with atopic dermatitis. Such colonization is often asymptomatic, but it can be associated with an acute weeping dermatitis or crusted, impetiginized lesions or pustules. Herpes simplex can cause extensive local or widespread infection. In the adolescent and adult stages of the disease, tinea pedis may be superimposed on a foot dermatitis.

PROGNOSIS

Atopic dermatitis is primarily a disease of children. Approximately one-third of cases resolve completely, one-third continue into adult life, and in one-third the skin disease is replaced by either asthma or hay fever. The disease tends to be one of remissions and exacerbations.

TREATMENT

The current management of atopic dermatitis is empirical, with treatment decisions dependent on the severity of the skin disease at any given time (Table 2).

TABLE 2. **General Management**

Address psychosocial issues
Modify diet (where indicated)
Avoid aggravating factors
Avoid primary irritants and allergens
Antihistamines
Topical corticosteroids
Antimicrobials (when indicated)

Psychosocial Issues

As with any chronic illness, families can become invested in the child's disease, and the child can use the disease for secondary gain. Although the parents and patients should be reminded that the disease is not caused by stress, stress management and biofeedback can sometimes help control itching and scratching. Parents and patients should be educated about the prognosis, particularly with regard to the natural waxing and waning of the disease. In most cases, they can be reassured that, in later life, the eczema will either become localized or go into remission. However, it is important not to be overly optimistic as fullblown atopic dermatitis does persist into adult life in some patients.

Diet

In spite of numerous articles expounding both points of view, the controversy about the relationship of atopic dermatitis to food allergies has not been resolved. Approximately 80% of patients with atopic dermatitis react on skin testing to more than one of a large number of environmental allergens including a multitude of foods. However, the relevance of a positive skin test to the pathogenesis of the lesions in atopic dermatitis remains to be determined, and the usefulness of skin testing for food intolerance has repeatedly been questioned. Nevertheless, if parents are insistent that their child is allergic to a specific food, it is prudent to withhold it and readminister it at a later date. However, even the most enthusiastic advocates of dietary manipulation claim that it is a suitable approach in only about 10% of children with eczema.

Lubrication

Attention to dryness of the skin is an important aspect in the treatment of many patients with atopic dermatitis. The dryness is best treated with a bathing regime using nonperfumed bath oils and possibly adding oatmeal (oilated Aveeno) to soothe the skin. After bathing, the child's skin should be patted dry and then covered with a lubricating ointment such as petrolatum USP, Eucerin, or Aquaphor. Lubricants should be applied two to three times a day on a regular basis. Humidifiers are useful in maintaining skin hydration in the winter.

Antihistamines

Antihistamines are routinely used to control pruritus in atopic dermatitis. Most studies suggest that their effectiveness is due to their sedative effect rather than to any specific antipruritic effect. Sedating antihistamines such as hydroxyzine (Atarax, Vistaril) or diphenhydramine (Benadryl) are probably more effective than nonsedating types. In adults, hydroxyzine can be started at 10 mg twice daily to 25 mg four times daily; the dose can be increased if adequate relief of pruritus is not achieved. Diphenhydramine can be started in doses of 25 mg two to four times daily. With both of these antihistamines, the dosage increase is limited by potential sedative side effects. Newer antihistamines that affect eosinophils, such as ceterizine (Reactin),* may prove beneficial in some patients.

Topical Corticosteroids

The mainstay of management of the inflammatory skin lesions of atopic dermatitis is the use of topical corticosteroids twice daily. The choice of agents depends upon the age of the patient and the location and extent of the skin lesions. Generally the lowest potency corticosteroid that is effective should be used. Potent topical steroids should not be used on areas such as the face or intertriginous areas because of the increased risk of side effects. The potential local side effects of long-term use of potent topical steroids include thinning of the skin with associated striae, telangiectasiae, and purpura. Young children are at increased risk of systemic side effects, including suppression of the hypothalamic-pituitary-adrenal axis and growth retardation due to their larger surface area relative to body weight, which permits approximately a threefold increase in systemic dose due to increased absorption.

In infants, the weakest topical corticosteroids (group 7), such as hydrocortisone acetate 1% or 0.25% methylprednisolone cream (Medrol), should be used. However, when indicated, more potent topical corticosteroids can be used for short periods of time, even in young children. Group 5 topical corticosteroids, including hydrocortisone valerate 0.2% cream (Westcort cream) or triamcinolone acetonide 0.1% cream (Aristocort A cream) can be safely given to all ages. In the adolescent and adult age groups, more potent topical steroids may be necessary. Betamethasone valerate 0.1% (Valisone cream) is commonly used in these patients. In localized disease, such as hand eczema, seen in the older age group, even more potent topical corticosteroids, such as fluocinonide cream 0.05% (Lidex) or halcinonide cream 0.1% (Halog cream), may be required. On the face and flexural areas, mild creams, such as 1% hydrocortisone or desonide cream 0.05% (Tridesilon), are indicated. Some patients do better with the corresponding ointment rather than the cream because of the increased hydration obtained by using the ointment base.

Treatment of Complications

Bacterial Infection

The skin lesions of atopic dermatitis are frequently colonized by *Staphylococcus aureus,* and the severity of the skin lesions appears to parallel the degree of colonization. Infectious complications may be trivial at the outset but can develop into systemically serious and occasionally life-threatening conditions. Typically, a child who has been doing fairly well suddenly gets much worse with widespread pustules or bullous impetigo. In very young children, staphylococcal scalded skin syndrome can supervene.

It is of some interest that potent corticosteroids have recently been shown to reduce the density of *Staphylococcus aureus* in patients with atopic dermatitis. However, when clinical infection supervenes, topical or systemic antibiotics are indicated. Localized infection can be treated with topical antibiotics such as mupirocin (Bactroban) or fusidic acid (Fucidin),* while more severe infections are generally treated with systemic antibiotics. Erythromycin is commonly used as a first-line systemic antibiotic. The recommended dosage is 250 to 500 mg four times daily for adults and 250 mg four times daily for children aged 6 to 12. Under age 6 years, dosage is calculated by weight. At the onset of antibiotic therapy, it is important to take cultures, as an increasing percentage of organisms are becoming resistant to erythromycin. In such cases, alternative therapy includes dicloxacillin (Dynapen) and oral cephalosporins. The recommended dosage of dicloxacillin is similar to that of erythromycin.

Herpes Simplex Infections

In patients with atopic dermatitis, herpes simplex infections can become widespread because areas of the skin are open and autoinoculation occurs from scratching. This results in a disseminated herpetic infection known as eczema herpeticum. The patient presents with widespread eczema and multiple small, uniform, punched-out erosions, ulcerations, or intact blisters that spread quickly over the skin surface. These patients may become toxic fairly quickly. The diagnosis can be confirmed by a Tzanck smear or by viral cultures. Widespread lesions of eczema herpeticum can be treated with oral acyclovir; however, patients with more severe disseminated disease should be admitted to the hospital for parenteral acyclovir therapy.

Severe Resistant Atopic Dermatitis

In spite of our best care, some patients are resistant to conventional therapy. More aggressive

---

*Not available in the United States.

*Not available in the United States.

or experimental therapy for resistant atopic dermatitis should be used based on the severity of the skin disease and the training of the physician.

Hospitalization

The least aggressive option for patients resistant to therapy is hospitalization. In many cases, the removal of the patient from the home environment and potential stress factors, along with education concerning the disease and assurance of compliance with therapy, results in a sustained reduction in the disease process.

Systemic Corticosteroids

Systemic corticosteroids are generally not indicated in atopic dermatitis. They produce prompt relief of symptoms, but because of the chronic nature of the disease, long-term use is contraindicated. Nevertheless, in severe resistant atopic dermatitis, short courses of oral steroids, starting at 30 mg of prednisone and tapering fairly rapidly over a few weeks, will often break the itch/scratch cycle. Although their use is somewhat controversial, intramuscular deposteroids such as triamcinolone acetonide 40 mg per mL (Kenalog) in a dosage of 40 to 60 mg can be given as a deep intramuscular injection no more frequently than every 6 to 8 weeks. Once the disease is brought under control, deposteroids should be abandoned.

Photochemotherapy

Photochemotherapy has been used in severe recalcitrant atopic dermatitis. Most studies demonstrate that a combination of UVA and UVB gives a better result than UVB alone. However, neither treatment produces a long-term response. Psoralens plus UVA (PUVA) therapy induces complete clearance, and in some cases, long-term remissions.

Cyclosporine

Cyclosporine* (Sandimmune, Cyclosporin A) reduces the number of dermal CD4+ cells and decreases their secretion of interleukins in addition to inhibiting the function of Langerhans cells. These effects appear to be dose dependent. In most trials, the action of oral cyclosporine in moderate doses induces a rapid and constant improvement in the skin disease. However, the risk of serious side effects and the reappearance of progressive disease after stopping treatment limits the indications for this drug.

Thymic Hormone: TP5 and TP1

Thymic hormone extract* has been used in an attempt to repair the deficit in cellular immunity found in these patients. Thymopentin (TP5) influences the immune system by promoting the differentiation of thymocytes and affecting the function of mature T cells. In a double-blind, placebo-controlled study of 100 patients, TP5 produced significant relief of pruritus and erythema due to atopic dermatitis without serious side effects. However, most patients relapsed after the seventh week of treatment. Similarly thymostimulin (TP1) in a double-blind controlled study showed a 20% reduction in clinical severity as compared with placebo-treated patients.

Topical Cromoglycate Solution (Cromolyn)

The effect of topical cromolyn ointment† on atopic dermatitis is a subject of some controversy with reports showing both efficacy and nonefficacy. Studies have shown that topical use of cromolyn nebulizer solution may be effective in treating severe facial atopic dermatitis in some patients.

Treatment of Fungal Skin Infections

Recently it has been demonstrated that hypersensitivity to *Pityrosporon* may play a significant role in flaring atopic dermatitis. In an open study on a small number of patients with atopic dermatitis confined primarily to the face, neck, and shoulders, treatment with 200 mg of ketoconazole (Nizoral) per day improved pruritus within 3 days and skin lesions within 2 weeks. These studies should be confirmed by a controlled trial involving more patients.

Recombinant Interferon-Gamma

Interferon-gamma can inhibit IgE synthesis induced by interleukin-4 in humans. The use of subcutaneous recombinant interferon-gamma in resistant cases of atopic dermatitis significantly improved inflammatory skin lesions. In some patients, serum IgE levels gradually decreased during therapy and spontaneous IgE production in vitro was reduced. Side effects included transient headaches, myalgia, and nausea, particularly with higher doses, and the disease rapidly relapsed when therapy was discontinued.

Interferon-Alpha

Although reports suggest that interferon-alpha inhibits IgE synthesis, there is disagreement about its efficacy in the treatment of atopic der-

---

*This use of cyclosporine is not listed in the manufacturer's official directive.

---

*Investigational drug in the United States.
†Not available in the United States.

matitis. Relevant studies included only small numbers of patients.

Interleukin-2

In a small study, human recombinant interleukin-2 was injected intravenously in six children, aged 2 to 11 years, suffering from severe atopic dermatitis. Lichenification and pruritus improved 5 days after commencing therapy. However, the dermatitis flared up in all cases 2 to 6 weeks after discontinuation of interleukin-2. As the therapeutic effect was transient and interleukin-2 therapy was rather toxic (chills, malaise, hepatomegaly, weight gain, edema, pleural effusions), it is unlikely to gain much favor in the treatment of atopic dermatitis except in severe, unremitting disease.

Allergen-Antibody Complexes

Clinical evidence has recently emerged showing that at least some forms of atopic dermatitis are exacerbated by exposure to airborne allergens in house dust. In many patients with atopic dermatitis, there is serologic evidence of immune sensitization to house dust mites, in particular *Dermatophagoides pteronyssinus*. In a recent study, 20 adult patients suffering from chronic atopic dermatitis were treated with regular injections of complexes made of *D. pteronyssinus* allergens and specific autologous antibodies. Preliminary results suggest that 73% of patients improved when treated with complexes, with a mean improvement of more than 70% after 4 months.

ERYTHEMA MULTIFORME AND OTHER ERYTHEMATOUS DISORDERS

method of
JOSEPH A. MUCCINI, M.D., and
ROBERT S. STERN, M.D.

Harvard Medical School
Boston, Massachusetts

Erythema (redness) is seen in virtually all inflammatory dermatologic conditions and in many disorders that involve blood vessel proliferation. An example of transient erythema is urticaria, which is most often an immune phenomenon. However, in some dermatoses a unique and characteristically recognizable type or configuration of erythema is the predominant feature, and in these cases, the condition is reasonably considered to be a distinct clinical entity. Among these disorders are erythema multiforme, erythema nodosum, and the figurate erythemas.

ERYTHEMA MULTIFORME, STEVENS-JOHNSON SYNDROME, AND TOXIC EPIDERMAL NECROLYSIS

Erythema multiforme is an acute and frequently recurrent cutaneous reaction that has numerous etiologies. Historically, the term "erythema multiforme" has been applied to a wide spectrum of diseases, and there has been substantial debate about its nosologic boundaries. For purposes of this article, we have divided the entire spectrum of erythema multiforme (EM), Stevens-Johnson syndrome (SJS), and toxic epidermal necrolysis (TEN), into five categories based on clinical features: (1) EM minor, (2) SJS, (3) overlap SJS-TEN, (4) TEN with spots, and (5) TEN without spots (Table 1).

Causes of EM, and perhaps SJS, include viral infections (herpes simplex infection, either type 1 or type 2), mycoplasmal (respiratory *Mycoplasma pneumoniae*) and bacterial infections, lupus erythematosus, deep x-ray therapy, carcinoma, sarcoidosis, and drug reactions (especially antibiotics, such as penicillins and sulfonamides, anticonvulsants such as phenytoin and phenobarbital, and nonsteroidal anti-inflammatory agents). TEN is usually associated with drugs.

As the name implies, erythema multiforme's characteristic lesions have several presentations. In differentiating these processes, it is important to correctly classify the so-called "target," or "iris," lesion. True target lesions have three distinct zones and two concentric rings around a central disc. The central disc may just be an area of pallor, or in more severe eruptions, a vesicle or bulla. The rings may be raised. Atypical (or targetoid) lesions can be flat or raised. They contain only one ring around a central disc and their borders may be poorly demarcated. The "spots" that can appear in association with TEN are usually macular spots or flat atypical target lesions. When mucosal lesions occur, they usually begin as smaller erythematous macules that can rapidly enlarge to form erosive plaques with pseudomembrane formation.

In EM minor, new crops of lesions may develop for a few days, but the eruption usually resolves within 1 to 2 weeks without scarring but sometimes with residual hyper- or hypopigmentation. EM minor may be accompanied by prodromal symptoms, including sore throat and fatigue. Although substantial involvement of multiple mucous membranes usually indicates a more severe bullous EM reaction (historically, EM major or SJS), limited mucosal lesions may also be present in EM minor. Typical target lesion are frequently observed.

Severe EM and SJS are typically associated with a more debilitating prodrome than EM mi-

TABLE 1. **Erythema Multiforme Spectrum Disorders**

Eruption Category	Constitutional Symptoms	Mucous Membranes Involved	Body Surface Area Detached	Presence of Typical Target Lesions*	Presence of Atypical Target Lesions†	Presence of Erythematous Spots
EM minor	Sore throat, fatigue, fever, malaise (variable)	None, or only one mildly involved	Minimal (but ≤20% BSA may be erythematous)	Often	Often raised	No
Stevens-Johnson syndrome	Fever, malaise, ± myalgia, arthralgia, diarrhea	Usually	<10%	No	Usually flat	Often
Overlap SJS-TEN	All of the above	Usually	10–29%	No	Flat	Often
TEN with spots	± Skin tenderness	Usually	≥30%	No	Flat	Often
TEN without spots	± Nikolsky's sign	Usually	≥10% (skin may exfoliate in large sheets)	No	No	No

*Typical target lesions are characterized by having two concentric rings around a central disc.

†Atypical lesions are flat or raised but contain only one ring around a central disc or with a poorly delineated border.

EM = erythema multiforme; SJS = Stevens-Johnson syndrome; TEN = toxic epidermal necrolysis; BSA = body surface area.

Adapted from Bastuji-Garin S, Rzany B, Stern RS, et al: A clinical classification of cases of toxic epidermal necrolysis, Stevens-Johnson syndrome and erythema multiforme. Arch Dermatol 129:92–96, 1993. Copyright 1993, American Medical Association.

nor. Symptoms include fever, malaise, and prostration. Following the prodrome, cutaneous and mucosal lesions develop rapidly. True target lesions are infrequent, and flat atypical targets are most often seen. The constitutional symptoms already present may worsen, and additional systemic complaints including myalgia, arthralgia, and diarrhea may develop. Even if relatively few cutaneous lesions are present, mucosal involvement may be widespread, affect any mucosal surface, and be debilitating. Patients may complain of photophobia, dysphagia, and esophagitis. Urinary retention is seen occasionally. Conjunctivitis, severe keratitis, uveitis, and iritis impair vision. The skin may become secondarily infected.

Overlap SJS-TEN and *TEN* (with and without spots) are more common in adults than in children and represent the most severe conditions within this spectrum. Drugs are almost always implicated. The prodrome may include conjunctival burning, skin tenderness, fever, headache, and malaise often lasting 1 to 2 days. This is followed by the rapid development of a generalized or morbilliform erythematous eruption or macular erythema. Although the face and extremities may be involved early on, the upper trunk is often most severely involved. The generalized erythema can occur de novo, or it can infrequently evolve rapidly from atypical target lesions, and for this reason, it may be difficult to distinguish between early TEN and SJS. Blisters can develop rapidly and coalesce to cover large areas of the body. In severe TEN, full-thickness epidermal necrosis is widespread with resultant loss of epidermis in large sheets. A positive Nikolsky sign can be elicited by exerting pressure

on red skin, with resultant skin separation. Mucosal involvement is generally severe and can involve any site. In addition, patients may lose the nails. Other manifestations include high fever, peripheral leukocytosis, elevated transaminases, and fluid and electrolyte imbalances. Mortality can exceed 50%. Age and extent of skin detachment are the most significant predictors of mortality. The most frequent cause of death is sepsis.

As originally described by Lyell in 1956, TEN had both a superficial (subcorneal) and a deep (subepidermal) variant, but it is now generally accepted that the subcorneal variant is a separate entity, presently called staphylococcal scalded skin syndrome (SSSS, or Ritter's disease). SSSS can appear clinically similar to TEN, but the cause is a staphylococcal exotoxin (most commonly from a phage group 2 strain). Unlike the full-thickness epidermal sloughing seen in TEN, only the stratum corneum is lost in SSSS.

Because of the numerous causes of EM reaction patterns, diagnostic evaluation should include documentation of any infections and exposure to drugs, especially within 3 weeks of the onset of the eruption. The patient's medical history should be reviewed, with attention to diseases and drugs known to cause this eruption. Throat or wound cultures for *Streptococcus* or other bacteria; serologic tests for hepatitis, *Mycoplasma,* and deep fungi; chest radiography for tuberculosis, *Mycoplasma,* and sarcoid; skin antigen testing for tuberculosis and *Mycoplasma* generally have low yield unless the clinical history suggests infection. Skin biopsy may help to exclude other diagnoses. Immunofluorescence tests are nonspecific and not generally helpful.

Treatment

Identification of underlying causes is desirable and should be followed by treatment of precipitating infections and discontinuation of all nonessential and any possibly causative drugs; however, in many cases, the underlying etiology is never established. Once a precipitating factor has been addressed, or if none is found, there are few treatment options for EM spectrum disorders. If the illness is mild, only supportive measures are required. Nonsteroidal anti-inflammatory medications may provide symptomatic relief in EM but do not significantly affect the course of the disease. Oral pain, with associated difficulty in eating and drinking, can be treated with topical analgesics such as viscous lidocaine (Xylocaine), dyclonine hydrochloride solution (Dyclone), or diphenhydramine hydrochloride (Benadryl elixir) alone or mixed with Kaopectate. If the oral mucosa is involved, fluids or soft diet can help maintain nutrition. If the EM reaction pattern is recurrent and possibly herpes associated, a trial of oral acyclovir, 200 mg two to five times daily, should be undertaken as prophylaxis. If there is mucosal eye involvement, an ophthalmology consultation is mandatory. In cases of SJS or TEN, intravenous fluids and nasogastric (if possible) or intravenous feedings may be required.

Antibiotics may also be necessary, but should usually be reserved for cases in which a specific infectious agent is suspect, since the indiscriminate use of prophylactic antibiotics can result in additional morbidity.

The role of systemic steroids and other immunomodulating agents is controversial, and we do not generally support their use. In bullous EM and SJS, steroids may provide initial symptomatic improvement but ultimately increase morbidity. In TEN, systemic corticosteroids increase morbidity and mortality and should not be used.

Patients with severe TEN should be cared for in a burn unit with specialized skin care, infection control, and fluid and electrolyte management. In cases in which significant denuding of the skin has occurred, porcine xenografts or human allografts can be used to reduce pain and the risk of infection. Topical antiseptics should be used with caution. Silver sulfadiazine (Silvadene) may cause neutropenia or inhibit re-epithelialization. Silver nitrate wet dressings inhibit infection but increase wound desiccation and can cause severe pain during dressing changes.

ERYTHEMA NODOSUM

Erythema nodosum (EN) is an erythematous eruption most common in young women. It is characterized by round or oval, nonulcerating, variably tender nodules, usually localized to the anterior distal lower extremities, but occasionally seen on the upper extremities or trunk. If the lesions are oval, their long axis usually follows the long axis of the limb. Individual nodules do not usually exceed 6 cm in diameter. Because of edema, erythema, and pain, early EN can be mistaken for cellulitis. Ankle swelling is common. Individual lesions resolve within 2 to 3 weeks, but new crops develop. Single episodes are more common than recurrent or chronic eruptions.

Conditions associated with EN include exposure to drugs (sulfonamides, halides, oral contraceptives), infections (especially upper respiratory infections with beta-hemolytic streptococci, gastrointestinal *Yersinia* infections, tuberculosis, blastomycosis, histoplasmosis, psittacosis, cat-scratch disease, lymphogranuloma venereum, and coccidioidomycosis), enteropathies (ulcerative colitis, regional ileitis), sarcoidosis, Hodgkin's disease, and pregnancy. Nonspecific upper respiratory syndromes, fever, malaise, and arthralgia may precede the eruption by up to 8 weeks. For about half of all cases no cause is identified. When erythema nodosum occurs with hilar adenopathy, fever, cough, and arthralgia, it is known as Löfgren's syndrome, which is considered an early sign of sarcoidosis.

Diagnostic evaluation of a patient presenting with EN should include a complete blood count and differential, erythrocyte sedimentation rate, antistreptolysin-O titer, throat culture, urinalysis, chest x-ray, and intradermal tuberculin test. If suspected, viral or *Yersinia* serologies or skin tests for fungal antigens may be performed. Accurate histologic evaluation requires a deep skin biopsy, including the subcutaneous fat; punch biopsies may be inadequate. Histologically, a septal panniculitis characterized by a lymphohistiocytic infiltrate, with few neutrophils in acute cases and with granuloma formation in the rarer, more chronic cases, is seen. Small vessels are most often involved. The septal panniculitis and absent or limited vasculitic component aid in differentiating EN from other entities that feature nodules of the legs, such as periarteritis nodosa, nodular vasculitis, lobular panniculitis (erythema induratum), and secondary inflammatory or vasculitic processes associated with underlying malignancy or connective tissue disorders.

Treatment

The condition is usually self-limited. Helpful supportive measures include treatment of any underlying condition that may have triggered the eruption, bed rest, leg elevation, wet dressings, and support stockings or bandages. Oral nonsteroidal anti-inflammatory agents, including salicylates (600 mg four times a day) or indomethacin also help to reduce discomfort and edema. If oral contraceptives are implicated, a trial of a lower dose alternative contraceptive may be helpful. Pulse therapy with oral prednisone (40 to 60 mg per day tapered over 2 to 4 weeks) may be helpful, but should be reserved for those cases in which the etiology of EN has been determined and the severity is sufficiently great to justify the risks of steroid therapy. Potassium iodide, with slow escalation up to doses of 300 mg three to four times per day for several weeks, has also been effective in some idiopathic cases. Parotitis may complicate treatment with potassium iodide.

THE FIGURATE ERYTHEMAS

The figurate erythemas include several cutaneous eruptions that may be annular, polycyclic, or irregular in shape. Individual lesions often migrate and tend to extend peripherally, but some variants may be fixed. The classification of the figurate erythemas is controversial. Subtypes may share histologic features. The figurative erythemas usually are classified on the basis of clinical and histopathologic characteristics as well as underlying cause.

Erythema chronicum migrans (ECM) is the cutaneous manifestation of early Lyme disease (Lyme borreliosis) and is frequently the first sign of infection. The causative organism is the spirochete *Borrelia burgdorferi,* which is transmitted by ticks, especially members of the *Ixodes* genus. Several vector species have been identified in different parts of the world. In the United States, the vector is *I. dammini* (the deer tick) in the northeast and midwest, *I. scapularis* in the southeast, and *I. pacificus* in California. *I. persulcatus* has been identified as a vector in Asia, whereas *I. ricinus* is more common in Europe.

The eruption begins as an erythematous papule at the site of the tick bite within days to weeks of the bite. The tick is small and may escape detection; only one-third of affected patients remember a tick bite. Over several days, the lesion may enlarge and clear centrally. The erythematous edge of the lesion may be flat or raised. A burning sensation in the lesion is sometimes reported. Nonspecific systemic complaints include headache, myalgia, arthralgia, fatigue, fever, and chills. In about half of patients, secondary lesions that are smaller but otherwise clinically similar to the original lesion develop at distant sites.

Detection of the spirochete either with silver stain of tissue or by cultures is often not possible. The most frequently employed diagnostic tests are serologic, generally ELISA or indirect immunofluorescence assays. Serum titers may not be elevated for up to 6 weeks following the infection. There is a high incidence of false negative tests. Therefore, if negative serology is obtained but clinical suspicion is high, the test should be repeated in 3 weeks. The eruption and other early features of Lyme disease (Stage 1 disease) generally subside within 3 to 4 weeks if the infection is not treated. However, weeks to months after the initial symptoms have resolved, serious neurologic or cardiac (Stage 2) disease may develop. Neurologic symptoms include meningitis, cranial neuritis (Bell's palsy), and radiculoneuritis. Cardiac manifestations include conduction defects, pancarditis, and ventricular dysfunction. Chronic (Stage 3) disease can develop weeks to years after the initial onset of the illness and is predominantly characterized by generalized fatigue and skin atrophy.

Tetracycline, previously a recommended therapy, has fallen into disfavor. The preferred treatment for Stage 1 disease in nonpregnant adults is doxycycline, 100 mg twice a day for 21 days. Alternative treatments include amoxicillin, 500 mg three times a day for 10 to 21 days, or erythromycin, 250 mg four times a day for 10 to 21 days. If *arthritis* is a predominant feature, 100 mg of doxycycline twice a day for 30 days is often recommended. Alternative regimens are amoxicillin and probenecid, 500 mg each four times a day for 30 days; penicillin G, 20 million units daily intravenously (IV) in divided doses for 14 to 21 days; or ceftriaxone, 2 grams IV daily for 14 to 21 days. The recommended treatment for *Lyme carditis* is ceftriaxone, 2 grams daily IV by single dose for 14 days (preferred); or, alternatively, penicillin G, 20 million units daily IV in divided doses for 14 days, doxycycline, 100 mg twice a day for 14 to 21 days, or amoxicillin, 500 mg three times a day for 14 to 21 days. Recommended treatment for *Lyme meningitis* is ceftriaxone, 2 grams daily IV by single dose for 14 to 21 days (preferred); or, alternatively, penicillin G, 20 million units daily IV in divided doses for 10 to 21 days, doxycycline, 100 mg twice a day for 14 to 21 days, or chloramphenicol, 1 gram IV every 6 hours for 10 to 21 days.

Stage 1 disease in pregnant or lactating women and children under 8 years of age can be treated with amoxicillin, 500 mg three times a day for 21 days, or erythromycin, 250 to 500 mg four times daily for 21 days. Disseminated early disease or late disease in these populations should be treated with penicillin G, 20 million units IV daily in divided doses for 14 to 21 days.

Recent studies suggest that if a patient is bitten by an *Ixodes* tick in endemic areas (especially where *I. dammini* and *I. pacificus* are found), empirical treatment may be more cost effective than waiting for symptomatic or serologic evidence of infection. In suspect cases of ECM associated with exposure in an endemic area, antibiotic therapy is almost certainly warranted.

Erythema annulare centrifugum is the name given to an eruption characterized by one or more lesions that initially start as small erythematous papules that enlarge peripherally into ringed or polycyclic figures. As the lesions expand, the center flattens and clears. The most commonly affected sites are the buttocks and surfaces of the proximal arms and legs. The edges of the lesions may advance by several millimeters per day. Lesion edges may be flat or raised and either smooth or scaly. Unlike the characteristic leading edge of scaling seen in dermatophyte infections, scale, when present, is usually found on the trailing edge. Lesions typically last days to weeks. A waxing and waning pattern of recurrence or persistence may be observed. The etiology in most cases of EAC remains obscure, but several triggering causes have been suggested, including infections with fungus, yeast, and *Ascaris,* drug hypersensitivity, thyroid or liver disease, underlying carcinoma, and Sjögren's syndrome. Management consists of treatment of the underlying cause when identified.

Erythema gyratum repens is a rare distinctive eruption characterized by a rapidly moving, whirling erythematous rash that resembles the grain of wood. This eruption is almost always found in association with an underlying malignancy, mandating a work-up for undiagnosed neoplasms.

Necrolytic migratory erythema is characterized by superficial migratory arcuate lesions, most commonly on the extremities and trunk and sometimes seen in perigenital and perioral locations. The lesions are often associated with peripheral blistering, desquamation, and necrosis. This condition occurs most often in patients with glucagon-secreting pancreatic tumors, infantile zinc deficiency, and zinc deficiency associated with hyperalimentation.

Figurate erythemas are also encountered in lupus *(annular eruption of lupus erythematosus),* in female carriers of chronic granulomatous disease, in mycosis fungoides (cutaneous T cell lymphoma), and in association with rheumatic fever *(erythema marginatum).*

BULLOUS DISORDERS

method of
N. FRED EAGLSTEIN, D.O.
University of Florida College of Medicine
Jacksonville, Florida

The most important bullous diseases are pemphigus vulgaris, bullous pemphigoid, and dermatitis herpeti-

formis. Other bullous disorders include cicatricial pemphigoid, herpes gestationis, epidermolysis bullosa acquisita, linear IgA dermatosis, bullous lupus erythematosus, and bullous drug reactions. Proper diagnosis is imperative as the prognosis and therapy will vary. Differentiation is established by the clinical presentation, histopathologic findings, and results of direct and indirect immunofluorescence.

PEMPHIGUS VULGARIS

Pemphigus is an autoimmune disorder in which antibodies of the IgG class attach to the intracellular space of epidermal cells, resulting in acantholysis (cell to cell separation). The resulting blister that develops occurs within the epidermis. This disease usually begins as superficial erosions in the mouth, disseminating to all body surfaces after 6 to 12 months. Superficial bullae on normal or erythematous skin rapidly erode and display little tendency towards self-healing. Variants of this disease are usually less severe, but often harder to control and include pemphigus vegetans, pemphigus foliaceous, Brazilian pemphigus (fogo-selvagem), and pemphigus erythematous (Senear-Usher syndrome).

Treatment

Systemic corticosteroids in large doses are the mainstay of therapy. Before the introduction of this therapy, most cases resulted in death. When adequate doses are given (prednisone 100–400 mg per day) new lesions are suppressed and erosions begin to heal. Once the disease is controlled, systemic steroids can be gradually tapered while monitoring patient response. Recent studies show that the serum titer of pemphigus antibodies is a reflection of disease activity. When the titer falls, therapy can be tapered and when the titer increases, therapy is increased.

In order to reduce side effects from prolonged corticosteroid therapy, the immunosuppressive agents can be utilized as "steroid sparing" agents. Antimetabolites include cyclophosphamide* (Cytoxan), azathioprine* (Imuran), and methotrexate.* Once therapy is initiated, the "steroid sparing" is demonstrable by 3 to 4 weeks at which point prednisone can be further reduced. Eventually the antimetabolite can be tapered.

Azathioprine is given at a dose of 1 to 2 mg per kg per day. Side effects include bone marrow suppression and hepatoxicity. Cyclophosphamide is used at 1 to 2 mg per kg per day. Side effects include bone marrow suppression, hemorrhagic cystitis, bladder fibrosis, sterility, and increased

---

*These uses of cyclophosphamide, azathioprine, and methotrexate are not listed in the manufacturers' official directive.

risk of malignancies. Methotrexate is given at a dose of 25 to 30 mg once a week. If prolonged therapy is required, pretreatment liver biopsies should be done and repeated whenever the cumulative dose reaches 1000 to 1500 mg. The use of these immunosuppressive agents requires close monitoring of complete blood count, liver function tests, renal function tests, serum chemistries, and urinalysis.

Gold therapy* (Myochrysine, Solganal) is used for mild to moderate cases or in combination with prednisone in severe cases. Side effects of these drugs include nephritis, bone marrow suppression, drug eruptions, and pruritus. A test dose of 10 mg intramuscularly is given. If the drug is well tolerated, 50 mg intramuscularly is given in 1 week and weekly thereafter. When the disease comes under control, the dosage is slowly reduced. A complete blood count and urinalysis must be obtained prior to each dose. Additionally, renal function, liver function, and serum chemistries should be closely monitored.

Recent reports show that plasmapheresis in conjunction with immunosuppressive drugs, cyclosporine (Sandimmune), and pulse steroid therapy is beneficial in severe recalcitrant disease.

Topical skin therapy utilizes high-potency topical steroid ointments. Lukewarm soaks or baths are beneficial in débriding crusts and dead skin. Close attention must be paid to electrolyte balance, nutrition, soft diet, antacid therapy, latent tuberculosis, and deep fungal infection.

Special consideration must be paid to oral lesions. With significant involvement, only liquids and soft foods are tolerated. Topical therapy with viscous lidocaine and saline mouth washes or dilute H_2O_2 offers symptomatic relief. Lesions in the mouth can be treated with intralesional triamcinolone (Kenalog) injections and topical triamcinolone acetonide (Kenalog in Orabase).

BULLOUS PEMPHIGOID

Pemphigoid is an autoimmune disorder in which antibodies of the IgG class attach to the basement membrane zone of the epidermis, resulting in subepidermal bullae. This disease is more prevalent than pemphigus and usually occurs in elderly patients. It begins as pruritic, erythematous, edematous plaques progressing to tense bullae on either normal or reddened skin. Unlike in pemphigus vulgaris, the bullae and subsequent erosions have a tendency toward self-healing. Overall, this disease has a better prognosis than pemphigus vulgaris.

Treatment

Application of potent topical corticosteroids or intralesional triamcinolone (Kenalog) is usually effective when the disease is mild and localized. The lesions should be débrided with wet compresses and systemic antibiotics given for secondary bacterial infections.

Moderate to severe disease requires systemic corticosteroids in dosages equivalent to 40 to 60 mg of prednisone per day. Regression usually occurs after several weeks to months, at which point the dose should be slowly tapered. If treatment with prednisone cannot be discontinued altogether, alternate day steroids can be used.

As mentioned, immunosuppressive agents can be used as "steroid sparing" agents. These drugs are used in the same fashion as for pemphigus vulgaris. Recent reports indicate that erythromycin* or tetracycline* (1 to 2 grams per day) plus nicotinamide* (1500 to 2500 mg per day) is effective in some patients. This approach can be utilized in moderate disease or when there are contraindications to systemic corticosteroids.

Dapsone,* 100 mg per day, is effective for dermatitis herpetiformis, but only a few cases of bullous pemphigoid will respond favorably, especially when there is a dense neutrophilic infiltrate on biopsy. Dapsone is used in the same fashion as described for dermatitis herpetiformis. Recent reports indicate that plasmapheresis, pulse steroid therapy, and cyclosporine* are of benefit in severe, recalcitrant disease.

DERMATITIS HERPETIFORMIS

Dermatitis herpetiformis is an immune mediated, extremely pruritic disease that presents as tiny vesicles, papules, and excoriations. Herpetiform grouping of lesions usually occurs on the elbows, knees, shoulders, and lumbosacral areas. This is a chronic disorder and spontaneous remission occurs in only 15% of patients. Diagnosis is confirmed by a skin biopsy and direct immunofluorescence of perilesional skin, which shows deposition of IgA in the dermal papulary tips. Ninety percent of patients have an asymptomatic gluten-sensitive enteropathy.

Treatment

Dapsone is the most effective drug in controlling this disease and usually works in 3 to 4 days. The lesions rapidly recur when the drug is stopped. Baseline laboratory tests include a com-

---

*These uses of gold compounds are not listed in the manufacturers' official directive.

*These uses of erythromycin, tetracycline, nicotinamide, dapsone, and cyclosporine are not listed in the manufacturers' official directive.

plete blood count, chemistry profile, and a glucose-6-phosphate dehydrogenase (G6PD) determination. Dapsone* is not used if the G6PD enzyme is absent. The initial dose of 25 mg per day is increased until there is a clinical response. If the disease is not controlled on 300 mg per day, the diagnosis should be reconsidered. The goal of treatment is to maintain the patient on the lowest possible dose that keeps the skin almost totally clear of lesions. Complete blood counts and clinical signs of cyanosis are closely monitored as dapsone invariably produces a hemolytic anemia and methemoglobulinemia. Other side effects include cholestasis, toxic hepatitis, toxic psychosis, neuropathies, hypersensitivity reactions, and rarely agranulocytosis. Renal and liver function tests must be checked initially, at 2- to 3-week intervals, and every 3 months thereafter.

In most cases, a strict gluten-free diet reduces or eliminates the need for dapsone after 6 to 12 months. However, most patients will not be able to comply with this diet as many staples such as breads, cakes, and cereals are disallowed. Oral antihistamines and potent topical corticosteroids can be used for patients with limited disease. Alternative therapies include oral cholestryramine or colchicine for patients who cannot tolerate standard therapy.

---

*This use of dapsone is not listed in the manufacturer's official directive.

CONTACT DERMATITIS

method of
DON C. HARTING, M.D.
Cleveland, Tennessee

Contact dermatitis is an acute or chronic inflammatory dermatosis due to primary irritants or contact allergens.

Primary irritant contact dermatitis can follow any of a large variety of exogenous insults. Chemicals, acids, alkalis, solvents, surfactants, and even mild irritants can induce inflammation depending upon the concentration of the irritant, the duration of exposure, and the cutaneous area involved. Previous exposure or an immunologic reaction is not necessary to elicit dermatitis.

Allergic contact dermatitis is a T cell mediated immune response. When exposed to a small amount of antigen, previously sensitized individuals may develop a mild to severe inflammatory reaction. The most common allergens are poison ivy, oak, and sumac, as well as nickel, preservatives, rubber compounds, fragrances, formaldehyde, and dyes.

Occupational contact dermatitis is discussed in a separate article.

DIAGNOSIS

The history and physical examination will help to differentiate irritant and allergic contact dermatitis. The etiology of acute irritant dermatitis is usually self evident. A traumatic event involving the skin causes acute inflammation with erythema, edema, vesicles, or moderate to severe burns.

Acute contact allergic dermatitis occurs within 1 to 5 days of exposure. The typical patient has pruritic, linear, erythematous, edematous papules, plaques, vesicles, or larger serum-filled bullous lesions. Weeping, crusting, and purulent exudate from secondary infection may also be present.

The lesions of chronic irritant and allergic contact dermatitis are pruritic, erythematous, scaling, lichenified (thickened) papules and plaques, often with fissures or excoriations. Differentiating between the two requires an extensive and detailed history and ultimately patch testing to make a definitive diagnosis.

TREATMENT

Neutralization or copious aqueous cleansing is required in cases of acute irritant dermatitis due to chemicals or other irritants. Treatment as for a first, second, or third-degree burn may be required.

Acute allergic contact dermatitis with minor lesions and limited involvement is treated topically with cool compresses, topical steroid creams, lotions, or gels, or calamine lotion. Low- to medium-potency topical steroids are used on the face or intertriginous areas and high potency topicals on the trunk and extremities (Table 1). Oint-

TABLE 1. **Topical Corticosteroids**

High Potency	Medium to Low Potency
Clobetasol propionate (Temovate)	Fluticasone propionate (Cutivate)
Halobetasol propionate (Ultravate)	Hydrocortisone valerate (Westcort)
Betamethasone dipropionate (Diprolene)	Hydrocortisone butyrate (Locoid)
Diflorasone diacetate (Psorcon)	Mometasone furoate (Elocon)
Fluocinonide (Lidex)	Betamethasone valerate (Valisone)
	Alclometasone dipropionate (Aclovate)
	Desonide (DesOwen)
	Hydrocortisone (Hytone 2½%)

TABLE 2. **Oral Prednisone Therapy**

Children
Example: 0.75 mg per kg per day
          40 to 80 lb child
          20 to 30 mg initially, tapered over 12 to 21 days
Adults
Example: 0.75 to 1.0 mg per kg per day
          120 to 170 lb adult
          40 to 70 mg initially, tapered over 12 to 21 days

SKIN DISEASES OF PREGNANCY

method of
MARILYNNE McKAY, M.D., and
ROBERT A. SWERLICK, M.D.
Emory University
Atlanta, Georgia

ments are occlusive and should be avoided in acute dermatitis.

Oral antihistamines such as diphenhydramine (Benadryl), hydroxyzine (Atarax), or cyproheptadine (Periactin) may be used for their antipruritic or sedating effects.

Moderate to severe allergic contact dermatitis is characterized by involvement of 30 to 50% or more of the total body surface area, extensive vesicular or bullous lesions with weeping and oozing, or extensive involvement of the face, hands, feet, or genitals.

Oral prednisone is given in an initial dose of 0.75 to 1.0 mg per kg per day, which is 40 to 70 mg initially for most adults. Depending on the severity of involvement, prednisone is tapered over a period of 12 to 21 days, as shorter periods of tapering often result in a rebound of the initial dermatitis (Table 2).

Weeping and oozing bullous lesions are treated with cool or tepid wet compresses or bathtub soaks for 20 to 30 minutes every 3 to 6 hours. Domeboro powder or Aveeno oatmeal bath may be added to relieve pruritus and hasten drying of the lesions. Calamine or other bland shake lotions are applied after the soaks. After the lesions have begun to dry, topical steroids are applied two to four times a day.

Patients should be monitored for signs of secondary infection and treated with appropriate antibiotics. Those with severe involvement should be examined frequently and carefully followed to prevent secondary infection, sepsis, scarring, and the rebound phenomenon.

A patient with chronic dermatitis, either irritant or allergic, requires extensive education on the principles of skin care and the avoidance of, or protection from, the offending agents. Topical steroids are used judiciously for inflammation and pruritus.

As many as one in five patients may complain of itching during pregnancy. When itching occurs in association with a rash, it may be the result of (1) a flare of a pre-existing skin disorder, (2) a coincidentally acquired problem, or (3) a dermatosis specifically related to pregnancy. The dermatoses of pregnancy are relatively rare (except for pruritus gravidarum), and the pregnant patient with a rash is much more likely to have a skin problem unrelated to her physiologic state. Consider common problems first, especially allergic rashes (urticaria, drug reactions, and contact dermatitis). The next diagnostic considerations are atopic dermatitis, nummular eczema, insect bites, scabies, pityriasis rosea, and even secondary syphilis.

The significance of a skin eruption relates primarily to the effect it may have on maternal and fetal health. The characteristic skin lesions of a pregnancy-related dermatosis may not be present the first time the patient complains of itching; if a rash is evolving, frequent follow-up visits should be scheduled to monitor disease progression. If one of the dermatoses of pregnancy is a consideration, a skin biopsy is the best way to make the diagnosis. A lesion should be biopsied for routine histologic examination; perilesional skin is best for direct immunofluorescence (for which Michel's medium, a special laboratory-supplied fixative, is used, rather than formalin.) Consultation with a specialist is recommended: immunofluorescence biopsies, for example, are best submitted to a laboratory that routinely performs these tests.

PRURITIC URTICARIAL PAPULES AND PLAQUES OF PREGNANCY (PUPPP)

PUPPP is a self-limited, highly pruritic eruption that usually occurs late in pregnancy (typically the third trimester of a first pregnancy). Red, blanchable, urticarial papules and plaques usually begin on abdominal striae, lower abdomen, and thighs. Erythema multiforme–like polycyclic and target lesions and tiny (2 mm) vesicles are seen, but the palms, soles, and face are rarely involved. Lesions can spread to the back, buttocks and proximal extremities. Though patients complain of itching, excoriations are rare. Histologically, there is a lymphohistiocytic infiltrate with variable numbers of eosinophils. Direct immunofluorescence differentiates PUPPP from herpes gestationis, which has a characteristic pattern (see next section).

PUPPP has no related systemic symptoms or laboratory abnormalities, nor are there associations with any known maternal or fetal problems.

The eruption clears promptly after delivery and successful therapy consists of controlling symptoms. High-potency corticosteroids such as fluocinonide (Lidex) 0.05% cream or gel, applied every 6 to 8 hours, and diphenhydramine (Benadryl), 25 to 50 mg every 6 to 8 hours, help to control itching. Patients with PUPPP only rarely require oral steroids to control the eruption.

HERPES GESTATIONIS

Herpes gestationis (HG) is a rare, recurrent vesiculobullous disease related to pregnancy and the puerperium. (The name reflects only the grouped appearance of the vesicles, for there is no evidence of an association with the herpes virus. HG should not be confused, either, with "impetigo herpetiformis," which is considered to be a variant of pustular psoriasis occurring in pregnancy.) In some cases, HG begins with a prodrome of malaise, fever, nausea, headache, chills, burning, and pruritus, but this clinical presentation is not consistent enough to be pathognomonic. The skin eruption is characteristic. Urticarial papules and polycyclic wheals evolve into target lesions and vesicles, finally becoming large, tense bullae—a process that takes an average of 4 weeks.

The diagnosis of HG is best made by biopsy: histologic findings (similar to those seen with bullous pemphigoid) include a subepidermal blister associated with variable infiltration with neutrophils and eosinophils. Biopsy of perilesional skin for direct immunofluorescence microscopy shows linear deposits of C3 at the basement membrane zone of the dermal-epidermal junction.

HG can begin as early as the first trimester, but some cases do not become apparent until after delivery, probably because an immediate postpartum flare is extremely common. The intensity of symptoms varies: some patients have severe, widespread vesiculation, while in others the skin spontaneously clears, even during pregnancy. After delivery, the disease usually resolves entirely, but it often recurs in subsequent pregnancies. Rare patients continue to have periodic eruptions, particularly after menstruation resumes, and some have exacerbations of HG after ingestion of oral contraceptives. Rarely, a transient cutaneous eruption occurs in children born to mothers with HG, but it requires no therapy. A much more controversial point is whether maternal HG carries an increased risk of fetal morbidity or mortality. Widely disparate results have come from different studies, but at least one study suggests an increased incidence of fetal complications, especially prematurity, in these infants.

Therapy of HG is directed at control of symptoms. Topical medications are the first line of treatment, since they are less likely to be harmful to the fetus. Triamcinolone acetonide (Kenalog, Aristocort), 0.1% cream, or fluocinonide (Lidex), 0.05% cream or gel, applied as often as every 4 to 6 hours, may control disease activity. Oozing lesions respond to application of compresses soaked in tap water or aluminum acetate (Domeboro, 1 tablet or packet in a pint of tap water, mixed fresh daily) before steroid applications. Diphenhydramine (Benadryl), 25 to 50 mg every 6 to 8 hours, usually controls pruritus.

Topical medications may not be effective in patients with severe, widespread disease; if so, systemic corticosteroids are the next choice. In these cases, 20 to 40 mg of prednisone are given daily as a single morning dose. Corticosteroids should certainly be used with caution during pregnancy, but experience with pregnant steroid-dependent asthmatics suggests that the risks are not significant if the patient is monitored closely for complications. When the eruption is controlled, the steroid regimen should be tapered to the lowest possible dose needed to control disease activity. Topical steroids may still be required as an adjunct to allow reduction of the systemic dose. Alternate-day doses are better tolerated, especially if several weeks of therapy are anticipated. Because HG often flares postpartum, systemic corticosteroids are often increased then.

PRURIGO GRAVIDARUM

This is the term used for the generalized itching that can occur during pregnancy without skin pathology. It is generally considered a mild, anicteric form of recurrent cholestasis of pregnancy. Liver function tests are helpful only in severe cases. Serum bilirubin may be only slightly increased, but levels of bile acids in the skin correlate well with the pruritus.

The main maternal complication is postpartum hemorrhage, a result of abnormal clotting times. Mild cases respond to topical triamcinolone acetonide 0.1% cream and diphenhydramine, 25 to 50 mg every 4 to 6 hours, and cholestyramine has been helpful in more severe cases. Intramuscular vitamin K reverses prolonged prothrombin time and partial thromboplastin time.

PRURITUS ANI AND VULVAE

method of
STEPHEN P. STONE, M.D.
Southern Illinois University School of Medicine
Springfield, Illinois

Pruritus ani and vulvae can be considered as symptoms or as disease entities. As symptoms, pruritus ani

TABLE 1. **Causes of Anogenital Pruritis**

Infection
Fungus
Dermatophyte
Yeast (*Candida*)
Bacteria
Parasites
Pinworms (anal area)
Pediculosis (vulvar area)

Local Manifestations of Generalized Cutaneous Disease
Psoriasis
Atopic eczema
Lichen planus

Manifestations of Systemic Disease
Lymphoma or other systemic malignancy
Diabetes

Other Local Disease Processes
Extramammary Paget's disease
Lichen sclerosus et atrophicus
Hemorrhoids
Fissures and fistulas
Eczema with or without lichenification

"Neurodermatitis"

and pruritus vulvae are fairly common and have multiple external causes. As disease entities, pruritus ani and pruritus vulvae are actually diagnoses of exclusion.

In approaching the patient with anogenital pruritus, it is most important to determine whether there is a specific treatable cause (Table 1). Most commonly, pruritus ani and vulvae are chronic and well established by the time the physician is consulted, and regardless of the degree of itching they are frequently intractable and resistant to the physician's and the patient's approaches.

Evaluation of the patient with pruritus ani and vulvae must include a careful examination of the skin, Scotch tape test for pinworm infestation, cultures for fungi, yeast, and bacteria, and in the case of visible change in the skin beyond excoriation, a punch biopsy.

TREATMENT

In the case of pruritus ani, cleanliness is extremely important. The patient should cleanse the area after each bowel movement and several times a day, as fecal soiling and mucus seepage during the day can cause an irritant reaction. Cleansing can be accomplished with Tucks cloth pads, water without soap, or a cleansing lotion such as Cetaphil or Balneol applied with a cotton ball and then gently rinsed with cool water. Toilet tissue should be white and unscented; it may be helpful to substitute a soft white facial tissue. I personally recommend avoiding paper entirely and using only Tucks cloth pads.

Some foods can exacerbate pruritus ani, possibly due to direct contact with the affected area. Some physicians theorize that caffeine and alco-

hol cause mild relaxation of the anal sphincter, allowing fecal leakage. Hence, the patient should avoid alcoholic beverages, coffee, tea, colas, chocolate, and highly spiced foods, particularly those containing peppers and pepper derivatives. Chronic use of antibiotics and laxatives has also been associated with pruritus ani. Finally, common food allergens have been associated with pruritus ani, and milk, pork, tomatoes, corn, and nuts might be avoided as a therapeutic trial.

If yeast is suspected, ketoconazole* (Nizoral), 200 mg daily, or nystatin oral tablets may be surprisingly effective in patients without objective evidence of yeast infection.

In the case of pruritus vulvae, the presence of skin disease must be determined both by close visual examination and by biopsy of any abnormal area that appears. In this site, infection is a common cause of itching, and bacterial, trichomonal, and candidal vaginitis must be ruled out. Even without clinical evidence of infection, I frequently administer a sequential trial of metronidazole, ketoconazole, and erythromycin or one of the better absorbed tetracyclines for 2 weeks. Subclinical allergic contact dermatitis to condoms, the scents in tampons and sanitary napkins, douches, and other medicaments used in the vaginal area must be ruled out.

Here, too, cleansing is very important. I recommend washing the affected area twice daily with a cleansing lotion such as Cetaphil or Balneol. Some patients find that switching from synthetic to cotton underwear is helpful, and others find that avoidance of fabric softeners will relieve some itching to some degree.

Oral antipruritics, such as hydroxyzine, trimeprazine (Temaril), or cyproheptadine (Periactin), are usually ineffective, but they should be tried because some patients do show remarkable improvement. In some elderly women with chronic pruritus vulvae, amitriptyline (Elavil) will sometimes produce striking improvement. It should be tried for a minimum of 2 weeks.

Topical steroids are useful in both pruritus ani and pruritus vulvae. The more potent steroids should be avoided, but triamcinolone ointment (0.025%) and fluocinolone (Synalar) ointment (0.025%) in a formulation that is free of parabens and other preservatives may be used. Because of the susceptibility of the anogenital area to atrophy when potent steroids are used, hydrocortisone ointment should be substituted as early as possible after improvement is noted.

Grenz ray therapy, 1 to 2 Gy (100 to 200 R) per week for 3 to 4 weeks, can be used as a second

---

*This use of ketoconazole is not listed in the manufacturer's official directive.

line therapy. This treatment is often sufficient to break the itch/scratch cycle and provide a long remission. If grenz ray is not available, or if the patient is phobic about the use of radiation therapy, then an intramuscular injection of triamcinolone acetonide (Kenalog), 40 to 60 mg every 3 to 4 weeks for 2 to 3 months, may provide prolonged suppression of symptoms.

URTICARIA AND ANGIOEDEMA

method of
CLIVE E. H. GRATTAN, F.R.C.P.
Norfolk and Norwich Hospital
Norwich, Norfolk, England

The urticarias are a heterogeneous group of skin disorders resulting from transient plasma leakage into skin, subcutaneous tissue, or both. Dermal edema is called a "weal;" subcutaneous or submucosal involvement is known as "angioedema." Angioedema is most commonly recognized by swelling of the mouth or eyelids but can affect any part of the skin. The gastrointestinal or respiratory mucosa may be affected in C_1 esterase inhibitor deficiency.

Plasma exudation from capillaries and postcapillary venules is usually mediated by histamine and other vasoactive mediators released from mast cells, but mechanisms involving activation of the complement, fibrinolytic, and kinin pathways may be important in special circumstances.

CLASSIFICATION

Five major patterns of urticaria/angioedema can be recognized on the basis of clinical, histological, and immunological features.

Ordinary Urticaria. Recurrent weals can last as long as 24 hours, but they sometimes subside in as little as 1 to 2 hours in patients with mild or partially controlled disease. They subside without bruising. When severe, the attacks may be associated with systemic symptoms such as shivering, aching, and lassitude, but long-term complications do not occur. Although associated angioedema is common, it rarely presents as a life-threatening emergency. Ordinary urticaria is often subdivided into two groups, acute and chronic, depending on how long it has been present. This is not a very useful distinction because acute urticaria can graduate into chronic urticaria, but it may be helpful in defining groups for therapeutic studies. Acute urticaria (resolving within days or weeks) is more often caused by immediate hypersensitivity reactions involving the binding of an allergen (e.g., nuts, shellfish, fish, fruit) to allergen-specific IgE on mast cells than is chronic urticaria, in which the cause usually remains uncertain. However, at least some of

these "idiopathic" cases may be due to histamine-releasing autoantibodies directed against the Fc fragment of cytophilic IgE or the FcεRI itself, which can be detected in vitro by a functional histamine release assay using heterologous basophils.

Physical Urticarias. The diagnosis can usually be suspected from the history, as the weals appear within minutes of the stimulus application and fade within an hour, except in delayed pressure urticaria and vibratory angioedema, in which deep weals develop several hours after the pressure stimulus and last up to 24 hours. Anaphylaxis may develop rarely. Physical urticarias are defined by the nature of the triggering stimulus, which can be pressure (delayed pressure urticaria), sweating (cholinergic urticaria), ultraviolet radiation (solar urticaria), cold (cold urticaria), heat (localized heat urticaria), water (aquagenic urticaria), and vibration (vibratory angioedema). A combination of physical stimuli may be required to initiate wealing in some patients (summation urticaria), and this can cause difficulties in reproducing the rash in a clinic setting and make the diagnosis harder to establish. Physical urticarias can coexist with ordinary urticaria. An association between delayed pressure urticaria and chronic idiopathic urticaria is well recognized.

C_1 Esterase Inhibitor Deficiency. Although C_1 esterase inhibitor deficiency is a very uncommon cause of angioedema, its recognition is essential because swellings of the throat and respiratory submucosa can be fatal. Bowel involvement may present as an acute abdomen. It can be defined by laboratory tests and treated effectively. Deep painful swellings can occur anywhere on the body surface but typical urticarial weals are not seen and itch is not a feature. It can be hereditary or acquired.

Urticarial Vasculitis. This systemic disease tends to present to rheumatologists rather than dermatologists because joint symptoms often predominate. Patients can also show evidence of renal, gastrointestinal, pulmonary, or central nervous system involvement. The skin presentation ranges from weals that are indistinguishable from those of chronic urticaria to papules, erythema multiforme–like plaques, and angioedema. The diagnosis should be suspected if individual weals persist for more than 2 days or show hemorrhage. They may cause burning discomfort rather than itch. Histologically there is a small vessel vasculitis. The erythrocyte sedimentation rate is nearly always raised, and there may be evidence of early complement pathway activation with anaphylatoxin generation and immune complex formation. Serum IgG antibodies to C_{1q} have been found in some patients. The hypocomplementemic presentation of urticarial vasculitis tends to be associated with more severe systemic complications, including nephritis.

Contact Urticaria. This type is usually diagnosed and managed easily because the stimulus (often of plant or animal origin) elicits an immediate weal and can therefore be recognized and avoided. Both immunologic and nonimmunologic stimuli of mast cell degranulation are recognized.

TREATMENT

The cause of urticaria should be identified and avoided whenever possible. The therapeutic op-

Mr. Ian Small, Pharmacy Manager, BUPA Hospital, Norwich, England provided helpful criticism of the manuscript.

tions are summarized in Table 1. Antihistamines are the mainstay of treatment for all patterns of urticaria except C_1 esterase inhibitor deficiency and urticarial vasculitis. Although stabilization of mast cells should theoretically offer the most rational approach to the therapy of the mast cell–mediated urticarias, currently available drug treatments are relatively ineffective. This paucity of safe and effective agents explains the wide range of therapeutic avenues that have been explored and the difficulty in achieving complete disease suppression in many patients.

Ordinary Urticaria. Exposure to stimuli that encourage cutaneous vasodilatation, such as heat and alcohol, should be minimized. Aspirin and nonsteroidal anti-inflammatory drugs should in general be avoided, although tolerance may develop with repeated exposures. Urticaria patients requiring opiates may need an alternative analgesic. Trace levels of penicillin in dairy products may be a contributory factor in urticaria patients shown to be hypersensitive to penicillin by patch or intracutaneous testing. A diet free of food coloring, antioxidants, and benzoate, should be advised for highly motivated patients. Other exclusion diets are generally unhelpful if a precipitant is not obvious from the history. Oral challenge with a food additive series may be performed but is seldom successful in revealing the cause of

TABLE 1. **Therapeutic Interventions**

Mediator Antagonists and Inhibitors
Antihistamines
   H_1 receptor antagonists (nonsedating, sedating, or combinations of both)
   Combination of an H_2 receptor antagonist and an H_1 receptor antagonist
Nonsteroidal anti-inflammatory drugs*,†

Mast Cell Stabilizers
Terbutaline (increases intracellular cyclic AMP)
Nifedipine (modifies calcium flux)

Therapies for C_1 Esterase Inhibitor Deficiency
Tranexamic acid, Σ-aminocaproic acid (antifibrinolytics)
Stanozolol, danazol (attenuated androgens)
C_1 esterase inhibitor concentrate (steam-treated lyophilized human blood product)
Fresh-frozen plasma

Adrenaline

Oral Corticosteroids*,†

Immunosuppressive Protocols
Plasmapheresis*,‡,§

Miscellaneous
Dapsone*
Colchicine*
Hydroxychloroquine*

*Urticarial vasculitis.
†Delayed pressure urticaria.
‡Severe "autoimmune" chronic urticaria.
§Solar urticaria.

chronic idiopathic urticaria in the author's experience.

Antihistamines should be taken regularly in full doses. Several effective and well-tolerated nonsedating H_1 antagonists are now available, including astemizole, loratadine, terfenadine, and acrivistine. Cetirizine, a metabolite of hydroxyzine, is classed as a minimally sedating antihistamine. Only astemizole, loratadine and terfenadine are currently available in the United States. Astemizole (Hismanal) differs from the others in having a notably longer half-life (1 to 3 days for the parent drug, 12 days for the active metabolite) and a more prolonged onset of action. It is taken in a 10 mg daily dose. Adverse effects include appetite stimulation and weight gain in some individuals. Loratadine (Claritin) is also taken as a 10 mg daily dose but has a shorter half-life (14 hours for the parent drug, 19 hours for the metabolite). Clinical comparisons suggest that terfenadine (Seldane), 60 mg twice daily, is probably the least effective of the newer nonsedating antihistamines for urticaria symptom control. Administration should be avoided in patients with hepatic impairment or QT interval prolongation and in those taking erythromycin, other macrolides, or azole antifungals, including ketoconazole (Nizoral), and itraconazole (Sporanox), because ventricular arrythmias have been reported. Combining a nonsedating with a sedating antihistamine at night, such as hydroxyzine (Atarax, Vistaril), 10 to 75 mg, or chlorpheniramine, 4 to 12 mg, can be helpful for patients whose sleep is disturbed by nocturnal weals. Tricyclic antidepressants with H_1 antagonist properties, such as doxepin (Sinequan)*, 10 mg three times daily, can be as effective as sedating antihistamines in this respect. Addition of an H_2 receptor antagonist, such as ranitidine (Zantac)*, 150 mg two times daily, or cimetidine (Tagamet)*, 400 mg two times daily, sometimes improves urticaria control in patients who respond insufficiently to H_1 antagonists alone. H_2 antagonists are ineffective as monotherapy.

A mast cell stabilizing drug should be considered if urticaria symptoms cannot be controlled with antihistamines alone. These act by modifying calcium influx or raising intracellular cyclic AMP levels. Nifedipine (Adalat, Procardia)* 10 to 20 mg three times daily, has been shown to be useful both as monotherapy and in combination with antihistamines. Oral terbutaline (Brethaire)*, 1.25 to 5.0 mg three times daily, benefits some patients but palpitations and tremor tend

---

*These uses of doxepin, ranitidine, cimetidine, nifedipine, and terbutaline are not listed in the manufacturers' official directives.

to be dose limiting. Sodium cromoglycate (cromolyn sodium [Gastrocrom]), has not been shown to benefit chronic urticaria patients, probably due to its poor absorption from the bowel, although it may offer some protection against adverse reactions to foods.

"Second-line" therapies, including systemic steroids, immunosuppressive protocols, and antifibrinolytic agents should be reserved for patients with severe refractory disease. The beneficial effects of systemic steroids are anti-inflammatory rather than immunosuppressive at the relatively low doses required for chronic urticaria control in most patients (10 to 40 mg prednisolone daily). Anti-IgE–induced histamine release from basophils is also inhibited in vitro. Long-term steroid therapy should not be used in the routine management of chronic urticaria patients since the adverse effects nearly always outweigh the benefits. Plasmapheresis has been shown to induce temporary remission or improvement in selected chronic urticaria patients showing histamine releasing activity in their blood, but it is expensive and not without potential morbidity. Combined immunotherapy protocols, such as plasmapheresis with systemic steroids and azathioprine,* may result in more sustained remissions with fewer adverse effects, but careful clinical studies need to be performed before this approach can be recommended. The antifibrinolytic agent tranexamic acid* appears to be beneficial for some patients with chronic idiopathic urticaria, presumably by inhibiting plasmin-induced vasopermeability.

Epinephrine is invaluable for the emergency treatment of angioedema and severe acute urticarial reactions associated with asthma or anaphylaxis, but it has no place in the routine management of chronic urticaria. Patients with recurrent severe angioedema can be taught to self-administer 0.5 ml of 1:1000 epinephrine by subcutaneous or intramuscular injection.

Unsubstantiated reports of success have been attributed to a wide range of other therapies including anticoagulation with warfarin, photochemotherapy, relaxation therapy, and autologous blood injection but further controlled studies are required to define whether these interventions have any place in the routine management of chronic urticaria.

Physical Urticarias. The management of physical urticarias should follow the same principles detailed in the preceding section on ordinary urticaria. Many patients find antihistamines helpful in conjunction with lifestyle changes. Delayed pressure urticaria presents the most difficult therapeutic problem since antihistamines are usually ineffective. Indomethacin*, 25 to 50 mg three times daily, has been used with occasional success but the response is unpredictable when delayed pressure is associated with chronic idiopathic urticaria, which may be worsened by nonsteroidal anti-inflammatory drugs. Systemic steroids probably offer the most effective treatment but need to be maintained at relatively high doses. Solar urticaria has been treated successfully with plasmapheresis, photochemotherapy, and narrow waveband ultraviolet B phototherapy desensitization programs. Cold desensitization therapy for cold urticaria is more of theoretical than practical interest.

C_1 Esterase Inhibitor Deficiency. Treatment of hereditary C_1 esterase inhibitor deficiency should be based more on the patient's wellbeing than on absolute inhibitor levels, which tend to correlate poorly with clinical disease activity. Type 1 disease (inhibitor levels are reduced to 5 to 30% of normal) and Type II disease (normal antigenic levels of dysfunctional inhibitor) should be managed in the same way. Patients with the Type II variant remain able to produce small amounts of functional as well as the dysfunctional inhibitor in response to attenuated androgens.

The antifibrinolytic drugs tranexamic acid (Cyklokapron),* 0.5 to 1.0 gram daily, and ε-aminocaproic acid (Amicar),* 8 to 10 grams daily, are effective for long-term prophylaxis in many patients but are contraindicated when there is a history of thrombosis. Regular ophthalmic examinations and monitoring of liver function are recommended with use of tranexamic acid. Stimulation of endogenous C_1 inhibitor production by the attenuated androgen danazol (Danocrine), 200 to 600 mg daily, is now the treatment of choice except during pregnancy. Menstrual irregularities and mild virilizing effects such as hirsutism can be minimized by maintaining the dose as low as possible. Many patients can be controlled on as little as 200 mg daily 5 days a week. Liver function needs to be checked periodically and serial measurements of C_1 esterase inhibitor can be valuable in monitoring the response to treatment. Stanozolol (Winstrol), 1 to 5 mg daily, is also effective and less expensive.

Short-term prophylaxis for patients undergoing traumatic procedures such as dental work can be achieved with antifibrinolytic drugs, attenuated androgens, or inhibitor replacement with purified C_1 esterase inhibitor concentrate infusion† or

---

*These uses of azathioprine and tranexamic acid are not listed in the manufacturers' official directive.

*These uses of indomethacin, tranexamic acid, and ε-aminocaproic acid are not listed in the manufacturers' official directive.

†Available in the United Kingdom on a named patient basis from Immuno, Vienna, Austria.

fresh-frozen plasma (FFP) if the concentrate is unavailable. Angioedema attacks should be treated in an emergency with purified C_1 esterase inhibitor concentrate infusion or FFP. Theoretically FFP, which contains the substrates for activated C_1, C_2, and C_4 as well as C_1 esterase inhibitor could cause an initial worsening of the angioedema but in practice this is not a serious limitation. Adrenaline and intravenous hydrocortisone can be given but are relatively ineffective. There is no place for the prophylactic or emergency use of antihistamines. Patients with upper airway obstruction or dysphagia should be hospitalized without delay as they may require intubation or tracheostomy.

Elderly patients presenting with acquired C_1 esterase inhibitor deficiency should be investigated and treated for an underlying paraproteinemia.

Urticarial Vasculitis. There are no ideal treatments for this uncommon systemic disease. Antihistamines are widely used for the urticarial component but are often disappointing because histamine is not the major mediator of the edema. Systemic steroids (up to 1 mg per kg per day prednisolone) may be required to suppress disease activity and prevent relapse. As the majority of patients with urticarial vasculitis follow a chronic but benign course, it is preferable to explore alternative therapies to minimize long-term adverse effects. Indomethacin*, 25 to 50 mg three times daily, dapsone*, 50 to 150 mg per day, colchicine*, 0.5 mg two to three times daily, and hydroxychloroquine (Plaquenil)*, 200 to 400 mg daily, may be helpful for some patients.

Patients taking dapsone must be monitored for anemia, which can be rapid and severe if they are deficient in glucose-6-phosphate dehydrogenase. Treatment with immunosuppressive agents including plasmapheresis, pulsed cyclophosphamide, azathioprine, and gold should probably be given under the supervision of clinicians experienced in their use.

---

*These uses of indomethacin, dapsone, colchicine, and hydroxychloroquine are not listed in the manufacturers' official directive.

PIGMENTARY DISORDERS OF THE SKIN

method of
JOEL E. BERNSTEIN, M.D.
Lincolnshire, Illinois

Normal skin color is dependent on melanin pigmentation (brown), oxygenated and reduced hemoglobin (red and blue), and carotenoids (yellow). Of these, melanin is by far the most important color determinant, and racial and ethnic differences in skin color depend on the number, size, shape, and distribution of melanin-containing structures, the melanosomes. Although many factors can produce local or general changes in the color of the skin (including hemosiderin and metallic pigments), disorders of melanin pigmentation are both the most common and the most important and constitute what is generally meant by the term "pigmentary disorders."

Disorders of melanin pigmentation are of two varieties: (1) increased melanin in the skin (hypermelanosis or hyperpigmentation); or (2) decreased melanin in the skin (hypomelanosis or hypopigmentation).

While the underlying causes of these disorders may vary, the clinical consequences are identical—either hyper- or hypopigmentation.

DISORDERS INVOLVING REDUCED PIGMENT IN THE SKIN

Vitiligo

Vitiligo is characterized by a loss of cutaneous melanocytes and resulting depigmentation. This idiopathic disorder affects from 1 to 3% of all races, is often familial (30 to 40%), and is associated with a variety of disorders considered to be of autoimmune etiology. A number of chemicals, including phenolic household cleaning solutions, can produce similar depigmentation.

Treatment

Treatment of vitiligo has been less than satisfactory. The dermatologic armamentarium for repigmenting skin is small. Some patients have very limited disease and may require little more than reassurance about the benign nature of the disorder and instruction in the use of cosmetic camouflage preparations for lesions on exposed areas. Effective preparations include cosmetic makeup (Covermark) and temporary skin dyes (Vitadye, Dy-O-Derm). In sunny climates, a protective sun screen should be recommended to reduce the contrast between amelanotic and adjacent normal skin.

In patients with less than 25% skin involvement, several treatment approaches have been effective. If lesions are small and of recent onset, a short course of a moderate to potent topical corticosteroid (betamethasone valerate [Valisone], fluocinonide [Lidex], clobetasol propionate [Temovate]) may be beneficial. Intralesional injections of a corticosteroid (Kenalog) are to be avoided as they frequently exacerbate the situation due to their atrophogenic effects. For localized, long-standing areas of vitiligo two other approaches have produced good therapeutic results. Improvement is seen with topical daily application (TID) of 0.025% capsaicin cream (Zostrix) to affected areas followed by very short bi- or tri-weekly exposure to an artificial source of ultraviolet B radiation (UVB = 290 to 320 nm). Repigmentation is observed in more than 50% of patients so treated over a 4 to 16 week period. The only side effect of consequence is transient burning or stinging at sites of application, which occurs in about 40% of patients and can be severe enough to limit the course of therapy.

A second approach is the topical application of psoralens coupled with exposure to an artificial source of ultraviolet A radiation (UVA = 320 to 400 nm). This therapy, topical PUVA, has proved useful in a number of patients, although the therapeutic to toxic ratio is low and undesirable phototoxic responses are common. A frequently employed regimen is to apply a 1.0% solution of methoxsalen (Oxsoralen), wait 30 minutes and then expose the skin to UVA. The initial UVA dose is 0.12 to 0.25 joules per cm², increased weekly to up to 2.0 joules per cm² depending upon the patient's skin type. After moderate asymptomatic erythema is achieved, the weekly UVA dosage should be maintained at a level necessary to retain this degree of erythema. Severe blistering and reversible border hyperpigmentation are common side effects. Exposure to sunlight should be avoided since phototoxic reactions are frequent.

For more extensive involvement (>25% of the skin surface) or when the previously described localized approaches have failed or are impractical, a combination of oral psoralens and exposure to UVA (PUVA) is often utilized. PUVA induces melanocyte proliferation at borders of vitiliginous lesions as well as melanocyte migration into depigmented areas. Standard treatment protocols call for an oral dosage of 0.3 to 0.45 mg per kg of 8-methoxsalen 1 to 1½ hours before exposure to UVA. Treatment is initiated with 1 to 2 joules per cm² on the initial visit and increased 1 joule every other visit until moderate but asymptomatic erythema develops. Significant repigmentation is usually apparent following 3 to 5 months of bi-weekly or triweekly treatments. One hundred or more treatments may be required, and those who have demonstrated no evidence of repigmentation following 20 treatments are considered treatment failures. Before initiating PUVA treatment, a baseline eye examination is performed, which is repeated every 6 to 12 months to monitor the development of cataracts. A prior history of photosensitivity or collagen vascular disease are contraindications for PUVA.

When repigmentation fails or cannot be attempted in patients with very extensive lesions (>50% of the skin surface), depigmentation of remaining melanized skin with topical applications of 20% monobenzyl ether of hydroquinone (Benoquin) is sometimes utilized. Twice daily applications are continued for 1 year or longer and may result in irreversible depigmentation. Such an approach has many risks both medically and psychosocially and should be carefully considered before being employed as a last resort.

Repigmentation by surgical implantation of autologous punch grafts of pigmented skin in the depigmented areas has had some reported success. Such procedures should be performed only by practitioners highly experienced in such techniques.

Postinflammatory Hypopigmentation

Hypomelanotic areas can be associated with or follow the resolution of a wide variety of inflammatory dermatoses, most commonly eczema and psoriasis. The intensity of the inflammatory reaction does not necessarily correlate with the degree of subsequent hypopigmentation. Generally, areas of postinflammatory hypopigmentation repigment slowly over weeks or months. Twice-a-day application of a low potency corticosteroid cream or lotion (Hytone, Texacort) may accelerate resolution.

Idiopathic Guttate Hypomelanosis

This entity is characterized by sharply defined porcelain-white macules (2 to 6 mm) occurring most frequently on the sun-exposed limbs. These lesions usually appear after age 20 and may increase in number and size with age. No treatment is necessary for this benign dermatosis. However, if lesions are numerous and the patient is concerned about the cosmetic deformity, intralesional triamcinolone (Kenalog), gentle freezing with liquid nitrogen, or camouflage makeup can provide some cosmetic improvement.

Albinism

Albinism is a genetically inherited disorder of the pigmentary system in which melanin synthesis is reduced or absent. The disorder affects melanocytes of the skin, hair, and eyes, manifests in a number of different variants, and varies in prevalence in different races. In all races, there is a marked diminution of pigment in skin, hair, and eyes. While prognosis for the albino is good in temperate climates, it is much poorer in tropical climates, where most albinos develop severe solar damage at an early age, and some die young from squamous cell carcinomas and melanomas. There is no specific treatment, and management focuses on vigorous use of photoprotective preparations and the avoidance of sun exposure.

DISORDERS INVOLVING INCREASED PIGMENT IN THE SKIN

Melasma (Chloasma)

Melasma is a common acquired circumscribed hypermelanosis characterized by brownish macules with a predilection for the cheeks, forehead, upper lip, nose, and chin which become more apparent following sun exposure. It is far more common in females and is frequently observed during pregnancy. It is also common in women using oral contraceptives and in patients of both sexes taking phenytoin (Dilantin). Melasma usually fades slowly following delivery or termination of the offending medicament.

Avoidance of sun exposure is critical. In all seasons, patients should use an opaque broad-spectrum sunscreen (A-Fil, RVPaque) every morning. The radiation that stimulates hyperpigmentation is not only found in the UVB range, but also in the UVA and visible range, and therefore, colorless UVB absorbing sunscreens are of limited value. Topical application of preparations containing from 2% (Eldopaque, Eldoquin) to 4% hydroquinone (Eldopaque Forte, Solaquin Forte) provide fair to good bleaching. The addition of 0.05% to 0.1% retinoic acid or hydrocortisone 1% to 2.5% to this regimen can provide greater benefit. The prolonged use of hydroquinone is not recommended. The monobenzyl ether of hydroquinone (Benoquin) should never be used in melasma therapy since it can cause irreversible depigmentation in disfiguring confetti-like spots both at sites of application and at distant sites.

Postinflammatory Hyperpigmentation

Hypermelanosis commonly follows acute or chronic inflammatory processes in the skin. The degree of inflammation does not always correlate with the degree of hyperpigmentation, being frequent and severe after some conditions and uncommon and mild after others. The most common skin conditions associated with postinflammatory hyperpigmentation are acne, eczemas, drug eruptions, lichen planus, and traumas such as burns or dermabrasion. Topical hydroquinone-containing bleaching agents are not very effective in postinflammatory hyperpigmentation, and management is directed at control of the primary skin problem.

Lentigines

Lentigines are benign pigmented macules that contain increased numbers of melanocytes. They are usually first noted after age 40 and occur on light-exposed areas such as the face and hands. These are often referred to as senile lentigines or popularly as "liver spots." The term "lentiginosis" is utilized when lentigines are present in exceptionally large numbers, and such abundance may suggest a clinical syndrome associated with a variety of medical abnormalities. Sun avoidance and use of sunscreens may delay or prevent emergence of such lesions. Regular application of 2 to 4% hydroquinone-containing creams may induce temporary lightening. Topical retinoic acid (Retin-A) preparations have been used recently with some success to decrease the intensity of pigmentation. The retinoic acid preparation is generally applied with a frequency that varies from once daily to two to three times per week according to the tolerance of the patient. Freezing lentigines with liquid nitrogen is a very common office-based technique that produces temporarily beneficial results.

Ephelides (Freckles)

Freckling is a genetically determined benign condition characterized by numerous 3- to 5-mm light-brown macules in sun-exposed areas. It is most common in redheads or blondes with blue eyes. Histologically characteristic of ephelides, in contrast to lentigines, are melanocytes that are long and rod-shaped but not increased in number. Freckles may be cosmetically disfiguring if numerous, but are otherwise benign. Broad-spectrum sunscreens (A-Fil, RVPaque) have been tried with mixed success. Ephelides can be peeled off after brief freezing with liquid nitrogen.

OCCUPATIONAL DERMATITIS

method of
ELIZABETH F. SHERERTZ, M.D.
Bowman Gray School of Medicine of Wake Forest University
Winston-Salem, North Carolina

The most common skin disease in the work place is contact dermatitis, which can be caused by irritants (e.g., direct or cumulative skin damage due to chemicals, water, soaps) or allergens (i.e., immunologic reaction to specific allergic substance). The most common site (80%) for occupational dermatitis is the hands. Any skin sites that are affected by work exposures, including airborne exposures, protective gear, or ultraviolet light, may be involved.

Occupations at risk for contact dermatitis include a variety of jobs in which the hands are frequently in and out of water or liquid chemicals. Housekeeping, health care, food processing, hairdressing, metal working, and machine tool production are examples of wet-work situations. Industrial processes in which there is exposure to potential allergens (e.g., nickel-plated metals, rubber chemicals or products, formaldehyde or formaldehyde resins, epoxy, chromate) are also associated with higher risks of occupational contact dermatitis. An accurate history of job tasks and exposure is key in evaluating a patient with suspected job-related dermatitis.

Irritant contact dermatitis represents 80% of occupational skin diseases. The nature of the irritating chemical, its concentration, and the duration or frequency of skin contact contribute to the clinical appearance, which can range from a blistering chemical burn at contact sites to a mild chapped, red or glazed appearance in the finger webs. Allergic contact dermatitis (e.g., poison ivy or oak in a forestry worker, glove dermatitis in a health care worker) presents acutely with pruritic vesicular eruptions at the contact sites, but it can subsequently spread to sites adjacent to and beyond areas of direct contact with the allergen. Secondary infection with *Staphylococcus aureus* or group A beta-hemolytic streptococci commonly occurs in fissured or crusted acute dermatitis. Chronic contact dermatitis is often manifested as thickened, scaling hyperkeratotic skin that may develop painful fissures.

Contact urticaria is an immediate reaction that is increasingly reported, particularly among health care workers using latex gloves. It presents as immediate redness, edema, and hives when gloves are worn. The lesions can evolve into vesicular hand dermatitis.

MANAGEMENT

Acute Dermatitis

Identification of irritant or allergic triggering factors in the work place should be sought through history and a description of job tasks. Skin patch testing with available allergens can document contact allergy, but there is no simple skin test to document irritant causes.

For acute vesicular dermatitis, temporary removal from job exposures is often indicated. Astringent dressings with tap water or Burow's solution (Domeboro, Bluboro) compresses are helpful.

Topical corticosteroids applied once or twice daily are often used. Ointment bases for the corticosteroids are preferable to creams, which have more vehicle ingredients and preservatives, to minimize additional chemicals in contact with the damaged, inflamed skin. Midpotency or high-potency corticosteroids, such as triamcinolone (Aristocort, Kenalog) or fluocinonide (Lidex) may be used on the hands. Less potent types, such as hydrocortisone (Hytone) or desonide (Tridesilon), are preferable for the face. Early in the course of severe, acute dermatitis, systemic corticosteroids (e.g., 40 to 60 mg of prednisone orally in a single morning dose for 2 to 3 weeks, with optional tapering) may be helpful. Shorter treatment courses of steroids often lead to a rapid rebound

of the dermatitis. Evaluation to clarify the precipitating events (e.g., patch testing) should be done after the patient has completed systemic corticosteroid treatment. Systemic antihistamines are often prescribed to help control itching, but many types have sedating effects that may interfere with safe job performance.

If significant pain, pustules, or golden-crusting occurs within the dermatitis, bacterial infection (e.g., impetigo, cellulitis) should be suspected and treated with appropriate oral antibiotics, such as dicloxacillin (Dynapen), cephalexin (Keflex), or erythromycin (Ethril), usually in doses of 1 gram daily administered in divided doses. Amoxicillin-clavulanic acid (Augmentin), in doses of 250 mg orally every 8 hours, is also useful. Neomycin-containing topical antibiotics and medicated petrolatum should be avoided, because these products cause contact allergy in a few patients. Caution should be used in recommending rubber gloves for protection until it is determined if a rubber allergy has contributed to the original problem. Vinyl gloves with cotton liners should be suggested for hand protection.

Chronic Dermatitis

For dry, thickened skin, hydration and emollients or lubricants are the most important therapeutic modalities. Plain white petrolatum (Vaseline) or mineral oil with polyethylene (Plastibase) should be applied after the skin has been soaked in water (e.g., after bathing). Other moisturizing creams or lotions have additional ingredients, such as fragrance or preservatives, that may further irritate the skin and prolong the healing time.

Protection and Education

Job modification or medical leave of absence may be indicated during the period of active dermatitis. However, a declaration of the "need to change jobs" should not be made lightly, because this may have devastating economic consequences and often does not solve the dermatitis problem. If contact dermatitis is diagnosed, appropriate impervious gloves that prevent skin contact from the offending chemicals may be helpful. Barrier creams are not usually beneficial. A change of industrial process to reduce direct skin contact with the offending agent(s) is sometimes indicated, particularly if more than one worker is affected. It is important to educate the patient or employee, business personnel, and medical caregivers about the nature of the problem and the need to avoid potentially aggravating exposures at work, at home, through hobbies, or by the topical treatment. Rapid recovery should not be predicted, because occupational contact dermatitis carries a poor prognosis: 75% of patients need continued medical management, even after a job change.

Other Occupational Dermatoses

Although contact dermatitis is by far the most important type of occupational skin disease, several others are worthy of mention. Acne may develop or pre-existing acne may worsen with some job exposures, particularly to oils, tars, or other petroleum distillates. Mechanical factors, such as friction of clothing or protective gear, may also contribute to acne lesions. The distribution may be on the arms and under clothing even more so than on the face. Treatment is aimed at reducing skin exposure to the irritant by protective and hygienic measures. Routine acne therapy with topical retinoic acid (Retin-A) and topical or oral antibiotics (e.g., erythromycin) is helpful.

Outdoor occupations (e.g., agriculture, road maintenance, construction) put workers (especially whites) at risk for ultraviolet radiation exposure, which produces sunburn and photoaging (e.g., wrinkles, thickened skin, actinic keratoses). Basal cell carcinoma and squamous cell carcinoma of the skin are associated with cumulative ultraviolet exposure. Protective clothing (e.g., hats, long sleeves) and daily sunscreen use can have a major impact.

SUNBURN AND PHOTOSENSITIVITY

method of
BERNHARD ORTEL, M.D.
University of Vienna
Vienna, Austria

The publicity regarding the potentially harmful effects of solar radiation has increased in the last few years. The growing incidence of malignant melanoma and the frightening reduction of the stratospheric ozone layer have attracted the interest of scientists and the public.

Sunlight contains a small fraction of radiation below 400 nm wavelength, the ultraviolet (UV) radiation. UVC (190 to 290 nm) is absorbed in the stratosphere and therefore does not reach the earth's surface. UVB (290 to 320 nm) is only partly absorbed by ozone and plays a biologically important role. UVA (320 to 400 nm) and UVB cause skin damage with greatly different efficiency. The knowledge that UV radiation is responsible for the development of skin cancer has made some people more cautious about sun bathing. The fact that the skin aging is closely related to UV exposure has done even more to raise public concern about excessive sun exposure.

SUNBURN

Virtually all light-skinned people experience a sunburn at some time. Sunburn is an erythematous skin reaction to solar UV exposure. Depending on skin type and the history of previous sun exposure, 10 to 50 mJ/cm^2 of UVB result in skin reddening. Assessment of endogenous pigmentation and hair and eye color may help in estimating individual sun sensitivity, but these parameters are not always reliable.

Individual UV sensitivity is defined by the minimal erythema dose (MED). This is the smallest radiation dose that suffices to induce a clearly visible erythema reaction. Higher UV doses result in edema, blister formation, and even skin necrosis. The time course of erythema depends on the peak intensity of the reaction and may even start during sun exposure. UVB erythema peaks around 24 hours after exposure and fades slowly over the next 3 days. With exposures to several MEDs, skin reactions persist longer. During the fading time of the erythema, pigmentation begins to develop. The tanning reaction depends on the skin type and the tanning history of the exposed area; previously exposed and tanned areas will develop more intense pigmentation.

For many years sunlight and UVB were considered synonymous. However, the role of UVA is becoming increasingly recognized. UVA is also erythemogenic and pigmentogenic but UVA MEDs lie three orders of magnitude above the UVB values. In the past few years, the public has become more aware of UVA for two reasons. First, commercially available tanning equipment use UVA sources to induce tan without the risk of UVB burn (these radiation sources emit 0.1% or less of UVB), and this may result in UVA exposure levels that would be impossible to reach with natural sunlight. The second reason for increased UVA exposure is, paradoxically, the development of sunscreen products with high sun protection factors (SPFs). The SPF value represents the factor by which the MED of an individual is expanded by adequate use of the product. This factor, however, is determined in the UVB range. Although some products contain UVA absorbers, the SPF in the UVA range never reaches the same magnitude as in the UVB range. This means that people using sunscreens may expose themselves to higher UVA doses than they otherwise might.

Little is known about the processes by which UV causes erythema. It has been shown that arachidonic acid and eicosanoids play a role in the early phase of erythema formation. Interleukin-1 and 6 are also associated with systemic effects of severe sunburn.

Treatment

Topical steroids and cool compresses are helpful in the management of moderate sunburn. Aspirin and indomethacin can be employed for more extensive sunburn, but the use of systemic steroids is controversial. Severe sunburns resemble first to second degree burns and can be accompanied by fever, malaise, and dehydration. Hospitalization may be required in such cases and the treatment should follow guidelines for thermal burns.

It is important to remember that even a severe sunburn will soon be forgotten by the patient. But no matter how well a sunburn is treated, the UV-induced DNA damage can remain in the cells for many years and may become a source of skin cancer. Therefore, use of topical sunscreens and a sensible attitude toward recreational sun exposure are recommended.

PHOTOSENSITIVITY

Photosensitivity is an abnormal reaction to nonionizing radiation. It can be classified according to etiology into four groups: (1) genetic and metabolic photosensitivity (e.g., xeroderma pigmentosum, Bloom's syndrome, porphyrias, pellagra); (2) light-induced reactions to exogenous sensitizers (phototoxicity and photoallergy); (3) idiopathic sun sensitivity (polymorphous light eruption, hydroa vacciniforme, solar urticaria); and (4) conditions that are precipitated or aggravated by sunlight (e.g., lupus erythematosus, herpes simplex, atopic dermatitis, Darier's disease).

Photosensitivity can be suspected by the patient, suggested by the history, or evident because of typical distribution of skin lesions. The upper eyelids, the submental and retroauricular areas, and areas covered by heavy clothing are usually spared.

The most common photodermatosis is polymorphous light eruption (PMLE), an idiopathic condition with a preference for young women. Despite variation in presentation among different individuals, a single patient will develop the same kind of skin lesions with repeated outbreaks. PMLE is common among people who travel from moderate climate to sunny countries where they receive relatively high amounts of radiation without benefit of prior adaptation. Within hours or days this can provoke an outbreak of mostly papular or papulovesicular lesions accompanied by intense pruritus. In most patients the V-shaped area of the neck, the face, and the dorsa of the hands are involved, but usually not all sun-exposed skin.

In mild cases, sunscreens and greater caution at the beginning of sun exposure may be preventive. However, most patients are sensitive in the UVA range and derive no benefit from topical sunscreens. Beta-carotene, nicotinamide, and chloroquine have been used but are of little more use than placebo treatment. In severe cases, phototherapy and photochemotherapy have been most effective for the prevention of PMLE.

Manifest disease is usually treated satisfactorily with topical steroids and oral antihistamines. More severe outbreaks are managed with oral steroids. After several years of repeated outbreaks, spontaneous remission is common.

In the differential diagnosis of PMLE it is necessary to exclude photosensitive lupus erythematosus (LE). Usually, the history and clinical presentation are sufficient to rule out LE. If doubt remains, it is mandatory to take biopsies for histology and direct immunofluorescence, and to perform serologic tests for antinuclear, anti-Ro/SSA, and anti-La/SSB antibodies.

Exogenous photosensitizers can induce a phototoxic reaction or a photoallergic response. Phototoxicity is more common and represents a dose-dependent phenomenon. The wide spectrum of clinical manifestations includes mostly erythema and increased pigmentation but can include everything from sunburn to sclerodermiform changes.

Antibiotics (e.g., tetracyclines, sulfonamides), nonsteroidal anti-inflammatory drugs, and diuretics are among the systemic agents that can cause phototoxicity. Plant-derived psoralens are known to cause a phototoxic reaction called phytophotodermatitis after accidental localized contact, with such sources as weeds, celery, lime peel, and figs.

Photoallergy is a delayed-type hypersensitivity that is induced as well as challenged only by the simultaneous exposure to the sensitizer and radiation. Antimicrobial agents that were notorious for inducing photoallergy have mostly been superseded by newer drugs. Some of them, however, have been reused recently in animals and have caused photosensitization in cattle breeders. Fragrances such as musk ambrette and 6-methylcourmarin are common photoallergens. The increased use of sunscreens has demonstrated that PABA, benzophenones, and cinnamates are allergenic and also photoallergenic.

In photosensitivity disease, light testing is an important diagnostic tool. First, threshold radiation doses with UVB, UVA, and sometimes visible light are determined. In solar urticaria, this first exposure can also be diagnostic. Phototesting with repeated doses aims at the reproduction of lesions under artificial conditions. Photopatch testing (a UVA-exposed patch test) helps to identify phototoxic and photoallergenic sensitizers.

Primary therapy of photosensitivity follows the guidelines for treatment of the clinically presented lesions, which means that (photoallergic) dermatitis is treated with topical steroids and (solar) urticaria with antihistamines. However, once the sensitizer is identified, it must be eliminated whenever possible. If this is impossible (e.g., in genetic or idiopathic photosensitivity disease), protection from solar and artificial radiation sources is required to prevent relapses and delayed cumulative effects.

BRAIN ABSCESS

method of
ALLAN R. TUNKEL, M.D., PH.D.
Medical College of Pennsylvania
Philadelphia, Pennsylvania

Brain abscess is one of the most serious complications of head and neck infections. Despite the introduction of antibiotics, mortality rates (40 to 60%) from brain abscess remained stable until recently. The current mortality rate is between 5 and 10%, an improvement that is probably due to advances in diagnosis with computed tomography (CT) and magnetic resonance imaging (MRI) and treatment during the last decade. The incidence of brain abscess varies geographically, with about 4 to 10 cases seen annually in active neurosurgical services in developed countries.

Microorganisms can reach the brain by several different mechanisms. The factors predisposing to the development of brain abscess and the etiologic agents for each circumstance are shown in Table 1. Knowledge of these pathogenic mechanisms is helpful in initiating empirical antimicrobial therapy after a brain abscess has been diagnosed. The most common mechanism is spread from a contiguous focus of infection, usually from the middle ear, mastoid cells, or paranasal sinuses. Hematogenous dissemination to the brain from a distant focus of infection (e.g., lung, cardiac valves, bone, skin, abdomen, pelvis) may also occur; these abscesses are usually multiple and multiloculated and have a higher mortality rate than abscesses that arise from a contiguous focus of infection. Trauma is a third pathogenic mechanism. Brain abscess can occur after an open cranial fracture with dural breech, after neurosurgery, or after foreign body injuries. Brain abscess is cryptogenic in approximately 20% of cases.

Among bacterial species causing brain abscess formation, streptococci (e.g., aerobic, anaerobic, microaerophilic) are most commonly isolated (60 to 70%). These bacteria (particularly *Streptococcus milleri*) normally reside in the oral cavity, appendix, and female genital tract and have a proclivity for abscess formation. *Staphylococcus aureus* accounts for 10 to 15% of bacterial isolates, although this frequency is increased among patients with bacterial endocarditis or cranial trauma. Attention to proper culture techniques has increased the isolation frequency of anaerobic organisms, particularly *Bacteroides* species, which are isolated in 20 to 40% of cases, often in mixed culture. Enteric gram-negative bacilli (e.g., *Proteus* species, *Escherichia coli, Klebsiella* species, *Pseudomonas* species) are isolated in 23 to 33% of cases, most commonly in patients with an otitic source of infection.

Isolation frequencies of certain bacterial pathogens are different in infants and children; streptococci were isolated in 16%, staphylococci in 23%, gram-negative aerobic bacilli in 35%, and anaerobes in 23% of pediatric cases. Other bacterial species that occur less commonly (<1%) as etiologic agents of brain abscess include *Haemophilus influenzae* and *Streptococcus pneumoniae*.

Listeria monocytogenes and *Nocardia asteroides* have a predilection for the immunocompromised host (i.e., patients with T lymphocyte or mononuclear defects), although as many as 48% of patients with nocardial infection have no obvious immunocompromising condition. Brain abscess due to *Actinomyces* species is commonly associated with a pulmonary or odontogenic focus of infection. Space-occupying lesions due to *Mycobacterium tuberculosis* were thought to be rare, but focal lesions (tuberculomas) have been observed on CT scans for a minority of cases of tuberculous meningitis.

Fungi are important etiologic agents of brain abscess due to the increased numbers of immunocompromised patients; mortality rates in patients with fungal brain abscesses remain extremely high. Patients with neutropenia or neutrophil defects are predisposed in infections with *Candida, Aspergillus,* and *Rhizopus.* Patients with diabetes mellitus and ketoacidosis are predisposed to the development of rhinocerebral mucormycosis; cerebral mucormycosis with abscess formation also occurs in intravenous drug abusers. *Cryptococcus neoformans* usually causes meningitis when it invades the central nervous system, but mass lesions due to this organism have also been observed. *Pseudallescheria boydii* may enter the central nervous system by direct trauma, hematogenous dissemination from a pulmonary source, through an intravenous catheter, or by direct extension from infected sinuses.

Various protozoa and helminths may cause brain abscesses. The incidence depends on the geographic locale and underlying conditions. The acquired immunodeficiency syndrome (AIDS) has become an important predisposing condition for the development of intracranial protozoal infections. *Toxoplasma gondii* is the leading cause (2.6 to 30.8%) of focal central nervous system disease in patients with AIDS. *Entamoeba histolytica* is the ameba most likely to cause a brain ab-

TABLE 1. **Empiric Antimicrobial Therapy for Bacterial Brain Abscess**

Predisposing Condition	Usual Bacterial Isolates	Antimicrobial Regimen
Otitis media or mastoiditis	Streptococci (anaerobic or aerobic), *Bacteroides* species, Enterobacteriaceae	Penicillin + metronidazole + a third-generation cephalosporin*
Sinusitis (frontoethmoidal or sphenoidal)	Streptococci, *Bacteroides* species, Enterobacteriaceae, *Staphylococcus aureus*, *Haemophilus* species	Vancomycin + metronidazole + a third-generation cephalosporin*
Dental sepsis	Mixed *Fusobacterium* and *Bacteroides* species, streptococci	Penicillin + metronidazole
Penetrating trauma or after neurosurgery	*Staphylococcus aureus*, streptococci, Enterobacteriaceae, *Clostridium*	Vancomycin + a third-generation cephalosporin*
Congenital heart disease	Streptococci, *Haemophilus* species	Penicillin + a third-generation cephalosporin*
Lung abscess, empyema, bronchiectasis	*Fusobacterium, Actinomyces, Bacteroides* species, streptococci, *Nocardia asteroides*	Penicillin + metronidazole + a sulfonamide†
Bacterial endocarditis	*Staphylococcus aureus*, streptococci	Vancomycin + gentamicin

*Cefotaxime or ceftriaxone; ceftazidime is used if *Pseudomonas aeruginosa* is suspected.
†Sulfadiazine or trimethoprim-sulfamethoxazole; include if *Nocardia asteroides* is suspected.

scess. Cysticercosis due to *Taenia solium* larvae is a major cause of brain lesions in the developing world.

TREATMENT

Antimicrobial Therapy

After a diagnosis of brain abscess is made presumptively by radiologic studies (CT or MRI) or by stereotactic CT-guided aspiration of the abscess, antimicrobial therapy should be initiated. Aspiration may provide an etiologic diagnosis on Gram's stain examination, but empirical antimicrobial therapy should be initiated based on the likely etiologic agent if a predisposing condition can be identified (Table 1). Due to the high rate of isolation of streptococci (particularly *S. milleri*) from brain abscesses, high-dose intravenous penicillin G or a third-generation cephalosporin, either cefotaxime (Claforan), or ceftriaxone (Rocephin), active against this organism should be included in the initial therapeutic regimens.

Penicillin G is also active against most anaerobic species (e.g., *Fusobacterium, Actinomyces*) with the notable exception of *Bacteroides fragilis*,

TABLE 2. **Antimicrobial Therapy for Brain Abscess**

Organism	Standard Therapy	Alternative Therapies
Actinomyces species	Penicillin G	Clindamycin
Aspergillus species	Amphotericin B*	Itraconazole†
Bacteroides fragilis	Metronidazole	Chloramphenicol, clindamycin
Candida species	Amphotericin B*	Fluconazole†
Cryptococcus neoformans	Amphotericin B*	Fluconazole
Enterobacteriaceae	Third-generation cephalosporin§	Aztreonam, trimethoprim-sulfamethoxazole, fluoroquinolone
Fusobacterium species	Penicillin G	Metronidazole
Haemophilus species	Third-generation cephalosporin§	Aztreonam, trimethoprim-sulfamethoxazole
Listeria monocytogenes	Ampicillin or penicillin G‖	Trimethoprim-sulfamethoxazole
Mycobacterium tuberculosis	Isoniazid, rifampin, pyrazinamide	
Nocardia asteroides	Trimethoprim-sulfamethoxazole or sulfadiazine	Minocycline, imipenem, a third-generation cephalosporin,§ fluoroquinolone
Pseudallescheria boydii	Miconazole	Fluconazole†
Pseudomonas aeruginosa	Ceftazidime‖	Aztreonam, fluoroquinolone
Staphylococcus aureus		
Methicillin-sensitive	Nafcillin or oxacillin	Vancomycin
Methicillin-resistant	Vancomycin	
Streptococcus milleri, other streptococci	Penicillin G	Third-generation cephalosporin,§ vancomycin
Toxoplasma gondii	Pyrimethamine + sulfadiazine	Pyrimethamine + clindamycin, azithromycin†

*Addition of flucytosine should be considered.
†Efficacy not yet proven in brain abscess due to this organism.
§Cefotaxime or ceftriaxone.
‖Addition of an aminoglycoside should be considered.

which is isolated in 20 to 40% of brain abscess cases. If *B. fragilis* is suspected, metronidazole (Flagyl) should be added; chloramphenicol (Chloromycetin) or clindamycin (Cleocin) is reserved if metronidazole cannot be used. The advantages of metronidazole over these other agents include its bactericidal activity against *B. fragilis* and its high concentrations in brain abscess pus, and its entry into cerebral abscesses is not affected by concomitant corticosteroid administration. Metronidazole, when substituted for chloramphenicol, may lead to more rapid healing and lower mortality in patients with anaerobic brain abscesses.

If *S. aureus* is a likely infecting pathogen (e.g., as a result of cranial trauma or after neurosurgery), nafcillin (Unipen) should be used, with vancomycin (Vancocin), which penetrates well into brain abscess fluid, reserved for the patient allergic to penicillin or when methicillin-resistant *S. aureus* is suspected or documented. For empirical therapy when members of the Enterobacteriaceae family are suspected (e.g., abscesses of otitic origin), a third-generation cephalosporin (cefotaxime or ceftriaxone) or trimethoprim-sulfamethoxazole (Bactrim) should be used. If *P. aeruginosa* is a likely infecting pathogen, ceftazidime (Fortaz) is the third-generation cephalosporin of choice. However, the regimen must also include penicillin G to treat a possible streptococcal infection, because ceftazidime has unreliable gram-positive activity. Direct instillation of antibiotics (usually bacitracin or penicillin) into the abscess cavity during aspiration has frequently been employed, although the efficacy of this practice has never been established. When a brain abscess due to *Nocardia* is suspected or proven, the sulfonamides, with or without trimethoprim, are a reasonable first choice for treatment.

After the infecting pathogen is isolated, antimicrobial therapy can be modified. Recommendations for therapy, with alternative agents, are shown in Table 2. Dosages of these agents for adults with central nervous system infections are shown in Table 3. High-dose intravenous antibiotics for bacterial brain abscess should be continued for 4 to 6 weeks and are often followed by oral antibiotic therapy for 2 to 6 months if an appropriate agent is available. Shorter courses of therapy (3 to 4 weeks) may be adequate for patients who have undergone surgical excision of the abscess. Some form of surgical therapy is often required for the optimal management of brain abscess, although certain subgroups of patients usually receive nonoperative management. These include patients with medical conditions that increase the risk of surgery, multiple abscesses, abscesses in a deep or dominant location, concomitant meningitis or ependymitis, early abscess reduction with clinical improvement after

TABLE 3. **Recommended Dosages of Antimicrobial Agents for Central Nervous System Infections in Adults**

Antimicrobial Agent	Total Daily Dosage*	Dosing Interval (hours)
Amikacin	15 mg/kg	8
Amphotericin B	0.6–1.0 mg/kg†	24
Ampicillin	12 gm	4
Aztreonam	6–8 gm	6–8
Cefotaxime	8–12 gm	4–6
Ceftazidime	6 gm	8
Ceftriaxone	4 gm	12
Chloramphenicol	4–6 gm	6
Ciprofloxacin	800 mg	12
Clindamycin	1200–4800 mg‡	6
Ethambutol§	15 mg/kg	24
Fluconazole	400 mg	24
Flucytosine§	150 mg/kg	6
Gentamicin	3–5 mg/kg	8
Isoniazid§	300 mg	24
Metronidazole	30 mg/kg	6
Miconazole	1.5–3.0 gm	8
Nafcillin	9–12 gm	4
Oxacillin	9–12 gm	4
Penicillin	24 million U	4
Pyrazinamide§	15–30 mg/kg	24
Pyrimethamine§	25–100 mg‡	24
Rifampin§	600 mg	24
Sulfadiazine§	4–6 gm	6
Tobramycin	3–5 mg/kg	8
Trimethoprim-sulfamethoxazole	10 mg/kg‖	12
Vancomycin	2 gm	12

*Patients with normal renal and hepatic function. Unless indicated, intravenous administration is used.

†Dosages up to 1.5 mg/kg/day may be used for aspergillosis or mucormycosis.

‡Higher dosages utilized in AIDS patients with toxoplasmic encephalitis.

§Oral administration.

‖Dosage based on trimethoprim component.

antimicrobial therapy, and an abscess smaller than 3 cm. Antimicrobial therapy for nocardial brain abscess has ranged from 3 to 12 months, although in immunocompromised patients, therapy should probably be continued for up to 1 year, with careful follow-up to monitor for relapse.

The optimal management of the human immunodeficiency virus (HIV)-infected patient with a focal central nervous system lesion remains controversial. Despite the broad range of possible etiologic infectious agents in this patient population, toxoplasmosis remains as the most common cause of abscess, especially if multiple enhancing lesions are observed on CT or MRI. In HIV-infected patients serologically positive for *Toxoplasma,* empirical therapy with pyrimethamine (Daraprim) plus sulfadiazine (Cremodiazine) is often employed; a clinical response is usually observed within 14 days of initiation of therapy. Brain biopsy should be performed immediately for serologically negative patients, for CT or MRI findings atypical for toxoplasmic encephalitis, and for patients who have evidence of dissemination of a different infecting pathogen.

Surgical Therapy

Most patients with bacterial brain abscess require surgical management for optimal therapy. The two procedures judged equivalent by outcome are aspiration of the abscess after burr hole placement and complete excision after craniotomy; the choice of procedure must be individualized for each patient. Aspiration may be performed by stereotactic CT guidance, affording the surgeon rapid, accurate (within 1 mm), and safe access for virtually any intracranial point; aspiration may also be used for rapid relief of increased intracranial pressure. A major disadvantage of aspiration is incomplete drainage of multiloculated abscesses, and these patients frequently require excision of the abscesses. Risks of aspiration include abscess rupture into the ventricle and leakage of pus into the subarachnoid space, leading to ventriculitis or meningitis.

Complete excision after craniotomy is most often employed for a patient with a stable neurologic condition. Some surgeons advocate excision if abscesses exhibit gas on radiologic evaluations and for posterior fossa abscesses. Surgery should be performed emergently in patients with worsening neurologic deficits, including deteriorating consciousness or signs of increased intracranial pressure. Excision is contraindicated in the early stages before a capsule is formed and occasionally due to abscess loculation. Excision is usually indicated for fungal brain abscesses because available drug treatment is unsatisfactory.

ALZHEIMER'S DISEASE

method of
VICTOR W. HENDERSON, M.D.
University of Southern California
Los Angeles, California

For years after the initial descriptions by Alois Alzheimer in 1907 and 1911, Alzheimer's disease (AD) was viewed as an uncommon dementing disorder with onset before age 65 years characterized by histopathologic findings of neurofibrillary tangles within cell bodies of vulnerable cerebral neurons and neuritic plaques within the cortical neurophil. It is now apparent that presenile and senile forms of the illness are not readily distinguished by clinical or pathologic features, and the term "Alzheimer's disease" is used without regard to the age at which the symptoms first appear.

An estimated 5 to 10% of persons older than age 65 years show moderate or severe dementia. AD is the most prevalent cause of dementia, accounting for at least one-half and perhaps three-quarters of all cases in most clinical or pathologic series; its incidence may be higher among women than men. About 85% of women and 70% of men in this country live to age 65 years or older. In the decades ahead, the trend toward increasing longevity will be exacerbated by the demographic bulge of aging post–World War II "baby boomers." Because the prevalence of AD increases dramatically with advancing age—even after age 65 years—the medical and societal importance of AD cannot be underestimated. Already, AD is represented as the fourth leading cause of death in this country.

The pathogenesis and etiology of AD remain obscure. Cytoskeletal abnormalities are prominent within vulnerable neurons in the cerebral cortex and elsewhere; in particular, an abnormally phosphorylated microtubule-associated protein *(tau)* seems to be an important constituent of the paired helical filaments. Paired helical filaments, in turn, are found within the neurofibrillary tangles and within the distended nerve processes of the neuritic plaques. A protein termed "beta-amyloid," derived from a normal chromosome 21 gene product, can also be found within plaque cores and within the cerebral vasculature. The relation between paired helical filaments and beta-amyloid is unclear. Abnormal neurites within the plaques may arise from tangle-containing neurons, and some pathologic features of AD appear to be transsynaptically mediated. The tangle formation and neuronal loss in AD affect cholinergic, noradrenergic, and serotonergic neurons that project widely to various brain regions.

Careful questioning will reveal a history of dementia consistent with AD in a first-degree relative of about one-half of AD cases. A positive family history is a significant risk factor for this disorder, although illnesses affecting more than one family member are not necessarily genetic, and the unambiguous differentiation of familial from nonfamilial AD can be formidable. The pedigree of some families strongly suggests an autosomal dominant pattern of inheritance. For several rare families, a missense point mutation in the chromosome 21 gene encoding the beta-amyloid precursor protein has been identified, but this gene is normal in other phenotypically similar families, some of whom have a defect on chromosome 14. For twins concordant for AD, the age at which dementia first appears can differ widely, and a number of identical twin pairs are discordant for this diagnosis. Although specific environmental determinants of AD have yet to be identified, it is almost certain that environmental factors will prove important in the pathogenesis of AD, at least in some instances.

DETERMINATION OF DEMENTIA

The term "dementia" refers to a decline in cognitive functioning of sufficient severity so as to interfere significantly with activities of daily living or with interpersonal, vocational, or avocational activities. Persons who are demented almost always have prominent memory deficits, as well as other cognitive disturbances. These can affect language, visuospatial skills, emotion and personality, or reasoning and judgment. The criteria for dementia determination are deficits in at least two cognitive domains; memory difficulties almost always represent one area of disturbance.

Dementia is more a symptom than a diagnosis, and the dementia determination depends on the clinical examination. Evaluation is directed both toward the documentation of dementia and the diagnosis of its cause. Most forms of dementia are treatable, and some are fully reversible.

The physician's assessment should include a careful medical, neurologic, and psychiatric history, a general physical examination, and a neurologic examination. Evaluation must also include mental status testing, more formal neuropsychologic evaluation (usually by a psychologist), or both. Dementia cannot be determined when consciousness is impaired by delirium, lethargy, or coma. The mental status assessment should include both behavioral observations and cognitive assessment. A bedside mental status examination or a short, formal cognitive screening instrument may overlook mild deficits that more extensive testing could uncover. Conversely, overreliance on scores from standardized tests can be misleading if the effects of education, primary language, motivation, distractions (e.g., as from a blaring television set in a common day room), or unrelated medical problems (e.g., headache that impairs concentration, arthritis that hinders responses on timed motor tasks, or poor hearing that impedes speech comprehension) are not considered.

DIAGNOSIS

Hippocampal and parahippocampal brain regions essential for the learning of new information are severely affected by AD pathology, and poor recall after an interval of several minutes or longer is an early and prominent sign of AD. Cortical association areas of the left and right cerebral hemispheres are also prominently involved, and language abnormalities (e.g., word-finding difficulty during spontaneous speech and on naming tasks) and visuospatial deficits (e.g., poor performance on line-drawing tasks) are commonly observed during mental status testing. Behavioral symptoms occur in many patients with AD. These include depression, agitation, delusions, or hallucinations.

The neurologic examination is usually normal in AD. Mild parkinsonian features, however, are found in some patients with otherwise typical AD. Bradykinesia and rigidity may be seen, but the resting tremor of Parkinson's disease is not characteristic of patients with dementia due to AD. For some patients with AD myoclonus or seizures can occur late in the disease course.

"Definite" AD

A certain diagnosis of AD in the demented patient, or "definite AD," requires histopathologic confirmation of characteristic brain alterations, almost always at the time of autopsy. Neuritic plaques, and to a lesser extent neurofibrillary tangles, are the diagnostic features most relied on by neuropathologists. It is important to recall, however, that tangles, plaques, and other pathologic and biochemical alterations of AD are not completely specific for this disorder. Tangles and

plaques, for example, can be seen in other diseases and in some nondemented older persons without evidence of dementia. It is the distribution and severity of the histopathologic features that best distinguish the AD-affected brain from changes that accompany so-called normal aging.

"Probable" and "Possible" AD

In the absence of histologic brain studies, the clinician is limited to a diagnosis of "probable AD." The criteria for probable AD (Table 1) prove to be accurate vis-à-vis postmortem validation about 70 to 90% of the time. Symptoms of AD usually begin insidiously and worsen gradually over time. This progressive course helps to distinguish AD from the second most prevalent cause of dementia, multiinfarct dementia, in which symptoms typically begin abruptly and cognitive deterioration occurs in a stepwise—not gradual—manner. When the clinical history is incomplete and the progressive nature of the symptoms is unclear, the physician may wish to reassess the patient in 6 to 12 months to see whether the cognitive skills evince a progressive decline over time. Plateaus in symptom progression are consistent with AD. It is important to recognize that caregivers occasionally report an abrupt onset of the symptoms occurring around the time of a stressful event, such as a surgical operation or the death of a spouse. Careful questioning in these instances usually reveals that some cognitive difficulties antedated the apparent precipitating event and confirm that symptoms have progressed since that time.

Short of a brain biopsy, there is yet no valid laboratory test for AD. Laboratory tests must be individually tailored to confirm or eliminate other systemic or neurologic illnesses that could account for the patient's dementia and to seek other medical conditions that might contribute to or exacerbate dementia symptoms. Laboratory investigations commonly ordered in the demented patient with suspected AD are given in Table 2. The cerebrospinal fluid is usually normal in AD. The electroencephalogram may be normal or show nonspecific slowing of the background rhythm. Brain imaging (computed tomographic scan or magnetic resonance imaging scan) may be normal or reveal atrophy. Atrophy, however, need not be present in AD, and some healthy older persons also show atrophy. The presence of punctate, hyperintense changes within the periventricular white matter on T2-weighted magnetic resonance images is of uncertain pathologic significance

---

TABLE 1. **Criteria for the Clinical Diagnosis of Alzheimer's Disease ("Probable" Alzheimer's Disease)**

Dementia, with cognitive deficits documented to affect memory (i.e., the learning and subsequent delayed recall of new information) plus at least one other cognitive domain

The insidious onset of dementia symptoms in the fifth decade of life or later, most often after 65 years of age

A progressive course of gradual worsening for memory and other cognitive deficits

The absence of systemic medical illnesses or other neurologic diseases that might account for the progressive dementia

TABLE 2. **Laboratory Investigations Usually Requested for Patients Suspected of Having Alzheimer's Disease**

Blood Tests
Complete blood count
Serum chemistries (including electrolytes, calcium, glucose, and tests of liver and renal function)
Thyroid functions
Vitamin B_{12} level
Treponemal serologic test for syphilis (fluorescent treponemal antibody-absorption test or microhemagglutination assay for antibodies to *Treponema pallidum*)
Human immunodeficiency virus antibody (especially for high-risk persons)

Urinalysis

Brain Imaging
Computed tomographic scan or magnetic resonance imaging scan; a contrast-enhanced scan is often unnecessary

Others, as Indicated
Chest x-ray
Digoxin level (for persons using this medication)
Electrocardiogram
Electroencephalogram
Erythrocyte sedimentation rate
Lumbar puncture with cerebrospinal fluid examination

and need not deter the clinician from a diagnosis of probable AD.

"Possible AD" is diagnosed in patients who would otherwise meet criteria for probable AD, except for the following: there are significant variations in the onset, manifestation, or clinical course of their illness; there is an associated systemic or neurologic illness that is sufficient to cause dementia but does not appear to be the primary cause of the patient's dementia; or there are progressive deficits limited to a single cognitive domain.

TREATMENT

Treatment of AD remains symptomatic; preventive interventions and rational therapy to slow, halt, or reverse the underlying disease course may await better elucidation of the pathogenesis of AD. Symptomatic pharmacologic treatment can be considered for cognitive symptoms and for behavioral symptoms. Nonpharmacologic environmental manipulations and supportive services are also important. In general, medications should be initiated at the lowest dose possible, increased cautiously, monitored closely, and reduced or discontinued as soon as feasible.

Treatment of Cognitive Symptoms

The symptomatic treatment of memory loss or other cognitive disturbances has met with limited success. The most common treatment strategy is derived from the cholinergic hypothesis of AD. Experimentally, it is known that manipulations

that reduce central cholinergic transmission impede new learning, and markers for the neurotransmitter acetylcholine are reduced within the cerebral cortex of the AD-affected brain. Cholinergic input to the hippocampus and cerebral cortex arises from the basal forebrain neurons, which are prominently affected in AD. Experimental treatment strategies have included precursor loading to increase acetylcholine synthesis (e.g., nonprescription dietary lecithin), anticholinesterases to prolong acetylcholine availability (e.g., physostigmine [Antilirium]), and cholinergic agonists that act directly at muscarinic receptor sites (e.g., arecoline).

The preponderance of evidence suggests negligible benefit from currently available drugs whose usage is derived from cholinergic strategies. One exception, however, appears to be tacrine (Cognex), also referred to as tetrahydroaminoacridine (THA). Food and Drug Administration (FDA) approved this long-acting anticholinesterase in 1993. The results of several large, double-blind, placebo-controlled studies of tacrine imply a modest, temporary symptomatic amelioration for some, perhaps a minority, of demented patients with AD. The dose of tacrine ranges from 10 mg to 40 mg four times a day. Hepatotoxicity, which may be dose-related, is a major problem. Weekly monitoring of serum transaminase levels has been recommended, and liver enzyme elevations have been reversible when tacrine was discontinued. A need for weekly monitoring of liver enzymes in serum would require a sustained commitment by patients, caregivers, and physicians who might decide to initiate treatment with tacrine.

Ergoloid mesylate (Hydergine) is FDA approved for the cognitive symptoms of dementia. The putative mechanisms of action include vasodilatation and metabolic enhancement. The side effects at dosages of 1 to 2 mg three times per day are minor, but most studies have failed to confirm any therapeutic benefit for this medication.

Treatment of Behavioral Symptoms

Behavioral changes—including depression, agitation, hostility, violent outbursts, delusions, and visual hallucinations—are common in AD, can often be ameliorated by nonpharmacologic interventions, and do not necessarily mandate treatment. Psychopharmacologic effects are often limited by adverse reactions. Central anticholinergic effects are of particular concern and might impair cognitive functioning. Exogenous factors should be considered, because behavioral symptoms are more common during intercurrent illnesses (e.g., urinary tract infection) or in new environments (e.g., while in a hospital or during a family vacation). Delusions sometimes represent perceptual misinterpretations (e.g., a patient who mistakes his or her reflection in the mirror for that of another person in the room) or paranoid misinterpretations (e.g., a woman who cannot recall where she has placed her purse or hidden her jewelry and who then claims that others have robbed her).

Neuroleptic medication is of modest benefit for symptomatic behaviors in some patients with AD, although extrapyramidal symptoms (e.g., parkinsonian rigidity and bradykinesia, akathisias, dystonia), sedation, and other side effects are frequently encountered. Sedation and extrapyramidal features can contribute to falls and hip fractures in elderly patients. The anticholinergic effects of some neuroleptics are likely to increase confusion and may lead to urinary retention in men with prostate enlargement. Constipation is another peripheral anticholinergic side effect, and narrow-angle glaucoma may be precipitated or exacerbated. Thioridazine (Mellaril), a low-potency phenothiazine with anticholinergic properties but a lower incidence of extrapyramidal side effects, can be initiated at dosages of 10 mg one to three times daily, with total daily dosages usually not exceeding 100 mg. The butyrophenome haloperidol (Haldol) has minimal anticholinergic effects, but extrapyramidal reactions are more common. The dosages of haloperidol should be kept low, beginning with 0.5 mg one to three times daily and usually not exceeding 3 mg per day. Neuroleptic therapy is problematic for patients with AD who manifest extrapyramidal signs on their pretreatment neurologic examination, but thioridazine may prove less troublesome for these patients than haloperidol. Neuroleptics, such as haloperidol or thioridazine, can be useful for nocturnal confusion, but as with all neuroleptics, tardive dyskinesia is a concern with long-term usage.

In small clinical series, it has been claimed that other drugs benefit aggressive, assaultive, or hostile behaviors in patients with dementia. These agents include the anticonvulsant carbamazepine (Tegretol) and the beta-adrenergic blocker propranolol (Inderal), but convincing empirical evidence of efficacy is wanting. Hypnotics for insomnia should usually be avoided. A small dose of a benzodiazepine, such as lorazepam (Ativan), 0.5 mg at bedtime, can be tried on an occasional basis. Low doses of a benzodiazepine can also be considered for occasional agitation when extrapyramidal side effects preclude the use of neuroleptics.

Depression, in and of itself, occasionally results in the symptoms of dementia. Depression, however, is also a common accompaniment of AD. As such, it often responds to standard antidepressant medications after 4 or more weeks of therapy. The choice of drugs is usually dictated by adverse effects, and the doses employed are typically lower than those for younger adults with major depression. The adverse effects of tricyclic antidepressants include sedation, attributed in part to antihistaminic effects; orthostatic hypotension related to alpha-adrenergic blockade; and the effects of anticholinergic activity. The cardiac rhythm can also be affected. The side effects are relatively less bothersome with desipramine (Norpramin) or nortriptyline (Aventyl, Pamelor) than with many of the other tricyclic antidepressants. Desipramine may be preferred for patients who need a more activating antidepressant and nortriptyline, for the more agitated patient. Desipramine is usually begun with a morning dose of 10 or 25 mg, with usual daily dosages of up to 75 mg in divided doses. Nortriptyline can be initiated with a bedtime dose of 10 or 25 mg; the usual daily dosages are up to 75 mg given at bedtime or in divided doses. Anticholinergic effects are also less of a problem with atypical antidepressants such as fluoxetine (Prozac) or bupropion (Wellbutrin). For fluoxetine, treatment can be initiated at 10 or 20 mg per day as a single morning dose, with usual daily dosages of up to 40 mg. Treatment with bupropion is initiated at 75 mg at breakfast time, with usual dosages of 150 to 300 mg per day.

Nonpharmacologic Management

Behavioral interventions are often effective in ameliorating such symptoms as agitation, confusion, or hostility. A simplified structured environment and a stable routine are important. Intercurrent medical problems should be assiduously sought. For example, the nocturnal awakenings that are distressing to caregivers might be related to a urinary tract infection or prostate enlargement leading to nocturia; the resultant drowsiness the next day might be associated with confusion or other behavioral consequences. Treating the underlying cause of nocturia would be more efficacious than bedtime sedation for sleep or neuroleptics for daytime confusion.

Day care centers and caregiver respite services can be crucial in allowing the caregiver a much-needed break and thereby prolonging the time that a patient can remain at home. Family support groups also help the family cope with the stress and frustration of caring for a loved one who may no longer even recall the caregiver's name. Ultimately, the physician may be asked to provide advice on chronic placement. The local chapter of the Alzheimer's Association can be an excellent source of family-oriented information on these and related topics.

The physician should also educate the caregiver about the illness and its likely progression. Caregivers cope much better when they can anticipate the clinical course. Legal guardianship or the durable power of attorney are important issues for family members to consider. In some states, health care workers are required to report patients with AD to the local health department, and physicians must inform the patient and family that such mandated reporting will likely result in the loss of driving privileges. Even when reporting is not mandatory, the patient with AD will likely be unable to operate a motor vehicle safely, and the physician may be in the best position to offer counsel in this regard.

PARENCHYMATOUS BRAIN HEMORRHAGE

method of
R. B. LIBMAN, M.D., and
J. P. MOHR, M.D.
The New York Neurological Institute
New York, New York

Intracerebral hemorrhage (ICH) accounts for 10% of all strokes. Its fatality rate remains high, ranging from 21% for small hematomas to 80% for larger hematomas. Chronic hypertension accounts for most parenchymatous hemorrhages, but the importance of nonhypertensive diseases is increasingly recognized. Management remains controversial and depends on the clinical scenario. Hematoma location, size, and underlying cause are crucial determinants of treatment.

Chronic hypertension causes fibrinoid necrosis of the walls of small, deep cerebral arteries, leading to mural disruption and hematoma formation. The vessels affected are mainly the small penetrating arteries arising from the circle of Willis, known as the lenticulostriates and thalamoperforants, and the paramedian branches of the basilar artery. The brain locations served by these vessels are the sites of the hemorrhage: the putamen (35 to 50% of cases), the thalamus (10 to 15%), the cerebellum (16%), and the pons (5 to 12%). ICH also occurs in the subcortical white matter of the cerebral lobes (30%), but many nonhypertensive causes are represented in lobar hemorrhage.

The period of active bleeding in hypertensive ICH is thought to last only minutes. By the time the patient arrives at the hospital, bleeding has usually ceased. Rebleeding in the acute period is unusual, in contrast to subarachnoid hemorrhage, in which rebleeding represents a major cause of morbidity and mortality. An exception to this rule is that of thalamic ICH, which has been associated with rebleeding in patients with uncontrolled hypertension. Further pathologic evolution is usually due to edema.

Cerebellar hemorrhage is almost uniquely amenable to surgical therapy. Cerebellar hemorrhage usually occurs in a hemisphere, originating in the dentate nucleus. The bleeding causes abrupt onset of headache, dizziness, nausea and vomiting, and an inability to walk, symptoms that may appear in isolation and mimic inner ear disease. Only vague lightheadedness and gait instability may be the presenting features. If the mass dissects laterally into the cerebellar hemisphere, ipsilateral appendicular ataxia is added to the symptoms, and brain stem displacement is suggested by ipsilateral gaze palsy and facial weakness. The clinical course is notoriously unpredictable; sudden worsening, from vomiting and ataxia to coma or death, may occur with little warning.

TREATMENT

Hypertensive Hemorrhage

Life-saving surgical evacuation of the cerebellar hematoma is undertaken if the lesion is larger than 3 cm and/or there is ventricular extension, but surgery is not performed based only on initial syndrome severity. Careful observation and medical management are recommended for the remainder of patients, with a plan for surgical decompression when extensor plantar responses appear or consciousness deteriorates.

Hypertensive hemorrhage in the other locations is not so clearly a neurosurgical emergency. Putaminal hemorrhage usually presents with an acute onset of hemiparesis accompanied by visual, sensory, and behavioral disturbances. There is a propensity to worsen over the first hours after the initial ictus, particularly the level of consciousness. Delayed deterioration may occur 3 to 5 days after the ictus secondary to the development of cerebral edema. The prognosis is directly related to hematoma size; flaccid hemiparesis, coma, and clinical progression after presentation correlate with large hematoma size and poorer outcome. Most cases of putaminal hemorrhage are managed medically. Studies have failed to show any benefit from surgery, but the number of patients in these studies has been small, and definitive conclusions have been difficult.

Caudate hemorrhage causes more ventricular than parenchymatous hemorrhage, with symptoms of headache, vomiting, stiff neck, stupor, and amnestic states. The degree of parenchymatous involvement is reflected in the extent of hemiparesis and gaze paresis, varying from mild to severe. The hydrocephalus created by the ventricular extension of the hemorrhage produces the stupor, which may persist for many days. Shunting is rarely required. Because the primary brain injury is mild, the long-term outcome is usually favorable, although this prognosis may seem optimistic during the initial phase of amnesia, somnolence, and incontinence.

Thalamic hemorrhage is usually large enough to trigger an abrupt sensorimotor deficit, with vomiting but surprisingly little headache. When the mass is large enough to depress the midbrain immediately below the thalamus, Parinaud's syndrome of upward gaze palsy with small, unreactive pupils occurs. The patient may exhibit "wrong-way" eyes, in which the eyes are deviated away from the side with the lesion; in contrast, deviation toward the lesion is seen with most supratentorial lesions. Aphasic or hemineglect syndromes may occur, depending on the side of the lesion. Ventricular extension is common because the thalamus is surrounded on three sides by spinal fluid spaces, but clinically disabling hydrocephalus is uncommon, and shunting or temporary ventricular drainage is infrequently required. For acute, severe hydrocephalus, emergency ventriculostomy occasionally results in dramatic clinical improvement. Very small hemorrhages mimic the syndromes of small infarcts and may come as a surprise on computed tomography (CT) scans. The prognosis is related to hemorrhage size; those larger than 3.3 cm are usually fatal.

Pontine hemorrhage is the most dramatic and least treatable of the parenchymatous hemorrhages. The usual site is in the ventral portion of the brain stem. It may cause an abrupt onset of stupor or coma, vomiting, abnormal respirations, pinpoint pupils, absent corneals, gaze palsies, internuclear ophthalmoplegia, ocular bobbing, and skew deviation. Quadriparesis with posturing and bilateral Babinski's signs complete the clinical picture. Death occurs within hours for patients with larger hemorrhages. Smaller lesions may mimic infarcts, especially those in lateral or posterior locations, and have a better prognosis. As for the larger lesions, there is no effective surgical or medical treatment, and the prognosis is poor.

Lobar hemorrhages usually occur in the subcortical white matter, with a predilection for the parietal and occipital regions. These hematomas may produce little motor deficit or change in consciousness if they are far from the central structures, and they cause seizures at onset more frequently than deep hemorrhages. Although hypertension accounts for many of these hemorrhages, nonhypertensive causes are more frequently implicated than in deep hematomas. The focal signs reflect the lesion location and are not readily differentiated clinically from those of infarction. The prognosis is much better than for other forms of ICH. Survival and functional recovery are related to the size of the hematoma. Those larger than 40 ml have a uniformly poorer outcome than those smaller than 20 ml. Surgical drainage is a controversial option and may be helpful for superficial, medium, or large hematomas if neurologic deterioration occurs after diagnosis.

Nonhypertensive Hemorrhage

Anticoagulants and Bleeding Disorders. Anticoagulant-related hemorrhages constitute approximately 1.5% of the bleeding complications of anticoagulant use. These hemorrhages have been characterized by a slower evolution, lobar location, and a tendency to have delayed and continued bleeding after diagnosis. They occur more frequently in patients in whom the prothrombin time is greater than one and one-half to two times the control value. Early recognition leads to definitive treatment of the coagulopathy, which should begin as soon as an anticoagulated patient suspected of having a cerebral event presents to an emergency room. Therapy includes cessation of the offending medication, infusion of fresh-frozen plasma, injection of phytonadione (Aquamephyton, vitamin K, 20 to 40 mg intravenously) in the case of warfarin (Coumadin)-related hemorrhage, and careful monitoring of the prothrombin and partial thromboplastin times. Rapid correction reduces bleeding and prepares the patient for surgical evacuation of the clot.

Hemorrhage due to hemophilia or other factor deficiencies should be similarly approached with the infusion of the deficient factor as soon as it is available. Platelet transfusions, sometimes requiring as many as a dozen units, may be needed for treating thrombocytopenia.

Drugs. Numerous medications have been implicated in spontaneous ICH, usually based on their effect on blood pressure. The hypothesis is that a rapid rise in systemic blood pressure leads to arterial, venous, or capillary bleeding. A drug-induced vasculitis has also been suggested. Examples include sympathomimetic agents such as amphetamines, cocaine ("crack"), phenylpropanolamine, ephedrine, and pseudoephedrine. An accurate history, which is not always forthcoming, is essential for the diagnosis. Abstention from further drug use is recommended.

Structural Lesions. Structural lesions such as arteriovenous malformations (AVM), aneurysms (berry and mycotic), and tumors may present as ICH. Recognition is important because rebleeding risks are high. Suspicion is raised if a hemorrhage presents in a superficial or lobar location with no history of hypertension, drug abuse, or trauma. Clues are further provided by an enhanced CT scan showing calcifications, unusual patterns of enhancement, or abnormally enhancing vessels. Repeat scanning after 7 to 10 days may allow blood resorption to eliminate the confounding mass effect. Transcranial Doppler ultrasonography has emerged as a highly sensitive and noninvasive method for the detection of AVMs. Magnetic resonance imaging may delineate the lesion in the hematoma, and angiography is usually definitive. Tumors that are more likely to hemorrhage include glioblastoma multiforme and metastases from renal cell carcinoma, melanoma, bronchogenic carcinoma, and thyroid carcinoma. Surgical therapy can be planned if the patient is clinically stable. In the case of mycotic aneurysms, intravenous antibiotic therapy is also required.

Amyloid Angiopathy. Recognized as an important cause of ICH in the elderly, amyloid is deposited in the walls of blood vessels in the cortex and subarachnoid space. This may lead to rupture of the arterial wall. There is no association between cerebral amyloid angiopathy and systemic amyloidosis. The frequency of amyloid angiopathy increases dramatically with age: autopsy series have shown an 8% prevalence for those in their seventies and a 60% prevalence for those older than 90 years. Nonhypertensive lobar hemorrhage in an elderly patient is the most common clinical presentation. The location is usually in the posterior aspects of the hemispheres. Hemorrhages due to amyloid angiopathy tend to be recurrent or multiple, and it is the recurrence within months in other lobar locations that supports this diagnosis. Cerebral biopsy is the only definitive way to establish the diagnosis during life, but it is usually not indicated. Because of the friable nature of blood vessels in amyloid angiopathy and their propensity for oozing, surgical evacuation of the hematoma may trigger more bleeding and is usually deferred unless the mass is life-threatening.

Medical Therapy

Medical therapy for ICH is aimed at prevention of complications and careful management of blood pressure. Sustained hypertension may alter cerebral autoregulation and cause additional neurologic deterioration, and hypotension may result in cerebral hypoperfusion, especially in the setting of increased intracranial pressure. Short-term diastolic blood pressures of up to 110 mmHg can be tolerated, particularly in the setting of a previous history of hypertension. Long-term hypertension requires treatment, usually with the patient's prior medical regimen, but often it may call for more vigorous measures. Sublingual or oral nifedipine (Procardia), oral or intravenous propranolol (Inderal), and oral captopril (Capo-

ten) are reasonable alternatives for treatment. Hypertension refractory to these measures may require infusion of intravenous labetalol (Trandate, Normodyne), or angiotensin-converting enzyme inhibitors, with arterial line monitoring, titrating to systolic pressures of 140 to 160 and diastolic pressures of 90 to 100 mmHg. Sodium nitroprusside (Nipride) and other nitrates should be avoided because of their propensity to raise intracranial pressure. Very low pressures, which cause neurologic deterioration, should be treated with fluid challenges and possibly pressors (dopamine, norepinephrine). Any intervention aimed at altering blood pressure requires careful neurologic monitoring to ensure that deterioration is not the result of overaggressive treatment.

There is a higher incidence of seizures with intracranial bleeding, more so with lobar hemorrhages and those that abut the cortex than those in the basal ganglia. Some physicians have recommended the prophylactic use of anticonvulsants, but it is justified to withhold anticonvulsants until clinically indicated. Phenytoin (Dilantin) is the drug of choice, using 1000 to 1500 mg for a loading dose and 300 mg per day as a maintenance dose. If given intravenously, slow administration with normal saline at no faster than 50 mg per minute with close blood pressure and cardiac monitoring (watching for widening of the QRS complex) is the correct method; 500 mg given orally every 3 hours for three doses serves as an adequate oral loading route.

Prevention and treatment of respiratory complications are important to survival. Prophylactic intubation with respirator support is often required if brain stem respiratory centers are involved or there is a markedly depressed level of consciousness. Suctioning and chest physical therapy to help prevent atelectasis and adequate oxygen therapy based on the arterial blood gas readings are standard measures. If respirator support is required for more than 10 days, a tracheostomy is preferred.

Infections are often responsible for worsening and should be sought if fevers are recorded. Pneumonia, urinary tract infections, line sepsis, and phlebitis are frequent sources. Central fevers should only be diagnosed by exclusion after exhaustive attempts to ascertain a systemic reason for the fever are persistently negative. Maintenance of adequate nutritional support is also a mainstay of therapy, requiring early institution of nasogastric tube feedings with graduated increases in caloric intake or, in the case of gastrointestinal dysfunction, total parenteral nutrition. Cardiac monitoring is sometimes necessary to detect centrally mediated arrhythmias, particularly ventricular and supraventricualar tachycardia and bradyarrhythmias.

Patients who survive the initial ictus should be started on an early physical therapy and rehabilitation program to prevent contractures and maximize functional recovery. Range-of-motion exercises, a sling, and wrist supports are early measures. As the patient improves, more progressive training and support devices can be arranged.

Treatment of Increased Intracranial Pressure

If a mass effect from the hemorrhage, resulting edema, or hydrocephalus causes a critical rise in intracranial pressure (ICP), herniation syndromes become evident. Swift intervention may alter the course and should begin while the patient is prepared for an emergency CT scan to identify the cause of the deterioration. The head of the bed should be raised to 30 degrees to help reduce ICP. Intubation is required to hyperventilate the patient to decrease the P_{CO_2} to 25 to 30 mmHg. After inserting a Foley catheter, mannitol is infused in a bolus dose of 100 grams over 20 minutes, and subsequent doses of 0.5 gram per kg are given every 6 hours for the next 24 hours and then slowly tapered. Careful monitoring of serum chemistries is required, especially sodium concentration, and serum osmolality should be maintained at 300 to 310 mOsm. Isotonic saline solutions may be infused slowly to maintain hydration, but hypotonic solutions (e.g., 5% glucose) should be avoided because of the risk of causing increased cerebral edema. The use of steroids is to be discouraged, because they have not improved neurologic outcome, and morbidity is increased because of infectious and diabetic complications.

Effective administration of these medications calls for titration to the ICP using a pressure transducer implanted in the subarachnoid, epidural, or intraventricular regions. Although an intraventricular catheter is usually preferred for other lesions, it can be dangerous for hematomas because rebleeding is a risk. Medical management of increased ICP may enable the patient to survive the critical 24 to 48 hours after the ictus, but often it is a temporizing maneuver in preparation for surgery.

Surgical Therapy

The role of surgery in the treatment of ICH depends mainly on the size and location of the hematoma. Prompt surgical attention is recommended for large cerebellar hemorrhage (> 3 cm in diameter), and surgical intervention may be needed for medium-sized or large lobar hemor-

rhage if there is progressive clinical deterioration. An operation performed within 24 hours is technically easier because of the liquidity of the clot. After 24 hours, solidification and organization of the clot necessitates a larger incision. In the case of lobar hemorrhage, evacuation mitigates additional damage from the mass effect, but in cerebellar hemorrhage, surgical intervention is lifesaving.

Before embarking on an operation, the risk/benefit ratio must be considered. Cardiac and pulmonary co-morbidity, other medical problems, and advanced age may cause unacceptably high operative mortality and morbidity. Severe neurologic disability may be unavoidable, despite lifesaving surgery. The wishes of the patient and the family should be explored before considering an aggressive approach.

FOCAL ISCHEMIC CEREBROVASCULAR DISEASE

method of
JOSEPH P. HANNA, M.D., and
ANTHONY J. FURLAN, M.D.
Cleveland Clinic Foundation
Cleveland, Ohio

Focal ischemic cerebrovascular disease is the most common subtype of stroke. The treatment of impending or recent-onset focal cerebral ischemia has made notable advances in the past several years. However, stroke prevention, supportive care, and rehabilitation are still the mainstays of management.

Focal ischemic cerebrovascular disease is often classified on the basis of duration of neurologic deficits. The transient ischemic attack (TIA) is defined as focal neurologic deficits occurring abruptly and lasting less than 24 hours. Most TIAs, however, are much briefer, lasting less than 15 minutes. The longer the TIA lasts, the more likely an appropriate lesion will be found on neuroimaging studies. The term "RIND" (reversible ischemic neurologic deficit) is sometimes used to signify a neurologic deficit lasting more than 24 hours but resolving without residua. A "stroke-in-evolution" denotes focal neurologic deficits referable to a vascular territory that are fluctuating or progressing. A cerebral infarction defines neurologic deficits referable to a vascular territory that last more than 24 hours.

RISK FACTORS

The prevention of focal cerebral ischemia is based on three strategies: elimination or minimization of risk factors, antiplatelet or anticoagulant therapy, and surgery. Risk factors for stroke may be divided into those that are not treatable (e.g., male sex and age) and those that are amenable to medical management.

Hypertension is by far the most important risk factor for stroke at any age. Both systolic and diastolic hypertension are strongly and independently related to focal cerebral ischemia. Even isolated systolic hypertension in elderly patients is associated with an increased risk for stroke. Diabetes predisposes patients to the development of cerebral atherosclerosis and is associated with an increased stroke risk. Hyperlipidemia has an uncertain independent significance for focal cerebral ischemia. However, the association of hypercholesterolemia with coronary atherosclerosis, which is associated with an increased stroke risk, merits control. Obesity predisposes patients to both hypertension and hyperlipidemia, leading to stroke.

Cigarette smoking is highly correlated with focal cerebral ischemia, especially in young patients. Young women who are smokers and use oral contraceptives are at an increased risk for stroke in comparison with their nonsmoking peers who do not take oral contraceptives. Excessive ethanol use has also been linked to stroke.

Cardiac diseases are not true risk factors, but they are best considered to be organ dysfunctions predisposing to stroke. Atherosclerotic coronary artery disease, congestive heart failure, and atrial fibrillation are stroke precursors.

In young adults with stroke, there are often other predisposing risk factors and conditions, including stimulant abuse, oral contraceptive use, migraine headaches, hypercoagulable states, and congenital heart disease.

DIAGNOSIS

The diagnosis of focal cerebral ischemia should be considered in any individual presenting with the abrupt onset of focal neurologic deficits. The differential diagnosis includes migraine headache, seizure, mass lesions (tumor, subdural), and demyelinating disease.

The evolution and constellation of symptoms help to differentiate among focal ischemia, seizure, and migraine. The symptoms and signs of focal ischemia appear abruptly and are usually negative phenomena (e.g., weakness, visual loss). Seizures and migraines produce predominantly positive symptoms (e.g., scintillating scotoma, migrating paresthesia), progressing over seconds and minutes, respectively. Tumors and subdural hematomas sometimes manifest abruptly with neurologic deficits. Demyelinating disease may manifest with sudden neurologic dysfunction, sometimes related to temperature increases.

INVESTIGATION AND TREATMENT

Focal cerebral ischemia, like myocardial ischemia, warrants urgent evaluation. The timing of the event with respect to the presentation, presumed vascular territory, viable tissue at risk for further ischemia, and concurrent physical condition of the patient help guide the physician in tailoring both investigations and therapy.

Patients with any new unexplained neurologic deficit should undergo the following minimal investigations at the time of presentation: complete blood count, routine serologic studies, urinalysis, prothrombin time/partial thromboplastin time studies, electrocardiography, and cranial computed tomography. The laboratory studies are essential for defining a baseline and screening for potential causes of stroke and intercurrent illnesses. The electrocardiogram identifies two important cardiac precipitants of stroke: atrial fibrillation and myocardial infarction. The computed tomogram aids in excluding intracranial hemorrhage, permitting the initiation of anticoagulation if indicated.

A division into focal ischemia subtype and presumed vascular territory is beneficial before the investigation proceeds further. A treatment plan based on the vascular territory at risk for further ischemia, acuity and severity of deficits, underlying medical problems, and stroke risk factors is then initiated.

Both anterior and posterior circulation brain ischemia result from intrinsic and extrinsic vascular causes. Intrinsic causes include atherosclerosis, lipohyalinosis, dissection, vasculitis, amyloid angiopathy, and venous infarction. Extrinsic causes are usually embolic. The sources of the emboli include the heart, aorta, and deep veins (paradoxical). Emboli can be composed of thrombus, platelet-fibrin, calcific debris, fat, tumor, air, or nitrogen.

Atherosclerosis of the intracranial and extracranial arteries is treated both surgically and medically. Carotid endarterectomy is significantly better than aspirin alone in preventing strokes in patients with symptomatic extracranial atherosclerotic narrowing of the internal carotid artery of more than 70%. Symptomatic carotid stenosis of less than 30% stenosis is better managed medically. The benefit of endarterectomy for both symptomatic carotid stenosis between 30 and 70%, as well as asymptomatic stenosis greater than 60%, is uncertain and under investigation. The extracranial-intracranial bypass procedure, once popular for inaccessible occlusive lesions, is of no proven benefit and is now rarely performed.

Posterior circulation atherosclerosis is much more difficult to approach surgically. In medically refractory cases of vertebrobasilar insufficiency, extracranial vertebral artery surgical procedures or endovascular balloon angioplasty is sometimes attempted.

The medical management of acute focal cerebral ischemia consists of the prevention of further ischemia and supportive care. Two goals are paramount: to maintain the cerebral blood flow above the infarction threshold (> 10 mL per 100 gm per minute) and to enhance the cellular resistance to a metabolic insult. The blood pressure should be kept in the mildly hypertensive range, approximately 180/100, as long as coronary ischemia does not occur. When it is necessary to lower the blood pressure acutely, a short-acting intravenous agent, such as labetalol (Normodyne, Trandate) or sodium nitroprusside (Nipride), should be used. Hyperglycemia should be limited to prevent lactic acidosis in ischemic tissue. Fever should be controlled because of the increased metabolic demand on the ischemic brain.

The benefit of anticoagulation in acute stroke remains unproven. Heparin is often used for embolic infarcts and atherothrombotic strokes-in-evolution. Completed atherothrombotic infarcts, hemorrhagic infarcts, and large infarcts should not be immediately anticoagulated. Heparin bolus doses should be avoided, because they may cause hemorrhagic conversion of a bland infarct. A constant heparin infusion of 1000 units per hour is begun with subsequent adjustment of the activated partial thromboplastin time to twice the control level.

The high risk of aspiration precludes oral intake for the first several days. Puréed food is then introduced. Dehydration is prevented with intravenous normal saline to prevent the development of hyperviscosity, hyponatremia, and hyperglycemia. Bed rest is advocated for avoiding orthostatic pressure fluctuations for the first several days. Support stockings, range-of-motion exercises, pneumatic compression devices, and subcutaneous heparin prevent development of deep venous thrombosis.

Large infarcts in both the anterior and posterior circulation develop significant edema, which can cause neurologic deterioration from a mass effect. Intensive care management is often necessary to prevent further deterioration and herniation. The initial therapy includes free water restriction, head elevation, and correction of hyponatremia if present. Hyperventilation to a carbon dioxide partial pressure of 30 mmHg decreases the intracranial pressure by decreasing the blood component of the intracranial compartment. Impending herniation is treated with intravenous furosemide (Lasix) and mannitol. Cerebellar infarcts that have not responded to these techniques may require emergent posterior fossa decompression.

Cytoprotective therapy with ionic channel blocking agents, glutamate receptor antagonists, oxygen free-radical scavenging 21-aminosteroids, and other agents is under investigation. The goal of these therapies is to widen the reversible ischemic window and salvage threatened neurons. Acute thrombolytic therapy with tissue plasminogen activator (Activase), urokinase (Abbokinase), and streptokinase (Streptase) is also under study. Low-molecular-weight heparinoids are being developed to maintain vessel patency after thrombolysis and to lower bleeding risks associated with anticoagulation in acute strokes. Endovascular techniques, such as angioplasty, are evolving to address the residual luminal stenosis after thrombolysis.

PREVENTION

Prevention of focal cerebral ischemia is accomplished with both antithrombotic and antiplatelet agents. Warfarin (Coumadin) is used when focal cerebral ischemia is due to cardioembolism, especially atrial fibrillation. The warfarin dosage is adjusted to attain a prothrombin time of 16 to 18 seconds (International Normalized Ratio [INR], 2.0 to 3.0). Prothrombin times of 18 to 22 seconds (INR, 3.0 to 4.0) are used for recent cardioembolism, mechanical prosthetic cardiac valves, and recurrent ischemia with lower prothrombin times.

Two antiplatelet agents, aspirin and ticlopidine (Ticlid), are commonly used for stroke prophylaxis in high-risk patients. Aspirin remains the initial choice for many patients, especially men with a prior TIA. The best dosage of aspirin for stroke prophylaxis is controversial. Higher doses (1300 mg daily) may work better but cause more side effects. Currently, we favor 650 mg daily of enteric-coated aspirin as initial therapy. Lower doses can be used in aspirin-intolerant patients, and higher doses can be considered if the symptoms recur.

Ticlopidine affects the platelet–fibrinogen interactions and was 47% better than aspirin in preventing recurrent ischemia during the first year of the Ticlopidine Aspirin Stroke Study (TASS) trial. A dosage of 250 mg twice a day is used. The most common reason for discontinuation is diarrhea. Patients must be monitored for neutropenia every other week for the first 3 months of therapy. Neutropenia, occurring in 2.4% of patients but severe in fewer than 1%, necessitates discontinuation of therapy, and the number of neutrophilic leukocytes usually normalizes within 1 to 3 weeks after cessation of therapy. Ticlopidine is preferred in aspirin-intolerant patients and can be considered for primary therapy in women with TIAs or for secondary prevention in patients with large strokes.

Dipyridamole (Persantine) monotherapy has not been demonstrated to prevent focal cerebral ischemia and probably adds little benefit to aspirin alone. Recurrent cardioemboli from mechanical prosthetic valves are decreased when dipyridamole is added to warfarin therapy that has failed at a therapeutic dosage.

REHABILITATION OF PERSONS WITH STROKE

method of
RAMON VALLARINO, M.D.
State University of New York
Health Science Center
Brooklyn, New York

The initial efforts in the treatment of stroke are oriented toward maintaining the life of the patient. Stroke victims may die as a direct result of the neurologic insult when, because of its extension or location, it severely affects a vital function (e.g., respiration and arterial blood pressure). More frequently, however, patients die as a result of the grave complications that follow the loss of alertness, mobility, perception, coordination, sensation, praxis, and cognition. Some typical complications that end the life of stroke victims within 1 to 2 weeks are pneumonia, related to the pooling of secretions in the lungs of patients kept supine for prolonged periods of time or secondary to aspiration of food, when swallowing is affected and coughing is deficient (dysphagia); deep venous thrombosis, which results from venous stasis in a lower limb affected by a lack of voluntary motion, followed by pulmonary embolism; and intestinal obstruction, secondary to reduced peristalsis associated with bed rest.

To prevent the first of these complications, the physician must ascertain that the patient is not aspirating food. It may be necessary to request expert assistance by means of radiologic testing of a barium swallow or by consulting with gastroenterology or otorhinolaryngology practitioners. Inadequate swallowing may require simple measures, such as thickening the consistency of fluids, or more drastic measures, such as passing a nasogastric catheter or surgical performance of a feeding gastrostomy. Approximately 80% of cases of dysphagia resolve within a few weeks. The practitioner must attentively watch for this development in order to stop, at that point, the measures that are no longer necessary.

The next concern of the physician must be to prevent deep venous thrombosis and pulmonary embolism. Anticoagulation or antiplatelet medication must be considered if not contraindicated. Lower limb blood stasis must be avoided by encouraging the patient to move the lower limbs as much as possible, by compressing those limbs intermittently with an automatic pneumatic pump, and by making sure that the patient wears compressive hose at all times. These strict measures can be progressively relaxed once the patient starts standing up to practice ambulation.

The patient must be taken out of bed as soon as the vital functions are stable. Exercises and activities are better performed out of bed. This is probably the best way to assist maintaining an adequate level of intestinal mobility to prevent constipation and obstruction.

Both when the patient is in bed and when he or she is sitting in a chair, extreme attention must be given to changing the patient's position not less frequently than every 2 hours. Remaining still in the same position results in the formation of a pressure sore at the point of contact with the surface on which it rests, particularly over bony prominences (such as the sacrum, the trochanters, and the heels) and cartilage (such as the ears). Even resting on soft surfaces, such as foam, water, gel, or air mattresses, results in a pressure sore if a sufficient time of immobility is allowed. The use of an indwelling urinary catheter, on the assumption that it is imperative to keep the skin dry to prevent pressure sores, is discouraged. Indwelling catheters usually result in a urinary tract infection, whereas wetness on the skin does not result per se in pressure sore formation. The incontinence of stroke patients, which occurs when the sensorium or the cognition are severely affected, is better handled with a condom catheter or a large-size disposable diaper, which is changed in a timely fashion by the nurse or a family member. Maceration of the skin occurs if these diapers are neglectfully left unchanged. The presence of pressure sores is always indicative of suboptimal care.

Rehabilitation prescriptions are appropriate from day 1. A consultation with a physiatrist, a physician specializing in the rehabilitation of the disabled patient, is absolutely pertinent. The physiatrist has the knowledge and the vocational calling to implement and supervise these measures and focuses efforts on helping the patient regain the maximal possible level of physical, mental, emotional, social, and vocational function. The role of the physiatrist, otherwise to be played by the primary care physician, includes taking a detailed history to determine the premorbid level of function and conducting a comprehensive physical examination to identify functional losses and their etiopathogeneses. The rehabilitation prescription takes into consideration the roles of rehabilitation experts, principally physical therapists, occupational therapists, and speech and audiology therapists. These professionals, ideally working under the leadership of the physiatrist, implement the therapeutic regimens of their training. The physical therapists provide exercises and apply physical modalities such as heat, electricity, and hydrotherapy. The occupational therapists use therapeutic activities and tasks to be performed by the patient to restore or enhance a function and train the patient in the activities of daily living, such as self-feeding, dressing, toilet use, and cooking. The speech therapists train the patient affected by aphasia, dysarthria, or dysphonia in communication skills, including the intense search for avenues of communication and the use of substitution modalities, such as gesturing, picture pointing, spelling boards, or computarized conversational equipment. These therapists also treat dysphagia.

It is a misunderstanding to equate therapy with strenuous or dangerous exercising or contraindicated activity. Professionally administered rehabilitative measures are never contraindicated. If the patient is comatose, lethargic, or confused to the point of being unable to follow instructions, the therapist provides passive exercises and postural care. These are not helpful for the restoration of function because only active exercise can do that. However, they prevent the previously mentioned complications and the development of contractures, which are caused by stiffening of the periarticular structures with resulting deformity, such as equinus deviation of the foot, flexed knee and hip, and clenched hand. The therapists seek the opportunity of implementing active exercises for ambulation, coordination, balance, range of motion, strength, and endurance. They use modalities to re-educate the muscles, including biofeedback equipment to enhance awareness and to provide a reward for an effort, and special techniques to attempt to reduce spasticity and improve sensation. Therapy sessions usually take a total of 3 hours per day in an acute hospital setting, particularly if the patient is placed in a rehabilitation unit. More or less time can be given, depending on the tolerance of the patient, who should not become unduly fatigued. Nurses and family members must continue providing the patient with range-of-motion exercises, postural care, and simple exercises and activities, as tolerated, the rest of the day.

The prognosis after a stroke depends on the severity of the neurologic damage, the time elapsed since the onset of the stroke, and the amount of functional return at the time of the examination. A comatose patient tends to have a worse prognosis than one who has remained alert. Severe paralysis usually suggests a worse outcome than mild paresis. Early after the onset of a stroke, the patient has many chances of recovering from hemiplegia; these chances diminish as time passes. Massive areas of brain infarct confer a worse prognosis than do small lacunar defects. Finally, the loss of cognition, perception, or praxis predict a worse outcome than the loss of volitional motion.

The physician is frequently challenged by questions about the patient's outcome. Early after the onset, there must be a statement about the seriousness of this life-threatening illness and the inability to predict at such an initial stage what course the events will follow. It is quite pertinent to express satisfaction about the patient's survival. It is helpful to keep the patient and other interested parties informed about positive and negative developments, giving them any good news in a timely fashion and not concealing the presence of disappointing events, such as a persistent lack of return of function. Although the physician must maintain the morale of those affected by this trying illness, he or she must not allow the presence of false expectations.

The sooner and greater the return of function is, the better is the prognosis, and vice versa. "Will the patient walk?" the physician is asked. Most likely, he or she will, if the patient is able to move (even slightly) the lower limbs early after the onset of the stroke. "Will the patient use the hands again?" Probably not as skillfully as before unless there is a return of very high magnitude within days after the onset. "Will the patient talk again?" Patients with aphasia and dysarthria tend to improve with time and training. Quite seldom does the patient remain permanently unable to communicate. However, speech disorders that do not improve rapidly tend to leave significant sequelae.

Lack of return of function by the end of the first month affects the prognosis negatively, because most of the crucial gains usually occur during that period of time. Nevertheless, functional improvement can continue during a period of many months, by surges or at a subtle, but steady, pace.

Rehabilitation works toward the return of focal function, such as the use of a hand or a leg, and furthermore, toward regaining the function of the patient as a whole. To regain the movement of a limb implies the reactivation or substitution of complex nervous system functions. Very little is known about this subject, and the ability of physicians to intervene at such a level is quite limited. Rehabilitation identifies as early as possible any return of function, frequently at such a subtle level that not even the patient has noticed it. Then, rehabilitation enhances the return with exercises and therapeutic activities. How exercise and therapeutic activities enhance the return of function is the subject of intense scientific research. It is established, however, throughout the literature, that although rehabilitation cannot trigger the return of function, it can perfect such a return. Rehabilitation can demonstrate its beneficial effect whether it is implemented early after the stroke onset or later on. Naturally, late programs must surmount complications that may have resulted from the patient's lack of mobility, as described earlier in this article.

When there is no return, or when its magnitude is insufficient for the performance of a task, rehabilitation trains the patient to perform the task in a different way and provides aids to facilitate such a function. Examples of such aids are orthotic braces or splints, walkers and canes, a crane lift to take the patient out of bed, a raised toilet seat to facilitate standing up, a commode to be placed at the bedside when ambulation is limited, grab bars in areas where the patient may lose balance, kitchen utensils and silverware to be used with one hand, a wheelchair, and a firm cushion over a seat to raise the patient and help him or her stand up. The list of ways in which the environment around a patient can be modified to facilitate the performance of functional tasks goes on and on and keeps growing at a fast pace.

To benefit from rehabilitation, a patient must participate actively. Active participation requires adequate mentation, motivation, and vigor from the patient. Adequate mentation consists of the patient's being able to maintain sufficient alertness and awareness to follow commands and to learn at least simple techniques. A person who does not meet this basic requirement cannot be rehabilitated and is in need of total nursing care. Motivation means the desire of the patient to be rehabilitated. A person with depression or with a behavioral disorder may refuse to be treated. In such cases, the physician may consider proper medication or seek the assistance of a psychiatrist or psychologist. Vigor is the level of tolerance to the demands of a process of training. No significant participation can be expected from a patient with very little vigor, such as one with a fever, marked anemia, or dehydration. However, properly administered rehabilitative techniques help build up tolerance to exercise, if there is a minimal level at the outset.

Rehabilitation is a team effort. In addition to physicians, therapists, nurses, and other health professionals, the team must include the patient, his or her family, and when available, relatives and friends. These people provide valuable insights in reference to premorbid skills and interests, hopes and expectations, concerns, suggestions, and requests. Of great relevance, they are expected to understand the therapeutic program and give the therapists approval and support.

The inpatient phase of poststroke rehabilitation varies in length, according to the patient's condition. For example, a comatose patient must stay in an acute ward until consistently stable. Then, if still comatose, he or she must be transferred to a long-term skilled nursing facility or is discharged home with around-the-clock services. The second option can often be accomplished without the use of skilled personnel but just by having two or three shifts of aides or responsible, caring helpers.

If the patient is alert, stable, and able to participate actively in rehabilitation, an early transfer to an acute rehabilitation unit or facility is ideal for intense comprehensive rehabilitation, with no less than 3 hours of therapy per day and no less than 5 days per week. The patient stays in this setting for about 1 month or less time if the goals are achieved, no further gains are foreseen, or comparable gains are predicted with the therapy given at a lesser level of intensity. Some more time may be needed if the patient keeps showing significant progress. From here, the patient goes home, with or without orders for more therapy under a home care agency or as an outpatient.

To supervise postdischarge therapy properly, the physician must realize that meaningful restorative therapy must be given three times per week for 30 minutes per session. Lesser intensity is usually applicable if the program is geared only to the maintenance of skills. Stroke survivors go to long-term facilities as permanent residents when they have no cognitive, physical, social, or financial means of returning to the community. Others go to those facilities to receive rehabilitative or nursing care as an interim situation while they are expected to reach a level that allows a safe return to the community. Long-term facilities, except those labeled as rehabilitation centers or brain trauma centers, are not expected to offer rehabilitation services of a magnitude comparable with those rendered in an acute setting. Brain trauma centers usually include stroke as a qualifying admitting diagnosis. They are usually strong in their programs of cognitive rehabilitation, implemented in particular by psychologists, occupational therapists, and speech therapists with the intense collaboration of rehabilitation nurses.

The practitioner has two other challenges in the area of stroke rehabilitation. The first is what to do when a program is not producing results. Under these circumstances, the physician must re-evaluate the potential of the patient and watch the implementation of the program. The patient may have less potential than initially thought, may have an intercurrent problem affecting his or her ability to participate, or may have reached a plateau. Perhaps the type of therapy is no longer adequate because the circumstances have become different, or insufficient time is allocated to the therapeutic session. Reacting to his or her findings, the physician can change the goals or can change the program. The second challenge is to decide when to discontinue a program. Programs may go on forever, particularly when otherwise welcome and necessary, warm, affectionate ties develop between the patient and the rehabilitation professional. Under these circumstances, the program becomes a maintenance one. Nothing is wrong with this if financial resources suffice to pay for it and if false hopes are not being sustained. Normally, a program is to be discontinued when sufficient time has elapsed without the patient's showing significant gains in function. Usually, 3 weeks of adequate therapy without any gains justify stopping a program. The patient must not be abandoned, though. Maintenance exercises and activities must continue on a permanent basis under the supervision of the physician. The physician must be alert to signs of renewed potential, which will call for the reactivation of a restorative program of therapy.

The physician must give advice in reference to the need to modify the patient's environment and on the subject of a possible return to gainful employment. A patient may function better if some alterations are performed in his or her dwelling, such as improving the lighting, enlarging a bathroom, or changing the height of the kitchen furniture. Sometimes, the physician must request that the patient be accommodated in a different dwelling, perhaps at street level or in a building with an elevator. Physical, cognitive, perceptual, and behavioral changes may require the patient to give up gainful employment. On many occasions, however, the patient may return to work if certain modifications are made in the place of employment, he or she is trained to perform the same job in a different way, or a new job that the patient is capable of performing is secured. The physician must identify realistic expectations and establish a program to help the patient return to work when possible. Assistance in this task can be obtained from vocational counselors. The physician who treats stroke victims should be familiar with the legislation that is pertinent to the employment of handicapped individuals, namely, The Americans with Disabilities Act.

The prevention of recurrences is a major task in the hands of internists, general and family practitioners, neurologists, geriatricians, and cardiovascular experts. Its discussion does not belong in this article. It can be said only that prevention must be actively pursued with judicious use of medication (i.e., antiplatelet aggregation drugs, antihypertensive medication) and lifestyle modification aimed at reducing risk factors.

EPILEPSY IN ADOLESCENTS AND ADULTS

method of
BASIM M. UTHMAN, M.D., and
B. J. WILDER, M.D.
Department of Veterans Affairs Medical Center
Gainesville, Florida

Epilepsy is a disorder characterized by recurrent episodes of central nervous system (CNS) electrochemical dysfunction that results in involuntary movements and/or various sensory experiences with or without convulsions, impairment of consciousness, or inappropriate changes in ongoing behavior. With the exception of certain rare disorders, such as LaFora's disease and Baltic myoclonus, epilepsy should not be considered a disease entity in itself. Every effort to differentiate epilepsy from seizures associated with other underlying illnesses should be made as decisions for management and treatment are taken. Epilepsy is the second most common neurologic disorder after stroke. Different sources indicate that the prevalence of epilepsy ranges between 0.6 and 3.4% in the general population (more conservative estimates are 0.5 to 1%). The incidence of epilepsy may be age specific, with an estimate of 20 to 40 new cases per 100,000 per year through maturity and middle life. In combination with the incidence rates for isolated seizures with those for epilepsy, it is estimated that 5.9% of the total population may experience at least one nonfebrile seizure in their lifetime.

DIAGNOSIS

Before a patient is labeled epileptic, every effort to rule out nonepileptic seizures should be made. A seizure of any type could be a symptom of an underlying disease process or a systemic derangement, which may or may not be directly related to CNS pathology and thus may be treated differently. These processes include cardiogenic causes, electrolyte imbalance, metabolic derangements, drug withdrawal, drug and metallic intoxication, infections, hyperthermia, and pseudoseizures (Table 1).

The diagnosis of epilepsy is established when seizures recur without an associated illness that could have directly caused convulsive or nonconvulsive seizures (e.g., fever). However, some illnesses and physiologic states, such as sleep deprivation, may be factors in precipitating an epileptic seizure. In more than 50% of patients, the cause of epilepsy cannot be determined. Neuroimaging studies often fail to show structural abnormalities in epileptic patients. Neurophysiologic studies, such as the electroencephalogram (EEG), sometimes show no interictal abnormalities. This should not exclude the diagnosis of a seizure disorder. Although the EEG is an important tool in diagnosis, abnormal findings, such as paroxysmal discharges and focal sharp waves, do not make the diagnosis of epilepsy, but when coupled with a seizure history, they indicate a seizure disorder. Focal and generalized EEG abnormalities associated with partial or generalized

TABLE 1. **Causes of Nonepileptic Seizures**

Cardiogenic
Simple syncope
Transient ischemic attack
Arrhythmias
Sick sinus syndrome

Electrolyte Imbalance
Hypocalcemia
Hyponatremia and water intoxication
Hypomagnesemia

Metabolic
Hypoglycemia
Hyperglycemia
Thyrotoxic storm
Pyridoxine deficiency

Acute Drug Withdrawal
Alcohol
Benzodiazepines
Cocaine
Barbiturates
Meperidine

Drug Intoxication
Cocaine
Dextroamphetamine
Theophylline
Isoniazid
Lithium
Nitrous oxide anesthesia
Acetylcholinesterase inhibitors

Metals
Mercury
Lead

Infections
Gram-negative septicemia with shock
Viral meningitis
Bacterial meningitis (gram-negative or syphilitic)

Hyperthermia

Pseudoseizures (Psychogenic)

Idiopathic (isolated unprovoked seizure)

seizures represent brain electrical dysfunction and do not indicate an etiologic factor. In general, focal EEG abnormalities correlate well with seizures of partial onset, and generalized paroxysmal discharges are correlated with primary generalized seizure disorders. The best correlation between EEG findings and seizures occurs in absence epilepsy, in which the EEG shows 3 Hz (range, 2.5 to 4) paroxysmal generalized spike and wave discharge.

With a careful history, clinical observation, and EEG findings, an accurate classification of seizure type can be made in most patients. The International Classification of Epileptic Seizures (Table 2) pivots around the onset of the seizures (i.e., whether it is generalized or focal and whether there is associated loss or impairment or no impairment of consciousness). "Partial" seizures denote seizures beginning locally, and they may be either simple or complex. Simple partial (SP) seizures indicate elementary signs or symptoms without impairment of consciousness. These symptoms may be somatic motor (e.g., jacksonian seizures), somatosensory, special sensory, or autonomic. Often, patients re-

port having "just auras and no seizures." These "auras" usually represent SP seizures with somatic and special sensory symptoms that may be isolated or may precede a complex partial seizure (CPS). The physician should carefully ask about these symptoms, because patients may disregard these experiences and inadvertently not volunteer this information.

CPS (partial seizures with complex symptoms), also known as temporal lobe or psychomotor seizures, denote seizures beginning locally with impairment of consciousness (e.g., awareness, cognition). Impairment of consciousness only as manifested by staring is a common symptom that is frequently described by witnesses as "glassy eyes." Other symptoms may be cognitive, affective, "psychosensory," or "psychomotor" with semipurposeful automatisms. Not infrequently, partial seizures may spread and become secondarily generalized. Generalized seizures are associated with a loss of consciousness at the onset and are bilaterally symmetric without focality. Generalized seizures may be convulsive or nonconvulsive. The convulsive generalized seizures predominantly seen in adolescents may be tonic-clonic (GTC, grand mal), clonic, clonic-tonic-clonic (GCTC), or myoclonic. Nonconvulsive general-

TABLE 2. **The International Classification of Epileptic Seizures**

Partial (Focal, Local) Seizures
　Simple Partial Seizures (Consciousness Not Impaired)
　　With motor symptoms
　　With somatosensory or special sensory symptoms
　　With autonomic symptoms
　　With psychic symptoms
　Complex Partial Seizures (with Impairment of Consciousness)
　　BEGINNING AS SIMPLE PARTIAL SEIZURES AND PROGRESSING TO IMPAIRMENT OF CONSCIOUSNESS
　　　With no other features
　　　With features as in I.A.1 to I.A.4
　　　With automatisms
　　WITH IMPAIRMENT OF CONSCIOUSNESS AT ONSET
　　　With no other features
　　　With features as in I.A.1 to I.A.4
　　　With automatisms
　Partial Seizures Evolving to Secondarily Generalized Seizures
　　Simple partial seizures evolving to generalized seizures
　　Complex partial seizures evolving to generalized seizures
　　Simple partial seizures evolving to complex partial seizures to generalized seizures

Generalized Seizures (Convulsive or Nonconvulsive)
　Absence Seizures
　　Absence seizures
　　Atypical absence seizures
　Myoclonic Seizures
　Clonic Seizures
　Tonic Seizures
　Tonic-Clonic Seizures
　Atonic Seizures (Astatic Seizures)

Unclassified Epileptic Seizures
Includes all seizures that cannot be classified because of inadequate or incomplete data and some that defy classification in hitherto-described categories; this includes some neonatal seizures (e.g., rhythmic eye movements, chewing, and swimming movements)

ized seizures may include absence (petit mal), atonic, and akinetic seizures. The classification of seizures is important for communication among treating physicians, the treatment of specific seizure types, and the prognosis. Some common seizure types may be difficult to differentiate clinically. The majority of patients who report their seizures as "petit mal" do not have typical absence or petit mal seizures, but they turn out to have CPS.

Absence (petit mal) and CPS are commonly confused and misdiagnosed. An accurate diagnosis can often be made on the basis of history, the duration of the seizure, the presence of an aura and/or postictal confusion, the pattern of automatic behavior, and the EEG. In absence seizures, minor clonic activity (eye blinks or head nodding) is present in up to 45% of cases, the mean duration is about 10 seconds, and the EEG shows the typical bilateral symmetrical 3 cycles per second spike and wave that may be easily provoked by hyperventilation. There is no aura or postictal confusion. In contrast, CPS may be preceded by an aura, are followed by postictal confusion, last longer (1 to 3 minutes), and are associated with more complex automatisms and less frequent clonic components. The EEG tends to show focal slow or sharp and slow wave activity. The differentiation between these two types of seizures is important. Absence seizures tend to disappear in adulthood, but CPS do not. Furthermore, phenytoin (Dilantin) and carbamazepine (Tegretol) are effective in treating CPS but not absence attacks.

Another important distinction is between the primarily GTC seizure and secondarily GTC seizures. The former denotes loss of consciousness from the onset of the attack and is more common in the idiopathic epilepsies. The latter denotes focality of onset with subsequent spread of activity to involve both hemispheres; it is more common in the symptomatic group. These two types respond differently to different antiepileptic drugs (AEDs). In addition, the manifestation of certain seizure types may localize the firing focus that may not otherwise show on neuroimaging or EEG studies.

The classification of the epilepsies and the epileptic syndromes (Table 3) is a further effort to categorize epileptic patients who have seizures of similar type, behavior, and natural history. The classification depends on the seizure types, specific EEG abnormality, age at onset, family history, and neurologic findings.

From the etiologic point of view, symptomatic (or secondary) and idiopathic (or primary) epilepsy must be differentiated (Table 4). Symptomatic epilepsy is usually caused by recent or remote focal or diffuse injury to the brain, malformations, tumors, or residua of infection. Idiopathic epilepsy results from a genetic predisposition. The signs of this injury are usually structural abnormalities that can often be detected by neuroimaging studies. The most common types of seizures seen in symptomatic epilepsy are SP, CPS, and secondarily generalized seizures. The idiopathic type entails epilepsies of unknown etiology without underlying CNS structural abnormalities or history of brain injury. These epilepsies tend to run in families, and the mode of inheritance is variable. Seizure types in the idiopathic group of adolescent and adult epileptic patients are usually primary generalized convulsive or nonconvulsive seizures. The classic absence type is not

TABLE 3. International Classification of Epilepsies and Epileptic Syndromes

Localization-Related (Focal, Local, Partial) Epilepsies and Syndromes
Idiopathic (with Age-Related Onset)
  Benign childhood epilepsy with centrotemporal spike
  Childhood epilepsy with occipital paroxysms
Symptomatic
  Syndromes of great individual variability

Generalized Epilepsies and Syndromes
Idiopathic (with Age-Related Onset; in Order of Age at Appearance)
  Benign neonatal familial convulsions
  Benign neonatal convulsions
  Benign myoclonic epilepsy in infancy
  Childhood absence epilepsy (pyknolepsy, petit mal)
  Juvenile absence epilepsy
  Juvenile myoclonic epilepsy (impulsive petit mal)
  Epilepsy with grand mal seizures (generalized tonic-clonic) on awakening
Idiopathic and/or Symptomatic (in Order of Age at Appearance)
  West's syndrome (infantile spasms, Blitz-Nick-Salaam Krampfe)
  Lennox, Gastaut syndrome
  Epilepsy with myoclonic-astatic seizures
  Epilepsy myoclonic absences
Symptomatic
  NONSPECIFIC ETIOLOGY
    Early myoclonic encephalopathy
  SPECIFIC SYNDROMES
    Epileptic seizures may complicate many disease states; include diseases in which seizures are the presenting or predominant feature

Epilepsies and Syndromes Undetermined as to Whether They are Focal or Generalized
With Both Generalized and Focal Seizures
  Neonatal seizures
  Severe myoclonic epilepsy in infancy
  Epilepsy with continuous spikes and waves during slow-wave sleep
  Acquired epileptic aphasia (Landau-Kleffner syndrome)
Without Unequivocal Generalized or Focal Features

Special Syndromes
Situation-Related Seizures (Gelegenheitsanfalle)
  Febrile convulsions
  Seizures related to other identifiable situations, such as stress, hormones, drugs, alcohol, or sleep deprivation
Isolated Apparently Unprovoked Epileptic Events
Epilepsies Characterized by Specific Modes of Seizure Precipitated
Chronic Progressive Epilepsia Partialis Continua of Childhood

common in this age group. When present in these patients, absence attacks are often accompanied by GTC, GCTC, or myoclonic attacks. The main causes for epileptic seizures with onset in the adolescent age group (10 to 18 years) are idiopathic and traumatic. In early adulthood, trauma, vascular malformation or bleeding, and idiopathic causes are common. In middle age (35 to 60 years), trauma, neoplasm, and vascular disease become more common, and in late adulthood (> 60 years), vascular disease, tumor, and degenerative disease take precedence.

TABLE 4. **Possible Causes of Epileptic Seizures in Adolescents and Adults**

Symptomatic (Secondary Epilepsy)
Head Trauma
   Perinatal
   Postnatal
   Acute head trauma
Encephalopathy
   Hypoxic (cardiac arrest, carbon monoxide poisoning,
      perinatal ischemia, suffocation, or respiratory arrest)
   Hypertensive
   Infectious:
      Viral (herpes simplex, Jakob-Creutzfeld disease)
      Bacterial
      Fungal
      Parasitic (neurocysticercosis)
   Neoplasia
   Primary brain tumors (astrocytoma, glioblastoma
      multiforme)
   Metastatic
Temporal Mesial Sclerosis
Phakomatoses
Vascular
   Malformations
   Aneurysms
   Hemorrhage (intraparenchymal, superficial siderosis)
   Stroke (thrombotic or embolic infarcts)
   Thrombotic thrombocytopenia purpura
   Cortical phlebothrombosis or thrombophlebitis
Degenerative
Idiopathic (Primary Epilepsy)
   Juvenile myoclonic epilepsy
   Juvenile absence
   Myoclonic
   Primary generalized tonic-clonic or clonic-tonic-clonic

ACUTE MANAGEMENT OF SEIZURES

In situations of acute seizures, the treating physician should observe the clinical manifestations from the onset, if possible with attention to any localization-related signs and the patient's degree of awareness and responsiveness. This is done with the goal of classifying the seizure type. First-aid measures should be taken to secure a patent airway, breathing, and circulation. No acute treatment with intravenous AEDs is necessary unless the seizure is prolonged or recurs repetitively within 1 hour. Every effort should be made to rule out nonepileptic seizures. Blood should be obtained for a complete blood count; measurements of serum glucose, electrolytes, calcium, albumin (to estimate the free Ca^{2+}), magnesium, blood urea nitrogen, and creatinine; liver function tests; and AED levels. Urine for urinalysis microscopy and drug screening should be collected. The patient's temperature and vital signs should be monitored. An alcoholic breath odor and signs of trauma (such as batter sign and raccoon eye) should be sought. A careful history from witnesses, family members, inmates, or life squad should be taken. A history of seizures should be entertained. A lumbar puncture for cerebrospinal fluid cell count, glucose, protein, Gram stain, and culture may be obtained. Pleocytosis is seen sometimes acutely after prolonged convulsive generalized seizures without an underlying infection. However, when it is present, infection must be ruled out.

In some situations, the patient may be admitted to the hospital for 24-hour observation. Later on, an EEG and a computed tomographic scan or magnetic resonance image of the head should be obtained even if the neurologic examination shows no abnormality. The patient should be advised to undertake seizure precaution (e.g., no driving, diving, or operating heavy machines) for several months, up to 1 year. Treatment with AEDs may not be initiated if the seizure was isolated and no possible etiology was identified. Before a patient is committed to long-term therapy with AEDs, the diagnosis of epilepsy should be established. For better compliance and treatment success, the patient should be educated about his or her seizures, and the treatment plan should be shared with him or her.

MANAGEMENT OF PATIENTS WITH A HISTORY OF RECURRENT SEIZURES

When a patient is referred with documented history of recurrent seizures and the diagnosis of epilepsy is established, a careful history about seizure types, the age at onset, the duration and frequency of the seizures, the time of occurrence of the seizures, trends of clustering or cyclicity, and precipitating factors should be taken. The longest seizure-free period and the history of the best control with certain AEDs with adequate documented serum AED levels should be evaluated. Appropriate studies should be considered if a prior work-up was judged to be incomplete. If a patient is already being treated and is taking more than one AED, every effort to treat with only one drug should be made. Patients are often receiving unnecessary multiple pharmaceuticals. Polypharmacy-type therapy is more expensive, more difficult to comply with, and may produce more side effects. Above all, because of drug interactions, one may not achieve adequate effective AED levels with the usual doses. This may result in toxicity and poor seizure control. The main principle in the treatment of epilepsy is to classify the seizure type and the epilepsy and treat with the most appropriate drug. Before considering another drug, monotherapy should be pursued until seizure control is achieved or toxicity occurs, whichever comes first. Often, serum AED levels above the upper "therapeutic" range may be necessary to achieve seizure control. Serum AED levels should be considered as a guide only, and the dosages should be modified as dictated by the response of the patient.

TREATMENT

The goal of treatment should be complete seizure control with minimal or no side effects. Therefore, after identifying the seizure type, therapy should be started with the least toxic single drug that is likely to produce long-term seizure control. A total daily dose may be individually "tailored" and "fine tuned," according to the patient's response. The serum levels serve as a guide to dosing and avoiding toxicity. They may be obtained periodically to ensure compliance. A trough serum AED level is preferable to have a consistent method of comparison at different intervals. The physician must be aware that different AEDs interact with each other when given together, and the serum levels may change. AEDs may interact with other medications too, such as antacids, antimicrobial agents (erythromycin), antifungals, oral contraceptives, isoniazid, disulfiram (Antabuse), propoxyphene (Darvon), calcium channel blockers, and H_2 blockers.

The interactions can be pharmacokinetic or pharmacodynamic. Pharmacokinetic interactions may occur at the stage of absorption, protein binding, or clearance and metabolism. Protein binding is an important property of the most commonly used AEDs. For example, phenytoin is 90 to 95% protein bound, and if another highly protein-bound compound is added and 10% of the protein-bound phenytoin is knocked off its protein sites, the serum free (unbound) phenytoin level would double, and the patient may experience toxic side effects. Some AEDs are inhibitors (e.g., valproate [Depakote]), and some are inducers (e.g., phenytoin and carbamazepine) of hepatic enzymes and, thus, may increase or decrease the serum levels of other drugs used concomitantly. Pharmacodynamic interactions are the effects of drugs that may potentiate or antagonize the effects of the other drugs on receptor sites.

The four major AEDs used at the present time are phenytoin, carbamazepine, valproate, and ethosuximide (Zarontin). Adjunctive AEDs include clorazepate (Tranxene), clonazepam (Klonopin), phenobarbital, primidone (Mysoline), and acetazolamide (Diamox). Ethosuximide or valproate is the drug of choice for absence seizures. Valproate is the drug of choice for the treatment of absence with tonic-clonic, absence with myoclonus (e.g., juvenile myoclonic epilepsy), GTC, and GCTC seizures. Carbamazepine and phenytoin may be as effective as valproate in the convulsive generalized seizures, such as grand mal (GTC)

seizures. Tonic and atonic seizures respond poorly to therapy; however, valproate remains the drug of choice, and clonazepam is an alternative. Phenytoin and carbamazepine are the drugs of choice in the symptomatic epilepsies of adolescence and adults, including seizures of partial onset. Valproate may be effective in the treatment of seizures of partial onset and, in particular, those that become secondarily generalized.

When the first AED is pushed to its maximal tolerated dosage without complete control of seizures, a second AED may be added. The first drug should be continued temporarily. After obtaining good seizure control with combination therapy, the first AED may be gradually withdrawn to see whether seizure control can be maintained using monotherapy with the second drug. The first AED should be tapered slowly over several weeks to prevent the occurrence of withdrawal seizures. If seizures recur, combination therapy with the first and second AEDs may be necessary. The patient should be advised not to drive during the process of AED withdrawal. When two-AED combination therapy fails to control seizures, a third AED may be added with the understanding that the first or second AED will be gradually withdrawn to minimize drug interactions and side effects.

A common question by patients is whether they have to receive AEDs for the rest of their lives or not. Often, patients may experiment by withdrawing their own AEDs to test whether they need them or not. Sometimes, the patient may remain seizure free without medications; however, most of the time, the withdrawal of AEDs is either sudden or too fast, and the patient may experience recurrence of seizures. In that case, it is difficult to differentiate whether the recurrent seizure was a withdrawal seizure or not. If seizures recur after appropriate slow AED withdrawal (approximately 25% of the total daily dose every 2 weeks), the chances are that AED therapy should be resumed to obtain seizure control. It is important to discuss the long-term plans with the patient and share the probable prognosis to the best of the physician's knowledge. It is highly recommended that AED therapy be continued for 2 to 5 years after the last seizure. At the end of that seizure-free period, an EEG is obtained and the continuation of AED therapy is re-evaluated.

Antiepileptic Drug Treatment and Pregnancy

Patients with child-bearing potential are advised of the teratogenic risks associated with the use of AEDs during pregnancy. Most AEDs have some teratogenic effects; however, these should be weighed against the risks of having seizures. The comparative teratogenicity of AEDs has not been well established. Each patient should be treated on an individual basis. As a general rule, if a pregnancy is planned ahead of time and the patient has been seizure free for 2 to 5 years, slow tapering of AEDs may be contemplated; otherwise, the lowest effective dose of the most effective AED may be administered. When a patient taking AEDs seeks advice during the second trimester of her pregnancy, discontinuation of AEDs may not be a wise decision, because most of the teratogenic effects tend to occur during the first trimester. Because of some pharmacokinetic changes during pregnancy (e.g., increased metabolism, decreased absorption, increased volume of distribution), close serum AED level monitoring (e.g., every 4 to 6 weeks) is advised, and periodic modification of the dosage may be necessary. AEDs may increase the risk of third-trimester and neonatal hemorrhage. Pregnant women receiving AEDs are advised to take folic acid and multivitamins, and 1 to 2 weeks before delivery, oral vitamin K, 20 mg per day should be administered. The newborn should also be treated with vitamin K to prevent hemorrhage. Most of the AEDs have been reported to cause a fetal anticonvulsant syndrome characterized by hypoplastic nails, short distal phalanges, and wide-set eyes. In pregnant women treated with carbamazepine, valproate, or a combination of both, follow-up with ultrasonography at 16 weeks' gestation is recommended in order to rule out neural tube defects.

Another concern that, fortunately, is reaching layman awareness is the use of generic forms of certain AEDs. The bioavailability of some generic forms of AEDs is not the same as that of the brand-name drugs in some cases, in particular, phenytoin and carbamazepine. There may be several generic products of the same AED, and the bioavailability among them may vary considerably.

Methods of Treatment

Phenytoin

Phenytoin is a choice drug for the treatment of partial (SP or CPS) seizures and primarily and secondarily GTC seizures. The maintenance dosage is 4 to 7 mg per kg per day. A loading dose of 15 to 20 mg per kg can be given either orally in three equal doses at 2- to 4-hour intervals, or intravenously at a rate not to exceed 50 mg per minute. Phenytoin is also available in a 125 mg and 30 mg per 5-mL oral suspension in 8-ounce bottles and in 5-mL unit-dose cups. For paren-

teral use, it is available in 5-mL ampules containing a sterile solution of 50 mg per mL of phenytoin sodium. Rapid intravenous administration may cause severe hypotension. Phenytoin should not be given intramuscularly, because the injections are painful and absorption is erratic by this route. Muscle biopsy at the site of phenytoin injection shows crystal formation of phenytoin and muscle fiber necrosis. The usual phenytoin dose of 4 to 5 mg per kg per day can be taken once daily in most adults. The average half-life of phenytoin is 22 to 24 hours, and it may take 1 week or more to reach a steady-state level if a loading dose was not given.

Some patients are naturally fast metabolizers of phenytoin and may need a dose higher than usual. The therapeutic serum levels denote the serum AED level usually associated with a significant reduction in seizures or complete seizure control without evidence of toxicity. The usual therapeutic range for phenytoin is 10 to 25 µg per mL of serum. However, some cases may be well controlled with serum levels less than 10 µg per mL or greater than 25 µg per mL without toxicity.

Phenytoin toxicity may be manifested as ataxia, dysarthria, nystagmus, cognitive impairment, dystonic posturing, and, in some cases of extremely high serum levels, increased seizure frequency. Allergic or idiosyncratic reactions are rare and include Stevens-Johnson syndrome, hepatitis, nephritis, lymphoma-like syndromes, agranulocytosis, thyroiditis, and systemic lupus erythematosus. The side effects associated with chronic phenytoin use include gingival hyperplasia, hirsutism, and coarse facial features. Peripheral neuropathy is rarely seen.

Phenytoin 100-mg capsules are almost completely absorbed through the gastrointestinal tract over a 1-day period with peak levels at 8 to 12 hours after the dose. The drug is 90 to 95% protein bound in the serum and is metabolized mainly in the liver. One may not be able to predict accurately the serum phenytoin concentration at a certain dose from the serum concentration taken at a different dose. Phenytoin has dose-dependent pharmacokinetics, which may change from first-order kinetics at lower doses to zero-order kinetics at higher doses. This change may occur at serum levels that are in the therapeutic range. Therefore, if a change in dose is desired when the serum levels are in the therapeutic range, fine tuning of the dose with smaller increments or decrements should be practiced. For this reason, phenytoin is also available in 50-mg tablets (Infatabs), which have the advantage of prompt absorption and the disadvantage of toxic side effects associated with the serum peak level. A 30-mg capsule that is similar to the 100-mg ones is also available. Periodic trough phenytoin levels are recommended, and sometimes, a determination of serum unbound (free) phenytoin may be necessary in patients with hepatic diseases or drug interactions. Drugs that are known to increase serum phenytoin level include carbamazepine, cimetidine (Tagamet), and chloramphenicol (chloromycetin), isoniazid, chlorpromazine (Thorazine), disulfiram, and propoxyphene. Phenytoin may lower the serum levels of concomitant oral contraceptives and other steroids, digoxin (Lanoxin), and thyroid hormone. Salicylates and ethanol may lower the serum phenytoin level.

Carbamazepine

According to the Veterans Affairs Cooperative double-blind AED efficacy study, carbamazepine and phenytoin showed no statistically significant difference in their effect on reducing GTC seizures or seizures of partial onset. Both were superior to primidone and phenobarbital. The usual maintenance dose is 10 to 20 mg per kg per day given orally. Because of its relatively short half-life (8 to 20 hours) and toxic effects associated with peak levels (2 to 3 hours after ingestion), administration in two to four divided daily doses is recommended. Carbamazepine is supplied as 100-mg chewable and 200-mg scored tablets, which can be divided easily for initiation of therapy. Carbamazepine is also available in a 100-mg per 5 mL oral suspension. The initial dosage should be small (100 to 200 mg in two daily doses for adults) to prevent gastrointestinal and other unpleasant side effects. This dosage can be increased in daily increments of 200 mg every 3 to 5 days until seizure control or therapeutic serum levels are attained. Usually, patients cannot tolerate taking the full maintenance daily dose initially, and titrating up is recommended; otherwise, carbamazepine treatment may be dropped and prematurely considered as a failure.

Carbamazepine is approximately 75% protein bound. Valproate may compete for its binding sites. Carbamazepine is metabolized in the liver to carbamazepine-10, 11-epoxide and carbamazepine-10, 11-dihydroxide. The former is pharmacologically active and has an anticonvulsant activity and toxicity similar to the parent compound. The usual therapeutic range of serum carbamazepine level is from 6 to 12 µg per mL; however, higher levels may be necessary in some cases for seizure control. With long-term carbamazepine therapy epoxide concentrations range between 15 to 50% of the carbamazepine serum concentrations.

Carbamazepine is a hepatic enzyme inducer and may reduce the effects of co-administered drugs, such as oral anticoagulants and contracep-tives. Other hepatic enzyme-inducing drugs, such as phenobarbital and phenytoin, may reduce the effects of carbamazepine, and higher doses of carbamazepine may be necessary to achieve the same serum levels. Cimetidine, calcium channel blockers, fluoxetine (Prozac), propoxyphene, erythromycin, and chloramphenicol co-administration may raise the serum carbamazepine concentrations and may result in toxicity. Carbamazepine causes autoinduction of its metabolism that results in a decrease in its half-life. This process may take many weeks (8 to 15) before stable steady-state serum levels of carbamazepine can be achieved; thus, close monitoring of serum carbamazepine levels in the first 2 to 4 months is advisable. A baseline complete blood count, serum electrolytes, and liver function tests are recommended, to be followed up periodically every 2 to 3 months initially for the first 6 to 12 months and, then probably, biannually thereafter.

Carbamazepine was reported earlier to have serious hematologic toxicity; however, this is rare, and the toxicity of carbamazepine is probably no greater than that of other AEDs. The side effects of carbamazepine include gastrointestinal disturbances, drowsiness, diplopia, blurred vision, and headache. These side effects are more common with higher serum carbamazepine levels, and dose adjustment usually alleviates those symptoms. The side effects are sometimes intermittent and coincide with the peak serum levels. In these situations, spreading and dividing the total daily dose over a longer period of time may alleviate the symptoms. Most of the adverse reactions are usually experienced in the first few weeks of therapy and often clear in a few days to weeks without dosage adjustment. Acute overdosage of carbamazepine may result in nausea, vomiting, nystagmus, drowsiness or coma, restlessness, agitation, confusion, tremor, abnormal reflexes, mydriasis, flushing, and urinary retention. Allergic reactions to carbamazepine may include various forms of dermatitis and skin eruptions or rashes.

Carbamazepine administration should be avoided in patients with history of serious blood dyscrasias or known sensitivity to tricyclic compounds. Carbamazepine should be used with caution in patients with cardiac irregularities or coronary artery disease. Carbamazepine may have an antidiuretic effect that may result in water intoxication, hyponatremia, and an increase in seizure activity. Neural tube defects have been reported in children of mothers receiving carbamazepine during pregnancy. The risks and benefits of carbamazepine treatment during pregnancy have to be weighed, and the serum carbamazepine levels should be closely monitored to avoid excessive concentrations and exposure to the fetus.

Ethosuximide

Ethosuximide is very effective in the treatment of absence (petit mal) seizures and is well tolerated by patients. The common side effects include drowsiness and gastrointestinal upset. Leukopenia may occur in a minority of patients and is reversible if detected early and ethosuximide is withdrawn. The maintenance dose is usually 15 to 30 mg per kg per day given in two equal doses. Therapy is started initially at 500 mg per day followed by 250-mg daily increments every few days to 1 week until seizure control is achieved or intolerable side effects result. Ethosuximide is available in 250-mg capsules. It is absorbed through the gastrointestinal tract almost completely, and its binding to serum protein is minimal. Ethosuximide does not have significant interactions with other AEDs, and if toxicity associated with the peak serum levels occur, the total daily dosage should be divided into three or four equal doses.

Valproate

Sodium divalproex has the same efficacy as ethosuximide in the treatment of absence seizures. Either AED may be used as a first choice; however, in some cases, a combination of both valproate and ethosuximide may be necessary to control petit mal seizures. Valproate is as effective as phenytoin and carbamazepine in the treatment of primarily GTC seizures. Valproate is the drug of choice in the treatment of absence associated with myoclonic or GTC seizures, in particular, juvenile myoclonic epilepsy. Valproate is also effective in the treatment of seizures of partial onset, especially those that are secondarily generalized. A controlled double-blind study comparing carbamazepine and valproate in the treatment of partial seizures has shown a slightly increased efficacy for carbamazepine, and more side effects were reported with valproate.

The usual maintenance dosage is 15 to 60 mg per kg per day in three to four divided doses. The initial dosage is 10 to 15 mg per kg per day with 4 to 10-mg per kg per day increments every week until seizure control is achieved or side effects occur. The therapeutic serum level range is 50 to 140 μg per mL. The common side effects include gastrointestinal upset, drowsiness, tremor, and weight gain. Other side effects may include platelet dysfunction, hyperammonemia, and elevated serum transaminase levels. Idiosyncratic side effects may include pancreatitis, thrombocytopenia, hepatitis, coma, and hair loss. Fatal hepatic failure may occur, and the greatest risk is in

TABLE 5. Status Epilepticus Flowchart: Suggested Guidelines for Initial Treatment

Critical Primary Care
Airway, oxygen, ventilation
Vital signs
Intravenous line
Initial tests:
  2 red-top* tubes (glucose, electrolytes, Ca²⁺, AED levels)
  1 purple-top tube (CBC)
  ABGs, if possible
  urine for toxic screen

General Treatment (IV therapy)
100 mg of thiamine
25–50 ml of 50% glucose (if blood glucose is low)
50–100 ml/h of normal saline

Anticonvulsant Therapy
Lorazepam (Ativan) 0.1 mg/kg total dose at 2 mg/min or diazepam (Valium) 0.15 mg/kg at 3–5 mg/min
Simultaneous loading with phenytoin (Dilantin) 20 mg/kg at 50 mg/min (use slower rates for small, cardiac, or old patients); monitor BP and HR

If Status Persists
Intubate and administer phenobarbital 15 mg/kg at 100 mg/min
Transfer to ICU
Call a neurologist

Caution
Intravenous phenytoin may cause hypotension
Diazepam, lorazepam, and phenobarbital can cause sedation and cardiorespiratory depression
Do not give any of these drugs if the patient is known to be allergic to them

*Save one for further testing that is initially not expected.
Abbreviations: AED = antiepileptic drugs; CBC = complete blood count; ABG = arterial blood gases; BP = blood pressure; HR = heart rate; ICU = intensive care unit.

young children receiving multiple AEDs. At particular risk are those younger than 2 years of age who are receiving other AEDs. Gastrointestinal side effects are more frequent with valproate (Depakene) and are much less frequent with the enteric-coated divalproex sodium formulation (Depakote).

Divalproex sodium is available in 125-mg, 250-mg, and 500-mg tablets. Valproate is not available for parenteral use at the present time. A slow-release 125-mg "sprinkle" formulation is available for children. The absorption of divalproex sodium is delayed, with the peak concentration occurring 3 to 4 hours after oral administration. Valproate can be given in two to three divided daily doses. Valproate is almost completely absorbed, and it is 75 to 90% protein bound (less protein binding percentage at higher serum levels). Valproate is primarily metabolized in the liver, and minimal amounts are lost in the urine or feces. Active metabolites are formed. A Δ^2-valproate metabolite is an anticonvulsant and may account for the increasing efficacy noted in some patients over a 4 to 6-week period after the initiation of therapy. Neural tube defects are reported in 1 to 1.5% of the offspring of epileptic mothers who receive valproate during the first trimester of pregnancy.

Other Drugs

Other AEDs that may be used as adjunctive therapy include phenobarbital, primidone, clorazepate, mephenytoin (Mesantoin), methsuximide (Celontin), ethotoin (Peganone), and clonazepam. Phenobarbital continues to be widely used in treating seizures; however, high doses are associated with impaired cognitive function. Phenobarbital is a sedative, reduces the attention span, and may impair learning. Primidone may be effective in symptomatic epilepsy. It should only be used in monotherapy. It is partially metabolized to phenobarbital in the liver. These adjunctive AEDs may be tried when the four major AEDs are ineffective or cause intolerable and serious side effects. Diazepam (Valium) or lorazepam (Ativan) may be used orally or rectally for intermittent home treatment to stop clusters of seizures and avoid unnecessary and expensive hospitalization. Phenytoin, phenobarbital, diazepam, and lorazepam may also be administered intravenously in the treatment of acute seizures, including status epilepticus. Status epilepticus is not discussed in this chapter; however, it is a medical emergency which requires adequate and prompt management and treatment. Guidelines for the initial treatment of status epilepticus are listed in Table 5.

Currently, there are more than 10 experimental AEDs under study, and a few have proven to be very promising. Three of these drugs (felbamate, lamotrigine, and gabapentin) are expected to be licensed in the United States in 1993.

EPILEPSY IN INFANTS AND CHILDREN

method of
KEVIN FARRELL, M.B., Ch.B., and
MARY B. CONNOLLY, M.B., B.Ch.
University of British Columbia
Vancouver, Canada

Epileptic seizures occur commonly in children and present diagnostic as well as treatment challenges. The incidence of educational and psychosocial difficulties is also higher among children with epilepsy, and the diagnosis of epilepsy may have a profound impact on the child and other family members, leading to secondary emotional difficulties. Consequently, a clear understanding of the factors that influence the diagno-

TABLE 1. **Steps in the Management of Epilepsy in Children**

Establish if the episodes are epileptic seizures.
Determine the type of seizure.
Look for the etiology of the epilepsy.
Decide if the child has an epileptic syndrome.
Decide whether to use antiepileptic medication.
Choose an antiepileptic drug and use appropriately.
Look for evidence of educational or social problems.
Educate the child and parents about epilepsy.
Decide when to discontinue medication.
Consider surgery if the seizures are intractable.

sis and treatment of epilepsy in childhood is important in the management of the child and family. This article describes a series of steps that permit a comprehensive approach to the management of epilepsy in children (Table 1).

EPILEPTIC OR NONEPILEPTIC SEIZURES

An epileptic seizure is a clinical event that occurs as a result of an abnormal, paroxysmal electrical discharge within the cerebral cortex. Many paroxysmal clinical events that resemble epileptic seizures are due not to epilepsy but to some other cause. Indeed, 20 to 25% of patients referred to one epilepsy clinic did not have epileptic seizures. The description of the episode is the most important clue to the diagnosis of nonepileptic events in childhood. Many of the episodes that mimic epileptic seizures occur in the first few years of life when the patient is least able to describe the symptoms. It is important to speak to someone who has witnessed an episode. In particular, it is important to ask about provoking factors and what was occurring before the event and to obtain a good description of the onset of the episode. The more common nonepileptic episodic phenomena are listed in Table 2.

The diagnosis of an epileptic seizure is based largely on the clinical history and, to a lesser extent, on the electroencephalogram (EEG). The clinical onset of an epileptic seizure is abrupt. If an aura occurs, it lasts for 1 or 2 seconds and not as long as the prodrome of migraine or the premonitory signs of a faint. If consciousness has been lost, there is a period of postictal confusion.

TABLE 2. **Paroxysmal Events That Can Resemble Seizures**

Breath-holding attacks
Syncope
Paroxysmal vertigo
Migraine and periodic syndrome
Hyperventilation syndrome
Pseudoepileptic seizures
Paroxysmal sleep disorders
Night terrors
Somnambulism
Movement disorders
Tics
Paroxysmal choreoathetosis

Role of EEG in the Diagnosis of Epilepsy

The EEG plays an important role in the diagnosis of epilepsy but is neither a sensitive nor a specific method of diagnosis in most children with epilepsy. Routine EEG recordings are performed for approximately 40 minutes, and it is uncommon for seizures to occur during the recording. Although the EEG nearly always demonstrates epileptiform abnormalities during an epileptic seizure, the interictal EEG is frequently normal in children with epilepsy, particularly in the very young. Conversely, epileptiform abnormalities may be observed in children without seizures. Thus, as with any laboratory test, the results of the EEG should be interpreted in relation to the clinical history. For example, in children younger than 10 years of age with absence seizures, the EEG always demonstrates 3 cycle per second spike and wave activity, particularly during hyperventilation. Similarly, generalized bursts of spike and wave activity are usually observed in the interictal recordings of patients with myoclonic seizures. In contrast, the interictal EEG is often normal in patients younger than 1 years of age who have generalized tonic-clonic or partial seizures. Focal EEG abnormalities are often seen only during sleep, and it is important that the child be asleep for at least some of the recording. For this reason, the parent should be instructed to deprive the child of at least 3 hours of sleep during the night before an EEG examination.

In addition to its role in the establishment of a diagnosis of epilepsy, the EEG is also important in the recognition of specific epileptic syndromes. Recognition of a specific epilepsy syndrome may be particularly useful with respect to the prognosis and treatment. The more common epileptic syndromes and their EEG characteristics are discussed subsequently.

TYPES OF SEIZURES

Seizures are classified according to whether they arise from a focal area of the brain or are generalized from the onset (Table 3). Seizure classification is based on the clinical description of the seizure, the EEG abnormalities during the seizure, and the EEG abnor-

TABLE 3. Classification of Epileptic Seizures

Partial Seizures
Simple partial seizures
Complex partial seizures
Partial seizures evolving to secondarily generalized seizures

Generalized Seizures
Absence seizures
Myoclonic seizures
Clonic seizures
Tonic seizures
Tonic-clonic seizures
Atonic seizures

Unclassified Seizures
Infantile spasms

Modified from Dreifuss, FE: Proposal for revised clinical and electroencephalographic classification of epileptic seizures. Epilepsia *22*:489–501, 1981.

TABLE 4. Influence of Seizure Type, Epileptic Syndrome, and Specific EEG Abnormalities on Choice of Drug

Type or Syndrome	Drug
Seizure Type	
Tonic-clonic	**Carbamazepine, valproic acid,*** phenytoin, phenobarbital
Partial	**Carbamazepine,** phenytoin, valproic acid
Absence	**Ethosuximide, valproic acid,** clonazepam
Myoclonic	**Valproic acid,** clonazepam,
Atypical absence	corticosteroids
Atonic	
Epileptic Syndrome	
Neonatal seizures	**Phenobarbital,** phenytoin
Febrile convulsions	Rectal diazepam, phenobarbital
Infantile spasms	**ACTH,** prednisolone, valproic acid, clonazepam
Lennox-Gastaut syndrome	**Valproic acid,** clonazepam
Childhood absence	**Ethosuximide,** valproic acid, clonazepam
Juvenile myoclonic epilepsy	**Valproic acid,** clonazepam
EEG Abnormalities	
Focal discharges	**Carbamazepine,** phenytoin
Generalized spike-wave	**Valproic acid,** clonazepam

*Drugs listed in **bold print** reflect the authors' choice.
Abbreviations: EEG = electroencephalogram; ACTH = adrenocorticotropin.

malities between seizures. In most patients, the physician has to rely on the history and the interictal EEG. Consequently, seizure classification can sometimes be difficult.

Seizure classification is important in the determination of the possible cause of the seizure, the diagnosis of specific epilepsy syndromes, and in the choice of the antiepileptic drug. Certain seizure types respond differently to particular antiepileptic drugs (Table 4). Thus, whereas ethosuximide (Zarontin) is very effective in the prevention of absence seizures, it is ineffective in the treatment of partial seizures. Conversely, carbamazepine (Tegretol) is effective in the prevention of partial and generalized tonic-clonic seizures, but it is not effective in the treatment of absence seizures and, indeed, may exacerbate this type of seizure.

ETIOLOGY OF THE EPILEPSY

Epileptic seizures are a manifestation of an underlying neurologic disorder. In most patients, several factors contribute to the occurrence of a seizure. Genetic factors are particularly important in many forms of epilepsy. The epilepsies with a strong genetic basis, such as childhood absence epilepsy, often occur during a specific age range and can be recognized by the positive family history or because they conform to the description of a particular epileptic syndrome.

Abnormalities of brain development (cerebral dysgenesis) are probably the next most important cause of seizures in children. The presence of neurocutaneous abnormalities or dysmorphic features suggests the possibility of cerebral dysgenesis. Magnetic resonance imaging (MRI) is a more sensitive method than computed tomographic (CT) head scan for the detection of cerebral dysgenesis, but many abnormalities cannot be detected by current neuroimaging techniques.

Brain tumors are an uncommon cause of seizures in childhood, but they must be considered in children with intractable partial or tonic-clonic seizures, particularly in those who have a normal neurologic examination and no other obvious cause of seizures. The tumors that cause seizures in children are usually very slow growing and the presence of a normal CT head scan does not exclude such a diagnosis.

In many children, the underlying cause cannot be demonstrated. In children with a benign epileptic syndrome, a strong family history of epilepsy, or features of primary generalized epilepsy, a CT or an MRI head scan is of little clinical value unless there are atypical features or seizures are difficult to control.

EPILEPTIC SYNDROMES

An epileptic syndrome is an epileptic disorder characterized by a cluster of signs and symptoms that usually occur together. Identification of an epileptic syndrome can be particularly important in the treatment and investigation of the child and in the prognosis given to the parents. For example, children between 6 months and 5 years of age, who have tonic-clonic seizures associated always with fever, are almost certain to have febrile convulsions and are highly unlikely to have seizures in later life. In contrast, teen-agers of normal intelligence with tonic-clonic seizures on awakening and myoclonic seizures are likely to have juvenile myoclonic epilepsy. The seizures in this type of epilepsy are easily controlled with valproic acid (Depakene, Depakote), but the tendency to seize is lifelong. Although primary care physicians have recognized certain epileptic syndromes for many years, e.g., febrile convulsions, infantile spasms, and the Lennox-Gastaut syndrome, several other epileptic syndromes occurring in childhood have now been described. In particular, several benign epileptic syndromes have been recognized, and the knowledge of their natural history has influenced both their management and the social development of these children.

The factors used to classify the epileptic syndromes include the age of onset of the seizures, precipitating factors, type of seizure, anatomic localization, diurnal and circadian rhythms, and prognosis. A review of the different epileptic syndromes is beyond the scope of this article, and only several of the syndromes that either occur commonly or have important management implications are described.

Several epileptic syndromes occurring in childhood carry a good prognosis for seizure remission and/or for normal development. These include benign familial neonatal convulsions, febrile convulsions, benign rolandic epilepsy, childhood absence epilepsy, and juvenile myoclonic epilepsy. These benign epileptic syndromes occur in specific age ranges, are associated with normal development, and often have a family history of self-remitting epilepsy. The importance of the recognition of such syndromes is in the reassurance that can be given to the parents and child and in the avoidance of expensive and unnecessary investigations. Thus, CT, MRI, and metabolic studies are not necessary in these children.

Neonatal Seizures

Seizures in the neonate are different from seizures in the older child, both in terms of their clinical manifestations and etiology. The characteristic clinical manifestations of seizures in the newborn reflect the immaturity of the neonatal brain and the difficulty in the recognition of clinical abnormalities that do not involve motor activity. Generalized tonic-clonic seizures are uncommon, and the most common seizure types are subtle, multifocal clonic, focal clonic, tonic, and myoclonic seizures. Subtle seizures, which are the most common type, can be difficult to recognize and may involve abnormal eye movements, oral buccal and lingual movements, rowing or cycling movements of the limbs, and apneic spells. The clonic, tonic, and myoclonic seizures are usually easy to recognize. It is important to differentiate seizure activity from jitteriness, which is stimulus sensitive, ceases with passive flexion of the limbs, and is never associated with abnormal eye movements.

Seizures are one of the most common manifestations of an acute neurologic problem in the neonatal period, and the underlying cause can be demonstrated in 75% of affected neonates. Determination of the etiology of neonatal seizures is critical because certain disorders necessitate specific treatment urgently (e.g., hypoglycemia, hypocalcemia, and central nervous system infection). The common causes of neonatal seizures and their typical time of onset are outlined in Table 5. Metabolic disorders associated with neonatal seizures include hypoglycemia, hypocalcemia, hypomagnesemia, hyperammonemia, amino acidopathies, organic acidopathies, and pyridoxine dependency. Seizures caused by hypocalcemia or hypomagnesemia are associated usually with an excellent prognosis.

Approximately 5% of newborns with seizures present around day 4 or 5 of life with an idiopathic self-limiting seizure disorder. Such infants are born at term without obvious problems and

TABLE 5. **Etiology of Neonatal Seizures and Time of Onset**

Etiology	Time of Onset	
	0–3 Days	> 3 Days
Hypoxic ischemic encephalopathy	+	
Intracranial hemorrhage	+	
Hypoglycemia	+	
Developmental defect	+	+
Drug withdrawal	+	+
Intracranial infection		+
Hypocalcemia		+
Benign idiopathic convulsions		+

appear normal during the first few days of life. The seizures are multifocal clonic and/or apneic seizures, and they may occur repeatedly over several hours or days. These infants have an excellent prognosis. It is important to recognize that this diagnosis is retrospective and that metabolic disorders, central nervous system infections, and congenital abnormalities of the brain may present in a similar fashion. A rare familial syndrome of neonatal seizures has also been described in which seizures begin typically on day 2 or 3 of life, and the infants appear well between seizures. This disorder is inherited in an autosomal dominant fashion with a high degree of penetrance and should be considered when there is a family history of idiopathic neonatal seizures. The gene for this disorder has been localized to chromosome 20.

The investigations that should be performed in newborns with seizures include blood glucose, calcium, magnesium, and sodium measurements and lumbar puncture to exclude bacterial or viral central nervous system infection. Other metabolic investigations which may be indicated include plasma and cerebrospinal fluid measurements of amino acids, plasma lactate, plasma ammonia, and urine organic acids. There are no clear guidelines for neuroimaging in neonatal seizures, but CT of the brain should be performed if there are persistent focal seizures affecting one limb or side of the body, because of the high incidence of focal ischemic cerebral lesions that are frequently not demonstrated by cerebral ultrasound examination. The EEG may help to distinguish if abnormal behavior or motor activity is a seizure. The EEG may also be helpful in the recognition of focal brain abnormalities and in the prognosis. However, interpretation of the EEG in the neonatal period is difficult and requires an electroencephalographer with experience in this area. In neonates who are critically ill and difficult to assess clinically (e.g., infants who require paralysis for maintenance of ventilation), intermittent EEG examinations should be performed to look for evidence of seizures.

The acute management of neonatal seizures consists of the specific treatment of the underlying disorder and antiepileptic medication. Phenobarbital is currently the medication of choice, and the loading dose is 20 mg per kg intravenously. If this is ineffective, a further 5 to 20 mg per kg can be administered intravenously, in aliquots of 5 mg per kg, to a total of 40 mg per kg. In view of the risk of respiratory and cardiac depression, the infant must be monitored closely. Because the metabolism of drugs varies widely among sick newborns, the maintenance dose of anticonvulsant drugs is usually based on blood levels. The usual maintenance dose of phenobarbital is 3 to 4 mg per kg per day.

If phenobarbital is ineffective, phenytoin (Dilantin) can be administered intravenously. The loading dose is 20 mg per kg, and the maintenance dose is 3 to 4 mg per kg. There is no well-established treatment for seizures which are intractable to a combination of phenobarbital and phenytoin at serum concentrations at the upper end of the therapeutic range. Primidone (Mysoline) has been demonstrated to be effective at serum concentrations above 6 µg per mL. Paraldehyde and diazepam (Valium) have also been used but can be associated with serious toxicity in this age group.

Pyridoxine dependency is a rare but treatable cause of intractable neonatal seizures. If the seizures do not respond to the previous treatment, 50 mg of pyridoxine should be administered intravenously under EEG control, and oral pyridoxine (100 mg daily) should be continued for at least 2 weeks.

The duration of antiepileptic drug treatment for neonatal seizures remains controversial. The risk of subsequent epilepsy in children who had neonatal seizures ranges from 10 to 20%. The principal determinants of increased risk include abnormal neurologic examination, seizure etiology, and abnormal EEG.

Febrile Seizures

Two of every three children with seizures have febrile convulsions. A knowledge of the natural history of this disorder is fundamental to the appropriate management. Febrile convulsions occur between 6 months and 5 years of age and are associated with a family history of febrile seizures in 25% of patients. The risk of a further seizure with fever is 30% when the first seizure occurs between 1 and 3 years of age, 50% when it occurs first at other ages, and 50% after a second febrile seizure. The prognosis for normal school progress and for seizure remission is excellent in children with febrile seizures. Both the intelligence quotient (IQ) and early academic progress of children with febrile seizures do not differ from those of siblings. Similarly, 98% of children with febrile seizures have no further seizures after 5 years of age. Factors associated with a high risk of later epilepsy include the presence of severe developmental delay or of cerebral palsy. Other factors known to influence the risk of later epilepsy include abnormal neurologic development; a history of epilepsy in a parent or sibling; and a seizure which has a focal onset, lasts longer than 15 minutes, or recurs in the same febrile illness. The risk of developing an afebrile seizure is 6 to 8% with one risk factor, 7 to 22% with two risk factors, and 49% with three risk factors. In contrast, the risk of developing afebrile seizures is not influenced markedly by the number of febrile seizures.

It is important to emphasize that the treatment of children with febrile convulsions using an antiepileptic drug does not alter the prognosis for mental development and does not influence the risk of developing epilepsy. Thus, prophylactic treatment is used to prevent recurrences of febrile seizures and not to prevent later epilepsy. When informed of these facts and of the side effects of the effective drugs, most parents elect not to treat their child with an antiepileptic drug. However, there may be certain situations in which treatment is advisable. Factors that may influence the decision to treat include whether the seizure was prolonged, whether the family live at a location remote from medical care, and the degree of parental anxiety.

Oral phenobarbital, oral valproic acid, and diazepam administered rectally during fever are the only drugs that have been demonstrated to reduce the risk of recurrent febrile seizures. The high incidence of fatal hepatotoxicity associated with valproic acid treatment in children younger than 3 years of age precludes its use as a prophylactic medication for febrile seizures. Phenobarbital is effective in the prevention of febrile convulsions when it is administered on a continuous basis but not when administered only during episodes of fever. A major drawback to the use of phenobarbital is the high incidence of neurobehavioral side effects and concern that its use in this age group may lower the ultimate IQ of the child. An alternative approach preferred by the authors is the rectal administration of diazepam solution, which is effective in both the acute treatment and the prevention of febrile seizures. When used prophylactically, diazepam is administered at a dose of 5 mg every 8 hours when the rectal temperature is greater than 38.5° C. Diazepam is absorbed fairly rapidly when administered rectally and diazepam (0.5 mg per kg; maximum, 10 mg) administered by this route may also be used by the parent at home to treat a seizure which persists for more than 5 minutes. In that situation, the authors recommend that the child be brought to the emergency department in case the seizure restarts when the medication effect wears off. The use of rectal diazepam at home to stop a seizure not only increases the chance of preventing prolonged febrile seizures but also gives the parent a sense of control over the situation. Such empowerment of the parent is an important aspect of management.

The degree of anxiety engendered in the family by a seizure can be considerable and is often just as great in children in whom the prognosis is good. Thus, education of the parents and caregivers on the excellent prognosis and on the management of both fever and seizures are important aspects of the management of febrile seizures.

Benign Rolandic Epilepsy

Benign rolandic epilepsy manifests between 4 and 10 years of age and is the most common cause of partial seizures in childhood. There is often a family history of epilepsy, and the developmental history and neurologic examination are normal. The seizures occur more often at night and have a characteristic pattern in most patients. Clonic jerking involves one side of the face and, often, the ipsilateral hand and leg. Involvement of the oropharyngeal muscles is common and manifests as dysarthria and excessive drooling. Patients are usually conscious during the initial phase, but the seizures may become secondarily generalized. The characteristic EEG features are a normal background and central temporal spikes, which have a dipole field and occur much more frequently during sleep.

The prognosis for seizure remission and normal development is excellent, even when seizures are initially difficult to control. All children outgrow their seizures before 16 years of age. The diagnosis of this disorder can be made in most patients on the basis of the clinical description of the episode, normal neurologic examination, and typical EEG features. In these patients, further investigations, such as CT head scan, are unnecessary. Because these seizures may occur during the day when the child is at school, anticonvulsant medication is often used. There is no evidence, however, that treatment alters the ultimate outcome, and it is perfectly reasonable to observe these patients without drug treatment.

Childhood Absence Epilepsy

Absence seizures can be seen in several different epileptic syndromes. Childhood absence epilepsy occurs in apparently normal children in whom the seizures begin between 4 and 10 years of age. The seizures are characterized by staring, unresponsiveness, eyelid fluttering, and occasional clonic movements of the limbs. The EEG demonstrates 3 cycle per second spike and wave discharges, and this abnormality is reliably present in all untreated children with childhood absence seizures if adequate hyperventilation is performed. Staring spells may be the clinical manifestation of, not only typical absence seizures, but also atypical absence seizures and complex partial seizures. These different seizure types respond to different antiepileptic drugs. Table 6 outlines the clinical and EEG features that help to distinguish these different seizure types. The prognosis for remission of absence seizures is good in children with childhood absence epilepsy. Although absence seizures remit by 20 years of age in most children with childhood absence epilepsy, 30 to 50% of these children have generalized tonic-clonic seizures. The onset of absence seizures after 10 years of age, the presence of mental or neurologic abnormality, and the occurrence of other seizure types are factors that increase the risk of developing tonic-clonic seizures later.

Juvenile Myoclonic Epilepsy

Juvenile myoclonic epilepsy presents for the first time around puberty in otherwise normal adolescents. Generalized tonic-clonic seizures, which often occur during sleep or shortly after waking, may be the only manifestation of the syndrome initially. Brief, symmetric, myoclonic jerks, which occur particularly after awakening and are provoked by sleep deprivation, are often not reported unless the patient is questioned directly. The EEG demonstrates generalized polyspike and wave complexes associated with a normal background.

Valproic acid is the treatment of choice for this seizure disorder and seizures are usually controlled easily. However, the risk of teratogenicity associated with valproic acid should be discussed with adolescent girls. Although the seizures are controlled easily with valproic acid in most patients, there is a lifelong high risk of seizure recurrence if medication is withdrawn.

Infantile Spasms

Infantile spasms are a type of seizure characterized by a sudden, bilateral, and symmetrical contraction of the muscles of the neck, trunk, and extremities. They occur in clusters, particularly on awakening. The EEG demonstrates hypsarrhythmia in most patients, and the occurrence of infantile spasms and hypsarrhythmia defines West's syndrome. Infantile spasms present in the first year of life and can be caused by a wide range of prenatal, perinatal, and postnatal disorders. The investigation of a child with infantile spasms should include structural neuroimaging with a CT or preferably an MRI head scan and studies to rule out an inborn error of metabolism and intrauterine infection. In addition, careful examination of the skin, including Wood's light examination, should be performed to exclude a diagnosis of a neurocutaneous syndrome. The retinas should be examined after pupil dilatation for evidence of congenital abnormalities.

Unlike other epilepsy syndromes, adrenocorticotropin (ACTH) and prednisone are effective in the treatment of infantile spasms. ACTH is the current treatment of choice. Nitrazepam (Mogadon, not available in the United States), valproic acid, and pyridoxine are also effective in the treatment of infantile spasms. Vigabatrin appears to be particularly effective in the treatment of infantile spasms due to tuberous sclerosis, but approval for its use in North America has not yet been obtained.

The prognosis for normal neurologic development in children with infantile spasms is extremely poor, and cerebral palsy (50%), mental retardation (75%), and epilepsy (60%) are common sequelae. The most important factor influencing the prognosis for mental and neurologic development is the underlying pathology. The prognosis appears to be better in those patients in whom an underlying cause cannot be demonstrated. A delay in starting treatment may be associated with a poorer prognosis. Consequently, early recognition of this disorder is important.

Lennox-Gastaut Syndrome

Lennox-Gastaut syndrome is characterized by the occurrence of certain seizure types between 1 and 8 years of age and by the presence of specific

TABLE 6. **Differential Diagnosis of Absence Seizures**

Features	Typical Absence	Atypical Absence	Complex Partial
Onset	Abrupt	Gradual	May have aura
Offset	Abrupt	Gradual	Gradual
Postictal state	Clear	Confused	Confused
Usual duration	1–15 s	5–60 s	>30 s
Neuro-development	Normal	Abnormal	Variable
EEG background	Normal	Abnormal	Variable

Abbreviation: EEG = electroencephalogram.

EEG abnormalities. The classic seizure types are tonic seizures and "drop" seizures, but atypical absence, atonic, and myoclonic seizures also occur. The EEG demonstrates an abnormal background rhythm associated with diffuse slow spike and wave discharges that become more prominent during sleep. The tonic seizures occur most frequently during sleep, may be very subtle, and may be difficult to recognize.

In children with Lennox-Gastaut syndrome, the seizures are often difficult to control, and progressive mental retardation occurs in the majority of patients. Onset before 3 years of age, a previous history of infantile spasms, and a history of status epilepticus are indicators of a poor prognosis. Investigations should be performed to rule out an underlying metabolic, neurodegenerative, or structural disorder but often do not demonstrate an underlying cause.

WHETHER TO USE AN ANTIEPILEPTIC DRUG

The decision whether to use an antiepileptic drug involves an analysis of the benefits and disadvantages of treatment. Because there is often a value judgment to be made, it is important to involve the parents and the older child in the decision. The factors which should be considered include the risk of seizure recurrence, the risk associated with a further seizure, and the possible side effects of the drug.

Many children only have a single seizure and do not require prophylactic medication. The rate of recurrence after a first unprovoked seizure is between 30 and 50%. Factors increasing the risk of recurrence include evidence of previous neurologic abnormality, a history of epilepsy in a sibling or parent, and epileptiform discharges on the EEG. The risk of a recurrence is much higher after a second seizure.

Recognition of certain epileptic syndromes may also influence the decision to treat. For example, most children with febrile seizures are not treated with prophylactic medication, because it is recognized that recurrent febrile seizures do not alter the natural history of the disorder. Similarly, the benefit of treating those children with benign rolandic epilepsy who only have nocturnal seizures may be extremely limited. In contrast, early control of seizures may have a significant impact on the neurodevelopmental outcome of children with those epileptic syndromes associated with a poor prognosis, such as infantile spasms and Lennox-Gastaut syndrome.

HOW TO CHOOSE AND USE AN ANTIEPILEPTIC DRUG

Monotherapy

In most newly diagnosed patients with epilepsy, the seizures can be controlled with a single antiepileptic drug. In addition, monotherapy is associated with fewer dose-dependent side effects. Clearly, when only one drug is used, it is important to choose a drug that is likely to be effective.

How to Choose an Antiepileptic Drug

The choice of antiepileptic drug should be influenced by the epilepsy syndrome, the seizure type, the EEG abnormalities, and the potential side effects (see Table 4). Recent studies suggest that the major antiepileptic drugs, carbamazepine, phenytoin, and valproic acid, are equally effective in the prevention of partial and tonic-clonic seizures. Consequently, the risk of side effects has become a more important factor in the choice of antiepileptic drug. This explains the diminishing role of phenobarbital in the treatment of childhood epilepsy. The epilepsy syndrome may also influence the choice of drug. Thus, although phenytoin and carbamazepine are effective normally in preventing tonic-clonic seizures, they are not effective in the prophylaxis of tonic-clonic seizures occurring as a manifestation of febrile convulsions. Similarly, valproic acid is the treatment of choice in the prevention of tonic-clonic seizures in patients with juvenile myoclonic epilepsy. Finally, the choice of drug may be influenced by the EEG findings. The presence of generalized spike and wave discharges may indicate that the seizures are more likely to respond to valproic acid or to a benzodiazepine. Table 4 describes how the seizure type, the epileptic syndrome, and the EEG may influence the choice of drug.

How to Use an Antiepileptic Drug

Most antiepileptic drugs produce intolerable, neurotoxic side effects if the maintenance dose is used immediately. An exception is phenytoin, which can be started at the estimated maintenance dosage. The dosage of other medications should be increased gradually every 5 to 7 days up to the maintenance dose. This permits the development of tolerance to the adverse effects of the drug.

The optimal drug dosage is that which prevents seizures without causing side effects. The required dosage depends partly on the severity of the epileptic tendency and varies widely between patients. This explains why seizures are controlled in many patients at serum drug concen-

TABLE 7. **Pharmacokinetics of Antiepileptic Drugs**

Drug	Half-Life (h)	Time to Steady State (Days)	Therapeutic Range (μg/mL)
Phenobarbital	60–100	12–21	10–40
Phenytoin	See text	5–21*	10–20
Ethosuximide	15–68	3–14	30–100
Carbamazepine	15–24	3–5	4–12
Valproic acid	10–18	2–4	30–100
Clonazepam	20–30	4–6	Not established

*The upper end of the range of time to reach steady state occurs at higher phenytoin concentrations (see text).

trations below the "therapeutic range." Conversely, it is important to appreciate that patients whose seizures are not controlled at serum drug concentrations in the middle of the therapeutic range may achieve seizure control at a higher serum concentration. Thus, in patients with more severe epilepsy, the dosage should be increased gradually until the seizures are controlled or the patient develops unacceptable side effects.

The pharmacokinetic properties of the commonly used antiepileptic drugs are outlined in Table 7. The metabolism of phenytoin differs from that of other antiepileptic drugs in that, at higher concentrations, small dosage increases may result in a disproportionately large increase in the blood level. For that reason, dosage increases should be limited to 25 mg per day when the blood level is in the therapeutic range.

Drug interactions are common with antiepileptic drugs. Phenobarbital, phenytoin, and carbamazepine induce the hepatic microsomal system and may result in lower blood levels and a decreased efficacy of the following drugs: corticosteroids, oral contraceptives, theophylline, chloramphenicol (Chloromycetin), warfarin (Coumadin), vitamin K, digoxin (Lanoxin), quinidine, haloperidol (Haldol), and cyclosporine (Sandimmune). Valproic acid inhibits the clearance of phenobarbital and ethosuximide, resulting in higher blood levels.

Therapeutic Drug Monitoring

The objective of treatment is to control seizures without side effects, not to obtain a serum concentration within the so-called therapeutic range. Thus, serum drug concentrations should only be measured when there is a particular problem to solve (Table 8). The timing of the blood sample is important and is determined by the problem. For example, if drug toxicity is suspected, the blood sample should be taken at the time of day when the patient is manifesting symptoms or when the serum concentration is likely to be highest. Con-

versely, if poor seizure control is the indication for measurement of the blood level, it is important to obtain a trough level, which is usually that level obtained before the morning dose.

Adverse Effects of Antiepileptic Drugs

The adverse effects of a drug may be concentration dependent or idiosyncratic. Concentration-dependent side effects tend to occur more commonly, improve when the dose is reduced, and are generally not life-threatening. In contrast, idiosyncratic side effects are rare but may be life-threatening.

The concentration-dependent side effects of the commonly used antiepileptic drugs are described in Table 9. These occur at high serum concentrations or if the drug dose is increased too rapidly. Serum drug concentrations may fluctuate markedly during the day, and the occurrence of symptoms at a specific time each day suggests a drug side effect. The use of a sustained-release formulation or the administration of the drug at more frequent intervals may diminish the side effects occurring as a consequence of the marked diurnal fluctuations in the blood level. It is important to appreciate that concentration-dependent side effects can occur at concentrations within the therapeutic range. Consequently, the common side effects should be discussed with the patient and parents prior to treatment. Providing a printed information sheet on the drug is extremely useful, because patients and their parents often forget what the physician has said. Furthermore, a record in the patient chart that such a handout has been supplied demonstrates evidence that the patient has been advised of the potential side effects of treatment.

Serious drug reactions include exfoliative dermatitis, Stevens-Johnson syndrome, bone marrow failure, and hepatitis, but they are very rare. Aplastic anemia and agranulocytosis complicate carbamazepine therapy in 1 in 200,000 and 1 in 700,000 patients, respectively. The risk of severe valproate hepatotoxicity is higher in children. Children younger than 3 years of age who are receiving valproate polytherapy have a 1 in 800 risk. Between 3 and 20 years of age, the risk of

TABLE 8. **Indications for Antiepileptic Drug Monitoring**

Lack of seizure control
Compliance
Possible side effects
Suspected drug interactions
Management of status epilepticus

TABLE 9. **Common Side Effects of Antiepileptic Drugs**

Drug	Side Effect
Phenobarbital	**Hyperactivity, sleep disturbance, aggression, drowsiness, poor school performance,*** depression, dysarthria, and movement disorders; mildly raised SGOT levels occur commonly in children and are rarely of clinical significance
Phenytoin	**Gingival hyperplasia, acne, hirsutism, coarsened facial features; nystagmus, ataxia, sedation, poor school performance,** drowsiness, movement disorders, exacerbation of seizures; mildly raised SGOT levels occur commonly in children and are rarely of clinical significance
Carbamazepine	**Nausea, vomiting, diplopia, drowsiness, ataxia,** movement disorders, exacerbation of seizures; mild leukopenia and mildly raised SGOT levels occur commonly in children and are rarely of clinical significance
Valproic acid	**Nausea, epigastric discomfort, excessive weight gain, tremor,** drowsiness, coma, thrombocytopenia, hypofibrinogenemia, hyperammonemia
Ethosuximide	**Nausea, anorexia, epigastric discomfort, drowsiness,** psychiatric disturbance, headache, movement disorders
Clonazepam	**Drowsiness, ataxia, behavioral change, drooling, hypotonia,** weight gain

*Those written in **bold print** occur most often.
Abbreviation: SGOT = serum glutamic oxaloacetic transaminase.

valproate-associated hepatic failure is 1 in 20,000 to 1 in 50,000 for those receiving monotherapy and 1 in 8,000 to 1 in 17,000 for those receiving polytherapy.

Although routine monitoring of serum liver enzymes and blood count at periodic intervals is recommended by the pharmaceutical companies, there is little evidence that this practice is helpful in predicting serious drug reactions. The onset of an idiosyncratic reaction is relatively rapid and not likely to be predicted by the measurement of laboratory tests at 3-month intervals. Furthermore, raised serum glutamic oxaloacetic transaminase (SGOT) activity has been demonstrated in at least 10% of children receiving phenobarbital, carbamazepine, phenytoin, and valproic acid and is a very nonspecific finding. Furthermore, the detection of an abnormal laboratory test result usually leads to repeated blood sampling from the child and to undue worry for the parent and child. Finally, the financial cost of routine laboratory monitoring is extremely high. Indeed, it has been calculated that the cost of measuring a complete blood count, platelet count, and SGOT on three occasions per year in all patients with epilepsy in North America would be $400,000,000. For these reasons, it is our practice to measure the blood count and SGOT before treatment in all children. Thereafter, the authors monitor laboratory tests only when the patient is symptomatic or if the patient is in a particularly high-risk group, e.g., an infant receiving valproic acid polytherapy. However, the patient, parents, and caregivers are educated with regard to the possible adverse effects and important drug interactions. This education involves both discussion with the parents and child and providing a printed information sheet on the drug.

EDUCATIONAL AND SOCIAL PROBLEMS

Cognitive Dysfunction

The intelligence in children with febrile convulsions and the benign epileptic syndromes is similar to that in the general population. However, there is a higher incidence of cognitive dysfunction in other children with epilepsy. Thus, a formal educational or neuropsychological evaluation should be performed at an early stage in those epileptic children with a history of developmental delay or educational difficulties.

Several factors may contribute to cognitive dysfunction in children with epilepsy: the presence of an underlying abnormality of the brain, the effect of repeated seizures, and the antiepileptic medications. Improvement in seizure control and early recognition of adverse drug effects are factors which the physician may influence. Cognition may be affected significantly by antiepileptic drugs, and this side effect can be difficult to recognize. Thus, it is important to have a high index of suspicion and to ask the parents to report promptly any change in mental function or deterioration in school performance.

Social Aspects of Epilepsy

For many epileptic patients and their families, the social aspects of epilepsy are a greater handicap than are the seizures. The lack of social skills and unemployment are perceived by adults with intractable seizures to be more of a problem than are the seizures. Many children with refractory epilepsy have extremely limited social skills and form few friendships. In addition, they have lower self-esteem, and there is a higher incidence of psychiatric disturbances. The underlying brain abnormality and the seizures may contribute to these difficulties. However, there are other factors, which may be amenable to therapy in childhood, that influence the social outcome. Overprotection by the parent, the attitude of the public toward epilepsy, and the fear of having a seizure in public may be important factors that contribute to these difficulties. Thus, management of these problems in childhood may play an important role in the patient's social development.

The attitude of the parents is also very important in the adaptation that the child makes to the diagnosis of epilepsy. Thus, the emotional dependence and social isolation of some children with epilepsy may relate to the tendency of parents to overprotect the child. The impact of the parents' behavior has been demonstrated in children with benign rolandic epilepsy. The emotional and social development in children diagnosed before the excellent prognosis for this syndrome was appreciated differed significantly from that in children whose parents were advised of the excellent prognosis. Thus, among the children whose parents had not been advised of the good prognosis, there was a higher incidence of emotional, social, and educational difficulties. This experience highlights the importance of parental attitudes. The authors believe that it is important for children to be allowed to take the necessary social and emotional risks to develop independent living skills.

PATIENT AND PARENT EDUCATION

The education of the parents and child is one of the most important aspects in the management of epilepsy. Many of the fears that parents have about epilepsy relate to misconceptions. Providing the family with information about epilepsy is the best method of allaying these fears.

It is important for parents to know what they should do if their child has another seizure. Similarly, the etiology, prognosis, and proposed treatment should be discussed with the parents and child. In most children with epilepsy, few restrictions are necessary with respect to sports. However, when the child is bathing at home or swimming, there should always be another person who is aware that the child might have a seizure. It is important that the parents and child fully understand how the medications should be used. The potential side effects and possible drug interactions should be reviewed. We find it useful to give the parents a written information sheet for each medication prescribed. Finally, it is important for the parents to appreciate that most children outgrow their epilepsy.

The educational process can rarely be achieved in one visit. Thus, it is helpful to have a checklist of educational points which can serve as a reminder and also as evidence that teaching has been performed (Table 10).

DISCONTINUING TREATMENT

Most children with epilepsy outgrow the tendency to have seizures. The decision to stop antiepileptic drug treatment should be based on a discussion of the risk of seizure recurrence with the parents and child. Factors that influence the risk of recurrence include the length of time since the last seizure, the presence of an associated neurologic abnormality, the initial degree of difficulty in controlling the seizures, and the presence of epileptiform abnormalities on the EEG. Recognition of an epileptic syndrome may suggest the natural history of the condition. Thus, seizures tend to remit spontaneously in children with benign rolandic epilepsy, and withdrawal of medication should be considered early in these children. In contrast, although seizures are controlled easily in most patients with juvenile myoclonic epilepsy, the risk of seizure relapse after discontinuing medication is very high, and a prolonged period of treatment is indicated.

There is an increasing tendency to stop treatment earlier in children whose seizures are controlled. The authors recommend discontinuation of an antiepileptic drug after a seizure-free period of 2 years if the child is normal neurologically, the EEG demonstrates no epileptiform abnormalities, and the seizures were controlled rapidly with treatment. If one of these adverse factors is present, they tend to recommend treatment for an additional year.

TABLE 10. **Checklist for Epilepsy Education**

General Information
Cause of epilepsy
Prognosis
Rationale for treatment
What to do if a child has a seizure
Recommended activity
Community resources

Safety Precautions
Bathtub and swimming
Driving
Medic Alert bracelet

Medications
Side effects
Drug interactions
Laboratory monitoring
Therapeutic drug levels
Dosage schedule

ROLE OF EPILEPSY SURGERY

Epilepsy surgery has previously been performed mainly in adolescents and adults. There is increasing evidence that delaying the surgery until adolescence or later may interfere seriously with the emotional and social development of the child. Thus, children whose seizures are intractable to medical therapy should be reviewed by a child neurologist to determine whether surgery may play a role.

Focal corticectomy, corpus callosotomy, and modified hemispherectomy are the most established forms of epilepsy surgery. Focal excision of an epileptogenic area is considered if the epileptic focus can be identified reliably and excision of that area of the brain can be accomplished without significant neurologic handicap to the patient. The indications for corpus callosotomy are less well established. The drop seizures which occur in patients with Lennox-Gastaut syndrome or other forms of secondary generalized epilepsy may be controlled, particularly if there is a unilateral frontal focus. Hemispherectomy can be considered in hemiparetic patients with severe unilateral disease in whom the seizures cannot be controlled by focal excision. Hemispherectomy at an early age may be particularly beneficial in patients with Sturge-Weber syndrome. Recent surgical developments have included the removal of epileptogenic tubers in patients with tuberous sclerosis, the surgical removal of focal abnormalities detected by positron emission tomography in patients with intractable infantile spasms, and multiple subpial transsection in patients in whom the epileptogenic lesion lies in unresectable cortex.

GILLES DE LA TOURETTE SYNDROME

method of
JACOB KERBESHIAN, M.D.
University of North Dakota
Grand Forks, North Dakota

In 1886, the French neurologist Georges Gilles de la Tourette described a complex neurologic and behavioral syndrome. By custom, the condition has come to be called Gilles de la Tourette syndrome (TS). Once thought to be quite rare, TS has a prevalence of about 1 per 2000. In the past, TS has been characterized as a chronic, severe, and debilitating tic disorder. More recent data indicate that TS is a neuropsychiatric developmental disorder with a broad spectrum of severity, and a natural history that may include improvement and stabilization of tics by late adolescence to early adulthood. The condition is heritable, with at least obsessive compulsive disorder (OCD) being an alternate phenotypic expression of the underlying genetic diathesis. Attention deficit hyperactivity disorder (ADHD) also concurs in a substantial number of individuals with TS. Studies of TS have indicated that there is aberrant neurotransmission of dopaminergic, noradrenergic, and/or serotonergic fibers in the corpus stratial or midbrain structures.

DIAGNOSIS

TS is defined by the not necessarily concurrent presence of multiple motor tics and one or more vocal tics with at least 1 year's duration. A nonorganic causation is presumed; criteria for diagnosis include a duration of at least 1 year and onset before age 21 years. A tic is a rapid, repetitive, recurrent, spasmodic, seemingly involuntary movement or vocalization, which may be temporarily suppressible. Tics appear to be migratory anatomically and wax and wane in intensity and frequency. It is characteristic of tics that they interrupt the flow of normal motor activity or of normal discourse. Motor and vocal tics may be either simple or complex. Simple motor tics may include eye blinking, head shaking, nose wrinkling, finger flicking, or foot tapping. Complex motor tics may include gesturing, jumping, touching of self or others, or self-injurious behaviors. Simple vocal tics may include grunting, coughing, or barking. Complex vocal tics may include the repetitive utterance of words or phrases out of context. Coprolalia is the interruptive utterance of a profanity. Coprolalia is infrequent in TS and need not be present to make the diagnosis. Echolalia is a vocal tic in which the individual automatically repeats a word or phrase of another. Palilalia is a vocal tic in which the individual automatically repeats his or her own utterances, often in a whisper.

Chronic motor tic disorder and chronic vocal tic disorder are believed to be on a continuum with TS. In the case of the former, the criteria for TS are met, with the absence of vocal tics; in the case of the latter, the criteria for TS are met, with the absence of motor tics. Transient tic disorder describes a tic syndrome in which symptoms are present for at least 2 weeks but for less than 1 year.

There are no intensity or impairment criteria in making a diagnosis of TS. Often, tic symptoms may be inconsequential in individuals who appear for treatment of co-morbid other developmental or behavioral problems, such as ADHD or OCD. In an individual with a characteristic clinical presentation, course, and family history, a complete history and routine physical and neurologic examination with routine screening laboratory studies, such as a hemogram, urinalysis, metabolic panel, and perhaps, thyroid function studies may be all that are required. If the presentation is atypical, particularly if there is the presence of other subcortically mediated abnormal involuntary movements or if there is the question of a toxic cause such as cocaine or other stimulant drug abuse, then a more comprehensive diagnostic work-up should be pursued.

TREATMENT

The critical decision to be made in the treatment of TS is whether pharmacologic management is necessary, or whether education, support, and/or judicious follow-up are the primary interventions. Although the presence of tic symptoms is necessary and sufficient to make a diagnosis of TS, it is less clear whether alternate expressions of the condition, such as OCD, or commonly co-morbid conditions, such as ADHD, are included within the boundaries of the disorder. Frequently, it is these other conditions which serve as the focus of intervention. The decision to treat medically the tic symptoms per se should be based on whether the tics are causing a disturbed sense of integrity of the individual in terms of the flow of motor activity, the ability to sustain attention, or the sense of continuity of the self; the presence of tics is leading to ostracism by peers; or the vigilance required to suppress tics or to engage in other compensatory maneuvers is emotionally depleting. The most effective medications used in treating TS tic symptoms per se include the neuroleptics, clonidine (Catapres), and clonazepam (Klonopin).

Neuroleptics

Haloperidol (Haldol) is a neuroleptic drug that has been the mainstay of treatment for TS. As with pimozide (Orap) and fluphenazine (Prolixin), its efficacy has been linked to its property of blocking postsynaptic dopamine-2 receptor sites. Because of the low but real possibility of neuroleptics in TS causing tardive dyskinesia, an abnormal involuntary movement disorder, they are being used less often as drugs of first choice. In children, a starting dose of haloperidol of 0.25 mg per day, with weekly increments of 0.25 to 0.5 mg per day to a maximum of 3 to 5 mg per day, is generally sufficient to bring about adequate suppression of the tic symptoms. In adolescents and adults, a starting dose of 0.5 mg per day, with weekly increments of 0.5 mg per day to a maximum of 6 to 8 mg per day, is sufficient. Complete tic suppression is not desirable, because the therapeutic strategy should be to increase doses during the waxing phases of the condition and to decrease doses during the waning phases. Single bedtime dosing minimizes sedation and improves compliance. With a slow upward titration of doses, one is not likely to encounter significant extrapyramidal side effects, such as tremor, motor restlessness, or rigidity. Infrequently, antiparkinsonian medications such as benztropine (Cogentin) may be required to mitigate these effects. Other side effects may include anxiety states, including school phobia in children, depression, and weight gain. Haloperidol should be discontinued over a period of at least weeks to minimize a withdrawal tic exacerbation.

Treatment recommendations, including the doses for fluphenazine, are similar to those for haloperidol. The side effect profile is also similar. Because fluphenazine has greater properties as an alpha-adrenergic blocker, there is a greater possibility of orthostatic hypotension than with haloperidol.

Pimozide is not a first-line neuroleptic for treating the tics of TS due to the possibility of its inducing electrocardiographic changes. Of particular concern is the possibility of prolongation of the QTc interval. A baseline electrocardiogram should be obtained before pimozide is initiated, with follow-up electrocardiograms after the initiation of treatment and after significant dosage increases. Pimozide may be less sedating than haloperidol and may be less likely to induce weight gain. Other side effects are similar to those for haloperidol. In addition to its ability to block dopamine-2 receptors, pimozide has calcium channel blocking properties, which may enhance its effectiveness as a tic suppressor. Once-per-day bedtime dosing is desirable. In children, a starting dose of 0.5 mg per day is usual, followed by weekly increments of 0.5 mg per day to a maximum of 5 to 8 mg per day. In adolescents and adults, a starting dose of 1 mg per day is usual, followed by weekly increments of 1 mg per day to a maximum of 10 to 15 mg per day. As with haloperidol, discontinuation should be gradual.

Clonidine

Clonidine is an alpha$_2$-adrenergic presynaptic receptor agonist that has the effect of decreasing noradrenergic neurotransmission from the brain stem to subcortical and cortical structures. It has been shown to be somewhat effective in tic suppression in TS, may be helpful in attenuating compulsive symptoms if present, may help with co-morbid ADHD symptoms, and may diminish impulsivity. Because of the risk of tardive dyskinesia with neuroleptics, clonidine is often used as a first-line drug. Its side effects include sedation, headache, abdominal discomfort, hypotension, depression, and irritability.

Doses three to four times per day are required for a continuity of therapeutic effect and to minimize sedation. In children, a starting dose of 0.025 mg twice per day is usual. Dividing the 0.1-mg tablet into quarters requires creative handiwork on the part of the parents. After 1 week to 10 days, the dosage may be increased to 0.025 mg four times per day. At 7- to 10-day intervals thereafter, divided increments of 0.05 mg are added evenly to the four-times-per-day schedule to a maximum of 0.4 mg per day. In adolescents and adults, a starting dose of 0.025 mg four times per day is customary; increases of 0.1 mg in four divided doses are added every week to 10 days to a maximum of 0.6 mg per day. The full therapeutic effect may not be evident until 1 to 3 months after a dose has been stabilized. Clonidine should be tapered and discontinued over a few days to 1 week, depending on the dose, to avoid rebound hypertension. Clonidine may also be administered in a transdermal patch form, with each administration lasting 5 to 7 days. The patches may be cut into halves to titrate doses more gradually. A starting dose of one-half a 0.1-mg patch would be usual for a child, with a maximum of two 0.2-mg patches after gradual titration upward. In adolescents and adults, one might start with a 0.1-mg patch with a gradual upward titration to a maximum of two 0.3-mg patches.

Clonazepam

Clonazepam is a benzodiazepine derivative which has been used increasingly in TS, particularly in adults. In children, there may be a propensity for the worsening of hyperactivity if ADHD is present. In older adolescents and adults, a starting dose of 0.25 mg twice per day is usual. A final dose as high as 2.5 mg twice per day is a typical ceiling. Dysphoria, sedation, and decreased reaction time may be side effects. Clonazepam may also be helpful if there is an associated anxiety disorder. The medication should not be used in individuals who show a potential for addiction.

TREATMENT OF CO-MORBIDITIES

OCD is fairly common in individuals with TS. Treatment with fluoxetine (Prozac), sertraline (Zoloft), or clomipramine (Anafranil) is often effective, with tic symptoms being exacerbated rarely. These medications may be combined successfully with clonidine and with the neuroleptics should differential treatment of tic symptoms also be necessary. ADHD in isolation is typically treated with stimulants such as methylphenidate (Ritalin), pemoline (Cylert), and dextroamphetamine (Dexedrine). There has been concern that stimulants may precipitate or exacerbate TS, although there is also convincing data to the contrary. If necessary, the stimulants may be successfully combined with the neuroleptics or with clonidine in individuals with both TS and ADHD. Initial treatment with clonidine may successfully treat both TS and ADHD. Desipramine (Norpra-

min), a tricyclic antidepressant, may successfully treat ADHD without exacerbating tics. Electrocardiogram monitoring is advised in children, because rare cases of sudden cardiac death have been reported with desipramine. Fluoxetine may also be beneficial in treating ADHD symptoms.

Novel or less frequently used treatments for the tics of TS include opiate blockers, calcium channel blockers, and nicotine augmentation of neuroleptics.

In conclusion, it should be emphasized that treatment of TS often goes beyond targeting specific tic symptoms. Psychological, educational, occupational, and social issues often come into play. The physician often must function as a member of a team in conjunction with professionals from other helping disciplines.

HEADACHE

method of
NINAN T. MATHEW, M.D.
Baylor College of Medicine
Houston, Texas

Headache disorders can be divided into two major categories: primary headache disorders and secondary headache disorders (headache due to structural and metabolic causes). The International Headache Society has reclassified headache disorders recently mainly for the purposes of epidemiologic and drug evaluation research studies. Table 1 gives a practical classification of primary headache disorders.

MIGRAINE

Migraine can occur with and without aura (warning symptoms). The most common aura is visual in nature, even though neurologic aura, such as hemisensory disturbances, hemiparesis, dysphasia, and changes in memory and state of consciousness, can occur occasionally. Migraine without aura is far more common than migraine with aura. Only approximately 20% of migraine attacks are associated with aura. The same person can have migraine with aura and migraine without aura at different times. Migraine is predominantly a disease of female patients. Identification of the trigger factors for attacks of migraine helps in the diagnosis. The trigger factors are listed on Table 2. The severity and frequency of attacks can vary from time to time. Cyclical exacerbations of migrainous episodes are possible during the patient's lifetime.

Migraine attack is typically episodic, occurring one to two times a month, and it manifests itself in many phases. The prodrome phase, consisting of symptoms of excitation or inhibition of the central nervous system, which include elation, excitability, irritability, increased appetite, craving for sweets or excessive yawning, depression, sleepiness, and fatigue, occurs in 30%

TABLE 1. Classification of Primary Headache Disorders

Migraine
Migraine without aura (common migraine)
Migraine with aura (classic migraine)
Complicated migraine (migraine with prominent neurologic symptoms)
  Basilar migraine
  Hemiplegic migraine
  Ophthalmoplegic migraine
Cluster Headache
Episodic
Chronic
Episodic Tension-Type Headache
Chronic Daily Headache
Chronic tension-type headache
Migraine, tension-type headache complex (mixed or combined headache)
  Usually evolved from migraine
Analgesic/ergotamine rebound headache

Modified from the International Headache Classification. Reprinted from Headache Classification Committee of the International Headache Society. Classification and diagnostic criteria for headache disorders, cranial neuralgias and facial pain. Cephalalgia 8(Suppl 7)1–96, 1988, by permission of Scandinavian University Press.

of patients. These may precede the attack by 12 to 24 hours. The prodrome phase may be followed by the aura phase which consists of specific visual or neurologic symptoms. The headache phase is the most prominent of the migraine attack. The headache is predominantly unilateral in at least 50% of the patients, even though it can be bilateral. It may start on one side and may switch to the other side. A pulsating quality of the head pain occurs in approximately 50% of patients. Nonpulsating headache does not exclude migraine. The headaches usually last from 4 to 72 hours, occasionally more. They are associated with gastrointestinal symptoms, such as nausea and/or vomiting and diarrhea, in 90% of patients. Heightened sensory perception, including phonophobia, photophobia, and increased sensitivity to smell, occur during the attacks. Patients usually want to be left alone, and the attacks can be very disabling in some patients.

The headache of migraine is of moderate or severe intensity (inhibits or prohibits daily activities) as opposed to episodic tension-type headache where the intensity is mild to moderate (may inhibit but does not prohibit activities). The headache of migraine is aggravated by any activity which increases the stroke volume or intracranial pressure, such as walking stairs, jogging, running, bending down, and coughing. During the headache, at least one of the following characteristics, namely nausea and/or vomiting, photophobia, and phonophobia, should be present to make a diagnosis of migraine. It should be noted that physical and neurologic examination should rule out any other structural or metabolic condition which would cause headache.

Menstrual Migraine

Migraine without aura can occur almost exclusively at a particular time of the menstrual cycle. True menstrual migraine occurs between 2 days before menses and the last day of menses. Migraine can also occur as a part of the late luteal phase dysphoric disorder (premenstrual tension). Migraine attacks are not uncommon during ovulation. Menstrual migraine is less responsive to prophylactic drug therapy.

"Status migrainosus" indicates a prolonged migraine attack usually lasting for more than 72 hours associated with nausea, vomiting, and dehydration. The patients are usually extremely sick and dehydrated and may have to be hospitalized. By the time they come to the emergency room, they may have already tried large quantities of analgesic medications and/or ergotamine with no benefit.

CLUSTER HEADACHE

Cluster headache is predominantly a disease of male patients. The headaches are almost always unilateral and short-lived, usually about 45 minutes to 1 hour. Multiple episodes occur on a daily basis for periods of 2 or 3 months with remissions lasting for a number of months to years, only to return in a cluster fashion again for 2 or 3 months. The cluster pattern and remissions are characteristics of the disease, even though, in approximately 10% of patients, there are no remissions (chronic cluster headache). Associated with the pain, there are autonomic features, such as watering of the eye, redness of the eye, and congestion of the conjunctiva, and ipsilateral congestion of the nostril during the attack.

EPISODIC TENSION-TYPE HEADACHE

The most common type of headache is the episodic tension-type headache for which the patients rarely consult a doctor. The headache is usually pressing or tightening in quality, bilateral, mild to moderate in severity, and occasionally associated with very mild nausea, photophobia, or sonophobia. There is no vomiting, and the patients are able to carry on their activities. The headache is not aggravated by physical activity.

CHRONIC DAILY HEADACHE

Even though this term is not included in the International Classification, from a practical point of view it is important. The "chronic tension-type headaches" form one of the types of chronic daily headache. The

TABLE 2. Triggers of Migraine

Common Factors	Less Common Factors
Stress, worry, anxiety	High humidity
Menstruation	Excessive sleep
Oral contraceptives	High altitude
Certain food stuffs and alcohol	Excessive vitamin A
Hunger	Drugs, nitroglycerin, reserpine, estrogens, hydralazine (Aprosoline), Ranitidine (Zantac)
Lack of sleep	
Glare, dazzle	
Weather or ambient temperature changes	Pungent odors
	Fluorescent lighting
Physical exertion, fatigue	Allergic reactions
Head trauma	Cold foods
	Refractory errors

clinical features of chronic tension-type headache are essentially the same as those of episodic tension-type headache, except that they occur for more than 180 days a year. The co-morbid factors often seen in chronic tension-type headache are anxiety, depression, excessive intake of pain medications, abnormal personality profiles, inadequate personality, and repressed anger. Both episodic and chronic tension-type headache could be associated with pericranial muscle tenderness and a low pain threshold. Digital palpation of the pericranial muscles, including the neck muscles, will show increased stiffness and tenderness. "Migraine, chronic tension-type headache complex" (mixed headache) manifests as daily or near-daily headaches showing features of migraine and chronic tension-type headache in a mixed form. Many patients have episodes of severe headache with migrainous features with interictal tension-type headache occurring very frequently. It sometimes becomes difficult to identify the termination of one type of headache and the beginning of the other type. There are two forms distinguishable in this variety of headache: those associated with analgesic and ergotamine overuse and those unassociated with drug overuse. It is now well known to specialists in headache that daily or near-daily use of analgesics and ergotamine in patients with migraine can lead to a chronic daily intractable headache condition which is referred to as an "analgesic/ergotamine rebound headache." It is important to look for this disorder in any patient who presents with chronic headaches. Analgesic/ergotamine rebound headache is refractory to regular treatments. The patients show many associated features, such as early-morning awakening with severe headaches, sleep disturbances, tolerance to pain medications over a period of time requiring a larger quantity of medications, and manifestation of withdrawal symptoms when the medications are stopped. In addition, the prophylactic antimigraine medications become ineffective as long as the patients are receiving daily pain medications or ergotamine.

Post-Traumatic Headache. This headache can follow a relatively minor head and neck trauma. Previously dormant migraine can be aggravated by such trauma. Patients with posttraumatic headache usually manifest a mixed form of migraine and tension-type headache with considerable detectable neck muscle spasm and pericranial tenderness.

TREATMENT OF MIGRAINE

Abortive Treatment of Acute Attacks of Migraine

Abortive treatment of acute attacks is aimed at interfering with the attack early so that the suffering is minimized. The treatment is aimed at reducing the head pain as well as the associated symptoms, such as nausea and vomiting. The medication chosen depends on the severity of the head pain and associated symptoms.

Mild to Moderate Episodes of Migraine

Mild to moderate episodes of migraine can be managed by simple analgesics, such as aspirin or acetaminophen. Either 650 mg of acetaminophen or aspirin may be all that is required for mild to moderate headaches if taken early. Aspirin is absorbed rapidly with a time to peak plasma concentration (t_{max}) of less than 0.5 hour in normal persons. During migraine attacks, there is a relative gastroparesis and delayed absorption of aspirin. Antiemetics may have to be combined with analgesics in the majority of patients with migraine, because they become nauseated during the attack. The antiemetic of choice in the treatment of acute attacks is metoclopramide (Reglan), because it enhances the gastric motility and aids in the absorption of analgesics. On the other hand, phenothiazines may delay the gastric emptying, thereby delaying the proper absorption of analgesics. Metoclopramide (10-mg) tablets may be combined with two tablets of aspirin.

Nonsteroidal Anti-Inflammatory Drugs (NSAIDs)

NSAIDs have been demonstrated to be useful both in the abortive as well as the prophylactic treatment of migraine. Table 3 lists the NSAIDs and indicates the agents that have been shown to be useful in migraine.

In general, carboxylic acids are more useful than enolic acids. Table 4 gives the recommended doses of commonly used NSAIDs in the abortive treatment of migraine. In the treatment of acute

TABLE 3. **Nonsteroidal Anti-Inflammatory Drugs and Their Efficacy in Migraine**

Carboxylic Acids	
Acetic Acids	
Indole acetic acids	Indomethacin (Indocin)
Phenylacetic acid	Diclofenac (Voltaren)*
	Fenclofenac†
Other heterocyclic acetic acids	Sulindac (Clinoril)
	Tolmetin (Tolectin)
Salicylic Acids	Aspirin*‡
	Benorylate†
Propionic Acids	Fenoprofen (Nalfon)‡
	Ibuprofen (Motrin, Advil, Nuprin)*
	Ketoprofen (Orudis)*‡
	Naproxen (Naprosyn)*‡
	Naproxen sodium (Anaprox)*‡
	Indoprofen†‡
	Flurbiprofen (Ansaid)*
	Pirprofen*†
Anthranilic Acids	Flufenamic acid†
	Meclofenamic acid
	Meclofenamate sodium (Meclomen)
	Mefenamic acid (Ponstel)‡
	Tolfenamic acid*†‡
Enolic Acids	
Pyrazolones	Phenylbutazone (Butazolidin)
	Azapropazone†
Oxicams	Piroxicam (Feldene)

*Demonstrated to be effective for acute attacks of migraine.
†Not available in the United States.
‡Demonstrated to be effective for prophylaxis of migraine.

TABLE 4. Commonly Used NSAIDs in Headache and Their Dosages

Medication	Dosage
Ibuprofen (Motrin, Advil, Nuprin)	800 mg at the onset, repeat 400 mg within 2 h
Naproxen sodium (Anaprox)	750 mg at the onset, repeat 375 mg within 2 h
Naproxen (Naprosyn)	750 mg at the onset, 250 mg within 2 h
Meclofenamate sodium (Meclomen)	200 mg at the onset, 100 mg within 2 h
Ketoprofen (Orudis)	150 mg at the onset, 75 mg within 2 h
Ketorolac (Toradol tablets)	20 mg at the onset, 10 mg within 2 h
Ketorolac (Toradol injections)	60 mg IM at the onset

Abbreviations: NSAIDs = nonsteroidal anti-inflammatory drugs.

migraine attacks, the important pharmacokinetic parameter is the speed of absorption. Most of the NSAIDs are absorbed rapidly after oral administration with a t_{max} within 2 hours. Naproxen (Naprosyn) and its sodium salt (Anaprox) have risen to a position of prominence in the treatment of migraine because of their efficacy, tolerance, and record of safety. The t_{max} for naproxen sodium is less than 1 hour compared with that of naproxen which has a t_{max} of 2 hours. The plasma levels increase linearly with doses up to 750 mg; at higher doses, the plasma levels continue to rise but with lesser increments. Thus, for an acute attack, a dose of at least 750 mg of naproxen sodium, if tolerated, should be considered. At our clinic, naproxen sodium, meclofenamate sodium (Meclomen), and ketorolac (Toradol) are preferred. In one study, tolfenamic acid (not available in the United States, comparable preparation is meclofenamate) was shown to be as effective as 1 mg of ergotamine. Ketorolac is effective, particularly in the injectable form (60 mg intramuscularly) for the abortive treatment of acute migraine and is an excellent alternative to narcotics. Many emergency room physicians are using intramuscular ketorolac for migraine.

The mechanisms of action of NSAIDs in migraine are not clear. Their antiprostaglandin effect, antiplatelet aggregation property, blockage of neurogenic inflammation at the trigeminal vascular system, and pure analgesic effect are the possible modes of action. While the precise role of prostaglandins in the pathogenesis of migraine is inadequately understood, they may play a more prominent role in menstrual migraine, accounting for the beneficial effect of NSAIDs in menstrual migraine.

Isometheptene Mucate Combination

An isometheptene mucate combination (Midrin, containing isometheptene mucate 65 mg, dichloral phenazone 100 mg, and acetaminophen 32 mg) is effective in mild to moderate attacks of migraine. Midrin is fairly well tolerated except for slight drowsiness in occasional patients.

The dosage of Midrin is two capsules at the onset of the attack followed by one capsule repeated every 0.5 hour up to about four to six capsules per attack. Isometheptene mucate is a sympathomimetic agent and should not be combined with monoaminoxidase inhibitors. It is also contraindicated in patients with hypertension and renal or liver disease.

Moderate to Severe Episodes of Migraine

Serotonin Agonists

Moderate to severe episodes of migraine should be treated with ergotamine or sumatriptan (Imitrex), both of which are vasoconstrictors acting as serotonin receptor (5-HT$_1$) agonists (Table 5).

ERGOTAMINE

Ergotamine tartrate has been in use since 1928 and is effective in approximately 60% of patients during the acute attack. The earlier it is used, the better the effect is. Three forms of ergotamine tartrate are available at the present time: oral, rectal, and sublingual (rectal suppositories of 2 mg, oral tablets of 1 mg, and sublingual tablets of 2 mg). Oral and rectal forms are combined with 100 mg of caffeine. Ergotamine given by these routes of administration is associated with poor and variable bioavailability, resulting in a wide variation in individual treatment response. The bioavailability is less than 5% for the oral dosage form, but it is considerably higher after rectal administration. Peak plasma concentrations are reached about 1 hour after oral or rectal dosing, but plasma levels after rectal administration are higher. The biologic effects of the drug last much longer than its short elimination half-life of 2 to 3 hours would suggest, possibly because of the action of one or more metabolites, which have an elimination half-life of approximately 20 hours. If the patient is not nauseated or not vomiting from the beginning, the oral tablets are useful; two tablets of Wigraine or Cafergot (caffeine in combination with ergotamine) followed by one tablet every 0.5 hour for a total of six tablets (6 mg of ergotamine) are recommended. If patients do not respond to 6 mg, it is unlikely that they will respond to higher doses, and they may have to resort to some other medication. Ergotamine can be combined with NSAIDs. The recommended combination is one tablet of Wigraine or Cafergot with 200 mg of meclofenamate sodium or 550 mg of naproxen sodium given early. This can be repeated within 1 hour; two doses are usually suf-

TABLE 5. **Serotonin Agonists**

Medications	Preparations	Dosage
Ergotamine tartrate	Oral (with caffeine) (Cafergot, Wigraine)	Two tablets at onset, may repeat with 1 tablet q 0.5 h up to 6/day, 10/week
	Rectal (with caffeine) (Cafergot, Wigraine)	One suppository at onset, may repeat with one suppository in 1 h up to two/day, five/week
	Sublingual (Ergomar, Ergostat)	One tablet at the onset, may repeat with one tablet 0.5 h up to three/day, five/week
Dihydroergotamine	DHE 45 for parenteral use	1 mL IM at onset, may repeat up to 3 mL/day, 5 mL/week
		0.5 mL IV initially, may repeat q 6 h for 48 h to break the cycle of status migrainosus (May be combined with IV prochlorperazine or metoclopramide)
Sumatriptan	Imitrex	6 mg subcutaneously initially, may repeat within 24 h or 100-mg oral tablet initially, may repeat within 24 h

ficient. The associated nausea can be managed by the addition of metoclopramide 10 mg or promethazine (Phenergan) 25-mg tablets or suppositories.

Rectal suppositories of ergotamine tartrate are more rapidly absorbed, and this route is preferred by some patients. A suppository of Cafergot or Wigraine in combination with a suppository of an antiemetic, such as prochlorperazine (Compazine) or promethazine, is adequate in many of the moderate to severe episodes of migraine. Because ergotamine may itself produce nausea in some patients, they may be advised to find a subnauseating dose of the suppository, when they are without headache, by dividing the suppository into smaller portions and administering it. Many patients may require only a portion of the whole suppository to abort the attack.

Ergotamine is a powerful and selective vasoconstrictor of the external carotid arterial system due to its direct effect on the arterial serotonin receptors. In addition to its arterial serotonin receptor action, ergotamine may influence central serotonin neurotransmission by depressing the firing rate of serotonergic neurons of the brain stem raphe.

Not more than 4 to 6 mg of ergotamine tartrate should be given in any 1 week, and it should only be given for two attacks preferably with a 4-day hiatus. The continuous use of ergotamine tartrate may give rise to ergotamine rebound headache. This headache occurs every day, it is only relieved by further doses of ergotamine tartrate, and it is very much like the migraine headache in that it is associated with nausea, vomiting, and a general feeling of illness. These headaches improve when the patients stop taking ergotamine tartrate.

Excessive use of ergotamine can result in symptoms of vasoconstriction, such as cold clammy extremities, intermittent claudication of the legs, chest pain, and transient cerebral ischemic symptoms. Peripheral numbness and cerebral symptoms of ergotism can also occur.

SUMATRIPTAN

Sumatriptan (a 5-HT$_1$ receptor agonist) is a specific drug for acute attacks of migraine with and without aura. The introduction of sumatriptan has proved to be a major advance in the treatment and understanding of the pathophysiology of migraine. Oral and subcutaneous preparations are available. Clinical trials have shown that 6 mg of subcutaneous sumatriptan reduces the pain of migraine attacks in 77% of patients after 1 hour and 83% after 2 hours. Subcutaneous sumatriptan is available as an autoinjector and is extremely convenient for the patients to self-inject. Studies using oral sumatriptan show that there is an improvement in headache in more than 50% of patients in 2 hours after ingestion. Sumatriptan has a short half-life and is rapidly absorbed. It is a quick-acting drug, and more than one dose may be necessary. Not only is the pain relieved rapidly within 1 hour, but it also reduces the associated symptoms of nausea, vomiting, photophobia, and phonophobia. It is effective against migraine headache when taken early or later in an attack, unlike ergotamine, which is only effective if taken early. The advantage of sumatriptan over ergotamine is that, by itself, it does not produce nausea, which in itself is a bothersome symptom of migraine. On the other hand, it reduces associated nausea. Sumatriptan does not cause grogginess, drowsiness, or hangover, and therefore, the patients can return to full functioning after the injection. This is a great advantage over other abortive agents for migraine.

The drug of choice for severe to extremely severe attacks of migraine is sumatriptan. Six milligrams of subcutaneous sumatriptan produces relief of migraine within 1 hour. Even though approximately 30% of patients may show recurrence of head pain within a 24-hour period, recurrence can also be treated effectively by repeating the sumatriptan dose.

Sumatriptan has very few side effects compared to ergotamine or dihydroergotamine. A burning or stinging sensation at the site of injection and a transient feeling of fullness or heaviness of the upper chest and neck area are the most common side effects. Sumatriptan should be used very cautiously in patients with known coronary artery disease or those who have increased risk factors for coronary artery disease, because it can cause vasospasm in diseased coronary arteries. Sumatriptan should not be combined with ergotamine or dihydroergotamine.

DIHYDROERGOTAMINE MESYLATE

Dihydroergotamine (DHE) is effective in the treatment in acute severe episodes of migraine. DHE can be administered intramuscularly or intravenously. In an emergency room situation, intravenous administration of DHE in conjunction with metoclopramide is highly effective and has been shown to be superior to meperidine (Demerol) and butorphanol (Stadol). A test dose of 5 mg of metoclopramide with 0.33 mg (0.33 ml) of DHE slow intravenous push is recommended. After waiting for about 10 minutes, the balance of the 1 mg of DHE with metoclopramide 5 mg can be given slowly. Approximately 30 to 40% of patients may become nauseated; however, the relief of headache is very striking. The effect of intravenous DHE is known in less than 15 minutes, because the peak plasma levels are obtained in 2 to 11 minutes. Intramuscular DHE is also effective, with the peak levels obtained in 30 minutes to 1 hour. Intramuscular DHE can be combined with intramuscular promethazine or metoclopramide. The maximal dose of DHE, intramuscularly or intravenously, should not exceed 3 mg per day. Monthly use should not exceed 12 headache events or 20 mg (20 ampules).

DHE, a chemical derivative of ergotamine, is better tolerated than ergotamine. Despite the close similarities in chemical structure, DHE is a relatively milder peripheral arterial constrictor compared to ergotamine. On the other hand, it is a powerful venoconstrictor, allowing for its usefulness in the treatment of orthostatic hypotension. As with ergotamine, the pharmacologic effect of DHE correlates poorly with the plasma levels of the parent drug. On the other hand, it may correlate with the plasma levels of the metabolites of DHE, which have an elimination half-life of about 20 hours. Its pharmacodynamic efficacy persists for hours to days after the drug is withdrawn and in the absence of measurable levels of the drug. Both DHE and its major metabolites bind selectively to brain serotonin receptors and act as agonists to 5-HT_{1A} and 5-HT_{1D} receptors. The minimal peripheral arterial constriction and central receptor binding indicate that the mechanism of action of DHE in migraine is at least partly central. The common side effects of DHE are nausea, vomiting, diarrhea, leg cramps, and abdominal discomfort. The diarrhea which occurs, especially on repeated doses, can be effectively controlled with a diphenoxylate and atropine combination (Lomotil). The leg muscle pain and abdominal discomfort usually disappear with a dosage reduction. The associated nausea and vomiting may interfere with its effective use in some patients despite concomitant use of metoclopramide or prochlorperazine. In this respect, sumatriptan is superior to DHE. Like ergotamine, idiosyncratic hypersensitivity reactions can occur with DHE, resulting in rare instances of severe peripheral and coronary arterial spasm. Patients with coronary artery disease and a history of Prinzmetal's angina should be excluded from treatment with DHE. It should not be used during pregnancy and should never be combined with sumatriptan.

Alternative Therapy for Acute Migraine

PHENOTHIAZINES

For those patients who are not responsive to sumatriptan or intravenous or intramuscular DHE, an alternate choice is intravenous prochlorperazine. A dose of 5 to 10 mg of prochlorperazine can be given intravenously in an emergency room setting. Dystonic reactions are possible in some of the patients who receive prochlorperazine and can be counteracted by an intramuscular injection of 1 mg of benztropine mesylate (Cogentin). Intravenous chlorpromazine (Thorazine) may also be worth trying in patients who do not satisfactorily respond to sumatriptan or DHE. A dose of 12.5 to 25 mg (0.1 mg per kg) of chlorpromazine given in piggyback fashion intravenously is effective in many patients with acute migraine. Repeat dosing every 15 minutes up to a total of three doses may become necessary. Orthostatic hypotension is a distinct side effect, and patients have to be monitored for a while before they are allowed to get up and walk around or go home. They have to be warned about the orthostatic hypotension.

NARCOTICS AND SEDATIVES IN ACUTE MIGRAINE

The majority of migraine attacks can be managed without using narcotics, with the medications mentioned previously. The reasons narcotics are not preferred in migraine are the following. First, serotonin mechanisms are disturbed in migraine, and medications such as sumatriptan, ergotamine, and dihydroergotamine are 5-HT_{1D} receptor agonists which reduce the neurogenic inflammation associated with migraine attacks, whereas narcotics reduce the pain without any specific effects on the neurogenic inflammation. Second, the narcotics and analgesics with sedatives may in fact produce a rebound headache phenomena and perpetuate the chronicity of migraine. Third, with frequent use, habituation occurs. For these reasons, narcotics are very rarely recommended for acute attacks of migraine. However, in a person who is totally nonresponsive to sumatriptan, ergotamine, DHE, and phenothiazines, one may use parenteral narcotics such as meperidine in a limited way; however, it should not be prescribed on a routine basis.

A number of preparations are available that contain butalbital with acetaminophen or aspirin and caffeine with or without codeine (e.g., Fiorinal, Fiorinal #3, Fioricet, Fioricet with Codeine, Esgic, Esgic with Codeine, Esgic Plus, and Phrenilin). While these preparations are useful for a person with occasional migraine, they are certainly not recommended for patients with frequent episodes of migraine or tension-type headache. Not only do these medications have a potential for abuse, they also invariably produce rebound headache phenomena if used frequently. The excessive use of medications containing butalbital results in lethargy, sleepiness, lack of concentration, and an overall sedated feeling. One of the other major dangers in the use of butalbital-containing medications is that abrupt discontinuation of the medication may result in withdrawal phenomena, such as increased headache, nausea, irritability, sleeplessness, and even seizures. Because of these problems with the combination medications containing butalbital, the author does not recommend them for routine use. If one has to use a narcotic oral pain medication, a combination of acetaminophen with 30 mg of codeine is probably the least controversial.

Prophylactic Treatment of Migraine

If a person has repeated episodes of migraine, which are interfering with lifestyle and work, and if those attacks cannot be effectively controlled with abortive treatment, he or she should be considered for prophylactic pharmacotherapy. It should be remembered that the medications used for prophylactic migraine may have side effects which have to be weighed against the benefits obtained by long-term prophylactic treatment. The general principles of treatment with prophylactic agents include: explaining the side effects versus the potential benefits to the patient before the medications are started; discontinuing the chronic frequent use of analgesics and ergotamine, because continuation of these drugs concomitantly with prophylactic agents will nullify the effects of prophylactic agents; starting the medications in smaller doses and gradually increasing them, depending on the ability of the patient to tolerate the medications and the side effects; continuing the medications for a reasonable period of time, approximately 6 weeks to 3 months before they are discontinued, because the majority of the medications used in the prophylaxis have a lag time before the beneficial effects are known; and when the medications are discontinued, doing it gradually over a period of a few days so that the acute effects of sudden withdrawal are avoided.

Every effort should be made to give an adequate and structured trial of abortive medication before prophylactic medications are prescribed. The need for prophylactic pharmacotherapy will depend to a great degree on the frequency and severity of the migraine attacks and the completeness of the response to abortive agents. In general, patients with more than two episodes of migraines per month who do not respond adequately to abortive agents may require prophylactic therapy. Common medications used in the prophylactic treatment of migraine are given in Table 6.

Beta-Adrenergic Blocking Agents

Beta-adrenergic blocking agents are the first line of drugs used in the prevention of migraine. Propranolol (Inderal) and timolol (Blocadren) are the only two beta blockers approved by the Food and Drug Administration specifically for the prophylactic treatment of migraine. However, other beta-adrenergic blocking agents, such as nadolol (Corgard), atenolol (Tenormin), metoprolol (Lopressor), and pindolol (Visken)* have been found to be effective in some patients with migraine. The effective dose of propranolol is about 80 to 160 mg. Some patients may require larger doses. It is recommended to start with small doses and gradually increase them. A long-acting preparation of propranolol is available (Inderal LA) which has the convenience of once-daily dose. However, the cost factor has to be taken into consideration. The short-acting propranolol is equally effective. We recommend using 20 mg of propranolol twice a day and gradually increasing it to 80 mg twice a day. The long-acting preparation can be started at 60 mg to be increased to 160 mg. The most common side effects of beta blockers are fatigue, lethargy, and depression. Patients have to be warned about these symptoms so that they can be recognized early. Some patients complain of muscular weakness involving the lower extremities. Exercise tolerance is

---

*This use of Visken is not listed in the manufacturer's original directive.

TABLE 6. **Prophylactic Pharmacotherapy for Migraine**

Medication	Dosage
Beta-Adrenergic Blocking Agents	
Propranolol (Inderal)	40–160 mg/day in divided doses
Propranolol long-acting (Inderal LA)	60–160 mg once daily
Nadolol (Corgard)	40–160 mg once daily
Timolol (Blocadren)	Up to 20 mg twice daily
Metoprolol (Lopressor)	50–100 mg/day
Pindolol (Visken)	10–30 mg/day
Atenolol (Tenormin)	50–100 mg/day
Antidepressants	
Tricyclic Antidepressants	
Amitriptyline (Elavil, Endep)	25–100 mg at bedtime
Doxepin (Sinequan, Adapin)	10–100 mg at bedtime
Nortriptyline (Aventyl, Pamelor)	10–50 mg at bedtime
Imipramine (Tofranil)	25–150 mg at bedtime
Desipramine (Pertofrane, Norpramin)	25–50 mg at bedtime
Selective Serotonin Uptake Inhibitors	
Fluoxetine (Prozac)	20 mg daily in the morning
Sertraline (Zoloft)	50 mg at bedtime
Monoamine Oxidase Inhibitors	
Phenelzine (Nardil)	15 mg three times daily
Isocarboxazid (Marplan)	10 mg four hours daily
Calcium Channel Blockers	
Verapamil (Calan, Isoptin, Verelan)	80–360 mg/day
Flunarizine (Sibelium)*	10–30 mg/day
Diltiazem (Cardizem)	60–90 mg three times/day
Nicardipine (Cardene)	20 mg three times/day
Nimodipine (Nimotop)	30 mg three times/day
Serotonin Antagonists	
Methysergide (Sansert)	4–8 mg/day
Cyproheptadine (Periactin)	8–16 mg/day
Pizotifen (Sandomigran)*	
Anticonvulsants	
Valproate (Depakote)	500–1500 mg/day
Phenytoin (Dilantin)	100–300 mg/day
Alpha-Adrenergic Agonist	
Clonidine (Catapres)	0.1–0.2 mg three times a day

*Not available in the United States.

reduced. The fact that beta blockers reduce the pulse rate has to be explained to patients who exercise regularly so that they will not base their exercise tolerance according to their pulse rate. Weight gain is a concern with beta blockers in women, who form the majority of patients with migraine. Weight gain has to be explained to the patients before they are given the medication. Lack of an adequate penile erection and subsequent impotence is a matter of grave concern in some male patients receiving propranolol.

The main contraindications for beta blockers include active asthma, congestive cardiac failure, atrioventricular conduction disturbances, and hypotension. Patients who have relatively low blood pressures do not appear to tolerate beta blockers well. Patients with a family history of asthma or a previous history of asthma will have to be warned about the possibility of asthmatic tendencies returning when they start to receive beta blockers. The use of beta blockers should be avoided in diabetic patients who are insulin dependent or receiving oral hypoglycemia agents. If a person does not respond adequately to one beta blocker, for example, propranolol, another beta blocker may be tried, because the patient may respond to the new compound more effectively. In other words, a lack of response to one particular beta blocker compound does not exclude the use of other beta blockers. Beta blockers should not be withdrawn abruptly in patients with coronary artery disease, because they may exacerbate the ischemia and induce arrhythmias. Beta blockers can be combined with tricyclic antidepressants very effectively in patients with frequent migraine episodes of migraine and mixed migraine, tension-type headache syndromes.

The mechanism of action of beta blockers in migraine is not clear. Beta-blockade is unlikely to be responsible for the therapeutic action in migraine. These drugs are thought to block the dilatation of cranial arteries and arterioles caused by a low concentration of serotonin. They also have an antianxiety effect. Because beta-adrenergic blocking agents are effective antihypertensives, they are the drugs of choice in patients with migraine and hypertension. They are also particularly effective in migraine sufferers with anxiety.

Antidepressants

TRICYCLIC ANTIDEPRESSANTS

Tricyclic antidepressants, particularly amitriptyline (Elavil, Endep) are effective in the prophylactic management of chronic headaches, especially mixed forms of migraine and tension-type headaches. Tricyclic antidepressants block serotonin uptake from the central synapse and have been shown to have central analgesic effects, because they reduce the firing rates of the spinal tract of the trigeminal nuclei, which is the converging point of craniofacial pain sensation in the central nervous system. The antiheadache effect of tricyclic compounds is independent of its antidepressant effect, although the antidepressant properties certainly help patients with chronic migraine who are also depressed and have associated sleep disturbances. Monitoring of blood levels, as is done in the treatment of depression using tricyclics, may not be necessary while treating a headache patient with amitriptyline.

Headache patients require only small doses of tricyclics. Usually 25 to 50 mg of amitriptyline at night is all that is required. It is recommended that one starts with small doses and gradually builds the dose up, so that the patient will not be too drowsy or groggy during the first few days of using the medications. A dose of 25 mg of amitriptyline at night plus propranolol during the day is a good combination.

A number of factors, such as the anticholinergic, sedating, and appetite-increasing effects of tricyclics, have to be considered while selecting the agents. The secondary compounds, such as nortriptyline (Pamelor), have less anticholinergic effects, thereby producing less of the symptoms, such as dryness of the mouth, blurred vision due to dilatation of the pupils, and dysuria. A dose of 25 mg of nortriptyline at night is recommended.

SELECTIVE SEROTONIN UPTAKE INHIBITORS

Selective serotonin uptake inhibitors, such as fluoxetine (Prozac) and sertraline (Zoloft), are useful adjuncts in the treatment of chronic headaches. While it has not been shown that they have a specific antimigraine effect, they are useful in patients who are not able to tolerate tricyclics, because of excess weight gain, sedation, or anticholinergic side effects, such as blurred vision, dysuria, and dry mouth. A dose of 20 mg of fluoxetine a day in combination with beta blockers is useful in some patients. Fluoxetine has to be administered in the morning, because it may keep some people awake if given at night. The side effects of fluoxetine include tremor, excitement, and hypomanic and manic reactions. Sertraline can be administered at a dose of 50 mg at bedtime.

Other antidepressants, such as trazodone (Desyrel) and bupropion (Wellbutrin), have not been shown to be particularly effective in patients with frequent headaches. In fact, the main metabolite of trazodone, namely meta-chlorophenyl piperazine (MCPP), has been shown to be an inducer of migraine experimentally.

Calcium Channel Blockers

Calcium channel antagonists have a place in the prophylactic treatment of migraine; however, the effectiveness of calcium channel blockers in migraine is not as striking as that of beta blockers. The calcium channel blockers may be particularly effective in migraine disorders associated with neurologic symptoms, such as basilar artery migraine, hemiplegic migraine, migraine with frequent visual and neurologic aura, and migraine with prolonged aura. The antivasospastic effect may be responsible for the effectiveness in these forms of migraine. Calcium channel antagonists also block serotonin release, alter slow potential shifts, and prevent spreading depression, all of which have been hypothesized to be mechanisms of migraine. Verapamil (Isoptin, Calan, Verelan) is the drug of choice. Verapamil 120 to 480 mg is the recommended dose, depending on the individual tolerance. Long-acting verapamil dosage forms, such as Calan SR or Isoptin SR, are recommended. Calcium channel blockers can be combined with tricyclic antidepressants. Edema and constipation are the most common side effects of verapamil. It should be noted that calcium channel blockers are not specifically approved by the Food and Drug Administration for use in migraine prophylaxis. Flunarizine, a calcium channel antagonist not available in the United States, is extensively used in other countries for migraine prophylaxis with reasonably good results.

Serotonin Antagonists

METHYSERGIDE

Methysergide (Sansert) is probably the most effective antimigraine agent available; however, the side-effect profile makes it one of the last choices in the prophylactic treatment of headache. The average dose is about 6 mg a day in divided doses. Some patients require 8 to 10 mg a day.

Its most common acute side effects are muscular pain involving the lower extremity, edema of the ankles, and discoloration of the ankles. The muscular pain may become severe enough to interfere with walking in some patients. Other less common side effects include gastric irritation and diarrhea. Those who tolerate the medication well do extremely well; however, the effectiveness may wane after about 4 to 5 months.

Because of the potential fibrotic reactions which may occur during long-term use, this medication is recommended for continuous use only for about 6 months. After using the drug for 6 months, a drug holiday is recommended for at least 2 to 3 months before the medication is resumed. The fibrotic reactions consist of the slow growth of fibrous tissue in the retroperitoneal area, lungs, and cardiac valves. The retroperitoneal fibrosis, if undetected, can result in ureteral obstruction, hydronephrosis, and renal failure. If one has to use methysergide repeatedly, it is recommended that the development of any fibrotic reaction be monitored from time to time using such tests as the echocardiogram, chest x-ray, intravenous pyelography, computed tomography or magnetic resonance imaging of the abdomen specifically to look for signs of fibrous tissue growth. Patients have to be warned about these symptoms very carefully. Written warnings have to be given to protect the physician medicolegally. The vasoconstrictor potential of the drug dictates it not be used in patients with primary peripheral vascular disease or ischemic heart or cardiovascular disease. Despite the potential dangers, methysergide is very useful for some of the more severe forms of migraine.

CYPROHEPTADINE

In addition to its antihistaminic properties, cyproheptadine (Periactin) is a serotonin antagonist with less vasoactivity than methysergide. Children respond to cyproheptadine more than do adults, and it is the drug of choice in them. Drowsiness and increased appetite with resulting weight gain are common side effects. The usual effective dose is 4 to 12 mg per day. A dose of 4 mg at bedtime with a gradual increase in the dose may help to cope with drowsiness.

Valproate

Valproate (Depakene, Depokote) has been found to be effective in the prophylactic treatment of migraine and chronic headaches in recent years. Valproate, a gamma-aminobutyric acid mimetic anticonvulsant, exerts its antimigraine effect probably through its action on serotonergic neurotransmission at the dorsal raphe nuclei and also by counteracting the excessive activity of glutamate, an excitatory amino acid which has recently been implicated in migraine pathogenesis. The effective dose of valproate is 500 to 1000 mg per day in divided doses. The therapeutic blood levels have to be kept between 50 and 100 μg per ml. Like other prophylactic agents, it is recommended that valproate be started in small doses and gradually increased to the effective tolerable dose. The usual side effects include asthenia, tremor, weight gain, and hair loss. Hepatotoxicity due to valproate is extremely rare in healthy adults; however, periodic monitoring of the blood chemistry and complete blood count is recommended. Valproate should not be used in patients with active liver disease. Barbiturate-containing medication should be avoided while the patient is receiving valproate. A recent double-blind study has shown valproate to be as effective as beta blockers in the prophylactic treatment of migraine. Valproate may become a second-line drug in the prophylactic treatment of migraine in the future.

NSAIDs

NSAIDs can be used in the prophylactic treatment of migraine. The drug which has been studied in a double-blind trial is naproxen, which can be used on a daily basis in the dose of 375 mg twice a day. However, gastroenteropathy after long-term use limits its usefulness. When used 6 months or longer, more than two-thirds of patients develop subclinical intestinal inflammation and occult blood loss. Up to one-fifth of them have bile acid malabsorption, and thus, diarrheal illness may develop. Naproxen can also be combined with other prophylactic agents in more resistant cases. Apart from the long-term gastrointestinal effects, the renal effects have to be monitored if this drug has to be used long term.

Treatment of Menstrual Migraine

Approximately 60 to 70% of female patients with migraine report worsening of their headaches around the menstrual time. About 15% have pure menstrual migraine. Cyclical treatment using a combination of ergotamine and NSAIDs, starting 2 to 3 days before the expected day of the headache and continued until the end of menstrual flow, is recommended. In those who have their headache immediately after the menstruation, they may be started on the combination medications toward the later one-half of menstrual flow and continued for 2 to 3 days after the expected headache. Cafergot or Wigraine (one tablet twice daily) with naproxen 500 mg twice daily is the recommended dose.

Hormonal manipulations are generally unsuccessful. However, some patients may respond to very small doses of estradiol (Estraderm patch, 0.2 mg) applied about 1 week before the expected menstrual cycle. This prevents the precipitous fall in estradiol in the late luteal phase of the cycle.

TREATMENT OF CLUSTER HEADACHE

Abortive Treatment of Acute Attacks of Cluster Headache

In the treatment of acute attack of cluster headache, oxygen is the preferred agent. Oxygen inhalation 8 liters per minute for 10 minutes using a mask will abort the attacks of cluster headache in approximately 70% of patients. Our patients with cluster headaches rent portable oxygen tanks. Oxygen may simply delay the headache in some patients, which returns after 1 hour or so.

Oxygen inhalation can be combined with ergotamine in a form which will be absorbed very rapidly. Ergotamine inhalation, which results in rapid plasma peak levels, is no longer available; therefore, one has to rely on sublingual, suppository, or oral preparations. The slower plasma peak levels after oral administration take a longer time for the drug to be effective in acute attacks of cluster headache. Sublingual preparations are rather erratic in their absorption pattern and, hence, are not very reliable. Suppositories are rather inconvenient for administration in cases of cluster headache, because their effect comes on rapidly without any warning and leaves rapidly. Despite these disadvantages, some patients do respond to a combination of oxygen and ergotamine in either oral, sublingual, or rectal forms. A dose of 1 mg of ergotamine tablets, 2 mg of sublingual tablets, or 2 mg of the suppository may be tried.

Sumatriptan is the drug of choice for acute episodes of cluster headache. Sumatriptan is available in 100-mg tablets and 6 mg by subcutaneous injection. Subcutaneous sumatriptan gives dramatic effect within 15 minutes of its administration. It can also be combined with oxygen. With this combination, the patient should obtain relief almost immediately, and acute attacks are aborted totally. Repeat administration of sumatriptan is possible and has not shown to produce any tolerance even after repeated use for more than approximately 1 year in patients with chronic cluster headache. Injectable sumatriptan is available in an autoinjector form, and it is very easy for the patient to self-administer. The advantages of sumatriptan are its lack of adverse effect, especially lack of nausea and vomiting, because it is specific 5-HT$_{1D}$ agonist without any

effects on any other neurotransmitter receptors. It is devoid of the side effects that are seen with the use of medications like DHE.

Upper chest discomfort, a burning sensation at the site of injection, and a hot feeling in the body for a short period of time are the relatively minor side effects of sumatriptan. Because the majority of patients with cluster headache are men, usually heavy smokers, their cardiac status has to be evaluated before drug therapy is started. Sumatriptan and ergotamine should not be used in patients with proven coronary artery disease and those who have multiple risk factors for coronary heart disease. Appropriate investigations to exclude ischemic heart disease have to be done before ergotamine, sumatriptan, and DHE are prescribed. DHE administered intramuscularly will relieve the cluster headache attack effectively, but it has a slower onset of action than does sumatriptan. Since cluster headache occurs one to three times per day on average, repeated intramuscular injections are painful and rather impractical. A nasal spray of DHE is under trial.

Analgesics and narcotics have no real place in the treatment of cluster headache. It should be noted that the total period of pain from each cluster headache is approximately 45 minutes, and by the time any oral narcotic gets absorbed and takes effect, the pain is usually already over. The prescription of narcotic medications will simply lead to excessive use with habituation without any major benefit as far as pain relief is concerned. Combination analgesics containing a barbiturate and caffeine (Fiorinal-type preparations) have no place in the treatment of acute cluster headaches.

Prophylactic Treatment of Cluster Headache

General Principles

Since cluster headache can occur many times a day and the suffering is extreme, it is important to use prophylactic medications to try to prevent the attacks. Medications have to be started early in the cluster period so that the total period can be shortened. It is always better to start with small doses over a period of a few days and build up to an optimum level that is tolerated well. Combinations of medications may become necessary. The selection of medications used for prophylactic treatment of cluster headache would depend on a number of factors, including the timing of the attack, the age of the patient, the type of cluster headache (episodic versus chronic), contraindications to particular medications (for example, coronary artery disease), and the patient's response to previous medications. Table 7 lists

TABLE 7. **Prophylactic Pharmacotherapy of Cluster Headache**

Medication	Dosage
Verapamil (Calan, Isoptin, Verelan)	120–480 mg per day
Lithium carbonate (Lithobid, Eskalith, Lithane)	600–900 mg per day
Methysergide (Sansert)	4–8 mg per day
Ergotamine (Wigraine, Cafergot)	1–2 mg per day
Prednisone†	40 mg per day to start with, 2–3 weeks course in decremental doses
Valproate (Depakote)	500–1500 mg per day
Indomethacin (Indocin)‡	50–150 mg per day

*Recommended for chronic cluster headache.
†Recommended only as short courses to break the cycle, if unresponsive to other prophylactic agents.
‡Useful only in chronic paroxysmal hemicrania.

the medications used for the prophylactic treatment of cluster headache.

Verapamil

Of all the medications used for the prophylaxis of cluster headache, verapamil appears to be the most effective and is the drug of choice. The usual dose is 120 mg three to four times a day. The dosage may have to be increased further in some patients. Verapamil should be continued at least for 2 to 3 weeks after the patient becomes totally free of headaches in the episodic variety. In chronic cluster headache, the length of treatment has to be determined by a trial-and-error method. The majority of the patients with chronic cluster headache will require verapamil for an indefinite period of time.

Ergotamine

Combinations of ergotamine and verapamil are known to give very good results in patients with cluster headache. The dosage of ergotamine is 1 mg twice a day. It should be noted that, unlike in migraine, ergotamine in cluster headache does not appear to result in a rebound phenomena. However, caution should be taken in regard to the use of daily ergotamine in patients with risk factors for cardiovascular disease. The majority of cluster headache patients are heavy smokers and some have hypertension; therefore, they have an increased risk of vascular disease.

Lithium Carbonate

Lithium carbonate is useful for both episodic and chronic cluster headache prophylaxis. Lithium is administered in divided doses of 300 mg two to three times a day. The effect of lithium is known in less than 1 week. If it is to be continued, monitoring of the lithium level to keep the level at the low therapeutic range of about 0.5 to 0.6 mEq per liter is necessary. The plasma level of lithium should never exceed 1.2 mEq per liter. Lithium is reasonably well tolerated by the majority of patients. While receiving lithium, the patients should not be taking sodium-depleting diuretics, because hyponatremia will lead to lithium toxicity. The common side effects of lithium include nausea, vomiting, tremor, and lethargy. Neurotoxicity occurs at higher plasma levels, resulting in ataxia, blurred vision, confusion, and altered consciousness. Lithium can be combined with verapamil or ergotamine tartrate. Combinations of lithium and verapamil are the drugs of choice in the treatment of chronic cluster headache.

Methysergide

Methysergide is useful in patients with episodic cluster headache, whereas patients with chronic cluster headache are less responsive to it. One tablet (2 mg) three to four times a day is the standard dose. The side effects of methysergide are described in the section on treatment of migraine.

Corticosteroids

Corticosteroids, particularly prednisone, have a definite place in the prophylactic treatment of cluster headache. The effect is usually dramatic, and the patients stop having cluster headache attacks within 1 to 2 days. However, when the corticosteroids are discontinued, the headache may come back with an equal frequency as before. Because of the exacerbation after the discontinuation of prednisone and because of the possibility of hypercorticism developing after frequent and prolonged use, prednisone should be reserved for short courses to break the cycle of headache when other agents, such as verapamil, ergotamine, lithium, and methysergide, are not helpful. The usual dose of prednisone is 20 mg two to three times a day to start with, which will be reduced gradually over a period of 2 to 3 weeks and then discontinued. The mechanism of action of corticosteroids in cluster headache is not clear. Corticosteroids may suppress the synthesis or release of humoral agents that mediate an attack of cluster headache or they may influence neurotransmitters involved in the headache. Corticosteroids modulate serotonergic pathways in the brain and may affect the hypothalamic biologic clock that is disrupted in patients with cluster headache.

Some headache specialists use prednisone at the onset of the cluster period along with verapamil. Then, the prednisone is tapered off after 2 weeks, and the verapamil is continued for the duration of the cluster period. This is a reasonable alternate approach; however, as mentioned previously, exacerbation of the headache can occur after the prednisone is discontinued, even though the chances of that happening are less while the patients are continued on verapamil.

Indomethacin

Indomethacin (Indocin) is specific for and always successful in the treatment of chronic paroxysmal hemicrania, which is a variant of cluster headache, occurring mostly in women. The attacks are short-lived, on average 5 to 10 minutes, as opposed to cluster headache, which lasts for 45 minutes to 1 hour. Multiple attacks (15 to 20 per day) occur, and autonomic symptoms may accompany the headache. It is always unilateral and there are no remissions, resembling the pattern seen in chronic cluster headache. The therapeutic response to indomethacin can be used as a diagnostic test for chronic paroxysmal hemicrania. The usual dose of indomethacin is 25 to 50 mg three times a day. Like other nonsteroidal anti-inflammatory agents, gastric side effects are common with indomethacin. Misoprostol (Cytotec) may help to protect the upper gastrointestinal tract from the effects of indomethacin in patients with chronic paroxysmal hemicrania who need to continue indomethacin for an indefinite period of time. Those receiving long-term indomethacin should have renal function tests done periodically.

Beta Blockers and Antidepressants

Some of the medications which are proved to be effective in the prophylaxis of migraine, such as beta-adrenergic blocking agents and tricyclic antidepressants, are not particularly useful in the treatment of cluster headache. However, there may be an occasional patient who may respond to these medications. In patients with chronic cluster headache who are also depressed, antidepressants may be of value as an adjunct.

DHE

DHE is useful to break the cycle of headache in those with intractable cluster headache attacks who do not respond to regular prophylactic therapy. DHE given intravenously every 6 hours will invariably break the cycle in 2 to 3 days. The remission obtained by DHE gives the physician an opportunity to adjust the prophylactic therapy. A course of DHE may put a patient into remission for a considerable period of time.

Surgical Treatment of Chronic Cluster Headache

About 10% of patients with chronic cluster headache are totally resistant to all known abor-

tive and preventive medications. These patients have frequent severe cluster headache attacks occurring four to five times a day without remissions for more than 1 year. They are usually totally disabled. Radiofrequency trigeminal gangliorhizolysis (radiofrequency lesion of the trigeminal nerve ganglion) has been shown to be useful in such patients with chronic medically resistant chronic cluster headache. Of 80 patients who underwent this procedure at the Houston Headache Clinic, 75% showed satisfactory control of their chronic cluster headaches.

TREATMENT OF TENSION-TYPE AND CHRONIC DAILY HEADACHE

Episodic tension-type headaches require very little treatment with medications. Simple analgesics, such as acetaminophen or aspirin, are all that are required in the majority of patients. NSAIDs, such as ibuprofen (Motrin), are used by many patients with satisfactory results. Chronic tension-type headache and chronic daily headache have to be evaluated carefully before treatment is initiated. The majority of patients with chronic headaches are receiving analgesic medications or ergotamine on a daily basis. The analgesic/ergotamine rebound phenomenon has to be recognized before prophylactic treatment is initiated. Patients have to be withdrawn from daily analgesics and ergotamine. Hospitalization may become necessary in some of the patients who have daily persistent headache while receiving daily analgesics. Withdrawal reactions resulting in increased headache, nausea, vomiting, restlessness, and sleeplessness can occur. Seizures have been reported in patients suddenly withdrawn from butalbital, caffeine, and aspirin combinations (Fiorinal). A clonidine (Catapres) patch 0.1 mg may be applied to minimize the withdrawal effects while the patients are undergoing withdrawal from narcotics.

Amitriptyline

Once the offending medications are withdrawn, patients with chronic tension-type headache may be started on prophylactic treatment. The drug of choice is amitriptyline or one of the tricyclic compounds which has been shown to be beneficial in more than one way in these patients. In addition to reducing the severity of the headache, they help the patients sleep better and also are effective in the management of the associated depression. Other antidepressants such as fluoxetine and sertraline can also be used.

Repetitive Intravenous DHE

Patients with chronic daily headache who have usually a mixed pattern of migraine and tension-type headache do respond to intravenous DHE. These patients are usually given intravenous DHE repetitively every 6 hours for a period of 48 to 72 hours to break the cycle of headache. Concomitantly, they should undergo detoxification from analgesics. Once the daily cycle of headache is broken, they can be started on prophylactic pharmacotherapy. Any of the drugs mentioned previously for the prophylaxis of migraine can be used for chronic daily headache.

Despite breaking the cycle of headache and reducing the frequency of headache, these patients will continue to have episodes during which they need abortive treatment. Any of the medications mentioned in the abortive treatment section on migraine can be used in these patients, depending on the severity of individual attacks. They should be discouraged from going back to their original analgesic/narcotic/sedative medications for symptomatic relief.

CRANIAL NEURALGIAS

Trigeminal Neuralgia

Trigeminal neuralgia or tic douloureux is the most common form of primary cranial neuralgia and occurs usually in patients older than age 50 years. The pain is excruciating and lancinating in character and manifests as sharp short-lived jabs lasting typically 20 to 30 seconds. It is unilateral, mostly confined to the second and third divisions of the trigeminal nerve. Most of the pain is felt in the circumoral area of the angle of the mouth. There may be "trigger zones" on the face, and as a result, the patient avoids touching, washing, or shaving the face, biting or chewing, or any other maneuver that could stimulate the pain site. Many patients with trigeminal neuralgia lose weight because they avoid eating, for fear of the pain brought on by chewing. There may be some periodicity in trigeminal neuralgia, manifesting itself in cycles.

Carbamazepine is the first-line drug for trigeminal neuralgia. The initial dose of 200 mg per day may be increased to 800 to 1200 mg daily in divided doses. Carbamazepine is fairly well tolerated in the majority of patients. However, drowsiness and lethargy are frequent side effects. In higher doses, dizziness, ataxia, and confusion can occur. Blood dyscrasias may occur on rare occasions as a result of carbamazepine. Periodic complete blood count monitoring is recommended. The therapeutic level is 6 to 8 μg per mL.

Phenytoin (Dilantin), up to 400 mg per day may be added to the carbamazepine regimen if the patient is unresponsive. Phenytoin levels should be kept at 10 to 20 μg per 100 mL. Higher levels of phenytoin will result in drowsiness, severe ataxia, confusion, double vision, and cerebellar signs. Hemopoietic change may also occur.

Baclofen (Lioresal) is the third-line drug for trigeminal neuralgia. It can be added to carbamazepine and/or phenytoin. The initial dose should be small (10 mg per day), gradually increased up to 60 mg per day. Drowsiness, weakness, nausea, and vomiting are common side effects.

If the patient is totally refractory to triple therapy using carbamazepine, phenytoin, and baclofen, surgery should be considered. Surgery, which is directed toward reducing trigeminal nerve pain transmission, includes trigeminal radiofrequency rhizotomy, glycerol injection into Meckel's cave, and microvascular decompression of the trigeminal nerve root (Jannetta procedure). The later requires a posterior form of craniotomy, whereas the former two are stereotaxic procedures done under fluoroscopic control and require no craniotomy.

NONPHARMACOLOGIC TREATMENT OF HEADACHE

It is extremely important that medications be combined with nonpharmacologic approaches in patients with recurrent headaches. Trigger factors should be identified and avoided.

Dietary Management

Approximately 20% of patients with migraine have dietary factors that precipitate their headache attacks. Tables 8, 9, and 10 summarize the dietary management. Patients should avoid the items listed as much as possible. Skipping meals should be avoided. Hypoglycemia can induce attacks of headache in those who are prone to migraine.

TABLE 8. **Diet in Migraine: General Hints**

Avoid dietary substances acting directly on blood vessels:
   Amines
      Tyramine (e.g., aged cheeses, meats)
      Phenylethylamine (chocolate)
   Nitrites (e.g., hot dogs)
   Monosodium glutamate (e.g., Chinese food)
   Alcohol
   Aspartame (NutraSweet, Equal)
Eat three well-balanced meals each day; may include
   between-meal snacks as needed
Avoid skipping meals
Avoid prolonged fasting

TABLE 9. **Low-Tyramine, Low-Caffeine, Low-Preservative Diet**

Type	Foods to Avoid
Beverage	Chocolate, cocoa, alcoholic beverages, asparatame (NutraSweet, Equal), diet drinks
Meat, fish, poultry	Aged, canned, cured, or processed meat, including ham or game; pickled herring, salad, and dried fish; chicken livers; bologna; fermented sausage; any food prepared with meat tenderizer, soy sauce or brewer's yeast; any food containing nitrates, nitrites, or tyramine
Dairy products	Cultured dairy products (buttermilk, sour cream); chocolate milk; and cheeses: blue, Boursin, brick, Brie types, Camembert types, cheddar, Gouda, Stilton, Swiss (Emmentaler), Roquefort, mozzarella, parmesan, provolone, romano
Bread, cereal	Fresh homemade yeast bread, bread or crackers containing cheese; fresh yeast coffee cake, doughnuts, sourdough bread; any produce containing chocolate or nuts
Vegetable	Beans such as pole, broad, lima, Italian, fava, navy, pinto, garbanzo; snow peas, pea pods, sauerkraut, raw onions, olives, pickles
Fruit	Avocados, figs, raisins, papaya, passion fruit, red plums
Soup	Canned soup, soup or bouillon cubes, soup base with autolytic yeast or monosodium glutamate (read labels)
Dessert	Chocolate ice cream, pudding, cookies, cake, or pies, mincemeat pie
Sweets	Chocolate candy or syrup, carob
Miscellaneous	Pizza, cheese sauce, monosodium glutamate in excessive amounts, yeast, yeast extract, meat tenderizer, Accent, seasoned salt; mixed dishes (macaroni and cheese, beef Stroganoff, cheese blintzes, lasagna, frozen dinners); nuts (peanuts, peanut butter); seeds (pumpkin, sesame, sunflower) (read labels on snack items); any pickled, preserved, or marinated food

Chronobiologic Management

Patients with migraine are known to trigger their headaches if they break their usual daily routines. Too much sleep and too little sleep in relation to which they are accustomed may bring on the headaches. Extreme alterations in the timing of daily activities will also trigger headaches. The regulation of these chronobiologic factors should be attempted. Prolonged periods of concentration without a break and improper lighting and ventilation at the work place are other factors which influence the occurrence of headache.

Physical Exercise

For people with chronic recurrent headaches, physical exercise, preferably aerobic exercise, is recommended at our clinic. They are advised to do so on a regular basis. Physical exercise relaxes the nervous system, reduces the sympathetic tone, and reduces blood pressure, and all these factors are important in the overall control of headaches.

Relaxation Exercises and Biofeedback Therapy

Relaxation exercises and biofeedback techniques are extremely useful to people with recurrent headaches. At the Houston Headache Clinic, biofeedback training is given in an intensive fashion approximately for a total of 10 hours. Patients are encouraged to practice biofeedback daily as a preventative for their headaches. It may be too late for the patient to abort an attack of migraine with a biofeedback technique. It is better that they practice it outside the headache phase.

Behavioral Counseling and Psychotherapy

Behavioral counseling and psychotherapy are required in some patients, especially in those with frequent headaches and associated co-morbid factors such as anxiety, extreme stress, and depression. The family environment and other psychosocial factors might be of importance in the

TABLE 10. **Monosodium Glutamate***

Partial List of Food Categories That Usually Contain Large Amounts of MSG

Frozen food (especially dinner entrees)
Canned and dry soups
Potato chips and prepared snacks
International foods
Most diet foods and weight-loss powders
Cured and luncheon meats (i.e., salami, bologna, pepperoni)
Most sauces in jars and cans (i.e., tomato and barbecue)
Most salad dressings and mayonnaise

FDA-Approved Food Label Terms Indicating MSG Content

MSG
Hydrolyzed vegetable protein (HVP)
Hydrolyzed plant protein (HPP)
Natural flavor (almost always)
Flavoring (almost always)
Kombu extract

*MSG, an established headache trigger, has become far more prevalent in canned, packaged, and prepared foods over the past decade. The presence of MSG in food may be difficult to detect since the terms "natural flavor," "flavoring," or "hydrolyzed vegetable protein (HVP)," all may appear on food labels and may refer to MSG, according to current FDA food labeling codes. HVP typically contains 10 to 30% MSG.

Cases are reported in which the elimination of all food sources of MSG resulted in decreased headache frequency. When patients are put on an MSG-free trial diet, attention needs to be given to the identification of the wide variety of food containing MSG and HVP.

Abbreviations: FDA = Food and Drug Administration; MSG = monosodium glutamate.

precipitation of headaches in some patients. These have to be identified in individual patients and treated appropriately. At the Houston Headache Clinic, individual counseling as well as family therapy are instituted as and when needed.

HEADACHE CLINICS VERSUS PAIN CLINICS

The essential difference between headache clinics and pain clinics which deal with chronic back pain is in the pharmacologic approaches. Pharmacotherapy is very important in a headache clinic, because primary headache disorders are spontaneous pain disorders which have been shown to be due to changes in the biology of the neurovascular system of the head. The pharmacologic approaches are of prime importance, followed by behavioral approaches, such as relaxation exercises, biofeedback, and behavioral counseling. The physical methods of treatment, such as physical therapy and nerve blocks, are of least importance in the management of chronic headache. On the other hand, physical methods are of prime importance in a pain clinic, and there is very little pharmacotherapy. Because of these reasons, a referral to a pain clinic may not be the most beneficial thing for a patient with chronic headaches. They have to be referred to a headache clinic which undertakes a comprehensive approach to the treatment of headache utilizing pharmacologic, behavioral, and if necessary, physical methods of treatment.

HOSPITALIZATION

Patients with headache may have to be hospitalized under certain special circumstances for a short period of time. The indications for hospitalization are listed in Table 11. After discharge from the hospital, patients with chronic recurrent headaches need long-term continuity of care. Combinations of pharmacologic and nonpharmacologic approaches have the best chance for success.

TABLE 11. **Admission Criteria for Inpatient Headache Treatment**

Status migrainosus: prolonged unrelenting headache with associated nausea, vomiting, and dehydration
Dependency on analgesics, caffeine, narcotics, barbiturates, or tranquilizers; withdrawal from these agents may have to be undertaken in an inpatient setting
Habituation to ergots; ergots taken on a daily basis, when stopped, will cause rebound headache
Headache accompanied by serious adverse reactions or complications from therapy
Headache associated with significant medical disease
Headache associated with significant psychiatric illness, such as extreme depression, severe anxiety, and panic attacks
Chronic cluster headache unresponsive to regular treatment
Patients who require continuance with drugs that may cause drug interactions necessitate careful observation within a hospital, for example, concomitant therapy using monoaminooxidase inhibitors and tricyclic antidepressants
Patients with accompanying organic disease

EPISODIC VERTIGO

method of
STEPHEN E. THURSTON, M.D.
Neurological Associates, Inc.
Richmond, Virginia

Vertigo is a symptom characterized by abnormal perceptions of motion or of spatial orientation. It results from physiologic or pathologic mismatches between various sensory systems (mainly visual, vestibular, and proprioceptive). These systems subserve stabilization of vision during head movements, spatial orientation, and maintenance of posture and locomotion. They also connect with autonomic centers in the medulla. Although many different disorders involving any of these systems may produce symptoms, vestibular dysfunction is the most common cause of clinically significant vertigo.

Vestibular vertigo may result from disease of the semicircular canals that sense angular rotation of the head or of the otoliths that sense linear translations of the head and static head position. Involvement of the canals or their central connections produces illusions of turning, spinning, or rotational movement. Disease of the otoliths or their central connections produces illusions of tilt, levitation, sway, or linear movement.

Vestibular vertigo is typically associated with nystagmus, postural imbalance, and autonomic symptoms of nausea, vomiting, pallor, diaphoresis, and generalized weakness. Nystagmus may result in blurred vision and oscillopsia, which is the illusory motion of objects due to the movement of their images on the retina.

The treatment of vertigo is based on establishing a vestibular cause of symptoms as distinct from the numerous other causes of "dizziness." The therapy may be divided into "general," with the goal of correcting the vestibular dysfunction, and "specific," aimed at the underlying cause of dysfunction. Causes of acute vertigo are summarized in Table 1. It should be noted that most causes of acute vertigo may also produce vertigo episodically. Many forms of vertigo can be positionally induced, particularly those due to benign paroxysmal positional vertigo (by definition), labyrinthine concussion, alcohol, multiple sclerosis, Arnold-Chiari malformation, and various other structural lesions in the posterior fossa.

TREATMENT

General Therapy

The general therapy of vertigo is aimed at alleviating acute autonomic symptoms and promot-

TABLE 1. **Causes of Acute Vertigo**

Physiologic vertigo: motion sickness, height vertigo, head extension vertigo

Benign paroxysmal positional vertigo (cupulolithiasis, canalolithiasis)

Infection of labyrinth and/or vestibular nerve: viral (including zoster), bacterial, syphilitic, fungal

Keratoma (cholesteatoma)

Drug toxicity: alcohol, aminoglycosides, anticonvulsants, salicylates, chemotherapeutic agents, heavy metals

Trauma: labyrinthine concussion, temporal bone fracture, perilymph fistula, barotrauma, postsurgical

Meniere's disease

Otosclerosis

Autoimmune inner ear disease

Cerebellar, brain stem, or labyrinthine ischemia (vertebrobasilar insufficiency); infarction; or hemorrhage

Migraine: Bickerstaff's basilar artery migraine, Slater's "benign recurrent vertigo"

Multiple sclerosis

Tumors of middle or inner ear, eighth cranial nerve, brain stem, or cerebellum

Neurovascular compression

Arnold-Chiari malformation and other posterior fossa anomalies

Paroxysmal ocular tilt reaction

Syringobulbia

Congenital anomalies of the inner ear

Cogan's syndrome

Benign paroxysmal vertigo of childhood

Familial periodic vertigo, ataxia, and nystagmus

Vestibular epilepsy

Paget's disease

Diabetes mellitus

Hyperviscosity syndrome

Vasculitis

---

limited and vestibular disorders encompass pathology in a variety of different anatomic, physiologic, and neurochemical systems. Vestibulosedative drugs decrease vertigo by decreasing vestibular function bilaterally—on both the normal and abnormal side—and, therefore, may produce ataxia. Additionally, experimental studies suggest that various central nervous system sedating agents actually inhibit vestibular compensation or produce decompensation. Drug therapy, therefore, should be restricted to the acute phase of the illness and used to relieve only the more severely disabling symptoms. In such settings, parenteral therapy is often necessary.

Prochlorperazine (Compazine) and trimethobenzamide (Tigan) are effective antiemetics with relatively less sedation than promethazine (Phenergan). Promethazine in combination with ephedrine is less sedating and more effective against autonomic symptoms. Scopolamine (Transderm-Scop), which can be administered transdermally with fewer side effects, is a convenient and effective method of preventing motion sickness and is also helpful in acute vertigo due to vestibular tone imbalance. Dextroamphetamine (Dexedrine) significantly potentiates the benefit of scopolamine, but has a high abuse potential and is not generally recommended for routine use. The use of papaverine, histamine, betahistamine, nylidrin (Arlidin), and other vaso-

ing restoration of normal vestibular function. Although some forms of vertigo may be either very mild or self-limited, requiring only limited intervention, the following approach is applicable to most acute peripheral or central vestibulopathies. In acute episodes, patients are kept at bed rest for a day or two and allowed to assume their most comfortable head position. Sudden head movements are avoided. Intravenous hydration may be beneficial in patients with protracted vomiting. A clear liquid diet is begun and advanced as tolerated. When indicated, the patient is reassured that the symptoms will improve, and every effort is made to decrease anxiety without using anxiolytic drugs.

A wide variety of vestibulosedative and antiemetic drugs are available for the symptomatic treatment of vertigo. Some of the more commonly used agents are listed in Table 2. Although considered helpful empirically, their effectiveness has rarely been evaluated by objective measurement of vestibular function. The variety of agents is indicative of the variability of effectiveness. It is often difficult to predict which patient will be helped by which drug, because our understanding of vestibular neuropharmacology is relatively

TABLE 2. **Drugs Commonly Used to Treat Vertigo**

Drug	Dose
Anticholinergic	
Scopolamine (Transderm-Scop)	0.6 mg PO q 4–6 h or 0.5 mg transdermally by patch q 3 days
Antihistamine	
Dimenhydrinate (Dramamine)	50 mg PO or IM q 4–6 h or 100 mg rectally q 8 h
Meclizine (Antivert, Bonine)	25 mg PO q 4–6 h
Promethazine (Phenergan)	25 or 50 mg PO or IM or rectally q 4–6 h
Cyclizine (Marezine)	50 mg PO or IM q 4–6 h or 100 mg rectally q 8 h
Trimethobenzamide (Tigan)	250 mg PO or IM q 6–8 h
Antidopaminergic	
Prochlorperazine (Compazine)	5 or 10 mg PO or IM q 4–6 h or 25 mg rectally q 12 h
Droperidol (Inapsine)	2.5 or 5 mg IM q 12 h
Haloperidol (Haldol)	1 or 2 mg PO or IM q 8–12 h
Benzodiazepines	
Diazepam (Valium, Valrelease)	5 or 10 mg PO, IM, or IV q 4–6 h
Sympathomimetic amines (adjunctive)	
Ephedrine sulfate	25 mg PO q 6 h with promethazine
Dextroamphetamine	5 mg PO q 6 h with scopolamine

dilators to improve blood flow to the labyrinth and brain stem is of unproven benefit. Vestibulo-sedative drugs should be used only in acute peripheral and central vestibulopathies and in the prophylaxis of motion sickness. There is no indication for the use of these drugs chronically.

The symptoms of an acute vestibulopathy usually improve significantly within a few days. While drug therapy and immobilization decrease symptoms, they also alter the sensory feedback that the central nervous system requires in order to restore vestibular balance. Experimental studies indicate that immobilization following unilateral peripheral vestibular lesions both prolongs adaptation and limits the ultimate degree of adaptation achieved. It has also been shown that enforced activity increases adaptation. Thus, pharmacotherapy and immobilization, if necessary, are restricted to only the very acute phase of illness, and an active program of vestibular rehabilitation is begun as soon as possible. This consists of exercises to elicit the visual and vestibular interactions necessary to promote recovery. In addition to vestibular adaptation, the exercises develop maximal use of other overlapping and compensatory systems. Since these same interactions (mismatches) produce an increase in the offending symptoms, patients will resist therapy. They must be reassured by explaining the rationale for treatment.

Physical therapy is begun as soon as possible after the severe autonomic symptoms subside. Cawthorne-Cooksey exercises or modifications (Table 3) are most commonly used. The patient progresses through the various levels of difficulty as rapidly as possible given the limitations of his or her particular illness. Corrective lenses should be worn during the exercises. Care should be taken with maneuvers done with the eyes closed or when the patient is particularly unstable. The series of exercises is repeated at least three times a day as long as vertigo persists.

In addition to formal exercises, the patient is encouraged to seek out offending head positions and movements, rather than to avoid them, and to engage in them actively as much as possible. Since adaptation tends to be rather stimulus specific, these movements should be practiced over a wide range of frequencies and velocities, particularly those that cause the most symptoms during the patient's daily routines.

Persistent vestibular deficits may occur with peripheral vestibular disease or with involvement of central structures important to adaptation, such as the cerebellum and the vestibular commissures in the brain stem. In the case of multiple sensory deficits, spatial orientation may be improved by supplementing proprioceptive and visual function through the use of such devices as canes or refractive correction. Only very rarely is surgical intervention, such as vestibular nerve section or labyrinthectomy, necessary.

TABLE 3. Modified Cawthorne-Cooksey Exercises

A. In bed—sitting up if possible
  1. Head stationary
    a. Look up and down (approximately ± 30 degrees)
    b. Look from side to side (approximately ± 45 degrees)
    c. Repeat a and b, focusing on finger moving up and down, side to side, slowly, then quickly
  2. Head moving—slowly, then quickly while fixating a stationary target
    a. Up and down (pitch)
    b. Rotating head side to side (yaw)
    c. Tilting head side to side (roll)
    d. Repeat a and b, fixating finger on outstretched arm as head and arm move together, then in opposite directions
B. Sitting
  Repeat 1 and 2
  3. Lean forward and pick up objects from floor
  4. Rotate head, shoulders, and trunk
C. Standing
  5. Practice standing with feet side by side with eyes open, then closed
  6. Change from sitting to standing with eyes open, then closed; repeat 1, 2, and 3
  7. Toss ball from hand to hand above eye level
  8. Pass ball from hand to hand under knees
  9. Change from sitting to standing and turn around in between; repeat 4
D. Walking
  10. Walk across room with eyes open, then closed
  11. Practice making sudden turns while walking
  12. Walk up and down slope with eyes open, then closed
  13. Stand on one foot with eyes open, then closed
  14. Tandem walking with eyes open, then closed
  15. Tandem walking backwards with eyes open, then closed

Specific Therapy

Specific therapy of vertigo is aimed at the underlying pathologic process (Table 1). Benign paroxysmal positional vertigo is the most common cause of positional vertigo. It is believed to be due to detached otoconia from the otoliths adhering to the cupula or floating within the endolymph of the posterior semicircular canal, making it gravity sensitive. It can usually be distinguished from positional vertigo due to central nervous system disease by a careful examination that includes Nylen-Barany positional testing. A vigorously performed variation of Nylen-Barany positional testing will reposition otoconial debris within the posterior canal and may be curative. Brandt and Daroff have demonstrated the effectiveness of head positioning exercises in treating benign paroxysmal positional vertigo. The exercises mechanically disperse the misplaced otoconial debris to a less sensitive portion of the labyrinth and promote adaptation.

Patients first tilt laterally from the seated position to lying on their affected side and hold that position until the evoked vertigo subsides. They then sit back upright 30 seconds before assuming the opposite head-down position for another 30 seconds. This sequence is repeated until the vertigo subsides, usually after several repetitions. These sessions are carried out every 3 hours while the patient is awake until he or she is free of vertigo for 2 consecutive days. The symptoms usually resolve in 1 to 2 weeks. Very rarely, symptoms will persist and surgical section of the posterior ampullary nerve or plugging the canal may be considered. In such a case, vestibular exercises should first be tried for at least 2 to 4 weeks. There is no indication for vestibulosedative drugs in benign paroxysmal positional vertigo.

Some vestibulotoxic agents such as alcohol, salicylates, and anticonvulsants produce predominantly reversible effects that resolve with reducing the dose or discontinuing the drug. Other vestibulotoxic agents, such as the aminoglycoside antibiotics (streptomycin, gentamicin, tobramycin, kanamycin, neomycin), produce more permanent effects, and the drug must be promptly discontinued at the first sign of toxicity.

Anticoagulation may be indicated in some unequivocal cases of vertebrobasilar ischemia. Episodic vertigo in isolation, without other evidence of posterior circulation ischemia, is not likely due to vertebrobasilar insufficiency. Cerebellar infarction or hemorrhage requires hospitalization and possible surgical decompression; anticoagulation is contraindicated.

Acute and chronic bacterial, syphilitic, or fungal infections of the middle or inner ear or meningeal spaces are treated with appropriate antibiotics. Myringotomy and culture may be necessary in bacterial labyrinthitis secondary to acute otitis media. Viral infections of the vestibular nerve, ganglion, or labyrinth are usually treated with the general measures described previously. Analgesics and specific antiviral therapy may prove useful in herpes zoster oticus, which is typically associated with ear pain, followed in several days by a vesicular eruption in the external auditory canal.

Most perilymph fistulas spontaneously resolve, especially with bed rest and avoidance of Valsalva maneuvers. Surgical repair after definitive diagnosis by exploratory tympanotomy may be necessary if symptoms persist for longer than 3 to 4 weeks. Temporal bone fractures with cerebrospinal fluid otorrhea require close monitoring for the possible development of meningitis. The use of prophylactic antibiotics is now questioned by many.

Meniere's disease is discussed separately. Otosclerosis is suggested by conductive or mixed hearing loss, tinnitus, and vestibular symptoms when examination of the tympanic membrane does not reveal middle ear disease. The recommended treatment has been calcium gluconate, 500 mg orally twice a day (before meals); sodium fluoride, 20 mg orally twice a day (after meals); and vitamin D, 400 units orally daily; however, the necessity for the calcium and vitamin D has been questioned, and the benefit of fluoride therapy must be weighed against the risk of fluorosis.

Tumors involving vestibular pathways often require surgical resection. The use of radiation therapy and/or chemotherapy depends on tumor location and type. Symptoms due to Arnold-Chiari malformation may improve with suboccipital decompression.

Cogan's syndrome (deafness, tinnitus, episodic vertigo, and interstitial keratitis) may respond to steroids and cyclophosphamide (Cytoxan).* Certain focal temporal and parietal seizures (vertiginous epilepsy) are rare causes of vertigo that respond to anticonvulsant therapy. Migraine (see the article Headache) may cause vertigo, not necessarily in association with headache. Since there is some anecdotal evidence that vasoconstricting agents may increase the ischemic complications of migraine, these agents should probably be avoided in treating migraine without headache. Familial periodic ataxia and nystagmus are controlled with acetazolamide (Diamox). Idiopathic vertigo of childhood does not need to be treated, given its benign course and the brief duration of symptoms.

In a large number of patients with episodic vertigo, no cause can be found. Although Meniere's disease or some other cause may be identified later, most resolve spontaneously. General therapy and follow-up is appropriate in these cases.

---

*This use is not listed in the manufacturer's directive.

MENIERE'S DISEASE

method of
FRED D. OWENS, M.D.
Dallas, Texas

Meniere's disease is characterized by the triad of symptoms: episodic vertigo, sensorineural hearing loss, and tinnitus. The symptoms are believed to be caused by excessive endolymph in the inner ear. The pathophysiology is believed to be either an overproduction of endolymph or an underabsorption of endolymph; it may have an immunologic basis. If the hydrops affects only the vestibular system, the characteristic symptoms are episodic vertigo, fullness in the ear, and nausea and/or vomiting. In this case, the hearing might be normal. On the other hand, if the fluid is excessive only in the cochlear system, the expected symptoms are fluctuation of hearing with tinnitus and aural fullness. The patient may begin with either cochlear or vestibular symptoms or both. However, to be classified as Meniere's disease, the patient must exhibit episodic vertigo, fluctuation of hearing, and tinnitus.

DIFFERENTIAL DIAGNOSIS

The differential diagnosis includes: vestibular neuronitis, acoustic neuroma, benign paroxysmal vertigo, syphilis, autoimmune disorders, and vertebrobasilar migraine.

DIAGNOSIS

History and Physical Examination

As in most illnesses, the patient history is the most important tool for diagnosing Meniere's disease. The typical history of Meniere's disease is episodic vertigo, tinnitus (which usually increases with the episodic vertigo), a sensorineural hearing loss (which is usually fluctuating), aural fullness, nausea and vomiting during the more severe episodes, and even sweating or diarrhea, or both, on occasion. The first attack is frequently the most severe and, because of the severity, is often mistaken for a heart attack, even though there is no pain associated with the episodes. The physical examination findings are often perfectly normal. In the beginning, the patient may exhibit no sensorineural hearing loss, but with repeated attacks, one will usually develop a sensorineural hearing loss, especially in the lower frequencies. Occasionally, lateral gaze nystagmus is observed during the physical examination, especially if the examination is during or shortly after an acute attack.

Diagnostic Testing

Audiologic Testing. Audiologic tests should include pure tones, discrimination, impedance, short increment sensitivity index, and electrocochleography. The pure tones are usually found to exhibit a low-tone sensorineural hearing loss with a slight inner ear conductive component in the lower frequencies. Discrimination scores will vary from normal to deteriorating. Impedance is generally normal in the patient with Meniere's disease. The short increment sensitivity index is frequently positive in this disease. Electrocochleography in the last few years has become a more acceptable test for diagnosing the disease.

Additional auditory tests to rule out central lesions should be performed in unilateral sensorineural hearing loss. These include auditory-evoked responses, tone decay, reflex decay, and roll over.

Vestibular Testing. Vestibular tests should include an electronystagmogram with pendulum tracking, visual suppression, optokinetics, spontaneous and positional nystagmus, and cold and warm calories. Other vestibular tests that might be considered are posturog-

raphy or rotational testing, but most examiners believe these tests are not definitive for Meniere's disease.

X-Rays. X-rays should include, at a minimum, petrous pyramid x-rays. A magnetic resonance image with gadolinium is the definitive imaging necessary to rule out the presence of an acoustic neuroma, which in some cases can present similar symptoms to those in Meniere's disease. In patients who cannot undergo magnetic imaging, either because of metal implants or claustrophobia, a computed tomography scan with contrast should be performed.

Other Tests. Other tests to consider are the glycerol tests, allergy testing, and blood tests, including the 5-hour glucose tolerance test; complete blood count; syphilis tests; levels of triglycerides, cholesterol, thyroxine, and triiodothyronine; and the thyroid index.

MEDICAL MANAGEMENT

Acute Medical Management

Acute medical management may include promethazine (Phenergan) suppositories, droperidol (Inapsine) intravenously, diazepam (Valium), intravenous histamine, and bed rest.

Long-Term Medical Management

The methods for long-term medical management of Meniere's disease vary greatly. Management methods to consider include low-salt diet, diuretics, vasodilators, and vestibular suppressants. The goal of medical management in almost all cases is to block the vestibular nerve or the central pathways of the vestibular system and/or to decrease the accumulated endolymph. A reduction in endolymph may be accomplished either by increasing blood flow or by changes in endolymph pressure accomplished by a low-salt diet or diuretics.

SURGICAL MANAGEMENT

Surgical management of Meniere's disease may be either nondestructive or destructive. Nondestructive procedures to consider are the endolymphatic subarachnoid shunt or the endolymphatic mastoid shunt. These procedures are performed by otolarynogologists and otologists across the country. The subarachnoid shunt was performed almost exclusively until the late 1970s. Since that time, many operators have opted to shunt the endolymph into the mastoid space.

Destructive procedures to consider in patients with serviceable hearing are selective vestibular nerve sections, either middle fossa or retrolabyrinthine. If the hearing is not serviceable and the patient has hearing in the contralateral ear, the surgeon may perform either a labyrinthectomy or labyrinthectomy and vestibular nerve section. If a destructive procedure is to be performed, the surgeon must be certain that the opposite labyrinth is functional.

ONE PHYSICIAN'S METHOD OF MANAGEMENT

The method of treatment of Meniere's disease in our office begins with vasodilators and vestibular suppressants. Occasionally, diuretics and a low-salt diet are utilized as well. Frequently, patients who are examined in the office have already had trials of numerous medications, which have failed. If the patient has not responded to medical management before being examined in our office, surgical options are offered. If the patient has had no medical treatment, our medical treatment is instituted and, if possible, given for 3 months before success or failure is determined. If the patient has incapacitating vertigo or rapidly progressive hearing loss, surgery is offered before the conclusion of the 3-month trial. If the medication is effective, the patient continues to receive all medications for a minimum of 3 months. The medications are then discontinued one by one over a period of months. It is our experience that a high percentage of patients with Meniere's disease can be controlled with medical therapy. The medications utilized include the following: diazepam (Valium) 2 mg three times a day; diphenhydramine (Benadryl) 25 mg at bedtime, propantheline (ProBanthine) 15 mg twice a day, histamine phosphate solution* 1:10,000 two drops under the tongue twice a day, niacin in subflushing dosages, and lipoflavonoids. For the acute case, frequently, histamine is given intravenously at a dose of 2.75 mg in 250 mL of normal saline once daily for 3 or 4 consecutive days. The histamine may cause severe flushing or headaches. For that reason, the histamine is first given at a rate of 15 drops per minute, and after 10 to 15 minutes if there are no severe headaches or flushing, the rate is advanced to as much as 30 drops per minute and continued at this rate until the intravenous solution has been completely administered.

Should the patient not be controlled by medication, surgery is indicated. The type of surgery is dependent on the residual hearing in the affected ear and the hearing in the contralateral ear. If the patient has serviceable hearing, an endolymphatic shunt is recommended. Serviceable hearing in our practice is defined as a value consisting of the speech reception threshold plus the reciprocal of the discrimination score. For example, if the speech reception threshold is 30 and the discrimination score is 60, then the value used to determine the serviceability of hearing is 30 + (100 − 60) = 70. If this number is 100 or above, it is believed that the hearing is not serviceable. However, the ultimate determination as to whether the hearing is serviceable will depend on the patient. Some patients, although their hearing is extremely poor, will determine that they would prefer to have some procedure performed that would not destroy their remaining hearing.

Our experience with shunt surgery is that severe vertigo attacks are controlled approximately 70% of the time although hearing is stabilized in 70% of the cases. Tinnitus is improved in 50% of the cases undergoing endolymphatic shunt surgery. The fullness in the ear is relieved 70% of the time as well. There is a 5% chance of hearing improvement and an equal chance that the hearing will deteriorate to total sensorineural hearing loss. During the first 3 months after the endolymphatic shunt procedure, the patient may have some slight degree of dizziness. If the shunt has been successful, however, they should not have severe episodes.

If the shunt procedure does not control the vertigo and the patient has incapacitating symptoms, further surgery is advised. The surgery recommended if the patient has serviceable hearing is either a retrolabyrinthine vestibular nerve section or a middle fossa vestibular nerve section. There is less danger of a sensorineural hearing loss and less danger of injury to the facial nerve with the retrolabyrinthine vestibular nerve section. This is usually recommended as opposed to the middle fossa approach. However, the experience of this surgeon is that the retrolabyrinthine vestibular nerve section is slightly less effective than the middle fossa nerve section. The vestibular nerve section can be expected to relieve the symptoms of vertigo in approximately 90% of the cases. However, the vestibular nerve section has no effect on the fluid imbalance within the inner ear, and the patient will continue to have the aural fullness and fluctuating hearing loss as well as the tinnitus.

If the hearing after the shunt is not serviceable, a labyrinthectomy and vestibular nerve section with or without section of the cochlear nerve is the operation of choice. This procedure is effective 95% of the time. With this procedure, the patient will have no residual hearing. If the age or physical condition of the patient precludes a labyrinthectomy and nerve section, a labyrinthec-

---

*The use of histamine is not listed in the manufacturer's official directive.

tomy is preferred and is 80% effective in controlling vertigo.

With either medical or surgical intervention, Meniere's disease can usually be controlled if the disease is unilateral. Meniere's disease is bilateral in as many as 30% of the cases. Bilateral shunts are performed, but seldom is a bilateral nerve section performed. If the patient has bilateral Meniere's disease and does not respond to medical therapy or endolymphatic shunt surgery, streptomycin can be utilized as a vestibular toxic medication with almost total destruction of the labyrinth bilaterally. One should attempt to control the destructive process with streptomycin to a point where there is still enough function left to prevent Dandy's syndrome. This is usually accomplished by giving 1 gram of streptomycin twice a day for 5 days and then performing vestibular testing. If the patient is not relieved of symptoms, as much as 20 grams of streptomycin, given using a regimen of 1 gram twice daily over a period of 10 days, is the usual dosage. In some cases, it is necessary to administer further streptomycin.

Controlling bilateral Meniere's disease with medicine, surgery, or both is extremely difficult. However, one should always inform the patient with unilateral Meniere's disease that there is an excellent chance of controlling the vertigo either by medical or surgical means. The patient should be encouraged that treatment is available and the disease can be controlled when it is unilateral.

VIRAL MENINGITIS AND ENCEPHALITIS

method of
NORMAN J. KACHUCK, M.D., and
LESLIE P. WEINER, M.D.
Department of Neurology, University of Southern California
Los Angeles, California

VIRAL MENINGITIS

The patient presenting with an acute meningitis syndrome complains of headache, stiff neck, photophobia, and nonspecific constitutional signs, such as fever, nausea, and malaise. An evaluation on an urgent basis is needed for signs and symptoms of systemic illness and for any neuropsychological aberration or abnormal findings on the neurologic examination. Evidence of alteration of mental status or personality, seizures, or any fo-

cality of deficit points to parenchymal involvement and potentially more serious disease.

The uncomplicated acute aseptic meningitis is predominantly caused by the non-polio enteroviruses or arbovirus species. Table 1 demonstrates the usual etiologic agents in their order of incidence. The summer phasic peaks of incidence for aseptic meningitis (as reported to the Centers for Disease Control) reflect the seasonal variation of these two most common agents.

Routine laboratory studies, including a complete blood count with differential, human immunodeficiency virus status, and assessment of immune cells, blood chemistries (including liver function studies), urinalysis, and chest x-ray may be useful in ruling out nonviral infections and the complications of immunoincompetence.

Examination of the cerebrospinal fluid (CSF) is critical in the differential diagnosis to evaluate for nonviral causes of the acute meningitis syndrome. Brain imaging should precede the CSF examination, and barring evidence of hydrocephalus, massive cerebral edema, or a shift of midline structures, a lumbar puncture should be performed. The possibility that an acute febrile meningitis is pyogenic necessitates that this be done with some speed. A noncontrast computed tomographic scan is usually sufficient for the purpose, and it and the lumbar puncture should be done within 1 hour of presentation. Broad-spectrum antibiotic coverage should be instituted if

TABLE 1. **Viral Etiologies of the Aseptic Meningitis Syndrome and Their Relative Incidence Rates**

Common
Enteroviruses (e.g., coxsackievirus and echovirus)
Arboviruses (epidemic and sporadic, e.g., St. Louis, California, and Colorado tick fever)
Herpes simplex virus type 2
Uncommon
Mumps
Lymphocytic choriomeningitis virus
Human immunodeficiency virus
Rare
Herpes simplex virus type 1
Varicella-zoster virus
Cytomegalovirus
Epstein-Barr virus
Influenza A and B virus
Parainfluenza virus
Measles
Rotavirus
Coronavirus
Encephalomyocarditis virus
Mollaret's recurrent meningitis (? herpesvirus type 6)

(Adapted from Rotbart HA: Viral meningitis and the aseptic meningitis syndrome. *In* Scheld WM, Whitley RJ, and Durack DT [eds]: Infections of the Central Nervous System. New York, Raven Press, 1991, pp 19–40.)

delay is inevitable. Parenchymal lesions should trigger further investigation, including magnetic resonance imaging and potentially neurosurgical consultation for definitive diagnosis. There is literature to support the contention that lumbar puncture without imaging can be safely done if no focal neurologic signs are present. The most important to exclude would be those findings signifying increased intracranial pressure and a herniation syndrome, such as coma, an abnormal breathing pattern, loss of normal pupillary reflexes, third or sixth nerve palsies, or posturing.

Viral meningitis and meningoencephalitis usually present with a clear colorless CSF under normal to moderately increased pressure (normal < 25 cmH$_2$O). A leukocytosis may be predominantly polymorphonuclear on the first tap in up to 75% of patients, but in the next 24 to 48 hours it should evolve to a monocytic/lymphocytic picture. CSF white cell counts range between 100 and 1000 per mm^3, but they are usually less than 300 cells per mm^3. In as many as 5% of patients, there may be no cells on the initial examination. The leukocytosis usually normalizes in several days, but it may persist for some months. Red blood cells and xanthochromia are not expected in viral meningitis; their presence in encephalitis suggests the necrotizing vasculitis of herpes simplex infection. CSF protein in meningitis and encephalitis is usually elevated but rarely exceeds 250 mg per dL. The normal CSF sugar value, roughly two-thirds of that in the serum, is a critical value. Serum and CSF glucose must both be tested within several hours of each other to control for sugar intake and serum/CSF equilibration. The ratio of CSF sugar to blood sugar is usually normal to slightly depressed in uncomplicated viral meningitis. Mumps and lymphocytic choriomeningitis virus are associated with lower CSF glucose values along with a marked pleocytosis.

Viral culturing from CSF as well as from blood, feces, urine, and throat washings should be attempted, although, in most cases of uncomplicated disease, these may only turn positive after the crisis has passed. Positive results will vary depending on the agent's predilection for route of entry. Ambiguous results in the evaluation of an acute meningitis may be clarified with testing for serum and CSF titers of virus-specific antibody repeated for greater than fourfold increases during the acute infection. Additionally, an index of the CSF to serum antibody production against specific agents, as directed by the survey titers obtained by complement fixation, may be performed by a competent laboratory.

Patients with equivocal CSF results may need coverage for bacterial infection until Gram's stain, culture, or repeat CSF examination can elucidate the etiology. CSF levels of tumor necrosis factor have been reported to differentiate bacterial from viral meningitis, being present in at least 74% of bacterial meningitides, and absent in patients with aseptic meningitis.

Treatment

With an otherwise unremarkable general workup, a nonfocal neurologic examination, and no evidence of alteration of mental status or of seizures, patients with viral meningitis may be managed conservatively but under close observation in the hospital until they are clearly in a recuperative phase of the illness. Fluid balance becomes especially important in the nauseated patient, or in those who suffer the rare complications of brain edema or the syndrome of inappropriate antidiuretic hormone secretion. Seizures may occur due to fever alone, especially in the younger patient; their presence should alert the physician to possible parenchymal involvement (encephalitis). Enterovirus and the other common viruses causing aseptic meningitis are cleared from the host by an antibody-mediated mechanism, and patients with defects in immunoglobulin G production or function may profit from exogenous gamma globulin treatment.

Although these illnesses are usually of short duration and self-limited, care should be taken to evaluate for the progression of symptoms, in which case, it is prudent to repeat studies for alternative etiologies for the primary event as well as for bacterial or other superinfection. A postviral asthenic state may last for days to weeks following the acute infection, preventing an expeditious return to premorbid levels of activity and employment. In a very few patients, a postviral chronic fatigue state may cause long-term disability.

VIRAL MENINGOENCEPHALITIS AND ENCEPHALITIS

A patient with an acute-onset headache, fever, an alteration of consciousness with delirium, behavioral or speech disturbance, with or without obtundation, and a mononuclear cell pleocytosis should be considered to have viral encephalitis. Such a presentation must be viewed as a medical emergency. Nonviral causes should be ruled out (Table 2). Several conditions have clinical presentations that may mimic that of viral encephalitis; infrequently, an inflammatory process with a lymphocytic or monocytic pleocytosis in the CSF may accompany, and confuse the diagnosis of, diseases such as cryptic brain tumors, brain abscesses, cerebrovascular accidents, and subarachnoid hemorrhage. Acute confusional states with

TABLE 2. **Diseases That Simulate Viral Meningoencephalitis**

Bacterial Processes	*Plasmodium falciparum*
Tuberculosis	Amebiasis
Mycoplasma pneumonia	Trichinosis
Listeriosis	Schistomiasis
Brucellosis	*Toxocara*
Typhoid fever	*Rickettsia*
Syphilis	Typhus
Leptospirosis	Rocky Mountain spotted fever
Lyme disease	**Noninfectious Disease**
Bacteria Related	Neoplasms
Parameningeal infections	Carcinomatous and leukemic meningitis
Partially treated meningitis	Diffuse gliomatosis
Brain abscess	Vasculitis
Mycotic aneurysms	Collagen vascular disease
Fungi	Granulomatous angiitis
Cryptococcosis	Sarcoidosis
Candidiasis	Behçet's syndrome
Coccidioidomycosis	Vogt-Koyanagi-Harada syndrome
Histoplasmosis	**Others**
North American blastomycosis	Multisystem disease with secondary encephalopathy
Parasites	Toxic encephalopathy due to cocaine, amphetamine,
Toxoplasmosis	phencyclidine use
Cysticercosis	Antineoplastic agents and immunosuppressants
Echinococcosis	Chemical meningitis due to nonsteroidal anti-inflammatory
Trypanosomiasis	agents or trimethoprim ± sulfonamides

or without secondary seizures, fevers, and pleocytosis may be associated with cocaine, amphetamine, or phencyclidine abuse.

The involvement of the gray matter of the brain by the infecting agent makes viral encephalitis a far more severe problem than the "pure" meningitides. Pathologically, acute viral encephalitis is associated with perivascular and parenchymal infiltration by cellular elements of the immune response along with cytokines, lymphokines, and other inflammatory mediators, with resulting neuronal and glial cell injury and death, as well as edema with possible increased intracranial pressure. Table 3 lists the common causes of viral encephalitis in order of incidence; regional variations should be noted. Therapy in most cases is limited to supportive care; exceptions to this are noted in Table 4.

Although it can be said that the majority of patients with viral meningoencephalitis will have a benign outcome, the percentage of patients left with significant morbidity is high (Table 5). Any clinical evidence of focal neurologic deficits points to the possibility of herpes simplex type 1 encephalitis (HSE), which if left untreated, carries a grim prognosis (Table 6). (Note that while herpes simplex type 2 is a frequent cause of a meningitis, it rarely causes encephalitis except in patients with acquired immune deficiency syndrome.) Although only 10% of viral encephalitides are due to HSE, more than one-half of deaths of viral encephalitis can be attributed to it. Given the sensitivity of this virus to available medical therapy, any suspicion of HSE is an indication for early treatment. The important corollary to this statement, however, is that, when the signs and symptoms of patients with biopsy-proven HSE were compared with those of patients with other

TABLE 3. **Causes of Viral Encephalitis and Virus-Related Encephalopathies**

Sporadic
Mumps
Herpes simplex viruses
Lymphocytic choriomeningitis virus
Cytomegalovirus
Epstein-Barr virus
Adenovirus
Rabies
Epidemic
Arboviruses (e.g., Eastern, Western, St. Louis, California [in particular, the LaCrosse agent], Venezuelan equine, Colorado tick fever, and Japanese B)
Enteroviruses (e.g., coxsackievirus and echovirus)
Postinfectious Encephalomyelitis
Measles
Varicella-zoster
Mumps
Rubella
Influenza
Viral Infection in Immunocompromised Patients
Human immunodeficiency virus
Cytomegalovirus
Herpes simplex viruses
Enteroviruses
Adenoviruses
Measles
Papovavirus (JC virus) and progressive multifocal leukoencephalopathy
Virus-Associated Encephalopathy
Reye's syndrome

TABLE 4. **Viral Meningoencephalitides for Which Specific Treatment Other than Support Is Available**

Organism	Treatment
Herpes simplex	Acyclovir 10 mg/kg q 8 h intravenously × 10–14 d or vidarabine 15 mg/kg/day × 10 d continuous intravenous drip
Cytomegalovirus	Ganciclovir 5 mg/kg q 12 h used for retinitis; dosage or duration for encephalitis not established
Varicella-zoster	Acyclovir as per herpes simplex protocol
Rabies	Rabies immune globulin 20 IU/kg intravenously and rabies vaccine into the wound and intramuscularly

TABLE 6. **Mortality and Morbidity Rates for Selected Encephalitides**

Selected Agent	Mortality	Moderate to Severe Morbidity
Herpes simplex 1	Up to 80% untreated; 20% treated	30–40%
Eastern equine encephalitis	70%	Up to 30%
St. Louis encephalitis	2–20%	Rare, emotional disturbance
Measles virus (postinfectious)	15%	25%
Western equine encephalitis	< 5%	Low in adults, up to 50% in children
Enteroviruses	Rare	Low in general, but higher in areas of poliomyelitis undervaccination
California encephalitis	Rare	Low in adults; 15% of children have recurrent seizures, personality problems

viral encephalitides, no distinguishing exclusive characteristics could be identified. HSE and the other encephalitides have additionally been associated with choreoathetosis, tremor, cranial nerve palsies, ataxia, and cortical blindness. So, although HSE is the most common necrotizing focal encephalitis, viruses that usually cause diffuse disease may localize in a similar manner and thus mimic it.

The diagnosis of viral encephalitis is dependent on epidemiologic, clinical, and laboratory data. A history of recent disease contacts at home, the work place, or social gatherings, as well as documentation of recent travel, can be helpful. Risks, such as contact with pets or other domestic animals, any wild animals, rodents, or ticks, should be identified, particularly because they may suggest treatable entities, such as Lyme disease; life-threatening entities, such as rabies; or benign conditions, such as that associated with infection by lymphocytic choriomeningitis virus. Regional activity for the epidemic viruses (the arboviruses

and the enteroviruses), as well as the season of onset, provide further valuable information. Late summer and early fall are associated with arbovirus and enterovirus infections, whereas spring is associated with mumps. An immunization history for the patient as well as the presence of recently immunized contacts (especially polio and mumps) may also be helpful.

The diagnosis of encephalitis may be aided by associated clinical signs. These include the following: a rash that might indicate a childhood exanthem or an enterovirus infection; oral thrush and other signs of possible immunocompromise; pneumonitis, suggesting lymphocytic choriomeninigitis virus, cytomegalovirus, or *Mycoplasma* and other nonviral infections. Pleurodynia and herpangina may be seen with different serotypes of coxsackievirus (a common enterovirus).

TABLE 5. **Neurologic Signs in Biopsy-Proven Herpes Encephalitis**

Alteration of consciousness
Fever
Personality change
Headache
Seizures (focal or generalized)
Vomiting
Hemiparesis
Memory loss
Language dysfunction
Autonomic dysfunction
Ataxia
Cranial nerve deficits
Visual field loss
Papilledema

(Based on data from Whitley RJ, et al. and the NIAID Collaborative Antiviral Study Group: Herpes simplex encephalitis: Clinical assessment. JAMA 247:317–320, 1982.)

POSTINFECTIOUS ENCEPHALOMYELITIS

A condition that may need to be differentiated from viral encephalitis is the syndrome of postinfectious encephalomyelitis. It is distinguished by a perivenular inflammatory autoimmune response, which in measles and postvaccinia infection has been shown to be directed against components of CNS myelin, with lesions of cerebral, brain stem, and spinal cord white matter. Pathologically, this process is similar to that found in an animal model for multiple sclerosis, i.e., experimental allergic encephalomyelitis. There may be a history of a flu-like illness that occurs as early as 6 weeks prior to but usually within 7 to 10 days of an acute onset of fever, obtundation, focal neurologic deficits, and seizures. If the illness is associated with an identifiable childhood exanthem or systemic viral illness, such as measles, the diagnosis is less difficult to make. In most instances, however, the antecedent syndrome is less well defined and poorly documented. It often is impossible to differentiate clinically between a case of direct viral invasion or relapse and the immune-mediated postinfectious demyelinating condition. Magnetic resonance imaging showing white matter inflammatory lesions, evoked potentials showing prolonged latencies, or the presence of myelin basic protein in the CSF may be useful in suggesting the latter. An open brain biopsy may be required in a patient whose condition continues to deteriorate.

Treatment

High-dose intravenous corticosteroid therapy has been recommended for patients with documented cases of postinfectious encephalomyelits. We utilize intravenous methylprednisolone 500 mg per day for 5 days with a posttreatment oral tapering dose over 1 to 2 weeks, with a H_2 blocker and potassium prophylaxis.

HERPES SIMPLEX VIRUS ENCEPHALITIS

HSE has no antecedent illness nor is there a seasonal variation. A history of or the concurrent finding of herpes labialis has no diagnostic value in implicating this virus as the etiologic agent of the encephalitis, in contrast to the clear correlation of meningitis to primary or recurrent herpes simplex type 2 infection. Typically, in addition to fever, headache, and malaise, behavioral abnormalities may be prominent during the early stages, prompting an inaccurate psychiatric diagnosis. The mental changes include withdrawal, agitation, hallucinations, and confusion. These may progress over hours or several days and gradually result in decreasing levels of consciousness. There may be an abrupt onset of major motor or focal seizures, or a more slowly evolving aphasia or focal motor or sensory deficit.

Although it is clear that herpesviruses can remain latent in sensory ganglia and reactivate, causing recurrent symptoms, the pathway and pathogenesis of HSE remains obscure. Evidence exists linking it to spread through the olfactory system, and perhaps this proximity to the underside of the brain explains the common adult distribution of necrotizing hemorrhagic lesions in the medial temporal lobes and orbital frontal regions, including insular cortices, olfactory tracts, and hippocampi.

The routine serum and CSF studies previously profiled should be performed. Although HSE is necrotizing, the presence of xanthochromia or of red blood cells in the CSF is inconstant and not diagnostic. The intrablood-brain barrier synthesis of antibodies against the virus can be determined by a specific antibody index comparing levels of immunoglobulins in the serum to CSF levels by antibody-capture enzyme immunoassay. Eighty percent of patients with biopsy-proven HSE have been shown to have increases of their viral antibody index 7 to 10 days after the onset of illness, and essentially all have increases by day 11. A negative result, however, does not rule out the diagnosis. Immunoblotting techniques can be used to detect viral antibodies more than 3 days after the onset of illness. In situ hybridization techniques can detect herpes simplex virus in CSF from the onset of symptoms, but these are less reliable when specific intrablood-brain barrier immunoglobulin G synthesis begins. Polymerase chain reaction amplification and identification of the viral genome is highly sensitive, even in the presence of antibodies, and sufficient virus may be present in the CSF for current techniques to identify. We are still far short, however, of the promise of this technology to replace brain biopsy in the definitive diagnosis of central nervous system diseases such as HSE.

Computed tomography may show areas of low attenuation and localized edema in the temporal lobes; magnetic resonance imaging is far more sensitive, especially when an enhancement agent is used, demonstrating localized increases in parenchymal water content and permeability of the blood-brain barrier. In the absence of a focal temporal lesion on brain imaging, electroencephalography (EEG) is perhaps the most sensitive test available. HSE, along with status epilepticus, represents one of the few indications for emergent EEG, and it should be done in the first hours of admission, especially if the imaging results are nondiagnostic. The EEG in encephalitis can show etiologically nonspecific generalized background slowing, but importantly, in HSE, it may show focal slowing, or even more dramatically, periodic unilateral or bilateral epileptiform discharges over the frontotemporal regions. The demonstration of such discharges is diagnostic for HSE, and immediate treatment is warranted.

Treatment

In a patient presenting with personality changes, fever, focal seizures, and lateralizing signs of acute onset, the diagnosis of HSE is strongly suggested. If there is a mass effect on imaging, with a midline shift or signs of increased intracranial pressure, lumbar puncture is contraindicated, and a biopsy of the temporal lobe should be performed as soon as possible. Treatment using acyclovir (Zovirax) should be instituted as soon as the diagnosis of HSE is seriously considered, at a dosage of 30 mg per kg intravenously, divided into three daily doses, for 10 days. Recently, there have been recommendations for increasing this to 14 days at the same daily dose, because of evidence of increasing numbers of resistant strains and reports of decreased relapse rates with the extended regimen. Acyclovir should be given as the biopsy preparations are being made.

If the CSF can be evaluated, the indications for biopsy can be approached differently. The indications for brain biopsy in acutely ill patients do not so much confirm the diagnosis as help one diagnose a process for which a delay of treatment will result in a disastrous outcome. The lack of a depression of the CSF sugar level is our best indication that only a few conditions need be considered that would require an immediate change in therapy. On the other hand, if there is a depression of CSF sugar, it is estimated that as many as 35% of patients presenting with neurologic signs will have a lesion for which treatment must not be delayed. These conditions include bacterial cerebritis or abscess, tuberculoma, cryptococcal abscess, and an infectious vasculitis, such as syphilis. The Collaborative Antiviral Study Group reported a diagnosis of HSE in 45% of 432 patients undergoing biopsy for encephalitis; no diagnosis in 33%; and another diagnosis of 22%, of whom nearly one-half had treatable conditions. Their estimated rate of complications from brain biopsy, such as hemorrhage or infection, was 1.4%, with no deaths or long-term sequelae arising from the procedure itself.

In those patients in whom focality has been demonstrated clinically but not by imaging or EEG initially, magnetic resonance imaging and/or EEG should be repeated in 48 to 72 hours. If there is no evidence of focality or mass effect, the CSF should be re-examined for alterations in the nature of the pleocytosis or the CSF sugar. Alterations in viral titers should be looked for, with at least 3 to 4 days between studies. If the patient's condition is deteriorating, a biopsy is indicated, guided by imaging or electrodiagnostic evidence, even in the absence of focal signs.

Thus, if there is a focal temporal lobe mass on the patient's imaging scan and CSF cannot be safely acquired, a biopsy should be performed immediately. If the CSF can be examined and the sugar is normal, the biopsy may not be necessary; if the sugar is reduced, then the biopsy should be performed as soon as possible to rule out non-HSE disease.

The biopsy should be done in the area of most disease, as established by signs and symptoms, imaging, and electrodiagnostic studies. The best diagnostic yield in our hands has been obtained by craniotomy, not by stereotactic biopsy. Of the greater than 2000 stereotactic biopsies done at our institution, although the accuracy with which brain tumors are diagnosed runs greater than 90%, inflammatory lesions are diagnosed at perhaps a 25% rate. Ninety percent of patients with a diagnosed inflammatory lesion have human immunodeficiency virus-related diseases, including toxoplasmosis, progressive multifocal leukoencephalopathy, and cryptococcosis. In addition to the improved diagnostic yield, the open craniotomy allows decompression of an edematous temporal lobe. The biopsy protocol should involve neurosurgeons, neurologists, infectious disease specialists, and pathologists. The processing of the specimen should be prioritized, with a portion fixed in formaldehyde for routine histologic examination; frozen samples for immunohistochemical staining, including complement fixation and fluorescent antibody assays; and adequate amounts sent for culturing for aerobic and anaerobic organisms, fungi, and viruses. Electron microscopy should be done and, as available, polymerase chain reaction studies.

Unless a specific alternative diagnosis has been made possible by the biopsy, the acyclovir should be continued for the full course, even in the face of an unrevealing biopsy. The drug's minimal toxicity, even in patients with human immunodeficiency virus, makes its empiric use reasonable in this setting. If a patient's course continues to deteriorate in the face of therapy but without a biopsy, the biopsy should be done immediately. If there is biopsy-proven herpes simplex type 1, then establishing acyclovir resistance on the cultured biopsy specimen, or even a re-biopsy to assess for persisting active infection, should be considered. A course of vidarabine (Vira-A) 15 mg per kg per day by continuous intravenous drip for 10 days may be administered, but not as an alternative to biopsy. Most deterioration in our experience has been less a problem of ongoing infection than a problem of intractable seizures, complications of increased intracranial pressure, or complicating medical conditions, such as fluid and electrolyte derangements and cardiorespiratory dysfunction. Relapse has been reported in cases treated with either acyclovir or vidarabine within several weeks of 10-day initial therapy.

General Supportive Therapy

Close observation is required for all cases of encephalitis. Standard infectious disease precau-

TABLE 7. Laboratory Study Abnormalities in Viral CNS Diseases in Immunocompetent Patients

Result	Possible Etiologies
Leukopenia	LCM virus, Colorado tick fever, Epstein-Barr virus
Thrombocytopenia	LCM virus, Colorado tick fever, St. Louis encephalitis (rare)
Atypical lymphocytosis	Epstein-Barr virus, cytomegalovirus
Renal dysfunction	St. Louis encephalitis
Abnormal liver function	LCM virus, Epstein-Barr virus, cytomegalovirus, arboviruses (some), mumps
Increased creatine kinase and aldolase	St. Louis encephalitis
Increased amylase and lipase	Mumps, enteroviruses (rare), LCM virus (rare)
Hyponatremia	St. Louis encephalitis

Abbreviation: LCM = lymphocytic choriomeningitis virus.
(Adapted with permission from Rubeiz H and Roos RP: Viral meningitis and encephalitis. Semin Neurol *12:*165–177, 1992, Thieme Medical Publishers, Inc.)

tions should be observed. Epidemic disease should be appropriately reported, and isolation measures instituted if a viral exanthem is present. Regular assessment of electrolytes, glucose, and renal and pulmonary function should be done, along with stool guaiac for stress ulceration. Table 7 lists frequent systemic complications of the encephalitogenic viruses. Inappropriate antidiuretic hormone secretion is a frequent complication of encephalitis, and urine output and electrolytes should be checked. In comatose patients, nutritional needs should be met using nasogastric tube feedings and converting to gastrostomy access for patients in prolonged coma. Due to the thermolability of viruses, a low-grade fever may be of some benefit in the patient's recovery and should not be too vigorously treated.

We routinely prescribe anticonvulsants for patients with HSE, with or without clinical seizures, using a loading dose of phenytoin (Dilantin) of 18 mg per kg and a maintenance dose of 3 to 5 mg per kg per day. Recurrent seizures are treated as per status epilepticus. Patients with encephalitides other than HSE, and who have no evidence of clinical seizures and lack focal signs or EEG changes, do not routinely receive anticonvulsants. All patients who have undergone biopsy receive anticonvulsants for a minimum of 6 months.

If there is evidence of increased intracranial pressure, endotracheal intubation may be indicated to ensure proper oxygenation, to control ventilatory rates, and protect against consequences of sudden respiratory failure from brain stem compression. Hyperventilation aimed at a partial pressure of carbon dioxide of 26 mmol/L will provide temporary treatment of increased intracranial pressure by constriction of the intracranial vasculature, but this technique loses its efficacy after about 24 hours. Tracheostomy is indicated in patients with prolonged coma. Other measures to be considered for treatment of increased intracranial pressure include a fluid restriction to one-half to two-thirds of the calculated daily requirement. Mannitol 0.25 to 1 grams per kg can be administered in repeated doses, with a limitation of a serum osmolality of 310 mOsm per liter. We routinely use high-dose intravenous corticosteroid therapy for high intracranial pressure in HSE; methylprednisolone 500 to 1000 mg per day for 3 to 5 days may be lifesaving in preventing the consequences of herniation syndromes, without having an impact on the antiviral therapy. Its prolonged use can result in immunosuppression and other complications and should be avoided.

REYE'S SYNDROME

method of
JOHN C. PARTIN, M.D.
State University of New York at Stony Brook
Stony Brook, New York

Reye's syndrome (RS) is a metabolic encephalopathy that is easily confused with medium chain acyl coenzyme-A dehydrogenase deficiency (MCAD) and related genetic metabolic encephalopathies of infancy and early childhood. Because of the likelihood of recurrent and potentially fatal encephalopathy in MCAD, a common recessive genetic defect, MCAD must be excluded in every suspected case of RS.

The onset of RS is signaled by the onset of persistent vomiting within 1 week of the onset of varicella or an influenza-like illness. Vomiting most often begins 3 to 5 days after the beginning of the prodromal viral illness. About one-third of RS cases progress through a dramatic stage of agitated delirium to severe coma; of these, about one-third die or sustain severe brain damage despite appropriate treatment.

During the 1970s and early 1980s, there were many community-wide outbreaks of RS associated with influenza and varicella epidemics. Most of these cases involved school-age children who had taken aspirin during the prodromal illness. Aspirin is now a recognized risk factor for developing RS. Concomitant with the elimination of aspirin as an antipyretic agent for children in the United States, there has been a great reduction in the occurrence of RS. It is not yet certain whether the reduction in RS is coincidental with reduced aspirin use or whether there is a cause-and-effect relationship. It must be stressed that RS can occur in the absence of aspirin use, and a negative history of aspirin ingestion does not exclude the diagnosis of RS. RS does occur, although rarely, among adults.

Many children younger than the age of 36 months whose disease was diagnosed as RS have been shown to have RS "mimickers." This has been particularly true of "recurrent" cases of RS and "familial" cases. RS mimickers, in addition to MCAD deficiency, include disorders of urea production, such as ornithine transcarbamylase deficiency; disorders of carnitine metabolism; and isovaleric acidemia and related defects. Bacterial meningitis and viral encephalitis are sometimes misdiagnosed as RS. Older children and adolescents with RS in agitated delirium have been mistaken for substance abusers.

The pathophysiology of RS is a severe, potentially reversible, injury of the brain and liver mitochondrial systems that oxidize fatty acids during the fasting stress of varicella and influenza. Because the children are vomiting, they are denied exogenous carbohydrate. When the liver cells and the neurons run out of stored carbohydrate (glycogen), the cells lose power, and toxic metabolites of fatty acids accumulate. The early administration of intravenous glucose may protect against progression of the disease by providing a substrate for energy metabolism and by suppressing the release of fatty acids from the adipose tissue.

TREATMENT

Treatment of Noncomatose (CDC Stage 0 and I) Cases

Prompt, vigorous treatment of early RS with intravenous 10% glucose and maintenance water and electrolytes can restore tissue glycogen, reduce lipolysis, and may prevent progression of Stage I cases to coma. Noncomatose cases are identified by a history of the unexpected onset of vomiting within 1 week of the onset of an appropriate antecedent illness, alanine aminotransferase (ALT) level greater than 200 IU (mean, 900 IU), normal or prolonged prothrombin time, and normal or elevated blood ammonia level. Noncomatose patients are treated with 2000 mL per M^2 of intravenous fluids containing 10% glucose, 50 mEq sodium chloride, 40 mEq potassium chloride. This treatment is started immediately in the emergency room. Initial urine should be examined for ketones and saved for gas chromatographic-mass spectrographic analysis for fatty acid metabolites. The blood sugar should be measured 4 to 6 hours after glucose infusion is begun to ensure that the blood sugar is maintained in the high normal range. Serum ALT and blood ammonia levels and the prothrombin time should be measured every 12 hours for the first 36 hours or more frequently if neurologic signs advance. Noncomatose children admitted with blood ammonia concentrations greater than 100 μg per dL and prolonged prothrombin times are at greater risk of progressing to coma and should

be kept under particularly close observation. The return of good appetite is a reliable sign of recovery.

Treatment of Comatose (CDC Stage II, III and IV) Cases

Patients who present with agitated delirium or more advanced coma should be managed in a qualified intensive care unit. We do not use prolonged deep sedation with barbiturates or morphine or protracted muscle paralysis, because these methods make meaningful neurologic examination impossible and they have been associated with unacceptable morbidity. We use moderate doses of pentobarbital (Nembutal) or morphine and intermittent pancuronium (Pavulon) to control patients during endotracheal intubation, lumbar puncture, or during performance of painful procedures and when their struggling against the respirator adversely affects intracranial pressure (ICP).

The goals of management are (1) to ensure adequate brain oxygenation by early elective endotracheal intubation, (2) to restore tissue glycogen and reduce lipolysis, (3) to prevent severe hypophosphatemia, (4) to maintain physiologic intravascular volume to sustain cerebral perfusion pressure (CPP), and (5) to control cerebral edema if present.

Lumbar puncture (LP) should be performed soon after the airway is secured to exclude bacterial meningitis, viral encephalitis, and cerebral hemorrhage and to determine ICP. We have experienced no adverse complications of LP in more than 250 RS cases. Patients are nursed in a 30-degree, neutral, head-up position on a cooling blanket to control hyperpyrexia, if present, and with a nasogastric tube in place. Urine output is monitored hourly by an indwelling urinary catheter. In severe cases, central venous catheters and arterial cannulas are placed to monitor blood pressure and CPP. An ICP monitor may be of help in managing increased ICP.

Most comatose cases of RS demonstrate centrally mediated hypercapnia and respiratory alkalosis often with a blood pH of 7.5 and a partial pressure of carbon dioxide (PCO_2) of 24 mmHg. Those requiring mechanical ventilation should have the PCO_2 maintained at about 24 mmHg. Blood sugar should be measured frequently to maintain the blood glucose concentration near the renal tubular transport maximum for glucose, i.e., 110 to 140 mg per dL. Dehydration should be corrected if present initially, and intravenous fluids should be administered at a rate of 1600 to 1800 mL per M^2 (normal maintenance water and electrolytes in most cases). Extreme dehydration and hypovolemia through excessive fluid restriction must be avoided. Hypophosphatemia may occur when glucose repletion is begun; it can be prevented by adding 20 mEq per liter of phosphate to the infusion mixture.

Cerebral edema is usually not present at the time of admission in comatose RS patients, but it is a frequent complication when the metabolic encephalopathy becomes severe. Cerebral edema is managed initially by hyperventilation to reduce the PCO_2. When this is not sufficient, mannitol is used beginning with a dose of 250 mg per kg given over 5 to 15 minutes. The "bolus" administration of mannitol can produce a fatal surge of ICP. Larger doses of mannitol may be required, but extreme hyperosmolarity must be avoided. The serum osmolarity should be maintained between 312 and 320 mOsm. In situations refractory to mannitol, furosemide (Lasix) has been tried, and some have advocated the use of 20% intragastric glycerol.

One large series of comatose RS patients with an 80% survival rate was treated by exchange transfusion using fresh whole blood in addition to the previous measures. Although unproved, exchange transfusion with fresh whole blood may be beneficial in selected cases with very high aspirin or toxic metabolite concentrations in the blood. Cranial decompression has been advocated as a lifesaving measure in RS complicated by uncontrollable ICP but at the cost of significant residual brain damage.

Deep barbiturate coma with or without hypothermia appears to be associated with unacceptable morbidity and mortality in RS. Corticosteroids have not been useful and may increase the likelihood of serious gastrointestinal bleeding. The use of citrulline to enhance ureagenesis or carnitine (Carnitor) to facilitate the detoxification of unesterified fatty acids has been suggested, but these modalities are of unproved safety or efficacy.

MULTIPLE SCLEROSIS

method of
WALLACE W. TOURTELLOTTE,
    M.D., PH.D., and
ROBERT W. BAUMHEFNER, M.D.
UCLA School of Medicine
Los Angeles, California

The target of the multiple sclerosis (MS) disease process is cells in the central nervous system (CNS), oligodendrocytes, which fabricate and maintain myelin sheaths, the covering of axons necessary for the normal conduction of nerve impulses. Destruction of oligodendrocytes occurs in clusters and is accompanied by loss of oligodendrocytes as well as their myelin sheath appendages with axon sparing (primary demyelination).

The cluster destruction of oligodendrocytes-myelin sheaths forms plaques, the pathologic hallmark of MS, which are multifocal with the majority in the white matter. The center of a plaque is composed of a watery gliotic scar, astrogliosis, which replaces oligodendrocytes-myelin sheaths; as plaques age, axons also drop out. At the edge of plaques, the site of the MS disease process, there can be found polyphasic inflammation. No evidence of intense inflammatory demyelination can be found in 40% of plaque edges, suggesting the body has a defense against the MS disease process. Further, 50% of plaque edges show varying degrees of active demyelination, and 10% show microglia nodules, the earliest lesion.

Accordingly, the plaque is a site of disconnection of conducted action potentials (nerve impulses) as well as cross-stimulation from a demyelinated axon to an adjacent one. It is this pathophysiologic event that accounts for the symptoms and signs of MS.

In chronic/progressive more than relapsing/remitting MS, serial magnetic resonance images (MRI), which reveal plaques in vivo, have shown that the MS disease process is dynamic, some plaques forming and disappearing in unpredictable and variable fashion with a prevalence of progression. This process is related to active demyelination at the plaque edge and is shown often by gadolinium enhancement, an MRI marker for an abnormal blood-brain barrier (BBB). It is probably the pathologic basis for clinical relapses and the variable course, even though many more MRI lesions come and go in a patient than a patient has relapses. That is, the clinical symptoms and signs are the tip of the iceberg of the MS disease process.

Almost all patients fall into one of the following courses based on symptoms and signs: 90% of all cases after first symptom have relapses followed by remissions and 60% of relapsing/remitting cases switch to a progressive course about 5 years after the first symptom. Ten percent have progressive disease from the onset. Some say up to 20% are benign, with one or two relapses and then good recovery. They are proven to have multifocal plaques at autopsy without evidence of an inflammatory demyelinating reaction. There is a very rare type termed "acute MS of the Marburg type" with rapid progression to death in several years or less.

MS is the number one disabling disease of young adults; 250,000 to 350,000 persons in the United States in 1990 had physician-diagnosed MS. There is an ethnic racial predilection (whites much more than blacks or Asians), an age/gender preference (female to male adult ratio of 2:1), and an environmental influence (latitude and migration reports). Multigenetic factors involve immune system function (histocompatibility antigen or HLA), which is manifested in phenotype expression as follows. The frequency of concordance for identical twins is 500 per 1000; for MS in a family in which a father, mother, brother, sister, or fraternal twin also has MS, 35 per 1000; and no MS, in a family, 1 per 1000.

There are reports that indicate that there are risk factors for relapses. There is a consensus that, 3 months post partum, the relapse rate can be increased. One report found that a viral type of respiratory infection precedes 40% of relapses by 7 weeks, but only about 10% of all infections are followed by a relapse. There are controlled studies that indicate that the following are not risk factors: trauma, surgery, vaccination, and stress. The etiology of MS is unknown.

DIAGNOSTIC CONSIDERATIONS

The mainstay of the MS diagnosis is the clinical evaluation. There are three clinical features that are common in the majority of patients with MS, even though no two patients are alike: age, multiple areas of the white matter lesions, and relapses and remission. In young adults (range, 15 to 50 years of age; average, 30 years), the symptoms and signs reflect the involvement of multiple areas of white matter of the CNS, which include visual loss, diplopia, weakness, sensory abnormalities, and unexplained paresthesias. Additionally, ataxia, bladder dysfunction, fatigue, and worsening with hyperthermia can be present. Furthermore, the history usually reveals multiple relapses and remissions varying in severity, duration, and frequency. Recovery after each relapse is unpredictable, but the overall level of disability tends to increase with sequential attacks. After about 5 years, 60% of patients will enter a progressive phase of the disease with infrequent relapses and remission. Patients older than 50 years of age often present with a progressive myelopathy, primarily manifested by spastic paraparesis. It is important to rule out other possible causes, such as intoxications, infections, trauma, metabolic (vitamin B_{12} deficiency), hereditary ataxias, neoplasms, vascular diseases, especially vasculitides, and late-onset developmental disorders.

The clinical diagnosis can be supported by three laboratory tests. Multifocal areas of demyelination can be imaged by MRI in almost every case. The block in the centrally conducted action potential can be detected by evoked-potential tests, especially of the visual system in about 80% of cases. The inflammation of the CNS can be assessed by a cerebrospinal fluid examination. In more than 99% of clinically definite patients with MS, intrathecal immunoglobin (Ig) G synthesis rate and IgG oligoclonal bands are abnormal. Rarely is the leukocyte count (all mononuclear cells) more than 50/cmm, and the leakage rate of albumin across the BBB is usually less than 75 mg per day. Furthermore, MRI gadolinium enhancement, a marker for the break in the BBB, is probably evidence of an inflammatory process.

As imperfect as the Kurtzke disability rating scale may be, it is recommended that when the clinical diagnosis and the results in the three supportive laboratory tests are recorded along with the type of MS, a disability rating should be included in the diagnosis (Table 1).

PREDICTING PROGNOSIS

Based on Metropolitan Life Insurance survival tables, the longevity of an affected patient's life is shortened by only a few years. However, the range of clinical severity encompasses so mild as to be detected only at autopsy to so severe that death occurs within several years, referred to as acute MS of the Marburg type. Fortunately, the latter is a very rare type of MS.

Accordingly, with the life expectancy affected minimally, the major consideration of the prognosis relates to predicting the effect of the MS disease process on the patient's quality of life. That is, when will functional disability and interference with independence of activities of daily living and employment appear, and how severe will it be? It is generally stated that, at the time of the first symptom/sign, one-third of patients will have a favorable; one-third, a poor; and one-third, an intermediate quality of life. On average, 20 to 25 years after first symptoms, 50% will be moderately disabled but ambulatory without aids, with the remainder distributed from mild to severe.

The period 10 years after the first symptoms provides a convenient point to predict later prognosis with reasonable accuracy. The majority of patients who will have progressive MS will have done so by this time, and those who subsequently will convert to progressive MS will remain at the lower end of the disability scales, i.e., minimal interference with all aspects of daily living, especially motor function.

The guidelines to predict the late prognosis for the first 10 years after the first symptoms, when the majority of patients are in the relapsing phase are as follows:

1. The number or frequency of the relapses does not significantly influence the course, but benign disease usually has very infrequent relapses.
2. A long-term favorable course correlates with the duration of the first remission, and a first remission, lasting 5 years or more, carries a favorable prognosis.
3. There is a correlation between disability and the duration of the attack; e.g., patients with symptoms present for more than 1 year do not usually recover.

The sites affected in any episode can correlate with the prognosis and disability. The common sites producing disability are as follows (worst to best): cervical cord, spinocerebellar tracts, corticospinal tracts, optic nerves, and sensory systems. A most important factor is the age at onset; an older age at onset increases the probability of disability.

The following laboratory abnormalities do not predict the clinical course:

1. Level of intrathecal IgG synthesis.
2. HLA phenotype.
3. Abnormal lymphocyte subpopulations.
4. Abnormal evoked potentials.

However, there are reports that progression of the MS disease process, as shown by serial MRI with gadolinium enhancement, correlates with a worse prognosis.

RESPONDING TO COMMON INQUIRES

A number of inquires arise concerning MS. Some of the common ones are listed in Table 2.

TREATMENT

Despite the fact there is no treatment that has been proven to eradicate or to ameliorate the MS

TABLE 1. **Self-Rated Overall Function Scale**

Listed below are a number of statements that might be used to describe the overall function of patients with MS. These statements are arranged in order from least severe (0) to most severe (9)

Instructions
1. First locate the category that best describes your ability to walk.
   • If you are able to walk without limitations, please choose a statement from Category I.
   • If you are able to walk only a limited distance, please choose a statement from Category II.
   • If you require aid(s) or assistance to walk or are unable to walk, please choose a statement from Category III.
2. Once you have found the Category that applies to you, circle the number of the *one* statement that *best* describes your overall condition at the present time.
3. In selecting your answer, refer back to your rating of the neurologic categories.
Remember to choose only *one* of the statements in Category I, II, or III.

Category I. Able to Walk
0.0 Essentially normal.
1.0 Abnormality in *one* of the neurologic categories but with no difficulty in function.
1.5 Abnormality in *more than one* of the neurologic categories but with no difficulty in function.
2.0 Minimal difficulty in *one* of the neurologic categories.
2.5 Minimal difficulty in two of the neurologic categories.
3.0 Moderate difficulty in *one* of the neurologic categories but able to walk.
3.5 Moderate difficulty in *one* of the neurologic categories and minimal difficulty in *one or more* of the neurologic categories but able to walk.

Category II. Able to Walk Only a Limited Distance
4.0 Able to walk without aid or rest at least seven city blocks (500 m or 1625 ft). Self-sufficient, up and about some 12 hours a day. (Relatively severe difficulty in one neurologic category or moderate difficulty in several of the neurologic categories.)
4.5 Able to walk without aid or rest at least four city blocks (300 m or 975 ft). May need minimal assistance; able to work a full day but may have some limitation of full activity. (Relatively severe difficulty in one neurologic category or moderate difficulty in several of the neurologic categories.)
5.0 Able to walk without aid or rest at least two and one-half city blocks (200 m or 650 ft). Disability is severe enough to *limit* full daily activities, for example, to work a full day without job modifications.
5.5 Able to walk without aid or rest at least one city block (100 m or 325 ft). Disability is severe enough to *prevent* full daily activities. (Very severe difficulty in one of the neurologic categories or moderate difficulty in several of the neurologic categories.)

Category III. Aid(s) Required or Unable to Walk
6.0 Assistance on one side (cane, crutch, or brace) is required to walk approximately one city block (approximately 100 m or 325 ft), with or without resting. (Moderate difficulty in more than two neurologic categories.)
6.5 Constant assistance on both sides (canes, crutches, braces, or walker) is required to walk about 20 m (65 ft). (Moderate difficulty in more than two neurologic categories.)
7.0 Unable to walk more than about 5 m (16 ft) even with aid. Essentially restricted to wheelchair. Can wheel self in standard wheelchair and can transfer alone. Up and about in wheelchair some 12 hours a day. (Severe difficulty in more than one neurologic category or severe weakness only.)
7.5 Unable to take more than a few steps. Restricted to wheelchair. Can wheel self in standard wheelchair and may need aid to transfer. Cannot remain in wheelchair for a full day. May require motorized wheelchair. (Severe difficulty in more than one neurologic category.)
8.0 Essentially restricted to bed much of the day. Has limited use of arms. Retains some self-care functions. (Severe difficulty in several neurologic categories.)
8.5 Essentially restricted to bed much of the day. Has limited use of arms. Retains some self-care functions. (Severe difficulty in several neurologic categories.)
9.0 Restricted to bed. Cannot use arms. Can speak and can eat if fed by others. (Severe difficulty in several neurologic categories.)

Table continued on following page

disease process, the MS disease process has only a small effect on the life expectancy. Accordingly, the primary goals in management are to control symptoms, avoid complications, and improve the quality of life. Solutions to obtain these goals can be divided into 10 general categories: treatments directed at the MS disease process, symptomatic treatment (medical and nonmedical), keeping cool, exercise for life, pursuit of wellness, a positive attitude, education (be MS smart), self-help/people support, financial assistance, and the Americans With Disabilities Act.

Treatments Directed at the MS Disease Process

Corticosteroids

The anti-inflammatory and immunosuppressant properties of corticosteroids do not alter the long-term course of MS, but they expedite recovery from some acute attacks. Because there is no way to predict if a patient will respond, clinical judgment prevails whether to go ahead or not.

When a patient has an acute worsening, it is important to determine that this is not due to an

TABLE 1. **Self-Rated Overall Function Scale** *Continued*

Neurologic Categories

Circle
one

Mild Mod Severe	1. Pyramidal Symptoms may include weakness, fatigue, spasticity, clonus, and limited walking distance.
Mild Mod Severe	2. Cerebellar Symptoms may include incoordination, tremor, and walking as if drunk.
Mild Mod Severe	3. Brain Stem Symptoms may include difficulty with speaking or swallowing, double vision, and facial pain.
Mild Mod Severe	4. Sensory Symptoms may include diminished sensitivity to touch or pain and paresthesia.
Mild Mod Severe	5. Bowel/bladder Symptoms may include hesitancy, urgency, and incontinence.
Mild Mod Severe	6. Visual Symptoms may include poor visual acuity, even with glasses, and blind spots.
Mild Mod Severe	7. Mental function Symptoms may include slowed thinking and forgetfulness.

From the Department of Neurology, Einstein Medical Ctr, Bronx, NY, verison of Kurtzke's disability scale.

infection with or without a fever or other intercurrent illness, such as an electrolyte imbalance or depression; appropriate treatment should follow immediately. If an acute attack is mild, i.e., it does not produce significant disability, it can go untreated. Mild symptoms are unlikely to benefit from any intervention other than coping, positive attitude, and a wellness lifestyle.

Acute attacks producing significant disability are treated on an outpatient basis with prednisone and supplements (Table 3), if there are no contraindications, such as positive tuberculin test results, diabetes mellitus, hypertension, or osteoporosis, especially of the femoral neck. It is important that patients have an appropriate exercise prescription.

If the patient is a prednisone responder, an improvement is usually seen by day 4. If there are no major adverse effects, we recommend a 7-day course before the taper starts. If the prednisone treatment is ineffective, a course of intravenous methylprednisolone (Solu-Medrol) can be tried (Table 4), but experience and some reports have shown that this treatment is no more effective than the prednisone treatment described. If intravenous methylprednisolone is ineffective, no further treatment is given; the patient is a corticosteroid nonresponder.

A recent controlled study by the Optic Neuritis Treatment Trial (ONTT) of acute optic neuritis, a frequent monosymptomatic presentation of MS, revealed intravenous methylprednisolone was effective, whereas oral prednisone and placebo were not. In fact, prednisone was reported to make MS symptoms worse. Even though this report is worrisome, based on our extensive experience and that of others, numerous successes have resulted using the protocol presented in Tables 3 and 4. On the other hand, a taper of 2 weeks, as used in the ONTT, in our experience can lead to a worsening of improved symptoms and signs. Furthermore, optic neuritis is not MS; it is demyelination of a nerve within a sheath that passes through a foramen. In view of the low dose of prednisone and short taper used, abandoning the protocols presented in Tables 3 and 4 is not warranted.

The chronic use of corticosteroids has not been submitted to controlled clinical trials, but based on experience, their use can be valuable. When a patient is physically conditioned, is following an exercise prescription, and is motivated and when there are no contraindications, a course of prednisone, as outlined in Table 3, can produce improved function. Maintenance of this improved function is possible for an undetermined period when the prednisone is given as a single daily morning dose every other day. A taper of 20 mg once a week will determine the maintenance dose. Using this schedule, the patient is usually better on the off day. Alternate-day dosing minimizes the hypothalamic-pituitary-adrenal axis,

TABLE 2. **Responding to Common Inquiries**

Inquiry	Response
What is MS?	See text
Making the diagnosis	See text
Informing patient of MS diagnosis	Honesty; Americans With Disabilities Act (ADA) attempts to prevent employment discrimination and improved physical environment for handicapped individuals.
Informing children	Honesty. Give them as much information as they need; emphasize that longevity is near normal, and the parent will not die before his or her time; regarding heredity, see text
Heredity	See text
Prognosis	See text
Contagiousness	No evidence
Migration	From high-risk region for MS (Northern Europe and Northern United States/Southern Canada, and Southern Australia) to low-risk region (nearer the equator) before the age of 15 years, an individual acquires low-risk frequency; from low-risk region to high-risk before the age of 15 years, an individual acquires high-risk frequency; after the age of 15 years, migration has no effect on the incidence rate
Marital discord	Psychosocial intervention is important
Temperature sensitivity and fever	80% of patients with MS have immediate worsening with an elevation in body temperature; accordingly, dress cool, eat cool, eat less, consume iced drinks and ice chips, take a cool shower/bath, and have a strong room air conditioner in the bedroom; if physically well conditioned, body temperature is less likely to become elevated
	A fever is an emergency; cool with antipyretics, alcohol sponges, cooling blanket, and wet T-shirt; immediately go to an emergency room for diagnosis in a cooled state
Immunization and prophylaxis against contagious diseases	Controversy; according to our experiments and experience, there is no risk for annual pneumococcal or influenza vaccination; if fever and malaise develop, cool with antipyretics. Avoid multiple vaccinations required for tropical travel.
Injuries	Controversy about making MS symptoms/signs worse; we recommend that every effort be made to keep rest as a treatment to a minimum; rest in a chair is a compromise between active and passive exercises; consider low-dose heparin as prophylaxis against pulmonary emboli
Pregnancy, contraception, and abortion	No contraindications to pregnancy, but if patient is moderately to severely disabled, it will be necessary to have assistance in caring for the baby; there is a postpartum risk of worsening; no additional risks to contraception or abortion; consult your obstetrican/gynecologist
Obstetric anesthesia	The method of delivery should depend on the indications; any type of anesthesia is not without risk, although there is some evidence that general anesthesia is better than caudal or spinal anesthesia, which add further dysfunction to lower extremities and bladder/bowel
Surgery and the appropriate anesthesia	There is some controversy that surgical procedures worsen MS; in our experience, if the procedure is indicated, do it; use the appropriate anesthesia, but avoid caudal or spinal anesthesia, which add further dysfunction to lower extremities and bladder/bowel
Emotional stress	Controversial; immediate worsening of short duration is frequent, but induction of a relapse is not an expected result in our experience and that of published reports
Diet	No diet has been proven to be of value; however, a low animal fat diet with high fiber, as recommended by wellness experts, is in order; in addition, 2 tbsp of canola oil per day (high in poly unsaturated fatty acids, such as linoleic) has some experimental support
Megavitamins	There is a trend for high daily dosing of antioxidant vitamins, such as beta carotene, 15 mg; vitamin C, 4 gm; and vitamin E (alpha-tocopherol), 3000 m units; furthermore, 100% of the recommended daily dose of vitamin B complex is also part of the trend
Calcium	Most individuals do not ingest enough calcium; accordingly, we recommend 900 mg of calcium per day (e.g., three calcium carbonate tablets, such as Tums 300 mg of Ca^{++} per tablet per day)
Cranberry juice	There is evidence that a substance in cranberry juice prevents *Escherichia coli* from binding to the bladder wall; 1 to 3 cups per day is recommended
Alcoholic beverages	Most patients with MS cannot tolerate alcohol because it makes the cerebellar signs worse; however, if tolerated, wellness experts recommend 1 to 2 cups (250–500 mL) of wine per day, preferably red
Silicone breast implants	Does silicone cause autoimmune disease? Controversial at present; hence, waiting for peer-reviewed publication for scientific basis for removal
Smoking	
Cigarettes	Adverse to health
Marijuana	Produces temporary mood elevation and pleasant withdrawal; adverse to health
Mercury in dental amalgam	No risk

TABLE 3. **Prednisone Protocols**

Prednisone, 40 mg qid for 7 Days
Prednisone Taper
8th day, no prednisone
9th day, 160 mg of prednisone in a single daily morning dose
   on alternate days 3 times
Each 3 times decrease the dose of prednisone by 20 mg, for
   example, 140 mg qod 3 times, then 120 mg qod 3 times,
   etc., to 20 mg qod 3 times, then 10 mg 3 times, then 0 mg.
Hold taper if the patient's condition worsens.
Supplements and Advice
Potassium (K-Lyte) 25 mEq bid
Sodium restriction (no added salt; no salted foods)
Tums extra large (300 mg Ca^{++}) in between meals and at
   bedtime
Daily weight gain of about 4 lbs indicates water retention.
   Treat with further salt restriction and diuretics.
Indigestion and black stools should be reported immediately.
Appropriate Exercise Prescription
Should include power walking tid, and severely afflicted
   patients should get up and move around 10 minutes each
   hour

weight gain, cushingoid appearance, and hypertension but probably not osteoporosis, cataracts, or diabetes. Therefore, an ongoing effort should be made to taper the dose to zero, with consideration of the lowest dose to maintain the best activities of daily living, exercise program, and employment efficiency. Our experience has shown that adrenocorticotropic hormone (ACTH) gel or intravenous ACTH is no better than the prednisone treatment described.

Beta Interferon

Beta interferon (Betaseron [Berlex]) has been approved by the U.S. Food and Drug Administration for relapsing-remitting ambulatory MS patients and will be available in late 1993. Forty-five million units are taken by subcutaneous injection every other day. The treatment lessens the frequency and severity of exacerbations for many relapsing-remitting patients, with minor side effects. In addition, the plaque burden and the number of new lesions were reduced.

Cytotoxic Immunosuppressants

Based on clinically controlled studies and our experience, we do not use azathioprine (Imuran), cyclophosphamide (Cytoxan), or cyclosporine (Sandimmune). However, there is regional enthu-

TABLE 4. **Methylprednisolone Protocol**

Methylprednisolone is mixed with 500 mL of dextrose 5% in
   water and administered over 30 min, preferably in the
   morning. Give 1 gm daily × 5 days
Taper: Use prednisone (see Table 3).
Supplements and advice (see Table 3).
Appropriate exercise prescription (see Table 3).

siasm for intermittent cyclophosphamide pulse therapy in progressive MS.

Other Experimental Treatments

The following putative treatments are being tested in formal clinical trials: to down-regulate the immune response to myelin destruction: copolymer 1 (COP 1), intravenous immunoglobulin therapy, desferrioxamine, total lymphoid irradiation, intravenous methylprednisolone (low versus high dose), oral myelin basic protein, beta interferon for chronic progressive MS, and T-lymphocyte peptide VB, receptor fragment vaccine and antibodies against T-lymphocyte receptors; to enhance nerve signal conduction: 3,4-diaminopyridine and digitalis.

Symptomatic Treatments

Until the cause of MS can be found and a specific therapy proven, the relief of symptoms and signs as they arise remains the primary goal in the management of patients. Symptoms in MS can be classified as "primary symptoms," which are those that directly result from plaques in various areas of the CNS (e.g., spasticity, numbness, and bladder dysfunction); "secondary symptoms," which are the results of the primary symptoms (e.g., cystitis, decubitus ulcers, and contractures); and "tertiary symptoms," which are related to the primary and secondary symptoms and the resultant disability and handicap they cause (e.g., depression, marital problems, and loss of employment). The first two are amenable to medical therapy, while the last requires psychosocial intervention. The symptomatic treatment of patients with MS rests almost entirely on advances in psycho- and neuropharmacology, medicine, surgery, psychology, and physical medicine. Table 5 lists, in alphabetical order, the symptoms and signs of MS. Based on experience and some clinical trials, nonmedical and medical treatments are noted. The dosage of the medications and the adverse effects are as cited in the *Physicians' Desk Reference*; so these are not included for brevity's sake. Experience indicates that one should commence with low doses and work upward slowly.

Keeping Cool

It has been reported that a cool suit that lowers the normal ear drum temperature 1° F (brain temperature) in 1 hour used twice a day for 1 to 2 months with an exercise prescription can improve neurologic function in some patients with MS compared with those just carrying out the same exercise prescription (Tables 2 and 3). One-third definitely improved, one-third probably improved, and one-third had no change. Hence, this

Text continued on page 904

TABLE 5. **Symptomatic Treatment of Multiple Sclerosis**

Symptoms (In Alphabetical Order)	Nonmedical Treatments & Comments	Medications	Adverse Side Effects
Balance sense dysfunction (incoordination of lower extremies and/or truncal ataxia)	Balance/coordination exercises, weighting, hydrotherapy, cooling, aids of ambulation. Education on safe walking.	Corticosteroids Inderal Klonopin	
Bladder dysfunction 1. Failure to store (small capacity, spastic urgency, frequency, and dribbling). 2. Failure to empty (large capacity, infrequency, and hesitancy; frequency and urgency when bladder stretched). 3. Combination of 1 and 2. 4. Detrusor sphincter dyssynergia (combination of 1 and 2). 5. Antisepsis 6. Cystitis	Classification of the type of dysfunction by measuring residual volume is necessary for proper diagnosis. This is best carried out by a urologist with special training in neurogenic bladders. Urination or intermittent catheterization schedule. Credé maneuver. Rectal stimulation. Condom catheter for men. Protective underpants with adult diapers. Surgical enlargement of the bladder and bypass procedures. Indwelling catheters should be used in only extreme cases, and then great care should be taken to avoid infections; they are more tolerable in women. To encourage, reduce the residual urine. Cranberry juice and fluid intake at 6–8 glasses/day. Proper peritoneal hygiene for women. Avoid indwelling catheters. If used, keep a closed system and practice asepsis of the catheter meatus junction and drainage apparatus, changing the catheter monthly and the bag, every 2 weeks. For cystitis, see antisepsis. Maintain adequate bladder drainage, force fluids, reduce fever. Intravenous pyelography or sonography studies of bladder dynamics if infections are frequent plus culture to determine antibiotic sensitivities, then use the appropriate antibiotic. Broad-spectrum antibiotic prior to culture results.	1. Failure to store: Oxybutynin choloride (Ditropan), propantheline bromide (Pro-Banthine), flavoxate HCl (Urispas), hyoscyamine (Cystospaz), and imipramine (Tofranil). Polypharmacy. Medically paralyze the bladder and use intermittent catheterization. 2. Failure to empty: Credé maneuver. Rectal stimulation. Bethanechol (Urecholine), phenoxybenzamine (Dibenzyline). Medically paralyze bladder (see 1) and use intermittent catheterization. 3. Combination of 1 and 2: See 2. 4. Detrusor sphincter dyssynergia: Credé maneuver. Imipramine, baclofen (Lioresal), terazosin HCl (Hytrin). Intermittent catheterization with or without medically paralyzing bladder. 5. Antisepsis: Ascorbic acid (4 gm/day), methenamine mandalate (Mandelamine), and co-trimoxazole (Bactrim or Septra) once/day. 6. Cystitis: Co-trimoxazole, norfloxacin (Noroxin).	Glaucoma is a contraindication to anticholinergics. Anticholinergic, dry mouth, blurred vision, tachycardia, drowsiness, and constipation. Indwelling catheter causes infection and bladder calculi.

Table continued on following page

TABLE 5. **Symptomatic Treatment of Multiple Sclerosis** *Continued*

Symptoms (In Alphabetical Order)	Nonmedical Treatments & Comments	Medications	Adverse Side Effects
Constipation with or without urgency with or without incontinence	Exercise. Six to 8 glasses of fluid per day. High-fiber diet (23 gm/day) with adequate fluid intake. Bowel program stressing regular evacuations, enemas, and digital stimulation or removal, especially if urgency results in incontinence. Disimpaction. Protective underpants and adult diapers. Rarely, colostomy for uncontrollable obstipation.	Metamucil, another bulk former. Stool softeners, such as docusate sodium (Colace). Milk of magnesia with or without cascara. Bisacodyl (Dulcolax) orally the night before and suppositories at the time of defecation. Sodium phosphate (Fleet) enemas.	Avoid bowel incontinence or leaking due to stool too soft. Gas from too rapid increase of fiber.
Contractures	Range-of-motion and stretching exercises. Cooling. Night splints, bivalved casts. Surgery includes motor nerve blocks, rhizotomies, tendonotomies, myelotomy, and arthrodesis.	Baclofen, diazepam (Valium), clonazepam (Klonopin), dantrolene (Dantrium). Protective underpants and adult diapers, Cyclobenzaprine HCl (Flexeril), intrathecal baclofen pump.	
Convulsive seizures	Search for other causes of seizures because only about 10 times more frequent in MS.	Carbamazepine (Tegretol), valproic acid (Depakene), phenytoin (Dilantin). After 6 months without seizures, taper anticonvulsants over 3 months if no other cause present.	Avoid overmedication to reduce sedation and ataxia.
Depression and behavioral problems	Fostering a good doctor-patient relationship. Psychotherapy. Suicide preventive measures.	Amitriptyline (Elavil), desipramine (Norpramin), fluoxetine (Prozac), imipramine, lithium (Eskalith), carbamazepine.	Commence low dose and individualize; gradual increase to optimize dosage.
Diarrhea/bowel incontinence	Unusual in MS, check for secondary causes, e.g., impaction, infection. Avoid dietary irritants. Bowel program stressing regular evacuations, enemas, suppositories. Protective underpants and adult diapers. In extreme cases, colostomy.	Attapulgite (Kaopectate), diphenoxylate HCl with atropine sulfate (Lomotil), anticholinergics (see Bladder, Failure to Store).	
Decubitus ulcers	See Pressure Ulcer.		
Diplopia	Use alternating patch. Teach to gaze in the direction least affected. Cooling.	Corticosteroids	
Dysarthria	Read aloud and talk a lot, slowly and distinctly. Speech therapist. Chew gum. Cooling. Alternative communication devices.		
Dysarthria paroxysmal	Cooling.	Carbamazepine, valproic acid (K), phenytoin, acetazolamide (Diamox).	

TABLE 5. **Symptomatic Treatment of Multiple Sclerosis** *Continued*

Symptoms (In Alphabetical Order)	Nonmedical Treatments & Comments	Medications	Adverse Side Effects
Dysphagia	Deep breath before swallowing. Chew gum. Food thickeners (Thick-It). Cooling. Stand-by aspirator. With fever, dysphagia can worsen and result in aspiration; cool immediately. See Pulmonary Infections. For severe ongoing dysphagia, percutaneous endoscopic gastrostomy for long-term enteral feeding.	Anticholinergics to dry salivary secretions with or without gastrostomy.	Aspiration followed by pneumonia, a major cause of death.
Fatigue	Positive attitude to "fight" fatigue; fatigue begets fatigue. Rest in chair. Plan day in detail and do it. Pace activities. Progressive exercise program. Aids of ambulation to conserve energy. Cooling.	Amitriptyline HCl, fluoxetine, pemoline (Cylert), amantadine (Symmetrel), methylphenidate HCl (Ritalin), selegiline HCl (Eldepryl), isoniazid with pyridoxine 2 mg.	Avoid overdose of pemoline and methylphenidate HCl, because insomnia may result with high doses.
Flexor spasm	Frequently occurs on falling asleep. Cooling.	Baclofen, diazepam, clonazepam, dantrolene, cyclobenzaprine HCl, carbamazepine (Tegretol). Timing: extra medication 30 min prior to sleep if nocturnal spasms.	
Hypoventilation	This is an emergency. Usually with fever. Respiratory assistance with or without intubation. Cooling.	Oxygen	
Intellectual impairment	Impairment of recent memory, sustained attention, conceptual reasoning, verbal fluency, and speed of informational processing; intelligence and language functions are relatively spared. Sometimes difficult to distinguish depression and fatigue as the main factors. *Education:* Read and recite. Read aloud. Social stimulation and talk a lot. Adaptive computers. Cognitive retraining. Use notebooks and pocket data books. Cooling. In severe cases, confinement with full-time caregivers.	Amitriptyline, fluoxetine, pemoline, amantadine, methylphenidate HCl.	Avoid overdose of pemoline and methylphenidate HCl, because insomnia may result with high doses.
Intention tremor	Made worse with stress. Physical and occupational therapy. Weighted bracelets and utensils. Cooling. Cryothalamotomy in extreme cases with good strength and mild dementia.	Diazepam, chlordiazepoxide HCl (Librium), hydroxyzine HCl (Atarax), propranolol (Inderal), hydroxyzine pamoate (Vistaril), clonazepam, chlorpromazine (thorazine), baclofen, isoniazid with pyridoxine 2 mg, haloperidol (Haldol).	Avoid excess sedation. Isoniazid, check for hepatic toxicity. Cryothalamotomy, a serious complication is corticospinal weakness.

Table continued on following page

TABLE 5. **Symptomatic Treatment of Multiple Sclerosis** *Continued*

Symptoms (In Alphabetical Order)	Nonmedical Treatments & Comments	Medications	Adverse Side Effects
Labile emotions	Stress can enhance. Cooling.	Amitriptyline, diazepam, carbidopa-levodopa (Sinemet), bromocriptine mesylate (Parlode).	Avoid overmedication.
Oscillopsia	Can produce low vision; so use refraction. Can be dissociated; so use patching. Cooling. Low vision clinic. Glasses with converging prisms.	Isoniazid with pyridoxine 2 mg, clonazepam, baclofen, anticonvulsants, anticholinergics. Corticosteroids.	Isoniazid, check for hepatitis.
Pulmonary infections	This is an emergency. Usually secondary to aspiration, the most common cause of death. Cool aggressively. Respiratory assistance with or without intubation.	Oxygen. Broad-spectrum antibiotics. IV fluids.	Most common cause of death.
Pain Neckache	Rule out surgically treatable spondylosis. Neck brace. Physical therapy. Exercises. Local heat. Massage. Ultrasound. Hydrotherapy.	Minimal analgesics, nonsteroidal anti-inflammatory drugs, and muscle relaxants.	
Backache	See Neckache. Rule out surgically treatable spondylosis. Bed rest with firm mattress.	Minimal analgesics, nonsteroidal anti-inflammatory drugs, and muscle relaxants.	
Headache	Rule out migraine.	If migraine, treat with antimigraine medication. If not migraine, use headache analgesics and antidepressants.	
Muscle cramps	Physical therapy. Range of motion.	Baclofen, diazepam, quinine sulfate (Quinamm), calcium carbonate (Tums).	
Paroxysmal extremity burning pain and dysalgesia	Persistent burning, predominantly in lower extremities, worse at night, aggravated by heat and walking. Cooling. Transcutaneous nerve stimulation. Biofeedback. Meditation. Acupuncture. Phenol nerve root blocks, posterior root section, or cordectomy in rare refractory cases.	Carbamazepine, valproic acid, phenytoin, amitriptyline, desipramine, nortriptyline (Pamelor), haloperidol, chlorpromazine, capsaicin (Zostrix topical analgesic cream, rub in lidocaine ointment first).	
See trigeminal neuralgia			
Paresthesias	Medically treat only if painful. Cooling.	Amitriptyline, desipramine, carbamazepine.	
Pressure ulcer	Prevention and vigilance: cushions, pads, special mattresses. Prevent wetness. Turning using circuloelectric beds and low air loss bed. Good nutrition. Debride. Expose to air. Heat lamps. Surgical cleansing. DuoDERM covering. Wet to dry dressings. Full-thickness skin grafting.	Tincture of benzoin, povidone-iodine (Betadine), hydrogen peroxide 3%.	

TABLE 5. **Symptomatic Treatment of Multiple Sclerosis** *Continued*

Symptoms (In Alphabetical Order)	Nonmedical Treatments & Comments	Medications	Adverse Side Effects
Sexual dysfunction	Sex therapy and psychotherapy. Treat spasticity and bladder and bowel dysfunction.	Treat spasticity, bladder and bowel dysfunction. See appropriate sections in this Table.	
Libido	Sex therapy and psychotherapy.	Testosterone, yohimbine.	
Erection dysfunction	Manual stimulation of penis. Vacuum pump. Penile prosthetic devices surgically implanted.	Inject penis with papaverine hydrochloride; consult urologist.	Priapism: This is an emergency requiring emergency room visit to reverse with intracorporeal injection of epinephrine, norepinehrine, or metaraminol (Aramine). Consult urologist in emergency room.
Ejaculation dysfunction	Treat spasticity, bowel and bladder dysfunction, fatigue. Prostatic stimulation.	Treat spasticity, bowel and bladder dysfunction. See appropriate sections in this Table.	
Female orgasmic dysfunction	Stimulation: manual or vibrator. Water-soluble lubrication. Treat spasticity, bladder and bowel dysfunction, fatigue.	Treat spasticity, bowel and bladder dysfunction, see appropriate sections in this Table. Painful genital sensations, see Pain treatment in this Table.	
Spasticity	Physical therapy: stretching, range of motion. Cooling. Aids of ambulation, braces. Daily exercises. Hydrotherapy. Prevent contractures.	Diazepam, baclofen, dantrolene, clonazepam. Combinations of above. In extreme cases, intrathecal baclofen, lidocaine (Xylocaine) blocks, if successful follow with phenol nerve blocks.	Dantrolene, check for hepatitis. Overmedication produces flaccidity and interferes with ambulation.
Tonic seizures	Avoid the movement or touch which precipitates them. Avoid hyperventilation.	Carbamazepine, acetazolamide, phenytoin, valproic acid. Attempt taper in 6 months over 3-month period.	Avoid overmedication.
Trigeminal neuralgia	Avoid the trigger point. If medical failure, surgery; such as percutaneous radiofrequency rhizotomy.	Carbamazepine, gradually increase; phenytoin, valproic acid, clonazepam, baclofen, amitriptyline HCl, perphenazine (Trifapon, Etrafon). Avoid analgesics.	
Vertigo	Avoid sudden changes in posture or find lying head position that dampens spin sensation. IV fluids if vomiting severe.	Dimenhydrinate (Dramamine), meclizine HCl hydrochloride (Antivert), chlorpromazine, fentanyl plus droperiodol (Innovar), diphenhydramine (Benadryl), corticosteroids	Avoid overmedication.
Visual loss Acute optic neuritis		High-dose IV methylprednisolone (Solu-Medrol)	

Table continued on following page

TABLE 5. **Symptomatic Treatment of Multiple Sclerosis** *Continued*

Symptoms (In Alphabetical Order)	Nonmedical Treatments & Comments	Medications	Adverse Side Effects
Acuity	Check for cataracts and uveitis. After best refraction, use magnifier with optimal lighting. Cooling. Low-vision books, computers, talking books. Low-vision clinics. Rule out uveitis.	Uveitis: mydriatics and local corticosteroids.	
Fixed defects	Engineer's triangular ruler. Cooling. Braille system of reading.		
Weakness	Check for infection, fever, heat exposure, calcium and electrolyte disturbances, malnutrition, overuse of muscle relaxants, overexercise, overexertion. Physical therapy. Hydrotherapy (walking, deep knee bends). Aids of ambulation. Braces. Cooling.	Corticosteroids; 4-aminopyridine (experimental).	

type of device offers some heat-sensitive patients an immediate improvement as well as a long-term benefit. There is no way of predicting who will improve; so, it is necessary to try it. Additionally, the cooling suit is easy to put on.

Exercise for Life

Exercise has special benefits for patients with MS. A regular exercise prescription helps overcome fatigue, enhances endurance, induces a feeling of well-being, and benefits every organ.

The cornerstone of the fitness program is a hydrotherapy prescription, a conditioning program of exercises performed in water at a temperature of about 80° F to help the patient build strength and endurance. Why a hydrotherapy exercise program? Regular exercise should be a part of everyone's lifestyle, whether the individual is a man or a woman, healthy, mildly disabled, moderately disabled, or severely disabled. Additionally, it is part of every wellness program, but not everyone, especially not the patient with MS, can start out in a regular fitness program by walking, power walking, jogging, bicycling, or swimming. The hydrotherapy exercise plan provides an alternative for those who are not able to participate in a conventional land exercise program, because of disability or intolerance to heat. It is a stepping stone to a regular program of first water exercises, then swimming, walking, and ultimately, power walking and stationary bicycling.

Doing progressive water exercises, such as walking, deep knee bends, one-legged standing, and swimming (use of a life preserver for safety is recommended when necessary) will help the patient to develop the stamina needed to participate in a conventional exercise program. Water exercises will also help the patient to develop strength, flexibility, and the endurance needed to develop cardiovascular fitness. The weightlessness achieved in water will provide an opportunity for the patient to exercise comfortably. Most important, with water exercises, the patient will not suffer from the heat effects associated with other types of exercises. Hydrotherapy thus provides the patient an opportunity to exercise for life. After a vigorous hydrotherapy session, it is necessary to prevent physiologic hyperthermia due to the exercise. We recommend sitting in the cool pool water or cool shower for 30 minutes.

Consult with a physical therapist to plan a program of exercise that is right for the patient. It should be emphasized to the patient that an exercise prescription is a way to fitness and a better quality of life.

Pursuit of Wellness and a Positive Attitude

Health maintenance to combat the aging process should be emphasized, because almost all patients' longevity is minimally affected. This includes regular visits to the neurologist and family doctor for a thorough checkup with appropriate screening tests and treatments. Furthermore, we recommend a low-fat, high-fiber diet, daily cranberry juice, multivitamins with extra antioxidants (beta carotene, C, and E), calcium daily, low-dose aspirin (81 mg) per day, ideal weight

TABLE 6. **Positive One-Liner Type of Paradigm That Reminds Patients with MS of Their Daily Strategy Against a Negative Self-Image and Depression**

TURN FROM DISABILITY TO ABILITY
Self-help (PACE & FIGHT*)
Significant Others (Support)
Education: Be MS Smart
Support Research and Development

*Positive Attitude Changes Everything & Fun in your job, Ingenuity, Goals, Hustle, Thoroughness

Reminder: Your patients' lives will not be shortened or their minds affected significantly by MS. Here is a method to turn from disability to ability on a daily basis.

It is always easier if significant others support the patient. Read, listen, and ask questions, the basis of all education, so you can be MS SMART.

And finally support research and development, the scientific method to find the cause and treatment of MS.

"What do we live for, if not to make life less difficult for each other?"

—George Eliot

"I expect to pass through life but once. If therefore there be any kindness I can show or any good thing I can do to any fellow human being, let me do it now, and not defer or neglect it, as I shall not pass this way again."

—William Penn

maintenance, and regular sleep, with naps only as necessary.

Optimism is a powerful tool. A positive attitude will influence every aspect of the patient's life and enhance developing new interests (Table 6). Encourage your patients to look and feel their best. Exercise their bodies and minds daily (read and tell stories). Have your patient use a computer. A new computer industry for handicapped people is developing rapidly; it focuses on assistive technology, computer access, communication, and literacy.

Education: Be MS Smart

The patient should be an expert in MS. They should learn the medical terminology, the hypotheses about the MS disease process, and the symptoms/signs and complications so that they can understand their condition. Encourage patients with MS to read, listen, and ask questions, the basis of all education, so they can be MS smart.

I recommend they read four books:

Schapiro RT: Symptom Management in Multiple Sclerosis. New York, Demos Publications, 1987.

Schapiro RT: Multiple Sclerosis: A Rehabilitation Approach to Management. New York, Demos Publications, 1991.

Kalb RC and Scheinberg LC: Multiple Sclerosis and the Family, 2nd ed. New York, Demos Publications, 1992.

Sibley WA: Therapeutic Claims in Multiple Sclerosis, 3rd ed. New York, Demos Publications, 1992.

In addition, two journals are useful: *Paraplegic News*, published by the Paralyzed Veterans of America, 5201 North 19th Avenue, Suite 111, Phoenix, AZ 85015-9986; and *Rehab Management*, published bimonthly by Allied Health Care Publications, 4676 Admiralty Way, Suite 202, Marina del Rey, CA 90292. Three newsletters are available: *Inside MS* published by the National Multiple Sclerosis Society, 205 East 42nd Street, New York, NY 10017-5706; *Motivator*, published by the Multiple Sclerosis Association of America, 601 White Horse Pike, Oaklyn, NJ 08107; and a wellness newsletter; there are many, such as the *Mayo Clinic Health Letter*, PO Box 53889, Boulder, CO 80322-3889.

Support

It starts with self-help. Patients have to have a positive attitude, set goals, and commit themselves.

It is easier if significant others support the patient, but in addition, the National Multiple Sclerosis Society has support groups where patients with MS can talk about what matters to them. They can share their concerns and successes and explore solutions to everyday problems. These meetings are facilitated by people who have MS. The goal is to learn to live with MS by conversing with other patients. The names of selected groups are as follows: Newly Diagnosed Education Information Meetings; Invisible or Minimal Symptoms Group, 10-Plus Group (for people who have had MS for 10 plus years), Friends and Family Support Group, Men to Men Workshop, Caregivers Workshop, Support Group for Employed People with MS, and One-Day Job Search Seminars. Additionally, there are respite programs, occupational/physical therapy referrals, hydrotherapy sessions, yoga classes, and information on handicap transportation. Of greatest importance, experts associated with the National Multiple Sclerosis Society chapters can help with Medicare, Social Security, and the rights and benefits that are provided in the new Americans With Disabilities Act.

MYASTHENIA GRAVIS

method of
EDWARD L. ARSURA, M.D.
University of California School of Medicine
Los Angeles, California

Myasthenia gravis (MG) is an autoimmune disorder characterized by fluctuating weakness and abnormal fatiguability. The clinical aspects of the disease for the most part are related to antibody and complement-mediated destruction of the acetylcholine receptor (AChR), a 250-kilodalton protein, located on the postsynaptic region of the neuromuscular junction.

CLINICAL FEATURES

MG is not a rare disorder, having an incidence ranging from 1 in 200,000 to 1 in 500,000 and a prevalence of 1 in 20,000 to 1 in 30,000. MG may present at any age. In younger age groups, female patients predominate; in patients older than age 50 years, the male sex is overrepresented.

Although the weakness in MG may be highly individualized with respect to the muscle groups that are involved and the rapidity at which the disease progresses, several general trends are noted. Weakness of the extraocular, facial, and/or bulbar muscles is usually the first symptom. Extraocular muscle involvement leading to diplopia and ptosis is almost invariable during the course of the disease and may be the initial symptom in approximately 40% of patients. As with other signs and symptoms, weakness of these muscle groups tends to fluctuate from day to day and during the day. Weakness generally improves after a period of rest and tends to be more severe as the day progresses or with increased exertion. Weakness of the facial muscles is present in a significant portion of patients. Orbicularis oculi weakness deserves special mention, because these muscles are involved in perhaps 99% of patients during the course of illness. Bulbar muscle weakness, producing pharyngeal and laryngeal weakness, results in nasal speech and nasal regurgitation of liquids, dysphagia, and aspiration of food or secretions. Chewing may be difficult, and at times, there may be complete fatigue of the jaw muscles. Weakness of the neck extensors and, to lesser extent, the flexors is not unusual. Fortunately, weakness of the respiratory muscles is less common; however, this occurrence remains an ever-present problem. Limb weakness may also present in a significant proportion of patients.

Signs of MG tend to be asymmetrical, although there are exceptions. Exacerbations can be provoked by menses, emotional disturbances, extremes of temperature, concomitant medical illnesses, and various medications. Among the most notorious medications are type IA antiarrhythmics (quinidine and procainamide [Procan-SR, Pronestyl]), aminoglycoside antibiotics, beta-blocking agents, narcotics, chlorpromazine (Thorazine), quinine, and diuretics (induction of hypokalemia).

The course of MG has been well described. Patients may have disease limited to the extraocular muscles or the disease may be generalized in nature. Although 40% of patients present with findings limited to the extraocular muscles, the majority (85%) develop more extensive involvement. If the disease becomes generalized, this occurs within the first 3 years after the onset of symptoms. The mortality rate of MG has been reduced from perhaps 90% or greater at the beginning of the twentieth century to less than 3% in recent years. This is related to newer therapeutic modalities, both specific and supportive (e.g., antibiotics and nutrition), modern intensive care units, and improved methods of mechanical ventilation. The mortality in MG is highest in the first 2 to 3 years of illness when the disease is less predictable and the symptoms tend to be more severe and refractory to therapy. The disease then progresses toward an improved steady state, and in some instances, it may enter a remission. The incidence of remission is increased by appropriate therapy.

DIAGNOSIS

The diagnosis of MG is based on the characteristic clinical history and physical examination, pharmacologic tests, electromyographic investigations, and AChR antibody titer determination. The most important component of the diagnosis of MG resides in the history and physical examination.

Pharmacologic tests rely on the ability of anticholinesterase (anti-AChE) medications to improve symptoms by inhibiting the enzyme acetylcholinesterase that catalyzes the degradation of acetylcholine (ACh). For diagnosis, edrophonium (Tensilon), an ultra-short-acting anti-AChE drug, is injected intravenously in increments of 2, 3, and 5 mg (total, 10 mg) at 60 to 120 second intervals. In using edrophonium, it is important to chose a muscle group in which objective improvement can be measured. The severity of ptosis measured by the width of the palpebral fissure is one example. The effect of intravenous edrophonium is evident within 60 seconds and lasts 5 to 10 minutes. Many patients are aware of the presence of edrophonium and may complain of symptoms of cholinergic excess. The ready recognition of the effects of edrophonium by patients may impede objective interpretation. The test can perhaps be improved by prior administration of atropine and performing it in a double-blind fashion. If atropine is not preadministered, it should be available, and intravenous access should be secured prior to administration of edrophonium, because adverse cardiovascular effects, including bradycardia or complete heart block, have been reported, especially among elderly patients. In lieu of edrophonium, intramuscular injection of neostigmine (Prostigmin) 0.5 mg or pyridostigmine (Mestinon) 30 to 60 mg orally may be used. The onset of action with neostigmine is apparent in 15 to 30 minutes and that of pyridostigmine, in 60 minutes. Using these agents prolongs the observation period and the total time for the evaluation.

Electromyographic studies will support the diagnosis of MG; these give positive findings in approximately 90% of patients with generalized MG. A typical myasthenic pattern is progressive decrement in the amplitude of the compound muscle action potential after repetitive stimulation.

Also useful in the evaluation of patients with MG is the determination of the titer of antibodies directed against AChR. These immunoglobulin G antibodies can be detected in 80 to 90% of patients with generalized MG. In patients with ocular MG only, 50% of the patients will have elevated antibody titers. Antibodies to AChR have a high degree of specificity and are seen in only a limited number of conditions other than MG. It is important to remember that approximately 15% of patients with definite MG never demonstrate elevated antibody titers.

Once the diagnosis is confirmed, every patient with MG should undergo a radiologic examination of the chest, including standard chest x-rays and computed tomography (CT) of the superior mediastinum to detect thymic hyperplasia or thymoma. Additional investigations include an assessment of precipitating factors (e.g., fever, medications, or electrolyte imbalance) and exclusion of those associated conditions that occur in MG with a greater frequency than in the general population. These include thyroid disease, both hypo- and hyperthyroidism, and collagen vascular disorders (including systemic lupus erythematosus, polymyositis, and rheumatoid arthritis).

TREATMENT

Supportive Measures

Once the patient's condition is diagnosed as MG, instructions should be provided to avoid situations that are known to precipitate or exacerbate weakness. Adequate amounts of rest and avoidance of overexertion are important as is the provision of appropriate nutritional supplementation, especially in patients who have difficulty in chewing or dysphagia. Avoidance of extremes of temperature and infection in patients whose disease is not in remission or who are unstable is wise counsel. Influenza and pneumococcal vaccine should be administered to appropriate candidates. Hypokalemia may exacerbate weakness, and an occasional patient may improve after administration of potassium supplementation, even if the patient is not hypokalemic. Other agents historically that have been used as adjuvants (ephedrine, theophylline, and spironolactone [Aldactone]) are generally not needed in the properly regulated patient. Various drugs, including alcohol, that are known to precipitate weakness should be eschewed. Patients should be reminded to communicate with their treating physician before initiating any prescription medication.

Therapeutic Options

Multiple options are available in patients with MG, and several therapeutic strategies may be used concomitantly. Anti-AChE drugs are useful in mild disease. However, in disease of moderate or greater severity, their efficacy is less than ideal. Therapeutic options for more severe disease are directed at influencing the abnormal immune response and include thymectomy, corticosteroids, nonsteroidal immune suppression, plasmapheresis, and intravenous immunoglobulin.

Anti-AChE Agents

Many patients with mild to moderate disease find that the addition of anti-AChE agents produces improvement in symptoms, allowing nearly normal resumption of activities. The most commonly used agent is pyridostigmine. Pyridostigmine is generally given orally. Less frequently, pyridostigmine may be administered by nasogastric tube or parenterally to patients who have difficulty swallowing. Another agent, neostigmine, is also available, if parenteral administration is warranted. Ambenonium (Mytelase) is infrequently used and will not be discussed further. Pyridostigmine generally produces improvement in strength after approximately 30 to 60 minutes and has a duration of activity of 3 to 6 hours. All anti-AChE agents may produce muscarinic signs of cholinergic excess. These include salivation, sweating, lacrimation, cramping, fasciculations, nausea, vomiting, diarrhea, adverse cardiovascular effects, and bronchospasm. The latter can be clinically relevant. Pyridostigmine is usually started in doses of 30 to 60 mg on a 4- to 6-hourly basis. The dose can be gradually increased until no further improvement occurs or troublesome signs of cholinergic excess appear. Patients who have severe disease or rapidly progressing disease may not respond to anti-AChE medication, and their condition is considered refractory. The refractory state may tempt the treating physician to administer even higher doses of anti-AChE medication, which paradoxically leads to blunting of the therapeutic response even further.

Patients who require greater than 120 to 180 mg of pyridostigmine every 3 to 4 hours should have additional therapeutic options examined. If no alternatives exist, further cautious dose increases may be considered. Patients who experience cholinergic symptoms may be given anticholinergic medications. Historically atropine 0.4 mg orally has been the most commonly used agent. However, in recent years, the supply of this medication has diminished, and other anticholinergic medications are equally effective. If the patient notices significant weakness in the morning because of the waning effect of pyridostigmine, a long-acting preparation of sustained-release pyridostigmine (Mestinon Timespan) may be administered prior to retiring. This preparation contains 180 mg of pyridostigmine, which is released more slowly and has a duration of action of two to two and one-half times that of regular pyridostigmine. Due to the erratic absorption and release of the Timespan dosage form, it is inadvisable to use this drug during the daytime. In the injectable form, pyridostigmine comes in 2-mL ampules that contain 5 mg per mL. Approximately 2 mg of injectable pyridostigmine is equivalent to 60 mg of oral pyridostigmine.

Neostigmine is used mainly in patients who require parenteral anti-AChE medications. Intramuscular injection (0.5 mg) of neostigmine is equivalent to 60 mg of pyridostigmine orally. The half-life of neostigmine is relatively short, and it should be administered every 2 to 3 hours. Increases in dosage may be made in 0.1- or 0.2-mg increments after evaluation of the peak response 45 to 60 minutes after injection.

Cholinergic side effects may be particularly prominent with neostigmine. Parenteral atropine 0.4 mg every 6 hours or other anticholinergic drugs may be useful.

Adjustment of the dose of anti-AChE medication relies on the assessment of the maximal improvement obtained, duration of the improvement, rapidity of the decrement in muscle strength, evaluation of whether some muscle groups are being overdosed, and evaluation of cholinergic excess. One must realize that titrating the dose of the anti-AChE medication upward to eradicate all symptoms may be unwise and may only yield increasing muscle weakness and signs of cholinergic excess. The dose of pyridostigmine is generally increased in 30-mg increments, allowing adequate time to transpire between future dose adjustments. Patients who have difficulty with meals should take their medication approximately 0.5 hour prior to mealtime.

Assessment of whether a patient is suffering from anti-AChE overdose or whether worsening symptoms reflect an exacerbation of MG is a vexing clinical problem. This task is made more difficult, because various muscle groups may be affected by the drug in differing fashions and one muscle group may have optimal muscle strength while another may be either underdosed or overdosed. Certain muscle groups tend to be relatively resistant to overdose, such as the extraocular muscles and the muscles of lower extremities. In addition to searching for other signs of cholinergic excess, the presence of fasciculations may be an important clue to overdosage. Weakness appearing shortly after a dose suggests overdosage, whereas weakness appearing later on is suggestive of underdosage or myasthenic weakness. Occasionally, injection of edrophonium may be useful as an aid in deciding whether the patient is overdosed or underdosed. In this situation, a smaller dose, 1 to 2 mg of edrophonium, is given approximately 1 hour after pyridostigmine, and an assessment of muscle strength is made before and after the injection of edrophonium. Although this may have utility, some are reluctant to give additional anti-AChE medication to patients who are potentially toxic from these agents. Furthermore, it is my belief that patients who need such careful titration with anti-AChE medication have truly refractory disease and the importance of additional therapeutic modalities becomes much more marked.

Immune Modulating Therapies

Therapies directed against the abnormal immune response in patients with MG include thymectomy, corticosteroids, nonsteroidal immune suppressive agents, plasmapheresis, and intravenous immunoglobulin.

THYMECTOMY

The majority of patients with MG have an abnormality of the thymus gland. Approximately 70% of patients have an overabundance of thymic germinal centers (thymic hyperplasia), and approximately 10% have thymoma. Conversely, in 10 to 20% of patients with thymoma, MG may develop. It is believed that the thymus contains myogenic cells that express AChR and represents the site where immune tolerance is broken. The incidence of thymic hyperplasia and thymoma varies in different age groups. Younger patients commonly have thymic hyperplasia, whereas the incidence of thymoma increases with advancing age. Most clinicians who follow large groups of patients with MG believe in the efficacy of thymectomy; yet thymectomy has never been subjected to a double-blind trial. Prospective trials have demonstrated that the majority of patients who undergo thymectomy (even those without thymic abnormalities) have disease remission. However, the remission may be delayed from several weeks to up to 2 to 5 years.

The exact timing of thymectomy is not certain, although in the appropriate candidate, early thymectomy is advocated by most. A consensus would recommend that all but the very elderly patient, those with seronegative MG, most patients with purely ocular disease, and those with severe complicating medical illnesses should undergo thymectomy. Patients should be appropriately prepared for thymectomy with the utilization of anti-AChE medication and additional modalities to gain the maximal strength possible. Patients should be examined prior to thymectomy by a physician knowledgeable in the muscle groups that may be involved in MG. Specifically, the function of the muscles of swallowing and respiratory function should be evaluated. Minimal or absent bulbar weakness should be sought. A vital capacity greater than 15 to 18 mL per kg and a negative inspiratory pressure of 40 cmH$_2$O are desirable. The importance of appropriate consultation between anesthesiologist, surgeon, and physician cannot be overemphasized. Four to 6 hours prior to surgery, anti-AChE agents should be omitted. Patients with MG are extremely sensitive to the effects of neuromuscular-blocking agents. If these agents are to be utilized, extremely low doses of succinylcholine (Anectine) and only one-third to one-fourth the dosage of short-acting non-depolarizing agents (atracurium [Tracium] or vecuronium [Norcuron]) should be given. The presence of thymoma adversely affects the course of MG, which tends to be of greater severity and increased mortality. In contradistinction to the results of thymectomy in non-thymomatous glands, the effects of thymectomy on the course of MG in patients with thymoma is less certain. The tumor, however, should be removed, because local invasion and, rarely, metastatic spread can lead to the patient's demise. Fortunately, in 75% of patients, the tumor is encapsulated, and it can be removed in its entirety. In the remaining 25%, local extension is evident.

Two surgical procedures have been offered: transcervical and the transsternal thymectomy. In 1994, the pendulum seems to have swung toward transsternal thymectomy with complete removal of the thymus and surrounding mediastinal tissue. Shortly after the procedure, there may be an unstable short-lived improvement, and careful management of anti-AChE medication is needed. Patients who have a remission after thymectomy and then a disease relapse or patients who do not respond to thymectomy should be reassessed for persistent thymic tissue. Reoperation in these patients may result in significant improvement. In patients older than age 30 years, some clinicians repeat CT scans of the chest at 3- to 5-year intervals, because patients with MG may develop thymomas years after the onset of the disease. Patients with thymoma, in addition to having AChR antibodies, may also have another antibody directed against components of striated muscle, antistriational muscle antibodies. They are present in approximately 84% of patients with thymoma and are of uncertain significance. Patients with thymoma who have had the tumor removed may develop MG as many as 12 years after thymectomy. It is believed that pathogenic lymphocytes with a half-life of up to 10 to 12 years still circulate after thymectomy.

CORTICOSTEROIDS

Corticosteroids lead to improvement of muscle strength in 90% of patients with MG. However, improvement is delayed, with the onset appearing approximately 13 days after the initiation of therapy and becoming maximum as late as several months after the start of therapy. In MG, corticosteroid therapy has a relatively unique hazard: improvement in strength is frequently preceded by deterioration of the patient's clinical status. This decrease in muscle strength generally appears several days after the administration of these drugs and may persist for 10 days or more. After improvement of muscle strength is apparent, no further decline is expected. Patients with MG can develop the familiar complications of high-dose prolonged corticosteroid use, such as increased incidence of peptic ulcer, glucose intolerance, hypertension, weight gain, infectious and psychological complications, cataracts, osteoporosis, aseptic necrosis, and steroid myopathy. Critically ill patients, or patients with a history of gastrointestinal bleeding, should have prophylaxis considered. Adequate exercise, calcium, and perhaps, supplementation with vitamin D are advisable. In anticipation of the mineralocorticoid effects of some corticosteroid preparations, one should monitor serum potassium levels and administer potassium chloride if needed. No one corticosteroid preparation is clearly superior to another. Unfortunately, there are no randomized trials of these drugs in MG. However, their use is almost universally believed to lead to improvement in the clinical status.

The usual doses in moderate to severe disease are in the range of 60 to 100 mg of prednisone. The patient with moderate to severe generalized MG should be observed closely in the hospital prior to administration of corticosteroid therapy. This precaution is taken to manage the corticosteroid-induced exacerbation properly. In critically ill patients, particularly those receiving mechanical ventilatory support, high-dose intravenous methylprednisolone (Solu-Medrol, 2000 mg) every 3 days for total of three doses can be administered. In general, the administration should be prolonged over a 12-hour period. This can be followed by maintenance oral prednisone at a dose of 30 to 60 mg daily. Improvement occurs more rapidly, and exacerbation of weakness occurs somewhat earlier. In patients who are considered candidates for corticosteroid therapy who are only mildly to moderately ill, one may attenuate some of the decrement in muscle strength from these drugs by starting with low-dose alternate-day therapy with 10 to 20 mg daily of prednisone and increasing the dose by 5 to 10 mg at weekly intervals while carefully observing the patient. With this method, improvement begins in approximately 10 to 30 days after corticosteroid therapy is initiated.

Most patients should receive such therapy for a minimum of 1 year. Patients will have relapses if the maintenance dose is reduced too rapidly and are more likely to maintain improvement if the daily dose is reduced slowly by 5 mg every other week until 20 mg daily is reached. At this point, if the patient has had a remission and has been thymectomized, it may be prudent to taper the dose further. If the patient has had neither a remission nor a thymectomy, continuation of the drug for another year prior to attempting to withdraw it would be suggested. Thymectomy should be considered.

NONSTEROIDAL IMMUNE SUPPRESSION

The most widely used nonsteroidal immune suppressive drug in MG is azathioprine (Imuran) given at a dosage of 1 to 3 mg per kg per day orally. A host of other agents have been utilized, and the next most frequent is cyclophosphamide (Cytoxan). Approximately 80 to 90% of patients achieve an improved steady state with azathioprine. The onset of improvement is delayed for approximately 2 to 6 months after the initiation of therapy. Azathioprine would be recommended for patients with moderate to severe disease who do not have adequate improvement while receiving doses of corticosteroids that have the potential to produce significant side effects. Additionally, after obtaining clinical improvement with combined corticosteroid/azathioprine therapy, azathioprine may be continued alone and lead to prolonged improvement after the corticosteroids have been stopped. Prior to the onset of improvement, an increase in red blood cell mean corpuscular volume is noted. Major toxicities with azathioprine include leukopenia, pancytopenia, pancreatitis, and hepatotoxicity. Complete blood counts should be monitored weekly after initiation of the drug, and then, once a stable dose has been achieved, biweekly would be adequate.

Cyclosporine (Sandimmune) has been the subject of several trials and yields improvement earlier than one sees with azathioprine and is somewhat more delayed in comparison with corticosteroids. However, its significant toxicity, which includes nephrotoxicity, hepatotoxicity, hypertension, hirsutism, and tremor, limits its use. Cyclosporine is generally given in a dose of 3 to 5 mg per kg per day orally. Because the toxicity is correlated with elevated trough plasma levels, these should be monitored as should serum creatinine, electrolytes, and transaminases. Trough plasma cyclosporine levels should be followed.

PLASMAPHERESIS

The removal of plasma from patients with MG and its replacement with saline and albumin is useful in the short-term control of MG. Plasmapheresis is used (usually in combination with other therapeutic modalities) in severely ill patients who require mechanical ventilation or whose disease is refractory to other forms of therapy. Plasmapheresis is also useful for preoperative preparation in patients undergoing thymectomy. In general, 2 to 3 liters of plasma are removed every other day.

Improvement usually occurs by the end of the first week of therapy. However, it may appear as early as after the first treatment, or it may be more delayed. Improvement is correlated to a decline in AChR titer, although other reasons for improvement have been postulated. Improvement can be prolonged by concomitant use of immunosuppressive agents (corticosteroids and azathioprine) that prevent re-elevation of the AChR antibody titer. Unfortunately, plasmapheresis is an expensive labor-intensive procedure and may lead to further immunosuppression in patients who are already immunocompromised. Infectious complications, hypotension, hypocalcemia, and vascular access difficulties may be noted. Immunoabsorption is a modification of plasmapheresis using an affinity gel resin or a column with a staphylococcal protein A that adsorbs immunoglobulin G, including AChR antibody. Although theoretically more specific, in clinical practice, the exact role of these latter modalities and whether they are more advantageous than plasmapheresis is not known.

INTRAVENOUS IMMUNOGLOBULIN

Intravenous immunoglobulin (IVIG) has appeal in the treatment of MG, because the toxicities of many of the aforementioned immunosuppressive therapies overlap, particularly with regard to infectious complications. IVIG has a different side-effect profile and does not expose patients to the same infectious risks. With this procedure, commercially prepared IVIG in a dose of 400 mg per kg per day for 5 consecutive days or 1 gram per kg per day on days 1 and 3 of therapy is administered. Response to this therapy may occur after approximately 4 days. The duration of response varies from 30 to 60 days. The response to IVIG is more durable if patients receive concomitant corticosteroid therapy. In general, 75% of patients respond, and repeated doses may be administered. As is the case with many of the therapies to date, there are no prospective randomized trials with IVIG. Because the hallmark of MG is fluctuation, it is uncertain whether the improvement that has been noted is IVIG induced or spontaneous. A major disadvantage of this form of therapy is the expense and the concern about injecting human blood products. Furthermore, as has been described with corticosteroids, a mild short-lived decreased in strength may occur. Volume overload, anaphylactic reactions, and headaches are additional complications.

NEONATAL MG

Twelve to twenty percent of infants born to mothers with MG will develop weakness shortly after birth, generally within the first few hours of life. The symptoms may appear as a weak suck or cry. The infants may have more generalized weakness and may, unfortunately, manifest respiratory difficulty. Interestingly, mothers who have relatively mild disease may give birth to an infant who is severely afflicted and mothers with severe disease may have a normal infant.

Originally, it was hypothesized that maternal-fetal transfer of immunoglobulin precipitated the disease in the infant; however, in afflicted infants, the specificities of the antibodies differ from those of their mothers. It is believed that the antibody production occurs in the infant. The disease is generally managed by support of vital functions, and in the case of respiratory difficulty, endotracheal intubation and ventilatory assistance may be needed. The diagnosis may be supported by the administration of 0.1 mg of edrophonium. Neostigmine 0.03 mg per kg intramuscularly may be given every 3 hours and titrated by observing the response, as described in the section on titration of anti-AChE medication.

PREGNANCY

Pregnancy may have no effect on muscle strength in MG; however, in some patients, there may be improvement, or there may be worsening of symptoms. The latter may be most marked after delivery. Patients with severe disease before the onset of pregnancy are more likely to suffer an exacerbation. Therapy may continue as in the nongravid state. The major exception being avoidance of medications having teratogenic effects, in particular nonsteroidal immunosuppressive agents. Because many patients are young women in their childbearing years who may be receiving drugs such as azathioprine, appropriate discussion of contraception or referral to a physician who would assist with birth control is indicated. If a Caesarean section is necessary (MG is not an indication for Caesarean section), general or spinal anesthesia would be preferred. The large volumes of local anesthetics needed for epidural anesthesia may exacerbate weakness. Many agents used in MG may be discovered in breast milk, and breast-feeding may be contraindicated.

OCULAR MYASTHENIA

Fifteen percent of patients have MG limited to the extraocular muscles. The diplopia and ptosis may significantly interfere with activities of daily living. Troublesome diplopia may require the administration of corticosteroids. Rarely is thymectomy advocated. Ptosis is generally controlled by anti-AChE medications. Eyeglasses with props may be helpful in ptosis. If acceptable to the patient, patching the eye may relieve diplopia.

MANAGEMENT OF MYASTHENIC CRISIS

One of the most dreaded complications of MG is myasthenic crisis. This is characterized by increased weakness, often with accentuated bulbar weakness and fatigue of the respiratory muscles. For the most part, patients have had an unstable clinical course for a period of time, or they have been on a downward trend over several weeks to months when an acute precipitating event prompts the crisis. Occasionally, respiratory failure may develop in a patient whose disease has been relatively stable. Although this latter event may happen unexpectedly, there is usually a significant precipitating event. Notable precipitating factors include infection, surgery, and other significant stresses. In some patients, a recent history of increasing doses of anti-AChE drug therapy may be obtained. Increasing the dosage of these agents may accelerate the deterioration by desensitizing the AChR to ACh. In addition, these agents may promote the accumulation of secretions that may be aspirated. Anti-AChE agents may cause bronchospasm, which reduces pulmonary compliance and heightens respiratory muscle fatigue. In this situation, a rapid assessment of the patient's clinical status should be carried out. These patients should be cared for in an intensive care unit to monitor their course closely.

General guidelines for the intubation of patients in myasthenia crisis include a vital capacity of less than 15 mL per kg (it should be mentioned that patients with facial weakness may not be able to comply with the spirometric measurements due to their inability to form a seal around the spirometer) and a negative inspiratory pressure of less than 40 cmH$_2$O. Undue dyspnea, with no other explanation, inability to handle secretions, and a respiratory rate of greater than 35 breaths per minute are all cause for concern. Once the patient retains carbon dioxide, one should be prepared for incipient respiratory arrest. In these circumstances, it is better not to delay intubation, because the course can abruptly worsen with the sudden supraimposition of respiratory failure. One should ascertain whether there are any reversible components to the weakness, such as hypokalemia. This should be rapidly treated. Once the airway is secured, it may be appropriate to sedate the patient and control the ventilation to rest the neuromuscular junctions. Anti-AChR medications should be omitted completely and may be reinstituted after 48 to 72 hours, initially in small dosages. Correction of electrolyte disturbances and treatment of infection should be a priority at this point. Once anti-AChR medications are reintroduced, voluminous amounts of secretions may be present, and appropriate suctioning should be ensured. Anticholinergic drying agents may be utilized. Prophylaxis for gastrointestinal hemorrhage and deep venous thrombosis should be administered. Patients in crisis are generally managed by the administration of multiple therapeutic modalities. Corticosteroids, either in high doses or in pulse therapy, may be given. Either plasmapheresis (preferably) or IVIG should also be considered. In general, with these measures, within 7 to 10 days, patients may be weaned from mechanical ventilatory support. In patients without significant pulmonary disease, the same parameters that were used for intubation may be applied for extubation. As a rough guideline, if the patient is still intubated at the end of 14 to 21 days, a tracheostomy should be considered. This should also be considered in patients whose secretions cannot be managed with an endotracheal tube.

TRIGEMINAL NEURALGIA

method of
SETH M. ZEIDMAN, M.D., and
RICHARD B. NORTH, M.D.
The Johns Hopkins University School of Medicine
Baltimore, Maryland

Trigeminal neuralgia is a painful condition of the face characterized by paroxysmal, transient, lancinating pain confined to the trigeminal sensory territory on one side of the face. Ordinarily, there is no associated sensory loss. It can be triggered by innocuous mechanical stimuli, including a breeze on the face, brushing the teeth, chewing, and swallowing. Patients frequently report specific trigger zones. It often presents in a series of exacerbations and remissions.

Trigeminal neuralgia is an entirely clinical entity. Performance of a focused history and neurologic examination is both necessary and sufficient to confirm the diagnosis; this should be directed toward excluding patients with posterior fossa tumor, arteriovenous malformation (AVM), or multiple sclerosis (MS). Although 5% of patients with MS initially present with trigeminal neuralgia, nearly all have concurrent clinical symptoms of MS.

Computed tomography and magnetic resonance imaging (MRI) rarely disclose a lesion as the source of the trigeminal neuralgia. Patients with posterior fossa tumor or AVM occasionally present with classic trigeminal neuralgia. Most have atypical, constant facial pain, trigeminal sensory or motor deficits, or a neurologic deficit outside of the trigeminal distribution. Aberrant blood vessels compressing the trigeminal root, considered to be responsible for the trigeminal neuralgia, are nearly always beyond the resolution of angiography or MRI. Prolonged trigeminal nerve latency during evoked-potential measurement is not reliable for diagnosis or as a prognostic indicator of the treatment outcome.

TREATMENT
Medical Therapy

Trigeminal neuralgia is unresponsive to conventional analgesics. Response to specific medical therapy, in fact, can be useful in diagnosing trigeminal neuralgia. Some investigators consider the patient response to carbamazepine (Tegretol) to be diagnostic in an adequate trial uncompromised by allergy or toxicity. Appropriate medical therapy results in a 90% initial resolution rate, but most patients eventually do not respond. Medical therapy may fail due to breakthrough pain or undesirable side effects, including bone marrow suppression and hepatotoxicity. The three most effective drugs, in order of preference, are carbamazepine, baclofen (Lioresal), and phenytoin (Dilantin). Our protocol calls for the following starting doses and maximal dosages: carbamazepine 100 mg twice daily (maximum, 1200 mg per day), baclofen 10 mg every 8 hours (maximum, 80 mg per day), and phenytoin 100 mg every 8 hours (maximum determined by levels).

The doses are titrated to efficacy or toxicity. Limitations to carbamazepine include hypersensitivity reactions precluding the use of the drug, e.g., dizziness, drowsiness, mental dullness, and ataxia. Baclofen is not usually helpful for refractory trigeminal neuralgia in patients who tolerate high doses of carbamazepine. Drug combinations may be useful; however, before beginning pharmacotherapy, a baseline white blood cell count should be obtained, because leukopenia can result from medical treatment. Non-dose-dependent and idiosyncratic bone marrow suppression can occur, necessitating close follow-up early in treatment.

If a patient fails to obtain satisfactory pain relief and/or experiences significant side effects from medical therapy, referral for surgery is warranted.

Surgical Therapy

Surgical approaches to trigeminal neuralgia are highly effective. The procedures can be divided into three general categories: simple neurectomy, percutaneous rhizotomy (PR), and microvascular decompression (MVD). Surgical therapy should be limited to patients with typical trigeminal neuralgia.

Simple Neurectomy

Simple peripheral neurectomy or alcohol neurolysis is effective in certain cases of trigeminal neuralgia. Supraorbital and supratrochlear nerve procedures play a limited role in patients with trigeminal neuralgia confined to the V1 distribution but sparing the cornea. The recurrence rate following simple neurectomy is greater than that after either PR or MVD. Infraorbital neurolysis and neurectomy have been supplanted by PR.

Percutaneous Rhizotomy

PR has been the most widely utilized technique for the treatment of trigeminal neuralgia because of its applicability to elderly patients who constitute the majority of those seeking surgical treatment. PR is indicated for patients older than age 60 years, patients in whom craniotomy is contraindicated, patients with trigeminal neuralgia associated with MS, and patients with trigeminal neuropathy attributable to infiltrating carcinoma. It can generally be performed with only an overnight stay in the hospital. PR is performed in the operating room utilizing fluoroscopy. Penetration of the foramen ovale is usually signaled by a wince and a brief masseter contraction, indicating stimulation of the mandibular nerve with irritation of the medially situated motor branch. Positioning the needle within the trigeminal cistern allows free flow of cerebrospinal fluid in most patients, except those with previous PR. The needle can then be advanced under fluoroscopic guidance to the affected division. Stimulation allows more precise localization.

The risks of the procedure are minimal. Carotid puncture occurs rarely, and although it has been associated with ischemic complications (including hemiparesis), this was reported only when radiofrequency lesion generation was attempted with the electrode positioned inside the artery. The risk of death from these procedures is close to zero, and the associated morbidity is minimal.

If the patient continues to have pain following a percutaneous procedure, the procedure can be repeated with a substantial success rate. Alternatively, patients who have not responded to PR may benefit from MVD.

Percutaneous Glycerol Rhizolysis

Håkanson (1981) serendipitously discovered percutaneous retrogasserian glycerol rhizotomy. The injection of glycerol into the cistern bathing the trigeminal ganglion in cerebrospinal fluid has since become the treatment of choice for most cases of trigeminal neuralgia. This can be performed with a smaller needle than the one used for thermocoagulation and is generally well tolerated. Accurate puncture of the cistern through the foramen ovale yields cerebrospinal fluid and permits the introduction of radiographic contrast material or glycerol. Sterile anhydrous glycerol introduced in this manner relieves trigeminal neuralgia with little or no sensory loss in the majority of cases.

Immediately after glycerol injection, many patients experience a transient but, occasionally, profound bradycardia and hypotension due to a presumed trigeminal-vagal brain stem reflex. Many patients require a second injection several months later, and few are unresponsive to repeat glycerol rhizotomy. Reports of 98% initial pain relief with occasional recurrence and an overall 86% complete relief with one or two injections are typical.

The risks of glycerol rhizotomy are lower than those of the other surgical procedures for trigeminal neuralgia. Occasionally, a slight zone of diminished pinprick sensation can persist on the cheek or nose, but loss of the corneal reflex is unusual and most often temporary. Postoperative herpetic eruptions on the lips have been reported in up to 50% of patients. These can be well controlled with topical antiviral ointments.

Percutaneous balloon microcompression is an alternative technique for performing rhizolysis.

Percutaneous Radiofrequency Rhizotomy

Radiofrequency neurolysis is based on temperature-dependent selective destruction of poorly myelinated or demyelinated fibers. The lesion must be created in the portion of the trigeminal ganglion proximal to the unipolar ganglion cells to prevent regeneration or recurrence, and so it is termed "retrogasserian rhizotomy." Radiofrequency rhizotomy inherently diminishes normal facial sensation.

Recent technical advances including temperature monitoring, curved electrode tips, and smaller-caliber insulated electrodes increase the procedure's safety and allow selective coagulation of the divisions involved in the patient's pain.

Lesions are generated by beginning at 60° C for 90 seconds. Initial lesions are made under anesthesia. Subsequent lesions are generated in 5° C increments. Sensory assessment of lesion progress performed between lesioning allows fine control of the denervation. The goal is anesthesia in the primarily affected divisions and hypalgesia in the divisions secondarily affected or harboring trigger zones.

Microvascular Decompression

Dandy (1934) was the first to implicate microvascular compression of the trigeminal sensory root by aberrant arteries and veins as a cause of trigeminal neuralgia. MVD of the trigeminal nerve was first performed successfully by Miklos and Gardner (1959) and gained rapid acceptance. Many series confirming the efficacy of MVD have been reported. The significant recurrence rate following MVD indicates that the etiology of trigeminal neuralgia may be more complex than that explained by current hypotheses. MVD may have an ablative quality, which has been the common factor in all successful surgical remedies for this disorder. Many surgeons think that MVD is the preferred method if there is no medical contraindication to craniotomy and the patient accepts the risks of the procedure.

Sensory preservation by anastomotic and intermediate fibers makes these lesions remarkably well tolerated. The risks of MVD include major stroke or death (about 1%) and ipsilateral hearing loss (about 3%).

The trigeminal sensory root is separate from the motor rootlets laying on its cephalad border. The sensory root and the root entry zone of the pons must be explored for vascular compression by arteries and/or veins. The vessels are frequently in proximity, and judgment must be exercised as to whether they are compressive, in contact, or uninvolved. The veins may be coagulated and divided. The arteries are cushioned from both the nerve and brain stem by a sculptured Ivalon sponge or Teflon pledget. When insignificant or no vascular involvement is found, we sometimes perform a partial rhizotomy near the root entry zone.

If MVD fails to relieve pain, a percutaneous procedure can be performed after a recovery interval. This is likely to relieve the pain.

Results of Surgical Therapy

The best way to compare the outcome of pain-relieving procedures is to determine the median time to the recurrence of symptoms. The initial efficacy for these procedures is good. Many series report more than 90% of patients to be pain-free after any of these procedures.

The median pain-free interval after glycerol PR is approximately 2 years. Radiofrequency PR or balloon compression yield slightly longer-lasting results. The median pain-free interval from MVD is approximately 10 years. The selection of a specific procedure in an individual case should consider these results and the associated risks, in the context of a patient's age, overall medical condition, and functional capacity.

OPTIC NEURITIS

method of
JERRY F. DONIN, M.D.
Pomona Valley Hospital Medical Center
Pomona, California

A patient who has unilateral acute optic neuritis is usually female (the male-to-female ratio is 1:2), about 30 years of age, and in apparent good health. The eye on the affected side is tender, and there is orbital pain, often aggravated by eye movements. Blurring of vision quickly ensues and worsens, reaching its nadir within about 1 week. This visual plateau is maintained for a varied interval, averaging about 2 weeks, following which, visual improvement usually begins. Such improvement may continue for 3 to 4 months thereafter, sometimes longer. Spontaneous recovery of good visual function is the rule. Careful testing usually reveals that the improvement is, in fact, incomplete. A patient may achieve a visual acuity of 20/20 but may demonstrate impaired color perception, depth perception, and contrast sensitivity. A few patients will experience no visual return following an episode of optic nerve inflammation.

In a patient who is in the throes of an episode of acute optic neuritis, the optic disk is either normal or it is elevated and congested, depending on whether the inflammatory and/or demyelinating foci are located distally (papillitis) or well behind the disk (retrobulbar neuritis). Visual acuity and color vision are decreased; brightness sense and contrast sensitivities of high spatial frequencies are diminished. There may be a variety of visual field defects, (e.g., central, cecocentral, arcuate, or altitudinal), alone or in combination with one another. Even when the reduction of visual acuity is modest, a relative afferent pupillary defect can be readily elicited.

A time-honored approach to the patient with acute optic neuritis has been to schedule a comprehensive medical examination, often including a neurologic evaluation. This should still be considered the order of the day. Appropriate laboratory studies should include a complete blood count, erythrocyte sedimentation rate, rheumatoid factor, and antinuclear antibody level. The results of the two latter tests may help to identify patients with immune-mediated optic nerve inflammation, a special category of optic neuritis. To this basic list, one should add a sensitive serologic test for syphilis (like the fluorescent treponemal antibody absorption test) and possibly tests for sarcoidosis, Lyme disease, and acquired immune deficiency syndrome, if indicated by the specific features of a particular case. I am reluctant to order computed tomography or magnetic resonance imaging of the skull or to perform a lumbar puncture in garden-variety cases of acute optic neuritis.

THE ROLE OF MULTIPLE SCLEROSIS (MS)

It has been long recognized that an episode of acute optic neuritis may be a harbinger of MS. Attempts to quantify the frequency of that relationship over the years have led to widely varying conclusions. The results of a 15-year follow-up study prompted two conclusions by its authors; i.e., that the clinical features of idiopathic optic neuritis and MS-related optic neuritis are identical and that an episode of acute optic neuritis represents prima facie evidence of MS.

In view of these conclusions, it would seem tempting to pursue vigorously the earliest possible confirmation of a diagnosis of MS. This would entail a search for areas of high-intensity signal in the cerebral white matter on T2-weighted magnetic resonance imaging and for oligoclonal banding in the cerebrospinal fluid. One should be reminded that such findings do not provide an absolute confirmation of a diagnosis of MS and that such findings do not necessarily predict the occurrence of or possible dimensions of future neurologic problems. In the absence of any proved, effective treatment for MS, I see no justification in telling patients prematurely that they have MS. Following an isolated episode of acute optic neuritis, if a patient were to ask specifically about the probability of MS, I would make the content of my reply bland, hopeful, and sufficiently noncommittal to obviate or minimize undue anxiety.

"TYPICAL" VERSUS "ATYPICAL" OPTIC NEURITIS

Unlike typical cases of acute optic neuritis, some atypical cases may indeed call for magnetic resonance imaging, lumbar puncture, and other tests deemed inappropriate for the idiopathic and clearly MS-related varieties. Optic neuritis has been properly characterized as more a clinical syndrome rather than a topical disease. Within the spectrum of this syndrome may lie optic nerve inflammation secondary to inflammation of the paranasal sinuses, meninges, and brain. There may be granulomatous inflammations like sarcoidosis. The need for more extensive testing, including brain scanning, in such cases becomes readily evident.

Optic neuritis in children is often bilateral, and there may be an accompanying retinitis with macular star formation. It is often associated with viral illnesses, such as measles, chicken pox, or mumps, affecting either the patient or other household members.

TREATMENT

The treatment of acute idiopathic and MS-related optic neuritis has until recently lacked crisp definition. When corticosteroids became available for clinical use about 40 years ago, they were soon the mainstay of treatment for this entity. In the years that followed, doubts as to their efficacy arose. There were suggestions that adrenocorticotropic hormone might be more effective.

During the past decade and longer, a majority of experienced clinicians had concluded that corticosteroid therapy probably did not improve the ultimate visual outcome of patients affected by acute optic neuritis. Despite this collective conclusion, many continued to prescribe corticosteroids for fear of being criticized by colleagues, particularly in those instances where there was ultimately little or no visual recovery. Some of these cases became the basis of malpractice actions.

The results of the Optic Neuritis Treatment Trial (ONTT) were published in 1992. This was a prospective, randomized, controlled study conducted at 15 clinical centers, which was designed to compare the efficacy of oral prednisone and intravenous methylprednisolone, each compared with an oral placebo for acute unilateral optic neuritis in adults. The two treatment schedules utilized were oral prednisone (1 mg per kg per day) for 14 days and intravenous methylprednisolone (1 gm per day) for 3 days, followed by oral prednisone (1 mg per kg per day) for 11 days.

The ONTT study determined that oral prednisone, as prescribed, was not only ineffective but also increased the risk of new episodes of optic neuritis. Also, it concluded that intravenous methylprednisolone followed by oral prednisone hastened the recovery of visual loss due to optic neuritis and resulted in slightly better vision at 6 months. Intravenous therapy did not predispose patients to recurrences.

After 40 years of varying uncertainty, the ONTT study has now provided clinicians with a firm underpinning, both medical and medicolegal, for their approach to the treatment of acute optic neuritis. Oral prednisone is not only not indicated, it is contraindicated. If a clinician feels compelled to prescribe treatment, I would recommend the ONTT intravenous/oral regimen. If such is being considered, the clinician should be aware of the limited visual benefits that may be gained as well as the small but real risk of serious side effects.

GLAUCOMA

method of
M. ROY WILSON, M.D., M.S., and
JASON BACHARACH, M.D.
UCLA School of Medicine
Los Angeles, California

Glaucoma comprises a family of diseases characterized by progressive damage to the optic nerve resulting in characteristic visual field deficits. Elevated intraocular pressure (IOP) is the most important risk factor for this condition. However, it is not the only risk factor and does not even necessarily have to be present for glaucoma to occur.

Glaucomas have traditionally been classified as primary or secondary and as open-angle or closed-angle types. The primary glaucomas (open-angle [POAG], closed-angle, and congenital) are generally defined as those in which the pathophysiologic events that lead to the IOP elevation and optic nerve damage are unknown. With the secondary glaucomas, a clearly recognized, underlying, predisposing condition is responsible for the pathologic condition. The primary glaucomas are by far the most common and will be the focus of this review. Primary congenital or developmental glaucoma will not be discussed.

PRIMARY OPEN-ANGLE GLAUCOMA

POAG is the most common form of glaucoma. As such, it is the most important from a public health perspective. By conservative estimates, 2.25 million Americans 40 years of age or older have POAG. The prevalence of POAG is known to increase with age and differs among races. Recent epidemiologic studies indicate the prevalence of POAG in the United States to be approximately 1.3% among whites 40 years of age and older and 4.7% among blacks in the same age group. Among those 70 years of age and older, these estimates increase to more than 2.5% and 8.5% for whites and blacks, respectively. POAG is the third leading cause of blindness among white Americans and the leading cause of blindness among black Americans.

Additional risk factors for developing POAG include the presence of diabetes mellitus, myopia, and a family history of the disease. Because glaucoma is symptomless until the advanced stages of the disease, it is important that persons with known risk factors be examined by appropriate eye care providers at routine intervals. Current recommendations are that, in the absence of symptoms or other indications, individuals should generally undergo a comprehensive eye examination, including checking for glaucoma every 1 to 2 years for those 65 years or older and every 2 to 4 years for those between the ages of 40 and 64 years. Because blacks have a higher prevalence, younger age of onset, and more aggressive disease course, blacks between the ages of 20 and 39 years should undergo a comprehensive examination every 3 to 5 years.

The importance of appropriate eye examinations is underscored by the fact that current screening methods are poor. The traditional method of testing the IOP suffers from having both a low sensitivity and specificity. Of note is that at least one-half of individuals with POAG will be missed by glaucoma screenings utilizing pressure measurements alone.

Clinical Features and Treatment

The diagnosis of POAG has traditionally been based on a triad of increased IOP (≥ 21 mmHg), optic nerve atrophy, and visual field defects. However, as already stated, IOP does not necessarily have to be elevated, and there is now a de-emphasis on IOP in the definition of POAG. The disease is characterized by a chronic insidious course with symptoms of tunnel vision occurring only in the very advanced stages. Detailed examination of the optic nerve typically reveals an increased area of central cupping. Focal notching and generalized pallor of the optic nerve head are also commonly seen. Asymmetry in the size or contour of the central cups is a highly suspicious sign of glaucomatous damage. Disk hemorrhages are also often present but are often not seen because of their transient nature.

Patients with glaucoma exhibit characteristic visual function deficits. In the early and moderate stages of glaucoma, these deficits are not noticed by the patient and can only be elicited by careful visual field testing. In the advanced stages, only a central island of visual field may remain, but the patient may have 20/20 Snellen visual acuity. Finally, in the end stages, the central island of vision is also abolished, and the patient will be without central visual acuity.

Treatment involves lowering the IOP to a level that will prevent further optic nerve damage. Initially, several classes of pharmacologic agents are used (Table 1) to attempt to achieve this "target pressure." Argon laser trabeculoplasty is usually the next line of treatment. Although high success rates can be achieved with laser trabeculoplasty, the effect of this treatment is typically temporary, and a loss of IOP control is often experienced after a few years. Surgical treatment is usually undertaken when medical and laser therapies fail. In the most common type of surgery, a trabeculectomy, the obstruction to outflow is circumvented by creating a fistula at the limbus between the anterior chamber and the subconjunctival space. Episcleral fibrosis and scarring are the primary causes of failure in this procedure. In eyes thought to be at high risk of surgical failure, adjunctive antimetabolites, such as 5-fluorouracil and mitomycin* (Mutamycin), are used to inhibit scar formation. Alternatively, these high-risk eyes undergo a different surgical procedure involving the use of valves or other devices implanted to shunt aqueous humor posteriorly to a reservoir. Ciliary body ablation procedures to decrease the amount of aqueous production can also be utilized in the treatment of refractory cases.

PRIMARY ANGLE-CLOSURE GLAUCOMA (PACG)

There are considerable differences in the prevalence of angle closure in different racial and ethnic groups. Although PACG accounts for only about 10% of glaucoma cases in the United States, it is the predominant form of glaucoma among Eskimos and many Asian populations. Predisposing factors for PACG relate primarily to the configuration of the eye. In brief, those at greater risk for PACG have small, crowded anterior segments. Thus, hyperopic eyes with small corneal diameters, shallow anterior chamber depths, and thick lenses are particularly predisposed to PACG. Additional risk factors include increased age, female sex, and positive family history of angle closure.

Clinical Features and Treatment

PACG is characterized by closure of the drainage angle of the eye due to pupillary block. With pupillary block, there is relative impedance of the aqueous humor from the posterior chamber to the anterior chamber, thereby resulting in forward bowing of the iris and angle closure. Subtypes of PACG include acute, chronic, and subacute (intermittent).

In acute PACG, the anterior chamber angle is obstructed suddenly. This results in a rapid rise

---

*This use of 5-fluorouracil and mitomycin is not listed in the manufacturers' official directives.

TABLE 1. **Pharmacologic Agents Available for Treatment of Primary Open-Angle Glaucoma**

Class	Drug	Form	Common Dosage and Concentration	Action	Systemic Side Effects	Ocular Side Effects
Beta-adrenergic blocking agents (nonselective)	Timolol (Timoptic)	Solution	bid (0.25, 0.5%)	Suppress aqueous production	Headache, arrhythmia, fatigue, syncope, heart block, stroke, congestive heart failure, nausea, depression, rash, bronchospasm, masks hypoglycemia, impotence	Burning, stinging, blepharo-conjunctivitis, decreased corneal sensitivity
	Levobunolol (Betagan)	Solution	bid (0.25, 0.5%)			
	Metipranolol (Optipranolol)	Solution	bid (0.3%)			
	Carteolol (Ocupress)	Solution	bid (0.1%)			
Beta-adrenergic blocking agents (Beta-1 cardioselective)	Betaxolol (Betoptic-S)	Solution	bid (0.25, 0.5%)	Suppress aqueous production	Same as above, less reactive airway distress	Same as above
Epinephrine compounds	Epinephrine (Epifrin)	Solution	bid (0.25, 0.5, 1, 2%)	Decrease aqueous inflow, improved aqueous outflow	Systemic hypertension	Stinging, browache, conjunctival hyperemia, adrenochrome deposits, allergic lid reaction
	Dipivefrin (Propine)	Solution	bid (0.1%)			
Cholinergic agents	Pilocarpine (IsoptoCarpine, Adsorbcarpine, A Karpine)	Solution	qid (0.5, 1, 2, 3, 4, 6%) qHs(4%)	Improve aqueous outflow	Salivation, syncope, cardiac arrhythmia, gastrointestinal cramping, vomiting, asthma, diarrhea, frequent urge to urinate, sweating	Burning, stinging, conjunctival hyperemia, blurring of vision, miosis, headache
	Pilocarpine	Gel	qHS			
	Ocusert	Controlled-release system	Once weekly			
	Carbachol (IsoptoCarbachol)	Solution	tid (1.5, 3%)			
	Echothiophate (Phospholine Iodide)	Suspension	bid (0.125, 0.25%)			Same as above, also cataract, retinal detachment
Carbonic-anhydrase inhibitors	Acetazolamide (Diamox)	Tablet, capsules	qid (125, 250 mg) bid (500 mg)	Suppress aqueous production	Sulfonamide reactions, including Stevens-Johnson syndrome, blood dyscrasias, urolithiasis, metabolic acidosis, decreased libido, paresthesias	
	Methazolamide (Neptazane)	Tablet	tid (25, 50 mg)			

of IOP to very high levels, often to levels of 60 mmHg or higher. The signs include marked conjunctival injection, corneal edema, and a sluggishly reactive or fixed, mid-dilated pupil. The patient experiences pain, blurred vision, and colored halos around lights. Nausea and vomiting often accompany these attacks.

Because of the extremely high IOP, considerable damage to the optic nerve may result within a short time. Thus, an attack of acute PACG must be considered a medical emergency, and immediate referral to an ophthalmologist must be made. Management consists of two parts. Initially, medical treatment is employed to lower the IOP (Table 2). Definitive treatment, however, consists of a laser iridotomy to relieve the pupillary block. Because of the tendency for angle closure to occur bilaterally, the fellow, uninvolved eye should also receive an iridotomy prophylactically. If treated early, angle closure can be reversed with no or minimal damage to the optic nerve.

Chronic PACG is characterized by a slowly progressive closure of the angle. With sufficient closure of the angle, a substantial elevation of IOP results. Because of its slowly progressive nature, the symptoms are usually absent until the advanced stages of visual field loss. Laser iridotomy is performed for treatment. However, the angle may have become permanently closed, and pressure-lowering medications, and perhaps even surgery, are often necessary.

In subacute or intermittent PACG, the symptoms are usually modest or absent. Patients often report having had intermittent, self-limited episodes of mild discomfort, blurred vision, and halos around lights. The IOP during these episodes is high, and the angle is at least partially closed. Between episodes the IOP is generally

TABLE 2. **Medical Treatment to Lower Intraocular Pressure in Angle-Closure Glaucoma**

Class	Example	Dose
Carbonic-anhydrase inhibitor	Acetazolamide (Diamox)	500 mg IV or PO
Topical beta blocker	Timolol (Timoptic)	One drop
Osmotic agent	Isosorbide* Mannitol	50–100 gm PO† 1–2 gms/kg IV over 45 min
Topical steroid	Prednisolone acetate 1%	1 drop q 30 min × 2 then q 1 h
Cholinergic agents	Pilocarpine 1–2% Pilocarpine 1/2%	1 drop q 15 min × 2 1 drop to fellow eye

*This use of isosorbide is not listed in the manufacturer's official directive.

†Exceeds dosage recommended by the manufacturer's official directive.

normal. Subacute angle closure may progress to either an acute attack or chronic PACG. Eyes with this condition should therefore be treated with laser iridotomy.

ACUTE PERIPHERAL FACIAL PARALYSIS
(Bell's Palsy)

method of
GORDON B. HUGHES, M.D.
The Cleveland Clinic Foundation
Cleveland, Ohio

Acute facial palsy can result from many causes, including tumor, trauma, infection, and stroke. When there is no obvious acquired cause and the patient is otherwise healthy, the most common cause is "idiopathic" Bell's palsy. Bell's palsy is acute weakness or paralysis of the face due to peripheral facial nerve dysfunction with no readily identifiable cause and with some recovery of function within 6 months.

The symptoms of Bell's palsy may include general malaise, facial pain, dry eye, dysacusis, dysgeusia, and facial hypesthesia; other cranial nerves also can be involved. Whether there is a prodrome or not, acute disease implies that the palsy progresses over several days or weeks, with the first day of visible weakness defined as day 1. It is presumed that maximal nerve injury usually occurs within the first 2 weeks of the disease.

Physical examination excludes lesions that can mimic Bell's palsy. The clinician should document four points in the chart: (1) all facial nerve branches are involved diffusely, (2) the otoscopic examination findings are normal, (3) there are no skin blebs or blisters (herpes zoster), and (4) there are no ipsilateral parotid

masses. These points distinguish idiopathic Bell's palsy from infection, tumor, trauma, and stroke. The absence of skin blebs or blisters suggests that the diagnosis is not herpes zoster oticus (Ramsay Hunt syndrome) for which acyclovir (Zovirax) is helpful; however, some cases of palsy result from herpesvirus infections without skin lesions.

No diagnostic tests are needed when paralysis is acute and peripheral in origin and there is no systemic disease, provided the patient is followed every 2 or 3 months until recovery is evident. On the other hand, the author prefers to obtain an enhanced computed tomographic (CT) or magnetic resonance imaging (MRI) scan of the ipsilateral temporal bone and adjacent areas if the face is paralyzed to reassure the patient further and support the presumptive diagnosis. CT or MRI scans also should be obtained if there is ipsilateral sensorineural hearing loss. Radiographic studies are not required if the audiogram is normal, the face is weak but not paralyzed, and the presumptive diagnosis is Bell's palsy. In paralyzed patients, a presumptive diagnosis of Bell's palsy must be supported by some degree of recovery within 6 months.

TREATMENT

Eye care is of paramount importance in all but very mild cases and may require many months until recovery is adequate. The author prescribes sterile ophthalmic lubricant solutions during the day, sterile ophthalmic lubricant ointment at night, and a moisture chamber over the eye at night. One convenient, inexpensive chamber can be created by applying a small square of clear plastic wrap to the face with gentle hair setting tape. Tape should not be placed directly on the eyelid to avoid scratching the globe. Temporary tarsorrhaphy, eyelid weights, and springs are rarely required.

If there is no contraindication and the patient is seen before 3 weeks have passed, the author recommends prednisone 1 mg per kg per day each

TABLE 1. **House-Brackmann Facial Nerve Grading System**

Grade	Description	Measurement	Function (%)	Estimated Function (%)
I	Normal	8/8	100	100
II	Slight	7/8	76–99	80
III	Moderate	5/8–6/8	51–75	60
IV	Moderately severe	3/8–4/8	26–50	40
V	Severe	1/8–2/8	1–25	20
VI	Total	0/8	0	0

(From Hughes GB: Acute peripheral facial nerve paralysis. *In* Britton BH [ed]: Common Problems in Otology. St. Louis, Mosby Yearbook, 1991, pp 229–246.)

morning and acyclovir* (Zovirax) 1 to 4 grams per day orally in five divided doses depending on age and body weight whether the face is slightly weak or paralyzed. Acyclovir is not yet approved in infants. Treatment is continued during the first 2 to 3 weeks of palsy; then, it is tapered and stopped. Preliminary studies suggest that acyclovir improves the final recovery. A recent controlled, randomized, double-blind study by Kedar K. Adour, M.D., and colleagues determined that final recovery was better with prednisone plus acyclovir than with prednisone plus placebo (p < 0.05) when treatment was started within the first 3 days. They administered prednisone 1 mg per kg per day for 5 days with a rapid taper over 5 days plus acyclovir 400 mg orally five times daily for 10 days. The results supported their hypothesis that some cases of idiopathic Bell's palsy are caused by reactivation of herpes simplex virus.

Medical treatment after 3 weeks probably is not helpful. The author does not routinely treat beyond this point. The author does not use facial massage or other physical therapy unless the patient requests it.

Presently, surgical decompression of the facial nerve should not be performed unless it is part of an established research protocol. In the near future, the results of a prospective, controlled study by Bruce J. Gantz, M.D. (personal communication) and colleagues will determine whether middle cranial fossa decompression is helpful in carefully selected patients.

The American Academy of Otolaryngology-Head and Neck Surgery recommends that recovery be measured and reported according to the House-Brackmann grading system (Table 1). Grade I is normal function; grade VI is paralysis; and grades II to V are intermediate. "Measurement" refers to observed voluntary movement of the mouth and eye. A centimeter scale is divided into four equal parts. On the involved side, the maximal voluntary lateral movement of the corner of the mouth and elevation of the eyebrow are each measured on a scale of 0 to 4. The resultant sum is 0 to 8, with 0 being paralyzed; 2 to 7, intermediate; and 8, normal.

With no treatment other than eye care, 84% of patients will have normal or near normal recovery, usually within 3 weeks. Maximum recovery occurs by 9 months in all patients. Hopefully, medical treatment will improve the 16% of patients who otherwise have less optimal results. Pending further research, the author believes that prednisone plus acyclovir is the treatment combination of choice.

---

*This use of acyclovir is not listed in the manufacturer's official directive.

PARKINSON'S DISEASE

method of
PETER A. LeWITT, M.D.
Wayne State University School of Medicine
Detroit, Michigan

THERAPY

Once the diagnosis of Parkinson's disease (PD) has been established, the clinician has several options for symptomatic therapy. The easiest choice may be no medication at all. This option is generally desirable when parkinsonism presents little or no disabilities. In many instances, the signs and symptoms of PD can persist in a mild form for months to years. At this stage of the illness, the most important therapeutic intervention is often an open and supportive discussion of PD to counter any unrealistic perceptions of this disorder held by patients or their families. When needed, medications can be used to achieve sometimes dramatic symptomatic relief of most parkinsonian disabilities. This chapter will review the variety of available drugs. The outcomes from their use may be similar, although their impact in terms of costs, side effects, and the complexity of the medication schedule can differ greatly. For this reason, determination of what is best for patients with Parkinson's disease is both an art and the rational application of pharmacologic principles.

Levodopa (Larodopa) and other antiparkinsonian agents can be so potent as to erase virtually all traces of parkinsonism. No treatment is currently known to halt the advance of the disease or to promote the recovery of neurons lost from the substantial nigra. However, this drawback of symptomatic treatment can be easily overlooked by the majority of patients who will achieve substantial improvement of disability from levodopa. Sometimes good symptomatic control of parkinsonism lasts for 10 years or more, with no perception of changes in the underlying disorder. Even the most potent medications for PD often lose some effectiveness over time, or else start to produce dose-limiting side effects. Little is known about ways to maintain the high degree of responsiveness to levodopa, which is generally experienced in the first few years after the start of treatment. The issue of improving long-term outcomes of levodopa-treated patients has become one of the greatest needs for future research in PD therapeutics.

Another direction of clinical investigation has been directed at therapies that might offer neuroprotection against the advance of the underlying disorder. The deleterious effects of oxidative stress have been hypothesized to contribute to the progressive loss of dopaminergic neurons in PD. Much attention has focused on mechanisms of dopamine metabolism and reactivity. Catabolism of dopamine by monoamine oxidase type B (MAO-B) results in the generation of hydrogen peroxide and an ensuing cascade of oxygen-derived free radicals. Several clinical trials have investigated whether an inhibitor of oxidative deamination, selegiline (Eldepryl), might lessen the progression of this disorder. Although there were promising preliminary results, more recent analyses have argued against a conclusion that a neuroprotective outcome was achieved from the use of selegiline. Similarly, administration of the free radical quencher, alpha-tocopherol (vitamin E), in high doses was ineffective. Other antioxidant strategies targeted at the possible causative mechanisms of PD are likely to be undertaken in the near future. At present, patients need to be aware that there are no known factors that slow or accelerate the course of PD. Employment and other lifestyle issues need to be assessed from the point of view of the marked variability that occurs with response to medications and in the progression of disability among patients.

There are several general principles that can help to guide the optimal management of PD. One is to recognize that not every patient needs treatment. Subtle and nondistressing features of parkinsonism generally do not necessarily call for treatment with medication. For example, mild tremor at rest is rarely disabling, because it tends to be suppressed during action. Although cogwheeling and decreased arm swing are also characteristic signs of parkinsonism, there is no need to abolish these features with medication as long as the patient is otherwise free of disability. The available medications for PD vary greatly in their effectiveness, price, and possible adverse effects. The price of medication is such that it can become a major expenditure for a family living on a fixed income (and an important factor in compliance). For this reason, the choice of appropriate medications should be tempered by considerations of cost effectiveness.

When medications are needed to relieve the emergence of disability, a conservative approach to the use of levodopa is warranted. Although symptomatic control of virtually every parkinsonian sign and symptom can be achieved with levodopa, other medications can also be effective. The use of levodopa for 3 or more years is often associated with a declining efficacy of the drug and the onset of problems, such as inconstant dose-by-dose effects (motor fluctuations) and involuntary movements (dyskinesias). These problems are not necessarily avoided by the strategy to delay the use of levodopa until a more advanced stage of PD has evolved. However, many experienced clinicians have concluded that starting treatment at the point of disability is the best policy for levodopa. There are also indications that using the smallest effective dose of the drug will lessen the chances for motor fluctuations or dyskinesias.

The choice of antiparkinsonian medication should be linked to specific therapeutic outcomes. In mildly affected patients, alternatives to levodopa, such as amantadine (Symmetrel) and anticholinergics, can be effective. If symptomatic relief of tremor is desired, good control can be achieved with trihexyphenidyl (Artane) 2 to 6 mg per day or benztropine (Cogentin) 1 to 4 mg per day. Amantadine (100 to 300 mg per day) also can be effective against tremor and other signs of parkinsonism. These drugs can also be helpful for other parkinsonian features, such as decreased dexterity, slowed walking, and excessive oral saliva content. Each of these drugs is a good choice for initial therapy. These drugs tend to be useful only for mild parkinsonian disabilities, and they are not effective for all patients. However, they can continue to add benefit to regimens involving levodopa. Ultimately, levodopa is needed by most patients with Parkinson's disease to attain optimal control of bradykinesia, decreased dexterity, imbalance, and the other disabling features of the disorder, which tend to increase with time.

Both amantadine and anticholinergics can be used in elderly patients, especially if they are introduced gradually and attention is given to possible side effects that might occur. A periodic discontinuation of these drugs is appropriate to determine if they are providing tangible benefits. Anticholinergic drugs can cause urinary retention, difficulty in focusing, and dryness of the mouth and eyes. Some patients experience sedation, confusion, forgetfulness, depression, or other psychic effects from these drugs. Amantadine also produces dryness of the mouth, although it does not act by an anticholinergic action. Rarely, it can cause vivid dreams or hallucinations. Livedo reticularis and limb edema can result from amantadine but do not call for its discontinuation. Anticholinergics and amantadine are usually my first choice for treating mild parkinsonism, although they are not effective for all patients. Amantadine seems to lose effectiveness for some patients after use for several months. In others, efforts to withdraw the drug years later will demonstrate its continuing benefits.

Whenever a new course of antiparkinsonian medications is tried, this clinical "experiment" may or may not prove successful. "Confessing" this to patients on a frequent basis is one way to maintain their confidence in the fickle business of pharmacotherapy. Sometimes, side effects at the institution of therapy are the problem; in such situations, very gradual introduction of medications can ensure that tolerance to adverse reactions will develop. Levodopa is the most likely drug to provide relief of parkinsonian signs and symptoms. Usually, as little as 200 mg per day of levodopa (in the form of carbidopa/levodopa [Sinemet]) will relieve most features of parkinsonism within days. Even patients not needing levodopa for relief of disability can benefit from a short trial of levodopa for confirmation of the diagnosis and to provide reassurance that this disorder can be controlled. Sometimes, patients might wish to use levodopa solely on special occasions, even though they might regard the regular use of this drug as unnecessary.

Eventually, most patients with Parkinson's disease will begin to use levodopa on a regular basis. The benefit usually derived from this drug is such that patients starting this drug should re-assess the additional benefits that amantadine or anticholinergics might be contributing. Often, the maximal effectiveness of levodopa treatment takes several weeks to assess, even though its actions may be evident within 1 hour after the first dose. There is a wide range of optimal doses for levodopa. It is usually administered in the form of levodopa plus carbidopa in a combination tablet. Until the recent release of generic forms, Sinemet has been the only brand name of this product, which is currently available in four formulations. Two of them (Sinemet 10-100 and Sinemet 25-100) contain 100 mg of levodopa. Sinemet 25-250 contains 250 mg, and the sustained-release preparation, Sinemet CR, contains 200 mg. The reason for adding carbidopa is to block the peripheral decarboxylation of levodopa to minimize the peripheral adverse effects from peripherally generated dopamine. For maximal blockade of decarboxylation, daily intake of carbidopa needs to be in excess of 50 to 75 mg. Using the 10-100 form of carbidopa/levodopa, five or more tablets per day would be needed to prevent the peripheral synthesis of dopamine. The ratio of carbidopa to levodopa in these tablets is of no consequence, because it is intake of carbidopa in excess of the amounts needed for inhibiting peripheral decarboxylation. Patients who experience nausea or symptomatic postural hypotension after taking a carbidopa/levodopa tablet may benefit from taking supplemental carbidopa 0.5 hour earlier. The 25-mg carbidopa preparation (Lodosyn) is available from Merck Sharp & Dohme only by mailed request.

Levodopa therapeutics are best guided by the relief of disability. Some patients need no more than a total of 200 mg (in the form of carbidopa/levodopa) to achieve the full effect. Others may require 600 to 800 mg per day in divided doses.

The ideal way to introduce this drug is by a gradually increasing schedule, stopping as soon as adequate relief of disability is achieved. Usually, dosing no more two to three times per day is effective for patients starting this medication. Because symptom relief is not needed during sleep, the early and midday times are most appropriate for dosing. Taking a late evening dose is essentially a waste of the drug and can result also in disruption of sleep as a result of the common side effect of vivid dreams. Some patients can benefit from just one-half tablet (50 mg of levodopa) at each dose. Levodopa can be taken with meals, and this spacing may be optimal to improve compliance. With food, there may be less tendency for the drug to cause nausea, but many, if not most, patients can ultimately change to schedules involving dosing at times other than meals.

Some general principles apply to the determination of the optimal levodopa dosage. Peak absorption of the drug occurs within 15 to 45 minutes after ingestion. Initially, patients do not experience variability in the effects of levodopa after a morning dose is taken. After 3 years or longer, however, more than one-third of all levodopa-treated patients with Parkinson's disease will start to experience problems, such as a perceived wearing-off in antiparkinsonian effects 3 hours after a dose was taken. The wearing-off of the medication effect is common in chronically treated patients with Parkinson's disease. Studies that have compared the peripheral pharmacokinetics of levodopa and the timing of wearing-off events have suggested that the rise and fall in the rates of drug delivery to the brain are closely related to this phenomenon.

The dose-by-dose variation in the onset and wearing-off of levodopa's action indicates that the storage or "buffering" capacity of the brain with respect to levodopa changes with chronic therapy (even though the drug's peripheral pharmacokinetics stay the same). In this situation, it seems that the blood concentration of levodopa becomes a major determinant governing the clinical effects of levodopa. To manage the dose-by-dose variability, efforts to stabilize the levodopa concentrations in the circulation can be undertaken. Smaller, more frequent doses taken at the drug's approximate half-life of 3 hours can be beneficial. Some patients need to take medication even closer together than at 3- to 4-hour intervals. The sustained-release form of levodopa can be helpful because of its extended and more gradual decline in plasma levodopa concentrations. This 200-mg preparation of levodopa has 1 to 2 hours of effect greater than the action of conventional carbidopa/levodopa preparations. With the use of this form, patients can attempt to smooth out the abruptness of the rise and fall in the blood concentrations of levodopa. The sustained-release form can be substituted for conventional carbidopa/levodopa with attention to its longer half-life and somewhat decreased bioavailability (approximately 80% of the fast-acting forms). Many patients receiving it need to take supplementary levodopa in conventional forms to achieve an optimal effect. Because the onset of peak action for the sustained-release form is delayed 1 to 1.5 hours longer than conventional carbidopa/levodopa's effects, some patients need to boost the first dose of the day with a concomitant faster-acting form.

There are other strategies for extending the actions of levodopa. Some patients find that taking levodopa with meals may retard the absorption of the drug (and thereby extend its action), although mealtime dosing may also add a factor of irregularity in the effect. In other instances, meals interfere with the clinical effects of levodopa. The key factor in this relatively uncommon situation is the protein content of the meal. Because levodopa is taken up in the gut and crosses the blood-brain barrier by L-neutral amino acid-facilitated transport mechanisms, this situation can sometimes be improved by limiting protein intake during the earlier hours of the day. Other pharmacologic measures can improve the duration of action. Selegiline blocks the breakdown of dopamine in the brain by inhibiting MAO-B, the main route of dopamine catabolism. A dosage of 5 mg twice a day has been advocated, although because of the irreversible nature of this drug's inhibition, lower doses might be just as effective at completely blocking MAO-B. Amantadine, 100 to 300 mg per day, can also extend the effects of levodopa.

The strategies that can extend the duration of levodopa action also need to be assessed in regard to another phenomenon that commonly occurs after chronic use of levodopa (sometimes in the same patients experiencing wearing-off problems). This problem is one of involuntary movements, i.e., choreic or writhing movements that can range from the appearance of restlessness or fidgeting to an exhausting thrashing or sustained dystonic posturing. The occurrence of dyskinesias seems to be the result of supersensitivity to levodopa's dopaminergic effects. Often, their occurrence coincides with the timing of benefit against parkinsonism. Therapies that enhance the peak effects of levodopa, such as selegiline or increasing levodopa intake, usually exacerbate the involuntary movements. In contrast, switching to a controlled-release preparation of levodopa can, in some instances, lessen the abruptness and magnitude of the onset of dyskinesia. The improvement with a sustained-release preparation may be the result of its more flattened pharmacoki-netic profile in comparison with those of conventional levodopa forms. For many patients, these involuntary movements are dose-limiting features of antiparkinsonian therapy.

Dystonic features (especially equinovarus posturing of the feet) can be painful accompaniments of peak-effect dyskinesia. These problems are particularly common in patients whose parkinsonism began before the age of 45 years. Often, levodopa exacerbates dystonic phenomena at its peak action or when the benefits of the drug wear off. Some patients awaken in the early morning hours with foot or leg spasms as a reflection of this problem. In some situations, adjustments of levodopa intake can be useful to control dystonia. These problems can also be responsive to baclofen (Lioresal) in conventional doses or to drugs with anticholinergic properties. Recently, botulinum toxin (Botox) has become available for selective denervation of muscles contributing to parkinsonism-related foot dystonia. The use of dopaminergic agonists can also be helpful.

Two dopaminergic agonists, pergolide (Permax) and bromocriptine (Parlodel), are marketed in the United States, and several others are under development. These drugs have an increased potency of effect over the natural neurotransmitter, dopamine. Unlike levodopa, the dopaminergic agonists are not prodrugs requiring conversion to an active form, and they are not catabolized in the central nervous system. The main application for these drugs is as adjuncts to levodopa. In situations where the effectiveness of levodopa has declined, the addition of bromocriptine or pergolide can greatly improve antiparkinsonian control even when increases of levodopa do not. These drugs have longer pharmacologic half-lives and can extend the dose-by-dose duration of effects achieved with levodopa. Their potential to improve motor fluctuations may be related in part to less variability in their peripheral pharmacokinetics compared with levodopa.

Pergolide and bromocriptine can be useful for sudden episodes of hesitancy or immobility, which patients may describe as "freezing." Such experiences can be regular or intermittent events. They can occur when patients with Parkinson's disease start to walk, or when they pass through doorways. Although there are certain psychological "tricks" that can be used to overcome these sudden "off" states (such as stepping over imaginary obstacles), the dopaminergic agonists can sometimes improve greatly the effects achieved by levodopa alone. Another application for pergolide and bromocriptine is for partial substitution of levodopa intake to lessen the severity of dyskinesias and other types of involuntary movements. Substitutions of up to 50% or more of the previous levodopa regimen sometimes result in an improved therapeutic "window" between too little and too much medication effect. The dopaminergic agonists are an alternative to selegiline, amantadine, or sustained-release levodopa in efforts to smooth out the dose-by-dose variability from levodopa. Another application is the use of these drugs at night to lessen the occurrence of dystonic muscle spasms that can wake patients from sleep.

The dopaminergic agonists have a much wider range of optimal dosages than does levodopa. Pergolide has approximately 10 to 15 times the per milligram potency of bromocriptine, and so, its optimal dose range is typically between 0.75 and 4 mg per day. The usual dose range for maximal benefit from bromocriptine can range from 7.5 to 80 mg per day (and rarely, more). Typically, dosing divided into three to five times per day is appropriate for the dopaminergic compounds, which can be taken together with levodopa and other antiparkinsonian medications. The introduction of these drugs should be extremely gradual. For bromocriptine, a starting dose of 1.25 mg twice a day, increased by additions of no more than 2.5 mg per week, offers the best chance for lessening adverse effects at introduction. With pergolide, the options for gradually increasing the drug are somewhat greater, because a 0.05-mg tablet (which can be halved) is available. Weekly increments of no more than 0.2 mg per day are advisable. Using this gradual build-up, several weeks will typically elapse before a dose range is reached at which the benefits will be evident. Sometimes, the lowest doses of these drugs will produce an exacerbation of parkinsonian features. The slow build-up schedule requires patience but offers one way to avoid an extremely common problem in managing parkinsonism, i.e., the loss of enthusiasm for continuing on with a medication that, at least initially, has led to adverse effects. Nausea, hallucinations, hypotension, and sedation are among the initial side effects to which patients can develop tolerance so that they no longer experience them.

Other forms of medication are available for managing many common parkinsonian problems. Drooling can be lessened by drugs producing dryness of the mouth. Although anticholinergics and amantadine have this property, a peripherally acting anticholinergic, such as glycopyrrolate (Robinul) 1 to 3 mg per day, can also be used for this purpose. Postural hypotension is common in medicated patients with Parkinson's disease, although it usually is not a feature of the disease. Some patients have an orthostatic drop of 20 mmHg or more without any associated symptoms. In some instances, this measured orthostatic change is most likely a peripheral phenomenon in which measurements in the arm do not reflect the core blood pressure. If the blood pressure drop does produce lightheadedness or the faintness is symptomatic and calls for treatment, a reduction in the amount of dopaminergic medication taken each time can be one strategy. Augmentation of daily salt intake or the use of fludrocortisone (Florinef) can be helpful. Another medication that for unclear reasons can counteract orthostatic hypotension is indomethacin, taken in conventional doses.

Managing PD can be complicated, and it is a good principle to make changes gradually and in only one medication at a time. Although polypharmacy adds complication and expense, it is sometimes the most effective way to manage the range of parkinsonian symptoms and disabilities. Furthermore, efforts to lessen the quantity of levodopa intake may be in the patient's best interest over the long term, even though this goal may result in the addition of one or more medications. Several uncontrolled studies have suggested that addition of a dopaminergic agonist to levodopa lessens the long-term chances of the occurrence of involuntary movements or motor fluctuations, such as wearing-off. This claim needs to be substantiated. If the use of dopaminergic agonists or other measures can eliminate the risk of dyskinesias or wearing-off problems, then it might be possible to use levodopa therapy earlier and in higher doses without the concerns that currently call for a conservative approach with this drug.

Another goal for current PD research is for therapies that might retard the progression of disability. Of great interest is the possibility that an available medication, selegiline, might protect against the progression of PD. Several large-scale studies with chronic monotherapy regimens have shown that the apparent progression of parkinsonian disability can be lessened by the use of selegiline 10 mg per day. However, the basis for these conclusions is unclear, because selegiline has some mild symptomatic effects against parkinsonism that can take weeks to be eliminated after the drug is discontinued. The potential for this or other MAO inhibition approaches in the control of PD awaits further study.

In summary, management of PD requires familiarity with the preparations of levodopa, the drugs capable of enhancing its actions, and the several principles guiding changes in medication. The response patterns to drugs and the prognosis of PD vary greatly from patient to patient. Despite the availability of levodopa for more than 30 years, there has been no definitive answer to the issue of whether this drug should be used conservatively (i.e., only when substantial disability has evolved), as is currently the policy of many neurologists. No new forms of treatment for parkinsonism have been introduced in the past 2 decades. However, a new class of drugs that block glutamate receptors has been proposed as an alternative therapy, which does not act through activation of dopamine receptors. Glutamate antagonists and other novel approaches under development (such as fetal dopaminergic tissue implants to striatum and thalamic stimulators for tremor) could conceivably become as important as the medications currently available, but to do so, they will have to match the efficacy and cost of drugs like levodopa, which is still the "gold standard" for treating PD.

PERIPHERAL NEUROPATHIES

method of
S. H. SUBRAMONY, M.D.
University of Mississippi Medical Center
Jackson, Mississippi

The definitive therapy of peripheral nerve diseases is to identify and eliminate the causative factors. Other therapies include rehabilitation of neurologic deficits and treatment of symptoms related to the neuropathies. Classification systems that facilitate etiologic diagnosis are listed in Table 1.

MONONEUROPATHIES

Trauma is the most common cause of mononeuropathies. However, mononeuropathies and focal neuropathies can occur in nontraumatic settings.

Entrapment Neuropathies

Carpal tunnel syndrome (CTS) is the most common entrapment seen in clinical practice. Patients, often women in their forties, complain of hand paresthesias, typically, with nocturnal exacerbation. It should be pointed out that the pain related to CTS often will extend into the forearm and elbow area and, occasionally, into the shoulder. Hand pain alone is an uncommon manifestation of CTS. Sensory and motor deficits in the median nerve distribution occur late. Provocative maneuvers, like Tinel's and Phalen's signs, are not reliable and lack specificity and sensitivity. Very often CTS is misdiagnosed as cervical radiculopathy, thoracic outlet syndrome, or a variety of other disorders. The danger of not diagnosing CTS in its early stages is the later occurrence of wasting, atrophy, and weakness of the thenar muscles, leading to hand dysfunction. Electro-

Acknowledgment: The author thanks Dr. V. V. Vedanarayanan for his help in editing the chapter and Mrs. Trissy Crosswhite for her patience in the preparation of this manuscript.

myography and nerve conduction studies are excellent tools to document CTS, although in a very small proportion of patients with early CTS, these test results may be normal as well. When encountering a patient with CTS, one should rule out underlying predisposing factors, especially hypothyroidism, diabetes, and rheumatoid arthritis. Previous trauma to the wrist and repetitive hand motions are other risk factors. Weight reduction and adequate control of hypothyroidism or diabetes alone may reverse early and mild CTS. If these treatments do not reverse the symptoms, carpal tunnel release by an experienced hand surgeon becomes mandatory.

Other entrapment neuropathies commonly seen include ulnar nerve lesions at the elbow and entrapment of the lateral cutaneous nerve of the thigh under the ilioinguinal ligament (meralgia paresthetica). The latter leads to paresthesias and sensory loss in the anterior lateral aspect of the thigh. Weight reduction will help this situation. The value of surgery has not been clearly established. Ulnar nerve lesions at the elbow are difficult to localize with electromyographic studies and the entrapment often occurs in different areas, including the retrocondylar groove and the cubital tunnel. Progressive ulnar neuropathies in this area need surgical correction. Other common compression neuropathies seen in clinical practice include radial nerve compression in the spiral groove, leading to wrist drop, and peroneal nerve compression at the fibular head, leading to foot drop. These can be readily documented as such by electromyography and, usually, resolve spontaneously. Acute ulnar nerve compression may also occur at the elbow. One should be aware that acute ulnar compressive neuropathies at the elbow as well as peroneal palsies located at the fibular head can be iatrogenic, resulting from faulty positioning of the limbs during surgery or intensive care, and adequate preventive measures need to be taken.

TABLE 1. **Classification of Peripheral Nerve Diseases**

Based on Pattern of Nerve Involvement
Mononeuropathy (affliction of large, anatomically defined single nerves) and mononeuropathy multiplex (affliction of several anatomically defined nerves), e.g., traumatic lesions, carpal tunnel syndrome
Polyneuropathy (generalized affliction of nerves with no restriction to anatomically defined nerves), e.g., diabetic and uremic neuropathy

Based on Tempo of Evolution
Acute polyneuropathies (rapid evolution of neuropathic symptoms), e.g., Guillain-Barré syndrome, toxic neuropathies, porphyria
Chronic polyneuropathies, e.g., diabetic neuropathy and uremic neuropathy

Miscellaneous Mononeuropathies

Other rarer mononeuropathies encountered in clinical practice include neuralgic amyotrophy, which is characterized by painful paralysis of the shoulder girdle or other brachial plexus-innervated muscles, often following a nonspecific viral infection. If this diagnosis is established after excluding compression in the cervical area, adequate control of pain with drugs, including narcotics, for short periods is all that is needed. This disorder has an excellent prognosis with nearly 90% recovery over a period of about 3 years. The brachial plexus can also be involved by either tumor infiltration or following radiation. The important function of the clinician is to make an accurate diagnosis, because tumor infiltration needs to be treated with radiation therapy. There is no acceptable treatment for radiation plexopathy.

POLYNEUROPATHIES

The term "polyneuropathy" is used to describe a clinical syndrome that appears to involve all the nerves in the body in a generalized fashion due to a generalized metabolic, toxic, or genetic error. Even though the term indicates that all the nerves are involved, this is not strictly true, because most polyneuropathies have a specific pattern of involvement. This is related to the fact that many polyneuropathies behave as "distal axonopathies."

Their pathologic origin involves a "dying back phenomenon" in which the axons degenerate from the tip backward toward the cell body. Much of the synthetic apparatus of the neuron resides in the cell body; proteins, transmitters, and a variety of other substances that are made in the soma have to be transported the entire length of the axon by axoplasmic transport. Therefore, the very ends of the axons appear to be metabolically vulnerable, and in situations that lead to polyneuropathies, axons appear to "die backwards." The largest and longest axons in the body will be the earliest to degenerate. Such axons subserve sensory and motor function distally in the feet. This explains the typical clinical syndrome of polyneuropathy, which often begins with sensory dysfunction both positive (e.g., paresthesias, dysesthesias, and burning pain) as well as negative (e.g., numbness and sensory loss) in the feet.

The sensory dysfunction ascends up the lower extremities in a symmetrical fashion and is soon associated with motor dysfunction. The earliest muscles to be involved are the intrinsic foot muscles with inability to move the toes. Subsequently, a bilaterally symmetrical foot drop develops. By the time the motor and sensory dysfunction in the lower extremities reaches the lower one-third of the thigh, sensory loss and motor dysfunction appear in the hands. This is associated with reflex loss, beginning with the ankle reflex, subsequently the knee reflex, and finally, when the disorder becomes more severe, the upper extremity reflexes. This is the typical clinical syndrome of "glove and stocking" sensory loss and motor dysfunction in polyneuropathies.

There are variations in the theme of polyneuropathy, some being relatively purely sensory and others being predominantly motor in their nature. There is also considerable variability in the severity of this syndrome. The vast majority of patients with polyneuropathy have mild to moderate disability involving lower extremity muscles and often the intrinsic hand muscles. In others, polyneuropathies can be so severe as to lead to ventilatory failure. The severity of the polyneuropathy is often related to its etiology.

When faced with the syndrome of polyneuropathy, the clinician has to elucidate the cause accurately so that appropriate treatment can be applied. Two factors, in my experience, seem to be important in the probability of uncovering an etiology for polyneuropathies. The younger the age of the patient is, the more likely that one will uncover a cause for it. The more disabling the polyneuropathy is, the more likely one will be able to determine its cause. A mild polyneuropathy in an elderly person often will have no apparent cause.

Table 2 is a classification of polyneuropathies that is clinically based. It also details a diagnostic approach to these patients.

Acute Polyneuropathies

In this situation, a patient who has previously been in good health rapidly develops sensory loss as well as severe motor dysfunction over a period of a few days to a few weeks. The prototype of an acute polyneuropathy is Guillain-Barré syndrome (GBS). GBS is often preceded within the past 2 to 3 weeks by a nonspecific infectious illness or, occasionally, by surgery. The disorder often begins with sensory symptoms, such as paresthesias in the feet, but these sensory features are soon overshadowed by muscle weakness. The muscle weakness can have an ascending or descending pattern in GBS. This is related to the fact that the pathogenesis of this polyneuropathy involves a primary affliction of the myelin sheaths rather than the axons.

The symptoms usually will begin with lower extremity weakness, often evolving into bilateral foot drop, and then loss of ability to walk. Within a few days, there are problems with upper ex-

TABLE 2. **Etiologic Classification of and Diagnostic Approach to Polyneuropathies**

Classification	Clinical Clues	Laboratory Studies
Acute Polyneuropathies		
1. Guillain-Barré syndrome	Ascending areflexic paralysis, previous "viral" syndrome	CSF, EMG
2. Arsenic*	Hyperkeratosis, previous gastrointestinal syndrome	LFT, blood counts, urine, hair, and nail arsenic levels
3. Porphyria	Family history, change in urine color, abdominal pain, psychiatric manifestations	24-h urine for porphyrin metabolites
4. Solvent toxicity*	History of exposure (glue sniffing)	Nerve biopsy
5. Vasculitic*	Systemic organ disease	ESR, chest x-ray, nerve biopsy, mesenteric angiogram
Chronic Polyneuropathies		
1. Metabolic disease	Diabetes, renal failure, hypothyroidism	Blood sugar, BUN, creatinine, T_3, T_4, TSH
2. Toxic exposure	History of alcohol, drugs (Vinca alkaloids, cisplatin, vitamin B_6, amiodarone, perhexiline, disulfiram, industrial toxins	Urine for lead, thallium, LFT
3. Nutritional deficiency	Alcohol abuse, malabsorption, weight loss	Hematocrit, serum proteins, vitamin B_{12}, folate levels
4. Immune mediated or possibly immune mediated	Lupus, Sjögren, rheumatoid arthritis, myeloma, sarcoid	ANA, rheumatoid factor, serum/urine IEP, skeletal survey, EMG, chest x-ray
5. Infectious	HIV, leprosy, Lyme disease	Nerve biopsy, Lyme antibody, HIV
6. Paraneoplastic	Lung/ovarian cancer	Pelvic examination, chest x-ray
7. Genetic	High arched feet, family history, young onset	EMG

*May be chronic/subacute depending on tempo of exposure/disease.
Abbreviations: HIV = human immunodeficiency virus; CSF = cerebrospinal fluid; EMG = electromyography; LFT = liver function tests; ESR = erythrocyte sedimentation rate; BUN = blood urea nitrogen; T_3 = triiodothyronine; T_4 = thyroxine; TSH = thyroid-stimulating hormone; ANA = antinuclear antibody; IEP = immunoelectrophoresis.

tremity motor function extending into the shoulder girdle muscles. In about 50% of these patients, a variety of cranial nerve deficits appear, including facial weakness, oculomotor weakness, and pharyngeal palsy with resultant dysphagia. The muscle weakness is relatively symmetrical, and in about 20% of these patients, especially in those in whom there is involvement of the shoulder girdle muscles and bulbar muscles, respiratory failure develops. The patient loses all deep tendon reflexes. There is mild but definite sensory loss in the majority of patients. Typically, the illness does not progress beyond 4 weeks. Sphincter control is relatively preserved, although many patients can go through a short phase of urinary retention. When one encounters an acutely paraplegic or quadriplegic patient, it is essential to rule out spinal cord compression expeditiously. The clinical signs that distinguish GBS from acute spinal cord compression include the lack of a sensory level, the relative sparing of sphincters, and the lack of upper motor neuron signs, such as hyperreflexia and Babinski's signs. However, none of these may be absolute, and if suspicion exists, spinal imaging needs to be performed. In addition, other causes of an acute polyneuropathy need to be ruled out diligently in any person suspected of having GBS.

The treatment of GBS revolves around suppor-

tive care of patients who have varying degrees of quadriplegia, including respiratory failure and dysphagia. Specific therapies are directed at the immunologic mechanisms responsible for the disease. The more rapid the evolution of weakness is, the more likely it is that the patient will need ventilatory support. The patient needs to be monitored for the evolution of dysphagia and difficulty with handling secretions as well as progressive respiratory failure. Such monitoring includes repeated neurologic evaluations of these patients, assessing the need for frequent suctioning, including blind endotracheal suctioning, serial measurements of pulmonary mechanics, and pulse oximetry.

Vital capacity and negative inspiratory force, which can be measured at the bedside, are valuable tools. The frequency with which patients are monitored depends on the severity of the illness and the rate of progression at that time. Thus, patients who already are nonambulatory and have proximal upper extremity muscle weakness with or without mild bulbar symptoms need very frequent monitoring several times during the day and night. A vital capacity below 20 mL per kg, a negative inspiratory force that goes below -30 cmH$_2$O, inability of the patient to keep his or her pharynx clear of secretions, as well as the need for blind endotracheal suctioning are all indications for transfer of the patient to an intensive care setting. A further fall in pulmonary mechanics, such as a vital capacity of 15 to 18 mL per kg, a negative inspiratory force less than −25 to −22 cmH$_2$O, and inability to protect the airway are also indications for endotracheal intubation. It is essential that these patients be electively intubated and not in the setting of "Code Blue," which indicates frank respiratory failure with hypercapnia, hypoxia, confusion, and other central nervous system effects.

In patients with severe illness, supportive care includes care of the skin to prevent trophic ulceration; prophylaxis for venous thrombosis in the legs (using either subcutaneous heparin or pneumatic boots); care of nutritional requirements (with, if necessary, a Dobhoff tube); and monitoring for infection with frequent chest x-rays, urinalysis, and blood studies. Cardiac and blood pressure monitoring are essential in severely involved patients, because autonomic dysfunction is a frequent accompaniment of GBS. The prognosis for GBS is excellent, with 80% of patients making a complete recovery and about 20% having mild to moderate residual dysfunction. However, the mortality rate for this disease remains at about 2 to 3%, and the causes of death include infections, pulmonary embolism, and dysautonomia.

The specific treatment for GBS is undergoing evolution. Over the last 7 years, plasma exchange has become the treatment of choice for GBS. Exchanges are performed at the rate of 3 to 3.5 liters per session every other day for a total of three to five exchanges. Such therapy reduces the time spent on a ventilator and the number of days spent in the hospital and quickens the recovery of motor function. It prevents many patients from reaching a point of ventilatory support. Equally good results may be obtained by a simpler procedure involving the infusion of immunoglobulins* intravenously at a rate of 400 mg per kg per day for a total of 5 days. This therapy needs further confirmation of its usefulness.

Other illnesses can give rise to acute polyneuropathies. It is important to recognize them and differentiate them from GBS, because they need other types of specific therapies rather than plasma exchange or immunoglobulin infusion. Acute arsenical poisoning gives rise to a peripheral nerve syndrome that is identical to GBS with rapid evolution of ascending paralysis, elevation of cerebrospinal fluid protein, and in the early stages, electrodiagnostic abnormalities that are very similar. The diagnosis of arsenical neuropathy should be suspected if there is other evidence of systemic toxicity, such as abnormal liver function test results and abnormal bone marrow function indicated by leukopenia or thrombocytopenia. The diagnosis can be further substantiated by measuring 24-hour urinary levels of arsenic, although this may not be elevated for long periods of time after a single acute exposure, because of the short half-life of arsenic. Other tissues that are useful for measurement of arsenic include hair and nails, which retain arsenic for long periods after exposure. The treatment of acute arsenical intoxication includes all the supportive care mentioned in GBS. The role of chelation therapy either with British anti-Lewisite (BAL) or with D-penicillamine (Cuprimine) is unclear. Only small series of patients have been treated but none in a prospective randomized study. BAL may be given in a dose of 2.5 mg per kg four times a day for 2 days, two times a day for day 3, and once a day for 10 days. An alternative is to administer D-penicillamine in a dose of 250 mg four times a day and measure 24-hour urines for arsenic for the next 72 hours. If penicillamine increases the urinary arsenic level, the treatment is continued until the arsenic level falls below 25 µg per 24 hours. Recovery from arsenical neuropathy takes a long time, because of the severe axonal degeneration.

Still another cause of an acute rapidly evolving polyneuropathy is that related to inborn errors of porphyrin metabolism. The most common porphyria that causes an acute polyneuropathy is acute intermittent porphyria, which is related to the deficiency of an enzyme, porphobilinogen deaminase. The genetic defect is dominantly inherited, and there may be a positive family history in other members of the family with similar attacks of neuropathy. In the basal state, many of these patients do not have any symptoms. However, on exposure to pharmacologic agents or other precipitating factors that induce liver enzymes, the porphyrin metabolites, preceding the level of the block, increase in amount, resulting in a porphyric attack. The exact pathogenesis of porphyric neuropathy is not clear. Acute attacks of polyneuropathy often occur in combination with evidence of autonomic dysfunction, such as hypertension and abdominal cramping, and also central nervous system dysfunction, such as confusional state and psychosis. The neuropathy resembles GBS.

It is best to prevent attacks of acute porphyric neuropathy. Patients identified as having the enzyme defect should avoid all drugs that are known to precipitate such attacks, and an appropriate textbook should be consulted for a list of such drugs. In the case of new drugs, sufficient information often does not exist. Any drug that is

---

*This use of immunoglobulins is not listed in the manufacturer's official directive.

known to induce hepatic cytochrome P-450 enzyme systems should be avoided. In addition, a low intake of carbohydrates is also known to precipitate attacks, and patients should be encouraged to consume a high-carbohydrate diet. Acute attacks of porphyric neuropathy are treated with glucose infusions (500 grams per 24 hours). In addition, intravenous infusion of hemin at a dose of 1 to 4 mg per kg per day for 3 to 14 days is often useful in producing rapid remission of symptoms, presumably by suppressing the enzymes that have been induced during the attack. Drugs that are useful for treating pain and anxiety include chlorpromazine (Thorazine), meperidine (Demerol), and morphine.

An acute polyneuropathy can occur in patients who are admitted to critical care units for other reasons, such as sepsis, making weaning from the ventilator more difficult. In a proportion of such individuals, electrodiagnostic studies and sural nerve morphology suggest the presence of an axonal neuropathy that is quite distinct from GBS, and the term "critical illness polyneuropathy" has been applied to this syndrome. The pathogenesis of this syndrome is unclear and seems to involve the length of stay in the intensive care unit and, perhaps, may also be related to elevations of blood glucose and lowering of serum albumin during such critical care. It is important to identify this and distinguish it from GBS, because it will not respond to plasma exchange and there is no known treatment. It is also important to note that, in some individuals in critical care units, a primary muscle disease develops, such as rhabdomyolysis with myoglobinuria or a myopathy of uncertain etiology. Again, it is important to recognize this, because such a myopathy may have a better prognosis with quicker recovery than an axonal degeneration type of neuropathy.

Chronic Polyneuropathies

When confronted with a patient who has the clinical syndrome of a chronic or subacute polyneuropathy, two important tasks need to be accomplished. First, one should be certain that the syndrome is, indeed, a polyneuropathy. Illnesses that can mimic a polyneuropathy include multiple lumbosacral radiculopathies, due to diskogenic compression or lumbar canal stenosis, and cervical myelopathy, due to spondylotic disease of the cervical spine. An adequate physical examination and judicious use of laboratory tests, such as imaging and, particularly, electromyography, are useful in making the diagnosis of peripheral polyneuropathy. The second task of the clinician is to establish an etiology for the polyneuropathy. This often can be a daunting task. Important

causes of polyneuropathy have been listed in Table 2.

Diabetic Polyneuropathy

Diabetes is one of the most common causes of polyneuropathies in clinical practice. The most common peripheral nerve syndrome caused by diabetes is a distal symmetrical polyneuropathy, which is indistinguishable from many other causes of polyneuropathy. The prevalence of symptomatic diabetic neuropathy is related to the duration of the diabetes. About 50% of diabetic patients with a duration of diabetes for 25 years will have symptomatic polyneuropathy. In most of the patients, diabetic neuropathy remains a mild to moderate illness, although disabling sensory symptoms, such as pain and burning, may be found. The treatment of such diabetic polyneuropathy at the moment remains strict control of hyperglycemia. Studies have shown that peripheral nerve function improves with a stricter control of blood glucose levels by using continuous infusion methods than can be achieved with routine types of therapy. Other groups of drugs have been tried in diabetic polyneuropathy based on current hypotheses of the pathogenesis of diabetic neuropathy. Based on studies showing a reduction in *myo*-inositol levels in the nerves of animal models of diabetic polyneuropathy and studies demonstrating an accumulation of sugar alcohols, such as sorbitol, from the activity of aldose reductase, *myo*-inositol supplementation and drugs capable of inhibiting aldose reductase, such as sorbinil (not available in the United States), have been tried in diabetic polyneuropathy. Small studies have not revealed any significant beneficial effect of such modalities of treatment.

Diabetes can affect the peripheral nervous system in several other ways. Diabetic patients may be more prone to entrapment neuropathies, and such superimposed lesions need to be recognized and treated with appropriate surgery. Another fairly common clinical situation is one in which the patient presents with rapid evolution of pain and profound muscle weakness involving the proximal lower extremity muscles, often bilateral but nevertheless asymmetrical. Initially, the pain is severe and often nocturnal in character. As the pain gets somewhat better, the patient notices progressive weakness, particularly involving the thigh muscles, such as the quadriceps and iliopsoas. Although the term "femoral neuropathy" has been used to describe such an illness, in our experience, this illness has never been confined to the distribution of the femoral nerve but seems to involve primarily the muscles in the distribution of the lumbar plexus. The important task is to recognize that this is a complication of diabetes and exclude other causes of a similar nerve lesion, such as compression or infiltration of the same nerve roots, either at the level of the lumbosacral spine or at the level of the lumbar plexus. Adequate control of pain needs to be achieved. Strict diabetes control needs to be instituted. The patient can be reassured that this illness usually has a good prognosis with nearly complete recovery occurring over a period of 1 year or more. This entity has been variously described in the literature as "diabetic proximal neuropathy" and "diabetic amyotrophy."

Occasionally, patients with diabetes will present with pain, sensory loss, and discomfort in the distribution of a trunkal intercostal nerve. These patients often get worked up for intra-abdominal pathologic conditions before it is recognized that the problem may be along the intercostal nerves. Electromyography may be useful in establishing this diagnosis, and the term "diabetic truncal neuropathy" has been used to describe this entity.

Finally, autonomic symptoms may predominate in patients with diabetic neuropathy. The symptoms and signs include sexual dysfunction, orthostatic hypotension (OH), and a variety of gastrointestinal disturbances. OH may respond to physical measures, such as elastic stockings, high fluid intake, and occasionally, medications such as fludrocortisone (Florinef) 0.1 mg one to two times per day. Impaired gastric motility may respond to metoclopramide (Reglan) 10 mg 30 minutes before meals up to 4 times a day.

Uremic Neuropathy

Peripheral neuropathy is commonplace in patients with renal failure and, probably, occurs in nearly 100% of patients undergoing chronic hemodialysis or peritoneal dialysis. The pathogenesis of uremic polyneuropathy is unclear and may be related to retention of a variety of toxic molecules termed "middle molecules." Reversal of the metabolic abnormalities, either with peritoneal dialysis or with repeated hemodialysis, will reverse many of the symptoms of uremic neuropathy and prevent their progression. Renal transplantation reverses uremic polyneuropathy even better than does dialysis.

Alcoholic Neuropathy

Clinically, it is not possible to distinguish alcoholic polyneuropathy from other types of distal symmetrical polyneuropathies without a history of alcohol intake and nutritional deficiency. It is believed that much of the neuropathy in alcoholism is related to a deficiency of a variety of vitamins, particularly the B group. Treatment of alcoholic polyneuropathy includes strict abstinence and the improvement of nutritional status, including supplementation with the entire group of B vitamins, especially vitamins B_1, B_6, and B_{12}. Folic acid supplementation may also be needed.

Toxic Neuropathies

Barring alcohol, the most common examples of toxic neuropathies are drug-induced neuropathies. A careful drug history is very important in the evaluation of patients with polyneuropathy. Although it is recognized that several drugs may be related to polyneuropathies, the common drugs that do this include certain cancer chemotherapeutic agents (Vinca alkaloids, cisplatin, and taxol*), certain antibiotics (especially isoniazid), some of the newer cardiac-active drugs (amiodarone [Cordarone] and perhexiline maleate*), gold when used in the treatment of rheumatoid arthritis, disulfiram (Antabuse) used in the treatment of alcoholism, recreational use of nitrous oxide, and megadose use (doses exceeding 50 to 200 mg per day) of vitamin B_6. Other drug-induced neuropathies include those related to nitrofurantoin (Macrodantin), metronidazole (Flagyl), colchicine, and phenytoin (Dilantin). Toxic neuropathies due to industrial or accidental exposure include those related to hexacarbon solvents, such as n-hexane; acrylamide; and metals, such as arsenic, thallium, and lead. In each of these instances, it is important to identify the offending toxic agent (by utilizing a detailed history and, when applicable, appropriate laboratory measures) and to eliminate the toxic agent so that the peripheral nervous system can recover. Most toxic neuropathies are primarily axonal in type and will take a long time to recover once the offending agent is removed. Isoniazid-induced neuropathy can be prevented by co-administering pyridoxine 10 mg with each daily dose of isoniazid.

Immunologically Mediated Polyneuropathies

Many autoimmune disorders, readily recognized by internists and other primary care physicians, are associated with polyneuropathy as a complication. These disorders include systemic lupus erythematosus, rheumatoid arthritis, and Sjögren's syndrome. Sarcoidosis may also be associated with polyneuropathy. The treatment of

---

*Investigational drug in the United States.

these polyneuropathies is that of the underlying autoimmune disease and should be directed to the appropriate specialty.

It has become increasingly recognized that a variety of peripheral nerve syndromes of a subacute or chronic nature can be related to autoimmune mechanisms directed solely against the peripheral nervous system. An example of a presumed autoimmune disease of the peripheral nervous system is GBS. A more chronic disorder of the peripheral nervous system that is believed to have an autoimmune pathogenesis is known as chronic demyelinating inflammatory polyneuropathy (CDIP). This is an important polyneuropathy to be recognized, because it is eminently treatable. CDIP should be considered whenever a patient has a disabling polyneuropathy that does not appear to have any other cause using routine laboratory evaluation. The clinical recognition of CDIP is straightforward if adequate laboratory support is available. The illness resembles GBS in many respects. It evolves in the form often of ascending paralysis and is predominantly motor with more modest sensory loss. There is usually generalized areflexia just like in GBS. The cerebrospinal fluid protein shows a similar abnormality to GBS with a normal cell count. Electrodiagnostic testing reveals similar abnormalities, including severe slowing of conduction velocities and the presence of conduction blocks, because the pathogenesis of this neuropathy also involves primary demyelination.

CDIP differs from GBS in two important respects. The evolution of this illness is slower, and therefore, these patients often do not look very ill in the acute phase of the illness. On the other hand, spontaneous recovery does not occur in CDIP. Left untreated, patients with CDIP will gradually progress, and significant mortality and morbidity is associated with this illness. Accurate diagnosis depends on the recognition of the clinical syndrome and is supported by electrodiagnostic tests. A nerve biopsy occasionally helps.

The treatment of choice for CDIP is the use of high-dose corticosteroids. Prednisone is begun in a dose of 60 to 100 mg per day and continued for 8 to 12 weeks as the patient is monitored for improvement in muscle strength. Once this is achieved, a gradual tapering is begun. In my experience, the best results are achieved with an extremely slow tapering of prednisone at a rate of not more than 5 mg per week. This is begun with even-day doses until an alternate-day regimen is achieved in many patients. At any level of prednisone, if symptoms recur, the previous higher level of prednisone is utilized for a longer period. Patients who are unresponsive to prednisone may be treated with other immunosuppressive regimens. Experience with such regimens is

anecdotal, and my preference is to start with azathioprine (Imuran) at a dose of 2 mg per kg per day. It should be pointed out that the beneficial effects of azathioprine may take several months to occur. Both prednisone and azathioprine have numerous side effects that need careful monitoring. It has also been shown that CDIP will respond to plasma exchange. Certainly patients who are severely weak with CDIP may be subjected to plasma exchange as an initial approach; similarly, some patients may benefit from repeated courses of plasma exchange at periodic intervals to keep them functional. Intravenous immunoglobulin infusion may also help patients with CDIP.

A syndrome indistinguishable from CDIP can be triggered by many underlying illnesses. It is assumed that these underlying illnesses trigger the immune mechanisms responsible for the CDIP. Therefore, any time one encounters a patient with the syndrome of CDIP, it is essential that such underlying disorders be ruled out. These include malignancies, such as bronchogenic carcinoma; asymptomatic human immunodeficiency virus (HIV) infection; and a monoclonal gammopathy.

The presence of a monoclonal gammopathy related to a variety of illnesses can be associated with a polyneuropathy. It is believed that, at least in some instances, the monoclonal protein may be directed against peripheral nerve antigenic determinants and induce the neuropathy by autoimmune mechanisms. The causes of such monoclonal gammopathies that can be related to polyneuropathy include multiple myeloma, isolated plasmacytoma, Waldenström's macroglobulinemia, the Poems syndrome, and the so-called monoclonal gammopathy of undetermined significance. The polyneuropathy associated with monoclonal gammopathies may present with a variety of features, including a syndrome that closely resembles CDIP, one of pure sensory neuropathy, and one of mild to moderate sensory/motor neuropathy indistinguishable from other garden-variety neuropathies. In addition, a proportion of patients with monoclonal gammopathies and polyneuropathy have secondary amyloidosis as the pathogenic mechanism.

The method of choice for detecting monoclonal proteins in the setting of a polyneuropathy include immunofixation and immunoelectrophoresis rather than the routine serum protein electrophoresis. It is also important to search the urine for monoclonal protein, using similar techniques. Finally, if a gammopathy is suspected, it is important to obtain a metastatic skeletal survey to look for either isolated plasmacytoma or osteosclerotic multiple myeloma, which appears to be particularly associated with polyneuropathies. Isolated suspicious bone lesions should undergo biopsy. Bone marrow examination is also needed. The treatment of neuropathies associated with such gammopathies includes suppression of the monoclonal protein using a variety of chemotherapeutic agents. There is anecdotal evidence that some of these patients will improve by eliminating the monoclonal protein by utilizing plasma exchange.

Recently, a syndrome of progressive muscle weakness often of an asymmetrical nature, beginning in the upper extremities, and in the absence of sensory loss has been recognized. Such a syndrome has been associated with the presence of an electrophysiologic phenomenon known as "conduction block" along the peripheral nerves, which can be detected using careful nerve conduction studies. This illness often superficially resembles amyotrophic lateral sclerosis, but the distinction is made by detecting conduction blocks using nerve conduction studies. The illness may have an immune basis and has often been linked to the presence in the blood of a variety of antibodies, particularly antibodies against peripheral nerve gangliosides known as anti-GM1 antibodies. Routine immunosuppression with corticosteroids is often not helpful; treatment with cyclophosphamide* (Cytoxan) or immunoglobulin* infusion may be beneficial in patients with multifocal motor neuropathy conduction blocks.

Finally, vasculitis related to any cause can result in significant involvement of the peripheral nervous system. The basis for peripheral nerve damage in vasculitis is probably multiple nerve infarctions and, therefore, the disorder is strictly a mononeuropathy multiplex rather than a polyneuropathy. However, in its end stages, mononeuropathy multiplex can resemble a severe polyneuropathy. The underlying causes of vasculitis in this situation include systemic necrotizing vasculitis, such as polyarteritis nodosa and Wegener's granulomatosis, as well as other collagen disorders, such as rheumatoid arthritis and systemic lupus erythematosus. In an occasional patient, the vasculitis may be limited to the peripheral nervous system. It should not be forgotten that peripheral nerve involvement may be the earliest sign of vasculitis, and when the peripheral nervous system is involved, nerve biopsy is a very useful technique for establishing the diagnosis of vasculitis. The treatment of mononeuropathy multiplex related to vasculitis is that of the underlying systemic vasculitis. We utilize large doses of corticosteroids (prednisone 100 mg per day often in combination with daily oral cyclophosphamide at a dose of 2 mg per kg). Both

steroids and cyclophosphamide are used for several months before being tapered off. Careful monitoring for side effects is essential. With especially aggressive disease, an initial course of high-dose intravenous methylprednisolone (Solu-Medrol) may be given for several days. The prognosis of vasculitic neuropathy is often related to the underlying systemic complications of vasculitis.

Inherited Neuropathies

A variety of gene abnormalities can result in polyneuropathies. Most of these are uncommon and include porphyria; amyloidosis; a variety of neuropathies, such as pure sensory neuropathy and Dejerine-Sota's disease; as well as Refsum disease. The most common type of familial neuropathy in clinical practice is Charcot-Marie-Tooth disease (CMT). The CMT phenotype is characterized by the onset of a very slowly progressive polyneuropathy, often in the second or the third decade, with gradual evolution of bilateral foot drop, followed subsequently by hand muscle wasting and weakness. Sensory complaints tend to be uncommon with CMT; however, sensory loss can be readily documented, particularly involving proprioceptive function, and follows the typical stocking-and-glove pattern. The progression of this disorder tends to be almost imperceptible; only a small proportion of patients with CMT eventually lose ambulation. However, a significant proportion will need assistive devices for continued ambulation, such as appropriately fitted ankle-foot orthoses, canes, or walkers.

A genetically determined polyneuropathy, especially CMT, should be considered in any patient whose polyneuropathy has its onset during childhood or young adulthood. In the majority of patients with CMT, the pattern of inheritance is autosomal dominant. Therefore, one is able to identify other persons in the family, particularly one of the parents, as being affected. However, the disorder often tends to have extreme variability in its clinical expression in the same family. Thus, rarely, one encounters severe neuropathy in some members of the family, whereas others are often asymptomatic. The occurrence of skeletal deformities, such as high arched feet and kyphoscoliosis, can be a clue to the presence of genetic neuropathy, but these occur only in about 60% of these patients. One variety of CMT (CMT type I) is characterized by severe slowing of nerve conduction velocities, and this may be another clue. In fact, nerve-conduction studies are excellent tools to document the expression of the abnormal gene in asymptomatic individuals. The importance of recognizing familial neuropathy is

---

*This use of cyclophosphamide and immunoglobulin is not listed in the manufacturer's official directive.

that one is able to avoid an expensive laboratory work-up to uncover the causation of such a neuropathy.

In another variety of CMT (CMT type II), the clinical phenotype is very similar; however, the nerve conduction velocities are either not slowed at all or only minimally slowed. Both of these disorders are dominantly inherited. Occasionally, the same CMT phenotype can be inherited in other ways, including autosomal recessive and sex linked. In addition to the genetic heterogeneity of this syndrome suggested by the various inheritance patterns, emerging evidence suggests genetic heterogeneity even among a clinically homogeneous group of patients, such as CMT type I. At least two different gene locus abnormalities can give rise to an identical CMT type I clinical picture and electrophysiologic findings. Emerging genetic techniques will make more accurate presymptomatic identification possible in the near future, and prenatal testing may become feasible as well. However, ethical considerations regarding prenatal testing in a relatively benign disorder, such as CMT, have not been addressed.

At the moment, there is no specific treatment for inherited neuropathies of the CMT type. The patients need rehabilitative efforts, depending on the degree of their disability.

Infectious Neuropathies

Both HIV infection and Lyme disease can affect the peripheral nervous system. A variety of peripheral nerve syndromes can occur in the setting of HIV infection. Demyelinating polyneuropathies that clinically and physiologically resemble GBS as well as CDIP have been associated with HIV infection. These usually occur early in the course of HIV infection when the patients are otherwise asymptomatic. Such demyelinating neuropathies in the setting of HIV infection can be treated in a manner similar to GBS and CDIP in HIV I seronegative patients. However, there may be concerns regarding the use of long-term corticosteroids in patients with HIV I infections. A vasculitic mononeuropathy multiplex can occur in HIV-infected patients usually during the phase of acquired immune deficiency syndrome (AIDS)-related complex. Because of limited experience, the ideal way to treat such vasculitic neuropathy in the setting of HIV infection is unclear.

During full-blown HIV infection, a more garden-variety distal symmetrical predominantly sensory polyneuropathy occurs. The cause of this disorder is unknown. It may be related to direct HIV infection of the nervous system or to a variety of other factors, including nutritional deficiency and the use of a variety of drugs in patients with such severe illness. Finally, patients in the late stage of HIV infection (AIDS) can present with a subacutely evolving cauda equina syndrome, which is asymmetrical, painful, and predominantly motor. There is often bowel and bladder incontinence. This has been related to a cytomegalovirus-induced polyradiculitis. The spinal fluid reveals polymorphonuclear leukocytosis, low glucose, and elevated protein. Other tissues, such as the retina, blood, and urine, can reveal evidence of this virus. The antiviral drug, ganciclovir (Cytovene), may be effective in stabilizing and improving cytomegalovirus-related polyradiculitis.

Lyme disease is a multisystem disease caused by a tick-borne spirochete, *Borrelia burgdorferi.* Peripheral nerve lesions can occur both during the early disseminated stage (stage II) as well as during late stages of infection (stage III). During stage II, peripheral nerve involvement takes the form of cranial nerve lesions, especially seventh nerve palsy, which closely resembles Bell's palsy. Headache and meningismus often accompany such cranial neuropathies, and there is usually cerebrospinal fluid pleocytosis. In about 40% of patients with stage II infection, a peripheral radicular neuritis develops. This is a painful illness characterized by radicular pain, paresthesias, and spinal pain followed by asymmetrical muscle weakness, which is usually more common in the lower extremities than in the upper extremities. An occasional patient will develop a syndrome indistinguishable from GBS. Again, cerebrospinal fluid mononuclear pleocytosis is a common finding. In late stages of infection, a mild symmetrical polyneuropathy occurs, and often, paresthesias in the extremities are troublesome complaints. The diagnosis can be established by estimating immunoglobulin M and G antibodies to *B. burgdorferi* using a variety of immunologic techniques. Cerebrospinal fluid antibodies also become positive. In Lyme disease with such neurologic involvement, the treatment choices include penicillin G 20 to 24 million units per day for 10 to 14 days intraveneously or intravenous ceftriaxone (Rocephin) 2 grams per day for 2 to 4 weeks. Other regimens, including cefotaxime (Claforan) and doxycycline (Vibramycin), have been described as well.

TREATMENT OF PAIN IN PERIPHERAL POLYNEUROPATHIES

A variety of painful and unpleasant positive sensory symptoms occurs in patients with polyneuropathies. These include paresthesias and unpleasant dysesthesias, such as burning and tingling, as well as sharp, lancinating, and stabbing pains. Often, there is exaggeration of the response to otherwise innocuous stimuli in patients with peripheral nerve lesions. In a typical patient with polyneuropathy, such symptoms are the most troublesome in the distal lower extremities. Other features include the interpretation of a nonpainful stimulus as being painful and the perception of a normally noxious stimulus as being more painful than it should be. In general, I treat the pain associated with peripheral polyneuropathy only if it is incapacitating. The specific treatment for the polyneuropathy involved will usually eventually relieve the pain as well. In patients who require it, pharmacotherapy may be tried with the full understanding that some degree of trial and error is involved in finding the right agent. For sharp, burning, and diffuse pain, I use tricyclic antidepressants, starting with amitriptyline (Elavil), doxepin (Sinequan, Adapin), or trazodone (Desyrel). The dosage employed varies from 75 to 150 mg per day. If there is a significant lancinating component to the pain, an anticonvulsant, such as carbamazepine (Tegretol), may be the drug of first choice; alternatively, phenytoin (Dilantin) may be used. The carbamazepine dosage ranges up to 800 mg per day, and the phenytoin dosage ranges up to 300 to 400 mg per day. It should be pointed out that, in elderly patients with peripheral polyneuropathies, the added central nervous system balance difficulties created by these anticonvulsants may be particularly troublesome. Topical capsaicin (Zostrix), a cream containing 0.025% or 0.075% of the active agent, is being reported to be effective in the treatment of painful dysesthesias. Finally, in an occasional patient, I have found temporary use of a transcutaneous electrical nerve stimulator to be useful in controlling pain without the side effects noted with pharmacotherapy.

REHABILITATION IN PATIENTS WITH PERIPHERAL POLYNEUROPATHIES

Patients with significant neurologic deficits related to peripheral polyneuropathies can receive considerable benefit from a good physical medicine and rehabilitation consultation. Physical and occupational therapists can advise patients regarding exercising the muscles that are still functional for optimal performance and stretching and other methods for keeping physically fit. Patients can be equipped with the right type of rehabilitative devices, such as ankle-foot orthoses, canes, and walkers, with the help of physical therapists. In more severely disabled patients, a variety of other devices may be helpful, such as raised toilet seats, shower benches, deltoid assists, and modifications in the home and at the place of work, which can be suggested by specialists in physical medicine and rehabilitation.

ACUTE HEAD INJURY IN ADULTS
method of
J. C. STEVENSON, M.B.,
A. D. MENDELOW, M.D., Ph.D.,
A. J. JENKINS, M.D., and
N. V. TODD, M.D.
University of Newcastle upon Tyne
Newcastle upon Tyne, United Kingdom

A head injury occurs every 15 seconds in the United States. As a result of these injuries, approximately 44,000 people per year will die. In the United Kingdom, 1 million patients attend accident and emergency departments each year with head injuries, of whom more than 5000 die and 1500 are left with permanent neurologic sequelae.

Trauma is the most common cause of death in patients younger than 35 years of age, and head injury is the most common of these accidental deaths. In trauma, the mortality is three times higher in patients with head injury, and death is the direct result of the head injury in two-thirds of patients.

The majority of these deaths result from severe primary brain damage sustained at the time of impact. However, a significant number die of brain damage, which can occur as a result of a secondary intracranial complication, such as a hematoma or hypoxic/ischemic brain damage, often due to a secondary extracranial insult (Table 1). Hypoxic/ischemic damage can be reduced by early resuscitation and intensive monitoring and by limiting the transfer of patients between units to those who are well oxygenated and hemodynamically stable.

Not all hospitals have computed tomographic (CT) imaging, and in the United Kingdom, the availability

TABLE 1. **Classification of Mechanisms of Brain Damage Following Trauma**

Intracranial Mechanisms
Primary Brain Damage
Diffuse axonal injury
Lacerations
Contusions
Secondary Brain Damage
Hemorrhage
Extradural
Intradural
Brain swelling
Venous congestion
Edema
Infection
Meningitis
Abscess
Extracranial Mechanisms
Hypoxia
Hypotension

of CT in different regions varies considerably. Guidelines for head-injury management have been developed using risk factors from large epidemiologic studies.

The main causes of head injury are road traffic accidents, falls, and assaults. Many are alcohol related. Gunshot wounds are a common cause of fatal head injuries in the United States, but they are rare in the United Kingdom.

PATHOPHYSIOLOGY OF HEAD INJURY

The mechanisms of brain damage that occur as a result of head injury can be divided into primary and secondary ones (Table 1). Primary brain injury occurs at the time of impact and consists of diffuse axonal injury, cerebral contusions, and lacerations. Diffuse axonal injury results from the sudden deceleration of the brain, leading to the disruption of axonal pathways. It may cause prolonged unconsciousness, and the outcome is often poor. Primary brain damage is responsible for immediate unconsciousness, and prolonged coma from the time of the accident suggests severe primary impact damage to the brain. Secondary brain injury occurs at a variable time after the impact. Extracranial complications tend to occur early, although intracranial events may be responsible for delayed deterioration in the level of consciousness with or without the development of a focal neurologic deficit.

The intracranial causes of secondary brain damage include hematomas, brain swelling, and infection. Hematomas may be extradural, subdural, or intracerebral. Extradural hematoma is the least common but critically important, because of a frequent lack of primary damage and, therefore, preserved consciousness in the initial stages. It is usually associated with a fracture in the temporal region with bleeding from a meningeal artery, but bleeding from the fracture or from meningeal veins can also result in a hematoma. Subdural hemorrhage is usually due to cortical disruption in more severe injuries, although it may result from tearing of the bridging veins running from the cortex to the dura. Intracerebral hemorrhage is common and may consist of scattered contusions or an isolated hematoma. Contusions in the frontal region are particularly dangerous and may result in delayed deterioration.

Brain swelling is due to vascular engorgement or brain edema and may cause raised intracranial pressure (ICP). Compound depressed skull fractures and penetrating missile injuries may be associated with the complication of a brain abscess and meningitis. Basal skull fractures with cerebrospinal fluid rhinorrhea or otorrhea may also result in meningitis.

Secondary brain damage particularly in patients with multiple trauma may occur as a result of either hypotension or hypoxia, causing ischemia, which may be global or may affect the arterial boundary zones. Adequate resuscitation within the first hours of injury will avoid some of the long-term consequences of hypoxia or hypotension.

ASSESSMENT OF HEAD INJURY

Emergency departments have to handle many cases of minor head injury. It is difficult for the duty doctor to decide which patients require a skull x-ray, which patients should be admitted for observation, and which patients require neurosurgical consultation. A good history is essential to ascertain the mechanism of injury. This should be followed by direct questioning concerning the neurologic symptoms: headache, nausea, vomiting, drowsiness, diplopia, confusion, and focal neurologic deficits. Then, a quick neurologic examination can be done, which includes assessment of the level of consciousness on the Glasgow coma scale (Table 2).

Guidelines have been established and widely distributed in the United Kingdom to aid the emergency room doctor in the decision-making process (Table 3). In the United States, where CT scanners are more widely distributed, most head-injured patients (except the most minor) will be scanned.

RELATIVE RISK OF DEVELOPING A HEMATOMA

Most of the many head-injured patients who attend the accident and emergency departments every year will have minor injuries, but all have the potential for a hematoma to develop. The difficulty is to decide which of these minor head injuries is more likely to cause an intracranial hematoma. There is no single clinical picture associated with a traumatic hematoma. Although delayed neurologic deterioration following head injury suggests the development of an intracranial hematoma, many patients will have no history of deterioration. Risk factors for hematoma have been identified and used to select patients for CT scanning before neurologic deterioration takes place. These relative risks have been quantified by epidemiologic studies (summarized in Table 4).

Adult patients in emergency departments with alterations of conscious level and a skull fracture have a high risk of hematoma (1:5). Altered consciousness without skull fracture or a persisting neurologic deficit carries a risk of hematoma of 1:180. A skull fracture without a change in conscious level has a risk of hematoma of 1:45. This means that patients at high risk of

---

TABLE 2. **The Glasgow Coma Scale**

Eye-Opening Response
4 = Spontaneous
3 = To speech
2 = To painful stimuli
1 = None
Best Motor Response in Upper Limbs
6 = Obeys commands
5 = Localizes
4 = Withdraws (normal flexion)
3 = Flexes abnormally (spastic flexion)
2 = Extends
1 = None
Verbal Response
5 = Oriented
4 = Confused
3 = Inappropriate words
2 = Incomprehensible sounds
1 = None

TABLE 3. **Criteria for Skull X-Ray After Recent Head Injury**

Skull x-ray is not necessary if computed tomography is to take place. Clinical judgment is necessary, but the following criteria are helpful:
Loss of consciousness or amnesia suspected at any time
Neurologic symptoms or signs (including headache and/or vomiting)
Cerebrospinal fluid or blood from the nose or ear
Suspected penetrating injury
Scalp bruising or laceration (to bone or > 5 cm long)
Falls from height (> 60 cm) or onto a hard surface
Suspected nonaccidental injury
Tense fontanelle
Inadequate history

Criteria for Admission to Hospital
Confusion or any other depression of the level of consciousness at the time of the examination (< 5 years at any time following injury)
Skull fracture
Neurologic symptoms or signs even if minor, particularly in children (headache or vomiting)
Other medical conditions (e.g., coagulation disorders)
Difficulty in assessing the patient (e.g., suspected drugs/glue/alcohol/nonaccidental injury)
Patients sent home should be accompanied by a responsible adult who should receive written advice to return immediately if there is any deterioration.

Criteria for Consultation with a Neurosurgical Unit (The first five categories require urgent computed tomographic scanning)
Deterioration in the level of consciousness or other neurologic signs
Confusion or coma continuing after adequate resuscitation
Tense fontanelle
Skull fractures
Sutural diastasis
Compound depressed skull fracture of the skull vault
Suspected fracture of the skull base

---

hematoma can be identified for early CT scanning before neurologic deterioration occurs. CT must be performed when a significant risk factor has been identified and should not await neurologic deterioration.

TREATMENT

The Unconscious Patient

Initial assessment of the unconscious patient should start with ensuring airway patency and adequate respiration. Control of the cervical spine with a collar is essential until a cervical injury is excluded by radiography. All unconscious patients should receive 100% oxygen by mask. An open chest wound or a pneumothorax should be excluded. Arterial blood gases should be taken early in the initial assessment and repeated frequently. Indications for ventilation include: (1) inability to maintain an airway or poor respiratory effort, (2) oxygen saturation less than 90% or an arterial oxygen tension of less than 60 mmHg, and (3) an arterial carbon dioxide tension greater than 45 mmHg.

Intravenous access must be achieved early during the initial assessment of the patient. If hypotension is identified, then adequate fluid resuscitation should begin without delay. Hypotension following head injury is usually due to hypovolemia and is almost always due to blood loss from extracranial causes. However, blood loss from the scalp in infants, compound depressed skull fractures involving a major venous sinus, pituitary trauma, and spinal injury may rarely cause hypotension. In the presence of hypotension or persistent tachycardia, it is likely that an extracranial cause has been missed and a further search must be made. Early correction of arterial hypotension and hypoxia substantially decreases the mortality and morbidity rates from head injury.

During the initial assessment, a detailed history from people present at the time of the accident can be helpful in identifying the mechanism

TABLE 4. **Estimated Number of Patients Attending Hospitals with Head Injury per Year per Million Total Population and the Absolute Risk of Traumatic Intracranial Hematoma**

	Adults	
	Number Attending	Risk (1:n)
No Fracture		
Conscious	10,700	7866
Impaired consciousness	630	180
Coma	75	27
Fracture		
Conscious	150	45
Impaired consciousness	49	5.1
Coma	46	3.6

Based on data in Teasdale GM, Murray G, Anderson E, et al: Risks of acute traumatic intracranial haematoma in children and adults: Implications for managing head injuries. BMJ *300*:363–367, 1990.

of injury and the time course of changes in conscious level.

The Glasgow coma scale is widely accepted for the assessment of conscious level in head-injured patients. It is based on eye opening, the best motor response, and the best verbal response (Table 2). Initial responses should be recorded and the coma scale reassessed at regular intervals.

A hematoma can present with focal lateralizing signs. Localizing signs include a nonreacting dilated pupil, facial weakness, or a hemiparesis.

A full neurologic examination is often neither possible nor suitable in a head-injured patient, because it may delay urgent diagnostic measures or treatment. It is essential to assess the level of consciousness, the pupillary response, and any limb weakness prior to further diagnostic procedures. The progression of the clinical picture is important.

Investigation

Skull X-Ray

Guidelines for skull x-ray have been formulated (Table 3). Fully conscious patients with significant trauma should undergo x-ray examination. An adult patient who is fully conscious in the emergency room following head injury and who does not have a skull fracture can be sent home with a head-injury information card.

CT Scan

A patient with impaired consciousness or focal neurologic signs requires urgent CT. If CT is not available locally, then plans must be made for the transfer of the patient to a neurosurgical unit. A skull x-ray need not be done if a CT is to be performed immediately. If the CT shows an intracranial hematoma, then urgent referral to a neurosurgical unit is essential. Figure 1 gives an algorithm for head-injury management, which has

been proposed in the United Kingdom. Where CT imaging is easily available, early scanning is recommended in all those patients with head injuries with any impairment of consciousness (skull x-ray can be omitted in this group) and in those with a skull fracture, even if they remain oriented. (This group has a hematoma risk of 1:45 for adults.)

FURTHER MANAGEMENT OF HEAD INJURY

If accepted by a neurosurgical unit, personnel able to insert and reposition an endotracheal tube should accompany the patient for transfer. Scalp lacerations should be cleaned and sutured.

Careful fluid management will be required to maintain systolic blood pressure. A urinary catheter should be passed prior to transfer. Finally, the notes, trauma charts, and x-rays should accompany the patient. Observation should continue during the transfer.

Management of Specific Problems

Scalp Lacerations

Wounds should be thoroughly examined for foreign bodies and nonviable tissue fragments. The wound edges should be shaved and irrigated with normal saline, and the wound itself débrided. When closing the wound, it is essential to repair the galea if a subgaleal hematoma is to be avoided.

Compound Depressed Skull Fractures

These fractures require surgical débridement to remove foreign bodies and nonviable tissue fragments. It is important to examine for dural tears. Prophylactic antibiotics and a tetanus booster (if required) are given to protect against infection.

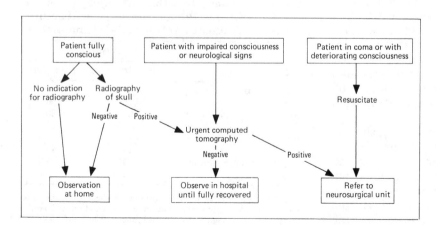

Figure 1. Algorithm for management of head-injured patients in a district general hospital with a computed tomographic scanner. (From Teasdale GM, Murray G, Anderson E, et al: Risks of acute traumatic intracranial haematoma in children and adults: Implications for managing head injuries. BMJ *300*:363–367, 1990.)

Basal Skull Fractures

Basal skull fractures may not be apparent using skull x-rays. The diagnosis is made on clinical grounds. Retromastoid bruising (Battle's sign) or bilateral orbital bruising (raccoon eyes) may be present, and the patients may have either otorrhea or rhinorrhea. Although many recommend that antibiotic therapy should be started immediately, there is some evidence from clinical trials that an expectant policy can be adopted. Persistent rhinorrhea or otorrhea requires further investigation and surgical repair.

Intracranial Hematomas

EXTRADURAL HEMATOMA

Most patients with an extradural hematoma, and all who deteriorate suddenly, will require urgent surgery. Satisfactory decompression is not possible through burr holes, and a craniotomy is required. The bleeding point can then be identified and cauterized.

SUBDURAL HEMATOMA

Surgery is indicated if there is a large hematoma with evidence of a mass effect. A craniotomy is required to evacuate these hematomas.

INTRACEREBRAL HEMATOMA

Again, if there is a significant mass effect and a decrease in the conscious level, then an intracerebral hematoma should be evacuated. Otherwise, it is reasonable to monitor ICP in these patients. Where the ICP is more than 30 mmHg, the risk of neurologic deterioration is high, and evacuation of the hematoma should be undertaken. An ICP less than 20 mmHg is seldom associated with clinical deterioration.

Diffuse Axonal Injury

Nothing can be done to reverse primary brain damage. However, the development of brain edema or an intracranial hematoma will lead to increased ICP, which can be measured with a catheter introduced into the ventricle, the subdural space, or the brain parenchyma. Normal values for ICP are less than 15 mmHg. By simultaneously measuring the blood pressure, one can calculate and monitor the cerebral perfusion pressure (CPP). Maintenance of a CPP greater than 70 to 80 mmHg has been shown to improve the outcome. ICP monitoring is especially useful with ventilated patients in whom muscle paralysis masks neurologic changes.

The medical management of increased ICP involves the use of mannitol, diuretics, and hyperventilation. There is no evidence for benefit from the routine use of barbiturates, high-dose corticosteroids, or calcium antagonists in the management of head injury. Mannitol (0.5 to 1.0 gram per kg as a bolus) and diuretics (furosemide [Lasix]) produce a diuresis that can help lower the ICP. These diuretics will "buy time" for the severely head-injured patient being transferred or awaiting surgery, but they do not benefit patients when used over a longer period of time, because they lead to hypovolemia with a fall in CPP.

Hyperventilation aims to keep the patient mildly hypocapnic (partial pressure of carbon dioxide of 30 to 35 mmHg). Hypercapnia leads to cerebral vasodilatation, increased cerebral blood flow, and increased ICP. In the initial stages of resuscitation, it is far better to err on the side of hyperventilation rather than hypoventilation, but prolonged hyperventilation may not be as beneficial as was once thought.

Careful fluid balance is important in head-injured patients, because overhydration may exacerbate cerebral edema. Normal saline or Ringer's lactate is the fluid of choice. Dextrose 5% may diffuse out of the intravascular compartment very quickly and exacerbate the cerebral edema. Fluid restriction and excessive use of diuretics can lead to hypovolemia and hypotension with a reduced CPP.

LATE COMPLICATIONS OF HEAD INJURY

Epilepsy

Epilepsy can occur following head injury. Patients particularly at risk are those with a compound depressed skull fracture or an intracerebral hematoma. Additional risk factors that make the development of late epilepsy more likely are a dural tear, early epilepsy, and post-traumatic amnesia for more than 24 hours. A loading dose of phenytoin (Dilantin) can be given with safety following a seizure (20 mg per kg injected at a rate of 50 mg per minute). The patient should then continue to receive a maintenance dose of phenytoin for up to 1 year (300 mg daily). If no further seizures occur, the anticonvulsant can be reduced gradually and discontinued. If seizures recur, then anticonvulsants can be given for a further period.

Chronic Subdural Hematoma

These hematomas are occasionally difficult to diagnose and differentiate on CT scan when they may appear isodense with the brain. Magnetic resonance imaging is excellent for differentiating between a chronic hematoma and a cerebral infarction. Patients with a chronic subdural hematoma who are symptomatic require burr-hole drainage of the hematoma. However, small chronic subdural hematomas without a mass effect can be treated conservatively with dexamethasone (Decadron).

DIAGNOSIS OF BRAIN STEM DEATH

In the United Kingdom, brain stem death is a clinical diagnosis. Once it is clear that there is irreversible structural brain damage following a head injury and the patient is in an apneic coma (on a ventilator and unresponsive), then specific tests of brain stem death are carried out. These tests are done by two senior medical staff. The first test is performed when all sedative and paralyzing pharmacologic agents have been reversed and the second, some hours later. Two positive brain stem death tests are required before the family is approached and the ventilator turned off. In the United Kingdom, most regions have a transplant co-ordinator who will approach the relatives and discuss the possibilities of organ donation.

ACUTE HEAD INJURIES IN CHILDREN

method of
ROBIN P. HUMPHREYS, M.D.
University of Toronto
Toronto, Canada

Trauma remains the most common killer of children younger than 18 years of age. A traumatic insult of the central nervous system is directly responsible for the child's demise in 79% of cases. Although physician statements and legislated requirements as well as consumer protection measures have had some impact on the injuries caused by falls, cycling, and motor vehicles, other events, such as nonaccidental injuries and gunshot wounds, are now taking an increasing toll. Those who dedicate themselves to the care of children's traumatic injuries must also act vigorously for the child's protection.

Children may suffer head injuries in a huge variety of ways, some of which causes might border on the bizarre. In this regard, nothing should surprise the examiner. Moreover, a history of head injury lurks in every child's background, so that the physician will be challenged to match the child's clinical condition with the historic information. The governing principle is that the stated cause of the child's present injury matches the clinical findings. It is inappropriate to reconcile a somewhat innocuous explanation for an infant's severe head injury. A useful maxim is that 90% of severe accidental head injuries in children occur as a result of falls or motor-vehicle trauma. A child who is severely injured from unwitnessed causes other than these should be regarded as the victim of a nonaccidental injury.

PHYSICAL ASSESSMENT OF THE HEAD-INJURED CHILD

The triage physical examinations of the injured patient, i.e., airway, breathing, and circulation, apply to all children with head injuries. Children do not suffer hypovolemic shock from a head injury alone, but infants may become profoundly anemic from a surface hematoma (usually extradural). When assessing the child's level of consciousness, the physician must be aware if any paralyzing medications were administered during the initial resuscitation. If they have altered the child's early test results, then either the medication will have to be reversed or allowed to wear off so that an accurate measure of the child's level of consciousness and neurologic performance can be obtained. Similarly, children who have suffered an impact convulsion will have test results that are clinically worse than they really are. Certain postictal events (such as a dilating pupil) can even mimic neurologic deterioration and tentorial herniation.

Coma scale ratings (i.e., the Glasgow coma scale), although potentially incomplete in children younger than 5 years of age, are still valuable with regard to early motor performance. Ideally, the scoring is carried out at 6 hours postinjury when the child's condition is stabilized. The head injury is regarded as "minor" if the score is 13 or better. Focal deficits of vision, ocular mobility, facial movement, or hearing, often reversible in time, are nonetheless noteworthy in the child.

CHILDHOOD CONCUSSION SYNDROME

The majority of head injuries in children are ultimately minor in nature. Their characteristics of "concussion" differ from those occurring in adults. For example, loss of consciousness is not a mandate for every child's concussion syndrome, but if it has occurred, it is typically of short duration. The child is more likely to be stunned after the impact and then appears well. Within the next 90 minutes, drowsiness occurs, and the subsequent repeated episodes of vomiting alarm the parents. The latter spurs medical evaluation. When increasing stupor follows, it suggests the presence of an intracranial hematoma. It is at this stage that the physician must match the historic facts with the clinical findings.

Although the history of the child's injury may be unimpressive and the neurologic and computed tomographic (CT) examinations likewise, it is most expedient to admit the child to a hospital for overnight observation. The vomiting always resolves on its own, and during that time, specific intravenous fluid replacement therapy is optional. Characteristically, the child's behavior reverts to normal within 24 to 36 hours. Late consequences, such as headache, altered memory, or cognitive performance, occur infrequently in this particular group of children.

NONACCIDENTAL HEAD INJURY

It is the legislated requirement in many jurisdictions for the primary care physician to report injuries that a child may have received as a result of nonaccidental trauma. It is believed that upwards of 2000 children die annually in the United States from such abuse. The suspicious physician must seek out the many features typical of the syndrome. In terms of head trauma, these include (1) an uncertain history in which the history of trauma is ever changing or, particularly, appears to be at odds with the clinical picture, and/or the event was unwitnessed; (2) unexplained seizures in association with (3) retinal hemorrhages; and (4) radiologic imaging (CT scan), which shows intradural surface hemorrhages and possibly also unexplained rib or extremity fractures. It is usually the primary care physician who initiates the first alert to the local child protection agency, although resolution of the matter may take days to months after that.

RADIOLOGIC IMAGING STUDIES

Skull radiographs are recommended for all head-injured children (1) younger than 2 years of age; (2) with changed consciousness at the time of injury or with persistent vomiting; (3) with impact seizures; (4) with multiple trauma, especially if facial injuries are present; (5) with a suspected depressed skull fracture, and (6) in whom nonaccidental injury is suspected. It is further advised that a CT scan be obtained in all patients with altered consciousness (past or present) or in those with focal and/or deteriorating neurologic deficit or cerebrospinal fluid leak, as well as in children with depressed skull fracture or penetrating skull wound.

A contentious issue is whether all children with confirmed head injuries require cervical spine radiographs. The incidence of an unstable cervical injury occurring in the head-injured child is low indeed (just under 1%). Nonetheless, it is recommended that all children with severe head injury or those injured by a mechanism that might also place the cervical spine at risk (e.g., falls) have routine cervical spine x-rays taken as part of their early trauma evaluation.

SKULL FRACTURES

The presence of a scalp hematoma in an infant who is injured as the result of a fall almost always equates with an underlying skull fracture.

Linear

Linear skull fractures most commonly occur in the parietal bone in infants and run between adjacent vault sutures. Although there might be difficulty distinguishing such fractures from rudimentary sutures or wormian bones, the suspect fracture, when compatible with the site of trauma and the overlying scalp swelling, is indeed genuine.

There is no correlation between the sometimes startling display of the skull fracture(s) and the child's immediate needs or outcome. In this instance, it is the child's condition and not the x-ray that dictates the treatment path. Unless the fracture is several days old, the child should be admitted for continuing hospital evaluation. No specific therapy is required for the fracture, and the intent of hospitalization is to seek complicating intracranial phenomena.

Skull Base (Basal)

The diagnosis of the child's skull base fracture is more often made for inferential reasons than on the basis of radiologic definition. The clinical signatures of a periorbital hematoma (racoon's eye) or hemotympanum raise one's suspicions about the presence of a fracture that runs through the floor of the anterior or middle cranial fossae, respectively. Specialized CT techniques may be required to define such a fracture. These children must be followed closely for evidence of a cerebrospinal fluid leak and/or hearing impairment.

The leakage of cerebrospinal fluid through the nose (rhinorrhea) or ear (otorrhea) is absolute evidence that a basal skull fracture has occurred. The leakage usually halts spontaneously within 7 to 10 days, but its very occurrence demands a neurosurgical evaluation. The decision for operative treatment of such an injury is based on the severity and duration of the leak, the degree of bony disruption seen on the CT scan, and other regional damage to the brain's structures.

Depressed

The palpation of a scalp laceration or cephalohematoma is not the manner by which a depressed skull fracture is diagnosed. The latter can only be detected by skull radiographs in which the depression is noted in two differing views. The depressed segment is elevated in all children in whom the injury is compound or in whom the degree of depression is greater than the thickness of the skull vault.

A variation of this type of injury is the Ping-Pong fracture that occurs in the infant. So named because it resembles the depression that can be created in a Ping-Pong ball, this fracture is usually encountered in an infant younger than 6 months of age. The patient is seldom harmed by the injury and not rendered susceptible to seizures. Although some of these fractures may reduce spontaneously, the reality is that they have to be elevated by an operation, because their very appearance creates considerable anxiety in the family.

EXITS FROM THE EMERGENCY ROOM

There are three distinct paths from the emergency room which the child with a head injury may take. Given the most innocent circumstances, particularly if there is question that the head was even injured at all and when the child has normal test results and responsible guardians, then the patient may be discharged directly home. If the features of the childhood concussion syndrome (especially vomiting) are obvious and the child's parent expresses unease, however, then the child is admitted for a period of 24 to 48 hours for observation. The same policy is adopted for all children with suspect or proven skull fractures, impact seizures, or who are suspected of being a victim of a nonaccidental injury.

Clearly, children with more consequential injuries will have to be admitted, but their routes from the emergency room may take them first to the radiology department, the operating room, and/or the intensive care unit. A decision concerning the transfer of the child to the operating room or intensive care unit is sometimes only made after the imaging studies are completed.

TREATMENT

Protocol Management of Severe Head Injuries in Children

The treatment of a child with a severe closed head injury (by definition, a Glasgow coma scale rating of eight or less) usually follows an established institutional protocol. When the clinical and neuroimaging examinations are completed, the child is transferred to an intensive care unit where all efforts are directed at preventing the secondary insults of cerebral hypoxia and ischemia. Ventilation is controlled, and intracranial pressure is monitored by an indwelling sensor. The aim of therapy, which is continued for at least 5 days, is to maintain intracranial pressure at or below 20 mmHg, arterial carbon dioxide tension at or below 25 mmHg, and cerebral perfusion pressure above 50 mmHg.

Pharmacologic Management of Pediatric Head Trauma

There are very few rationalized medication choices for the head-injured child. The airway may have to be secured with endotracheal intubation to guarantee its patency and to allow controlled ventilation for patient transport or other early remedial measures. Pancuronium (Pavulon) (0.1 mg per kg dose intravenously every 30 minutes as needed) will be given under these circumstances, but such treatment blurs the entire neurologic examination, except for the pupillary responses.

An anticonvulsant drug is perhaps the most frequently used medication for the head-injured child. The incidence of early seizures in such children is 6.5 to 10%, and because more than 90% of the convulsions occur in the first 12 hours, the prophylactic administration of anticonvulsants that require substantially more time to achieve satisfactory blood levels serves no purpose. However, the physician may have to halt early repetitive seizures and for that purpose lorazepam (Ativan)* (0.05 mg per kg per dose, intravenously; may repeat once; maximal dose, 4 mg per dose) will be required. Longer-term protection can be provided with phenobarbital (4 to 6 mg per kg per

day) in the child younger than 5 years age. For those older, phenytoin (Dilantin) (5 to 6 mg per kg per day) may be used. The regimen should be maintained for a minimum of 6 months and up to a period of 2 years after the child's last convulsion.

The hyperosmotic agent mannitol is held in reserve for any crisis that arises during the patient's initial assessment. If there is clear evidence that the child's coma scale rating is deteriorating and that other features of the neurologic testing are also worsening, then 20% mannitol may be given (0.5 to 1.0 mg per kg intravenously over 30 to 45 minutes). Having initiated therapy, the physician is then obligated to a subsequent course of action, i.e., to determine whether it is patient transfer to a specialized hospital or transport within such from the emergency room to imaging or operative facilities. The drug buys time for these maneuvers.

As a rule, no sedating or pain relief medication should be administered until much more is known about the child and the neurologic status. The anxious, restless patient may be reacting to hypoxia, undiscovered painful injuries, or uncomfortable treatments already applied. The indiscriminate use of sedation could be dangerous. The same holds for the administration of narcotics for pain relief. Such are given only when the child's ventilation is mechanically supported, after imaging studies have been completed, and an intracranial pressure monitor has been placed. Otherwise, the narcotics given to the child even with a seemingly minor injury will confuse the continuing evaluations of consciousness, respiration, and pupillary characteristics.

For the most part, antibiotics will not be required in the management of a child's head injury. There is no evidence that they protect the child with a known or suspected cerebrospinal fluid leak. They are not required for the patient with a compound, depressed skull fracture unless the dura is torn and the brain is herniating through the wound.

The use of corticosteroid medication (dexamethasone [Decadron]) is not indicated for the treatment of a child's head injury.

Operative Care for the Child's Head Injury

Children are less likely than adults to have an operable intracranial lesion associated with severe head trauma. A surface collection of blood or parenchymal damage that requires débridement occurs in no more than 30% of such children. Hence, the need for early surgery will be dictated by the child's clinical profile and CT scan.

There are very few circumstances that will dic-

---

*This use of parenteral lorazepam in children <18 years old is not listed in the manufacturer's official directive.

tate the child's direct transfer from the emergency room to the operating room without an intervening stop in the radiologic suite. It is recommended that children who have obvious operative conditions (e.g., compound depressed skull fracture or clinical evidence suggesting an extradural hematoma) undergo preoperative imaging studies. In the unique situation when the clinical events (i.e., lucid interval, headache, deteriorating pulse rate, and consciousness with unilateral expanding pupil) indicate that a child's rapid deterioration can be due only to an extradural clot, a child should be transferred directly to the operating room for operative evacuation of the surface hematoma (which usually lies on the side of the dilated pupil and scalp bruise). Otherwise, the surgeon, after reviewing the CT, will decide if the subdural or intracerebral hematoma requires immediate or delayed release and/or whether an intracranial pressure monitor needs to be inserted.

The incidence of post-traumatic chronic subdural hematoma has lessened during the past 15 years. A problem occurring primarily in the child younger than 2 years of age, these collections of xanthochromic fluid confined by membranes produce unexplained irritability and craniomegaly in the previously injured child. The diagnosis is confirmed in the infant by percutaneous subdural taps and, in all children, by positive CT scan findings. The fluid is relieved by craniotomy and/or placement of a drainage subdural to peritoneal shunt.

OUTCOMES AFTER PEDIATRIC HEAD INJURY

The child's prognosis after receiving a head injury is clearly determined by the nature and severity of that injury. For example, the childhood mortality rate from a severe injury equivalent to Glasgow coma scale ratings of 3 to 4 is 59%. However, the child treated promptly for a life-threatening extradural hematoma can be expected to return to normal. The duration of a coma associated with diffuse axonal injury if less than 24 hours is associated with a better prognosis than one that lasts more than 7 days. The majority of children who have suffered the childhood concussion syndrome will recover without incident.

There are certain covert consequences of pediatric head injury of the moderate type (Glasgow coma scale ratings of 9 to 12). These include nightmares, social timidity, and for the first 6 to 12 months after return to school, poor concentration, lowered attention span, and impaired recent memory. This group of children must not be allowed to flounder, because they require neuropsychological testing and guidance.

BRAIN TUMORS

method of
EDWARD J. DROPCHO, M.D.
*The University of Alabama at Birmingham
Birmingham, Alabama*

There is a wide variety of histologic types of brain tumors, and any type of brain tumor can occur among patients of all ages, but in practical terms, a small number of tumor types account for the majority of tumors affecting children and adults.

MEDULLOBLASTOMA

Medulloblastoma is the most common brain tumor of childhood, most often arising in or near the cerebellar vermis. Among primary brain tumors, medulloblastoma is the most likely to disseminate in the subarachnoid space and to metastasize outside the central nervous system (CNS). Several prognostic factors separate patients into "average-risk" and "poor-risk" subgroups: (1) Nearly all studies have shown a relatively poor prognosis for younger patients, especially children younger than 4 years of age at diagnosis. This is partially confounded, however, by the tendency for younger patients also to have other poor prognostic features. (2) The preoperative size and extent of the tumor has had prognostic significance in some studies but not in others. It seems clear, however, that tumor invasion of the brain stem carries a poor prognosis. (3) Leptomeningeal dissemination of the tumor at diagnosis (identified by cerebrospinal fluid [CSF] cytology plus myelography or spine magnetic resonance imaging [MRI] is probably the single most important prognostic factor. Leptomeningeal spread (generally asymptomatic) is present in 20 to 30% of patients at diagnosis and in an even higher percentage in younger children.

The importance of the extent of surgical resection of medulloblastoma (gross total resection versus subtotal resection) as an independent predictor of patient outcome remains controversial, although all studies show that patients do poorly if a biopsy is merely performed on the tumor, or only a small amount of tumor is resected. Postoperative radiation therapy (RT) consists of 5500 cGy to the posterior fossa and 3600 cGy to the whole brain and spine. Following surgery and craniospinal RT, the reported 5-year disease-free survival for children with medulloblastoma in large series is 50 to 60%.

At the present time, there is insufficient evidence to justify the use of post-RT chemotherapy for all children with medulloblastoma, but several studies have shown a survival benefit for "high-risk" patients who receive chemotherapy (most commonly lomustine [CeeNU] and vincristine [Oncovin] in addition to RT. Chemotherapy probably also has a role (as yet experimental) in very young patients, especially younger than 2 years of age, in whom it is given as the primary therapy in an effort to delay the need for RT. Finally, chemotherapy (usually including cisplatin [Platinol]) may be useful for patients with recurrent CNS disease or systemic metastases.

BRAIN METASTASES

Parenchymal brain metastases are present in 10 to 20% of patients with cancer at autopsy; in 60 to 75% of these patients, the metastases are symptomatic during life. In the United States, the incidence of clinically evident brain metastases is at least 20,000 and perhaps as high as 100,000 cases annually. Any malignant neoplasm is capable of metastasizing to the brain, but bronchogenic carcinomas, breast carcinoma, and malignant melanoma together account for approximately 75% of affected patients.

Whole-brain radiation therapy (WBRT) remains the mainstay of treatment for brain metastases. The most frequently used WBRT regimen delivers a total dose of 3000 cGy in 10 to 15 daily fractions. The whole brain is irradiated even in patients with seemingly localized lesions because computed tomography (CT) or MRI probably fails to detect a significant number of small metastases and it is difficult to give a second course of treatment following focal RT. Giving a "coned-down" focal dose of RT to the area of a single or prominent metastasis has not been shown to yield better results than conventional WBRT. Several large studies have shown that a number of WBRT regimens using different fraction sizes and total doses (2000 to 5000 cGy) produce equivalent response rates and duration of improvement. Recent evidence regarding the long-term neurotoxicity of WBRT suggests that patients whose anticipated survival is longer than 12 months should receive daily dose fractions of 200 cGy or less.

The results of RT for brain metastases vary significantly among various primary tumor types and also vary (somewhat unpredictably) between individuals with similar tumors. Overall, from 30 to 80% of all patients with brain metastases respond to WBRT by clinical and/or neuroimaging criteria. Lymphomas are generally quite radiosensitive, as are germ cell tumors, breast cancer, and small cell lung carcinoma. Considerably lower response rates are seen with brain metastases from non–small cell lung cancers, melanoma, colorectal carcinoma, and other solid tumors, but some patients with these radioresistant tumors do have significant, objective responses to RT.

Two-thirds of patients irradiated for brain metastases maintain an improved level of neurologic function until death is caused by systemic disease. These patients represent clinical neurologic "cures" even though most patients whose metastases shrink or disappear on imaging studies still have residual microscopic tumor at autopsy. Approximately one-third of patients who initially respond to WBRT suffer a "CNS relapse," either progression of pre-existing lesions or the appearance of new metastatic foci. The median survival of patients following WBRT is 3 to 6 months, with only 10 to 20% of patients surviving 1 year. Among patients with solid-tumors, breast cancer tends to carry the best 1-year survival outlook, whereas patients with melanoma have a particularly poor prognosis. These statistics are somewhat misleading because the main determinant of survival is the patient's systemic cancer and not the brain lesions. Only in metastatic melanoma do a majority of patients die neurologic deaths, although progressive neurologic disability in nonresponders with any primary tumor may contribute to early mortality.

The majority of patients with brain metastases have multiple lesions, so the role of surgery is restricted to making a tissue diagnosis (in patients without a previous cancer diagnosis) or to debulk a life-threatening lesion that is very large or located in the posterior fossa. For patients with a single brain metastasis (documented by gadolinium-enhanced MR scan) from melanoma, non–small cell lung cancers, or other radioresistant tumors, resection of the metastasis followed by WBRT reduces the risk of local tumor recurrence, prolongs a good quality of life, and reduces the likelihood of a "neurologic death" compared with WBRT alone.

To date, chemotherapy has played a very minor role in the treatment of brain metastases. The entry of chemotherapy drugs into the brain is limited by local blood flow and by the integrity of the blood-brain (blood-tumor) barrier; the ability to achieve cytotoxic drug concentrations probably varies among primary tumor types, among individual patients, and even among different regions within a single metastasis. The most important limiting factor for chemotherapy, however, is probably the inherent resistance of many of the primary tumors to currently available agents. Despite these theoretical and practical problems, chemotherapy for brain metastases is useful in a number of settings. The best results have been reported for brain metastases from germ cell tumors; combinations of vincristine, bleomycin (Blenoxane), methotrexate, and cisplatin have produced durable responses in metastatic nonseminomatous tumors. Given the high level of chemosensitivity of these tumors and the anticipated long duration of survival, a case can be made for using chemotherapy as the front-line treatment for brain metastases and reserving WBRT for chemotherapy failures. A similar approach has been advocated for gestational trophoblastic tumors. Systemic multiagent chemotherapy occasionally produces objective improvement in patients with brain metastases from breast cancer or small cell lung carcinoma. A small proportion of patients with metastatic melanoma responds temporarily to cisplatin or to a nitrosourea. To date, intra-arterial chemotherapy for brain metastases has not been particularly worthwhile, although there are anecdotal reports of patients with bilateral brain metastases in whom the lesion(s) ipsilateral to intra-arterial (IA) carmustine (BiCNU) or cisplatin infusion regressed, while lesions in the contralateral hemisphere showed progression despite being exposed to the drug via the systemic circulation.

LOW-GRADE GLIOMAS

As a group, gliomas are the most common primary intracranial tumors of adults and are diagnosed in approximately 8000 persons in the United States every year. The majority of these lesions are histologically malignant and clinically aggressive; unfortunately, a "benign" glioma can often be equally devastating. The management of low-grade glial tumors is complicated by the absence of well-designed clinical trials on which to base treatment decisions. There have been no prospective or controlled studies to address key treatment questions such as: What is the desired extent of surgical resection? Which patients should be given RT after surgical diagnosis? What are the optimal doses and ports of RT? What is the quality of life of patients following treatment? MRI has significantly improved the ability to diagnose these tumors early, but it has also presented the dilemma of how best to manage patients with a single seizure or well-controlled seizure disorder, normal neurologic examination results, and an abnormal MRI scan.

Astrocytomas

A distinction should be made between *pilocytic* astrocytomas and the more common *fibrillary* tumors. Pilocytic astrocytomas occur most commonly in the cerebellum or diencephalon of children and young adults but can arise at any age and in any location. The tumors often consist of a gross cyst with a mural tumor nodule, and they are characterized histologically by elongated (pil-

ocytic) tumor cells, microcystic change, and Rosenthal fibers. Gross total surgical resection is possible in many patients and results in very long survival or even cure; the outlook is also quite favorable even for patients with less than total tumor resection. RT is therefore generally not recommended unless a postoperative tumor burden remains or tumor progression occurs after surgery.

Several tentative conclusions regarding low-grade ("benign" or "Grades I and II") fibrillary astrocytomas can be derived from the existing literature, despite the obvious hazards of basing treatment recommendations on nonrandomized, retrospective data:

1. There is probably a survival advantage for patients who undergo extensive surgical resection compared with those who have only biopsy or partial tumor excision.

2. There is a consensus that patients who receive postoperative RT have modestly better 5-year and 10-year survival rates than patients undergoing surgery alone, although some studies suggest that RT delays tumor recurrence but does not actually affect the eventual long-term (greater than 10-year) survival. The optimal RT dose and ports are not known, although "standard" treatment generally consists of 5000 to 5500 cGy given focally to the tumor plus a 2- to 4-cm "margin" as defined by CT or MRI. For patients who have a gross total resection, a case can be made for withholding RT and monitoring the patient with serial imaging studies.

3. At the time of recurrence, 50 to 75% of initially low-grade astrocytomas show progression to a higher grade of histologic malignancy. There are no data to address the question of whether RT prevents, or even accelerates, the malignant transformation of these tumors, nor is it known whether RT given "up front" at the initial diagnosis or deferred until the time of tumor recurrence would yield a better quality of life and duration of survival.

4. Almost no published studies have addressed the issue of neurologic impairment and long-term quality of life following RT. There is growing recognition that a significant proportion of patients develop cerebral atrophy and cognitive impairment, sometimes severe, after doses of cranial irradiation (especially WBRT) previously believed to be safe.

Oligodendrogliomas

As with tumors of astrocytic derivation, oligodendrogliomas exhibit a spectrum of histologic malignancy. Postoperative survival of more than 10 years is not at all unusual for histologically benign oligodendrogliomas. Gross total or subtotal resection, when feasible, should be the goal of surgery. The published studies addressing the usefulness of postsurgical RT for oligodendrogliomas are all retrospective and nonrandomized, and they arrive at conflicting conclusions regarding the impact of RT on the time to tumor progression and the total survival. At present it seems reasonable to give focal RT (5000 to 5500 cGy) to patients with a significant postsurgical tumor burden and to defer RT in patients who undergo complete or nearly complete tumor excision.

MALIGNANT GLIOMAS

Large cooperative studies have supported the usefulness of classifying malignant astrocytic neoplasms into two main groups, anaplastic astrocytoma (AA) and glioblastoma multiforme (GBM). The heading "malignant gliomas" also includes anaplastic oligodendroglioma and gliosarcoma. There are three major prognostic factors for malignant gliomas that are useful as independent predictors of individual patient outcome, and they are critically important in designing and interpreting clinical trials. (1) Patient age is probably the single most powerful predictor of outcome; the median survival is inversely proportional to age throughout all decades of adult life. (2) Tumor histologic findings are also important; the median survival of patients with intratumoral necrosis (which distinguishes AA from GBM) is less than one-half that of patients without necrosis. With standard multimodality treatment, only about 10% of patients with GBM survive 24 months, whereas the 24-month survival rate for those with AA approaches 50%. (3) Patients with a better performance status at the time of diagnosis have a better survival outlook than patients who present with severe neurologic impairment.

Surgery

The rationale for extensive surgical resection of malignant gliomas includes the alleviation of increased intracranial pressure, removal of necrotic tissue, "buying time" for subsequent therapy, and cytoreduction, which leaves behind fewer tumor cells to become resistant to RT or chemotherapy. Although this has never been subjected to a prospective randomized trial, the weight of evidence indicates that the amount of residual tumor remaining after surgery is an important independent predictor of survival. The goal of surgery should therefore be the maximal tumor resection consistent with preservation of neurologic func-

tion; a "biopsy-only" approach should be restricted to tumors located in deep or critical locations. Surgery also has an important role at the time of tumor "recurrence" or progression. In selected patients with a relatively young age, good performance status, and accessible lesions, a second debulking or resection can "set up" further chemotherapy and has a good chance of improving neurologic function and prolonging survival.

Radiation Therapy

The addition of external RT to surgery doubles the median survival of patients with malignant gliomas from 14 months to 36 months. Standard RT regimens deliver 4000 cGy WBRT and an additional focal boost so that the "tumor volume" receives 6000 cGy. Tumor doses less than 6000 cGy yield inferior survival rates, whereas doses exceeding 6000 cGy are more neurotoxic and do not improve the survival outlook.

Malignant gliomas occasionally spread through the leptomeninges or recur far from the initial tumor site, but for the majority of patients the ultimate cause of death is tumor recurrence at the primary site. In addition, as many as 30 to 40% of patients with malignant gliomas who survive longer than 18 or 24 months after WBRT have cognitive impairment, sometimes progressive, associated with diffuse cerebral atrophy and abnormal hemispheric white matter on neuroimaging studies. These observations have led some to question the need for WBRT in all patients and to recommend limited-field RT with "generous margins" based on CT or MRI scans. On the other hand, the ability of glioma cells to infiltrate the "brain around the tumor" well beyond the area of enhancement on CT or MRI scans makes it difficult to outline the true "tumor margin" with any certainty. Until the controversy is resolved by a randomized comparison between focal and WBRT, it seems prudent to continue to give the WBRT plus tumor-boost regimen to patients with large or clearly diffuse tumors and to use limited-field RT (5500 to 6000 cGy with wide margins) for patients with unusually small or "well-circumscribed" lesions.

There have been many attempts to increase the effectiveness of RT for malignant gliomas, including the use of hyperfractionated RT, radiosensitizing drugs, and heavy particle irradiation, but to date, none have yielded a convincing advantage over conventional RT. Stereotactic irradiation or "gamma knife" RT can deliver a focused high dose of RT to a small area, but most malignant gliomas are too large and poorly circumscribed to permit this approach. Brachytherapy using interstitial radionuclides consists of stereotactic placement into the tumor of one or more removable catheters that are then afterloaded with high-activity iodine-125 sources; the implants deliver a very high radiation dose to the tumor with a rapid dropoff in the dose absorbed by surrounding normal brain. Nonrandomized studies of brachytherapy in highly selected patients with recurrent gliomas have shown encouraging results, but tumors that are large, bilateral, irregularly shaped, or located in critical areas are generally not suited for brachytherapy. A major problem following brachytherapy is the high incidence of focal necrosis, which confounds the assessment of response and causes clinical deterioration requiring surgical debulking in up to 50% of patients. The proper role of brachytherapy (including proper patient selection and possible combination with external RT for newly diagnosed patients) is currently under study.

Chemotherapy

The large number and wide diversity of published chemotherapy trials for malignant gliomas attest to the absence of a regimen with dramatic effectiveness and acceptable toxicity. The therapeutic resistance of gliomas to chemotherapy is probably due to a combination of factors, including limited drug delivery into tumors, the relatively low tolerance of normal brain tissue, and to the poorly understood intrinsic resistance of the tumor cells to currently available agents.

Postoperative RT plus systemic nitrosourea chemotherapy remains the "conventional" treatment for malignant gliomas against which newer therapies should be compared. A large randomized study by the Brain Tumor Study Group has demonstrated statistically significant increases in the median survival (from 36 weeks to 51 weeks) and in the proportion of "long-term survivors" (24% at 18 months) for patients receiving intravenous carmustine in addition to surgery and RT. The modest effect on total median survival is due to the fact that only a minority of patients clearly respond to this drug; in a larger number of patients, the chemotherapy probably has little or no effect on tumor progression or survival.

Intravenous carmustine (200 mg per M^2 infused over 1 to 2 hours) for newly diagnosed patients is generally begun during the first week of RT and administered every 8 weeks, depending on the recovery of blood counts. The drug is also effective in some patients with recurrent tumors. The only common acute toxicity of carmustine is mild to moderate nausea and vomiting, and most patients tolerate outpatient treatment quite well. The most frequent (and often dose-limiting) side effect is delayed, cumulative myelosuppression. Progressive interstitial pulmonary fibrosis is a serious concern but is rare unless patients have preexisting lung disease or receive a cumulative dose exceeding 1400 mg per $M^{2;}$ the drug should be discontinued if serial pulmonary diffusion capacities fall below 60 to 70% of the predicted value. Oral procarbazine (Matulane), given in monthly courses is probably as effective as carmustine and is a reasonable alternative for patients who cannot receive nitrosoureas.

The search for better chemotherapy regimens for malignant gliomas has included trials of single agents, multiple agents, and improved delivery techniques. Several agents, most notably including cisplatin and the lipid-soluble drug diaziquone (investigational), have shown some effectiveness in patients with recurrent tumors, but no single agent has been proven to be superior to carmustine for newly diagnosed patients. There have been numerous trials of multiagent regimens, generally combining cell cycle–nonspecific drugs (such as the nitrosoureas or cisplatin) with cycle-specific drugs (such as hydroxyurea [Hydrea], vincristine, or 5-fluorouracil), but to date, none has been convincingly shown to be superior to carmustine or to other single agents, either for newly diagnosed patients or for recurrent tumors.

IA chemotherapy is capable of delivering several times more drug into the infused tumor (and normal brain) than is the same dose of drug given systemically. Carmustine has pharmacokinetic properties that are particularly well suited to IA therapy, but IA carmustine has never been proven to be more effective than conventional intravenous carmustine, and IA carmustine can produce severe, often fatal, leukoencephalopathy. Intracarotid cisplatin has shown promising efficacy in some patients with newly diagnosed or recurrent tumors; the side effects include visual and/or hearing loss, seizures, and acute neurologic deterioration after infusion, but to date, the devastating delayed neurotoxicity seen with carmustine has not been reported with cisplatin.

At the present time, patients with AA, GBM, gliosarcoma, or mixed anaplastic glioma are treated in the same fashion, although GBM and gliosarcoma are probably inherently less chemosensitive. It has been shown recently that anaplastic oligodendrogliomas are significantly more sensitive than these other gliomas to regimens such as intravenous melphalan (Alkeran) or a combination of procarbazine, lomustine, and vincristine.

PRIMARY CNS LYMPHOMA

Lymphoma occurring in the brain without systemic involvement is seen in three distinct patient populations: (1) patients with iatrogenic immunodeficiency, particularly recipients of organ transplants, in whom the risk of developing CNS lymphoma is more than 100-fold higher than in the general population; (2) patients with acquired immune deficiency syndrome, in whom the incidence of CNS lymphoma approaches 3%; and (3) patients without any apparent immune deficiency, in whom the incidence of CNS lymphoma is increasing.

Several clinical features of primary CNS lymphoma deserve mention. (1) The tumors have a predilection for deep or midline brain structures and are multifocal (at least by neuroimaging studies) in 30 to 50% of patients. (2) Lymphomatous infiltration of the posterior vitreous and/or retina occurs in 10 to 20% of patients. (3) Leptomeningeal dissemination occurs at some time in 10 to 40% of patients. The diagnosis of leptomeningeal dissemination often requires special immunocytochemical studies of CSF cells to demonstrate lymphoma-specific cell surface markers.

CNS lymphoma is unique among primary brain tumors in that corticosteroids not only reduce peritumoral cerebral edema (see subsequent discussion) but also have a direct oncolytic effect and often produce significant (but temporary) clinical and radiographic improvement. CNS lymphoma is also unusual in that there is no real benefit in attempting a surgical resection; the role of surgery is only to provide a diagnostic biopsy. RT should deliver at least 5000 cGy to the tumor area(s); patients generally also receive 4000 cGy to the whole brain, but the optimal doses are not precisely known. Routine spinal irradiation does not prolong survival and compromises the ability to administer chemotherapy. These tumors are quite radiosensitive but recur quickly; the median survival after RT alone is less than 18 months. Systemic and/or intrathecal chemotherapy probably prolongs survival over that seen with RT alone, but most published studies are small, and the optimal drugs, doses, and routes of administration are not known. Most regimens include multiple systemic agents (such as cyclophosphamide [Cytoxan], doxorubicin [Adriamycin], vincristine, and a corticosteroid) plus an agent administered to reach tumor cells in the CSF; this includes either methotrexate given via an intraventricular Ommaya reservoir or high-dose intravenous methotrexate or cytarabine (Cytosar-U).

SUPPORTIVE THERAPY

The mainstay of supportive treatment of patients with brain tumors is the use of corticosteroids to control cerebral edema. Corticosteroid treatment must be individualized for each patient, but several general guidelines apply. Adult patients are generally begun on 8 to 16 mg dexamethasone (Decadron) per day prior to surgery and the dose is escalated as necessary. "Generalized" symptoms, such as headache and altered mental status, tend to improve more dramatically than focal symptoms. The effects of beginning or changing the dose of steroids are generally seen within 48 to 72 hours. Continual efforts should be made to taper the dose of steroids gradually, although most patients require at least a low dose to minimize the acute side effects of radiation therapy (headache, nausea, worsening of focal symptoms). In patients with recurrent tumors unresponsive to treatment, the daily dexamethasone dose may be increased to 60 mg or more to maintain (although transiently) neurologic function. For obtunded patients with terminal disease, serious consideration should be given (in consultation with families) to abrupt discontinuation of steroids.

The cumulative incidence of seizures among patients with gliomas or brain metastases is approximately 20 to 50%. The basic principles of anticonvulsant pharmacokinetics and seizure management apply to patients with brain tumors just as to other patients with epilepsy. Prophylactic anticonvulsants (usually phenytoin [Dilantin]) are often begun in patients prior to craniotomy, but there is no hard evidence to support the efficacy of this practice. Retrospective reviews have not shown prophylactic anticonvulsants to be effective in preventing "late" seizures, but a prospective randomized study of prophylactic anticonvulsants (with diligent monitoring of blood levels) has never been done. A practical problem of anticonvulsant therapy for patients with brain tumors is that there are mutual interactions between the metabolism of dexamethasone and phenytoin (or most other anticonvulsants). This often results in difficulties in maintaining therapeutic blood levels using conventional doses of anticonvulsants. Conversely, patients receiving anticonvulsants may require unexpectedly high doses of corticosteroids to control cerebral edema. In addition, erythema multiforme or Stevens-Johnson syndrome may occur as a rare but life-threatening complication in patients taking phenytoin or carbamazepine (Tegretol) and tapering doses of dexamethasone during or shortly after receiving cranial RT. Until solid evidence to the contrary becomes available, the consensus is that anticonvulsants should be withheld in patients with primary or metastatic brain tumors until a seizure occurs. Patients with metastatic melanoma are an exception to this approach; the high incidence of seizures in these patients (up to 50%) justifies prophylactic anticonvulsant use.

Section 14

The Locomotor System

RHEUMATOID ARTHRITIS

method of
RUTH DITZIAN KADANOFF, M.D., PH.D.
Mount Sinai Hospital
Chicago, Illinois

Rheumatoid arthritis (RA) is a systemic, inflammatory disease occurring in about 1% of the population, involving mainly the synovium-lined joints. RA affects predominantly females in a ratio of 3:1 and can strike at any age. The course of RA is characterized by exacerbations superimposed on chronic disease. RA severity is extremely variable, from mild joint swelling with no effect on function to erosive, severely and rapidly crippling disease. Total remissions, both spontaneous and in response to therapy, occur but are rare. Pain and disability can be successfully reduced in most patients by appropriate treatment. Systemic manifestations, reduced function, and lower education level all decrease survival, underscoring the importance of patient education and the need for physical and occupational therapy.

Although the cause is still unknown, family studies had long indicated a genetic predisposition. Now the major histocompatibility complex (MHC) molecule gene portion that confers the predisposition has been sequenced. This sequence is present in the RA susceptible HLA-DR4 and HLA-DR1 subtypes. Patients with RA and two such genes are likely to have more severe disease. Although being female increases the risk of disease, pregnancy usually induces a temporary partial remission. Rheumatoid factor (RF), which is an autoantibody, mainly IgM, to the constant part of the human IgG molecule, is present in about 75% of RA patients. High titers of RF are usually associated with more severe disease, the presence of rheumatoid nodules, and poorer prognosis. Abnormalities in the immune system, both cellular and humoral; uncontrolled synovial proliferation; and inflammation are all present and play a role in producing the damage of RA.

DIFFERENTIAL DIAGNOSIS

Many conditions can resemble early RA, and making the correct diagnosis is crucial. Waiting until erosions are clearly seen in radiographs delays treatment of aggressive disease, allowing avoidable irreversible loss of function. Second-line drugs, now referred to as slow-acting antirheumatic drugs, are not risk free and should not be prescribed inappropriately. The formal criteria for RA, devised to standardize clinical studies and not individual diagnoses, require 6 weeks of unremitting symptoms. This avoids inclusion of viral diseases that cause a self-limiting arthritis, such as rubella, the prodrome of hepatitis B, and parvovirus B19. Subacute bacterial endocarditis (SBE), Lyme disease, tuberculosis arthritis, acute rheumatic fever, Whipple disease, and septic polyarthritis in acquired immune deficiency syndrome (AIDS) patients can mimic RA.

All the autoimmune diseases, the vasculitides, and the spondyloarthropathies can present with peripheral joint symptoms. Late gout can result in symmetrical finger deformities with tophi resembling rheumatoid nodules, but radiographs differentiate the two diseases. Pseudogout has a pseudorheumatoid presentation too, but, in contrast to RA, joints tend to flare out of phase with each other. Erosive osteoarthritis resembles RA, especially when Bouchard nodes are present, but sparing of the metacarpophalangeal (MCP) joints and wrists, the presence of Heberden nodes, and radiologic appearance distinguish the two diseases. One should remember that RF is positive in 1 to 5% of normal subjects, particularly the aged, and is elevated in SBE, tuberculosis, and all autoimmune diseases. The standard RF test measures only IgM titers, and some patients have RF that is only IgA or IgG. Therefore, although an important criterion, positive RF does not make the diagnosis of RA, nor does its absence rule it out.

CLINICAL MANIFESTATIONS AND PATHOLOGY

In most patients, the disease has an insidious start with nonspecific symptoms, such as fatigue and malaise, accompanied by arthralgias and sometimes low-grade fever. Later polyarticular, mostly symmetrical, joint swelling starts involving the proximal interphalangeal, MCP, wrist, elbow, shoulder, knee, ankle, and metatarsophalangeal but commonly sparing the distal interphalangeal joints. Cervical spine involvement at C1-2 is common, but the remainder of the spine is usually spared. Joint stiffness in the morning lasting more than 1 hour and returning after prolonged inactivity is characteristic of RA; its duration is used in diagnosis and in assessing disease response to therapy. Acute onset of RA occurs in about 20% of patients.

The course of the disease is generally a slow progression punctuated with flares. Cartilage destruction and ensuing joint space narrowing are irreversible. Unrelieved chronic pain and inflammation lead to joint immobility and contractions. The synovium, normally two cell layers thick, proliferates and erodes adjacent cartilage and bone. Cytokines, particularly interleukin-1

(Il-1) and tumor necrosis factor-alpha (TNF-α), secreted by macrophages in the synovium are responsible for some of the systemic effects of RA, such as fever and anemia. These cytokines also cause cartilage and bone destruction by stimulating chondrocytes and osteoclasts and increase inflammation by promoting prostaglandin secretion and endothelial activation. CD4 helper T cells promote the inflammation early in the disease and are abundant in the synovium and synovial fluid.

Early radiographic changes are periarticular osteoporosis and soft tissue swelling of affected joints, progressing to marginal erosions adjacent to the synovium and joint space narrowing. Later joint space obliteration and even fusion can occur, and osteoarthritis changes may be added to the picture. Rheumatoid nodules, inflammatory cells organized similarly to foreign body granulomas, can occur anywhere and are often seen on extensor surfaces and elbows.

Mild, normochromic, normocytic anemia of chronic disease with low to normal iron and iron-binding protein and normal to high erythropoietin is common in RA and improves with successful RA treatment. Ferritin, an acute phase reactant, is usually elevated in RA, which can mask iron deficiency. Synovial fluid from affected joints is characteristically thick and opalescent, with 2000 to 50,000 white blood cells per mm³, low viscosity, low glucose, and low complement. There is a tendency for increased infection in RA, so a newly highly inflamed joint should be aspirated and the fluid sent for Gram's stain and culture. One should culture for mycobacteria and fungi if appropriate risk factors are present. Markers of inflammation, such as platelet count, sedimentation rate, and C-reactive protein, tend to be elevated.

COMMON JOINT-RELATED COMPLICATIONS

Carpal tunnel syndrome, causing morning tingling and numbness of the first three digits and half of the fourth is treated with night splinting of the wrist in 30 degrees extension, steroid injections, and surgical release if conservative measures fail.

Baker's cysts are large knee effusions expanding a bursal sac posteriorly and down into the calf. Aspiration and steroid injection in the knee can prevent reaccumulation. Synovial fluid leaking into the gastrocnemius muscle produces severe inflammation and pain. Ultrasonography reveals a fluid-filled mass distinguishing it from thrombophlebitis.

Atlanto-occipital and atlantoaxial subluxation owing to erosion are uncommon but dangerous complications. Neurologic deficits usually start in the lower extremities. Surgical fixation is reserved for severely symptomatic patients because surgical morbidity and mortality are high. Protection of the neck with a collar is advisable. Cervical spine x-rays in flexion and extension should be performed in preparation for any surgery requiring intubation.

SYSTEMIC COMPLICATIONS

Sjögren's syndrome, manifested by dry mucous membranes, is treated symptomatically with conservation and addition of moisture (artificial tears, such as Tears Naturale, every 2 to 3 hours and Lacrisert at night).

Felty's syndrome (splenomegaly, neutropenia, and positive RF) usually occurs late in the disease. Treating the RA aggressively may reverse the neutropenia. Recurrent infections or severe abdominal pain and hematologic abnormalities secondary to splenomegaly require splenectomy.

Vasculitis is rare, commonly manifesting with nonhealing ulcers in the malleolar areas, but mesenteric vasculitis or mononeuritis multiplex similar to polyarteritis nodosa occurs.

Fibrinous pericarditis is present in 40% of RA autopsies and is usually asymptomatic, but constricting pericarditis can occur and also, extremely rarely, life-threatening tamponade. Pleural effusions occur. Both pericardial and pleural fluids exhibit low glucose and complement levels and high lactate dehydrogenase and protein levels. Rheumatoid nodules can be found in the heart, where they can cause conduction disturbances, and in the lung, where they can cavitate or become infected. Diffuse interstitial fibrosis, causing reduced diffusion with restrictive pattern on pulmonary function tests and a honeycomb pattern on chest x-ray, is more common in patients with secondary Sjögren's syndrome or those treated with gold. Florid pneumonitis with respiratory failure is rare but has been reported. Aggressive treatment of the underlying RA is recommended.

Hematopoietic malignancies, lymphomas in particular, are increased in RA patients.

TREATMENT

Education

The nature of the disease and the need to comply with a lifetime regimen of rest, exercise, and medication should be made clear to the patient and the family. Success of therapy is maximized when the patient is part of the team consisting of the physician, nurse, physical and occupational therapists, and psychosocial professionals. Job and family responsibilities should be altered to fit the patient's limitations. Independence, however, is important to self-esteem, and a "learned helplessness" pattern of behavior leads to depression, noncompliance, and functional loss.

Physical and Occupational Therapy

The goals of physical therapy are maintaining joint range of motion, strengthening muscles, and preventing disuse atrophy by appropriate exercises while avoiding articular trauma and fatigue. Occupational therapy offers alternative approaches to difficult tasks in daily living activities, for instance, large soft holders for utensils; hand dexterity exercises; and pain reduction modalities such as ice packs on inflamed joints, warming hand immersions, and wrist splints (in 30 degrees extension) to be worn at night and during repetitive activities.

Drug Therapy

Salicylates and Nonsteroidal Anti-Inflammatory Drugs

The mainstay of RA therapy is the use of nonsteroidal anti-inflammatory drugs (NSAIDs), which in mild disease may suffice. They diminish the pain indirectly by reducing the inflammation and provide quick, excellent analgesia. They do not stop the disease process but when used in anti-inflammatory doses reduce the damage fueled by the prostaglandins.

Acetylsalicylic acid (Aspirin, ASA) has the advantage of low price and measurable serum levels. The anti-inflammatory dose is 2.5 to 5 grams per day (serum levels 20 to 30 mg per dL). ASA has great gastrointestinal toxicity; causes severe bronchoconstriction in many asthmatics; and irreversibly disables platelets, thereby increasing the risk of gastrointestinal bleeds. Tinnitus is a common effect of all salicylates, reversible by lowering the dose. Enteric-coated preparations are less distressing to the stomach but have variable absorption. ASA often causes asymptomatic liver enzyme (liver function test [LFT]) elevation, but rarely liver failure can occur.

Nonacetylated salicylates (Trilisate, salsalate [Disalcid]) are anti-inflammatory without being cyclooxygenase inhibitors and therefore have no interfering effect on platelets and little gastrointestinal or kidney toxicity. Their anti-inflammatory and analgesic properties are often less than NSAIDs or aspirin. A dosage of 45 mg per kg per day should be used, divided in two or three daily doses.

Individual response to the NSAIDs varies and often changes with time. A common practice is to have the patient try NSAIDs for a week or two at an intermediate dose and assess improvement of joint pain and inflammation and tolerability of side effects. One should then attempt to increase efficacy (if needed) by raising the dose once, without exceeding maximum, before switching NSAIDs. Mixing NSAIDs increases toxic side effects and not efficacy and is to be discouraged. Regular dosing, not as needed, is required for anti-inflammatory levels (when well controlled on methotrexate, which is a potent anti-inflammatory, ASA or NSAIDs can be used as analgesics only).

NSAIDs reduce glomerular filtration in patients with impaired kidney perfusion, further reducing creatinine clearance. One should therefore keep the doses low and monitor renal functions frequently in diabetics and hypertensives with mild creatinine elevation. Short-acting preparations should be used in the elderly and the renal impaired owing to the risk of drug accumulation in the serum. Some patients also prefer frequent analgesic boosts, whereas longer acting preparations, such as piroxicam (Feldene) and nabumetone (Relafen), with their once-a-day dosing have an advantage for compliance in the young. Patients should have their kidney functions tested 1 to 2 weeks after initiation of therapy. Central nervous system side effects, especially with indomethacin; confusion in the elderly; and headache in women are reported. LFT elevation is seen in about 15% of patients on NSAIDs and should be checked 4 weeks after therapy is started, particularly with diclofenac (Voltaren).

The principal side effect of NSAIDs is gastrotoxicity. They should be administered with food or antacids. Misoprostol (Cytotec) has been shown to reduce the gastric mucosal damage from NSAIDs. In patients at risk for peptic ulcers who cannot tolerate nonacetylated salicylates and have to be on NSAIDs, it is the protective drug of choice at a dose of 100 µg every 6 to 8 hours. Although 200 µg every 6 hours is slightly more effective, the main side effect, diarrhea, is ubiquitous. The drug can cause miscarriage; contraception is required.

Steroids

Intra-articular steroids are extremely effective in reducing inflammation in the injected joints with hardly any systemic ill effects. Steroid injection is contraindicated in the presence of infection and is more effective without the inflammatory effusion. So aspirating the joint dry and visually assessing the synovial fluid before changing syringe and injecting is standard practice. Aseptic technique is required. A long-acting steroid crystalline suspension, such as triamcinolone hexacetonide (Aristospan) or prednisolone tebutate (Hydeltra), 5 to 40 mg, is mixed with 5 mL local anesthetic (1 or 2% lidocaine) to provide sufficient volume to distribute well in the joint. In finger joints, the dose is 0.2 to 0.3 mL with no anesthetic owing to space limitation. Spraying the skin with ethyl chloride reduces the needle prick pain. The frequency of any joint injection should be limited to at most every 3 months to avoid possible cartilage damage. Anesthetic relief is within minutes, lasting an hour. Anti-inflammatory effects are to be expected only 4 to 48 hours after the injection and can last for weeks to months.

Oral corticosteroids, usually prednisone, are used for a short term in low dose, 5 to 10 mg per day, as bridging therapy when starting or changing to a slow-acting antirheumatic drug to provide rapid relief of inflammation and morning stiffness. Osteopenia is a complication of long-term steroid treatment, and calcium supplementation is often suggested. Vitamin D has also been used, but the possibility of increased bone resorption and hypercalcemia is worrisome. Both may contribute to renal stone formation and should not be used in patients who have had calcium stones. In elderly patients, an RA variant that resembles polymyalgia rheumatica with high erythrocyte sedimentation rate and marked hand stiffness, responsive to low-dose prednisone, has been described.

Other Steroids

Osteoporosis is present in RA patients, and the risk of fractures is doubled and further increased by corticosteroid use in men and postmenopausal women. The standard estrogen therapy (Premarin, 0.625 mg for 21 days a month, with 10 mg Provera for at least 10 days if the uterus is present) should be considered in all postmenopausal women with RA in the absence of contraindications but particularly if they are taking corticosteroids. In men with documented low serum testosterone, the arthritis as well as the hormone levels improve with long-acting testosterone esters intramuscularly 200 mg every 2 weeks, and testosterone increases bone density.

Second-Line Drugs, Slow-Acting Antirheumatic Drugs

Gold, D-penicillamine, antimalarials, sulfasalazine, and dapsone used to be called disease-modifying antirheumatic drugs. These drugs have an 8 or more week delay to the onset of therapeutic effect. There is a high rate of rashes to all but the antimalarials. Often there is a poor response; only 30% of patients are still taking the drug and doing well a year later. In patients who respond, good partial remissions are obtained.

After a test dose of 10 mg, gold, in the form of aurothioglucose (Solganal) or gold sodium thiomalate (Myochrysine), 50 mg, is injected intramuscularly weekly. Complete blood count (CBC) and urinalysis are checked before each shot for proteinuria or drop in white count or platelets.

Bone marrow suppression and membranous glomerulonephritis can occur. After a cumulative dose of 1 gram, the injections are usually given biweekly for a few months, then reduced to every 3 weeks, and then monthly subsequently.

Oral gold, auranofin (Ridaura), is less effective but less likely to cause side effects than intramuscular gold. Its dose is 3 mg twice a day. CBC and urinalysis should be performed monthly.

D-Penicillamine (Cuprimin, Depen) is started with one 250-mg tablet daily, increasing gradually by one tablet a day every 4 to 6 weeks to 750 mg if tolerated. CBC and urinalysis should be performed a week after each change, monitoring for neutropenia, thrombocytopenia (common), and proteinuria. Then the tests can be done every 2 weeks for a couple of months, then monthly. Intestinal discomfort, loss of appetite, and general intolerance are common. Rarer side effects are bronchiolitis obliterans, gynecomastia, myasthenia gravis, and polymyositis.

Hydroxychloroquine (Plaquenil) is the most studied and best tolerated of the antimalarials. In patients with overlap of RA and lupus, it is a very helpful drug. Ophthalmologic checkups to monitor for retinal deposits and red desaturation are done routinely at 6-month intervals, but at the current dose of hydroxychloroquine (200 mg twice a day), the occurrence is rare. It causes occasional gastrointestinal intolerance and skin discoloration, mostly with sun exposure.

Sulfasalazine (Azulfidine) is started at one 500-mg tablet a day and increased slowly up to four. Urinalysis and CBC should be followed.

Immunosuppressives

Methotrexate (MTX) has been given in the last few years with increasing enthusiasm, often before gold, when rapid aggressive therapy is needed. This is due to a high rate of clinical response, about 90 to 95%, and rapid onset of response, about 3 weeks. Cirrhosis is not seen in RA patients, and liver biopsy currently is not recommended at any cumulative dose. LFTs are followed monthly (but did not correlate with liver damage in psoriatics). Chronic active hepatitis B and C flare on MTX, progressing rapidly to cirrhosis, and should be excluded before starting MTX. Bone marrow suppression requiring leucovorin rescue can occur when the kidneys do not excrete the drug well; in dialysis patients, the drug is lethal, so CBC and kidney functions should be checked before initiating treatment. Mouth sores are an early sign of toxicity and, if CBC and renal functions are normal, can be healed with added folate.

Pneumocystis carinii pneumonia and increased infection rates, particularly of the skin, have been seen in patients on MTX even without corticosteroids. Pneumonitis with fever and a diffuse pattern on chest film occurs in about 1 to 2% of patients and requires drug cessation. MTX is an abortifacient. Although healthy infants were born to mothers who took it, the risk of malformations is not excluded, and patients should use an effective method of birth control. Morbid obesity and alcohol abuse are relative contraindications owing to liver problems. Trimethoprim-sulfamethoxazole (Septra, Bactrim) should not be used in conjunction with MTX because folate inhibition may become excessive. Average starting dose is 7.5 mg orally once weekly (three 2.5-mg tablets), and the dose can be increased up to 25 mg with increased efficacy. Parenteral administration reduces gastrointestinal toxicity.

Azathioprine (Imuran) is an effective drug. No increase over the already increased risk of lymphoma in RA patients has been seen in a number of clinical studies. Starting dose is 50 mg a day increased up to 1 to 2 mg per kg per day while following white blood cells and platelets. The effects on bone marrow are dose dependent and are usually reversible.

Third-Line Drugs

Cyclophosphamide (Cytoxan) is recommended for vasculitis not responding to more conservative treatment. Monthly bolus (intravenous or oral) or daily oral medications have been used. The risk of overdosing, causing lethal infections, cannot be overstated. The rheumatologist follows urinalysis, CBC, and platelets. Bone marrow suppression is reversible. The risk of hematopoietic malignancies 10 to 20 years later is up to 1%. Infertility occurs in both sexes and in women depends on total dose. Hemorrhagic cystitis on oral Cytoxan is common, and the risk of fibrosis and cancer of the bladder is increased. Hydration, frequent bladder emptying, and bolus therapy may help reduce this risk.

Cyclosporine

Cyclosporine* (Sandimmune) is quite effective at doses of 2.5 to 5 mg per kg per day, but the mean serum creatinine may rise 30%, even in absence of NSAIDs, and may remain elevated after drug cessation. Both therapeutic effect and nephrotoxicity are dose related. It should be reserved for failures of other therapies. Hypertrichosis and hypertension are common side effects.

Combination Therapy

Synergy has not been found in combinations. Gold and hydroxychloroquine together yield a small benefit added to single drug effect, but the incidence of toxicity increases. MTX and hydroxychloroquine may offer some improvement over MTX alone and possibly protect the liver. Combination triple drug therapy including cyclophosphamide has been tried in a few patients with success but also with some fatal malignancies. Of note, hydroxychloroquine and D-penicillamine together are less effective than either one alone.

Experimental Therapies

A remarkable and long-lasting improvement is seen with total lymphoid irradiation, but deaths from infection have occurred. Other promising future therapies are biologic molecules. Under study are antibodies and competing soluble receptors to interleukins (IL-1 and IL-2) and a soluble adhesion molecule (sICAM-1). Studies with antibodies directed against T-lymphocyte markers CD4 (OKT4A), CD2, CDw52 (CAMPATH-1), some coupled with toxins (CD5Plus), are also in progress.

Surgery

Knee and hip total joint arthroplasties have become technically excellent and can restore function if the muscles are not atrophied. The osteoporotic bone of RA renders the implantation more difficult, sometimes requiring bone grafts. Synovectomy can restore pain-free function for months in a joint that failed other therapy, but eventually the synovium grows back. Finger extensor tendons can be repaired or preferably repositioned to avoid rupture. In painful wrists with little movement, fusion can eliminate pain with no significant loss of function. Silastic joint prostheses can restore function to deformed, damaged finger joints.

JUVENILE RHEUMATOID ARTHRITIS

method of
BALU H. ATHREYA, M.D.
University of Pennsylvania School of Medicine
Philadelphia, Pennsylvania

Juvenile rheumatoid arthritis (JRA) is one of the important chronic disorders and is the most common rheumatic disorder in children in the United States. The incidence is approximately 0.1 to 0.2 in 1000 and prevalence approximately 0.5 to 1 in 1000. There are three major subvarieties of JRA: systemic, pauciarticular, and polyarticular. This division is based on the behavior of the disease during the first 6 months after onset. On long-term follow-up, however, the course may change (Table 1).

---

*This use of cyclosporine is not listed in the manufacturer's official directive.

TABLE 1. **Course of Juvenile Rheumatoid Arthritis**

Onset	Course
Systemic	Remission
	Oligoarthritis
	Polyarthritis
Pauciarticular	Remission
	Extended pauciarticular
	Polyarticular
	Monarticular
Polyarticular	Remission
	Polyarticular
	Oligoarticular

The definition of systemic-onset JRA is based on the clinical features of generalized involvement, such as fever, rash, hepatosplenomegaly, lymphadenopathy, and serositis. Pauciarticular JRA is characterized by involvement of four or less than four joints. This is again subdivided into two subgroups: one group seen mostly in girls, younger than 4 years of age, with circulating antinuclear antibody (ANA) and high incidence of iridocyclitis, and another group seen in older boys, which may evolve into one of the spondyloarthropathies, particularly if associated with HLA-B27. More subvarieties are being recognized within pauciarticular JRA with characteristic HLA markers. Polyarticular JRA is characterized by involvement of five or more joints. A subgroup of children with this type of JRA may have circulating rheumatoid factor (RF) in their serum. They resemble adults with RF-positive arthritis, with severe erosive disease, and are HLA-DR4 positive. Children with RF-negative JRA carry a better prognosis.

GENERAL MANAGEMENT

JRA is a chronic disease. Although certain forms carry a good prognosis, recent studies indicate that up to 58% of children with the systemic variety, 71% with the pauciarticular variety, and 50% with the polyarticular variety have active disease even after 10 years. These children require multiple medical consultations (ophthalmology and orthopedics); services of therapists (physical and occupational); and counseling on school life, sports, and education. Family members often need support and counseling. During adolescence, these children need help with vocational, sexual, and transitional issues. The financial burden of caring for a child with a chronic disease is heavy. Therefore care of these children is ideally provided by a tertiary center that has on its staff a pediatric rheumatologist and that can also provide other subspecialty and allied health services. At the same time, overall management should be family centered and community based, with the family physician or the pediatrician providing primary care and coordination of care.

TREATMENT

A general approach to treatment of children with JRA is given in Table 2. The main goals of therapy are to control inflammation of the joints and systemic disease (if present), prevent deformities, maintain strength and endurance, and encourage as normal a life as possible.

Nonsteroidal Anti-Inflammatory Drugs

Although a number of nonsteroidal anti-inflammatory drugs (NSAIDs) are available (Table 3), it is best to be familiar with one or two of them and understand their pharmacology and toxicity thoroughly. Recent studies have shown that more than half the children respond to one of the NSAIDs. Some children respond to one NSAID and not to another. Some children may take 8 to 12 weeks for good response, but the average response time is approximately 1 month. Other considerations in choice of NSAIDs are (1) availability of liquid preparation, (2) two to three doses per day rather than every 4 hours or once-a-day dosage, and (3) relative safety.

Acetylsalicylic acid (aspirin) is still one of the most important NSAIDs. It is usually given in three to four divided doses, preferably with some food or milk. If "baby aspirins" are given, children should not be allowed to chew them because this practice leads to erosion of surfaces of the teeth. It is adequate if the dosage is distributed through the waking hours of the day, and it is not necessary to wake the children at night to give a dose. The author's usual practice is to obtain serum levels of salicylate 4 to 5 days after starting therapy and adjust the dosage to obtain serum salicylate levels of 20 to 25 mg per dL. Liver function tests should be monitored, particularly during the first few months of therapy. Although small elevations of aspartate transaminase (AST) and alanine transaminase (ALT) are not indications for stopping therapy, elevations of three to four times the normal values warrant cessation of therapy, particularly if prothrombin time and

TABLE 2. **General Management of Children with Juvenile Rheumatoid Arthritis**

Complete evaluation—psychosocial history, developmental needs, plan for growth and development
Nonsteroidal drugs
Slow-acting antirheumatic drugs
Physical/occupational therapy
Orthopedic surgery
Treatment of extra-articular features
  Systemic: nonsteroidal; steroids; intravenous gamma globulin (?)
  Eye disease: topical steroid; intraocular steroid; immunosuppressive therapy

TABLE 3. **Nonsteroidal Anti-Inflammatory Drugs Used in Children with Arthritis**

Generic Name	Dose*	Usual Frequency Given Daily	Maximal Dose
Aspirin	60–80 mg/kg/day	3–4	2500 mg/day (for 25 kg)
Tolmetin Na	15–30 mg/kg/day	4	1800 mg/day
Ibuprofen	30–50 mg/kg/day	4	3000 mg/day
Ketoprofen	100–200 mg/m²/day	4	300 mg/day
Meclofenamate Na†	3–7.5 mg/kg/day	4	300 mg/day
Fenoprofen	900–1800 mg/m²/day	4	2600 mg/day
Naproxen	10–20 mg/kg/day	2	750–1000 mg/day
Sulindac	± 6 mg/kg/day	2	400 mg/day
Flurbiprofen†	3–5 mg/kg/day	3–4	300 mg/day
Diclofenac	3 mg/kg/day	4	200 mg/day
Piroxicam	0.3–0.5 mg/kg/day	1	20 mg/day

*Doses shown are taken from studies. For most children, the dose is in mid to upper portion of the range, but lowest effective dose should be used.

†This use of meclofenamate Na and flurbiprofen is not listed in the manufacturer's official directive.

Reproduced from Fink CW: The clinical features, course, prognosis and treatment of juvenile arthritis. Rec Progr Med *82*:552–560, 1991.

partial thromboplastin time are also abnormal. In addition to this hepatotoxicity, which at times can be serious, there is also the association between Reye's syndrome and aspirin. Every pediatrician and family physician's office has a poster warning about this danger. It is no wonder that most parents are aware of this association. It is best to stop therapy with aspirin if the child has any sickness associated with vomiting or if he or she has influenza or chickenpox. Indeed the American Academy of Pediatrics recommends yearly influenza virus vaccine for children on long-term salicylate therapy. In children who are allergic to aspirin or who cannot tolerate aspirin, choline salicylate or choline magnesium trisalicylate may be tried.

Because of all of the aforementioned problems, the author has all but given up using aspirin as the first NSAID. The author usually starts with tolmetin (Tolectin) or naproxen (Naprosyn) or ibuprofen. If there is no response after therapy using full doses of one of these NSAIDs for 2 to 3 months, another NSAID can be tried for 2 to 3 more months.

Periodic monitoring of these children should include complete blood count (CBC), AST, ALT, and urinalysis. There is increasing concern about renal toxicity of NSAIDs. Soon after initiation of therapy, some children develop a mild edema probably secondary to the effects on glomerular blood flow. This is transient. Some children, however, develop more serious problems, such as interstitial nephritis.

Gastric irritation is less common with NSAIDs other than aspirin. Some children on any one of these drugs, however, develop gastric ulcer associated with severe bleeding or silent perforation. Fortunately, this is relatively rare in children. In the author's center, with experience in treating more than 800 children with JRA, only five children with NSAID-induced gastric ulcer have been seen. Because even normal children complain of abdominal pain often, it is important to obtain a good history and perform an abdominal examination during every visit. Treatment with mild antacids is adequate in most situations.

Slow-Acting Antirheumatic Drugs

This group of drugs (also called disease modifying antirheumatic drugs) includes gold (oral and parenteral), hydroxychloroquine sulfate (Plaquenil), D-penicillamine, and sulfasalazine (Azulfidine). One of these compounds is added when a fully satisfactory result is not achieved with the basic regimen of NSAID therapy. The timing of this addition varies depending on the type of arthritis, adequacy of response to NSAID, and aggressiveness of the disease (rapid increase in number of joints involved or rapid progression of the disease). These drugs are not usually effective in controlling systemic features, and the possibility of serious adverse reactions is more common when used in systemic-onset JRA.

Hydroxychloroquine sulfate (Plaquenil) is used only for children older than 6 years of age. It is easy to give (once a day) and easy to monitor (no frequent blood tests). In the pediatric collaborative multicenter trial comparing hydroxychloroquine sulfate , penicillamine (Cuprimine, Depen), and placebo, hydroxychloroquine sulfate was found to be slightly more effective. The disadvantages are (1) bitter taste, (2) lack of smaller dosage forms, and (3) inability of younger children to report visual loss and to cooperate with visual testing.

The usual dose is 6 mg per kg per day (maximum is 400 mg per day). Before starting therapy, a complete ophthalmologic examination, including field of vision and color vision, must be performed. This should be repeated at least twice a year. Although retinal toxicity is unusual at this dose, the use of hydroxychloroquine sulfate should be discontinued at the first sign of retinopathy because its effect on macular vision is cumulative. It is the author's policy to check the status of glucose-6-phosphate dehydrogenase also before starting therapy.

Gold

The oral preparation is triethylphosphine gold (auranofin), and the usual dose is 0.1 to 0.2 mg per kg per day (maximum, 9 mg per day). It is given in one dose at bedtime, and the dose can be reduced if the child develops loose stools (a common side effect). Although this drug is relatively less toxic compared with parenteral gold, its effectiveness is questionable. Monitoring during therapy should include CBC and urinalysis before starting therapy and every 1 to 2 months thereafter.

Parenteral gold is a time-honored drug for the treatment of JRA, although there are no controlled studies to document its efficacy. Two preparations are available: sodium aurothiomalate (Solganal) and sodium aurothioglucose (Myochrysine). Anaphylactoid reactions may occur, particularly with aurothiomalate. Therefore the first injection must be given only under medical supervision, and first-aid measures should be available. The test dose is usually 0.1 mg per kg (maximum, 5 mg). If there are no reactions, the first full dose can be given the following week. Injections are given weekly. The dose is increased gradually over a period of 3 to 4 weeks (0.25 mg per kg, week 1; 0.5 mg per kg, week 2; 1 mg per kg, week 3) until the maximal weekly dose of 1 mg per kg is reached (maximal weekly dose is 50 mg).

Before starting therapy and before each weekly dose, a CBC and urinalysis must be obtained. If the child has no adverse reactions, such as rash, oral ulcers, fall in hemoglobin (more than 1 gram), leukopenia or drop in counts of more than 3000 per mm³ from earlier values, eosinophilia, low platelets (drop of 25% or more), proteinuria, or red blood cells in urine, the injections are continued weekly for 4 to 6 months. If objective improvement is noted, the weekly dosage level is maintained, but the frequency is reduced gradually (once in 2 weeks for three doses; once in 3 weeks for two doses). Finally, the child is maintained on monthly injections for varying periods of time, depending on response and tolerance. If there is no response after 4 to 6 months or if there are adverse reactions, gold injections are discontinued.

Approximately 25% of children receiving gold injection develop toxic reactions, particularly those with systemic disease. Therefore careful monitoring and checking the patient and laboratory results *before* each injection are mandatory. Adverse reactions may be controlled by stopping therapy or with steroids or chelating agents depending on the severity.

D-Penicillamine

The usual starting dose of D-penicillamine is 5 mg per kg per day increased gradually to 10 mg per kg per day if there is no response at the initial dose. The maximum dose is 750 mg per day. It is usually given in the morning on an empty stomach. In addition to its effects on bone marrow and kidney, D-penicillamine is also associated with lupus-like syndrome and myasthenia. Therefore, careful clinical and laboratory monitoring is essential. CBC and urinalysis are obtained weekly during the first month of therapy. The frequency of monitoring can be gradually reduced to once a month or once in 2 months after the first 6 months.

Sulfasalazine

This drug is being used increasingly for the treatment of adults and children with arthritis, although it has not been approved by the Food and Drug Administration for this use. Sulfasalazine has been found to be particularly effective in treating asymmetrical polyarticular arthritis, reactive arthritis, and ankylosing spondylitis. The response, if any, is usually seen within 6 to 8 weeks. The toxicity list is long and includes dermatitis, gastrointestinal irritation, suppression of bone marrow, hemolytic anemia, Stevens-Johnson syndrome, and hepatotoxicity. Children with systemic-onset JRA are particularly prone to develop toxicity.

The suggested initial dose for children is 40 to 50 mg per kg per day in three to four divided doses (maximum dose 2 grams per day), taken with food or milk. After appropriate response is achieved, the dose may be gradually reduced to a maintenance dose of 25 mg per kg per day, provided that the improvement is sustained at this lower dose. Careful monitoring of CBC, urine, and liver functions is essential.

Immunosuppressives

Immunosuppressives have only a limited role in JRA, at least in the United States. Because

JRA is not a "killing disease," the author prefers not to use drugs with a high toxicity profile, such as cyclophosphamide (Cytoxan). In Europe and England, where amyloidosis associated with JRA is higher (7 to 16%), one can consider drugs such as chlorambucil. In the United States, use of azathioprine (Imuran), cyclophosphamide, and chlorambucil should be restricted to children with severe life-threatening complications or after all other treatments have failed. Thus such therapy should be administered only in a pediatric rheumatology center.

Methotrexate*

Among all the drugs tested for use in JRA, methotrexate (MTX) is clearly the best. In a recently published randomized, placebo-controlled, double-blind study, approximately 62% of children on 10 mg per m^2 per week of MTX responded according to a composite index of several response variables compared with 36% of the placebo group. At the dosages used, it is more anti-inflammatory than immunosuppressive. It is easy to administer (once a week). The toxicity profile at dosages used is low, although some of them can be life-threatening. Drug levels are also easy to monitor. Liver toxicity, the most common adverse effect, has not been found to be severe or irreversible. There is only one report of MTX-associated liver fibrosis in a child with JRA. In one other study, no significant structural abnormalities of the liver were seen on liver biopsy in 12 children after 815 to 2980 mg of cumulative dose.

Disadvantages include: (1) Although MTX is effective in controlling systemic features it is not effective in controlling synovitis. (2) It controls the disease but does not induce true remission, as shown by the recrudescence of symptoms after withdrawal. (3) Consequent concerns exist about prolonged use of a potentially hepatotoxic drug in growing children.

The only other concern is that MTX, although not oncogenic, can cause congenital malformation if taken during pregnancy. Therefore it is essential to advise sexually active adolescents against getting pregnant. It is also essential to advise adolescents regarding alcohol consumption because the risk of hepatotoxicity increases with other factors.

The use of MTX should be avoided in children with malnutrition, viral hepatitis, obesity, diabetes, and alcoholism. Baseline studies to be obtained before start of therapy should include

CBC; urinalysis; liver function profile, including AST, ALT, serum albumin, and renal function (serum creatinine); and a chest roentgenogram. These are repeated (except x-ray) every 2 weeks for 2 months, every month for 4 months, and every 1 to 2 months throughout the period of therapy.

Based on the placebo-controlled study on the use of MTX in JRA, we recommend a starting dose of 10 mg per m^2 per week given orally. If kidney functions are not normal, a lesser dose should be used and drug level monitored. After initial improvement, some children require gradual increase in dosage to maintain the improvement. The dosage may then be increased to 15 to 20 mg per m^2 per week. Higher dose may not be absorbed orally in the expected manner or may not be tolerated orally. Intramuscular injection may be necessary in these children.

If mild abnormalities of AST and ALT occur, it is first advisable to re-check the results. If these abnormalities are reproducible, it is often worthwhile withdrawing the NSAID rather than stopping the MTX because the half-life of the NSAID may be prolonged and clearance delayed by MTX. If the liver function abnormalities are persistent or severe (over three times normal), it is prudent to withhold MTX and reassess the situation. It is also best to stop MTX if the child develops chickenpox, although in at least one study, children with JRA on MTX handled this infection without serious consequences.

Once the disease is under complete control clinically and by laboratory criteria, it is advisable to taper the dose of MTX gradually (2.5 mg per week) over a period of 2 to 3 months before stopping it. In the author's experience, only 4 out of 33 children taking MTX for JRA entered remission. Only one, however, was able to come off MTX completely. All the others had good control of the disease. This indicates that MTX does not alter the basic pathophysiology and that the long-term dependence on this hepatotoxic agent for children may not be acceptable.

Corticosteroids

Pediatric rheumatologists usually have high respect for prednisone. It is the treatment of choice for children with acute, severe systemic disease (e.g., pericarditis and macrophage-activation syndrome) and localized disease (uveitis). It is also associated, however, with well-known complications, such as growth retardation, osteoporosis, increased susceptibility to infection, hypertension, and ulcer disease.

Some strategies to minimize the risks of side effects of corticosteroids are:

---

*This use of methotrexate in children is not listed in the manufacturer's official directive.

1. Start with every-other-day steroids, if at all possible.

2. If not possible, start with daily steroids, but switch to every-other-day steroids as soon as possible.

3. Facilitate switch to every-other-day steroids in older children by using one dose of indomethacin (Indocin) (if tolerated) on the evenings of nonsteroid days.

4. Use "pulse" methylprednisolone, and use this cover to reduce daily steroids.

Recently an oxazolone derivative of prednisone (deflazacort) has been introduced in Europe. This compound has been shown to have lower negative effects on calcium balance, bone turnover, and skeletal growth. Once it is available in the United States, this may be the ideal corticosteroid for maintenance therapy.

Children on corticosteroids require monitoring of their weight and blood pressure frequently. In addition, they need monitoring of their eyes (for cataract) and lipid profiles, serum potassium, and blood glucose. They should be advised regarding symptoms of ulcer and gastrointestinal bleeding, exposure to infections such as chickenpox, and reduced salt intake.

The usual dose of prednisone is 0.5 to 1 mg per kg per day in a single dose. In severe disease, one may use 2 mg per kg per day given in divided doses. Intravenous "pulse" methylprednisolone may be helpful in acute situations and may also help minimize the need for continuous long-term therapy. The dose is 30 mg per kg per dose (maximum, 1 gram) of methylprednisolone (Solu-Medrol) administered over a period of 30 to 45 minutes through a "soluset" with 50 to 100 mL of D5W. In acute conditions, this usually is given daily or on alternate days for three doses. The maintenance dose is often given once a month. Frequent monitoring of blood pressure and heart rate is essential during the infusion. Serious and fatal complications involving electrolyte imbalance and cardiac arrhythmias have been reported.

Intra-articular use of steroids (in the form of prednisolone tertiary butylacetate or triamcinolone hexacetonide) is indicated in the presence of monarticular arthritis that is difficult to control. The dose varies between 5 and 40 mg depending on the size of the joint. In older children, local anesthesia is adequate. In younger children, one may need general anesthesia or deep sedation. Therefore it may be preferable to have an orthopedic surgeon help with intra-articular steroids in the younger age group. It is important to make sure that aseptic precautions are taken before injection. After injection, rest in the form of splinting for 2 to 3 days is said to improve results.

The author generally does not inject the same joint more than three times and gives an interval of at least 3 months between injections, although there are no strong data to support such recommendations.

Eye Disease

Treatment of eye disease (uveitis) of JRA should be supervised by an ophthalmologist. Initial therapy includes steroid eye drops and mydriatic drops. After acute inflammation is controlled, a short-acting mydriatic drug may be administered once a day in the evening so pupillary dilation does not interfere with school activities. In severe and unremitting inflammation, systemic steroids, intraocular steroids, or both may be needed. Occasionally immunosuppressives, such as cyclosporine (Sandimmune), are used. Surgical management of glaucoma, corneal opacity, and cataracts may also be indicated.

Physical Therapy and Occupational Therapy

Children with JRA may require physical or occupational therapy (or both) to relieve pain, improve range of motion, increase muscle strength, and maintain activities of daily living. In addition, they may require splints to rest joints in proper position or serial splints to correct flexion deformities. Morning stiffness is controlled by sleeping in a sleeping bag or waterbed. In the morning, a warm bath should help reduce the stiffness.

Orthopedic Surgery

Synovectomy may be indicated in selected children with severe unremitting synovitis and consequent mechanical impairment of joint motion. Because recurrence of synovial growth is common, this procedure was given up a few years ago. The arrival of arthroscopy, however, has revived the interests of rheumatologists in this procedure. Arthroscopic synovectomy is much easier with less morbidity and does not require prolonged immobilization. Indications for arthroscopic synovectomy include persistent arthritis of a single joint that is not controlled with adequate medical management or intra-articular corticosteroid.

Soft tissue releases, capsulotomy, and muscle lengthening may be indicated to relieve flexion contractures. Fusion of joints is indicated in the presence of severe subluxation at the wrist and pain in the foot owing to inflammation and erosions of the subtalar joint.

Reconstructive surgery has assumed an all-important role in the rehabilitation of older patients with JRA. Total joint replacement is indicated in the presence of severe pain or limitation of range of motion interfering with rehabilitation. There is good experience with replacement of the hips and knees in children. In general, this type of surgery is considered only after growth has ceased (i.e., after 16 to 18 years of age).

ANKYLOSING SPONDYLITIS

method of
MUHAMMAD ASIM KHAN, M.D.
Case Western Reserve University
Cleveland, Ohio

Ankylosing spondylitis (AS) is a chronic systemic inflammatory rheumatic disorder that primarily affects the axial skeleton, and sacroiliac joint involvement (sacroiliitis) is its hallmark. Involvement of the limb joints other than hips and shoulders is uncommon. The disease is strongly associated with a genetic marker HLA-B27 and may show familial aggregation. The inflammatory process involves the synovial and cartilaginous joints as well as the osseous attachments of tendons and ligaments, frequently resulting in fibrous and bony ankylosis. The disease may occur in association with reactive arthritis (Reiter's syndrome), psoriasis, or chronic inflammatory bowel disease ("secondary" AS), but most patients have no evidence of these associated diseases ("primary" or "pure" AS).

CLINICAL FEATURES

Clinical manifestations of the disease usually begin in late adolescence or early adulthood. The disease can begin in childhood, but onset after age 40 is uncommon. The disease is three times more common in men than in women, and its clinical and roentgenographic features seem to evolve more slowly in women. The diagnosis is based on clinical features; the best clues are offered by the patient's symptoms, the family history, the articular and extra-articular physical findings, and the roentgenographic evidence of bilateral sacroiliitis. The most common and characteristic early complaint is chronic low back pain of insidious onset, dull in character, difficult to localize, and felt deep in the gluteal or sacroiliac region. The pain may be unilateral or intermittent at first; however, within a few months, it generally becomes persistent and bilateral, and the lower lumbar area becomes stiff and painful. Pain in the lumbar area rather than the more typical buttock-ache may be the initial symptom in some patients. The second common early symptom is back stiffness, which is worse in the morning and is eased by mild physical activity or hot shower. Prolonged periods of inactivity worsen back pain and stiffness; the patient often experiences considerable difficulty in getting out of bed in the morning. At times, the pain may awaken the patient from sleep; some patients have difficulty sleeping well or find it necessary to wake up at night to move about or exercise for a few minutes before returning to bed. The back symptoms may be absent or mild in an occasional patient, whereas some may complain only of back stiffness, fleeting muscle aches, or musculotendinous tender spots. These symptoms may be worsened on exposure to cold or dampness, and such patients may occasionally be misdiagnosed as having "fibrositis."

Extra-articular or juxta-articular bony tenderness may be an early feature of the disease and is due to enthesitis (inflammatory lesions of entheses) at costosternal junctions, spinous processes, iliac crests, ischial tuberosities, or heels. Involvement of the costovertebral and the costotransverse joints and occurrence of enthesitis at costosternal areas may cause chest pain that may be accentuated on coughing or sneezing. Some patients may complain of inability to expand the chest fully on inspiration. Stiffness and pain in the cervical spine and tenderness of the spinous processes may occur in early stages of the disease in some patients, but generally this tends to occur after some years. The reported frequency of hip joint involvement varies from 17 to 36%; it is usually bilateral, insidious in onset, and potentially more crippling than involvement of any other joint of the extremities. Some degree of flexion contractures at the hip joints is not uncommon at later stages of the disease, giving rise to a characteristic, rigid gait with some flexion at the knees to maintain erect posture. Involvement of peripheral joints, other than hips and shoulders, is quite infrequent in primary AS; it is rarely persistent or erosive and tends to resolve without any residual joint deformity. For example, intermittent knee effusions may occasionally be the presenting manifestation of AS of juvenile onset. Involvement of the temporomandibular joint with resultant pain and local tenderness may occur in about 10% of patients. Mild constitutional symptoms, such as anorexia, malaise, or mild fever, may occur in some patients in early stages of their disease and may be observed relatively more commonly among patients with juvenile onset.

A thorough physical examination, particularly of the axial skeleton, is critical in making an early diagnosis of AS; there is often some limitation of motion of the lumbar spine, most easily recognized on hyperextension, lateral flexion, or rotation. The ability of a patient to touch the floor with fingertips, keeping the knees fully extended, should not be solely relied on for evaluation of spinal mobility because a good range of motion of the hip joints can compensate for considerable loss of mobility of lumbar spine. Direct pressure over the inflamed sacroiliac joints frequently elicits pain, but sometimes the sacroiliac tenderness may be absent because these sacroiliac joints are surrounded by strong ligaments that may allow only minimal motion or in late stages of the disease when inflammation is replaced by fibrosis and bony ankylosis. The chest expansion becomes restricted, the breathing becomes primarily diaphragmatic, and the abdomen becomes protuberant. The entire spine becomes increasingly stiff after many years of disease progression, with progressive flattening of lumbar spine and gentle thoracic kyphosis. Involvement of the cervical spine results in progressive limitation of neck motion and a forward cervical stoop. The diagnosis is readily apparent at this advanced stage because of the characteristic gait and posture and the way the patient sits or rises from the examining table. Spinal ankylosis develops at a variable rate and pattern; sometimes the disease may remain confined to one part of the spine. Typical deformities tend to evolve after 10 or more years.

The most common extraskeletal involvement is acute anterior uveitis (acute iritis), and it occurs in 25 to 30% of patients at some time in the course of their disease. The eye inflammation is typically unilateral and has an acute onset; symptoms include pain, increased lacrimation, photophobia, and blurred vision. Rare extraarticular involvements or complications include aortitis (leading to slowly progressive aortic valve incompetence and conduction abnormalities, sometimes requiring a pacemaker), apical pulmonary fibrosis and cavitation, amyloidosis, and IgA glomerulonephropathy. There is a lack of convincing evidence for involvement of skeletal muscles; the marked muscle wasting seen in some patients with advanced disease results from disuse atrophy. Neurologic involvement may occur owing to fracture-dislocation, atlantoaxial subluxations, or cauda equina syndrome. The fracture can follow a relatively minor trauma in patients with ankylosed spine; it usually occurs in the lower cervical spine; and the resultant quadriplegia is the most dreaded complication, with a high mortality rate.

DIAGNOSIS

The absence of a known cause of AS provides a hurdle to its early diagnosis; one has to depend primarily on the patient's clinical history and the clinical and roentgenographic findings. Low back pain and stiffness are the most common presenting symptoms, although a variety of other presentations may antedate back symptoms in some patients. Restriction of spinal mobility and a decreased chest expansion further support the diagnosis. There are no diagnostic or pathognomonic tests. An elevated erythrocyte sedimentation rate is seen in up to 75% of patients, and a mild to moderate elevation of serum IgA concentration is also frequently observed. There is no association with rheumatoid factor and antinuclear antibodies, and the synovial fluid or synovial biopsy do not show markedly distinctive features as compared with other inflammatory arthropathies.

The characteristic radiographic changes of AS may evolve slowly over many years but are usually present by the time the patient seeks medical attention. They are primarily seen in the axial skeleton, especially in the sacroiliac joint. Radiographic evidence of sacroiliitis is required for diagnosis and is the most consistent finding. A simple anteroposterior roentgenogram is usually sufficient for its detection. The changes are bilateral and symmetrical and consist of blurring of the subchondral bone plate, followed by erosions (similar to postage stamp serration) and sclerosis of the adjacent bone. These are first noted and are more prominent on the iliac side of the joint, later progressing to "pseudowidening" followed by gradual narrowing owing to interosseous bridging and ossification. Ulti-

mately (usually after many years) there may be complete bony ankylosis of the sacroiliac joints and resolution of the juxta-articular bony sclerosis.

The inflammatory lesions in the vertebral column affect the superficial layers of the annulus fibrosus, at their attachment to the corners of vertebral bodies, resulting in reactive bone sclerosis, seen roentgenographically as highlighting of the corners and subsequent bone resorption (erosions). This leads to "squaring" of the vertebral bodies and gradual ossification of the superficial layers of the annulus fibrosus that form intervertebral bony "bridging" called syndesmophytes. There are often concomitant inflammatory changes resulting in ankylosis of the apophyseal joints and ossification of the spinal ligaments, ultimately resulting in a virtually complete fusion of the vertebral column ("bamboo spine") in patients with severe AS of long duration. Spinal osteoporosis is also frequently observed as a result of ankylosis and lack of spinal mobility. In patients with early disease in whom standard roentgenography of the sacroiliac joints may show normal or equivocal changes, computed tomography appears to be more sensitive but equally specific when compared with conventional roentgenography but is rarely needed. Magnetic resonance imaging can produce excellent but costly imaging without ionizing radiation and is especially useful in cauda equina syndrome. Quantitative radioactive scintigraphy may be too nonspecific to be useful.

HLA-B27 typing can occasionally be used as an aid to the diagnosis of AS, but an overwhelming majority of patients with AS can be readily diagnosed clinically on the basis of history, physical examination, and roentgenographic findings, and they do not need the B27 test. It is not a routine, diagnostic, confirmatory, or screening test for AS in patients with back pain, even though the test in some ethnic and racial groups is highly sensitive for AS (90% sensitivity among whites compared to 50% among African-Americans). HLA-B27 is present in 8% of the normal population (2% of African-Americans).

NATURAL HISTORY

The course of AS is highly variable, characterized by spontaneous remissions and exacerbations, but it is generally favorable; earlier studies suggesting a generally unremitting course primarily involved patients with severe disease studied in hospitals. It has become apparent in the last decade that a number of HLA-B27–positive individuals, not previously recognized as having AS, manifest clinical features that are often relatively mild or self-limited. Good functional capacity and the ability to work are maintained in most patients, even in cases of protracted disease. Although it is difficult to predict the ultimate prognosis for an individual patient, those with hip involvement or completely ankylosed cervical spine with kyphosis are more likely to be disabled. Fortunately, the results of total hip arthroplasty in recent years are gratifying in preventing partial or total disability. Some studies have suggested a slightly reduced life expectancy of patients with AS, but because of the selection bias for severe disease inherent in those studies, it is likely that patients with relatively milder disease have normal life expectancy.

MANAGEMENT

There is currently no preventive measure or cure for AS, but most patients can be well managed. A concerned physician providing continuity of care can be most valuable. Patient education is crucial for successful management. The patient should thoroughly understand that although pain and stiffness can often be well controlled by appropriate use of nonsteroidal anti-inflammatory drugs (NSAIDs), regular therapeutic exercises to minimize and prevent deformity and disability are the single most important measure in medical management. The patient should walk erect; do back extension exercises regularly; and sleep on a firm mattress, without a pillow if possible. It is better to sleep on the back or in a prone position with an extended and stretched back and avoid sleeping curled up on one side. The patient should stop or avoid cigarette smoking and do regular deep breathing exercises to preserve normal chest expansion. Swimming is the best overall exercise for patients with AS, and use of snorkel and face mask may permit even those with considerable cervical flexion deformity to do freestyle swimming under observation.

Aspirin seldom provides an adequate therapeutic response. Phenylbutazone (Butazolidin) is probably the most effective NSAID for AS patients and offers good symptomatic relief, but because of its potentially greater risk of bone marrow toxicity, other NSAIDs should be tried first, such as indomethacin (Indocin), naproxen (Naprosyn), diclofenac (Voltaren), or sulindac (Clinoril). There are additional NSAIDs that may be equally effective in AS, but they may not be currently approved by the U.S. Food and Drug Administration for such clinical use. Some patients may respond better to one NSAID than another.

Sulfasalazine may be effective for peripheral arthritis in some AS patients whose symptoms are not adequately controlled by NSAIDs; because of its efficacy in inflammatory bowel disease as well, it would appear to be especially useful in enteropathic AS or for those intolerant to NSAIDs. Antimalarial drugs, D-penicillamine, and immunosuppressants have not been well studied in AS. Oral corticosteroids have no therapeutic value in the long-term management of the musculoskeletal aspects of AS because of their potential for serious side effects, and they do not halt the progression of the disease. Recalcitrant enthesopathy and persistent synovitis may respond quite well to a local corticosteroid injection.

In extreme cases in which the disease has progressed to a severe stage, surgery is helpful. Total hip replacement gives good results and prevents partial or total disability from severe hip disease. Vertebral wedge osteotomy may be needed for correction of severe kyphosis in some patients, although it carries a relatively high risk of paraplegia. Acute anterior uveitis can be well managed with dilatation of the pupil and use of corticosteroid eye drops. Systemic steroids or immunosuppressives may be needed for rare patients with severe refractory uveitis. Cardiac complications may require aortic valve replacement or pacemaker implantation. Apical pulmonary fibrosis is not easy to manage; surgical resection may rarely be required. It is the general consensus that radiotherapy has no role in the modern management of patients with AS because of the high risk of leukemia and aplastic anemia. Splints, braces, and corsets are generally not helpful in the management of AS. There is no special diet, and there is no evidence that any specific food has something to do with the initiation or exacerbation of AS.

Many patients may have difficulty driving because of the impaired neck mobility, and special wide-view mirrors can be helpful for such patients. Similarly, special prism glasses can help improve visibility of those rare patients who are so kyphotic that they cannot look ahead while walking. There are many AS patient support groups in various countries that, in addition to enlisting enthusiastic cooperation of the patients, also provide useful pamphlets and information about the disease and its management and advice about life and health insurance, jobs, working environment, wide-view mirrors, and other useful items.

TEMPOROMANDIBULAR DISORDERS

method of
CHARLES C. ALLING III, D.D.S., M.S., D.Sc.(Hon)
Brookwood Medical Center
Birmingham, Alabama

Temporomandibular disorders are frequently and often inaccurately referred to as TMJ (temporomandibular joint) disorders, syndromes, or dysfunctions. The confusion in terms has resulted in dentists, physicians, and other health professionals embracing a concept that "TMJ" is a disease entity; this has resulted in both a profusion of treatments based on *symptoms* of chronic pain in all areas above the neck and in a few practitioners' even espousing the "TMJ" being the cause of disorders in distant anatomic areas, e.g., the gastrointestinal tract, spinal column, neurologic speech center, central nervous system, cardiovascular system, and urologic system. To emphasize that the temporomandibular joint is merely a portion of the musculoskeletal system, the author refers to it as the TM joint, not the TMJ.

TM disorders are often several clinical problems involving either the TM joint or the major and minor muscles of mastication. The patients' complaints may include facial pain, pain in muscular areas, earaches, headaches, limitation of mandibular movements, TM joint sounds, and TM joint pains. TM disorders, which occur in the musculoskeletal system, may be either augmented by or mistaken for diseases and disorders of the psychogenic controls of the vascular and nervous systems and occult inflammatory and neoplastic lesions of the nasoantral and dentoalveolar structures. The trend in the medical and dental professions has been to avoid determining precise diagnoses for TM joint and facial myofascial pains and instead to create nomenclatures for all-encompassing syndromes and disorders. These have been referred to as Costen's syndrome, TMJ syndrome (or disorder), TMJ, TMJ pain dysfunction syndrome, myofascial pain dysfunction syndrome, TM disorders, and craniomandibular disorders.

It is likely that many patients who cannot cope with facial myofascial pains and TM joint disorders are biologically different from other individuals, who have similar lifestyles, personalities, emotional stresses, and medical backgrounds but who either do not suffer or able to cope. Facial myofascial pains and TM joint disorders are a subset in chronic pain categories that afflict patients. For example, it is possible that when the ultimate therapies for tension (muscle contraction) and migraine (vascular instability) headaches are established, the treatment for the vast majority of facial myofascial pains will likewise be found.

Patients who cannot cope with chronic pains are not well understood by many physicians and dentists and may be subjected to surgical procedures and other therapies, directed at symptoms and not causes, that may do harm. In time, chronic pain that is influenced by subtle disturbances of the brain, biochemistry, and general physiology on a molecular biologic level will be clearly identified. For the present, it is important for patients with facial myofascial and TM joint pains that physicians and dentists identify and treat discrete somatic maladies and the overwhelming influences of the psyche.

PREVALENCE

Epidemiologic studies of cross sections of specific populations revealed that 33% have at least one painful symptom in the craniomandibular area and that 75% have at least one TM joint sign, such as TM joint noise, that may be interpreted as TM joint dysfunction. The majority of patients with facial pain, which includes the TM joints and masticatory and facial myofascial disorders, are between 15 and 45 years of age. Of patients seeking care, women predominate. Significantly among individuals not seeking care, the signs and symptoms are about equal between the genders.

ETIOLOGY

For clinical accuracy in defining the cause, establishing a diagnosis, and developing a prudent, logical treatment plan, the complaints, symptoms, history, and physical findings of the patient should point to the facial pain complaints and TM joint disorders as having a cause in one of several major systems or categories: psychogenic, musculoskeletal and TM joint, vascular, neurologic, and occult pathology in the oral cavity or the nasal and sinal areas. As a rule, there are overlapping and reinforcing etiologic factors.

The TM joint may be implicated as the cause of disorders in the oral and maxillofacial region when, in fact, it is injured as a result of other factors. The delicate TM joint is a stress-bearing structure with a complex movement; the complex movement is possible owing to the meniscus that divides the joint space into superior and inferior compartments. A patient, often a women in the second or third decade of life who is subjected to psychosocial stresses, may unwittingly introduce unusual stresses and relationships into the TM joint by abnormal and noxious habits of posturing the mandible, for example, by clenching the teeth in full or a modified occlusion. An unusual TM joint movement may result that may be painful. The movement may feature a subluxation (clicking) or dislocation (closed lock) position of the disk. A treatment regimen may ensue that features a variety of somatic treatments, including adjusting the occlusion, inserting splints between the teeth, and even surgery to the TM joint.

Somatoform Pain Disorders

Somatoform pain disorders, manifested in the facial tissues, are identified if there are no physical or pathofunction causes and if contributing psychogenic and psychological factors are present. The pain may be manifested in tensions and trigger points in the major and minor muscles of mastication and in the cervical muscles. The resultant abnormal muscle activity may produce a disorder within the TM joint. The patient and physician may focus on the TM joint disorder as a priority rather than the cause: that is, the psyche of the patient. Treatment of a noisy, abnormal functioning, and possibly painful TM joint, in many social settings, is more acceptable to the patient than undergoing behavior modification treatment. For many physicians who treat TM disorders, a comfortable treatment focus may be on the muscular pain and the TM joint dysfunctions rather than recognizing the anxieties and depressions of the patient. One clinician after another may subject the patient to a favorite treatment procedure that has relieved pain in other patients. Patients with facial pain with a psychosomatic cause may pressure clinicians to provide somatic treatments even when the probability of restoration of function is minimal. The attempts at treatment may become a series of worsening failures and mutilations when the primary problem is undiagnosed as a psychogenic pain disorder. The problem is fueled when a clinician does not appreciate the power of a patient's mind over the body, and the patient is unwilling to discuss or to admit to having a somatoform pain disorder.

Musculoskeletal Disorders

Musculoskeletal disorders may be either the etiologic factor or, as in the case of psychogenic maladies, secondary manifestations for facial pain. Trigger points may arise in musculature secondary to mandibular abusive posture habits, trauma, or as a factor of psychogenic stress. The major muscles of mastication (the masseter, temporalis, and internal and external pterygoid muscles) may have pain trigger points within the muscles, and the trigger points may produce referred pain. As a representative masticatory muscle, trigger points in the temporalis muscle may, for example, refer pain to the TM joint or the maxillary teeth in the form of a temporal headache. As a representative cervical muscle, trigger points in the sternocleidomastoid muscle may, for example, produce referred pain in the form of an earache, a frontal headache, or pain to the eye and cheek. The clinical diagnosis of various referred myofascial pains from the sternocleidomastoid muscle are labeled atypical facial neuralgia, myofascial pain dysfunction syndrome, tension headache, and cervicocephalalgia.

The TM joint has a unique design. Most of the freely movable joints have articular surfaces of hyaline cartilage that function directly against one another and with an incomplete intervening cartilaginous meniscus. The TM joint meniscus is all the tissues between the mandibular condyle and the temporal bone articular fossa and eminence; the meniscus has an avascular disk that is positioned around the superior and anterior curve of the condyle and extends anteriorly below the temporal articular crest. In healthy TM joints, the anterior attachment of the disk is to the sphenomeniscus muscle (the superior head of the external pterygoid muscle), the posterior is to fibers of the bilaminar zone, and the lateral and medial attachments are to poles of the condyle. The thinnest and most compact part of the disk is in its central zone and is positioned, when the mouth is either in the rest position or closed in a full intercuspal position of the dental arches, between the posterior incline of the articular eminence and the anterior-superior surface of the condyle. As the mandible moves, embrasures of varying dimensions are created between the condyle and the temporal bone. The volume of the flexible disk is adequate to fill the potential superior and inferior TM joint spaces during all functional positions of the condyle and thus to provide stabilization for the mandible relative to the temporal bone. If there is laxity of the posterior, medial, or lateral attachments of the disk or if there is a muscular dysfunction at the anterior attachment, there is a disharmonious movement between the condyle and the disk, and a subluxation of the disk occurs, producing a clicking sound. It is noted that TM joint sounds occur as either transient or permanent physiologic variations of normal in the majority of individuals. If the greatest bulk of the disk should be positioned anterior to the condyle, the disk is dislocated, and a block, expressed

as a closed lock, of the mandible occurs. By inspection of mandibular movements and by auscultation, a diagnosis is possible of the painful and painless disk subluxations and dislocations. Other disk problems include perforations, which may be a normal physiologic finding in some individuals; degenerative changes associated with TM joint arthritis; and fractures or tears of the disk following acute trauma.

Inspection, palpation, and auscultation of the TM joints identify anterior subluxations and dislocations of the disks. Anterior subluxations of the disks usually occur during the opening movements of the mandible or may also occur as a reciprocal click on the closing movements. Dislocations of the disks (not the mandible) usually occur at about a 25-mm opening as measured between the incisal edges of the anterior teeth when a definite blocking movement is reported by the patient and is observed by the physician. Definitive subcategories of pathofunctions of the disk are established by clinical evaluations that indicate the type of treatment, usually splint therapy. After an accurate diagnosis is established, a series of clinical tests is performed to establish the probability of responsiveness to nonsurgical therapy. In rare instances, surgery may be indicated if there is more of a painful medial than an anterior displacement of the disk; then open TM joint surgery is performed to reposition and stabilize the disk.

Psychogenic stress, facial skeletal deformities, trauma, and deflective occlusal relationships are more likely to produce a disk movement discoordination in women. This may be explained in part by the fact that many women may have less stable and sturdy musculoskeletal systems compared with men. Any definitive treatment, as discussed later, should include preoperative, intraoperative, and postoperative physical therapy to stabilize the TM joint.

Vascular Disorders

Vascular disorders and abnormalities may produce painful sensations to the face by referral from intracranial vessels, temporal arteritis, and migraine and migrainous instabilities of the carotid systems. Emotional stress is a frequent precipitant of migrainous attacks, although no evidence is apparent that migraine patients are subjected to greater stress than nonmigraine subjects. Migraine headaches usually are clearly identified and are not mistakenly labeled TM joint disorders.

Two recurring disorders of vascular origin have been labeled as being "TMJ." Patients with lower half headaches that affect the facial tissues, usually with periorbital manifestations, have been referred for treatment with a transfer diagnosis of "TMJ." As with chronic facial myofascial pain problems, there may be a dysfunctioning of the TM joint, often including the signs of disk subluxation (clicking), and this finding may be mistaken for the cause of a lower half headache. The other unusual manifestation that erroneously may be thought to originate in the TM joint is neurovascular odontalgia (atypical odontalgia). The closed, confined spaces of the dental pulp chambers in each individual tooth are rich in nociceptors, and stimulation from changes in the vascular system may be manifested as toothaches. Resultant unusual posturing of the mandible, which produces TM joint signs and symptoms, may give the clinician the impression that the TM joint is awry, producing the malocclusion and hence the toothaches. Neurovascular odontalgia often has been successfully treated by physicians specializing in neurology.

Neurologic Disorders

Neurologic disorders are usually clearly identified by the patient in the area of distribution of the affected nerve. Pains are characteristically of short duration but of great intensity. The second and third cervical nerves innervate areas at the angle of the mandible. Pain of cardiac muscle ischemia can be referred to both angles of the mandible, but more frequently it is referred to the left; the only complaint of an ischemic heart attack may be a complaint of pain in the mandibular area. It is rare, but not surprising, when patients are referred with "TMJ," and the final diagnosis is commensurate with variations of major and minor trigeminal neuralgias, central cranial lesions, or cardiac ischemia.

Occult Pathology

Occult pathology of the dentition and nasal and sinal passages may result in a diagnosis of "TMJ" and in the provision of a variety of intraoral procedures or the placement of devices on the occlusal surfaces of teeth. Occult pathology of teeth includes impacted teeth destroying contiguous tissues, teeth with scarely detectible cracks, pulp stones, and other anomalies. The pain is often diffuse along the applicable branch of the trigeminal nerve, and it may be referred to a distant site while the pathologic tooth is relatively pain free. Pathology in the sinal or nasal passages may be manifested as pain in dentition or as pain referred to a distant site.

TREATMENT

The management of TM joint disorders, as a portion of the locomotor system, must include a precise diagnosis. The human face is the most expressive portion of the body, and the TM joint, masticator muscles, and muscles of facial expression are key portions. At the onset of the evaluation, the patient is asked to point with one finger to the area of pain. If the pain is psychogenic in origin, the patient may insist on pointing to bilateral areas rather than a single area, pointing to widely diverse locations, and waving fingers in the air around the face and cranium. If pain is vascular in origin, the patient may point around the eyes; if neurologic, along a branch of a trigeminal nerve or the second or third cervical nerves; if locomotor, that is, actually a TM joint or a muscle problem, the involved muscle or the TM joint.

Occult pathology results in a wide variety of indications.

Physical evaluation includes inspection, palpation, auscultation, and percussion, as indicated, of the TM joint and cervical spine; the facial, cervical, and masticatory muscles; intraoral structures; movements of the TM joint as recorded by mandibular excursions; the cranial and cervical nerves; and the vascular structures. Assuming, as often occurs, that the patient's history and physical examination reveal a strong psychogenic element underlying the TM joint and muscle pain, a prudent, rational treatment would be centered on a psychiatrist or psychologist. If the subsequent examinations reveal neurologic or vascular origins as the cause of the patient's complaints, definitive care is often with a general medical practitioner or a neurologist who specializes in managing headaches.

In the facial musculoskeletal system, the factors of stress, trauma, iatrogenesis, and malocclusion predispose the TM joints and masticator and facial expression musculature to myofascial dysfunctions. Initiating factors of TM joint dysfunctions, especially in women, are repetitive loading traumas to the TM joint. The initiating trauma may be from sustained, repetitive loading of the TM joints by clenching, bruxism, stress and anxiety, and medications. Perpetuating factors that sustain the TM joint and muscle disorders include social, emotional, and cognitive difficulties. There may be a social gain for the patient to have pain that attracts and holds attention. An emotional perpetuating factor may be depression, seen in many chronic pain patients. Cognitive factors of confusion and misunderstanding are often seen in chronic pain patients because of the varied and opposing diagnoses and recommendations for therapy. Often these patients have an unrealistic expectation that the physician can provide complete and immediate pain relief.

Imaging should not substitute for responsible clinical evaluation but may be indicated to confirm or enhance the clinical findings. In general, imaging studies should be ordered when the results of the imaging have the probability, not a mere possibility, of altering the treatment plan; unfortunately, nonmedical reasons may prevail and dictate the ordering of imaging: a routine of the practice, medical-legal considerations, and documentation for insurance companies. For osseous abnormalities of the TM joint, transpharyngeal, panoramic, and transorbital radiographs with the usual equipment in outpatient dental clinics provide surveys and, in some cases, final diagnostic views of the TM joint osseous structures. Definitive views of the TM joint osseous structures are obtained with either computed tomography or polycyclic tomograms corrected for the long axis of the mandibular condyle. For soft tissue imaging, TM joint arthrography uses radiopaque materials in the superior and inferior potential TM joint spaces to outline the position of the meniscus. Arthrography demonstrates a perforation, which may be a normal physiologic change, of the TM joint disk portion of the meniscus. Magnetic resonance imaging displays the soft tissues of the TM joint and confirms the location of the disk, which is usually already ascertained by history and physical evaluation.

Arthroscopy is confined by most of the currently used procedures to delivering clear images of only the superior joint space, and it should be noted that degenerative arthritic and other pathologic changes, often associated with the mandibular condyle, occur in the inferior joint space. The flushing of fluids through the superior joint space that accompanies an arthroscopic examination results in increased joint mobility; this phenomenon has been observed in the past with the injection of anesthetics and antibiotics and other solutions, including radiopaque media, when performing arthrographic examinations.

The treatment plan includes controlling pain, decreasing adverse loading, restoring function, and restoring the normal activities of life. Nonsurgical therapy, such as behavior modification, physical therapy, and short-term intraoral splint devices, is indicated first instead of a nonreversible changing of the occlusal relationships or performing TM joint surgery. The success rate in studies that included up to 10 years' follow-up of nonsurgical therapy ranged between 85.5% and more than 90%. If there has not been a structural change of the TM joint, which may require surgery to correct, the usual TM joint and muscle pain patient can be treated by an integrated program that includes patient education, behavior modification, physical therapy, palliative home care, and pharmacotherapy. Some patients require occlusal therapy, as a form of physical therapy, and a few patients are benefited by surgery.

Patient Education

Patient education is a fundamental aspect of care. The responsible physician should tailor a one-on-one conference with the patient to ensure that the patient understands the applicable anatomy, physiology, and pathology. One of the key items to be learned by the patient is that the relationship of the mandible to the maxilla in health is the rest position with a separation of the maxillary and mandibular teeth. This position relieves most pains in the TM joint and muscles. A patient who has been thoroughly indoctrinated by a dentist striving for perfect occlusion

in the fully *closed position* of the mandible to the maxilla may be initially frustrated by the information on the physiologic desirability of the *rest position* of the mandible and the muscles of mastication. For a receptive patient who wishes to be rid of facial myofascial pain and TM joint dysfunction, the use of visual aids helps illustrate how the rest position is the normal healthy relationship of the mandible to maxilla and that full, closed occlusion is not; the patient needs to understand that the rest position both removes internal compressive strains in the TM joint space and relaxes muscle that may be ladened with painful trigger points.

Behavior Modification

Behavior modification may be necessary through stress management and counseling programs. These may embrace biofeedback, progressive relaxation, and changes in lifestyle. This type of treatment may be administered by a psychiatrist or a psychologist informed on TM joint and muscle disabilities. Chronic pain patients are often laden with anxieties, depressions, and anger associated with the chronicity of their disorder. Somatic direct treatments to the dentition or to the TM joints should await stabilizing of the patient under the care of a mental health professional who is informed on TM joint and muscle disabilities. In many cases, no somatic direct treatments to the dentition or to the TM joints is necessary after behavior modification treatments.

Physical Therapy

Physical therapy alters sensory inputs and strengthens coordinated muscle activity and is especially indicated for female patients who may have loose, unstable TM joints. For patients who are to undergo intraoral treatments or TM joint surgery, physical therapy ideally should be prescribed from the preoperative through the postoperative phases of treatment. One objective of physical therapy is to obtain mandibular posture training, with the mandible in the correct anatomic rest position without contact of the dentition except when swallowing. Exercise therapy of mandibular movements to establish coordinated muscle functions, isotonic exercises to increase range of motion, and isometric exercises to strengthen the muscle are goals and modalities in most physical therapy regimens. In many cases, no direct somatic care to the teeth or to the TM joints is necessary after physical therapy.

Palliative Self-Care

Palliative self-care, in combination with physical therapy, may consist of the application of thermal packs to the TM joint and muscle areas, modification of abusive habits, avoidance of functions that strain the TM joint and muscles, control of clenching, and practicing prescribed mandibular exercises calculated to strengthen muscle groups.

Pharmacotherapy

Pharmacotherapy for patients with chronic TM joint and muscle pains and disabilities should be adjunctive to patient education, physical therapy, palliative self-care, and behavior modification procedures. When used as a part of a comprehensive management program, pharmacotherapy can be a powerful catalyst for the comfort and rehabilitation of the patient. The medications should be for a short term and be discontinued as physical therapy, palliative self-care, and behavior modification become effective. The agents used in various circumstances include non-narcotic analgesics, low-dose antidepressants, anti-inflammatory drugs, occasionally corticosteroids, and, for specific short-term goals, narcotic analgesics.

Interocclusal Splints

Interocclusal splints are effective in reducing pain in TM joints and muscle and for repositioning most of the subluxated TM joint disks. There are many varieties of splints for either stabilizing the mandible in the rest position or repositioning of the mandible as related to the maxilla and hence altering the relationships within the TM joint space. Splints should be used for short prescribed periods of time lest they cause irreversible changes in the relationships of the maxillary and mandibular dental arches.

Occlusal Therapy

Occlusal therapy, which irreversibly alters the occluding surfaces of the dental arches, should follow, when indicated, the successful management of a patient's facial myofascial pain and TM joint disorders. The maxillomandibular relationship, neuromuscular activity, and psychosocial problems should be normal or under control before initiating occlusal therapy.

Orthognathic Surgery

Orthognathic surgery, similar to occlusal therapy, should await normalization of a painful and malfunctioning TM joint and muscles. Abnormal facial skeletal relationships may have been the exciting cause for TM joint and muscle pain, but the painful episode should be resolved and controlled before instituting orthognathic surgery.

Orthognathic surgery to alleviate ongoing chronic and acute TM joint and muscle pains and dysfunctions is not indicated.

Temporomandibular Joint Surgery

TM joint surgery for painful TM joint and muscles caused by an internal joint derangement should be decided on with the following considerations: (1) assurance that effective behavioral therapy has been given the patient and that the patient has a sound psyche; (2) positive evidence that the cause of the myofascial and TM joint pain is due to the disk displacement or other joint disorder; (3) appropriate imaging documentation of TM joint disk displacement or other pathology; (4) disabling pain or dysfunction is present and due to a somatic TM joint etiology; (5) prior nonsurgical treatments that included sound physical and possible interocclusal splint therapies; (6) control of oral parafunctional habits or conditions that would adversely affect the outcome of the surgery; and (7) patient informed consent and request for surgery.

The surgical approaches are numerous and may be grouped as arthroscopic and open surgery of the TM joint. Arthroscopic surgery, using both mechanical and laser modalities, has a high success rate for managing persistent, nonreducing displaced TM disks; for revising procedures following earlier surgery by removing intracapsular fibrosis; for biopsies; and for débridement and lavages. Interestingly the distention of the joint space, usually *only the superior joint space* with commonly used techniques by the lavaging flood of fluid that accompanies arthroscopic procedures, is beneficial in freeing adhesions and increasing joint mobility even, inexplicably, when the pathologic changes, as with most arthritides, are on the mandibular condyle in the inferior joint space.

OTHER TEMPOROMANDIBULAR JOINT MALADIES

The TM joint is subject to the usual array of arthritides and joint maladies. These include degenerative, rheumatoid, psoriatic, infectious, systemic lupus erythematosus–induced, and traumatic arthritides; synovial chondromatosis; neuropathic joint disease; and other maladies, including neoplasms and hemarthrosis secondary to hemophilia. In this group, the degenerative arthritides have pathogeneses that are unique to the TM joint. There is a monarticular reversible degenerative TM joint arthritis that occurs in young women in the first 10 to 20 years after the menarche. The disease goes through four stages and, after 18 to 48 months, resolves with a normally functioning joint. The painful episodes are managed with patient (and sponsor, if indicated) education; interocclusal splints to relieve TM joint intracapsular pressures; physical therapy; and antidepressant, if indicated, and anti-inflammatory medications. In some patients, arthroscopic TM joint procedures are beneficial in relieving painful episodes. Irreversible TM joint degenerative arthritis occurs in the elderly, as with other joints.

The oral and maxillofacial manifestations of TM joint rheumatoid arthritis include a progressive apertognathism (anterior open bite) and usually are bilateral in the TM joints. The systemic general management of the TM joint is the same as for other joints. The onset of a fibrous ankylosis may require surgical intervention; in some cases, after the disease becomes quiescent, orthognathic surgical correction or TM joint reconstruction may be considered.

Infectious arthritides of the TM joint may result in an ankylosis that is treated by surgical TM joint reconstruction following the cessation of the disease.

A variant of traumatic arthritis is an acute hypertranslation of the TM joint, a so-called whiplash injury of the TM joint. In the twentieth century, millions of patients have been treated for maxillofacial fractures and injuries incurred in violent accidents, altercations, and warfare; however, only in the past 20 years have TM disorders and so-called TM joint whiplash been diagnosed as incurred by the trauma. In many cases, patient awareness of a clicking or other actual internal derangement of a TM joint and a history of an episode of trauma may have been combined with a hope of the benefits of legal recourse. Individuals with either a normal or an abnormal TM joint clicking sound and experiencing myofascial facial pains may be diagnosed by a physician as having either a TM disorder or one of the synonymous disorders. The individual with the preceding combination of symptoms and a diagnostic label may seek legal recourse by citing as the cause acute trauma; general anesthetic intubation; and intraoral, transoral, and pharyngeal surgical procedures. In the area of imaginative legal gamesmanship, it is helpful to recall the words of the orthopedic surgeon, H. M. Frost: "In my time, I have seen for diagnosis and/or treatment more than 10,000 patients with unresolved liability from a real or imagined injury. Yet in the same period, I have seen only three patients desiring help or advice for just injury after the liability was closed."*

*Mahan PE, Alling CC: Facial Pain, 3rd ed. Philadelphia, Lea & Febiger, 1991, 103.

BURSITIS, TENDINITIS, MYOFASCIAL PAIN, AND FIBROMYALGIA

method of
ROBERT M. BENNETT, M.D.
Oregon Health Sciences University
Portland, Oregon

The muscular apparatus is the largest organ in the body, accounting for 40% of body weight. There are 696 individual muscles, most of which are attached to tendons, which merge with the periosteum; some attach directly to the periosteum through a musculoperiosteal junction. The smooth functioning of muscles is aided by the encasement of some tendons by synovial tendon sheaths and the development of bursae where muscles and tendons have close proximity to bony prominences or where major muscle bundles rub over each other. Some 80 paired bursae have been described in various anatomic texts. The majority of patients who present to their physician with rheumatic pain have a disorder of the muscle-tendon-bursa apparatus rather than a true arthritis. Commonly encountered syndromes involving bursae, tendons, and muscles are shown in Tables 1 through 3. There has been an increasing awareness over the past decade that some patients, mainly women, have a history of widespread musculoskeletal pain often in association with profound fatigue and many other somatic symptoms; this is now called the fibromyalgia syndrome (Table 4).

MANAGEMENT

The effective management of these four conditions demands an accurate analysis as to the anatomic structure(s) involved. Most patients presenting with bursitis, tendinitis, or myofascial pain have a predisposing cause for the initiation of the problem. In many cases, perpetuation of the problem is due to repetitive activities that irritate the involved structures. The most difficult part of treatment is to identify precisely and eliminate these aggravating factors. Biomechanical dysfunction may be an important contributory factor (e.g., genu valgus or unequal leg length). In some patients, there is an underlying systemic disease, such as rheumatoid arthritis, gout, or Reiter's disease. In patients with septic bursitis or septic tenosynovitis, there is usually a history of a penetrating injury. In cases in which this is not apparent, one should search for a focus of blood-borne sepsis, such as staphylococcal skin lesions, gram-negative sepsis from urogenital instrumentation, or gonococcemia from pelvic inflammation.

There are several points that are important in the overall treatment plan of these conditions:

TABLE 1. **Commonly Involved Bursae**

Site	Symptom	Findings
Subdeltoid	Shoulder pain	Tender subcutaneous swelling
Olecranon	Elbow pain	Tender subcutaneous swelling
Trochanteric	Lateral hip pain	Tenderness over greater trochanter
Ischial (Weaver's bottom)	Pain on sitting	Tenderness with pressure over ischium
Prepatellar (housemaid's knee)	Painful knee	Subcutaneous swelling over patella
Infrapatellar (clergyman's knee)	Painful knee	Subcutaneous swelling below patella
Anserine	Painful knee	Tenderness over medial aspect of knee
Iliopectineal	Painful groin	Tenderness over inguinal triangle
Achilles (pump bump)	Painful heel	Subcutaneous swelling at back of Achilles tendon
Calcaneal	Painful heel	Tenderness on pressure over calcaneum

1. Explain to the patient why he or she has the condition and the expected results of therapy, including the time course for recovery and possible complications.

2. Provide information on the avoidance of aggravating factors.

3. If the patient is in a work situation that is aggravating or perpetuating the condition, provide appropriate time off work for recovery and counsel on modification of job description.

4. Provide biomechanical rest when appropriate, e.g., splinting, slings, instruction in the use of a cane.

5. Provide pain relief.

6. Provide anti-inflammatory treatment.

7. Prescribe a long-term plan of stretching and muscle-strengthening exercise to minimize recurrence of the problem.

Bursitis

When inflammation of a bursa is superficial, such as the shoulder, knee, elbow, and Achilles tendon, the diagnosis is usually obvious. Deeper bursa, such as those around the hip joint and the ischial tuberosity, do not present with obvious swelling; a diagnosis must be inferred from local tenderness and exacerbation of pain by activation of the associated muscles. Bursitis seldom shows up on plain x-rays and expensive imaging studies, such as magnetic resonance imaging or radio-

contrast studies are not routinely advocated if a nonarticular cause of pain is suspected. If possible, one should aspirate the bursa because the finding of synovial fluid helps confirm the diagnosis of bursitis. If the fluid is not clear (as is the case in most instances of "irritated" bursitis), it should be sent for culture and examined for the presence of crystals.

Non-infective bursitis is treated as follows: The involved areas should be rested if feasible, e.g., the provision of a sling for subdeltoid bursitis or instruction in the use of a cane in the contralateral hand for trochanteric bursitis. The quickest and usually most complete relief is obtained by an appropriately placed corticosteroid injection. After aspirating the bursa, a mixture of 1% procaine (about 3 mL) containing 1 to 2 mL of a long-acting corticosteroid preparation, such as triamcinolone hexacetonide (Aristospan), prednisolone tebutate (Hydeltra TBA), betamethasone acetate (Celestone Soluspan), methylprednisolone acetate (DeproMedrol), or dexamethasone acetate (Decadron LA), can be instilled. Prompt amelioration of discomfort within about 5 minutes of giving this injection (due to the effect of the local anesthetic) gives some reassurance that the injection has been accurately placed and the diagnosis is correct. Patients should be warned that the initial response to the local anesthetic wears off within about an hour and that they may have more pain over the next 12 to 24 hours until the

TABLE 2. **Commonly Involved Tendons**

Site	Symptom	Findings
Supraspinatus	Shoulder pain	Painful arc
Bicipital	Shoulder pain	Local tenderness anteriorly
Infraspinatus	Shoulder pain	Pain on internal rotation
Extensor pollicis brevis and abductor pollicis longus (de Quervain's tenosynovitis)	Wrist pain	Pain on ulnar deviation of wrist
Lateral epicondyle muscle attachments	Elbow pain	Tenderness just below lateral epicondyle
Patellar tendon	Knee pain	Local tenderness
Finger flexors	Trigger finger	"Catching" on extension of finger
Tibialis posterior	Ankle pain	Local pain under medial malleolus
Peroneal tendons	Ankle pain	Local pain under lateral malleolus

TABLE 3. **Commonly Involved Sites of Myofascial Pain**

Location of Trigger Point	Symptoms
Trapezius (most commonly upper portion)	Shoulder and neck pain, often headache
Sternomastoid (often multiple trigger points)	Atypical facial pain, headache
Masseter	Temporomandibular pain syndrome
Suboccipital	Headache—occipital, retro-orbital, forehead
Levator scapulae	Stiff neck
Gluteus medius (upper portion)	Pain in low back and buttock
Muscles inserting into greater trochanter	Lateral hip and thigh pain
Tensor fasciae latae	Lateral thigh pain
Muscles inserting into upper border of patella	Knee pain

corticosteroid preparation takes effect. In some cases, the injection of a long-acting corticosteroid preparation, which is usually microcrystalline, provokes an acute inflammatory response akin to gout. This is almost always averted if the patient is prescribed concomitant nonsteroidal anti-inflammatory drugs (NSAIDs) (e.g., Indocin SR, 75 mg twice daily), ibuprofen (Motrin or Rufen, 800 mg three times a day), ketoprofen (Orudis, 75 mg twice daily), sulindac (Clinoril, 200 mg twice daily), naproxen (Naprosyn, 500 twice daily), etodolac (Lodine, 750 mg twice daily), or nabumetone (Relafen, 500 mg twice daily). Therapy with NSAIDs should be continued for approximately 1 week after all symptoms have subsided and the patient has embarked on a program of gentle return to normal activity. If aggravating factors have been eliminated, the patient seldom needs repeated injections. A recurrence of the bursitis within 7 days of injection should always be of a concern regarding possible septic bursitis, and a re-aspiration should be performed.

Septic bursitis is usually due to a penicillin-resistant *Staphylococcus aureus*; the physician should always consider the possibility of the patient being diabetic, an intravenous drug abuser,

TABLE 4. **Clinical Features of Fibromyalgia**

Nearly Always Present	Often Present
Total body pain	Recurrent headaches
Multiple tender points on examination	Irritable bowel syndrome
Severe fatigue	Atypical paresthesias
Nonrestorative sleep (alpha-delta sleep)	Cold sensitivity (often Raynaud's)
Post-exertional increase in muscle pain	Restless leg syndrome
Reduced functional ability	Aerobic deconditioning

or immunocompromised owing to human immunodeficiency virus (HIV) infection. It is important to note that septic bursitis is *not* treated with local antibiotics. In many patients, systemic treatment with oral dicloxacillin (Dynapen, 500 mg four times a day for 10 days) is an effective regimen. Patients who have a serious underlying illness should be treated more vigorously with intravenous antibiotics, such as oxacillin (Prostaphlin), 2 grams four times a day for 7 days, followed by oral dicloxacillin. In patients who are allergic to beta-lactams, the appropriate antibiotic is dictated by the culture report. At the initiation of therapy, it is most important that the bursal contents be drained through a 16- to 18-gauge needle. This drainage often has to be repeated two or three times over the course of the first week of treatment. In those rare cases in which re-accumulation of infected bursa fluid is recurrent, despite appropriate antibiotics, the possibility of open surgical drainage needs to be discussed with an orthopedic surgeon.

Tendinitis

Tendons may tear or be partially ruptured but are never truly inflamed. The term "tendinitis" refers to an inflammation of the peritendinous tissues or synovial sheaths (tenosynovitis). Awareness of this distinction is not purely academic because the injection of corticosteroids into a tendon, particularly if repeated, may lead to its subsequent rupture. Most instances of tendinitis result from overuse or unaccustomed activity; hence rest or splinting (or both) is an important ingredient in successful treatment. As in the case of nonseptic bursitis, an accurately placed injection of corticosteroids provides the quickest symptomatic relief. Effective injection of tendons is an acquired skill. A knowledge of the relevant anatomy is essential to the success of such injections. Tendons are not injected; rather the small space between the exterior surface of the tendon and the peritendinous sheath is infiltrated with a mixture of corticosteroids and local anesthetic (as noted for the injection of bursitis). To avoid snagging the tendon, it is important that the bevel of the needle be face downward and parallel to the long axis of the tendon. Local corticosteroids should not be used in patients with Achilles tendinitis because of its propensity to rupture. In competitive athletes, peritendinous injections should be avoided in relation to the infrapatella tendon and the supraspinatus muscle, for similar reasons.

Myofascial Pain

Minor muscle tears consequent on injury, unaccustomed activity, or repetitive use may cause a painful irritative focus in a muscle—commonly referred to as a "trigger point." In the author's experience, this is the most common cause of non-articular rheumatic pain; it presents as a regional musculoskeletal pain syndrome (see Table 3). Many patients who have myofascial pain are initially misdiagnosed as having bursitis, tendinitis, or even a more serious condition, such as a nerve entrapment syndrome, fracture, or tumor. Trigger points are not visualized on routine imaging studies; as such, patients may have significant dysfunction not amenable to routine testing and may be erroneously labeled as malingering or having a "functional syndrome." Many patients with a bonafide tendinitis/bursitis develop biomechanical imbalance, which leads to a secondary myofascial pain syndrome. Failure to recognize the evolution of such a myofascial pain syndrome results in apparent treatment failures.

The finding of a single or several trigger points should suggest the diagnosis of a myofascial pain syndrome. The characteristics of a trigger point are as follows:

1. Symptoms of regional musculoskeletal pain.
2. Local pain on pressure of the trigger point, often with centrifugal referral.
3. Pain on stretching the involved muscle.
4. Pain on contraction of the involved muscle.
5. Functional shortening of the involved muscle.
6. The finding of an increased consistency of muscle on palpation of the trigger point area.
7. A temporary relief of pain by the precise injection of 1 to 3 mL of 1% procaine hydrochloride into the trigger point area.

The essential prerequisites of myofascial therapy are as follows:

1. Identification and elimination of aggravating factors.
2. The accurate injection of the myofascial trigger points as detailed subsequently.
3. Passive stretching of the involved muscle after the local anesthetic has taken effect; this is often aided by spraying the overlying skin with Fluori-Methane spray before passive stretching.
4. The application of a hot pack while the patient remains in a relaxed position for 30 minutes after the injection.

In most patients, this treatment regimen needs to be repeated over a period of several weeks and occasionally over several months. Recalcitrant cases are usually due to failure to eliminate an aggravating factor, imprecise injection of the trigger point, or failure to inject satellite trigger points. Trigger points are usually injected with 3 to 5 mL of 1% procaine. Whether the addition of a small amount of local corticosteroid (e.g., 0.25 mL of Hydeltra TBA) provides increased benefit has not been carefully studied. There is certainly no rationale for injecting concentrated corticosteroids into a myofascial trigger point; furthermore, insoluble corticosteroid preparations may leak back into subcutaneous tissues and cause an unsightly area of skin atrophy.

The technique for injection is as follows: After cleaning the skin, a 24- to 26-gauge needle is inserted only as far as the deep dermis. The needle is then slowly advanced into the area of the trigger point, and the patient is instructed to tell the physician when an acute increase of pain is noted. There are two reliable signs that a trigger point has been entered: (1) the patient's experience of a sudden pain, often with a centrifugal pattern of referral, and (2) a feeling of increased resistance to the progression of the needle tip. In superficial muscles, a transient "twitch response" of the muscle may be observed. Approximately 0.5 mL of fluid is injected and the needle then reinserted (without it leaving the original skin puncture) into an adjacent area of muscle. This "peppering" procedure is repeated until no more pain is experienced. For the average sized trigger point, the total amount injected is between 3 and 5 mL. Typically the beneficial effects from such an injection occur within 2 to 4 days. Patients should be informed that they may experience an immediate relief of the pain from the effects of the local anesthetic, but there may be a temporary increase in pain for 1 to 3 days. There are often several trigger points responsible for myofascial pain syndrome; hence more than one trigger point may need to be injected at the same time. Because large volumes of local anesthetic (more than 15 mL) may cause light-headedness, tinnitus, muscle fasciculations, bradycardia, hypertension, and rarely convulsions or cardiorespiratory arrest, the number of injections should be limited in any one day to three. Repeat visits for the injection of other satellite trigger points are scheduled at 1- to 2-week intervals. Anaphylaxis is a rare complication from all local anesthetics, and physicians doing these procedures should have a ready availability of airway oxygen, 1:1000 epinephrine, and intravenous diazepam. Injections in the upper back and other locations close to the thorax may result in a pneumothorax if the needle penetrates the pleura or lung. An awareness of this potential problem and the entering of trigger points at an oblique angle to the surface of the chest wall minimize the likelihood of this complication.

Fibromyalgia

Over the past decade, there has been an increasing realization and acceptance that many patients presenting with widespread musculoskeletal pain can best be classified as having the fibromyalgia syndrome. Simplistically fibromyalgia can be thought of as widespread myofascial pain, in that such patients have multiple myofascial tender points. Indeed, the American College of Rheumatology has defined the fibromyalgia syndrome in terms of widespread musculoskeletal pain (defined as pain in three or more quadrants of the body plus axial pain) and the presence of 11 or more out of 18 specifically designated tender points. In reality, most fibromyalgia patients present with a syndrome of complicated somatic distress (see Table 4). A treatable cause for the sleep disturbance should always be sought. For instance, a small number of patients have sleep apnea and benefit from continuous positive airway pressure therapy. Other patients have nocturnal myoclonus associated with a restless leg syndrome and may often be helped by the prescription of clonazepam (Klonopin), 0.1 mg at bedtime or carbidopa-levodopa (Sinemet), 10/100 at bedtime. In the majority of patients, the sleep disturbance seems to be rooted in psychological distress or due to pain itself. For instance, a regional myofascial pain syndrome consequent to a whiplash injury may cause a persistent sleep disruption, which eventually leads to the appearance of widespread musculoskeletal pain consistent with the fibromyalgia syndrome; this transition from regional pain to widespread pain typically occurs over a period of 6 to 18 months. In some patients, trochanteric bursitis or subacromial bursitis/tendinitis causes a sleep disruption every time the patient turns over onto that side, and appropriate treatment of the bursitis (see previous section) may lead to a more restorative sleep pattern. In many fibromyalgia patients, the sleep disturbance may be helped by the judicious prescription of a low-dose tricyclic antidepressant (TCA). It should be stressed that the doses required to promote restorative sleep in fibromyalgia are usually not in the range required to treat depression. Currently there seems to be no logical way of knowing which TCA to prescribe. The ideal medication would produce restorative sleep with a feeling of being refreshed on awakening with no side effects. In reality, some patients are excessively sensitive to TCAs and have a severe sense of "morning hangover"; this may be helped by switching from one of the more sedative agents to a more stimulant TCA. Other patients find TCAs unacceptable owing to anticholinergic side effects, such as tachycardia, dry mouth, and constipation. Most TCAs cause some weight gain, but in certain patients this may amount to 20% of their initial body weight and is thus unacceptable. The author often initiates TCA therapy with

a trial of four medications taken for 6 days each with a 1-day washout between. Patients can be advised to start medication on a Friday evening to minimize the inconvenience of a possible hangover the next morning. If the patient has not taken a TCA before, the following drugs and dosages can typically be used: amitriptyline (Elavil, Endep), 10 mg at bedtime; doxepin (Sinequan, Adapin), 10 mg at bedtime; nortriptyline (Pamelor, Aventil), 10 mg at bedtime; and trazadone (Desyrel), 25 mg at bedtime. Depending on their reactions to these medications three or four more different TCAs may be prescribed if a suitable efficacy or side effect profile has not been found. Unless the patient has a concomitant major depressive illness, the author does not routinely advocate fluoxetine (Prozac) because this often exacerbates insomnia and causes agitation. When fluoxetine is used in patients with concomitant major depression, the author routinely employs a low-dose TCA, such as trazadone, 50 mg at bedtime.

There is currently no cure for fibromyalgia, and most patients persist with chronic problems of somatic distress, which at best can be only partially ameliorated by therapy. Bearing this in mind, it is important to provide educational literature; some patients benefit from well-run support groups (which should be supervised by a health care professional with the aim of concentrating on positive coping strategies and minimizing "whining"). There is evidence that fibromyalgia patients benefit from increasing aerobic conditioning, but many are reluctant to exercise on account of increased pain and fatigue. Most patients, however, can be motivated to increase their level of fitness if they are provided realistic guidelines for exercise and have regular follow-up. The use of NSAIDs in these patients is usually disappointing; it is unusual for fibromyaglia patients to experience more than a 20% relief of their pain, but many consider this to be worthwhile. The severity of pain and the location of "hot spots" typically varies from month to month, and the judicious use of myofascial trigger point injections is worthwhile in selected patients. Many fibromyalgia patients develop a reduced functional ability, and the treating physician should act on their behalf in sanctioning a reduced or modified load at work and at home. The overall philosophy of treating fibromyalgia patients, however, is to provide them with realistic expectations of what can be done to help and de-emphasize the role of medications. Frequent visits to physical therapists, masseurs, and chiropractors and a dependence on repeated myofascial trigger point injections should be discouraged. Unless the patient has an obvious psychiatric illness, referral to psychiatrists is usually nonproductive. Psychological counseling, particularly the use of techniques such as cognitive restructuring and biofeedback, may be of benefit in some patients who are having difficulties coping with the realities of their illness and associated problems.

OSTEOARTHRITIS

method of
KENNETH E. SACK, M.D.
University of California–San Francisco
San Francisco, California

Osteoarthritis refers to a degeneration of articular cartilage, typically accompanied by sclerosis of subchondral bone and the formation of marginal osteophytes. Although not primarily an inflammatory disease, osteoarthritis occasionally presents with an accompanying synovitis, particularly in menopausal women. Synovial inflammation also may occur late in the disease, presumably as a response to severe degeneration of cartilage.

Osteoarthritis characteristically affects the distal and proximal interphalangeal and first carpometacarpal joints of the hands as well as the hips, knees, first metatarsophalangeal joints, and movable portions of the spine. When degeneration of cartilage is especially severe or occurs in atypical locations, other forms of degenerative joint disease should be considered (Table 1).

TREATMENT

Patient Education

Patients should receive reassurance that osteoarthritis is a common condition that rarely

TABLE 1. **Other Forms of Degenerative Joint Disease**

Inflammatory Joint Diseases
Rheumatoid arthritis
Infectious arthritis

Physical Factors
Trauma
  Joint injury
  Obesity
  Biomechanical derangement
  Neuropathy
Avascular necrosis of bone

Endocrine Disorders
Diabetes mellitus
Acromegaly

Metabolic Disorders
Hemochromatosis
Wilson's disease
Ochronosis
Crystal diseases (e.g., gout, pseudogout).

cripples. Thus the focus of treatment is to relieve symptoms in the safest way possible. Local chapters of the Arthritis Foundation can provide names of nearby rheumatologists, exercise programs, and appropriate support groups.

Diet

Dietary manipulation does not induce or cause progression of osteoarthritis. There is, however, a correlation between obesity and osteoarthritis in the knees. In such patients, a weight-reduction program may alleviate pain.

Physical Modalities

Exercise helps maintain the integrity of cartilage and improves the strength of joint stabilizing muscles. The ideal exercise program avoids harmful impact loading on joints and emphasizes relatively atraumatic isometric exercises (contraction of the muscle without movement of the joint). Taking a warm shower or applying heat to a painful joint may make exercising less stressful by increasing tendon distensibility and raising the pain threshold. By contrast, massaging the affected joint with ice relieves pain in some patients.

Low-impact aerobic exercises are not harmful and may be beneficial to cartilage. If joint pain increases and persists for more than an hour after completing an exercise, the activity should be modified or discontinued. Water exercise may benefit markedly obese patients or those with severe disease in weight-bearing joints. A physical or occupational therapist can assist in tailoring the treatment program to the patient's particular needs (Table 2).

Drug Therapy

Many patients with osteoarthritis require only a simple analgesic, such as acetaminophen or a nonsteroidal anti-inflammatory drug (NSAID) in low dosage. Higher dosages may be necessary for some patients, suggesting that inflammation is somehow contributing to the symptoms. Unfortunately, patients with osteoarthritis are often elderly and therefore are more susceptible to the serious toxicity (e.g., gastropathy, renal failure) of NSAIDs. It is prudent therefore to use NSAIDs sparingly in this disorder.

For patients with osteoarthritis and unrelenting joint pain, injection of a corticosteroid (Table 3) into the affected joint often gives prolonged relief, presumably by reducing associated inflammation. The dose of corticosteroid that suppresses the production of degradative enzymes

TABLE 2. **Physical Modalities for Treating Patients with Osteoarthritis**

Problem Area	Treatment
Fingers	Work modification
	Heat
	Gentle stretching
Neck	Rest (use of modified pillow, cervical collar)
	Heat (including ultrasound)
	Gentle stretching (including traction)
	Isometric strengthening exercises
Low back	Rest (bed rest on firm mattress, posture training, corset)
	Gentle stretching (including traction)
	Heat (including ultrasound)
	Isometric strengthening exercises
Hip	Rest (mobility-assisting devices)
	Heat (including ultrasound)
	Gentle stretching
	Isometric strengthening exercises
Knee	Rest (mobility-assisting devices)
	Heat
	Gentle stretching
	Isometric strengthening exercises
Foot	Rest (shoe modification)
	Heat

probably does little harm to the cartilage. Triamcinolone hexacetonide gives the most prolonged response and is appropriate for large joints, such as the knee. Use of a more soluble preparation, such as triamcinolone acetonide, for smaller joints reduces the risk of causing atrophy in the overlying skin. Mixing the steroid with an equal volume of 1% lidocaine not only provides analgesia, but also dilutes the concentration of corticosteroid and may lower the incidence of a post-injection flare in pain.

TABLE 3. **Intra-Articular Steroid Doses**

Preparation	Dose for Large Joint (e.g., knee)* (mg)
Triamcinolone hexacetonide (Aristospan), 20 mg/mL	20–30
Triamcinolone acetonide (Kenalog), 10 and 40 mg/mL	30–40
Prednisolone tebutate (Hydeltra TBA), 20 mg/mL	30–40
Methylprednisolone acetate (Depo-Medrol), 20, 40, and 80 mg/mL	30–40
Dexamethasone acetate (Decadron-LA), 8 mg/mL	3–4
Dexamethasone sodium phosphate (Decadron and Hexadrol), 4 mg/mL	3–4
Betamethasone sodium phosphate and acetate suspension (Celestone Soluspan), 6 mg/mL	5–6

*Use approximately half this dose for medium size joints (e.g., wrist) and one-tenth for small joints (e.g., metacarpophalangeal).

Surgery

Consultation with an orthopedic surgeon is indicated when pain, stiffness, or instability of the affected joint substantially limits its function. Such joints may require surgical remodeling or replacement; this is especially true for the hip and knee. Fortunately, some patients with osteoarthritis in the lower extremity have less pain as they get older, even though the physical or radiographic appearance of the joint is unchanged.

Other effective surgical procedures include extraction of a loose bony or cartilaginous fragment (typically through an arthroscope), resection of painful metatarsal heads, and removal of degenerative disk material or bone to relieve impingement on a spinal nerve root.

POLYMYALGIA RHEUMATICA AND GIANT CELL ARTERITIS

method of
MATTHEW O. SWARTZ, M.D.
Prince William Hospital
Manassas, Virginia

Much is written about the conditions polymyalgia rheumatica (PMR) and giant cell arteritis (GCA), but little has changed in diagnosis and treatment. Both are common conditions of the sixth decade of life and beyond; may present concurrently, sequentially, or independently; and demonstrate unusual sensitivity to systemic corticosteroid therapy. Although the treatment of these conditions is considered separately, it is critical that the reader know of and appreciate the controversy and varied experience with the unique interrelationship that exists between the two.

The coexistence of PMR and GCA has been known for more than 30 years. Similarity in presenting complaints led to the biopsy of asymptomatic temporal arteries and the findings of temporal arteritis in 10 to 30%. Despite this, the controversy of whether all patients with typical PMR should undergo temporal artery biopsy is unsettled. It is further complicated by the well-described observation that a negative biopsy result does not always rule out GCA on the contralateral side or involving other branches of the aortic arch, even becoming symptomatic later in the course. Epidemiologic studies suggest an ethnicity with reports from Scandinavia and, in the United States, of populations of Scandinavian descent approaching 20%. In more heterogeneous populations, positive biopsy results are rarely found. Thus the decision to perform a temporal artery biopsy and when to perform the biopsy must be in each case individualized. It seems prudent to share this controversy with the patient. Although most are naturally reluctant to undergo "unnecessary testing," they are usually willing to be carefully monitored and immediately report changes in status or new symptoms that might change a previous decision regarding biopsy. In this way, patients have done well with "pure" PMR.

The complaints at presentation are what one expects from a systemic illness superimposed on those that strongly suggest a rheumatologic process. Almost always of abrupt onset, patients report the disabling pain in their upper back, shoulders, and hips began "that morning" and the incapacitating stiffness that failed to respond to over-the-counter analgesics, prescription anti-inflammatory agents, or even narcotics. There is an understandable hopelessness conveyed by the patient and the family with an attendant anxiety that previous independence has been permanently lost, or the diagnosis of neoplasia must have been missed. Anorexia, weight loss, and malaise make this possibility seem likely. Historical clues, however, including the dramatic onset, absence of localizing symptoms on review of systems, and previous vigorous good health, are helpful. It has been said that jaw claudication may be the sine qua non of GCA.

The physical examination, frequently devoid of significant findings, nonetheless is important. Scalp or temporal artery tenderness should be sought both at the time of initial evaluation and thereafter throughout the treatment course. Large joint synovitis, clinically appreciable in shoulders, wrists, and knees, can yield inflammatory, but sterile, Class II synovial fluid. Provided that pain does not interfere, muscle strength should be normal and not weaken with simple repetitive movements. Neurologic examination should be free of focal or lateralizing signs.

Laboratory data should include a measure of acute-phase reactants (elevation of erythrocyte sedimentation rate, C-reactive protein, and globulin fraction on serum protein electrophoresis are expected), complete blood count (which might demonstrate a normochromic, normocytic anemia and moderate thrombocytosis), and automated chemical profile (often showing elevation in alkaline phosphatase). An intermediate-strength purified protein derivative, with a control to rule out anergy, should be considered in light of the implications for long-term systemic corticosteroids. Depending on geographic location or travel history, antibodies directed against the *Borrelia burgdorferi* spirochete may be required to rule out Lyme disease. A recent report has identified anticardiolipin antibodies in both PMR and GCA with a statistically significant predilection for the latter.

TREATMENT

Polymyalgia Rheumatica

As dramatically as PMR appears, it seems to respond to treatment just as quickly. Doses of less than 20 mg daily of prednisone, as a single dose, are generally sufficient to eliminate all traces of disease activity within the first 2 weeks of treatment. Should there fail to be substantial improvement in the patient's global assessment, the possibility of an alternative diagnosis should be raised. With subjective improvement, confirmed by fall in the acute-phase reactants measured before treatment, reduction in prednisone dose can be initiated.

There is no fixed pattern for tapering the corticosteroid dose. Decrements in the daily dose of prednisone, 2.5 mg, every week are generally well tolerated after the first 2 weeks of treatment. A more gradual rate of 1 mg per week to establish the "lowest dose necessary" should be titrated against any recrudescence of patient symptoms and every 6 to 8 weeks' monitoring of the acute-phase reactants (usually the erythrocyte sedimentation rate). One should be satisfied with a maintenance dose of 5 to 7.5 mg prednisone daily, and at that point, careful documentation of the patient's stability over time takes precedence. If recurrence is suggested, reverting back two dose levels is usually sufficient to recapture control, provided that this adjustment is made promptly. Delay in identifying the flare may make it more difficult and require even greater dose increases. Use of nonsteroidal anti-inflammatory drugs is not worth the increased risk of ulcer disease, and alternate-day dosing is generally not adequate to maintain control and adds little to reduce untoward effects of these small corticosteroid doses.

Frequent monitoring of the acute-phase reactants during treatment seems limited because what the patient relates is usually confirmed. Marked increases should be viewed as evidence of possible crossover to GCA. Stability in the test while a patient's symptoms are worsening requires treatment, so literal interpretation of the test result out of context of the patient's status should be avoided.

Giant Cell Arteritis

GCA is diagnosed by temporal artery biopsy. In the face of an adequate (no less than 5 cm) sampling and exhaustive histopathologic search for changes that may "skip" segments of the biopsy, failure to demonstrate the characteristic mononuclear cell infiltrates into the muscular layer of the vessel wall does not preclude treatment in certain circumstances. Jaw claudication, the unmistakable, acute fatigue in the muscles of mastication with prolonged, vigorous chewing, has been considered pathognomonic. A careful ophthalmologic examination may show changes of ischemia, which, with elevated erythrocyte sedimentation rate in a patient with characteristic headache would be compelling for a clinical diagnosis of GCA. Failure to make the diagnosis may result in irreversible retinal damage and permanent visual loss, making clinical judgment crucial for optimal outcome.

Once the diagnosis has been considered likely, prompt treatment should begin, even while awaiting temporal artery biopsy or the report. Prednisone, 1 mg per kg given as a single daily dose, is preferred. Divided equally and given twice daily is acceptable, but the former schedule aids in minimizing toxicity. Subjective response rates vary, but overall improvement, including constitutional symptoms, such as fever, are generally noted to subside in 2 to 4 weeks and should be expected to resolve completely. So, too, should the acute phase reactants. Despite this, the temptation to begin rapid tapering of the corticosteroids should be avoided. It should be viewed that vascular injury has occurred in branches of the aortic arch, including the intracranial system, and adequate time must be allowed for control of the initiating process as well as repair of damage. An interval of 1 year has been suggested but probably is excessive. A consistent 3 to 6 months, however, should be targeted.

Although most cases seem to resolve after 1 year, reports of activity after more than 2 years of treatment are not rare. If the patient is subjectively free of symptoms and other established parameters have responded, tapering of the prednisone dose may proceed by 5 mg monthly to a daily dose of 20 mg. At that point, one should proceed more slowly, perhaps 2.5 mg monthly to 10 mg. This should roughly coincide with 1 year of treatment, and further tapering by 1 mg per week can be followed because recurrent vasculitic phenomena will usually break through at higher doses.

The length of time the corticosteroid treatment is required, total daily doses, and the age group being treated all contribute to the potential morbidity of treatment for GCA. Rapid worsening of existing cataracts, accelerated loss of bone density, myopathic weakness, impairment of sodium and water metabolism, hypertension, and glucose intolerance are all to be anticipated. Regular eye examinations, detailed discussion of calcium and vitamin D intake, supplementing dietary sources if necessary, restricting sodium and fluid intake as needed while avoiding diuretics, and careful calorie counts should all be part of the treatment plan. Confusion or frank psychosis may necessitate gentle sedation during the initial phase of therapy. Other immunosuppressive agents have not been shown to be helpful in reducing these toxicities or providing a therapeutic option in treating GCA.

OSTEOMYELITIS

method of
JON T. MADER, M.D.,
JOSE A. COBOS, M.D., and
JASON H. CALHOUN, M.D., M.ENG.
The University of Texas Medical Branch
Galveston, Texas

Osteomyelitis may be acute or chronic. The acute disease is characterized by a suppurative infection accompanied by edema, vascular congestion, and small vessel thrombosis. The vascular supply to the bone is compromised as the infection extends into the surrounding soft tissue. Large areas of dead bone (sequestra) may be formed when both the medullary and the periosteal blood supplies are compromised. Viable colonies of bacteria may be harbored within the necrotic and ischemic tissues even after an intense host response, surgery, or therapeutic antibiotics. Once the antibiotics are discontinued or the host response declines, the organisms may again proliferate and lead to a recurrence of the infection. The hallmarks of chronic osteomyelitis are a nidus of infected dead bone or scar tissue, an ischemic soft tissue envelope, and a refractory clinical course.

HEMATOGENOUS OSTEOMYELITIS

Hematogenous osteomyelitis occurs mainly in infants and children. The metaphyses of the long bones (tibia, femur) are most frequently involved. A single pathogenic organism is almost always recovered from the bone in hematogenous osteomyelitis. Polymicrobic hematogenous osteomyelitis is rare. In the infant, *Staphylococcus aureus,* group B streptococcus, and *Escherichia coli* are the most frequently recovered bone isolates. In children older than 1 year of age, *S. aureus, Streptococcus pyogenes,* and *Haemophilus influenzae* are most commonly isolated. After age 4, however, the incidence of *H. influenzae* osteomyelitis decreases. In the adult, *S. aureus, S. epidermidis,* and aerobic gram-negative organisms account for the majority of the bone or blood isolates.

VERTEBRAL OSTEOMYELITIS

Vertebral osteomyelitis in the adult patient population is usually hematogenous in origin but may occur secondarily to trauma. Clinically the patient usually presents with vague symptoms and signs consisting of dull constant back pain and spasm of the paravertebral muscles. More specific complaints may localize to a soft tissue abscess. The presence of point tenderness over the involved vertebral body is a characteristic finding. Fever may be low grade or absent.

The infection is usually monomicrobic when hematogenous in origin. The most common organism isolated is *S. aureus.* Aerobic gram-negative rods, however, are found in 30% of the cases. *Pseudomonas*

The authors wish to thank Joan Mader, M.S.N., for manuscript research, editing, and preparation.

aeruginosa and *Serratia marcescens* have a high incidence of isolation among intravenous drug abusers.

CONTIGUOUS-FOCUS OSTEOMYELITIS WITH NO GENERALIZED VASCULAR INSUFFICIENCY

In contiguous-focus osteomyelitis, the organism may be directly inoculated into the bone at the time of trauma or may extend from adjacent soft tissue infections. Common predisposing conditions include open fractures, surgical reduction and internal fixation of fractures, chronic soft tissue infections, and radiation therapy. In contrast to hematogenous osteomyelitis, multiple bacterial organisms are usually isolated from the infected bone. The bacteriology is diverse, but *S. aureus* remains the most commonly isolated pathogen. In addition, aerobic gram-negative bacilli and anaerobic organisms are frequently isolated. Bone necrosis, soft tissue damage, and loss of bone stability occur, often making this form of osteomyelitis difficult to manage. The long bones are most frequently involved.

CONTIGUOUS-FOCUS OSTEOMYELITIS WITH GENERALIZED VASCULAR INSUFFICIENCY

The small bones of the feet are commonly involved in this category of osteomyelitis. Inadequate tissue perfusion predisposes the patient to the infection by blunting the local inflammatory response. The infection commonly develops following minor trauma to the feet, infected nail beds, cellulitis, or trophic skin ulceration. Multiple bacteria are usually isolated from the infected bone. The most common organisms are *S. aureus, S. epidermidis, Enterococcus* spp, gram-negative rods, and anaerobes. Although cure is desirable, a more attainable goal of therapy is to suppress the infection and maintain the functional integrity of the involved limb. Even after presumed successful treatment, recurrence or reinfection occurs in the majority of patients. Eventually resection of the infected area is almost always required.

CHRONIC OSTEOMYELITIS

Both hematogenous and contiguous-focus osteomyelitis can progress to a chronic bone infection. No precise criteria distinguish acute from chronic osteomyelitis. Clinically newly recognized bone infections are considered acute, whereas a relapse of a treated infection represents a chronic process. This simplistic classification, however, is clearly inadequate. A staging system developed by Cierny and Mader overcomes many of the problems in classifying osteomyelitis (Tables 1 and 2). As mentioned, the hallmark of chronic osteomyelitis is the simultaneous presence of organisms, necrotic bone, and a compromised soft tissue envelope. The infection cannot resolve until the nidus for the persistent contamination is removed. Persistent drainage and sinus tract(s) are common. Antibiotic therapy alone is usually unsuccessful in the treatment of chronic osteomyelitis.

Multiple species of bacteria are usually isolated from biopsy specimens of infected granulations from deep within the wound. Chronic hematogenous osteomyelitis is the exception to this statement inasmuch as a single organism is often recovered from these patients even after years of intermittent drainage. The possibility of attenuating the infection is reduced when the integrity of the soft tissue surrounding the infection is poor or the bone itself is unstable secondary to an infected non-union or a septic joint.

DIAGNOSIS OF BACTERIAL OSTEOMYELITIS

The bacteriologic diagnosis of long-bone bacterial osteomyelitis rests on the isolation of the causative bacteria from the bone or the blood. In hematogenous osteomyelitis, positive blood cultures can often obviate the need for a bone biopsy when there is associated radiographic or radionuclide scan evidence of osteomyelitis. Chronic osteomyelitis is rarely associated with a bacteremia, unless there is an acute extension of the infection into the soft tissues. Sinus tract cultures are not reliable predictors of a causative organism(s). Therefore, antibiotic treatment of osteomyelitis should be contingent on deep bone biopsy cultures and specific antimicrobial susceptibilities.

Radiographic changes in acute hematogenous osteomyelitis are often equivocal and lag at least 2 weeks behind the onset of infection. The earliest radiographic changes are soft tissue swelling, periosteal thickening or elevation, and focal osteopenia. These findings are subtle and may be overlooked. Detectable diagnostic

TABLE 1. **Cierny and Mader Classification System for Osteomyelitis**

Anatomic Type
Stage 1: Medullary osteomyelitis
Stage 2: Superficial osteomyelitis
Stage 3: Localized osteomyelitis
Stage 4: Diffuse osteomyelitis
Physiologic Class
A Host: Normal host
B Host: Systemic compromise (Bs)
Local compromise (Bl)
C Host: Treatment worse than the disease

TABLE 2. **Systemic or Local Factors That Affect Immune Surveillance, Metabolism, and Local Vascularity**

Systemic (Bs)	Local (Bl)
Malnutrition	Chronic lymphedema
Renal, liver failure	Venous stasis
Diabetes mellitus	Major vessel compromise
Chronic hypoxia	Arteritis
Immune deficiency/ suppression	Extensive scarring Radiation fibrosis
Malignancy	Small vessel disease
Extremes of age	Complete loss of local sensation
Autoimmune disease	
Tobacco abuse	
Intravenous drug use	

lytic changes are delayed and often associated with an indolent infection of several months' duration. Later, when the patient is receiving appropriate antimicrobial therapy, radiographic improvement may lag behind clinical recovery. In contiguous focus and chronic osteomyelitis, the radiographic changes are even more subtle, often seen in association with nonspecific radiographic findings, and require careful clinical correlation to achieve diagnostic value.

An earlier diagnosis of osteomyelitis may be achieved with radionuclide imaging. The actual mechanism of labeling bone with radiopharmaceuticals, however, is still unclear. The technetium polyphosphate (^{99m}Tc) scan demonstrates increased isotope accumulation in areas of increased blood flow and reactive new bone formation. It is usually positive in biopsy-confirmed cases of hematogenous osteomyelitis as early as 48 hours after the initiation of the infection. Negative ^{99m}Tc scans reported in documented osteomyelitis may reflect impaired blood supply to the infected area.

A second class of radiopharmaceuticals used for the evaluation of osteomyelitis includes gallium citrate and indium chloride. Gallium/indium attaches to transferrin, which leaks from the blood stream into areas of inflammation. Gallium/indium scans also demonstrate increased isotope uptake in areas of concentrated polymorphonuclear leukocytes, macrophages, and malignant tumors. Because these scans do not show bone detail well, it is often difficult to distinguish between bone and soft tissue inflammation; a comparison with a ^{99m}Tc scan helps resolve this difficulty. In contrast to gallium citrate, indium chloride is more heavily concentrated by hematopoietic tissue and is not found to accumulate in areas of reactive bone. During the initial evaluation of a suspected case of osteomyelitis, x-rays, technetium bone scans, and gallium or indium scans are selectively ordered to assist in the diagnosis, assess the extent of involvement, and guide the site selection for the bone biopsy.

Indium-labeled leukocyte scans are less beneficial in the evaluation of osteomyelitis. Indium leukocyte scans are positive in approximately 40% of patients with acute osteomyelitis and 60% of patients with septic arthritis. Patients with chronic osteomyelitis, bony metastases, and degenerative arthritis often have negative scans.

Computed tomography (CT) may play a role in the diagnosis of osteomyelitis. Increased marrow density occurs early in the infection, and intramedullary gas has been reported in patients with hematogenous osteomyelitis. The CT scan is also useful in identifying areas of necrotic bone and assessing the extent of soft tissue involvement. In a recalcitrant infection, the CT scan may identify the surgical approach and augment a thorough débridement. One disadvantage of this study is the scatter phenomenon, which occurs when metal is present in or near the area of bone infection. This scatter effect causes a significant loss of image resolution.

Magnetic resonance imaging (MRI) is a useful modality for differentiating between bone and soft tissue infection. Initial MRI screening usually consists of a T1-weighted and a T2-weighted spin-echo pulse sequence. In a T1-weighted study, tissue edema is dark, and fat is bright. In a T2-weighted study, the reverse is true. The typical appearance of osteomyelitis is a localized area of abnormal marrow with decreased signal intensity on T1-weighted images and increased signal intensity on T2-weighted images. On occasion, there may be decreased signal intensity on T2-weighted images. Post-traumatic and surgical scarring of the bone marrow shows a region of decreased signal intensity on T1-weighted images with no change on the T2-weighted image. Sinus tracts are seen as areas of high signal intensity on the T2-weighted image extending from the marrow and bone through the soft tissues and skin. Differentiation of infection from neoplasm on the basis of the MRI may be difficult; therefore, clinical and radiographic correlation is mandatory. Metallic implants in the region of interest may produce focal artifacts, decreasing the utility of the image.

Sedimentation rates and leukocyte counts are frequently elevated before therapy in the acute disease. The white blood cell count rarely exceeds 15,000 per mm³. The leukocyte count is usually normal in patients with chronic osteomyelitis. The sedimentation rates and leukocyte counts may fall with appropriate therapy. Both values, however, may elevate contemporaneously around each débridement surgery. A sedimentation rate that returns to normal during the course of therapy is a favorable prognostic sign. This laboratory determination, however, is not reliable in the compromised host because these patients are constantly challenged by minor illnesses and peripheral lesions that may elevate this index.

A conclusive diagnosis of vertebral osteomyelitis requires isolation of a causative organism from the infected vertebral body, disk space, paravertebral abscess, or blood. A closed biopsy for culture and histology may be performed under fluoroscopy or CT guidance. An open biopsy is indicated when a closed biopsy carries a high risk of possible complications. Tissue must be sent for both cultures and histologic confirmation because the differential diagnosis includes metastatic or primary tumors, mycoses, and tuberculosis. The earliest radiographic change is a subtle rarefaction of the vertebral end-plate. Narrowing of the adjacent joint and involvement of the vertebral body occur in advanced disease.

The technetium scan is useful in vertebral infections and is usually positive in biopsy-confirmed cases of axial osteomyelitis. The gallium/indium scans are difficult to interpret because of the high concentrations of hematopoietic tissue in the vertebral bodies. CT and MRI are used to assess the extent of vertebral, paravertebral, and soft tissue involvement.

THERAPY

Acute Hematogenous Osteomyelitis

In children, acute hematogenous osteomyelitis is primarily a medical disease. In the adult, débridement surgery and incision and drainage of soft tissue abscesses are often required. Identification of the causative pathogen is essential. The infection is usually responsive to specific antimicrobial therapy. Mismanagement with an inappropriate antibiotic(s) encourages disease extension, sequestra formation, and development of a refractory infection. Surgical intervention is indicated if the patient has not responded to specific antimicrobial therapy within 48 hours, has evidence of a persistent soft tissue abscess, or is diagnosed with or suspected of having joint sepsis. Initially appropriate culture material must be obtained. A bone biopsy is necessary unless the patient has positive blood cultures along with x-ray or bone scan findings consistent with osteomyelitis. Following cultures, a parenteral antimicrobial regimen is begun presumptively to cover the clinically suspected pathogens. Table 3 outlines initial antibiotic therapy choices. Once the specific organism is identified, the antibacterial activity of different antibiotic classes can be determined by appropriate sensitivity methods. The disk diffusion method is often a sufficient guideline for antibiotic therapy. Quantitative antibiotic sensitivity testing by the macrodilution or microdilution technique on all aerobic bone isolates, however, is a prerequisite to determine the minimum concentration of the antibiotic to inhibit (minimum inhibitory concentration [MIC]) and kill (minimum bactericidal concentration [MBC]) the pathogenic organism(s). It is best to choose an antibiotic or antibiotic combination that has a low MIC/MBC relative to its expected serum concentration. The initial antibiotic regimen may be continued or changed on the basis of sensitivity results. The patient is treated for 4 to 6 weeks with appropriate parenteral antimicrobial therapy dated from the initiation of therapy or after the last major débridement surgery. The goal of therapy is to prevent a refractory infection. If the initial medical management fails and the patient is clinically compromised by a recurrent infection, medullary or soft tissue débridement is required in conjunction with another 4- to 6-week course of antibiotics.

Occasionally oral antibiotic therapy can be used for treatment of childhood osteomyelitis. It is recommended, however, that the patient initially receive 2 weeks of parenteral antibiotic therapy before changing to an oral regimen. In addition, the patient must be compliant and agree to close outpatient supervision. Absorption and activity of the orally administered antibiotic should be monitored by measurement of the serum bactericidal activity against the causative pathogen. A peak bactericidal dilution of at least 1:8 or greater should be established and maintained. Oral therapy is possible in pediatric hematogenous osteomyelitis because of an increased bone blood flow and the aggressive mesenchymal and immunologic responses found in this age group. Patients under the age of puberty cannot be given oral antimicrobial therapy with the quinolone class of antibiotics.

Vertebral Osteomyelitis

The therapy of vertebral osteomyelitis requires parenteral antibiotics and may include early sur-

TABLE 3. **Initial Choice of Antibiotics for Therapy of Osteomyelitis (Adult Doses)**

Organism	Antibiotics of First Choice	Alternative Antibiotics
Staphylococcus aureus	Nafcillin, 2 gm q 6 h, or clindamycin, 900 mg q 8 h	Vancomycin, cefazolin
Methicillin-resistant Staphylococcus aureus	Vancomycin, 1 gm q 12 h	SXT + rifampin, imipenem-cilastatin (Primaxin)
Staphylococcus epidermidis	Vancomycin, 1gm q 12 h, or nafcillin, 2 gm q 6 h	Cefazolin, clindamycin
Group A streptococcus	Penicillin G, 2 million U q 4 h	Clindamycin, cefazolin
Group B streptococcus	Penicillin G, 2 million U q 4 h	Clindamycin, cefazolin
Enterococcus species	Ampicillin, 2 gm q 6 h, ± gentamicin, 5 mg/kg/day q 8 h	Vancomycin, ampicillin-sulbactam (Unasyn)
Escherichia coli	Ampicillin, 2 gm q 6 h	Cefazolin, tobramycin
Proteus mirabilis	Ampicillin, 2 gm q 6 h	Cefazolin, gentamicin
Proteus vulgaris Proteus rettgeri Morganella morganii	Cefotaxime (Claforan), 2 gm q 6 h ± gentamicin, 5 mg/kg/day q 8 h	Mezlocillin (Mezlin) + gentamicin
Serratia marcescens	Cefotaxime (Claforan), 2 gm q 6 h ± gentamicin, 5 mg/kg/day q 8 h	Ciprofloxacin (Cipro), mezlocillin (Mezlin), + gentamicin
Pseudomonas aeruginosa	Piperacillin (Pipracil), 3 gm q 4 h or ceftazidime, 2 gm q 8 h, + tobramycin, 5 mg/kg/day q 8 h	Ciprofloxacin (Cipro), amikacin (Amikin)
Bacteroides fragilis group	Clindamycin, 900 mg q 8 h	Metronidazole, ampicillin-sulbactam (Unasyn)
Peptostreptococcus species	Penicillin G, 2 million U q 4 h	Clindamycin, metronidazole, ampicillin-sulbactam (Unasyn)

Abbreviation: SXT = sulfamethoxazole-trimethoprim.

gery and stabilization. The choice of an antibiotic(s) is guided by the biopsy or débridement culture results. The antibiotic(s) is given for 4 to 6 weeks and is usually dated from the initiation of therapy or from the last major débridement surgery. The indications for surgery include impending vertebral instability or neurologic deterioration. Fusion of adjacent infected vertebral bodies is a major goal of therapy. The decision to advise an orthosis as opposed to internal fixation or bed rest is best individualized. The failure rate with bed rest alone is not statistically different from that for patients stabilized with a cast, corset, or brace.

Osteomyelitis Secondary to Contiguous-Focus Infection; Chronic Osteomyelitis

These types of osteomyelitis share the common denominators of infected necrotic bone and poorly perfused soft tissue enveloping the bone. Adequate drainage, thorough débridement, obliteration of dead space, wound protection, and specific antimicrobial coverage are the mainstays of therapy. Following diagnostic evaluation, a bone biopsy is performed. Aerobic and anaerobic cultures are taken from these bone samples. Generally the patient receives antibiotics only after the results of the cultures and their sensitivities are known. If immediate débridement surgery is required, however, the patient is treated presumptively with antibiotics appropriate for the suspected pathogens before the bacteriologic data are reported. These antibiotics may be modified, if necessary, when results of the débridement cultures and sensitivities are determined.

When possible, débridement surgery is delayed until after specific antibiotic therapy has begun. Antimicrobial therapy initiated before surgery decreases the risk of bacteremia at surgery, helps marginate the wound, and produces more supple soft tissues at the time of surgery. Surgical exposure is direct, atraumatic, and designed to avoid unnecessary devitalization of bone and soft tissue. If necessary, the wound is débrided every 48 to 72 hours until all nonviable tissue and superfluous hardware have been removed. The cortical and cancellous bone remaining in the wound after débridement surgery must bleed uniformly to ensure antibiotic perfusion and avoid progressive sequestration.

Appropriate management of the dead space created by débridement surgery is mandatory to arrest the disease and maintain the integrity of the skeletal part. The goal of dead space management is to replace dead bone and scar tissue with durable vascularized tissue. For this reason, secondary intention healing is discouraged because the scar tissue that fills the defect may later become avascular. Suction irrigation systems are not recommended because of the high incidence of associated nosocomial infections and the unreliability of these set-ups. Complete wound closure should be attained whenever possible. Local tissue flaps or free flaps may be used to fill dead space. An alternative technique is to place cancellous bone grafts beneath local or transferred tissues where structural augmentation is necessary. Careful preoperative planning is crucial to make efficient use of the patient's limited cancellous bone reserves. Open cancellous grafts without soft tissue coverage are useful when a free tissue transfer is not a treatment option and local tissue flaps are inadequate. Antibiotic-impregnated acrylic beads are occasionally used to sterilize and temporarily maintain a dead space. The beads are usually removed within 2 to 4 weeks and replaced with a cancellous bone graft. The evolution of local antibiotic therapy is rapidly taking place. Finally, if movement is present at the site of infection, measures must be taken to achieve permanent stability of the skeletal unit.

Most recently, bone reconstruction of segmental defects and difficult infected non-unions has been accomplished using the Ilizarov external fixation method. This method uses distraction or compression histogeneses, a process of bone regeneration to fill bone defects or to compress non-unions and correct malunions. In one clinical series, reconstruction was successful in 92% of patients with chronic osteomyelitis with segmental defects ranging from simple non-unions to 8-cm gaps. The technique is labor intensive and requires a long period of treatment (average of 8.5 months in the device).

Antibiotics are used to treat live infected bone and to protect bone undergoing revascularization (see Table 3). Because it takes bone 3 to 4 weeks to revascularize after débridement surgery, the patient is treated with 4 to 6 weeks of parenteral antimicrobial therapy usually dated from the last major débridement surgery. The optimal length of antibiotic administration for osteomyelitis remains arguable. Outpatient intravenous therapy is now a feasible option. The long-term intravenous access catheters (Hickman, Broviac, Groshong catheters) make outpatient intravenous treatment possible and decrease hospitalization time. A responsible patient or visiting nurse can administer the antibiotic at home via the implanted catheter. Outpatient intramuscular antibiotic administration is also feasible. Oral therapy using the quinolone class of antibiotics is currently being evaluated in adult patients with osteomyelitis. Effective oral therapy would make the treatment of adult osteomyelitis less confining and expensive for the patient.

Osteomyelitis Secondary to Contiguous-Focus Infection with Vascular Disease

Osteomyelitis associated with vascular insufficiency is difficult to treat owing to the relative inability of the host to participate in the eradication of the infection process. Because these infections are insidious, they are often beyond simple salvage by the time the patient seeks medical therapy.

The determination of the vascular status of the tissue at the infection site is crucial in the evaluation of these patients. Several methods can be used to determine the vascular status. The measurement of cutaneous oxygen tensions and pulse pressures, however, is most commonly employed. Cutaneous oxygen tensions are obtained by a modified Clark electrode that is applied to the skin surface. These tensions provide guidelines for determining the location of adequate tissue perfusion. The values are helpful in predicting the benefit of local débridement surgery and in selecting surgical margins where healing can be expected to occur. Hyperbaric oxygen therapy may facilitate healing in areas where marginal tensions are present.

The patient may be managed by suppressive antibiotic therapy, local débridement surgery, or ablative surgery. Judgment regarding which type of treatment to offer the patient depends on tissue oxygen perfusion at the infection site, extent of the osteomyelitis, and the preference of the patient.

The patient may be given long-term suppressive therapy when a definitive surgical procedure would lead to unacceptable patient morbidity or disability or in cases in which the patient refuses local débridement or ablative surgery. Even with suppressive antibiotic therapy, most of these patients eventually require an ablative surgical procedure.

Local débridement surgery and a 4-week course of antibiotics may be employed in the patient who has localized osteomyelitis and good tissue oxygen perfusion. Unless these criteria are present, the wound will fail to heal and ultimately lead to an ablative procedure.

The patient with extensive osteomyelitis and poor tissue oxygen perfusion usually requires some type of ablative surgery. Digital and ray resections, transmetatarsal amputations, midfoot disarticulations, and Syme amputations permit the patient to ambulate without a prosthesis. The amputation level is determined by the vascularity of the tissues proximal to the site of infection and the requirements of a thorough débridement. The patient is given 4 weeks of antibiotics when infected bone is surgically transected. Two weeks of antibiotics is given when the infected bone is completely removed, but there is still some residual soft tissue infection. When the amputation is performed proximal to the bone and soft tissue infection, the patient is given standard prophylaxis.

COMMON SPORTS INJURIES

method of
JACK HARVEY, M.D.
Orthopedic Center of The Rockies
Fort Collins, Colorado

and

GREG GUTIERREZ, M.D.
St. Joseph Hospital
Denver, Colorado

Musculoskeletal sports injuries are generally divided into acute and traumatic injuries and overuse injuries. The mechanism of injury in acute traumatic injuries is the single application of enough force to disrupt anatomic structures to some degree. Included in this classification are contusions, lacerations, sprains, dislocations, and fractures. History taking in these injuries is straightforward because the patient can readily relate how and when the injury occurred. The mechanism of injury and a thorough knowledge of anatomy are essential to making the proper diagnosis. Overuse injuries conversely occur because of the repetitive application of a small amount of force or microtrauma. Here the history is not so clear cut, and the patient may have a difficult time relating exactly when the injury started because it usually comes on gradually. One or more activities produce a repetitive stress to muscle, tendon, or bone with a resulting myositis, tendinitis, or stress fracture, to catalog a few of the common overuse injuries.

DIAGNOSIS

First aid and initial diagnosis of acute traumatic injuries should be performed as soon as possible. Early in the injury, there is less pain, swelling, and muscle spasm, allowing for examination that is easier than an hour or so later when these are all present. Inspection, palpation, and tests for the integrity of bone, muscle, or ligament are usually employed. Sprains and strains are graded as mild, moderate, or severe (grades I, II, and III). Mild sprains result from minor forces and usually have only microtrauma or slight stretching of the ligament. Moderate injury produces a partial macroscopic tear, and a severe or grade III injury results in a complete tear of the ligament. In children, occasionally the stronger ligament avulses an epiphysis or opens a growth plate, the diagnosis of which is aided by plain and stress radiographs.

TREATMENT

First aid of these injuries starts with immediate rest or nonweight bearing of the injured limb. If there is gross instability, taping or splinting of the injured limb is performed along with neurovascular checks before transporting the patient. The limb should be splinted in a position of function or comfort; for example, the knee is usually best immobilized with a posterior splint or hinged brace at 15 to 20 degrees of flexion, not at full extension as is customarily done with a straight leg immobilizer or cylinder cast. Circumferential casting or taping the knee is discouraged early because of ensuing swelling of the injured limb.

The next step is the application of ice and gentle compression with an elastic wrap to limit some of the swelling and provide hemostasis. A couple of wraps of wet elastic are applied over the skin and then the ice bag. Finally, the limb should be elevated slightly if comfortable to the patient. The ice is left in place for 20 to 40 minutes and then removed and the elastic wrap replaced. This process is repeated several times over the first 24 to 48 hours post-injury. Contusions of muscles should receive the same treatment. The next phase is to re-establish normal range of motion as tolerated by the patient. On regaining a majority of the range of motion, light resistance exercises are initiated, and following the acceptance of these, heavier strength training is started. The final phase is the use of functional exercises that mimic what the athlete will be required to do on return to practice and play. Heat is not used in any of these stages; however, anti-inflammatory drugs may be helpful. Strong analgesics can be used in the first few days but must be discontinued on initiation of the rehabilitation phase. The first aid sequence is easily remembered by *r*est, *i*ce, *c*ompression, and *e*levation (RICE).

Overuse injuries also can be graded as mild, moderate, and severe with the mild variety usually responding to a decrease or cessation of the offending activities for a few days or a couple of weeks. The use of an ice pack or ice massage a couple of times a day for a period of 20 to 60 minutes followed by a short period of gentle stretching or movement of the injured limb often accelerates the healing process. If the injury is near the surface, such as an Achilles tendon, 20 minutes suffices. A muscular shoulder with a deeper rotator cuff tendinitis, however, requires 40 to 60 minutes of icing. More severe overuse injuries may require a short period of splinting or taping to limit or restrict painful movements. Anti-inflammatory medications, such as the nonsteroidals, are helpful adjuncts to treatment. Steroid injections should be used sparingly and never in load-bearing tendons, such as the Achilles or patellar tendons. Physical therapy modalities are also helpful in reducing inflammation and can be employed initially in more severe cases or to minor injuries that do not respond to the initial treatment of rest and cryotherapy. After the inflammation is in remission, rehabilitation of the injury should be performed to prevent recurrence of the injury when the athlete returns to training, which of course should be done gradually when rehabilitation is complete.

Rehabilitation should start with stretching and progress to concentric and eccentric exercises that meet and exceed the demands that will be placed on the structure when return to play is permitted. Occasionally an orthotic device is helpful to correct a biomechanical problem seen in an analysis of the athlete's training schedule and biomechanics. These measures are used for recalcitrant and chronic cases and should not be included in the initial approach to the vast majority of overuse injuries.

Section 15

Obstetrics and Gynecology

ANTEPARTUM CARE

method of
MYOUNG OCK AHN, M.D., Ph.D, M.P.H.
YonSei University, College of Medicine
Seoul, Korea

and

JEFFREY P. PHELAN, M.D., J.D.
Pomona Valley Hospital Medical Center
Pomona, California

PRECONCEPTION CARE

As a rule, pregnant patients come to visit obstetric care providers after conception has taken place. However, modern improvements in prenatal care reveal that the optimal time to assess, manage, and treat many pregnancy conditions and complications is before pregnancy even occurs. The best time for women to seek prenatal care is when they are considering pregnancy. At that time, much of the risk assessment can be performed, as well as the basic physical and laboratory evaluation, particularly for women whose health histories place their pregnancies at risk. Prenatal counseling should occur before conception. The content of the preconceptional visit should include assessment of social, demographic, medical, and obstetric risk factors. This assessment should be combined with appropriate physical and laboratory evaluations.

Although every pregnancy should be preceded by preconceptional counseling, some of the most common indications are illustrated in Table 1.

The first preconceptional counseling visit is the time to evaluate patients for the potential of inherited, genetic, or infectious disease. For example, a rubella titer can be drawn to determine a patient's susceptibility to rubella. If she is susceptible, rubella vaccine can be given to immunize her. Once she is immunized, contraception is recommended for 3 months. Similarly, appropriate populations can be screened for carrier status of genetic diseases, such as Tay-Sachs disease, or for the presence of hemoglobinopathies, such as sickle cell disease or Bartz anemia. Early resolution of these issues is much easier and less harried without the time constraints imposed by an advancing pregnancy. Medical conditions such as anemia, urinary tract infections, and hypothyroidism can be fully evaluated, treated, and controlled before conception.

At the preconceptional visit, the importance of determining gestational age can be discussed with the patient. Great precision in observation and treatment can be achieved with an accurate menstrual calendar predating pregnancy. Women taking oral contraceptives should be advised to stop taking the pills at least a month before attempting pregnancy.

In the United States, the incidence of birth rates among women over 35 years of age is increasing. Women within this age group are more likely to have medical complications, such as hypertension and diabetes mellitus, and chromosomally defective offspring. For example, if a woman gives birth at age 35, her risk of having a child with Down's syndrome or any chromosomal abnormality is 1 in 365 or 1 in 178, respectively. By age 40, this risk has risen to 1/109 or 1/50, respectively. Once carrier status has been determined, the patient with a genetic disorder can be counseled with regard to the risk of having an

TABLE 1. **Preconception Care**

Advanced Maternal Age
  Risk of genetic disorders
  Previous congenital and/or chromosomal abnormalities
  X-linked disease
  Inborn errors of metabolism
  Increased risk of neural tube defects
Maternal Medical Illnesses
  Diabetes mellitus
  Cardiac disorders
  Chronic hypertension and/or renal insufficiency
  Collagen vascular disease (e.g., systemic lupus
    erythematosus)
  Convulsive disorders
  Chronic infections
  Hematologic disease (e.g., immune thrombocytopenic
    purpura)
Prior History of Neural Tube Defect
Isoimmunization
Drug Exposure
Previous Cesarean Delivery
History of Preterm Delivery
Unusual Dietary or Exercise Regimens

affected child as well as the availability of options such as ovum or sperm donation and gene therapy. Thus preconceptional counseling can provide women with the information required for them to make intelligent family planning decisions before pregnancy and to assist them in approaching pregnancy with a positive mental outlook.

Another example of women at risk for complications is insulin-dependent diabetic patients. Preconceptional counseling enables clinicians to control diabetes in a patient before conception and thus lessen her chances of having a child with structural anomalies. For example, major congenital malformations such as sacral agenesis, anencephaly, and congenital heart disease are the most common causes of neonatal morbidity and mortality among diabetic pregnancies. The rate is three to four times that found among nondiabetic pregnancies. Most of all, strict diabetic control before conception and throughout pregnancy lessens these risks as well as perinatal mortality rates.

Neural tube defects (NTDs), namely, anencephaly and meningomyelocele, occur in 1 per 1000 births in the United States. Although the cause of this disorder is not known, the recurrence risk is 2 to 3% in this country. Recent evidence has indicated that folic acid supplementation before and during the first 3 months of pregnancy can reduce the incidence of recurrent NTDs. Thus in patients who have previous children with an NTD, 4 mg of folic acid each day is recommended for 1 month before conception and the first 3 months of pregnancy.

ASSESSMENT OF PREGNANCY AND ACCURATE GESTATIONAL AGE

Early diagnosis of pregnancy permits an earlier appraisal of potential medical and obstetric problems and assists in the establishment of a more reliable estimated due date, or date of confinement (EDC). An accurate EDC is helpful for subsequent obstetric decision making.

Diagnosis of Pregnancy

Early pregnancy diagnosis relies on the presence of human chorionic gonadotropin (hCG) in the maternal urine or blood. Tests to rapidly determine hCG levels are readily available and can be divided into three major groups: (1) The latex agglutination test is based on the presence of hCG in the urine and has a sensitivity of 1.5 to 3.0 IU per mL. This test, however, does not distinguish between luteinizing hormone (LH) and hCG. Thus false-positive results may occur in perimenopausal women, whose LH levels are fre-

quently elevated. (2) The radioreceptor assay technique is more sensitive but, like the latex agglutination test, cannot distinguish LH from hCG. (3) Radioimmunoassay of the beta subunit of hCG (hCG-beta) is the most sensitive and reliable technique. This method detects serum levels of 1 to 5 mIU per mL of hCG. This specific assay for hCG-beta does not cross-react with LH and does not produce false-positive results. Because of its high sensitivity, pregnancy can be established within 8 days of conception.

Pregnancy can also be confirmed with ultrasonography. Identification of a gestational sac within the uterus is frequently possible 5 weeks after the beginning of the patient's last period. Earlier identification can also be achieved with vaginal ultrasonography. Early confirmation of an intrauterine pregnancy is helpful in identifying patients at high risk for an ectopic pregnancy.

Establishing a Reliable Due Date

The cornerstone of obstetric care is a reliable EDC. The primary basis for determining a woman's EDC is her last menstrual period (LMP). Because of menstrual irregularities, the menstrual history may be helpful in establishing an EDC. In that circumstance, however, additional confirmation is frequently necessary.

Confirmation of EDC may be achieved by early pregnancy evaluation and an estimation of the uterine size. If the length of gestation according to LMP corresponds with the uterine size in the first trimester of pregnancy, the accuracy of the EDC is reasonably certain. However, additional corroboration of the EDC can be done with DeLee auscultation of the fetal heart rate (at 20 weeks' gestation) and when the pregnant woman first perceives fetal movement (usually around 16 to 19 weeks' gestation).

If there are discrepancies in these clinical landmarks, ultrasonography should be used to supplement the clinical findings. Sonographic accuracy of fetal gestational age, however, diminishes with advancing gestation. For example, first-trimester sonographic measurements of the fetal crown-to-rump length constitute the most accurate determination of gestational age; the margin of error is ±1 week. By the third trimester, the margin of error has risen to ±3 weeks, or a range of 6 weeks. In clinical circumstances in which late prenatal care is an issue, serial sonographic evaluations may be obstetrically necessary to ensure accuracy of the EDC.

ANTEPARTUM CARE

Prenatal care demonstrably reduces the incidence of low birth weight and improves perinatal outcome. Although the optimal prenatal care package has yet to be defined, recent work has focused on fine-tuning prenatal care so that it will be more effective and better able to serve the future individual needs of each family. Suggested clinical considerations for the first antepartum visit are presented in Table 2. Additional considerations are reflected in Table 3 and consist primarily of a number of socioeconomic factors.

TABLE 2. **The First Prenatal Care Visit**

Goals
To define health status of mother and fetus
To determine gestational age of fetus
To initiate plan for continuing obstetric care

History
Medical, surgical, and reproductive history
Family history; include genetic
Review of system; consider sexual history, family
    relationship, nutrition, drug and alcohol use, smoking

Physical Examination
Breast
Abdominal
Pelvic; include Papanicolaou smear, gonorrhea culture,
    chlamydia test

**Laboratory Tests to Consider During Pregnancy and
    Initial Prenatal Visit**

First Visit
Hemoglobin/hematocrit
Urinalysis and culture
Blood group, Rh, and antibody screen
Serology test for syphilis
TB skin test
Rubella screen
Sickle cell screen, if needed
Blood glucose screen, if indicated, then or in third trimester
Maternal serum alpha-fetoprotein test at 16 weeks
Hepatitis B screen

Subsequent Tests Based on Initial Visit Test Results
Genetic evaluation
Ultrasonography
HIV test

**General and Preterm Labor Risk Assessment
Prenatal Care Instructions for Patient**
Vaginal bleeding
Swelling
Blurring of vision
Severe or continuous headache
Abdominal pain
Persistent vomiting
Chills or fever
Dysuria
Escape of fluid from the vagina
Marked change in frequency or intensity of fetal movements

Referral Considerations
Maternal-fetal medicine specialist (perinatologist) or other
    members of health care team
High-risk pregnancy center
Delivering hospital
Dental care

Abbreviations: TB = tuberculosis; HIV = human immunodeficiency virus.

TABLE 3. **Antenatal Care Components**

Medical Assessment
Hygiene of Pregnancy
Exercise
Bathing
Coitus
Employment
Travel
Housework
Rest
Sleep
Clothing
Alcohol use
Smoking
Use of narcotics and other drugs
Dental hygiene
Personal hygiene

Nutrition
Effect of inadequate diet in pregnancy
Groups at special risk
Antenatal management
Special problems
    Obesity and excess weight gain
    Underweight

Social Aspects of Pregnancy

Social Deprivation

Etiology and Effects
Personal characteristic
Economics
Accomodation
Malnutrition

Special Problem Groups
Unsupported mother
Immigrant
Third World background
Marital stress
Immaturity
Inadequate coping ability
Handicapped child at home

First Obstetric Visit

Antenatal care should begin as soon after conception as is practical for patients. Thus when a patient suspects that she is pregnant, she should seek prenatal care within a reasonable time. The purposes of the initial visit are to establish a trusting relationship between the physician and the patient, to document the medical history, to perform a complete physical examination, to estimate if possible the patient's present risk status, to counsel her as to lifestyle during the pregnancy, to provide her with educational material as well as information about prenatal classes, and to discuss the available choices regarding types of childbirth experiences. Out of this initial visit should come a plan for management during the pregnancy, as well as assessment of any known risks that could adversely affect pregnancy outcome.

Prenatal laboratory tests recommended at the time of the initial visit are listed in Table 2. Some physicians prefer to screen for gestational diabetes at the initial prenatal visit by administering 50-gram glucola solution and drawing blood 1 hour later. A value of 140 mg per dL or higher suggests the need for a 3-hour glucose tolerance test. However, the test can be delayed to the third trimester.

At the initial prenatal care visit, a genetic history should be obtained from each patient. This assessment should include, but is not limited to, chromosomal or structural abnormalities in previous offspring, chromosomal abnormalities in either parent, family history of sex-linked conditions, inborn errors of metabolism, NTDs, the presence of hemoglobinopathies, and advanced maternal age (≥35 years at the time of delivery, not conception). If abnormalities are identified or suspected, referral to a prenatal diagnostic center is a reasonable consideration.

Education of patients at the time of the first visit is important because the physician can provide reassurance, if possible, to the patient of the normalcy of her pregnancy. If a number of risk factors are present, she can be advised of them and of plans for their clinical management. This plan could include referral to a maternal-fetal medicine specialist or perinatologist.

In addition, the patient should be instructed on the hazards of smoking and of alcohol and drug use. Principles of an adequate diet should be discussed, as should the various warning signs and symptoms about which the patient should contact the physician (see Table 2). Finally, she should be encouraged to take childbirth education classes.

Return Visits

At present, there are no established guidelines for return prenatal visits. In general, the frequency of return visits in an uncomplicated pregnancy is every 4 weeks for the first 28 weeks of pregnancy, every 2 to 3 weeks until 36 weeks of gestation, and weekly thereafter. Women with obstetric risk factors or medical or surgical disease may need to be seen more frequently, but the frequency and number of visits depend on the medical or obstetric condition at issue. During subsequent visits, a brief interval history, the patient's weight, blood pressure, and uterine fundal height measurement, fetal presentation, and fetal heart rate are usually documented. At these follow-up visits, urinalyses for protein, glucose, and ketone levels are often taken.

Sometime during the pregnancy, risk factors should be reassessed. For example, in indicated patients, gestational diabetes screening should be considered if not done previously. A repeated test for sexually transmitted diseases should be considered if the patient is a member of a high-risk population. A repeated antibody screen should be done to evaluate for Rh sensitization or atypical antibodies. In Rh-negative gravid women with a negative Rh-antibody screen, antenatal Rh_o (D) immune globulin (e.g., RhoGAM) should be given at around 28 weeks' gestation. The physician and the patient should have final discussions concerning plans for hospital admission, labor, and delivery. These discussions can take into account changes in the patient's risk status or other relevant findings during the prenatal period.

NUTRITION DURING PREGNANCY

The diets of pregnant women have been the subject of endless discussions that often resulted in considerable contradiction and confusion. However, there is general agreement about weight gain during pregnancy and about requirements such as recommended dietary allowances and intake of nutrients during pregnancy and lactation.

The American College of Obstetricians and Gynecologists and other organizations have recommended that pregnant women gain 10 to 12 kg (22 to 27 pounds) during pregnancy. Of the recommended weight gain, approximately 9 kg comprise the normal physiologic events and features of pregnancy. These include the fetus, placenta, amniotic fluid, uterine hypertrophy, increase in maternal blood volume, breast enlargement, and dependent maternal edema as the consequence of mechanical factors. The remaining 1 to 3 kg appear to be mostly maternal fat. Poor weight gain may be associated with intrauterine growth retardation (IUGR). Rapid weight gain should lead the clinician to suspect pregnancy-induced hypertension.

The energy requirements during pregnancy are 15% higher than in the nonpregnant state. Most authorities therefore recommend an additional 300 kcal per day throughout pregnancy. In addition to the increased caloric requirements, 65 grams of protein per day should be included. In following these guidelines, the average gravid patient will gain an additional 20 to 30 pounds. In most instances, pregnant patients may be counseled to eat three balanced meals per day and salted to taste. Sodium restrictions during pregnancy have not proved to be effective in reducing the incidence of hypertension.

Because most women are unable to meet the minimal nutritional requirements, the use of prenatal vitamins is recommended during pregnancy. Supplementation with 30 to 60 mg per day of elemental iron is commonly recommended. Thirty milligrams of iron per day should also fulfill the iron requirements for lactation. Additional iron supplementation with 60 to 100 mg of iron per day or 1 to 2 mg of folic acid per day should be considered in obese patients, patients with a multiple gestation, and patients with documented anemia. As mentioned earlier, folic acid supplementation is recommended before conception in patients with prior offspring with NTDs, to reduce the incidence of recurrent NTDs.

HIGH-RISK PREGNANCY

A normal, uncomplicated pregnancy is a retrospective diagnosis. Approximately 50% of patients, however, have normal pregnancies. This percentage is based on the presence of antenatal, intrapartum, or postnatal complications. This percentage drops considerably if patients with such minor disorders such as morning sickness, heartburn, cramps, varicose veins, and hemorrhoids are excluded.

The concept of high-risk pregnancy has evolved over the past two decades and may be defined as any gestation in which the mother or the fetus has a disorder predisposing one or both to increased risk of morbidity or mortality. Special attention must be paid to the welfare of both mother and fetus. Therefore, pregnancy-related disorders necessitate the special attention of a perinatal team that includes a maternal-fetal medicine specialist who can identify and manage the mother and fetus at risk so as to improve, if possible, pregnancy outcome.

Relatively few major obstetric complications are associated with high-risk pregnancy, but those complications nevertheless belong to significant clusters. They include (1) pre-existing medical illness; (2) previous poor pregnancy outcomes, such as perinatal mortality, prematurity, fetal growth retardation, fetal malformations, placental accidents, and maternal hemorrhage; and (3) evidence of maternal malnutrition. For instance, placental abruption occurs in fewer than 1% of pregnancies and carries a perinatal mortality rate of 25%. This statistic reveals the fetal significance of this complication, but it does not reflect the maternal complications associated with abruption, such as hypovolemic shock, renal failure, consumption coagulopathy, and postpartum hemorrhage. Another example of a serious obstetric complication is multiple pregnancy, which is often associated with preeclampsia, anemia, malpresentations, premature labor, and postpartum hemorrhage.

Identification of High-Risk Pregnancies

In the past, the efforts of investigators were directed toward the objective identification of a high-risk population of obstetric patients. By reassessing risk factors during pregnancy and again during labor, the ability to identify patients at highest risk increases. None of these assessment methods, however, provided for reassigning patients to a low-risk status when the alleged high-risk factor did not materialize.

Nonetheless, it is important to individualize care of patients. This type of conscious effort to identify at-risk patients has led to heightened awareness and sensitivity on the part of obstetricians that have resulted in improvements in perinatal care. Although completing a detailed list of risk factors for each individual patient is no longer uniformly believed to be necessary, the concept of the high-risk pregnancy has been advanced and remains an integral part of prenatal care. Careful history taking and compilation of problem lists for each patient help identify those who may require heightened scrutiny during pregnancy. When a high-risk pregnancy is identified, prompt referral to a maternal-fetal medicine specialist to manage or comanage the pregnancy is beneficial.

For purposes of this chapter, selected complicated pregnancies are briefly reviewed.

Hypertensive Disorders During Pregnancy

Eight to ten percent of all pregnancies are complicated by hypertension, including chronic hypertension (occurring before 20 weeks' gestation), pregnancy-induced hypertension (PIH) (occurring after the 20th week), and PIH superimposed on chronic hypertension.

Chronic hypertension, newly diagnosed in pregnancy, necessitates medical therapy when the blood pressure is above 140/90 mmHg. The antihypertensives most commonly used during pregnancy are methyldopa and hydralazine. Both have been used extensively in obstetrics. Before therapy is initiated, the following laboratory tests are suggested, but which ones are chosen may vary, depending on the circumstances: 24-hour urine collection for measurement of creatinine clearance and total protein; serum blood urea nitrogen, creatinine, and electrolyte measurements; electrocardiogram; and chest x-ray (the abdomen must be shielded), if appropriate. If those studies and the physical examination results are normal, the patient is presumed to have essential hypertension. Medical therapy may be instituted with methyldopa in doses of 250 mg twice daily and increased to a maximum of 2 grams per day to achieve an acceptable blood pressure.

Pregnant patients with chronic hypertension are at risk for the development of IUGR, intrauterine fetal death, abruptio placentae, and superimposed PIH. The last is manifested by worsening blood pressure, increasing proteinuria, and deteriorating renal function. In these patients, fetal surveillance is recommended, beginning at 34 weeks or earlier, depending on the circumstances, and continuing until delivery.

Preeclampsia can be defined as a blood pressure of 140/90 mmHg, a 30-mmHg rise in the systolic blood pressure, or a 15-mmHg rise in the diastolic blood pressure over prepregnant (baseline) levels. Generalized edema and proteinuria are variably present. The treatment for preeclampsia at term is delivery, generally with anticonvulsant therapy with parenteral magnesium sulfate. In preterm patients, bed rest with serial testing of renal function and of fetal well-being is reasonable. Worsening hypertension, deteriorating renal function, and abnormal fetal heart rate are indications for delivery. Severe preeclampsia is defined as a blood pressure elevation to 160/110 mmHg or higher, 5 grams per 24 hours of proteinuria, headache, epigastric pain, oliguria, abnormal liver function, or fetal growth retardation. When severe preeclampsia is diagnosed, patients should be considered for delivery.

A variant of preeclampsia characterized by hemolysis, elevated liver function, and low platelet counts has been described and called the HELLP syndrome. Even though many of the patients with this disorder do not meet the blood pressure criteria for the diagnosis of severe preeclampsia, these patients should be considered to have it. The subsequent management of these patients should be consistent with the management of a patient with the diagnosis of severe preeclampsia.

In gravid patients with severe preeclampsia, especially in the presence of oliguria, pulmonary edema, or poorly controlled hypertension, central hemodynamic monitoring with a flow-directed pulmonary artery catheter may be of significant assistance in directing therapy.

Most authorities recommend continuing magnesium therapy until 24 hours post partum or until clinical improvement occurs. This is usually heralded by pronounced diuresis.

Diabetes Mellitus

Because of the high frequency of latent diabetes mellitus during pregnancy, some authorities have recommended that all pregnant patients be screened for gestational diabetes. Of the numerous diabetic screening tests available, screening with the 1-hour glucola test is the simplest. In this test, a glucose determination is made 1 hour after oral ingestion of a 50-gram glucose load without reference to the time of the patient's previous meal. Any serum value greater than 140 mg per dL warrants a 3-hour glucose tolerance test (GTT). Some indications for early diabetic screening for diabetes mellitus include, but are not limited to, persistent glycosuria, prior delivery of an infant weighing more than 4000 grams (8.8 pounds), family history of diabetes mellitus, prior unexplained stillbirth with or without congenital anomalies, and history of gestational diabetes (see Table 3). If two or more values of a GTT are abnormal (Table 4), the diagnosis of gestational diabetes (Class A) should be made. Once a diagnosis of diabetes is established, the patient should undergo dietary counseling and be placed on an American Diabetes Association (ADA) diet consisting of 25 to 35 kcal per kg, depending on her body weight. This diet should include 1.5 grams of protein per kg of actual body weight.

During pregnancy, frequent glucose assessment to determine the adequacy of diabetic control is necessary. In insulin-dependent diabetic patients, glucose assessment four times a day is usually necessary. Patients with gestational diabetes require frequent assessment of fasting and 2-hour postprandial glucose levels.

The primary goal in diabetic pregnancies is to maintain euglycemia, if possible. In insulin-dependent diabetic patients, this means serum glucose levels below 105 mg per dL and all other glucose levels below 140 mg per dL. The underlying rationale for strict glucose control is its known association with reduced perinatal morbidity and mortality. When strict glucose control was initiated before pregnancy in insulin-dependent diabetic patients, the incidence of structural anomalies of the fetus was demonstrably reduced. If possible, ketoacidosis and hypoglycemia should be avoided.

In addition to frequent glucose assessment, antepartum fetal surveillance is an integral part of the clinical management of the diabetic pregnancy. As such, nonstress tests should be initiated at 40 weeks' gestation in patients with gestational diabetes. In patients with insulin-dependent diabetes mellitus, testing should be initiated at 32 weeks' gestation. In patients with significant underlying vascular disease, prior

TABLE 4. **Threshold Serum Glucose Values***

Time	Glucose Value (mg/dL)
Fasting	105
1 h	190
2 h	165
3 h	145

*For 3-h glucose tolerance test during pregnancy.

stillbirth, or evidence of preeclampsia, earlier testing may be obstetrically necessary.

In the absence of complications that necessitate early delivery, the timing of delivery varies with the type of diabetes. Typically, patients with gestational diabetes deliver at term but no later than 42 weeks, whereas insulin-dependent diabetic patients usually deliver at approximately 37 to 38 weeks and after confirmation of fetal lung maturity. In the absence of fetal macrosomia, oxytocin induction of labor and vaginal delivery may be considered. If ultrasonographic or clinical estimates of fetal weight exceed 4000 grams, elective primary cesarean delivery is a reasonable but not mandatory consideration in diabetic pregnancies.

Isoimmunization

At the initial prenatal visit, pregnant women should undergo blood typing, Rh determination, and antibody screening. Repeat antibody testing should be done in both Rh-positive and Rh-negative gravid women in the second or third trimester. The underlying rationale is to detect Rh sensitization and to screen for atypical antibodies such as anti-Kell. Because of the widespread use of Rh_O (D) immune globulin (RhoGAM), the incidence of sensitization to the D-antigen appears to be decreasing, whereas antibodies to other blood group antigens (e, E, c, C, Duffy, and Kell) are being seen more frequently. The presence of an antibody titer is an indication for evaluation by a maternal-fetal medicine specialist.

If the antibody titer is significant, amniocentesis to detect the presence of bilirubin pigments in the amniotic fluid or ultrasonography to evaluate for pericardial or pleural effusion is done. These studies indicate whether an intrauterine fetal transfusion is medically necessary.

Nonsensitized Rh-negative women should receive antenatal Rh_O (D) immune globulin prophylaxis with 300 μg at approximately 28 weeks' gestation. This approach is designed to prevent the sensitization that occurs in approximately 1% of Rh-negative patients before delivery. Finally, each physician should be familiar with the indications (Table 5) for Rh_O (D) immune globulin administration.

Urinary Tract Infection

Because of the known association between acute pyelonephritis and untreated asymptomatic bacteriuria (ASB), defined as more than 100,000 colonies per mL in a clean-catch urine specimen, pregnant women should be screened for ASB at the initial prenatal visit. If indicated, subsequent treatment should be based on the

TABLE 5. **Recommendations for Rh_O (D) Immune Globulin Administration in Rh-Negative Women to Prevent Subsequent Rh Sensitization**

Antenatal administration at or around 28 weeks' gestation
After delivery of Rh-positive infant
After spontaneous abortion, therapeutic abortion, or ectopic pregnancy
After amniocentesis or chorionic villi sampling
After external cephalic version
If bleeding during pregnancy
After blunt abdominal trauma

sensitivity report. Nitrofurantoin, cephalosporins, and ampicillin are reasonable antibiotics for treating ASB in nonallergic patients. Once they are treated, periodic urine cultures should be performed.

If recurrent ASB is found on a follow-up culture, repeated treatment with an appropriate antibiotic should be initiated. Subsequently, the patient should be considered for prophylactic antibiotics with nitrofurantoin, 100 mg nightly, or a similarly effective agent.

Acute pyelonephritis is an indication for hospitalization and parenteral antibiotic therapy. Initially, cephalosporins or ampicillin is used to combat the infection. This treatment may change once the sensitivity report is available. Aminoglycosides, because of their toxicity, should be reserved for serious or unresponsive infections. After completion of parenteral antibiotic therapy, prophylaxis with nitrofurantoin as previously suggested should be considered and continued until delivery. It is necessary to monitor follow-up urine cultures for possible recurrent infection.

Preterm Delivery

Premature birth occurs in 7 to 10% of all pregnancies and accounts for more than 60% of the perinatal morbidity and mortality. The more common risk factors for prematurity are listed in Table 6. A patient who has one or more of these risk factors should be counseled with regard to the signs and symptoms of preterm labor. In addition, she should alter her lifestyle and work habits and increase her bed rest and pelvic rest. In selected circumstances, home uterine activity monitoring for the early detection of premature labor is an available option.

TABLE 6. **Most Common Risk Factors for Premature Birth**

Prior preterm birth
Uterine malformation
Multiple gestation
Three or more abortions

If premature labor develops, as defined by recurrent uterine contractions at least 10 minutes apart and not necessarily accompanied by cervical change, the patient should be evaluated for possible tocolytic therapy. Once clinical evaluation confirms the presence of premature labor and the absence of any contraindications to tocolysis (Table 7), tocolytic therapy with a beta-mimetic, such as ritodrine or terbutaline, or with magnesium sulfate is a reasonable consideration. Because both agents are equally efficacious, the decision to use a beta-mimetic or magnesium sulfate depends primarily on the presence of any contraindications to the use of the agent chosen. For example, patients with underlying cardiac disease (with or without an arrhythmia), diabetes mellitus, thyrotoxosis, or third-trimester bleeding from placenta previa or abruption are not initially treated with a beta-mimetic. In these circumstances, beta-mimetics may exacerbate the underlying maternal medical condition. Therefore, magnesium sulfate or a different tocolytic agent is typically used. If the magnesium sulfate at maximal dosages fails to stop the premature labor, beta-mimetic or indomethacin therapy is obstetrically reasonable in an effort to prevent preterm birth. If a beta-mimetic is selected in the four circumstances previously enumerated, heightened scrutiny of the patient is medically necessary.

If a second agent at maximal dosage fails to stop the premature labor (e.g., if magnesium sulfate and a beta-mimetic fail), short-term indomethacin therapy in euhydramnic patients is reasonable. Typically, indomethacin is used as an adjunct to the last agent used. During indomethacin therapy, frequent assessment of the amniotic fluid volume is necessary in order to monitor for the potential development of oligohydramnios. If oligohydramnios develops, the indomethacin should be discontinued. As a rule, the amniotic fluid volume returns to normal. Finally, during the course of active therapy to inhibit premature labor, combination chemotherapy with parenteral magnesium sulfate and a beta-mimetic should be avoided because of its known association with myocardial ischemia and pulmonary edema.

Once the premature labor has been arrested, parenteral tocolytics are continued for an extended period of time. Then the patient is gradually weaned or abruptly discontinued from the tocolytic. Once the tocolytic has been discontinued, prophylactic tocolysis with an oral beta-mimetic or magnesium sulfate is usually recommended in order to reduce the incidence of recurrent premature labor. Most recently, terbutaline pump therapy has been used for this purpose.

Beta-mimetic therapy can produce maternal

TABLE 7. Commonly Cited Reasons for Not Using Tocolytic Therapy to Arrest Preterm Labor

Advanced labor
Fetal demise
Chorioamnionitis
Obstetric indication for delivery
Advanced gestational age
Premature membrane rupture

and fetal side effects, but these are usually transient and rarely necessitate discontinuation. These side effects, such as tachycardia, reflect beta$_1$ activity of the agent. Nevertheless, if major side effects develop in the patient or the fetus (Table 8), the beta-mimetic should be discontinued.

Premature rupture of the membranes (PROM), defined as rupture of the membranes before the onset of labor, occurs in 10% of all pregnancies. PROM is suggested by pooling of the amniotic fluid in the posterior fornix on sterile speculum examination, a history of spontaneous loss of fluid from the vagina, or a significant reduction in the amniotic fluid index. PROM is clinically confirmed by the finding of an alkaline pH on nitrazine paper testing or the finding of ferning on a microscope slide specimen.

When PROM is confirmed, the subsequent clinical management depends on the gestational age. In a term pregnancy, reasonable clinical approaches include induction of labor or awaiting the onset of spontaneous labor.

In patients with confirmed preterm PROM, expectant management is used more often to permit enhancement of fetal lung maturity. Delivery is recommended whenever there is evidence of fetal compromise, chorioamniotinitis, labor, or sufficient maturity of the fetus. Therefore, in patients with PROM, vaginal cultures for group B streptococci and *Chlamydia* are a reasonable consideration. The decision to use amniocentesis (to identify amnionitis), tocolytics, antibiotic prophylaxis, or steroids (to enhance fetal lung maturity) depends on the physician's clinical judgment. At present, there is literature to support the use or nonuse of these approaches.

Once the clinical evaluation of the preterm

TABLE 8. Major Side Effects of Beta-Mimetic Tocolytic Therapy That Necessitate Discontinuation of Beta-Mimetic

Maternal heart rate > 150 bpm
Fetal heart rate > 200 bpm
Diastolic blood pressure < 40 mmHg
Premature ventricular contractions > 6 per minute
Persistent chest pain
Pulmonary edema

PROM patient is complete, continuous electronic fetal monitoring is used for a prolonged period to assess fetal condition. Because oligohydramnios can occur in PROM patients, the primary focus is on the development of variable decelerations during fetal heart rate monitoring. After the initial monitoring period, fetal heart rate monitoring and ultrasonography to quantify the amniotic fluid volume are used to assess fetal condition on a periodic basis. Persistent variable decelerations or the development of oligohydramnios suggests the need for continuous electronic fetal monitoring in a labor and delivery setting.

Intrauterine Growth Retardation

IUGR is a complex fetal complication that occurs in 5% of pregnancies. Two basic etiologic theories for its development have been proposed. To account for these theories, two types of IUGR have been identified. Symmetrical IUGR, so called because the fetal head and abdomen are similarly affected, is more common. This type of IUGR is encountered in circumstances that affect the overall development of the fetus, such as congenital infections or chromosomal anomalies. Asymmetrical IUGR is believed to be caused by uteroplacental dysfunction and is characterized by normal head growth (head sparing) but abdominal wasting, as exemplified by a smaller abdominal circumference. The development of an hourglass figure, or head/abdomen disproportion, in the fetus is associated with higher perinatal morbidity and mortality rates.

Nevertheless, IUGR goes undetected before delivery in as many as 40 to 50% of all neonates who are small for gestational age. With the increasing use of ultrasonography, this incidence will decrease. Associated risk factors for IUGR include, but are not limited to, multiple gestation, maternal vascular disease, and congenital or chromosomal anomalies in the fetus. Clinical suspicion may be aroused when the uterine fundal height lags behind the fetus's gestational age for a prolonged period of time or when oligohydramnios is suspected. In uncommon circumstances, the sonographic finding of symmetrical IUGR may indicate end-stage asymmetrical IUGR.

In patients considered at risk for IUGR, ultrasound examinations should be considered in order to determine the adequacy of fetal growth. No single ultrasound parameter is reliable in the detection of IUGR. Thus multiple measurements that include but are not limited to the biparietal diameter, head circumference, abdominal circumference, and femur length are necessary for evaluating fetal growth. The evaluation should include an assessment of the amniotic fluid volume and an anatomic survey. Both types of IUGR are an indication for antepartum fetal heart rate testing. When IUGR is complicated by fetal heart rate abnormalities or amniotic fluid volume abnormalities, an evaluation for delivery should be considered. Delivery results depend on the clinical circumstances and the gestational age at the time of diagnosis.

Abnormal Presentation

With advancing gestational age, the fetus assumes a longitudinal lie and a cephalic presentation. At term, approximately 4 to 5% of pregnancies are in a noncephalic presentation. Thus fetal presentation is assessed during prenatal visits. The presence of a breech presentation or a transverse lie at 37 weeks or beyond should prompt an evaluation for its etiology. Abnormal presentations are associated with placenta previa, uterine malformations, and fetal anomalies. If these are not identified sonographically, the patient's subsequent management depends on a variety of factors such as the type of breech and the gestational age at the time of diagnosis.

Clinical management of term pregnancies with breech presentations includes external cephalic version, elective cesarean delivery, or selected vaginal breech delivery. If attempted vaginal delivery is acceptable to the patient, she should be instructed to report to the hospital promptly after labor begins or membrane rupture occurs. If this and external cephalic version are unacceptable to her, strong consideration should be given for elective primary cesarean delivery.

External cephalic version has a reported success rate of 70 to 75% and is a reasonable consideration. If successful, it may obviate the need for cesarean delivery and lower the chances of umbilical cord prolapse. Version is typically performed in an outpatient or inpatient setting at 36 weeks' gestation or later. Before an attempted version, the patient is screened with ultrasonography and a nonstress test to determine her candidacy for the procedure. With the patient's permission, external cephalic version is accomplished with or without tocolysis. During the version, the fetal heart rate is assessed periodically. After an attempted external cephalic version, a second nonstress test is performed. In Rh-negative women, Rh_0 (D) immune globulin is given. The patient is then discharged with a recommendation for weekly nonstress tests.

Multiple Gestation

Twin pregnancies occur in 1% of all pregnancies. Because of the marked increase in prema-

TABLE 9. **Indications of Increased Likelihood of Multiple Pregnancy**

Size-date discrepancy
Ovulation induction
Preeclampsia at <20 weeks
In vitro fertilization

turity and perinatal mortality among undiagnosed twins, early diagnosis is essential; however, it is not always possible. Although routine ultrasonography would improve the rate of antenatal detection, ultrasonography is not routinely performed in the United States. Nonetheless, consideration should be given for ultrasound evaluation in patients considered at high risk for a multiple pregnancy (Table 9). Twin pregnancies are more likely to be complicated by anemia, glucose intolerance, pregnancy-induced hypertension, IUGR, prematurity, and postpartum hemorrhage. To reduce the likelihood of prematurity, patients with twin gestations should be encouraged to increase the amount of bed rest in the early third trimester. The efficacy of this approach, however, is controversial. Antepartum care must also include frequent ultrasound assessment to monitor fetal growth and fetal surveillance testing to assess fetal well-being.

Postdate

When pregnancy has exceeded 42 weeks from the first day of the last menstrual period, the pregnancy is considered to be postdate. Approximately 10% of all pregnancies extend beyond 42 weeks.

Investigators have also shown that among pregnancies that extend beyond 41 completed weeks, morbidity increases remarkably. Thus several authorities have recommended that antepartum fetal surveillance tests begin at 41 weeks' gestation, or 7 days after the EDC. However, current recommendations for the management of the postdate pregnancy conflict. Some authors recommend fetal surveillance testing and selective induction of labor, whereas others prefer routine induction of labor at 42 weeks. Several reports have failed to demonstrate an advantage of one approach over the other. If the former approach is elected, patients with an inducible cervix (Bishop score of 5 or greater) or with evidence of fetal macrosomia should be considered for delivery. If the patient does not meet these criteria, fetal well-being should be assessed. Recent evidence suggests that combination fetal surveillance with the amniotic fluid index is the optimal approach. This approach, however, is not readily available outside the university hospital environment. In patients undergoing fetal surveillance testing, the subsequent management is based on the results of the fetal surveillance tests and the inducibility of the cervix.

ANTENATAL FETAL SURVEILLANCE

With the development of fetal heart rate monitoring and ultrasonography, clinicians can now visualize the intrauterine environment and conduct a fetal physical examination. Moreover, newer techniques such as fetal acoustic stimulation and the development of biophysical profile and the amniotic fluid index (AFI) have helped physicians to more effectively evaluate fetal status.

Ultrasonography

Routine ultrasound assessment of every pregnancy is not currently recommended, even though there is no clinical evidence of an increased risk to mother or fetus from the use of ultrasonography. Nevertheless, ultrasound evaluations are used for diagnostic purposes and to assess fetal well-being. Indications for diagnostic ultrasonography include, but are not limited to, diagnosis of early pregnancy, size-EDC discrepancy, confirmation of adequate fetal growth, diagnosis of anomalies, guidance of amniocentesis, evaluation of placental location, estimation of fetal weight, documentation of fetal viability, documentation of fetal lung maturity, evaluation of adnexal masses, uterine tumors or anomalies, and confirmation of EDC.

In addition, ultrasonography is used as an adjunct to current fetal monitoring techniques to assess fetal well-being. For example, it is used to monitor the amniotic fluid with the AFI or to assess fetal condition with the biophysical profile (Table 10). The AFI in normal pregnancies is 16.2 ± 5.3 cm. An AFI of 5.0 cm or less is indicative of oligohydramnios and a consideration for delivery. Whenever the AFI is 25 cm or more, polyhydramnios is considered.

A score of 8 or 10 on the biophysical profile is

TABLE 10. **Fetal Biophysical Profile Scoring System**

Component	Score
NST-reactive	2
Fetal breathing movement for 1 min	2
Three fetal movements	2
Fetal tone	2
Amniotic fluid index > 5.0 cm	2
Maximal score	10

Abbreviation: NST = nonstress test.

considered normal. Retesting in this circumstance depends primarily on the indication for testing. A score of 6 is considered suspicious, and the patients are retested in 12 to 24 hours. Patients with a biophysical profile score of 4 or less are admitted to the hospital for continuous fetal surveillance and evaluation for delivery.

Antepartum Fetal Heart Rate Testing

The primary method of fetal surveillance testing is the nonstress test. Indications for testing include, but are not limited to, postdate pregnancies, hypertensive disorders, IUGR, multiple gestation, isoimmunization, diabetes mellitus, and a history of prior stillbirth. A test is considered reactive if there are two or more spontaneous or evoked fetal heart rate accelerations of at least 15 beats per minute, each beat lasting at least 15 seconds from the time the heart rate leaves baseline until it returns, in a 10-minute moving window. If these criteria are not satisfied in a 40-minute monitoring period, the test is considered nonreactive. In this circumstance, acoustic stimulation can be used to reduce the incidence of nonreactivity. A patient's nonreactive test requires additional assessment of fetal health with the biophysical profile, the contraction stress test, or an additional testing modality. The clinical management of patients with the various biophysical profile scores has been discussed earlier. When the contraction stress test result is negative, a repeated test is indicated in 1 week. Patients with a positive test result are admitted to the hospital for continuous fetal monitoring and evaluated for delivery.

The presence of variable decelerations during fetal surveillance testing should alert the clinician to possible oligohydramnios. This is especially true in patients with growth-impaired or postdate pregnancies. If a decreased amniotic fluid volume is identified, these patients should be admitted to the hospital and evaluated for delivery.

ECTOPIC PREGNANCY

method of
SANTIAGO L. PADILLA, M.D.
Greater Baltimore Medical Center
Baltimore, Maryland

Ectopic pregnancy is defined as a gestation outside of the endometrial cavity. Although the rate of maternal mortality from this condition has progressively dropped to a low of 0.05%, ectopic pregnancy is the leading cause of maternal death in the first trimester of pregnancy and is the second major cause of maternal mortality overall for all trimesters. An estimated 80,000 to 90,000 cases per year represent approximately 1.5% of all pregnancies in the United States. The site of the ectopic gestation is most commonly the fallopian tube, although implantations can occur in the abdomen, ovary or cervix.

Ectopic pregnancy is a phenomenon that appears to be unique to the human species. Disease and surgery of the fallopian tubes are the most common causes of ectopic pregnancy. Although patients with an abnormal fallopian tube are at increased risk of ectopic pregnancies, most of the fallopian tubes that contain ectopic pregnancies are morphologically normal. History of pelvic inflammatory disease, intrauterine contraceptive devices, and previous ectopic pregnancy are some of the risk factors associated with ectopic pregnancy. However, 42% of all patients with documented ectopic pregnancy do not have an identifiable risk factor. Patients undergoing advanced reproductive techniques such as in vitro fertilization and ovulation induction may be at a higher risk than is the general population. When multiple embryos or multiple oocytes are transferred, the incidence of heterotopic pregnancy—simultaneous intrauterine and ectopic pregnancies—is increased.

HISTORY AND PHYSICAL EXAMINATION

The clinical manifestations of ectopic pregnancy can mimic those of many abdominal and pelvic diseases. During the early stages, an unruptured ectopic pregnancy manifests most commonly with unilateral abdominal pain. Abnormal vaginal bleeding associated with a history of missed or abnormal menstrual period is also reported. Patients may present with nausea and low-grade fever. Careful evaluation of patients at high risk has demonstrated that many patients have no symptoms during the early stages of an ectopic pregnancy.

Physical findings may range from a normal physical examination result to clear-cut signs of peritoneal irritation and intraperitoneal bleeding. Adnexal tenderness and fullness as well as minimal enlargement and presence of an adnexal mass may be detected. Cervical motion tenderness is a key sign in patients with an ectopic gestation. In advanced cases of ruptured ectopic pregnancies, patients present with acute abdominal pain and may be hemodynamically unstable.

DIAGNOSIS

The key to diagnosis is clinical suspicion. The patient at an increased risk for an ectopic pregnancy should be carefully counseled with regard to the early signs and symptoms of an ectopic pregnancy. Patients with a previous ectopic pregnancy can usually tell when another ectopic pregnancy is occurring. A quantitative human chorionic gonadotropin (hCG) assay by radioimmunoassay or enzyme-linked immunoassay is the most important initial step of diagnosis. This assay usually detects hCG at levels above 5 mIU per mL. Some very rare cases have been reported with negative hCG levels; for all practical clinical purposes, however, a negative hCG finding in serum excludes the diagnosis of ectopic pregnancy.

The goal at diagnosis is to detect the ectopic pregnancy before rupture. A combination of the level of the hCG in serum with pelvic ultrasound findings is the best way of assessing presence or absence of an ectopic pregnancy. Several authors have reported a "discriminatory zone" of hCG levels. In the early 1980s, studies with transabdominal ultrasonography demonstrated that 96% of normal pregnancies had a gestational sac when the hCG level was above 6000 mIU per mL. With the recent use of endovaginal ultrasonography, this discriminatory zone has been established at approximately 1500 to 2000 mIU per mL, although in some preliminary studies the lower limit may be as low as 1000 mIU per mL. These levels are in accordance with the First International Reference Preparation, which is the old standard for hCG assays. A Second International Standard has been developed, and because some laboratories may use this standard, the discriminatory zone should be clarified with the laboratory conducting the study.

In a normal pregnancy, hCG titers increase logarithmically; during the first 6 weeks after conception, the level doubles every 48 hours. In some normal pregnancies the doubling time may be as long as 72 hours, but certainly no more than that. Inappropriately rising, plateauing, or decreasing hCG titers should raise suspicion of an ectopic pregnancy, and ultrasound evaluation should be performed to verify the diagnosis. Although ultrasound resolution has improved significantly, the direct diagnosis of ectopic pregnancy is confirmed by ultrasonography in only 15 to 20% of the cases. Direct diagnosis requires visualization of a gestational sac on the adnexa. In many ectopic pregnancies, adnexal findings are normal. Ultrasound diagnosis is usually indirect when there is absence of an intrauterine gestational sac with adequate levels of hCG. With the exception of patients undergoing assisted reproductive techniques, the demonstration of an intrauterine gestation virtually excludes ectopic pregnancy inasmuch as heterotopic pregnancy occurs in only 1 per 30,000 pregnancies.

If the exact time of conception is known, as it is in patients who are undergoing inseminations or assisted reproductive techniques, a gestational sac should be visualized approximately 3 to 3.5 weeks after conception has occurred. A true gestational sac can be differentiated from a pseudodecidual sac by the presence of a double-lined ring that surrounds the real gestational sac. A fetal pole and fetal heart activity can be seen 5 weeks after conception. Serum progesterone levels below 15 ng per mL are commonly found in ectopic pregnancies, but they are not as discriminatory as the hCG levels; patients undergoing miscarriage also have lower progesterone levels. Short of direct ultrasound diagnosis, the diagnosis of ectopic pregnancy is usually confirmed surgically by diagnostic laparoscopy.

MANAGEMENT

Management is dictated by the clinical condition of the patient, the amount of damage from the ectopic pregnancy, and her desire regarding future pregnancy. A patient who presents to the emergency room and is in unstable condition requires emergency surgery. Most gynecologists recommend immediate laparotomy to control the bleeding. Although some very experienced endoscopic surgeons have approached ruptured ectopic pregnancies by laparoscopy, the delay in diagnosis may put the patient at significant risk; therefore, only highly skilled endoscopic surgeons should attempt laparoscopy. In most such ectopic pregnancies, a fallopian tube has ruptured, and the chances of saving the fallopian tube are very low. In occasional cases in which the rupture occurred at the level of the isthmus, a segmental resection allows the possibility of a future reanastomosis.

In stable patients, there are three possibilities for management: (1) salpingectomy, (2) conservative surgery of the fallopian tube, and (3) pharmacologic treatment with methotrexate.* The usual surgical procedure for most of the twentieth century has been salpingectomy. Originally, cornual resection was recommended, but this has been shown not to be necessary. There is no reason to remove the ipsilateral ovary because patients may undergo in vitro fertilization in the future.

Conservative surgery of the fallopian tube is frequently used. Recent data suggest that the incidence of ectopic pregnancy after conservative surgery of the tube is no different or only minimally elevated over the incidence of ectopic pregnancy on the contralateral tube. The procedure depends on the location of the ectopic pregnancy. If the ectopic pregnancy is in the isthmus, a segmental resection is usually performed. The author recommends reanastomosis at a subsequent operation rather than at the time of removal of the ectopic pregnancy. If the ectopic pregnancy is in the ampulla, a linear salpingostomy is the treatment of choice. Originally this procedure was performed by laparotomy, but an endoscopic approach has proved to be the optimal way. Conservative surgery by laparoscopy results in lesser morbidity, short hospital stay, lower costs, and an earlier return of the patient to full activity. The incision on the fallopian tube can be closed by secondary intention without need of suture material; this may actually reduce the incidence of adhesion formation.

Every patient who undergoes conservative surgery should be monitored with weekly hCG measurements until the levels become negative. Pregnancies on the ampulla should not be "milked out." Delayed postoperative bleeding and persistent trophoblast are two complications that can

---

*This use of methotrexate is not listed in the manufacturer's official directive.

occur with conservative management, as opposed to a salpingectomy. The incidence of persistent trophoblast is 5% in most series. A 3% incidence of delayed bleeding has also been reported in these patients.

A new but as yet controversial approach to treatment of ectopic pregnancy is the use of pharmacologic treatment with methotrexate. This agent is usually used in combination with citrovorum rescue. Side effects include stomatitis, gastritis, elevation of hepatic enzymes, and hematopoietic suppression. Currently most centers administer pharmacologic treatment only in cases of persistent trophoblast after conservative surgery. Several centers administer methotrexate as a primary therapy for ectopic pregnancies, especially abdominal and cervical pregnancies. Long-term studies need to be conducted on the future fertility and the tubal patency rate of patients who undergo methotrexate therapy as primary therapy for their ectopic pregnancy. Rh-negative women who are unsensitized should be given Rh_O (D) immune globulin (RhoGAM). During early gestation (<12 weeks), 50 μg of RhoGAM should be given; for older gestations, 300 μg.

VAGINAL BLEEDING IN LATE PREGNANCY

method of
MARLA S. EGLOWSTEIN, M.D.
Albany Medical Center Hospital
Albany, New York

The most important issue in management is differentiating between causes such as cervicitis and postcoital trauma and causes associated with high morbidity and mortality, such as placenta previa and abruptio placentae (premature separation of the placenta).

LOCAL CAUSES

Many patients report vaginal bleeding in late pregnancy. Physicians should attempt to estimate the amount of bleeding; one method of doing so is to ask a patient how the amount of bleeding compares with her normal menstrual flow. Because patients often have difficulty assessing blood loss, a thorough evaluation is always essential, including a history of trauma and infection, recent Papanicolaou (Pap) smear results, time of recent intercourse, and a physical examination.

Eversion of the endocervical glands is often observed in pregnancy, leading to an increased susceptibility to trauma during intercourse. The columnar epithelium is easily infected by normal vaginal bacterial flora; sloughing of the epithelium of the endocervical glands

as a result of minor infections may be seen. Cultures should be obtained in symptomatic women to identify specific organisms, especially if abnormal discharge is present. Active infection should be treated with an appropriate antibiotic considered safe in pregnancy. Most of these infections respond to erythromycin (the estolate [Ilosone] should not be used during pregnancy) or to penicillins or cephalosporins. The common antifungal agents used for candidiasis in nonpregnant women may also be used during pregnancy.

The pelvic examination may reveal a cervical lesion suggestive of neoplastic disease. Regardless of previous Pap smear results, any suspicious lesion should be sampled with biopsy. During colposcopy, any abnormal areas that are revealed by application of 3% acetic acid should undergo biopsy. The entire cervix, especially the squamocolumnar junction, must be examined. In pregnancy, the cervix may bleed vigorously after biopsy, but direct pressure and application of Monsel's solution (ferric subsulfate) or silver nitrate usually control the bleeding. Management of dysplasia or malignancy depends on the severity of the lesion and the gestational age and is discussed elsewhere in this book.

Mild vaginal bleeding may be associated with cervical dilation; it may occur in the absence of perceived labor and is sometimes referred to as "bloody show." Minor vaginal bleeding occasionally occurs in women who are in preterm labor and are not aware of uterine contractions. Their symptoms are commonly attributed to either gastrointestinal or genitourinary irritability or infection; however, vaginal bleeding in the context of such complaints definitely should be regarded as a possible indicator of preterm labor. Preterm labor, in and of itself, may be associated with abruptio placentae (to be discussed).

DIFFERENTIAL DIAGNOSIS: ABRUPTIO PLACENTAE AND PLACENTA PREVIA

Abruptio placentae and placenta previa constitute the two most worrisome and potentially lethal causes of antepartum bleeding. In both, coagulopathy may result from excessive consumption of coagulation products of hemorrhage, including platelets, fibrinogen, and other clotting factors. In abruption, an initial disruption at the maternal-fetal surface produces a space-occupying lesion, which may enlarge by dissection along the planes of least resistance. Increased pressure associated with further extravasation of blood can result in rupture of the decidua cells. This in turn induces elaboration of prostaglandins, which may produce pain and uterine contractions. Occult abruption may be seen with uterine fundal or posterior placental implantation, and the clinician should always bear in mind that clinical abruption need not be associated with severe vaginal bleeding.

In placenta previa, a space-occupying lesion often does not develop, because blood can pass more directly from a disrupted region of the maternal-fetal surface to the cervix. Because the decidua is less developed in the lower uterine segment than in the fundus, and because no mass lesion develops, there is less stimulation of prostaglandin elaboration leading to labor. Therefore, affected patients commonly report painless vaginal bleeding with placenta previa. Uterine irritability is commonly seen at presentation. Shock or hemodynamic instability out of proportion to blood loss is sometimes seen in occult abruptio placentae. However, this usually is not true of placenta previa, in which the patient's hemodynamic status is likely to correspond more closely to the apparent amount of blood loss. In abruptio placentae, the uterus tends to be irritable so that, even in the absence of contractions, a contraction can be induced by palpation of the uterus. In classic severe abruption, the uterus has a boardlike feeling. This is seldom true with placenta previa. The clinical similarity in appearance of these two conditions necessitates close monitoring while further evaluation and possible delivery of the fetus are planned.

MANAGEMENT

Both placental abruption and placenta previa require intensive maternal and fetal monitoring, evaluation for coagulopathy, and preparation for hemodynamic resuscitation. Extensive replacement of blood and clotting factors, with fresh-frozen plasma or cryoprecipitate, may be necessary.

Placenta Previa

Placenta previa occurs in 0.5 to 1% of all pregnancies after 20 weeks. The earlier in pregnancy, the higher the incidence seems to be. Placenta previa may be classified according to whether the placenta completely overlies the cervix (complete) or whether merely an edge of the placenta is near the cervix (marginal or partial). Vaginal ultrasonography has proved safe and has made more accurate localization of the placenta possible. Additional clues that might suggest the diagnosis of placenta previa include a fetal malpresentation, such as a transverse lie or a breech presentation. Placenta previa is associated with a twofold increase in congenital fetal malformations. In addition, many investigators believe that intrauterine growth retardation is common in this condition.

The most common presenting symptom of placenta previa is painless vaginal bleeding. The prognosis for maternal and fetal outcome is less favorable when bleeding occurs early; specifically, the risk of preterm birth increases greatly. Active bleeding in a patient with placenta previa requires admission to the hospital. At the time of admission, a large-bore intravenous line should be inserted and fluids started. Intake and output must be monitored precisely. This may be facilitated by inserting a Foley catheter if the patient appears unstable. Initial blood work should include hemoglobin, hematocrit, and fibrinogen measurement; platelet count; and coagulation profile. The initial evaluation results may be mis-

leading because hemoconcentration and vasoconstriction caused by severe hemorrhage could mask even a significant blood loss. Therefore, blood work should be repeated at frequent intervals until the patient's stability is ensured. Blood pressure and pulse should be taken at frequent intervals (e.g., every 15 minutes until stable, every half hour for 2 hours, and then hourly). Orthostatic blood pressure and pulse measurements are useful. Again, compensatory vasoconstriction can temporarily mask volume depletion and hypotension, especially if preeclampsia is also present. If the patient is hemodynamically unstable at any time, central venous pressure monitoring, Swan-Ganz catheter monitoring, or both may be necessary.

Close fetal monitoring is critical in this setting. Electronic fetal monitoring may reveal evidence of instability such as fetal tachycardia, absence of reactivity, and late heart rate decelerations. If there is brisk bleeding, tocolysis is contraindicated. If there is no active bleeding after a few hours of observation, inhibition of uterine irritability can be considered. Should the patient stabilize with no evidence of fetal or maternal distress, the use of steroids to accelerate maturation of fetal pulmonary function can also be considered. It has been demonstrated that respiratory distress is increased in the presence of fetal asphyxia and is secondary to prematurity, and thus the use of steroids is warranted. If placenta previa is documented between 28 and 32 weeks, such a management plan would be indicated. Patients in the author's unit are given weekly doses of betamethasone until 32 to 34 weeks. Few data support the use of steroids after 34 weeks.

Vasa Praevia

Vasa praevia is a variant of placenta previa. This entity occurs most often with marginal insertion of the umbilical cord and is more common in multiple gestations. The most frequent finding on pathologic examination involves cord insertion at the lateral aspect of the placenta and exposure of the umbilical vessels in the fetal membranes, instead of being invested in Wharton's jelly; the vessels are therefore subject to trauma and rupture. This represents a potentially catastrophic situation for the fetus, and the diagnosis of vasa praevia at the time of actual bleeding is very difficult to make unless there is a high index of suspicion on the part of the clinician.

Vasa praevia may be found on ultrasound scans with careful evaluation. The vaginal probe examination may be helpful in making the diagnosis. The presence of fetal red blood cells in vaginal blood as documented by either an alum-precipitated toxoid test or a Kleihauer-Betke test supports this diagnosis. If the diagnosis of marginal or partial placenta previa is made, the possibility of vasa praevia should be considered. This diagnosis necessitates increased surveillance beyond that associated with placenta previa. Delivery by cesarean section should be strongly considered as soon as the diagnosis is made, especially after 34 weeks. Steroid therapy for pulmonary maturation can be used in this situation if the gestational age is less than 34 weeks.

Double–Set-Up Examination

If the pregnancy is 36 weeks or more at the time of third-trimester bleeding, if bleeding is light, and if the physician is unable to determine the exact location of the edge of the placenta by ultrasonography, double–set-up examination is justified. The double–set-up examination is performed to determine whether vaginal delivery is possible; preparation is made for immediate cesarean delivery if it is not. After the patient's current laboratory values and adequate blood products are obtained, the patient may be examined with caution in the operating room. Nursing, anesthesia, and pediatric personnel should be immediately available. The first examination is done by speculum for evaluation of the cervix. On occasion, the presenting part may be seen if the cervix is dilated; in this case, one may then proceed with expectant management, allowing the fetus to act as a tamponade for the low-lying or marginal placenta previa. If the placenta can be seen or felt through the dilated cervix, cesarean section is indicated. If bleeding is light and the cervix appears to be undilated, gentle palpation can be accomplished; a boggy mass felt in the anterior vaginal or lateral fornices of the portio vaginalis confirms the diagnosis of placenta previa. The double–set-up examination should not be performed in circumstances in which bleeding is extremely brisk, if the ultrasonogram clearly demonstrates placenta anteriorly and posteriorly over the cervical os, and, of course, if there is any evidence of fetal or maternal instability.

The primary cause of perinatal morbidity and mortality in the setting of placenta previa is prematurity. The goal of the management plan should be enabling the patient to reach 36 to 37 weeks of gestation. To achieve this, hospitalization and bedrest with bathroom privileges and diminished activity is recommended. The patient must avoid coitus. Iron stores should be replaced with 300 mg of ferrous sulfate orally one to three times daily, depending on the hematocrit. Type and hold specimens should be sent as often as necessary to keep blood available until delivery. Hematocrit should be measured at frequent in-

tervals. Many of these patients require hospitalization until delivery; outpatient management is not recommended unless bleeding stops completely. In placenta previa, the magnitude of bleeding can be unrecognized, and insidious blood loss can lead to severe anemia within several days. Weekly nonstress testing is indicated; more frequent testing is necessary if bleeding increases. In the current literature, however, exact guidelines for the optimal frequency of testing in a changing situation do not exist. Fetal growth assessment biweekly is recommended, in as much as intrauterine growth restriction is sometimes seen.

Outpatient management in chronic abruption and placenta previa is suitable for some patients. However, strict criteria should be employed, in writing. The patient must live less than 15 minutes away from the hospital, and transportation must be available 24 hours a day. When the amount of bleeding changes, the patient should be re-examined at the earliest possible time, and her hemodynamic situation and need for delivery should be reassessed before continued outpatient care is allowed. At cesarean section, the operator should try to avoid the placenta if possible. Repeated ultrasound examination before surgery may be helpful. The position of the fetus should also be established by ultrasonography before cesarean section, because one of the difficulties encountered with a low transverse uterine incision may be related to malpresentation of the fetus. Because transverse and breech presentations are more often found in association with placenta previa, there is a greater possibility that extension of the incision may be necessary. In this situation, the operator might prefer to use a vertical uterine incision and should advise the patient of this possible need regardless of the intended initial incision.

Abruptio Placentae

Abruptio placentae occurs in approximately 1 in 80 pregnancies. Associated findings include the presence of chronic hypertension; vascular diseases such as systemic lupus erythematosus; pregnancy-induced hypertension; preeclampsia; and tobacco or cocaine use. Multiple pregnancy is also commonly associated with abruption.

The classic manifestation of placental abruption is in the patient with significant vaginal bleeding, a rigid abdomen, and a dead fetus. Although there are different degrees of severity in abruption, there is often less opportunity for expectant management. In this condition, in comparison with placenta previa, fetal compromise may be extremely rapid. Assessment of hemodynamic stability and laboratory tests is similar to that outlined earlier for placenta previa. The most rapid method of assessing coagulability is to draw an extra tube of blood without additives and look for clotting, which normally occurs within 2 to 3 minutes. Continuous fetal and maternal monitoring is critical.

The goal in management of patients with abruption when there is no evidence of fetal distress is vaginal delivery, as this route would be safer for a mother with a coagulation deficit. However, cesarean section is performed in approximately 40 to 50% of all cases, either because of deteriorating fetal status or because of rapidly changing maternal status remote from anticipated vaginal delivery. Ultrasound examination to rule out placenta previa is mandatory. Uterine contractions occurring at frequent intervals and a rigid abdomen strongly suggest the diagnosis. Hypertonicity between contractions is commonly seen on external tocodynamometry. On speculum examination, the cervix usually appears dilated, with bleeding coming from inside the uterus. At that point, membranes should be ruptured, and an internal scalp electrode and an internal uterine pressure catheter should be applied. The absence of fetal heart rate variability or the presence of bradycardia or tachycardia mandates immediate delivery. If fetal heart rate variability is adequate, fetal heart rate is normal, and decelerations are absent, expectant management is indicated. If adequate progress does not occur, a dilute solution of oxytocin (Pitocin) should be administered. High doses of oxytocin may be needed under these circumstances. Any delay in progress of labor, manifested by lack of either cervical dilation or descent, should lead to cesarean section.

At the time of cesarean section, the uterus occasionally appears mottled and purple. This condition, Couvelaire's uterus, arises from bleeding into the myometrium. The incision can safely be made through such an area, if necessary, despite the presence of extravasated blood. The uterus should contract well after the cesarean section is performed. However, it is critical to close the incision only after hemostasis is ensured, because coagulopathy may not appear until after the surgery is begun. Although in most cases removal of the placenta relieves the coagulopathy, intraoperative transfusion of packed red blood cells and coagulation factors may be necessary and should be made available before surgery, if possible. Patients in shock who may have been hypotensive before surgery could begin to manifest evidence of additional bleeding or preeclampsia during or after surgery as a more stable hemodynamic situation is achieved. These patients should be monitored closely in the postpartum period for evidence of hypertension or bleeding; further treatment with antihypertensive drugs, magnesium sulfate, or blood products is sometimes necessary.

In summary, the potentially life-threatening causes of bleeding in late pregnancy necessitate detailed evaluation of these patients. The possibilities of occult abruption and previa should always be foremost in the examiner's differential diagnosis. History, physical examination, laboratory parameters, fetal monitoring, and ultrasonography should be included in the work-up of all such patients.

HYPERTENSIVE DISORDERS OF PREGNANCY

method of
WAYNE KRAMER, M.D., and
BRIAN KIRSHON, M.D.
Baylor College of Medicine
Houston, Texas

The hypertensive disorders of pregnancy remain one of the most common medical problems encountered in pregnancy. The management of hypertension antedating pregnancy as opposed to blood pressure elevation occurring during pregnancy, as well as the different impacts on both mother and fetus, necessitate a classification to differentiate the two. Numerous definitions have been proposed by the American College of Obstetricians and Gynecologists (ACOG) (1972), the World Health Organization (1987), the International Society for the Study of Hypertension in Pregnancy (1987), and the National High Blood Pressure Council (1990). The classification recommended by ACOG is used at the authors' institution:

1. Chronic hypertension.
2. Preeclampsia-eclampsia (pregnancy-induced hypertension [PIH]).
3. Preeclampsia superimposed upon chronic hypertension.
4. Gestational (late) or transient hypertension.
5. Unclassified.

CHRONIC HYPERTENSION

Chronic hypertension is defined as hypertension that is present and observed before pregnancy or that is diagnosed before the 20th week of gestation. Hypertension is a blood pressure higher than 140/90 mmHg. Hypertension diagnosed during pregnancy and persisting beyond 6 weeks post partum is also classified as chronic hypertension.

PREECLAMPSIA-ECLAMPSIA

Preeclampsia-eclampsia is defined as the onset of hypertension with proteinuria, edema, or both at 20 weeks or more of gestation. It may also be defined as a rise in systolic blood pressure of more than 30 mmHg or a diastolic blood pressure that is more than 15 mmHg over baseline blood pressure on more than two occasions more than 6 hours apart. A mean arterial pressure of 105 mmHg and above is considered indicative of hypertension.

Proteinuria (+1 or greater on dipstick testing) is defined as excretion of more than 300 mg of protein in 24 hours. Edema is classified as nondependent swelling, usually involving hands and face, with a rapid weight gain (>5 pounds in 1 week).

Preeclampsia is further subdivided into mild and severe forms. Severe preeclampsia is diagnosed when the following criteria are met:

1. Systolic blood pressure higher than 160 mmHg systolic or diastolic pressure higher than 110 mgHg on more than two occasions more than 6 hours apart.
2. Proteinuria (excretion of >5 grams of protein in 24 hours, or 3 to 4 + on dipstick testing).
3. Oliguria (excretion of 500 mL of urine or less in 24 hours) or renal failure.
4. Visual disturbances.
5. Epigastric pain.
6. Pulmonary edema.
7. Eclampsia (occurrence of seizures in a patient with preeclampsia).
8. Coagulopathy.
9. HELLP syndrome (hemolysis, elevated liver enzyme levels, thrombocytopenia, proteinuria).

PREECLAMPSIA SUPERIMPOSED UPON CHRONIC HYPERTENSION

The diagnosis can be made on the basis of an increase in blood pressure (>30 mmHg systolic and >15 mmHg diastolic, or >20 mmHg mean arterial pressure) associated with proteinuria or edema.

GESTATIONAL (LATE) HYPERTENSION

Gestational hypertension occurs in the second half of pregnancy or in the first 24 hours post partum without edema or proteinuria and with a return to normal blood pressure within several days of delivery.

PREECLAMPSIA-ECLAMPSIA

Epidemiology

Preeclampsia, a disorder unique to pregnancy, occurs in 5 to 10% of pregnancies in the United States and is severe in less than 1%. Eclampsia occurs in approximately 0.1% of all pregnancies. At least two-thirds of patients with preeclampsia are nulliparous. There is no clear relationship between preeclampsia and race or socioeconomic status. There is a genetic association: the daughters of eclamptic mothers have a greater chance of having preeclampsia. Among patients with certain medical disorders, including diabetes, renal disease, and chronic hypertension, there is an in-creased incidence of preeclampsia. Certain pregnancy-associated conditions are also associated with an increased incidence of preeclampsia and include multiple pregnancies (14 to 30% incidence); nonimmune hydrops fetalis (up to 50% incidence) and hydatidiform mole. Patients who exhibited preeclampsia in a previous pregnancy are at increased risk of developing preeclampsia in subsequent pregnancies. Patients who had severe preeclampsia in a prior pregnancy have up to a 66% chance of developing preeclampsia in the next pregnancy.

Pathophysiology

Studies of the decidual vessels supplying the placental site in mothers with preeclampsia indicate that there is failure of trophoblastic tissue to invade the maternal spiral arteries, resulting in less dilatation of these vessels. This indicates that preeclampsia may be a disorder of placentation and thus difficult to prevent. It has also been shown that there is a lack of adrenergic innervation at the base of the spiral arteries. More recently, it has been suggested that increased endothelial cell injury disrupts the arachnidonic acid pathway, leading to decreased production of prostacyclin and elevated thromboxane levels.

The major systems targeted by preeclampsia are cardiovascular (manifested by increased blood pressure), renal (proteinuria), and placental (intrauterine growth retardation).

Diagnosis

Blood Pressure

Hypertension develops as a result of vasospasm and hyperdynamic circulation. As many as 40% of patients with chronic hypertension are normotensive in the second trimester, and blood pressure therefore returns to baseline levels in the third trimester and is misinterpreted as preeclampsia. It is advisable to monitor the first, fourth, and fifth Korotkoff sounds while a patient is in the sitting position with the cuff arm resting on the desk or in the left lateral recumbent position, so that the arm is not raised above the level of the patient's heart. The patient's blood pressure may be falsely elevated if the cuff size is too small. The systolic blood pressure must rise 30 mmHg or more or the diastolic pressure must rise 15 mmHg or more from early pregnancy in order to be classified as preeclampsia.

Proteinuria

Either voided or catheterized specimens may be used for diagnosis. Strenuous activity, urinary tract infections, or dehydration may increase the number of red or white blood cells in the urine and cause a falsely elevated protein level. The amount of proteinuria may also be underestimated as a result of dilution. As many as 13% of patients with preeclampsia may not have proteinuria.

Symptoms

A multitude of symptoms may occur; however, those associated with poor perfusion are important indicators of the severity of the disease. These include headache, dizziness, drowsiness, blurred vision, scotoma, amaurosis, nausea, vomiting, epigastric pain, anuria, and oliguria.

Laboratory Evaluations

Hematologic Assessment. Intravascular depletion may result in an increase in hematocrit as a result of hemoconcentration. Thrombocytopenia complicates approximately 10% of cases of severe preeclampsia, and the lowest count may occur only 24 to 48 hours after delivery. When thrombocytopenia is present, a full coagulogram should be obtained because disseminated intravascular coagulation (DIC) may develop. Delivery should of course be accomplished in the presence of thrombocytopenia and DIC. If the platelet count is less than 50,000 per mm³ before anticipated surgery (i.e., cesarean section), a platelet transfusion of 6 to 10 units of platelets should be given immediately preoperatively. Accordingly, fresh-frozen plasma, cryoprecipitate, or both should be given for prolonged prothrombin time, prolonged partial thromboplastin time, and low fibrinogen levels, respectively.

Liver Function Tests. Elevations of liver enzyme levels are seen in patients with severe preeclampsia, and marked elevations are associated with a subcapsular hematoma and potential hepatic capsule rupture.

Renal Function Tests. A uric acid level of more than 5 mg per dL is abnormal in pregnancy and may be a sensitive indicator of preeclampsia. Blood urea nitrogen levels higher than 10 mg per dL and creatinine levels higher than 1 mg per dL are abnormal in pregnancy. The creatinine clearance is frequently decreased in preeclampsia. The 24-hour urinary calcium excretion is also markedly decreased in preeclampsia.

Management

Antepartum Management

Mild preeclampsia can occur any time after 20 weeks' gestation but usually occurs late in pregnancy. The patient with mild preeclampsia may be managed conservatively to allow for fetal lung maturation when appropriate. Initial laboratory tests should include a complete blood count, measurements of liver enzymes and uric acid, a coagulation profile, and a 24-hour urine sample for protein. Biweekly antepartum fetal surveillance (consisting of biophysical profile or nonstress test) with daily fetal kick counts should be performed. Ultrasound assessment of growth and fluid volume should be assessed. In patients at less than 32 weeks' gestation, the authors administer weekly steroid therapy (Celestone, 12 mg intramuscularly) through 34 weeks to reduce the incidence of respiratory distress syndrome in the advent of a premature delivery.

If the disease becomes severe, if evidence of fetal compromise is apparent, or if there is appropriate fetal lung maturity, the infant should be delivered. The authors usually perform an amniocentesis at 36 weeks in patients with mild preeclampsia and every week until a mature profile is obtained, at which time the infant is delivered.

Intrapartum Management

If the patient is at less than 34 weeks' gestation, she should be referred to a tertiary care center. Appropriate laboratory data, including complete blood count, coagulation profile, serum chemistry studies, uric acid measurements, and liver battery, should be obtained. Patients should undergo labor in the left lateral position with electronic fetal heart rate monitoring.

Seizure Prophylaxis. All patients with preeclampsia-eclampsia should receive magnesium sulfate for seizure prophylaxis during labor and for at least 24 hours post partum. An intravenous loading dose of 4 to 6 grams is given and followed by a maintenance dose of 2 grams per hour. A mild transient decrease in blood pressure is seen soon after magnesium sulfate therapy is commenced. Serum levels should be checked every 6 to 8 hours during the infusion to obtain the desired therapeutic range of 5 to 7 mEq per dL. The patient should be monitored for deep tendon reflexes every hour, respiratory rate, and urinary output. If a decrease in any of these occurs, the magnesium level should be measured; the infusion may have to be decreased or discontinued. If the patient has a seizure while receiving magnesium sulfate, diazepam, 5 to 10 mg intravenously, or pentothal is recommended. Magnesium sulfate overdose can be treated with 10 mL of 10% calcium gluconate or chloride intravenously.

Blood Pressure Management. Women with a diastolic blood pressure of 110 mmHg or higher are treated with antihypertensive agents. The goal is not to obtain a normal blood pressure but to reduce the diastolic blood pressure to a level that will provide a margin of maternal safety (95 to 100 mmHg). Intravenous hydralazine, 5 mg

TABLE 1. **Postpartum Hypertensive Agents**

Drug Name	Dosage
Alpha-methyldopa	500–1000 mg IV followed by 500 mg PO q 6 h
Hydralazine	25–75 mg PO qid
Nifedipine	10–20 mg PO q 6 h prn

over 2 to 4 minutes, is given initially. If this does not stabilize the blood pressure within 20 minutes, an additional 5 mg is given and so on until the desired control is obtained. If after administration of 20 mg of hydralazine blood pressure control is not adequate, the patient may need pulmonary artery catheterization and nitroglycerin or nitroprusside therapy.

Fluid Management. This is an area of controversy. Intravenous fluids of a balanced salt solution are administered at a rate of 100 to 125 mL per hour. Urine output is monitored closely, and a Foley catheter is placed. Oliguria, defined as less than 0.5 mL of urine per kg over 2 consecutive hours, should be managed by giving a fluid bolus of 500 to 1000 mL of a balanced salt solution. If oliguria persists, central monitoring through a pulmonary artery catheter should be instituted. Most patients with oliguria in preeclampsia are intravascularly depleted and require more fluid, but a small subset require vasodilator therapy for renal artery vasospasm. A small group have congestive heart failure and require inotropic agents and diuretics.

Epidural Anesthesia. The use of epidural anesthesia in preeclampsia-eclampsia is controversial because declines in blood pressure can occur if volume contraction is not corrected before epidural placement. If the coagulation profile is normal, volume loading is employed, and fetal wellbeing is confirmed, epidural anesthesia is used.

In most academic units, a pulmonary artery catheter is placed if an epidural is used in a patient with severe preeclampsia.

Postpartum Management

Approximately 33% of seizures occur in the postpartum period. The majority of seizures that occur post partum occur within 24 hours, and virtually all occur within 48 hours. The authors continue magnesium sulfate therapy for 24 hours post partum or until the patient has entered the diuretic phase (>100 mL of urine per hour in 3 consecutive hours) The hypertension may last for up to 6 weeks post partum. If the blood pressure remains above 150/100 mmHg during this 6-week period, therapy is initiated with alpha-methyldopa, hydralazine, or nifedipine either alone or combination (Table 1).

CHRONIC HYPERTENSION

Patients with chronic hypertension usually have a history of elevated blood pressure as well as a strong family history. The differentiation of chronic hypertension from preeclampsia is difficult but important because the progression and management of each varies considerably. A fundoscopic examination may demonstrate changes in chronic hypertension that are absent in preeclampsia. Antithrombin III is lowered, whereas uric acid, fibronectin, and atrial naturetic peptide levels are elevated, in preeclampsia. None of these laboratory parameters are affected by chronic hypertension.

The goals of obstetric management of chronic hypertension include early recognition of superimposed preeclampsia, monitoring of fetal wellbeing, and prevention of intrauterine growth retardation. The authors obtain a baseline 24-hour urine collection to measure creatinine clearance

TABLE 2. **Commonly Used Antihypertensive Agents**

Drug Name/Group	Fetal/Neonatal Effects	Usual Dosage
Direct Vasodilators		
Hydralazine	Thrombocytopenia	25–75 mg bid–qid
Alpha- and Beta-Blocking Agents		
Propranolol	Intrauterine growth retardation, bradycardia, respiratory distress syndrome, impaired autonomic nervous system, hypoglycemia	20–40 mg bid–qid
Labetalol	Possible bradycardia	100 mg bid–tid
Sympatholytic Agents		
Methyldopa	Tremor, hypotension, decreased head circumference	250–500 mg bid–qid
Clonidine	Not known	0.1 mg bid–qid
Diuretics		
Furosemide	Not known	20–40 mg/day
Thiazides	Hypokalemia, thrombocytopenia	25–100 mg/day
Calcium Channel Blockers		
Nifedipine	Not known	10–20 mg qid

and total protein as well as blood urea nitrogen, creatinine, and uric acid. A baseline ultrasound study is obtained between 18 and 24 weeks' gestation to confirm dates and is repeated at 28 weeks and then every 4 weeks until delivery to aid in the diagnosis of intrauterine growth retardation. After 26 weeks, patients are seen every other week; after 30 weeks, they are seen weekly. Fetal evaluation is begun between 30 to 32 weeks and can be performed weekly or biweekly. A nonstress test or biophysical profile is performed with addition of fetal activity counts. More than six movements in a 1-hour observation period is considered normal. It is also advantageous for the patient to monitor her own blood pressure at home and to test her urine for protein at these daily recordings in order to aid in the diagnosis of early preeclampsia.

Antihypertensive Therapy

For patients with mild hypertension (blood pressure <150/100 mmHg), the use of antihypertensive agents is controversial. However, therapy can be used safely when indicated by maternal condition. Antihypertensives reduce the maternal risk of markedly elevated pressures, may delay or prevent preeclampsia if started early in pregnancy, and appear to reduce the rates of perinatal morbidity and mortality. The authors treat a persistently elevated diastolic pressure of 90 mmHg or higher. Various antihypertensive agents have been used in pregnancy (Table 2); however, alpha-methyldopa, a central alpha$_2$-adrenergic agonist, has been more completely studied than any other drug during pregnancy. The authors initiate therapy with 250 mg twice daily and increase the dosage as needed to a maximum of 2 grams per day. Hydralazine, in doses up to 300 mg per day, may have to be added if alpha-methyldopa alone is insufficient. Diuretics are usually added only if salt and water retention become extreme and alpha-methyldopa's effect is becoming impaired. Third-trimester antepartum surveillance is employed.

The authors allow patients with uncomplicated mild hypertension to enter labor spontaneously but induce labor if there is any evidence of fetal compromise. They do not allow chronically hypertensive patients to go post dates. In severely hypertensive patients, infants are delivered as clinically indicated (i.e., intrauterine growth retardation, fetal distress, superimposed severe preeclampsia, oligohydramnios). Post partum, patients continue antihypertension therapy. Table 2 outlines the various antihypertensive agents with the fetal and neonatal effects.

GESTATIONAL HYPERTENSION

Patients presenting late in pregnancy with gestational hypertension are managed in the same way as those with preeclampsia.

OBSTETRIC ANESTHESIA

method of
GLENN K. SHOPPER, M.D.
University of Missouri School of Medicine
Kansas City, Missouri

and

MARK D. JOHNSON, M.D.
University of Texas
Dallas, Texas

Obstetric anesthesia is complicated by the parturient's altered physiology and the unpredictable nature of her peripartum course. Obstetric emergencies occur frequently, necessitating rapid, decisive action and sophisticated technical skills. Medications administered to the mother affect the fetus by altering maternal physiology and by direct effects on placental perfusion, on uterine contractility and the progress of labor, and on the fetus itself. Labor pain, in addition to being unpleasant to the mother, is not beneficial to the fetus. Stress hormones released in response to pain can have a deleterious effect on placental perfusion. The development of regional anesthetic techniques has significantly reduced maternal suffering and improved fetal and maternal safety.

PHYSIOLOGIC CHANGES OF PREGNANCY

The increased metabolic demands of the developing fetus are met with a rise in cardiac output of up to 40% at term. This increase is attributed to an increase in heart rate and a decrease in afterload. Stroke volume increases of as much as 30% have also been reported. Increases in cardiac output immediately after delivery occur after autotransfusion of 500 to 750 mL of blood from the contracted uterus.

Platelet count and levels of clotting Factors VII, X, and XII and of fibrinogen are increased with pregnancy. At term, maternal blood volume has increased by 35%. The increase in plasma volume exceeds that of the red cell mass, resulting in the physiologic anemia of pregnancy. Despite a normal gravid hematocrit of 32 to 35%, oxygen delivery to tissues does not suffer, because the increase in cardiac output restores oxygen delivery.

The gravid uterus provides a high-flow, low-resistance arterial-to-venous shunt, with uterine blood flow of up to 40 times the nonpregnant rate, accounting for 20% of cardiac output. This dramatic decrease in afterload results in a slight fall in blood pressure during pregnancy despite increased cardiac output.

At term, when the parturient is supine, the gravid uterus is capable of compressing the aorta and the vena cava, leading to decreased venous return to the heart and systemic hypotension. Supine hypotension is most commonly seen with conditions involving a large uterus (e.g., multiple gestations, polyhydramnios), a loss of sympathetic tone (i.e., regional anesthesia), or inadequate intravascular volume. As the normal uterine vasculature is near-maximally dilated, any significant decrement in systemic blood pressure cannot be met with an autoregulatory decrease in uterine vascular resistance, and uterine perfusion is thus jeopardized. Left uterine displacement with a wedge or cushion under the right hip is imperative, especially when a regional anesthetic is administered.

The enlarged uterus may also indirectly cause difficulties in administering an epidural anesthetic. Increased intra-abdominal pressure may be transmitted to the lumbar epidural space, where a positive intraepidural pressure may render the "hanging drop" method inappropriate for locating the epidural space. Venous engorgement of the epidural venous plexus increases the possibility of cannulation of an epidural vein, with resultant intravascular injection of local anesthetic.

The increased oxygen demands of the developing fetus are met by the respiratory system with a 50% increase in minute ventilation secondary to an increased respiratory rate and increased tidal volume. Arterial blood gas analysis demonstrates a respiratory alkalosis with a compensatory metabolic acidosis. Although total lung capacity is unchanged, the gravid uterus causes a resting elevation of the diaphragm, decreasing functional residual capacity (FRC). The decrease in FRC is significant because conditions that further decrease FRC (e.g., obesity, Trendelenburg's positioning, general anesthesia) can cause FRC to decrease below closing capacity, leading to ventilation/perfusion mismatching and arterial oxygen desaturation. Because FRC represents the oxygen stores during periods of apnea (e.g., during induction of general anesthesia), hypoxia can be expected to ensue much sooner. Additional changes within the respiratory system include capillary engorgement of the nasal and pharyngeal mucosa, causing decreased airway diameter and making insertion of nasal airways and nasal intubations relatively contraindicated.

Glomerular filtration rate is increased 50% during pregnancy, as is tubular resorption of water and solutes, leading to a normal water and sodium balance with decreased creatine and blood urea nitrogen (BUN). "Normal" BUN and creatine values in a parturient may indicate renal pathology.

Gastric emptying is decreased during pregnancy secondary to hormonal and mechanical factors. The placenta secretes gastrin, stimulating gastric acid secretion. The net result is an increased likelihood that gastric contents will exceed 30 mL and the pH will be less than 2.5, both of which are risk factors for pulmonary aspiration of gastric contents.

The actions of general and local anesthetics are potentiated during pregnancy. Minimal alveolar concentration (MAC), the concentration of volatile anesthetic necessary to inhibit response to a surgical stimulus, is decreased 25%. Decreased doses of local anesthetics are required for spinal and epidural blocks, reflecting an increased sensitivity to local anesthetics and possibly a compression of the epidural space by the gravid uterus.

ANESTHESIA FOR VAGINAL DELIVERY

Systemic Medications

Although systemically administered analgesics have potentially untoward effects on the mother and fetus, they have the advantages of rapidity of onset, sureness of effect, and minimal hemodynamic effects. They are particularly appropriate if regional analgesia techniques are contraindicated by coagulopathies, hemorrhage, sepsis, infections at site of regional block, or the patient's refusal. If coagulopathy is suspected (e.g., liver disease, preeclampsia), a regional anesthetic may be contraindicated if the prothrombin time, partial thromboplastin time, fibrinogen level, and bleeding time are not within normal limits or if the platelet count is less than 100,000.

Because of the intermittent nature of pain from contractions, a constant level of analgesia may be insufficient to give satisfactory relief of pain during the peak of contraction, while causing excessive sedation between contractions. The hazards imposed by systemic analgesics include maternal respiratory depression, hypercapnia, and hypoxia; obtundation of airway reflexes and risk of aspiration; decreased maternal consciousness and cooperation with voluntary expulsive efforts; decreased beat-to-beat variation of the fetal heart rate; and neonatal respiratory depression. All commonly used systemic medications (e.g., narcotics, barbiturates, benzodiazepines, phenothiazines, scopolamine) rapidly equilibrate across the placenta. Fetal narcotic levels are approximately one-third of maternal peak levels, and when narcotics are used in large doses, the possibility of neonatal resuscitation must be considered.

Narcotics. Narcotics are the most popular systemic analgesics for labor. They are efficacious and predictable. Naloxone is available in the event of maternal or neonatal respiratory depression. Although narcotics are frequently administered intramuscularly, the intravenous route is preferable because it allows more rapid onset and facilitates titration of effect, reducing the incidence of overdosing or underdosing. In obese patients, attempts at intramuscular injections may actually result in subcutaneous administrations with erratic absorption kinetics. Patient-controlled analgesia (PCA), although relatively unexplored for labor analgesia, appears well suited for this indication and may prove to be an effective mode of narcotic administration. Meperidine (Demerol) is one of the most popular narcotics because its pharmacokinetics provide a rapid onset with an intermediate duration of action. Tachycardia is a common side effect of meperidine administration. Doses of 12.5 to 50 mg intravenously are effective, with a peak effect after 5 to 10 minutes; 50 to 100 mg intramuscularly can also be used. Morphine is less frequently used because it has a slower onset and longer duration and because the side effects of nausea, vomiting, and vasodilation (causing hypotension) occur frequently. With meperidine and morphine, neonatal respiratory depression is most frequent if the narcotics are administered 2 to 3 hours before delivery.

Other narcotic analgesics commonly used are fentanyl (Sublimaze) and sufentanil (Sufenta). Both are highly potent agents with very rapid onset and short duration of action. Agonist-antagonist agents such as butorphanol (Stadol) and nalbuphine (Nubain) are also used. Nalbuphine has profound sedative properties and should be administered if additional sedation is advantageous. One potential advantage of butorphanol and nalbuphine is their ceiling for respiratory depression. Additional doses of drug beyond 1 to 2 mg of butorphanol or 10 to 20 mg of nalbuphine (equivalent to 10 to 20 mg of morphine) do not cause additional side effects or analgesia. One precaution to be considered when these drugs are used is their antagonist effect if a potent narcotic has previously been administered; both butorphanol and nalbuphine can precipitate withdrawal symptoms in a parturient who has become dependent on the administration of narcotics.

Sedatives. Neuroleptics are also frequently used for their antiemetic and sedative properties. Used alone, they have no analgesic qualities. Sedatives, although they produce the outward appearance of tranquility, are no substitute for emotional support and psychological preparation for childbirth. Most anxiety is caused by pain or the anticipation of pain; in these cases, the need for sedation is obviated by adequate analgesia. Promethazine (Phenergan) and propiomazine (Largon) are commonly used in doses of 50 and 20 mg, respectively, given intravenously or intramuscularly. When an antiemetic agent that has minimal sedating properties is desired, 10 mg of metoclopramide (Reglan) intravenously or intramuscularly is very effective. Metoclopramide has the additional advantage of increasing gastric emptying, thereby reducing the risks of aspiration of gastric contents.

Regional Techniques

Although most techniques for regional anesthesia and analgesia are technically more demanding, they have many advantages over systemic techniques:

1. Pain relief is unsurpassed.
2. The mother is able to participate actively in the birth process with a clear sensorium.
3. The possibility of fetal drug exposure is minimized.
4. In the absence of hypotension, a properly administered spinal or epidural analgesic, by reducing the levels of circulating catecholamines, can improve uterine perfusion, especially if uterine perfusion is jeopardized (e.g., preeclampsia).
5. Although regional anesthesia does not obviate the need for airway management, an epidural analgesic administered during labor can be rapidly extended to provide excellent surgical conditions without necessitating general anesthesia.
6. Regional anesthesia can provide greater hemodynamic stability. Epidural blocks can be titrated slowly to achieve a slow onset of a sympathectomy, with adequate opportunity to rectify any incipient changes. During general anesthesia, significant hemodynamic aberrations can occur during tracheal intubation, extubation, and skin incision.

The disadvantages of regional techniques are few: because technical skill is essential, failure of blocks are more frequent when administered by inexperienced physicians. Onset time is longer than with general anesthesia. Although controversial, epidural analgesia administered during labor may prolong Stage II of labor and has been associated with an increased incidence of instrumental deliveries.

The minimal preparation for regional analgesia and anesthesia involves a brief history directed toward obstetric, cardiac, respiratory, and neurologic pathology; contraindications to regional anesthesia should be ruled out. Physical examination should include evaluation of the airway, lumbar spine, and venous access and must include evaluation of any pathology elicited by the history. Laboratory tests are necessary only if specific pathology dictates. Before initiating a block, 30 mL of a nonparticulate antacid, 0.3 M sodium citrate (Bicitra), is given orally; 500 to 1000 mL of warmed Ringer's lactate or normal saline is instilled intravenously to decrease the incidence of hypotension during the onset of the sympathectomy. Because of the possibility of loss of consciousness or of airway reflexes during the performance of the block, resuscitative equipment, including materials for tracheal intubation, should be readily available.

Epidural Analgesia. Lumbar epidural analgesia is particularly suited for vaginal deliveries; it affords easy titration and can be rapidly extended for operative and instrumental deliveries. With dilute solutions of local anesthetic, minimal motor block is possible, allowing effective expulsive efforts.

After the decision has been made to administer an epidural analgesic, the patient is placed in the lateral decubitus or sitting position; the latter facilitates placement if technical difficulties (e.g., obesity, scoliosis) are anticipated. The patient is encouraged to arch her back. The back is prepared and draped to maintain sterility. Because the spinal cord ends above L1–2, the interspace L2–3 or L3–4 is appropriate for placing a block. A skin wheal is made, and the epidural needle is inserted until it is anchored in the supraspinous or intraspinous ligaments. It is then advanced into the epidural space by using the loss of resistance to air or saline. A catheter is advanced 2 to 3 cm through the needle (after the patient is warned of the possibility of paresthesias), and the needle is removed.

The use of epinephrine (1:200,000) in test doses of local anesthetic is controversial. In nonlaboring patients, a 15-μg dose of epinephrine in 3 mL of local anesthetic will cause an increase in heart rate when administered intravascularly. However, during labor, maternal heart rate fluctuations are frequent, rendering the test dose of epinephrine ineffective. Epinephrine in the local anesthetic can increase the incidence of motor block, and epinephrine administered intravascularly can increase uterine artery resistance.

The catheter should be aspirated before any drug is administered, but the inability to aspirate blood or cerebrospinal fluid does not rule out intrathecal or intravascular placement. The best method of identifying intravascular injections is to watch closely for symptoms of systemic local anesthetic effects (e.g., tinnitus, perioral numbness, dizziness, lightheadedness) and effects of intrathecal injections (e.g., hypotension, a dense, abrupt motor and sensory block) after giving any drug through the catheter. Incremental dosing is essential to avoid administering a toxic bolus of drug, with resultant seizures or cardiovascular collapse.

An appropriate local anesthetic is one that has a rapid onset, provides reliable analgesia without undue motor block, and has a maximal margin of safety in the event of an intravascular injection. A 0.75 to 1% solution of lidocaine (Xylocaine) fulfills these criteria and is an excellent choice for initiating a block. Alkalinization with bicarbonate (1 mL of 8.4% sodium bicarbonate to 10 mL of lidocaine) further decreases onset time. Although 0.25% bupivacaine (Marcaine) has the disadvantages of slower onset and greater cardiotoxicity in the event of an undetected intravascular injection, some clinicians prefer its use for the initiation of epidural block, because the motor blockade with dilute bupivacaine is minimal. Despite the rapid onset of chloroprocaine (Nesacaine), its antagonism of epidural narcotics and amide local anesthetics can lead to disappointing results when it is used to initiate a block. Although chloroprocaine's short plasma half-life would make it appear an attractive choice for a test dose, it is inappropriate because intrathecal chloroprocaine has been associated with adhesive arachnoiditis.

Volumes of 12 to 15 mL of local anesthetic usually result in a block extending to T10. Because afferent nerves from the contracting uterus and dilating cervix enter the spinal cord at T10–L1, an epidural block that extends to these dermatomes provides analgesia during the first stage of labor. The second stage of labor involves stretching of structures innervated by the pudendal nerve (S2–4). Sacral spread of local anesthetic can be facilitated by using larger volumes of local anesthetic solution and positioning the patient with her head up.

Hypotension is a relatively frequent occurrence during the onset of a sympathectomy. Because placental perfusion depends on maternal blood pressure, avoidance of hypotension is essential. Blood pressures should be checked every 2 minutes during the initiation of a block and every 15 minutes thereafter. Nausea and vomiting frequently herald hypotension; prior administration of metoclopramide can mask this early warning. Acute volume expansion before initiating the block decreases the frequency and severity of hypotension. Left uterine displacement must be maintained. Ephedrine, 5 to 10 mg given intravenously, is an appropriate vasopressor and should be used aggressively, accompanied by additional intravenous fluid administration as a trend toward hypotension develops. Because preeclamptic patients have an exaggerated response to vasopressors, an initial dose of 2.5 mg ephedrine is appropriate. In addition to increasing vascular tone, ephedrine increases cardiac output, and tachycardia is a frequent side effect. As maternal heart rate increases, the usefulness of ephedrine diminishes. Phenylephrine (Neo-Synephrine) can increase uterine artery resistance when it is used to increase blood pressure above normal levels; however, when it is used to restore normotension during a sympathectomy, the placental constrictive effect is minimal. It should not be withheld during periods of hypotension, because untreated hypotension has a far greater deleterious effect on uterine perfusion.

Infusions are frequently used for maintaining an epidural block. When epidural blockade has been established with lidocaine, its short duration of action mandates early reinforcement with bupivacaine before the infusion is initiated. Many recipes for infusions have been espoused; the authors have found that 0.125% bupivacaine with 2 μg of fentanyl per mL of diluent at an initial rate of 10 mL per hour usually provides excellent analgesia with minimal side effects. If analgesia is insufficient, the block should be evaluated for bilateral coverage of dermatomes appropriate to the stage of labor. A regressing block should always alert the anesthesiologist to the possibility of an intravascular migration of the catheter; a progressively dense block should arouse the suspicion of an intrathecal migration. If the dermatomal spread is adequate and increased depth of block is needed, additional local anesthetic (e.g., 0.25% bupivacaine) or narcotic (e.g., 50 μg of fentanyl) is appropriate. Fentanyl should be administered with a large volume (10 to 20 mL) of diluent, because this is associated with increased quality and duration of analgesia. The most common side effects of epidural fentanyl are pruritus, nausea, and urinary retention; these can be treated with 10 to 20 μg per hour of naloxone (Narcan), given intravenously, or a narcotic agonist-antagonist, such as 0.5 to 1 mg of butorphanol, given parenterally. Oral naltrexone (Trexan), 25 mg, is also effective. Pruritus can also be treated with 25 to 50 mg of diphenhydramine (Benadryl), given intravenously.

Spinal Anesthesia. Spinal anesthesia has a long history in labor analgesia, although limited by its relatively short duration of action and frequent motor block. Because most spinal blocks are single-shot techniques, they are generally reserved for Stage II of labor or episiotomy repairs. For these indications, a sacral distribution (i.e., saddle block) is sufficient and can be achieved with hyperbaric lidocaine, 20 to 50 mg, or 5 to 7 mg of bupivacaine. Although the onset of sympathectomy and associated hypotension is more rapid with spinal anesthesia, the limited extent of a saddle block usually results in a low incidence of hypotension.

One further disadvantage to spinal techniques is the need to penetrate the dura with its attendant risk of post-dural puncture headache (PDPH). Also called spinal headache, PDPH is more common among young, female, or pregnant patients. Needle size is also influential; in parturients, the incidence of PDPH after puncture with a 27-gauge needle is 4 to 6%, and the incidence of PDPH after puncture with a 17-gauge needle is approximately 75 to 90%. Orientation of the bevel of the needle parallel with the dural fibers reduces the incidence of PDPH, as does the use of a pencil-point (Whitacre and Sprotte) needle; with the use of a 25-gauge Whitacre needle, PDPH incidence is reduced to approximately 2%.

The diagnosis of PDPH is made from a patient's history. A headache occurring in the upright position and relieved in the supine position after a dural puncture indicates PDPH. The headache is self-limiting; conservative therapy includes analgesics, bedrest, increased fluid intake, and methylxanthines (caffeine or theophylline). If the headache is severe, is slow to resolve, or impairs the patient's ability to care for her newborn, she may elect to have an epidural blood patch. This procedure involves the injection of 20 mL of autologous blood into the epidural space at the site of the dural puncture. A blood patch has a success rate of over 95%; failures generally indicate misdiagnosis of the headache or improper identification of the epidural space.

Occasionally, accidental dural punctures may occur during attempts at epidural placement. In these instances, consideration should be given to placement of an intrathecal 19-gauge catheter. For Stage I of labor, an isobaric local anesthetic in low concentration can be titrated to provide analgesia with minimal motor blockade. Stage II of labor requires hyperbaric solutions to titrate sacral anesthesia. Intrathecal narcotics can also be used as adjuncts, alone or with local anesthetics.

Intrathecal meperidine has the unusual property of possessing narcotic (mu agonist) and local anesthetic properties. At low concentrations, its narcotic effects predominate; in high concentrations, its block is similar to that of lidocaine. Preservative-free meperidine in concentrations of 50 mg per mL is isobaric. Initially, doses of 10 mg can be titrated to achieve analgesia for Stage I of labor. Sacral anesthesia for Stage II of labor can be achieved with a dose of 20 mg made hyperbaric with dextrose. Doses of 75 mg of hyperbaric meperidine delivered intrathecally have been used successfully as the sole agent for cesarean sections.

Peripheral Nerve Blocks. Peripheral nerve blocks have been used extensively in the past for labor analgesia. Paracervical block provides analgesia for Stage I of labor without hypotension or motor block. However, the high incidence of fetal bradycardia and hypoxia and occasional trauma to the fetal head has resulted in a decline in its popularity. Because most cases of fetal distress after paracervical block are associated with high blood levels of local anesthetic, chloroprocaine is the local anesthetic of choice if this technique is to be used.

Pudendal block can provide analgesia for the second stage of labor without motor or sympathetic block. Untoward fetal effects are rare. However, the success rate is low; even when administered by experienced obstetricians, the rate of bilateral block is 50 to 60%. The transvaginal approach has been associated with a significant infection rate.

Retained Placenta

Manual extraction of a retained placenta can be accomplished with sedation or with epidural, low spinal, or general anesthesia. A retained placenta can precipitate significant postpartum bleeding, and restoration of intravascular volume must be accomplished before a regional anesthetic is instituted. Uterine relaxation is frequently necessary. Deep inhalation anesthesia provides excellent relaxation, but tracheal intubation is mandatory. An effective alternative is 50 to 100 µg of nitroglycerin given intravenously, with a maximal dose of 500 µg.

Uterine relaxation occurs within 3 minutes and has a duration of approximately 5 minutes. Narcotics should be administered because headache is a frequent side effect of nitroglycerin.

Instrumental Deliveries

If a epidural catheter has been previously placed during labor, an epidural block can easily be extended to include the sacral dermatomes to facilitate forceps delivery. Otherwise, spinal blocks are ideal; a saddle block can be achieved with 30 to 40 mg of hyperbaric lidocaine. The obstetrician should be consulted before anesthesia is administered; if success is considered unlikely with a significant probability of cesarean section, a block to T4 should be established. Forceps deliveries can also be performed with intravenous sedation. Small boluses of 25 to 50 µg of fentanyl, 0.5 to 1 mg of midazolam (Versed), and 5 to 10 mg of ketamine provide analgesia and amnesia. However, it is essential that maternal consciousness and airway reflexes not be compromised, and the obstetrician and patient must understand that heavy sedation will not be administered. If the delivery cannot be accomplished with judicious doses of medications, a regional or general endotracheal anesthetic must be administered.

ANESTHESIA FOR CESAREAN SECTION

General Anesthesia

Although general anesthesia is rarely indicated for vaginal deliveries, it is occasionally appropriate for emergent instrumental deliveries, uterine relaxation, or manual extraction of a retained placenta. More frequently, general anesthesia is indicated for cesarean sections in patients who are volume depleted (e.g., hemorrhage), if there are other contraindications to regional anesthesia, or if fetal distress mandates emergency surgery. Preparation for general anesthesia includes routine hemodynamic monitoring (e.g., blood pressure, electrocardiogram), pulse oximetry, capnography, and a peripheral nerve stimulator.

Induction of Anesthesia. The possibility of pulmonary aspiration of acidic gastric contents is a real threat, and meticulous attention must be given to reducing this risk. A nonparticulate antacid (e.g., sodium citrate) is given before induction of anesthesia; metoclopramide or an H_2 blocker is administered if it is likely that sufficient time for these agents' effects will elapse before anesthesia; and a rapid-sequence induction is performed.

Until the fetus is delivered, left uterine displacement must be maintained with a roll or wedge under the right thigh. Denitrogenation (preoxygenation) is performed during the abdominal preparing and draping, allowing the parturient to breathe pure oxygen at high flow rates to wash out the nitrogen from her lungs. Denitrogenation increases the time between the start of apnea and the onset of arterial desaturation. Ideally, 3 minutes of normal breathing of 100% oxygen allows adequate denitrogenation; if time constraints mandate, four vital capacity breaths can suffice.

Anesthetic induction is performed, if tracheal intubation is anticipated to be successful. A rapid-sequence induction is mandatory, unless severe maternal pathology (e.g., cardiac failure) mandates otherwise. Induction is achieved with 3 to 5 mg of sodium pentothal per kg or 0.75 to 1 mg of ketamine per kg if hypovolemia or bronchospasm is considered likely. Succinylcholine, 1 mg per kg, provides superb conditions for intubation within the shortest time. Although all induction agents cross the placenta, neonatal respiratory depression is minimal at the recommended doses. Succinylcholine and nondepolarizing agents can affect the fetus. However, succinylcholine is highly metabolized by maternal and fetal plasma pseudocholinesterase; nondepolarizing agents are highly polarized and cross the placenta only in minimal amounts. A defasciculating dose of non-depolarizing muscle relaxant before succinylcholine is not necessary. Such agents increase succinylcholine requirements (1.5 mg per kg for induction), and if magnesium has been given preoperatively, the combination may act synergistically to precipitate respiratory failure. There is no evidence that defasciculation decreases the barrier pressure across the lower esophageal sphincter. The pregnant patient does not fasciculate to the same extent as do nonpregnant patients, and postoperative muscle pain has not been a common complaint.

At the start of induction, cricoid pressure must be maintained by an experienced assistant and not interrupted until tracheal intubation with a cuffed endotracheal tube has been unequivocally established. Proper cricoid pressure occludes the esophagus between the cricoid cartilage and the body of the vertebra posteriorly. Intubation must be performed by a skilled anesthesiologist, and the time between induction and intubation must be minimal. A wide selection of laryngoscope blades and handles (including a short handle) and endotracheal tubes (diameters from 7.0 to 5.0 mm) should be styletted and readily available; the parturient frequently has capillary engorgement of the airways, and a smaller endotracheal tube may be a necessity. The patient is not ventilated by mask during induction unless failure to intubate necessitates mask ventilation with continuous application of cricoid pressure. Because failure of intubations is an unfortunate reality, a structured, logical plan must be established in advance of the event.

Management of the Difficult Airway. The leading cause of maternal mortality associated with obstetric anesthesia is airway catastrophe. It has been estimated that the incidence of difficult intubations in pregnancy is 1 in 100, and the incidence of failed intubation may be as high as 1 in 300.

Ideally, an airway that poses a difficult intubation is best recognized preoperatively; direct laryngoscopy in the awake, topically anesthetized patient is well tolerated and allows assessment for intubation. If a difficult intubation is predicted, a fiberoptic intubation should be performed while the patient is awake after adequate topical anesthesia. Sedation should not be withheld if it expedites control of the airway. A retrograde wire technique, although invasive, is appropriate if a fiberoptic bronchoscope is not available. Blind nasal intubations are relatively contraindicated because the friable, engorged nasal mucosa is likely to bleed profusely after nasal instrumentation. Because these techniques are relatively time consuming, the anesthesiologist

may be requested to "put the patient to sleep" immediately, especially if there is fetal distress. Under no circumstances should time constraints force an anesthesiologist to jeopardize the mother and fetus by rendering the patient apneic and paralyzed and then being unable to guarantee airway control.

Nonetheless, even the most experienced clinician encounters an unexpected, difficult intubation. If intubation is unsuccessful, repositioning the patient's head or changing laryngoscope blades or endotracheal tubes often meets with success. However, after more than one attempt at intubation, arterial hypoxia mandates ventilating the patient. If positive-pressure ventilation is attempted by mask, the maintenance of cricoid pressure is of paramount importance. Some anesthesiologists recommend the placement of a cuffed endotracheal tube in the esophagus with the cuff inflated to act as an obturator; mask ventilation can be attempted with the esophageal tube protruding past the side of the mask. Gastric suction can be performed through the esophageal tube. If upper airway obstruction is encountered, insertion of an oral airway or changing head position may relieve the obstruction. Although nasal airways can precipitate bleeding, their use may be necessary to clear an upper airway obstruction; topical 0.5% phenylephrine instilled into the nares can reduce the occurrence of bleeding. If intubation is unsuccessful but ventilation can be achieved, three options are available; all should be considered in consultation with the obstetrician:

1. Proceeding with surgery and ventilating by mask (with cricoid pressure) may be appropriate in cases of fetal distress.

2. Allowing the patient to awaken, and performing an oral intubation as described earlier.

3. Allowing the patient to awaken, and administering a regional anesthetic (e.g., spinal or epidural block), or, depending on the skill of the obstetrician, performing the cesarean section with the use of local anesthesia. Although successful, especially for thin parturients, the risks are formidable. These problems include inadequate anesthesia and maternal distress and the need for near-toxic volumes of local anesthetic.

The scenario that holds the gravest consequences is that in which neither mask ventilation nor tracheal intubation can be achieved. After a reasonable number of unsuccessful attempts, if ventilation does not occur, arterial hypoxia rapidly ensues. Hypoxia, not hypoventilation and acidosis, is the most deleterious consequence; therapy must be aimed at introducing oxygen into the lungs, and surgical access to the airway must be obtained. After this, the obstetrician should immediately deliver the fetus by cesarean section. Because the fetus derives its oxygen from the maternal circulation, maternal hypoxia begets fetal asphyxia. The fetus is a metabolic parasite, causing increased maternal oxygen demand, and delivery of the infant improves maternal pulmonary mechanics.

One form of access to the trachea is a needle cricothyroidotomy. A large-bore intravenous catheter is inserted through the cricothyroid membrane and connected to an oxygen jet ventilator or the breathing circuit of the anesthesia machine. Although it is difficult to provide positive-pressure ventilation and maintain normocapnia, sufficient oxygen to prevent hypoxia can be instilled into the lungs until the muscle relaxation wears off and spontaneous ventilation returns. Disadvantages of this technique include the inability to protect the airway from gastric aspiration and the possibility of barotrauma.

An alternative technique is to make an incision across the cricothyroid membrane large enough to accommodate a small endotracheal tube. Skin hooks or a Kelly clamp are used to retract the distal portion of the trachea to expose the tracheal lumen, and the tube is inserted into the trachea. This technique, although more invasive, allows insertion of a cuffed endotracheal tube to protect the airway from gastric aspiration and provide tidal volumes sufficient to avoid atelectasis. A device (Pertrach) has been developed that allows insertion of a cuffed tube on a dilating obturator by a splittable needle; this system is self-contained and should be less invasive than a cricothyroid membrane incision.

Maintenance of General Anesthesia. After anesthesia is induced and tracheal intubation has been verified, the order to proceed with the surgical incision can be given to the obstetrician. Anesthesia is maintained with 50% nitrous oxide in oxygen, with low doses of volatile agents (approximately one-half MAC); muscle relaxation can be maintained with a succinylcholine infusion or with a short-acting nondepolarizing agent. After delivery of the infant, 20 units of oxytocin (Pitocin) per liter is added to the intravenous fluids to facilitate uterine contraction; the concentration of nitrous oxide is increased to 70%; the volatile agent is decreased or discontinued; and maintenance is continued with a narcotic (e.g., 50 to 100 µg of fentanyl). Although volatile agents increase uterine relaxation and pose a potential risk for uterine atony and subsequent hemorrhage, the authors have not found this to occur at low concentrations (e.g., 0.2% isoflurane). Benzodiazepines (e.g., 1 to 2 mg of midazolam) can be used to ensure no recall if volatile anesthetics are discontinued entirely. An orogastric catheter should be placed to evacuate the stomach. At the conclusion of surgery, the patient should not be extubated until awake, cooperative, and free from residual neuromuscular blockade.

Epidural Anesthesia

Epidural anesthesia is appropriate if operative delivery is performed on a parturient with an epidural placed previously for labor analgesia. The gradual onset of epidural anesthesia is also indicated if abrupt onset of sympathectomy and the resultant hypotension would be poorly tolerated (e.g., preeclampsia, cardiac disease, volume depletion). The use of a catheter is warranted if surgical time may be long.

The technique is similar to that for labor analgesia; antacids, left uterine displacement, intravenous volume loading, and monitoring are identical except that maternal heart rate monitoring may be desirable. In the nonlaboring parturient, baseline maternal heart rate fluctuations are infrequent, and 15 µg of epinephrine in the test dose of local anesthetic can facilitate identification of an intravascular injection. A 2% lidocaine solution with epinephrine (alkalinized with sodium bicarbonate 4.2 mEq per liter in a 1:10 dilution) is an excellent choice of agent, with a rapid onset of dense anesthesia lasting 75 to 90 minutes. A 0.5% bupivacaine solution provides an adequate block lasting 90 to 120 minutes with a slow (45-minute) onset; however, the quality of anesthesia is often inferior to that provided by lidocaine. Bupivacaine should not be alkalinized, because it precipitates. A 50-µg dose of fentanyl epidurally improves the quality of sensory block, especially during peritoneal traction; it is particularly appropriate with 0.5% bupivacaine. A block from S5 to T4 is necessary to ensure adequate anesthesia; this is usually accomplished with volumes of 20 to 30 mL of local anesthetic solution. Many instances of inadequate anesthesia can be ascribed to inadequate volumes of local anesthetic. A portion of the dose should be given with the patient in the sitting position to facilitate sacral spread.

A 3% chloroprocaine solution provides excellent surgical anesthesia. Its disadvantages are tachyphylaxis and a short duration of action (30 minutes), which can complicate redosing schedules; antagonism of subsequently administered amides and narcotics, decreasing their usefulness for postoperative analgesia; and back pain, especially after administration of large quantities of chloroprocaine. Chloroprocaine's usefulness lies in its speed of onset, which makes it the ideal agent for use in urgent cesarean sections; onset is hastened when pH is increased with bicarbonate. Chloroprocaine is also the safest agent to administer if there is fetal distress. Local anesthetics can be sequestered in an acidotic fetus, and chloroprocaine has the lowest rate of placental transfer and the shortest half-life in the systemic circulation. If 20 to 25 mL of chloroprocaine is administered in sequential 4-mL boluses immediately after the decision to perform a cesarean section, a surgical level of anesthesia is usually achieved in the time it takes to transfer the patient to the operating room and prepare the operative site. Like any other local anesthetic, dosing must be performed incrementally, with adequate time between doses to avoid intravascular or intrathecal boluses. Maternal blood pressure monitoring should be available during transit. Oxygen should be administered during emergency transport.

Spinal Anesthesia

Spinal anesthesia is an excellent technique for operative and instrumental deliveries, providing a rapid, reliable, dense block with minimal systemic drug levels. Preparation is similar to that for an epidural block, except that intravenous volume expansion with 1 to 1.5 liters is performed before initiating the block. Lumbar puncture is performed below L2. If the spinal anesthesia is initiated with the patient in the right lateral decubitus position, subsequent left uterine displacement results in a bilateral block. If anatomic anomalies (e.g., obesity, scoliosis) impair the ability to perform lumbar puncture, a paramedian approach may facilitate intrathecal access. The lumbar spine can be further flexed in the sitting position. Although difficult, fetal monitoring is essential. The abrupt and extensive sympathectomy is impressive, mandating frequent blood pressure measurements and early, aggressive treatment of hypotension. Some clinicians advocate prophylactic intravenous ephedrine in a dose of 5 mg immediately after initiation of the block (in the absence of contraindications).

Solutions of 0.75% hyperbaric bupivacaine and 5% lidocaine provide anesthesia for durations of 90 to 120 minutes and 45 to 75 minutes, respectively. A level of blockade to T4 is necessary. Dosages are influenced by height; for bupivacaine, 1 mL (7.5 mg) is used if the patient is 5 feet tall, and 0.1 mL is added for each inch of height, to a total dose of 15 mg. Dosing is similar for lidocaine, 50 to 75 mg, based on height. A dose of 10 to 15 μg of fentanyl intrathecally improves the quality of the block, especially during peritoneal traction.

Morbid Obesity

Morbid obesity significantly increases the morbidity and mortality of pregnant patients undergoing cesarean delivery. For the elective patient, epidural anesthesia is often successful but may be technically difficult because of obscuration of bony landmarks and poor spread of local anesthetic within the epidural space. Although spinal analgesics generally produce in a consistent, predictable block, the dermatomal spread may be unpredictable in morbidly obese patients. Success of the block is essential because morbidly obese patients frequently have redundant upper airway tissue, making laryngoscopy and intubation difficult. Because morbid obesity can prolong surgical duration and cause an exaggerated hypotensive response to sympathectomy, a continuous spinal technique with an intrathecal catheter allows gradual, precise titration of a spinal block. Small, incremental dosing results in a slow, controlled onset of the sympathectomy, and redosing through the catheter can extend the duration of anesthesia. Although spinal microcatheters that can pass through needles as small as 27 gauge have been developed, they are currently not available, as they have been associated with cases of cauda equina syndrome. However, a 19-gauge intrathecal catheter passed through a 17-gauge Tuohy needle is appropriate for use with morbidly obese patients.

The risk of PDPH associated with the larger needles used for continuous spinal anesthesia is seen by some clinicians as a contraindication to this technique. In the authors' experience, morbidly obese patients develop PDPH infrequently after continuous spinal anesthesia, even with a 17-gauge dural puncture. Furthermore, PDPH is relatively benign, and if a continuous spinal technique can preclude a more serious complication, it should not be withheld.

POSTPARTUM CARE

method of
ALEXANDER REITER, M.D.
Baylor College of Medicine
Houston, Texas

The postpartum period or puerperium, or the so-called fourth trimester of pregnancy, begins after the delivery of the newborn and the placenta and empirically ends 6 weeks afterwards. At that time, most of the anatomic and physiologic changes that occurred during the pregnancy have reversed. Some of the most dreadful obstetric complications, such as hemorrhage, eclamptic seizures, thromboembolic phenomena, and severe infections, may occur during the postpartum period. Immediate recognition and adequate management of these complications are essential for intact maternal survival.

PHYSIOLOGY AND MANAGEMENT

After the vaginal delivery of the newborn, the uterus becomes smaller and harder. The amount of vaginal bleeding is normally between 150 and 300 mL. The birth canal can be inspected while separation of the placenta is awaited. The examiner introduces two fingers into the vagina and applies gentle downward pressure on the perineum. To visualize the vaginal walls, the cervix is moved from side to side with a sponge stick. In order to inspect the cervix, the author applies a ring forceps on both the anterior and posterior cervical lip and gently pulls out until visualization is adequate. If lacerations of the birth canal are noted to bleed heavily, constant pressure over the bleeding area is applied with a sponge stick or a pad until the placenta separates and final repair can be achieved. On rare occasions, hemostatic sutures must be placed in order to control the bleeding before the placenta separates. As long as the uterus is firm and there is no abnormal bleeding, the examiner can wait for the spontaneous separation of the placenta. There is no consensus with regard to the length of time before intervening. The author considers 1 hour a reasonable period, because chances of spontaneous separation afterward are minimal. The examiner manually removes the placenta, if necessary (under appropriate anesthesia), by placing a hand inside the uterus and dissecting the edge of the placenta from the uterine wall until it is completely loose. The separated placenta is then pulled out. The bladder needs to be empty because a full bladder may interfere with the delivery of the placenta.

The following are signs of spontaneous separation of placenta: the uterus becomes harder and globular in shape and rises higher in the abdomen as the placenta drops down into the lower uterine segment; there is a sudden increase in the amount of vaginal bleeding; and the umbilical cord protrudes farther out of the vagina. Once the separation occurs, the patient is asked to push down. The physician can facilitate the expulsion by expressing mild pressure on the fundus of the uterus. Twisting the placenta several times as it appears in the vagina and at the vulva causes the membranes to separate completely. If the membranes start to tear apart from the placenta, they

should be grasped with a ring forceps and gently pulled out. Once delivered, the maternal surface of the placenta should be inspected for possible missing fragments, in which case the surface appears asymmetrical and rough. The presence of accessory vessels on the lateral margins of the fetal membranes may indicate a succenturiate lobe that might have been retained in the uterus. The placental fragments are removed either manually or by curettage.

After the delivery of the placenta, the episiotomy and other possible lacerations of the birth canal are repaired. At this time, the uterus is firm, and the fundus reaches the level of the umbilicus. Routine administration of oxytocin has been shown to reduce the overall blood loss. Oxytocin is usually administered intravenously at a concentration of 10 or 20 units in 1000 mL of a crystalloid solution. The rate of infusion is about 200 mL per hour. Intravenous bolus doses of oxytocin should be avoided because they may cause hypotension and arrhythmia.

Postpartum hemorrhage, defined as blood loss in excess of 500 mL in the first 12 hours after the delivery, is encountered in about 4% of cases. This is a significant complication in that hemorrhage accounts for about 10% of the non–abortion-related maternal mortality in the United States. Fifty percent of the cases of postpartum hemorrhage are caused by uterine atony; 20% are secondary to birth canal trauma; 20% are related to uterine rupture, placenta previa, or uterine inversion (after excessive traction of the umbilical cord); and 10% occur late in the postpartum period and are related to retained products of conception or to coagulopathies.

Aggressive management of postpartum hemorrhage is critical. Large-bore intravenous lines should be started immediately while blood products are made available. Clotting studies are obtained, and the patient's vital signs and urinary output are carefully monitored. The birth canal should be methodically inspected, and any source of bleeding should be repaired. If atony is suspected, the uterus is massaged through the abdominal wall. Ergot preparations such as ergonovine maleate (Ergotrate) or methylergonovine (Methergine), 0.2 mg, can be administered intramuscularly in patients who do not respond to oxytocin. Ergot drugs cause sustained uterine contractions that start shortly after administration and last for several hours. They may cause high blood pressure and should not be used in patients with a history of cardiac disease or hypertension. An alternative drug is intramuscular prostaglandin 15-methyl-F2-alpha (0.25 mg every 30 to 60 minutes).

A surgical approach is undertaken whenever the pharmacologic management fails to control the postpartum hemorrhage. The first step is the postpartum curettage, meant to remove possible products of conception. The author recommends that this procedure be done under continuous ultrasound guidance in order to minimize the risks of uterine perforation. Laparatomy with ligation of uterine or hypogastric arteries or hysterectomy is occasionally needed in the most difficult cases of postpartum hemorrhage.

During the first 1 or 2 hours after the delivery, the vital signs are monitored every 30 minutes, and the patient is observed carefully for signs of excessive blood loss (more than 500 mL). Pelvic and birth canal hematomas can enlarge rapidly, causing intense pain (never to be overlooked in this situation) and significant hemodynamic changes that are disproportional to the amount of external bleeding. Pelvic examination and inspection of the birth canal are performed, and hematomas, if present, are opened and drained. Sites of bleeding need to be controlled, but if they are not easily identified, hemostatic sutures are applied over the bleeding area. On occasion, a patient is unable to void spontaneously because of a combined effect of local edema and anesthetic drugs. The urethra can be catheterized in order to decompress an overdistended bladder that interferes with uterine contraction and causes pelvic pain and pressure.

During the first few days after the delivery, the patient might experience pain related to the episiotomy, and mild analgesics might be required. Normal healing is expected to be complete in 2 to 3 weeks. Extensive episiotomies or those complicated by lacerations of the sphincter or the wall of the rectum are usually more painful and necessitate stronger analgesic treatment. However, intense pain unresponsive to analgesics needs to be evaluated for the possibility of hematoma or perineal infection. Prolapsed hemorrhoids (especially if thrombotic) might be another cause of sustained perineal pain.

The pain associated with the physiologic uterine contractions usually decreases in intensity and becomes mild by the third or fourth postpartum day. Significant lower abdominal pain, especially if associated with fever, suggests the possibility of endometritis or urinary tract infection.

The most common sites of postpartum infection are the uterus (endometritis), the birth canal, the urinary tract, and the breasts (mastitis). The vaginal bleeding (lochia rubra) decreases over the first 3 to 4 postpartum days and becomes pale and thinner (lochia serosa between days 3 to 10). Then it becomes thicker and white-yellowish (lochia alba) and might persist for about 3 to 5 weeks. Foul-smelling lochia suggests endometritis. The author does not recommend the use of tampons during the postpartum period because of the risk of infection. They can, however, be used in patients who do not have lacerations of the birth canal and who change their tampons regularly every 3 to 4 hours.

The duration of the postpartum confinement varies between 12 hours and 3 days for patients with uncomplicated vaginal deliveries and is 4 to 5 days for patients with uncomplicated cesarean deliveries. This period is important not only for ascertaining the patient's hemodynamic stability but also for providing education and help in areas such as breast-feeding and care of the newborn.

The early discharge from the hospital, more and more encouraged by third-party payers, should be allowed only after the vaginal bleeding is carefully evaluated and a stable hematocrit is available. Other laboratory tests to be assessed before the discharge are the blood type, the Rh factor (anti-Rh prophylaxis must be administered in the appropriate cases), and the rubella immune status. Prenatal vitamins and iron supplements are recommended for another 4 to 6 weeks. Upon the discharge from the hospital, the patient should receive specific instructions regarding her immediate lifestyle. Physical activity is not restricted, and the patient may return to normal activities and exercise whenever she desires. Persistent complaints of lethargy and fatigue must be evaluated for severe anemia and for hypothyroidism.

Postpartum psychological reactions (postpartum "blues") in the form of anxiety, restlessness, and extreme irritability occur in up to 70% of postpartum patients. These reactions usually resolve without therapy within 10 to 15 days. The more severe condition of postpartum depression is less common and has a strong association with previous psychological problems. This condition necessitates medical treatment.

Sexual activity may be resumed when the bleeding has subsided, the lacerations have healed, and the perineum is comfortable. The libido is, however, very much decreased in the postpartum period. Patients may return to work 6 weeks after delivery. This is regarded as the postpartum "disability" period.

Suppression of lactation, if desired, can be achieved by applying breast binders and ice packs, using mild analgesics, and avoiding nipple stimulation. In cases of extreme breast engorgement, when the conservative methods have failed, oral bromocriptine (Parlodel), which is a dopamine receptor agonist, can be used in a dosage of 2.5 mg twice daily for 14 days. This is successful in about 90% of the cases. This drug should be avoided, however, in patients with hypertension or pregnancy-induced hypertension.

At the end of the postpartum period, the patient should have a gynecologic examination and a Papanicolaou smear. Contraceptive methods should be discussed on this occasion.

NEONATAL RESUSCITATION

method of
WILLIAM R. SEXSON, M.D.
Emory University School of Medicine
Atlanta, Georgia

Although the need to resuscitate can be anticipated in some situations, in many others infants who require resuscitation are born with no prior warning that such intervention is needed. Anticipating the unexpected is always wise in dealing with neonates who potentially require resuscitation. In a number of situations, however, resuscitation should be anticipated and planned for. Table 1 details the antepartum and intrapartum events that place infants at high risk. In these situations, the physician responsible for an infant should be notified before delivery, so that there is time to plan for the resuscitation.*

In nurseries at the author's institution, this list has been further refined to include a smaller number of "critical deliveries" (Table 2). In these situations, a resuscitation team is assembled in the delivery room, and all aspects of the resuscitation are reviewed before the birth of the infant.

The delivery of a nondistressed term infant by scheduled, elective, repeated cesarean section is not considered a high-risk situation in nurseries at the author's institution.

EQUIPMENT FOR RESUSCITATION

All equipment needed to accomplish a complete resuscitation must be immediately available in the delivery room and should be fully operational at all times. The equipment should be checked daily (or more often for busy services) to be certain that all equipment is in place and is functioning properly.

PERSONNEL FOR RESUSCITATION

Every delivery should be attended by at least one person who can perform a complete resuscitation. This person may be a physician, nurse, midwife, anesthetist, or respiratory therapist. Having such a person on-call for resuscitation either elsewhere in the hospital or from home is not adequate.

In general, most persons with designated involvement in neonatal resuscitation should have successfully completed the course in Neonatal Resuscitation developed by the American Heart Association and the American Academy of Pediatrics. In addition, by performing regular skill checks and resuscitation drills,

---

*Several published references detail all the components necessary for performing an adequate resuscitation. These references have become the current standards by which the adequacy of planning and implementation of resuscitation are judged. See *Guidelines for Perinatal Care, Third Edition,* Copyright 1992 by the American Academy of Pediatrics and the American College of Obstetricians and Gynecologists; and *Textbook of Neonatal Resuscitation,* published in 1990 by the American Heart Association and the American Academy of Pediatrics.

TABLE 1. Situations Placing an Infant at Increased Risk for Needing Resuscitation

Antepartum Factors
Ongoing medical problems
Diabetes mellitus
Drug abuse
Sexually transmitted disease
Lack of prenatal care
Hypertension
Prior Rh/ABO disease
Abnormal amniotic fluid volume
Multiple gestation
Growth retardation
Thrombocytopenia
Severe anemia

Intrapartum Factors
Emergency cesarean section
Pre-/postterm
Abnormal presentation
Hypertension
Evidence of fetal distress
    Scalp pH < 7.2
    Meconium
    Heart rate abnormality
    Decreased fetal movement
Suspected placental abruption or placenta previa
Maternal age < 16 or > 35
Chorioamnionitis
Abnormal fetal ultrasonogram
Prolapsed umbilical cord
Hydrops fetalis
Membranes ruptured for > 24 hours (> 12 hours if preterm)

the hospital and service chiefs should ensure that the skills of all designated personnel are current.

Although the presence of a trained and prepared staff member at the delivery of a high-risk infant is essential, a trained and prepared team may also be invaluable. Although many resuscitations can be handled by one person skilled at intubation, others require a much more aggressive approach. A full resuscitation on an infant with one of the conditions listed in Table 2 might take four people working closely together (specifically, one person to ventilate, one to perform cardiac compressions, one to establish vascular access, and one to draw medications). The author and colleagues have found it desirable to have a designated team in the hospital at all times. This team can then be assembled quickly by the person responsible for initiating the resuscitation.

TABLE 2. Critical Deliveries

Estimated birth weight < 1000 gm but > 500 gm
Estimated gestational age > 23 weeks and < 28 weeks
Multiple gestation < 32 weeks, total weight < 1500 gm
Hydrops fetalis
Diaphragmatic hernia
Obstetric evidence of profound asphyxia
Umbilical cord accidents (prolapse)
Malformations affecting the heart or lungs
Other situations as requested by obstetrics

TABLE 3. Common Reasons for Inadequate Chest Expansion During Ventilation

Ventilation with Bag and Mask
Blocked airway (secretions vs. positioning)
Inadequate seal around face mask
Inadequate pressure
Pneumothorax

Ventilation with Endotracheal Tube
Tube in the esophagus
Tube down main bronchus
Inadequate pressure
Pneumothorax

PREPARATION FOR RESUSCITATION

When a resuscitation is anticipated, the person responsible for resuscitation should accomplish the following:

1. Discuss the potential problems with the obstetric team.

2. Discuss with the parents the need for resuscitation, the potential problems, the outcome, and the parents' wishes.

3. Check all the equipment to be certain that it is present and working.

4. Determine the need for additional team members and assemble them as necessary.

5. Review with each team member his or her responsibility.

The events during resuscitation must focus on adequately ventilating and oxygenating the infant, restoring adequate pulmonary and systemic blood flow, and reversing any acidosis present. During a resuscitation, the decisions are based not on the Apgar score but rather on an evaluation of the infant's respiration and heart rates, the degree of cyanosis, and the adequacy of perfusion. Successful resuscitation is generally accomplished when all of these signs are normal. One of the signs that are most difficult to assess in newborns is the status of perfusion. In neonates vasoconstriction is such that the blood pressure may appear nearly normal despite inadequate cardiac output. In this situation, assessment of capillary refill is important: The examiner presses on the infant's skin over the sternum; after the examiner lifts the finger, there should be return of capillary perfusion where the skin was pressed within 3 seconds. If the capillary refill takes longer than this, conditions causing decreased cardiac output (e.g., hypovolemia, sepsis) should be suspected.

Hypothermia is a common and dangerous finding after resuscitation. In hypothermic neonates, hypoxia, hypoglycemia, and acidosis generally develop as consequences of the hypothermia. These secondary metabolic phenomena compound the hypoxia, acidosis, and cellular injury that occur with asphyxia. The prevention of heat loss and accentuation of heat gain is a first and essential part of every resuscitation. At the beginning of each resuscitation, the infant should be placed on a radiant warming bed and dried. The wet towels or blankets should be removed quickly to prevent further evaporative heat loss. For very tiny infants (those weighing less than 1000 grams), the author and colleagues generally use a thermal blanket, which circulates warm water through the mattress under the infant. This provides a source of conductive warmth to compliment the radiant warmer.

At this point, the resuscitation should proceed in the classic "ABCD" (i.e., establish Airway, Breathe, support Circulation, consider Drugs) manner. After placement on the warmer and drying, the infant should be placed in the "sniffing" position, and first the mouth and then the nose should be gently suctioned. The clinician must be careful not to overextend or underextend the infant's neck; either of these actions may occlude the airway and impede ventilation. (See later discussion of situations necessitating immediate intubation.) A wash cloth rolled up and placed under the infant's shoulders (not the neck) may help maintain the proper position of the infant. If additional stimulation is needed to assist the infant in initiating breathing, the stimulation should be gentle. The most appropriate methods for doing this are slapping the soles of the feet and rubbing the infant's back. All of the resuscitative activities just described should be completed within approximately 20 seconds.

Next, the respiration and heart rates are evaluated. The heart rate can usually be best evaluated either by feeling the umbilical cord or by auscultation. If respiration is absent or if the heart rate is below 100, bag-and-mask ventilation is initiated and continued for 15 to 30 seconds, and then the infant is reassessed. Oxygen administration alone in the infant who is not breathing is of little value and may only delay more appropriate management. If there is a possibility of drug depression from opiates (e.g., morphine, meperidine hydrochloride [Demerol], or fentanyl), 0.1 mg per kg of naloxone (Narcan, 0.4 mg per mL concentration) is administered either as an intramuscular injection or, if the infant is intubated, down the endotracheal tube. The reasons for inadequate chest movement and inadequate ventilation are listed in Table 3.

Most neonatal resuscitation can be successfully accomplished through the use of bag-and-mask ventilation. Because there are many different types of resuscitation bags and masks, it is essential that resuscitation skill training include hands-on practice and intimate familiarity with the equipment present in each specific hospital. At a minimum, the neonatal resuscitation bag should be able to deliver 80 to 100% oxygen and should have some mechanism to ensure that too much pressure is not delivered. This mechanism may either be a pressure pop-off valve or a manometer. A soft-rimmed mask is usually advisable, and the mask should be of a size that easily covers the area between the nasal bridge and the chin without being either too large or too small.

Ventilation should be started with a pressure of 20 to 40 cmH$_2$O; with subsequent breaths, pressures of 20 cmH$_2$O or as much pressure as needed to move the chest should be used. The rate of ventilation should be approximately 40 to 60 breaths per minute. The best ways to assess the adequacy of ventilation are to observe the infant for chest movement and to determine the response of the heart rate. The infant should appear to take shallow, "easy" breaths in response to bag-and-mask ventilation, and the heart rate should generally stabilize above 100 beats per minute. An 8-French orogastric catheter may need to be inserted if gastric distention is noted.

If after the initial period of bag-and-mask ventilation the infant is breathing, has a heart rate of over 100 beats per minute, but is still cyanotic, administration of oxygen is appropriate. Only enough oxygen to alleviate the cyanosis should be given. Once the infant's normal color is restored, the oxygen should be gradually withdrawn. At this point, pulse oximetry should be considered. If the oxygen is being administered via a tube without a face mask, it should be remembered that the concentration of oxygen delivered to the infant decreases rapidly once the tube is farther than 1 to 2 inches from the nares. Although an anesthesia bag may be used to administer oxygen when bag-and-mask ventilation is not used, the self-inflating bag generally does not deliver oxygen except during bag-and-mask ventilation.

If after 15 to 30 seconds of bag-and-mask ventilation the infant is still apneic or the heart rate is less than 100, the ventilation should be continued. Cardiac compressions should be started if the heart rate is less than 60 or is between 60 and 100 and not increasing. The lower portion of the infant's sternum should be compressed 1.5 to 2 cm. Compressions may be accomplished by using either the tips of two fingers of one hand or by grasping the infant's trunk with both hands and using both thumbs to compress. In practice, the two-finger method is generally easier and provides greater access to the patient when other therapies (e.g., umbilical catheterization) are needed. The rate of compression should be 120 times per minute.

Compressions and ventilation do not have to be provided in a synchronized manner. They should be provided for an additional 1 to 2 minutes, and then the heart rate should be reassessed. If the

TABLE 4. **Endotracheal Tube Size and Length of Insertion Based on Estimated Weight**

Weight (gm)	Tube Size (mm)	Insertion Distance (cm)
500–750	2.5	6.0
750–1000	2.5	6.0–6.5
1000–1250	3.0	6.5–7.0
1250–1500	3.0	7.0–7.5
1500–2000	3.0	7.5–8.0
2000–3000	3.5	8.0–9.0
3000–4000	3.5	9.0–10.0

heart rate is still less than 100 beats per minute, intubation should be considered and the second "law" of neonatal resuscitation recalled: The most common reason for failed resuscitation is inadequate ventilation. The corollary to this law is, If you are ventilating and doing compressions and are still not winning, you are probably doing something wrong! At this point, the clinician should reassess what is being done and should be sure that everything is being done as planned.

If the baby is meconium-stained, if a congenital diaphragmatic hernia is suspected, when prolonged ventilation is anticipated, or when bag-and-mask ventilation is ineffective, immediate endotracheal intubation should be done. The size of the tube and the distance of insertion are critical in ultimately achieving adequate ventilation and are based on the estimated weight of the infant (Table 4).

SITUATIONS NECESSITATING IMMEDIATE INTUBATION

Meconium-Stained Amniotic Fluid

Meconium is a common finding in amniotic fluid. Because this finding may be associated with aspiration pneumonia, the presence of meconium should always be viewed as a possible danger sign. In the majority of infants who are vigorous at delivery, small amounts of thin, watery meconium in the amniotic fluid probably do not cause significant problems. Special management of such infants is probably not indicated. Thick particulate meconium or meconium in the amniotic fluid of unresponsive infants is of much greater concern. The management of these infants requires suctioning of the nasopharynx before complete delivery of the infant (while the infant's head is on the mother's perineum) and nasopharyngeal and endotracheal suctioning as soon as the infant is on the radiant warmer. The endotracheal suctioning should occur before drying or stimulation of the infant.

Thick meconium is often difficult to remove with a small-bore catheter; the preferred method of endotracheal suctioning is to apply the suction through the endotracheal tube. This may be accomplished by using a suction adapter. This commercially available adapter allows suction tubing to be joined to an endotracheal tube. Because of the risk of the spread of infection, devices involving orally applied suction are currently not recommended. Repeated intubation and suctioning may be needed if significant amounts of meconium are obtained. This repeated suctioning may be needed even if the infant's heart rate is slow. Once the trachea has been suctioned, a suction catheter should be passed into the stomach to aspirate the stomach contents so as to prevent possible reflux and aspiration of meconium from the gastric contents.

Congenital Diaphragmatic Hernia

Infants with this condition may be very critically ill. If the condition is diagnosed in utero, efforts should be made to deliver the infant to a tertiary center where extracorporeal membrane oxygenation is available. Because bag-and-mask ventilation can cause gastric distention, which in turn may cause lung compression, immediate intubation is essential.

MEDICATIONS

Most neonatal resuscitation can be successfully accomplished without the need for medications. Drugs do have a distinct role and should be considered if an infant has not responded, after approximately 3 to 5 minutes, to adequate ventilation and compressions. The indications, dosages, and routes of administration for drugs commonly used in neonatal resuscitation are listed in Table 5. In general, the author and colleagues use epinephrine as the first-line drug; sodium bicarbonate is reserved for the infant in whom documented acidosis persists despite adequate ventilation. Volume expanders should be used cautiously in asphyxiated premature newborns because of the risk of intracranial hemorrhage. In general, volume expanders should be given over 5 to 30 minutes so as to minimize this risk.

CONDITIONS FOR NONRESUSCITATION

The author and colleagues are frequently confronted with situations in which the outcome of the baby is such that resuscitation may not be indicated. For example, many infants weighing 400 to 600 grams do not survive, and the parents may wish to limit the care to a lower level of

TABLE 5. Medications for Neonatal Resuscitation

Medication	Indication	Dose	Route
Naloxone (Narcan), 0.4 mg/mL	Opiate depression	0.1 mg/kg	IM, IV, ETT
Epinephrine, 1:10,000	Persistent bradycardia	0.1–0.3 mL/kg	IV, ETT
Sodium bicarbonate, 4.2% (0.5 mEq/mL)	Metabolic acidosis	2 mEq/kg	IV
Volume expanders: 5% albumin or Ringer's lactate	Hypovolemia	10 mL/kg	IV slowly
D10W	Hypoglycemia	1–2 mL/kg	IV

Abbreviations: IM = intramuscularly; IV = intravenously; ETT = endotracheal tube.

humane support. These decisions should be made after communication among the parents, the obstetric and pediatric teams, and other involved persons. Nonresuscitation can be considered when an infant is vegetative without hope of recovery or if the resuscitation would be futile because the underlying conditions cannot be corrected and would imminently cause the death of the infant.

CARE OF THE HIGH-RISK NEONATE

method of
HERB KOFFLER, M.D.
University of New Mexico School of Medicine
Albuquerque, New Mexico

Almost four million infants are delivered annually in the United States, and 2 to 4% require some form of special care in the immediate neonatal period.

Approximately 10% of pregnancies are considered to be high risk. If all of the compromised newborns came from this population, it would be simple to anticipate and identify the problems that caretakers of the infant would have to deal with. Unfortunately, not all the 2 to 4% of infants who require special care come from the 10% of high-risk pregnancies. As many as 40% of the problems for which infants are admitted to special care units are not expected or detected before labor and delivery.

EXTRAUTERINE ADAPTATION

After delivery, the infant makes numerous physiologic adjustments that are geared toward survival. A successful transition depends primarily on the transfer of respiratory function from the placenta to the newborn's lungs in concert with changes in the cardiovascular system.

Pulmonary Adaptation. The anatomic and biochemical status of the fetal lungs at birth are the primary determinants of independent survival. Fetal lungs are filled with a fluid that differs chemically from amniotic fluid. During gestation, the pulmonary fluid from the fetal lung contributes to the volume of amniotic fluid. With vaginal delivery, fluid in the airway is squeezed out through the infant's nose and mouth. The thoracic squeeze occurs only minimally with cesarean delivery. Any remaining lung fluid is reabsorbed into the circulation as the infant makes a successful adaptation to the extrauterine environment.

Immediately after delivery, the newborn infant's first inspiratory effort generates a very large transpulmonary pressure, thereby overcoming increased pulmonary tissue resistance, alveolar surface tension, and fluid viscosity within the lung. If mature lung surfactants are present, each succeeding breath requires less distending pressure. In any infant with respiratory distress soon after delivery, awareness of the infant's gestational maturation plays an important part in the differential diagnosis. The more immature the infant, the less likely it is that the surfactant system is functioning adequately. The term infant with respiratory distress should not be considered to have surfactant deficiency disease. Other causes must be considered.

Cardiovascular Adaptation. In the fetus, the organ of respiration is the placenta rather than the lungs. Consequently, distribution of the circulation in the fetus differs from that in the newborn. In the fetus, blood with the highest oxygen content courses from the umbilical vein through the ductus venosus and across the foramen ovale into the left side of the circulation. Blood with a lower oxygen content in the right side of the circulation bypasses the lung through the ductus arteriosus and returns to the placenta through the umbilical arteries.

At birth, clamping the umbilical cord eliminates blood flow through the lower resistance placental circuit. A series of changes must then occur. As the lungs fill with air, pulmonary vascular resistance drops, and pulmonary blood flow increases. Left atrial pressure increases and exceeds right atrial pressure, functionally closing the foramen ovale. In the more mature infant, the ductus arteriosus closes by 48 to 96 hours after delivery. The ductus venosus begins to close with cessation of umbilical venous blood flow.

Role of Other Organ Systems in Adaptation. After birth, survival critically depends on the integration of cardiac and pulmonary functions. However, these adaptations are influenced by other organ systems. Abnormal development of the gastrointestinal system, kidneys, or brain may contribute to faulty neonatal adaptation. During gestation, the fetal gastrointestinal tract and kidneys regulate the volume and composition of amniotic fluid. Renal agenesis or obstruction of the fetal urinary tract results in paucity of amniotic fluid (i.e., oligohydramnios) and its consequences: pulmonary hypoplasia, late intrauterine growth retardation, deformities of the extremities, and abnormal facies (i.e., oligohydramnios tetrad). Pulmonary hypoplasia results in early acute pulmonary failure because hypoplastic lungs do not aerate effectively. Excessive amniotic fluid (i.e., polyhydramnios) results from upper gastrointestinal obstruction, such as esophageal or duodenal atresia; dysfunctional swallowing arising from abnormalities of the central nervous system; fetal heart failure secondary to anemia, myocardial abnormalities, or other abnormalities; multiple fetuses; or congenital chylothorax. Other impairments to the adaptation process may be due to heart failure, aspiration pneumonias, lung compression, anemia, or polycythemia.

Thermoregulation. Immediately after birth, the infant's rectal temperature is the same or slightly higher than that of the mother. Because the infant is wet and the delivery room is cool, the infant's body temperature begins to fall immediately. Cold stress evokes a series of events that can compromise the infant's adaptation significantly. There are no specific guidelines for delivery room temperatures other than what is comfortable for the adults in the room. A delivery room temperature of 24° to 27° C (75° to 80° F) is recommended to reduce cold stress to the infant. After delivery, the infant should be dried with a warm towel and placed in a warm environment. Attention to the thermoregulatory status must be included in the infant's evaluation in the delivery room even in the "heat" of extensive resuscitation procedures. After transfer to the nursery, temperature stability should be maintained because the infant's metabolic rate increases when exposed to wide swings in environmental temperature. The neutral thermal environment, the environmental temperature at which oxygen consumption is minimal, contributes to an efficient adaptive response.

Assessment of Adaptation. The Apgar score is a clinical standard for evaluating the newborn's response to labor and delivery and the fetus's early adaptation to extrauterine life. The more immature the infant, the less applicable the Apgar score. This reflects the immature neuromuscular status of the preterm infant. However, skin color and the two vital signs of heart rate and respiratory rate are valuable indicators.

An attempt to standardize the approach to neonatal resuscitation has been made by the American Academy of Pediatrics and the American Heart Association. Any hospital or facility with a delivery service should require that the neonatal resuscitation program be taken by personnel involved in the delivery service. Additional information is provided in the section on neonatal resuscitation.

Every infant should have a brief examination in the delivery room to ensure that extrauterine adaptation is occurring without compromise and to ascertain that no major anomalies exist. The placenta should be examined to determine whether there are any gross changes or abnormalities. If there is any question about the status of the newborn, the placenta should be appropriately labeled and sent to the pathology laboratory with specific requests regarding the examiner's concerns, or stored until the infant is discharged.

While in the delivery room, the physician or midwife delivering the infant must decide about whether the infant will go to the normal nursery, transition nursery, or intensive care unit. Even the infants admitted to the routine nursery must be observed closely until their adaptation to the extrauterine environment has been successful. The medical and nursing staff should keep in mind that the newborn continues to make physiologic adjustments during the first postnatal day. The period of initial transition is well defined (Figure 1). After it has been determined that the infant may not go to the routine care nursery, the care plan should include the infant and the infant's family.

So that they are not lost in the confusion of the delivery room, prophylactic procedures, such as the administration of vitamin K and eye care, should not be done in the delivery room. This should be part of the standing orders on admission to the special care nursery.

ASSESSMENT OF PATIENT

History

The first comprehensive medical evaluation of the newborn should be performed as soon after birth as possible. The examination begins with a thorough review of the history of the pregnancy, labor, delivery, and the medical histories of the parents and their families. This information usually is included in the obstetric record, a copy of which should be sent routinely to the nursery. When complete, the record should contain the following information:

1. Ages of the mother and father.
2. Marital status.

3. Mother's obstetric history, including number of previous pregnancies, birthweights and gestational ages of the previous pregnancies, and their outcome.
4. The last normal menstrual period and expected date of delivery.
5. Prenatal care during the current pregnancy.
6. Prepregnant weight and weight gain during the current pregnancy.
7. Medications (prescription and nonprescription).
8. Exposure to infectious diseases.
9. Habits (drugs, alcohol, smoking).
10. Family and genetic diseases.
11. Maternal systemic diseases.
12. Maternal blood type and serologic tests.
13. Mode of feeding preferred (breast or formula).
14. Circumcision (yes or no).

If any of this information is missing or incomplete, it is necessary to question the obstetrician or interview the parents. The medical history of the newborn infant is complex because it encompasses genetics, embryology, obstetrics, and the developmental physiology of the fetus and newborn. It is imperative for the examiner to have open communication with his or her obstetric colleague about anticipated problems.

Maturational Assessment

As part of the initial physical examination, gestational maturation should also be evaluated. In the nursery, the author uses the New Ballard Score (Figure 2) for maturational assessment. The appearance of the anterior vascular capsule of the lens is evaluated by direct ophthalmoscopic examination. Maturation can be roughly assessed by the infant's weight: 1000 grams, 28 weeks' gestation; 1500 grams, 32 weeks' gestation; 2500 grams, 36 weeks' gestation; 3500 grams, 40 weeks' gestation. By convention, gestational age is expressed as completed weeks from the last menstrual period. A term gestation is 38 to 42 completed weeks. A post-term infant is older than 42 weeks. A preterm infant is younger than 38 weeks. The assessment of gestational maturation is an integral part of the examination and evaluation of each newborn.

Gestational age is a nomenclature based on time. When the last normal menstrual period dating is unknown and early ultrasound assessment of the gestation has not been obtained, the determination of gestational age must be estimated. The timetable of growth and maturation varies for each fetus and is based on factors such as nutrition, heredity, metabolism, and acute and

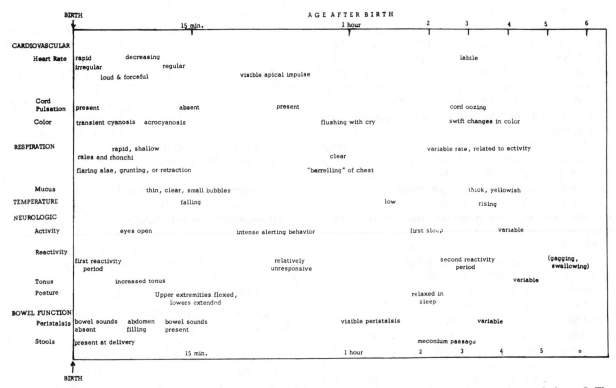

Figure 1. Newborn adaptations following birth. (From Desmond MM, et al: The clinical behavior of the newly born. I. The term baby. J Pediatr *63*:307, 1963.)

chronic stress. For example, chronic intrauterine stress secondary to chronic hypertensive disease of the mother may result in rapid fetal maturation. An infant whose mother had non–insulin-dependent diabetes mellitus sometimes has slow fetal maturation but a high birth weight.

Preterm Infant. By definition, an infant who is delivered before 37 completed weeks' gestation is preterm. The word "premature" implies biologic behavior rather than weeks of gestation and is incorrect nomenclature for describing an infant's gestational age. The key to the initial care of a sick preterm infant is anticipation and preparedness. The obstetric history and clinical scoring techniques for evaluating an infant's gestation and maturational age should be applied. With experience, it becomes apparent that all low-birthweight infants (2500 grams or less) are not necessarily preterm and that not all term infants necessarily weigh more than 2500 grams.

The cause of the preterm delivery may be secondary to maternal diseases (e.g., preeclampsia or infection), placental problems (e.g., rupture of the fetal membrane or retroplacental hemorrhage), fetal abnormalities, inaccurate obstetric determination of gestational age, or undetermined factors. In each case, a specific cause for the preterm delivery should be sought because it

clarifies the treatment plans for the newborn. It is essential to identify conditions that predispose the infant to sepsis.

The behavior of the near-term infant is frustrating for the hospital staff because they expect the infant to feed and behave like a term infant. It is a challenge to identify preterm infants in the range of 35 to 37 weeks' gestation who are not distressed and appear mature. The telltale signs of their biologic maturity are their sluggish feeding behavior, other behavioral aberrations, and their need for thermal support. The parents often sense this frustration and, with their own frustration, become apprehensive. The hospital staff can help the parents by explaining the peculiarities of the near-term infant. The parents should be supported and reassured that their infant's behavior is normal.

Post-Term Infant. Approximately 10% of all pregnancies are post-term (i.e., exceeding 294 days or 42 weeks' gestation). Although the words "post-mature" and "post-term" are frequently used interchangeably, "post-term" is more precise because it is defined by age. "Dysmature" is another term used to describe the post-term infant, but this nomenclature also may be applied to the preterm or term infant who is scrawny and small for gestational age and whose skin is desquamat-

Neuromuscular Maturity

	-1	0	1	2	3	4	5
Posture							
Square Window (wrist)	>90°	90°	60°	45°	30°	0°	
Arm Recoil		180°	140°-180°	110°-140°	90°-110°	<90°	
Popliteal Angle	180°	160°	140°	120°	100°	90°	<90°
Scarf Sign							
Heel to Ear							

Physical Maturity

	sticky friable transparent	gelatinous red, translucent	smooth pink, visible veins	superficial peeling &/or rash. few veins	cracking pale areas rare veins	parchment deep cracking no vessels	leathery cracked wrinkled
Skin							
Lanugo	none	sparse	abundant	thinning	bald areas	mostly bald	
Plantar Surface	heel-toe 40-50mm:-1 <40mm:-2	>50mm no crease	faint red marks	anterior transverse crease only	creases ant. 2/3	creases over entire sole	
Breast	imperceptible	barely perceptible	flat areola no bud	stippled areola 1-2mm bud	raised areola 3-4mm bud	full areola 5-10mm bud	
Eye/Ear	lids fused loosely:-1 tightly:-2	lids open pinna flat stays folded	sl. curved pinna; soft; slow recoil	well-curved pinna; soft but ready recoil	formed &firm instant recoil	thick cartilage ear stiff	
Genitals male	scrotum flat, smooth	scrotum empty faint rugae	testes in upper canal rare rugae	testes descending few rugae	testes down good rugae	testes pendulous deep rugae	
Genitals female	clitoris prominent labia flat	prominent clitoris small labia minora	prominent clitoris enlarging minora	majora & minora equally prominent	majora large minora small	majora cover clitoris & minora	

Maturity Rating

score	weeks
-10	20
-5	22
0	24
5	26
10	28
15	30
20	32
25	34
30	36
35	38
40	40
45	42
50	44

Figure 2. Expanded New Ballard Score (NBS) includes extremely premature infants and has been refined to improve accuracy in more mature infants. (From Ballard JL, et al: New Ballard Score, expanded to include extremely premature infants. *J Pediatr* *119*(3):417–423, 1991.)

ing and has poor turgor. The cause of post-term delivery is poorly defined. Delivery may be thought to be late because of miscalculated dates; otherwise, post-term deliveries may be associated with conditions that include anencephaly, sulfatase deficiency, and poor initiation of labor, especially in an older mother. The post-term infant usually appears very alert. Approximately two of three are overgrown. Thirty percent have evidence of significant placental insufficiency, and morbidity is subsequently increased, manifested by intrauterine growth retardation, hypoglycemia, asphyxia, meconium aspiration, and the polycythemia hyperviscosity syndrome.

The delivered infant can be classified into nine categories. The infant is small, appropriate-sized, or large for gestational age and is preterm, term, or post-term. Each of these classifications has its own associated rate of morbidity (Figure 3).

Physical Examination

A careful physical examination should be performed. The infant's color, breathing pattern, morphology, level of activity, and responsiveness should be recorded.

Head. The shape and contour of the head at birth are influenced by the mode of delivery. The ossification of the cranial bones may vary. Laceration, bruises, puncture marks, and petechial hemorrhages should be identified during inspection of the head. Soft-tissue swellings or bony prominences produce asymmetrical contours. A caput succedaneum can be differentiated from a cephal-

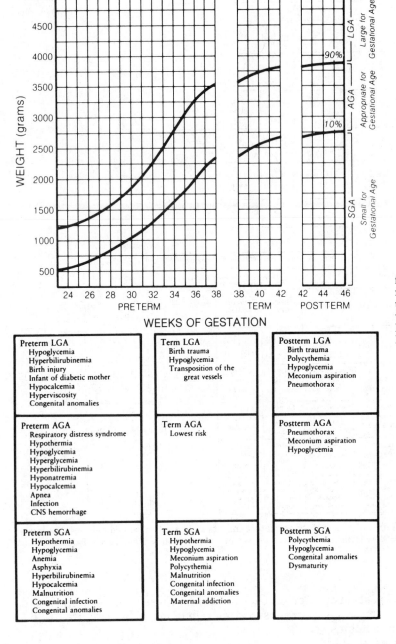

Figure 3. Neonatal morbidity risk. (Adapted from Lubchenco LO, et al: Neonatal mortality rate: Relationship to birth weight and gestational age. J Pediatr *81:*818, 1972; reprinted with permission from Coen RW, and Koffler H: Primary Care of the Newborn. Boston, Little, Brown and Company, 1987, p. 60.)

Preterm LGA
Hypoglycemia
Hyperbilirubinemia
Birth injury
Infant of diabetic mother
Hypocalcemia
Hyperviscosity
Congenital anomalies

Term LGA
Birth trauma
Hypoglycemia
Transposition of the
   great vessels

Postterm LGA
Birth trauma
Polycythemia
Hypoglycemia
Meconium aspiration
Pneumothorax

Preterm AGA
Respiratory distress syndrome
Hypothermia
Hypoglycemia
Hyperglycemia
Hyperbilirubinemia
Hyponatremia
Hypocalcemia
Apnea
Infection
CNS hemorrhage

Term AGA
Lowest risk

Postterm AGA
Pneumothorax
Meconium aspiration
Hypoglycemia

Preterm SGA
Hypothermia
Hypoglycemia
Anemia
Asphyxia
Hyperbilirubinemia
Hypocalcemia
Malnutrition
Congenital infection
Congenital anomalies

Term SGA
Hypothermia
Hypoglycemia
Meconium aspiration
Polycythemia
Malnutrition
Congenital infection
Congenital anomalies
Maternal addiction

Postterm SGA
Polycythemia
Hypoglycemia
Congenital anomalies
Dysmaturity

hematoma by palpation. The network of cranial sutures and fontanelles should also be identified. The major sutures include the sagittal, coronal, lambdoidal, and frontal. Widened sutures should raise the suspicion of intracranial pathology.

Eyes. It is often quite difficult to examine the eyes in the acutely ill newborn. However, an attempt to obtain a red reflex should never be omitted. Cataracts, for instance, may identify the presence of an infectious or metabolic process.

Ears. The attachment of the helix of the ear to the scalp at a point horizontal to the lateral angle of the eye is the landmark that determines whether the ears are "low set."

Nose. The nasal passages normally are symmetrical. Flaring of the nasal alae occurs when the infant is having respiratory distress. Bilateral choanal atresia is diagnosed in the delivery room because it causes acute respiratory distress. Unilateral choanal atresia should be suspected in any newborn who has respiratory difficulties not explained by other etiologies. Nasal obstruction is excluded by passing a No. 8 French catheter through the external nares along the floor of the nose into the nasopharynx.

Mouth. The lips and mouth are observed for symmetry at rest and during movement. If the infant is to be intubated, the palate should be inspected. Inspection of the buccal mucosa, palate, and posterior pharynx should be performed before inserting the endotracheal tube if possible.

Neck. The neck is inspected for symmetry, sinuses, and clefts and to identify that the trachea is in the midline. The thyroid gland usually is not felt unless very enlarged, regardless of the gestation. No other masses should be present.

Chest. The chest is inspected for obvious deformities, particularly in the area of the nipples, clavicles, and sternum. Auscultation of the lungs shortly after birth often discloses adventitious sounds, such as rales or rhonchi. These may be produced by pulmonary fluid that has not been absorbed completely. In addition, noises made by secretions in the upper airway, especially the nose, are transmitted to the lung fields. The normal respiratory rate ranges from 30 to 60 breaths per minute. Because the neonatal respiratory cycle normally is variable, counting respirations for 15 seconds rather than a full minute may yield a falsely low or high result. While listening to the lung fields, the examiner should carefully auscultate the heart. The normal heart rate is from 120 to 160 beats per minute but may range between 80 and 180 beats per minute. The rhythm may vary with the phase of respiration, increasing during inspiration and decreasing during expiration. The second heart sound splits during inspiration and closes with expiration. This splitting of the second sound is the best evidence of normal pulmonary circulation. If the physical examination does not reveal that the heart is in the left thoracic cavity, the examiner must determine whether the infant's situs is totally abnormal or the heart has been displaced for other reasons. Both anteroposterior and lateral radiographs are required.

Abdomen. The configuration of the abdomen is inspected to determine whether it is symmetrical, distended, or sunken (i.e., scaphoid). Then the umbilical cord is examined to determine that two arteries and one vein show through the cut end. Normal kidneys are not readily palpable. However, if the kidneys are easily palpable, they may be enlarged. The liver edge may be felt approximately 2 to 3 cm below the right costal margin in the midclavicular line. If more readily palpable, the examiner should suspect that it is being pushed down from something above the diaphragm, pushed out from an intra-abdominal mass behind the liver, or enlarged for some other reason. Only rarely is the normal spleen palpable. Enlargement of the spleen and liver indicate a hemolytic process or an infectious process. Femoral pulses are palpable in the femoral triangle. Within the first 24 hours, in the presence of patent ductus arteriosus, femoral pulses may be palpable even in the presence of coarctation of the aorta.

Genitalia. Examination of the genitalia requires only inspection and palpation. In female newborns, if the abdomen is distended, it should be determined whether the vaginal orifice is patent in order to rule out hydrometrocolpos. Any evidence of inguinal masses must be considered gonads until proved otherwise. Inspection of the male genitalia reveals that the more mature the infant, the more likely it is that the testicles are down in the scrotum. If neither testis is palpable, the infant should not be assigned a male gender until bilateral cryptorchidism is proved.

Anus. The anus should be inspected to determine its patency, its position on the perineum, and the relationship of the sphincter to the anal orifice. A digital examination is rarely indicated. Noninvasive techniques may provide as much information with much less trauma.

Skeleton. As the fetus matures, flexor tone overcomes extensor tone. The passive range of motion of all extremities and the hips should be checked. While the number of digits is counted, the ridge patterns on the fingers and hands should also be examined. There may be clues to the diagnosis of chromosomal disorders and syndromes. Intrauterine positioning may deform the lower extremities. These deformities should not be confused with congenital malformations. In extremely sick preterm infants, the hip examination is often passed over. It should be done before the umbilical catheter is placed so that the catheter does not get dislodged during the examination. Examination of the back in critically ill infants is also often overlooked. Because of the possibility of midline neurologic abnormalities, it should not be omitted.

Neurologic System. The most important aspect of examining the neurologic system is careful observation. The state of alertness appears to be the most sensitive of all indicators of neurologic function. Changes in the state of alertness depend on gestational maturity, chronologic age, feeding schedules, and environmental stimuli. The neurologic examination is influenced significantly by changes in the behavioral state. Newborns display six behavioral states: two sleep states and four waking states. Basic motor functions involve tone, posture, and reflex activity. Deep tendon reflexes are spinal reflexes that involve peripheral, sensory, motor, and proprioceptive nerve fibers. Unsustained clonus may be a normal response when the Achilles tendon is tapped or when the ankle is flexed rapidly.

Laboratory Assessment

Routine laboratory evaluations in the author's special care nursery include a hematocrit, a glucose determination, a serologic test for syphilis, blood typing, and Coombs' test.

Hematocrit. A hematocrit for the distressed infant helps determine whether the complications of polycythemia or anemia are present. If the hematocrit levels determined from a capillary specimen are greater or less than the normal limits, the hematocrit should be performed again on blood from a venipuncture specimen. A central venous hematocrit value less than 40% indicates moderate to severe anemia that often is secondary to hemolysis or acute or chronic blood loss. A central hematocrit of greater than 65% indicates polycythemia and potential hyperviscosity.

Glucose. The serum glucose concentration in the fetus approximates that of the mother. After the umbilical cord is clamped, there is a rapid fall in the infant's serum glucose concentrations to a mean value of 50 mg per dL during the first few hours. Subsequently, the blood glucose concentration rises and equilibrates. Hypoglycemia is defined as a whole blood glucose concentration of less than 30 mg per dL during the first 72 hours in the full-birthweight baby. It is 10 mg per dL lower in the low-birthweight infant. The blood glucose concentration is assessed for every infant at the time of admission to exclude hypoglycemia. An approximation of the blood glucose concentration can be obtained rapidly by using reagent strips for glucose testing on whole blood if the test instructions are followed precisely. The chemicals in these strips are sensitive to oxidation, and the container should be kept tightly closed. If the color reaction indicates a low blood glucose value, a blood sample should be drawn and sent to the chemistry laboratory for confirmation and documentation of the hypoglycemia. Therapy should begin immediately while these results are awaited.

Fluid and Electrolytes

Fluids. In the author's nursery, treatment of infants less than 1000 grams at birth is begun with 100 to 120 mL of fluid per kg per day. The dextrose concentration of that fluid is typically 5% glucose. Infants weighing between 1000 and 1500 grams begin with 80 to 100 mL of fluid per kg per day, and larger infants begin with 60 to 80 mL of fluid per kg per day (Table 1). An infant who requires intubation, umbilical catheterization, and placement of a peripheral intravenous line should be weighed before and after the procedures are accomplished. The infant should lose 1 to 2% of body weight per day for the first 3 to 4 days. Weight is the most accurate indicator of an infant's fluid status in the absence of third spacing. It should be measured every 12 hours or more often when the status is changing rapidly. The intravenous fluid rate should be advanced by approximately 20 to 30 mL of fluid per kg per day as long as the infant is following the expected weight curves, including the initial loss.

Factors that increase fluid needs are extreme immaturity (due to increased evaporation and the inability to concentrate urine), use of a radiant warmer, phototherapy, third spacing, tachypnea, hyperthermia, increased convective losses, and excessive nasogastric chest tube or stool output. Factors that decrease fluid needs include use of a plastic shield or blanket, use of a humidified isolette, use of a humidified ventilator, and renal insufficiency. The last occurs with acute tubular necrosis and indomethacin therapy. Acceptable urinary output is 1 to 4 mL of urine per kg per hour. Urine-specific gravity is not as helpful as it is in older children. Immaturity of the kidneys impairs their concentrating ability. Signs of fluid overload include hyponatremia, excessive weight gain (particularly in association with inadequate caloric intake), high-volume dilute urine, puffiness, rales, hepatomegaly, and a "wet" chest radiograph. Signs of dehydration include hypernatremia, excessive weight loss, decreased urine output and tachycardia, poor perfusion, and hypotension. The latter three signs are late signs of significant dehydration. Initial treatment of infants begins with 10% glucose water without any electrolytes if they require intravenous access soon after delivery. Treatment of infants weighing less than 1000 grams begins with 5% glucose.

Electrolytes. Because an infant's electrolyte status reflects the mother's, it is unnecessary to measure the infant's serum electrolytes on admission unless there is a predisposing factor causing the mother to have electrolyte imbalance. After the infant is voiding, it is safe to consider adding potassium to the intravenous fluid. Otherwise, the infant is at risk for hyperkalemia. The dose of maintenance potassium is 2 mEq per kg per day. This is not done on a per volume of intravenous fluid basis.

Maintenance sodium is also begun at the same time at 3 mEq per kg per day. Very-low-birthweight infants (<1500 grams) may need more sodium as a result of increased renal losses. In the authors' nursery, an infant with a serum sodium level of less than 130 mEq per liter is considered hyponatremic. The etiology includes iatrogenic causes, syndrome of inappropriate antidiuretic hormone, renal failure, congestive heart failure, and pseudohypoaldosteronism (associated with normal to high serum potassium levels). Hypernatremia is defined as a serum sodium level of greater than 150 mEq per liter. Causes include dehydration, renal disease, and iatrogenic factors.

TABLE 1. **Guidelines for Starting Fluids**

Infant Size	Day 1	Day 2	After Day 2*
<1000 gm	100–120 mL/kg/day	140–160 mL/kg/day	140–200 mL/kg/day
1000–1500 gm	80–100 mL/kg/day	110–130 mL/kg/day	110–180 mL/kg day
1500–2500 gm	60–80 mL/kg/day	90–110 mL/kg/day	90–160 mL/kg/day

*Advance fluids by 20 to 30 mL per kg per day until up to full fluids *as long as baby is following expected weight curve* with initial loss.

In each instance, the object of therapy is to treat the underlying cause. Because the patient may be exposed to many screening procedures, it is important to get as much information on the least amount of blood in the fewest number of specimens that can be obtained throughout the infant's hospitalization. For instance, the manager of the chemistry laboratory can relate the volumes and types of tests that can be obtained with their automated systems. More value for the patient's dollar can be obtained by being aware of the capabilities of the chemistry laboratory. The author measures sodium and potassium concentrations at least every 12 hours until they are stable. They are then checked on a daily basis until the infant's condition is extremely stable or feedings have been established. When introducing diuretic therapy or pharmacologically treating a patent ductus arteriosus, serum electrolytes must be closely monitored.

Calcium. Hypocalcemia is a common problem in preterm infants, asphyxiated infants, and infants of diabetic mothers. If ionized serum calcium cannot be measured, a total serum calcium measurement is quite acceptable. A total serum calcium of less than 7 mg per dL is considered consistent with hypocalcemia. The serum calcium level usually reaches its lowest point during the second postnatal day. If calcium is to be added to intravenous fluids, it can be given as a slow intravenous push of 100 to 200 mg per kg of calcium gluconate or as part of the daily intravenous infusion. If calcium is given over a short period of time, the heart rate should be closely monitored in case bradycardia is a complication. If an infant is being treated with sodium bicarbonate, calcium should not be mixed in the same line.

Nutrition

If it appears that the infant's condition cannot permit enteral therapy within the first few days, beginning the infant on parenteral nutrition should be considered. This includes a protein and carbohydrate solution and a fat emulsion. At least 50 calories per kg per day is necessary for protein sparing. The author begins with 90 to 100 kcal per kg per day and with protein concentrations of about 1 to 2 grams per kg per day. Any

glucose concentration greater than 12.5 mg per dL requires central access. The author begins intravenous fat infusion at a concentration of 0.5 to 1 gram per kg per day. The goal is to increase the protein concentration to 3 grams per kg per day and the fat concentration to approximately 3 grams per kg per day.

Small feedings are begun at very slow rates, even in the most immature infant. Infants with low Apgar scores and potential compromise of gut perfusion around the time of delivery are not fed aggressively. In that situation, the author usually waits 3 to 5 days before beginning enteral feedings. The eventual goal is to obtain an intake that will achieve 120 calories per kg per day. For infants less than 38 weeks' gestation, the preterm proprietary formulas are used. The preterm formulas are continued until the infant reaches term or is discharged or special needs have been resolved. The advantage of the proprietary preterm formulas is that 40 to 50% of the total fat is in the form of medium-chain triglycerides. They also have a ratio of whey to casein of 60:40, which is similar to that in human milk. The carbohydrate in these formulas is designed to respond to the limited intestinal lactase in the preterm infant. The osmotic load is only 300 mOsm per liter even in the formulas with 24 calories per ounce. The formulas are fortified with extra vitamins and minerals to meet most of the infant's recommended requirements.

The author begins feedings after the infant's condition is stable or improving on assisted ventilation or in infants without lung disease who have successfully made the transition to extrauterine life. The first feeding is sterile water to ensure patency of the upper gastrointestinal tract. Glucose water is not an acceptable alternative; aspiration of glucose water can cause pneumonitis similar to formula aspiration. For the most part, the author does not dilute the caloric density of the formula that we use. For infants weighing less than 1200 grams, continuous feedings are begun at 0.5 to 1 mL per hour. An infant weighing more than 1200 grams is started at 5 mL per kg per hour, or about one-third of the total fluid rate that is calculated to provide sufficient fluids for the infant. The author sometimes uses bolus feedings in infants weighing less than 1200 grams who do not tolerate continuous feedings, and nipple feeding is not tried until about 32 to 34 weeks' gestation, when suck and swallow coordination becomes mature. After reaching full volume feedings, the infant may be switched to a formula with 22 or 24 calories per ounce. Breast milk fortifiers are given to the stable preterm infant who may need caloric enhancement.

Acid-Base Status

In addition to monitoring the infant's laboratory values, the author monitors the cardiorespiratory status, acid-base balance, and adequacy of oxygenation and ventilation. If an infant is identified as being acidotic, it must be determined whether acidosis is respiratory, metabolic, or mixed. Because inadequate ventilation is one of the most common causes for admission to a special care nursery, assisted ventilation should be considered while the cause is being determined. An infant with an arterial pH that is falling and a carbon dioxide tension of greater than 50 mmHg should be intubated and treated with assisted ventilation. If an appropriate support system to maintain assisted ventilation is not in place, the infant should be transferred. If the acidosis is of metabolic origin, the anion gap may suggest the underlying condition. In the acute situation soon after delivery, the most common causes are associated with impaired oxygen delivery (hypoxia), sepsis, hypothermia, congenital heart disease, hypovolemia, or inborn errors of metabolism that can be differentiated by whether the serum ammonia concentration is elevated or normal. In the case of a metabolic acidosis, sodium bicarbonate therapy and increased fluid rates are indicated. If the infant has a pure respiratory acidosis, therapy with bicarbonate is not indicated and may be contraindicated. The objective of therapy for respiratory acidosis is to establish adequate ventilation and oxygenation and effective carbon dioxide elimination. Because infants weighing less than 1500 grams may waste bicarbonate in their urine and tend to have a mild metabolic acidosis, the author often substitutes sodium acetate for sodium chloride in their parenteral nutrition. The acetate is converted to bicarbonate in the liver and acts as an appropriate substitute without causing precipitation in the tubing.

SPECIAL PROBLEMS

Respiratory Distress

Common pulmonary causes of respiratory distress include transient tachypnea, meconium aspiration, pneumonia, pneumothorax, and primary pulmonary hypertension in the full-term infant. In addition to these causes, surfactant deficiency disease must be considered in the preterm infant. Extrapulmonary causes include hypothermia, cyanotic congenital heart disease, anemia, shock, hyperviscosity syndrome, and central nervous system abnormalities. Therapy must be linked to correcting the underlying cause of the problem. For the preterm infant with surfactant deficiency disease, surfactant preparations are now available. This therapy is not without complications and should not be undertaken unless personnel and support systems are immediately and consistently available.

Heart Disease and Cyanosis

Faced with a cyanotic infant, the differential diagnosis is not limited to the heart or the lungs. A central nervous system or hematologic cause should also be considered. The infant may have congenital methemoglobinemia. A much more common abnormality is polycythemia and resultant hyperviscosity. Central nervous system causes of cyanosis include intracranial hemorrhage, perinatal asphyxia, neonatal seizures, and respiratory depression secondary to maternal medications that cross the placenta. The differential diagnosis of cyanotic congenital heart disease includes five lesions that begin with the letter T: transposition of the great vessels, tetralogy of Fallot, truncus arteriosus, tricuspid atresia, and total anomalous pulmonary venous return (TAPVR). Hypoplastic left heart syndrome is the other major diagnosis to consider. Because a palliative procedure can be carried out for an infant with transposition of the great vessels, it is important that these infants be diagnosed as soon after birth as possible.

Infants who are grunting and whose nares are flaring and retracting with or without cyanosis in the immediate neonatal period may be cold stressed, may be polycythemic, or may have pneumothorax. All three conditions are readily treatable in most nurseries and do not necessitate transfer or admission to a special care nursery. An infant admitted directly from the delivery room and found to have a metabolic acidosis frequently responds to a bolus of 10 to 20 mL per kg of volume expander. If cardiac output is adequate and renal perfusion is sufficient, the acidosis may clear spontaneously and the infant may not require any bicarbonate therapy. When reviewing the chest radiograph to determine whether the infant has cyanotic or pulmonary disease, the examiner must pay specific attention to thoracic and abdominal situs, cardiac size, cardiac configuration, pulmonary vascularity, and aortic arch position. If there are markedly increased pulmonary vascular markings, the examiner must consider transposition of the great vessels, TAPVR, truncus arteriosus, or hypoplastic left heart syndrome. If the pulmonary markings are significantly reduced, the examiner must think of reasons for pulmonary ischemia such as tetralogy of Fallot, pulmonary stenosis, pulmonary atresia, Ebstein's disease, tricuspid atresia, or double-outlet right ventricle. A right aortic arch is seen in less than 0.5% of the normal population.

Patent Ductus Arteriosus

Every infant has a patent ductus arteriosus (PDA) in utero. However, in the infant weighing less than 1750 grams, it may become hemodynamically significant after delivery. About 20% of infants weighing less than 1750 grams may have a clinically significant PDA. This incidence is more than double among infants with extremely low birthweights (<1000 grams). The author has identified PDA as being a significant problem in many infants treated with surfactant. Treatment should not be undertaken without confirming the diagnosis. This should be done noninvasively with echocardiographic technique. After the diagnosis has been confirmed, the examiner must be sure that the fluid infusion rate has not been excessive. The author has been able to pharmacologically close most of the PDAs with intravenous indomethacin (Indocin) therapy. Supportive care and monitoring are an integral part of this therapy.

Blood Pressure

Hypotension is a common problem precipitating admission to special care nurseries. While the underlying cause is sought, volume therapy should be initiated. This can be done with a 5% albumin or plasmanate solution or even with whole blood. If there are reasons why the infant cannot be given large amounts of intravenous fluids, inotropic therapy should be considered. Hypertension is not a common diagnosis in the special care nursery, and if it occurs after the initial few days, it is often secondary to complications of umbilical artery catheters.

Seizures

Seizures are the most frequent manifestation of central nervous system dysfunction in the newborn. The underlying problem may be a primary central nervous system disorder or acute brain injury. Reported incidence of seizures is 1 to 14 per 1000 live births; 50% occur within the first 24 hours after delivery and 85% occur within the first 2 weeks.

As care of sick newborns has become increasingly sophisticated, the relative importance of various causes of central nervous system dysfunction in newborns has continued to evolve. The concept of what constitutes a clinical seizure has gradually changed. The author accepts that varied, poorly organized, and often subtle episodic and stereotypic motor activities and behaviors represent seizures, presumably epileptic in nature. Subtle seizures or motor automatisms consistently associated with hypoxic-ischemic insults are not associated with abnormal electroencephalographic (EEG) patterns. Because they probably represent brain stem release phenomena, controversy exists regarding the use of antiepileptic therapy. That is why it is preferable to obtain an EEG before considering therapy. After treatable causes of neonatal seizures, such as hypocalcemia, hypomagnesemia, hypoglycemia, and infection, have been excluded, specific anticonvulsant therapy may be initiated. Phenobarbital (Luminal) is the initial drug used for the treatment of neonatal seizures. The loading dose is 20 mg per kg intravenously. If seizure activity continues, an additional 5 mg per kg can be given every 5 minutes for four more doses. Maintenance therapy is 3 to 4 mg per kg in two divided doses or once daily. Serum levels should be followed. Most seizures are controlled with the blood level of 20 to 40 µg per mL.

Hypoxic-Ischemic Encephalopathy

The clinical and neuropathologic findings that occur in the full-term infant after a significant episode of intrapartum or neonatal asphyxia represent the most important perinatal cause of neurologic morbidity in full-term infants. The frequency of hypoxic-ischemic encephalopathy (HIE) is approximately 4%, and this rate has remained fairly constant over the past decade. To confirm this diagnosis, there must be a history of perinatal distress and the infant must have an abnormal neurologic examination result shortly after birth. In the past, the clinical management of infants with HIE focused on the treatment of central nervous system dysfunction. It is now recognized that such infants may have variable injury or global injury to multiple organ systems, particularly pulmonary, cardiovascular, renal, and metabolic systems. Most neonatal deaths can be attributed to complications arising from the severe compromise of organ systems other than the central nervous system.

The goal of therapy is to mitigate further brain and other system injury. The usual pattern of clinical seizure activity begins within 12 to 24 hours after delivery. These seizures are poorly responsive to anticonvulsant therapy, and the seizures stop spontaneously 5 to 7 days after they begin. This may be because the seizures have a subcortical origin, representing a lack of cortical inhibition rather than excessive cortical activity. However, until more data are available, anticonvulsive treatment of clinical seizures is recommended.

Periventricular-Intraventricular Hemorrhage

A condition of the preterm infant, the incidence of periventricular-intraventricular hemorrhage (PIVH) in infants weighing less than 1500 grams is approximately 30 to 35%. Most hemorrhages occur within a few days after delivery, and virtually all occur within the first week. An inverse relationship exists between gestational age and PIVH; the most immature infants have the highest risk. The reported mortality figures range from 27 to 50%. However, only 50% of preterm infants with severe hemorrhage are expected to die because of their hemorrhage. The most accurate and reliable method for detecting this abnormality is noninvasive cranial imaging. The clinical signs associated with PIVH are not very specific. PIVH may be identified in preterm infants who have no demonstrable neurologic lesions whatsoever, and approximately 50% of preterm infants in whom PIVH is detected do not have clinical signs or symptoms of hemorrhage.

INFECTIOUS DISEASES

The incidence of neonatal sepsis is about 1%. It increases to more than 30% if certain predisposing factors are present. Maternal factors include premature rupture of the membranes, prolonged rupture of the membranes, maternal infection (e.g., amnionitis, urinary tract infection), vaginal or cervical bacterial colonization, or complications during labor and delivery. Neonatal factors include prematurity, male gender, an underlying disease process, instrumentation, difficult resuscitation at birth, and physical anomalies. The clinical signs that lead to the consideration of the diagnosis are nonspecific. They include temperature instability, lethargy, poor tone, feeding intolerance, poor perfusion, mottling or pallor, apnea, respiratory distress, and jaundice. A total leukocyte count of less than 5000 or greater than 30,000 is beyond the normal range. Platelet counts of less than 100,000 often accompany infection. If an infant has an absolute neutrophil count of less than 1500, the diagnosis of neonatal sepsis must be entertained and antibacterial therapy must be instituted. Infections are ac-

quired in utero by the transplacental route or through a tear in the fetal membranes. Hematogenous spread through the placenta is unusual but does occur in viral infections, tuberculosis, syphilis, and listeriosis. A direct relationship exists between the rupture of membranes and contamination of the amniotic fluid. Bacteria have been recovered from the fetal environment in more than 80% of cases in which the membranes were ruptured longer than 24 hours. When membrane rupture is accompanied by labor, the percentage of cases with bacterial isolates increases to 90%.

The infant may acquire an infectious organism during passage through the birth canal. The most virulent of these include group B streptococci, herpes simplex virus, pathogenic *E. coli, Neisseria gonorrhoeae, Chlamydia trachomatis,* and *Listeria monocytogenes.* The spectrum of organisms that cause infections postnatally is remarkably wide and includes agents that usually are not pathogenic in older patients.

After colonization in the newborn, an organism may gain entry through the umbilicus, punctures and abrasions in the skin, or mucous membranes. After it gains access to the bloodstream, it spreads to remote, secondary foci and to organs, tissues, and fluids.

Although the newborn's leukocytes respond to the organisms by chemotaxis, phagocytosis, and bactericidal activities, their overall function is impaired by maturational factors and by the infection itself. In addition to the cellular response, the normal infant activates complement and immunoglobulins in response to infection. The more immature the infant, the less likely the infant can generate a response. The diagnosis of overwhelming sepsis is not difficult, but recognition of sepsis in its earliest stages requires knowledge, skill, and experience.

Bacterial cultures should be obtained for all patients before antibiotic therapy is instituted. Evaluation of the infant's urinary tract is not immediately necessary unless there is evidence of a developmental abnormality. Suprapubic aspiration, the method of choice for obtaining a specimen, probably is unnecessary when infants are investigated for sepsis immediately after birth because the yield of positive cultures is extremely low. Other sites to be cultured are the skin, nasopharynx, stool, and drainage from any lesion. Lumbar puncture should be performed in infants whose mothers were febrile during labor and delivery and in any infant who is foul smelling at birth and displays central nervous signs or symptoms. In some cases in which some fetal membranes are ruptured for about 24 hours and the mother and infant pair are asymptomatic, a lumbar puncture may be deferred, although deferment carries risk. In these cases, a peripheral total and differential leukocyte count, platelet count, blood culture, and prudent observation of the infant are mandatory. Early discharge is contraindicated in this situation. Appropriate radiographs should be obtained. Blood gases may document a metabolic acidosis, an early sign of sepsis.

Antibiotic therapy should be started immediately after specimens are obtained for culture. A penicillin derivative to cover the gram-positive spectrum and an aminoglycocide derivative to cover the gram-negative spectrum are usually instituted and continued until the culture results and antimicrobial sensitivity are known (Table 2). The duration of treatment is predicated on the diagnostic findings, culture results, and the infant's response to therapy. If an infant is highly suspected of being infected and improves with therapy, but the cultures prove to be negative, antibiotics should be continued for approximately 1 week. If an infection is suspected, but the infant is well and stable, the antibiotic may be discontinued after 3 to 5 days if the cultures are negative. With proven pneumonia, omphalitis, gastrointestinal infection, and septicemia, antibiotics should be continued for 7 to 14 days. Serious, deep-seated infections such as meningitis or osteomyelitis are treated with antibiotics intravenously for an extended period. Bacterial spread from infant to infant in the nursery is rare, but when it occurs, it is usually secondary to poor hand-washing techniques of the staff.

Infants whose mothers have received antenatal antibiotics present a problem. The term asymptomatic infant may be merely observed. The term or preterm symptomatic infant should get a full course of antibiotics whether the cultures are positive or not. The preterm asymptomatic infant needs at least a few days of antibiotic therapy and observation.

HEMATOLOGIC SYSTEM

An infant born with a hematocrit of less than 40% has a significant anemia. If the reticulocyte count is low, a congenital hypoplastic marrow should be considered. If it is normal or high, a direct Coombs' test should be obtained to rule out immunohemolytic anemia. If the Coombs' test is negative, blood loss, hemolysis secondary to infection, or hemolysis secondary to abnormalities of the erythrocyte membrane should be considered.

Polycythemia and associated hyperviscosity occur in approximately 5% of newborns. Some of the predisposing factors include maternal diabetes, placental insufficiency, maternal-fetal transfusion, twin-to-twin transfusion, and placental-fetal transfusion resulting from factors such as delayed cord clamping or milking the cord into the infant at the time of delivery. Remarkably,

TABLE 2. **Antibiotics**

	Postconceptual Age	Dose (IV or IM)	Interval
Ampicillin			
For use with suspected sepsis and meningitis.			
Suspected sepsis	<1 week	50 mg/kg/dose	q 12 hr
Meningitis	<1 week	100 mg/kg/dose	q 12 hr
Suspected sepsis	>1 week	50 mg/kg/dose	q 8 hr
Meningitis	>1 week	100 mg/kg/dose	q 8 hr
Cefotaxime			
For use with gram-negative neonatal meningitis and sepsis caused by susceptible gram-negative organisms (e.g., *E. coli, H. influenzae, Klebsiella,* and *Pseudomonas*).			
	Preterm infants <1 week	50 mg/kg/dose	q 12 hr
	Preterm infants >1 week and term infants <1 week	50 mg/kg/dose	q 8 hr
	Term infants >1 week	50 mg/kg/dose	q 6 hr
Gentamicin			
Loading dose 4 mg/kg/dose IV or IM (IV preferred) **1st Dose Only.** This includes anuric infants as one-time dose. Maintenance dose is based on infant's gestational age.			
	<30 weeks	2.5 mg/kg/dose	q 24 hr
	30–37 weeks	2.5 mg/kg/dose	q 18 hr
	38–42 weeks	2.5 mg/kg/dose	q 12 hr
Vancomycin			
For use with *Staphylococcus aureus* or *S. epidermidis* infections.			
	≤29 weeks	18 mg/kg dose*	q 24 hr
	30–36 weeks	15 mg/kg/dose*	q 12 hr
	37–44 weeks	10 mg/kg/dose*	q 8 hr
	≥45 weeks	10 mg/kg/dose*	q 6 hr

*IV only.
Abbreviations: IV = intravenously; IM = intramuscularly.

the infant may appear normal, plethoric, pale, or cyanotic. The infant may be asymptomatic. Polycythemia rarely occurs in the preterm infant. If the infant is symptomatic, neurologic signs range from lethargy to irritability and seizures. Tachypnea, tachycardia, respiratory distress, hypoglycemia, and poor feeding are associated findings. The chest radiograph shows increased pulmonary vascularity and cardiomegaly. The diagnosis should be suspected if the hematocrit from a warmed heel sample at 4 to 6 hours after delivery exceeds 65%. Polycythemia then is confirmed if a central venous hematocrit exceeds 65%.

Polycythemia should be treated with an isovolemic partial exchange transfusion, not simple phlebotomy. During the exchange transfusion, the infant's whole blood, drawn in 15- to 20-mL aliquots from a catheter in the umbilical vein, is replaced with an equal volume of 5% albumin, fresh-frozen plasma, or commercially available human plasma protein fraction. The latter may be preferable because it is prepackaged and requires no mixing, and there is no risk of hepatitis or acquired immune deficiency syndrome (AIDS). The volume to be replaced equals the observed hematocrit minus the expected hematocrit times the blood volume divided by the observed hematocrit. The observed hematocrit is a central value obtained at 4 to 6 hours. The expected hematocrit is 55%. The blood volume is calculated by multiplying the birthweight in kilograms by 80.

The prognosis depends on the factors predisposing to polycythemia and whether the infant is symptomatic. Symptomatic polycythemic infants should undergo partial exchange transfusion. Some authorities believe that asymptomatic infants also should undergo partial exchange transfusion if the hematocrit value exceeds 65%. Others would delay the procedure until the hematocrit exceeds 70%.

BILIRUBIN

Jaundice is a frequent problem in well and sick newborns. Bilirubin levels in the fetus, as indicated by cord blood levels, rarely exceed 1 to 2 mg per dL because fetal bilirubin, which is unconjugated, freely crosses the placenta to the mother where it is conjugated and excreted. Even in severe hemolytic conditions, the cord bilirubin concentration at birth seldom exceeds 6 mg per dL. Jaundice in the first 24 hours or jaundice that rises progressively to a level of greater than 12 mg per dL in the first 24 hours is abnormal and necessitates investigation. The basic clinical and laboratory data that are sought in the evaluation of hyperbilirubinemia include a review of the ma-

ternal and family history for evidence of jaundice, anemia, gallstones, or splenectomy. The infant is examined for bruising or entrapped hemorrhages, signs of infection, hepatosplenomegaly, and general state of well-being. The laboratory evaluation includes the determination of the serum bilirubin level, blood group typing of mother and infant, an indirect Coombs' test on the mother and a direct Coombs' test on the infant, a complete blood count, a platelet count, hematocrit, a reticulocyte count, and a peripheral blood smear for the determination of erythrocyte morphology and leukocyte differential. Serial bilirubin determinations are necessary every 4 to 6 hours in the icteric infant whose bilirubin is rising.

If the clinical jaundice is yellow-orange, it can be assessed by serially checking only the total serum bilirubin concentration. However, if the jaundice is a greenish hue, such as that observed with biliary obstruction in adults, the direct bilirubin fraction and total bilirubin concentration should be evaluated. Elevation in the direct reacting bilirubin fraction is seen in gram-negative bacterial infections and in hepatitis and biliary obstruction. These processes rarely are evident in the first week. If jaundice is persistent and no specific cause is discernible, blood and urine should be tested to exclude the diagnosis of galactocemia. Thyroid function tests should be obtained to exclude hypothyroidism.

Breast-feeding is associated with persistent low-grade jaundice. Physiologic hyperbilirubinemia of the newborn is a diagnosis made by exclusion. The diagnosis may not be considered if the jaundice occurs in the first 24 hours, the total serum bilirubin concentration is increasing more than 5 mg per dL per day, the total serial bilirubin concentration exceeds 12 mg per dL, the direct serum bilirubin concentration exceeds 1.5 to 2 mg per dL, and clinical jaundice persists longer than 1 week in a full-term infant and 2 weeks in a preterm infant.

The primary aim of treatment of neonatal jaundice is the prevention of bilirubin encephalopathy, including kernicterus. Each case of hyperbilirubinemia must be evaluated carefully and managed individually. For example, if a hemolytic process such as an Rh incompatibility is present, the infant should be evaluated for thrombocytopenia, hypoglycemia, and anemia. If the hemolytic process is secondary to sepsis, antibiotics should be administered. Reduction of the serum bilirubin, regardless of the cause, can be accomplished by the use of phototherapy or exchange transfusion. Both treatments carry risks. Exchange transfusion is invasive and requires technical experience and the administration of blood products. Phototherapy, although of low risk, may cause eye damage, apnea by displacement of the eye patches and obstruction of the nares, increased incidence of insensible water loss, and difficulties with thermoregulation. The author begins phototherapy when the serum bilirubin concentration reaches a level of 3 to 5 mg per dL below what would normally be considered for an exchange transfusion. If the underlying condition producing anemia and hyperbilirubinemia is secondary to a hemolytic process, hematocrits must also be followed. During phototherapy, bilirubin is expected to fall 2 to 4 mg per dL over a 24-hour period, provided that the production of bilirubin is not continuing or accelerating and that the phototherapy lights are working properly. Extensive use of phototherapy has led to a dramatic decrease in the number of exchange transfusions performed in a nursery. With that, however, has come a significant decrease in the number of trainees and pediatricians who have experience with exchange transfusions. An exchange transfusion is a complex procedure that may result in significant changes in the infant's blood chemistry profile and cardiac performance. Therefore, it should be performed with cardiorespiratory monitoring and with experienced personnel. It also may be necessary to transfer the infant to another facility that has experience with the procedure.

NECROTIZING ENTEROCOLITIS

Necrotizing enterocolitis is a disease occurring in ill preterm infants, usually within the first week. It is rare for it to occur in infants who have never been fed or who are fed breast milk. Because of sensitivity to the problems associated with feeding intolerance, the author screens stools for the presence of blood. Guaiac-positive stools often are caused by maternal blood swallowed during delivery. In this situation, the infant has stable vital signs and appears healthy except for the guaiac positivity. The blood can easily be diagnosed as maternal by performing an Apt test on the stool to identify adult hemoglobin. If the infant appears ill, there may be a coagulation disorder secondary to sepsis, shock, or necrotizing enterocolitis. Anal and rectal fissures are a benign cause of rectal bleeding in the newborn.

INFANTS OF DIABETIC MOTHERS

Infants of diabetic mothers require special mention. As a result of hyperinsulinemia in the infant, the infant's blood glucose concentration declines rapidly after delivery, reaching a nadir by 1 to 2 hours. The celerity of this response is directly related to the maternal glucose concen-

tration at delivery. As a rule, the higher the glucose concentration in the mother before delivery, the more rapid the fall in the newborn's serum glucose after delivery. The management of hypoglycemia in the infant of the diabetic mother is identical to that outlined earlier in the section on glucose. Infants of diabetic mothers may have additional problems, including hypocalcemia, hyperbilirubinemia, polycythemia, hypomagnesemia, respiratory and cardiac problems, sepsis, and an increased incidence of congenital abnormalities.

SURGICAL EMERGENCIES

Those responsible for the medical care of infants should be familiar with the most common problems requiring surgery. The final outcome is often determined by how quickly the diagnosis is made and the effectiveness of the initial supportive care in preventing infection and metabolic derangements. All conditions necessitating major surgery should be referred to a pediatric surgeon. Many common conditions are presented in Table 3.

Some general principles of management bear mentioning. An orogastric or nasogastric tube should be placed appropriately and attached to

TABLE 3. **Neonatal Problems Requiring Surgery**

Cardiopulmonary Systems
Congenital heart disease
Choanal atresia
Intrinsic or extrinsic neck mass
Tracheoesophageal fistula
Pneumothorax (tension)
Congenital chylothorax
Lobar emphysema
Cystic adenomatoid malformation

Gastrointestinal System
Diaphragmatic hernia
Intestinal atresia
Malrotation
Midgut volvulus
Gastroschisis
Omphalocele
Meconium ileus
Hirschsprung's disease
Imperforate anus
Duplication
Meckel's diverticulum

Genitourinary System
Exstrophy of the bladder
Meningomyelocele
Encephalocele
Hydrocephalus

Others
Sacrococcygeal teratoma
Neuroblastoma

Reprinted with permission from Coen RW, and Koffler H: Primary Care of the Newborn. Boston, Little, Brown and Company, 1987.

suction when a diagnosis of diaphragmatic hernia, esophageal atresia, or bowel obstruction is suspected or confirmed. Exposed viscera should be covered with a sterile, warm, saline wrapping. Acute respiratory distress secondary to a tension pneumothorax or congenital chylothorax requires immediate thoracentesis or thoracotomy and placement of a chest tube. Hydration must be maintained with intravenous fluids such as 10% dextrose solution at an initial rate of at least 100 mL per kg per day. Electrolytes should be added to the intravenous solution as soon as the infant is urinating.

INFANTS OF SUBSTANCE-ABUSING MOTHERS

For the most part, infants of mothers who abuse alcohol or drugs do not necessarily require treatment in a special care nursery. However, they do require a staff and social service system that can best provide support for the infant and the infant's family.

MULTIPLE BIRTHS

The incidence of naturally occurring multiple births is estimated to be 1 in 80 pregnancies for twins, 1 in 80^2 for triplets, and 1 in 80^3 for quadruplets. Twins are the most frequent type of multiple birth encountered in the nursery. In the first 24 hours, if the many physiologic adjustments that are necessary to ensure each infant's immediate survival do not occur, the infants qualify for the special care nursery. Changes in an infant's condition become apparent if the vital signs are checked and recorded frequently. The second-born twin often has more problems making an efficient transition to the extrauterine environment.

PERINATAL LOSS

Unfortunately, neonatal death is also one of the things experienced in the special care nursery. When a fetal or neonatal death occurs, profound grief follows. The grief of the family is shared by the caretakers. The same grief process occurs when an infant is born with a serious congenital malformation or illness. Similar feelings may develop in a woman who has a stillborn baby or who gives up her newborn for adoption. Discussions with the parents regarding the process about to envelop them may temper their grief. Shock or disbelief, mourning, and recovery constitute the major grief phases. In the initial phase, fear, anger, guilt, and sadness are the overwhelming feelings. Denial can be prevented and the grieving process facilitated if the parents see and hold their dead or dying infant. Sometimes the family is so immobilized that they cannot cope with this experience. A photograph of the infant that is shared with the family at a later date often helps them cope with their grief. The second phase of grief, the mourning phase, is a much more extended process. It is the period of adjustment to living without a loved one. Recovery, the third phase, is a time of resolution of the grief. The three phases often overlap, and backsliding may occur months after the infant's death. In general, the phases are handled differently by the mother and the father. A follow-up appointment with parents 4 to 6 weeks after the infant's death affords an opportunity to assess their adaptation, discuss any unresolved questions and feelings, and review the results of autopsy or other premortem or postmortem studies. The hospital staff also needs a support system.

DISCHARGE

Although medical care in the nursery is extremely important, it is only a prelude to what the infant will receive in the following years. In addition to providing general medical support, the role of the physician should be to provide anticipatory guidance in child rearing. Some parents may have participated in prenatal courses, but they were not anticipating that their infant would have a difficulty. The education of parents as caretakers must not be ignored because the infant is totally dependent on the parents and because the concepts and abilities in rearing a child are neither innate nor an inalienable right.

NORMAL INFANT FEEDING

method of
SIMON S. RABINOWITZ, PH.D., M.D., and
LAURENCE FINBERG, M.D.
Children's Medical Center of Brooklyn
Brooklyn, New York

The most dramatic growth and development in a person's life occurs during infancy. Infants usually double their birthweight by 6 months of age and triple it by 1 year. Length and head circumference increase by one-half and one-third, respectively, by the age of 1 year. The increase in head circumference reflects the development of the child's brain. The nutrients consumed provide the building blocks for rapidly dividing somatic and neurologic tissue.

The first year of life is a period not only of unparalleled growth but also of discovery and learning. Food-related activities represent important ways in which the infant learns to interact with the environment and with others. One important skill that the infant acquires during the middle third of the first year is eating from a spoon. As coordination improves, the child attempts to begin feeding itself. Toward the end of the first year, the child is exposed to the socialization of eating with other family members. Parents are forced to deal with their children's attempts to assert themselves through food preferences.

While the infant is growing as a whole organism, there is a rapid and controlled development of many organs and tissues. Ideally, the eating habits and nutritional content of the infant's diet should support growth and contribute to a healthy and full life. Investigators are now considering what role the diet of the infant plays in the development of diseases that become clinically apparent in later childhood or during adult life. Until these and other questions are answered, a prudent diet guided by good judgment is the best recommendation that can be given.

INFANT FEEDING

Human Milk

The aphorism that the "breast is best" has much anthropologic and biologic merit. From a historical perspective, the species has evolved into its present state from a long history of breast-feeding that has only recently been varied. There still exist many cultures in which infants are exclusively breast-fed and receive human milk until well past infancy. Similar feeding behavior is observed in other mammalian species.

The macronutrient composition of breast milk, simulated by commercial formula manufacturers, provides its most compelling basis for suitability. The carbohydrate source is the disaccharide lactose, a synthesis of glucose and galactose molecules. The enzyme needed to digest this sugar is found in the mucosa of the small intestine. The concentration of this enzyme is highest in infancy; in certain races, it gradually diminishes until it is found only in very small amounts during later childhood and beyond. The protein source is a mixture of 70% whey, the portion remaining after the curd has settled, and 30% casein, the insoluble portion that contains much of the calcium and phosphorus as complexed mineral. The fat source is a combination of saturated and unsaturated fatty acids, including adequate amounts of the essential fatty acids linoleic and linolenic acids.

Numerous investigations of undernourished women in the Third World and in economically deprived areas of developed nations have confirmed the adequacy of their milk and its similarity to the milk obtained from well-nourished women. The caloric content of mature human milk is always very close to 0.7 kcal per mL. Fat provides 51% of the energy. The composition of the fatty acids found in a mother's milk is influenced by her dietary intake. The protein provides about 8% of the total calories; the remainder comes from lactose. Except for the most malnourished nursing mothers, breast milk provides all of the essential amino acids in proper ratios and adequate essential fatty acids.

The whey portion of human milk contains lactalbumin and other proteins that contribute most of its immunologic benefit. Immunoglobulins, mainly IgA, are passed from the mother to the suckling infant and provide immediate protection from foreign antigens. Lysozyme is a hydrolytic enzyme that can break down bacterial walls. Lactoferrin is an avid binder of iron that competes with iron-requiring bacteria. Complement sensitizes other arms of the immune system and directly assists in phagocytosis. Interferons are a class of immunologic mediators involved in the response to viruses. Together, these proteins protect against microbial infections. Although technically not part of the whey protein, human milk contains white blood cells, including T and B lymphocytes, macrophages, and polymorphonuclear leukocytes, which also contribute to immune protection.

An assortment of other peptides that are believed to benefit the suckling infant are found in the whey portion of human milk. These include hormones such as thyroxin, thyroid-stimulating hormone, corticosteroids, adrenocorticotropic hormone, insulin, erythropoietin, and calcitonin; growth factors such as epidermal growth factor, insulin growth factor, nerve growth factor, and somatomedin C; the digestive enzymes amylase, lipase, and esterase; and the anti-inflammatory agent alpha$_1$-antitrypsin. These components beneficially influence the postnatal development of the human gastrointestinal tract and other organ systems.

Although the normal term infant does not require these components for normal maturation, various investigators have speculated that breast milk feeding protects against the development in later life of certain diseases, such as inflammatory bowel disease and alpha$_1$-antitrypsin deficiency. Conversely, milk protein intolerance occurs in infants fed human milk, but the incidence is substantially lower than in infants receiving formula.

Human milk provides a standard for the macronutrient, vitamin, and mineral content of infant formulas. Vitamins A, E, and K (fat soluble), thiamin, riboflavin, niacin, pyridoxine, pantothenate, folacin, B$_{12}$, biotin, and C are present in human milk. However, there have been reports of hemorrhagic disease of the newborn resulting from vitamin K deficiency in breast-fed infants. Therefore, 1 mg of vitamin K is given in the delivery room. The concentrations of the water-soluble vitamins reflect the mother's diet and the concentration of the fat-soluble vitamins reflect diet and storage. The breast-feeding mother who does not follow a balanced diet should continue taking her prenatal vitamins. For full-term infants, the mineral content of human milk, including calcium, phosphorus, magnesium, sodium, potassium, chloride, and sulfur, is optimal and forms the basis for infant formulas and infant parenteral nutrition.

Human milk is also a source of trace elements, including iron, zinc, copper, manganese, selenium, chromium, nickel, and iodine. The unique properties of human milk allow for higher bioavailability of certain minerals, such as iron and zinc, so that a lower concentration is required in human milk than in infant formulas to prevent deficiency in the first 3 to 4 months, when the milk is the sole feeding.

Human milk requires little supplementation. It does not contain adequate vitamin D, and a supplement of 400 IU per day is recommended. Although not necessary if the infant is exposed to sunlight, pigmented skin increases the requirement and urban smog vitiates sunlight. A fluoride supplement containing 0.25 mg per day is recommended in areas without fluoridated water, starting at about 6 months of age, to prevent later dental caries.

Unlike the composition of mature human milk, which appears toward the end of the second week after birth, the initial expressed milk, colostrum, contains more of the immunologic proteins, especially IgA, and less fat and calories. The protein component contains a unique amino acid composition, rich in arginine and tryptophan. There are also higher concentrations of some vitamins and minerals and of leukocytes.

Frequent suckling by the newborn infant of the less calorically dense colostrum increases the amount of breast milk expressed and stimulates the gradual change to transition milk and then to mature milk. Even after breast-feeding has been successfully established, the expressed milk is heterogeneous. The initial part of the feeding, fore milk, is closer to colostrum than most of the milk, known as hind milk. In determining the composition of mature human milk, these two components are averaged together. Determinations of the nutritional content of human milk are based on pooled samples because there is slight variability from mother to mother.

Human milk is recommended for full-term infants by a variety of sources, including the American Academy of Pediatrics. Women who are considering breast-feeding for the first time should receive encouragement and information before delivery. Although this is a "natural activity," a certain amount of orientation is often necessary. Infants should be allowed to stay with their mothers immediately after delivery and should be fed on demand to ensure success. A lactation assistant or a supportive and knowledgeable obstetric nurse should be available for consultation.

It is crucial for ultimate success that the physiologic letdown reflex be initiated as soon as possible. Care should be taken to properly position the infant and mother. It is also important to ascertain that the infant takes in enough of the breast to begin suckling the nipple. After feeding at one breast for 10 to 15 minutes, the infant should be put on the second breast. This should be repeated every few hours. There is variability in the aptitude that newborns have for breast-feeding, and a mother should not become discouraged if there are initially some difficulties.

The stimulus of suckling the nipple results in two neuroendocrine responses. The first results in prolactin release from the anterior pituitary, which stimulates milk secretion. The second, or letdown reflex, results in oxytocin release from the posterior pituitary, which causes contraction of myoepithelial cells in the mammary glands, resulting in the ejection of milk. As these reflexes are subjected to behavioral influences the new mother should be given support and guidance in her efforts. After feeding has been initiated, the lower caloric content of colostrum causes the newborn to suck more vigorously, further promoting the maternal neuroendocrine stimuli. This increases the yield of milk.

It is rarely necessary to supplement human milk with additional formula. By providing an alternative source of nutrition that is more easily obtained, the newborn can become confused and suck less vigorously at the breast. After about 7 to 10 days, when the colostrum has given way to mature human milk, the caloric requirements for growth should be met by breast-feeding. In the next few days, the infant should begin to gain weight and exceed its birthweight. One way to roughly gauge adequacy of breast-feeding is whether the infant has at least five or six wet diapers during the day. If there is a concern about sluggish weight gain and adequate time has elapsed, the first intervention is to document the amount of milk being produced. If supplementation is thought to be necessary, it is preferable to offer the supplement after the infant has fed on both breasts, rather than in place of a breast-feeding. Many of the immunologic virtues of human milk are vitiated when other foods are introduced in the early months.

The mother who has decided to breast-feed her infant should be reminded to eat a balanced diet, including supplemental vitamins, high-energy foods, calcium, and phosphorus; to take additional fluids; and to get adequate rest. Nipple discomfort is not uncommon and can usually be treated with warm compresses and dry heat supplied by a 60-W lamp or a hair dryer. A sturdy, well-fitting nursing brassiere is often helpful. Mastitis is almost always due to a blocked duct rather than an infectious process and is not a contraindication to continuing feeding.

Although many medications are secreted into human milk, very few preclude breast-feeding. The product insert or *Physicians' Desk Reference* usually supplies this information. Medications that should be avoided include cytotoxic drugs, immunosuppressive agents, radioactive isotopes, certain antithyroid drugs, sulfonamides in the first weeks, and drugs that suppress lactation, such as bromocriptine (Parlodel) and chlorothiazide (Diuril).

A commonly encountered source of concern among parents is the variability in the frequency and consistency of breast-fed infants' stools. Because of the predominance of whey protein, which has less complex salts, it is not unusual for these infants to produce small, loose movements after each feed. However, certain infants absorb almost all of their low-residue feedings and may pass only one stool in 7 to 10 days. As long as the abdomen is not distended and the stools are soft, there is no cause for concern and the parents should be reassured. Discomfort related to colic is frequently misinterpreted as pain from constipation.

The duration that women choose to breast-feed their infant varies. Human milk is able to supply all of the needed nutrition until 3 to 4 months. If a working mother decides to continue breast-feeding, human milk can be collected in thoroughly washed bottles and refrigerated for 24 hours. For longer periods of storage, freezing and gradual thawing is recommended. Microwave ovens are inappropriate for thawing human milk. This allows the infant to safely receive human milk when its mother is not available. If a woman finds that it is not possible to breast-feed for 6 months, she should be encouraged to switch to infant formula rather than unmodified cow milk.

Human milk is not suitable as a sole feeding for low-birthweight infants because the levels of protein and phosphorus are too low for them. Supplements are available for mothers of premature infants wishing to breast-feed.

Infant Formula and Evaporated Milk Formula

Infant formulas are the best alternative for mothers who do not wish to breast-feed. Several basic products are available in the United States for the healthy full-term infant. They are all based on human milk and are constantly being subtly modified to even closer approximate human milk. All contain lactose as the carbohydrate source, long-chain fatty acids with essential fatty acids as the lipid source, and various ratios of casein and whey as the protein source. These products are supplemented with vitamins and minerals, according to recommendations of the Committee on Nutrition of the Academy of Pediatrics as specified in the Infant Formula Act of the U.S. Congress.

The adequacy of infant formulas is apparent from the fact that about half of the infants born in the United States are fed formula when they leave the hospital, and 20 years ago, almost 75% of infants received this form of nutrition. Infant formula can be purchased in the United States as a ready-to-feed product, as a concentrated liquid, and as a powder. Physicians should review with the new mother these various preparations to avoid errors that may harm the neonate.

Because there is no physiologic mechanism to regulate formula intake, as with breast feeding, guidelines are appropriate. Infants should begin with about 60 mL per feeding every 2 to 3 hours and be gradually increased to a maximum of about 1 liter per day. Water that is not from a municipal water supply and is used to prepare formula should be boiled. The temperature of a bottle should be checked before it is given to the baby. The practice of giving a bottle to the infant every time he or she cries should be discouraged.

For a variety of unsubstantiated reasons, including cow milk protein allergy, colic, and intercurrent enteritis, soy protein formulas are frequently substituted for cow-milk-derived formulas. Because soy is a whole protein itself, the infant who has a true milk protein allergy is liable to develop an allergy to soya beans as well. Colic is a self-limited condition that has been found in all parts of the world and has not been convincingly shown to improve with soy formula. Improvement during intercurrent enteritis is more likely due to the absence of lactose in the soy formulas than to the protein. However, investigators have documented that adequate growth and development can be achieved in the full-term infant fed soy formula for about 6 weeks. The authors do not recommend sole feeding of these products for a longer period.

One nutrient whose concentration varies significantly among human milk, infant formula, and whole cow milk is iron. Formula must contain greater quantities because of its substantially higher bioavailability in human milk. However, infant formula provides adequate amounts of iron, in combination with iron-fortified foods, for the older infant. This is not the case for cow milk, which is not fortified with iron and can cause microscopic blood loss in the gastrointestinal tract. It can cause a relative iron deficiency, reflected in worse hematologic indices and in central nervous system and developmental compromise. Children who begin taking cow milk before 1 year of age should always have iron-containing foods included in the diet. Cow milk should provide no more than 60% of calories.

The advantage of using evaporated milk as the basis for infant formula is reduced expense. The greatest disadvantage is the inconvenience of mixing the formula at home. Cow milk has high protein, high salt, and high phosphate levels, making it hazardous for some infants. To minimize these ill effects, a carbohydrate source is added to dilute the protein and mineral. In practice, a 12-ounce (360-mL) can of evaporated milk is diluted with 16 ounces (480 mL) of water, and 2 tablespoons of corn syrup or sucrose or 4 tablespoons of dextromaltose are added to provide 15 grams of carbohydrate. This mixture contains approximately 0.67 kcal per mL, with 17% of energy as protein, 50% as carbohydrate, and 33% as fat. Vitamin C, 30 mg per day, must be supplemented until the infant begins taking juices or alternative sources of ascorbate.

Human milk and standard infant formulas are comparable in their ability to support growth and development during the first year of life. The rate of weight gain in breast-fed infants is significantly less than in those fed formula, and this trend continues even after the addition of solid foods to the diet. Immunologically, human milk is superior to formula, but there is very little clinical significance to the additional protection in normal infants growing up in Western countries. However, factors that are not fully delineated, including the added nurturing and bonding that are derived from breast-feeding, make this the best choice.

Weaning

Weaning or the introduction of solid foods, beikost, to the infant's diet should be thought of as a gradual process. Several factors determine the appropriate time to begin this process. Usually the infant signals the parent when the right time comes, and parents should be dissuaded from initiating weaning prematurely. The infant should be able to hold his or her head well and to coordinate swallowing from a spoon. Adding cereal to the bottle before this time is unnecessary.

Frequently, the infant's first signals are hunger. An infant should not have to receive more than 1 liter of milk per day. If an infant is having trouble sleeping through the night or not gaining weight appropriately on this quantity of milk, weaning should be considered. All of these changes usually occur between 3 and 6 months of age. At this same time, the gastrointestinal tract matures, and the likelihood of developing food allergies from new antigens is significantly decreased.

Because the healthy, full-term newborn has adequate stores of iron only for the first 3 months of life, the first food to be introduced should be iron-fortified single-grain cereal. After several days of increasing amounts, other types of fortified cereals may be introduced. Depending on how early cereals are introduced, several weeks or a month later, fruits and vegetables can be sequentially offered. Only one new food should be offered every few days so that it is easier to detect any that causes an adverse reaction. Fruits and vegetables can be bought as baby food jars or prepared at home, as long as they have a soft and smooth consistency. Protein-containing foods can be added in accordance with the same suggestions. Juices, a source of vitamin C, can be introduced after the infant can drink from a cup.

Foods that should be avoided during the first year of life include those with added sugar and salt and those that require anything more than minimal chewing, such as whole pieces of meat, fish, uncooked vegetables, grapes, nuts, and hard candies. Certain feeding practices can also be problematic. Offering the infant a bottle of milk or juice to sleep with should be discouraged because it can lead to dental caries. Infants should not be fed egg white and potent antigens until 9 to 10 months of age.

Behavioral Aspects of Infant Nutrition

One of the main ways that the infant and parent bond is during feeding. Breast-feeding may offer some benefits in this regard, but bottle-fed infants also quickly attach to those providing sustenance. During the initial visits with new parents, physicians should explore their feelings concerning feeding. Undue pressure from other members of the extended family that may result in overfeeding should be addressed. Eating should always be thought of as a pleasurable and satisfying experience for the infant and parent. As long as weight gain is adequate and basic guidelines are being adhered to, parents should be encouraged in their efforts.

When the child enters into the second half of infancy, he or she becomes a more active participant during meal times. Beikost should be given on a spoon so that eating becomes both a physical skill and a social means of interaction. Individual foods should be given separately to make eating a more gratifying experience. Older infants should be encouraged in their early efforts to feed themselves by a spoon, to eat finger foods such as soft vegetables, fruit, and meats, and to drink from a cup, even though this makes mealtimes messy.

Parents, especially new parents, should understand that the development of eating skills during infancy is a complex process that they must guide. The younger infant is fed on demand, but the older infant eats scheduled meals. This gradual transition requires the primary caretaker to balance the infant's hunger with the ability to postpone eating. This can usually be effectively accomplished by the judicious use of snacks. Parents should also understand that the infant's approach to eating is inconsistent. On some days they are more interested in eating than on others; foods that are readily taken one day may be refused the next.

Parents should be encouraged to look for and respond to subtle cues provided by their children. The infant may become interested in some other stimuli during meals and stop eating before being satiated. The patient parent joins the child in this diversion and then returns to eating. Conversely, stringent attempts to "clean the plate" can lead to overfeeding infants. If the normal infant is offered nutritional foods in a supportive and interactive manner, the likelihood of eating or growth problems is substantially minimized.

Most parents rely on the advice of family members and friends more than on that of their health care providers for feeding guidelines. This is even more likely in less educated, more socioeconomically disadvantaged families. Certain experts have theorized that this situation is in part accountable for the relatively high proportion of infants who are considered to be overweight, have nonorganic failure to thrive, or have less evident disordered eating patterns. Primary physicians caring for children can play a greater role in nutritional issues by addressing the character, amounts, and sequence of foods and by discussing the behavioral aspects of infant nutrition.

Future of Infant Nutrition

The goal of the formula companies is to manufacture a product that is identical to human milk. Recent additions have included taurine, a sulfur-containing amino acid that binds bile salts and aids in retinal development of kittens; carnitine, a carrier molecule needed for the intracellular transport and oxidation of fatty acids; nucleotides, precursors of DNA and RNA that are theorized to have immunomodulating and growth-stimulating properties; and increased concentrations of essential fatty acids. As long as researchers become more sophisticated in analyzing human milk and producing individual components, the composition of infant formulas will continue to evolve.

A more difficult issue to approach is whether aspects of an infant's diet can prevent or encourage disease processes that become clinically apparent years later. There is a retrospective study that indicates the incidence of inflammatory bowel disease is higher among children who were formula fed than those who were breast-fed as infants. The recommendation that follows is that infants who are at risk for developing inflammatory bowel disease should receive human milk. Although this observation may be verified in the future and universally endorsed, there is no harm in suggesting this to mothers who have inflammatory bowel disease or first-degree relatives who suffer with this condition.

Perhaps because of the wide dissemination of medical literature abstracts in the lay press, ill-founded and potentially deleterious pediatric nutritional practices are becoming more widespread. The issue of dietary cholesterol and fat content is a good example. The observation was made that fatty streaks, potential precursors to atherosclerotic plaques, were found in very young children. The reaction was to withhold fatty foods from certain children. Ironically, this practice may be more common among more educated parents who read newspapers and become frightened by these implications. The end result is that certain children became undernourished because of the reactions of overzealous parents. Central nervous system myelination requires fatty acids, and parents should be cautioned against giving their infants skim milk or 2% milk in an effort to prevent heart disease.

There are few convincing data that any novel dietary manipulations during infancy can produce future benefits. It is therefore necessary to discuss feelings about infant nutrition with new parents and to explore any unorthodox practices. The best method of ensuring optimal infant feeding remains an ongoing dialogue between the primary care physician and the new parents.

DISEASES OF THE BREAST

method of
ROGER S. FOSTER, JR., M.D.
Emory University
Atlanta, Georgia

Breast cancer is the most prevalent of all breast diseases. Breast cancer can be expected to develop in one in nine women in the United States. Death from breast cancer currently reduces the life expectancy of the average woman by approximately one-half year. The risk of death from breast cancer can be reduced both by earlier detection and by effective primary treatment.

SCREENING FOR BREAST CANCER

In the screening of asymptomatic women for breast cancer, breast palpation and mammography are the two techniques of proven value. There are no convincing data to establish the worth of thermography, transillumination, or sonography as screening procedures.

Mammographic screening of asymptomatic women aged 50 to 74 years has been demonstrated in several controlled trials to reduce breast cancer deaths by about one-third. The benefits of screening mammography for average-risk women under the age of 50 years are less and are the subject of considerable debate. The density of normal breast tissue makes imaging more difficult in younger women, and faster tumor growth rates may make it more difficult to get a screening benefit, particularly if mammograms are performed at intervals longer than annually. The recommendations of the U.S. National Cancer Institute are for mammographic screening of all women aged 50 years and over; screening mammography for younger women is recommended to be limited to those with a personal history of breast cancer or an immediate relative with breast cancer. The American Cancer Society recommends that mammographic screening of average-risk women begin at age 40.

Factors that place a woman at increased risk for breast cancer include family history, early menarche, late menopause, nulliparity, first full-term pregnancy after the age of 30, and exposure to ionizing irradiation. It is estimated that 5% of breast cancers in the United States occur in women who have inherited a strong genetic susceptibility. A positive family history of breast cancer is of particular significance when the patient's mother, aunt, or daughter has had breast cancer diagnosed before the age of 50 or when a relative has had bilateral breast cancer. The two most important risk factors, however, are female gender and increased age. Fewer than 1% of all breast cancers occur in women under the age of 30, 2% occur in women under 35, and more than 70% occur in women over the age of 50. No factors can define a set of women over the age of 30 who are not at significant risk of breast cancer; therefore, breast cancer screening is important in all women.

On the basis of currently available data, the breast cancer screening program that the author recommends is as follows:

1. Women aged 20 to 39 years with no personal or significant family history of breast cancer: breast self-examination (BSE) monthly and clinical breast examination (CBE) every 2 to 3 years.
2. Women aged 40 to 49: BSE monthly and CBE yearly. For women under 50 years of age who decide to have mammographic screening, the author advises annual mammograms because of the more rapid growth rate and shorter time to reach a palpable size in younger women.
3. Women aged 50 to 75: BSE monthly, CBE yearly, and mammography every 1 to 2 years.
4. Women with a strong family history of premenopausal breast cancer or a personal history of breast cancer: BSE monthly, CBE twice yearly, and mammography yearly beginning at age 35 or after treatment of first breast cancer.
5. Women aged 75 and older: CBE yearly, monthly BSE if they are capable. Any mammography screening should be restricted to those in general good health with a long life expectancy, because the benefits of screening probably take 5 or more years to become evident.

BENIGN BREAST PROBLEMS

The most important aspect of the management of benign breast problems is to exclude the possibility of malignancy.

Physiologic Nodulation and "Fibrocystic Breast Disease"

The breasts of premenopausal women undergo repeated cyclic hormonal stimulation, and physiologically induced breast nodulations, or lumpiness, develop in many women. Such nodulations typically increase during the premenstrual period and regress afterward. Accompanying symptoms are variable, but for some women there may be fairly severe premenstrual pain, swelling, and tenderness. The term "fibrocystic breast disease" for a condition that occurs to some degree in the majority of women is inappropriate and frightening. There is no associated increased risk for breast cancer. Treatment is careful physical examination (best performed during the postmenstrual interval) and reassurance, with the suggestion that analgesics such as aspirin be used if the symptoms interfere with physical or sexual activity.

The degree of breast nodulation is probably not related to the ingestion of methylxanthines (caffeine, theophylline, theobromine), but in some women the degree of breast tenderness may be related. For the rare patient whose problem does not respond to simple measures, there is a limited role for treatment with antiestrogen medication such as tamoxifen (Nolvadex); bromocriptine (Parlodel), which inhibits pituitary prolactin; or an impeded androgen such as danazol (Danocrine), which inhibits the release of pituitary gonadotropins. Attempts at treating these patients with subcutaneous mastectomies have resulted in symptomatic failures and complications, and such treatment is inappropriate.

Women with asymmetrical areas of breast nodulation may require additional investigation. Fine-needle aspiration biopsy (to be described) of such areas occasionally demonstrates malignant cells even in the absence of a distinct mass or a mammographic abnormality. If the fine-needle aspiration biopsy demonstrates an adequate number of normal ductal cells, there is considerable reassurance that the area is benign, and open breast biopsy is not necessary.

Gross Cysts

In contrast to physiologic breast nodulations, true breast masses, which are distinguished as being discrete, dense, dominant, and different from the rest of the breast tissue, should receive surgical attention. All palpable true breast masses are aspirated with a fine needle (e.g., 21-gauge). Gross cysts, which can occur in patients of any age but are most common in the 15 years before menopause, are completely evacuated and the fluid is discarded; cytologic examination is obtained only if the fluid is bloody.

Fibroadenomas

Fibroadenomas are benign fibroepithelial neoplasms that occur most commonly in women under the age of 30. Fibroadenomas tend to be very firm, mobile, nontender, and well delineated, and some resistance to withdrawal of the needle occurs after attempted aspiration. Cytologic examination is obtained on material aspirated with a fine needle from any solid lesion in which malignancy is deemed a possibility. Fibroadenomas and other true discrete breast masses are excised on an outpatient basis, usually under local anesthesia, to remove the mass because fine-needle aspiration cannot rule out malignancy when there is a true mass.

Nipple Discharge

Nipple discharge is of clinical significance only if it is spontaneous. Self-induced nipple discharge has no importance, and patients should be taught not to squeeze the nipples as part of BSE. Spontaneous serous and bloody discharges are most commonly caused by an intraductal papilloma, but mammographic evaluation followed by excision of the distal duct or ducts is necessary in order to rule out the possibility of a carcinoma. Nonlactational milky discharge should be evaluated with a test for serum prolactin because of the possibility of a pituitary adenoma.

Infection

Most of the infections that occur in other areas of the body can occur in the breast. Infections from *Staphylococcus aureus, Staphylococcus epidermidis,* and *Streptococcus* spp. are particularly common in lactating breasts and can usually be managed with antibiotics; breast-feeding can be continued during treatment. A nipple shield or breast pump may be used if a nipple fissure makes breast-feeding painful. If a breast abscess is present, breast-feeding should be discontinued, the abscess drained, and biopsy of the abscess wall performed. Recurrent periareolar abscess in nonlactating women is commonly caused by squamous metaplasia of the lactiferous ducts. Treatment is by surgical excision of the abnormal distal duct or ducts, usually after the acute process has been controlled by drainage of the abscess and antibiotics.

COSMETIC SURGERY

Cosmetic surgery may be desired by women who have asymmetrically sized breasts, whose breasts have not developed to an acceptable size or have involuted after pregnancy, or whose breasts have developed to an abnormally large size. The augmentation mammoplasty operation, involving the use of a submusculofascial Silastic bag implant, is relatively simple and usually provides good cosmetic results, but there has been recent controversy as to safety. Reduction mammoplasty for excessively large and heavy breasts is a more complex procedure in which the breast is resized and the nipple-areolar complex is repositioned. When the volume of breast tissue is satisfactory but stretching of skin has led to marked ptosis, a mastopexy operation, in which excess skin is removed and the nipple-areolar complex is repositioned, can be performed.

PRIMARY BREAST CANCER

Diagnosis and Staging of Breast Cancer

The diagnosis of a palpable breast cancer can be established by fine-needle aspiration biopsy, by core-cutting needle biopsy, by open incisional biopsy, or by excisional biopsy. The diagnosis of nonpalpable breast cancers that are detectable only on mammography is usually made by open biopsy after the area to be examined is localized by the tip of a needle, which is placed at the site from which the specimen is to be taken under mammographic control. Fine-needle aspiration biopsy is of particular value because it can be performed as an office procedure. Although this procedure is conceptually a simple technique, the operator must be able to obtain an adequate sample, and the cytopathologist must be experienced in providing reliable interpretation. Fine-needle aspiration biopsy of mammographic lesions may sometimes be done with ultrasound guidance or by using a stereoscopic mammography technique.

Excisional biopsy studies of lesions known or suspected to be cancer should be performed as formal partial mastectomies—that is, a small margin of apparently normal breast tissue surrounding the lesion is also excised, and the pathologist paints the external surface with India ink before sectioning—so that it can be established that there are tumor-free margins. If tumor-free margins are obtained and the patient's definitive treatment is to be partial mastectomy, no further resection of breast tissue is needed; the cosmetic results are better than when a second resection of breast tissue must be performed after an excisional biopsy. In addition to establishing a histologic diagnosis of cancer, the pathologist should immediately obtain and freeze material for later analysis for estrogen and progesterone receptors.

The histologic type of the breast cancer has a bearing on both the prognosis and the management. The most important distinction in terms of biologic behavior is between invasive breast cancer, which has a relatively high likelihood of systemic metastases, and noninvasive or in situ cancer, which has a very low likelihood of systemic metastases. Unfortunately, the noninvasive cancers are much less common than the invasive cancers; they are, however, being increasingly recognized with screening mammography.

The two different types of noninvasive breast cancer are (1) ductal carcinoma in situ (DCIS, or intraductal carcinoma), which usually involves only one breast, and (2) lobular carcinoma in situ, sometimes referred to as lobular neoplasia, which commonly involves both breasts. With the passage of time, noninvasive carcinomas frequently but not inevitably develop into invasive cancer. A coexistent invasive carcinoma has been reported in about 20% of patients whose predominant lesion is an intraductal carcinoma. In 15 to 50% of patients with small areas of intraductal carcinoma who have undergone only a limited biopsy, invasive ductal carcinoma develops in the same site over a median interval of 10 years. In about 25% of patients with lobular carcinoma in situ who have undergone only biopsy, invasive carcinoma develops over a median interval of 20 years; the risk is relatively even for both breasts.

Invasive ductal carcinoma is the most common type of invasive breast carcinoma, accounting for about 70% of these cancers. Invasive ductal carcinomas frequently cause a productive fibrosis, which is responsible for much of the hardness that is felt on palpation and the grittiness that is felt when the tumor is cut with a knife or entered with a needle. Lobular invasive carcinoma accounts for 5 to 10% of invasive breast cancers. The biologic behavior and prognosis of lobular carcinoma are similar to those of invasive ductal carcinoma. Medullary carcinomas account for 5% of invasive cancers, and it has been suggested that they carry a somewhat more favorable prognosis. Their biologic behavior is not much different from that of invasive ductal carcinoma. Colloid, tubular, adenocystic, and papillary carcinomas are relatively rare types and generally carry much better prognoses than do the more common types of invasive carcinoma.

Once a diagnosis or even strong presumptive diagnosis of breast cancer has been made, the clinical stage, or extent of disease, should be established. Clinical TNM (tumor, node, metastases) staging is based on the size of the primary cancer and any invasion of skin or underlying muscle or chest wall, on clinical evidence of involvement of regional nodes (axillary, supraclavicular, or infraclavicular), and on any evidence of more distant metastases. In addition to physical examination, the clinical evaluation of all patients should include chest x-ray and a serum alkaline phosphatase assay to screen for hepatic involvement. Routine bone scans, liver scans, and computed tomographic scans are not indicated unless the patient is symptomatic, has evidence of locally advanced disease on physical examination, or has an abnormal alkaline phosphatase level.

Pathologic staging of breast cancer is more definitive than clinical staging. For surgically operable invasive breast cancers, the presence or absence of histologically documented regional node metastases (axillary nodes) and the determination of the absolute number of nodes involved by metastases provide the most important information for prognosis and for decision making in relation to the use of systemic adjuvant chemotherapy. The levels of estrogen and of progesterone receptor proteins in the tumor provide additional prognostic and management information; high levels of receptor proteins indicate both a slightly more favorable prognosis and a greater likelihood of response to hormonal therapy when there are metastases.

Treatment

Local-Regional Treatment

The majority of patients are probably candidates for breast-conserving surgery; currently in the United States, however, the most common local-regional treatment for surgically operable carcinoma of the breast is total mastectomy and axillary dissection with preservation of the chest wall muscles (modified radical mastectomy). Radiotherapy to the regional lymph nodes after mastectomy and axillary dissection does not improve survival and increases morbidity. Breast-conserving surgery (lumpectomy and radiotherapy) is increasingly being used.

In the author's practice, most patients with primary cancers less than 4 to 5 cm in diameter are treated by partial (segmental) mastectomy followed by radiotherapy (5000 rad to the breast delivered through two tangential ports without any radiation boost to the tumor bed); an axillary dissection is usually performed through a separate incision. This technique is the partial mastectomy technique that has been demonstrated by the National Surgical Adjuvant Breast Project (NSABP) studies to provide 10-year survival rates similar to those obtained with modified radical mastectomy and to permit preservation of the breast in most of the patients.

A small percentage of patients treated by partial mastectomy demonstrate recurrence of tumor in the breast and subsequently require a total mastectomy. The expertise required for properly delivering the radiotherapy may not be available in all hospitals. Most women whose disease is unsuited to partial mastectomy are offered either immediate or delayed breast reconstruction. The author and colleagues find that in many patients the breast is appropriately reconstructed with a submuscular tissue expander and a Silastic implant. Some patients are better served by procedures that transfer the abdominal or latissimus dorsi muscles with overlying fat and skin.

Noninvasive breast cancers present particular difficulties in relation to the amount of breast tissue that needs to be removed. In contrast to most invasive cancers, many intraductal carcinomas involve the breast so diffusely that they cannot be excised by partial mastectomy, and thus many women with these prognostically favorable tumors are treated by total mastectomy, which may be followed by reconstruction. Patients with localized intraductal carcinoma may be treated by a combination of partial mastectomy and breast irradiation, which has been shown to decrease recurrence.

Appropriate management of lobular carcinoma in situ is even more poorly defined; because this disease is diffuse and bilateral, any management policy should be the same for both breasts. Most patients with lobular carcinoma in situ are managed with a conservative policy of repeated physical and mammographic examinations; selected patients may elect bilateral total mastectomy and breast reconstruction.

Systemic Adjuvant Treatment

Although in 95% of patients the disease is apparently localized to the breast and regional nodes at the time of initial treatment, systemic metastases develop over a 10-year period in nearly half the patients receiving only local regional therapy (surgery with or without radiotherapy). In the era before systemic adjuvant therapy, 75% of the patients with metastases to the axillary nodes had recurrences and were dead at 10 years. Patients with palpable tumors but without axillary node metastases have a recurrence rate of more than 40% at 10 years. For patients with invasive tumors less than 1 cm in diameter, which are frequently detected by screening mammography, 90% are expected to be free of recurrence at 10 years. For patients with noninvasive cancers, who should be recurrence free if resection is complete, the 10-year recurrence rate is 1 to 2%, presumably because an invasive component was present.

It has been shown that systemic adjuvant therapy can produce modest but very meaningful reductions in recurrence and improvements in survival in both premenopausal and postmenopausal patients with breast cancer. Benefit has been seen in both node-positive patients and in the higher risk node-negative patients. The relative magnitudes of the benefits of systemic adjuvant therapy are similar in high-risk and low-risk patients. Because a higher portion of the low-risk patients are destined never to have a recurrence,

the absolute benefits of systemic therapy are less for them. A larger portion of the lower risk patients bear the cost and toxicity of treatment without benefit. Outside of the context of a formal clinical trial, systemic adjuvant therapy is not recommended for patients with invasive tumors less than 1 cm in diameter or for patients with the smaller pure tubular, papillary, or typical medullary histologic findings, and it is not recommended for noninvasive cancers. Systemic adjuvant therapy is given to almost all patients with primary breast cancer with metastases to the regional nodes and to most patients with tumors 3 cm in diameter and larger.

Patients with node-negative tumors in the 1-to-3–cm range are problematic; overall, recurrences can be expected in approximately 30% of these patients. The ability to distinguish the majority of patients who will not benefit from chemotherapy from the minority who will is imperfect. Some clinicians rely on histologic specimens (well differentiated) and estimates of growth rates (S-phase fraction) to select patients who are less likely to benefit from adjuvant systemic therapy. For some patients, the effect of systemic therapy on reducing in-breast recurrence after lumpectomy and reducing the incidence of contralateral breast cancers may be factors weighing in favor of treatment.

When premenopausal patients are treated with systemic adjuvant therapy, a cytotoxic chemotherapy protocol is most often used. Postmenopausal patients are most commonly treated with the antiestrogen tamoxifen. For postmenopausal patients between the ages of 50 and 70 years, many clinicians prescribe cytotoxic chemotherapy in addition to tamoxifen, particularly for higher risk patients or if the tumor is estrogen- or progesterone-receptor negative.

METASTATIC BREAST CANCER

Metastatic breast cancer is rarely cured, which is the reason for the emphasis on systemic adjuvant therapy given at the time of diagnosis of the primary tumor. In recent years there has been an attempt to cure metastatic breast cancer in younger women with the use of very intensive cytotoxic chemotherapy programs that require special support of the bone marrow through transplantation of bone marrow cells, peripheral blood progenitor cells, or both along with the administration of blood cell growth factors. The preliminary data are encouraging, but the data from the controlled trials currently under way are not yet available.

The common sites for breast cancer metastases include bone, the liver, the lungs, the brain, and the chest wall. Although a limited number of patients remain free of disease after resection of solitary lung, brain, or cutaneous metastases, treatment of metastatic breast cancer is for the most part palliative. Therapy for metastatic breast cancer includes both cytotoxic chemotherapy and hormonal manipulations, as well as site-specific local therapy.

Patients with oncologic emergencies such as hypercalcemia, central nervous system metastases, unstable bone metastases, or pleural effusion need prompt therapy specific for the problem. Hypercalcemia usually responds to intravenous hydration and furosemide-induced diuresis. Brain and spinal cord metastases should be treated with high doses of corticosteroids, and immediate neurosurgical and radiotherapy consultations should be obtained. Patients with hip and leg pain should undergo bone scan and x-ray evaluations to determine whether lesions that may lead to pathologic fracture are present; impending fractures can be prevented by radiotherapy with or without insertion of a metal prosthesis as indicated. Large pleural effusions can be treated by insertion of a chest tube to evacuate the effusion, after which a sclerosing agent can be injected to create an adherence between the parietal and visceral pleura (pleurodesis).

About 50% of breast cancer patients are estrogen- or progesterone-receptor positive. Hormonal manipulations are preferred over cytotoxic chemotherapy in receptor-positive and receptor-unknown patients because the response durations tend to be longer and side effects are fewer. Older patients and patients with well-differentiated tumors are more likely to be receptor-positive. Initial hormonal therapies include antiestrogens, such as tamoxifen; progestational agents; and, for premenopausal patients, oophorectomy. The median duration of an endocrine response is about 12 to 18 months. After initial response to hormonal therapy and then further progression of disease, additional responses may be obtained by secondary hormonal manipulation. Patients whose disease is unsuited to hormonal manipulations or is no longer responsive are treated with combination cytotoxic chemotherapy. Response to current first-line combination chemotherapy occurs in 50 to 75% of patients, with a median duration of response of 6 to 12 months. Response to second-line chemotherapy regimens tends to be less.

ENDOMETRIOSIS

method of
ANTHONY A. LUCIANO, M.D.
University of Connecticut School of Medicine
Farmington, Connecticut

Endometriosis is a progressive, often debilitating disease that affects 10 to 15% of women, mostly during their reproductive years. It accounts for 25% of all laparotomies performed by gynecologists and, although not usually life-threatening, may significantly impair health and fertility potential.

J. A. Sampson introduced the first accurate description of endometriosis in 1921 when he defined the disease as "the presence of ectopic tissue which possesses the histologic structure and function of the uterine mucosa." Essential to the understanding of the pathophysiology and treatment of endometriosis is a thorough knowledge of the biologic actions of sex steroids on the endometrium (Table 1). Like normally implanted endometrium, endometriosis responds to the fluctuating blood levels of ovarian hormones during the menstrual cycle. At the end of each cycle, endometriosis breaks down and bleeds, causing pain and eliciting an inflammatory reaction with subsequent injury to the affected organs.

DIAGNOSIS

Although endometriosis is more commonly diagnosed in nulliparous women, usually white women in their late 20s or early 30s, it is by no means rare in teenagers, blacks, multiparous women, or indigent women. Therefore, regardless of age, parity, race, or socioeconomic status, endometriosis should be suspected in any patient with the clinical triad of progressive dysmenorrhea, dyspareunia, and infertility. Because it is a progressive and potentially crippling disease, a definitive diagnosis of endometriosis must be established as early as possible so that therapy aimed at arresting the disease and preventing its complications may be instituted.

Symptoms

Although it occurs most frequently in the pelvis, endometriosis has been found in most areas of the body, including the abdominal wall, diaphragm, small and large bowel, pleura, lungs, and extremities. The symptoms (Table 2) typically reflect the areas of involvement and tend to be most severe at the time of menstruation. The most common physical findings of pelvic endometriosis are generalized pelvic tenderness, nodular induration of the uterosacral ligaments, ovarian enlargements, and fixed retroflexed uterus.

A definitive diagnosis of endometriosis can be made only by direct visualization, preferably by laparoscopy because it provides a panoramic or microscopic view of the pelvis and the entire abdomen and enables surgical resection of disease while being minimally invasive. Endometriosis lesions are easily identifiable by their typical "gunpowder burns" appearance—stellate-

TABLE 1. **Effects of Sex Steroids on Endometrial Tissue**

Hormonal Milieu	Effects on Endometrium	Effects on Endometriosis
Estrogen	Proliferation	Proliferation
	Hyperplasia	Hyperplasia
	Carcinoma	Carcinoma
Lack of estrogen	Atrophy	Atrophy and regression
Progesterone	Growth arrest	Growth arrest
	Secretory changes	Secretory changes
		Decidual reaction
	Decidual reaction	Necrobiosis
Androgens	Atrophy	Atrophy and regression

scarred lesions surrounded by reddish-blue implants on the ovaries or peritoneal surfaces of the uterus, bladder, or intestine. Atypical endometriosis, described as clear vesicles, pinkish implants, or white-erythematous areas on the peritoneum, is equally common and must be thoroughly investigated. Therefore, any apparent abnormality visualized in the pelvis at the time of laparoscopy should be excised and subjected to biopsy for histologic evaluation. The extent of the disease should be properly staged at the time of initial diagnostic laparoscopy according to the American Fertility Society Revised Classification (AFS-RC).

TREATMENT

In planning therapy, many variables must be considered, such as age of the patient, extent of disease, degree of symptoms, and desire for immediate or deferred fertility. In most instances, the indications for treatment are pain or infertility or both, and the treatment may be surgical or endocrinologic or both. In the following discussion, the role of hormonal and surgical therapy in the treatment of pelvic pain and infertility associated with endometriosis is reviewed.

Hormonal Therapy

On the assumption that the improvement and regression of endometriosis observed during pregnancy can be reproduced by simulating the hormonal milieu of pregnancy with oral contraceptives, R. L. Kistner introduced a pseudo-pregnancy regimen in 1956. This treatment involves giving one of the combination oral contraceptives uninterruptedly for 6 to 9 months. The patient usually takes one tablet a day until she experiences breakthrough bleeding, at which time the dosage is increased to two or more tablets a day until amenorrhea is established. Although combined estrogen and progestin therapy relieves dysmenorrhea and pelvic pain, the side effects are significant, leading up to 40% of patients to discontinue therapy. Abdominal swelling, mastalgia, increased appetite, and breakthrough bleeding occur in the majority of patients.

Progestins

A better option than oral contraceptives may be found in the progestational compounds, which obviate the adverse effects and risks associated with the high doses of synthetic estrogens present in the birth control pills. The parenteral route may consist of 100 mg of medroxyprogesterone acetate (Depo-Provera) intramuscularly every 2 weeks for four doses and then 150 mg monthly for 4 additional months. This therapy produces side effects similar to the effects such as bloating, weight gain, and mood swings that patients experience during pregnancy. If pregnancy is desired immediately after treatment, Depo-Provera should be avoided because hypothalamic suppression may persist for 6 to 12 months after treatment when this agent is discontinued.

Perhaps better tolerated is oral medroxyprogesterone acetate (Provera) at a daily dose of 30 to 50 mg for 4 to 6 months. After treatment with oral medroxyprogesterone, 50 mg daily for 4 months, the mean endometriosis (AFS-RC) scores decrease by more than 65% (from 18.2 ± 2 to 5.9 ± 1), symptoms improve in more than 80% of patients, and 50% of infertile patients conceive successfully. During treatment, menstrual cycles are interrupted, and the majority of patients either are amenorrheic or experience occasional breakthrough bleeding, which reflects decidualized atrophic endometrium. Ovulation is inhibited in all patients, but normal ovulatory cycles resume within 2 months of treatment termination. Side effects are usually benign and easily tolerated. Except for significant suppressions of

TABLE 2. **Symptoms Associated with Endometriosis***

Common	Less Common	Occasional	Rare
Dysmenorrhea	Dyschezia	Urgency	Hemoptysis
Dyspareunia	Premenstrual spotting	Rectal bleeding	Intestinal obstruction
Infertility	Dysfunctional uterine bleeding	Hematuria	Hydroureter-hydronephrosis
Pelvic pain	Dysuria	None	Cutaneous nodules

*Typically reflect the areas of involvement and tend to be most severe at the time of menstruation.

serum levels of luteinizing hormone (LH), sex hormone–binding globulin, and estradiol, no major alterations in the blood levels of other reproductive hormones, in serum chemistry, in liver enzymes, in lipids, or in lipoproteins occur during treatment with oral medroxyprogesterone acetate.

Androgens

Danazol (Danocrine), a synthetic isoxazol derivative of ethisterone, has mild androgenic and weak progestational effects but strong antiestrogenic action. In keeping with these pharmacologic actions, most patients receiving danazol therapy experience interruption of their menstrual cycles and hot flushes (antiestrogenic effects); acne, mild hirsutism, and, in rare instances, deepening of the voice (androgenic effects); and weight gain, water retention, and mood changes (androgenic/progestational effects).

After 6 months of danazol treatment at doses of 200 twice or thrice daily, 70% of patients report improvement of symptoms and demonstrate objective disease regression at laparoscopy. Symptoms recur in 5 to 15% of patients each year after treatment is discontinued.

The metabolic alterations reported to occur during danazol treatment include decreased glucose tolerance, increased bromosulfalene retention, decreased serum levels of high-density lipoprotein-cholesterol, and increased serum levels of low-density lipoprotein-cholesterol. However, these metabolic effects return to baseline within 2 to 3 months.

GnRH Analogues

The most effective treatment of endometriosis has been oophorectomy, which establishes a severe, albeit permanent, hypoestrogenemic state. The administration of long-acting gonadotropin-releasing hormone (GnRH) analogues induces down-regulation of GnRH receptors at the pituitary level, suppressing the release of LH and follicle-stimulating hormone (FSH). This results in decreased ovarian activity and a degree of hypoestrogenemia that is similar to that observed in postmenopausal women or in women who have undergone oophorectomy. Well-controlled prospective studies with the use of GnRH analogues have reported favorable effects on the symptoms of endometriosis and regression of the disease. Currently, long-acting GnRH analogues are available as injectable (leuprolide [Lupron]) or nasal spray (nafarelin [Synarel]) preparations. As expected, their adverse effects are similar to menopausal symptoms and include hot flashes,

atrophic changes of the reproductive organs, and bone loss, which may not be significant if treatment is limited to the recommended period of 6 months.

Radical Surgery

Definitive surgical treatment, which entails resecting endometriotic lesions as completely as possible and removing the uterus and both ovaries, should be reserved for patients with severe symptoms who have no further desire to become pregnant. Bilateral oophorectomy is essential for depriving the ectopic endometrium of the cyclic estrogen that sustains and stimulates its proliferation and growth. Failure rates of 13% at 3 and 40% at 5 years have been reported to occur when ovarian function is preserved. Consequently, in patients who have enough pain to justify hysterectomy, removal of both ovaries, regardless of age, offers the best hope for a permanent cure.

After radical surgery, these women require hormone replacement to avoid menopausal symptoms and to protect them from osteoporosis and the risk of cardiovascular disease. Hormone replacement therapy may be started shortly after surgery. For patients with diffuse disease that could not be completely resected, a single intramuscular injection of 100 mg of medroxyprogesterone acetate (Depo-Provera) administered on the second postoperative day suppresses hot flashes for up to 12 weeks and, in conjunction with the hypoestrogenemia that follows oophorectomy, results in regression of residual implants. Similar effects may be achieved with oral medroxyprogesterone acetate at the daily dose of 20 to 30 mg for the first 3 postoperative months. Thereafter, a combined estrogen and progestin regimen, which has been shown to inhibit endometrial proliferation, may be started and continued for up to 12 months after surgery. These patients may be treated with 0.625 mg of conjugated estrogen, 50 μg of transdermal estradiol (Estraderm) twice per week, or 1.0 mg of micronized estradiol (Estrace) daily, together with 5 to 10 mg of medroxyprogesterone acetate daily for the first postoperative year, to induce further regression of residual disease. Subsequently, the progestin may be discontinued, and the patient is treated with unopposed estrogen indefinitely, with minimal risk of endometriosis recurrence.

Conservative Surgery

Conservative surgical treatment is reserved for infertile women in whom the disease has advanced and who wish to conceive. Although seldom curative, it does improve the likelihood of pregnancy while temporarily relieving symptoms. Approximately 25% of patients who undergo conservative operations require a subsequent surgical procedure for disease recurrence. The reoperation rate is directly related to the extent of disease and is much higher in patients who fail to conceive (40%) than in those who achieve pregnancy (10%) after the initial surgery. In most instances, conservative surgery is cytoreductive, and the recurrence of symptoms may be attributable to progression of existing, microscopic disease that over time becomes evident and symptomatic. The rates of pregnancy after conservative surgery for endometriosis have been reported to be from 22 to 100%, a variability that depends not only on the extent of disease and therapeutic modality but also on the duration of follow-up and the methods by which pregnancy rates were determined, none of which have been standardized.

THERAPEUTIC OPTIONS

Conservative or radical surgery, sex steroids to induce pseudopregnancy, GnRH analogues to induce medical oophorectomy, and danazol are all being used to relieve the symptoms of endometriosis or to treat infertility that frequently accompanies it. The choice of therapy should be determined by the patient's symptoms, her childbearing desires, and the extent of the disease. The author's therapeutic approach for patients with endometriosis is as follows:

Young Patients Who Wish to Delay Childbearing. At initial laparoscopy, all visible endometriosis, adhesions, and any other pelvic pathologic processes are removed. Postoperatively, hormonal suppressive therapy is administered for 6 months; any of the GnRH analogues (the author administers leuprolide acetate [Lupron Depot], 3.75 mg intramuscularly every 28 days); medroxyprogesterone, 30 to 50 mg per day; or danazol 200 mg thrice daily, may be used to induce further regression of disease. Thereafter, the patient is encouraged to use low-dose oral contraceptives or the "mini-Pill" to inhibit endometrial proliferation and reduce the risk of disease recurrence, until the patient wishes to conceive.

Infertile Patients With Mild or Extensive Endometriosis. Removal of all adhesions, resection or ablation of all implants of endometriosis, and total excision of endometriomas are accomplished surgically. Immediately postoperatively, the patient is encouraged to attempt to conceive for 9 to 12 months. Patients who fail to become pregnant will be advised to undergo repeated laparoscopy to assess the need for further conservative surgical treatment. If further surgical treatment is unsuccessful or not indicated, the patient is offered Assisted Reproductive Technology procedures, such as in vitro fertilization, gamete intrafallopian transfer, or human menopausal gonadotropin superovulation with intrauterine insemination, which yield rewarding options when other treatment has failed.

Patients Who Do Not Desire Further Childbearing. If symptoms are severe and the quality of life is impaired, total hysterectomy and bilateral salpingo-oophorectomy may be curative. Patients who want to postpone or avoid a major operation may benefit from a course of hormonal-suppressive therapy.

Patients with Endometriosis Involving Organs Outside the Pelvis. Hormonal-suppressive therapy for 6 to 9 months has been reported to be successful in the treatment of patients with pulmonary, intestinal, and ureteral endometriosis. Patients desiring pregnancy may benefit from a course of such therapy. If pregnancy is not desired, total abdominal hysterectomy and bilateral salpingo-oophorectomy should be performed.

DYSFUNCTIONAL UTERINE BLEEDING

method of
CHAD I. FRIEDMAN, M.D.
Ohio State University Hospitals
Columbus, Ohio

The normal menstrual cycle is characterized by cyclic bleeding every 24 to 36 days, induced by the synchronized withdrawal of estrogen and progesterone. Menses normally persist for 3 to 7 days and are associated with a 20- to 80-mL blood loss. The fluid perceived by the patient is actually a combination of blood, transudate, and shed tissue. Hormones released by the ovary, uterus, and hypothalamus orchestrate the normal ovulatory menstrual cycle and result in a complex of moliminal symptoms heralding the onset of menstruation. The amount of cyclic bleeding and the severity of premenstrual symptoms are highly correlated with ovulatory function. Factors limiting the amount of menstrual bleeding include uterine contractions (cramping); normal coagulation; progesterone-induced vascular and stromal changes; and resumption of estrogen-induced endometrial proliferation and healing.

"Dysfunctional uterine bleeding" (DUB) refers to uterine bleeding resulting from irregular sloughing of the endometrium in association with ovulatory dysfunction. Lacking the normal hormonal changes that occur with ovulatory cycles, bleeding commonly begins in the absence of any premenstrual symptoms. For most cases of DUB, presenting complaints include erratic and prolonged uterine bleeding with intermittent spotting. Often a history of several missed menstrual periods precedes the complaints of irregular bleeding. The lack of progesterone in the presence of chronic estrogen stimulation results in thickening of the endometrium, which lacks the stromal support and vascular changes typically seen during the luteal phase. A nonsynchronized breakdown of endometrial regions results in the prolonged erratic bleeding clinically observed. The incidence of DUB is markedly enhanced at the extremes—menarche and menopause—of reproductive function.

Documentation of normal ovulatory function (biphasic basal body temperature chart, midluteal serum progesterone level greater than 10 ng per mL, or secretory endometrium on an endometrial biopsy) excludes the diagnosis of DUB. It is important to remember, however, that DUB, when present, can be observed with other common causes of abnormal uterine bleeding. Proper evaluation for the presumed diagnosis of DUB includes attempts to diagnose the cause of anovulation (polycystic ovarian disease, thyroid dysfunction, adrenal hyperplasia, hyperprolactinemia, stress) as well as to rule out other causes of abnormal uterine bleeding.

In rare cases, DUB manifests as profuse uterine bleeding. Rather than being a situation of endometrial overgrowth with irregular breakdown of the endometrium, profuse bleeding may imply a combination of abnormalities. This is perhaps best exemplified in perimenarchial girls with profuse vaginal bleeding, in whom coagulation defects are commonly observed. For many of these girls, menarche is the first challenge for their coagulation system. In the absence of the progesterone-induced stromal changes, the anovulatory bleeding commonly seen at menarche places these patients at significant risk for hemorrhage. Similarly, perimenopausal women with fibroids have a defect in uterine contractility and often exhibit profuse bleeding when the fibroid manifests in combination with anovulatory bleeding. Examples of other pathologic states associated with vaginal bleeding are shown in Table 1.

In addition to a careful history and physical examination, the clinical or laboratory studies shown in Table 2 should be considered in patients suspected of having DUB.

TABLE 1. Causes of Vaginal Bleeding

Hormonal
Dysfunctional uterine bleeding
Coagulation Defects
Platelet dysfunction, thrombocytopenia, factor deficiencies, vascular defects (e.g., Ehlers-Danlos syndrome)
Anatomic Abnormalities
Leiomyoma, endometrial polyps, uterine arteriovenous malformations, traumatic tear
Neoplastic Processes
Cervical carcinoma, uterine carcinoma, uterine sarcomas, choriocarcinoma
Early Pregnancy–Related
Abortion, cervical pregnancy, retained products of conception
Other
Adenomyosis, endometritis

TABLE 2. Evaluation of Dysfunctional Uterine Bleeding

Pregnancy test
Complete blood count ± platelet count, coagulation profile, bleeding time
Papanicolaou smear
Basal body temperature chart, serum progesterone measurement
Serum prolactin and thyroid-stimulating hormone measurements
Liver function studies
Endometrial biopsy
Hysterosalpingogram or hysteroscopy
Pelvic ultrasonography

MANAGEMENT AND TREATMENT

Management of DUB can be outlined according to the urgency imposed by the rate and amount of blood loss.

Profuse Acute Uterine Bleeding

Assessment of acute profuse uterine bleeding relies on monitoring the following characteristics:

1. Vital signs, including orthostatic changes and urine output.
2. Changes in hemoglobin and hematocrit in response to intravascular volume replacement.
3. Direct visualization of blood loss through repeated speculum examinations.

Speculum examination provides the opportunity to determine the source of bleeding and directly assess the amount of active bleeding. All blood within the vaginal vault and in the cervix should be removed to allow for an accurate assessment of the extent of bleeding between examinations.

In cases of profuse uterine bleeding, intravenous access should be established and appropriate fluid replacement begun. Blood for a pregnancy test, complete blood count, platelet count, clotting studies, and a type and crossmatch study must be obtained. Infusion rates of fluids, blood transfusions, and transfusions of platelets and coagulation factors are determined in accordance with the results of the initial evaluation and laboratory studies. In cases of presumed DUB, 25 mg of conjugated estrogens (Premarin) is administered intravenously every 4 to 6 hours until bleeding significantly decreases. In situations of unremitting profuse uterine bleeding, operative management should be considered. Vaginal ultrasonography should be performed before surgery, to evaluate for fibroids or other intrauterine masses as a cause of bleeding. In the absence of obvious uterine pathologic processes, suction curettage followed by gentle sharp curettage is frequently effective in reducing bleeding and in obtaining tissue for histologic evaluation. In cases of profuse bleeding, hysteroscopy, while desirable, is generally inadequate because blood compromises the visualization. In cases in which the bleeding fails to respond to dilatation and curettage (D & C) uterine tamponade can generally be accomplished by placement of an intrauterine Foley catheter into the cavity with inflation of the bulb. At this time, the possibility of proceeding with either uterine artery embolization or hysterectomy must be considered in the event that control of the bleeding cannot be adequately obtained with the Foley catheter or resumes once the Foley catheter is removed 24 hours later.

In most cases of profuse vaginal bleeding, bleeding is steady but can be easily compensated for by infusion of crystalloid and possibly limited transfusions of blood. Intravenous conjugated estrogens, 25 mg, can be repeated every 4 to 6 hours. Alternatively, oral conjugated estrogens (Premarin), 2.5 mg, can be administered every 6 to 12 hours if the patient is stable enough to take oral medications. If the bleeding is not life-threatening, conjugated estrogens typically are effective in significantly reducing the bleeding within 12 to 24 hours. The evaluation of the patient is identical to that already described, with the exception that an endometrial biopsy is likely to be substituted for the formal D & C. Hysteroscopy and D & C should be performed if a complete cessation of bleeding cannot be achieved within 24 to 48 hours of estrogen therapy in the absence of a documented coagulopathy.

In patients responding to estrogen therapy, the estrogen is continued for an additional 24 hours. After this, an oral contraceptive containing 50 μg of ethinyl estradiol is begun. One pill per day is administered for 21 days, after which treatment is stopped and another withdrawal bleed is initiated. Cyclic oral contraceptives, iron, and folate are continued until the hemoglobin and hematocrit approach the normal range. Once this is achieved, the treatment can be converted to a lower-dose oral contraceptive, or the patient can be reassessed for resumption of ovulatory function or treated with a cyclic progestational agent, as discussed in the following section.

Chronic Abnormal Uterine Bleeding

Most cases of dysfunctional uterine bleeding are treated in the physician's office rather than in the emergency room. Here, establishing the diagnosis is of equal concern as obtaining immediate control of the bleeding. In most cases, the history and results of the physical examination limit the differential diagnosis and lead to a cost-efficient selection of laboratory tests. In the absence of profuse bleeding, coagulation studies are seldom necessary. Hormonal evaluation in general is limited to measurements of thyroid-stimulating hormone and prolactin. Androgens may be considered when hirsutism is present, cortisol when Cushing's disease is suspected, or an estradiol if a granulosa cell tumor is suspected.

The presence of copious cervical mucus is commonly found and supports the diagnosis of DUB. Chronic estrogen stimulation in the absence of progesterone allows for mucus production. If pregnancy is ruled out, an endometrial biopsy and vaginal ultrasonography can be used to rule out other pathologic states. In the presence of active bleeding in which cervical mucus cannot be readily assessed, conjugated estrogens, 2.5 to 5.0 mg daily, are taken orally for 14 days. Medroxyprogesterone, 10 to 20 mg per day, or norethindrone acetate, 5 mg per day, is administered for the last 12 days of the estrogen therapy. If abundant cervical mucus is noted with minimal bleeding that is consistent with chronic estrogen stimulation, the estrogen therapy is omitted and only the progestin treatment given. The patient is carefully informed that a heavy menstrual bleed is to be expected after completing the hormonal therapy.

A return visit is scheduled for approximately 1 week after the hormones are discontinued. At that time, the clinical course, laboratory studies, and biopsy results are reviewed. If the diagnosis of DUB is confirmed, either the cause of anovulation is treated and corrected or a regimen for cyclic withdrawal bleeding is prescribed. Oral contraceptives are the simplest treatment for inducing cyclic endometrial sloughing. Alternatively, in sexually inactive women or in cases in which oral contraceptives are unsatisfactory, 10 to 14 days of a progestin (medroxyprogesterone, 5 to 10 mg per day, or norethindrone acetate, 5 mg per day) every 6 weeks is effective. If menstrual bleeding is observed between the proposed administration of progestins, the progestin is withheld for another 6 weeks, and a basal body temperature chart performed or a midluteal progesterone measurement is obtained in the next cycle. Findings consistent with a progestational rise before menstruation suggest resumption of ovulation and the lack of further need for pharmacologic therapy. Failure to document ovulation implies the need for continued progestational therapy.

Women suffering from DUB and yet desiring to conceive in the very near future are not candidates for long-term oral contraceptives. Many of these women require treatment with clomiphene citrate, menopausal gonadotropins, gonadotropin-releasing factor, or glucocorticoids to induce ovulation. However, these drugs are indicated only for those women actively wishing to conceive.

It must be acknowledged that failure to control what is presumed to be DUB necessitates additional studies. These studies include hysteroscopy and perhaps a repeated endometrial biopsy.

AMENORRHEA

method of
PAULO SERAFINI, M.D.
Huntington Memorial Hospital
Pasadena, California

The average age at menarche in the United States is 12.8 years. The initiation and maintenance of normal menstrual function requires a functional integration of the hypothalamic-pituitary-thyroid-adrenal-gonadal axis coupled with a patent genital outflow tract.

Primary amenorrhea is defined as either (1) lack of menses by age 16 years in the presence of normal pubertal growth and development or (2) lack of menarche by age 14 years in the absence of normal pubertal growth and development.

Secondary amenorrhea is defined by the absence of menses for 6 consecutive months or for three of the usual cycle intervals after the establishment of menstrual function. The differential diagnosis of amenorrhea is complex and requires knowledge of endocrine and non-endocrine pathology. Although amenorrhea may be physiologic (i.e., resulting from pregnancy), it could also represent the first sign of a serious underlying systemic disease. To make the subject more complex, several therapeutic interventions, including multiple combinations of drug regimens, are recommended. Finally, implementation of a definitive therapeutic intervention relies on the patient's desire to pursue parenthood. Therefore, the author proposes a simplified practical approach to the management of amenorrhea.

The evaluation of amenorrhea begins with a detailed history and meticulous physical examination, including weight, height, and neurologic assessment. A high-resolution pelvic sonographic examination is of utmost importance to evaluate the uterus, ovaries, and upper third of the vagina.

DIAGNOSIS AND MANAGEMENT

Primary Amenorrhea

Figure 1 outlines the work-up and basic treatment approach for primary amenorrhea.

Hypergonadotropic Hypogonadal Amenorrhea

Patients with this type of amenorrhea present with elevated serum gonadotropin levels, impaired ovarian folliculogenesis, and a consequent lack of breast development. Nevertheless, they have appropriate müllerian development; the examination discloses the presence of a normal uterus. Chromosomal abnormalities are common among these patients. Actually, the incidence of hypergonadotropic hypogonadism is increased fourfold among patients with primary amenorrhea in comparison with those with secondary amenorrhea. The most common abnormalities are variances of the 45,X syndrome.

Deficiency of 17α-hydroxylase is a rare cause of hypergonadotropic amenorrhea, but the recognization of this abnormality is very important. Women with this enzymatic deficiency present with hyponatremia, hypokalemia, and hypertension as a consequence of cortisol deficiency. Patients with autoimmune disturbances such as lupus, polymyositis, Hashimoto's thyroiditis, and related disorders may present in a similar manner.

Estrogen-progesterone (EP4) therapy is the treatment of choice. Daily oral administration of conjugated estrogens (Premarin, 0.625 to 1.25 mg, depending on the necessity to enhance secondary sexual characteristics, bone mass, or both) should be considered. Alternative forms of estrogen therapy may be considered; these include daily oral administration of 2 to 4 mg of micronized estradiol (E2, Estrace) or the application of 0.05 to 0.1 mg of transdermal E2 patches (Estraderm) every third day. Daily medroxyprogesterone acetate (Provera), 5 to 10 mg, or micronized oral progesterone, 300 mg, is added for a period of 13 days beginning in the first calendar day of the month. Cyclic midmonth menstruation occurs. Glucocorticoid therapy with hydrocortisone (Cortef) is used for patients with amenorrhea resulting from 17α-hydroxylase deficiency.

Hypogonadotropic Hypogonadism

Patients with this disorder present with reduced baseline serum levels of luteinizing hormone (LH) and follicle-stimulating hormone (FSH), hypoestrogenemia, and a consequent absence of secondary sexual characteristics and normal müllerian development. This condition may be brought about by brain tumors, infiltrative and infectious diseases, trauma, radiotherapy, or central nervous system infarctions. Craniopharyngiomas, pinealomas, teratomas, endodermal sinus tumors, gliomas, and metastatic disease are the most common neoplasias. Central nervous system sarcoidosis occurs in 5% of patients with systemic disease. Diabetes insipidus and hyperprolactinemia are common manifestations of central sarcoidosis. Tuberculosis, syphilis, histiocytosis, and hemochromatosis also cause this type of amenorrhea. Amenorrhea may also follow pituitary apoplexy.

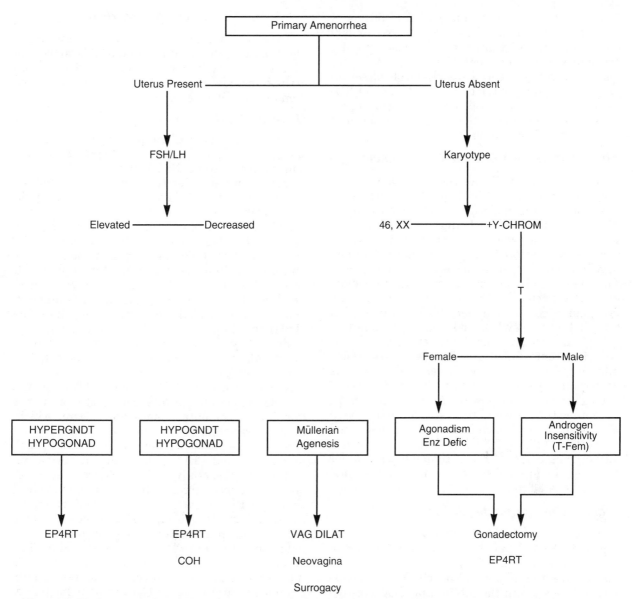

Figure 1. Work-up and treatment approach for primary amenorrhea. *Abbreviations:* E = estrogen; RT = replacement therapy; P4 = progesterone; Enz = enzymatic; COH = controlled ovarian hyperstimulation; Defic = deficiency; VAG = vaginal; DILAT = dilation; HYPERGNDT = hypergonadotropic; HYPOGNDT = hypogonadotropic; HYPOGONAD = hypogonadism; CHROM = chromosome; T = testosterone; T-Fem = testicular feminization.

Ideally, treatment should address the primary illness. Thyroid replacement, glucocorticoid therapy, and estrogen-progesterone replacement should be considered when indicated. Ovulation induction, after the eradication of primary disease in a patient who remains amenorrheic, can be initiated with the lowest dose of either pure FSH (urofollitropin [Metrodin], 75 IU) or human menopausal gonadotropin (menotropins [Pergonal], 75 IU), which is initially maintained for 5 days. After this period, a pelvic ultrasonogram and serum E2 determinations orient the clinician with regard to dosage adjustment to support follicle growth. Menotropin dosage should be increased cautiously because serious life-threatening complications such as ovarian hyperstimulation syndrome (OHSS) can arise. Patients with hypogonadotropic hypogonadism are at great risk for development of the severe form of OHSS.

Ovulation may be triggered with 5000 or 10,000 IU of human chorionic gonadotropin (hCG). Luteal phase support can be accomplished by administering 1500 IU of hCG therapy for three doses every third day.

Alternative therapy includes 12.5 to 50 mg of daily progesterone-in-oil intramuscularly or 300 mg of micronized P4 until the establishment of a pregnancy. Doses of progesterone should be adjusted according to serial weekly levels of serum progesterone during the early first trimester. Patients who become allergic or cannot tolerate intramuscular administration should use the oral progesterone formulation.

Abnormalities of Müllerian Development

Congenital anomalies of the müllerian system are common (1 in 200 to 1 in 600 reproductive-age women), the majority being fusion defects. These abnormalities are found in 15% of patients with primary amenorrhea. These women experience cyclic ovarian function and normal breast development without associated menstrual flow. The complete absence of müllerian duct development is reflected by the absence of the uterus, fallopian tubes, and upper third of the vagina (Mayer-Rokitansky-Kuster-Hauser syndrome).

Vaginal reconstruction by an experienced surgeon is recommended. Alternatively, progressive dilation of the vagina with serial dilators has been quite satisfactory. In vitro fertilization (IVF) surrogacy is the only way to maintain genetic parenthood. Because of the association of severe müllerian system anomalies with chromosomal aberrations (45,X, 47,XXX, and mosaic patterns), karyotyping before IVF is recommended in order to avoid impaired disjunction mechanisms and poorer assisted conception outcomes.

Male Pseudohermaphroditism

Patients with this disorder have a male karyotype (46,XY) and female phenotype with normal breast development. They lack a uterus, and many have a blind vaginal pouch. Serum testosterone levels aid in the differential diagnosis between testicular feminization (T-Fem) (male range) and gonadal/adrenal enzymatic deficiencies (female range). Patients with testicular feminization have normal testosterone production but lack androgen receptor activity and therefore do not respond to circulating testosterone. Patients with female-range serum testosterone levels have either gonadal and adrenal 17α-hydroxylase or 17,20-desmolase deficiency.

These patients are at great risk (20 to 25%) of developing gonadoblastomas and dysgerminomas and should therefore undergo gonadectomy, followed by EP4 replacement, soon after puberty. Although some authors advocate unopposed estrogen therapy, there is considerable evidence in favor of progestin administration to oppose estrogenic mitotic effect on the mammary glands.

Secondary Amenorrhea

An algorithm for the evaluation and management of secondary amenorrhea is shown in Figure 2. Physiologic causes of secondary amenorrhea include pregnancy, lactation, and perimenopausal syndrome.

Hyperprolactinemia

Anterior pituitary gland prolactin (PRL) secretion is under tonic inhibition of hypothalamic dopaminergic neurons. PRL levels vary with stress, breast examination, estrogenemia, sleep, feeding, presence of empty sella syndrome, medical conditions such as renal failure, and use of a large variety of antidopaminergic drugs; therefore, a second blood test should confirm an initial elevated PRL level (>20 ng per mL in the follicular phase and >30 ng per mL in the luteal phase). If serum PRL remains elevated (>30 ng/mL, inasmuch as the woman being evaluated is amenorrheic), the level of thyroid-stimulating hormone (TSH) should be measured to rule out hypothyroidism. Thyrotropin-releasing hormone is known to stimulate PRL production and is elevated in patients with primary hypothyroidism.

A normal serum TSH level should direct the clinician to obtain a pituitary magnetic resonance imaging or computed tomographic scan, whichever is available, to rule out the presence of an adenoma because adenomas can occur with mildly elevated PRL levels. Either a normal pituitary imaging study or the presence of microadenoma (<1 cm) warrants the initiation of medical therapy with a dopamine agonist such as bromocriptine (Parlodel). Dosing should begin at 2.5 mg per day, taken at bedtime, to avoid postural hypotension. A serum PRL measurement should be repeated after 2 weeks and the dose should be increased by 2.5 mg, as needed. Menses usually resumes within 6 weeks of treatment initiation. Intravaginal bromocriptine is a reasonable alternative for patients with intolerable gastrointestinal side effects. The same oral tablet is placed deep into the vaginal fornix.

Women undergoing controlled ovarian hyperstimulation should stop taking bromocriptine on the day of hCG administration. However, if they become pregnant spontaneously, they should discontinue bromocriptine as soon as they become aware of the establishment of pregnancy. Clomiphene citrate (Clomid), a synthetic antiestrogenic compound, can be started to induce ovulation. Therapy is initiated with a 50-mg dose taken orally for 5 days, beginning on day 3 to 5 of a spontaneous or progestin-induced menses. If ovulation does not occur, the dose may be increased by 50 mg per day each month to a maximum of

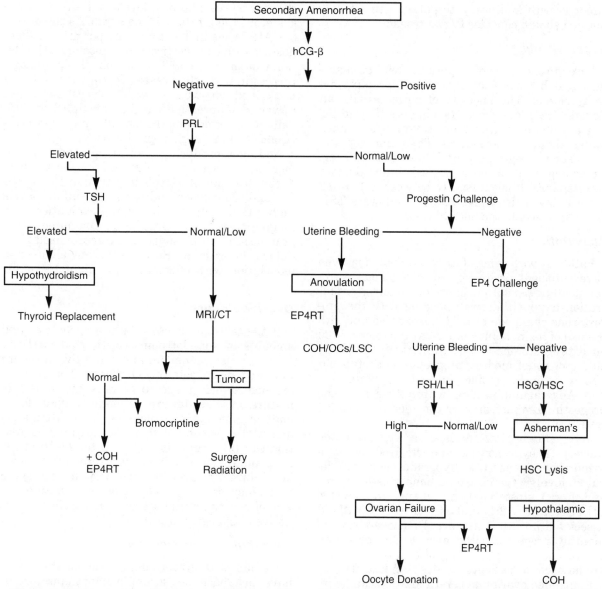

Figure 2. Work-up and treatment of secondary amenorrhea. *Abbreviations:* hCG-β = human chorionic gonadotropin-beta; PRL = prolactin; LH = luteinizing hormone; FSH = follicle-stimulating hormone; TSH = thyroid-stimulating hormone; COH = controlled ovarian hyperstimulation; HSG = hysterosalpingogram; MRI = magnetic resonance imaging; CT = computed tomography; E = estrogen; P4 = progesterone; RT = replacement therapy; HSC = hysteroscopy; LSC = laparoscopy; OCs = oral contraceptives.

250 mg* for 7 days. The use of menotropins should follow if ovulation or pregnancy fails to occur.

Although it appears that bromocriptine is not associated with an increased incidence of fetal malformations, there is no evidence to support the continuation of therapy during pregnancy even in the presence of an adenoma. Symptomatic patients who fail medical therapy should be considered for trans-sphenoidal removal of the

adenoma. In the presence of a pituitary macroadenoma, bromocriptine therapy should be initiated with consideration given to neurosurgery for women who desire pregnancy or radiation therapy for poor surgical candidates.

Mild elevations of serum PRL in the presence of macroadenomas are more frequently observed among patients with growth hormone–, adrenocorticotropic hormone–, TSH-, LH-, and FSH-producing tumors, and therefore a thorough endocrine investigation should be performed. Patients who fail surgical therapy or are at risk for

_____
*Exceeds dosage recommended by the manufacturer.

tumor growth and desire to pursue genetic parenthood should consider IVF surrogacy.

Hypothyroidism

Three to five percent of patients with galactorrhea and hyperprolactinemia have primary hypothyroidism. The majority of patients with an elevated TSH level have Hashimoto's thyroiditis, and antimicrosomal and antithyroglobulin antibodies should be evaluated. Thyroxine replacement should begin with daily doses of 0.05 mg, increasing by 0.05 mg at 2-week intervals to a maintenance dosage, usually between 0.1 to 0.2 mg per day. This dosage effectively lowers TSH and PRL levels to the normal ranges.

Anovulation

Patients with anovulatory amenorrhea who have sufficient production of endogenous estrogen (>40 pg per mL) to cause endometrial proliferation have withdrawal bleeding with the progesterone challenge test. This is carried out with the use of a single intramuscular injection of 200 mg of progesterone-in-oil. Alternatively, oral daily 10-mg doses of medroxyprogesterone acetate for 10 days is an acceptable pharmacologic intervention. Any vaginal bleeding within 2 weeks of the progestin administration is considered a positive response.

Polycystic ovarian disease, a very common cause of anovulation, is characterized by oligomenorrhea-amenorrhea, hyperandrogenism (elevated levels of androstenedione, testosterone, and free testosterone), hirsutism, an elevated LH:FSH ratio (>2:1), and obesity with or without associated insulin resistance. Diet, exercise, and monthly progestin withdrawal or low-dose oral contraceptives (30 to 35 μg of ethinyl estradiol) are advised for patients not desiring fertility.

Controlled ovarian hyperstimulation can be initiated with clomiphene citrate. A daily 0.5-mg dose of dexamethasone may be added to poor responders with elevated adrenal tone. Pure FSH (urofollitropin [Metrodin]) is the drug of choice for clomiphene-resistant patients. Laparoscopic creation of multiple ovarian electrocautery or laser "punctures" with diameters of 5 mm can be accomplished after failure of drug therapy. Cautious exercise is recommended because periadnexal adhesions with resultant infertility may ensue.

Adult-onset congenital adrenal hyperplasia (CAH) is caused by partial 21-hydroxylase deficiency. The clinical presentation is identical to that of polycystic ovary and is prevalent among Ashkenazi Jews, Hispanics, and descendants of Central European immigrants. A screening test that measures 8:00 A.M. levels of 17-hydroxyprogesterone higher than 3.3 ng per mL is suggestive of CAH; levels higher than 8 ng per mL are diagnostic. An adrenocorticotropin hormone stimulation test should be able to rule out this pathologic process in borderline cases. Therapy is similar as prescribed for women with polycystic ovaries; however, suppression can be accomplished with daily doses of dexamethasone (0.5 mg), hydrocortisone (15 to 20 mg), or prednisone (5 mg).

Androgen-producing ovarian and adrenal tumors are a rare cause of secondary amenorrhea. Serum testosterone levels higher than 150 ng per dL and dehydroepiandrosterone sulfate levels higher than 7 μg per dL require evaluation with magnetic resonance imaging or computed tomographic scan of the suggestive compromised glandular compartment. Surgical therapy alone or in association with chemotherapy might be necessary.

Ovarian Failure

Patients with ovarian failure have elevated amounts of gonadotropins (FSH, >30 mIU per mL), hypoestrogenemia, and a positive response to estrogen-progesterone challenge. The onset of menopause before age 40 years is known as premature ovarian failure. Genetic, immunologic, and hormonal evaluation should be conducted and EP4 replacement therapy instituted. Ovulation can be accomplished in up to 20% in some subpopulations of women with premature ovarian failure; however, the prognosis for achieving pregnancy is very poor. Oocyte donation for women with a normal uterus is an excellent alternative to biologic parenthood.

Hypothalamic Amenorrhea

Women with hypothalamic amenorrhea, who have low baseline serum gonadotropin levels, have idiopathic hypothalamic dysfunction and respond to the EP4 challenge. Abnormalities of gonadotropin-releasing hormone (GnRH) and consequently LH pulsatility are hallmarks of this dysfunction, which might be caused by a central nervous system neurotransmitter alteration or a hypothalamic derangement. Intravenous or subcutaneous administration of GnRH, via electronic pump designed to deliver GnRH pulses at 90- to 120-minute intervals with doses ranging between 5 and 10 μg per pulse, is the therapeutic modality of choice. Hypothalamic amenorrhea in conjunction with anosmia characterize Kallman's syndrome. Central nervous system–hypothalamic failure caused by tumors, sarcoidosis, and meningitis may also respond to GnRH treatment after establishment of the primary therapy.

Amenorrhea associated with excessive weight loss has a complex etiology, and it is difficult to isolate stress from weight loss as the sole cause of amenorrhea. The incidence of anorexia nervosa, a psychogenic cause of amenorrhea, is relatively high among high school–aged girls. These patients have severe weight loss, reduced gonadotropin levels, and reduced serum T3 levels, and evaluations also show elevated cortisol and reverse triiodothyronine levels. Dietary counseling and psychiatric treatment are mandatory because mortality rate may reach 10%.

Strenuous exercise and stress are other causes of hypothalamic amenorrhea that is usually associated with weight loss in athletes. Athletes whose amounts of body fat are below the tenth percentile for age are likely to manifest amenorrhea. Menses can be usually restarted by decreasing the amount of physical exercise and following behavioral modifications. Patients with the so-called post-Pill amenorrhea have normal gonadotropin and PRL levels. If menses does not resume within 6 months, a trial of clomiphene citrate is recommended for those desiring fertility. Amenorrhea in nonalcoholic chronic liver disease seems to be related to undernutrition, and the clinical picture appears quite variable. EP4 replacement therapy is recommended.

Uterine Adhesions

The lack of response to EP4 challenge in a eugonadotropic woman indicates the presence of intrauterine adhesions. Adhesions may result from previous uterine instrumentation or infection. Evaluation with either hysterosalpingogram or hysteroscopy with concomitant mechanical or laser adhesiolysis can be curative. Placement of an intrauterine stent, intrauterine device, or pediatric Foley catheter and administration of relatively high doses of conjugated estrogens (Premarin, 2.5 mg twice daily*), along with prophylactic antibiotics, have been successfully used.

Surgical repair of imperforated hymen can be easily accomplished to solve this type of outflow abnormality.

---

*This use of Premarin is not listed in the manufacturer's official directive.

DYSMENORRHEA

method of
LARRY BARMAT, M.D., and
JAY SCHINFELD, M.D.
Abington, Pennsylvania

Dysmenorrhea, or painful menstruation, is one of the most common gynecologic disorders. The incidence of painful menstruation is estimated to affect two-thirds of all postpubescent women. Socioeconomic and psychological consequences result from the impact of this disorder. Examples include increased absenteeism from work or school, poor work performance, and increased levels of depression and neuroticism.

Dysmenorrhea clinically is a cluster of symptoms composed of spasmodic abdominal, thigh, and low back labor-like pains. Associated systemic symptoms, including nausea, vomiting, diarrhea, fatigue, headache, syncope, and nervousness, may also be present. It is important to distinguish primary from secondary dysmenorrhea for effective therapy. The diagnosis of primary dysmenorrhea is reserved for women with no discernible organic pathologic processes, and secondary dysmenorrhea is the diagnosis when concomitant pelvic disease is discovered.

Primary dysmenorrhea occurs in ovulatory cycles. It may manifest at any age but generally begins at menarche or shortly thereafter. The syndrome starts with or before the onset of menstrual flow and typically lasts 48 to 72 hours. A careful history and physical examination fail to disclose a pathologic condition resulting in the menstrual discomfort. Therefore, therapy is directed at the proposed underlying cause of the menstrual pain.

Conversely, secondary dysmenorrhea is diagnosed when a concurrent organic pathologic process is clearly established. This pelvic pain of genital tract origin usually occurs at a later age and lasts longer into the menstrual period than does primary dysmenorrhea. The underlying pelvic condition may be endometriosis, myomas, adenomyosis, polyps, cervical stenosis, pelvic inflammatory disease, or the presence of an intrauterine device. Other causes that should be considered include urinary tract infections, inflammatory or spasmodic bowel disease, and appendicitis. These secondary causes should be discovered in the history and physical examination, and effective therapy should be directed at the underlying cause. Noninvasive as well as invasive studies may be required for proper diagnosis; such studies include pelvic ultrasonography, laparoscopy, hysteroscopy, hysterosalpingography, gastrointestinal studies, and, in rare instances, computed tomographic scan or magnetic resonance imaging.

The pathogenesis of primary dysmenorrhea appears to be increased production and release of endometrial prostaglandins during menstruation. This results in heightened and abnormal uterine activity. There is compelling evidence supporting the role of prostaglandins in primary dysmenorrhea. The administration of exogenous prostaglandins for induction of labor or midtrimester termination produces similar clinical side effects. Elevated levels of prostaglandins have been

TABLE 1. **Prostaglandin Synthetase Inhibitors**

Chemical Group	Drug	Dosage
Benzoic acid	Acetylsalicylic acid (aspirin)	500 mg q 6 h
Butyrophenones	Phenylbutazone (Butazolidin)	Not available
	Oxyphenbutazone	
Indole-3-acetic acid	Indomethecin (Indocin)	25–50 mg q 8 h
Fenamates	Flufenamic acid	500 mg initial dose, then 250 mg q 6 h
	Mefenamic acid (Ponstel)	
	Mebeverine	
Arylpropionic acid	Ibuprofen (Motrin)	400 mg q 6 h
	Naproxen (Naprosyn)	500 mg initial dose, then 250 mg q 4–6 h
	Naproxen sodium (Anaprox)	550 mg initial dose, then 275 mg q 6–8 h
	Ketoprofen (Orudis)	50 mg q 8 h
Miscellaneous	Piroxicam (Feldene)	20–40 mg once a day

found in endometrial samples from dysmenorrheic women. Finally, prostaglandin synthetase inhibitors have been shown to be effective treatment of primary dysmenorrhea. In the small group of primary dysmenorrhea sufferers whose pain is refractory to prostaglandin synthetase inhibitors, recent experiments have focused on leukotrienes, platelet activating factor, and vasopressin as alternative pathogenic causes.

The mechanism of pain is believed to be the product of uterine hyperactivity, uterine ischemia, and a lowered pain threshold of nerve terminals related to production of prostaglandins. The process begins after ovulation, when the production of progesterone by the corpus luteum is enhanced. If fertilization does not occur, the corpus luteum regresses, resulting in a decline of progesterone. Progesterone, which previously stabilized lysosomes, now causes lysosomal labilization. This results in release of phospholipase A_2, which converts endometrial cell phospholipids to arachidonic acid. The pool of arachidonic acid combined with the events culminating in menstrual flow stimulates the arachidonic acid cascade in the direction of prostaglandin production. These elevated levels of prostaglandin in the menstrual fluid stimulate myometrial contractions, ischemia, and increased sensitization to pain.

TREATMENT

Effective treatment of primary dysmenorrhea is accomplished in approximately two-thirds of sufferers with prostaglandin synthetase inhibitors or, if contraception is desired, the oral contraceptive pill. Other therapeutic options include gonadotropin-releasing hormone (GnRH) agonists,* presacral neurectomy, laparoscopic uterosacral nerve ablation (LUNA), transcutaneous electrical nerve stimulation (TENS), calcium-channel blockers,† beta-adrenergic stimulators,‡ and an experimental oxytocin antagonist.

---

*This use of GnRH agonists is not listed in the manufacturer's directive.

†This use of calcium channel blockers is not listed in the manufacturer's directive.

‡This use of beta-adrenergic stimulators is not listed in the manufacturer's directive.

The use of nonsteroidal anti-inflammatory drugs (NSAIDs) relieves primary dysmenorrhea by inhibiting prostaglandin production. This suppresses the menstrual fluid prostaglandin levels and counteracts the proposed cause of pain. The advantages of NSAIDs over hormonal therapy are that NSAIDs need be used only a few days each cycle and do not alter the hormonal milieu of the hypothalamic-pituitary-ovarian axis.

There are five major groups of prostaglandin synthetase inhibitors. All show significant relief of dysmenorrhea with few exceptions. Acetylsalicylic acid, which is inexpensive and widely available, unfortunately is not significantly more effective than placebo. Indomethacin and the butyrophenones are not generally prescribed because of poorly tolerated side effects. The fenamates and the arylpropionic acid derivatives are the most commonly used NSAIDs. Fenamates have an additional property of antagonizing prostaglandin receptors and decreasing the effects of preformed prostaglandins. They also significantly decrease menstrual blood loss in menorrhagic patients. All propionic acid derivatives have relatively equal effectiveness. Ketoprofen has been shown to possibly have a quicker onset of pain relief. The chemical group, drug, and dosages are shown in Table 1.

NSAIDs, if not contraindicated, are taken at the onset of menstrual pain, or just before if the pain is predictable, and are continued for a few days. If relief is not obtained, dosage and type should be altered. This regimen should be continued for at least 3 to 6 months; if it is unsuccessful, a laparoscopy is indicated in order to search for possible undiagnosed pathologic processes.

Oral contraceptive pills constitute another highly effective therapy, especially if contraception is desired. The pill's mechanism of action is through inhibition of ovulation and endometrial growth, causing a suppression in prostaglandin levels in menstrual fluid.

There are four basic formulations of oral contraception, as well as the recently marketed subdermal progestin implants. The pill formulations include monophasics, biphasics, triphasics, and a progestin-only pill. The monophasics contain constant estrogen and progestin doses and were the first developed. As the pill evolved, the biphasic, triphasic, and progestin-only forms were developed; they have a lower total hormonal content and subsequently less of an anovulatory effect. This decreased anovulatory effect also applied to the subdermal progestin implants.

Therapeutic management with the pill is similar to that of NSAIDs. If initial relief is not obtained, an oral contraceptive of another formulation is tried. The addition of an NSAID is also an option. If relief is not obtained in 3 to 6 months, an operative procedure is indicated in order to search for undiagnosed disease.

GnRH agonists, presacral neurectomy, LUNA, and TENS are valuable options for intractable dysmenorrhea. GnRH agonists have defined roles in secondary dysmenorrhea caused by endometriosis and in preoperative management for myoma surgery. Its role may extend to treatment of primary dysmenorrhea. A 4- to 6-month trial of GnRH agonist with the possible addition of a low-dose estrogen supplement may relieve the dysmenorrhea as well as combat the hypoestrogenic side effects of the GnRH agonist. These beneficial effects are generally short-lived, and symptoms recur when the medication is discontinued. Presacral neurectomy and LUNA are relatively effective operations for midline pelvic pain. LUNA offers the advantages of being an outpatient procedure and having a lower incidence of side effects than does presacral neurectomy. Finally, the TENS unit has been shown to provide pure analgesic relief by altering the patient's ability to perceive or receive the pain signal.

The use of beta-mimetic agonists has been shown to decrease uterine tone and contractions. Agonists such as terbutaline, ritodrine, and isoxsuprine have been used in the past, but unwanted side effects such as tremor and palpitations have been poorly tolerated. Calcium channel blockers, which can reduce uterine hyperactivity, also produce poorly tolerated side effects.

An oxytocin antagonist is also being investigated. Studies have shown significant reduction of symptoms, but currently no preparation for oral use is yet available.

With the success of current medical as well as operative therapies, dysmenorrhea may be relieved in the majority of sufferers. Consequently, the quality of their lives has improved, whereas previously it was hindered.

PREMENSTRUAL SYNDROME

method of
H. JANE CHIHAL, M.D., Ph.D.
Trinity Medical Center
Carrollton, Texas

Premenstrual syndrome (PMS) is a syndrome of unknown etiology that causes a recurrent profile of symptoms that are annoying for many women but can be debilitating for 1 to 5% of all women before menopause. The features of PMS are varied and may be physical, psychological, or both. The heterogenicity of these manifestations often causes difficulty in establishing the diagnosis (Table 1). The cyclical manifestation of these symptoms in rhythm with the menstrual cycle is pathognomonic of PMS. The criteria for diagnosis are that (1) symptoms are present to some degree in each menstrual cycle and begin at or after ovulation, (2) symptoms resolve near menses, and (3) the patient is symptom free from the cessation of menses until near the time of ovulation (at least 7 symptom-free days are present each cycle).

The diagnosis of PMS is one of exclusion based on a patient's history, a complete physical examination, and the patient's charting of symptoms. It is particularly important that the chart be kept by the patient on a daily basis for at least two and preferably three menstrual cycles. Retrospective charting of symptoms has been proved to be totally unreliable. Patients retrospectively exaggerate the extent of symptoms, especially in the premenstrual phase of the cycle. The patient should be asked to record, at bedtime, the severity of each day's symptoms. A simple chart with the months listed vertically on the left side and the days of the month horizontally on the top is preferred over more complicated charts. Scoring of the symptoms ranges from 10 (the most severe she has ever experi-

TABLE 1. **Symptoms of Premenstrual Syndrome**

Physical
Abdominal bloating
Edema
Weight gain
Constipation
Hot flashes
Breast pain
Headache
Acne
Rhinitis
Palpitations
Psychological
Anxiety
Depression
Irritability
Wide mood swings
Increased appetite
Aggression
Lethargy or fatigue
Forgetfulness/reduced concentration
Sleep disorders
Phobias

enced) to 0 (no problems that day). An X denotes the days of menstrual flow. The most common symptoms are listed on the back of the chart. The health care professional can then plot day of cycle versus degree of symptoms from 0 to 10 to construct a graphic representation.

It is very important to differentiate premenstrual exacerbation of an underlying psychiatric disorder from "true" PMS. Many patients with anxiety, depression, or a bipolar affective disorder experience premenstrual exacerbation of their symptoms. These patients do not consistently have the 7-day symptom-free period during the follicular phase. Approximately 40 to 50% of patients who present to a health care facility with self-diagnosed PMS do not have this syndrome; rather, they have another psychiatric diagnosis, most commonly endogenous depression. The treatment of PMS may continue for many years. To be effective, therapy obviously must begin with a correct diagnosis. Because the severity of PMS may vary significantly from cycle to cycle and depression often varies spontaneously, several cycles may have to be carefully studied in order to differentiate these disorders. Patients often prefer the diagnosis of PMS and resist the diagnosis of depression. Both of these disorders seem to be derangements of the central nervous system biochemistry. However, PMS is a more socially acceptable problem.

Perimenopausal problems caused by decreased estrogen production can also mimic PMS. Hot flashes, vaginal dryness, difficulty sleeping, and menstrual cycle irregularity often occur in the transition phase from normal-cycle menses to the cessation of menses. However, hot flashes also often occur in the luteal phase of the menstrual cycle during PMS symptoms, and there is often a concurrent sleep disorder. The manifestations of estrogen deprivation are most effectively treated with appropriate estrogen supplementation. The most common ages for PMS complaints are 25 to 40, the later years of which can also overlap with the perimenopause. If there is any question of the etiology of the symptoms, a follicle-stimulating hormone (FSH) level in serum on cycle days 2, 3, or 4 can be helpful in ruling out the climacteric as the cause of the symptoms. An elevation in FSH above 20 in the early follicular phase often indicates the start of the climacteric, and a level consistently above 30 is diagnostic. (The FSH level is always elevated at midcycle just before ovulation.)

The history and physical examination results sometimes indicate the need for other laboratory testing to rule out medical disorders such as lupus and other connective tissue disorders, thyroid disease, diabetes, and Cushing's syndrome. The routine use of laboratory screening tests is expensive and unrewarding. Laboratory testing should be ordered only if specific indications are found in the history and physical examination. For example, patients with a tremor, weight loss, anxiety, or an enlarged tender thyroid certainly need a complete thyroid evaluation. A woman with hypertension, depression, and truncal obesity should be screened with an overnight cortisol suppression test. Patients might perceive these symptoms as cyclical when they are really just randomly variable.

Dysmenorrhea and cyclical pelvic pain are not part of the PMS complex of symptoms. Patients often mis-take these pain syndromes as PMS. Dysmenorrhea may be functional, resulting from the overproduction of prostaglandins, or may be associated with endometriosis.

Undiagnosed pelvic pain syndromes should be completely evaluated by a pelvic examination, pelvic ultrasonography, and ultimately, if necessary, a diagnostic laparoscopy to rule out endometriosis, pelvic adhesions, and pelvic inflammatory disease.

It is often difficult to convince the patient of the importance of the 2 to 3 months of baseline studies necessary to make an accurate diagnosis of PMS. Everyone is interested in rapid diagnosis and a quick cure. It is important in the early phases of education of patients to emphasize that this diagnosis may significantly affect their well-being for many years. The diagnosis should be made carefully and completely. A patient may have been ridiculed or merely labeled "neurotic" by others from whom she has sought help. Taking her complaints seriously and instituting appropriate testing is often all that is needed to elicit cooperation. These early months of evaluation can also be used for education, lifestyle alterations, and counseling. If after the baseline history, physical examination, two- or three–menstrual cycle diary, and any indicated laboratory testing there is still a question of diagnosis, more sophisticated psychological testing should be done.

In addition, difficult cases can often be evaluated by making the patient temporarily menopausal with a gonadotropin-releasing hormone (GnRH) agonist such as leuprolide* (Lupron), which is injected every 4 weeks (3.75 or 7.5 mg), or nafarelin† (Synarel), which is a nasal spray used in each nostril twice daily. These GnRH agonists down-regulate the reproductive system to stop the menstrual cycle after an initial stimulation period of 2 to 3 weeks. A serum estradiol level of less than 40 after the second injection of leuprolide or after 4 to 6 weeks of nafarelin helps ensure adequate suppression. The patient experiences hot flashes. The medication can be continued for 6 months.

Any PMS symptoms should cease after 2 months of adequate suppression. If symptoms persist into the third month of therapy, it is highly unlikely that PMS is the cause of symptoms. The GnRH agonists are currently more helpful for diagnosis than for therapy. Long-term or repeated use of these medications could result in osteoporosis. In the future, the use of GnRH agonists with "add-back" therapy with estrogen and progestin may prove to be a good therapeutic approach for severe PMS that is unresponsive to other therapies. The efficacy and safety of this approach has not been determined. The GnRH agonists can be used as a trial for patients who are contemplating a hysterectomy and bilateral salpingo-oophorectomy as therapy for PMS. Such a radical surgical approach should obviously be reserved for severely affected patients whose symptoms do not adequately respond to other therapies. If the symptoms are not relieved by a trial of a GnRH

---

*This use of leuprolide is not listed in the manufacturer's directive.

†This use of nafarelin is not listed in the manufacturer's directive.

agonist, surgical castration will likely not be effective, and the patient should be more completely evaluated for other possible diagnoses.

THERAPEUTIC OPTIONS

Lifestyle Changes and Stress Reduction

No conclusive data show that PMS is caused by any nutritional deficiency or that the syndrome can be relieved by alteration of the diet or by nutritional supplements. However, reactive hypoglycemia can exacerbate PMS symptoms. Frequent, low-fat, high–complex carbohydrate meals with adequate protein can decrease fatigue and improve weight control. Regular aerobic exercise decreases depression and the symptoms of stress. Patients with PMS are more reactive to stressful situations. Generalized stress-reduction techniques can decrease symptoms. Many patients can link the start of symptoms to a stressful situation such as the birth of a child, death, divorce, or loss of employment.

Increased consumption of caffeine is correlated with increased risk of PMS. Patients should decrease caffeine intake and limit the use of alcohol. Patients with PMS are more likely to have a history of drug or alcohol abuse than are patients without PMS.

The empirical use of large doses of pyridoxine should be especially condemned because in high doses, this vitamin can cause permanent neurologic abnormalities. Patients should be warned not to take more than 100 mg daily.

Several studies have shown that vitamin E can decrease some PMS symptoms, especially breast tenderness. Usually 400 IU daily is recommended.

Medications

In most initial studies, investigators assumed that PMS was caused by an alteration in hormone levels during the menstrual cycle, and low progesterone production was the most commonly hypothesized problem. Several well-designed studies have failed to show any abnormalities in estradiol, progesterone, prolactin, dehydroepiandrosterone sulfate, testosterone, aldosterone, FSH, or luteinizing hormone in PMS patients in comparison with non-PMS controls.

The medication most commonly prescribed for PMS has been progesterone supplementation, either as a vaginal suppository or as an oral capsule. All PMS studies show a significant placebo effect, which often decreases if the study continues for three cycles. None of the well-designed, placebo-controlled studies have shown that progesterone suppositories are helpful in treating PMS; however, they have not been shown to be harmful, either. There are still significant numbers of PMS patients who believe that progesterone definitely improves their symptoms. Progesterone suppositories are usually used at doses of 800 to 1200 mg daily in three equal doses starting at least 3 days before anticipated symptoms.

Spironolactone, a potassium-sparing diuretic, has been extensively studied in the treatment of PMS. None of the well-designed, placebo-controlled studies show significant improvement. Other diuretics have not been shown to improve PMS and can cause significant side effects. Diuretic abuse is common. The abdominal bloating in the premenstrual phase is attributable more to fluid shifts than to actual increased body fluid.

In addition, there is no convincing evidence that bromocriptine (Parlodel) improves PMS. If a patient has galactorrhea, an appropriate work-up with prolactin levels should be obtained. Bromocriptine should be used in specific cases of well-documented hyperprolactinemia not caused by a thyroid disorder.

Prostaglandin inhibitors such as mefenamic acid (Ponstel) and naproxen sodium (Anaprox) are effective therapies for dysmenorrhea and have also been shown in some studies to decrease the symptoms of PMS, including depression and irritability.

Danazol* (Danocrine) in daily doses of 200 to 800 mg has been shown to significantly decrease PMS symptoms. However, the side effects of this mild androgen are often as frustrating as the PMS itself. The side effects are dose related and usually are not significant at the 200-mg level, which can be helpful in PMS. This dose does not inhibit ovulation, and a female fetus conceived while this medication was used can become masculinized. Effective contraception is very important.

Because PMS is associated with ovulation, the use of oral contraceptives seems like a logical therapeutic option. However, there are no placebo-controlled, double-blind studies to support this supposition. A recent trial of a tricyclic pill failed to show any improved response. Some patients with PMS who take oral contraceptives have symptoms the entire cycle, especially depression.

In women in whom depression is the main symptom, fluoxetine (Prozac) to treat PMS has been shown to be effective. Because it takes 10 to 14 days for a significant response to this medication to be seen, it should be used the entire menstrual cycle. The average dose is 20 mg daily as a one-time morning dose.

*This use of danazol is not listed in the manufacturer's official directive.

In women in whom the main symptom is anxiety, two medications have been shown to have significant therapeutic value: alprazolam (Xanax) and buspirone (BuSpar). Alprazolam should be started at the anticipated time of the onset of symptoms in an average daily dose of 2.25 mg. The starting dose of alprazolam should be 0.25 mg three or four times daily and titrated until symptoms are controlled. The medication is decreased by 25% each day after the start of menses. Tapering the medication can preclude many of the side effects of withdrawal, including anxiety, tremors, and palpitations. Alprazolam is an addictive medication and can cause significant drowsiness, making driving potentially hazardous. Because the incidence of drug abuse is increased among PMS patients, use of this medication must be carefully monitored.

Buspirone is not addictive and has no abuse potential. Drowsiness is minimal. Patients initially start on 5 mg three times daily for 4 to 5 days and then take 10 mg three times daily. An excellent response rate of over 80% has been reported among women in whom anxiety is the main PMS symptom. Because, as mentioned, the potential for abuse of alprazolam is high, buspirone is the drug of choice.

MENOPAUSE

method of
BRIAN W. WALSH, M.D., and
ISAAC SCHIFF, M.D.

Harvard Medical School
Boston, Massachusetts

Menopause is the permanent cessation of menses. It occurs when the ovaries, as a consequence of aging, become depleted of follicles and no longer produce estradiol. The average age at menopause has not changed since antiquity; as a result, increases in life expectancy mean that American women today will spend one-third of their lifetime after ovarian failure. Thus successful management of the problems related to the menopause will become increasingly important in the coming decades.

In this article, the authors review the pathogenesis and current approach to management of the major problems associated with the menopause: vasomotor flushes, osteoporosis, genital atrophy, and atherosclerosis. The use and potential complications of estrogen and progestin therapy are also discussed.

VASOMOTOR FLUSHES

Among the most frequent and troublesome symptoms at the climacteric are vasomotor flushes, or hot flashes, which occur in approximately 80% of women within 3 months of the menopause. This problem persists for more than 1 year in most cases.

A hot flash is the subjective sensation of intense warmth of the upper body, typically lasting about 4 minutes. This sensation is accompanied by a visible ascending flush of the thorax, neck, and face and is followed by profuse sweating. Hot flashes frequently awaken patients from sleep, causing insomnia and fatigue. This may then lead to secondary symptoms such as irritability, impairment of memory, and poor concentration.

Hot flashes result from the acute withdrawal of estrogens, either by menopause or by discontinuation of exogenous estrogen. For example, women with Turner's syndrome, who are hypoestrogenic, do not have hot flashes unless they discontinue exogenous estrogen treatment. Similarly, if men are prescribed estrogens, they may experience hot flashes if the medication is later discontinued. Estrogen appears to act via central neurotransmitters that stabilize the thermoregulatory center in the hypothalamus.

Treatment

The administration of estrogens is effective in relieving hot flashes in more than 95% of women. The benefit of estrogens is not seen immediately; a minimum of 2 to 4 weeks' treatment is usually necessary to relieve hot flashes. Thus the dose should not be increased before this time because of presumed resistance to therapy. If estrogens are to be discontinued, they should be tapered slowly to minimize recurrent symptoms.

Progestins are 70% effective in relieving hot flashes and are useful for women in whom estrogens are contraindicated. The usual dose of medroxyprogesterone acetate is 10 mg orally per day or 50 to 150 mg intramuscularly every 3 months. Progesterone, like estrogen, appears to act via central neurotransmitters, inasmuch as it is known to raise body temperature during the luteal phase in ovulatory women.

Another alternative, which is effective in 30 to 40% of cases, is clonidine, a centrally acting alpha-adrenergic agonist. Clonidine may act by inhibiting the binding of norepinephrine in the hypothalamus, the release of which may be the event that initiates hot flashes. This drug is associated with a high incidence of side effects, such as dizziness and dry mouth. Thus hypertensive patients are the best candidates for this agent if hormonal therapy is not being used. The initial dose of clonidine is 0.1 mg twice daily; this may be increased to 0.2 twice daily, if there are no side effects and the hot flashes persist.

OSTEOPOROSIS

Osteoporosis is a progressive reduction in bone mass without qualitative abnormalities. It affects trabecular bone earlier than cortical bone, and the major consequence is fracture. The most frequent sites of fracture are the vertebral bodies, the distal radius, and the femoral neck. The seriousness of postmenopausal osteoporosis, which is estimated to carry an annual health care cost in the United States of about $7 billion, can be appreciated from the following observations:

1. Vertebral fractures are demonstrated on x-ray in 25% of women over age 60 and in 50% of women over age 75.

2. Hip fractures occur in 25% of women beyond age 80; the annual incidence is 1.3% per year after age 65 and 3.3% per year after age 85.

3. One of six women with a hip fracture dies within 3 months of the event.

Peak bone mass is achieved in normal women at age 30 and then falls progressively at a rate of approximately 1 to 2% per year after age 40. However, the rate of bone loss increases to 4% per year for the 6 years after the menopause. Women with a lower peak bone mass before menopause are more likely to manifest significant osteoporosis; thus white women and Asian women are at higher risk than black women, and thin women are at higher risk than obese women. More rapid bone loss is also more likely in women who smoke, drink alcohol, are sedentary, or consume a low-calcium or a high-protein and high-phosphate diet. Family history of osteoporosis is also a significant risk factor.

Estrogen deficiency is the cause of osteoporosis of 95% of cases. Other etiologic factors include glucocorticoid or heparin use, chronic renal failure, hyperthyroidism, primary hyperparathyroidism, hyperadrenalism, dietary calcium deficiency, and surgery on the upper gastrointestinal tract. Because osteoporosis resulting from menopause is a diagnosis of exclusion, women with osteoporosis or osteoporosis-related fractures should be evaluated for these less common problems. Measurement of plasma calcium, phosphate, and alkaline phosphatase levels, the erythrocyte sedimentation rate, and serum protein electrophoresis may be helpful in diagnosing one of these disorders; results of all of these tests are normal in women with primary osteoporosis.

Treatment

Established osteoporosis cannot be significantly reversed. As a result, medical management must emphasize prevention rather than treatment. Measures such as stopping smoking, exercising regularly, and reducing dietary phosphate may be beneficial.

Of greatest efficacy, however, is the administration of estrogens. Estrogens decrease bone resorption, increase intestinal calcium absorption, and reduce urinary calcium excretion, all of which may serve to prevent osteoporosis. Conjugated equine estrogens (CEE), in a dose of 0.625 mg per day, have proved to minimize bone loss and diminish the incidence of fractures. CEE is maximally effective when begun shortly after the menopause to prevent the rapid bone loss that occurs at that time. CEE therapy should be continued for at least 6 years, to reduce the lifetime risk of fracture. There is as yet no ideal method to identify which women will manifest osteoporosis; thus postmenopausal women should discuss this therapy with their physicians, particularly if their baseline bone density is low.

Calcium supplementation can modestly reduce the rate of bone loss. Calcium is not a substitute for estrogen therapy, but it can serve as a useful adjunct that may allow use of a lower dose of estrogen. The amount of calcium required for maintaining positive calcium balance—1500 mg per day—exceeds that found in most diets; as a result, oral supplements are usually necessary. Caution should be used in administration of calcium supplements to patients with a history of kidney stones.

GENITAL ATROPHY

The tissues of the lower vagina, labia, urethra, and trigone are estrogen dependent and become pale and thin after the loss of estrogen at menopause. The local environment also changes at this time: Before menopause, the vaginal epithelial cells are rich in glycogen. Metabolism of this glycogen by lactobacilli creates an acid environment that protects the vagina from bacterial overgrowth. Loss of this protective mechanism after menopause leaves the thin, friable tissue vulnerable to infection and ulceration. Thus patients may experience vaginal discharge, burning, itching, or bleeding. They also may complain of symptoms secondary to vaginal dryness, such as dyspareunia, vaginismus, or diminished libido.

The urethra and urinary trigone undergo similar atrophic changes. Dysuria, urgency, frequency, and suprapubic pain may occur in the absence of infection. A proposed mechanism is that the markedly thin urethral mucosa allows urine to come in close contact with sensory nerves. In addition, loss of the resistance to urinary flow by a thick, well-vascularized urethral mucosa has been hypothesized to contribute to urinary incontinence.

Atrophic vaginitis can be diagnosed by its typical appearance; however, biopsy specimens of all atypical lesions should be obtained. If a discharge is present, the patient should be evaluated for pathogens such as *Candida,* gonorrhea, *Chlamydia, Trichomonas,* and *Gardenerella.* If *Candida* is found, the patient should be screened for diabetes mellitus, because the normally low glycogen content of unestrogenized vaginal epithelial cells ordinarily does not support the growth of *Candida.* Atrophic urethritis or trigonitis is diagnosed by ruling out the presence of infection.

Treatment

Estrogen is the only effective therapy for genital atrophy. The dose required generally is less than that needed for hot flashes or osteoporosis; as a result, treatment for these conditions is also adequate for genital atrophy. Daily estrogen use for a minimum of 2 to 12 weeks, followed by intermittent therapy two to three times a week, is required in order to reverse atrophy. Estrogens can be administered orally or vaginally; typical vaginal doses are 0.3 mg of CEE or 0.2 mg of micronized beta-estradiol. Although these estrogens predominantly act locally, a portion is absorbed systemically, which possibly leads to endometrial hyperplasia (described in the section "Side Effects of Estrogen Replacement"). Thus intermittent use of a progestin is recommended for patients with an intact uterus.

If estrogens are contraindicated, synthetic mucopolysaccharides or water-soluble lubricants can relieve dyspareunia. Vaginal stenosis can be improved by the use of graduated vaginal dilators.

ATHEROSCLEROSIS

Cardiovascular disease (CVD) is the leading cause of death among women in industrialized countries, including more than 50% of postmenopausal women. Estrogens have been thought to protect against atherosclerosis, because the incidence of CVD is quite low before the menopause. As an example, the rate of cardiovascular mortality in premenopausal women is approximately one-fifth that of age-matched men; after menopause, the rate rapidly rises to approach that of men. Similarly, among women who undergo a premature surgical menopause (after bilateral oophorectomy) and who do not use estrogen replacement, the rate of CVD is twice as high as that among age-matched premenopausal controls. There is, however, no increase in cardiovascular risk if estrogens are administered.

A protective effect of estrogens against CVD may be mediated in part by alterations in lipid metabolism. Before menopause, women have lower plasma levels of low-density lipoprotein (LDL) than do men; after menopause, however, LDL levels rapidly rise to exceed those of men. In contrast, the plasma concentration of high-density lipoprotein (HDL), which is cardioprotective, remains constant throughout a woman's lifetime and exceeds that in men. Estrogens may also protect against CVD by promoting vasodilatation.

Treatment

Exogenous estrogens have a favorable effect on the lipid profile: They raise HDL by 16 to 18% and lower atherogenic LDL by 15 to 19%. Both these actions serve to reduce cardiovascular risk and are mediated by estrogen-induced increases in HDL production and in LDL clearance from the circulation via enhanced hepatic uptake.

In comparison, progestins, particularly the androgenic 19-nortestosterone derivatives norethindrone and norgestrel, have the opposite actions: lowering HDL and raising LDL (discussed in the section "Progestins"). Progestins are usually given in combination with estrogen; the net effect of a particular regimen on lipid metabolism depends on the particular estrogen and progestin used, as well as the day of the cycle on which the measurements are obtained.

In a number of epidemiologic studies, the incidences of CVD among postmenopausal estrogen users and nonusers have been compared; in nearly all, estrogen users have been found to have less CVD. For example, the Nurse's Health Study found the relative risk of CVD among current estrogen users to be 0.56%. Although these analyses were controlled for many confounding factors, the results can also be explained by the fact that healthier women are more likely to seek and to be prescribed estrogens by their physicians. Definitive proof of the benefit of estrogens in reducing CVD may be provided by a long-term, large-scale, placebo-controlled clinical trial planned by the National Institutes of Health.

SIDE EFFECTS OF ESTROGEN REPLACEMENT

Estrogens can cause a number of symptoms, including nausea, mastalgia, headache, and mood changes. There are, in addition, a number of more serious concerns.

Endometrial Neoplasia

Unopposed estrogen use (i.e., without the addition of a progestin) can induce endometrial hyperplasia and, ultimately, adenocarcinoma. Unopposed estrogen use appears to increase the risk of endometrial cancer two- to four-fold, from 1 to 4 per 1000 women per year; the incidence is related to both the dose and the duration (minimum, 1 to 2 years) of estrogen use. Endometrial carcinomas associated with estrogen use are generally of early stage and low grade and are not likely to have deeply invaded the myometrium. The adjusted 5-year survival rate in affected women is 94%, possibly a result of earlier diagnosis in these closely followed patients.

The concurrent administration of progestins can both prevent and reverse hyperplasia; their use has been found to reduce the incidence of endometrial cancer to a level below that among women not receiving any hormonal therapy. The duration of monthly progestin use is important. Seven days' treatment per month lowers the annual incidence of hyperplasia to 3%, whereas 13 days' treatment reduces this risk to essentially zero.

Breast Neoplasia

The possibility that estrogen use might increase the risk of breast cancer was raised because of the following observations: (1) breast cancer can be an estrogen-sensitive tumor; (2) estrogens can induce mammary tumors in rodents; and (3) women with prolonged endogenous estrogen exposure (as occurs with early menarche, late menopause, and nulliparity) are at increased risk of breast malignancies. Despite these observations, most epidemiologic studies have not revealed an increased incidence of breast cancer in postmenopausal estrogen users. However, there does appear to be a small increase in risk among women who used estrogen for more than 10 years or who have a very strong family history of breast cancer.

The possibility that the addition of a progestin may protect against breast cancer has been suggested but remains unproved. As noted earlier, progestins do minimize or prevent endometrial hyperplasia and cancer; however, the use of these agents in women without a uterus is unnecessary and possibly detrimental in view of the adverse effect of progestins on lipid metabolism.

Gallbladder Disease

Estrogen replacement has been found to increase the incidence of gallbladder disease by 20% during the first year of use. This complication is presumably mediated by increased cholesterol saturation of bile, which leads to precipitation and stone formation.

Other Conditions

Estrogen replacement may possibly increase the risk of endometrioid cancer of the ovary (which constitutes 10 to 20% of all ovarian malignancies). It is not known whether progestin use reduces this risk, if it indeed exists. Use of oral contraceptives, particularly those with the highest estrogen content, has been linked to thromboembolic disease, hypertension, and glucose intolerance. These responses are dose dependent, and controlled epidemiologic studies of the use of less potent postmenopausal estrogen have revealed no increase in thrombotic events, hypertension, or glucose intolerance. Postmenopausal diabetic women treated with estrogen typically show no change or actually show an improvement in glucose tolerance, as evidenced by lower glucose levels in plasma and reduced requirements for insulin.

Contraindications to Estrogen Use

There are both absolute and relative contraindications to the postmenopausal administration of estrogens. Absolute contraindications include the following:

1. Known or suspected endometrial or breast cancer.
2. Genital bleeding of uncertain cause.
3. Active liver disease.
4. Active thromboembolic disease or a history of estrogen-related thromboembolic disease.

Relative contraindications include chronic liver dysfunction (the liver's ability to metabolize estrogen is impaired, which leads to excessive levels of estrogen), pre-existing uterine leiomyomata and active endometriosis (estrogen use may prevent the involution of these conditions, which typically regress after the menopause), poorly controlled hypertension, a history of thromboembolic disease, and acute intermittent porphyria (estrogens are known to precipitate attacks).

PROGESTINS

Progestins are used primarily to prevent estrogen-induced endometrial stimulation. They can also relieve hot flashes in patients who are not candidates for estrogen replacement. Medroxyprogesterone acetate, 10 mg per day, is effective against hyperplasia, with minor effects on serum lipids. A lower dose, 5 mg per day, can be used in patients in whom side effects develop, such as abdominal bloating, mastalgia, headaches, mood changes, and acne. This dose offers protection against hyperplasia, unless the patient is a poor absorber of medroxyprogesterone acetate. Alternative available progestins are megestrol acetate (Megace), 40 to 80 mg per day; micronized progesterone, 200 mg to 300 mg daily; and norethindrone, 1.05 mg per day. Because all progestins can decrease plasma levels of HDL-cholesterol, there is a concern that they may negate, in part, the protective effect of estrogen against cardiovascular disease. Thus progestins should be prescribed at the minimum dose needed to prevent endometrial cancer.

RECOMMENDATIONS

At present, data are insufficient to indicate that all postmenopausal women must be treated with estrogen replacement. For that reason, the benefits and risks, as they pertain to each patient, should be reviewed in detail. Ultimately, it is the patient who must make an informed decision.

Patients considered for hormonal therapy should provide a complete history and undergo physical examination, including blood pressure measurement, breast and pelvic examination, and Papanicolaou smear. Mammography should be performed initially to avoid estrogen administration in a patient with pre-existing, subclinical breast cancer; it should be repeated yearly after age 50. An endometrial biopsy should be performed if the patient is likely to have pre-existing endometrial hyperplasia (risk factors are obesity and the presence of abnormal vaginal bleeding). Endometrial sampling can be accomplished by endometrial aspiration or, if this is not possible, by fractional dilatation and curettage. Patients who will receive unopposed estrogens for an extended time should undergo biopsy before therapy is instituted and yearly thereafter regardless of bleeding, because the annual incidence of hyperplasia is 30%.

The most commonly used schedule of hormone replacement in the United States for women with intact uteri is cyclic. CEE is given in a dose of 0.625 mg per day, and medroxyprogesterone acetate is given in a dose of 10 mg per day for the first 13 calendar days of each month. On this regimen, many patients demonstrate withdrawal bleeding, usually occurring between days 11 and 20 of each month. An endometrial biopsy should be performed if bleeding occurs at any other time. Progestin therapy is not needed for women who have had a hysterectomy.

This schedule can be modified by substituting another estrogen for CEE, such as 1 mg per day of micronized estradiol, 1.25 mg per day of piperazine estrone sulfate (Ogen), or 0.05 mg twice a week of transdermal estradiol. A different progestin can also be substituted for medroxyprogesterone acetate.

A continuous rather than cyclic regimen is commonly used in women who want to avoid withdrawal bleeding. Medroxyprogesterone acetate is given in a dose of 5 mg per day with CEE, 0.625 to 1.25 mg per day, as needed to control symptoms. Most women have irregular vaginal bleeding for the first 2 to 3 months, but amenorrhea usually occurs by 1 year. Some women will not tolerate this bleeding and will discontinue treatment. The daily medroxyprogesterone acetate dose can be reduced to 2.5 mg after several months, especially if lower doses of CEE (0.625 mg) per day are used. If medroxyprogesterone acetate leads to unacceptable abdominal bloating and mastalgia, norethindrone (0.35 to 1.05 mg per day) can be given.

VULVOVAGINITIS

method of
LYNN BROOKS, M.D.
St. John Hospital—Nassau Bay
Houston, Texas

Vulvovaginitis is one of the most common gynecologic complaints seen in clinical practice. Vaginal discharge is one of the 25 most common reasons why women consult their physicians, and approximately 40% of those complaining of vaginal symptoms have some type of vaginitis. Symptoms may include vaginal discharge, itching, vaginal odor, vaginal discomfort, dysuria, and dyspareunia. Three types of vaginitis in women of reproductive age account for over 90% of all cases of infections: bacterial vaginosis (BV), vulvovaginal candidiasis (VVC) and trichomoniasis, which occurs less frequently than BV or VVC. Other causes include atrophic vaginitis, lichen sclerosus, atopic or allergic vulvovaginitis, and seborrheic dermatitis; additional causes are included in Table 1.

Diagnosis and treatment of vulvovaginitis are straightforward in most cases; however, many patients have persistent or recurrent infection, and others, who

TABLE 1. **Causes of Vulvovaginitis**

Bacterial vaginosis
Vulvovaginal candidiasis
Trichomoniasis vaginalis
Atrophic vaginitis
Postpartum atrophic vaginitis
Allergic or chemical reaction
Foreign body
Ulcerative vaginitis associated with Crohn's disease or *Staphylococcus aureus*/toxic shock syndrome
Desquamative inflammatory vaginitis
Beta-hemolytic streptococcal vaginitis
Collagen vascular disease
Scabies
Lichen sclerosus
Seborrheic dermatitis

have a less distinctive type of vaginitis, often receive inadequate or unsatisfactory treatment. Because the patient usually presents with a history of vulvovaginitis, the examination must include a detailed description of symptoms and their duration; the consistency, color, and odor of discharge; a sexual history (including recent change in sexual partners); a menstrual history; and a record of past therapy and response to therapy.

A thorough examination should include (1) careful inspection of the vaginal mucosa for vulvar erythema, excoriations or lesions, petechiae, ulcerations, edema, atrophy, and adherent discharge; (2) assessment of pooled vaginal secretions for color, consistency, volume, and odor; and (3) inspection of the cervix for eversion, friability, and color of mucus. The physician must perform a careful systematic inspection and palpation with a cotton-tipped swab of the vulva, including the vestibule, which often is overlooked. Vestibular gland adenitis (focal vulvitis, vulvar vestibulitis syndrome, vulvodynia) is not a form of vaginitis, although it is frequently misdiagnosed as one. The hallmark of vestibular gland adenitis is introital dyspareunia, although patients may complain of pain with tampon insertion, biking, or wearing of tight clothes.

The physician should obtain samples of the discharge from the middle third of the posterior vagina to perform the following tests:

1. pH: paper that distinguishes pHs in the range of 4.0 to 5.0 (Table 2).
2. Amine test: a fishy odor (positive amine or whiff test) is produced upon alkalinization of vaginal secretions when a drop of 10% potassium hydroxide (KOH) solution is added to a drop of vaginal discharge.
3. Saline preparation for identifying clue cells and trichomonads.
4. 10% KOH preparation for identification of hyphae and pseudomycelia.
5. Cultures for yeast and bacteria in the presence of negative microscopy.
6. Specimens for identification of *Chlamydia trachomatis*, *Neisseria gonorrhoeae*, and herpes simplex virus if cervicitis is suspected.

BACTERIAL VAGINOSIS

Previously called "nonspecific vaginitis," *Gardnerella vaginalis* vaginitis, or *Haemophilus vaginalis* vaginitis, BV is the most prevalent cause of vaginitis in sexually active women and is characterized by the overgrowth of several species of facultative anaerobes. The descriptive term, "vaginosis," is more appropriate than "vaginitis" because vaginal inflammation is not a feature of BV. Although there is massive overgrowth of anaerobes and of *Gardnerella*, *Mycoplasma*, and *Mobiluncus* spp., no single bacterial species is known to be responsible for BV. BV has been linked to preterm labor, premature rupture of the membranes, postoperative and postpartum infections, and pelvic inflammatory disease.

TABLE 2. **Diagnostic Findings with Normal Secretions and Vaginitis**

Condition	Symptoms	Appearance of Discharge	pH	Amine Test	Clue Cells	Trichomonads	Mycelia	Other Microscopic Findings
Normal	None or physiologic discharge	Clear or white; nonhomogeneous; scant to moderate amount	<4.5	Absent	Absent	Absent	Absent	Normal epithelial cells, predominance of lactobacilli
Bacterial vaginosis	Malodorous discharge	White or gray; homogeneous; ± bubbles, moderate amount	>4.5	Present	Present	Absent	Absent	Predominance of coccobacilli, few to no leukocytes
Vulvovaginal candidiasis	Pruritus, discharge	Thick white; homogeneous; clumped but variable; ± vulvar, introital, and vaginal edema and erythema; variable amount	<4.5	Absent	Absent	Absent	Present	Normal flora
Trichomoniasis	Pruritus, fishy odor, discharge	Gray, yellow-green, or white; thin; odorous; homogeneous; ± vulvar and vaginal erythema	>4.5	Absent	Absent	Present	Absent	Many polymorphonuclear leukocytes, large amount of cellular debris
Atrophic vaginitis	Pruritus; bleeding or spotting	Scant, purulent bloody discharge; smooth; pale; atrophic epithelium; ± submucosal hemorrhages	6–7	Absent	Absent	Absent	Absent	Moderate number of white blood cells; few lactobacilli

In women with BV, the numbers of lactobacilli present in the vagina are reduced. Increased substrate availability, increased pH, and loss of the normal lactobacillus-dominated vaginal flora are common theories explaining the development of BV. In normal women, lactobacilli, which usually produce hydrogen peroxide (H_2O_2), are the predominant organisms. Only 50% of women in whom BV is diagnosed have lactobacilli, and most of these lactobacilli do not produce H_2O_2. Anaerobes then predominate and, in turn, produce amines, which are responsible for the unpleasant fishy odor and elevation of the pH.

The cardinal symptom of BV is the malodorous vaginal discharge, which often appears after unprotected intercourse. Abdominal pain, pruritus, dysuria, and dyspareunia are not manifestations of BV. A homogeneous grayish-white adherent discharge often is visible at the introitus. There is much less vulvovaginal irritation with BV than with candidiasis or trichomoniasis. BV is diagnosed when (1) there is the characteristic homogeneous discharge, which is sometimes frothy, (2) the result of the amine test is positive, (3) the vaginal pH is greater than 4.5, and, most important, (4) clue cells are present on wet mount specimens. Clue cells are exfoliated vaginal squamous epithelial cells that are so heavily covered with *Gardnerella vaginalis* that a granular or stippled appearance is produced and clear cell borders are obscured. This is the most reliable predictor of BV. Epithelial cells with few bacteria and clear borders should not be misidentified as clue cells. In addition to clue cells on wet mount specimens, there is a lack of polymorphonuclear leukocytes (PMNs), a paucity of lactobacilli, and a predominance of coccobacillary organisms.

Treatment

A greater than 90% cure rate can be achieved with metronidazole (Flagyl), 500 mg orally twice daily for 1 week. Single-dose therapy with 2 grams of metronidazole achieves immediate clinical response, but recurrence rates are higher than with the longer treatment regimen. The efficacy of metronidazole vaginal gel, one applicatorful twice daily for 5 days, is similar to that of oral therapy. Clindamycin, administered as one applicatorful of 2% vaginal cream nightly for 7 nights, is an effective alternative in women who are allergic to or unable to tolerate metronidazole. Amoxicillin, 500 mg, plus clavulanic acid (Augmentin) three times daily for 7 days carries an 80 to 85% cure rate. Amoxicillin, 500 mg three times daily for 7 days, has moderate cure rates of 50 to 60%. Topical vaginal yogurt and hydrogen peroxide douches are not effective therapies for BV. Vaginal sulfa creams have not been proved effective in treating BV. In approximately 30% of patients who initially respond to a 7-day course of metronidazole, BV recurs within 3 months. Treatment of male sexual partners remains controversial, and the Centers for Disease Control do not recommend treating male partners of women with BV because concomitant therapy does not appear to decrease the rate of recurrence.

Although there are no data to suggest that metronidazole is a teratogenic agent and its designation as a U.S. Food and Drug Administration (FDA) category B drug indicates that it is "relatively safe," it is prudent to avoid its use in the first trimester of pregnancy.

VULVOVAGINAL CANDIDIASIS

It is estimated that 75% of women suffer from at least one episode of yeast vulvovaginitis, or moniliasis, during their childbearing years. About half of these patients have a recurrence, and some suffer from frequent relapses. The majority of these cases are caused by *Candida* spp., and approximately 90% of cases are caused specifically by *Candida albicans,* a dimorphic organism that is present in humans as both spores and mycelia. These two forms are generally responsible for different manifestations of the infection. The spore form is usually the form by which the infection is spread most readily and is commonly associated with asymptomatic colonization of the vagina. The mycelium form appears to be associated with symptomatic infections. *Candida* spp. gain access to the vagina predominantly from the adjacent perianal area. Many women carry yeast in the vagina without any symptoms.

During pregnancy, there is increased susceptibility to vaginal infection, a higher incidence of vaginal colonization and infection, and lower cure rates. The clinical rate of disease is highest during the third trimester. High levels of reproductive hormones result in a higher glycogen content in the vagina and provide an excellent substrate for the germination and growth of *Candida*. The role of oral contraceptives is controversial. Vaginal colonization with *Candida* is more common among diabetic women, and uncontrolled diabetes predisposes patients to symptomatic vaginitis. Although glucose tolerance tests have been recommended for women with chronic or recurrent VVC (at least four episodes in 12 months), the yield is low, and testing is not necessary in otherwise healthy premenopausal women.

Symptomatic VVC frequently is observed during or after courses of systemic antibiotics. Broad-spectrum antibiotics, such as the penicillins, tetracyclines, and cephalosporins, are mainly responsible for this problem by eliminating normal protective vaginal bacterial flora. The natural flora provide a colonization-resistant mechanism and prevent *Candida* germination. Other factors that contribute to the increased incidence of VVC include the use of tight, poorly ventilated clothing and nylon underclothing, which increase perineal moisture and temperature. Chemical contact, local allergy, and hypersensitivity reactions may also predispose the patient to symptomatic vaginitis. There is no evidence confirming that iron deficiency contributes to VVC. Oral ingestion of yogurt containing viable *Lactobacillus acidophilus* cultures as preventive therapy is controversial. Topical vaginal yogurt and *L. acidophilus*–containing milk products have not proved effective for treating VVC.

Recurrent VVC has been attributed to repeated fungal reinoculation or auto-inoculation of the vagina from a persistent intestinal source or to sexual transmission. Although penile colonization with *Candida* is present in approximately 20% of male partners of women with recurrent VVC, confirmation of sexual transmission is still lacking. Routine therapy for male partners of women with recurrent infections is unlikely to reduce recurrence rates substantially. Whether recurrence is due to vaginal reinfection or relapse, women with recurrent VVC differ from those with infrequent episodes by an inability to tolerate small numbers of *Candida* organisms. In patients who are susceptible to yeast infections, prophylactic local antifungals are appropriate when these patients are prescribed antibiotics for other infections.

Theories about the pathogenesis of recurrent disease include deficiencies in the normal protective vaginal bacterial flora and an acquired, often transient, antigen-specific deficiency in T lymphocyte function that permits unchecked yeast proliferation and germination. The presence of oral and vaginal candidiasis is strongly correlated with depressed cell-mediated immunity in debilitated or immunosuppressed patients. Vaginal candidiasis may be the first symptom of human immunodeficiency virus (HIV) infection in women. Women with refractory or recurrent VVC should be offered HIV counseling and testing by their physician.

Another theory is that of an acquired acute hypersensitivity reaction, as evidenced by an elevated vaginal titer of *Candida* antigen-specific IgE, severe rash, erythema, swelling, and pruritus with minimal discharge and low titers of organisms in these patients. After coitus with *Candida*-infected women, male partners have reported allergic responses involving the genitalia (acute onset of erythema, edema, severe pruritus, and irritation of the penis).

The most frequent symptom is vulvar itching; however, there may be complaints of vaginal soreness, irritation, vulvar burning, dyspareunia, and external dysuria. Vaginal discharge is not always present. The consistency of the discharge is variable, from watery to cottage cheese–like and thick. The odor is minimal and nonoffensive. Characteristic findings include reddening of the vulva or vaginal areas with vulvar scaling, edema, or excoriation and raised white or yellow adherent vaginal plaques. Involvement of the intertrigonal area is not uncommon. The cervix is normal. Symptoms are often exacerbated during the week before onset of menses.

The diagnosis is confirmed by noting mycelia or pseudohyphae on direct low-power microscopic evaluation in a 10% KOH preparation. For patients who have symptoms and a negative KOH preparation, a fungal culture with Nickerson's media should be obtained. It should not be assumed, however, that *Candida* is always responsible for the vaginal symptoms even when cultures are positive. There is no reliable serologic technique for the diagnosis of symptomatic candidiasis.

Treatment

Treatment of acute VVC results in symptomatic relief and eradication of yeast in 80 to 90% of cases; however, recurrence is common. Predisposing factors should be eliminated, if this has not already been done. A variety of antifungal agents are available for local use as creams, lotions, aerosol sprays, vaginal tablets, suppositories, and coated tampons. Local application of antifungal agents is often accompanied by local burning and discomfort. Increased compliance by patients with shorter courses and improved cure rates supports the use of single-dose therapy. The newer agents, miconazole and clotrimazole, have become increasingly popular and are relatively safe for use in pregnancy (FDA category B drugs). Terconazole (Terazol) is a relatively new triazole antifungal that has been shown in some studies to have a higher cure rate than miconazole. It is an FDA category C drug and probably should be avoided in the first trimester. Because single-dose suppository treatment is curative in most patients, it is appropriate therapy for patients with first episodes or infrequent recurrent episodes of VVC.

Other regimens include application of 1% gentian violet to the cervical and vaginal mucosa, but in addition to being messy and staining clothing, gentian violet can cause marked drying and itching. Intravaginal gelatin capsules containing 600 mg of boric acid powder (U.S.P.) inserted nightly for 2 weeks achieve a 92% cure rate. This inexpensive treatment regimen is not commercially available but can be compounded by a pharmacist. Emphasis must be made to the patient that this is intravaginal therapy, not oral, and care must be taken to keep boric acid capsules away from children. This therapy must be avoided during pregnancy. Antifungal agents commonly used in the topical treatment of VVC and recurrent VVC are listed in Table 3.

TRICHOMONIASIS

The protozoan *Trichomonas vaginalis* is responsible for approximately 25% of cases of clinically evident vaginitis, but *T. vaginalis* is also commonly found in asymptomatic women. Sexual transmission is the primary method of introducing *T. vaginalis* into the vagina, especially with multiple sexual partners, in the presence of other sexually transmitted diseases, and with the use of nonbarrier methods of contraception. *T. vaginalis* colonization is not associated with age, day of menstrual cycle, recent history of antibiotic therapy, frequency of coitus, or type of contraceptive used. Perinatal transmission has been reported in female infants born to infected mothers.

Recurrence of infection is common, and although low titers of serum antibody develop, these are insufficient to provide clinically significant protective immunity or to permit diagnostic serologic testing. The predominant host defense is evidenced by the proliferation of PMNs, which contributes to the copious vaginal discharge. Typically, a yellow-green or gray, frothy, homogenous, malodorous discharge with a pH greater than 4.5 is present. The "strawberry" or "flea-bitten" appearance of the cervix that is caused by punctate mucosal hemorrhages is not often seen with the naked eye but is easily identified with colposcopy. Diffuse vulvar erythema is common.

Diagnosis is confirmed with observation of the extreme activity of the flagellated trichomonads on a saline wet preparation sample. The trichomonads can easily be missed because of the heavy polymorphonuclear infiltrate. The slide should therefore be examined in an area with relatively few white blood cells.

Treatment

Treatment of the patient and her partner or partners with metronidazole or related 5-nitroimidazole derivatives (tinidazole,* ornidazole*) is the only effective therapy for trichomoniasis. Oral therapy is generally preferred to local vaginal therapy because of the frequency of urethral and periurethral gland involvement, which can provide a source for endogenous reinfection. Both oral metronidazole, 250 mg three times daily for 7 to 10 days, and a single dose of 2 grams orally have been shown to be equally effective, with a cure rate of 85 to 95%. The Centers for Disease Control recommend a single 2-gram dose as the regimen of choice for initial treatment. Higher doses ranging from 500 to 750 mg orally four times a day for 7 to 10 days are successful for treatment of persistent infection after compliance of the patient and her sexual partner or partners is ensured. Other medications, such as phenytoin or phenobarbital, induce production of microsomal liver enzymes and accelerate the elimination of metronidazole. With longer treatment regimens, the incidence of VVC increases; this is probably secondary to the alteration of normal vaginal flora. Patients should be counseled to either refrain from intercourse during treatment or use a condom to prevent reinfection.

Nausea and vomiting occur in approximately 4 to 5% of patients with a single-dose regimen. Occasionally patients may complain of a headache or a metallic or bitter aftertaste after ingestion of metronidazole. Alcohol should be avoided during and 1 day after treatment because of the disulfiram-like reaction. Blood dyscrasias with metro-

TABLE 3. **Commonly Used Treatment Regimens for Yeast Vulvovaginitis**

How Supplied	Regimen
Miconazole (Monistat)	
100-mg suppositories	qd × 7 days
200-mg vaginal suppositories	qd × 3 days
2% vaginal cream	qd × 7–10 days
2% topical cream	bid × 14 days
2% topical lotion	bid × 14 days
Clotrimazole (Gyne-Lotrimin, Lotrimin, Mycelex)	
100-mg vaginal tablets	qd × 7 days
500-mg vaginal tablets	Single dose
1% vaginal cream	qd × 7–14 days
1% topical cream	qd × 7–14 days
1% topical lotion	qd × 7–14 days
Terconazole (Terazol)	
80-mg vaginal suppositories	qd × 3 days
0.4% cream	qd × 7 days
Butoconazole (Femstat)	
2% vaginal cream	qd × 3 days
Nystatin (Mycostatin, Nilstat)	
100,000 U/gm vaginal tablets	bid × 14 days
100,000 U/gm topical cream	bid × 14 days
Ketoconazole (Nizoral)	
200-mg oral tablets	qd or bid × 14 days
2% topical cream	qd × 14 days
Boric acid	
600-mg in 0-size gelatin capsules (must be made)	qd or bid × 14 days

*Not available in the United States.

nidazole therapy are rare. However, if a second course is necessary or if a higher dose of metronidazole is used for persistent infection, a total and differential leukocyte count should be obtained before and after treatment.

Metronidazole should not be given during the first trimester of pregnancy, and its use in later gestation is controversial. Patients with symptomatic infection during this period can be provided symptomatic relief with local administration of clotrimazole (Gyne-Lotrimin).

ATROPHIC VAGINITIS

The majority of women with vaginal atrophy are asymptomatic, especially in the absence of sexual intercourse. Because of a reduction in endogenous estrogen, the vaginal epithelium becomes pale, thin, and smooth. Lacking in glycogen, the epithelium contributes to a reduction of lactic acid production. With the pH being only slightly acidic, there is an overgrowth of nonacidophilic coliform bacteria.

Patients with an inflamed atrophic vagina often complain of vaginal soreness, occasional spotting or discharge, dyspareunia, and burning, which often are precipitated by coitus. In addition, patients may report urinary urge incontinence. The scant vaginal discharge is often blood-tinged, and wet preparation samples show PMNs with small, round epithelial or parabasal cells. These immature squamous cells lack sufficient estrogen exposure to allow maturation into the more typical superficial squamous cells seen in a well-estrogenized vagina.

Bacterial cultures are usually not necessary but a Papanicolaou smear and bimanual examination must be performed to rule out genital tract carcinoma.

Treatment

Rapid relief of the burning, itching, and dyspareunia is accomplished with treatment consisting of topical vaginal estrogen cream, one-half to one applicatorful nightly for 1 to 2 weeks. If the patient is not already receiving oral hormone replacement therapy, she should be evaluated for possible initiation of therapy. Secondary infection can be treated by local sulfonamide preparations. Intercourse should be avoided during any treatment for vaginitis.

TOXIC SHOCK SYNDROME

method of
GREGORY A. GRANT, M.D., and
ANTHONY W. CHOW, M.D.
University of British Columbia
Vancouver, British Columbia, Canada

Toxic shock syndrome (TSS) is an acute illness characterized by hypotension, fever, desquamative skin rash, and multisystem involvement. TSS is associated with infection by certain strains of *Staphylococcus aureus,* although bacteremia is rare, and the syndrome is believed to be mediated by the effects of toxin elaboration rather than of bacterial invasion. TSS is accompanied by the sudden onset of high fever, myalgias, vomiting, diarrhea, and a scarlatiniform rash that over several days may lead to full-thickness desquamation of the hands and feet. Within a few hours, severe hypotension or shock associated with a generalized nonpitting edema, as well as hyperemia of the conjunctival, oral, and urogenital mucosa, may develop. Multiple organ system failure of the hepatic, neurologic, gastrointestinal, cardiovascular, respiratory, musculoskeletal, renal, and hematologic systems may ensue.

Although initially associated with the use of hyperabsorbent tampons, this syndrome has been recognized increasingly in nonmenstruating women and in men. Nonmenstrual TSS is associated with the use of contraceptive diaphragms or sponges, as well as with parturition, nasal packing, and surgical or nonsurgical wounds. Despite increased awareness of this condition, the mortality rate remains high (3 to 7%); a majority (75 to 90%) of patients report some form of late sequelae or long-term morbidity. Recurrence is common in both menstrual (15%) and nonmenstrual (22%) TSS and is associated with inadequate anti-staphylococcal therapy during the prior episode of TSS.

TSS should be considered in the differential diagnosis of any man, woman, or child with the triad of fever, hypotension, and skin rash. It is important to recognize the early manifestations of TSS and to identify the infected site from which toxin is being produced, especially in nonmenstrual TSS associated with a wound infection, in which the local inflammatory response may be minimal or absent. Because there is no definitive laboratory test for TSS, the diagnosis depends primarily on clinical findings (Table 1) and epidemiologic considerations of risk factors (Table 2). Features nearly always present are fever of at least 38.9° C; a skin rash described as a diffuse macular erythroderma that desquamates 1 to 2 weeks after the onset of illness; nausea or vomiting; and progressive hypotension. Multiorgan involvement is readily evident eventually. Laboratory findings, although striking, are nonspecific and are useful mainly for monitoring target organ dysfunction and the severity of complications. Blood should be drawn for baseline investigations, and cultures from blood, urine, wounds, and other body sites should be obtained. Although the distinction between TSS and other illness can be quite difficult at times, a careful history and physical examination in combination with

TABLE 1. **Multisystem Manifestations of Toxic Shock Syndrome**

Common (20–80%)	Uncommon (<20%)
Neurologic	
Headache, confusion or agitation, meningismus	Photophobia, seizures, cerebral edema
Musculoskeletal	
Myalgia, arthralgia, increased creatine phosphokinase level	Arthritis
Gastrointestinal	
Nausea, vomiting, increased aspartate transaminase and bilirubin levels	Hepatosplenomegaly
Hematologic	
Thrombocytopenia, leukocytosis with immature cells	
Dermatologic	
Pharyngitis, vaginitis, conjunctivitis, strawberry tongue	
Renal	
Azotemia, sterile pyuria	
Pulmonary	Lung infiltrates, adult respiratory distress syndrome
Cardiac	Pericarditis, cardiomyopathy

a strong index of suspicion and appropriate laboratory tests of exclusion usually provide the correct diagnosis (Table 3).

PATHOGENESIS

In contrast to gram-negative or pneumococcal sepsis, bacteremia is rarely seen in TSS. TSS appears to be mediated by a toxin or toxins produced by certain strains of *S. aureus*. A 24-kilodalton protein, toxic shock syndrome toxin-1 (TSST-1), is produced in more than 95% of *S. aureus* strains associated with menstrual TSS. Although not yet fully characterized, it appears that TSST-1 is a potent inducer of several monokines and lymphokines, including interleukin-1, interleukin-2, tumor necrosis factor, lymphotoxin, in-

TABLE 2. **Risk Factors for Toxic Shock Syndrome**

High
Absence of antibody to TSST-1
Infection with TSST-1, positive *Staphylococcus aureus* culture
Menstruation in a female <35 years of age
Continuous use of super-absorbency tampon during menstruation
Nasal surgery with packing
Moderate
Use of regular-absorbency tampons during menstruation
Alternating use of tampons and sanitary pads
Use of contraceptive sponge
Low
Use of contraceptive diaphragm
Presence of intrauterine contraceptive device
Surgical wound infections
Early postpartum state

Abbreviation: TSST-1 = toxic shock syndrome toxin-1.

TABLE 3. **Differential Diagnosis and Differentiation from Toxic Shock Syndrome**

Scarlet fever	Lack of hypotension, presence of group A streptococcus
Streptococcal toxic shock–like syndrome	Necrotizing fasciitis and bacteremia common
Staphylococcal scalded skin syndrome	Bullous skin lesions and positive Nikolsky's sign
Drug-associated scarlatiniform eruption	Fever, diarrhea, and hypotension uncommon
Kawasaki's disease	Affects young children; prominent lymphadenopathy, prolonged course
Rocky Mountain spotted fever	Presence of tick exposure, petechial lesions, and cerebrospinal fluid abnormalities; absence of diarrhea

terferon-gamma, and others, which ultimately lead to the clinical manifestations of TSS. The precise mechanism and specific roles of these mediators and TSST-1 in the pathophysiology of TSS is still unclear. It is suggested that the final pathway of tissue injury may be similar to that of endotoxin (lipopolysaccharide) in gram-negative sepsis, leading to the development of sepsis syndrome and irreversible shock. Patients in whom acute TSS develops are found to lack antibodies to TSST-1, which are present in high titers in the normal general population. Conversely, polyclonal and certain monoclonal antibodies to TSST-1 are protective in animal models of TSS. However, it is clear that TSST-1 is not responsible for all cases of TSS, inasmuch as up to 30% of *S. aureus* strains isolated from patients with nonmenstrual TSS do not produce TSST-1. Other toxins such as staphylococcal enterotoxins A, B, and C, which produce biologic effects similar to those of TSST-1, may be responsible for the clinical manifestations of TSS in such cases. A similar clinical picture, referred to as toxic shock–like syndrome and attributed to toxins produced by group A streptococci, has also been described. The final common pathway leading to the most important pathophysiologic event in TSS is massive capillary leakage of intravascular fluid into the interstitial space, resulting in rapidly progressive hypovolemia, tissue hypoperfusion, and multiple end-organ damage. In addition to these hemodynamic effects, TSST-1 or its mediators appear also to have direct toxic effects on the myocardium, kidneys, lungs, liver, muscles, lymphoid tissue, and possibly the central and peripheral nervous systems.

TREATMENT

The principles of treatment in TSS are (1) resuscitation and monitoring for hypovolemia and shock; (2) antimicrobial therapy directed at eradication of toxin-producing *S. aureus;* (3) removal or neutralization of preformed toxin or toxins; (4) neutralization or inhibition of host mediators that lead to the sepsis syndrome; and (5) treatment of complications.

Resuscitation and Monitoring

Immediate attention to the circulating volume and appropriate monitoring is essential for all hospitalized patients with suspected TSS (Table 4). Rapid infusion of large amounts of intravenous crystalloids or colloids may be required in order to counteract massive leakage of intravascular fluid into the interstitial space and to maintain tissue perfusion. Oxygen delivery should be maximized with supplemental oxygen, and urinary output should be monitored as a measure of end-organ function. If these simple measures do not quickly restore hemodymamic stability, consideration should be given to managing the patient in an intensive care facility with invasive hemodynamic monitoring and aggressive cardiovascular support (Table 5).

The initial hemodynamic changes in acute TSS consist of a markedly decreased systemic vascular resistance, decreased mean arterial pressure, and increased cardiac output. In some patients, however, after an initial phase of increased cardiac output, myocardial contractility decreases, presumably because of a toxin-mediated cardiomyopathy. This results in a decrease in cardiac output, an increase in pulmonary artery wedge pressure (PAWP), and an increase in central venous pressure (CVP). This stage of myocardial dysfunction may not be readily apparent from the nonspecific electrocardiogram findings but is quickly recognized from increases in CVP and PAWP readings, a decrease in cardiac index, and an abnormal echocardiogram. Early recognition of myocardial failure and potential arrhythmias should lead to changes in management, such as decreasing the amount of fluid volume administered and considering afterload reduction with dopamine or dobutamine.

Antimicrobial Therapy

The most important aspects of antimicrobial therapy are the identification of the site of infection and the institution of local surgical drainage, débridement, or removal of the focus of infection. Because it may be difficult initially to make a firm diagnosis of TSS, it is prudent to begin antimicrobial coverage with broad-spectrum antibiotics active against both gram-positive and gram-negative organisms until a diagnosis of TSS is clinically established or the presence of S. aureus is microbiologically confirmed. The choice of specific anti-staphylococcal agents depends on other factors such as history of penicillin hypersensitivity or pattern of local antibiotic resistance. Beta-lactamase–stable penicillins such as nafcillin or cloxacillin (100 mg per kg per day given every 6 hours) or cephalosporins such as cefazolin (500 to 1000 mg every 8 hours) are appropriate choices. In penicillin-allergic patients or in areas where methicillin resistance is common, vancomycin (Vancocin), 500 mg every 6 hours, is the preferred alternative. Clindamycin (Cleocin), 25 mg per kg per day every 8 hours, may also be very effective, even though it is considered a bacteriostatic antibiotic. Animal and in vitro studies suggest that clindamycin may decrease the production of toxins through its action on inhibition of bacterial protein synthesis at the ribosomal level. There are no clinical trials in which the relative efficacy of different anti-staphylococcal antibiotic regimens for the treatment of TSS has been compared or in which the issue of the optimal duration of antimicrobial therapy has been studied. However, most clinicians consider a 10- to 14-day course of anti-staphylococcal therapy appropriate.

Toxin Removal and Neutralization

The local removal of any foreign material such as infected prostheses, intravenous catheters, tampons, diaphragms, pessaries, and contraceptive sponges is essential. Some authors advocate the local irrigation of any potentially infected areas with saline or povidone-iodine solutions.

TABLE 4. **Monitoring of Patients with Toxic Shock Syndrome**

Initial
Clinical
Blood pressure
Urine output
Respiratory rate
Heart rate
Heart sounds
Pulmonary sounds
Temperature
Weight
Level of consciousness
Laboratory
Electrolyte and acid-base status
Serum calcium and phosphate levels
Chest x-ray
Electrocardiogram
Coagulation status
Blood urea nitrogen or serum creatinine level
Liver function tests
Stool guaiac level
Cultures of infected focus, blood, and urine
Prolonged Hypotension (>2 Hours)
Central venous pressure
Pulmonary artery wedge pressure
Mean arterial wedge pressure
Cardiac index
Measurement of arterial blood gases
M-mode and two-dimensional echocardiogram

From Chesney PJ: Toxic shock syndrome. *In* Rakel RE (ed): Conn's Current Therapy 1992. Philadelphia, WB Saunders, 1992, p 1024.

TABLE 5. **Supportive and Symptomatic Therapy**

Hypovolemia and Hypotension	Other Systems
Initial Resuscitation	
Oxygen, intubation, PEEP	ADULT RESPIRATORY DISTRESS SYNDROME (ARDS)
Large-bore intravascular catheter	Anticipate ARDS
Rapid administration of 20–40 mL/kg of crystalloid over 1 h to stabilize BP and achieve urine output of ≥2 mL/kg/h	ELECTROLYTE AND ACID-BASE STATUS Correct initial hyponatremia and acidosis; anticipate and correct hypocalcemia and tetany
Methylprednisolone (Solu-Medrol), 30 mg/kg q 6 h for 2 doses	
If No Response After 1 h	
Transfer to ICU	ACUTE RENAL FAILURE
Continue crystalloid infusion at 20 mL/kg/h; more may be required to restore BP	Avoid nephrotoxic drugs Monitor and dialyze if necessary
Establish CVP line	THROMBOCYTOPENIA AND DIC
Correct electrolyte/calcium/acid-base status	Administer fresh-frozen plasma and platelets if needed
If No Response After 2–4 h	EDEMA, PERICARDIAL AND PLEURAL EFFUSIONS
Place pulmonary artery Swan-Ganz and arterial catheters	Maintain adequate intravascular volume before administering diuretic to mobilize extravascular fluid
Establish status of myocardium and lungs	
Consider use of dopamine (Dopastat) or dobutamine (Dobutrex) for afterload reduction	HEPATIC DYSFUNCTION Avoid drugs conjugated in the liver
Appropriate therapy for myocardial dysfunction if needed	
Look for sources of bleeding	
If BP Remains Unstable After 12–24 h	CENTRAL NERVOUS SYSTEM DYSFUNCTION
Look for continued source of toxin production and consider other methods of toxin removal (see text)	Anticipate irrational behavior; manage seizures with anticonvulsant therapy

Abbreviations: PEEP = positive end-expiratory pressure; BP = blood pressure; ICU = intensive care unit; CVP = central venous pressure; DIC = disseminated intravascular coagulation.

Modified from Chesney PJ: Toxic shock syndrome. *In* Rakel RE (ed): Conn's Current Therapy 1992. Philadelphia, WB Saunders, 1992, p 1025.

There are no data to support the effectiveness of this local measure. Furthermore, povidone-iodine is readily absorbed from the vagina after only a 2-minute application, leading to five- to fifteenfold increases in the total iodine and inorganic iodide concentrations in serum within 15 minutes. Thus although saline irrigations are unlikely to be harmful, use of povidone-iodine should be considered with caution.

Antibodies to TSST-1 are absent in the majority of people in whom acute TSS develops but are present in high titers in the population at large and in pooled normal immunoglobulin. Because antibodies to TSST-1 are found to be protective in animal models of TSS, the use of intravenous immunoglobulin (IVIG) in an attempt to remove toxin from the circulation has been advocated. The use of immunoglobulin involves the theoretic risk of the possible transmission of blood-borne diseases, inasmuch as it is a human-derived product, but the major drawback is the significant cost. IVIG has been administered to several patients with acute TSS in an intensive care setting with no apparent adverse effects. In patients who are severely ill with TSS, the administration of IVIG may be considered. Unfortunately, because TSS is a relatively uncommon disorder, it will be difficult to implement a controlled clinical trial to study the effect of IVIG on the outcome of TSS.

Treatment of Sepsis Syndrome

Some patients with TSS progress into full-blown sepsis syndrome or septic shock. In a number of clinical trials, investigators have examined possible treatment of these disorders with agents directed at the host responses to the toxin. High-dose corticosteroids—for example, methylprednisolone (Solu-Medrol), 10 to 30 mg per kg every 6 to 8 hours—have been tried. Although there are no prospective data, retrospective analysis indicated some benefit if treatment is administered within the first 2 to 3 days of illness. Naloxone and ibuprofen have also been suggested for the treatment of refractory shock. In addition, several large clinical trials in humans are under way to examine the role of monoclonal antibodies against tumor necrosis factor alpha, soluble tumor necrosis factor inhibitors, or interleukin-1 receptor antagonists in the treatment of sepsis syndrome and septic shock. Their application in the treatment of acute TSS must be considered investigational at this time.

Management of Complications

It is difficult to establish whether complications following TSS result from the direct effects of the toxin or from multiorgan system failure. Electrolyte and acid-base disturbances such as hyponatremia, hypocalcemia, hypercalcemia, hypomagnesemia, and acidosis may be severe and necessitate attention. Acute neurologic complications such as seizures may necessitate anticonvulsant therapy, and late complications such as neuromyasthenia, memory loss, recurrent headaches, and impaired consciousness, although uncommon, may necessitate continued treatment, support, and psychological counseling. Cardiomyopathy may persist or may slowly resolve and may result in considerable morbidity, as may pulmonary fibrosis secondary to adult respiratory distress syndrome.

PREVENTION

Primary prevention is difficult because the pathogenesis of TSS is not fully understood. After the outbreak of TSS in the early 1980s, it was thought that the use of superabsorbent tampons was the major factor contributing to the increased incidence. Since the removal of such tampons from the market and the requirement of absorbency labels by all tampon manufacturers, there appears to have been a decline in the incidence of menstrual TSS cases. Other preventive strategies include general education about tampon use, promotion of the use of sanitary pads at night, and immediate tampon removal when symptoms suggestive of TSS develop. Prevention of nonmenstrual TSS should be directed at the reduction of postoperative wound infections through the judicious use of prophylactic antibiotics, improved surgical techniques, and general wound care. Because recurrence of both menstrual and nonmenstrual TSS is more common (15 to 25%) among patients who received inadequate anti-staphylococcal therapy, early recognition and effective antimicrobial treatment are essential for reducing both acute morbidity and recurrence. Such patients may remain at risk as long as they continue to be colonized with TSST-1–producing strains of *S. aureus* and have no antibody to TSST-1. Thus determination of antibody titers and repeated vaginal cultures several months after the initial episode may help to identify persistent carriers who remain at risk. Such patients should discontinue tampon use until antibody to TSST-1 is present. A course of oral antibiotics (e.g., clindamycin [Cleocin], 600 mg every 8 hours) for 7 to 10 days to eliminate cervicovaginal *S. aureus* may be indicated.

Despite considerable efforts in public health measures and improved therapeutic modalities, TSS continues to be a significant clinical problem. Many more advances are clearly needed, particularly in screening for those at risk, in early and definitive diagnosis, in specific antitoxin therapy, and in more effective treatment of refractory shock or multiorgan system failure associated with sepsis syndrome.

CHLAMYDIA TRACHOMATIS INFECTION

method of
UDELE V. TAYLOR, M.D., and
JOSEPH J. APUZZIO, M.D.
New Jersey Medical School
Newark, New Jersey

Chlamydia trachomatis is an organism referred to in writings from ancient Egypt and Greece. It is a common cause of blindness in adults in developing countries. Although there are no accurate statistics, it is now believed to be the source of the most common sexually transmitted disease in the United States; over 4 million cases are estimated to occur annually. *Chlamydia* is a common organism involved in acute pelvic inflammatory disease, the sequelae of which may result in infertility, ectopic pregnancy, and chronic pelvic pain. *Chlamydia* may also complicate pregnancy and be transmitted to the newborn during the birth process, resulting in conjunctivitis, pneumonia, and possibly otitis media. The medical and economic implications of infection with this organism are therefore enormous.

MICROBIOLOGY

The genus *Chlamydia* contains two species: *C. psittaci* and *C. trachomatis*. These bacteria contain both RNA and DNA but are unable to carry out oxidative phosphorylation. Therefore, they are obligate intracellular parasites and require live host cells in order to replicate. There are 15 serotypes of *C. trachomatis*. Types A, B, and C cause endemic trachoma. Serotypes D to K cause oculogenital infection. Serotypes L1, L2, and L3 cause lymphogranuloma venereum, which is discussed in another article.

EPIDEMIOLOGY

The oculogenital serotypes of *C. trachomatis* are probably the most common sexually transmitted disease in the United States. *Chlamydia* infections are more prevalent in populations in which there is sexual promiscuity. Risk factors for infection include those listed in Table 1. At University Hospital, Newark, New Jersey, the carriage rate of *Chlamydia* from the endocervix in the authors' prenatal clinic is 27%. Most of these infections are asymptomatic.

TABLE 1. **Risk Factors for *Chlamydia***

1. Teenager
2. Multiple sexual partners
3. Unmarried pregnant patient
4. Inner-city population
5. Consort with nongonococcal urethritis

CLINICAL MANIFESTATION

Chlamydial infection is often asymptomatic, especially in females (Table 2). Therefore, members of the populations at risk for genital tract carriage or infection should be screened when they enter the health care system. For example, the prenatal clinic population at University Hospital consists mostly of indigent, inner-city patients. These are at high risk for *Chlamydia* and are routinely screened with specimens obtained from the endocervix at the time of the first prenatal visit and again in the third trimester. Patients with positive test results are treated with erythromycin, and their sexual consorts are referred for treatment.

ACUTE PELVIC INFLAMMATORY DISEASE

Most cases of acute pelvic inflammatory disease are caused by several organisms, including *C. trachomatis.* Therefore, antibiotic treatment of acute salpingitis must include coverage for *Chlamydia* as well as other common pathogens.

MUCOPURULENT CERVICITIS

This entity is caused by *Chlamydia* but may also be caused by other organisms. The cervix appears hypertrophic and eroded, with a yellow-appearing discharge. Criteria for diagnosis include a yellow or green endocervical discharge, more than 10 polymorphonuclear cells per high-power field, and friability of the cervix. The cervix should be cultured for *Chlamydia* and gonorrhea, and treatment with oral antibiotics should be based on the culture results.

ACUTE URETHRAL SYNDROME

In patients who complain of dysuria and frequency of urination but who have a negative urine culture and pyuria, *Chlamydia* may be the causative organism. *C. trachomatis* does not grow in the standard urine culture. These patients may benefit from antibiotic therapy specifically directed at *C. trachomatis.*

NEONATAL INFECTION

Transmission of *C. trachomatis* to the fetus may occur at the time of delivery. It is estimated that in up to 50% of infants born through an infected birth canal, conjunctivitis develops within 1 to 3 weeks after delivery. Although neonatal chlamydial conjunctivitis is usually self-limiting, it should be treated with parenteral antibiotics to prevent colonization of the respiratory passages and eustachian tubes. Colonization of these areas may lead to pneumonia, which may occur 4 weeks after delivery, or to otitis media.

Neonatal chlamydial conjunctivitis may be prevented by routine placement of erythromycin ointment in the newborn's eyes after delivery. However, topical erythromycin at the time of delivery does not prevent nasopharyngeal complications from occurring. Therefore, many hospitals still use silver nitrate drops to prevent gonorrhea conjunctivitis and observe the neonate for signs of chlamydial conjunctivitis. They then treat the neonate with parenteral antibiotics if these signs appear.

DIAGNOSIS

The gold standard for the diagnosis of chlamydial infection is isolation of the organism in tissue culture. However, obtaining the specimen with the proper technique, specimen transport, and processing is crucial for the recovery of the organism. It is important to obtain infected cells for the specimen because the organism resides inside cells. Therefore, a vaginal specimen for *Chlamydia* does not reveal the organism because the squamous cells of the vagina do not allow the organism to attach to them. Specimens for culture should be plated immediately into tissue culture (usually McCoy cells) or frozen at $-70°$ C until plated.

Because of the expense and the cumbersome method of obtaining specimens for culture, a number of indirect tests have been developed. These antigen-detection tests are an alternative to culture, but their reliability in a population in which *Chlamydia* prevalence is low is questionable. The commonly used methods are direct immunofluorescent assay and the enzyme-linked immunosorbent assay (ELISA).

The ELISA method for detecting *C. trachomatis* antigen has a 90% sensitivity and 90% specificity when the prevalence of *Chlamydia* in the population is 7% or more. When the prevalence rate is lower, a positive ELISA result agrees with culture results in only 50% of cases (false-positive ELISA test). Therefore, in populations with a low prevalence rate of *Chlamydia* infection, these tests should be used with caution, especially when used as a screening test.

Other, newer tests for *Chlamydia* use monoclonal antibodies to detect elementary bodies of *Chlamydia.* Again, however, when the prevalence of *Chlamydia* is above 7%, the sensitivity and specificity are greater than 90%. When the prevalence is lower, the tests may not be as reliable.

TREATMENT

The chlamydial organism is sensitive to few antibiotics, and some of these are poorly tolerated by patients because of adverse reactions. Tetracycline is the mainstay of treatment in nonpregnant patients (Table 3). Doxycycline (Vibramycin) may be a more desirable drug of choice because

TABLE 2. **Spectrum of Genital Chlamydial Infection**

1. Cervicitis
2. Urethritis
3. Salpingitis
4. Proctitis
5. Conjunctivitis
6. Pharyngitis
7. Neonatal conjunctivitis
8. Neonatal pneumonia
9. Neonatal otitis media

TABLE 3. Antibiotic Treatment for Uncomplicated Urethral, Endocervical, or Rectal Chlamydial Infection

Recommended
Tetracycline, 500 mg orally qid for 7 days
or
Doxycycline, 100 mg orally bid for 7 days

Alternative
Erythromycin base, 500 mg orally qid for 7 days
  (or equivalent salt)
or
Azithromycin, four 250-mg capsules as one dose
or
Sulfisoxazole, 500 mg orally qid for 10 days

During Pregnancy
Erythromycin base or stearate, 500 mg orally qid for 7 days;
  if patient is intolerant of erythromycin, amoxicillin, 500 mg
  orally tid for 7 days

its twice-a-day dosage allows for better compliance by patients.

Pregnant patients with chlamydial infections should be treated with erythromycin base or stearate, 500 mg four times a day, or erythromycin ethylsuccinate (E.E.S.), 500 mg four times a day. Erythromycin estolate (Ilosone) should not be used during pregnancy because drug-related hepatotoxicity can result. A second-line alternative for pregnant patients who are intolerant of erythromycin is amoxicillin, 500 mg three times a day for 7 days.

The new fluoroquinolone group of antibiotics has shown antichlamydial activity in female patients. Further research is needed to clarify their position. Azithromycin (Zithromax) is a new macrolide antibiotic. A 1-gram dose (four 250-mg capsules) taken on an empty stomach is as effective as the doxycycline regimen.

Clindamycin (Cleocin), although not a drug of first choice for *Chlamydia* infections, is effective when used in the appropriate dose. The dose of clindamycin when used intravenously for acute pelvic inflammatory disease is 600 mg every 6 hours or 900 mg every 8 hours, combined with gentamicin (Garamycin), 1.5 mg per kg every 8 hours. When clindamycin is prescribed orally, the dose is 450 mg four times a day for 7 to 10 days. Peak and trough levels of gentamicin are needed in order to guide dosage.

The sexual partners of patients with chlamydial infection should be evaluated and treated. Follow-up tests of cure should be obtained 3 to 4 weeks after treatment. It is important not to repeat the test for cure too soon when using the nonculture methods for diagnosis, because the antigen may remain in the genital tract after the organism has been eradicated and produce a false-positive result.

Tests for other sexually transmitted diseases, such as syphilis, gonorrhea, and the human immunodeficiency virus (HIV), should also be obtained from the patient and her partner or partners.

PELVIC INFLAMMATORY DISEASE

method of
SHERWOOD C. LYNN, JR., M.D.
University of South Alabama
Mobile, Alabama

Acute inflammation of the serosal surfaces of the female pelvic organs, prototypically caused by ascending infection by *Neisseria gonorrhoeae*, is descriptively labeled "pelvic inflammatory disease" (PID). This term is used synonymously with salpingitis or acute salpingitis. However, because the inflammatory response may be observed over the uterus, broad ligaments, ovaries, peritoneal surfaces of the bladder, rectum, and pelvic sidewalls, as well as the oviducts, it is, in fact, pelvic peritonitis. Although chronic pelvic infections may result from tuberculosis and actinomycosis, most sequelae of acute PID are a result of tissue damage caused by the inflammatory response and resultant adhesions. Thus the term "chronic PID" is being abandoned in favor of more descriptive terminology. Furthermore, "PID" is more commonly used in reference to sexually transmitted infections than with surgically associated infections such as septic abortion or post–cesarean section endometritis or parametritis.

The cost of medical services produced by the epidemic of sexually transmitted disease (STD) seen in the United States since the mid-1960s was estimated at $3.5 billion in 1990, a 17% increase over the 1980 cost. These estimates of the cost of treating STD and PID and its sequelae must be added to the economic burden of missed work and the agonizing psychological strain of infertility, ectopic pregnancy, and pain. One-fourth of women who have PID are destined to experience subsequent problems, including a 10% risk of infertility (20% after a second and 50% after a third episode of PID), a six- to 10-fold increase in ectopic pregnancies, and a 15 to 20% risk of chronic pelvic pain and/or dyspareunia.

ETIOLOGY

PID is the result of infection of the upper genital tract through an ascending infection from the vagina and cervix. The offending organism is introduced into the vagina and cervix by the penis or ejaculate, perhaps adherent to sperm or even trichomonads, and sequentially invades the mucosa of the endometrium and endosalpinx. This invasion incites an inflammatory response that involves the submucosa, then the muscularis, and finally the serosa. Although 85% of these infections are spontaneous, 15% are associated with instrumentation of the uterus: for example, endometrial biopsy, dilatation and curettage, intrauterine contraceptive device (IUD) insertion, and hysterosalpingography.

It is clear from modern culturing techniques that PID is polymicrobial. *N. gonorrhoeae,* an extensively studied early isolate, has provided much of the descriptive terminology used today. This organism is a gram-negative diplococcus requiring a carbon dioxide–enriched environment in order to survive outside the body. It produces a rapid and intense inflammatory response associated with dramatic cellular and tissue destruction in the tube. Both piliated and nonpiliated strains elaborate a lipopolysaccharide that acts both as a chemotactic agent for polymorphonuclear leukocytes and a toxin that desquamates the ciliated mucosal cells. Many of the recent isolates have been found to produce beta-lactamase, which renders the penicillins ineffective. Up to 6% of sexually active women of reproductive age have cervical cultures positive for *N. gonorrhoeae* and about 25% of those have cultures positive for *Chlamydia* as well. In 10 to 20% of the women with "gonococcal cervicitis," PID develops. Of the women with the clinical manifestations of PID who have positive cervical cultures, only about 22% have *N. gonorrhoeae* isolated from the peritoneum as the sole organism. In 78% of cases it is found in combination with other organisms or not at all.

With the advent of suitable transport and culturing techniques for *Chlamydia* first put into clinical use in Scandinavia, there has been a huge surge in interest in this organism. *Chlamydia trachomatis* (serotypes D to K) has surpassed the gonococcus as the primary cause of STD. The clinical entity produced by this organism is much more insidious and there appears to be considerably less tissue destruction than with *N. gonorrhoeae.* As an obligate intracellular parasite, the elementary body attaches to specific receptors on columnar cells inducing phagocytosis. The elementary body then transforms into the reticulate body, which uses the host synthetic mechanism to reproduce itself. The reticulate body then reorganizes into the elementary body, which fills the cell and causes its rupture some 48 to 72 hours after phagocytosis. Perhaps because of this protected intracellular reproductive mechanism, it appears that much of the tissue damage is induced by antigen-antibody complexes.

Whether *Mycoplasma* incites PID is controversial. *Mycoplasma pneumoniae, M. hominis,* and *Ureaplasma urealyticum* have all been isolated from patients with documented PID. Although colonization of the lower genital tract with *M. hominis* and *U. urealyticum* frequently occurs at birth, it tends to clear with age. However, these organisms are not cultured from the normal upper genital tract. Nonetheless, experimental evidence from primate research indicates that *Mycoplasma* does produce a mild inflammatory reaction in the oviduct.

Many other organisms have been isolated from the endocervix, endometrium, tubes, and cul-de-sac, primarily according to the point in the disease process at which the cultures are taken. Cultures positive for the aerobic nonhemolytic streptococci, *E. coli,* group B streptococci, coagulase-negative staphylocci, anaerobic *Bacteroides* species, *Peptococcus, Veillonella,* and *Peptostreptococcus* have all been reported from simultaneous samples taken for various isolates and may or may not confirm the presence of *N. gonorrhoeae* and/or *Chlamydia.* Although unusual, *Actinomyces israelii* may be associated with PID when an IUD is in place, and *Mycobacterium tuberculosis* may be the causative agent in a more chronic clinical picture.

RISK FACTORS

Women between the ages of 18 and 25 with multiple sexual partners and whose initial sexual encounter was at an early age are at particularly high risk for PID. Black and other nonwhite women are at higher risk than whites, although white teenagers are at an ever-increasing risk. Women who have experienced a previous episode of PID are at an increased risk. Instrumentation of the endometrial cavity is a risk factor. Although oral contraception may protect against *N. gonorrhoeae* by rendering the cervical mucus progestational, it may produce ectopy of the cervix, which increases the risk of chlamydial infection. Barrier methods of contraception, especially if used with spermicidal agents, should be most protective. Isthmic tubal ligation blocks the channel of bacterial spread, thus dramatically reducing the risk of PID.

SYMPTOMS AND SIGNS

The most common symptom of PID is lower abdominal and pelvic pain of relatively short duration, usually within 1 week of menses. Other symptoms include vaginal discharge, abnormal bleeding, dysuria, nausea, vomiting, tenesmus, and fever. Upper abdominal pain is usually relatively late and may represent Fitz-Hugh-Curtis syndrome. Gonococcal PID generally has a rapid course, whereas chlamydial PID is slower with less pain and fever.

Although most patients are febrile, all have lower abdominal and pelvic tenderness to direct palpation, and many exhibit rebound tenderness in the lower abdomen. Tenderness of the right upper quadrant should be carefully assessed, and if it is present, hospitalization for treatment should be considered. The pelvic examination demonstrates a purulent cervical discharge and exquisite tenderness of the cervix to motion. Bimanual examination confirms cervical, uterine, and adnexal tenderness with bilateral parametrial fullness, although a definite mass may not be palpated. The sensation of a full or bulging cul-de-sac may also be appreciated without palpation of a specific mass. If an inflammatory mass is defined or suspected, the patient should be admitted for treatment.

DIAGNOSIS

Twenty-three percent of women in whom PID is diagnosed have been reported to have normal pelves at laparoscopy. Twelve percent had other entities, such as appendicitis, hemorrhagic corpus luteum, ectopic pregnancy, endometriosis, and pyelonephritis. Despite the laparoscopic confirmation of PID in only 65%, it remains a clinical diagnosis. A history of abdominal and pelvic pain centered around menses, associated with abdominal and pelvic tenderness, fever, and leukorrhea, is highly suspicious. For confirmation, it is important to culture the cervix for *N. gonorrhoeae*. The presence of *Chlamydia* should be assessed by either direct culture or an antigen detection test. A Gram's stain of the cervical mucus should be obtained in order to look for gram-negative, intracellular diplococci in an inflammatory background. Blood from venipuncture should be obtained for complete blood count (leukocytosis greater than 10,000 per mm³), erythrocyte sedimentation rate (more than 20 mm per hour is correlated with severity), and beta–human chorionic gonadotropin (to rule out pregnancy). Liver function studies should be obtained as indicated. Urine should be obtained for urinalysis and held for culture and sensitivity as indicated. Pelvic ultrasonography is used only to measure the size of a pelvic mass or to assess the pelvis if a mass is suspected. Laparoscopy is reserved for cases in which the diagnosis is uncertain or that are not responding promptly to therapy.

TREATMENT

Treatment of PID is directed at rapid resolution of symptoms, reflecting improvement of the inflammation and its resultant sequelae. Because of the expense of hospitalization, many patients are treated in emergency departments, offices, and clinics. Table 1 lists the 1989 Centers for Disease Control (CDC) recommendations for outpatient treatment. This regimen consists of a single intramuscular injection of cefoxitin (Mefoxin) or ceftriaxone (Rocephin) followed by oral doxycycline or tetracycline for 10 to 14 days. Ceftriaxone may be the best choice today because of the rapid emergence of cefoxitin-resistant *N. gonorrhoeae*. The course of the tetracycline is necessary for adequate therapy of *Chlamydia*. The patient should be re-examined in 2 to 3 days to assess treatment. If symptoms persist, the patient should be hospitalized for inpatient therapy.

Criteria for admission and inpatient therapy at the initial evaluation include high fever or leukocytosis, peritoneal signs, an adnexal mass, an

TABLE 1. Recommended Regimen for Ambulatory Management

Cefoxitin (Mefoxin), 2 gm IM, plus probenecid, 1 gm PO, concurrently, or ceftriaxone (Rocephin), 250 mg IM, or equivalent cephalosporin

plus

Doxycycline (Vibramycin), 100 mg PO bid for 10–14 days

or

Tetracycline, 500 mg PO qid for 10–14 days

Alternative for Patients Who Do Not Tolerate Doxycycline

Erythromycin, 500 mg PO qid for 10–14 days, may be substituted for doxycycline or tetracycline; this regimen, however, is based on limited clinical data

Abbreviations: IM = intramuscularly; PO = per os (orally).
From Centers for Disease Control. 1989 Sexually transmitted diseases treatment guidelines. MMWR *38*(S-8):31–35, 1989.

TABLE 2. Recommended Regimen for Inpatient Treatment

One of the following:

Regimen A

Cefoxitin (Mefoxin), 2 gm IV q 6 h, or cefotetan* (Cefotan), 2 gm IV q 12 h

plus

Doxycycline, 100 mg q 12 h PO or IV

This regimen is given for at least 48 h after the patient improves clinically

After discharge from hospital, continuation of doxycycline, 100 mg PO bid for a total of 10–14 days

Regimen B

Clindamycin (Cleocin), 900 mg IV q 8 h

plus

Gentamicin (Garamycin), loading dose IV or IM (2 mg/kg) followed by a maintenance dose (1.5 mg/kg) q 8 h

This regimen is given for at least 48 h after the patient improves clinically

After discharge from the hospital, continuation of doxycycline, 100 mg PO bid for 10–14 days total

*Other cephalosporins, such as ceftizoxime (Cefizox), cefotaxime (Claforan), and ceftriaxone (Rocephin), which provide adequate gonococcal coverage, may be utilized in appropriate doses.
Abbreviations: IV = intravenously; PO = per os (orally); IM = intramuscularly.
From Centers for Disease Control. 1989 Sexually transmitted diseases treatment guidelines. MMWR *38*(S-8):31–35, 1989.

IUD in place, and an uncertain diagnosis. Table 2 lists the CDC recommendations for treatment of inpatients with PID. Regimen A consists of cefoxitin or an equivalent cephalosporin given in combination with doxycycline and covers both *N. gonorrhoeae* and *Chlamydia*. Regimen B, consisting of clindamycin and gentamicin, is probably better for more complicated cases involving IUDs, instrumentation, or inflammatory masses. Both regimens should be administered for at least 4 days and at least 48 hours after the patient has improved. Both regimens should include the completion of 10 to 14 days of doxycycline.

A number of new antibiotics, highly efficacious for treatment of PID, have been developed in response to the emergence of resistant strains of *N. gonorrhoeae*. Included among them are second- and third-generation cephalosporins (CDC Regimen A) and the beta-lactam–protected antibiotics (e.g., ampicillin-sulbactam [Unasyn] and ticarcillin–clavulanic acid [Timentin]). These should be administered parenterally in combination with doxycycline for at least 4 days and at least 48 hours after the patient improves and followed by completion of 10 to 14 days of oral doxycycline.

The majority of cases of PID respond to aggressive medical management, but there is one life-threatening situation that necessitates surgical intervention: the ruptured tubo-ovarian abscess. Other situations that may benefit by surgical management include removal of a persistent symptomatic mass, removal of a unilateral adnexal mass to preserve reproductive function, drainage of a cul-de-sac abscess via colpotomy, and hysterectomy with bilateral salpingo-oophorectomy for a persistent mass in older women who no longer desire fertility.

LEIOMYOMAS OF THE UTERUS

method of
W. SCOTT TAYLOR, M.D.
Washington Hospital Center
Washington, D.C.

The most common pelvic tumors of genital origin in women are the leiomyomas. Often referred to as uterine fibroids, these tumors are thought to arise from a single smooth muscle cell. As growth of such a tumor continues, fibrous or connective tissue material becomes incorporated into the tumor mass. Thus the terms "leiomyoma," "myoma," "fibromyoma," and "fibroid" can be used interchangeably.

Although a single uterine fibroid tumor may be identified, the most common clinical manifestation by far is one of multiple tumors of varying size and location. These tumors occur in at least 20% of white women and nearly 50% of black women. The factors that stimulate or impede growth of these tumors have not been completely identified, but it is reasonable to assume that variability of blood supply is somehow related both to growth rate and to the degenerative processes to which these tumors are prone. It is also reasonable to assume that many of these tumors are hormone dependent inasmuch as they are rarely seen before the menarche, are known to grow rapidly during pregnancy, and are known to regress during the menopause. A number of secretory and metabolic functions of fibroids, including estrogen metabolism and production of catechol estrogens, prostaglandins, prolactin, and erythropoietin, have been identified. The consequences of these functions remain to be elucidated. In addition, reports indicate a higher concentration of estrogen receptors in the cells of leiomyomas than in normal myometrial cells.

PATHOLOGY

These tumors undergo a variety of degenerative processes that are readily identified on gross examination (Table 1).

Degeneration is a benign process and is likely related to the duration or severity or both of compromised blood supply and to growth rate. The literature also refers to a process called "sarcomatous degeneration." This unusual occurrence is marked by finding an area of sarcomatous change within a benign leiomyoma. This lesion is clinically distinct from a leiomyosarcoma of the uterine wall, which is a diffuse process. It is thought that both processes are very uncommon, if not rare. It has been reported that among cases in

TABLE 1. **Degenerative Processes of Uterine Fibroids**

Edematous
Hyaline
Pseudomyxomatous
Fatty
Cystic
Carneous (red)
Calcific

which there is no extension of the sarcomatous process beyond the pseudocapsule in a benign myoma, the cure rate approaches 80 to 90%. For this reason, it is important to distinguish between uterine leiomyosarcoma and sarcomatous change within a benign leiomyoma.

Although the histologic picture of benign leiomyomas is usually uncomplicated, unusual cell types are seen on occasion (Table 2). In general, a leiomyoma is determined to be benign if microscopic evaluation reveals fewer than 5 mitotic figures (MF) per 10 high-power fields (HPF). If there are more than 10 MF per 10 HPF, the lesion is histologically malignant; if there are between 5 and 10 MF per HPF, the lesion is said to represent leiomyoma of uncertain malignant potential. Unfortunately, the number of mitotic figures present depends on variation and timing of histologic processing. Other factors such as the patient's age, invasiveness and size of the tumor, presence of necrosis, and cytologic atypia must be taken into consideration when a histologic diagnosis is made. The mitotic count is the best diagnostic criterion of clinical behavior.

Besides microscopic variability, some benign tumors behave erratically (Table 3). Although these conditions are unusual, their clinical manifestations can be confusing, and it may be difficult to establish the pathologic diagnosis.

SYMPTOMS

Abnormal bleeding and pelvic pain are the symptoms most commonly associated with uterine fibroids. Bleeding patterns of progressively heavier and then longer menstrual periods are common and are occasionally accompanied by intermenstrual bleeding of variable degree. Excessive blood loss may be subtle, protracted, and well-compensated, leading to surprisingly severe chronic anemia. Cramping pain generally occurs with menstruation and may be related to passage of large blood clots, degenerative processes within a myoma, or both. Acute pain is generally caused by torsion of a pedunculated fibroid or by carneous (red)

TABLE 2. **Unusual Cell Types of Benign Leiomyomas**

Variants of Benign Leiomyoma	Microscopic Characteristics
Cellular myoma	Small cells
Symplastic myoma	Large, hyperchromatic cells
Hemorrhagic cellular myoma	Dense cellularity and hemorrhage

TABLE 3. **Behavior of Benign Leiomyomatous Conditions**

Benign Tumor Classification	Behavioral Characteristics
Peritoneal leiomyomatosis	Benign smooth muscle masses on peritoneal surfaces, especially related to pregnancy
	Metaplastic
Metastasizing leiomyoma	Benign smooth muscle masses found in distant sites
	May be related to hormonal factors
	Metastatic
Intravenous leiomyomatosis	Nodules of benign smooth muscle protruding into pelvic veins

degeneration. Other symptoms include a feeling of pelvic heaviness, pelvic pressure, bladder symptoms, constipation, and, in some cases, dyspareunia. The size of uterine fibroids characteristically bears little relationship to the severity of symptoms.

Although the majority of women with uterine fibroids experience no impairment in fertility or fecundity, some tumors, depending on location or size or both, interfere with normal tubal function or with implantation. In addition, uterine fibroids may be linked to premature labor, abnormal placentation, dysfunctional labor, postpartum hemorrhage, malpresentation, and intrauterine growth retardation. Overall, the incidence of obstetric complications relating to uterine fibroids is approximately 10%.

DIAGNOSIS

The diagnosis of uterine fibroids is made from a complete history and results of thorough physical examination that are suggestive of a pelvic mass. The examination may be complemented by imaging techniques such as ultrasonography and magnetic resonance imaging. Such confirmatory studies are especially important when relationship to fertility is being considered. Specific localization and definition may well indicate both further diagnostic modalities and surgical approaches. The differential diagnosis must include benign and malignant neoplastic masses, infectious masses, and congenital anomalies of any pelvic structure.

TREATMENT

Observation

The mere presence of uterine fibroids without symptoms or disturbance of normal function does not warrant treatment. Indications for treatment include abnormal bleeding, pelvic pain, enlargement to a degree that may disturb the normal anatomy or function of other pelvic structures (generally conceded to be greater than 12 weeks' gestational size), or the presence of fibroids in association with reproductive disorders. Under most circumstances, therefore, because uterine fibroids tend to be small and asymptomatic, periodic examinations every 6 months to determine symptoms and growth rate are all that is necessary. Uterine fibroids tend to decrease in size after the menopause and, fortunately, are generally not responsive to the usual low doses of exogenous estrogens used for hormone replacement therapy. These tumors may grow rapidly during pregnancy or in response to high doses of estrogens in some oral contraceptives.

Medical Treatment

Currently, no medication safely causes complete regression or disappearance of uterine fibroids. Although progestational agents and danazol* (Danocrine) have been used to decrease fibroid size, results have not been consistent. In the past few years, gonadotropin releasing hormone (GnRH) agonists such as leuprolide acetate† in its depot form (Lupron-Depot) have been used successfully by many investigators and clinicians to decrease fibroid size and alleviate symptoms. These agents selectively abolish estrogen production by the ovary and secondarily decrease the volume of both normal uterine musculature and fibroid masses. The usual dose of (Lupron-Depot) is 3.75 mg intramuscularly, monthly.

Patients should be informed of the menopausal-like symptoms that result from the use of GnRH agonists. In general, clinical studies indicate that approximately 50% of patients experience a decrease in total uterine volume by about 50%. This effect can usually be achieved by 12 weeks of treatment. Rapid regrowth occurs when medication is discontinued. Therefore, this method of therapy should be reserved for infertile patients, women nearing the menopause, patients scheduled for myomectomy, and patients who might be candidates for vaginal hysterectomy if total uterine volume could be sufficiently reduced. Additional benefits of increasing hematocrit and hemoglobin concentrations result from the amenorrhea produced by this treatment. When used for long periods of time (longer than 6 months), the risks of hypogonadism, especially osteoporosis, must be strongly considered.

Surgical Treatment

Hysterectomy is the only definitive cure for uterine fibroids, and a diagnosis of fibroids is the

---

*This use of danazol is not listed in the manufacturer's official directive.

†This use of leuprolide acetate is not listed in the manufacturer's official directive.

most common given for this procedure. This operation is warranted in the presence of persistent or recurrent signs and symptoms not controllable by conservative means in women for whom childbirth is no longer a consideration.

At present, myomectomy should be performed when there is reasonable indication that uterine fibroids are likely related to reproductive failure. Some studies have shown a rate of recurrence over 10 years as high as 27%. Myomectomy can be accomplished transabdominally by traditional laparotomy or by operative video-laparoscopy with or without laser. Myomectomy can also be performed transvaginally by operative hysteroscopy with the use of a resectoscope for submucous tumors. The approach used is dependent on the location of the tumors to be removed, the operative experience of the surgeon, anticipated goals of surgical therapy, and desires of the patient. Postoperative adhesion formation in these patients remains a serious concern. Because of the rapidly improving technology of operative endoscopy, it is possible that with further clinical evaluation, myomectomy may replace total hysterectomy in selected patients, even those for whom fertility is not an issue.

ENDOMETRIAL CANCER

method of
JEFFREY M. FOWLER, M.D., and
LEO B. TWIGGS, M.D.
University of Minnesota
Minneapolis, Minnesota

It was estimated that 31,000 new cases of endometrial cancer were diagnosed in the United States in 1992. Endometrial cancer is the most common gynecologic malignancy and the fourth most common malignancy in women, after breast, colorectal, and lung cancer. Although this is the most common gynecologic malignancy (46%), most patients present in the early stage; there were only 5700 deaths in 1992, accounting for 17% of deaths from gynecologic cancer.

Endometrial cancer affects mainly postmenopausal women. The average age at diagnosis is 58 years. Seventy-five percent of the cases occur after age 50, and fewer than 5% occur before age 40. No genetic marker for endometrial cancer is known, although a small percentage of the cases may be associated with a hereditary syndrome. The incidence of endometrial cancer is also higher among women with a history of breast, endometrial, or ovarian malignancies. Women with endometrial cancer tend to belong to a high socioeconomic status, and the frequency of this malignancy is higher in industrialized countries. Both these factors may be related to a high intake of dietary fat.

Women at high risk for endometrial cancer tend to

TABLE 1. **Risk Factors for Endometrial Cancer**

Obesity
Nulliparity
Late menopause
History of ovarian, breast, or colorectal cancer
Polycystic ovary syndrome
Hormone secretory tumors
Unopposed exogenous estrogens
Pelvic irradiation
Endometrial hyperplasia

be menopausal and obese and to have a large body frame. The most significant risk factor for endometrial cancer is obesity; the risk ratio is 1:10 in women who are at least 50 pounds overweight. The overwhelming risk factor for endometrial cancer in women is the presence of unopposed estrogen: that is, high circulating levels of estrogen with low or no levels of progesterone. This hormonal milieu may be realized by unopposed estrogen replacement therapy, obesity, or other conditions that result in overall excess estrogen production (Table 1).

PATHOLOGY

Most cases of endometrial carcinoma are associated with a precursor lesion termed "endometrial hyperplasia." The classification of endometrial hyperplasia is based on the presence or absence of cytologic atypia and the degree of complexity of the architectural pattern. Cytologic atypia is the most predictive for the likelihood of progression to carcinoma (Table 2). These precursor lesions may be treated with progestins or surgery, depending on the complexity of the lesion and the patient's desire for further childbearing.

Approximately 80% of endometrial carcinoma is endometrioid adenocarcinoma. The differentiation of endometrial carcinoma is expressed in grades and the aggressiveness of the malignancy is related to its grade. Architectural criteria are used in the International Federation of Gynecology and Obstetrics (FIGO) classification of tumors and are easily applied to most cell types (Table 3). The higher the grade of tumor, the more likely there is deep myometrial invasion, pelvic or para-aortic lymph node metastases, or extrauterine spread.

Most cases of endometrial cancer are associated with endometrial hyperplasia and occur in patients with one or more risk factors. However, there is a subgroup of

TABLE 2. **Classification of Endometrial Hyperplasia**

Type of Hyperplasia	Progression to Cancer
No Cytologic Atypia	
Simple (cystic)	1%
Complex (adenomatous)	3%
Cytologic Atypia Present	
Simple (cystic)	8%
Complex (adenomatous)	29%

TABLE 3. **International Federation of Gynecology and Obstetrics (FIGO) Classification of Carcinoma of the Corpus Uteri (1988)**

Stage	Characteristics
IA G123	Tumor limited to endometrium
IB G123	Invasion to less than one-half the myometrium
IC G123	Invasion to more than one-half of the myometrium
IIA G123	Endocervical glandular involvement only
IIB G123	Cervical stromal invasion
IIIA G123	Tumor invades serosa or adnexa, or positive peritoneal cytologic finding
IIIB G123	Vaginal metastases
IIIC G123	Metastases to pelvic or para-aortic lymph nodes
IVA G123	Tumor invasion of bladder or bowel mucosa
IVB	Distant metastases, including intra-abdominal and inguinal lymph nodes

Degree of histopathologic differentiation: Cases of carcinoma of corpus should be classified (or graded) according to degree of histologic differentiation, as follows: GI = 5% or less of a nonsquamous or nonmorular solid growth pattern; G2 = 6–50% of a nonsquamous or nonmorular solid growth pattern; G3 = more than 50% of a nonsquamous or nonmorular solid growth pattern.

From Yoshimitsu K, Nakamura G, and Nakano H: Dating sonographic endometrial images in the normal ovulatory cycle. Int J Gynecol Obstet 28:33–39, 1989.

patients who do not fit the stereotype and have cell types other than endometrioid adenocarcinoma that are associated with a poor prognosis. These poor prognostic cell types include serous, clear-cell, undifferentiated, and adenosquamous carcinoma. These types are uncommon but nevertheless are very aggressive and are associated with a high incidence of extrauterine disease; they are also not easily graded architecturally. Any patient with these cell types, regardless of the grade, should have complete surgical staging, and adjuvant therapy should be considered.

DIAGNOSIS

Abnormal vaginal bleeding is the cardinal symptom of endometrial cancer. More than 90% of patients with endometrial carcinoma have this symptom. Although very good for cervical cancer, the Papanicolaou smear is not accurate in the detection of endometrial malignancies. Routine cervical cytologic studies only occasionally lead to the diagnosis of endometrial cancer. Any abnormal vaginal bleeding in an anovulatory premenopausal, perimenopausal, or postmenopausal woman should lead to further investigation. The physician should be amenable to performing an endometrial biopsy. Many devices are available for outpatient biopsies and are very accurate in comparison with the standard dilatation and curettage. Ninety percent of women who need an endometrial sampling can successfully undergo this procedure in the physician's office. If outpatient sampling techniques fail to provide sufficient diagnostic information, a formal fractional dilatation and curettage with hysteroscopy should be performed. Transvaginal ultrasonography may also assist in the evaluation of abnormal uterine bleeding. Before endometrial biopsy, an endometrial stripe of less than 5 mm in diameter in a postmenopausal pa-

tient is rarely associated with a neoplastic abnormality.

Once a histologic diagnosis of endometrial carcinoma is obtained, pretreatment evaluation should be performed. Routine serum chemistry studies, liver function tests, and a complete blood count, as well as chest x-ray and electrocardiogram, are obtained in all patients. Additional endoscopic and radiologic studies may be performed when indicated but certainly should not be routine. Pelvic and abdominal computed tomography may be helpful if extrauterine or metastatic disease is suspected.

TREATMENT AND STAGING

Over the past decade, the surgical-pathologic spread pattern of endometrial cancer has been re-evaluated. In a significant number (10 to 20%) of patients with clinical Stage I cancers, disease has spread outside of the uterus. The most common sites of metastatic disease are the adnexa and the pelvic and para-aortic lymph nodes. Increasing tumor grade and myometrial invasion are associated with an increasing risk for pelvic and para-aortic lymph node metastases, adnexal metastases, positive peritoneal cytologic findings, and recurrence. Cytologic type and grade can be assessed before a hysterectomy, but in up to 20% of patients, the histologic grade is worse at hysterectomy than reported at curettage. Also, the findings from endocervical curettage have a false-positive rate of 50% and a false-negative rate of about 10%. Myometrial invasion is best assessed after a hysterectomy with either frozen or permanent sections.

The inaccuracy in clinical staging of endometrial carcinoma impedes optimal therapy and analysis of treatment results. The treatment of a malignancy should conform to the perceived spread patterns of the disease. Fortunately, most patients with endometrial cancer have early-stage disease. Unless metastatic or systemic disease is identified, the initial approach for all medically fit patients should be a total abdominal hysterectomy/bilateral salpingo-oophorectomy (TAH/BSO). In 1988, FIGO determined that endometrial cancer should be surgically staged (see Table 3). As a result of this international consensus, staging is dependent on the findings at the time of surgery and histologic differentiation. This classification allows for a more accurate assessment of disease spread and enables the development of comparable statistics between institutions. The staging procedure should include an adequate abdominal incision in order to obtain sampling of peritoneal fluid for cytologic evaluation, as well as abdominal and pelvic exploration with biopsy or excision of any extrauterine lesion suspected of being a tumor. Any pelvic and para-aortic lymph nodes under suspicion should be removed for pathologic evaluation and should be routinely sampled in high-risk situations, even if no retroperitoneal nodes are under suspicion.

In early-stage endometrial cancer, the risk of pelvic and para-aortic lymph node metastases ranges from 3 to 25% and from 2 to 16% respectively for grades 1 to 3. The incidence of lymph nodes metastases increases to as high as 40% with increasing depth of invasion. In patients with Stage I grade 1 disease without deep myometrial invasion, the probability of lymph node metastases is less than 2%. Therefore, most clinicians agree that routine pelvic and para-aortic lymph node sampling is not necessary in these patients unless palpable nodes are present. The rate of positive lymph nodes increases in grades 2 and 3 disease and deeply invasive grade 1 disease; therefore a pelvic and para-aortic lymph node sampling is recommended in patients with these forms of the disease.

Adjunctive therapy, if needed, can be planned, depending on whether the surgical-pathologic findings indicate intrauterine only or extrauterine disease. The patient may receive 4000 to 5000 cGy of external beam radiation to the pelvis if pelvic nodes are positive and 4500 cGy of external beam radiation to the para-aortic fields if those nodes are positive. Patients with other sites of extrauterine disease may require whole abdominal irradiation. Some patients may need systemic therapy in addition to radiation therapy, depending on sites of spread.

The necessity of adjuvant radiation therapy in surgically staged patients without evidence of extrauterine disease is controversial. In this setting, irradiation has not been shown to improve survival for patients with endometrial cancer, although it has been shown to decrease the incidence of both pelvic and vaginal recurrences. Morbidity secondary to radiation therapy increases with increasing field size and after surgery. Information obtained from surgical staging enables 50 to 75% of patients with Stage I disease to forgo postoperative irradiation. Prospective clinical trials are now ongoing to define the role of adjuvant treatment in this setting.

Patients with Stage II disease are at higher risk for having extrauterine disease and recurrence. Several options for treatment are appropriate in this setting. If the cervix is of normal size and grossly normal, one approach is an extrafascial TAH/BSO with complete surgical staging followed by postoperative irradiation. With gross cervical involvement, two options are available. The first is whole pelvic irradiation followed by one intracavitary implant, which is then followed by a TAH/BSO and para-aortic lymph node sampling. The second option is a radical hysterectomy, BSO, and pelvic and para-aortic lymphade-

nectomy with irradiation tailored to the surgical findings, if necessary.

Fortunately, most patients with endometrial cancer do not present with advanced disease. In surgical Stage III disease, primary surgery with the use of a TAH/BSO with tumor debulking may be attempted. Extrapelvic disease, depending on the site and extent, may necessitate extended field irradiation, systemic chemotherapy, or hormone therapy. Patients with Stage III disease, by virtue of vaginal or parametrial extension, need a thorough metastatic survey and then irradiation. A TAH/BSO may be indicated after this therapy is completed. Patients with clinical Stage III disease on the basis of an adnexal mass should undergo exploratory laparotomy.

Most patients with Stage IV disease are best treated with systemic therapy, which includes hormones or chemotherapy. Pelvic irradiation or hysterectomy is reserved for palliative control purposes.

TREATMENT OF RECURRENT DISEASE

Patients with recurrent endometrial cancer in the pelvis may be treated with radiotherapy. Unfortunately, the majority of these patients also have distant metastases as well. Isolated central recurrences in the pelvis after irradiation are rare. However, if this situation does occur, selected patients may be candidates for pelvic exenterative surgery. The majority of patients with recurrent disease are treated with hormones or chemotherapy.

Progestins have been used for decades to treat recurrent endometrial cancer. The overall response to progestins is approximately 25%, although recent trials demonstrate lower response rates, in the range of 15 to 20%. Patients with endometrial carcinoma with progesterone-positive and estrogen-positive receptors have a better response to endocrine therapy. Most patients with positive receptors respond to progestins, whereas only 15% with negative receptors respond. Receptor positivity is related to the grade of the tumor inasmuch as well-differentiated lesions are more likely to be positive and poorly differentiated lesions are more likely to be negative. Medroxyprogesterone acetate (Provera) and megestrol acetate (Megace) are the agents most commonly used. Tamoxifen (Nolvadex) has also been used to treat patients with recurring endometrial cancer, and responses are usually seen in patients who have previously responded to progestins.

Several cytotoxic agents have activity for endometrial cancer, but responses are short-lived, and the treatment for advanced and recurrent disease is considered palliative. The two most active single agents are doxorubicin and cisplatin. Many combinations of cytotoxic agents have been used, but the results of multiagent chemotherapy do not appear to be significantly better than those of single-agent chemotherapy.

CARCINOMA OF THE UTERINE CERVIX

method of
DAVID G. MUTCH, M.D.
Washington University School of Medicine
St. Louis, Missouri

Carcinoma of the uterine cervix is the fourth most common cancer in women. In 1991, there were 13,000 new cases of this disease and more than 50,000 cases of preinvasive carcinoma of the cervix. The incidence of cervical cancer is substantially higher in women of low socioeconomic status, in women who had first intercourse at an early age, and in women who have a history of multiple sexual partners. Many have said that cervical cancer is essentially a sexually transmitted disease, because of its high association with the human papillomavirus (HPV). Although more than one-half of women with more than one sexual partner have evidence of HPV infection, no actual cause and effect have been established.

Squamous cell carcinoma of the cervix is associated with premalignant abnormalities (dysplasia), which precede it by 10 to 20 years. About 30% of patients with carcinoma in situ of the cervix will develop invasive cancer by the 10th year. This incidence continues to increase over 30 years. Squamous cell cancer tends to arise from the squamocolumnar junction and initially involves the cervix. Spread tends to be lateral into the parametrial tissue, down the vagina, or to regional lymph nodes.

SCREENING

The incidence in the United States of invasive carcinoma of the uterine cervix has decreased substantially over the last 50 years, although the incidence of preinvasive disease has increased. This is presumably due to the fact that premalignant abnormalities can be identified by cytologic screening. Regular screening programs have been in effect since the 1950s.

Although the mortality rate from cervical cancer in the United States has decreased significantly over the last 50 years, presumably because of Pap smear screening, the cost of this screening is significant. Approximately 75,000 Pap smears are needed to detect one invasive cancer. For this reason, it is important to consider optimal screening intervals. The American College of Obstetricians and Gynecologists has recommended that Pap smears be obtained on a yearly basis after the age of 18 years or after first intercourse. The American Cancer Society has recommended that asymptomatic low-risk women be screened for 3 consecutive years then at least every 3 years thereafter until the age of 65 years. Women with more than one sexual partner or other risk factors are considered to be at high risk and should be screened at more frequent intervals.

Pap smears should be obtained from patients prior to vaginal examination with lubricants and should consist of an endocervical specimen obtained with a moistened cotton swab or cytobrush and a second specimen obtained with a spatula. There is evidence that cytobrushes increase the sensitivity of the Pap smear and, therefore, should probably be used in place of cotton swabs if possible. Despite its apparent effectiveness, the Pap smear is only a screening test, with false-negative rates of 10 to 40% reported. The Pap smear must be used in conjunction with good visual inspection of the cervix, especially in patients who report symptoms of vaginal discharge or postcoital bleeding.

Abnormal smears are reported in a variety of ways, e.g., the Bethesda system and the Standard Class system (Table 1). Once a patient has an abnormal Pap smear, colposcopic evaluation is mandatory. Simply repeating the Pap smear is not a sufficient means to follow these patients, because invasive lesions can be missed. Colposcopy is a technique in which the cervix is visualized using a magnifying lens. Abnormal patterns are identified by staining the cervix with acetic acid and visualizing it under magnification. There are four abnormal patterns that can be identified by the colposcopist: (1) white epithelium, (2) mosaic patterns, (3) punctation, and (4) atypical vessels. Atypical vessels represent cancer until proven otherwise by biopsy. The colposcopist must visualize the entire transformation zone, visualize the entire lesion, and obtain endocervical curettings. If these criteria are met and the cytologic findings are not disparate from the histologic ones, then the colposcopy is considered adequate. Inadequate colposcopic evaluations must be followed by a cone biopsy or other extirpative procedure, because invasion cannot be entirely ruled out (Figure 1). Preinvasive lesions may be treated by cryotherapy or laser or electrical loop excision (LEEP).

DIAGNOSTIC EVALUATION

Once the diagnosis of invasive cancer is made, the extent of the disease must be determined so that appropriate treatment plans can be initiated. Mandatory tests consist of a physical examination (if there is any

TABLE 1. **Abnormal Cervical Cytologic Findings**

Bethesda System	Classic System
Squamous carcinoma	Carcinoma in situ
High-grade squamous intraepithelial lesion	Severe dysplasia
Low-grade squamous intraepithelial lesion	Moderate dysplasia Mild dysplasia Koilocytosis

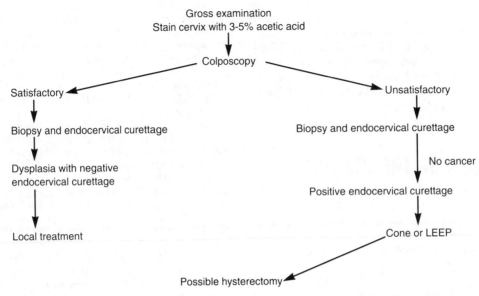

Figure 1. Management of abnormal Pap smear. LEEP = laser or electrical loop excision.

question of the extent of disease, an examination under anesthesia should be performed jointly by the radiation oncologist and gynecologic oncologist), chest x-ray, and intravenous pyelography (IVP). If the patient undergoes an examination under anesthesia, cystoscopy and proctoscopy are usually appropriate. Additional tests, such as computed tomography, magnetic resonance imaging, and barium enema may be performed at the discretion of the physician but are not necessary in the staging of the patient. The International Federation of Gynecology and Obstetrics staging of cervical cancer is a clinical one and is based on physical examination, chest x-ray, and IVP (Table 2).

Cervical cancer usually spreads in an orderly fashion from the cervix to the surrounding tissues or to the pelvic lymph nodes and then to the periaortic nodes. Evaluation of patients with advanced disease for lymph node metastases, although not necessary for staging, may be useful in determining the best treatment. Lymphangiograms of the retroperitoneal nodes may be helpful in determining if there is disease spread to the pelvic or periaortic areas. More invasive staging has been proposed in the form of retroperitoneal staging laparotomies. Whereas this procedure is helpful in determining the prognosis and establishing treatment, no survival advantage has been demonstrated in patients undergoing this more thorough metastatic evaluation.

PROGNOSTIC FACTORS

Many prognostic factors have been identified as affecting the survival of patients with cervical cancer. Some reports indicate that younger patients do more poorly than older patients. However, most studies show no difference in survival based on age. Black patients tend to present at a later stage and, therefore, tend to do worse than whites; a similar difference occurs between patients of lower and higher socioeconomic status.

Increasing tumor volume is associated with a worse outcome. Many studies show that the larger the lesion, the greater the stromal invasion; or the higher the stage, the worse the outcome (Table 3). Endometrial tumor extension is also associated with decreased survival. Numerous reports show that patients who have lymph node involvement have a worse prognosis. There is a 90% survival rate for patients treated by surgery for Stage Ib disease. This falls to 50 to 60% for patients with positive pelvic nodes and to 25 to 30% for patients with positive periaortic nodes. Also, decreasing survival has been noted as the number of positive nodes increases.

TABLE 2. **Staging of Cervical Cancer**

	Carcinoma in situ
I	Cervical cancer confined to the uterus
Ia	Preclinical invasive cancer, only microscopic diagnosis possible
Ia1	Microscopic stromal invasion
Ia2	Tumor with invasive component 5 mm or less in depth taken from the base of the epithelium and 7 mm or less in horizontal spread
Ib	Tumor larger than one in stage Ia2
II	Cervical cancer invades beyond the uterus but not to the pelvic sidewall or to the lower third of the vagina
IIa	Vaginal involvement but no parametrial disease
IIb	Parametrial involvement
III	Cervical cancer extends to the pelvic sidewall, involves the lower third of the vagina, or causes hydronephrosis
IIIa	Tumor involves the lower third of the vagina without extension to the pelvic sidewall
IIIb	Tumor involves the pelvic sidewall or there is evidence of hydronephrosis
IV	Disease beyond the pelvis or invasion into surrounding structures
IVa	Cervical cancer invades into rectum, bladder, or outside the true pelvis
IVb	Distant metastases

TABLE 3. **Five-Year Survival with Respect to Stage in Patients with Cervical Cancer**

Stage	5-Year Survival
I	85%
II	66%
III	35%
IV	7%

Lymphovascular space involvement has been identified as a poor prognostic factor and may be as bad as positive lymph node involvement. Also, many authors have shown that there is no significant difference in survival based on differentiation, although some have shown that adenocarcinomas do worse than squamous tumors. Small cell cervical carcinoma is a very poor histologic type with almost no survivors at 5 years. Other factors that affect survival are anemia, hypertension, diabetes, and a history of pelvic inflammatory disease.

PATHOLOGIC FINDINGS

Squamous cell cancers comprise approximately 85% of all cervical cancers. These cancers may show keratinization and have been subclassified according to their cell type or degree of differentiation. These are commonly reported as large cell nonkeratinizing, large cell keratinizing and small cell. Other variants of squamous cell cancers include verrucous cell carcinoma, papillary squamous cell carcinoma, and lymphoepithelial-like carcinoma. Other histologic types are adenocarcinoma. These cancers frequently arise in the endocervical canal, and therefore there may be no gross lesion identified on the surface of the cervix. Simple adenocarcinomas arising from the endocervix account for approximately 70% of all adenocarcinomas of the cervix. There are a variety of other histologic types, which include clear cell carcinoma, endometrioid carcinoma, adenoid basal carcinoma, and mesonephric carcinoma. Generally, all these cancers are treated similarly, based on the stage, with the possible exception of small cell carcinoma, which carries such a very poor prognosis that a single-treatment modality is usually not sufficient therapy.

TREATMENT

Treatment planning of patients with cervical cancers is best done jointly by both a radiation oncologist and gynecologic oncologist. Most treatment planning involves radiation therapy, except in the early stages of the disease. Carcinoma in situ of the cervix may be treated conservatively with simple excision of the abnormal area. This can be performed by conization, laser therapy, cryotherapy, or LEEP. Occasionally, hysterectomy may be appropriate in patients who no longer wish to bear children or in women with recurrent disease.

Early-stage invasive disease (Stage Ia) may be treated with simple hysterectomy up to a depth of 3 mm. Once there is more than 3-mm invasion, the likelihood of lymph node involvement increases, and therefore more radical therapy is required. Stage Ia cancers of the cervix may be treated with intracavitary treatment alone in cases where the patient may not be able to tolerate a major surgical procedure. Stage Ib and IIa cancers of the cervix can be treated with either radical hysterectomy and lymph node dissection or radical radiation therapy. The choice of one therapeutic modality over the other is controversial, but in properly selected cases, the survival rate is equivalent for each treatment modality, approaching 90%. The choice of therapy should be based on the individual patient's needs. Generally, younger patients tend to benefit more from surgery, because the ovaries can be preserved. Older patients at high risk for complications from surgery benefit more from radiation therapy.

Stage IIb, III, and IVa cancers of the cervix are best treated with radiation therapy. This should consist of 2000 to 3000 cGy to the whole pelvis followed by 2000 to 3000 cGy of split-field radiation and two intracavitary implants or 5000 to 6000 cGy to the whole pelvis and one or two intracavitary implants. The survival rate is good with radiation alone: 60 to 70% for Stage IIb and 30 to 45% for Stage III disease. Occasionally, a simple hysterectomy is performed, and an invasive cancer of the cervix is found. Postoperative radiation therapy is generally indicated in these cases, and the survival rates of these patients parallels, stage for stage, the survival rates of those who were treated with radiation alone, although the complication rate is somewhat higher.

Treatment of cervical cancer may be complicated by pregnancy. If this occurs, the wishes of the patient regarding the timing of treatment relative to fetal viability, stage, and the duration of remaining gestation must be carefully considered. There is no evidence that pregnancy per se adversely affects the outcome of the cancer, and the survival rate (stage for stage) is the same. One may consider delaying treatment until there is fetal viability in certain cases if the patient wishes to accept the unknown risk of delayed treatment.

POST-TREATMENT SURVEILLANCE

Most treatment failures occur in the first 2 to 3 years after treatment. Vaginal bleeding, abnormal Pap smears, pain, or weight loss are signs of recurrent disease and should be evaluated promptly. If recurrent disease is diagnosed, a metastatic evaluation should be undertaken to determine the extent of the disease and aid in treatment planning.

If the patient has recurrent disease after radical hysterectomy and there is no evidence of distant disease, radiation therapy is the treatment of choice. For patients who have undergone previous radiation therapy, some additional radiation can frequently be given. If there is a central recurrence with no evidence of distant disease, a pelvic exenteration can be performed. The survival rate of patients who are able to undergo pelvic exenteration may approach 50%. Even though these patients have undergone a process that results in major alteration of body image, they seem to adjust well, and few psychological problems have been reported.

Patients who are not candidates for additional radiation therapy or an exenterative procedure may benefit from chemotherapy. Agents that demonstrate activity against cervical cancer include cisplatin (Platinol), carboplatin (Paraplatin), and ifosfamide (Ifex). Patients treated with chemotherapy for recurrent cervical cancer have a median survival of 6 to 8 months.

NEOPLASMS OF THE VULVA

method of
R. ALLEN LAWHEAD, JR., M.D.
Georgia Baptist Medical Center
Atlanta, Georgia

Vulvar neoplasms present serious challenges to body image, sexual function, life, and quality of life for women of all ages. A vulvar neoplasm is a new growth caused by abnormal cell proliferation occurring on the vulva. Anatomically, the vulva is defined as the female external genitalia, including the mons pubis, extending to the genitocrural folds laterally and the anus inferiorly, and surrounding the vaginal introitus.

The diagnosis of a vulvar neoplasm can only be established by a histologic evaluation of a biopsy or surgical specimen. Vulvar neoplasms may be classified as benign, of premalignant potential, or malignant (Table 1). Early detection is the most important single factor

in the successful treatment of vulvar neoplasms. Unfortunately, the medical literature confirms that the two major barriers to successful treatment of vulvar neoplasms are delayed patient presentation and delayed physician evaluation. Currently, it is recommended that all women have a complete physical examination, including pelvic examination with careful inspection of the vulva, at least annually. Women should also be taught to perform routine vulvar self-examination (VSE) with a hand-held mirror and adequate lighting. VSE should be performed monthly or whenever symptoms relating to the vulva appear.

Findings such as warts, bumps, ulcers, or pigmented lesions should be reported to the physician immediately. Women should be informed that most findings will not be cancerous, but they do warrant further evaluation.

BENIGN NEOPLASMS OF THE VULVA

Clinical Manifestation, Evaluation, and Diagnosis

Benign vulvar neoplasms generally present as a bump or swelling on the vulva, often causing pain or discomfort. Asymptomatic patients may present with growths detected during VSE.

Benign neoplasms of the vulva include leiomyoma, lipoma, and fibroma, which generally present as subcutaneous tumors. Because of their subcutaneous location and potential for deeper extension, these lesions may not be amenable to colposcopically directed biopsy and are frequently better suited for complete excision for definitive diagnosis and treatment.

Hemangiomas of the vulva are generally small, red, or purple lesions noted on the surface of the skin. Usually, no treatment is required other than observation. Lesions that are enlarging or producing symptoms may be excised. Tumors of neural origin, including granular cell myoblastoma or neurofibroma, are generally treated by excision because they rarely undergo malignant change.

Treatment

Complete surgical excision is the treatment of choice for benign vulvar neoplasms. Recurrence

TABLE 1. **Classification of Vulvar Neoplasia**

Benign	Premalignant Potential	Malignant
Lipoma	VIN	Squamous cell carcinoma (invasive)
Fibroma	VIN-1 (mild dysplasia)	Adenocarcinoma
Hemangioma	VIN-2 (moderate dysplasia)	Melanoma
Leiomyoma	VIN-3 (severe dysplasia/carcinoma	Sarcoma
Neurofibroma	in situ)	Verrucous carcinoma
Granular cell	Intraepithelial Paget's disease	Extramammary Paget's with underlying adenocarcinoma
myoblastoma	Condyloma acuminatum	Bartholin's gland carcinoma (squamous, adenocarcinoma, transitional cell carcinoma)
		Basal cell carcinoma
		Metastatic cancer

Abbreviation: VIN = vulvar intraepithelial neoplasia.

of benign tumors after complete excision is rare and occurs more frequently with granular cell myoblastoma and leiomyoma. Patients with recurrent benign tumors are also best treated by complete surgical excision. Surgical specimens of large vulvar tumors should be carefully sectioned to rule out malignancy.

NEOPLASMS OF THE VULVA WITH PREMALIGNANT POTENTIAL

Neoplasms of the vulva with premalignant potential are defined as neoplasms that are frequently associated with or antecedent to vulvar malignancy (Table 1).

Condyloma Acuminatum (Genital Wart)

Clinical Manifestation, Evaluation, and Diagnosis

Condyloma acuminatum is the most common neoplasm of the vulva. The incidence of condyloma acuminatum is increasing in epidemic proportions. Condyloma acuminatum is caused by the human papillomavirus, of which there are more than forty types.

Condyloma acuminatum frequently begins as a small cauliflower lesion on the vulva. Asymptomatic lesions may be detected early in their course by patients performing routine VSE or by a health care professional at the time of pelvic examination. Such early diagnosis often allows for successful conservative treatment.

Although the human papillomavirus is highly sexually transmissible, nonsexual transmission is possible. Many infected patients do not have condylomata acuminatum.

The presence of this virus in the lower genital tract is associated with an increase risk for cervical neoplasia. Currently, the presence of human papillomavirus may also represent a risk factor for developing vaginal or vulvar neoplasia, although most patients with clinical condyloma acuminatum will not have a malignancy.

Condyloma acuminatum may undergo malignant transformation, may occur in association with malignancy or vulvar intraepithelial neoplasia (VIN), and may resemble vulvar carcinoma in clinical appearance. Therefore, careful evaluation with vulvar colposcopy and appropriate biopsies is indicated for patients with condylomatous vulvar lesions. Colposcopy of the entire lower genital tract should be used to define the extent of the vulvar condyloma, select the proper site for biopsy, and rule out associated vaginal or cervical neoplasia.

Treatment

Following a biopsy diagnosis of condyloma acuminatum (if there is no suspicion of underlying malignancy), treatment may be carried out for the following indications: (1) patients with associated premalignant conditions, such as VIN; (2) large masses of warts causing pain or pruritus; or (3) smaller warts that present unacceptable cosmetic effects or anxiety to the patient.

In general, patients with known human papillomavirus infection who are asymptomatic without neoplasia do not require treatment merely for the presence of the virus in the lower genital tract. Currently, there is no known treatment that will conclusively eliminate the virus from the lower genital tract. In this regard, patients with minimal microscopic condyloma may undergo careful observation, because it is estimated that as many as one-third of condylomata will spontaneously regress.

Once a patient has been properly evaluated and found to have an indication for treatment, she may be treated by a variety of methods including chemical treatment with trichloroacetic acid or podophyllin, surgical therapy with excision, or carbon dioxide laser vaporization. Other available therapeutic options include cryotherapy, topical treatment with 5-fluorouracil (5% Efudex) cream, or intralesional interferon.

In general, we prefer to use 50 to 80% trichloroacetic acid for treatment of small condylomatous lesions of the vulva. If the lesions are larger or if the patient is unwilling to have topical therapy, then carbon dioxide laser vaporization after appropriate histologic confirmation of the diagnosis is very satisfactory. Should the patient have one large condyloma or a large mass of condylomata, surgical excision is also appropriate. Because an exophytic cancer can resemble condylomata, however, it is important to obtain the appropriate histologic specimens prior to treatment. Any condylomatous lesion suspicious for cancer should be excised rather than treated with laser vaporization. This is especially true for large masses of condylomata in postmenopausal women. Although we think that biopsy-related diagnosis of a condylomatous lesion is important prior to treatment, some clinicians prefer to treat a smaller condyloma with topical therapy without a pretreatment biopsy. If this approach is used, condylomata that fail to regress promptly should be evaluated by biopsy prior to further treatment.

Vulvar Intraepithelial Neoplasia

VIN is characterized by a spectrum of disordered maturation of the squamous epithelium on the vulva. It represents a continuum of pathologic change extending from mild dysplasia or VIN-1 to VIN-3, which includes severe dysplasia and carcinoma in situ. The histologic criteria for the diagnosis of VIN are listed in Table 2.

The incidence of VIN is increasing in all women but, especially, among younger women. This increase parallels and appears to be associated with the increasing incidence of human papillomavirus. This virus has been implicated as a possible etiologic factor in VIN. However, the exact role of human papillomavirus in the initiation and/or promotion of vulvar malignancy has not been documented.

Clinical Manifestation, Evaluation, and Diagnosis

VIN exhibits a wide variety of clinical manifestations. It may appear on the vulva as a red, white, brown, or black pigmented lesion and may exist in relatively normal-looking epithelium. VIN lesions may also be ulcerative, flat, exophytic, or condylomatous. Because of this, all patients with significant vulvar lesions require biopsy evaluation.

If a woman presents with findings of a vulvar lesion on self-examination or symptoms of pruritus or pain that lead to the finding of a vulvar lesion, the evaluation should include a careful physical examination with colposcopy of the vulva using 3 to 6% acetic acid followed by the biopsy of appropriate lesions. Either 2% lidocaine (Xylocaine) jelly or 1% local lidocaine injection may be used for anesthetizing the area to undergo a biopsy. The biopsy should then be done under colposcopic guidance and may be done with standard punch biopsy forceps or a Keyes punch as indicated by the clinical situation. Small lesions that can be completely excised in the office may also be excised by the scalpel technique. If the biopsy site defects are small, they can be treated with Monsell's solution for hemostasis. Patients are then instructed in the care of the biopsy sites by using sitz baths. The use of a hair dryer on a cool setting is encouraged to help dry the vulva after sitz baths.

When a relatively large lesion is excised in the office, suture closure with an absorbable suture may be appropriate. Small biopsy sites generally heal very well without suture closure.

Evaluation of vulvar lesions should be goal directed with the purpose of colposcopy being to identify and evaluate the extent of the vulvar lesions, select the most abnormal sites for biopsy, and rule out associated cervical or vaginal neoplasia. Patients with vulvar neoplasia appear to be at increased risk for cervical and vaginal neoplasia. Therefore, a Pap smear of the cervix (or, in the case of a posthysterectomy patient, a Pap smear of the vagina) should be taken.

The characteristics of abnormal epithelium under colposcopic visualization with 3 to 6% acetic acid include white epithelium with or without abnormal vascular changes, such as punctuation, mosaic changes, and bizarre vessel formation. Lesions with an abnormal surface contour should also be carefully evaluated. Colposcopic evaluation of a visible vulvar lesion is an invaluable technique to detect microscopic satellite disease. It is important to select the most colposcopically abnormal site for biopsy to maximize the detection of early occult invasive lesions.

Treatment

Currently, VIN-3 (severe dysplasia or carcinoma in situ) is generally treated with either wide excision or carbon dioxide laser vaporization following the appropriate evaluation to rule out occult invasive carcinoma. Treatment for VIN-3 should generally be undertaken with two objectives. The primary goal is to eradicate the lesion completely, but a second and equally important objective is to maximize preservation of female identity and sexual function. In this regard, complete vulvectomy or skinning vulvectomy for focal lesions is rarely (if ever) indicated.

We believe that most patients are best treated with wide excision, which allows for primary surgical closure with less postoperative pain and morbidity, as well as a thorough histologic evaluation of the specimen to rule out occult invasive disease. It is especially important to use wide local excision when treating exophytic lesions that are histologically shown to contain VIN-3 on biopsy, because of the possibility of occult invasive carcinoma.

Carbon dioxide laser vaporization, on the other hand, appears to be ideally suited for focal lesions on the labia minora or clitoris, which can be treated with the maximal preservation of architecture and function. Excisional therapy of lesions on the labia minora or clitoris often results

TABLE 2. **Classification of VIN**

Grade		Histologic Definition
VIN 1	Mild dysplasia	Neoplastic cells involve bottom 1/3 of epithelium
VIN 2	Moderate dysplasia	Neoplastic cells involve > 1/3 but < 2/3 of epithelium
VIN 3	Severe dysplasia/CIS	Neoplastic cells involve ≥ 2/3 of epithelium (full-thickness involvement constitutes CIS)

Abbreviations: VIN = vulvar intraepithelial neoplasia; CIS = carcinoma in situ.

in a less than ideal functional result; microscopic treatment using the carbon dioxide laser in these regions allows for optimal success and conservative therapy.

Because the goals of successful curative treatment and conservation of female sexual function and identity are important to women of all ages, occasionally, a combination approach is desirable with multifocal lesions, resulting in local excision of some lesions with laser vaporization of others. Treatment with wide excision or laser vaporization can generally result in a cure rate of 90% with a single treatment.

All patients should be instructed to perform regular VSE and continue careful clinical follow-up, because new sites of vulvar neoplasia may arise in other locations of the vulva. It is never appropriate to treat a lesion with laser vaporization without appropriate histologic confirmation of the diagnosis. With the availability of conservative therapy for early lesions, it is imperative that patients be taught the technique of monthly VSE using a hand-held mirror to inspect the vulva in between menstrual periods or whenever they have symptoms relating to the vulva. Patients presenting with lesions found during VSE should have prompt, colposcopic evaluation with biopsies as indicated to achieve early detection and successful conservative therapy.

Patients with recurrent VIN-3 or new primary lesions of VIN-3 should undergo evaluation and treatment as previously described here. For patients who perform regular VSE of the vulva and careful follow-up colposcopy and biopsy as indicated, vulvectomy can almost always be avoided. Patients with VIN-1 or VIN-2 should be treated with excision or laser vaporization if they have visible lesions. If VIN-1 or VIN-2 occurs in normal-appearing skin or if the patient does not desire treatment, she should receive careful follow-up with VSE and biopsies as indicated, because the progression rate of VIN-1 or VIN-2 to malignancy is not well documented.

Intraepithelial Paget's Disease

Clinical Manifestation, Evaluation, and Diagnosis

Extramammary Paget's disease of the vulva is a relatively rare clinical entity distinguished by the histologic finding of pagetoid cells in the epithelium and skin adnexa of the vulva. This generally occurs as an intraepithelial neoplasia. Approximately 10% of patients with intraepithelial Paget's disease will have an underlying adenocarcinoma. Patients with extramammary Paget's disease will usually have a visible lesion on the vulva that is pink or red-velvety in color and may complain of itching and burning.

Patients who present with such lesions or symptoms should be evaluated by colposcopy with biopsy. Those with a biopsy-related diagnosis of intraepithelial Paget's disease should undergo a careful evaluation to rule out underlying vulvar adenocarcinoma and also have a complete evaluation with mammography to rule out concurrent adenocarcinoma of the breast or gastrointestinal tract.

Colposcopic examination of the lower genital tract with biopsies as indicated is appropriate to rule out cervical or vaginal neoplasia as with VIN. Once an associated invasive malignancy is ruled out, treatment may be undertaken. Patients with an associated underlying adenocarcinoma of the vulva are generally treated as would be appropriate for their invasive disease.

Treatment

Extramammary Paget's disease may be treated by wide excision or laser vaporization. Wide excision is preferable to rule out an underlying adenocarcinoma. Laser vaporization is generally more appropriate in patients with lesions affecting the clitoris and labia minora in which the surgical cosmetic effect would be less than optimum. Sometimes, a combined modality may be required to achieve the most successful results and preserve optimal sexual function and female identity. All patients with a history of Paget's disease should be followed carefully, be taught to perform monthly VSE, and have a clinical evaluation with colposcopy as indicated.

MALIGNANT LESIONS OF THE VULVA

Invasive Squamous Cell Carcinoma

Clinical Manifestation, Evaluation, and Diagnosis

In concert with the general upward trend for VIN, the incidence of invasive squamous cell cancer of the vulva also appears to be increasing, especially among younger women. Recently, it has been reported that carcinoma of the vulva accounts for 5 to 8% of gynecologic malignancies.

Cancer of the vulva represents the ultimate challenge to female identity and sexual function. Over 95% of patients with vulvar cancer are symptomatic and present with complaints such as pruritus, bleeding, pain, irritation, discharge, or palpation of a mass or ulcer. Almost all invasive vulvar cancers are visible to the eye of the patient (using a mirror) and physician at the time of diagnosis. Early diagnosis is the most important factor for cure and conservative management of vulvar cancer. Despite these facts, the major obstacles to the successful treatment of vulvar cancer continue to be delayed patient presentation and delayed physician evaluation, which were originally described by Dr. Charles Meigs in 1854.

Recently, improved understanding of the clinicopathologic behavior of vulvar cancer has led to the development of successful conservative treatment strategies that preserve life, female identity, and sexual function. It has been shown that patients utilizing VSE can present to physicians for early diagnosis and successful conservative therapy of very early vulvar malignancies.

Squamous cell carcinoma of the vulva can present with a variety of appearances, including red, brown, black, yellow, pink, or white lesions, which may be ulcerative, exophytic, or condylomatoid in appearance. Patients with invasive vulvar carcinoma should have a thorough physical evaluation with colposcopy of the entire lower genital tract and biopsies as indicated. An essential part of this evaluation is careful palpation of the inguinal nodes. Usually, we prefer to evaluate clinically suspicious groin nodes at the time of definitive surgery and groin dissection. However, very elderly patients or patients who are not surgical candidates may benefit from a fine-needle biopsy technique. The presence of a negative fine-needle biopsy result, however, does not rule out malignancy in the lymph node.

Proctosigmoidoscopy or barium enema may be helpful in patients with adenocarcinoma of the vulva, in patients with lesions close to the anorectum, or in patients with gastrointestinal symptoms. Computed tomography of the abdomen and pelvis are recommended in patients with very large tumors or tumors believed to involve the bone or other pelvic structures.

Treatment

Currently, surgical excision of the tumor and regional lymph nodes is the therapy of choice. The current International Federation of Gynecology and Obstetrics (FIGO) staging system for carcinoma of the vulva utilizes surgical findings and is shown in Table 3. Continued improvements in our understanding of the clinicopathologic behavior of vulvar neoplasia have allowed for a rapidly evolving conservative approach to the treatment of women with vulvar carcinoma that recognizes the emphasis of contemporary women on the quality of life as well as survival.

Up until the last five years, the treatment for even the smallest invasive vulvar carcinoma was often radical vulvectomy and bilateral groin dissection. Current studies have demonstrated that the treatment of invasive squamous cell carcinoma of the vulva can generally be individualized, based on the location and extent of the lesion and the likelihood of involvement of underlying regional lymph nodes.

In the opinion of this author, one of the most significant improvements in the classification of vulvar malignancy is the definition of early stromal invasion (Stage Ia) established by the International Society for the Study of Vulvar Disease in 1989. Stage Ia (early stromal invasion) is defined as a vulvar malignancy less than or equal to 2 cm in diameter with stromal invasion of 1 mm or less as measured from the nearest adjacent dermal papilla.

Numerous studies confirm that this subset of patients may be treated successfully by wide excision only (without groin dissection), thus establishing a category of patients with vulvar malignancy that may truly receive conservative therapy with preservation of female identity and sexual function. This mandates careful attention to the biopsy specimens in all patients with early, small invasive vulvar carcinomas to identify patients for conservative therapy. Although Stage Ia as proposed by the International Society for the Study of Vulvar Disease is not recognized by FIGO, adopting and applying this key definition in the evaluation of patients with early vulvar carcinoma is essential for excellent care.

Because the treatment for invasive carcinoma of the vulva must be individualized and depends on a very meticulous evaluation, all patients with invasive malignancies of the vulva should be referred to a gynecologic oncologist for definitive evaluation and therapy. Patients with early stromal invasion, Stage Ia, may be expected to have a 90 to 100% cure rate when treated by wide radical excision, which often allows for preservation of female identity and sexual function. Currently, none of our patients treated in this fashion have developed recurrent invasive carcinoma of the vulva.

Patients with unilateral Stage I lesions and greater than 1 mm of stromal invasion and those with Stage II lesions may be treated with radical excision or hemivulvectomy and ipsilateral groin dissection. If the lymph nodes and the margins of resection are negative, treatment is considered complete. If the regional lymph nodes are positive, patients are generally treated with postoperative radiation therapy to the pelvis. If the lesion is bilateral or in the midline, a bilateral groin dissection is usually performed.

Some authorities prefer to treat Stages I and II unilateral lesions with radical vulvectomy and bilateral groin dissection. However, in our experience, this does not add to survival and certainly contributes to morbidity and a decreased quality of life even in patients who are cured.

TABLE 3. **International Federation of Gynecology and Obstetrics Staging for Primary Carcinoma of the Vulva**

Stage 0	Tis	Carcinoma in situ, intraepithelial carcinoma
Stage I	T1N0M0	Tumor confined to the vulva and/or perineum, 2 cm or less in greatest dimension, no nodal metastasis
Stage II	T2N0M0	Tumor confined to the vulva and/or perineum, more than 2 cm in greatest dimension, no nodal metastasis
Stage III	T3N0M0	Tumor of any size with adjacent spread to the lower urethra and/or the
	T3N1M0	vagina, or the anus, and/or unilateral regional lymph node metastasis
	T1N1M0	
	T2N1M0	
Stage IVa	T1N2M0	Tumor invades any of the following: upper urethra, bladder mucosa,
	T2N2M0	rectal mucosa, pelvic bone, and/or bilateral regional node metastasis
	T3N2M0	
	T4 Any N M0	
Stage IVb	Any T, Any N, M1	Any distant metastasis, including pelvic lymph nodes

In patients with Stages III and IV lesions, surgical therapy is often the initial therapy of choice in an effort to stage the tumor completely and resect the malignancy. Radical vulvectomy and bilateral groin dissection or primary pelvic exenteration with groin node dissection may be required for curative surgical therapy. Patients with large primary malignancies of the vulva may also be treated by primary radiation therapy or radiation therapy in combination with chemotherapy (chemoradiation).

Chemoradiation using such agents as mitomycin (Mutamycin) with 5-fluorouracil, or cisplatin (Platinol) with 5-fluorouracil has been shown to be effective at inducing complete remission in patients with large tumors. Chemoradiation presents a curative treatment option in patients with large tumors who are not candidates for exenteration or who do not desire ultraradical surgery.

Approximately 75% of patients with vulvar carcinoma will be cured. The overall 5-year survival rate for patients with Stages I and II disease is 90%. In the absence of regional lymph node involvement and distant metastasis (regardless of stage), 90 to 95% of patients with vulvar carcinoma will be cured. The presence of positive groin nodes significantly decreases the survival rate to the range of 45 to 65%, depending on the number of nodes involved. Patients with positive pelvic nodes and distant metastasis may expect a survival rate of 20% or less.

The treatment of recurrent carcinoma of the vulva must be individualized. Patients with a local skin recurrence may be treated with wide excision. Those with large recurrent tumors following surgery and/or radiation therapy may require radical excision or exenteration with the use of rectus abdominis or gracilis myocutaneous flaps for reconstruction as indicated. Radiation can also be used to treat local recurrences. Patients with distant metastasis may be treated with che-motherapeutic regimens, such as cisplatin and 5-fluorouracil or cisplatin, ifosfamide (Ifex), bleomycin (Blenoxane).

The follow-up for patients treated for vulvar carcinoma includes monthly VSE and physical examinations every 3 months during the 1st year, every 4 months during the 2nd year, and then every 6 months thereafter, with diagnostic studies as indicated.

Melanoma of the Vulva

Clinical Manifestation, Evaluation, and Diagnosis

Although relatively rare, melanoma of the vulva is the second most common malignancy occurring on the vulva. Melanoma accounts for 5 to 10% of malignant neoplasms of the vulva. Although the skin of the vulva accounts for approximately 1% of the total skin surface, approximately 4% of skin melanomas occur on the vulva. Because of this, many authorities have suggested that all vulvar nevi should be excised prophylactically to rule out melanoma as well as to prevent the subsequent development of melanoma.

In patients who have benign-appearing nevi on the clitoris or labia minora and who refuse prophylactic excision, we think it is mandatory that the patient learn careful VSE and report any changes in size, shape, or consistency of any nevi to the physician for immediate evaluation. Women using VSE to find new pigmented lesions or changes in previously pigmented lesions have presented for early conservative and curative therapy of vulvar melanoma.

As with squamous cell carcinoma, the most important factor for curative therapy and optimal lifestyle is early diagnosis. Patients with melanoma of the vulva should receive a presurgical evaluation similar to that for squamous cell carcinoma, and then they are generally treated surgically.

Treatment

Wide radical excision is the treatment of choice for primary lesions with the use of groin dissection in patients with clinically suspicious nodes. Some authorities also recommend doing a regional lymph node dissection for significantly invasive melanomas even though current data suggest this procedure is of prognostic value only.

The microscopic staging systems currently used in patients with vulvar melanoma are listed in Table 4. Although Clark levels have been the standard for melanomas of the skin in general, Chung levels offer a more accurate assessment of vulvar melanoma, because of the peculiar characteristics of vulvar skin.

The cure rate for surgically treated vulvar melanoma varies with the level of disease, ranging from a cure rate of almost 100% for patients with Level 1 lesions and decreasing to 25% or less with Levels 4 and 5 lesions.

Patients who have metastatic lesions outside the genital tract not amenable to surgery should have their treatment individualized. Cure is difficult to accomplish in these patients. Chemotherapy, immunotherapy, radiation therapy, or combinations of these modalities may be utilized. Currently, there is much investigational interest in the use of chemotherapy with immunotherapy to patients with advanced vulvar melanoma. As with squamous cell carcinoma, patients with a diagnosis of vulvar melanoma should be promptly referred to a gynecologic oncologist for definitive evaluation and therapy.

Vulvar Sarcoma

Clinical Manifestation, Evaluation, and Diagnosis

Primary sarcomas rarely occur on the vulva and are generally treated surgically with treatment individualized to the extent of the disease and the medical condition of the patient. The histologic grade of a sarcoma is one of the most important features in assessing the prognosis.

Treatment

Treatment is aimed at radical removal of the primary vulvar tumor with negative surgical margins. In patients with very low-grade sarcomas, wide excision only may suffice, whereas in patients with anaplastic or poorly differentiated tumors, groin dissection may be included. In patients with metastatic disease, postoperative radiation therapy or chemotherapy may be useful.

Verrucous Carcinoma (Giant Condyloma of Buschke-Lowenstein)

Clinical Manifestation, Evaluation, and Diagnosis

Verrucous carcinoma is a very well-differentiated squamous cell carcinoma. It has a clinical tendency for local invasion but generally does not produce regional lymphatic spread. It is often diagnosed under the synonym "giant condyloma of Buschke-Lowenstein" and may be confused with condyloma acuminatum. Avoiding this confusion is yet another reason for careful colposcopic evaluation with appropriate biopsies of patients with condylomatous lesions.

Treatment

Patients with giant condyloma of Buschke-Lowenstein (or verrucous carcinoma) are best treated by wide local excision. Those with negative surgical margins may generally expect a 90% or better cure rate. Inguinal node metastasis is extremely rare, even with large tumors, if the histologic diagnosis has been rigorously confirmed.

Basal Cell Carcinoma

Basal cell carcinoma presents as a small nodule with central umbilication or as an ulcer. These lesions may cause pruritus, pain, or chronic irritation. Colposcopic evaluation of the lower genital tract with an appropriate biopsy-directed diagnosis completes the evaluation of patients with localized basal cell carcinoma.

Treatment

Treatment is wide excision, which is curative in patients with negative surgical margins.

Bartholin's Gland Carcinoma

Carcinoma of the Bartholin's glands occurs in about 1% of patients with vulvar malignancy and

TABLE 4. **Two Methods for Microscopic Staging of Vulvar Melanoma**

Stage (Level)	Chung	Clark
I	In situ melanoma	Same
II	Invasion ≤ 1 mm from granular layer	Invasion into papillary dermis
III	Invasion > 1 mm, but ≤ 2 mm	Tumor fills papillary dermis, extends to but not into reticular dermis
IV	Invasion > 2 mm without extension to underlying fat	Invasion into reticular dermis
V	Invasion into subcutaneous fat	Same

generally occurs in postmenopausal women. Multiple histologic types have been observed, including squamous cell carcinoma, adenosquamous carcinoma, adenoid cystic carcinoma, and transitional cell carcinoma. Because of the location of these tumors, dyspareunia is often the initial presenting symptom. Approximately one-half of the Bartholin's gland carcinomas appear to be squamous cell in origin.

Treatment

A woman in the postmenopausal period with an enlarged Bartholin's gland should usually have this gland excised. Even premenopausal patients with persistent Bartholin's glands abscesses, masses, or infections should be considered for complete surgical excision of the Bartholin's gland if they have had two or more Bartholin's gland operations. The optimal treatment is surgical therapy, which includes complete resection of the malignancy and regional lymph node dissection.

Adenocarcinoma of the Vulva

Adenocarcinoma of the vulva is an uncommon entity and may be seen either as a primary adenocarcinoma involving the apocrine sweat glands or Bartholin's glands or associated with intraepithelial Paget's disease. In general, patients with primary adenocarcinoma of the vulva receive an evaluation and treatment that are similar to those in patients with primary squamous cell carcinoma.

Metastatic Tumors

Although tumor metastasis to the vulva occurs infrequently, it is essential to rule out metastasis in any patient presenting with a new vulvar malignancy. A thorough examination of the lower genital tract to rule out a metastasis from a primary cervical or vaginal tumor is essential. Endometrial, ovarian, or colon carcinomas also metastasize to the vulva. These etiologies should always be considered when the primary histologic finding of the vulvar lesion is adenocarcinoma.

Patients with melanoma of the vulva should undergo a complete skin survey and ophthalmoscopic examination to confirm the primary site of malignancy. The treatment for metastatic tumor deposits on the vulva should be individualized with primary attention being given to the relief of symptoms and the cosmetic and functional removal of the lesion. Because of the importance of the vulva to a woman's quality of life, it is imperative that the physician exercise the highest degree of judgment when dealing with metastatic tumors of the vulva. As with all cases of vulvar malignancy, patients should be referred to a gynecologic oncologist for definitive evaluation and therapy.

THROMBOPHLEBITIS IN OBSTETRICS AND GYNECOLOGY

method of
BARBARA BENNETT, M.D., and
PATRICK DUFF, M.D.
University of Florida College of Medicine
Gainesville, Florida

VENOUS THROMBOSIS

Venous thrombosis is a serious problem that is not confined to obstetric and gynecologic patients. However, patients in this population do harbor certain risk factors unique to their gender that result in a much greater incidence of thromboembolic disease than occurs in the general population. Two to 10% of women undergoing cesarean deliveries and 0.25 to 1% of women having vaginal deliveries will have some form of thromboembolic disease. Fortunately, only 0.4% of these will result in pulmonary embolus (PE). Untreated, PE is fatal in up to 12% of patients, underscoring the need for prevention, early diagnosis, and treatment of venous thrombosis.

Risk Factors

Venous stasis, hypercoagulability, and endothelial cell damage make up Virchow's triad of prerequisite factors for the development of thrombosis. Unfortunately, obstetric patients demonstrate all these prerequisites. During pregnancy, stasis occurs due to compression of the inferior vena cava by the gravid uterus. Blood becomes hypercoagulable due to the increased hepatic synthesis of fibrinogen and factors VII to X. As a result, thromboembolic events occur twice as often as in the nonpregnant state. The incidence of thromboembolic disease is even greater during the immediate puerperium, especially after surgical delivery, because vascular injury and infection are more likely to occur. Conditions such as connective tissue disease and antiphospholipid antibody syndrome also markedly increase the risk of thrombosis.

Patients with gynecologic conditions are also at increased risk of thromboembolic disease. Decreased blood flow in the iliac vessels during pelvic surgery, as well as increases in platelets and coagulation factors II, VIII, IX, and X, makes the average incidence of postoperative thrombosis in patients undergoing gynecologic surgery as high as 15%. The risk is also dependent on the duration and extent of surgery, amount of blood loss, and presence of malignancy. Other factors that increase the risk include age, obesity, prior history of deep venous thrombosis (DVT), prior radiation therapy, venous disease, history of hypercoagulability, leg edema, and poor ambulation. Antithrombin III, a natural anticoagulant, is decreased in women who take oral contraceptives, especially those who also smoke, and therefore these individuals also are at increased risk of thromboembolism.

Diagnosis

The diagnosis of superficial thrombophlebitis is usually obvious during the physical examination. In the upper extremities, thrombophlebitis is particularly likely to occur at the site of an intravenous catheter. The site may become tender, swollen, and erythematous, and the patient may have a fever. In the lower extremities, superficial varicose veins may become inflamed as a result of inactivity and venous stasis.

Symptoms of DVT are, unfortunately, absent in as many as one-half of cases. Calf tenderness, edema, and induration (a "cord") may be present, as may a low-grade fever and tachycardia. Homans' sign is found less than 20% of the time. DVT usually develops within 72 hours of surgery but may not present until after the patient's discharge. Any patient in whom there is suspicion of DVT must undergo intensive evaluation, because a fatal pulmonary embolus may result from untreated thrombosis in the lower extremities.

The "gold standard" for the diagnosis of DVT is venography. A venous thrombus is seen as a defect within the vessel, a cutoff of contrast, or nonfilling of a vessel in association with collateral flow to superficial veins. Although the technique allows evaluation of the entire lower extremity, drawbacks include its invasive nature, difficulty in distinguishing old from new clots, technical difficulty in cannulating pedal veins, contrast-induced phlebitis, and patient discomfort. These problems have given impetus to the development of other, noninvasive diagnostic tests. Venography during pregnancy should be performed with the abdomen shielded.

Impedance plethysmography (IPG) is a noninvasive technique that measures the reduction in venous outflow from a lower extremity caused by proximal DVT by detecting changes in electrical resistance. In some series, the overall sensitivity and specificity of IPG has exceeded 90%, and many investigators treat patients solely on the basis of IPG results. However, IPG cannot distinguish between old versus new clots and thrombotic versus nonthrombotic obstruction to venous outflow. In addition, because the veins of the calf are small and have multiple parallel collateral channels, thromboses cannot be detected by IPG until multiple veins are affected. Finally, the experience with IPG in pregnant women is still limited.

Another noninvasive means of evaluating the deep venous system is duplex Doppler ultrasonography. This technique combines an audible representation of blood flow with real-time B-mode visualization to assess the proximal deep veins. This technique is able to distinguish between acute versus chronic clot on the basis of echogenicity and occlusive versus nonocclusive clot. However, it is unable to evaluate the veins of the calf reliably. The accuracy of this test approaches that of venography and has replaced it in many centers. Triplex scanning includes color flow Doppler to provide information about the velocity of flow within the vessels.

Iodine-125–labeled fibrinogen scanning is a technique that measures fibrinogen incorporation into a developing thrombus. It is able to detect thrombi in the lower thigh and calf, but it is less reliable in assessing thrombi in the veins of the upper thigh, because of the close proximity of the bladder and large veins of the pelvis. The disadvantages of this technique include a decreased sensitivity in detecting an old clot and the need to wait for up to 72 hours for a positive result. The technique is contraindicated in pregnancy and lactation.

Another scintigraphic test uses indium- or technetium-labeled antifibrin monoclonal antibodies. This technique is still under study but appears to be more accurate in detecting acute and recurrent DVT. Other advantages include the ability to evaluate the lower extremities above and below the knee and the decreased time required for the diagnosis because of the rapid clearance of the labeled fibrin.

Treatment

The treatment of superficial thrombophlebitis consists of rest, elevation, and local heat. Nonsteroidal anti-inflammatory agents may be helpful; anticoagulation and antibiotics are rarely necessary.

The initial management of DVT includes rest and elevation until the pain and edema in the extremity resolve. Most physicians do not treat DVT with anticoagulation unless the clot extends above the popliteal veins, because calf vein thrombi rarely propagate to the lung. For clots that do extend above this level, anticoagulation with heparin prevents extension of the existing clot. Heparin combines with antithrombin III to inactivate factor Xa and inhibit thrombin formation. The normal fibrinolytic mechanism is responsible for lysis of the initial clot.

Intravenous heparin therapy should be initiated with a loading dose of 70 to 100 units per kg, followed by a maintenance infusion of 15 to 25 units per kg per hour, adjusting the dose to achieve an activated partial thromboplastin time (aPTT) of 1.5 to 2 times normal or a serum heparin level of 0.2 to 0.7 units per mL. The platelet count should also be monitored, because heparin can cause thrombocytopenia. The most serious complication of heparin use is hemorrhage; therefore, use of drugs that interfere with platelet function or blood clotting (e.g., aspirin or nonsteroidal anti-inflammatory agents) should be avoided during treatment. Other side effects of heparin include osteoporosis, paradoxical thrombosis, hypersensitivity, and skin necrosis.

Intravenous heparin should be administered for at least 5 days. In nonpregnant patients, oral anticoagulation with warfarin (Coumadin) should be continued for 4 to 6 months. Warfarin may be started at the same time as intravenous heparin, and the dose should be titrated to increase the prothrombin time (PT) to 1.5 times normal. Heparin should not be discontinued until the PT is therapeutic for at least 4 days. The initial rise in PT is due to an early drop in factor VII, but the complete antithrombotic effect is delayed until factors IX and X decline, usually after about 4 days.

Pregnant patients must be maintained on intermittent subcutaneous heparin injections instead of oral warfarin, because the latter is teratogenic. Warfarin does not pass into breast milk in significant amounts, so breast-feeding is acceptable. Subcutaneous heparin injections of 5000 to 10,000 units every 8 to 12 hours are usually sufficient to prolong PTT values. Heparin should be discontinued in labor and restarted several hours after delivery, and anticoagulation with either heparin or warfarin should be continued until at least 3 months post partum.

Fibrinolytic agents are seldom used in the treatment of DVT and are usually reserved for cases in which the clot has propagated beyond the origin of the femoral vein. These agents are contraindicated in pregnancy. Vena caval filters may be indicated in patients with recurrent pulmonary emboli despite anticoagulation or in patients who have a contraindication to anticoagulation. Complete iliofemoral occlusion may require thrombectomy to prevent propagation into the inferior vena cava and subsequent PE.

Complications

PE occurs in 8% of patients with calf vein thrombosis and up to 50% of patients with femoral vein thrombosis if the condition is left untreated. Although many patients who experience PE are asymptomatic, massive PE can be fatal. Clinically, patients usually complain of dyspnea, pleuritic chest pain, and apprehension. Rales, an increase in intensity of the second heart sound over the pulmonic area, and tachypnea are common signs. An electrocardiogram may show tachycardia, but the signs of right axis deviation and ST segment changes are rare except in cases of massive PE. Chest x-ray alone is not usually helpful in the diagnosis of PE but does rule out other pulmonary disorders and assists the radiologist with the interpretation of ventilation-perfusion studies (V/Q scan). The V/Q scan employs injection of radiocolloid particles into the circulation and ventilation scintigraphy using technetium or xenon gas. The results are usually reported in terms of the "probability" of a PE (low, moderate, high, or indeterminant). A low-probability or negative scan result effectively rules out PE. Conversely, a patient with a high-probability scan finding has an 85% chance of truly having a PE. An indeterminant or moderate probability scan result is nondiagnostic and should be followed by pulmonary arteriography, the "gold standard" for diagnosis. This latter study carries a 5% morbidity and 0.2% mortality rate and is usually reserved for patients in whom V/Q scanning is nondiagnostic. Treatment of PE is the same as that for DVT. Thrombolytic therapy may be used in patients with bilateral PEs or hemodynamic compromise due to a massive saddle embolism.

Another complication of DVT is the postphlebitic syndrome in which lower extremity edema, dermatitis, ulceration, and pain occur as a result of a distortion of the venous valves and endothelium due to the recanalization process. Stripping of these dilated veins may improve the condition.

Prevention

The best intervention for thromboembolic disease is to prevent its occurrence. Alteration of the reversible risk factors is the first step. A thorough history will identify those patients at highest risk and allow preoperative interventions, such as increased ambulation, weight loss, treatment of coexisting medical problems, treatment of pelvic infection, and discontinuation of oral contraceptives. Patients at moderate to high risk should wear graduated compression stockings or intermittent pneumatic compression stockings and be given minidose anticoagulation. Heparin in a dose of 5000 units subcutaneously 2 hours before and every 8 to 12 hours after surgery is standard; however, some advocate addition of dihydroergotamine (D.H.E. 45) to this regimen for improved prophylaxis. Use of this combination in pregnancy has not been reported. Other ergots are known uterotonic agents, and the vasotonic effects of dihydroergotamine may contraindicate its use in pregnancy.

SEPTIC PELVIC VEIN THROMBOPHLEBITIS

Septic pelvic vein thrombophlebitis is an uncommon but potentially life-threatening complication of soft tissue infections of the pelvis. It occurs in 2% or less of patients who have postoperative pelvic infections or pelvic inflammatory disease.

Septic pelvic vein thrombophlebitis occurs in two distinct forms. The most commonly described presentation is acute thrombosis of one or both ovarian veins. The right ovarian vein is more likely to be affected than the left. Affected patients typically have a high fever, chills, and lower abdominal pain. They also demonstrate abdominal tenderness, guarding, and an adynamic ileus. Approximately one-half to two-thirds of patients have a sausage-shaped, tender mass that originates near the uterine cornua and extends cephalad toward the midline. The principal elements in the differential diagnosis of ovarian vein thrombosis are pyelonephritis, nephrolithiasis, appendicitis, adnexal torsion, and pelvic abscess.

The second presentation of septic pelvic vein thrombophlebitis has been characterized as "enigmatic fever." Affected patients usually have a persistent febrile course after surgery but do not have a significant degree of abdominal pain or tenderness. Very few patients have a palpable mass. Presumably, these individuals have multiple thrombi in the smaller vessels of the pelvis rather than a single large thrombus. The other major disorders that must be considered in the differential diagnosis of enigmatic fever include drug fever, viral syndrome, connective tissue disease, and pelvic abscess.

In patients who present with signs of acute peritonitis, the diagnosis of septic pelvic vein thrombophlebitis must be established by laparotomy. In patients who are less severely ill, particularly those with a large thrombus in one of the major pelvic vessels, noninvasive tests, such as computed tomography (CT), magnetic resonance imaging (MRI), and ultrasonography, may be valuable in confirming the clinical diagnosis. In patients with enigmatic fever, CT, MRI, and ultrasonography usually have negative results, and an empirical trial of anticoagulation with heparin may be necessary to establish the correct diagnosis.

Once the diagnosis of septic pelvic vein thrombophlebitis is made, the patient should be treated with full anticoagulant doses of heparin. The drug should be administered by continuous or intermittent infusion in doses sufficient to prolong the aPTT to 1.5 to 2.0 times normal or to achieve a serum heparin concentration of 0.2 to 0.7 IU per mL. Parenteral anticoagulation should be continued for 7 to 10 days. Extended oral anticoagulation is indicated in patients who have had clear evidence of a large thrombus in one or several of the major pelvic vessels or who have sustained a septic pulmonary embolism.

In addition to receiving anticoagulation, patients should be treated with broad-spectrum intravenous antibiotics. Clindamycin (Cleocin) 900 mg every 8 hours or metronidazole (Flagyl) 500 mg every 6 hours plus penicillin 5 million units every 6 hours or ampicillin 2 grams every 6 hours plus gentamicin (Garamycin) 1.5 mg per kg every 8 hours or aztreonam (Azactam) 2 grams every 8 hours are regimens that have been tested extensively and shown to be effective in this clinical situation. Antibiotics should be continued for the 7 to 10 days that the patient is receiving heparin.

Once antibiotics and heparin are administered, most patients show a clear response to treatment within 48 to 72 hours. If no improvement occurs, two possibilities must be considered. The first is that of an incorrect diagnosis. The second is that the thrombotic process is so extensive that surgery may be necessary to ligate or excise the infected pelvic vessels.

CONTRACEPTION

method of
LOUISE B. TYRER, M.D.
Association of Reproductive Health Professionals
Washington, D.C.

During most of their lives sexually active women want to avoid pregnancy. Of the approximately 58 million women aged 15 to 44 years, 67% are at any given time at risk of unintended pregnancy. Despite the wide range of contraceptives available today more than one-half of the nearly 6 million pregnancies in the United States each year are unintended. About one-half of these pregnancies end in induced abortion, except among women 35 years of age and older who more often choose abortion than birth. To add to the problem, contraception is not always effective nor used appropriately. About 50% of women who come for abortion indicate they were using contraception at the time they conceived.

The woman's choice of a contraceptive method is greatly influenced by its effectiveness and whether she wants more children in the future. This explains in part why sterilization is the method used most commonly by American couples who do not want more children. Oral contraceptives are the most frequently used method of contraception among women who intend to have a child in the future, followed by barriers and spermicides.

In counseling women and couples about contraceptive choices, one must not only discuss the health benefits, risks, and effectiveness rates of all options, but also make an assessment as to whether or not the person will effectively use the method. It is also important to discuss how they might respond in the event the method fails. Women who find abortion unacceptable are usually candidates for methods with the lowest failure rates.

Another dimension has been added to the decision-making process for contraception, and this relates to the epidemic of sexually transmitted diseases (STDs), most particularly, human immunodeficiency virus (HIV) infection. It is essential that the health professional also assess with a patient their potential risk of contracting a STD. In the case of most STDs, women are at greater risk of becoming infected by men than vice versa, and it is often more difficult for them to be assertive about safer sexual practices. In any case, if the woman is or may be at risk for STDs, it is essential to recommend the addition of a barrier method to whatever other highly effective contraceptive method may be chosen. The latex condom offers the greatest protection, but female barrier and spermicide methods also afford some protection against contracting an STD.

The presently available contraceptives can be classified into the following categories: surgical methods (tubal sterilization and vasectomy); short-acting (oral contraceptives) and long-acting hormonal methods (injectables and implants); mechanical methods (intrauterine devices [IUDs]), some with adjunctive hormone; barrier/spermicide methods (condom, diaphragm, cervical cap, sponge, and spermicides); behavorial methods (periodic abstinence, lactation, and withdrawal); and postcoital methods (hormonal and IUD).

SURGICAL METHODS

Over one-third of all women in the United States who are at risk of pregnancy depend on sterilization; 25% of women have had tubal sterilization, and 11% rely on their partner's vasectomy. Laparoscopic tubal sterilization is the most commonly used technique in this country. Mini-laparotomy is preferred in the developing countries. No-scalpel vasectomy, a simplified technique that accesses the vas deferens through a small puncture wound, is increasing the acceptability of vasectomy worldwide. The risk to life with the surgical methods is low, and the very low failure rate coupled with its permanence make it the number one method of contraception worldwide. Its choice must be preceded by thorough counseling in regard to its intended permanence, and voluntary consent must be documented in writing.

HORMONAL METHODS

Hormonal methods are subdivided into short-acting (oral contraceptives) and long-acting (implants and injections).

Oral Contraceptives

Oral contraception is the most frequently chosen method of contraception by women in the United States who want to delay childbearing. The most commonly prescribed one is the combined formulation containing no more than 35 μg of estrogen along with a progestin. The active-hormone tablets are taken for 21 days of the 28-day menstrual cycle. Minipills containing progestin only must be taken daily.

As the doses of both estrogen and progestin have declined over the years, oral contraceptives have become safer and, consequently, available for use by many more women. The major risks, albeit rare, are related to potential adverse cardiovascular effects. Women with medical conditions that place them at significant risk can be screened out. Age alone (young or older) is no longer considered a contraindication, but smoking at age 35 years and older is a strong contraindication (Table 1). The reduced hormonal content has also minimized the undesirable side effects. If they do occur, most subside after 3 months of use. If not, they may be reduced by a change in formulation. The most common reason why women discontinue oral contraceptives is amenorrhea. However, this side effect can be readily controlled by changing to a less androgenic formulation or increasing the estrogen content of the prescribed medication.

There are significant health benefits for some women. Those that are well-documented are as follows: a decrease in menorrhagia, iron deficiency anemia, dysmenorrhea, premenstrual tension, benign breast disease, ovarian cysts, ovarian and endometrial cancer, and pelvic inflammatory disease with fewer ectopic pregnancies. One study found that women who had ever used oral contraceptives lived longer than those who had not. This suggests that incessant ovulation predisposes women to various pathologic conditions, which are reduced through the suppression of ovulation associated by use of these drugs.

Although there may be a slightly increased risk for earlier development of breast cancer among

TABLE 1. **Major Contraindications, Serious Sequelae, and Reported Side Effects of Combination Oral Contraceptives**

Major Contraindications	Serious Sequelae	Reported Side Effects
Thromboembolism (current or past)	Thromboembolism	Irregular bleeding
Stroke	Stroke	Amenorrhea
Coronary heart disease	Myocardial infarction	Nausea
Lipid disorder	Hypertension (reversible on discontinuation)	Weight gain
Estrogen-dependent tumor	Benign liver tumor	Breast tenderness
Breast or endometrial cancer	Cholelithiasis	Acne
Estrogen-related liver tumor		Mood changes
Impaired liver function		Headaches
Cholestasis of pregnancy		
Smokers aged 35 years and older		
Vascular or migraine headaches*		
Gallbladder disease*		
Lactation*		

*Relative contraindications.

women prone to this disease who initiate use at a young age (prior to their first pregnancy) and use the drugs for 5 years or more, the overall risk for the development of breast cancer is not increased. The Food and Drug Administration and the World Health Organization do not recommend changes in prescribing practices.

LONG-ACTING HORMONAL METHODS

Presently marketed long-acting methods vary from 3 months to 5 years in duration. Their effectiveness approaches that of sterilization. As they become more widely used, the rates of sterilization and also the incidence of sterilization regret should decline.

Levonorgestrel Implant (Norplant)

This implant system consists of six Silastic rods containing the progestin hormone levonorgestrel. They are implanted under the skin of the upper arm. The implants can be felt but not seen. They slowly release the hormone, thereby suppressing the endometrium, thickening the cervical mucus to make it less penetrable by sperm, and reducing ovulation to a minimum. The levonorgestrel implant is highly effective for its 5-year life and may be reimplanted at the time of removal. Once removed, fertility returns to normal in a matter of months.

The contraindications of use are similar to those for oral contraceptives. However, it may be used in some women for whom estrogen is contraindicated. The most significant side effect is disruption of the menstrual cycle. Although most women bleed less, its occurrence is irregular. When women are counseled in advance about what to expect and accept this effect, the continuation rate is high.

Medroxyprogesterone Acetate (Depo-Provera)

Depot medroxyprogesterone is a 3-month injectable progestin-only contraceptive. The dose is 150 mg intramuscularly. Its mode of action and effectiveness rates are similar to those of levonorgestrel, and the contraindications of use are generally the same. Depot medroxyprogesterone also disrupts the menstrual cycle, and after 6 months of use, there is a significant incidence of prolonged amenorrhea, which many women experience. Women need to be counseled in advance about its effects on the menses and also advised that the return of fertility may be delayed up to 18 months. Some bone loss may occur, but it is insignificant from a clinical perspective and appears to be reversible.

MECHANICAL METHODS (SOME WITH HORMONE)

IUDs

The copper-containing T380A (Paragard) is now approved for 8 years of use and Progestasert for 1 year. They are highly effective. Paragard is the least costly of the long-acting contraceptive methods. Unfortunately, IUDs have been significantly underutilized in the United States because of the adverse publicity and litigation surrounding the use of the Dalkon shield. Their main drawback has been an often inappropriate concern over an increased risk of pelvic infection with subsequent infertility. However, studies from the Centers for Disease Control have shown that, except for a very slight increased risk of infection in the first few months related to insertion, there is no additional risk of infection from the IUD itself. Rather, the risk is related to contracting STDs.

It is essential that a careful sexual history be taken prior to the decision about IUD use. In general, uninfected women in a mutually monogamous relationship do well with the IUD. Uterine bleeding is increased with IUD use. The IUD has been found to act mainly by blocking fertilization.

The Progestasert IUD releases progesterone hormone. This hormone suppresses the uterine lining, resulting in less blood loss. It may also reduce dysmenorrhea.

Hopefully, the IUD in time will regain its rightful place in the United States as a good contraceptive device for appropriate candidates.

BARRIER/SPERMICIDE METHODS

These methods, although not considered to be highly effective in preventing pregnancy, are the only contraceptive methods that offer any protection against contracting STDs, some of which, e.g., HIV, are fatal.

Condom

The "rubber remedy" is the most frequently used method after sterilization and oral contraceptives. Condoms now come in sizes, nonlubricated or lubricated (some with spermicide added), smooth or textured, with or without a reservoir tip, as well as in various colors. Latex condoms provide the best protection against infection. However, lambskin condoms are available, used mainly by men who want to increase their sensitivity or have an allergy to rubber products. In addition to primary use to prevent pregnancy, many men and women rely on them in conjunction with the more highly effective contraceptives to minimize their risk of contracting an STD— and well they should. Other advantages are that condoms are readily available and inexpensive.

Diaphragm

The diaphragm, the first female contraceptive method introduced into the United States, is used with a spermicide placed inside the cup prior to insertion. It requires careful fitting by a health professional, as well as a prescription. Training of the patient is essential, which should include a return visit with the diaphragm in place in 7 to 10 days to ensure the size is correct and the woman has mastered the technique. It may be inserted up to 6 hours prior to intercourse and must remain in place for at least 6 hours afterward. Repeated intercourse needs to be preceded by more applications of a spermicide. It should not be left in place longer than 24 hours because

of a possible increased risk of toxic shock syndrome. Some women cannot be fitted with a diaphragm. Allergy to rubber or spermicide is a contraindication.

Cervical Cap

This device is similar to the diaphragm. It fits snugly over the cervix, depending on suction to hold it in place. Because it comes in sizes, it must be fitted by a health professional. All the same caveats as for the diaphragm apply except that the cap is approved for wearing for 24 hours. It is significantly more difficult for a woman to learn to insert and remove, and some women cannot be fitted with the cap.

Sponge

The polyurethane sponge comes in one size, does not require fitting, and is available over the counter. It is impregnated with a sufficient dose of the spermicide nonoxynol-9 to last for a 24-hour wearing period, irrespective of the number of times intercourse takes place. It is disposable. The sponge has a wide range of effectiveness but is considered to be less effective than the medically prescribed methods. Some women note a burning sensation with use. Allergy to spermicides is a contraindication.

BEHAVORIAL METHODS

Periodic Abstinence

The use of these methods depends on attempting to predict ovulation prior to its occurrence and abstaining from intercourse during the designated unsafe times of the cycle. The various methods used to predict ovulation include the basal body temperature method, the mucus (Billings or ovulation) method, the calendar rhythm method, and the symptothermal method. Women who have irregular cycles are poor candidates for these methods. When studied in highly motivated couples, the failure rate is quite low.

Lactation

Women who are fully breast-feeding experience ovulatory suppression, which may last up to 6 months. However, once weaning is to begin or menses commence, some other form of contraception is indicated.

Withdrawal

Withdrawal is not a very effective method to use unless the male partner has perfect ejaculatory control. Furthermore, preejaculatory fluid can contain sperm and result in a pregnancy.

POSTCOITAL METHODS

Postcoital Contraception

The use of short-term higher-dose oral contraceptives initiated within 72 hours of a single act of unprotected coitus is highly effective in preventing conception. The regimen most researched is 100 μg of ethinyl estradiol and 1.0 mg of norgestrel (two Ovral tablets) immediately (within the 72-hour limitation) with two more tablets in 12 hours. High-dose estrogens are also effective, but nausea and vomiting are more common side effects.

Insertion of a copper IUD within 5 to 7 days of the unprotected intercourse is also a highly effective contraceptive.

Psychiatric Disorders

ALCOHOLISM

method of
MARGARET KOTZ, D.O., and
EDWARD C. COVINGTON, M.D.
Cleveland Clinic Foundation
Cleveland, Ohio

Our conceptualization of alcoholism has evolved from a moralistic, judgmental understanding of it as a form of inappropriate behavior, consisting predominantly of drinking too much, to that of an actual disease with associated signs and symptoms, natural history, and genetics. Although numerous signs and symptoms are required to confirm the diagnosis of alcoholism, the essence of the illness consists of three factors: preoccupation, loss of control, and continued use despite consequences.

Alcohol becomes the organizing principle of life for the alcoholic; it is his or her primary attachment. The alcoholic arranges his or her life so as to be where alcohol is available to the greatest extent possible and to avoid those places where it is unavailable. Thus, the alcoholic is not interested in outings with friends who do not drink, but finds them "boring." Maintaining access to a supply of alcohol becomes essential.

Loss of control can be difficult to confirm because the alcoholic usually (correctly) points out that he or she can often limit drinking to reasonable amounts. The point, however, is that the alcoholic is unable to predict when he or she will lose control, drink much more than intended, and perhaps suffer consequences.

People who suffer an adverse reaction to penicillin carefully avoid it thereafter. Nonalcoholics who have an adverse reaction to alcohol respond in a similar fashion. The alcoholic continues to drink despite hypertension, gastritis, pancreatitis, cirrhosis, divorce, convictions for driving while intoxicated, declining productivity at work, loss of friendships, and family conflict. To make the diagnosis, it is important to inquire about alcohol-induced effects on work, health, socialization, mood, and behavior. For example, has alcohol led to behavior that later produced remorse or shame? Have there been memory blackouts, mornings when the alcoholic has not recalled how he or she came home or where his or her car was?

Alcoholism, similar to any other illness, has a natural history. It is one of progression toward lethality, although there may be long periods or "plateaus" in which the quantity of drinking is relatively constant and vocational and health issues are not perceptibly impacted. The natural history of alcoholism has been most memorably documented by Jellinek, whose famous chart depicts the slow, inexorable progression of alcoholism from occasional loss of control with minor consequences; through increasingly frequent adverse incidents; to almost constant drinking with dissipation, severe health complications, and loss of family, friends, and job—a condition popularized as "hitting bottom." Following this, assuming the alcoholic does not die, there may be a progressive recovery toward, in many cases, normal function and health but never to the ability to drink socially with impunity.

ETIOLOGY

It is unclear why one individual drinks occasionally and responsibly throughout life, whereas another rapidly progresses into severe alcoholism. Certain factors, however, are known. There is a clear genetic component: Children and grandchildren of alcoholics, even when not reared at home, have a higher incidence of alcoholism than offspring of nonalcoholics. Age of onset of habituating substance use is also a risk factor; subjects who begin drinking in their early teens are much more likely to develop alcoholism than those who begin drinking later in life. There may be different varieties of alcoholism based on separate biologic foundations. In one variety, a cluster of findings, including sociopathy, early drinking, and rapid decline into severe alcoholism is present. This is in contrast with others in whom sociopathy is lacking and disease progression is much slower and more insidious.

PREVALENCE

Approximately 10% of all individuals who drink develop alcoholism. This represents approximately 8% of the population, or 20 million people in the United States. Alcoholism probably accounts for 15% of the health care dollars spent in the United States, not including the 28,000 motor vehicle fatalities annually in which it is thought to play a factor. Child and spouse abuse, physical and sexual, and much of the criminality that besets our society are also attributable to this disease.

DIAGNOSIS

The major obstacle to the diagnosis of alcoholism is the defense structure erected by the person who has the illness. Thus family problems are ascribed to puritanical spouses, hypertension is blamed on exploitative employers, and drunk driving convictions are because the police have a quota to meet. The myriad consequences suffered by the alcoholic are attributed to everything *except* the actual causative factor—alcohol. The alcoholic defends his or her denial vigorously, for it is essential because it permits the alcoholic to continue drinking. The diagnosis may also be hindered in homemakers, who can drink steadily throughout the day without coming to the attention of customers or employers.

Another obstacle to diagnosis lies in the attitudes of physicians. Diagnosticians are demonstrably more apt to diagnose conditions that they feel able to address than those that seem hopeless. There is a great deal of unwarranted nihilism regarding the treatment of alcoholism, which helps this epidemic to remain hidden. Alcoholism is similar to cancer: Early diagnosis, when there are minimal symptoms and slight findings, is difficult. Late diagnosis, when there are irreversible cognitive losses, varices, and liver failure, may be easy but of little value.

Unexplained macrocytosis and liver enzyme abnormalities are the most common laboratory clues that point to unsuspected alcoholism. Such medical complications as hypertension, gastritis, neuropathy, cardiomyopathy, and cerebellar dysfunction may also suggest covert alcoholism. Behavioral clues include irritability, depression, social deterioration, and irresponsible behaviors.

The CAGE questionnaire has been shown to be a highly reliable screening instrument that takes only a minute to administer. The questions are:

Have you ever:

thought about	**C**utting down on your drinking?
felt	**A**nnoyed when others criticize your drinking?
felt	**G**uilty about drinking?
used alcohol as an	**E**ye-opener?

A yes answer to two or more questions constitutes a positive test and should be followed up with further evaluation.

Perhaps the best diagnostic instrument in diagnosing alcoholism is the corroborative interview. Family members often provide information that the alcoholic has forgotten or seeks to suppress, which allows the diagnosis to be made with confidence.

TREATMENT

The prognosis for alcoholism is favorable. Even those sick enough to require inpatient treatment have a 60% chance of remaining sober more than 2 years after treatment in many programs. Persuading the alcoholic to accept treatment may be difficult and may require formal intervention in which the physician, together with family members, friends, and perhaps employers, firmly confronts the alcoholic with the reality of his or her behavior and its impact on others.

Detoxification is often required. Those with a history of major withdrawal symptoms in the past, such as severe tremulousness, delirium tremens, or seizures, require a formal period of detoxification with either a long-acting benzo-

diazepine or perhaps carbamazepine. Hepatic dysfunction may mandate the use of short half-life agents. It must always be borne in mind that detoxification only prepares the alcoholic for treatment of alcoholism and in no way constitutes treatment of the addictive disorder.

Alcoholics Anonymous (AA) was started by two men, a physician and a stockbroker who were themselves alcoholic. As a sole treatment, it assists many individuals to achieve and maintain sobriety. In addition, it is an essential component of aftercare for patients treated in professional settings. AA provides a caring, supportive, and nonjudgmental atmosphere that firmly confronts denial and encourages acceptance of the diagnosis of alcoholism. The individual is helped to recognize the unmanageability of his or her life, his or her powerlessness over alcohol, and the futility of efforts to control its use. For the alcoholic who has been struggling desperately trying to get his or her life under control, it offers a way to achieve serenity through surrender—"letting go" of all the efforts to control and "turning over" these unmanageable issues to a "higher power." AA members can be a valuable source of information as to which treatment facilities in the community provide good outcomes.

ROLE OF THE PHYSICIAN

It is critical to support the alcoholic's efforts at recovery and to help with relapse prevention. A prescription for disulfiram (Antabuse) does not guarantee sobriety but may help the alcoholic to protect himself or herself against an impulsive drink. It is helpful only if used as adjunctive therapy, however, in the context of a comprehensive behavioral/cognitive recovery program. Because the alcoholic has proved himself or herself incapable of using mind-altering chemicals in a healthy way, these chemicals should be avoided because they place sobriety at risk. For example, panic attacks are better treated with antidepressants than with alprazolam (Xanax). Similarly, if insomnia requires treatment (and prolonged sleep deprivation can promote relapse) antihistamines or antidepressants are preferable to hypnotics. Acute migraine can be managed with parenteral chlorpromazine* (Thorazine), or ketorolac (Toradol). Although acute pains, such as those surrounding surgery, require opiates (perhaps in higher than usual doses), there should be a rapid transition to oral medications, administration by the clock, and, whenever possible, complete detoxification before discharge.

---

*This use of chlorpromazine is not listed in the manufacturer's official directive.

The rewards of addressing the alcoholic's needs are substantial because these patients are typically grateful for their recovery and toward those who helped them attain it. This gratitude is shared by families and employers. Thus the physician who helps the alcoholic attain sobriety has benefited those with whom the alcoholic interacts and the community as a whole.

DRUG ABUSE

method of
DAVID J. ROBERTS, M.D.
North Memorial Medical Center
Minneapolis, Minnesota

Despite its legality, alcohol abuse overshadows all other forms of drug abuse in the United States. The cost of alcohol-associated absenteeism, loss of productivity, and alcohol-related accidents at home and work is enormous, and the associated human suffering is incalculable. Alcoholism is discussed elsewhere. This chapter focuses on the complications of recreational abuse of other legal and illegal drugs.

DIAGNOSIS OF DRUG ABUSE

The most common and easily recognized presentation of drug abuse is acute intoxication, with signs and symptoms such as obtundation, slurred speech (e.g., depressant drugs); agitation, tachycardia (e.g., stimulant drugs); and auditory or visual hallucinations (e.g., hallucinogenic drugs). The youth or adult who presents with obtundation and an obvious alcohol odor demands no diagnostic acumen. The patient who presents with a first seizure, however, may easily undergo a traditional work-up, and the diagnosis of cocaine abuse may be overlooked because no one thought to obtain a urine drug screen within the 4-day detection period for this drug. Table 1 lists the less common presentations of drug abuse.

Accidents are another common presentation of drug abuse. The physical examination is often limited to the injured extremity, and signs of drug abuse—easily detected by a more complete examination—are overlooked. Now that the legality of drug testing has been established, even mandated in some cases, more and more employers are requiring routine urine drug screening after workplace accidents. A study of Georgia Power Company employees between 1983 and 1987 showed that drug users had a significantly higher annual rate of lost time (0.008 per individual vs. 0.000) and vehicular accidents (0.23 vs. 0.109). In addition, drug users had significantly higher annual medical benefits usage ($1377 vs. $163 for matched controls) and higher annual absenteeism (165 hours vs. 47 hours). In 1987, the National Institute on Drug Abuse (NIDA) estimated that occupational drug abuse cost the United States $100 billion in lost productivity alone. Many trauma centers include a blood alcohol test in their routine screening for major trauma cases, but it is clear that any drug of abuse can affect judgment and the ability to operate a motor vehicle or any machinery.

URINE DRUG SCREENING

Urine is preferred to blood for routine qualitative screening for abused drugs. Most common drugs of abuse, with the exception of solvents, can be readily and inexpensively detected by immunoassay screening. Because of the enormous impact of a positive test, especially for employment, a positive test should always be confirmed by a second, unrelated technique, usually gas chromatography or mass spectrometry. Table 2 lists the average detection periods for drugs. In addition to a thorough physical examination, several readily obtainable studies can detect most complications of drug abuse: rhythm strip, complete blood count, electrolytes, glucose, blood urea nitrogen, and urinalysis.

STIMULANT DRUGS

Table 3 lists the commonly abused stimulant drugs. Most people using stimulant drugs achieve the desired effects of increased alertness and energy, decreased fatigue, euphoria, and anorexia, and they never present to an emergency department. What makes a user a patient is some undesired or frightening effect, either psychological (e.g., panic attack, dysphoric reaction) or physiologic (e.g., tachycardia, chest pain). Cocaine and amphetamines are the dominant drugs of abuse in this class, and their effects and toxicity are similar. Cocaine is rapidly metabolized by the liver, and its effects usually dissipate in minutes, but the effects of amphetamines can persist for hours. Either drug, depending on the dose and individual susceptibility, can precipitate acute anxiety states, paranoia, hallucinations, acute psychosis, and violent behavior.

In addition to undesired behavioral effects, patients may present with various unpleasant physiologic effects. A first seizure in an adolescent or young adult demands that cocaine and other stimulants be ruled out. The patient, fearing parental or legal consequences, often denies drug abuse. If initial history and testing are negative for common causes of seizure, such as previous or acute head injury, family history of seizure, metabolic derangement, or central nervous system (CNS) infection and disease, drug abuse should be pursued more aggressively. Other common causes for seizure, such as carbon monoxide and acute overdose of other medications, should not be overlooked. The attending physician should also consider withdrawal from a drug of abuse and look for supporting signs, such as tachycardia, diaphoresis, tremor, or agitation.

An especially dangerous presentation of co-

TABLE 1. **Less Common Presentations of Drug Abuse**

Presentation	Drug
Seizure	Cocaine, amphetamines, "designer drug," PCP, propoxyphene, solvent; withdrawal
Subcutaneous abscess, especially antecubital	Parenteral drugs, especially cocaine
Stains on face or hands	Solvents
Cyanosis	Nitrites (methemoglobinemia)
Accidents	All drugs of abuse
Unusual odors	Solvents, alcohol, chloral hydrate, ethchlorvynol, marijuana
Nystagmus	Alcohol, PCP, solvents, mescaline, sedative hypnotics
Miosis	Narcotics, PCP
Mydriasis	Amphetamines, cocaine, LSD, glutethimide, meperidine, hypoxia secondary to respiratory depression
Ischemic chest pain at unusually young age	Cocaine, amphetamines
Acute psychiatric disorders (e.g., hyperventilation, panic, dysphoria, psychosis)	Alcohol, amphetamines, cocaine, PCP, hallucinogens, marijuana
Neuropathy	Nitrous oxide, toluene
Myoglobinuria	Cocaine, amphetamines, PCP
Salivation, drooling	PCP (cholinergic effects)
Hyperthermia	Cocaine, amphetamines, PCP, withdrawal
Hypothermia	Alcohol, barbiturates, ethchlorvynol
Pulmonary edema	Narcotics, barbiturates, ethchlorvynol, meprobamate
Confusional state in elderly	Alcohol, sedative hypnotics, narcotics, withdrawal
Tachydysrhythmias	Stimulants, hallucinogens, propoxyphene
Neonatal withdrawal	Maternal abuse of alcohol, narcotics, cocaine, amphetamines

caine abuse is ischemic chest pain in the young, healthy-appearing patient. If the history of cocaine use is not volunteered or elicited, the patient is likely to be sent home with reassurance and an analgesic. Myocardial infarction is a recognized complication of cocaine abuse, even in the absence of traditional risk factors. Some risk management protocols suggest obtaining an electrocardiogram (ECG) in all cases of chest pain in patients older than 25, but if cocaine use is suspected, an ECG should be obtained at any age. Cardiac monitoring may reveal various dysrhythmias, such as sinus tachycardia, paroxysmal supraventricular tachycardia, premature ventricular contraction, ventricular tachycardia, and ventricular fibrillation.

Phencyclidine (PCP, "angel dust") is abused for its stimulant and mood-altering effects, but it is pharmacologically more complex than most other drugs of abuse. Because it affects multiple neurotransmitters in the brain, it can produce CNS stimulation and depression, hallucinations, analgesia, and cholinergic effects. Its behavioral effects include dysphoria, violence, psychosis, and catatonia. Because of a combination of hyperactivity and delusion of strength, PCP abusers may suffer serious injuries and rhabdomyolysis. Because of its analgesic effects, patients on PCP may not complain of pain, and a complete physical examination is indicated. Using a purely psychiatric approach in cases of drug abuse (i.e., interviewing the patient fully clothed) invites overlooking serious injuries and complications. A

TABLE 2. **Detection Periods for Drugs of Abuse in Blood and Urine**

Drug	Detection Period
Alcohol, ethyl	3–10 h
Amphetamine	1–2 days
Barbiturates	
Secobarbital	24 h
Phenobarbital	2–6 weeks
Benzodiazepines, heavy abuse	3–5 days
	3–6 weeks
Cocaine	5 h
Benzoylecgonine (cocaine metabolite)	2–4 days
Codeine	1–2 days
Heroin	1–2 days
Hydromorphone (Dilaudid)	1–2 days
LSD	8 h
Methaqualone (Quaalude)	2 weeks
Methadone (Dolophine)	2–3 days
Morphine	1–2 days
PCP (phencyclidine)	2–8 days
Propoxyphene (Darvon)	6 h
Propoxyphene metabolites	6–48 h
THC metabolite (marijuana)	
1 joint, urine	2 days
3 times weekly, urine	2 weeks
Daily, urine	3–6 weeks
Blood	8 h

With permission of Harry G. McCoy, Pharm.D., Clinical Director, Med Tox Laboratories, St. Paul, MN.

TABLE 3. **Commonly Abused Stimulant Drugs**

Amphetamines	Phencyclidine
Cocaine	Phenylpropanolamine
Caffeine	Ephedrine
Nicotine	Pseudoephedrine

combined psychiatric and medical approach is well rewarded.

Treatment

Milder panic or dysphoric reactions may respond to reassurance and the continuous presence of a friend, nurse, or counselor until the drug effect subsides. Other patients may benefit from a short-acting benzodiazepine, such as 0.25 mg of triazolam (Halcion), which may be given sublingually. Making the patient comfortable with a "downer" could be construed as enabling the drug abuse, so referral for chemical dependency evaluation and treatment should also be made.

Violent patients present an immediate threat to themselves and others. Initial restraint is most safely achieved by five staff members, one for each limb and one for the head. Physical restraints can then be applied. Many patients, however, continue to thrash dangerously after being restrained, and some form of chemical restraint is often needed. Chemical restraints bring their own risks of toxicity, such as respiratory depression, but their benefits usually outweigh their risks. The most popular drugs for chemical restraint have been short-acting benzodiazepines and haloperidol (Haldol), a butyrophenone. These drugs have a better safety profile than barbiturates and phenothiazines, and their use, dosage, and effectiveness have been well documented in the emergency medicine literature. A common protocol is 5 mg of haloperidol plus 2 mg of lorazepam (Ativan) intravenously or intramuscularly. Most other benzodiazepines are not well absorbed intramuscularly. The combined use of the two drugs obviates the need for an excessive dose of either drug alone. If necessary, the dose can be repeated in 30 minutes. Dystonic reactions occasionally complicate haloperidol use and are controlled by diphenhydramine (Benadryl), 50 mg four times daily, or benztropine (Cogentin), 1 to 2 mg twice daily. Use of chemical restraint obligates the physician to even closer physiologic monitoring.

Dysrhythmias range from mild sinus tachycardia to life-threatening ventricular arrhythmias. Sinus tachycardia is usually well tolerated and self-limited, and the associated anxiety may be treated with reassurance or a small dose of a short-acting benzodiazepine. Hemodynamically significant PSVT should be treated with an intravenous beta blocker, such as 5 mg of metoprolol (Lopressor), or a calcium channel blocker, such as 5 mg of verapamil (Isoptin). Each drug can be safely repeated in a few minutes if necessary. Drug-driven tachycardias are less likely to respond to vagal maneuvers, and the likelihood of recurrence of PSVT after adenosine is high. If the supraventricular tachycardia is associated with hypertension, labetalol (Normodyne, Trandate), which blocks both alpha and beta receptors, or verapamil makes the most sense. There have been some reports of hypertension worsening after the administration of other beta blockers, especially propranolol (Inderal), because of unopposed alpha effect. Hypertensive emergencies can also be controlled with nitroprusside (Nipride) infusions. Ventricular arrhythmias should be treated with lidocaine (Xylocaine), beta blockers, or cardioversion.

The toxicity of stimulant drugs is not limited to behavioral and cardiovascular effects. Other serious effects include seizures, cerebrovascular accidents, hyperthermia, rhabdomyolysis, and acute tubular necrosis. Seizures usually complicate *overdoses* of stimulant drugs, but they may also occur with recreational use. Seizures are best controlled with intravenous diazepam (Valium). If more seizures are expected, the patient should be loaded intravenously with phenytoin (Dilantin) at a rate of 25 to 50 mg per minute for a total dose of 15 to 18 mg per kg. Alternatively, phenobarbital (Luminal) can be loaded at 18 mg per kg. Seizures and hyperactivity can result in hyperthermia. Failing to measure body temperature is a common oversight in the setting of drug abuse or overdose. Rhabdomyolysis is suggested by a urine dipstick positive for blood when the microscopic examination shows no erythrocytes. If rhabdomyolysis is suspected, intravenous hydration should begin immediately. Alkalinization of the urine with intravenous sodium bicarbonate may offer additional benefit because myoglobin is more likely to precipitate and damage renal tubules in the normally acidic urine.

If the patient presents shortly after ingestion of a stimulant drug, gastric emptying (e.g., induced emesis, lavage) is worthwhile. If presentation is delayed beyond 1 hour, charcoal administration is more appropriate (initial dose, 50 grams). Repeat oral charcoal, 25 grams every 2 to 4 hours, is indicated in the asymptomatic cocaine body packer. Induced emesis or endoscopic attempts at removal may result in packet rupture and immediate lethal toxicity. Whole-bowel irrigation may also be helpful. Plain abdominal radiographs or contrast studies may help detect and quantitate the packets, although not all are radiopaque. Drugs other than cocaine, such as heroin, may also be smuggled by body packing, and clinical presentation may vary. Extracorporeal methods to remove stimulant drugs (e.g., hemodialysis, hemoperfusion, plasmapheresis, exchange transfusion) are ineffective.

Withdrawal

In contrast to withdrawal from alcohol and sedative hypnotic drugs, physiologic withdrawal from stimulant drugs is seldom severe or life-threatening, and events such as seizures are rare. Serious depression and suicidal ideation, however, may occur and require treatment with antidepressant medication.

HALLUCINOGENS

Table 4 lists the common hallucinogenic drugs. Hallucinations may be the desired effect sought by the user of these drugs, but occasionally the hallucinations are frightening, especially to the inexperienced user. A "bad trip" may bring a young user to the emergency department or crisis intervention center for treatment. The hallucinations may also be accompanied by a panic reaction or psychosis. The most commonly abused drug in this class is lysergic acid diethylamide (LSD). Known for its induction of vivid visual hallucinations, LSD may also demonstrate sympathomimetic effects, such as mydriasis, hypertension, and tachycardia, but these effects are usually mild and seldom require treatment. Mescaline is a less potent hallucinogen that is related chemically to epinephrine and exhibits sympathomimetic effects. Designer drugs, such as MDA, MDMA ("ecstasy"), MDEA, and others, have been synthesized in an effort to escape criminal designation. They are more potent stimulants and hallucinogens. Their adrenergic effects may be more pronounced, and seizures and death have been associated with their use.

Of all the illegal drugs of abuse, marijuana is the most popular. NIDA estimated in 1986 that there were about 18,000,000 users of this drug, outnumbered only by the users of alcohol, nicotine, and caffeine. Its widespread use among young people guarantees that it will remain a problem. According to the 1990 National School-Based Youth Risk Behavior Survey, almost one-third (31.4%) of all students in grades 9 through 12 had used marijuana at least once. In a 1987 to 1989 study of accidents by the Federal Railroad Administration, cannabinoids were the most commonly encountered single drug finding for years

TABLE 4. Commonly Abused Hallucinogens

Lysergic acid diethylamide (LSD)
Mescaline
Designer drugs (e.g., MDA, MDMA, MDEA)
Marijuana and hashish (tetrahydrocannabinol)
Peyote (cactus)
Mushrooms (psilocybin, psilocin)
Morning glory seeds

TABLE 5. Commonly Abused Narcotics

Heroin	Hydrocodone
Opium	Codeine
Morphine	Propoxyphene
Hydromorphone	Pentazocine
Methadone	Diphenoxylate
Oxycodone	Fentanyl

1 (61%) and 2 (47%). Although grouped here with the hallucinogens, marijuana does not usually cause hallucinations at the doses smoked or ingested. It is used for its mood-altering effects, and patients usually present as a result of accidents or dysphoric reactions.

Treatment

Those suffering "bad trips" and dysphoric reactions may be "talked down," as in the case of stimulant drugs. Those experiencing more severe reactions or psychosis may require sedation with benzodiazepines or haloperidol. Even if haloperidol is used only briefly, the doses required raise the risk of extrapyramidal reactions, and the author prescribes 50 mg of diphenhydramine every 6 hours or 2 mg of benztropine every day for 2 days after the last dose.

NARCOTICS

Table 5 lists the commonly abused narcotics. Although stimulants and hallucinogens generally cause CNS excitation, narcotics, sedative hypnotics, and solvents cause various degrees of CNS depression.

Narcotic abuse classically presents as miosis, respiratory depression, and CNS depression (i.e., narcotic toxidrome). Exceptions are meperidine (Demerol) and diphenoxylate (Lomotil), which produce mydriasis or no pupillary change because of their anticholinergic effect. Propoxyphene (Darvon), meperidine, and codeine can cause seizures. Nausea, vomiting, and hypotension also occur. Cardiac arrhythmias occur with propoxyphene, but they can follow any narcotic dose large enough to cause hypoxia or pulmonary edema, which is more likely after intravenous administration. Parenteral drug abuse is associated with a variety of infectious complications, such as subcutaneous abscesses, septic emboli, pneumonia, endocarditis, hepatitis, and acquired immune deficiency syndrome (AIDS).

Treatment

As with any drug abuse emergency, attention should be directed first to the basics of airway, breathing, and circulation because most drugs lack a specific antidote or antagonist. For the respiratory depression induced by narcotics, however, naloxone (Narcan) is a rapid, safe, and effective antidote. Narcosis is reversed within seconds. The initial dose should be 2 mg. Synthetic narcotics, such as codeine, methadone, pentazocine (Talwin), and propoxyphene, may require higher doses, and narcotic overdose is not ruled out until 10 mg have been given. Suddenly aroused narcotic abusers may become agitated and violent, and the staff should be prepared to restrain them. Because the duration of many narcotics exceeds that of naloxone, these patients require prolonged observation or admission. An intravenous naloxone infusion at an hourly rate equal to two-thirds of the arousal dose maintains normal respirations.

Withdrawal

Narcotic withdrawal is not as serious as that from alcohol and sedative hypnotic drugs, and many patients can withdraw without medication. Withdrawal symptoms begin soon after the first missed dose of narcotic, peak at about 48 hours, and subside in 7 to 10 days, depending on the half-life of the abused opioid. Early symptoms include lacrimation, rhinorrhea, and diaphoresis. Soon the patient becomes restless and irritable, and examination often shows sinus tachycardia, mydriasis, and tremor. Appetite and sleep are disturbed, and the patient often complains of abdominal cramps and general achiness. Nausea, vomiting, and diarrhea can be troublesome. Treatment is symptomatic: non-narcotic antidiarrheal agents, non-narcotic analgesics, and antiemetics. Clonidine (Catapres) has also been shown to mitigate the withdrawal syndrome. Narcotics, other than methadone for maintenance therapy in strictly supervised programs, should not be used for managing narcotic withdrawal.

SEDATIVE HYPNOTIC DRUGS

Table 6 lists the commonly abused sedative hypnotic drugs. This diverse class of drugs includes barbiturates, benzodiazepines, and non-barbiturate nonbenzodiazepines. They are all CNS depressants, and acute intoxication resembles that of alcohol and narcotics. Patients may present with slurred speech, ataxia, slowed mentation, impaired memory, and somnolence. Overdose can result in coma, respiratory depression, and hypotension. Lesser doses, as with alcohol, may cause emotional lability and acute dysphoric reactions. Their disinhibitory effect may also re-

TABLE 6. **Commonly Abused Sedative Hypnotic Drugs**

Benzodiazepines	**Piperidinediones**
Alprazolam	Glutethimide
Chlorazepate	Methyprylon
Chlordiazepoxide	
Clonazepam	**Quinazolines**
Diazepam	Methaqualone
Flurazepam	
Halazepam	**Barbiturates**
Lorazepam	Amobarbital
Midazolam	Barbital
Oxazepam	Butabarbital
Prazepam	Pentobarbital
Temazepam	Phenobarbital
Triazolam	Secobarbital
Alcohols	
Chloral hydrate	
Ethchlorvynol	
Propanediol Carbamate	
Meprobamate	
Ethinamate	

sult in aggressiveness and violent behavior. The clinical presentation may also be confused by the concomitant abuse of other drugs, as when a sedative hypnotic is used to counteract the unpleasant excitation of stimulant or hallucinogenic drugs. Sedative hypnotic drugs are abused by the old and young. Drug abuse should be considered in any elderly patient who presents with confusion or acute or chronic dementia.

Some sedative hypnotic drugs have important effects other than CNS depression. For example, barbiturates, especially in overdose, can cause hypotension, hypothermia, skin blisters, and pulmonary edema. Chloral hydrate can cause cardiac disturbances, such as atrial fibrillation, aberrant conduction, PVCs, and ventricular tachycardia. Glutethimide (Doriden) has anticholinergic activity and can cause mydriasis, urinary retention, tachycardia, and hypertension.

Treatment

Treatment of sedative hypnotic intoxication is usually supportive, with special attention to preserving the airway and ventilation. Traditionally unconscious patients are treated empirically with naloxone and glucose to rule out narcotics and hypoglycemia. No other specific antagonist is available except flumazenil (Mazicon), which rapidly and effectively reverses the CNS depression of benzodiazepines. For the treatment of overdose, the recommended initial dose is 0.2 mg intravenously over 30 seconds. If no arousal occurs, a second dose of 0.3 mg is given over 30 seconds. If necessary, further doses of 0.5 mg can be administered over 30 seconds, up to a total dose of 3.0 mg.

TABLE 7. **Commonly Abused Solvents and Inhalants**

Product	Solvent or Inhalant
Gasoline	Various hydrocarbons, tetraethyl lead
Typewriter correction fluid	Trichloroethane, trichloroethylene, perchloroethylene
Lighter fluid	Butane
Model glue or cement	Toluene, xylene
Adhesives	Toluene
Nail polish remover	Acetone, amyl acetate
Aerosol cans (paints, fabric protector)	Fluorocarbons
Paints, varnishes, lacquers	Trichloroethylene, toluene, methylene chloride
Spot remover, dry cleaning chemicals	Trichloroethane, trichloroethylene, tetrachloroethylene
Hair styling mousse	Propane, butane, isobutane
Anesthetic, whipped cream propellant	Nitrous oxide
"Aphrodisiac" inhalants	Amyl, butyl, and isobutyl nitrites

If a patient presents in an acute state of sedation, gastric decontamination is indicated. Activated charcoal should also be administered, and repeat doses may remove additional drug by "intestinal dialysis," shortening the half-life of the drug and its associated coma. Alkaline diuresis enhances excretion of phenobarbital but not the shorter acting barbiturates. Hemodialysis and hemoperfusion can also remove long-acting barbiturates, but expense and complications of these therapies should be considered because most patients recover with good supportive care. A regional poison center should be consulted for advice on specific drugs and problems.

Withdrawal

Withdrawal from these drugs is probably more dangerous than from other drugs of abuse. In contrast to withdrawal from alcohol and narcotics, which usually begins within hours to days after the last dose, withdrawal from long-acting sedative hypnotic drugs may be delayed for many days. Detoxification from alcohol is usually accomplished within a few days, but withdrawal from sedative hypnotics may require 2 to 3 weeks.

Signs and symptoms are similar to alcohol withdrawal. Patients are restless, tremulous, and diaphoretic. They frequently complain of nausea, vomiting, and abdominal pain. Hyperreflexia and myoclonic jerks may precede generalized seizures, which may be severe and prolonged. Hallucinations and delirium complicate severe cases. Withdrawal should be managed by toxicologists or experienced physicians in a hospital or other institutional setting. Withdrawal is usually ameliorated by slowly tapering doses of intermediate-acting to long-acting barbiturates or benzodiazepines.

SOLVENTS

No discussion of drug abuse would be complete without including solvents and other inhalants.

No dealer or pusher is needed to obtain these chemicals, which are in many household products. Table 7 lists the commonly abused solvents. They are generally abused by the most inexperienced drug seekers: adolescents and preadolescents.

Solvents are volatile, lipid-soluble substances that have CNS depressant effects. Abusers may sniff the open containers, "huff" rags soaked with the solvent, or "bag" the vapors from a plastic bag. Bagging is probably the most dangerous because the vapors are more concentrated and the abuser can lose consciousness and suffocate. Asphyxiation was commonly assumed to be the cause of death until it was appreciated that solvents, especially halogenated hydrocarbons, could sensitize the heart to catecholamines and cause ventricular tachycardia and fibrillation. All too often the presentation is sudden death; few successful resuscitations have been reported. More commonly, however, the patient presents with slurred speech, ataxia, and somnolence. A solvent, rather than alcohol, odor is usually conspicuous. Chronic abuse can result in toxicity to the bone marrow, liver, and peripheral nerves. Toluene is especially noxious, causing electrolyte imbalance, renal tubular acidosis, and neurotoxicity. Urine drug screens generally do not detect solvents. Physicians should alert the toxicology laboratory about what chemical is suspected.

Treatment

Treatment of solvent abuse is mainly supportive, assuring a stable airway and ventilation. Supplemental oxygen may be helpful. There is no other way to enhance excretion as with ingested drugs of abuse. The heart should be monitored initially for arrhythmias. Antiarrhythmic drugs, such as lidocaine and beta blockers, should be administered for life-threatening ventricular arrhythmias. A complete blood count, electrolytes, liver enzymes, and urinalysis should be obtained to rule out toxicity of solvents such as toluene. Toluene intoxication may require intravenous fluids, electrolyte replacement, and administration of sodium bicarbonate if acidosis is significant. Methemoglobinemia may complicate abuse of nitrites and require treatment with methylene blue. Peripheral neuropathy secondary to chronic nitrous oxide abuse may respond to vitamin B_{12} and thiamine.

Knowledge and therapies are continuously expanding in toxicology. When an unfamiliar drug is encountered, it is always wise to consult a toxicologist, regional poison center, or a standard reference such as *Clinical Management of Poisoning and Drug Overdose,* edited by Lester Haddad and James Winchester. As with all drugs of abuse, medical treatment of complications should be followed by psychiatric or chemical dependency evaluation and treatment.

ANXIETY DISORDERS

method of
J. DOUGLAS BREMNER, M.D., and
DENNIS S. CHARNEY, M.D.
Yale University School of Medicine
New Haven, Connecticut

The anxiety disorders are the most common of all psychiatric disorders. Anxiety can serve adaptive functions in removing the individual from life-threatening situations or enhancing performance at crucial times. When excessive or out of the proper context, however, anxiety can be debilitating and disabling.

Symptoms of anxiety are common to all of the anxiety disorders. Anxiety symptoms are best remembered by thinking about what occurs during a normally stressful event, such as taking an examination or delivering a speech in public. Subjective anxiety or worry is accompanied by the feeling of being on edge or irritable with physical manifestations of autonomic hyperactivity, including trembling, muscle tension, restlessness, shortness of breath, palpitations or rapid heart rate, sweating, dry mouth, dizziness, nausea, hot flushes, frequent urination, and trouble swallowing. Patients with anxiety disorders also have additional symptoms specific to the particular disorder (Table 1), which often determine the pharmacologic intervention that is appropriate for that disorder.

TREATMENT

Patients presenting with anxiety disorders should be treated following two important principles: altering the patient's environment when appropriate and ruling out medical causes of anxiety (Table 2). Medical conditions that present with anxiety as a chief complaint include cardio-vascular, pulmonary, and endocrine disorders. Some cardiovascular disorders that may masquerade as anxiety include acute myocardial infarction, congestive heart failure, and mitral valve prolapse. Pulmonary disorders that may cause anxiety include chronic obstructive pulmonary disease, pneumothorax, and pulmonary embolus. Hyperthyroidism, hypoglycemia, and Cushing's syndrome are endocrine disorders that can present with anxiety as the chief complaint. The importance of ruling out medical causes of anxiety becomes apparent on inspection of this list of potentially life-threatening disorders that can present with anxiety as a chief complaint often in an emergency room setting.

Several medications can produce anxiety as a side effect, which makes the taking of a careful medication history mandatory (Table 3). Medications that can cause anxiety include beta-receptor agonists, such as theophylline, and stimulants, including amphetamines and methylphenidate, thyroxine, steroids, caffeine-containing medications (such as Goody's powder or over-the-counter cold medications), and yohimbine.

Anxiety can also be the result of alcohol or substance withdrawal or intoxication. Substances that can cause anxiety symptoms during withdrawal or intoxication states include opiates, amphetamines, phencyclidine, cocaine, hallucinogens, marijuana, caffeine, and benzodiazepines (Table 4). Many anxiety disorder patients use drugs or alcohol to self-medicate their anxiety symptoms. Alcohol, however, may have the long-term effect of increasing anxiety, even though patients may feel some initial short-term relief. In addition, anxiety may be the presenting complaint of alcohol withdrawal or even delirium tremens. Patients with anxiety disorders should eliminate the use of alcohol, illicit substances, and caffeine. Most individuals are reticent to volunteer information about illicit substance use, making the taking of a careful substance abuse history mandatory.

Medications that have been found to be effective in the treatment of anxiety disorders include tricyclic antidepressants, monoamine oxidase (MAO) inhibitors, serotonin (5-HT) reuptake inhibitors, $5-HT_{1A}$ receptor agonists, and benzodiazepines. These medications are discussed in the context of the specific anxiety disorder for which they are prescribed.

Generalized Anxiety Disorder

Generalized anxiety disorder (GAD) is the most common anxiety disorder, with a lifetime prevalence of 9.1%. GAD is characterized by an excessive worry or preoccupation with life circum-

TABLE 1. **Diagnosis of Anxiety Disorders Based on *DSM–III–R* Criteria**

Generalized Anxiety Disorder

Unrealistic or excessive anxiety or worry about two or more life circumstances for a period of 6 months or longer

At least six of the following symptoms are often present when anxious: trembling, muscle tension, restlessness, easy fatigability, shortness of breath, palpitations, sweating, dry mouth, dizziness, nausea, flushes, frequent urination, trouble swallowing, feeling on edge, exaggerated startle, difficulty concentrating, sleep disturbance, irritability

Anxiety is not secondary to another psychiatric disorder, such as panic disorder or obsessive-compulsive disorder, does not occur during the course of a mood or psychotic disorder, and is not due to an organic factor

Panic Disorder

Presence of unexpected panic attacks of up to four in a 4-week period, or one attack followed by a period of 1 month of persistent fear of having another attack

Panic attacks are accompanied by at least four of the following physical symptoms: shortness of breath, dizziness, palpitations, trembling, sweating, choking, nausea, depersonalization, numbness or tingling, flushes or chills, chest discomfort, fear of dying, fear of going crazy

During some of the attacks, at least four of the physical symptoms develop within 10 minutes of the initiation of the attack

Panic attacks are not due to an organic factor

Obsessive-Compulsive Disorder

Either obsessions or compulsions:

Obsessions: Recurrent and persistent ideas, thoughts, impulses, or images that are experienced as intrusive and senseless. The person tries to ignore or suppress or neutralize the thoughts with some type of action. The contents of the thoughts are not related to some other psychiatric disorder

Compulsions: Repetitive, purposeful, and intentional behaviors that are performed in response to an obsession. They are designed to neutralize or to prevent discomfort or some dreaded event, although the individual recognizes that the behavior is excessive or unreasonable

The obsessions or compulsions cause marked distress, are time-consuming (take more than 1 hour in a day), or significantly interfere with the person's normal routine, occupational functioning, or relationships with others

Post-Traumatic Stress Disorder

Person experienced an event that is beyond the range of normal human experience and that would be markedly distressing to almost anyone

Symptoms of re-experiencing the traumatic event in at least one of the following ways: intrusive memories, nightmares, flashbacks, or feeling worse with reminders of the trauma

Avoidance of stimuli associated with the trauma, indicated by at least three of the following: avoidance of thoughts associated with the trauma, avoidance of thinking about the trauma, inability to recall details of the trauma, loss of interest in things that used to be important, feeling cut off from others, feeling unable to have caring feelings for others, sense of foreshortened future

Symptoms of increased arousal indicated by two or more of the following: sleep disturbance, irritability, difficulty concentrating, hypervigilance, exaggerated startle response, physiologic reactivity on exposure to events that resemble the traumatic event

Duration of symptoms of at least 1 month

Simple Phobia

Persistent fear of a circumscribed stimulus other than fear of having a panic attack or of being humiliated in social situations

Exposure to stimulus, at some phase of the disturbance, almost invariably provokes an immediate anxiety response

The object or situation is avoided or endured with intense anxiety

The fear or the avoidant behavior significantly interferes with the person's normal routine or with relationships with others

The person recognizes that the fear is excessive or unreasonable

The phobic stimulus is unrelated to the content of the obsessive-compulsive disorder or post-traumatic stress disorder

Abbreviation: DSM–III–R = Diagnostic and Statistical Manual of Mental Disorders, 3rd ed—Revised. Washington, DC, American Psychiatric Association, 1987.

stances. This can take the form, for instance, of worrying about one's finances, misfortune to one's children when there is no danger present, or problems with one's health when there is no cause for concern. It is normal to worry about these things, sometimes even when there is no reason, from time to time. GAD has therefore been defined as a preoccupation that bothers the individual more days than not and that has been going on for 6 months or more (see Table 1).

GAD is a chronic disorder that presents frequently to the general practitioner. The first line of treatment of GAD is to identify any stressors that may be the cause of the anxiety. When possible, the removal of the stressor or counseling,

support, and reassurance can prevent the initiation of any unnecessary pharmacologic treatment trials. In some cases, appropriate and time-limited medication trials can be beneficial when combined with a supportive interchange between the physician and the patient.

The two main classes of medications that have been found to have efficacy in the treatment of GAD are 5-HT_{1A} receptor agonists and benzodiazepines (Table 5). Several studies have demonstrated the efficacy of the 5-HT_{1A} agonist buspirone (Buspar). Buspirone has the advantage over benzodiazepines of being free of the side effects of sedation, ataxia, alterations in memory, and possible withdrawal effects. The disadvantages of

TABLE 2. **Examples of Important Medical Conditions in the Differential Diagnosis of Anxiety**

Cardiovascular Disorders
Congestive heart failure
Myocardial infarction
Mitral valve prolapse
Paroxysmal atrial tachycardia

Endocrine Disorders
Pheochromocytoma
Cushing's disease
Hyperthyroidism
Insulinoma
Carcinoid tumor
Hypoglycemia

Pulmonary Disorders
Chronic obstructive pulmonary disease
Asthma
Pulmonary embolus
Pneumothorax

TABLE 4. **Commonly Prescribed Medications That Can Have Anxiety as a Side Effect**

Beta agonists (e.g., aminophylline, theophylline, albuterol)
Stimulants (e.g., amphetamine, methylphenidate, diet medications)
Over-the-counter cold remedies containing caffeine or phenylephrine (e.g., Goody's powder)
Steroids (e.g., prednisone)
Thyroid replacement medications (e.g., thyroxine)
Neuroleptics
Yohimbine (used in the treatment of impotence)

buspirone include a delayed onset of action; a requirement for continuous dosing (it does not work on an as-needed basis); and a possible decrease in efficacy in comparison to benzodiazepines in selected patients, especially those who have been previously treated with benzodiazepines. Buspirone is started in a divided dose of 5 mg three times daily. Doses are generally increased gradually over a several-week period with a maximum daily dosage of 60 mg. The benzodiazepines have been shown to be a safe, rapidly effective treatment for anxiety with a low potential for overdose. The disadvantages of benzodiazepines include a potential for dependence and physiologic withdrawal, a potential for addiction, and a synergistic action with alcohol that can be dangerous.

It is generally recommended that a trial with buspirone precede that with a benzodiazepine in GAD patients who have not previously been treated with antianxiety medications. Benzodiazepines should be prescribed initially for patients who need immediate relief, when as-needed dosing (e.g., just before a predictable stressor) is most appropriate.

Panic Disorder

Approximately 0.4 to 2.5% of people, based on epidemiologic studies, develop panic disorder at

TABLE 3. **Substances of Abuse That May Cause Anxiety to Be the Chief Complaint in the Context of Intoxication or Withdrawal States**

Caffeine	Opiates
Phencyclidine	Benzodiazepines
Amphetamines	Marijuana
Alcohol	Hallucinogens
Nicotine	Cocaine

some time in their life. Patients with panic disorder experience discrete episodes of panic or severe anxiety associated with the feeling that they are going to die or go crazy or that something bad is going to happen. These episodes typically come from "out of the blue" at first and are not triggered by situations that would normally cause anxiety. Panic attacks are accompanied by physical symptoms of shortness of breath, dizziness, trembling, sweating, choking, nausea, numbness and tingling, flushes, and chest discomfort (see Table 1). These panic attacks can be extremely disabling, causing patients to make multiple visits to emergency rooms and to seek consultation with multiple cardiovascular specialists, often with the conviction that they are suffering from heart disease. Even with appropriate diagnosis, panic disorder patients often remain trapped in their homes and restricted in their activities by the fear that they will have a panic attack when they are in a vulnerable position. Panic disorder patients usually have accompanying agoraphobia. Agoraphobia, which literally means "fear of the marketplace," occurs when patients are afraid to go into places where they would be compromised if they had a panic attack. Typically these places include bridges; supermarkets; standing in line; or being in a bus, train, or car. Anticipatory anxiety occurs when patients develop anxiety associated with the fear of having another panic attack. Thus anticipatory anxiety and agoraphobia contribute to the psychopathology of patients with panic disorder.

The pathophysiology of panic attacks is unknown; however, several brain systems have been linked to anxiety states, including norepinephrine, serotonin, and benzodiazepine brain systems. Consistent with this, the medication classes that have been shown to be effective in treating panic disorder include antidepressants, which act on norepinephrine and serotonin brain systems, and benzodiazepines (Table 6).

Most of the tricyclic medications are efficacious in treating panic disorder, including imipramine (Tofranil), desipramine (Norpramin), and clomipramine (Anafranil). The potent, specific serotonin

TABLE 5. **Efficacy of Available Pharmacologic Agents in the Treatment of Generalized Anxiety Disorder**

Drug Class	Efficacy*	Replication†	Therapeutic Dose Range (mg/day)
5HT$_{1A}$ Agonists			
Buspirone (Buspar)	+ + +	+ + +	20–60
Gepirone	+ + +	+	Not yet available
Antidepressants with Mixed Actions			
Imipramine (Tofranil)	+ +	+	25–300
Benzodiazepines			
Diazepam (Valium)	+ + +	+ + +	5–20
Lorazepam (Ativan)	+ + +	+ +	2–6
Alprazolam (Xanax)	+ + +	+ + +	1–3
Chlordiazepoxide (Librium)	+ + +	+ + +	25–75

*Efficacy was rated as follows: NT, not tested; 0, ineffective; +, slightly effective; + +, moderately effective; + + +, very effective.
†Replication refers to the extent to which the efficacy of the agent has been investigated; it was rated as follows: +, only one or two controlled studies conducted; + +, several controlled studies conducted but further studies indicated; + + + highly replicated and consistent efficacy reported.

re-uptake inhibitors, including fluoxetine (Prozac) and fluvoxamine, are also therapeutic. In addition, MAO inhibitors phenelzine (Nardil) and tranylcypromine (Parnate) are useful in treating panic disorder. MAO inhibitors, however, need to be administered with a low tyramine diet, which has the disadvantage of requiring counseling and close monitoring. It should be emphasized that not all antidepressant medications are efficacious in the treatment of panic disorder. Specifically, trazodone (Desyrel) and buproprion (Wellbutrin) are ineffective. Benzodiazepine medications are widely used in the treatment of panic disorder. The benzodiazepines most commonly prescribed for panic disorder are alprazolam (Xanax) and clonazepam (Klonopin). The doses required for

TABLE 6. **Efficacy of Available Pharmacologic Agents in the Treatment of Panic Disorder**

Drug Class	Efficacy*	Replication†	Therapeutic Dose Range (mg/day)
5HT$_{1A}$ Agonists			
Buspirone (Buspar)	0	+	20–60
5HT Re-Uptake Inhibitors			
Fluvoxamine	+ + +	+	Not yet available
Fluoxetine (Prozac)	+ + +	+	20–80
Tricyclic Antidepressants with Mixed Actions			
Imipramine (Tofranil)	+ + +	+ + +	25–300
Clomipramine (Anafranil)	+ + +	+ +	25–250
Norepinephrine Re-Uptake Inhibitors			
Desipramine (Norpramin)	+ + +	+	25–300
Monoamine Oxidase Inhibitors			
Phenelzine (Nardil)	+ + +	+ + +	15–90
Tranylcypromine (Parnate)	+ + +	+ +	10–60
Atypical Antidepressants			
Trazodone (Desyrel)	0	+	150–450
Buproprion (Wellbutrin)	0	+	150–450
Benzodiazepines			
Diazepam (Valium)	+ + +	+ +	10–80
Lorazepam (Ativan)	+ + +	+ +	2–16
Alprazolam (Xanax)	+ + +	+ + +	1–8
Clonazepam (Klonepin)	+ + +	+ + +	0.5–4

*Efficacy was rated as follows: NT, not tested; 0, ineffective; +, slightly effective; + +, moderately effective; + + +, very effective.
†Replication refers to the extent to which the efficacy of the agent has been investigated; it was rated as follows: +, only one or two controlled studies conducted; + +, several controlled studies conducted but further studies indicated; + + + highly replicated and consistent efficacy reported.

treatment of panic disorder are generally twice that needed for treatment of GAD.

In patients who present with previously untreated panic disorder, the clinician should consider the initiation of tricyclic or serotonin reuptake inhibitor therapy, such as imipramine (Tofranil) or fluoxetine (Prozac). Patients should be started on these medications in doses that are initially small and increased gradually, because panic attacks can be provoked if the initial dose is too high. If no improvement is seen in a 4- to 6-week period, the clinician has several choices. A benzodiazepine may be added to the tricyclic or serotonin reuptake inhibitor medication. An alternative is to discontinue the tricyclic or serotonin reuptake inhibitor medication and initiate therapy with a benzodiazepine or MAO inhibitor. Patients who are particularly treatment resistant frequently require a combination of MAO inhibitor and a benzodiazepine.

Long-term follow-up indicates that tolerance does not develop with benzodiazepine or tricyclic antidepressant treatment in panic disorder patients. Patients with panic disorder should generally be maintained on medication for at least 6 months while symptom free before a medication taper, to prevent a relapse of panic attacks. Approximately 50% of patients with panic disorder require long-term medication maintenance, which may involve several years of treatment. In contrast to GAD, buspirone has not been found to be effective for panic disorder.

Behavioral treatment can be extremely effective in treating panic disorder when administered in a group setting. In fact, optimal treatment of panic disorder involves both medication and behavioral psychotherapy. Psychotherapeutic treatment in many cases may reduce the dose of medication required and the risk of relapse when it is discontinued. Some patients may require less medication or have no requirement for medication when administered this type of treatment.

Obsessive-Compulsive Disorder

About 2 to 3% of the general population will be diagnosed with obsessive-compulsive disorder (OCD) during their lifetime. OCD is characterized by the presence of obsessive and compulsive symptoms that cause marked distress, are time-consuming (take up more than 1 hour out of the day), or cause significant impairment in one's work or relationships with people. Obsessions are recurrent ideas, thoughts, or impulses that the individual experiences as intrusive or senseless and that the individual attempts to ignore or suppress. An example of an obsession is the repeated thought that the house is going to burn down,

which the individual realizes is senseless. Compulsions are repetitive behaviors, such as washing one's hands, which are designed to neutralize or prevent some discomfort or dreaded situation, such as perpetually having dirt on one's hands (see Table 1). OCD can potentially be a disabling and chronic disorder that causes serious impairments in functional ability and lifestyle.

Serotonin reuptake inhibitors are the only medications that result in substantial improvement in symptoms of OCD. Several well-designed placebo-controlled studies have confirmed the efficacy of fluoxetine (Prozac), fluvoxamine* (Floxyfral), and clomipramine (Anafranil) for OCD. Approximately 50% of patients show improvement of symptoms of OCD with administration of serotonin reuptake inhibitor medications, but even these patients usually have residual symptoms. Medications that do not potently block the reuptake of serotonin, such as imipramine (Tofranil), amitriptyline (Elavil), nortriptyline (Pamelor), desipramine (Norpramin), and trazodone (Desyrel), have little use in the treatment of OCD. In addition, benzodiazepines and neuroleptics given alone have not been shown to be efficacious. OCD patients with symptoms that border on the delusional, however, have been shown to respond to a combination of a neuroleptic and a 5-HT re-uptake inhibitor. Individual and group therapy with a behavioral orientation can reduce the dose of medication required and the risk of relapse after medications are discontinued.

Post-Traumatic Stress Disorder

Post-traumatic stress disorder (PTSD) currently afflicts about 1% of the population, with a rate of 17% reported in one high-risk urban youth population. PTSD is characterized by a constellation of symptoms that occur after exposure to an extremely stressful or traumatic event defined as being beyond the range of normal human experience. Examples of traumatic events include exposure to combat, life-threatening natural disasters, being held hostage, train wrecks, rape, or physical abuse. Symptoms of PTSD include flashbacks, nightmares, feeling worse with reminders of the trauma, sleep disturbance, avoidance of the trauma, physiologic arousal, exaggerated startle response, guilt, emotional numbing, and feeling cut off from other people. Flashbacks and intrusive memories of the trauma, when present on a recurrent basis, can often be the most disabling and problematic symptoms of PTSD.

Treatment of PTSD may be focused on a discussion of the traumatic event. In patients with

---

*Investigational drug in the United States.

chronic PTSD, group therapy can be directed toward reintegrating the traumatized individual back into the home, family, and societal context. More research is needed to identify effective medications for treatment of PTSD. In the two controlled studies that have been conducted in PTSD, imipramine (Tofranil), phenelzine (Nardil), and amitriptyline (Elavil) have been found to have some beneficial effect. Benzodiazepines appear to have some benefit, although no controlled studies have been conducted in this area, and caution should be taken owing to the high comorbidity of substance abuse disorders in this patient population with attendant risks of addiction and abuse.

Phobic Disorders

Phobic disorders include agoraphobia, with a lifetime prevalence of 2.9%; simple phobias, with a lifetime prevalence of 4% for males and 9% for females; and social phobia, with a current prevalence of 1.2 to 2.2%. Agoraphobia, the fear of being in open places, is increasingly recognized as being commonly associated with panic disorder and as being a consequence of the fear of having a panic attack in public. Phobias are commonly associated with what is known as anticipatory anxiety, or a persistent anxiety associated with the fear of encountering the phobic stimulus.

Simple phobia is defined as the persistent fear of a specific stimulus, such as animals, closed spaces, or heights (see Table 1). Individuals typically avoid situations in which they would encounter the phobic stimulus and experience marked anxiety when exposed to the stimulus. Behavior therapy is the treatment of choice for simple phobias. Behavior therapy uses desensitization techniques in which the aversive stimulus is presented gradually over repeated sessions in a non-anxiogenic setting. In desensitization therapy, the individual may be exposed daily to the phobic stimulus, perhaps at first in his or her mind, then approaching the stimulus gradually through representation, and then finally directly in such a manner that the patient does not become overwhelmed with anxiety. Medications generally have little role in the treatment of simple phobia.

Social phobia is the fear of being in public situations in which the person would come under scrutiny or be the subject of humiliation. Examples include the fear of eating in public, with the specific fear that something would happen that would be the source of embarassment. Individual and group therapy are currently used in the treatment of social phobia. Some preliminary evidence suggests that MAO inhibitors may also be of benefit in the treatment of social phobia.

Adjustment Disorder with Anxious Mood

Most patients presenting to the general practitioner with pathologic anxiety have an adjustment disorder with anxious mood. Adjustment disorders occur after exposure to a stressful life event and are characterized by an exaggerated or pathologic response to the event. Adjustment disorders are usually time-limited and resolve with changes in life circumstances. Appropriate treatment of the adjustment disorders consists of a discussion of the life events in a supportive context. The patient may need to be seen frequently until the stressors resolve. A short course of benzodiazepine treatment can be beneficial in conjunction with supportive contacts with the clinician.

BULIMIA NERVOSA

method of
PAUL E. GARFINKEL, M.D.
University of Toronto
Toronto, Ontario, Canada

The symptom of bulimia describes binge eating per se—the consumption of a large amount of food in a discrete period of time, with a sense of loss of control. Bulimia can be a symptom in a variety of medical disorders or a component of the anorexia nervosa syndrome. It is also encountered as a separate syndrome (bulimia nervosa) accompanied by relatively normal body weights or obesity. Some patients display the features of anorexia nervosa with bulimia or alternate between features of anorexia and bulimia nervosa.

The term "bulimia nervosa" refers to a psychiatric disorder that includes, but is not limited to, binge eating episodes. It is also characterized by distinct psychological preoccupations regarding fears of becoming fat, as occurs in anorexia nervosa. Accompanying the episodes of binge eating and fueled by the fears of obesity are feelings of loss of personal control and efforts to counter the effects of the ingested calories through a variety of purgative techniques. Bulimia nervosa is largely, but not exclusively, a disorder of females, typically between the ages of 16 and 35 years. It occurs in 1 to 2% of women in Western society.

DIAGNOSIS AND CLINICAL FEATURES

The diagnostic criteria as defined by the American Psychiatric Association are listed in Table 1. A morbid fear of fatness is the overriding psychological preoccupation in bulimia nervosa. Self-loathing and disgust with the body are marked. Extreme dieting is interrupted only by the eating binges. The latter may occur

TABLE 1. Bulimia Nervosa Diagnostic Criteria

Recurrent episodes of binge eating (rapid consumption of a large amount of food in a discrete period of time)

A feeling of lack of control over eating behavior during eating binges

Person regularly engages in self-induced vomiting, use of laxatives or diuretics, strict dieting or fasting, or vigorous exercise to prevent weight gain

A minimum average of two binge-eating episodes a week for at least 3 months

Persistent overconcern with body shape and weight

From American Psychiatric Association: Diagnostic and Statistical Manual of Mental Disorders, 3rd ed—Revised. Washington, DC, American Psychiatric Association, 1987.

habitually or may be triggered by unpleasant feelings: anger, anxiety, depression, or loneliness. During the minutes to hours of bingeing, patients frequently describe a sense of frenzy and may consume as many as 5000 calories. In severe cases, cycles of binge eating and vomiting may occur throughout the day. Guilt and dysphoria are common afterward, although some patients experience the binges themselves as soothing. The binges are typically followed by efforts to prevent weight gain. Most commonly this is by self-induced vomiting or occasionally by ingesting the potentially toxic syrup of ipecac. Laxative or diuretic misuse is also common, although these agents almost exclusively produce fluid rather than calorie loss. Some patients binge and do not purge but display extreme caloric restriction between episodes. They may exhibit wide fluctuations in weight or become obese.

Recently there has been recognition that bulimia nervosa encompasses a broad spectrum of psychopathology; for some patients, it is a relatively isolated but disturbing area of dysfunction. For others, it represents one aspect of poor impulse control and character pathology. A significant minority report impulsive stealing of food or of money to buy food. In some, it develops after an episode of anorexia nervosa or substance abuse.

Secrecy and shame associated with the disorder can result in social isolation and impaired vocational functioning. Depression frequently occurs in patients with eating disorders. Because starvation itself can cause cognitive, affective, and social changes that resemble depression, some have argued that the depression is purely based on nutritional factors. In many cases, however, depression appears before the eating disorder, and there is evidence of a high rate of major depression (more than 50% of patients), even after recovery. People with eating disorders also have high rates of anxiety disorders, including agoraphobia, social phobia, and panic disorder. Bulimic patients frequently develop substance abuse, especially misusing alcohol to modulate intense affects, as they do when binge eating.

ASSOCIATED MEDICAL FINDINGS

Patients with both bulimia nervosa and anorexia nervosa frequently display features associated with starvation. These include an emaciated appearance, la-

nugo hair growth, some loss of scalp hair, bradycardia and hypotension, and bruises from subsequent falls. Chronically ill patients may have osteoporosis. Others develop carotene pigmentation on the soles and palms.

Patients with bulimia nervosa at a normal weight generally do not exhibit such obvious signs. Many, however, exhibit parotid enlargement. This is likely due to overstimulation of the glands and is associated with elevated levels of salivary amylase in at least one-third of bulimic patients. Also common are calluses or erosions on the dorsum of the hand near the knuckles, caused by friction against the teeth while inducing vomiting. The acid content of vomitus has an erosive effect on dental enamel and can lead to dental decay and recession of the gums, so the diagnosis of bulimia nervosa may initially be made by dentists.

Patients who are repeatedly binge eating and purging often develop such complications as dehydration, hypochloremic alkalosis, and hypokalemia. Some patients require regular monitoring of serum potassium and potassium supplements. Bloating and edema are common, especially when severe diuretic and laxative use are abruptly stopped. Cardiac abnormalities occur secondary to starvation, hypokalemia, or the chronic ingestion of syrup of ipecac. The latter, an over-the-counter emetic, contains emetine, a muscle poison that produces significant peripheral myopathies and cardiomyopathy.

A variety of gastrointestinal complications may occur. These range from chronic constipation, or alternating constipation with diarrhea, to markedly delayed gastric emptying. Gastric and esophageal erosions and irritations may be secondary to chronic vomiting. Uncommonly gastric dilatation and rupture has been reported.

Many of the hormonal changes are secondary to weight loss and loss of body fat. Oligomenorrhea and amenorrhea are common, the latter especially at low body weights. The response of the thyroid is of conservation, with reduced levels of thyroxine (T_4) and triiodothyronine (T_3) and elevations of reverse T_3. Hypersecretion of cortisol occurs, independent of any weight loss. Levels of insulin and C-peptide are low in bulimia nervosa.

ETIOLOGY AND PATHOGENESIS

Bulimia nervosa can be viewed as an illness with a variety of predispositions. These may be considered to be in the culture, the family, and the individual. The risk factors are associated with an intense need in the individual to maintain self-worth through undue self-control in the area of weight control. These risk factors may be quite different from factors that initiate or precipitate the illness. These, in turn, may be quite different from circumstances that perpetuate the disorder.

Sociocultural Risk Factors

Culturally, prejudice against obesity is strong, and the idealization of thinness is high. Conflict between pressures on women to perform professionally and to be nurturing may highlight concerns about personal control that are manifest in weight regulation. Furthermore, some career choices link thinness and achievement, and these special populations—notably dancers and fashion models—have been shown to be at unusually high risk for the development of eating disorders. It is important to note, however, that these disorders were well described clinically long before thinness achieved its current high social desirability.

Familial Risk Factors

At the level of the family, a history of depression, alcoholism, obesity, or an eating disorder increases the risk for the development of bulimia nervosa, although the mechanism for this is not understood. At a genetic level, there is evidence for greater than an 80% concordance rate for bulimia nervosa among monozygous twins, versus a 30% concordance among dizygotic twins. Even here, however, it is difficult to separate issues of genetic vulnerability from obstacles to the establishment of individual psychological identity. Families may magnify dominant cultural attitudes or imbue food, weight, or shape with undue symbolic significance. For example, a recent study found that mothers of bulimic daughters differed from a non-disordered eating sample by having a greater frequency of an eating disorder or dieting behavior, greater preoccupation with their daughters' dieting, and greater dissatisfaction with the general functioning of the family system. Particular family patterns in which independence is discouraged may also be a contributor. This area is difficult to evaluate in the retrospective studies that have been conducted to date because it is difficult to know whether abnormal familial behavior patterns are a cause or a result of the eating disorder in the child.

Risk Factors in the Individual

At an individual level, predisposing factors include a sense of personal helplessness, fears of losing control, self-esteem highly dependent on the opinions of others, and an all-or-nothing thinking style. A history of premorbid obesity may also heighten risk. A systematic study of female juvenile-onset diabetics revealed an unusually high prevalence of eating disorders, although this may be due to a sampling bias of this study. An earlier history of abuse may also be a risk factor, through its effect on producing a feeling of helplessness and dissatisfaction with one's body.

Evidence shows an association between borderline personality disorder and bulimia, whether it is the bulimic form of anorexia nervosa or bulimia nervosa. This personality disturbance may be a risk for the eating disorder by virtue of problems such people have in separation and individuation, with self-esteem, and difficulty linking self-esteem to external phenomena.

Starvation and repeated bingeing and purging produce changes in neurotransmitter levels, which in turn can be responsible for some of the manifestations of anorexia or bulimia nervosa. Reduced norepinephrine synthesis occurs, and this contributes to the changes in the thyroid, a reduced metabolic rate, bradycardia and hypotension, and possibly a reduced core temperature and an impairment in temperature regulation.

There has been recent interest in the role of serotonin (5HT) in bulimia, with deficient central states possibly arising from repeated episodes of nutritional chaos and purging. A variety of indirect evidence—low 5-hydroxyindole levels in the cerebrospinal fluid, elevated platelet 5HT, blunted prolactin responses to serotoninergic challenges—supports such a link. Because there is evidence for the role of 5HT in inducing satiety, especially in regulation of carbohydrate-containing foods, a deficiency in central 5HT in bulimics has been suggested as a means of the perpetuation of the binge-purge cycle. This requires further study.

TREATMENT

People with serious eating disorders may be mistrustful of physicians, whom they see as being interested only in refeeding them or making them lose their will and becoming fat. The physician must encourage normal eating habits and weight without making this the only focus of treatment or a battleground. The physician must also emphasize that he or she will remain with the patient through difficult times and focus on many different issues as required. The goal is not control of the person but rather relief of suffering. It is helpful to have a firm, nonjudgmental attitude.

Education is of great value. Patients benefit from learning about body weight regulation and the effects of starvation. Dietary misconceptions can be clarified. Often a specific meal plan may be prescribed to avoid long intervals of deprivation that may facilitate episodes of binge eating. It is important to review the effects of vomiting and laxatives on bodily functions. The physician should have a frank discussion with the patient about how easily people can be manipulated by cultural phenomena. It is also important to discuss issues of self-esteem and how a person can relate self-worth entirely to a body size and weight and in doing so force herself to be something that is not natural for her.

Inpatient Treatment

Most patients can be treated entirely as outpatients. A minority may require admission to the hospital after failure to respond to adequate outpatient treatments or if anorexia nervosa is also present because of low body weight. Metabolic or suicidal crises may also require emergency admission. In the hospital, there is often merit in defining a fixed time interval, for example, 4 to 6 weeks, if weight restoration is not an issue. In this time, a schedule can be negotiated during which a normal eating pattern, without vomiting or purgative misuse, is initiated. This can be followed by exposure to so-called binge foods under supervised conditions.

Pharmacotherapies

A series of controlled evaluations have documented the benefits of a variety of antidepressant medications. Desipramine* and imipramine* (in doses of 150 to 300 mg per day) and fluoxetine* (Prozac) (20 to 60 mg) have all been shown to produce a reduction of bingeing and vomiting. The monoamine oxidase inhibitors isocarboxazid* (Marplan) and phenelzine* (Nardil) have also been shown to be useful in controlled studies. These, however, have been associated with high dropout rates, and caution must be exercised in selecting patients who can avoid the multiple interactions with these drugs. At present, there is no evidence for enhanced responses to any of the antidepressants, so selection is based on minimizing anticholinergic and antihistaminic side effects. Response to these medications cannot be predicted based on severity of depression or family history of depression, so bulimic patients who do not demonstrate initial improvement to psychotherapy should undergo a trial of an antidepressant. Further research is required to determine the long-term benefits and optimal duration of treatment. At present, there is evidence for a 70% reduction in bulimic symptoms, and about 35% of patients stop bingeing and purging entirely. After 6 months, about 30% of responders seem to relapse even on maintenance medication.

Psychological Therapies

The outpatient program involves (1) monitoring eating and weight; (2) monitoring appropriate biochemical indices (patients may require monitoring of potassium if hypokalemia has been a problem; for some, potassium supplements are necessary); and (3) ongoing psychotherapy, both for the individual and often for family members. Presently psychotherapy generally involves cognitive, behavioral, and psychodynamic components. Controlled treatment trials that have been conducted to date show that patients display improvements from all three psychotherapeutic methods; about 50% of patients have stopped bingeing and vomiting entirely at 1-year follow-up. Maintenance of change over the longer term requires further study, as does whether there is added benefit in combining antidepressant medication with the psychotherapy.

Eating and weight can be dealt with in the following way:

1. Patients should be encouraged to throw out their scales and be weighed regularly by their physician.

2. When encouraging weight gains, modest increases of 0.5 kg per week are reasonable.

3. The patient should continue eating three meals per day of moderate caloric intake, even if she is binge eating. Binge eating on one day should not be followed by a restriction of intake because this perpetuates the pattern.

4. Patients often benefit from record keeping of dietary intake for a period in treatment. This includes the patient recording what she has eaten, the time and the place when binge eating occurs, and the feelings and events associated with this.

5. Exercise should be limited (30 minutes per day); if it becomes compulsive, the patient should not be permitted to exercise at all.

6. The patient should know that if her weight falls below her goal range, the treatment will alter (this may involve more focus on nutrition in the treatment, addition of liquid supplements, and restricting activities).

The psychological treatment has a number of components:

1. An educative role as described earlier is important.

2. A focus on cognitive elements reduces the tendency to diet and helps in problem solving and in cognitive restructuring.

3. Re-interpretation of the patient's distortions regarding her body is needed. This involves having the individual learn to trust how others see her and to feel her body to be a source of comfort and pleasure.

4. The psychotherapy must involve the person learning to recognize different feeling states and responding appropriately to these (affective expression).

5. Self-esteem has been tied to weight and to a look. The person should gradually recognize that self-esteem can be built up by factors outside of this.

6. Identifying and addressing the major interpersonal problems associated with the illness is important.

7. Family therapy is useful as a primary treatment modality for adolescents and as an adjunct to the individual psychotherapy for older patients.

8. Group therapies are generally useful; they may take different forms, including psychodynamic, behavioral, feminist, or self-help orientations. The appropriate comparisons of these treatments alone with individual psychotherapies have not yet been completed, so for most patients they represent adjuncts to an individual therapy.

---

*This use of desipramine, imipramine, fluoxetine, isocarboxazid, and phenelzine is not listed in the manufacturers' official directives.

COURSE

Bulimia nervosa is often chronic when untreated, but some patients show significant improvements and later have recurrences at times of stress. They are also vulnerable to later depression, anxiety, and substance abuse disorders as well as a general impairment of social adjustment. Initial studies of treated patients show that one-half are well, one-quarter are improved, and one-quarter are unchanged. Mortality rates of bulimia nervosa are not yet known.

DELIRIUM

method of
PETER V. RABINS, M.D., M.P.H.
Johns Hopkins Medical Institutions
Baltimore, Maryland

Delirium is among the most common psychiatric disorders in the medically ill. Among the elderly, 10 to 30% of acutely hospitalized patients are admitted with or develop delirium. Prompt identification and evaluation are important because delirium is often caused by a treatable disorder, and the associated impairment is usually reversible.

RECOGNITION AND DIAGNOSIS

The two clinical hallmarks of delirium are (1) impaired cognitive function and (2) altered level of alertness or consciousness. Diminished cognitive performance can be subtle in mild delirium, but it is usually easy to identify with a standard mental status examination of cognitive performance, such as the Mini-Mental State Exam (MMSE) or the Short Portable Mental Status Examination. The MMSE is particularly useful because it measures nonmemory functions. Similar to all screening instruments, however, it can miss mild delirium. Altered level of consciousness and impaired attention have proved more difficult to operationalize. Generally delirious patients appear drowsy or inaccessible, and their ability to attend or participate in a conversation fluctuates. On occasion they are hyperalert or hypervigilant. Whether the patient is drowsy or alert, examiners find themselves repeating questions, explaining things several times, or repeatedly needing to awaken or alert the patient when assessing or talking with a delirious patient.

A number of associated symptoms should raise suspicion of delirium. These include (1) disorders of perception, i.e., hallucinations, illusions, or misinterpretations; (2) wide fluctuations in behavior; (3) disturbances in the sleep/wake cycle; and (4) activity level changes, either increased or decreased from usual level. Delirium usually develops acutely and is short-lived, lasting several days to several weeks. On occasion it becomes chronic. Pre-existing cognitive disorder (dementia), older age, and more severe medical illness are risk factors.

CLINICAL MANAGEMENT

Prompt early recognition is an important part of the management of delirium because correction of the underlying cause is the primary focus of management. Although delirium often has a treatable cause, it is frequently superimposed on a chronic condition.

Evaluation

As can be seen in Table 1, the differential diagnosis of delirium covers a wide variety of causes; disorders in almost every organ system can be a cause. After delirium has been identified, the first step in the evaluation is to review the physical examination, history, and recent medications. These often suggest one or several causes. These high likelihood causes should be assessed with the appropriate studies and clinical responses. For example, if drug withdrawal is suspected, a test dose of the agent thought to be involved would be a first step. If a toxic drug reaction is suspected, a blood level should be drawn if one is available and the potentially offending agent withdrawn if possible. Because metabolic and infectious causes commonly result in delirium, it is usually prudent to order a complete blood count, metabolic panel, urinalysis, and chest x-ray on all patients whenever delirium is suspected. When no specific cause is identified by the history, physical examination, or review of the medical record, the search for a cause should begin by focusing on the common infectious, metabolic, and toxic causes.

TABLE 1. **Common Causes of Delirium**

Metabolic
Electrolyte disturbances are most common. Hypoxia, calcium imbalance, liver failure, renal failure. Most endocrine disorders can present with delirium often due to excess or deficient actions of the hormone

Infectious
Any systemic infection can cause delirium, even upper respiratory and urinary tract infections. Fever is not always present, especially in the debilitated elderly

Vascular
Any condition leading to decreased brain perfusion (e.g., congestive heart failure, circulatory failure); anemia; stroke; hypertensive encephalopathy; autoimmune vasculitis

Toxic
Medications and psychoactive substances are most common. Drugs from many classes can cause delirium. Heavy metals. Drug withdrawal

Intrinsic Brain Disorders
Mass lesions (tumor, subdural hematoma), postictal state, sequelae of concussion and brain injury

Psychiatric
Severe depression and mania can mimic delirium. Hysterical fugue states can also mimic

If hypoxia is in the differential diagnosis, arterial blood gases should be obtained. Unsuspected alcohol and drug withdrawal are common causes of delirium, and a high level of suspicion is warranted; signs of vasomotor instability (orthostatic hypotension, tachycardia) are common indicators of withdrawal. Improvement in cognition, behavior, and vital signs after a single dose of short-acting benzodiazepine (e.g., lorazepam, 0.5 to 1 mg) suggests alcohol or benzodiazepine withdrawal. If central nervous system pathology is possible or has not been ruled out, computed tomography head scan or magnetic resonance imaging can identify subdural hematomas, acute stroke, or intracranial masses. A lumbar puncture should be done when there is no papilledema or evidence of intracranial mass.

Medications are among the most common causes because the majority of pharmacologically active substances can cause cognitive impairment. A high level of suspicion is warranted. Any change in a medication during the 30 days preceding the development of delirium should be closely reviewed as a potential cause. Anticholinergic toxicity is a common cause of delirium because a wide variety of pharmacologic compounds have anticholinergic activity. Table 2 reproduces an index of anticholinergic activity recently developed by Tune. Plasma blood levels (e.g., digoxin, quinidine, antidepressant, anticonvulsant) should be obtained whenever possible.

The electroencephalogram (EEG) can be helpful at several stages of assessment and management. The characteristic EEG change in delirium is generalized slowing. In a mild delirium, the EEG is helpful in confirming the diagnosis. Improvement from baseline of the EEG to normal is a helpful objective finding when the clinician is unsure whether there has been improvement. A diffusely slow EEG is also seen in moderate and severe dementia, so the EEG is not useful in distinguishing between delirium and dementia.

SYMPTOM MANAGEMENT

The associated symptoms—hallucinations, delusions, agitation—require treatment if they lead to dangerous behavior or are of significant distress to the patient. Although no well-designed trials of psychopharmacologic management have been published, most experts recommend haloperidol at beginning doses of 0.5 mg twice a day when pharmacotherapy is indicated. Some clinicians use low-dose benzodiazepines in this circumstance, but because they are more likely to cause sedation and respiratory depression, they are usually not recommended.

Environmental adjustments are also widely recommended but little studied. Lighting that is adequate but not too bright is thought to decrease misperceptions and illusions. Frequent orientation and frequent reassurance, as often as every 15 minutes, appear to be helpful to many patients.

It is important to explain, in lay language, to patients, their families, and attendants that delirium is the cause of the cognitive and behavior disorder. Delirium is often frightening to the patient and caregiver. Identifying and explaining it can relieve some of this concern.

TABLE 2. **Anticholinergic Properties of the 25 Most Commonly Prescribed Medications***

Medication†	Anticholinergic Drug Level (ng/mL of Atropine Equivalents)
Cimetidine	0.86
Prednisolone	0.55
Theophylline anhydrous	0.44
Digoxin	0.25
Furosemide	0.22
Nifedipine	0.22
Ranitidine	0.22
Isosorbide dinitrate	0.15
Warfarin	0.12
Dipyridamole	0.11
Codeine	0.11
Dyazide	0.08
Captopril	0.02

*All others have no anticholinergic properties.
†At a 10^{-8} Molar concentration.
From Tune L, Carr S, Hoag E, Cooper T: Anticholinergic effects of drugs commonly prescribed for the elderly: Potential means for assessing risk of delirium. Am J Psychiatry 149:1393–1394, 1992. Copyright 1992, the American Psychiatric Association. Reprinted by permission.

MOOD DISORDERS

method of
IRIS R. BELL, M.D., PH.D., and
ALAN J. GELENBERG, M.D.
University of Arizona College of Medicine
Tucson, Arizona

Mood disorders are an extremely common, often chronic or recurrent clinical problem in the general population (5.8%, 6-month prevalence) that occur in a high proportion of medically ill patients. Mood disorders include major depression; dysthymia; bipolar disorder; cyclothymia; depression not otherwise specified ("atypical"); and organic mood disorders secondary to brain lesions, medical conditions, or medication side effects. Approximately 5% of Americans experience major depression over a 1-year period; 5 to 45% of patients with severe medical illnesses have concomitant depression. Among depressed patients treated in medical and psychiatric outpatient settings, more than 65% have concomitant medical illnesses, notably hypertension and arthritis. Substance abuse, especially with alcohol, can be a cause or a result of mood disturbances. Depressed patients, especially older persons, experience greater morbidity and mortality from causes other than suicide than nondepressed patients, but suicide remains a significant risk for as many as 15% of untreated depressed patients of all ages; adolescent and elderly men are at a particularly high risk for suicide.

Mood disorders, even those without currently identifiable organic factors, probably have a significant genetic and biochemical component. These illnesses probably represent neurochemical and neurophysiologic dysfunctions in the brain that are exacerbated by psychosocial stressors, which may evolve over their chronic course into autonomous processes independent of life events. Depression is more than the simple sadness or "blues" from which anyone may suffer during periods of loss or distress.

From epidemiologic and genetic studies, we know that the relative risk of developing major depression in a first-degree relative of a person who has the illness is three times that of normals, and the risk of developing bipolar disorder is 24.5 times that of normals. More women experience major depression than men (5 to 9% versus 2 to 4%), but the sexes are equally affected by bipolar disorder (Type I, 0.4 to 1.2%). Depression can coexist with other psychiatric disorders, including personality disorders, such as borderline, histrionic, and dependent types, and organic mental disorders, such as the dementias associated with Alzheimer's disease, multi-infarct dementia, or Parkinson's disease.

TYPES OF MOOD DISORDER

Diagnosis of mood disorders depends primarily on thorough clinical history and exclusion of organic factors. Although laboratory studies, such as the dexamethasone suppression test and the thyrotropin-releasing hormone stimulation test, reveal abnormalities in endocrine regulation of many depressives, no test is sufficiently sensitive and specific for routine diagnostic purposes. Psychiatric terminology in the *Diagnostic and Statistical Manual of Mental Disorders, Third Edition—Revised (DSM–III–R)* describes mainly the phenomena, rather than causes, of psychiatric disorders, including mood disorders. Each patient presents with a unique cluster of affective, cognitive, and somatic features. Selection of appropriate treatment requires identification of target symptoms and signs and consideration of the biologic, psychological, and social context of each patient.

Major Depression

Major depression can commence at any age, but it most often presents in the third decade of life. It entails a single episode with full recovery in approximately 40% of cases but recurrence or chronicity in at least 60%. Untreated depressions can persist for as long as 2 years. Women are more prone than men to develop major depression. The diagnostic characteristics of major depression include at least five of the following nine symptoms for at least a 2-week period: depressed mood, diminished interest or pleasure in activities, significant change in weight or appetite, insomnia or hypersomnia, psychomotor agitation or retardation, fatigue or loss of energy, feelings of worthlessness or excessive guilt, diminished ability to concentrate or make decisions, or recurrent thoughts of death or suicide.

The major descriptive subtypes include psychotic, melancholic, and seasonal depression. The psychotic type of major depression frequently involves delusions of guilt, serious medical disease, and a sense of deserved punishment for self-perceived misdeeds. Auditory hallucinations and other types of delusions can also occur.

The melancholic type is a severe form in which at least five of nine symptoms are present: loss of interest in all activities, lack of ability to feel better even temporarily from good events, morning worsening of mood, early morning awakening (often 3 or 4 A.M.), observable psychomotor retardation or agitation, more than 5% weight loss in a month, no significant personality disturbance before the first depressive episode, one or more previous major depressions followed by complete recovery, or previous good response to somatic therapies such as antidepressant medications or electroconvulsive therapy.

The seasonal type shows at least a 3-year pattern of regular temporal relationships between the onset of mood disturbance and a specific 60-day period of the year, notably autumn, and between complete remission and a specific 60-day period of the year, notably spring, in northern latitudes. Symptomatically the seasonal type is characterized by hypersomnia, carbohydrate craving, and weight gain. Bipolar Type II patients often experience the seasonal form of major depression.

Elderly patients with onset of first mood disturbance late in life require careful attention to possible organic causes. Even without specific findings, vascular disease risk factors may be more common in late-life depressives than in matched controls.

Dysthymia

Many patients live with chronically dysphoric conditions, including dysthymia, and episodically develop major depression superimposed on their baseline mood. Studies suggest that pharmacologic treatment ameliorates the major depression and perhaps the dysthymia in certain persons.

The *DSM–III–R* defines dysthymia as a depressed mood (or irritable mood in children and adolescents) for most of the day, more days than not, for at least 2 years (1 year for children and adolescents). During this time, the patient must not be symptom free for more than 2 months. At least two of the following symptoms are experienced while depressed: poor appetite or overeating, insomnia or hypersomnia, low energy or fatigue, low self-esteem, poor concentration or difficulty making decisions, or feelings of hopelessness.

Bipolar Disorder

Bipolar disorder is a cyclical disorder characterized by a chronic course of episodic manias and major depressions. Between episodes, most bipolar patients are comparatively asymptomatic, although 25 to 33% experience impaired interepisode functioning. Approximately 60 to 80% of patients exhibit manias as the initial manifestation of their illness, with later episodes of major depression predominating. With age, mood episodes can occur more often and last longer. The bipolar nature of the illness is often missed in persons who present initially with major depression or with Type II bipolar disorder (i.e., those whose "highs" are less extreme than those of Type I patients). Patients who cycle into mood episodes four or more times per year are considered to have a rapid cycling form of the disorder, and their treatment needs may vary from those with classic presentations. Others can present with elements of mania and depression during the same episode (mixed).

Bipolar patients meeting the *DSM–III–R* criteria for a manic episode at some point in their illness have a distinct period of abnormally and persistently elevated, expansive, or irritable mood. During the period of mood disturbance, at least three of the following symptoms have persisted (four if the mood is only irritable) to a significant degree: inflated self-esteem or grandiosity, decreased need for sleep, more talkative than usual or pressure to keep talking, flight of ideas or subjective experience that thoughts are racing, distractibility, increase in goal-directed activity or psychomotor agitation, or excessive involvement in pleasurable activities that have a high potential for painful consequences (e.g., buying sprees, sexual indiscretions, unwise business investments).

During mania, according to the *DSM–III–R* criteria, the mood disturbance is sufficiently severe to cause marked impairment in occupational functioning or in usual social activities or relationships with others, or it necessitates hospitalization to prevent harm to self or others. For diagnosis of the less severe form, hypomania, this criterion is not required. At no time during the disturbance have there been delusions or hallucinations for as long as 2 weeks without prominent mood symptoms.

Cyclothymia

As in dysthymia, some persons with cyclothymia experience chronic mood disturbances of lesser severity than those seen in bipolar disorder. Cyclothymia occurs with a prevalence of 0.4 to 3.5% in the general population, and it may be more common among persons with a family history of bipolar disorder.

The *DSM–III–R* criteria for cyclothymia require at least 2 years (1 year for children and adolescents) of numerous hypomanic episodes and numerous periods of depressed mood or loss of interest or pleasure that do not meet criteria for major depression. During a 2-year period (1 year for children and adolescents) of the disturbance, the patient is never without hypomanic or depressive symptoms for more than a 2-month interval. No clear evidence of a major depression or mania exists during the first 2 years of the disturbance (1 year for children and adolescents).

Organic Mood Disorders

It is extremely important for the physician to be alert to the identification of mood disorders in the gen-

TABLE 1. **Medical Causes of Depression**

Deficiency States	**Malignant Disease**
Pellagra	Metastases
Pernicious anemia	Breast
Wernicke's encephalopathy	Gastrointestinal
	Lung
Drugs and Medication	Pancreas
Alcohol	Prostate
Amphetamines	Remote effect: pancreas
Antihypertensive agents	
Clonidine	**Metabolic Disorders**
Diuretics (hypokalemia or	Electrolyte imbalance
hyponatremia)*	Hypokalemia
Guanethidine	Hyponatremia
Methyldopa	Hepatic encephalopathy
Propranolol	Hypo-oxygenation
Reserpine	Cerebral arteriosclerosis
Birth control pills	Chronic bronchitis
Cimetidine	Congestive heart failure*
Digitalis	Emphysema
Disulfiram	Myocardial infarction*
Sedatives	Paroxysmal dysrhythmias
Barbiturates	Pneumonia*
Benzodiazepines	Severe anemia*
Steroids/ACTH	Uremia*
Endocrine Disorders	**Neurologic Disorders**
Acromegaly	Alzheimer's disease
Adrenal	Amyotrophic lateral sclerosis
Addison's disease*	Creutzfeldt-Jakob disease
Cushing's disease	Huntington's chorea
Hyper- and	Multiple sclerosis
hypoparathyroidism*	Myasthenia gravis
Insulinoma	Normal-pressure
Pheochromocytoma	hydrocephalus
Pituitary	Parkinson's disease
	Pick's disease
Infections	Wilson's disease
Encephalitis	
Fungal	**Trauma**
Meningitis	Postconcussion
Neurosyphilis	
Tuberculosis	

*Acute life-threatening disorders.
Abbreviation: ACTH = adrenocorticotropic hormone.
From Jenike MA: Depressed in the E. R. Emerg Med *16:* 102–120, 1984.

eral medical patient population and of the wide range of organic causes that can underlie mood disturbances. Tables 1 and 2 list the organic causes of depression and mania. In many clinical situations, the central nervous system shows subtle evidence of dysfunction before problems in other bodily systems become apparent; the manifestations of brain dysfunction are problems in the psychological and behavioral realms. The general classes of organic factors that can cause mood disorders include endocrine, metabolic, and nutritional disorders (often subclinical), neurologic disorders, malignancies, drugs, and infections. Many of these possibilities are common in medical patients and must be ruled out in the comprehensive evaluation of every patient with mood disturbance.

The initial medical evaluation of a manic or depressed patient should include a thorough personal and family medical and psychiatric history, blood levels of medications or toxic screens for drugs of abuse, a blood chemistry screening panel (e.g., electrolytes,

TABLE 2. **Organic Causes of Manic and Hypomanic Symptoms**

Drug-Related	**Infection**
Isoniazid*	Influenza*
Procarbazine*	Q fever*
Levodopa*	Neurosyphilis
Bromide*	Post–St. Louis type A
Decongestants	encephalitis*
Bronchodilators	"Benign" herpes simplex
Procyclidine	encephalitis
Calcium replacement	AIDS (HIV)
Phencyclidine	
Metoclopramide	**Neoplasm**
Corticosteroids and ACTH*	Parasagittal meningioma*
Hallucinogens	Diencephalic glioma*
Sympathomimetic amines	Suprasellar
Disulfiram (Antabuse)	craniopharyngioma*
Alcohol	Suprasellar diencephalic
Barbiturates	tumor*
Anticholinergics	Benign spheno-occipital
Anticonvulsants	tumor*
Benzodiazepines	Right-intraventricular
	meningioma
Metabolic Disturbance	Right-temporoparietal
Postoperative states*	occipital metastases
Hemodialysis*	Tumor of floor of fourth
Vitamin B_{12} deficiency	ventricle
Addison's disease	
Cushing's disease	**Other Conditions**
Postinfection states	Post-isolation syndrome
Dialysis	Right-temporal lobectomy
Hyperthyroidism	Post-traumatic confusion
	Post-electroconvulsive
Neurologic Conditions	therapy
Right-temporal seizure focus*	Deliriform organic brain
Multiple sclerosis	disease
Right-hemisphere damage	
Epilepsy	
Huntington's disease	
Postcerebrovascular accident	

*Meets criteria of Krauthammer and Klerman for secondary mania.
Abbreviations: ACTH = adrenocorticotropic hormone; AIDS = acquired immune deficiency syndrome; HIV = human immunodeficiency virus.
From Goodwin FK, and Jamison KR: Manic-Depressive Illness. New York, Oxford University Press, 1990.

blood urea nitrogen, creatinine, liver function tests), syphilis serology, blood count and sedimentation rate, thyrotropin-stimulating hormone and thyroid index (free thyroxine [T_4] and reverse triiodothyronine [rT_3] uptake), and serum folate and B_{12} levels (even with normal red blood cell indices, which are not an adequate screen). The clinical data may guide the clinician to consider computed tomography or magnetic resonance scan of the head, electroencephalograph (EEG), adrenal function studies, or more specialized tests. Specific treatment of the etiologic factor is always preferable to the symptomatic treatment that is afforded by current psychopharmacologic regimens.

TREATMENT

In addition to the medical evaluation of affective disturbed patients for etiologic factors, certain premedication laboratory tests are strongly indicated. Patients with any pre-existing cardiac condition and those older than 40 years generally require an electrocardiogram with attention to possible conduction defects and prolonged QT intervals. The complete blood count with white cell differential and platelet counts and the liver and renal blood chemistry panel mentioned earlier are important to establish the baseline status and safety for initiating a number of psychotropic medications. As part of the informed consent process, women of childbearing age should have a pregnancy test and careful counseling on the known and unknown risks of psychopharmacologic agents to fetal development during pregnancy, especially lithium (e.g., Epstein's anomaly). Psychotropic medications should be avoided during the first trimester of pregnancy, and electroconvulsive therapy (ECT) may be the treatment of choice in many pregnant women whose psychiatric condition necessitates intervention.

Depression

The treatment of mood disorders involves a systematic decision tree (Figure 1) that integrates knowledge of the neurochemical actions and side effects of the drug options with attention to the biologic, psychological, and social characteristics of the patient. The recent introduction of several newer agents has expanded the armamentarium for effective pharmacologic treatment of depression and mania. To avoid the risks of the anticholinergic and orthostatic side effects of the tertiary amine tricyclic antidepressants, such as amitriptyline (Elavil), that were once in favor, psychiatrists have shifted their first-line pharmacotherapy of depression to secondary amine tricyclics, such as nortriptyline (Pamelor) or desipramine (Norpramin), and to the recently introduced nontricyclics, such as fluoxetine (Prozac), sertraline (Zoloft), paroxetine (Paxil), and bupropion (Wellbutrin).

The tricyclic antidepressants exert multiple effects on central and autonomic nervous system pathways, partially by presynaptic blockade of norepinephrine or serotonin reuptake. Their common side effects include dry mouth, blurred vision, tachycardia, constipation (anticholinergic), orthostatic hypotension (alpha-adrenergic blockade), and weight gain. Owing to their quinidine-like actions, tricyclics at therapeutic doses can exert beneficial antiarrhythmic effects on atrial or ventricular premature contractions, but they increase cardiac risk for patients with second-degree and third-degree heart block or right-bundle or left-bundle branch block or for those who overdose. Excessive sedation occurs more often with the tertiary amine tricyclics, perhaps because of antihistaminic effects. Patients with treated

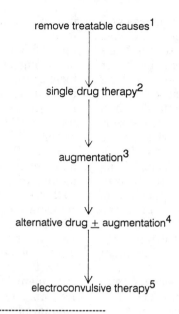

remove treatable causes[1]

single drug therapy[2]

augmentation[3]

alternative drug $\pm$ augmentation[4]

electroconvulsive therapy[5]

---

[1] See Tables 1 and 2.

[2] For sedation, choose nortriptyline; for activation, desipramine or fluoxetine or bupropion. Combine with antipsychotic agent if psychotic features present.

[3] Try lithium carbonate; possibly folic acid, T3, or T4.

[4] Select alternative agent of a drug class different from that of initial agent.

[5] Taper and stop certain drugs before starting ECT, e.g. lithium and benzodiazepines.

Figure 1. Decision tree for the treatment of depression.

open-angle, but not closed-angle, glaucoma can safely receive tricyclics. Blood levels to determine adequate treatment dose of the tricyclics are most useful in terms of suprathreshold levels, although there is some evidence that nortriptyline has a curvilinear relationship between blood level and response (50 to 150 ng per mL).

Newer antidepressants do not share the anticholinergic properties of the tricyclics and thus offer alternatives for many patients. Fluoxetine is a propylamine, selective blocker of serotonin reuptake. Many patients respond to the starting dose of 20 mg per day, but a substantial proportion need lower doses (e.g., 2.5 to 10 mg per day, now available in liquid form), and some require higher doses (up to 80 mg per day). One of the most striking properties of fluoxetine is the extremely long half-life of the parent drug (1 to 3 days) and its active metabolite norfluoxetine (7 to 15 days). Its most common side effects are agitation, insomnia, and gastrointestinal upset; in contrast to tricyclics, fluoxetine does not appear to be lethal in overdose. A small percentage of patients experience excessive drowsiness rather than agitation. The allegations from recent anecdotal reports about the capacity of fluoxetine to trigger suicidal or homicidal acts are not fully resolved, but large-scale, systematic reviews of records have failed to find an increased frequency of violent acts in patients treated with fluoxetine compared with other antidepressant medications. The ability of this drug to cause profound agitation in excessive doses may offer some explanation for violent or suicidal behaviors in a few patients.

Newer selective serotonin re-uptake inhibitors (SSRIs) that may be an alternative to fluoxetine are the shorter half-life drugs sertraline (Zoloft) (doses of 50 to 200 mg per day) and paroxetine (Paxil) (doses of 20 to 50 mg per day). Major side effects of the newer SSRIs are gastrointestinal distress, tremor, insomnia, somnolence, and dry mouth.

Bupropion, a unique newer antidepressant, has a structure similar to phenylethylamine but an unknown mechanism of action. It is often effective in cases for which tricyclics are not helpful or are potentially harmful, such as in bipolar depression. Similar to fluoxetine, bupropion is an activating drug whose side effects include agitation, insomnia, headache, and gastrointestinal distress. Despite initial concerns about its potential to cause generalized tonic-clonic seizures at a rate of 4 per 1000 patients, a recent extensive review of clinical records suggests that seizure risk is not greater for this drug than for other antidepressants except at higher doses (>450 mg per day or >150 mg per dose) and perhaps in bulimics. Otherwise, its shorter half-life than fluoxetine, the availability of small unit doses, and its low cardiac and orthostatic risk profile make it a valuable option, especially for the elderly. Usual treatment doses range from 75 mg twice daily to 150 mg three times daily. In contrast with tricyclics, both fluoxetine and bupropion have the additional advantage of not causing weight gain. The amount of weight loss, however, that occurs in some patients on these drugs is too small to justify their use in weight management programs per se.

Although most primary care physicians refer patients who need monoamine oxidase (MAO) inhibitors to a psychiatrist, it is important to be aware of these drugs. MAO inhibitors are effective antidepressants whose mode of action is to block irreversibly postsynaptic inactivation of epinephrine, norepinephrine, dopamine, and serotonin. MAO inhibitors benefit many patients who fail to respond to any of the previously discussed agents. For patients with concomitant anxiety and depression, the more sedating hydrazine, phenelzine (Nardil), in divided doses ranging from 45 to 90 mg per day, is appropriate. For those with anergic bipolar depression, the stimulant-like nonhydrazine, tranylcypromine (Parnate), is given in divided doses ranging from 10 to 30 mg per day.

MAO inhibitors do not exert the anticholinergic side effects seen with tricyclics. The most common side effects of these drugs are dizziness, orthostatic hypotension, sexual dysfunction, insomnia, and daytime sleepiness. The greatest risk is the occurrence of hypertensive crises and possible resultant strokes owing to the interaction of pressor substances with the MAO inhibitor–induced inability to inactivate them. Hypertensive crises are precipitated by ingestion of aged foods, such as aged cheese, sausage, smoked fish, beer, or red wine, and of stimulant or sympathomimetic drugs. Concomitant administration of meperidine (Demerol), fluoxetine, or clomipramine (Anafranil) with MAO inhibitors is contraindicated owing to the risk of a lethal serotoninergic syndrome with hypermetabolic crisis (i.e., hyperthermia, neuromuscular irritability, delirium). It is essential to discontinue other antidepressant drugs and impose at least a 1-week washout period (5 weeks for fluoxetine) of no antidepressant medications in switching from another class of antidepressant to an MAO inhibitor and a 2-week washout period in switching from an MAO inhibitor to another class of antidepressant. The treatment of hypertensive crises involves use of 2 to 5 mg of phentolamine (Regitine) intravenously or of 10 mg of nifedipine (Procardia) in capsules, bitten and swallowed. Dantrolene (Dantrium), the antispasticity drug that attenuates malignant hyperthermia, may be useful in the treatment of MAO inhibitor–related hypermetabolic crises.

Tricyclic-Resistant Cases. If the antidepressant medications described earlier fail as single agents, augmentation with low-dose lithium for 1 to 2 weeks is usually the next step. Some psychopharmacologists try cautious combinations of a tricyclic with fluoxetine (watching for excessive elevations of tricyclic levels) or an antidepressant with folic acid. Although early reports indicated benefit from T_3 or T_4 augmentation of tricyclic treatment in euthyroid depressives, clinicians do not consider this strategy to be generally reliable compared with, for example, lithium augmentation. The next alternative is to taper and stop other antidepressant drugs and initiate a trial of an MAO inhibitor, such as phenelzine or tranylcypromine, after an appropriate washout period. Limited evidence suggests that buspirone (BuSpar), a nonaddictive antianxiety agent, may be beneficial for single-drug therapy of agitated depression in divided doses up to 60 mg per day, but it is not currently a first-line agent for this indication. For medically ill patients with apathy and fatigue but not necessarily with major depression (e.g., AIDS or elderly hip fracture patients in rehabilitation), low doses (5 to 20 mg per day) of stimulant drugs, such as methylphenidate (Ritalin) or dextroamphetamine (Dexedrine), can act rapidly to mobilize participation in care.

Tables 3 and 4 summarize the dosing and properties of the preferred major agents. All of the usual antidepressant agents have a 2- to 8-week delay in onset of therapeutic action. Therefore, the decision to use a medication rather than ECT first is largely based on the acuity of the patient's overall condition and history.

Active suicidality, severe dehydration and malnourishment from the anorexia of depression, medical conditions complicating safe medication treatment, and a history of multiple failed antidepressant drug trials favor prompt use of ECT in most cases. The major side effects of ECT are headache and temporary impairment in short-term memory; investigators have not found evidence of brain damage or of lasting adverse effects on cognition. Contraindications for ECT include increased intracranial pressure, recent myocardial infarction, and an inability to tolerate brief anesthesia.

Definitive treatment of major depression with psychotic features requires combined antidepres-

TABLE 3. **Major Medications in the Treatment of Depression**

Agent	Trade Name	Initial Daily Dosage	Usual Therapeutic Dosage
Tricyclics			
Nortriptyline	Pamelor	20–40 mg	75–150 mg
Desipramine	Norpramin	25–75 mg	75–200 mg
Doxepin	Sinequan	25–75 mg	150–300 mg
Heterocyclics			
Fluoxetine	Prozac	20 mg	20 mg
Bupropion	Wellbutrin	75–100 mg bid	100–150 mg tid
Trazodone	Desyrel	50–100 mg	150–600 mg
Monamine Oxidase Inhibitors			
Tranylcypromine	Parnate	10 mg	10–30 mg
Phenelzine	Nardil	30 mg	45–90 mg

sant and antipsychotic medication or ECT. Some research suggests that seasonal affective disorder remits with exposure to 2 to 4 hours per day of bright white light administered in early morning or at dusk, without medications, but most of these patients also respond to customary antidepressants without light therapy.

The initial choice of an antidepressant is based on target symptoms, such as whether the patient has an agitated presentation (favoring the more sedative nortriptyline) or a psychomotor retarded one (favoring the more activating desipramine, bupropion, or fluoxetine). Patients with major depression superimposed on obsessive-compulsive disorder should receive medications with primarily serotoninergic properties (i.e., clomipramine [Anafranil] or fluoxetine). The tricyclics have the advantage of longer widespread clinical use and the availability of blood levels to assist assessment of compliance and appropriate dosing.

Medical factors also clarify the options. For example, although the tricyclic anticholinergic side effect of urinary retention may be problematic for male patients with benign prostatic hypertrophy, tricyclics are an optimal treatment for other depressed patients with stress or urge urinary incontinence. Nortriptyline is the tricyclic of choice in treating geriatric depression because of its relatively lower risks of orthostatic hypotension and anticholinergic side effects and its therapeutic window for blood levels (50 to 150 ng per mL).

Certain tricyclics, such as doxepin (Sinequan), although highly sedative, are at least as effective H_2 blockers as cimetidine (Tagamet) in healing peptic ulcers. Patients with severe cardiac conduction defects have a higher risk from the quinidine-like tricyclic drugs, and those with ventricular arrhythmias have a higher risk from trazodone (Desyrel). Bupropion, with the most benign reported cardiac profile, may be preferable in that situation. Fluoxetine is probably a good second choice for those with cardiac conduction problems, but some reports suggest occasional instances of fluoxetine-related sinus bradycardia, syncope, and hypotension. In patients with seizure disorders or bulimia, bupropion may—and maprotiline (Ludiomil) can—increase seizure risk to unacceptable levels.

Trazodone causes a relatively rare but significant side effect of priapism in men; a similar side effect occurs rarely in women. In patients on multiple medications, especially those tightly protein bound or metabolized by the liver, fluoxetine can prolong half-life or induce elevations and thus toxicity of certain drugs (e.g., coumadin, digitoxin, tricyclic antidepressants, thyroxine, diaze-

TABLE 4. **Comparison of Antidepressant Adverse Effects**

Antidepressant	Anticholinergic Effects	Orthostatic Hypotension	Sedation	Insomnia	Agitation/ Restlessness	Nausea	Headaches/ Migraine	Sexual Dysfunction
Tertiary Amine Tricyclics								
Amitriptyline (Elavil)	+ + +	+ + +	+ + +	0	0	0	+	+ +
Doxepin (Sinequan)	+ +	+ + +	+ + +	0	0	0	+	+ +
Imipramine (Tofranil)	+ +	+ + +	+ +	0	+	0	+	+ +
Secondary Tricyclics								
Nortriptyline (Pamelor)	+	+	+ +	0	+	0	+	+
Desipramine (Norpramin)	+	+ +	+	0	+	0	+	+
Other								
Fluoxetine (Prozac)	0	0	+	+ + +	+ + +	+ +	+ + +	+ + +
Trazodone (Desyrel)	0	+ + +	+ + +	0	0	+	+	+ +
Bupropion (Wellbutrin)	+	+	0	+ + +	+ + +	+ + +	+ + +	0
Sertraline (Zoloft)	0	0	+	+	+	+ +	+	+ +
Paroxetine (Paxil)	0	0	+	+	+	+ +	+	+ +

Abbreviations: + + + = occurs frequently; + + = intermediate frequency; + = minimal frequency; 0 = not reported.

Adapted from Gelenberg AJ: Introduction: New perspectives on the use of tricyclic antidepressants. J Clin Psychiatry 50(7, Suppl):3, 1989. Copyright 1989, Physicians Postgraduate Press.

pam) whose dosing was previously stable and within therapeutic range.

Patients with Parkinson's disease may benefit from single-drug therapy with the newer MAO inhibitor selegiline (Eldepryl), which may slow the progression of their neurologic disorder at lower doses (selective MAO B inhibition) but also act as an antidepressant at higher doses, at which selectivity is lost, and dietary and drug precautions are necessary. In patients whose medical treatment may involve the need for sympathomimetic drugs or meperidine (Demerol), however, the MAO inhibitors are contraindicated owing to the risk of hypertensive or hypermetabolic crises from drug interactions.

Combination agents with antipsychotics and antidepressants, such as perphenazine-amitriptyline (Triavil), may seem parsimonious, but they increase the difficulty of finding appropriate doses of each agent in patients who need both classes of drugs. For those who have agitation but not psychosis, a risky practice has been to use combination drugs, amoxapine (Asendin), a tricyclic antidepressant that is also an antipsychotic, or even thioridazine (Mellaril) for depression. With increased awareness of the risks of potentially irreversible tardive dyskinesia from cumulative exposure to antipsychotic drugs, it is no longer appropriate to expose a nonpsychotic patient to these agents under most circumstances. Older women with mood disorders have the highest risk of developing tardive dyskinesia from antipsychotic medications.

High-dose alprazolam (Xanax) is useful in the treatment of certain depressions, but it carries significant risks of inducing tolerance and dependence on an agent whose withdrawal is extremely difficult to manage. Alprazolam withdrawal is complex because of patient insomnia, agitation, and possible withdrawal seizures, even in nonepileptic patients.

Concomitant Sleep Disturbance. One of the pitfalls of overlooking the diagnosis of depression is that patients may receive only sedative hypnotics, such as benzodiazepines, for the insomnia component of their illness. Most benzodiazepines offer only short-term benefit (up to 2 weeks) for insomnia before tolerance develops. They are central nervous system depressants and can worsen the underlying depression.

It is preferable to treat the insomnia secondary to depression with a sedating antidepressant. If an activating antidepressant is needed for the rest of the clinical picture, some psychopharmacologists add the highly sedative antidepressant drug trazodone, in doses of 25 to 150 mg at bedtime, to an ongoing trial of another antidepressant, such as fluoxetine. Trazodone is more problematic to manage as an antidepressant by itself,

owing to its broad range of possible therapeutic doses (150 to 600 mg), strong propensity to cause orthostatic hypotension and extreme sedation at higher antidepressant doses, tendency to exacerbate ventricular arrhythmias, and the idiosyncratic risk of inducing priapism. In low doses for sedative purposes, however, its lack of anticholinergic, depressant, or addictive properties makes it a reasonable option for the initial treatment of many cases of depression-related insomnia. The need for sleeping medication can be re-evaluated after resolution of the depression.

After an adequate antidepressant response has been achieved, it is imperative to continue treatment with the antidepressant for an additional 4 to 6 months. These treatments control but do not cure the underlying neurochemical propensity toward depression during an episode, and premature discontinuation of drug treatment is a common cause of relapse or recurrence. This also applies to patients who have responded to ECT, after which maintenance antidepressant medications or maintenance ECT at regular intervals in drug-resistant situations is necessary.

Bipolar Disorder

The cyclical nature of bipolar disorder dictates the need for a mood-stabilizing agent for the chronic component of the condition. The first-line option remains lithium carbonate (Eskalith). In lithium-resistant cases, psychopharmacologists now use anticonvulsants with limbic nervous system activity, such as valproate (Depakote) or carbamazepine (Tegretol). Despite mood-stabilizing treatment, many patients suffer recurrent episodes of mania or depression. Others have difficulty accepting their need for maintenance medication, which leads to poor compliance and to relapse in 20 to 30% of patients. After an episode has begun, the patient is likely to require additional symptom-specific medication or ECT for the mania or depression.

Table 5 summarizes the usual doses and side effects for medications used in treatment of bipolar disorder. Lithium carbonate is a salt excreted by the kidneys with a narrow range between therapeutic and toxic blood levels. A prelithium work-up and annual monitoring include an electrocardiogram, complete blood count with white cell differential count, thyroid-stimulating hormone and T_4 index, serum calcium, blood urea nitrogen, and serum creatinine. One side effect of lithium is the elevation of the white blood cell count into the range of 12,000 to 15,000 cells per mm^3, with primary effects on neutrophils, which can confuse a practitioner evaluating blood counts for signs of acute infection. Lithium is

TABLE 5. **Major Medications in the Treatment of Mania**

Agent	Trade Name	Initial Daily Dosage	Usual Therapeutic Dosage	Common Side Effects
Mood Stabilizers				
Lithium	Eskalith	600–1200 mg	1200–2400 mg	Tremor, gastrointestinal upset, polydipsia, polyuria, weight gain
Valproate	Depakote	500 mg	1000–1500 mg	Gastrointestinal upset
Carbamazepine	Tegretol	400 mg	800–1600 mg	Gastrointestinal upset, sedation, ataxia
Sedatives or Anti-agitation Agents				
Lorazepam*	Ativan	1–2 mg	2–6 mg	Sedation, ataxia
Clonazepam	Klonopin	1–2 mg	2–10 mg	Sedation, ataxia
Antipsychotics				
Haloperidol*	Haldol	2–5 mg	5–15 mg	Stiffness, tremor, bradykinesia, akathisia, dyskinesia

*Lorazepam, which has a shorter half-life than clonazepam, is injectable. Haloperidol and many other antipsychotic agents have oral and parenteral forms for administration.

sometimes used to augment treatment in certain cancer patients with neutropenia.

Lithium is usually initiated in doses of 900 to 1200 mg per day (divided into doses three times per day), with weekly monitoring until a steady state is achieved, drawing blood levels 12 hours after the last dose. The target blood level is 0.8 to 1.2 mEq per liter. Monitoring can then be limited to monthly (ultimately every few months) blood levels. Recent studies suggest that, although use of lower maintenance blood levels of lithium (e.g., 0.4 mEq per liter) are better tolerated by patients, they result in a clinically greater risk of relapse than do blood levels at 0.8 or above.

The most common side effects of lithium include gastrointestinal upset, fine tremor, increased thirst and appetite, increased urination, and edema. Early toxicity is often heralded by vomiting or diarrhea, drowsiness, ataxia, and confusion. In less severe cases, treatment of lithium toxicity involves temporary discontinuation of the drug and fluid and electrolyte support as indicated. The narrow margin between therapeutic and toxic levels of lithium, however, increases the possibility of severe toxicity, which can cause lasting neurologic damage or death from central nervous system depression, cardiovascular collapse, or both. Aggressive treatment with hemodialysis is necessary at blood levels of 4.0 mEq per liter or greater and may be indicated at levels between 2.0 to 4.0 mEq per liter if accompanied by serious clinical deterioration. Several medications interact with lithium clearance to elevate blood levels and produce toxicity, most notably thiazide diuretics and nonsteroidal anti-inflammatory drugs.

Lithium does not adequately control cycling in some bipolar patients. These treatment-resistant cases often respond to one of the anticonvulsants mentioned earlier, alone or in combination with lithium. Valproate has achieved better patient acceptance with its less-sedating profile. Its most common side effect is gastrointestinal distress; its most serious risk of fatal hepatic toxicity appears to be limited to young children with epilepsy. Valproate doses begin with 250 mg twice daily, titrated to a blood range of 50 to 100 μg per mL. Carbamazepine doses begin with 200 mg twice daily, titrated to a blood range of 6 to 10 mg per liter. After 1 month of treatment, carbamazepine induces an increase in its own metabolism by the liver, and compensatory readjustment of dose is necessary. The major risks of carbamazepine treatment include sleepiness, gastrointestinal upset, ataxia, and neutropenia (discontinue at white counts below 3000 cells per mm^3) and aplastic anemia (1 of 125,000 cases).

In rapid cycling bipolar patients, some investigators have found subclinical hypothyroid conditions, with thyroid supplementation helpful in reducing the frequency of cycles. Carbamazepine also may be useful in conjunction with lithium. Initial evidence indicates that the antidepressant bupropion may assist in the stabilization of rapid cyclers. Definitive treatment of this form of the disorder is not yet well established.

Acute Mania and Depression

In acute mania, lithium adjusted into the high therapeutic range (1.0 to 1.3 mEq per liter) controls symptoms, but its onset of action is delayed 5 to 14 days or longer, and most acutely manic patients require adjunctive treatment. For sedation in psychotic or nonpsychotic agitated manics, high-potency benzodiazepines, such as lorazepam (Ativan) or clonazepam (Klonopin), in divided doses of 2 and up to 10 mg per day are effective and act rapidly. The ability to administer loraze-pam intramuscularly is an advantage in certain clinical situations. In patients with psychotic features, antipsychotic medications such as haloperidol (Haldol) in doses of 5 to 15 mg per day are useful. High doses of antipsychotics are no longer used because the risks of possible neuroleptic malignant syndrome or severe extrapyramidal side effects (e.g., stiffness, akathisic restlessness) outweigh their benefits. In selected treatment-resistant cases of chronic mania or schizoaffective psychoses, the unique antipsychotic medication clozapine (Clozaril) is being tried, with anecdotally reported benefits. Given the need for careful monitoring of hematologic status for agranulocytosis, the decision to employ clozapine in a bipolar patient should be made only after consultation with a psychopharmacologist.

Bipolar depressives often present with psychomotor retardation or with atypical depressions involving hypersomnia and hyperphagia. The treatment options outlined earlier for major depression apply to a bipolar patient in a depressed state. Some evidence, however, suggests that tricyclic treatment may accelerate the cycling process, and some psychopharmacologists prefer an MAO inhibitor, such as tranylcypromine, for its activating effects. Bupropion may have unique benefits in the treatment of bipolar patients, especially rapid cyclers, by minimizing the risk of manic episodes that otherwise can follow treatment for depression. Patients with a mixture of mania and depression appear to be more treatment resistant. ECT remains the most effective treatment for mania and depression, although its use is usually reserved for the specific indications outlined earlier.

OVERALL MANAGEMENT AND REFERRAL DECISIONS

Specific types of short-term, focused psychotherapy, such as cognitive-behavioral and interpersonal approaches, have equivalent efficacy to tricyclic medications for treating mild or moderate nonpsychotic depressive conditions. Many studies suggest that the combination of pharmacotherapy with psychotherapy is more effective, especially for long-term maintenance, than either treatment strategy alone. Medical practitioners are unlikely to be able to offer such specialized care in the setting of a busy outpatient practice, and referral to a qualified psychologist or psychiatrist for psychotherapy is indicated.

In the most severe cases, especially if psychiatric hospitalization is indicated for suicidality or socially disabling illness, rapid psychiatric referral is necessary. For a substantial subset of affec-tively ill patients who first present to their family physician, however, brief supportive interventions by the physician alone during medication management visits may be the most acceptable to the patient. Many patients still find psychiatric referral to be a socially stigmatizing event. Affirmation of the primary physician's plan of continued involvement and of the consultant role of the psychiatrist may assist patient acceptance.

There are many outpatients whose mood disorders simply fail to respond to single-drug therapy. In those cases, early consultation with a psychiatrist who has psychopharmacologic expertise can provide cost-effective treatment by identifying etiologic factors, determining adequacy of previous drug trials, or developing a strategy for adjunctive or alternative medications.

SCHIZOPHRENIA

method of
STEPHEN R. MARDER, M.D.
University of California, Los Angeles, School of Medicine
Los Angeles, California

Schizophrenia is a psychiatric illness that is characterized by (1) psychotic symptoms, such as hallucinations, delusions, bizarre behavior, and disorganized thought processes; (2) impaired emotional responses, particularly a blunting of emotional reactions; and (3) a deterioration in social and vocational functioning. The illness usually has its onset during late adolescence or the early twenties but can emerge at any time from childhood to old age. Schizophrenia affects about 1% of the world population. It exists in severe forms, which can lead to chronic institutionalization, or in relatively mild forms, which respond well to pharmacotherapy. Before a patient is assigned a final diagnosis of schizophrenia, other psychiatric disorders, such as bipolar illness, should be considered as well as organic mental disorders that can be associated with psychosis, such as stimulant intoxication, steroid psychosis, Huntington's disease, and many others.

Although the cause of schizophrenia remains controversial, a consensus has developed about some of its biologic underpinnings. There is compelling evidence that individuals can inherit a vulnerability to develop schizophrenia. A number of structural brain abnormalities, such as increased ventricular size and sulcal enlargement, are more common in schizophrenic patients. There is inconclusive evidence suggesting that schizophrenia may be associated with an abnormal dopamine system. There is clear evidence, however, that drugs that are dopamine agonists or increase dopamine turnover, such as amphetamine or cocaine, can worsen the illness, and drugs that decrease dopamine turnover or block dopamine receptors improve symptoms of schizophrenia.

An important characteristic of schizophrenia is that it affects nearly all aspects of a patient's life. As a result, patients often present to clinicians with considerably more than just psychotic thought processes. They may have impairments in social relationships, deterioration in work or educational performance, and disturbed family relationships. Because these problems occur in many different dimensions, it is understandable that there is, as yet, no single effective treatment that addresses all of the problems that torment schizophrenic patients and their families. Physicians who treat schizophrenia often combine pharmacologic treatments that address the signs and symptoms of the illness with psychosocial interventions, which address the secondary impairments.

DRUG TREATMENT OF ACUTE SCHIZOPHRENIA

Few clinical effects in medicine have been as clearly demonstrated as the advantage of an antipsychotic medication over a placebo for treatment of psychotic symptoms in acute schizophrenia. Findings from numerous studies as well as a vast amount of clinical experience have provided the justification for recommending that nearly all acutely psychotic schizophrenic patients receive antipsychotic drug treatment. The fact that antipsychotic drugs have been shown to be highly effective in groups of patients, however, does not mean that they work for every patient or that every patient should receive them. Schizophrenic patients differ markedly in the degree to which they improve on drugs and in their sensitivity to antipsychotic drug side effects. Moreover, patients also differ in the severity of their schizophrenic symptoms, which can be subtle and hardly debilitating in some patients and severe in others. As a result, the decision as to whether a particular patient should be treated with antipsychotic medications is based on an analysis of the possible benefits and the likely adverse effects.

All of the symptoms associated with schizophrenia are affected to some degree by antipsychotics. The so-called positive symptoms, which include hallucinations, delusions, and disorganized thoughts, are more responsive to drug treatment than are negative symptoms, such as blunted affect, emotional withdrawal, and lack of social interest. Frequently positive symptoms are eliminated by drug treatment, whereas negative symptoms are only modestly improved and continue to impair the patient's social recovery. A substantial proportion of schizophrenic patients—about 10 to 20%—fail to demonstrate substantial improvement when they are treated with neuroleptics. This subgroup of treatment-refractory schizophrenic patients often requires long-term institutionalization in state hospitals and similar facilities.

Selection of an Antipsychotic Drug

A large number of antipsychotic medications are available to clinicians treating schizophrenia. For the most part, all are equally effective against psychotic symptoms. Possible exceptions are clozapine, which has advantages for patients with illnesses that respond poorly to older antipsychotics, and newer drugs, such as risperidone and remoxipride, which may reach the U.S. market in 1993 or 1994. In the past, it was believed that different types of schizophrenia responded better to certain types of drugs. For example, it was believed that chlorpromazine, a drug with considerable sedative side effect, was better for agitated or excited patients, whereas haloperidol, a drug that is only minimally sedating, was better for more withdrawn patients. This has not been supported by empirical research, and it is currently believed that all of the classes of neuroleptics are equally efficacious for all of the different manifestations of the illness. These observations are based on the average responses of groups of patients and cannot be strictly applied to individual cases. It is possible that a particular patient may do well on one drug and be unimproved or even worsened by another. Thus a record of a good or poor response to a particular drug should be an important factor in selecting that drug.

The most important differences among antipsychotics are in their side effects (Table 1). For simplicity, these drugs are usually divided into two groups: high-potency drugs, including fluphenazine, haloperidol, thiothixene, and trifluoperazine, and low-potency drugs, including chlorpromazine and thioridazine. High-potency drugs are prescribed in much lower doses (as the result of their high potency) and tend to be more associated with neurologic side effects (see section on side effects later), such as stiffness, restlessness, and tremor. Low-potency drugs result in much less neurologic side effect but are associated with more anticholinergic side effects, such as dry mouth, constipation, and blurred vision, and more autonomic side effects, such as postural hypotension and sedation. Recently there has been a strong tendency to prescribe the high-potency drugs because their side effects are usually more manageable.

Route of Administration

Antipsychotics also differ in their available routes of administration. It is preferable to pre-

TABLE 1. **Classes of Antipsychotic Compounds**

Class	Example	Usual Daily Dose (mg)	Extrapyramidal Side Effects	Postural Hypotension
Phenothiazines	Fluphenazine	5–20	+ + +	+
	Chlorpromazine	300–1000	+ +	+ +
	Thioridazine	300–800	+ +	+ +
Thioxanthenes	Thiothixene	10–50	+ +	+ +
Butyrophenones	Haloperidol	5–20	+ + +	+
Dibenzoxazepines	Loxapine	25–100	+ +	+
Dihydroindolones	Molindone	25–100	+ +	+
Dibenzodiazepines	Clozapine	200–900	0	+ + +
Benzisoxazole	Risperidone*	4–16	+	+ +

+ = minimal; + + = moderate; + + + = severe.
*Not available in the United States.

scribe oral antipsychotics for most acutely psychotic individuals. There are occasions when clinicians may find it useful to administer short-acting intramuscular medications for patients who are agitated or for those who refuse medications. Because intramuscular medications are absorbed more rapidly than oral medications, the calming effect of antipsychotics may become apparent earlier. This calming effect on agitation, however, is different than the true antipsychotic effect of these medications, which may require several days and sometimes several weeks. Therefore patients should be started on a regimen of oral medications as soon as a decision is made to treat with antipsychotics.

Although most antipsychotics are available as short-acting injectables, some are not. In addition, fluphenazine and haloperidol are available as long-acting injectables. This form of drug delivery consists of an injection that is administered once every 2 to 4 weeks. The drug is slowly released from the injection site, resulting in a reasonably steady drug level for the entire interval between injections. This latter form of drug administration is usually used for patients who have been stabilized and are being maintained in long-term drug therapy. Long-acting depot drugs are poorly suited for treating acutely psychotic patients because these drugs take a long time—about 3 months—to reach steady state and are eliminated slowly. As a result, the clinician is unable to titrate dose against clinical response and side effects.

Drug Dose for Acute Treatment

There are large differences in the doses of antipsychotic drugs that are used to treat different individuals. For example, some patients have an adequate therapeutic response to 2 mg of haloperidol daily, whereas others require 40 mg or more. Similarly, some experience intolerable side effects on 2 mg, whereas others have no difficulty

tolerating 100 mg. Some of this variation can be explained by the fact that different patients have as much as a 20-fold variation in their blood levels of a drug after receiving the same amount of a neuroleptic.

Despite these large differences in the dose that patients tolerate, recent research has provided guidance to clinicians who are selecting a dose for acute treatment. Most acutely psychotic schizophrenic patients require 300 mg or more of chlorpromazine (or its equivalent if another antipsychotic is used) daily. Raising the dose above 1000 mg daily is unlikely to increase patients' chances of improving. Because 100 mg of chlorpromazine has equal antipsychotic potency to 2 mg of haloperidol or fluphenazine, this indicates that the effective dose range for these drugs is 6 to 20 mg daily. Several years ago, a number of authorities suggested that acutely ill patients responded better to "rapid neuroleptization," a practice that advocated the use of relatively high doses of injectable high-potency drugs, such as haloperidol or fluphenazine, during the first days of treatment. A number of carefully designed clinical trials have since indicated that this practice is no more effective than using conventional doses of oral drugs, and as a result it has fallen out of favor.

Time for Improvement

Improvement on antipsychotic medications may not occur for days or weeks after drug treatment is started. Patients who are experiencing psychotic agitation usually experience a calming effect that begins within hours of the start of drug treatment. Symptoms such as hallucinations, delusions, and disturbed behaviors, however, may not begin to improve until much later. Once patients begin to improve, it may take months before they achieve maximal benefit. This slow time course can become a problem if the clinician believes after a week or two that a patient is not responding because the wrong drug or dose was prescribed. This may result in a change in drug or an increase in dose that is unnecessary.

These observations suggest that a reasonable strategy for an acutely psychotic schizophrenic patient involves prescribing a moderate dose of an antipsychotic drug, such as 6 to 20 mg of haloperidol or fluphenazine daily. If the dose is well tolerated, the clinician should wait for 4 to 6 weeks before considering a change in drug or dose.

Side Effects of Antipsychotics

Neurologic side effects, also called extrapyramidal side effects (EPS), are the major problem in prescribing neuroleptics. The most common EPS is akathisia, a side effect consisting of a subjective feeling of restlessness. Patients who experience severe akathisia often pace continuously or move their feet restlessly while they are sitting. Some complain of a feeling that they are unable to feel comfortable, regardless of what they do. Severe akathisia can cause patients to feel anxious or irritable, and some reports suggest that severe akathisia can result in aggressive or suicidal acts.

Acute dystonic reactions are abrupt-onset, sometimes bizarre, muscular spasms affecting mainly the musculature of the head and neck but sometimes the trunk and lower extremities, leading to gait disturbances. These reactions usually appear within the first few days of therapy when patients are treated with large doses of high-potency neuroleptics, such as haloperidol or fluphenazine. Younger patients are more likely to develop dystonias. Dystonias almost always respond rapidly to antiparkinson medications and can usually be prevented either by pretreatment with antiparkinson medications or by limiting the neuroleptic dosage prescribed. Another manifestation of EPS is drug-induced parkinsonism, consisting of stiffness, tremor, and shuffling gait. Often patients with these symptoms also experience akinesia, a side effect consisting of difficulty initiating movement. In some cases, drug-induced parkinsonism can be nearly identical to Parkinson's disease.

For most patients, EPS are treatable. The anticholinergic antiparkinson drugs, such as benztropine (1 to 2 mg twice daily) or trihexyphenidyl (2 to 4 mg three times daily), are by far the most commonly used drugs for EPS. Many clinicians prescribe these drugs routinely for patients who are receiving high-potency antipsychotics. A number of studies indicate that prescribing antiparkinson medications before patients demonstrate EPS can prevent dystonias. Unfortunately,

these drugs also have side effects of their own, including dry mouth, constipation, urinary retention, and blurry vision.

Other drugs for treating EPS include amantadine, a drug that is effective against parkinsonism, and propranolol, which is effective in managing akathisia. Both of these drugs can be added to anticholinergic antiparkinson drugs.

Tardive dyskinesia is a movement disorder that may occur following long-term treatment with antipsychotic medications. Patients with tardive dyskinesia may have any or all of a number of abnormal movements. These frequently consist of mouth and tongue movements, such as lip smacking and puckering, as well as facial grimacing. Other movements may include irregular movements of the limbs, particularly piano player–like movements of the fingers and toes, and slow, writhing movements of the trunk. Although seriously disabling dyskinesia is uncommon, a small proportion may affect walking, breathing, eating, and talking. At least 10 to 20% of patients treated with neuroleptics for more than a year develop tardive dyskinesia. Certain populations are at a greater risk than others for developing tardive dyskinesia. Increasing age seems to increase risk, with elderly women being particularly vulnerable.

The neuroleptic malignant syndrome is a potentially fatal but rare complication of neuroleptic treatment. It presents initially as muscular rigidity and progresses to elevated temperature, fluctuating consciousness, and unstable vital signs. Mortality in well-developed cases has been reported as ranging from 20 to 30% and may be higher when depot forms are used. Clinicians should be concerned about any patient who demonstrates severe muscular rigidity and a rising temperature because early diagnosis and treatment can be lifesaving.

Other side effects that may be associated with antipsychotics are sedation; postural hypotension; weight gain; endocrine effects, including galactorrhea and amenorrhea in women; and erectile and ejaculatory disturbances in men.

Long-Term Maintenance Therapy

Antipsychotic medications are effective in preventing psychotic relapse in schizophrenic patients who are stable. If stabilized patients in the community have their antipsychotics discontinued, a large proportion—about 65 to 75%—relapse within 1 year. If patients are continued on their medications, fewer than 25 to 35% relapse. This large difference in survival between drug-treated and placebo-treated patients is the main reason why schizophrenic patients are commonly continued on long-term neuroleptic maintenance treatment after a schizophrenic episode.

The first 3 to 6 months after an acute episode is a period for stabilization when patients may not demonstrate acute symptoms but may nevertheless remain more vulnerable to relapse. Following this stabilization period, clinicians should consider gradually lowering the dose of antipsychotic. Reducing the dose is likely to decrease EPS and may decrease the patient's vulnerability to developing tardive dyskinesia. A maintenance dose may be as low as 2.5 mg of oral fluphenazine or haloperidol daily, 50 mg of haloperidol decanoate every 4 weeks, or 6.25 to 12.5 mg of fluphenazine decanoate every 2 weeks.

Atypical Antipsychotics

When the first atypical neuroleptic, clozapine (Clozaril), was introduced into clinical studies during the early 1970s, it was noted that this drug was highly effective and associated with negligible EPS. Unfortunately, clozapine was also associated with a relatively high rate (1 to 2% during the first year of exposure) of agranulocytosis. More recent studies have found that clozapine-induced agranulocytosis is reversible if it is diagnosed early. As a result, clozapine is currently indicated for certain schizophrenic patients. The available data suggest that patients who are most likely to benefit from clozapine treatment are those who have schizophrenic illnesses with severe positive symptoms, such as hallucinations, delusions, and thought disturbances, that are poorly responsive to conventional neuroleptic medications. Clozapine is also a reasonable choice for patients who may have neuroleptic responsive illnesses but who suffer from severe EPS at the doses that are needed to control the illness. Patients with severe tardive dyskinesia may also be candidates for clozapine treatment. A number of studies indicate that clozapine is associated with a substantially lower risk for tardive dyskinesia when compared with typical neuroleptics and that tardive dyskinesia may actually improve on clozapine.

Patients who receive clozapine are required to be enrolled in a monitoring system that assures that patients have their white blood cell counts monitored on a weekly basis. The drug should be discontinued if the white blood count drops below 3000 and the granulocyte count drops below 1500. At that time, patients should be carefully monitored for evidence of infections. If the white blood count and granulocyte count rise above these levels, clozapine treatment may be resumed. If the white blood count drops below 2000 and the granulocyte count drops below 1000,

however, clozapine should be discontinued, and patients should be carefully monitored by a hematologist and perhaps a specialist in infectious disease.

The advantages of clozapine—efficacy with minimal EPS—have led to intensive search for other atypical antipsychotic medications. Risperidone and remoxipride are the first two atypical drugs that are likely to be marketed in the United States. Both of these have some liability for causing EPS but substantially less than the traditional antipsychotics. Moreover, neither of these drugs has a substantial risk of agranulocytosis. As a result, these two compounds may be appropriate for a larger population of schizophrenic patients than clozapine.

When Patients Fail to Respond

When patients fail to improve after an adequate trial of an antipsychotic, a number of alternative strategies are available for clinicians. Increasing the dose of the current antipsychotic drug or changing to a drug from another class is sometimes helpful. As mentioned previously, clozapine may be helpful for patients who fail to respond to traditional antipsychotics. Patients are sometimes helped by adding lithium to their antipsychotics, particularly when there is an excited component to their illness. Patients who have had their psychotic symptoms well controlled on antipsychotics but remain depressed are often helped by the addition of an antidepressant medication. Other medications that have been tried as adjuncts to antipsychotics include carbamazepine, valproate, and propranolol. These treatments, however, are limited in what they can do and should be saved until after a dosage adjustment of a conventional drug or clozapine has had an adequate trial.

PSYCHOSOCIAL TREATMENTS FOR SCHIZOPHRENIA

When the goals of the clinician and the patient include more than the management of psychotic symptoms—perhaps work rehabilitation or improved socialization—the optimal treatment plan should include the use of other treatment modalities, such as psychotherapy, vocational rehabilitation, family therapy, or social skills training. These treatments are most effective during the outpatient phase of treatment, when psychotic thought processes and impairments in information processing are less likely to interfere with psychosocial treatments. In most cases, drug and psychosocial treatments are carried out in the context of a multidisciplinary treatment team.

PANIC DISORDER AND AGORAPHOBIA

method of
MARK H. POLLACK, M.D., and
JERROLD F. ROSENBAUM, M.D.

Massachusetts General Hospital
Boston, Massachusetts

Panic disorder is an important but often undiagnosed cause of distress for patients in the medical setting. Unrecognized and untreated, panic disorder may result in significant patient morbidity and mortality, exposure to unfruitful laboratory testing and potentially dangerous invasive procedures, and substantial patient and clinician frustration. Appreciation of diagnostic criteria, including differential diagnosis and co-morbidity with other psychiatric and medical illnesses, understanding of its purported underlying pathophysiology, and familiarity with available treatments are critical to the medical practitioner.

DIAGNOSTIC CONSIDERATIONS

Panic attacks are characterized by the sudden onset of intense feelings of anxiety, apprehension, fear, sense of impending doom, or loss of control, which early in the course of illness are typically spontaneous and unexpected, reach full intensity in seconds to minutes, may last for minutes or hours, and are associated with a number of physical symptoms of autonomic, primarily sympathetic, arousal (Table 1). As the disorder progresses, more attacks may be anticipated, preceded by the fear of having one, especially in certain settings where attacks are more threatening, embarrassing, or previously experienced.

For patients to meet criteria for panic disorder, they must have had at least one spontaneous or unexpected major panic attack (an attack, associated with four or more panic symptoms) and either four attacks within a 4-week period or followed by a period of at least a month of persistent anticipatory anxiety (apprehension of further panic). One of the critical defining features in assessment of panic disorder is the rapid onset of symptoms; anxiety that develops gradually over hours or days is not a panic attack. Patients may also experience attacks with fewer than four symptoms known as "limited symptom attacks." Limited symptom panic attacks may be more frequent than major panic attacks in some patients, a possible source of confusion in the medical setting, where patients may present with one or two panic symptoms, such as tachycardia, dizziness, or hyperventilation. These limited symptom panic attacks are important to recognize because they are associated with the same morbidity and complications as major panic attacks over time. Patients with limited symptom attacks are more likely to have symptoms attributed to another medical illness, delaying initiation of treatment.

Although initial panic attacks are usually spontaneous, some patients may develop agoraphobia and go on to associate panic attacks with specific situations and begin to fear and avoid them. Typical phobic situations are those from which easy escape may be difficult or embarrassing or help may not be readily available, such as driving in traffic or on highways or other settings of restricted escape. Some patients may continue to enter feared situations despite their anxiety, but others may become progressively more avoidant and restrict the scope of their activities because of fear of having another panic attack. Some become dependent on companions or may be unable to leave their home because of fear of having a panic attack. Other situations that patients may avoid include using public transportation, flying on airplanes, shopping in malls or large stores, going to restaurants or movie theaters, standing in line or in crowds, or being at home alone.

Agoraphobia may also occur without panic attacks, although most patients with predominant agoraphobic symptoms report a history of panic attacks if carefully questioned. Many patients report that feared situations are associated with emergent physical symptoms, such as respiratory distress, chest discomfort, headaches, palpitations, or bowel symptoms, which may be manifestations of limited symptom or major panic attacks.

Panic attacks are markedly distressing and frightening and when unrecognized lead patients to emergency rooms or other acute medical settings in fear of having suffered a myocardial infarction or stroke. The cardiopulmonary symptoms of panic may be of sufficient magnitude that an intensive care admission is required to rule out myocardial infarction, and patients may undergo unnecessary and potentially dangerous invasive diagnostic procedures if the panic disorder is unrecognized and extensive medical work-up is pursued. Studies of patients with atypical chest pain and normal coronary angiograms demonstrate that 40 to 60% of these patients may have panic disorder.

Patients with "masked or nonfearful panic" may experience paroxysmal physical symptoms, typically autonomic, without prominent associated anxiety and persist in medical evaluations despite an absence of objective findings, only to respond in time when antipanic treatment is initiated. Studies suggest that nonfearful panic is common among patients with atypical chest pain. Similarly, neurologic patients with paroxysmal symptoms such as dizziness may respond to typical antipanic treatments.

TABLE 1. Panic Attack Symptoms

Shortness of breath or smothering sensations
Dizziness, unsteady feelings, or faintness
Palpitations or tachycardia
Trembling or shaking
Sweating
Choking
Nausea or abdominal distress
Depersonalization or derealization
Numbness or tingling sensations
Flushes (hot flashes) or chills
Chest pain or discomfort
Fear of dying
Fear of going crazy or doing something uncontrolled

EPIDEMIOLOGY

One to two percent of people in the United States have panic disorder, and an additional 2 to 3% suffer agoraphobia with or without panic. As many as a third of college students report experiencing panic attacks in the preceding year. About two-thirds of panic disorder patients are female. Anxiety disorders, including panic, are relatively frequent in the medical setting. Up to 20% of primary care patients meet lifetime criteria for panic disorder and 13% for current panic disorder. Close to another 10% have occasional panic attacks. Forty percent of panic patients report visiting an emergency room for emotional problems in the prior year, and cardiologists, neurologists, and gastroenterologists may be particularly likely to see patients with symptoms stemming from panic disorder.

The onset of the disorder is typically in the third decade of life, although many patients report a history of significant anxiety dating back to childhood manifesting as separation anxiety, school phobia, shyness, or behavioral inhibition in unfamiliar circumstances. Many patients report that their panic attacks began within a year of a psychosocial stressor (such as a change in relationship, job loss, or medical illness), although once triggered, the disorder tends to persist even after the stress has disappeared. Panic attacks that occur for the first time after the age of 40 are less common and require more intensive efforts to search for an underlying organic cause.

ETIOLOGY AND PATHOPHYSIOLOGY

Family studies demonstrating increased risk of panic disorder in first-degree and second-degree relatives of panic patients and concordance for panic attacks in monozygotic as compared with dizygotic twin pairs point to an underlying genetic component for the disorder. Family genetic studies suggest that for some, the risk for panic disorder may be inherited as a single gene locus, although a multifactorial mode of transmission may also be possible.

Studies of children at risk for anxiety disorders provide further support for the notion that panic disorder may be a manifestation of a constitutional predisposition for anxiety. Retrospective studies of adult panic patients report high rates of childhood anxiety disorders in these patients. Direct observation of the children of panic disorder and agoraphobia patients reveals high rates of behavioral inhibition to the unfamiliar, a temperamental quality characterized by increased arousal, anxiety, and constricted behavior in the face of novel stimuli. These inhibited children demonstrate increased rates of anxiety and depressive disorders as do their first-degree relatives, consistent with the assertion that there is a familial vulnerability to the development of anxiety disorders.

Dysregulation in certain central nervous system functions may also be associated with panic disorder. Abnormalities in the brain's noradrenergic system have been implicated in anxiety; factors that increase rates of firing of the locus coeruleus, a retropontine nucleus producing more than 70% of total brain norepinephrine, provoke panic attacks. Other brain systems implicated in the neurobiology of panic disorder include serotonergic, endogenous benzodiazepine, and dopaminergic systems; cortisol-releasing factor; adenosine; and a variety of neuropeptides including cholecystokinin. A recent theory highlights abnormalities in the central control of respiratory function or a "suffocation alarm system" as a prominent symptom of panic disorder, which is a sense of suffocation, difficulty breathing, or air hunger.

CO-MORBIDITY AND DIFFERENTIAL DIAGNOSIS

Patients with panic disorder may also suffer other psychiatric disorders, including other anxiety disorders. *Generalized anxiety disorder (GAD)* is characterized by excessive worry about two or more life circumstances (e.g., finances or danger to loved ones) in excess of what is reasonable for a period of 6 months or longer. Although there may be some overlap, GAD symptoms tend to be more persistent and chronic without the rapid onset, intensity, and paroxysmal quality of panic attacks. Patients with *social phobia* fear scrutiny by others and believe they will experience humiliation or embarrassment. A *simple phobia* is the fear of discrete situations or objects, such as heights, animals, or the sight of blood. Patients afflicted with *post-traumatic stress disorder (PTSD)* have experienced a catastrophic event that would be considered distressing to anyone (e.g., a threat to one's life or witnessing a serious accident) and may re-experience the traumatic event; avoid stimuli associated with the trauma; become detached and estranged from others; and experience irritability, hypervigilance, and difficulty sleeping and concentrating. Although recognition of PTSD has been focused on combat veterans, it may also occur in civilians, and these patients have increased rates of panic attacks.

Up to two-thirds of panic disorder patients experience a *major depressive* episode at some point in their lives. Patients known to have significant anxiety should be assessed for the presence of depression. Panic disorder may carry an independent risk for suicidal behavior, but the presence of suicidal ideation, especially when accompanied by prominent symptoms of depressed mood, psychomotor retardation or agitation, early morning awakening, or hopelessness, should raise concerns about the presence of depression. Depressed patients with panic attacks are at increased risk for suicide attempts. It is critical to consider depression when evaluating an anxious patient because of the treatment implications: Benzodiazepines are effective anxiolytics, but depression responds best to treatment with antidepressants, and patients may continue to suffer persistent morbidity and risk of suicide if the diagnosis of depression is overlooked and treatment limited to benzodiazepines alone.

Panic disorder patients are at increased risk to develop alcohol and substance abuse, often as an attempt at self-medicating uncomfortable anxiety symptoms. Once substance abuse is established, it usually requires specific intervention, but treating the anxiety disorder may also be indicated and improve outcome. The use of benzodiazepines is relatively contraindicated for anxiety patients actively abusing alcohol or drugs.

Somatoform Disorders (Hypochondriasis and Somatization)

Somatization represents a tendency to amplify and focus on somatic symptoms. Patients with somatization disorder have a history of multiple, chronic physical complaints not accounted for by organic pathology that cause them to take prescription medication, seek medical treatment, or make other lifestyle changes. Hypochondriasis is characterized by patients' conviction that they have an illness, usually based on misinterpretation of physical signs and symptoms and persisting despite negative work-ups and reassurances.

The somatic symptoms of panic disorder typically lead patients to seek a medical explanation for their symptoms. Panic patients may fear that their attacks are manifestations of specific medical illness, but this fear may lessen when the anxiety disorder is diagnosed and, especially, effectively treated. Acceptance of the diagnosis may be enhanced by presenting the disorder as a medical illness with recognized symptoms, pathophysiology, and treatment rather than as purely psychological distress.

MEDICAL DISORDERS

In considering medical disorders that may present with anxiety symptoms, evaluation directed toward the somatic system (e.g., cardiac, neurologic) may provide the most fruitful yield from further diagnostic investigations. Systematic consideration of the characteristic features of panic disorder is critical: Onset of anxiety symptoms after the age of 40, a lack of personal or family history of anxiety disorders, negative childhood history of anxiety symptoms, an absence of significant life events triggering or exacerbating anxiety symptoms, lack of avoidance behavior, and poor response to standard antipanic agents all suggest that panic symptoms may be secondary to another condition. A review of conditions commonly associated with anxiety, such as arrhythmias, thyroid disease, caffeinism, and licit or illicit substance intoxication and withdrawal, should be undertaken even in apparently healthy individuals.

Hyperthyroidism

Hyperthyroidism may feature some of the same symptoms as panic disorder, including anxiety, tremor, nervousness, palpitations, labile mood, shortness of breath, and gastrointestinal distress. The prevalence of thyroid disease in panic patients is higher than in the general population, although the nature of this association is unclear. Symptoms associated with hyperthyroidism tend to be less episodic than those seen in panic disorder patients.

Hypoglycemia

Although hypoglycemia is often considered a potential cause for panic-like symptoms, clinical data suggest it is rather uncommon. Patients who report a history of hypoglycemia should be questioned carefully about the presence of panic disorder because they may inappropriately attribute their symptoms of tachycardia, anxiety, and lightheadedness to undocumented hypoglycemia rather than to panic.

Pheochromocytoma

Pheochromocytoma may present with panic-type symptoms, secondary to the release of massive amounts of catecholamines. Patients with pheochromocytomas do not, however, generally meet criteria for panic disorder or develop phobic avoidance, and they tend to have few psychological as opposed to physical symptoms of anxiety. Significant blood pressure abnormalities are more common in pheochromocytoma patients than those with panic disorder. Patients with a family history of pheochromocytoma or other endocrine abnormalities should be considered particularly at risk and receive appropriate work-up.

Cardiac Pathology

Panic attack symptoms, including chest pain, dyspnea, and palpitations, may overlap with those of angina as well as arrhythmias. Patients at risk should receive appropriate work-up, but patients with few risk factors such as younger female patients without personal or family cardiac histories should be carefully evaluated for the presence of panic disorder. Mitral valve prolapse and panic disorder sometimes coexist, although the nature and significance of this association are not clear.

Audiovestibular Dysfunctions

Patients with panic disorder may present with complaints of unsteadiness, vertigo, dizziness, and fears of falling that may mimic audiovestibular dysfunction; however, most patients with panic disorder when carefully tested have normal audiovestibular function.

Complex Partial Seizures

Patients with complex partial seizures may present with panic attacks or episodic symptoms of anxiety, including chest pain; tachyarrhythmias; syncope; abdominal distress; changes in levels of consciousness; staring spells; micropsia or macropsia; abnormal motor movements or twitching, and auditory, olfactory, gustatory, or visual hallucinations. Panic attacks characterized by atypical features, such as derealization, depersonalization, unilateral paresthesias or shock-like sensations, may be secondary to complex partial seizures.

Caffeinism

Excessive use of caffeine may produce symptoms of anxiety or panic attacks and may worsen anxiety symptoms in predisposed individuals. Thus attention to caffeine intake and recommendations for gradual reduction in use may improve the patient's condition.

TREATMENT

Patient education is a critical component of the treatment of panic disorder. Patients may be reassured that their symptoms reflect a known medical condition rather than being purely psychological. They should know that, once identified and treated, the disorder is not at all likely to be associated with catastrophic medical or psychiatric outcome. Patients impressed that their physical symptoms reflect a medical illness should be reassured that panic disorder is a medical illness and that they are receiving a definitive diagnosis for which appropriate treatment is available rather than false reassurance that "it's just nerves." Patients should be advised to reduce caffeine intake, which may exacerbate anxiety. Prescribed medications that may promote anxiety symptoms, such as theophylline derivatives, diet pills, or decongestants, should be reduced or discontinued if possible. Patients should be reminded to decrease use of alcohol, which may worsen anxiety symptoms over time, and to stop use of recreational substances, such as cocaine and marijuana, which may worsen symptoms. Patients who fail to respond robustly to treatment should be re-evaluated for presence of occult substance abuse. Patients should be encouraged to maintain normal levels of activity as much as possible to minimize their overattention to symptoms and to promote exposure to feared situations.

Although early intervention may prevent complications, many patients present for treatment after years of symptoms and disabilities. Despite the chronic nature of their symptoms, however, many patients achieve substantial improvement with available treatment, including antipanic pharmacotherapy and cognitive-behavioral therapy. For some patients, initiation of antipanic medication may result in remission of phobic anxiety and disability once panic attacks have ceased. For patients with residual phobic anxiety and avoidance, however, cognitive-behavioral strategies may be successfully employed. Cognitive-behavioral therapy may also be used initially if phobic symptoms are primary and panic attacks infrequent or if the patient declines initial pharmacotherapy; medication therapy may be subsequently employed if anxiety symptoms emerge or are exacerbated during or after the behavioral program.

Pharmacologic Treatment

Tricyclic Antidepressants

Tricyclic antidepressants (TCAs) were the first pharmacologic agents noted to be effective for the treatment of panic disorder. These agents include imipramine (Tofranil), desipramine (Norpramin), and nortriptyline (Pamelor). Imipramine is the agent most frequently studied, but all TCAs are similarly effective. Adequate dosing is critical, and most patients should receive at least 150 mg per day of imipramine or its equivalent to receive maximal therapeutic benefit, although some patients may respond at lower doses. Onset of therapeutic effect typically takes at least 3 to 4 weeks. Panic disorder patients or anxious depressed patients may experience marked increases in anxiety, panic, and jitteriness on initiation of TCA treatment, and for this reason treatment in these patients should be initiated at very low doses, e.g., 10 mg per day of imipramine, and the dose titrated up as tolerated over the next 2 to 3 weeks in 25-mg increments. Starting at lower doses initially often results in the patient ultimately being able to achieve higher therapeutic doses. Although clearly effective, use of the TCAs may be complicated by multiple treatment–emergent side effects, including anticholinergic effects, cardiac conduction disturbance, orthostatic hypotension, and weight gain, which are often dose-dependent and which may reduce patients' compliance with treatment. Up to half of panic patients followed long term for treatment with antidepressant medication may discontinue it because of side effects such as increased anxiety early on and weight gain over time.

Serotonin-Specific Re-uptake Inhibitors

Serotonin-specific re-uptake inhibitors, such as fluoxetine (Prozac), sertraline (Zoloft), and paroxetine (Paxil), although less well studied, are also clearly effective for treatment of panic disorder. They are often first-line agents for treatment of the anxiety disorders when an antidepressant is indicated because of their favorable side effect profile. These agents do not have significant anticholinergic or cardiac conduction effects nor propensity to cause orthostasis or weight gain. Early anxiety associated with their administration may be minimized by initiating treatment with low doses (e.g., 5 mg per day of fluoxetine, 25 mg per day of sertraline, 10 mg per day of paroxetine) and titrating up as needed over the first few weeks, although many patients may respond to these lower doses. In addition to 10-mg capsules, a liquid form of fluoxetine is now available for better titration of the starting dose. A patient can also make a solution of Prozac capsule contents and pour out appropriate aliquots on a daily basis.

Clomipramine (Anafranil) is a serotoninergic antidepressant also effective in the treatment of panic disorder in doses ranging from 25 mg per day up to 150 to 300 mg per day. It may sometimes be effective for patients refractory to other pharmacologic interventions. As a heterocyclic antidepressant, it shares a similar side effect profile to TCAs.

Monoamine Oxidase Inhibitors

Monoamine oxidase inhibitors, such as phenelzine (Nardil), tranylcypromine (Parnate), and isocarboxazid (Marplan), have demonstrated efficacy for treatment of panic disorder, and many clinicians believe they are potentially the most comprehensively effective agents for treating panic disorder, blocking panic attacks, relieving depression, and offering a "confidence enhancing" effect, of particular value for a patient recovering from marked vigilance and avoidance. Their use, however, is limited by their side effect profile, including orthostatic hypotension, weight gain, and sexual dysfunction and the potential for adverse drug and food interactions producing hypertensive crises. Thus they are often used as second-line treatment after safer and more easily tolerated agents fail. Of particular note in the medical setting, patients on monoamine oxidase inhibitors should never receive meperidine (Demerol) because of risk of delirium and cardiovascular collapse.

High-Potency Benzodiazepines

High-potency benzodiazepines, such as alprazolam (Xanax), clonazepam (Klonopin), and possibly lorazepam (Ativan), are effective for treatment of panic disorder and are well tolerated and safe with a rapid onset of effect. The initial dose of alprazolam is 0.5 mg two to three times a day with the dose titrated up after initial sedation remits. Patients should be warned not to drive or use machinery until they acclimate to the initial sedation. Total daily dose is usually 2 to 8 mg per day, and dosing is typically three to four times a day because of the relatively short half-life of the agent. One study reports a differential effect of dosing level on symptom relief with 3 mg per day effective in blocking panic attacks and 6 mg per day required to treat phobic avoidance.

Potential drawbacks of treatment include concerns about abuse and dependency, interdose rebound symptoms, and early relapse after discontinuation. As a relatively short half-life benzodiazepine, alprazolam may cause withdrawal symptoms and rebound anxiety, especially after long-term treatment is discontinued; such symptoms may be minimized by employing a gradual rate of taper (e.g., 0.25 to 0.5 mg per week). Abuse is rare in panic patients without a history of alcohol or substance abuse, although as with any benzodiazepine, inappropriate use may occur without controlled prescribing for target symptoms. Tolerance to the antipanic effects of benzodiazepines is uncommon, and most patients tend to decrease their dose over time despite continuation of symptoms because of moralistic concerns about reliance on medication. Except when panic attacks are infrequent, patients should be instructed to take the medication on a regular basis rather than as needed so anxiety symptoms may be prevented and the patient is less likely to experience panic attacks when in feared situations.

Clonazepam (Klonopin) is another high-potency benzodiazepine effective for treatment of panic disorder. Twice as potent as alprazolam, its dosing range is typically 1 to 5 mg per day. Sedation is a limiting factor in dose titration and is managed by initiating treatment with a low dose (e.g., 0.25 mg at bedtime) and titrating up to therapeutic doses as tolerated. As a longer acting agent with a half-life of 20 to 50 hours, it can be dosed on a twice-a-day basis with generally less interdose rebound anxiety associated with its administration than with shorter acting agents such as alprazolam. Some patients may develop depressive symptoms when taking clonazepam or alprazolam. Resolution of depressive symptoms may occur with lowering the dose or with the introduction of an antidepressant, and the patient may be treated with combination therapy or possibly on the antidepressant alone.

Other Agents

Certain antidepressants, such as bupropion (Wellbutrin), trazodone (Desyrel), and amoxapine (Asendin), appear not to be effective for treatment of panic disorder. Beta blockers, such as propranolol (Inderal), may reduce the tachycardia and autonomic overactivity associated with panic but are ineffective for blocking the cognitive and fear components of the disorder. Buspirone (Buspar) is sometimes used to treat generalized anxiety and residual anticipatory anxiety in panic patients but is not a primary treatment for panic disorder. Clonidine, an alpha-$_2$ receptor agonist, has been used to treat panic disorder owing to the demonstration of alpha-$_2$ receptor subsensitivity in panic disorder patients. Initial improvement with treatment, however, has not been maintained. A new class of agents, the reversible monoamine oxidase-A inhibitors, is currently under study and appears to be effective for treatment of panic disorder with a decreased risk of hypertensive crises and treatment-emergent adverse effects.

Cognitive-Behavioral Therapy

Cognitive-behavioral therapies may have direct antipanic efficacy and treat anticipatory anxiety and phobic avoidance. Behavior therapies typically involve repeated exposure to the feared situations aimed at reducing avoidant behavior. Newer strategies target reduction of the patient's fear of the anxiety sensations themselves by exposing the patient to elicited anxiety symptoms, such as lightheadedness, tachycardia, and hyperventilation. Cognitive therapies are aimed at reducing the negative, unwanted thoughts or catastrophization of symptoms associated with panic, such as "I'm dying or going crazy," and replacing these with more positive or neutral thoughts: "This will pass. I'll be fine in a minute." Some patients may benefit from behavioral therapy alone, whereas others with continued panic attacks and anticipatory anxiety require medication treatment for more complete symptom relief. Studies suggest that the effects of behavior therapy and medication therapy are synergistic and that behavior therapy may improve long-term outcome in medication-treated patients.

Duration and Discontinuation of Treatment

Studies suggest that 50 to 80% of patients relapse after discontinuation of treatment with benzodiazepines or antidepressants. This may be understood in the context of the naturalistically observed longitudinal course of the disorder, which is frequently chronic, and as further evidence that, for some patients, panic disorder is a manifestation of an underlying constitutional vulnerability to anxiety requiring ongoing treatment.

There are limited data regarding optimal duration of treatment, but recent evidence suggests that the risk of relapse may be lessened with a duration of treatment of at least 1 to 2 years. Patients who repeatedly fail attempts to discontinue treatment or relapse after discontinuation may be candidates for ongoing maintenance treatment similar to other chronic disorders, such as hypertension or asthma.

When treatment is to be discontinued, medications, particularly benzodiazepines, should be gradually tapered. Taper rates should be gradual (e.g., 0.25 to 0.5 mg per day of alprazolam) to minimize emergent withdrawal symptoms. A number of other interventions have been used to decrease withdrawal-related symptoms, including adding antidepressants; buspirone; or anticonvulsants, such as carbamazepine or valproic acid, but none have demonstrated robust effectiveness. Recently cognitive behavioral therapy administered during discontinuation has been demonstrated to decrease withdrawal symptoms and prevent re-emergence of symptoms after medication is discontinued.

Physical and Chemical Injuries

BURNS

method of
WILLIAM R. CLARK, Jr., M.D.
State University of New York
Health Science Center at Syracuse
Syracuse, New York

Accidents are the fourth leading cause of death for all age groups in the United States, and burns (excluding scalds) are the fourth most frequent cause of accidental death, with a mean rate of 2.0 per 100,000. Serious thermal injuries occur more frequently in economically and educationally disadvantaged people, who often live in substandard housing or use hazardous materials such as gasoline in a careless way. These injuries also tend to occur in those who cannot anticipate hazards or who do not respond appropriately once an accident occurs, such as children (0 to 4 years, death rate >4.0 per 100,000), the handicapped, and the elderly (>75 years, death rate 7.2 per 100,000). Burns that are not life-threatening result in significant morbidity because totally destroyed tissue cannot be restored and major economic losses because the acute illness is long and convalescence is often prolonged. Many burns are so inconsequential that no professional treatment or only outpatient care is needed; at the other extreme are the more serious injuries that necessitate an estimated 70,000 hospital admissions and cause about 5000 deaths annually in the United States. Hospitalization may be required for the optimal care of burn victims with small wounds because of a constellation of psychosocial factors, including alcoholism, drug addiction, abuse, the absence of a caregiver in the house, and low pain thresholds. Despite the complex nature of the illness in patients with major injuries, the critical element in all burn treatment is wound care; the fundamentals of wound care are cleanliness and adequate nutrition.

BURN SEVERITY

Assessing the patient from a global perspective in terms of the severity of the injury is critical to the process of making decisions about the appropriate level of care and the urgency with which burn-specific treatment needs to be instituted. The major elements in burn severity include the size of the burn, depth of the burn, age, presence of significant pre-existing illness, associated injuries, and burns of critical body parts. The first two are directly related to severity. Burn size is estimated using the "rule of nines," which assigns body proportions based on nine or multiples of nine: the head and upper extremities each make up 9% of the body surface area (BSA); the anterior trunk (neck to groin), posterior trunk, and lower extremities make up 18% of the BSA. In infants, the head makes up a larger proportion of the BSA, and this increment is subtracted from the portion allocated to the lower extremities.

To estimate burn depth, the most superficial burns, first degree, involve the epidermal layer of skin only; they are inflamed and painful but have no blisters. They evolve into a sensitive, peeling surface in 4 to 7 days. Burns that involve the dermal layer of skin, second degree, have a large range of absolute depth because the dermis has some grossly detectable thickness to it and varies significantly in thickness over the body surface. Thus, a given heat load applied to the back or the buttocks where the dermis is thickest may result in a second-degree injury, whereas the same heat load applied to the inner aspect of the upper arm where the dermis is thin may produce a full-thickness or third-degree injury. Superficial second-degree injuries are characterized by blisters; when the blisters are broken, the wound surface is moist and pink, and capillary refill is usually brisk. Because the nerve endings have not been destroyed, these wounds are painful. If these wounds remain perfused and do not become infected, they can be expected to heal in 2 to 5 weeks, depending on the depth of the burn, the density of epidermal appendages (hair follicles), and the adequacy of local blood supply. In deeper second-degree injuries, the wound surface tends to be dryer, white, or mottled, and capillary refill often is not demonstrable.

Deep dermal burns are often considered with full-thickness or third-degree burns because there is little difference in the clinical consequences of these two depths of burn. Full-thickness burns go all the way through the skin, which may be charred or dry and white, depending on the burning agent. The presence of thrombosed veins in the burn wound is unequivocal evidence for a third-degree injury. Third-degree burns usually are not painful; they evolve into a granulating surface when the eschar or burned skin sloughs off. They heal by contraction and epithelialization from the edges of the wound, unless they are closed with a skin graft. If a thermal load is applied to tissue for a prolonged interval, deeper burns into the muscle or down to the bone may occur. These are called fourth-degree or fifth-degree injuries, but because these terms are not standardized, it is better to describe the wounds.

Most burn wounds change in appearance during the first 2 to 3 postburn days in a way that depends on systemic factors, such as the adequacy of resuscitation and the patient's ability to resist infection, and local factors, such as the dryness of the wound surface and the development of edema. It is often useful to correlate the mechanism of the injury with the appearance of the wound in deciding about wound depth when this is not obvious at the initial examination. Thus, immersion scalds tend to produce larger and deeper injuries than spill scalds; flash burns, which result from an explosive type of ignition without continued combustion, produce large, relatively superficial injuries; hot contact burns are small but deep; and burns that result from the ignition of clothing are invariably full thickness.

Age acts as a surrogate for metabolic or physiologic reserve in assessing burn severity. Physiologic reserve peaks at the age of puberty; it is lower in infants because of visceral immaturity and, after puberty, decreases with advancing age, even though the visceral compromise that results may not reach clinical thresholds. This is the reason why a burn of any given size or depth in an octogenarian is more serious than a similar injury in an adolescent. When this deficit in visceral function reaches clinical thresholds, so it can be labeled as a pre-existing illness, the severity of the burn is increased. Associated injuries, such as fractures, smoke inhalation, or myocardial infarction, or injuries to the abdominal viscera represent an additional stress and thus increase the severity of any given size of burn. The critical body parts usually considered in assigning severity are burns to the mouth and nose as well as the perineum; injuries to these areas often increase the mortality risk. Burns to the remainder of the face, the eyes and ears, and the hands and feet increase the morbid potential of the injury.

PATIENT'S DISPOSITION

After the initial assessment has been completed and the stabilization process has begun, decisions should be made about where best to treat the patient. Important elements in this decision-making process include the patient's particular circumstances as well as the resources and the expertise available in the community. When there is uncertainty about the appropriate disposition of the patient, an individual experienced in burn care should be consulted. If transfer to a specialized burn care facility is elected, this is always executed most safely when it occurs in a controlled way within the first 12 to 24 hours after injury. If complications such as wound infection or visceral failure ensue, transfer of the patient is much riskier, and a successful outcome is jeopardized. After patients with smaller injuries have been stabilized, calmed down, and instructed in the principles of appropriate wound care, they can be discharged from the hospital and managed on an outpatient basis. Immediately after the accident, the burn wound requires little in the way of specific treatment, but eventually the way in which the burn wound will be closed needs to be considered and factored into the overall treatment plan. Wounds that heal in 10 to 18 days can usually be managed nonoperatively if the patient can tolerate the pain of wound care with the expectation that the cosmetic and functional result will be satisfactory. Deep dermal or full-thickness burns can be managed by operative excision with simultaneous autografting; in experienced hands, this tactic has the potential for shortening the illness and providing a better functional and cosmetic result. This method of closing the wound is also useful in patients who have burns of functionally important body parts, such as the hands, or cosmetically important parts of the body, such as the face. Patients who are considered candidates for this form of treatment should be referred to appropriate centers as soon as possible after their injury.

TREATMENT

Prehospital Care

Once extricated from the site where burning occurred, the burn patient should be treated like any victim of major trauma. The only exception to this general statement is that during the initial assessment, any sources of further thermal injury should be removed; smoldering clothing should be extinguished, and chemicals still in contact with the skin surface should be brushed or lavaged off. Otherwise, the burn wound has a low priority at this stage of management. The airway needs to be assessed and secured in much the same way as in any trauma victim. Fractures need to be splinted, lacerations need to be covered with a bulky pressure bandage, and the cervical spine may need to be stabilized. The patient's level of consciousness should be assessed in the usual way. The cardiac rate and rhythm should be assessed and, if indicated, intravenous access attained with a large-bore cannula. If an emergency department is less than 30 minutes away, it is rarely appropriate to delay transport for the purpose of establishing intravenous access. Ringer's lactate and normal saline without glucose are appropriate fluids for these patients. During field stabilization and transport, these patients should be kept warm; they frequently ventilate most efficiently in a sitting or semirecumbent position. Burn victims with large injuries or those who have been exposed to smoke should receive oxygen during transport.

Emergency Department

In the emergency department, the assessment process is repeated with the patient completely undressed. Maintaining the airway is of critical and prime importance. If time permits, the history should include information about the time and the mechanism of the injury, whether remedial measures such as the application of cold water were instituted, any pre-existing illness, the requirement for any medications on a regular basis, the possibility of addiction to alcohol or other drugs, and the possibility of assault or a self-inflicted injury. This information should all be sought before the patient needs to be intubated, which precludes direct communication. Oxygen should be administered to patients with large injuries.

If airway access is thought to be a likely requirement, as it frequently is in patients with massive injuries, deep burns of the face and neck, or smoke inhalation, it should be undertaken by the most experienced individual available soon after arrival, so the edema resulting from the burn, which increases dramatically once resuscitation is undertaken, does not render this procedure technically impossible. Intravenous morphine sulfate, 2 to 5 mg, or diazepam (Valium), 5 to 10 mg, may be required to facilitate this procedure. If systemic paralysis is necessary, a nondepolarizing agent such as atracurium besylate (Tracrium), 1.0 to 1.5 mg per kg,* or pancuronium bromide (Pavulon), 0.15 to 0.2 mg per kg,* is preferable, but succinylcholine chloride (Anectine), 2 mg per kg, may be used safely up to 24 hours after the burn. The endotracheal tube should be secured with straps or tape that encircles the patient's head above and below the ears; the tube should not be cut so short that it disappears when the facial swelling reaches its peak.

Initial venous access should be secured with a large-bore cannula in a peripheral vein to avoid the hazard of creating a pneumothorax in an attempt to establish central venous access in an unresuscitated patient. The fluid of choice is Ringer's lactate without glucose, given in accordance with the estimate provided by the Parkland formula: 4 ml per kg of body weight per percentage of BSA burn. Only second-degree and third-degree burn is used in this calculation; one-half of the calculated volume should be given during the first 8 hours from the time of injury. This formula allows an estimate of the average volume of fluid that will be required during the first 24 hours after injury. After resuscitation is under way, the rate of fluid administration should be changed, depending on the patient's response; individuals who are not responding should have the rate of fluid infusion increased, and those who seem to be well resuscitated should have the rate of fluid infusion decreased. The absence of restlessness; a stable, intact sensorium; a pulse rate

of 80 to 110 beats per minute; and an hourly urine output of 1 ml per kg all suggest that resuscitation is adequate. Most children with burns larger than 8 to 10% of BSA and adults with burns larger than 15% of BSA benefit from intravenous resuscitation. This is especially true if anxiety or the nausea caused by the use of narcotic analgesics precludes the use of the gastrointestinal tract for oral resuscitation. The presence of black or dark red urine indicates a very deep burn. Burn victims with this problem may require intravenous sodium bicarbonate, 44.6 mEq per 50 ml, to help alkalinize the urine, and the use of a diuretic, mannitol, 25 grams intravenously, or furosemide (Lasix), 10 to 20 mg intravenously, to stimulate urine flow in an effort to prevent the precipitation of myoglobin in the renal tubules. In these circumstances, the hourly rate of urine flow no longer reflects the adequacy of renal blood flow, so other ways of assessing the status of resuscitation must be sought. Situations in which larger than average resuscitative volume may be required include delay in initiation of resuscitation, a very deep injury, smoke inhalation, high-voltage electrical injuries, and other associated injuries. It is useful to keep accurate records of the patient's intake and output during the emergency room phase of treatment. This is especially important if the patient is to be transferred elsewhere because it helps the physicians responsible for the patient's definitive care establish their reference points for subsequent fluid management.

Pain medications in patients with large injuries should be given only by the intravenous route in small sequential doses (e.g., morphine sulfate, 2 to 5 mg). Patients who have received narcotics intramuscularly or subcutaneously before adequate resuscitation should be observed for the development of respiratory depression and the possible requirement for a narcotic antagonist, such as naloxone hydrochloride (Narcan), 40 μg intravenously, repeated at 30- to 45-second intervals until a response is obtained.

As patient assessment continues and treatment is initiated, the patient should be kept warm. Sterile precautions (gowns and gloves) consistent with optimal wound care should be used. As stabilization proceeds, a thorough assessment can be undertaken with more attention given to the burn wound. Conjunctival and corneal burns should be assessed before eyelid swelling makes this an impossible task. Singed eyelashes should be trimmed and irrigated out of the conjunctival sac with normal saline. Constricting jewelry should be removed from burned parts; burned extremities should be elevated in an effort to limit the formation of edema. Time may be taken to obtain a chest radiograph and electro-

---

* Exceeds dosage recommended by the manufacturer.

cardiogram, insert a nasogastric tube, and obtain blood for baseline laboratory determinations.

Attention may now be directed to the burn wound. This should be washed gently with warm water and soap; hair-bearing areas with burns should be shaved. The wounds should be dried and covered with a topical agent, such as silver sulfadiazine (Flint SSD, Silvadene), and either bandaged or left open. Deep, full-thickness, circumferential burns of the thorax or an extremity should be incised (escharotomy), so the edema that forms underneath this inelastic eschar does not restrict ventilation or impair circulation to the residual viable tissue in the core of an extremity. These escharotomies can usually be done with a scalpel without anesthesia because the nerve endings in burns this deep do not function.

All burn victims should have tetanus immunization status brought up to date with administration of a tetanus booster (tetanus toxoid), 0.5 ml subcutaneously or tetanus immune globulin (Hyper-Tet), 250 U intramuscularly, plus tetanus toxoid if they have never been immunized. Antibiotics appropriate for the treatment of beta-hemolytic streptococcus may be useful at this stage of the injury to prevent the rapid conversion of partial-thickness burns to deeper injuries if the patient harbors this organism in epidermal appendages or if the wound cannot be adequately cleaned. The prevention of wound infection is critical. No topical antibacterial agent eliminates the potential for wound infection in a wound that is not adequately perfused and has not been mechanically cleaned.

Small Injuries

The systemic management of patients who have small, non–life-threatening burn wounds is not dramatic, but it must not be neglected if one is to achieve optimal results. Attention to adequate hydration and the consumption of regular, well-balanced meals is important. Vitamin supplementation is useful with additional vitamin C (500 mg daily) and A (10,000 U daily). Smokers should be persuaded to stop or reduce cigarette consumption. Adequate rest is important. Patients should continue to exercise normally whenever possible; joints with an overlying burn should be put through a full range of motion at least three times a day. When possible, the burned parts should be elevated for substantial intervals during the day to limit the formation of edema.

The management of small burn wounds does not involve esoteric techniques, but it is time-consuming for the caregiver and painful for the patient. Immediately after the injury, the application of a cloth or towel soaked in cool tap water may provide the most effective form of pain relief. After the wound is cleaned and bandaged so air currents no longer impinge on it, the pain usually lessens somewhat, especially if the injured part is elevated enough to preclude the formation of significant edema.

Some patients may require premedication with a narcotic, such as oxycodone plus acetaminophen (Percocet) 1 or 2 tablets orally, to help them tolerate dressing changes, although often the problem is more one of anxiety and anticipation than of real pain. A confident, relaxed attitude on the part of the caregivers, especially if they are able to distract or even hypnotize the patient, is a big asset during dressing changes. These painful manipulations of the wound should not be prolonged. Patients usually tolerate dressing changes best if they are in a supine position, so they do not have to watch what is taking place. Although speed in executing wound care is helpful, gentleness is more important because it is most likely to ensure that the patient remains cooperative throughout the burn illness.

Warm water and soap should be used to wash the entire wound and the surrounding skin. Body hair in this region should be shaved so serous exudate does not coagulate in the hair, forming an impenetrable mat. The shredded epidermis of broken blisters should be débrided. Intact blisters may be left for 3 or 4 days if there is no sign of infection in them. The fluid in the intact blisters keeps the wound surface moist, which makes it more comfortable for the patient and establishes an environment compatible with rapid healing. Bulky blisters that are difficult to bandage can be decompressed by making a small hole at the base of the blister and expressing the fluid so the epidermis can be pressed down onto the wound surface. Topical antibacterial agents, such as silver sulfadiazine (Silvadene) or bacitracin ointment or a triple antibiotic ointment containing polymyxin B, bacitracin, and neomycin (Neosporin), can be spread on the wound surface in a thin layer after the wound has been dried.

Patients are usually most comfortable if a bandage is applied that protects the wound from mechanical trauma and helps them maintain the wounded part in a position of function. If the wound is wet, the bandage should be thick enough to wick the wound exudate away from the wound surface without producing a saturated bandage. Wounds of the face and ears are sometimes easier to manage if treated without a bandage. In these situations, the topical antibacterial agent lasts better if it has a petroleum base (bacitracin) than if it has a water-miscible base (Silvadene). The frequency of bandage changes depends on the circumstances of the particular injury, but in general bandages should be changed at intervals of 1 to 3 days. A significant increase in wound pain is often the earliest sign of infection and makes a bandage change mandatory. If the bandage is to provide a débridement function, as when the dry gauze is pulled off the wound surface, the bandage needs to be changed at more frequent intervals.

The use of effective antibacterial agents on small, deep wounds ensures that the eschar remains in place for a prolonged interval. If the decision has been made to treat such wounds nonoperatively, allowing them to heal by contraction and epithelialization over a granulating surface, this prolonged retention of the eschar serves no purpose. Controlled noninvasive proliferation of bacteria often helps digest the eschars, or they can be treated enzymatically (sutilains ointment, Travase) to hasten their removal by nonmechanical means. Patients with clean superficial wounds can be managed with biologic dressings (e.g., porcine xenograft, pigskin, Mediskin) or synthetic types of dressing (e.g., Biobrane, Epigard), which seem to allow healing to progress more rapidly and make the patient more comfortable if they adhere to the wound surface. In most situations, these adjuncts to wound care are not immediately available except in places where burn wound care is conducted regularly.

These temporary wound coverings should not be placed on dirty or infected wounds; to do so in a sense creates an abscess, which at the very least, retards wound healing, and at the worst, renders the patient systemically ill. Wounds covered with these temporary dressings should be inspected regularly to make sure that no fluid collects beneath them. If this happens, they should be removed, the wound washed, and the coverings reapplied, or another form of wound care should be selected.

Electrical Burns

Low-voltage injuries in the United States typically result from exposure to household current at 110 to 220 volts. Characteristically the victim is a child 2 to 3 years of age, and the injury is most often around the mouth or on the hands. These wounds often evolve into a crater with ragged surfaces. Most are managed nonoperatively using the principles of wound care outlined earlier. The possibility of a delayed vascular rupture with significant hemorrhage from the depths of the wound should be kept in mind and the parents or caregivers advised how to handle this situation. High-voltage electrical injuries, greater than 1000 volts, typically occur in young adult males, 18 to 30 years of age. Characteristically

there is a site of entry and an exit wound, often with little in the way of skin changes between these two wounds. Because the current generates heat and destroys cellular membranes as it passes through the tissues of the body, these skin wounds may represent a minute fraction of the total amount of tissue destruction; this means that victims of high-voltage electrical injuries need to be assessed and managed aggressively with the realization that they may have sustained a massive injury despite the outward appearance of the wounds.

Often muscle compartments need to be decompressed with a fasciotomy, so the pressure that develops in them does not result in ischemic necrosis of tissue that was not damaged. Cardiac arrest or other rhythm disturbances are not unusual after a high-voltage electrical injury; these should be assessed in the emergency department, and cardiac function should be monitored for a significant interval. High-voltage electrical current frequently results in significant neurologic injuries, which means that a sophisticated neurologic examination should be conducted as soon as possible after injury in an effort to establish a baseline. The tetanic muscular contractions that occur while the patient is in contact with the current can cause fractures or rupture of muscle bellies; skip injuries may occur as the current arcs across acutely flexed joints. These patients may also have standard contusions and fractures if they fell from a height after they were shocked and thermal burns of the skin if the electrical arc ignited their clothing.

Chemical Burns

Chemical injuries of the skin can be caused by a host of agents too numerous to list; they may be caused in such protean scenarios as prolonged contact with soft concrete or immersion in hydrocarbon fuels, or (at the other end of the spectrum) they may result from powerful acids and alkalis used in industrial processes. Although not all chemicals are soluble in water or saline, copious lavage of the injured part with either of these agents should be instituted quickly in an effort to remove as much of the chemical as possible. The exception to this is when the offending chemical is still in the dry state, in which case it should be brushed off the skin before lavage. The lavage should continue for a prolonged interval.

Even though attempts at neutralization of the chemical are not recommended, a concerted effort should be made to identify the offending agent in case systemic absorption with visceral toxicity is a potential hazard of that particular chemical. In general, acids do not penetrate the skin as deeply as alkalis, which may continue to destroy tissue because they cannot be effectively removed by lavage. It may not be possible to assess the depth of the injury accurately for several days after a chemical injury. Chemical injuries are managed using the same guidelines that one uses for a thermal injury.

Associated Injuries

Burn victims can have as many and as great a variety of visceral and parietal injuries in addition to their burn as any other trauma victim. In general, these associated injuries take precedence over definitive care of the burn wound and should be managed in the same way as if the burn did not exist. Fractures can be stabilized and abdominal operations conducted through burned skin. Because these patients frequently present complex problems, it is usually helpful to have a physician with experience in burn care available to assist in the process of setting priorities for the patient's needs and providing definitive care for the burn.

Significant smoke inhalation is a serious associated injury present in 10 to 20% of flame burn victims. The presence of smoke inhalation increases the mortality risk of any given patient and complicates the illness. Burn victims who have been exposed to smoke should be presumed to have inhaled large amounts of carbon monoxide, which combines with hemoglobin and reduces the oxygen-carrying capacity of the blood, even though the measured oxygen tension in the arterial blood remains normal. The hypoxia that results from high levels of carboxyhemoglobin may precipitate cardiorespiratory arrest, which is treated in the usual way. These patients have profound metabolic acidosis. All patients with smoke inhalation should receive 100% oxygen from the earliest possible moment throughout the interval of assessment and stabilization. This reduces the half-life for elimination of carbon monoxide from 4 to 5 hours to 1 hour. The heat and the tissue-damaging chemicals in the smoke may injure the hypopharynx, larynx, and proximal airway. Injuries distal to the trachea are due to inhaled chemicals, which may be volatile agents or which may be adsorbed on inert carbon particles or absorbed in water droplets.

The clinical consequences of such an injury are acute obstruction of the proximal airway and damage of the distal airway and pulmonary parenchyma with respiratory insufficiency. These injuries at different locations in the respiratory tract are not necessarily of equal severity and do not necessarily become obvious at the same time. It is not unusual for the pulmonary parenchymal consequences of an inhalation injury to have delayed onset.

The treatment for a significant injury to the proximal airway is endotracheal intubation, which should be undertaken as soon as possible before the facial swelling, which can be anticipated if the patient has a burn to the face, makes this an impossible task. If possible, the vocal cords should be visualized at the time of intubation so subsequent decisions about how long to leave the endotracheal tube in place may be based on an appreciation of the extent of the original laryngeal injury. If endotracheal intubation by a nasal or oral route is impossible, the preferred method of airway access is a cricothyroidotomy.

Intubated patients should be ventilated with humidified oxygen. Because atelectasis and alveolar collapse is such a prominent feature of the pulmonary portion of this injury, low levels of positive end-expiratory pressure are often useful, provided that these levels do not interfere with resuscitation. Patients with smoke inhalation of indeterminate severity should be observed for a prolonged interval because of the potential for delayed onset of serious consequences. During this interval, they should receive moist oxygen, vigorous pulmonary toilet, and bronchodilators as needed: aerosolized metaproterenol (Alupent), 0 to 3 ml per 2.5 ml normal saline every 4 to 6 hours, or intravenous aminophylline, 5 mg per kg loading dose, then 12 to 20 mg per hour. If the patient does not improve rapidly or seems to be wearing out from the effort of maintaining adequate ventilation with increasingly noncompliant and atelectatic lungs, he or she should be intubated and consultation obtained with a physician experienced in managing these problems. Corticosteroids are contraindicated in the management of patients with an inhalation injury.

DISTURBANCES DUE TO COLD

method of
THOMAS W. SHEEHY, M.D.
The University of Alabama at Birmingham
Birmingham, Alabama

The major entities arising from cold injury are frostbite, immersion foot, and hypothermia. Each of these entities may exist alone or in combination. Immersion foot results from cold stasis and ischemia. The involved tissue is not frozen. Frostbite results when the involved tissue is frozen. Hypothermia is a systemic manifestation of multifactorial etiology. It is defined as a core body temperature below 32° C (95° F).

LOCAL COLD INJURY

There are two major types of local cold injury: (1) acute freezing injuries, i.e., frostnip and frostbite, and (2) nonfreezing injuries, i.e., chilblains and immersion foot.

Frostnip and Frostbite

Frostnip is the mildest form of acute freezing injury. It tends to involve the ears, nose, feet, and hands. Individuals exposed to strong wind and cold for a considerable period of time are the usual victims, e.g., skiers, sledders, mail carriers, soldiers, and sailors.

Initially frostnip causes a feeling of severe cold in the affected area. This is soon replaced by feelings of numbness and pain. The skin is flushed and cold but is not distorted. Frostnip is readily reversed by simple treatment. Normally placing the patient in a warm area, warming the affected tissue, and removing wet clothing are sufficient.

Superficial frostbite affects the skin and upper subcutaneous tissue. Muscle is not involved. Deep frostbite involves skin, subcutaneous tissue, and muscle. Superficial frostbite causes the skin to become waxy white in appearance and cold to the touch. Progression from superficial to deep frostbite should be suspected when the patient's sensation of cold discomfort is replaced by a feeling of warmth in the affected tissue. With deep frostbite, the flesh is hard and cold to the touch, ashen gray or blue in appearance, and painless. As it progresses, the fingers and extremities become stiff and lose their dexterity. With continual cold exposure, they become paralyzed. Finally, as freezing occurs, cold-induced anesthesia obliterates all awareness of local sensation.

The clinical findings observed 24 to 48 hours after rewarming have been used to classify the severity of frostbite. First-degree frostbite is characterized by hyperemia and edema; second-degree frostbite by hyperemia, edema, and blister formation; third-degree frostbite by hyperemia, edema, and hemorrhagic vesicles; and fourth-degree frostbite by tissue necrosis and gangrene.

Pathology

The major pathophysiologic events leading to frostbite are cold-induced vasospasm and extracellular ice-crystal formation. Freezing temperatures induce the sympathetic nervous system to cause local and reflex arterial and venous vasoconstriction. As capillary perfusion decreases, capillary permeability increases, while plasma viscosity increases. Simultaneously endothial cell damage and erythrocyte sludging ensue, thereby setting the scene for thrombus formation and tissue anoxia. Meanwhile, extracellular ice-crystal formation increases the extracellular osmotic gradient, causing a diffusion of water from the intracellular space. This leads to cellular dehydration and to disruption of the cell membrane and, unless the condition is relieved, to cell death.

Contributing Factors

A number of factors contribute to the extent and severity of frostbite: (1) degree of cold exposure, (2) its duration, (3) wind speed, (4) immobilization, (5) race, (6) lack of acclimatization and proper clothing, (7) previous frostbite, and (8) age. Peripheral vascular disease and drugs (e.g., alcohol) have also been cited as contributing factors.

The Degree of Cold Exposure. Most cases of frostbite occur at temperatures ranging from $-4°$ to $10°$ F and after 6 to 12 hours' exposure.

Duration. The longer the exposure to subfreezing levels, the greater the chance for frostbite.

Wind Speed. As it increases, at a constant ambient temperature, the amount of body heat lost by convection increases. At an ambient temperature of $10°$ F, a wind speed of 20 miles per hour results in an equivalent temperature on exposed flesh of $-25°$ F. Wind speed is useful in predicting the risk of frostbite to exposed flesh.

Immobilization. Troops immobilized in cold climates are at increased risk for cold injury the longer the period of immobilization lasts. Immobilization by enemy fire, riding in open vehicles, or confinement to foxholes was reported as a contributory factor for 67% of 1000 cold injuries in the Korean conflict.

Race. Blacks appear to be more susceptible to cold injury than whites. Similarly, individuals who have suffered previous frostbite are more likely to develop it again on re-exposure.

Age. Age impairs both the hypothermic and the hyperthermic responses. In cold exposure studies, older men were less able than younger men to defend their core body temperature (CBT). Body temperature is governed by central receptors located in the hypothalamus and by peripheral receptors (postsynaptic endings) found in the skin. Both deteriorate with time. This is true for all sensory perception, including taste, smell, and hearing. In the elderly, peripheral vasoconstriction and involuntary muscle contractions (shivering) are impaired. These changes, along with a decrease of 10 to 15% in total body water, make them more susceptible to the osmolal diuresis caused by cold exposure. Peripheral vascular disease is also prevalent among the aged, making their extremities more susceptible to frostbite.

Drugs. Drugs are a risk for both hypothermia and frostbite. Among the more prominent are alcohol, phenothiazine, imipramine, diazepam, barbiturates, reserpine, and morphine. Studies of urban cold injuries in both London and Tokyo have shown that hypothermia and frostbite occur predominately in inebriated, single men in their forties and fifties exposed to outdoor temperatures below 5°C. Most had a blood alcohol level in excess of 2.5 mg per dl.

Lack of Acclimatization and Proper Clothing. Acclimatization, education, and proper clothing are essential to survival in arctic conditions. For example, headgear prevents significant heat loss by radiation from the head. Individuals who must work outdoors in frigid weather need to wear clothing in layers that can be vented when they perspire. Boots should be water-repellent, and exposed skin should be protected with face masks, gloves, and scarves.

Treatment

Frostbite is managed best in a facility that is capable of providing definite therapy. Field treatment is not advocated unless evacuation to a definite care center is imminent. Thawing in the field, when there is the possibility of refreezing, is dangerous because freeze-thaw-freeze injuries lead to extensive tissue loss.

Immediate treatment implies (1) removal of the patient from the cold environs, (2) rewarming the body to restore normal body temperature, and (3) immersion of the frozen part or parts in a circulatory water bath with a water temperature ranging from 38° to 40° C (101° to 109° F). If a circulating water bath is unavailable, a plain tub or basin can be used. If a thermometer is unavailable, warm water comfortable to the normal hand is adequate. Monitoring the water bath temperature to maintain the recommended temperature is important. This can be done by removing the affected part, adding warm water as needed, and reimmersing the frozen part. (4) Avoidance of weight bearing is important. Walking on frostbitten feet can lead to tissue fracture. Similarly, rubbing the frozen part with snow or exercising it to hasten rewarming is to be avoided. (5) Strict aseptic precautions are imperative during rewarming and while handling frozen or injured tissue. (6) Frostbite is considered a tetanus-prone injury, and prophylaxis is recommended. (7) Antibiotics are given if there is evidence of infection. (8) When rewarming is complete, the tissue is cleaned and dried carefully with fine-pore cell sponges. (9) As thawing begins, sensation starts to return to the frozen tissue. The pain is throbbing and may become intense, requiring narcotics for relief.

The return of sensation heralds re-establishment of circulatory flow, which is accompanied by the appearance of an erythematous blushing of the skin and onset of edema owing to vascular injury, thrombosis, or both. Rewarming usually requires about 30 to 60 minutes depending on the extent of injury.

To prevent progressive dermal ischemia during the next 24 to 48 hours, some use enteric-coated aspirin, 325 mg daily, to counteract platelet aggregation and to decrease thromboxane production. Others advocate using a combination of ibuprofen (Motrin, 12 mg per kg daily for 1 week), a systemic prostaglandin inhibitor, and topical aloe vera. Aspirin allergy and peptic ulcer disease are contraindications to either oral agent. Aloe vera, a topical antithromboxane, is used locally to inhibit dermal ischemia. It is reapplied to frostbite wounds every 6 hours. It is also applied to débrided clear blisters. Hemorrhagic blisters are indicative of severe, deep tissue injury and are not debrided unless they rupture spontaneously. A protective cradle is used to cover the frozen lower extremities. Bed rest is continued until the edema is gone, and vesicles and bullae have dried. This may require 2 or more weeks.

Daily hydrotherapy (37° C [90° F]) is used to cleanse the tissue and to débride superficial sloughing tissue. It aids circulation and encourages limb motion, thereby helping to avoid stiff joints and wound contraction. After whirlpool therapy, the tissue is gently blotted dry to avoid abrading it and to reduce the chance for wound infection. Lamb's wool, cotton pledgets, or sterile gauze is used to separate injured digits. Hands are bandaged with fluffy gauze, and arms are elevated in a functional position to decrease edema. Night-time splinting of the hand or digits, in the intrinsic plus position, may be helpful.

For fourth-degree frostbite, the final depth of tissue injury cannot be assessed with certainty until the appearance of gangrenous demarcation. Recently scintigraphy with technetium 99m pertechnate has been reported useful in helping to differentiate viable from nonviable tissue.

Treatment for severe frostbite is painful, expensive, and time-consuming. Débridement must be conservative to prevent premature removal of potentially viable tissue. Mummification or gangrenous demarcation may take 60 to 90 days. Although spontaneous amputation may occur, this is rare, and usually amputation is necessary. Reconstructive or plastic surgery is often needed and may necessitate continued rehabilitation and physiotherapy. Occasionally, compartmental syndromes develop and require fasciotomy. Such surgery usually requires the use of antibiotics for specific or cultured infections. Smoking is prohibited during treatment because it induces vasoconstriction. Intra-arterial drugs, early sympathectomy, and the use of heparin have added little to immediate improvement. Sympathectomy, however, may be helpful in alleviating the chronic vasospastic pain that often follows severe frostbite. Alcoholism is common in cold-injured patients; hence withdrawal needs to be anticipated.

Nonfreezing Injuries

Chilblain

Pernio, or chilblain, is a chronic, often recurrent, vasculitis that occurs with exposure to cold but not freezing temperatures. Usually it occurs in young to middle-aged women, who may have onset of the condition in their teens. During an attack, the skin assumes a bluish red hue and begins to swell. Soon a burning pain and feeling of warmth encompass the affected area, which blanches with local pressure. Pruritus is common.

Attacks may last for up to 10 days and then subside, sometimes leaving an area of residual pigment. Susceptible individuals often suffer repeated attacks, and eventually their condition becomes chronic. In these patients, the condition may improve in summer only to recur with return of cold weather and re-exposure.

Treatment consists of local heat and massage, along with application of lubricants to keep the skin soft and free of cracks. In a recent study, nifedipine, 20 to 60 mg daily, both reduced the pain and soreness of the lesions and hastened their clearing. Reportedly the drug improves cutaneous blood flow, whereas microscopically it appears to reduce both edema and perivascular infiltration. Nifedipine, however, can induce acute hypothermia in patients with spinal cord injuries and should not be used in paraplegics.

Immersion (Trench) Foot

This condition follows prolonged exposure of the feet to cold but not freezing cold water. The condition was common among soldiers in the trenches in World War I and the Korean war. In Vietnam, the term "warm water immersion foot" was used to describe involvement of the soles of the feet immersed in relatively warm water, 15° to 32° C (59° to 89° F), for up to 72 hours. The term "tropical immersion foot" denotes longer periods of immersion along with damage to the dorsum of the feet as well as the soles. Water conducts heat 23 times faster than air; hence the colder the water, the more rapid the onset.

Warm water immersion foot is due to waterlogging of the thick stratum corneum of the soles of the feet. Under ideal conditions, from 1 to 2 grams of water may be absorbed per hour by the foot. Fresh water is absorbed more readily than salt water. Although most of the absorbed water enters the circulation, enough is retained in the stratum corneum of the sole to cause waterlogging. Biopsy specimens of such skin show thickening and fragmentation of the stratum corneum along with edema, capillary narrowing, and a lymphocytic vasculitis in the dermis. Recently warm water immersion foot has been reported in increasing numbers of the homeless. Here the problem is exposure to a damp environment and wearing damp or wet sneakers for prolonged periods.

In contrast to warm water immersion foot, classic immersion foot requires exposure to cold water for prolonged periods. This condition leads to extensive tissue injury because it damages both the vascular and the sympathetic nervous system. Vasospasm is prominent and often severe enough to cause intravascular thrombosis, leading to nerve injury and to fat and muscle necrosis. In contrast to frostbite, venous thrombosis is more common than arterial thrombosis. Considerable variation exists in susceptibility to immersion foot. Predisposing factors include immobilization, dehydration, constrictive footwear, nutritional deficiency, prolonged dependency of the weight-bearing limbs, trauma, and a history of immersion foot.

Clinically the cold-water immersion foot is cool, painful, and tender to touch. The feet are blanched, and the soles are wrinkled. In severe cases, edema, pealing, maceration, and erythema are notable, and abrasions are common over pressure joints. The peripheral pulses may be barely palpable, whereas the pain may be excruciating. A hyperemic or second phase tends to follow cold water exposure and may last up to 10 weeks. Here the pulses are bounding, and the feet are red, swollen, and painful. Blister formation and petechiae are common. Subsequently a third or posthyperemic phase may develop and last for months or years. As sequelae to the nerve injury, the feet are warm but extremely sensitive to cold and may perspire profusely.

TREATMENT

Uncomplicated warm water immersion foot and tropical immersion foot are treated conservatively. Bed rest, elevation of the legs, and air drying at room temperature are usually adequate. Nonsteroidal anti-inflammatory agents generally suffice for pain. Prevention of warm water immersion foot is aided by adequate air drying of the feet. The military suggest at least 8 hours per day. Boots are more protective against warm water immersion foot than tennis shoes. Daily application of silicone grease to the soles appears to delay onset and to decrease the severity of this condition.

Rewarming of the feet of patients with cold water immersion foot is also carried out at room temperature. Overheating the injured tissue in the ischemic phase may induce thrombus formation and lead to extensive injury, even to gangrene. Blebs are left intact but are débrided if they rupture. Physiotherapy is encouraged for severe cases in hope of restoring muscular and vascular tone. Antibiotics are ordered if extensive tissue sludging is present because of the propensity for infection. Anticoagulants are ordered if thrombophlebitis develops. Surgical intervention is conservative and consists primarily of superficial débridement.

SYSTEMIC HYPOTHERMIA

Two forms of hypothermia have been distinguished etiologically: primary and secondary.

Primary (accidental) hypothermia occurs when cold stress exceeds maximum body heat production, e.g., inadequately clothed snow skiers, soldiers, utility workers, or the homeless exposed to extremely low temperatures and chilling winds or cold water. Primary hypothermia may be divided into immersion and nonimmersion types. A snow skier is an example of the latter, whereas a flier forced to ditch his or her aircraft in the North Sea exemplifies the former. As mentioned previously, the high thermal conductivity of water leads to rapid onset of immersion hypothermia. The colder the water, the more rapid its onset. Immersion in water with a temperature of 10°C (50°F) or less almost invariably causes hypothermia.

Secondary hypothermia may follow in the wake of a predisposing illness or prolonged surgery. Numerous diseases may cause it, including endocrine disorders, e.g., myxedema or Addison's disease; cerebrovascular disorders, e.g., myocardial infarction or stroke; gastrointestinal disorders, e.g., acute pancreatitis; infections, e.g., fulminating hepatitis, septicemia; and drugs, e.g., alcohol, barbiturates, phenothiazines, and antidepressants. Alcohol causes vasodilation, impairs shivering, and may induce a lack of concern for the weather. Age is another predisposing factor. It impairs recognition of decreased temperatures and decreases mobility, vasoconstriction, and shivering. Occasionally the elderly exhibit a paradoxical response to cold. They experience a feeling of warmth despite hypothermia and undress despite the cold.

Hypothermia is also a common intraoperative and immediate postoperative complication. Predisposing factors during surgery include large exposed body surface areas, open body cavities, prolonged exposure to low operating room temperatures, massive transfusions of cold blood, cold irrigating solutions, and vasodilation secondary to anesthesia.

Physiology

Physiologic responses to cold are governed by peripheral afferent thermoreceptors. These send stimuli through the spinothalamic tracts to the temperature regulatory center in the hypothalamus. This center coordinates and controls the CBT. From here, impulses are sent to the sympathetic nervous system, the extrapyramidal tracts, and the anterior pituitary gland. Stimulation of the autonomic nervous system increases the heart rate, vasoconstricts the dermal blood vessels, and vasodilates muscle blood vessels. Extrapyramidal tract stimulation causes shivering and leads to vasodilatation of muscular arteries. Stimulation of the anterior pituitary gland indirectly increases a release of thyroxine and adrenal steroids. The overall effect is an increase in heat production and a decrease in heat loss. All of these physiologic responses are disrupted by hypothermia.

Clinical Manifestations

Early Phase

In the "early" or "responsive" stage of hypothermia, the skin is pale and cold to the touch owing to vasoconstriction. Shivering is usually present except in the elderly. Diuresis is common. If the patient is in good health, he or she is still capable of adjusting physiologically to this phase of hypothermia. Supportive therapy and rewarming lead to a rapid recovery.

Slowing Phase

As the CBT falls further, the "slowing" phase of hypothermia ensues, manifested by a decrease in the respiratory rate, heart rate, cardiac output, and blood pressure. Muscles begin to stiffen, and shivering decreases. Disorientation and hallucinations and neurologic deficits, such as hyporeflexia and impaired pupillary reflexes, begin to appear at a CBT below 30°C (86° F) (Table 1). Bradycardia is common at a CBT of 32°C (90° F), whereas myocardial irritability becomes evident at 30°C (86° F). Atrial fibrillation with a slow ventricular response is common between 27° and 30° C (80° and 86° F). Ventricular fibrillation is likely to occur if the CBT falls further. Hypotension also becomes progressively worse as the CBT falls. Together or alone, the depressed cardiac output, hypotension, and arrhythmia may lead to congestive heart failure or cardiac arrest, the usual terminal events.

TABLE 1. **Clinical Findings in Accidental Hypothermia**

Core Body Temperature			
C°	F°	Findings	Diagnosis
36–37	97–99	Physiological responses to cold intact	Normal
35	95	Increased shivering Slurred speech Normal electrocardiogram	Mild hypothermia
33	91	Blood pressure falls Bradycardia Diuresis Confusion	
30	86	Respiration falls Cardiac rate falls Shivering stops Arrhythmia possible Confusion, stupor	
27	81	Weak, slow pulse Reflexes absent Slow respiration Dilated pupils Ventricular fibrillation possible	Severe hypothermia
24	75	Rigor mortis–like Pain absent Acid-base disturbance Hypotension Corneal reflex absent Semicomatose	
21	70	Barely palpable pulse	
18	65	Asystole Flat electro-encephalogram	
16	61	Lowest recorded temperature for an adult survivor	

Significant electrocardiographic changes develop in this phase. Initially the PR, the QRS, and the QT intervals lengthen, and occasionally the T wave inverts, mimicking a myocardial infarction. About 25% of hypothermic patients develop a J wave (Osborn's sign). This is an extra upward deflection at the end of the QRS complex (camel's hump sign). It often increases in amplitude as the CBT falls. Cardiac creatine phosphokinase levels may increase in this phase.

Hypoventilation becomes prominent because the respiratory rate and the ventilatory volume fall, and there is a shift to the left in the oxyhemoglobin dissociation curve. The respiratory rate declines by about one-half for every fall of 8°C (14.5°F) in CBT. To obtain accurate blood gas values in this phase, it is necessary to alert the laboratory to the patient's body temperature. As the CBT approaches 24° C (75° F), respiratory arrest becomes a major threat to life.

The gastrointestinal tract ceases to function effectively in hypothermia. Bowel sounds are decreased owing to hypomotility, and the abdominal muscles become rigid, often simulating an acute abdomen. Occasionally pancreatitis is precipitated by microvascular sludging. Gastric lesions begin to appear when the CBT reaches 10° C (50° F). These are cystic dilatations of the mucosal capillaries.

Coagulopathy is also observed with hypothermia. Coagulation tests carried out on normal human plasma at assay temperatures similar to those encountered in hypothermic patients revealed prolonged prothrombin and partial thromboplastin times. Platelet function and vascular response too are temperature dependent.

Poikilothermic Phase

This implies a CBT of 24° C (75° F) or less. Now the body has a rigor mortis–like appearance and feels cold and stiff to the touch. If still conscious, the patient is confused and lethargic and has slurred speech. Most are comatose, however, and at this point, it has been said, the only differential diagnosis is death. Heretofore the only criterion for "irreversibility" was failure to respond to appropriate treatment, although recently it was reported that a high serum potassium level, i.e., above 10 mmol per liter, indicates recovery is unlikely. In this phase, persistence is the therapeutic guide, and the old adage "No one is dead—until warm and dead" is apropos.

Treatment

Initial treatment for hypothermia in the field entails application of simple measures to stop heat loss. After rescue, the patient is sheltered in a warm place or vehicle and shielded from the wind. Wind cools the skin much faster than still air. The patient is inspected for evidence of trauma, bleeding, or infection, and the cardiopulmonary status is ascertained. The feet and hands are examined for the pale, hard skin of frostbite. If the patient is conscious and still shivering, the chance for survival is excellent. If wet clothes are present, they are removed by cutting them from the body because water conduction leaches heat from the skin four to five times faster than air. The patient is given dry clothing or covered with blankets or placed in a sleeping bag. The head is covered. Dry blankets, foam padding, or bags are placed under the patient to insulate him or her from a cold table or the ground.

The patient is kept at rest and not forced to walk or to exercise. These maneuvers may force cold acidic blood from the extremities into the body and further reduce the CBT. Gentle handling is essential. Attempting cardiopulmonary resuscitation (CPR) when it is unnecessary is dangerous. It can precipitate ventricular fibrillation. In the "slowing" phase of hypothermia, cardiac arrest may be misdiagnosed because the pronounced bradycardia and the vasoconstriction may so enfeeble the peripheral pulses that they appear to be absent. The patient's pulses must be checked thoroughly and repeatedly before diagnosing cardiac arrest.

Sometimes CPR is necessary in the field. The Wilderness Medical Society proposed that when CPR is deemed necessary, it be given unless (1) obvious lethal injuries are present; (2) chest wall depression is impossible, i.e., it is frozen rigid; (3) any signs of life are present; (4) rescuers are endangered by evacuation delays or altered triage conditions; or (5) a "do not resuscitate" status is documented or verified.

A rigor mortis–like state or fixed dilated pupils are not contraindications to CPR. Once started, CPR must be continued during transportation to a treatment facility, preferably in an ambulance or vehicle heated to 30° C (80° F). No fluids or solid foods are given by mouth.

En route to the hospital, however, warm, humidified oxygen, 10 liters per minute, is given using a nonrebreathing reservoir mask. If the patient is not breathing, ventilation is given with a bagvalve mask ventilator connected to a humidified oxygen source. The masks prevent loss of heat and moisture via respiration. Hyperventilation is avoided because it may induce an arrhythmia. Generally patients with severe hypothermia are best rewarmed in a hospital where proper physiologic monitoring and life-support equipment are available.

Hospital Management

Severe hypothermia is a medical emergency, best managed in an intensive care unit. Initially the patient's cardiopulmonary functions are assessed. If the respiratory rate is low, it still may be sufficient to support the lowered metabolic requirements induced by hypothermia. A blood gas analysis can provide evidence to ascertain the patient's need for oxygenation and intubation.

If the patient is not breathing, an airway must be established promptly. Manual ventilation is carried out before endotracheal intubation to improve oxygenation and to reduce the possibility of ventricular irritability during intubation. In a recent multicenter study, however, ventricular fibrillation was not observed among 117 hypothermic patients subjected to endotracheal intubation. Warm humidified oxygen is supplied while the face mask is used and after placement of the endotracheal tube. Warm humidified oxygen supplied by the endotracheal tube raises the CBT about 1.0° to 1.5° C every hour. External cardiac compression is maintained during intubation of the pulseless patient.

Additional care should include (1) a thorough physical examination and, if possible, a history to identify any precipitating factors, such as heart disease, trauma, infarction, or drug overdose (2) Careful and continuous monitoring of the pulse, arterial pressure, and CBT entails placement of a venous line for fluid replacement, an arterial line for repeated blood gas values, and a central venous line to evaluate the results of volume expansion and to prevent fluid overload. CBT is measured repeatedly with a thermometer that can give readings to 21° C. Inexpensive oral thermometers are now being manufactured that have a range from 21° to 38° C (69.8° to 100.4° F). Continuous rectal readings can be made with a thermistor probe placed 10 to 15 cm within the rectum and secured with tape. Rectal temperatures are accurate and easy to measure, but they lag during rewarming, and cold feces may distort their reading. (3) Cardiac monitoring is essential for early detection of any arrhythmias. Sinus bradycardia, atrial fibrillation, and flutter are usually innocuous except in the elderly. They seldom require treatment and with rewarming usually revert spontaneously to normal sinus rhythm. Ventricular fibrillation may be life-threatening and refractory to treatment until the patient is rewarmed. Electrical defibrillation should be tried. If this is unsuccessful, some have used bretylium tosylate (Bretylol), an antiarrhythmic agent, which retains its activity when cold. It may be administered rapidly intravenously (5 mg per kg) for immediate suppression. It must be diluted according to the manufacturer's instructions for continuous suppression. Pharmacologic manipulation of the blood pressure is usually not necessary. If severe hypotension is present and coronary disease is absent, however, dopamine hydrochloride (Dopastat, Intropin) infusions (5 μg per kg per minute) have been used.

CBT, cardiac function, and respiratory function decline during hypothermia. Failure of any one to decline should arouse suspicion of a problem. For example, if the CBT is 90° F and the pulse is 115 per minute, hypoglycemia, hypovolemia, or drug overdosage must be considered. Rapid respiration in the hypothermic patient should raise the question of an underlying acidosis (diabetic, lactic, or alcoholic) or a cerebral injury. (4) Baseline laboratory studies should include arterial blood gases, complete blood count, electrolytes, amylase, creatine kinase, isoenzymes, creatinine, lactic dehydrogenase isoenzyme, prothrombin time, partial thromboplastin time, blood glucose levels, urinalysis, fluid intake and output, renal and hepatic function studies, and toxicologic analysis and blood cultures if indicated.

Hypoglycemia occurs in 40% of patients with hypothermia, which also predisposes to hypovolemia. Blood volume expansion is achieved with 5% dextrose in normal saline. Three hundred to 500 mL is administered rapidly, followed by 100 to 200 ml per hour to maintain blood pressure. Ringer's lactate solution is not used because a hypothermic liver cannot metabolize lactate to bicarbonate. The crystalloid solution should be warmed, preferably to 45° C (115° F). Microwave ovens can heat a liter of fluid to a reasonable temperature within 2 minutes at high power, and plastic containers made of polyvinyl chloride can be heated safely in this manner. (5) Foley catheter placement allows monitoring of urinary output and provides urine for toxicologic studies. Because the bladder is located near major blood vessels, bladder irrigation with warm saline may be helpful during rewarming.

Rewarming Techniques

The most important therapy for the hypothermic patient is rewarming. Two general methods are available: passive and active rewarming.

Passive rewarming relies on the ability of the body to generate heat spontaneously when the precipitating cause of the hypothermia is removed. The longer the patient has been exposed to cold temperatures, the longer it takes to raise the CBT to normal. Passive rewarming is relatively safe. It avoids the rapid physiologic changes induced by active rewarming methods that may precipitate cardiovascular complications. It is the preferred method for treating mild hypothermia, i.e., 33° C (91° F) or above. It is also advocated for treating severe hypothermia (<33° C) when the cardiovascular system is stable. It is not recommended for patients with unstable vital signs or cardiovascular compromise.

Passive rewarming consists of placing the patient in a warm environment, 25° to 33° C (77° to 91° F) and covering him or her with warm blankets. Warmed intravenous fluids are given, but they seldom raise the body temperature significantly. Passive rewarming allows the patient to rewarm at his or her own pace by generating body heat at a rate of about 0.5° C (0.9° F) per hour. If under optimal conditions the hourly increase is less, suspect a complicating illness, such as hypothyroidism.

Active rewarming involves the use of heat internally or externally to raise the CBT. Active external rewarming employs electric blankets, hot water bottles, or immersion in hot water at 40° to 45° C (104° to 113° F). Unfortunately, this method is not without risk. The cutaneous vaso-

dilation that develops may precipitate hypotension, myocardial ischemia, or shock. In the course of vasodilation, cool stagnant blood from the periphery is shunted to the core, where it may increase cardiac irritability and precipitate ventricular fibrillation.

Active internal rewarming is more aggressive. Usually it is reserved for patients with severe hypothermia or those with cardiovascular insufficiency, persistent hypotension, or ventricular fibrillation. Proponents claim that active internal rewarming, by providing preferential rewarming of the myocardium, increases cardiac output, decreases cardiac irritability, and yields a rapid return of the CBT to normal, thus minimizing the chance for rewarming shock. Techniques for active internal rewarming are numerous and include peritoneal dialysis, extracorporeal bypass, mediastinal irrigation, gastrointestinal irrigation, and diathermy. Peritoneal lavage is used for severe hypothermia. It employs an isotonic dialysate warmed to 40° to 45° C (104° to 112° F). Usually, 2 liters are introduced into the peritoneal cavity and withdrawn after 20 to 30 minutes. Mediastinal irrigation is limited to patients with cardiac arrest or compromise. Following thoracostomy, the heart is bathed with 1 to 2 liters of a warm isotonic electrolyte solution for 5 minutes. The solution is then drained and fresh solution infused. Cardiopulmonary bypass is more practical. It has been used more extensively than mediastinal irrigation for patients with cardiac arrest or a compromised cardiovascular system. Blood is drawn from the femoral vein, warmed, and then returned through the femoral artery. This approach can raise the CBT by 1° to 2° C (1.8° to 3.6° F) every 3 to 5 minutes. The need for anticoagulation, however, limits its use to patients without trauma. Cardiopulmonary bypass has been used successfully in several series of patients with severe hypothermia.

Prognosis

Mortality among hospitalized elderly patients with hypothermia is high, varying from 20 to 80%. Elderly hypothermic patients with no serious underlying medical problems, however, should survive if treated properly. Mortality is related to several factors: (1) the severity of hypotension on admission; (2) its duration before treatment; (3) the temperature on admission; (4) associated diseases, particularly cardiovascular disease; and (5) the development of complications. Careful and detailed supportive care is as vital as the rewarming process. Variance in supportive care is probably the reason for the large differences in mortality found in reported studies.

DISTURBANCES DUE TO HEAT

method of
PETER HANSON, M.S., M.D.

University of Wisconsin
Madison, Wisconsin

Heat illness represents a continuum of morbid responses to heat exposure in which fluid and electrolyte balance, cardiovascular regulation, and central nervous system function are progressively impaired. Heat illness occurs most frequently in athletes, military personnel, and outdoor workers who perform sustained activity in warm, humid environments. Episodic heat illness is also associated with seasonal heat waves, which commonly affect the elderly, homeless, and patients taking medications with anticholinergic activity.

HEAT SYNCOPE

Heat syncope usually occurs in the setting of heat exposure and orthostatic stress, such as standing in military formation. Another cause is inappropriate use of jacuzzi and sauna baths, especially after exercise or alcohol ingestion. Cutaneous vasodilation, the absence of muscle venous pump activity, and moderate fluid loss owing to sweating all contribute to inadequate central venous return and low ventricular filling volumes. Syncope is probably mediated by activation of ventricular stretch receptors owing to inadequate filling, causing reflex bradycardia and loss of sympathetic vasomotor tone. Treatment is supportive: Vital signs should be monitored closely and the airway protected from tongue obstruction or emesis. Venous return is enhanced by raising of the lower extremities and cooling of the skin. Volume repletion may be required if orthostatic intolerance persists (see later discussion). Victims of heat syncope should be questioned about the possible role of drugs or alcohol or a history of recurrent orthostatic intolerance.

HEAT EXHAUSTION

Heat exhaustion is a syndrome of progressive volume depletion owing to sustained sweat loss and inadequate fluid replacement that typically occurs in athletes (football players, runners) who are inadequately acclimatized. Symptoms include fatigue, weakness, nausea, and dizziness. Rectal temperature is moderately increased (38° to 39.5°C), the skin is cool and vasoconstricted, and active sweating is present (Table 1). Supine heart rate is mildly elevated, and blood pressure is in the low normal or hypotensive range. With orthostatic stress, there is a marked decrease in blood pressure with systolic values below 90 mmHg. Laboratory studies reveal hemoconcentration, variable electrolyte patterns owing to sweat losses and hemoconcentration, and increased urine specific gravity. Initial treatment is similar to heat syncope but with added emphasis on active cooling and intravascular volume repletion using oral (e.g., 2.5 grams sodium chloride per liter) or intravenous electrolyte fluids. If intravenous fluids are required, 0.50 or 0.25 normal saline may be more appropriate because these approximate the sodium concentration of unacclimatized sweat. Glucose and water should be used with caution because hyponatremia may occur with excessive hypotonic fluid replacement. Intravenous fluid therapy should be guided by stabilization of vital signs and normalization of orthostatic hypotension, serum electrolyte values, and urine output. Extensive laboratory work is usually unnecessary, unless there is evidence of concomitant hyperthermia, as discussed next.

TABLE 1. **Clinical Findings in Heat Illness**

	Heat Exhaustion	Heat Stroke
Level of consciousness	Mild confusion Presyncope on standing	Marked alteration Delirium, coma
Skin	Vasoconstricted Active sweating	Vasodilated Dry or sweating
Rectal temperature	38–40°C	>42°C
Cardiovascular status	Heart rate 90–120 Systolic blood pressure usually <110 mmHg with marked orthostatic drop <20 mmHg	Heart rate >120 Systolic blood pressure varies— low if in shock Low vascular resistance
Laboratory studies	Hemoconcentration Variable electrolytes Mild increase in muscle enzymes	Multisystem abnormalities: ↑ muscle, hepatic enzymes ↑ uric acid, lactate, K⁺ ↓ coagulation factors ↓ platelets + myoglobinuria + hemoglobinuria

↑ = increase, ↓ = decrease, + = present (abnormal).

HEAT STROKE

Heat stroke is a critical extension of the heat exhaustion syndrome that may present in a classic or exertional form. Classic heat stroke occurs with prolonged heat exposure, progressive hyperthermia, and eventual cessation of sweating. Exertional heat stroke occurs over a shorter time and is associated with combined effects of heat exposure and high-intensity exercise. Sweating is usually present but is inadequate for effective cooling. In both forms of heat stroke, there is marked central nervous system impairment ranging from delirium to coma and convulsions. The rectal temperature exceeds 42°C but may be lower after transport to a medical facility. The skin is warm and flushed, unless cardiovascular collapse has occurred. There is moderate to severe tachycardia and variable blood pressure values depending on cardiac function and vasomotor tone.

Emergency treatment requires a multisystem management approach. Immediate lowering of body temperature is essential. Immersion in an ice bath is now discouraged because intense cutaneous vasoconstriction may inhibit heat loss. Alternate methods that are highly effective include application of ice packs to the neck, axillae, and groin (areas of vascular countercurrent exchange) and spraying of the skin with tepid water while fanning vigorously to promote evaporative cooling. Rectal temperature must be monitored continuously. Active cooling should be discontinued when body temperature falls to 39°C. Consciousness usually returns at this point. Insertion of large-bore intravenous catheter lines and a Foley catheter is also essential. The hemodynamic state resembles a low vascular resistance circulatory failure. Cardiovascular support may require the judicious use of vasopressors (dopamine or norepinephrine) along with inotropic agents (dobutamine) and intravenous fluids (saline). Fluid should be administered in small boluses of 250 to 500 ml, however, to avoid cerebral or pulmonary edema. Urine output should be monitored carefully and mannitol (25 grams) or furosemide (Lasix) (40 to 80 mg) administered intravenously to initiate diuresis. Comprehensive laboratory studies include complete blood count with platelet count, liver function panel, creatine kinase, coagulation panel, glucose, lactate, electrolytes, calcium, uric acid, blood urea nitrogen, creatinine, and arterial blood gases. The urine should be tested for presence of hemoglobin and myoglobin. Major complications include hypoglycemia, metabolic acidosis, renal failure owing to acute tubular necrosis, rhabdomyolysis, disseminated intravascular coagulation syndrome, and hepatic failure. Some recent studies suggest that endotoxemia from increased gastrointestinal permeability may play an additional role in the heat stroke syndrome. Patients with documented or suspected heat stroke should always be admitted for observation because these complications may not develop for 24 to 48 hours.

SPIDER BITES AND SCORPION STINGS

method of
PRENTICE A. TOM, M.D., and
PAUL S. AUERBACH, M.D., M.S.
Stanford University Hospital
Stanford, California

Although most species of spiders are venomous, spider bites in the United States are to a large extent medically insignificant and result only in local inflammation. Table 1 describes general guidelines for the wound management of all spider bites. Prophylactic antibiotics are not necessary in the initial management of spider bites.

Rarely spider bites may result in large painful inflamed lesions, low-grade fever, lymphangitis, and cellulitis. Although such a reaction is probably an immune-mediated inflammatory response, it may be impossible to distinguish from a secondary bacterial infection, and the patient should be started on both a glucocorticoid preparation and a broad-spectrum antibiotic with skin flora coverage.

Only two genera of spiders in the United States cause reactions that routinely require more aggressive medical intervention: *Loxosceles* and *Latrodectus*.

BROWN RECLUSE SPIDER BITES

Five of the 13 species of *Loxosceles* found in the United States are known to cause ulcerative lesions. The brown recluse, *Loxosceles reclusa,* is the most notorious member of the *Loxosceles* genus. It inhabits primarily the central, south, and southwestern United States; however, envenomations have been reported throughout the United

TABLE 1. **Wound Management for Spider Bites**

Clean the wound
Have the patient rest for 24–48 hours to decrease systemic effects of spider venom
Elevate and immobilize affected area
Apply cool compresses to the area
Use an antihistamine such as diphenhydramine (Benadryl) for inflammation and pruritus
Give nonsteroidal anti-inflammatory medication or a mild narcotic analgesic as needed for pain control
Give tetanus prophylaxis if the patient's immunizations are not up to date

States. *Loxosceles* spiders are fond of quiet, warm, and dry environments. In endemic areas, the brown recluse is a house dweller, typically found in closets and old boxes. It can be recognized by the characteristic dark, violin-shaped marking on its dorsal cephalothorax, hence its nickname, the "fiddleback" spider.

Initially the brown recluse bite may go unnoticed or present as a mild transient local irritation. It has been suggested that the large majority of bites do not progress beyond this point, and thus many victims may never seek medical attention. Depending on the amount of venom injected and the patient's immunologic response, the bite may become progressively painful, erythematous, and swollen over the ensuing 6 to 10 hours.

Loxosceles venom contains at least 12 to 15 separate proteins, including an esterase, lipase, ribonucleotide phosphorylase, and sphingomyelinase. The last enzyme is thought to be primarily responsible for the dermonecrosis that is characteristically associated with the brown recluse bite. A hemolysin within the venom causes the wound to become mottled with a violaceous, hemorrhagic center and an erythematous outer border. Within a few hours of the bite, a hemorrhagic bleb or blister may form at the center, and within 2 to 3 days, central necrosis occurs with the development of a black, necrotic center. Secondary bacterial infection, lymphangitis, and lymphadenopathy may result. Over the next few weeks, the center sloughs, leaving an ulcer that can take months to heal completely. Systemic loxoscelism is uncommon and usually mild. It typically occurs only with larger cutaneous lesions or in victims of smaller size and may mimic many generalized systemic processes. Effects include fever, chills, malaise, weakness, nausea, vomiting, morbilliform rash, and leukocytosis. Rarely hemolytic anemia with hemoglobinemia, hemoglobinuria, proteinuria, and even renal failure occurs. Cases resulting in disseminated intravascular coagulation and death have been reported.

Treatment

As with the treatment of any spider bite, the management outlined in Table 1 should be followed. Initial management is aimed primarily at decreasing inflammation and pain, and cold compresses or ice packs should be applied to the wound for the first 24 hours. Dapsone, 100 mg orally every 12 hours for 14 days, is currently considered the first-line treatment if skin ulceration develops. Its mechanism of action is believed to be related to inhibition of leukocytes and limitation of dermonecrosis. Patients to whom dapsone is prescribed should have the hematocrit followed because hemolysis may occur in glucose-6-phosphate dehydrogenase–deficient patients. Immediate surgical excision of the wound and steroid injections have not been proved to limit or decrease the resulting lesion. Once necrosis has occurred, the wound should be débrided, and regular wound care should be instituted. Large ulcers may require skin grafting. Systemic loxoscelism requires aggressive management with glucocorticoids and standard fluid management to protect the kidneys.

BLACK WIDOW SPIDER BITES

Four *Latrodectus* spider species are found in the United States, and all are venomous. The black widow, *Latrodectus mactans,* is the most notorious and is found in every state except Alaska. The black widow is most commonly found in shaded areas outside the home. The female is responsible for all venomous bites. She is two to five times the size of the male and averages 1 to 1.5 cm in length. The female spider is characteristically identified by its black coloration and the red hourglass marking on its ventral abdomen. The hourglass marking, however, may or may not be present, depending on the spider's maturity.

The black widow's bite is frequently initially painless, but within minutes the victim often complains of local pain and erythema. A red blush or halo may develop at the puncture site. In contrast to the brown recluse bite, however, the systemic manifestations, and not the local cutaneous reaction, are of medical importance. The venom is a neurotoxin that acts primarily by effecting release of acetylcholine from nerve terminals. The primary symptom described by victims of black widow spider bites is pain. Typically the pain begins in the associated extremity and then involves the other limbs and trunk. Muscle cramping and truncal and abdominal rigidity can occur within 1 hour of envenomation. Associated symptoms are variable and include anxiety, fever, headache, hyperesthesias and paresthesias, tremors, restlessness, dizziness, nausea, vomiting, bronchorrhea, sialorrhea, tachypnea, ptosis, facial edema, hypertension, and cardiac arrhythmias. Severe reactions may present with hyperreflexia, altered level of consciousness, seizures, and coma. At increased risk are infants and young children, who receive a larger amount of venom per kilogram of body weight.

Treatment

The mainstay of therapy for the systemic manifestations of black widow bites has been calcium gluconate 10%, 5 to 10 ml intravenously every 2 to 4 hours as needed for recurrent symptoms. A recent study, however, has shown that intravenous narcotic analgesics and benzodiazepines are significantly more effective in alleviating symptoms. Methocarbamol (Robaxin) has also been used, although its mechanism of action has not been established. Severe hypertension should be treated as any hypertensive urgency or emergency. In life-threatening and high-risk cases, antivenin derived from horse serum may be used. Antivenin, 2.5 ml, is diluted in normal saline and given intravenously over 15 to 30 minutes. This dose may be repeated in 60 to 90 minutes if no improvement occurs. One recent study showed that in patients with severe *Lactrodectus hesperus* envenomation, administration of antivenin provided the most prompt and lasting relief. Because allergic reactions, serum sickness, and anaphylaxis have occurred in patients receiving antivenin, it should be reserved for patients who present with signs of significant envenomation and who do not have risk factors for immediate hypersensitivity reactions.

Patients with severe symptoms; those younger than 14 or older than 65 years of age; pregnant patients; and patients with a history of hypertension, cardiac disease, or other significant medical problem should be admitted to the hospital. All others may be observed for 8 to 10 hours and discharged.

SCORPION STINGS

Scorpions of the *Centruroides* genus are found in the southern section of the United States from Florida to California. They are typically found outside above ground in shaded areas and under rocks and logs. Scorpions are easily recognized. The body is segmented and ends in a tail that contains the stinging mechanism, and the second pair of legs ends in a lobster-like claw.

The local effects of scorpion stings include pain, swelling, and occasionally a small amount of surrounding erythema. Paresthesias, hyperesthesia, and numbness may also occur. Scorpion venom has both adrenergic and cholinergic properties as well as the ability to cause the release of kinins. Systemic manifestations include tachycardia, hypertension, diaphoresis, hyperglycemia, excess salivation, tearing, muscle twitching, and nausea and vomiting. More severe symptoms include bladder and bowel incontinence and seizures. Anaphylactic reactions have been reported.

Treatment

The anticholinergic effects are usually short-lasting and require no treatment. Atropine sul-

fate, 0.5 to 2.0 mg intravenously, can be used for an excessive or prolonged parasympathetic response. Beta blockers can be used for tachyarrhythmias, and either an alpha blocker, such as phentolamine, or nitroprusside can be used to control extreme increases in blood pressure. Calcium gluconate 10%, 10 ml intravenously or 0.1 ml per kg in pediatric patients, may be used to control muscle twitching. Benzodiazepines or phenobarbital (or both) in conjunction with adequate airway management may be used in the rare occurrence of seizure activity. Opiate derivatives are believed to augment the effects of scorpion venom and are contraindicated.

A goat serum–derived *Centruroides* antivenin is available in Arizona from the Antivenom Reproduction Laboratory at Arizona State University. A recent study, however, showed more than 50% of patients to whom antivenin was administered suffered some type of allergic reaction. Further, because older children and adults generally do well with appropriate supportive care, antivenin should probably be used only in young children.

SNAKE VENOM POISONING
method of
TERENCE M. DAVIDSON, M.D.
University of California, San Diego
San Diego, California

It is commonly reported that within the United States annually there are an estimated 45,000 snake bites. Eight thousand of these involve venomous snakes. Twelve to 15 deaths are reported yearly. The vast majority of medically important venomous bites are inflicted by North American pit vipers, predominantly rattlesnakes. Water moccasins and cottonmouths also inflict a significant number of bites. The venom injected in these cases, although similar to that of rattlesnakes, is typically less in volume, and although the principles of treatment are the same, the severity of the bite and the treatment aggressiveness are far less.

North American pit viper venoms contain assorted proteolytic enzymes, and an untreated envenomation results in substantial local soft tissue destruction, infection, and tissue loss. For this reason, snake bite deserves prompt medical attention. In bites with severe envenomation, cardiovascular, hematologic, and even neurologic problems develop. Prompt treatment avoids these problems as well.

TREATMENT

Although the presentation varies by snake, by person, and by region, the basic treatment principles for managing North American pit viper envenomation remain the same. The mainstay of medical treatment is the neutralization of venom with the intravenous administration of antivenin. First aid is therefore designed to bring the patient to a medical facility expeditiously and to keep the venom localized in the bitten extremity. First and foremost, get the patient and others away from the snake. There is no need to have a second bite. There is no value to killing the snake, and none benefit by bringing a live or dead snake along with the bitten patient. Keep the patient calm, and keep the bitten extremity at a position level with the heart. Remove constricting jewelry, such as rings and bracelets, because the bitten extremity swells rapidly and impressively. A constricting band that retards lymphatic and superficial venous flow helps keep venom localized to the bite site. The ideal constricting band is a 1×18 inch Penrose drain as used for venipuncture. Tourniquets that obstruct deep venous flow or arterial flow are dangerous and should not be used. The patient should now be transported to a medical facility. In most cases, this is not a full-blown emergency, and assuming the patient can be brought without undue movement or other problem by ground transportation, helicopters and other risky evacuations are not indicated. Incision, suction, excision, cryotherapy, and electric shock have all been advocated at one time or another. None have scientifically proven value, and most carry their own injury and morbidity.

Once the patient reaches the medical facility, the first task is to determine that the individual has, in fact, been bitten by a venomous snake and has been envenomated. Signs and symptoms of envenomation are listed in Table 1. If there are no significant signs or symptoms of envenomation, the constricting band should be released, and the patient should be observed in a medical facility for 2 hours and then released for observation at home for another 24 hours. Twenty percent of North American pit viper bites are known as dry bites, bites in which venom is not injected.

For envenomated individuals, medical, physical, and laboratory evaluation should begin. A complete history should be taken, and an appropriate physical examination should be performed. Blood and urine should be collected for the tests listed in Table 2. An electrocardiogram is also required. An intravenous catheter should be placed using a 16- or 18-gauge catheter. Lactated Ringer's or other crystalloid should be rapidly infused to ensure a well-hydrated patient and, should antivenin treatment be required, one with a brisk diuresis.

At this point, the physician needs to determine whether or not to initiate antivenin treatment. The antivenin is made from horse serum. It is

TABLE 1. Signs and Symptoms of Envenomation

Sign or Symptom	Frequency
Fang marks	100/100
Swelling and edema	74/100
Weakness	72/100
Pain	65/100
Sweating and/or chill	64/100
Numbness or tingling of tongue and mouth or scalp or feet	63/100
Changes in pulse rate	60/100
Faintness or dizziness	57/100
Ecchymosis	51/100
Nausea, vomiting, or both	48/100
Blood pressure changes	46/100
Decreased blood platelets	42/100
Tingling or numbness of affected part	42/100
Fasciculations	41/100
Vesiculations	40/100
Swelling regional lymph nodes	40/100
Respiratory rate changes	40/100
Increased blood clotting time	39/100
Decreased hemoglobin	37/100
Thirst	34/100
Change in body temperature	31/100
Necrosis	27/100
Abnormal electrocardiogram	26/100
Increased salivation	20/100
Glycosuria	20/100
Sphering of red blood cells	18/100
Cyanosis	16/100
Proteinuria	16/100
Hematemesis, hematuria, or melena	15/100
Unconsciousness	12/100
Blurring of vision	12/100
Muscle contractions	6/100
Increased blood platelets	4/25
Retinal hemorrhage	2/100
Swollen eyelids	2/100
Convulsions	1/100

moderately antigenic. It is relatively expensive and should be used only when necessary. Table 3 lists the Arizona Poison Control Center's envenomation grades. In truly mild envenomation, treatment may not be required. In those with moderate and severe envenomation, treatment should be initiated. In some patients with mild envenomation but significant local reaction, antivenin, in the author's opinion, is indicated. Once

TABLE 2. Laboratory Evaluation

Complete blood count with differential and
    platelet count
Coagulation parameters:
    Prothrombin time
    Partial thromboplastin time
    Fibrinogen levels
    Fibrin degradation products
Serum electrolytes, blood urea nitrogen/creatinine,
    calcium, phosphorus, lactate dehydrogenase
    (with isoenzyme analysis)
Urinalysis
Electrocardiogram

TABLE 3. Grade of Envenomation for Pit Viper Bites

Minimal Envenomation
Manifestations remain confined to or around the bite area
No systemic symptoms or signs
No significant laboratory changes

Moderate Envomation
Manifestations extend beyond immediate bite area
Significant systemic symptoms and signs
Moderate laboratory changes; i.e., decreased fibrinogen and/or platelets and hemo concentration

Severe Envenomation
Manifestations involve entire extremity or part
Serious systemic symptoms and signs
Very significant laboratory changes

---

the decision to treat has been made, the patient is skin tested for horse serum sensitivity. An intradermal test is used, and assuming it is negative, antivenin therapy is initiated. The average treatment for most rattlesnake bites ranges from 15 to 20 vials. When originally developed, it was thought that most snake bites could be successfully managed with two, four, or six vials of antivenin, and the current Wyeth Polyvalent Crotalidae antivenin insert reflects these thoughts. Experience has taught us that this is an insufficient amount of antivenin for treating humans, and hence considerably more aggressive therapy is generally employed. Water moccasins and cottonmouths require less antivenin. Severe envenomations can require as many as 40 to 60 vials of antivenin. Reconstitute five vials of antivenin at a time. Reconstitute each vial in 10 ml of lactated Ringer's or other intravenous solution. Maintain a rapid lactated Ringer's infusion, and administer the antivenin as an intravenous piggyback at a rate of one vial every 7 to 10 minutes. Because each vial is reconstituted in 10 ml, this is a rate of approximately 1 ml per minute. Assuming the patient tolerates the infusion rate of 1 ml per minute, this can be gradually increased to a rate of 1.5 ml per minute.

The patient should be monitored. Once the antivenin infusion has been initiated, the constricting band can be removed and the patient monitored by the signs, symptoms, and laboratory measurements. The physician's task is to titrate the antivenin infusion against the signs and symptoms of envenomation until the signs, symptoms, and laboratory parameters have all been neutralized. Pain is an excellent sign to titrate against. Progression of swelling is another excellent sign. Circumferential measurements should be made at appropriate locations on the bitten extremity, and these can be serially measured during treatment. Once treatment is complete, the swelling regresses slowly, so one cannot use regression of swelling as an end point. Other signs and symptoms, such as fasciculations, cardiovascular changes, and hematologic changes, require aggressive antivenin infusion. Some signs and symptoms, such as circumoral tingling, although characteristic of snake bite, do not regress rapidly and are not good indicators for continued antivenin infusion.

Even in severe bites, the antivenin infusion should be completed within several hours. All of this should occur in the emergency room or in an intensive care environment. The patient should then be monitored for 24 hours in an intensive care environment. Once stable for 12 to 18 hours, the patient can be transferred to a regular hospital bed and soon thereafter discharged to home. Antibiotics are not required. Tetanus prophylaxis should be current. The bitten extremity should certainly be bathed. Under most circumstances, no additional wound care is required. If questions arise during the evaluation and treatment, consultation is generally available through the regional poison control centers, and it is wise to contact the local regional poison control center early.

Surgical excision of the bite site and fasciotomy are rarely if ever required. If the physician is concerned about a compartment syndrome, Wick measurements generally show that the swelling is all in the subcutaneous compartments and that the muscle compartments are not involved, nor are they subject to unsafe pressures.

Anaphylaxis is always a risk of antivenin treatment, and so appropriate materials and personnel should be available. Delayed allergic reactions are common and are treated with antihistamines and in some cases a short course of steroids.

The other venomous snake native to the United States is the coral snake. This snake is primarily neurotoxic and manifests few of the local signs and symptoms of pit viper envenomation. The Western coral snake is so small that envenomations are extremely uncommon. The Eastern coral snake is large enough to inflict a bite. Patients should be approached and monitored the same as for North American pit vipers. Signs and symptoms are predominantly neurologic. Specific antivenin is available, and in these cases the physician can follow the package insert.

There are a number of exotic snakes housed within the United States. Unless the bite occurs at a facility such as a zoo, which maintains antivenin for that snake, the treatment of these individuals can be extremely difficult. In these cases, physicians should request assistance through their regional poison control center.

INJURY RECEIVED FROM HAZARDOUS MARINE ANIMALS

method of
ERIC L. WEISS, M.D., D.T.M.&H., and
PAUL S. AUERBACH, M.D., M.S.
Stanford University School of Medicine
Stanford, California

The ocean is the earth's greatest wilderness. Covering nearly three-quarters of the planet's surface and home to four-fifths of all living organisms, the oceans hold numerous inhabitants that may pose a threat to humans. Marine hazards can be loosely categorized into four groups: those that "bite" (marine trauma), those that "sting" (marine envenomation), those that "poison" (toxic ingestion), and those that "shock" (electrical injury).

MARINE TRAUMA

The most vilified yet romanticized marine animal is the shark. Ocean inhabitants for at least 375 million years, predatory sharks are endowed with sophisticated sensory organs, including skin chemoreceptors, motion detectors, and a series of reflecting plates in the retina that effectively amplify light along the optical path. At least 32 of 350 species of these efficient hunters are dangerous, responsible for an estimated 50 to 100 reported attacks (6 to 10 deaths) per year worldwide. The most feared of these is the formidable great white *(Carcharodon carcharias),* which has been captured at a length of 16.5 feet and 3450 pounds, but other threats include the blue, mako, tiger, hammerhead, and gray reef sharks. With advancing jaws that can produce a crushing force measured at 18 tons per square inch, the great white generates a fatality attack rate of only 15 to 25%, probably because the sharks lack definitive interest in a meal tainted with fiberglass and neoprene. The most common causes of death are hemorrhage and drowning; therefore initial management of the shark bite victim mandates prompt standard resuscitation (begun, if necessary, while still in the water) and subsequent meticulous wound care. Shark bites are "dirty wounds"; in addition to contamination with seaweed, sand, and other particulate matter, bites can be contaminated by the unique microbiologic flora of ocean water. Antibiotic prophylaxis should be considered for anything more than a minor injury and should cover *Vibrio, Aeromonas,* and *Pseudomonas* species as well as *Staphylococcus* and *Streptococcus.* Recommended prophylactic regimens include trimethoprim-sulfamethoxazole, a third-generation cephalosporin, or an aminoglycoside. Tetanus prophylaxis is mandatory. Surgical débridement is usually essential.

MARINE ENVENOMATION

Marine animals capable of envenoming humans come in a dazzling array of sizes, colors, and forms. From the graceful stingray and colorful scorpionfish to the spiny sea urchin and dramatic Portuguese man-of-war, these creatures represent both the most common and most potentially lethal marine hazards. Despite the multiplicity of stinging organisms, one can use symptoms, wound appearance, and an understanding of the stinging mechanisms to identify two broad categories of injury and subsequent patient management (Fig. 1).

The first group to consider is venomous fish. Eleven species of stingray are found in U.S. coastal waters. These nonaggressive bottom feeders have one to four venom-containing spines positioned approximately at the middle of the caudal appendage. When a wing of the ray is touched, either when the animal is handled or trodden on, the spine is reflexively thrust into the victim, causing both a laceration and envenomation. The heat-labile venom regularly causes pain out of proportion to the physical injury. Symptoms peak after 30 to 60 minutes and may last for 48 hours. The wound is dusky and ischemic in appearance and shows rapid necrosis. Systemic manifestations include vomiting, seizures, paralysis, hypertension, and bradycardia.

Scorpionfish are bony fish found in both temperate and tropical waters. Their several hundred species may be divided into three groups in ascending order of toxicity: the ornate and colorful lionfish, the bottom-dwelling and superbly camouflaged scorpionfish, and the hideous and extremely toxic stonefish. These and others, including weeverfish and catfish, share characteristics of 12 to 13 dorsal, 2 pelvic, and 3 anal spines bearing heat-labile venom glands. Pectoral spines may or may not carry venom. Injury usually results from accidental contact. Patients complain of immediate intense pain with central radiation. The sting of a stonefish causes pain as severe as any induced by a member of the animal kingdom. The wound may become ischemic or cyanotic, with surrounding areas of erythema and edema. Systemic symptoms include vomiting, diarrhea, abdominal pain, headache, paresthesias, and cardiovascular collapse. Fatalities from stonefish stings are rare.

Sea snakes are the most abundant reptiles on earth. These nonaggressive creatures are frequently found in the waters of Southeast Asia, the Persian Gulf, and the Malay Archipelago but are not resident in the Atlantic Ocean or the Caribbean Sea. Sea snake venom is predominately neurotoxic. The initial bite causes little discomfort, with minimal local reaction. Neurologic

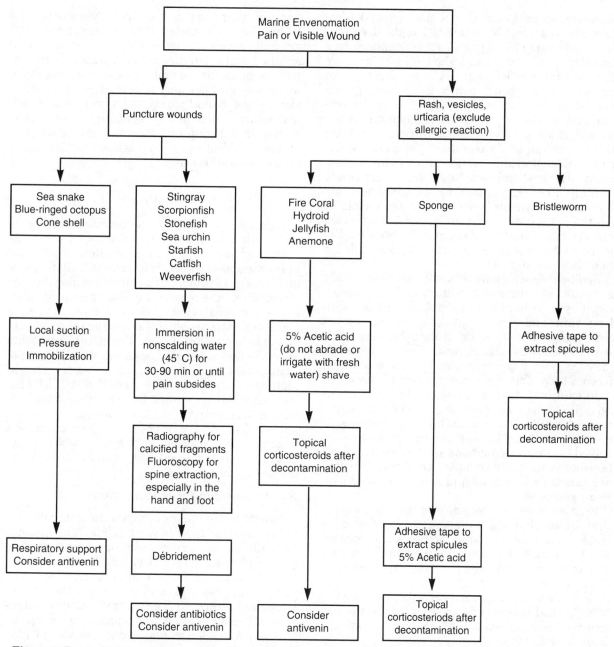

Figure 1. Types of injury and management of patients. (From Auerbach PS: Marine envenomations. N Engl J Med *325*:490, 1991. Reprinted by permission of the New England Journal of Medicine.)

symptoms usually occur within 2 to 3 hours and include painful muscle movement, ascending paralysis, and ophthalmoplegia. Despite these dramatic symptoms, death is rare.

Coelenterates are predators that feed on fish and crustaceans and share a sophisticated stinging mechanism using nematocysts. Members of this phylum include the Hydrozoa (fire coral, feather hydroid, and Portuguese man-of-war), Schyphozoa (box jellyfish, blue jellyfish, and sea wasp), and Anthozoa (stony coral and sea anemone). The nematocyst is a stinging organelle

consisting of a tightly coiled and sharply pointed injector tube within a venom sack. When triggered by either physical contact or chemical stimulation, venom is forcibly injected into the victim. Of note, nematocysts may be viable for months even after the animal dies or the tentacles become detached. In U.S. coastal waters, the most common coelenterate envenomation occurs from fire coral, feather hydroids, or small jellyfish exposure. More dramatic, but less common, are the Atlantic and Pacific Portuguese man-of-war *(Physalia physalis)*. These iridescent creatures measure up to 30 cm across the bell and have tentacles reaching 30 meters in length. Each tentacle may carry more than 750,000 nematocysts. Smaller (2 to 10 cm across the bell) but far more lethal is the box jellyfish *(Chironex fleckeri)*. An adult can carry enough venom to kill three grown men. Examination of sting fatalities in Australian and Southeast Asian waters suggest that the Indo-Pacific box jellyfish certainly poses a greater threat to humans than does the great white shark. Coelenterate envenomation yields a spectrum of signs and symptoms from immediate burning, itching, and mild urticaria to the rapid formation of wheals, vesicles, and red-purple or frosted whip-like "tentacle prints." Associated muscle spasm and paralysis may be present. Extensive *Chironex* envenomation has caused death in as little as 30 seconds.

Echinoderms include animals more commonly known as sea urchins and starfish. Easily recognized by their hard protective shell bristling with long, thin, and venom-containing spines, sea urchin stings result in immediate burning pain with associated erythema and edema. Purple dye may leach from the spines and mimic a retained foreign body. True spiny foreign bodies represent a difficult management problem. Spines may enter joint spaces causing severe synovitis or become the nidus for a sarcoid-like granuloma. If more than 15 to 20 sea urchin spines are involved, systemic symptoms (paresthesias, hypotension, respiratory collapse) are likely. Starfish are generally less toxic and rarely invoke a systemic response.

Bristleworms are segmented marine worms that are covered with numerous silky bristles, or "setae," resembling cactus spines. Skin contact results in multiple, small, retained foreign bodies and an intense urticarial reaction. The horny but elastic exoskeleton of members of the sponge family may also cause an allergic or irritant dermatitis. Typical bothersome species include the fire sponge *(Tedania ignis)* and poison-bun sponge *(Fibulia nolitangere)*.

Unsegmented soft-bodied mollusk invertebrates, which often secrete a calcareous shell, may also envenom. In shallow Indo-Pacific waters, the beautiful and seemingly harmless cone shells of the genus *Conus* house a mollusk that is able to inject its prey with a potent neurotoxin by means of a detachable, harpoon-like, venomous tooth. Usual symptoms are similar to a bee sting; however, severe envenomation may result in paresthesias, muscular paralysis, and bronchospastic respiratory failure. Another neurotoxin-producing mollusk is the Australian blue-ringed octopus *(Octopus maculosus)*. The octopus normally secretes its toxin into the water around its beak to subdue its prey but if handled by an unsuspecting diver may deliver a venomous bite. It has been estimated that a fully grown (25 grams) octopus carries enough venom to kill 10 adults. Local symptoms are conspicuously absent, with most victims complaining of oral and facial numbness and peripheral paresthesias. Progression to total flaccid paralysis and respiratory failure occurs. Mechanical respiratory support may be required during the venom's peak effect (4 to 10 hours). Most properly attended victims make an uneventful recovery.

Treatment

Treatment of marine envenomations may be divided into two broad categories based on symptoms and wound appearance. Remember that many victims of even minor envenomations panic and drown, so prompt attention to removal of the victim from the water and institution of basic ABCs is mandatory. Any victim complaining of an acute and extremely painful marine injury should be considered envenomed. The astute physician searches for evidence of envenomation in any patient pulled from the ocean suffering from unexplained collapse or altered mental status. The patient should be examined for evidence of puncture wound (stingray, sea snake, octopus, starfish, scorpionfish, or sea urchin sting) or cutaneous toxicity (rash, vesicles, or "tentacle whips," suggesting coelenterate injury). Patient care may be divided as follows:

Puncture Wound Envenomation

Puncture wound envenomation generally involves a toxin that is heat labile. The wounds typically cause pain out of proportion to the degree of physical injury. A gaping lower extremity laceration, particularly with cyanotic edges, suggests a stingray injury. Multiple punctures in an irregular pattern, with or without retained spines or purple discoloration, are typical of a sea urchin sting(s). A single ischemic puncture wound with rapid swelling and an erythematous halo suggests scorpionfish envenomation. Sea snake bites yield one to eight fang marks but minimal local symptoms. The site of a cone shell sting is punctate, painful, and ischemic in appearance. Painless punctures with paralysis suggest the bite of a blue-ringed octopus.

For all wounds except sea snake and blue-ringed octopus bites, the injury should be grossly débrided, quickly irrigated, and then immersed in water as hot as the patient can tolerate (non-scalding, 45° C) for 30 to 90 minutes or until the pain subsides. Narcotic pain control, regional nerve block, and other symptomatic therapy may be added as necessary. Vesicular fluid should be aseptically removed. Close attention should then be paid to foreign body removal. The purple dye from sea urchin spines may mimic retained spines, so x-ray examination should be used liberally. Deep or particularly dirty wounds should be débrided in the operating room. Tetanus prophylaxis is mandatory, as are antibiotics for prophylaxis (ciprofloxacin, trimethoprim-sulfamethoxazole) for any deep or dirty injury. Note that penicillin, erythromycin, and first-generation cephalosporins do not adequately cover *Vibrio* species. For selected neurotoxin envenomations (stonefish, sea snake), antivenin is available from certain centers. The minimal initial dose of sea snake antivenin is 1 to 3 vials; up to 10 vials may be required. The initial dose of stonefish antivenin is 1 vial per two stings. When required, early ventilatory support has the greatest influence on outcome following selected octopus and sea snake bites.

Coelenterate Injury

Coelenterate injury requires immediate intervention to prevent further envenomation by untriggered nematocysts. Wounds may exhibit only nonspecific, wheal-and-flare reactions, so clinical suspicion is mandatory. Rapid (within 24 hours) onset of skin necrosis suggests sea anemone sting. "Tentacle prints" with a frosted appearance or cross-hatching are pathognomonic for box jellyfish injury. Ocular or intraoral lesions may be caused by fragmented hydroids or coelenterate tentacles. Caretakers who attempt to remove attached tentacles by rubbing them with sand or irrigating with fresh water only increase envenomation. Unfired nematocysts may be inactivated with a solution of 5% acetic acid (vinegar), which should be applied continuously for at least 30 minutes or until symptoms are relieved. An alternative is 40 to 70% isopropyl alcohol. Other alleged detoxicants (none superior to vinegar or rubbing alcohol) include sodium bicarbonate, olive oil, sugar, and urine. After chemical inactivation, visible tentacles may be removed by forceps or double-gloved hand. Remaining nematocysts should then be removed by applying a layer of shaving foam or a paste of baking soda, flour, or talc and shaving the area gently. Topical steroid creams may provide additional symptomatic relief. Hot water immersion or prophylactic antibiotics are not indicated. For severe envenomation (box jellyfish), antivenin in a dose of 1 to 3 vials intravenously is available.

The dermatitis secondary to exposure to bristleworms or sponges is exacerbated by minute retained foreign bodies. These may be removed by the application and removal of adhesive tape or commercial facial peel material. Acetic acid irrigation should also be used because many sponges are also home to minute nematocyst-containing coelenterates. Again, topical or systemic corticosteroids may provide symptomatic relief.

TOXIC MARINE INGESTIONS

Ciguatera Fish Poisoning

Ciguatoxin is originally produced by tiny dinoflagellates in concentrations that are harmless to humans. By virtue of being concentrated by passage along the food chain, however, patients may receive a toxic dose by consuming large predator reef fishes, such as the snapper, jack, barracuda, or grouper. Ciguatoxic fish have no unusual odor, taste, or color, and toxicity is unaffected by heat or drying. Patients develop symptoms of abdominal pain, vomiting, and diarrhea, typically 1 to 3 hours postingestion. Neurologic complaints, including pathognomonic paresthesias with hot-cold reversal, may be described. Treatment is largely supportive, although intravenous mannitol has been described as effective for the neurologic symptoms. The gastrointestinal symptoms generally resolve within 24 to 48 hours, but patients may be bothered by intermittent paresthesias, myalgias, and pruritus for many months. It is estimated that some 50,000 persons may be affected by ciguatera poisoning each year.

Shellfish Poisoning

Common mollusks (clams, oysters, scallops, and mussels) filter large amounts of sea water to gather plankton and extract oxygen for survival. This causes the potential for concentration of both marine toxins and infectious agents. Common examples of the latter include polio, coxsackie, and hepatitis A viruses as well as the bacteria responsible for typhoid fever and cholera. Mollusks also concentrate small unicellular phytoplankton, which may produce numerous toxins, including saxitoxin. Ingestion of saxitoxin causes a syndrome known as paralytic shellfish poisoning. During certain times of the year, these plankton may multiply at enormous rates, actually discoloring the water to cause blue, red, yellow, or brown "tides" or "blooms." The consumption of mollusks taken from such waters can expose the patient to toxic levels of saxitoxin. Symptoms are primarily gastrointestinal (abdominal pain, nausea, vomiting, diarrhea) and neurologic. Within minutes to hours, patients complain of intraoral and perioral paresthesias and numbness. This may progress to flaccid paralysis with respiratory insufficiency. Treatment is supportive, involving most importantly mechanical ventilation. With such care, outcomes are generally good.

Scrombroid Poisoning

Large fish of the suborder Scrombroidei (albacore, mackerel, certain tuna, bonito, and mahimahi) have the potential to generate a toxic dose of histamine. This occurs when the normal piscine bacterial flora break down muscle histidine to histamine and saurine during times of poor refrigeration or storage. Histamine levels may increase by a factor of 400, causing a typical constellation of symptoms in the unwary diner. Within 15 to 90 minutes, patients complain of flushing, urticaria, vomiting, diarrhea, palpitations, and possibly bronchospasm. When questioned, patients may sometimes recall the fish having had a sharp, metallic, or peppery taste. Interestingly not all who eat the same fish become ill, perhaps owing to unequal distribution of the histamine cogeners. Therapy is antihistamine based, with other supportive measures used as necessary. Intravenous H_2 blockers may be effective in rapidly ameliorating symptoms.

ELECTRICAL MARINE INJURY

Despite public belief, there are only two groups of marine electric fish. These include the stargazer (Astroscopus) and the electric ray (Torpedo). Able to generate low amperage but relatively high voltage (8 to 220) to stun prey, these curious creatures rarely pose a health hazard to humans. The better known electric eel is a freshwater Amazonian animal.

CONCLUSION

Through an increased interest in scuba diving and international travel, more people are discovering the colorful and fascinating ocean world. Despite the myriad of potential hazards, it is not the authors' intent to discourage adventures. The vast majority of ocean creatures are nonaggressive and cause injury only if they perceive a threat to their well-being or that of their offspring. Using a cautious hands-off approach, even the recently initiated seafarer may safely explore the earth's greatest wilderness.

ACUTE POISONINGS

method of
HOWARD C. MOFENSON, M.D.,
THOMAS R. CARACCIO, Pharm.D., and
JOSEPH GREENSHER, M.D.
Long Island Regional Poison Control Center
East Meadow, New York

BASIC MANAGEMENT OF POISONINGS

The severity of the manifestations of acute poisoning exposures varies greatly with the age and intent of the victims. Accidental poisoning exposures make up 80 to 85% of all poisoning episodes and are most frequent in children under 5 years of age. Many of these episodes are actually ingestions of relatively nontoxic substances that require minimal medical care. Intentional poisonings constitute 10 to 15% of poisonings, and often these patients require the highest standards of medical and nursing care and the occasional use of sophisticated equipment for recovery. Suicide attempts represent a significant number of these poisonings, and the use of toxic substances is often involved. The majority of the drug-related suicide attempts involve a central nervous system (CNS) depressant, and "coma management" is vital to the treatment.

Sixty percent of patients who take a drug overdose do so with their own prescribed medication and 15% with drugs prescribed for relatives. The top poisoning categories for all ages are over-the-counter analgesics, sedative-hypnotics, benzodiazepines, cleaning agents and petroleum products, alcohol and substance abuse, pesticides, tricyclic antidepressants, plants, carbon monoxide, and opioids.

ASSESSMENT AND MAINTENANCE OF VITAL FUNCTIONS

Upper airway obstruction is the most common cause of death in intoxicated patients outside the hospital. Any patient who is comatose and has absent protective airway reflexes is able to tolerate an endotracheal tube (cuffed for those over ages 7 to 9 years) and should have it inserted as soon as possible.

Ventilation is required if the respiratory rate and depth are inadequate.

The circulatory status is best assessed by the blood pressure and heart rate and rhythm. The circulatory clinical status and tissue perfusion may be inferred from the skin temperature, the return of color after pressure blanching (capillary filling), and the urine output. Intra-arterial blood pressure measurements are essential for adequate monitoring.

If the circulation fails to improve after adequate ventilation and oxygenation, a 15- to 20-cm elevation of the foot of the bed may aid by increasing the venous return to the heart. A fluid challenge also may improve the circulatory status if hypovolemia is the cause. If these measures fail, plasma expanders and similar products may be required. As a last resort, vasopressors may be needed. If these measures fail to produce a response, a central venous pressure or a pulmonary artery wedge pressure (PAWP) line should be inserted to monitor for heart failure and fluid overload.

The level of consciousness of all intoxicated patients should be assessed and the time of assessment recorded. The Glasgow Coma Score used in head trauma is not useful in intoxications because alcohol, depressant drugs, and hypotension may give falsely lowered scores. The Reed Coma Scale is preferred (Table 1).

PREVENTION OF ABSORPTION AND REDUCTION OF LOCAL DAMAGE

Ocular exposure should be immediately treated with water or saline irrigation for 20 minutes with eyelids fully retracted. Do not use neutralizing chemicals. All caustic and corrosive injuries should be evaluated by an ophthalmologist.

Dermal exposure is treated immediately with rinsing, not a forceful flushing in a shower, which might result in deeper penetration of the toxic substance. The skin should be rinsed with copious amounts of water for at least 30 minutes. Hair shampoo, cleansing of fingernails and navel, and irrigation of the eyes are necessary in an extensive exposure. The clothes may have to be discarded. Leather goods are irreversibly contaminated and must be abandoned. Caustics (alkali) often require hours of irrigation until the "soapy" feeling of the burn is gone. Dermal absorption may occur with pesticides, hydrocarbons, and cyanide.

Injected exposures to drugs and toxins or those introduced by envenomation may require a proximal tourniquet and early suction. (See Antidotes 4 through 6 in Table 4.)

Inhalation exposures to toxic substances are treated by immediately removing the victim from the contaminated environment.

Gastrointestinal exposure is the most common route of poisoning, and an estimate of what, when, and how much of the toxic substance was ingested must be made. If there is a possibility of potential intoxication, gastrointestinal decontamination is performed rather than waiting for symptoms to develop.

Gastrointestinal Decontamination

To decrease gastrointestinal absorption, emesis should be induced or gastric aspiration and lavage performed. Neither of these methods is completely effective; each removes only 30 to 50% of the ingested substance. They are recommended up to 3 to 4 hours postingestion; however, there are few indications for induced emesis in the emergency department in an adult because it delays the administration of more effective activated charcoal.

Emesis

Relative contraindications to the induction of emesis are (1) petroleum distillate ingestion of high-viscosity agents; (2) agents that are likely to rapidly produce coma (short-acting barbiturates) or convulsions (propoxyphene, camphor, isoniazid, strychnine, tricyclic antidepressants) in less than 30 minutes and therefore may predispose to aspiration during emesis; and (3) prior significant vomiting.

Absolute contraindications to the induction of emesis are (1) caustic (alkali) or corrosive (acid) ingestions; (2) convulsions because of the danger of aspiration and possible induction of laryngospasm; (3) coma because of the possibility of aspiration with the loss of protective airway reflexes; (4) absence of a cough reflex—absence of the gag reflex is not a reliable indication of lack of airway protection because a number of healthy people lack gag reflexes; (5) hematemesis, in which vomiting may produce additional damage; (6) an infant under 6 months of age, because of immature protective airway reflexes; (7) foreign bodies—emesis is ineffective and risks obstruction or aspiration; and (8) absence of bowel sounds (when no bowel sounds are present, gastric lavage is preferred).

TABLE 1. **Level of Consciousness (Reed Coma Scale)**

Stage	Conscious Level	Pain Response	Reflexes	Respiration	Circulation
0	Asleep	Normal	Normal	Normal	Normal
1	Coma	Decreased	Normal	Normal	Normal
2	Coma	None	Normal	Normal	Normal
3*	Coma	None	None	Normal	Normal
4†	Coma	None	None	Abnormal	Abnormal

*Patients in Stages 3 and 4 require intubation and placement in an intensive care unit.
†Patients in Stage 4 need intervention to sustain life.

Inducing Emesis

Syrup of ipecac is the preferred agent but never fluid extract of ipecac, which is too potent, or salt water, which has produced fatal hypernatremia. Emesis is not recommended to be induced at home in children younger than 1 year of age but can be performed in a medical facility under supervision when indicated. The dose of syrup of ipecac in the 6- to 9-month-old infant is 5 mL; in the 9- to 12-month-old, 10 mL; and in the 1- to 12-year-old, 15 mL. In children over 12 years and in adults, the dose is 30 mL. The dose may be repeated *once* if the child does not vomit in 15 to 20 minutes. The vomitus should be inspected for remnants of pills or toxic substances, and the appearance and odor should be noted.

Apomorphine is a parenteral emetic that must be freshly prepared. Its use is fraught with complications, although it produces more rapid onset of emesis than syrup of ipecac. We do not recommend its use in the cooperative patient. Naloxone should be available to reverse CNS depression.

Gastric aspiration and lavage may be preferable to the induction of emesis in cooperative adolescents or adults because a large tube can be introduced through the oral cavity. Contraindications to gastric aspiration and lavage in intoxicated patients are (1) caustic (alkali) and corrosive (acid) ingestions because of the risk of esophageal perforation; (2) uncontrolled convulsions because of the danger of aspiration and injury during the procedure; (3) petroleum distillate products; (4) coma or absent protective airway reflexes, which require the insertion of an endotracheal tube to protect against aspiration; (5) significant cardiac dysrhythmias, which should be controlled first; and (6) hematemesis, which may be a relative contraindication.

The best results with gastric aspiration and lavage are obtained with the largest possible orogastric tube that can be reasonably passed (nasogastric tubes are not large enough for this purpose). In adults, use a large-bore orogastric Lavacuator hose or a No. 42 French Ewald tube; in children, use a No. 22–28 French orogastric-type tube.

The amount of fluid used varies with the patient's age and size, but in general, aliquots of 150 to 200 mL per lavage are used in adolescents or adults and 5 mL per kg or 50 to 100 mL per lavage in children younger than 5 years of age.

Continuous gastric suction has been used for substances that have an enterohepatic recirculation or are actively secreted into the gastrointestinal tract, such as tricyclic antidepressants (imipramine [Tofranil]) and local anesthetics such as mepivacaine (Carbocaine) (Table 2).

Activated charcoal is produced by combustion

TABLE 2. Substances with Enterohepatic Recirculation

Chloral hydrate
Colchicine
Digitalis preparations (digoxin, digitoxin)
Glutethimide
Halogenated hydrocarbons (DDT derivatives)
Isoniazid
Methaqualone
Nonsteroidal anti-inflammatory agents
Phencyclidine
Phenothiazines
Phenytoin
Salicylates
Tricyclic antidepressants

of organic material in the absence of air until the carbon particle is formed. There are few relative contraindications to the use of activated charcoal: (1) It should not be administered before, concomitantly with, or shortly after syrup of ipecac because it may adsorb the ipecac and interfere with its emetic properties; (2) it should not be given before, concomitantly with, or shortly after oral antidotes unless proved not to interfere significantly with their absorption; (3) it does not effectively adsorb caustics and corrosives and may produce vomiting or cling to the esophageal or gastric mucosa and falsely appear as a burn on endoscopy; and (4) it should not be given if there are no bowel sounds. Activated charcoal has no absolute contraindications, but it does not effectively adsorb alcohols, boric acid, caustics, corrosives, cyanide, metals, and drugs insoluble in aqueous acid solution (Table 3). Activated charcoal is a stool marker, indicating that the toxin has passed through the gastrointestinal tract and that no further significant absorption from the original ingestion will occur.

The dose of activated charcoal is 1 gram per kg per dose orally, with a minimum of 15 grams. The usual adolescent and adult dose is 60 to 100 grams. It is administered as a slurry mixed with water or by orogastric tube. A continuous nasogastric drip of activated charcoal, 0.25 gm per kg per hour, is an alternative in children. It should

TABLE 3. Substances Poorly Adsorbed by Activated Charcoal

C—caustics and corrosives
H—heavy metals (arsenic, iron, lead, lithium, mercury)
A—alcohols (ethanol, methanol) and glycols (ethylene glycols)
C—chlorine and iodine
O—other substances insoluble in water
A—aliphatic and poorly absorbed hydrocarbons
L—laxatives sodium, magnesium, sorbitol

not be mixed with milk, marmalade, or starch because these interfere with charcoal's adsorptive action. Charcoal is administered with a cathartic initially. Subsequently, cathartics should be given every 24 hours.

Activated charcoal may be administered orally every 4 hours as long as bowel sounds are present, and it may be especially beneficial in intoxications that have an enterohepatic recirculation (see Table 2). Repeated dosing with oral activated charcoal has been shown to increase the clearance of many drugs without enterohepatic recirculation (see individual poisonings).

Catharsis is used to hasten the elimination of any remaining toxin in the gastrointestinal tract. Cathartics are relatively contraindicated (1) when ileus is indicated by absence of bowel sounds, (2) in intestinal obstruction or evidence of intestinal perforation, and (3) in cases with a pre-existing electrolyte disturbance. Magnesium sulfate (Epsom salts) is contraindicated in renal failure; sodium sulfate (Glauber's salts), in heart failure or diseases requiring sodium restriction. Magnesium sulfate or sodium sulfate is administered in doses of 250 mg per kg per dose as 20% solutions. The adolescent and adult dose is 30 grams. Sorbitol is given at 2.8 mL per kg to a maximum of 214 mL of a 70% solution, for adults. The cathartic should be given with the initial dose of activated charcoal. Sorbitol in children younger than age 3 years should be used with caution and is not recommended under 1 year of age.

Dilutional treatment is indicated for the immediate management of caustic and corrosive poisonings but is otherwise not useful. Contraindications to dilution are (1) inability of the patient to swallow, resulting in aspiration of the diluting fluid, and (2) signs of upper airway obstruction, esophageal perforation, and shock. The administration of large quantities of diluting fluid—above 30 mL in children and 250 mL in adults—may produce vomiting, re-exposing the vital tissues to the effects of local damage and possible aspiration.

Neutralization has not been proved to be scientifically effective.

Whole-bowel irrigation uses bowel-cleansing solutions of polyethylene glycol with electrolytes. It may be indicated with substances that are poorly absorbed by activated charcoal, such as iron, lithium, or ingestions of sustained-release preparations. The procedure has been used successfully with iron overdose when abdominal x-rays revealed incomplete emptying of excess ingested iron. There are additional implications in other ingestions, i.e., body packers of illicit drugs, such as cocaine and heroin. The procedure is to administer, orally or by nasogastric tube, the so-

lution (GoLytely or Colyte), 0.5 liter per hour in children younger than 5 years of age and 2 liters per hour in adolescents and adults. The end point is when the rectal effluent is clear. This takes approximately 2 to 4 hours. These measures should not be used if there is extensive hematemesis, ileus, signs of bowel obstruction, perforation, or peritonitis.

USE OF ANTIDOTES

Antidotes are available for only a relatively small number of poisons. An available antidote should be administered only after the vital functions are established. Table 4 summarizes the commonly used antidotes and their indications and methods of administration. Most informational, so-called first aid measures, and antidotes on commercial product labels are notorious for their inaccuracy; it is preferable to contact the Regional Poison Control Center rather than follow recommendations on these labels.

ENHANCEMENT OF ELIMINATION

The medical methods for elimination of the absorbed toxic substances are diuresis, dialysis, hemoperfusion, exchange transfusion, plasmapheresis, enzyme induction, and inhibition. The methods to increase urinary excretion of toxic chemicals and drugs are being studied extensively, but the other modalities have not been well evaluated.

In general, these methods are needed in only a minority of instances and should be reserved for life-threatening circumstances or when a definite benefit is anticipated.

Diuresis

Diuresis increases the renal clearance of compounds that are partially reabsorbed in the renal tubules. Forced-fluid diuresis is based on the principle that it will shorten exposure for reabsorption at the distal renal tubules. The risks of diuresis are fluid overload, with cerebral and pulmonary edema, and disturbances in acid-base and electrolyte balance. Failure to produce a diuresis may imply prerenal or renal failure. If renal failure is present, dialysis should be considered.

Osmotic diuresis is meant to increase the osmotic gradient and prevent reabsorption from the proximal loop and distal tubules. Mannitol is used to initiate this type of diuresis, and then fluids are added in sufficient amounts to produce a diuresis similar to forced-fluid diuresis.

Acid and alkaline diuresis is based on the principle that to inhibit reabsorption of certain toxic agents, the urinary pH can be adjusted so the substance is maintained in its ionized form, which interferes with its passage back into the blood. Electrolyte and acid-base monitoring are necessary. Hypokalemia and hypocalcemia are frequent complications. Acid diuresis is accomplished by using ammonium chloride (Antidote 2, Table 4). Although it may enhance the elimination of weak bases, such as amphetamines and fenfluramine (Pondimin), it is not recommended. Ammonium chloride is contraindicated if rhabdomyolysis is present. Alkaline diuresis with sodium bicarbonate can be used in the therapy of weak acids, such as salicylates, and long-acting barbiturates, such as phenobarbital (Antidote 39, Table 4).

Dialysis

Dialysis is the extrarenal means of removing certain toxins from the body and can substitute for the kidney when renal failure occurs. Dialysis is never the first measure instituted; however, it may be lifesaving later in the course of the severe intoxication. It is needed only in a small minority of intoxications (Table 5). Peritoneal dialysis is only one-twentieth as effective as hemodialysis. It is easier to use and less hazardous to the patient but also less reliable in removing the toxin; thus it is seldom used. Hemodialysis is the most effective means of dialysis but requires experience with sophisticated equipment. The patient-related criteria for dialysis are anticipated prolonged coma and the likelihood of complications, renal impairment, and deterioration despite careful medical management. Most dialyzable substances have a Vd of less than 1 liter per kg and protein-binding of less than 50%.

Hemoperfusion

Hemoperfusion is the extracorporeal exposure of the patient's blood to an adsorbing surface (charcoal or resin). This procedure has extended extracorporeal removal to a large range of substances that were either poorly dialyzable or nondialyzable. Hemoperfusion may be used for agents that have high protein binding, low aqueous solubility, and poor distribution in the plasma water. In these cases, hemodialysis is relatively ineffective. Hemoperfusion has proved useful in glutethimide (Doriden) intoxication, barbiturate overdose even with short-acting barbiturates, theophylline, cyclic antidepressants, and chlorophenothane (DDT). Activated charcoal cartridges are the primary type that is currently available. In general, supportive care is all that is required. Analysis of studies with hemodialysis and hemoperfusion does not indicate that they reduce morbidity or mortality substantially except in certain cases (Table 6).

SUPPORTIVE CARE, OBSERVATION, AND THERAPY OF COMPLICATIONS

The comatose patient is on the threshold of death and must be stabilized initially by establishing an airway. Intubation should be accomplished in any comatose patient.

An intravenous line should be inserted in all comatose patients and blood collected for appropriate tests, including toxicologic analysis (10 mL of clotted blood, initial gastric aspirate, 100 mL of urine). The initial management of the comatose patient should include the administration of 100% oxygen, 100 mg of thiamine intravenously, 50% glucose as an intravenous bolus, and 2 to 10 mg of naloxone (Narcan) intravenously. Other causes associated with coma and mimicking intoxications should be eliminated by examination and laboratory tests (trauma, infection, cerebrovascular accident, hypoxia, and endocrine-metabolic causes).

Pulmonary edema complicating poisoning may be cardiac or noncardiac in origin. Fluid overload during forced diuresis may cause the cardiac variety, particularly if the drugs have an antidiuretic effect (opioids, barbiturates, and salicylates). Some toxic agents produce increased pulmonary capillary permeability, and other agents may cause a massive sympathetic discharge resulting in neurogenic pulmonary edema (opioids and salicylates). Management consists of minimizing the fluid administration; diuretics; and oxygen. If renal failure is present, dialysis may be necessary. The noncardiac type of pulmonary edema occurs with inhaled toxins, such as ammonia, chlorine, and oxides of nitrogen, or with drugs, such as salicylates, opioids, paraquat, and intravenous ethchlorvynol (Placidyl). This type does not respond to cardiac measures, and oxygen with intensive respiratory management using mechanical ventilation with positive end-expiratory pressure (PEEP) is necessary.

Hypotension and circulatory shock may be caused by heart failure due to myocardial depression, hypovolemia (fluid loss or venous pooling), decrease in peripheral vasculature resistance (adrenergic blockage), or loss of vasomotor tone caused by central nervous system depression.

Renal failure may be due to tubular necrosis as a result of hypotension, hypoxia, or a direct effect of the poison on the tubular cells (salicylate, paraquat, acetaminophen, carbon tetrachloride). Hemoglobinuria or myoglobinuria may precipi-

Text continued on page 1170

TABLE 4. **Antidotes***

Medication	Indications	Comments
1. **N-Acetylcysteine** (NAC, Mucomyst, Mead Johnson). Glutathione precursor that prevents accumulation and helps detoxify acetaminophen metabolites. **Dose:** *Adult,* 140 mg/kg PO of 5% solution as loading dose, then 70 mg/kg PO q 4 h for 17 doses as maintenance dose. *Child,* same as adult. **Packaged:** 10 and 20% solution in 4-, 10-, and 30-mL vials.	Acetaminophen toxicity. Most effective within first 8 h (to make more palatable, administer through a straw inserted into closed container of citrus juice). **AR:** Stomatitis, nausea, vomiting. See Acetaminophen in text. The full course of therapy is required in any patient whose level falls in the toxic range.	IV preparation experimental. The dose of NAC should be repeated if the patient vomits within 1 h after administration. Methods to stop vomiting of the NAC are: (a) placement of a tube in the duodenum, (b) slow administration over 1 h, (c) ½ h before NAC dose use metoclopramide (Reglan), 1 mg/kg intravenously over 15 min (max dose 10 mg) q 6 h; infants 0.1 mg/kg/dose IM, IV. Droperidol (Inapsine), 1.25 mg IV; for extrapyramidal reactions, use diphenhydramine (see 18).
2. **Ammonium chloride.**	Not recommended.	
3. **Amyl nitrate.**	See 14, Cyanide kit.	
4. **Antivenin,** black widow spider (*Latrodectum mactans*). **Dose:** 1–2 vials infused over 1 h. **Packaged:** 6000 U/vial with 2.5 mL sterile water and 1 mL horse serum 1:10 dilution.	Black widow spider; all *Latrodectus* species with severe symptoms. Most healthy adults survive with supportive care. Used in elderly or infants or if there is underlying medical condition causing hemodynamic instability. **AR:** Same as Antivenin polyvalent because derived from horse serum.	Preliminary sensitivity test. Supportive care alone is standard management.
5. **Antivenin Polyvalent** for Crotalidae (pit vipers), Wyeth, IV only. **Dose:** Depends on degree of envenomation: minimal: 5–8 vials; moderate: 8–12 vials; severe: 13–30 vials. Dilute in 500–2000 mL of crystalloid solution and start IV at a slow rate, increasing after the first 20 min, if no reaction occurs. **Packaged:** 1 vial (10 mL) lyophilized serum, 1 vial (10 mL) bacteriostatic water for injection, 1 vial (1 mL) normal horse serum.	Venoms of crotalids (pit vipers) of North and South America. **AR:** (Shock anaphylaxis) Reaction occurs within 30 min. Serum sickness usually occurs 5–44 days after administration. It may occur in less than 5 days, especially in those who have received horse serum products in the past. Symptoms include fever, edema, arthralgia, nausea, and vomiting, as well as pain and muscle weakness.	Consider consulting with regional poison control center and herpetologist. Administer IV. Preliminary sensitivity test. Never inject in fingers, toes, or bite site.
6. **Antivenin,** North American coral snake, Wyeth, IV only. **Dose:** 3–5 vials (30–50 mL) by slow IV injection. First 1–2 mL should be injected over 3–5 min. **Packaged:** 1 vial antivenin, 10 mL. 1 vial bacteriostatic water 10 mL for injection.	*Micrurus fulvius* (Eastern coral snake); *Micrurus tenere* (Texac coral snake). **AR:** Anaphylaxis (sensitivity reaction). Usually 30 min after administration. Signs/symptoms: Flushing, itching, edema of face, cough, dyspnea, cyanosis. Neurologic manifestations—usually involve the shoulders and arms. Pain and muscle weakness are frequently present, and permanent atrophy may develop.	Same as for Antivenin polyvalent: for Crotalidae. Will not neutralize the venom of *Micrurus euryxanthus* (Arizona or Sonoran coral snake).

Abbreviations: AR = adverse reaction to antidotes; MP = monitoring parameters; FDA = US Food and Drug Administration; Conc. = concentration; ECG = electrocardiogram; TIBC = total iron-binding capacity; G6PD = glucose-6-phosphate dehydrogenase; CNS = central nervous system; GI = gastrointestinal; AV = atrioventricular; EEG = electroencephalogram; RBC = red blood count; CBC = complete blood count.

*This is for information purposes and is not intended to subsitute for independent judgment. It is always advisable to review the package insert for the most up-to-date information. Contact Regional Poison Control Center for additional details on use.

†This dose may exceed the manufacturer's recommended dose.

Table continued on following page

TABLE 4. **Antidotes*** *Continued*

Medication	Indications	Comments
7. **Atropine** (various manufacturers). Antagonizes cholinergic stimuli at muscarinic recptors. **Dose:** *Adult,* initial dose 2–4 mg IV. Dose every 10–15 min as necessary until cessation of secretions. Severe poisoning may require doses up to 2000 mg. *Child,* initial dose of 0.02 mg/kg to a max of 2 mg every 10–15 min as necessary until cessation of secretions. Use preservative-free atropine if infusion. **Packaged:** 0.3 mg/mL; 0.4 mg/mL in 0.5-, 1-, 20-, and 30-ml vials; 1 mg/mL in 1- and 10-mL vials.	Therapy in carbamate and organophosphate insecticide poisonings. Rarely needed in cholinergic mushroom intoxication (*Amanita muscaria, Clitocybe, Inocybe* spp.). Lack of signs of atropinization confirms diagnosis of cholinesterase inhibition. **AR:** Flushing and dryness of skin, blurred vision, rapid and irregular pulse, fever, and loss of neuromuscular coordination. **Diagnostic Test:** *Child:* 0.01 mg/kg IV. *Adult:* 1 mg total.	If cyanosis, establish respiration first because atropine in cyanotic patients may cause ventricular fibrillation. If severe signs of atropinization, may correct with physostigmine in doses equal to one-half dose of atropine. If symptomatic, administer until the end point of drying secretions and clearing of lungs. Hallucinations, flushing of the skin, dilated pupils, tachycardia, and elevation of body temperature are not end points and do not preclude atropine administration. Atropinization should be maintained for 12–24 h, then taper dose and observe for relapse. Atropine has been administered successfully by IV infusion, although this method has not received FDA approval. **Dose:** Place 8 mg of atropine in 100 mL D5W or saline. Conc. = 0.08 mg/mL. Dose range = 0.02–0.08 mg/kg/h or 0.25–1 mL/kg/h. Severe poisoning may require supplemental doses of intravenous atropine intermittently in doses of 2–4 mg until drying of secretions occurs.
8. **BAL**	See 17, Dimercaprol.	
9. **Bicarbonate**	See 39, Sodium bicarbonate.	
10. **Botulism antitoxin,** Connaught Medical Research Labs. **Dose:** *Adult,* 1 vial IV stat, then 1 vial IM, repeat in 2–4 h if symptoms appear in 12–24 h. *Child,* check with state health department.	Prevention or treatment of botulism.	Contact local or state health department for full management guidelines.
11. **Calcium disodium edetate** (EDTA, Disodium Versenate, Riker). **Dose:** *Adult,* max 4 gm. *Child,* max 1 gm. Moderate toxicity, IM or IV, 50 mg/kg/day for 3–5 days. Severe toxicity: IV or IM, 75 mg/kg/day for 4–5 days. Doses divided into 3–6 doses daily. Dilute 1 gm in 250–500 mL saline or D5W, infuse over 4 h bid for 5–7 days. For lead levels over 69 µg/dL or if symptoms of lead poisoning or encephalopathy: Add BAL alone initially, 4 mg/kg, then combination BAL and EDTA at different sites. EDTA dose: 12.5 mg/kg IM. (See Lead in text for latest recommendations.) Modify dose in renal failure. **Packaged:** 200 mg/mL ampules.	For chelation of cadmium, chromium, cobalt, copper, lead, magnesium, nickel, selenium, tellurium, tungsten, uranium, vanadium, and zinc poisoning. **AR:** 1. Thrombophlebitis. 2. Nausea, vomiting. 3. Hypotension. 4. Transient bone marrow suppression. 5. Nephrotoxitiy, reversible tubular necrosis, (particularly in acid urine). 6. Fever 4–8 h after infusion. 7. Increased prothrombin time.	Hydrate first and establish renal flow. Avoid plain sodium EDTA because hypocalcemia may result. Procaine 0.25–1 mL of 0.5% for each mL of IM EDTA to reduce pain. Do not use EDTA orally. Limit use to 7 days (otherwise loss of other ions and cardiac dysrhythmias may occur). **MP:** Calcium levels, urinalysis, renal profile, erythrocyte protoporphyrin, blood lead, and liver profile. Contraindicated in iron intoxication, hepatic impairment, and renal failure.

Abbreviations: AR = adverse reaction to antidotes; MP = monitoring parameters; FDA = US Food and Drug Administration; Conc. = concentration; ECG = electrocardiogram; TIBC = total iron-binding capacity; G6PD = glucose-6-phosphate dehydrogenase; CNS = central nervous system; GI = gastrointestinal; AV = atrioventricular; EEG = electroencephalogram; RBC = red blood count; CBC = complete blood count.

*This is for information purposes and is not intended to subsitute for independent judgment. It is always advisable to review the package insert for the most up-to-date information. Contact Regional Poison Control Center for additional details on use.

†This dose may exceed the manufacturer's recommended dose.

TABLE 4. **Antidotes*** *Continued*

Medication	Indications	Comments
12. (A) **Calcium gluconate** 10%. **Dose:** IV 0.2–0.5 mL/kg of elemental calcium up to max 10 mL (1 gm) over 5–10 min with continuous ECG monitoring. Titrate to adequate response. **Packaged:** 10% in 10-mL vial.	Calcium channel blocker poisoning, e.g., nifedipine (Procardia), verapamil (Calan), diltiazem (Cardizem). It improves the blood pressure but does not affect the dysrhythmias. Hypocalcemia as result of poisonings. Black widow spider envenomation.	Repeat dose as needed. Monitor calcium levels. Contraindicated with digitalis poisoning.
(B) **Calcium chloride.** **Dose:** IV 0.2 mL/kg up to max 10 mL (1 gm) with continuous IV monitoring. Titrate to adequate response. Rate should not exceed 2 mL/min.	Hydrofluoric acid (HF) (if irrigation with cool water fails to control the pain). **AR:** IV bradycardia, asystole, necrosis with extravasation.	Infiltration with calcium gluconate should be considered if HF exposure results in immediate tissue damage and erythema and pain persist following adequate irrigation.
(C) **Infiltration of calcium gluconate.** **Dose:** Infiltrate each square cm of the affected dermis and subcutaneous tissue with about 0.5 mL of 10% calcium gluconate using a 30-gauge needle. Repeat as needed to control pain. **Packaged:** 10% in 10-mL vial.		
(D) **Calcium gel** 3.5 gm USP calcium gluconate powder added to 5 oz of water-soluble lubricating jelly.	Dermal exposure of hydrofluoric acid less than 20%.	Gel must have direct access to burn area; if pain persists, calcium gluconate injection may be needed. Placing a loose-fitting surgical glove over the gel when the fingers are involved helps to keep preparation in contact with burn area.
13. **Chemet.**	See 42, Succimer.	
14. **Cyanide antidote kit,** Lilly. Nitrite-induced methemoglobinemia attracts cyanide off cytochrome oxidase and thiosulfate forms nontoxic thiocyanate. **Doses:** *Adult,* amyl nitrite. Inhale for 30 sec of every min. Use a new ampule every 3 min. Reapply until sodium nitrite can be given. Then inject IV 300 mg (10 ml of 3% solution of sodium nitrite) over 20 min. Alternative: IV infusion, 300 mg in 50–100 mL of 0.9% saline over 20 min. Then inject 12.5 gm (50 mL of 25% sol) of sodium thiosulfate over 20 minutes. *Child,* use the following chart for children's dosage. **Packaged:** 2- to 10-mL ampules sodium nitrite injection; 2- to 50-mL ampules sodium thiosulfate injection; 0.3-mL amyl nitrite inhalant.	Cyanide poisoning. **AR:** Hypotension, methemoglobinemia.	*Note:* If a child is given the adult dose of sodium nitrite, a fatal methemoglobinemia may result. Do not use methylene blue for methemoglobinemia in cyanide therapy. Observe for hypotension and have epinephrine available. Cyanide kits should have amyl nitrite changed annually. Administer oxygen 100% between inhalations of amyl nitrite. Monitor hemoglobin, arterial blood gases, methemoglobin concentration (nitrite given to obtain a methemoglobin of 25%). Some add nitrite ampule to resuscitation bag.

Abbreviations: AR = adverse reaction to antidotes; MP = monitoring parameters; FDA = US Food and Drug Administration; Conc. = concentration; ECG = electrocardiogram; TIBC = total iron-binding capacity; G6PD = glucose-6-phosphate dehydrogenase; CNS = central nervous system; GI = gastrointestinal; AV = atrioventricular; EEG = electroencephalogram; RBC = red blood count; CBC = complete blood count.

*This is for information purposes and is not intended to subsitute for independent judgment. It is always advisable to review the package insert for the most up-to-date information. Contact Regional Poison Control Center for additional details on use.

†This dose may exceed the manufacturer's recommended dose.

Table continued on following page

TABLE 4. **Antidotes*** *Continued*

Medication	Indications	Comments

Chart should be used to determine dose of sodium nitrite and sodium thiosulfate in children on the basis of hemoglobin concentration on left. The average child with a normal hemoglobin requires 0.33–0.39 mL/kg of sodium nitrite up to 10 mL over 20 min.

Hemoglobin	Initial Child Dose of Sodium Nitrite 3% (do not exceed 10 mL)	Initial Child Dose of Sodium Thiosulfate (do not exceed 12.5 gm)
8 gm	0.22 mL/kg (6.6 mg/kg)	1.10 mL/kg
10 gm	0.27 mL/kg (8.7 mg/kg)	1.35 mL/kg
12 gm	0.33 mL/kg (10 mg/kg)	1.65 mL/kg
14 gm	0.39 mL/kg (11.6 mg/kg)	1.95 mL/kg

If signs of poisoning reappear, repeat above procedure at one-half the above doses. Each agent should be given at a rate of over 20 min.

15. **Deferoxamine mesylate** (DFOM, Desferal, Ciba). Has a remarkable affinity for ferric iron and chelates it.
   Therapeutic Dose: *Adult,* 90 mg/kg† IM or IV q 8 h to a max of 1 gm per injection; may repeat to maximum of 6 gm in 24 h. *Child,* same as adult. IV administration can be given by slow infusion at rate not exceeding 15 mg/kg/h.
   Packaged: 500 mg/ampule (powder).

DFOM is useful in the treatment of symptomatic iron poisoning or cases where the serum iron is greater than 500 µg/dL. If the DFOM challenge test is positive, it is not a definite indication that therapy is necessary in the asymptomatic patient. Oral DFOM is not recommended.
Iron intoxication.
Therapeutic—see dose in left column.
Diagnostic trial: Give deferoxamine, 50 mg/kg IM (up to 1 gm). If serum iron exceeds TIBC, unbound iron is excreted in urine, producing a "vin rose" color of chelated iron complex in the urine (pink-orange). However, may be negative with high serum iron exceeding TIBC.
AR: Flushing of the skin, generalized erythema, urticaria, hypotension, and shock may occur. Blindness has occurred rarely in patients receiving long-term, high-dose DFOM therapy. Continuous infusions of DFOM over 24 h has produced severe pulmonary manifestations such as adult respiratory distress syndrome.
Contraindicated in patients with renal disease or anuria.

Therapy is usually continued until serum iron < 100 µg/dL, or when positive "vin rose" urine turns clear, or when asymptomatic. Therapy is rarely required over 24 h.
Establish a good renal flow.
To be effective, DFOM should be administered in first 12–16 h.
In mild to moderate iron intoxication or shock, IV route only.
Monitor serum iron levels, urine output, and urine color.

16. **Diazepam** (Valium, Roche).
   Dose: *Adult,* 5–10 mg IV (max 20 mg) at a rate of 5 mg/min until seizure is controlled. May be repeated 2 or 3 times. *Child,* 0.1–0.3 mg/kg up to 10 mg IV slowly over 2 min.
   Packaged: 5 mg/mL; 2 mL, 10-mL vials.

Any intoxication that provokes seizures when specific therapy is not available, e.g., amphetamines, PCP, barbiturate and alcohol withdrawal.
Chloroquine poisoning.
AR: Confusion, somnolence, coma, hypotension.

Intramuscular absorption is erratic. Establish airway and administer 100% oxygen and glucose.

Abbreviations: AR = adverse reaction to antidotes; MP = monitoring parameters; FDA = US Food and Drug Administration; Conc. = concentration; ECG = electrocardiogram; TIBC = total iron-binding capacity; G6PD = glucose-6-phosphate dehydrogenase; CNS = central nervous system; GI = gastrointestinal; AV = atrioventricular; EEG = electroencephalogram; RBC = red blood count; CBC = complete blood count.

*This is for information purposes and is not intended to subsitute for independent judgment. It is always advisable to review the package insert for the most up-to-date information. Contact Regional Poison Control Center for additional details on use.

†This dose may exceed the manufacturer's recommended dose.

TABLE 4. **Antidotes*** *Continued*

Medication	Indications	Comments
17. **Dimercaprol** (BAL, Hynson, Westcott, and Dunning). **Dose:** Recommendations vary; contact regional poison control center. Prevents inhibition of sulfhydryl enzymes. Given deep IM only. *For severe lead poisoning*—see 11. EDTA. *For mild arsenic or gold*—2.5 mg/kg q 6 h for 2 days, then q 12 h on the third day, and once daily thereafter for 10 days. *For severe arsenic or gold*—3–5 mg/kg q 6 h for 3 days, then q 12 h thereafter for 10 days.† *For mercury*—5 mg/kg initially, followed by 2.5 mg/kg 1 or 2 times daily for 10 days. **Packaged:** 100 mg/mL 10% in oil in 3-mL ampules.	For chelation of antimony, arsenic, bismuth, chromates, copper, gold, lead, mercury, and nickel. **AR:** 30% of patients have reactions: fever (30% of children), hypertension, tachycardia, may cause hemolysis in G6PD deficiency patients. Doses greater than recommended may cause various adverse effects: nausea, vomiting, headache, chest pain, tachycardia, and hypertension.	Contraindicated in instances of hepatic insufficiency, with the exception of postarsenic jaundice. Should be discontinued or used only with extreme caution if acute renal insufficiency is present. Monitor blood pressure and heart rate (both may increase), urinalysis, qualitative urine excretion of heavy metal. Contraindicated in iron, silver, uranium, selenium, and cadmium poisoning.
18. **Dimercaptosuccinic acid** (DMSA).	See 42, Succimer.	
19. **Diphenhydramine** (Benadryl, Parke-Davis). Antiparkinsonian action. **Dose:** *Adult,* 10–50 mg IV over 2 min. *Child,* 1–2 mg/kg IV up to 50 mg over 2 min. Max in 24 h, 400 mg. **Packaged:** 10 mg/mL in 10- and 30-mL vials. 50 mg/mL in 1-, 5-, 10-, and 30-mL vials. Capsules, tablets 25 mg. Elixir, syrup 12.5 mg/5mL.	Used to treat extrapyramidal symptoms and dystonia induced by phenothiazines and related drugs. **AR:** Fatal dose, 20–40 mg/kg. Dry mouth, drowsiness.	Continue with oral diphenhydramine 5 mg/kg/day to 25 mg 3 times a day for 72 h to avoid recurrence.
20. **EDTA.**	See 11, Calcium disodium edetate.	
21. **Ethanol** (ETOH). Competitively inhibits alcohol dehydrogenase. **Dose:** *Loading*—administer 7.6–10.0 mL/kg of 10% ETOH in D5W over 30 min IV or 0.8–1.0 mL/kg 95% ETOH PO in 6 oz of orange juice over 30 min. While administering loading dose, start maintenance. *Maintenance:* Volume of 10% ETOH needed IV or 95% oral solution (not in dialysis). See chart on maintenance dose, below. If patient is on dialysis, add 91 mL/h in addition to regular maintenance dose. See comments to prepare 10% solution if not commercially available. **Packaged:** 10% ethanol in D5W 1000 mL; 95% ethanol. May be given as 50% solution orally.	Methanol, ethylene glycol. Ethanol infusion therapy may be started in cases of suspected methanol and ethylene glycol poisoning presenting with increased anion gap and osmolal gap, or if the urine shows the crystalluria of ethylene glycol poisoning or the hyperemia of the optic disk of methanol intoxication. **AR:** CNS depression, hypoglycemia.	Monitor blood ethanol 1 h after starting infusion and q 4–6 h. Maintain a blood ethanol concentration of 100–200 mg/dL. Monitor blood glucose, electrolytes, blood gases, urinalysis, and renal profile at least daily. Continue infusion until safe concentration of ethylene glycol or methanol is reached. Ethanol-induced hypoglycemia may occur. Dialysis, preferably hemodialysis, should be considered in severe intoxication not controlled by ethanol alone. To prepare 10% ethanol for infusion therapy. Remove 100 mL from 1 L D5W and replace with 100 mL of tax-free bulk absolute alcohol after passing through 0.22-μ filter, 50-mL vials of pyrogen-free absolute ethanol for injection are available from Pharm-Serv, 218–20 96th Avenue, Queen's Village, NY 11429. Telephone 718–475–1601.

Maintenance Dose:

Patient Category	mL/kg/h using 10% IV	mL/kg/h using 50% oral
Nondrinker	0.83	0.17
Occasional drinker	1.40	0.28
Alcoholic	1.96	0.39

Abbreviations: AR = adverse reaction to antidotes; MP = monitoring parameters; FDA = US Food and Drug Administration; Conc. = concentration; ECG = electrocardiogram; TIBC = total iron-binding capacity; G6PD = glucose-6-phosphate dehydrogenase; CNS = central nervous system; GI = gastrointestinal; AV = atrioventricular; EEG = electroencephalogram; RBC = red blood count; CBC = complete blood count.

*This is for information purposes and is not intended to subsitute for independent judgment. It is always advisable to review the package insert for the most up-to-date information. Contact Regional Poison Control Center for additional details on use.

†This dose may exceed the manufacturer's recommended dose.

Table continued on following page

TABLE 4. **Antidotes*** *Continued*

Medication	Indications	Comments
22. **Fab** (antibody fragment, Digibind). **Dose:** The average dose used during clinical testing was 10 vials. Dosage details are specified by the manufacturer. It should be administered by the IV route over 30 min. Calculate on basis of body burden either by known amount ingested or by serum digoxin concentration. *Calculation of dose of Fab:* 1. Known amount ingested multiplied by bioavailability (0.8) = body burden. Body burden divided by 0.6 = number of vials. 2. Known serum digoxin (obtained 6 h postingestion) multiplied by volume distribution (5.6 L/kg) and weight in kg divided by 1000 = body burden. Body burden divided by 0.6 = number of vials.	Digoxin, digitoxin, oleander tea with the following: 1. Imminent cardiac arrest or shock. 2. Hyperkalemia > 5.5 mEq/L. 3. Serum digoxin > 10 ng/mL at 6–12 h postingestion in adults. 4. Life-threatening dysrhythmias. 5. Ingestion over 10 mg in adults or 4 mg in child (0.3 mg/kg). 6. Bradycardia or second- or third-degree heart block unresponsive to atropine.	Contact regional poison control center. Preliminary sensitivity test. Administer through a 0.22-μ filter. It causes a rise in measured bound digoxin but a fall in free digoxin. 40 mg binds 0.6 mg digoxin.
23. **Flumazenil** (Mazicon, Roche Labs), Benzodiazepine (BZP) receptor antagonist. **Dose:** 1. *Management of BZP overdose:* (Caution) 0.2 mg (2 mL) IV over 30 sec; may repeat after 30 sec with 0.3 mg (3 mL). Further doses of 0.5 mg over 30 sec. If no response in 5 min and max of 5 mg, cause of sedation is unlikely to be BZP. 2. *Reversal of conscious sedation or in general anesthesia:* 0.2 mg (2 mL) IV over 15 sec. May repeat in 45 sec—0.2 mg (2 mL). Doses may be repeated at 60-sec intervals to max dose of 1 mg (10 mL). If resedation, repeated doses may be administered at 20-min intervals to max 1 mg (0.2 mg/min). Max 3 mg should be given in any 1 h. **Packaged:** 0.1 mg/mL in 5- and 10-mL multiple-use vials.	1. Reversal of the sedative effects of BZP general anesthesia. 2. Sedation with BZP for procedures. 3. Caution in management of overdose. **AR:** Convulsions, dizziness, injection site pain, increased sweating, headache and abnormal or blurred vision (3–9%).	Not treatment for hypoventilation. Caution with overdoses. Flumazenil is not recommended for cyclic antidepressant poisoning, if seizures or increased intracranial pressure are present. Flumazenil has been associated with seizures in long-term benzodiazepine use or dependency.
24. **Folic acid.**	See 28, Leucovorin.	
25. **Folinic acid.**	See 28, Leucovorin.	
26. **Glucagon.** Works by stimulating production of cyclic adenyl monophosphate. **Dose:** 50–150 μg/kg over 1 min IV followed by a continuous infusion of 1–5 mg/h in dextrose and then taper over 5–12 h. 2 mg of phenol per 1 mg glucagon. 50 mg is the maximum amount of phenol recommended; therefore, toxicity may result when high doses of glucagon are used. **Packaged:** 1-mg (1-unit) vial with 1-mL diluent with glycerin and phenol; also in 10-mL size.	Beta blockers, quinidine, and calcium channel blockers intoxication. **AR:** Generally well tolerated— most frequent are nausea, vomiting.	Do not dissolve the lyophilized glucagon in the solvent packaged with it when administering IV infusion because of possible phenol toxicity. Use 0.9% saline or D5W. Effects of single dose observed in 5–10 min and last for 15–30 min. A constant infusion may be necessary to sustain desired effects.

Abbreviations: AR = adverse reaction to antidotes; MP = monitoring parameters; FDA = US Food and Drug Administration; Conc. = concentration; ECG = electrocardiogram; TIBC = total iron-binding capacity; G6PD = glucose-6-phosphate dehydrogenase; CNS = central nervous system; GI = gastrointestinal; AV = atrioventricular; EEG = electroencephalogram; RBC = red blood count; CBC = complete blood count.

*This is for information purposes and is not intended to subsitute for independent judgment. It is always advisable to review the package insert for the most up-to-date information. Contact Regional Poison Control Center for additional details on use.

†This dose may exceed the manufacturer's recommended dose.

TABLE 4. **Antidotes*** *Continued*

Medication	Indications	Comments
27. **Labetalol hydrochloride** (Normodyne, Schering; Trandate, Glaxo). Nonselective beta and mild alpha blocker. **Dose:** IV 20 mg over 2 min. Additional injections of 40 or 80 mg can be given at 10-min intervals until desired supine blood pressure achieved. Max dose 300 mg. Alternative: Slow IV infusion: 200 mg (40 mL) is added to 160 or 250 mL of D5W and given at 2 mg/min. Titrate infusion according to response. **Packaged:** Solution 5 mg/mL in 20 mL.	Hypertensive crises secondary to cocaine. **AR:** GI disturbances, orthostatic hypotension, bronchospasm, congestive heart failure, AV conduction disturbances, and peripheral vascular reactions.	Concomitant diuretic enhances therapeutic response. Patient should be kept in a supine position during infusion. **MP:** Monitor blood pressure during and after administration.
28. **Leucovorin.** Dose for methanol poisoning: 1 mg/kg up to 50 mg IV q 4 h for 6 doses. **Dose:** See Comments. **Packaged:** 3 mg/mL (1 mL), 5 mg/mL (1 and 5 mL), 50 mg/vial.	1. **Methanol poisoning:** Active form of folic acid used to enhance metabolism of formic acid in animals to carbon dioxide and water. 2. **Methotrexate (MTX) overdose:** Supplies tetrahydrofolate cofactor, which is blocked by methotrexate. **AR:** Allergic sensitization.	For MTX overdose, initial dose can give IV or IM in MTX equivalent dose up to 75 mg. If a MTX blood level is measured 6 h postingestion, and is above 10^{-8} molar or is unavailable, give 12 mg q 6 h after the MTX level is below 10^{-8} molar. Alternatively, if GI function is adequate, may give orally 10 mg/M^2 q 6 h until MTX levels are lowered to less than 10^{-8} molar. Leucovorin in doses of 5–15 mg PO per day has also been recommended to counteract hematologic toxicity from folic acid antagonists such as trimethoprin and pyrimethamine.
29. **Methylene blue,** Harvey and others. Methylene blue reduces the ferric ion of methemoglobin, to the ferrous ion of hemoglobin. **Dose:** *Adult,* 0.1–0.2 mL/kg of 1% solution (1–2 mg/kg) over 5 min IV. Max adults 7 mg/kg. *Child,* same as adults. Max infants 4 mg/kg. **Packaged:** 1% 10-mL ampules. May repeat in 1 h if necessary. Repeat only once.	Methemoglobinemia. **AR:** GI (nausea, vomiting), headache, hypertension, dizziness, mental confusion, restlessness, dyspnea, hemolysis, blue skin, blue urine, burning sensation in vein when IV dose exceeds 7 mg/kg. Treatment is unnecessary unless methemoglobin is over 30% or respiratory distress.	Saliva, urine, and other body fluids may turn blue. Contraindications: Renal insufficiency, cyanide poisonings when sodium nitrite is used to induce methemoglobinemia; in G6PD deficiency patients. Monitor hemolysis, methemoglobin level, and arterial blood gases. Avoid extravasation because of local necrosis.
30. **Naloxone** (Narcan). Pure opioid antagonist. **Dose:** *Adult,* 0.4–2.0 mg IV and repeat at 3-min intervals until respiratory function is stable. Before excluding opioid intoxication on the basis of a lack of naloxone response, a minimum of 2 mg in a child or 10 mg in an adult should be administered. *Child,* initial dose is 0.1 mg/kg IV. **Packaged:** 0.02 mg/mL, 0.4 mg/mL ampule, 10-mL multidose vial.	1. Comatose patient (not just a lethargic patient). 2. Ineffective ventilationn or an adult respiratory rate <12. 3. Pinpoint pupils. 4. Circumstantial evidence of opioid intoxication, i.e., known drug abuser, track marks, opioid paraphernalia. **AR:** Relatively free of adverse reactions. Rare reports of pulmonary edema. Should be administered with caution in pregnancy.	Naloxone infusion therapy should be used if a large initial dose was required, repeated boluses are necessary, or a long-acting opiate is involved. In infusion therapy the initial response dose is administered every hour and may need to be boostered in a half-hour after starting. The infusion may be tapered after 12 h of therapy. Naloxone infusion: calculate out daily fluid requirements, add initial response dose of naloxone multiplied by 24 to the solution. Divide fluid by 24 h for naloxone infusion rate per hour. Does not cause CNS depression. Routes: IV or endotracheal are preferred routes. Pentazocine (Talwin), dextramethorphan, propoxyphene (Darvon), and codeine may require larger doses.

Abbreviations: AR = adverse reaction to antidotes; MP = monitoring parameters; FDA = US Food and Drug Administration; Conc. = concentration; ECG = electrocardiogram; TIBC = total iron-binding capacity; G6PD = glucose-6-phosphate dehydrogenase; CNS = central nervous system; GI = gastrointestinal; AV = atrioventricular; EEG = electroencephalogram; RBC = red blood count; CBC = complete blood count.

*This is for information purposes and is not intended to subsitute for independent judgment. It is always advisable to review the package insert for the most up-to-date information. Contact Regional Poison Control Center for additional details on use.

†This dose may exceed the manufacturer's recommended dose.

Table continued on following page

TABLE 4. **Antidotes*** *Continued*

Medication	Indications	Comments
31. **Nicotinamide,** various manufacturers. **Dose:** *Adult,* 500 mg IM or IV slowly, then 200–400 mg q 4 h. If symptoms develop, the frequency of injections should be increased to every 2 h (max 3 gm/day). *Child,* One-half suggested adult dose. **Packaged:** 100 mg/mL: 2-, 5-, 10-, 30-mL vials; 25- and 50-mg tablets.	Vacor poisoning: phenylurea pesticide intoxication. *Note:* Vacor 2% is now available only to professional exterminators. 0.5% Vacor is available to the general public and can be toxic to children if swallowed. **AR:** Large doses—flushing, pruritis, sensation of burning, nausea, vomiting, anaphylactic shock.	Nicotinamide is most effective when given within 1 h of ingestion. Do not use niacin or nicotinic acid in place of nicotinamide. Monitor liver profile.
32. **Oxygen** 100%. **Dose:** *Adult,* 100% oxygen by inhalation or 100% oxygen in hyperbaric chamber at 2–3 atm. *Child,* Same as adult.	Carbon monoxide, cyanide, methemoglobinemia. Any inhalation intoxication.	Half-life of carboxyhemoglobin is 240 min in room air 21% oxygen; if a patient is hyperventilated with 100% oxygen, half-life of carboxyhemoglobin is 90 min; in chamber at 2 atm, half-life is 25–30 min.
33. **Pancuronium bromide** (Pavulon). Nondepolarizing (competitive) blocking agent. **Dose:** *Adults and children,* initially, 0.1 mg/kg IV; for intubation, 0.1 mg/kg IV, repeated as required (generally every 40–60 min).† **Packaged:** Solution 1 mg/mL in 10 mL. 2 mg/mL in 2- and 5-ml containers.	Neuromuscular blocking agent. Used for intubation and seizure control, acts in 2 min, lasts 40–60 min. **AR:** Main hazard is inadequate postoperative ventilation. Tachycardia and slight increase in arterial pressure may occur due to vagolytic action.	The required dose varies greatly, and a peripheral nerve stimulator aids in determining appropriate amount. Should monitor EEG, because motor effect may be abolished without decreasing electrical discharge from brain.
34. **D-Penicillamine** (Cuprimine, Merck; Depen, Wallace). Effective chelator and promotes excretion in urine. **Dose:** 250 mg 4 times daily PO for up to 5 days for long-term (20–40 days) therapy; 30–40 mg/kg/day in children. Max 1 gm/day. For chronic therapy 25 mg/kg/day in 4 doses. **Packaged:** 125- and 250-mg capsules.	Heavy metals, arsenic, cadmium, chromates, cobalt, copper, lead, mercury, nickel, and zinc. **MP:** Routine urinalysis, white blood count differential, hemoglobin determination, direct platelet count, renal and hepatic profiles. Collect 24-h urine, quantify for heavy metal. **AR:** Leukopenia (2%); thrombocytopenia (4%); GI– nausea, vomiting, anaphylactic shock, diarrhea (17%); fever, rash, lupus syndrome, renal and hepatic injury.	This is not considered standard therapy for lead poisoning after chelation therapy. May produce ampicillin-like rash, allergic reactions, neutropenia, and nephropathy. Contraindication: hypersensitivity to penicillin.
35. **Physostigmine salicylate** (Antilirium, O'Neil). Cholinesterase inhibitor, a diagnostic trial is not recommended. **Dose:** *Adult,* 1–2 mg IV over 2 min; may repeat every 5 min to max dose of 6 mg. *Child,* IV, 0.5 mg (0.02 mg/kg) over paralysis, 2 min to a max dose of 2 mg q 30–60 min if symptoms recur.† Once effect accomplished, give lowest effective dose. **Packaged:** 1 mg/mL in 2 mL/ampule.	Not advised as a diagnostic test or for routine use in treating anticholinergic effects. Reserve for life-threatening complications. **AR:** Death may result from respiratory paralysis, hypertension/hypotension, bradycardia/tachycardia/asystole, hypersalivation, respiratory difficulties/convulsions (cholinergic crisis).	Do not consider for the following: antidepressants, amoxapine, maprotiline, nomifensine, bupropion, trazodone, imipramine. IV administration should be at a slow controlled rate, not more than 1 mg/min. Rapid administration can cause adverse reactions.

Abbreviations: AR = adverse reaction to antidotes; MP = monitoring parameters; FDA = US Food and Drug Administration; Conc. = concentration; ECG = electrocardiogram; TIBC = total iron-binding capacity; G6PD = glucose-6-phosphate dehydrogenase; CNS = central nervous system; GI = gastrointestinal; AV = atrioventricular; EEG = electroencephalogram; RBC = red blood count; CBC = complete blood count.

*This is for information purposes and is not intended to subsitute for independent judgment. It is always advisable to review the package insert for the most up-to-date information. Contact Regional Poison Control Center for additional details on use.

†This dose may exceed the manufacturer's recommended dose.

TABLE 4. **Antidotes*** *Continued*

Medication	Indications	Comments
36. **Pralidoxime chloride** (2-PAM, Protopam, Ayerst). Cholinesterase reactivator by removing phosphate. **Dose:** *Adults,* 1–2 gm IV infused in 100–250 mL saline IV over 15–30 min. Repeat in 1 h if needed. Repeat q 8–12 h when needed; if severe, can give 0.5 gm/h infusion. *Child,* 25–50 mg/kg IV over 30 min. No faster than 10 mg/kg/min. Max 12 gm/24 h. **Packaged:** 1 gm/20-mL vials.	Organophosphate insecticide (OPI) poisoning. Not usually needed in carbamate insecticide poisoning. Most effective if started in first 24 h before bonding of phosphate. **AR:** Rapid IV injection has produced tachycardia, muscle rigidity, transient neuromuscular blockade. IM: conjunctival hyperemia, subconjunctival hemorrhage, especially if concentrations exceed 5%. Oral: nausea, vomiting, diarrhea, malaise.	Should be used only after initial treatment with atropine. Draw blood for RBC cholinesterase level before giving 2-PAM. The use of 2-PAM may require a reduction in the dose of atropine. The end point is absence of fasciculations and return of muscle strength. **MP:** Monitor renal profile and reduce dose accordingly. Half-life = 1–2 h. Reversal of OPI effects at 4 μg/mL of 2-PAM. Start early because "aging" of PO_4 on Achase makes it more difficult to reverse.
37. **Protamine sulfate.** **Dose:** 1 mg neutralizes 90–115 U of heparin, max dose = 50 mg IV over 5 min at 10 mg/mL. **Packaged:** 5 mL = 50 mg; 25 mL = 250 mg.	Heparin overdose. **AR:** Rapid administration causes anaphylactoid reactions.	**MP:** Monitor thromboplastin times. Doses of up to 200 mg have been tolerated over 2 h in an adult.
38. **Pyridoxine** (Vitamin B$_6$). Gamma amino acid agonist. **Dose:** *Unknown amount ingested:* 5 gm over 5 min IV. *Known amount:* Add 1 gm of pyridoxine for each gram of INH ingested IV over 5 min. **Packaged:** 50 and 100 mg/mL; 10, 30 mL.	Isoniazid (INH), monomethyl hydrazine mushrooms. **AR:** Unlikely owing to the fact that vitamin B$_6$ is water-soluble. However, nausea, vomiting, somnolence, and paresthesia have been reported from chronic high doses up to 52 gm IV and up to 357 mg/kg have been tolerated.	Pyridoxine is given as 5–10% solution IV mixed with water. It may be repeated every 5–20 min until seizures cease. Some administer pyridoxine over 30–60 min. **MP:** Correct acidosis, monitor liver profile, acid-base parameters. Lethal dose of pyridoxine in animals is 1 gm/kg.
39. **Sodium bicarbonate.** **Dose:** IV 1–3 mEq/kg as needed to keep pH 7.5 (generally 2 mEq/kg q 6 h). When alkalinization is desired to correct acidosis to a pH of 7.3, use 2 mEq/kg to raise pH 0.1 unit. **Packaged:** 50 mL, 50-mEq ampule.	To promote urinary alkalinization for salicylates, phenobarbital (weak acids with low volume of distribution *excreted* in urine unchanged). To correct severe acidosis. To promote protein binding and supply sodium ions into Purkinje cells in cyclic antidepressant intoxication. **AR:** Large doses in patients with renal insufficiency may cause metabolic alkalosis. In patients with ketoacidosis, rapid alkalinization with sodium bicarbonate may result in clouding of consciousness, cerebral dysfunction, seizures, hypoxia, and lactic acidosis.	Alkaline diuresis. The assessment of the need for bicarbonate should be based on both the blood and urine pH. Maintain the blood pH at 7.5. Keep the urinary output at 3–6 mL/kg/h. May use a diuretic to enhance diuresis. Potassium is necessary to produce alkaline diuresis. Monitor electrolytes, calcium, pH of both urine and blood, arterial blood gases.
40. **Sodium nitrite.**	See 14, Cyanide antidote kit.	
41. **Sodium thiosulfate.**	See 14, Cyanide antidote kit.	

Abbreviations: AR = adverse reaction to antidotes; MP = monitoring parameters; FDA = US Food and Drug Administration; Conc. = concentration; ECG = electrocardiogram; TIBC = total iron-binding capacity; G6PD = glucose-6-phosphate dehydrogenase; CNS = central nervous system; GI = gastrointestinal; AV = atrioventricular; EEG = electroencephalogram; RBC = red blood count; CBC = complete blood count.

*This is for information purposes and is not intended to subsitute for independent judgment. It is always advisable to review the package insert for the most up-to-date information. Contact Regional Poison Control Center for additional details on use.

†This dose may exceed the manufacturer's recommended dose.

Table continued on following page

TABLE 4. **Antidotes*** *Continued*

Medication	Indications	Comments
42. **Succimer** (DMSA, Chemet, McNeil Consumer Products). **Dose:** 10 mg/kg or 350 mg/M^2 q 8 h for 5 days, then 10 mg/kg or 350 mg/M^2 q 12 h for 14 more days (see following chart). Therapy course lasts 19 days. **Packaged:** 100-mg capsule.	For chelation in children only whose blood lead is >45 µg/dL. **AR:** Rashes, nausea, vomiting, an elevation of serum transaminases occur in 6–10% of patients.	A minimum of 2 weeks between courses is recommended unless the venous lead indicates a need for more prompt therapy. Patients who have received CaEDTA or BAL may use succimer after an interval of 4 weeks. In young children the capsule can be opened and sprinkled on soft food. Monitor venous lead before therapy, day 7, and weekly for rebound. Monitor the following tests: CBC, platelets, ferritin, liver transaminases, renal function, calcium, glucose, total protein, albumin, and urinalysis.

Pediatric Dosing Chart

lbs	kg	Dose (mg)	No. of Capsules
18–35	8–15	100	1
36–55	16–23	200	2
56–75	24–34	300	3
76–100	35–44	400	4
>100	>45	500	5

Medication	Indications	Comments
43. **Vitamin K** (Aqua MEPHYTON, Merck). Promotes hepatic biosynthesis of prothrombin and other coagulation factors. Competitive antagonist of warfarin. It may be administered orally in the absence of vomiting. **Dose:** *Adult,* 2.5–10 mg IV, depending on potential for hemorrhage. Oral dose is 15–25 mg/day. Severe bleeding, 5–25 mg slow IV push. Rate 1 mg/min. Repeat q 4–8 h depending on prothrombin time. *Child,* 1–5 mg IV may be given orally when vomiting ceases at a dose of 5–10 mg/day. **Packaged:** 2 mg/mL in 0.5-mL ampules. 2.5- or 5-mL vials. Child oral dose 5–10 mg.	Warfarin (coumarin), superwarfarins, salicylate intoxication.	Fatalities from anaphylactic reaction have been reported following IV route. It takes 24 h for vitamin K to be effective. The need for further vitamin K is determined by the prothrombin time test. If severe bleeding, fresh blood or plasma transfusion may be needed.

Abbreviations: AR = adverse reaction to antidotes; MP = monitoring parameters; FDA = US Food and Drug Administration; Conc. = concentration; ECG = electrocardiogram; TIBC = total iron-binding capacity; G6PD = glucose-6-phosphate dehydrogenase; CNS = central nervous system; GI = gastrointestinal; AV = atrioventricular; EEG = electroencephalogram; RBC = red blood count; CBC = complete blood count.

*This is for information purposes and is not intended to subsitute for independent judgment. It is always advisable to review the package insert for the most up-to-date information. Contact Regional Poison Control Center for additional details on use.

†This dose may exceed the manufacturer's recommended dose.

---

tate in the renal tubules and produce renal failure.

Cerebral edema in intoxications is produced by hypoxia, hypercapnia, hypotension, hypoglycemia, and drug-impaired capillary integrity. Computed tomography may aid in diagnosis. Therapy consists of correction of the arterial blood gas and metabolic abnormalities and the hypotension. Reduction of the increased intracranial pressure may be accomplished by 20% mannitol, 0.5 gram per kg, run in over a 30-minute period, and hy-perventilation to reduce the PaCO$_2$ to 25 mmHg. The head should be elevated, and intracranial pressure monitoring should be considered. Fluid administration should be minimized.

Seizures are caused by many substances, such as amphetamines, camphor, chlorinated hydrocarbon insecticides, cocaine, isoniazid, lithium, phencyclidine, phenothiazines, propoxyphene, strychnine, tricyclic antidepressants, and drug withdrawal from ethanol and sedative-hypnotics. Recurring or protracted seizures require intravenous diazepam (Valium) and phenytoin and, if seizure persists, a neuromuscular blocking agent and assisted ventilation.

Cardiac dysrhythmias occur with poisoning. A wide QT interval occurs with phenothiazines, and a wide QRS interval occurs with tricyclic antidepressants, quinine, or quinidine overdose. Digitalis, cocaine, cyanide, propranolol, theophylline, and amphetamines are among the more frequent toxic causes of dysrhythmias. Correction of metabolic disturbances and adequate oxygenation correct some of the dysrhythmias; others may require antidysrhythmic drugs or a cardiac pacemaker or cardioversion.

TABLE 5. **Indications and Contraindications for Dialysis**

Immediate Consideration of Dialysis
Etyhlene glycol with refractory acidosis
Methanol with refractory acidosis and levels
    consistently over 50 mg/dL
Lithium levels consistently elevated over 4 mEq/L
Amanita phalloides

Incidations on Basis of Patient's Condition (coma greater than Stage 3 of Reed Coma Scale)

Alcohol*	Iodides
Ammonia	Isoniazid*
Amphetamines	Meprobamate
Anilines	Paraldehyde
Antibiotics	Potassium*
Barbiturates* (long-acting)	Quinidine
Boric acid	Quinine
Bromides*	Salicylates*
Calcium	Strychnine
Chloral hydrate*	Thiocyanates
Fluorides	(Certain other drugs also dialyzable)

Indicated for General Supportive Therapy
Uncontrollable metabolic acidosis or alkalosis
Uncontrollable electrolyte disturbance, particularly
    sodium or potassium
Overhydration
Renal failure
Hyperosmolality not responding to conservative
    therapy
Marked hypothermia
Nonresponsive Stage 3 or greater coma (Reed Coma
    Scale)

Contraindicated on Pharmacologic Basis Except for Supportive Care
Antidepressants (tricyclic and monoamine oxidase
    inhibitors)
Antihistamines
Barbiturates (short-acting)
Belladonna alkaloids
Benzodiazepines (Valium, Librium)
Digitalis and derivatives
Hallucinogens
Meprobamate (Equanil, Miltown)
Methyprylon (Noludar)
Opioids (heroin, Lomotil)
Phenothiazines (Thorazine, Compazine)
Phenytoin (Dilantin)

*Most useful.

TABLE 6. **Plasma Concentrations Above Which Removal by Extracorporeal Means May Be Indicated**

Drug	Plasma Concentration (mg/dL)*	Method of Choice
Phenobarbital	10	HP>HD
Other barbiturates	5	HP
Glutethimide	4	HP
Methaqualone	4	HP
Salicylates	80	HD>HP
Ethchlorvynol	15	HP
Meprobamate	10	HP
Trichloroethanol	5	HP
Paraquat	0.1	HP>HD
Theophylline	6 (chronic), 10 (acute)	HP
Methanol	50	HD
Ethylene glycol	Unknown	HD
Lithium	4 mEq/L	HD
Ethanol	500	HD

Abbreviations: HP = hemoperfusion; HD = hemodialysis.
*1 mg/dL = 10 μg/mL.
Modified from Haddad L, and Winchester JF (eds): Clinical Management of Poisoning and Drug Overdose. Philadelphia, W. B. Saunders, 1983, p 162.

Metabolic acidosis with an increased anion gap is seen with many agents in overdose. There is a mnemonic by which to remember these agents: MUD PILES (*m*ethanol, *u*remia, *d*iabetic ketoacidosis, *p*araldehyde and *p*henformin, *i*ron and *iso*niazid, *l*actic acidosis, *e*thylene glycol and *e*thanol, *s*alicylate and *s*tarvation and *s*olvents such as toluene). Assessment of the arterial blood gases, electrolytes, and osmolality may be a clue to the etiologic agent. Intravenous sodium bicarbonate may be needed when the pH is below 7.1 if there is adequate ventilation.

Hematemesis can be produced by caustics and corrosives, iron, lithium, mercury, phosphorus, arsenic, mushrooms, plant poisons, fluoride, and organophosphates. Therapy consists of fluid and blood replacement and iced saline lavage if there is no esophageal damage. Although controversial, antacids, H_2 blockers, sucralfate, or misoprostol may be used.

TOXICOKINETICS FOR THE PRACTICING PHYSICIAN

Toxicokinetics is clinical pharmacokinetics from the viewpoint of the toxicologist. Pharmacokinetics is a mathematic description of what the body does to a drug. Knowledge of the toxicokinetics of a specific toxic agent allows the physician to plan a rational approach to the definitive management of the intoxicated patient after the vital functions have been stabilized.

The LD_{50} (the lethal dose for 50% of experimental animals) and the MLD (the minimum lethal dose) are seldom relevant in human intoxications but indicate potential toxicity of the substance. Protein binding of toxic agents influences the volume distribution, elimination, and action of the drug. Diuresis and dialysis are usually reserved for drugs with less than 50% protein binding. The therapeutic blood range is the concentration of any drug at which the majority of the treated population can be expected to receive therapeutic benefit. The toxic blood range is the concentration at which this majority would be expected to have toxic manifestations. The range is not an absolute value. Blood concentrations are a quantitative aid in determining whether more specific measures need to be instituted in correlation with the clinical manifestations. The apparent volume distribution (Vd) is the percentage of body mass in which the drug is distributed. It is determined by dividing the amount absorbed by the blood concentration. When a substance has a large volume distribution, as in most lipid-soluble chemicals (above 1 liter per kg), and is concentrated in the body fat, it is not available for diuresis, dialysis, or exchange transfusion. Elimination routes of detoxification allow the physician to make therapeutic decisions, such as using ethanol to interfere with the metabolism of methanol and ethylene glycol into more toxic metabolites. Urine identification is usually qualitative and allows only the identification of an agent.

Never manage a poisoned patient solely by laboratory tests, and always treat according to the manifestations of poisoning, not the laboratory test results. The laboratory toxicology analyst should be given whatever historic information is available so the agent can be sought and identified as rapidly as possible. Toxicologic analysis is like a miniresearch project, unlike most other laboratory tests. Specimens for toxicologic analysis require the patient's name, date, time of exposure, time specimen was drawn, therapeutic drugs administered, patient's manifestations, and other relevant data. The toxicologic specimens that should be obtained for analysis are (1) vomitus or initial gastric aspiration; (2) blood, 10 mL (ask the analyst about the type of container and anticoagulant); and (3) urine, 100 mL. Acetaminophen plasma concentrations should be assessed in all suicide attempts.

COMMON POISONS AND THERAPY

Abbreviations Used in Following List of Common Poisons

t½ = half-life (time required for blood level to drop by 50% of the original value)

Vd = volume of distribution (liter per kg)

TLV = threshold limit value in air
TWA = time-weighted average
PPM = parts per million in air and water

Conversion Factors

1 gram	= 1000 milligrams (mg)
1 milligram (mg)	= 1000 micrograms (μg)
1 microgram (μg)	= 1000 nanograms (ng)
Standard International Units:	
1 mole	= mol wt in grams per liter
1 millimole	= mol wt in milligrams per liter
1 micromole	= mol wt in micrograms per liter
Blood levels:	
1 microgram per mL	= 100 micrograms per dL
	= 1 milligram per L
	= 1000 nanograms per mL
100 mg per dL	= 0.1 gram per dL
	= 1000 mg (1 gram) per L
	= 1 mg per mL

Acetaminophen, APAP (Tylenol). *Toxic dose:* Child, 3 grams or more; adult, 7.5 grams or more. Liver toxicity, 140 mg per kg. *Toxicokinetics:* Absorption time, 0.5 to 1 hour. Vd, 0.9 L per kg. Route of elimination by liver. Draw peak blood level after 4 hours in overdose. *Manifestations:* First 24 hours: malaise, nausea, vomiting, and drowsiness, followed by a latent period of 24 hours to 5 days; then hepatic symptoms, disturbances in clotting mechanism, and renal damage. *Management:* (1) Activated charcoal may be given when *N*-acetylcysteine is contemplated. In these circumstances, the loading dose of *N*-acetylcysteine is given twice. (2) *N*-Acetylcysteine for toxic overdose (Antidote 1, Table 4). Start and give a full course if a toxic dose has been ingested or if blood concentrations are above the toxic line on the nomogram shown in Figure 1. (3) In this instance, a saline sulfate cathartic is preferred to sorbitol. Treat at lower APAP plasma levels if patients have history of alcoholism or if on enzyme inducer medication, i.e., anticonvulsants. *Laboratory aids:* APAP level, optimally at 4 to 6 hours. Plot levels on nomogram in Figure 1 as a guide for treatment. Monitor liver and renal profiles daily.

Acids. See Caustics and Corrosives.

Alcohols

1. ETHANOL (grain alcohol). *Manifestations:* Blood ethanol levels over 30 mg per dL produce euphoria; over 50, incoordination and intoxication; over 100, ataxia; over 300, stupor; and over 500, coma. Levels of 500 to 700 mg per dL may be fatal. Chronic alcoholic patients tolerate higher levels, and the correlation may not be valid. *Management:* (1) Gastrointestinal decontamination. Caution: The rapid onset of CNS depression may preclude the induction of emesis. Activated charcoal and cathartics are not indicated. (2) Give 0.25 gram per kg of dextrose, 50%, intravenously if the blood glucose level is less

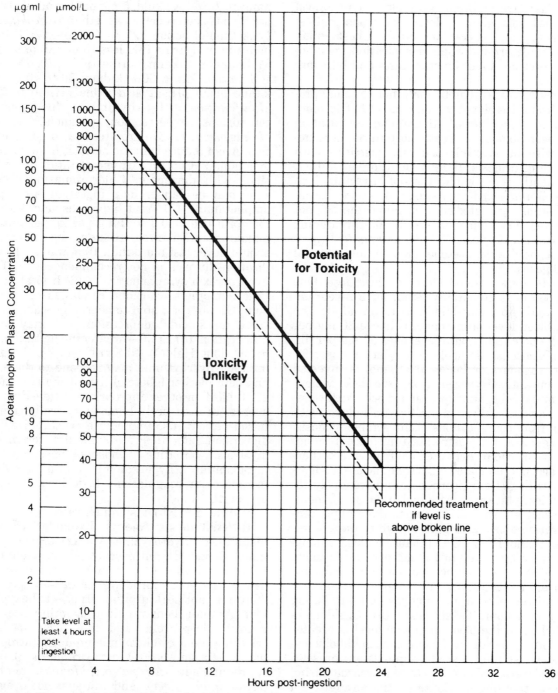

Figure 1. Nomogram for acetaminophen intoxication. Start *N*-acetylcysteine therapy if levels and time coordinates are above the lower line on the nomogram. Continue and complete therapy even if subsequent values fall below the toxic zone. The nomogram is useful only in acute, single ingestions. Serum levels drawn before 4 hours may not represent peak levels. (From Rumack BH, and Matthew H: Acetaminophen poisoning and toxicity. Pediatrics 55:871, 1975. Reproduced by permission of Pediatrics.)

than 60 mg per dL. (3) Thiamine, 100 mg intravenously, if chronic is suspected, to prevent Wernicke-Korsakoff syndrome. (4) Hemodialysis is indicated in severe cases when conventional therapy is ineffective (rarely needed). (5) Treat seizures with diazepam (Valium) followed by phenytoin (Dilantin) if unresponsive. (6) Treat withdrawal with hydration and chlordiazepoxide (Librium) or diazepam. Large doses of sedatives may be required for delirium tremens. *Labora-*

tory aids: Arterial blood gases, electrolytes, blood ethanol levels, glucose; determine anion and osmolar gap and check for ketosis. Chest radiograph to determine whether aspiration pneumonia is present. Liver function tests and bilirubin levels.

2. ISOPROPANOL (rubbing alcohol). Normal propyl alcohol is related to isopropanol but is more toxic. *Manifestations:* Ethanol-like intoxication with acetone odor to breath, acetonuria, acetonemia without systemic acidosis, gastritis. With worsening acidosis, there is multiorgan failure, with death from complications of intractable acidosis. *Management:* (1) Gastrointestinal decontamination. Activated charcoal and cathartics not indicated. (2) Hemodialysis in life-threatening overdose (rarely needed). *Laboratory aids:* Isopropyl alcohol levels, acetone, glucose, and arterial blood gases.

3. METHANOL (wood alcohol). *Toxic dose:* One teaspoonful is potentially lethal for a 2-year-old child and can cause blindness in an adult. The toxic blood level of methanol is above 20 mg per dL, the potentially fatal level over 50 mg per dL. *Manifestations:* Metabolism may delay onset for 12 to 18 hours or longer if ethanol is ingested concomitantly. Hyperemia of optic disk, violent abdominal colic, blindness, and shock. With worsening acidosis, there is multiorgan failure, with death from complications of intractable acidosis. *Management:* (1) Gastrointestinal decontamination up to 1 hour. Activated charcoal and cathartics are not indicated. (2) Treat acidosis vigorously with sodium bicarbonate intravenously. (3) If clinically suspect methanol because of metabolic acidosis, with an anion gap if methanol concentration above 20 mg per dL, immediately initiate ethanol IV or PO to produce a blood ethanol concentration of 100 to 150 mg per dL (Antidote 21, Table 4). (4) Folinic acid and folic acid have been used successfully in animal investigations. Administer leucovorin, 1 mg per kg up to 50 mg IV every 4 hours for six doses. (5) Consider hemodialysis if the blood methanol level is greater than 50 mg per dL or if significant metabolic acidosis or visual or mental symptoms are present. *Note:* The ethanol dose has to be increased during dialysis therapy. (6) Continue therapy (ethanol and hemodialysis) until blood methanol level is preferably undetectable, and there is no acidosis and no mental or visual disturbances. This often requires 2 to 5 days. (7) Ophthalmology consultation. *Laboratory aids:* Methanol and ethanol levels, electrolytes, glucose, and arterial blood gases.

Alkali. See Caustics and Corrosives.

Amitriptyline (Elavil). See Tricyclic Antidepressants.

Amphetamines (diet pills, various trade names). *Toxicity:* Child, 5 mg per kg; adult, 12 mg per kg has been reported as lethal. *Toxicokinetics:* Peak time of action is 2 to 4 hours. t½, 8 to 10 hours in acid urine (pH less than 6.0) and 16 to 31 hours in alkaline urine (pH, 7.5). *Route of elimination:* Liver, 60%; kidney, 30 to 40% at alkaline urine pH; at acid urine pH, 50 to 70%. *Manifestations:* Dysrhythmias, hyperpyrexia, convulsions, hypertension, paranoia, violence. *Management:* (1) Gastrointestinal decontamination. Avoid induced emesis because of rapid onset of action. (2) Control extreme agitation or convulsions with diazepam. Chlorpromazine (Thorazine) may be dangerous if ingestion is not pure amphetamine. (3) Treat hypertensive crisis with nitroprusside at 0.3 to 2 mg per kg per minute; maximum infusion rate 10 μg per kg per minute; should never last more than 10 minutes. (4) Acidification diuresis is not recommended. (5) Treat hyperpyrexia symptomatically. (6) If focal neurologic symptoms, consider cerebrovascular accident. Obtain computed tomography scan. (7) Observe for suicidal depression that may follow intoxication. (8) In life-threatening agitation, use haloperidol (Haldol). (9) Significant life-threatening tachydysrhythmia may respond to the alpha and beta blocker labetalol (Normodyne; Antidote 27, Table 4) or other appropriate antidysrhythmic agents. In a severely hemodynamically compromised patient, use immediate synchronized cardioversion. *Laboratory aids:* Monitor for rhabdomyolysis (creatine phosphokinase [CPK]), myoglobinuria, hyperkalemia, and disseminated intravascular coagulation. Toxic blood level, 10 μg per dL.

Aniline. See Nitrites and Nitrates.

Anticholinergic Agents. Examples are antihistamines—hydroxyzine (Atarax), diphenhydramine (Benadryl); antipsychotics (neuroleptics)—phenothiazines (Thorazine); antidepressant drugs (tricyclic antidepressants)—imipramine (Tofranil); antiparkinsonian drugs—trihexyphenidyl (Artane), benztropine (Cogentin); over-the-counter sleep, cold, and hay fever medicine (methapyrilene); ophthalmic products (atropine); plants—jimsonweed (*Datura stramonium*), deadly nightshade (*Atropa belladonna*), henbane (*Hyoscyamus niger*); and antispasmodic agents for the bowel (atropine). *Toxicokinetics:* See Table 7. *Manifestations:* Anticholinergic signs—hyperpyrexia, dilated pupils, flushing of skin, dry mucosa, tachycardia, delirium, hallucinations, coma, and convulsions. *Management:* (1) Gastrointestinal decontamination up to 12 hours postingestion. *Note:* caution with emesis if diphenhydramine overdose because of rapid onset of action and seizures. (2) Control seizures with diazepam. (3) Control ventricular dysrhythmias with lidocaine. (4) Physostigmine (Antidote 35, Table 4)

TABLE 7. **Toxicokinetics of Anticholinergic Agents**

Drug	Potential Fatal Dose	Peak Effect	Vd (L/kg)	Half-life (h)	Excretion Route (%)
Atropine	Child: 10–20 mg; adult: 100 mg	1–2 h, may be prolonged in overdose	2.3	2–3	Renal (30–50); hepatic (50–70)
Diphenhydramine	Child: 25 mg/kg; adult: 2–8 gm	2 h, may be prolonged in overdose	3.3–6.8	3–10	98% hepatic

for life-threatening anticholinergic effects refractory to conventional treatments. (5) Relieve urinary retention by catheterization to avoid reabsorption. (6) Treat cardiac dysrhythmias only if tissue perfusion is not adequate or if the patient is hypotensive. (7) Control hyperpexia by external cooling. No antipyretics.

Anticonvulsants. See Table 8. *Toxic dose:* Specific anticonvulsant blood levels and the clinical manifestations indicate toxicity. In general, the ingestion of five times the therapeutic dose is expected to have the potential for toxicity. *Management:* (1) Gastrointestinal decontamination up to 12 hours postingestion. Repeated doses of activated charcoal shorten t½ of carbamazepine, phenobarbital, primidone, phenytoin, and possibly others. Naloxone (Antidote 30, Table 4) may improve valproic acid–induced coma. (2) Monitor specific anticonvulsant blood levels. (3) The effectiveness of hemoperfusion and dialysis has not been established.

Antidepressants. See Tricyclic Antidepressants.

Antifreeze. See Alcohols (Methanol) and Ethylene Glycol.

Antihistamines (H₁ Receptor Antagonists). See Anticholinergic Agents. Newer nonsedating long-acting preparations—terfenadine and astemizole—may produce prolonged QT intervals and torsades de pointes.

Arsenic and Arsine Gas. *Toxic dose:* In humans, the inorganic arsenic trioxide toxic dose is

TABLE 8. **Anticonvulsants**

Drug	Peak Time of Action/h (Steady State)	Vd (L/kg)	Half-life (h)	Route of Elimination (%)	Protein Binding (%)	Blood Level (μg/mL)	Comment*
Carbamazepine (Tegretol)	8–24 (2–4 days)	1.0	18–54	Liver (98)	70	Therapeutic, 4–10	Related to tricyclic antidepressants, can cause dysrhythmias
Ethosuximide (Zarontin)	24–48 (5–8 days)	0.8	36–55	Liver (80–90)	0	Therapeutic, 40–100	
Phenytoin (Dilantin)	PO 6–12 IV, 1 (5–10 days)	1.0	24; varies in toxic doses: zero-order kinetics	Liver (95)	90	Therapeutic, 10–20; toxic, 20–30; nystagmus only, 30–40; ataxia, 40+; coma, convulsions	Dysrhythmias with parenteral use only
Primidone (Mysoline)	?3–4 days	0.6	Parent, 3–12; metabolites, 30–36	Liver	60	Therapeutic, 6–12 primidone and 15–40 phenobarbital (PB); toxic, over 50 primidone and over 40 PB (see Barbiturates)	Metabolized to active metabolites phenylethylmalonamide and PB; overdose gives white crystals in urine†
Valproic acid (Depakene)	? 1–2 days	0.4	5–15	Liver (80–100)	84–96	Therapeutic, 50–100	Produces nausea and vomiting, changes in liver function
Clonazepam (Clonopin)	?		20–60	Liver (98)	90	Therapeutic, 20–70 ng/mL	
Phenobarbital (Luminal)	3–6 h	0.75	50–120	Liver	30	Therapeutic, 15–40	

*Manifestations: The major manifestations of these agents are depression of consciousness and respiratory depression. Other significant manifestations are mentioned in this column.

†Primidone produces whorls of shimmering white crystals in the urine from precipitation of intact primidone in massive overdose.

5 to 50 mg; the potential fatal dose is 120 mg or 1 to 2 mg per kg. Sodium arsenite is nine times more toxic than arsenic trioxide. Organic arsenic is less toxic. The maximum allowable concentration for prolonged exposure is 0.05 PPM. See Table 9. Humans are more sensitive than rodents to arsenic. Acute poisoning results from accidental ingestion of arsenic-containing pesticides. (Ant traps sold in some states contain arsenic.) *Toxicokinetics:* Arsenates are water soluble and arsenite is lipid soluble. The soluble forms of arsenic are rapidly absorbed by inhalation and ingestion. Crosses placenta and can cause fetal damage. Distributes into spleen, liver, kidneys. *Excretion:* In urine, 90%. Following acute ingestion, it takes 10 days to clear a single dose; chronic ingestion takes up to 70 days. *Arsine gas:* Forms when active hydrogen comes in contact with arsenic. This may occur when zinc, antimony, lead, or iron is contaminated with arsenic and comes in contact with acid. This causes arsine inhalation intoxication characterized by a latent period of 2 to 48 hours and a triad of abdominal pain, jaundice (due to hemolysis), and hematuria. *Manifestations:* Gastroenteritis, neurologic and cardiac abnormalities, subsequent renal involvement. A garlic odor to the breath may be a clue. Smaller doses and prolonged low-level exposure produce subacute (stomatitis) and chronic (peripheral neuropathy) symptoms. *Management:* (1) Gastrointestinal decontamination. Activated charcoal is ineffective. Cathartics are not advised because of potential for diarrhea. Follow with abdominal radiographs because arsenic is radiopaque. Consider whole-bowel washout if usual methods fail to remove arsenic. (2) Intravenous fluids to correct dehydration and electrolyte deficiencies. (3) Treat shock with oxygen, blood, and fluids as needed. (4) In severe cases, administer BAL (dimercaprol) (Antidote 17, Table 4). (5) In chronic poisoning, D-penicillamine (Antidote 34, Table 4) may be used to chelate arsenic. Therapy should be continued in 5-day cycles until the urine arsenic is less than 50 μg per liter. (6) Treat liver and renal impairment. (7) Hemodialysis is effective in acute poisoning and can be used concurrently with chelation therapy in severe cases, especially if renal failure devel-

ops. (8) Arsine intoxication is treated by exchange transfusion and hemodialysis if renal failure occurs. BAL is ineffective. *Laboratory aids:* Blood arsenic and 24-hour urine arsenic levels. Excessive exposure is indicated by a level of 50 μg per liter of arsenic in urine, but persons whose diets are rich in seafood may excrete larger amounts. View values over 50 μg per day with suspicion. Monitor electrocardiogram (ECG) and renal function. A blood arsenic level above 1.0 mg per liter is toxic, and one of 9 to 15 mg per liter is potentially fatal (false values occur in inexperienced laboratories).

Aspirin. See Salicylates.

Atropine. See Anticholinergic Agents.

Barbiturates. See Table 10. *Management:* (1) Gastrointestinal decontamination up to 8 to 12 hours. Avoid emesis in short-acting barbiturates. Activated charcoal and a cathartic in repeated doses have been shown to reduce the serum half-life and increase the nonrenal clearance over 50%. Give every 4 hours while the patient is comatose. (2) Supportive and symptomatic care is all that is necessary in the majority of cases. (3) Alkalinization with sodium bicarbonate, 2 mEq per kg IV during the first hour, followed by sufficient sodium bicarbonate (Antidote 39, Table 4) to keep the urinary pH at 7.5 to 8.0, enhances excretion of long-acting barbiturates. Alkalinization is not useful for short-acting barbiturates. Forced diuresis should be used with caution because of fluid overload. At present, alkalinization without diuresis is advocated. (4) In severe cases that do not respond to conservative measures, consider hemodialysis and hemoperfusion. (5) Treat any bullae as a local second-degree skin burn. (6) Give intensive care monitoring to the comatose patient. *Treatment of withdrawal:* In an emergency, use pentothal or diazepam intravenously. If the patient is stable, a pentobarbital is given orally and the patient examined after 1 hour for signs of intoxication (nystagmus, slurred speech, and ataxia). If none is present, the dose is repeated every 3 hours until these signs develop. This is the stabilizing dose; the patient is maintained on this dose for 72 hours and then changed to phenobarbital, 30 mg substituted for each 100 mg of pentobarbital. The phenobarbital is tapered, decreasing by 10% or 30 mg every 3 to 5 days. *Laboratory aids:* Emergency plasma barbiturate concentrations rarely alter management.

Benzene. See Hydrocarbons.

Benzodiazepines (BZP). See Table 11. *Toxicity:* Low toxic potential. More than 500 mg has been ingested without respiratory depression. Benzodiazepines have an additive effect with sedatives, such as alcohol and barbiturates. Most patients intoxicated with benzodiazepines alone recover within 24 hours. Many of these agents have ac-

TABLE 9. **Comparative Acute Toxicities of Some Common Arsenicals**

Arsenic Compound	Lethal Dose
Arsenate	5–50 mg/kg
Arsenites	<5 mg/kg
Arsenic trioxide (insoluble)	120 mg total
Arsenic trioxide (soluble)*	13 mg total

*Nine times as toxic as insoluble form.

TABLE 10. **Features of Barbiturates***

Feature	Long Acting (Lab)		Intermediate (IAB)	Short (SAB)
Duration	>8 h		3–8 h	<3 h
Medical use	Anticonvulsants		Sedative-hypnotics	
Half-life	>50 h		<50 h	<50 h
DEA	Schedule IV		Schedule II	Schedule II

Barbiturate	Barbital	Phenobarbital†	Amobarbital	Pentobarbital	Secobarbital
Trade name	Veronal	Luminal	Amytal	Nembutal	Seconal
Slang name	—	Purple hearts	Blues	Yellows	Red devils
pKa	7.8	7.24	7.9	7.96	7.9
Elimination route	Renal 20%	Renal 30%	Hepatic 98%	Hepatic >90%	Hepatic >90%
	Hepatic 80%	Hepatic 70%			
Onset IV	22 min	12 min	—	0.1 min	0.1 min
Onset oral	1 h	20–60 min	13–30 min	15–30 min	10–30 min
Peak conc oral	12–18 h	6–18 h	3–4 h	2–4 h	1–2 h
Protein-bound	6%	20–40%	40–60%	40–65%	40–60%
Oral doses					
Fatal dose	10 gm	8 gm	5 gm	3 gm	3 gm
	75 mg/kg	65 mg/kg	40 mg/kg	50 mg/kg	30 mg/kg
Toxic dose	>8 mg/kg	15–35 mg/kg	>6 mg/kg	>6 mg/kg	>6 mg/kg
Adult nontol		300 mg	200–300 mg	200–300 mg	200 mg
Therap dose	2–6 mg/kg	2–6 mg/kg	2–6 mg/kg	2–6 mg/kg	6 mg/kg
Adult dose	300–500 mg	100–200 mg	100–200 mg	100–200 mg	100–200 mg
Blood Concentrations					
Therap	5–8 µg/mL	15–40 µg/mL	5–6 µg/mL	1–5 µg/mL	1–5 µg/mL
Toxic	>30 µg/mL	>40 µg/mL	10–30 µg/mL	>10 µg/mL	>10 µg/mL
Lethal‡	>100 µg/mL	>100 µg/mL	>50 µg/mL	>35 µg/mL	>35 µg/mL
Duration	16 h	6–8 h	6 h	6 h	6 h
t½ elimin	56–96 h	50–120 h	15–40 h	15–30 h	22–29 h
Vd		0.75 L/kg	0.5 L/kg	0.65 L/kg	1.5 L/kg
Available					
Cap (mg)		16	65, 200	50, 100	50, 100
Tab (mg)		16, 32, 65, 100	15, 30, 50, 100	—	100
Elixr (mg/5 mL)		15, 20	—	20	—
Supp (mg)				30, 60, 120, 200	—

Manifestations
Low dose: Euphoria, ataxia, incoordination, nystagmus on lateral gaze
High dose: Flaccid coma, hypotension, respiratory depression, pulmonary edema (particularly with the short-acting barbiturates), subcutaneous bullae (6%), dermatographia

Abbreviations: DEA = Drug Enforcement Agency; conc = concentration; nontol = nontolerant; therap = therapeutic; t½ = half-life; elimin = elimination; Vd = volulme of distribution; cap = capsule; tab = tablet; elixr = elixir; supp = suppository.
*Classification into long acting, intermediate, and short acting has no relationship to the duration of coma.
†The half-life (t½) in children is approximately 50% of adult.
‡These levels are not absolute, and tolerance occurs.

tive metabolites with a long plasma t½, so performance in skilled tasks, such as driving, may be impaired. Withdrawal may be delayed. *Manifestations:* CNS depression. Deep coma leading to respiratory depression suggests presence of other drugs. *Management:* (1) Gastrointestinal decontamination. (2) Supportive and symptomatic care. (3) Flumazenil is a recently approved specific benzodiazepine antagonist. It is not a treatment for hypoventilation and should be used in caution with overdose because of dependency and seizures (Antidote 23, Table 4). (4) Withdrawal, if it occurs, is treated with a long-acting benzodiazepine on a tapering schedule. *Laboratory aids:* Document benzodiazepines in urine. Quantitative blood levels are not useful.

Bleach. Household bleaches are 4 to 6% sodium hypochlorite. Commercial types are 10 to 20%. *Manifestations:* Difficulty in swallowing; pain in mouth, throat, chest, or abdomen. General household strength bleach does not produce burns; commercial strength bleach may. Inhalation of gases produced by mixing chlorine bleach with acids (toilet bowl cleaner and rust removers—chlorine gas) or with household ammonia (chloramine gas) is irritating to mucous membranes, eyes, and upper respiratory tract. *Management:* (1) Ingestion—avoid gastrointestinal decontamination procedures. Dilute with small amounts of water or milk. Avoid acids. (2) Esophagoscopy only if unusually large amounts have been ingested, the patient is symptomatic, or the

TABLE 11. **Benzodiazepines (BZP)**

Drug	Oral Dosage Range	Peak Oral Plasma Levels (h)	Half-life (h)	Major Active Metabolites (Half-life in h)	Elimination Rate
Anxiolytics					
Diazepam (Valium)	6–40 mg/day	1–2	20–50	Desmethyldiazepam (30–60)	Slow
Chlordiazepoxide (Librium, Libritabs, various others)	15–100 mg/day	2–4	5–30	Desmethylchlordiazepoxide, demoxepam, desmethyldiazepam	Slow
Clorazepate (Tranxene)	15–60 mg/day	1–2.5	30–60	Desmethyldiazepam	Slow
Prazepam (Centrax)	20–60 mg/day	6	78	3-Hydroxyprazepam, desmethyldiazepam	Slow
Halazepam (Paxipam)	60–160 mg/day	1–3	7	N-3-Hydroxyhalazepam, desmethyldiazepam	Slow
Oxazepam (Serax)	30–120 mg/day	1–2	3–10	None	Rapid to intermediate
Lorazepam (Ativan)	2–6 mg/day	2	10–20	None	Intermediate
Alprazolam (Xanax)	0.75–4 mg/day	0.7–1.6	12–19	α-Hydroxyalprazolam	Intermediate
Hypnotics					
Flurazepam (Dalmane)	15–60 mg	3–6	50–100	Desalkylflurazepam (50–100)	Slow
Midazolam (Versed)	5–30 mg/day IV	0.3–0.8	3–5	None	—
Flunitrazepam (Rohypnol— investigational, Roche)	1–2 mg	<1	—	7-Aminoflunitrazepam (23), N-desmethylflunitrazepam (31)	—
Tamazepam (Restoril)	15–30 mg	2–3	9–12	None	Intermediate
Triazolam (Halcion)	0.125–0.5 mg	0.5–1.5	2–3	α-Hydroxytriazolam	Rapid
Anticonvulsant					
Clonazepam (Klonopin)	1.5–20 mg/day	1–4	24–48	None	—

product was stronger than the average household bleach. (3) Inhalation—Remove from contaminated area. Observe for pulmonary edema. (4) Ocular exposure requires immediate gentle irrigation with water for at least 15 minutes, followed by fluorescein dye stain for damage.

Botulism. See article Food-Borne Illness in Section 2.

Brake Fluid. See Ethylene Glycol.

Calcium Channel Blockers. Used in treatment of effort angina, supraventricular tachycardia, and hypertension. See Table 12. *Manifestations:* Hypotension, bradycardia within 1 to 5 hours, CNS depression, and gastric distress. Manifestations are delayed after ingestion of slow-release preparations. *Management:* (1) Gastrointestinal decontamination. If long-acting preparation, consider whole-bowel washout. If symptomatic, obtain cardiac consult. May need pacemaker. (2) Treat hypotension and bradycardia with positioning, fluids, and calcium gluconate or chloride (Antidote 12B, Table 4). Dopamine or norepinephrine may be used if necessary. If calcium fails use sodium bicarbonate, glucagon, or both (Antidote 26, Table 4). (3) Heart block—may respond to intravenous calcium (Antidote 12B, Table 4) or atropine sulfate, 0.5 to 1 mg, if no response. (4) Ventricular pacing may be required in the severely intoxicated patient. (5) Patients receiving digitalis run the risk of toxicity and should be carefully monitored. (6) Extracorporeal measures are generally not considered to be useful. *Laboratory aids:* Specific drug levels, blood sugar and calcium, ECG.

Camphor (External analgesic rubs, Vicks Vaporub 4.8%, Campho-Phenique 11%). Many camphorated oil products were removed from the marketplace in September, 1982. Five milliliters of camphorated oil (20% camphor) equals 1 gram of camphor. *Toxicity:* More than 10 mg per kg may cause seizures. Adult, 5 grams; child, 1 gram has been fatal. *Toxicokinetics:* Onset of manifestations, 5 to 90 minutes. Readily and rapidly absorbed through the skin, mucous membranes, and gastrointestinal tract, and crosses the placenta. Route of elimination: Rapidly metabolized in liver to the glucuronide form, which is excreted in urine. Pulmonary excretion causes a distinctive odor on the breath. *Manifestations:* Nausea, vomiting, and burning epigastric pain. Seizures may occur suddenly and without warning within 5 minutes of ingestion. Apnea and vision disturbances may occur. *Management:* (1) Induction of emesis is contraindicated because of early seizures. (2) Remove residual drug by gastric lavage. (3) Administer activated charcoal and a saline

TABLE 12. **Kinetics of the Calcium Channel Blockers**

Parameter	Nifedipine	Verapamil	Diltiazem	Nicardipine	Nimodipine	Felodipine*
Class	Dihydropyridine	Phenylalkylamine	Benzothiazepine	Dihydropyridine	Dihydropyridine	Dihydropyridine
Trade name	Procardia	Calan, Isoptin	Cardizem	Cardene	Nimotop	Plendil
Preparations	10-, 20-mg cap	80-, 12-mg tab	30-, 60-, 90-, 120-mg tab	20-, 30-mg cap	30 mg	5 mg
Slow release	30-, 60-, 90-mg caps	240-mg tab	30-, 60-, 90-mg tab	None	None	None
Bioavailability	65–70%	20–30%	40%	35%	3–30%	20%
Mean toxic dose	340 mg	3.2 gm	? rare toxicity	NA	NA	NA
Serious toxic amount	Lowest 200 mg	40 mg/kg child 2–3 gm adult	Up to 300 mg well tolerated by adults	NA	NA	NA
Onset of action						
Oral	<20 min	30–120 min	<15 min	<20 min	<20 min	—
IV	<1 min	<3 min	<1 min	—	—	—
Sublingual	3–5 min	—	—	—	—	—
Peak action						
Oral	30–90 min	60–90 min	30–60 min	60 min	60 min	2.5–6 h
Sublingual	20 min	—	—	—	—	—
Sustained	—	4–8 h	3–4 h	—	—	—
Peak blood conc	30–60 min	90–120 min	120–180 min	60 min	NA	NA
Half-life	3–6 h	6–12 h	4–9 h	8 h	1–8 h	24 h
Duration	4–12 h	6–12 h	—	4–6 h	NA	—
Protein binding	92–98%	90–99%	70–85%	>95%	>95%	NA
Vd	1–5 L/kg	4.5–7 L/kg	3–5 L/kg	NA	—	—
Elimination	Renal 50–70%	Hepatic 60–65%	Renal 70–80%	Liver	—	—
Metabolite	Inactive	Active mild norverapamil	Active 50% parent diacetyldiltiazem	NA	NA	NA

Abbreviations: cap = capsules; tab = tablets; NA = no available information; conc = concentration.
*Anonymous: Felodipine—another calcium channel blocker for hypertension. Med Lett *33*:115–116, 1991.

cathartic. Avoid giving oils or alcohol. (4) Treat seizures with intravenous diazepam. (5) Treat apnea with respiratory support.

Carbon Monoxide (CO). This is an odorless gas produced from incomplete combustion; it is found also as an in vivo metabolic breakdown product of methylene chloride (paint removers). Observe for the symptoms described in Table 13. Contrary to popular belief, the skin rarely shows a cherry-red color in the live patient. *Toxicokinetics:* CO is rapidly absorbed through the lungs. The rate of absorption is directly related to alveolar ventilation. Elimination occurs through the lungs. The t½ in room air equals 5 to 6 hours; in 100% oxygen, 90 minutes; in hyperbaric oxygen, 20 minutes. The nomogram pictured in Figure 2 can be used to decide quickly whether serious CO intoxication is likely to have occurred and to select patients at high risk or who need early management in the intensive care unit or hyperbaric oxygen. *Management:* (1) Remove the patient from contaminated area and expose to fresh air. Establish vital functions. (2) Give 100% oxygen to all patients until the carboxyhemoglobin level falls to 5% or less. Assisted ventilation may be necessary. The exposed pregnant woman should

TABLE 13. **Carbon Monoxide (CO)**

CO in Atmosphere (PPM)	Duration of Exposure	Saturation of Blood (%)	Symptoms
Up to 0.01	Indefinite	1–10	None
0.01–0.02	Indefinite	10–20	Tightness across forehead, slight headache, dilation of cutaneous vessels
0.02–0.03	5–6 h	20–30	Headache, throbbing temples
0.04–0.06	4–5 h	30–40	Severe headache, weakness and dizziness, nausea and vomiting, collapse, leukocytosis
0.07–0.10	3–4 h	40–50	Above, plus increased tendency to collapse and syncope, increased pulse and respiratory rate
0.11–0.15	1.5–3 h	50–60	Increased pulse and respiratory rate, syncope, Cheyne-Stokes respiration, coma with intermittent convulsions
0.16–0.30	1–1.5 h	60–70	Coma with intermittent convulsions, depressed heart action and respirations, death possible
0.50–1.00	1–2 h	70–80	Weak pulse, depressed respirations, respiratory failure, and death

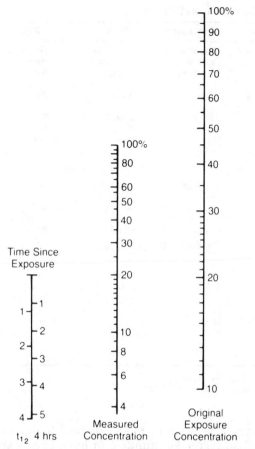

Figure 2. Nomogram for calculating carboxyhemoglobin concentration at time of exposure. The time since exposure is given on two scales to allow for the effects of previous oxygen administration on the half-life of carboxyhemoglobin (left-hand scale assumes a half-life of 3 hours). *Note:* The nomogram assumes a half-life of carboxyhemoglobin of 4 hours in a subject breathing room air. Most patients will not have received supplementary oxygen before admission, and at best this will have been administered via a face mask, giving a maximum fractional inspired oxygen concentration of 50 to 60% with little effect on carboxyhemoglobin elimination. The scale on the left side of the time column makes allowances for prior oxygen supplements by assuming a short half-life of 3 hours. The nomogram may help decide quickly whether serious carbon monoxide intoxication is likely to have occurred and may help select patients at high risk for early management in the intensive care unit. The nomogram may be an oversimplification because patients usually are not resuscitated with constant concentrations of oxygen, and many patients may hyperventilate, thus changing elimination characteristics. (Redrawn from Clark CJ, et al: Blood carboxyhaemoglobin and cyanide levels in fire survivors. Lancet *1*:1332, 1981.)

be kept in 100% oxygen for several hours after the carboxyhemoglobin level is zero because carboxyhemoglobin concentrates in the fetus and oxygen is needed five times longer to ensure elimination of CO from fetal circulation. CO or hypoxia may be teratogenic. (3) Monitor arterial blood gases and carboxyhemoglobin levels. Determine carboxyhemoglobin level at time of exposure by using nomogram. *Note:* A near-normal carboxyhemoglobin level does not rule out significant CO poisoning. (4) Only if pH is below 7.1 after correction of hypoxia and adequate ventilation, give sodium bicarbonate to correct acidosis. (5) Indications for 100% oxygen and if possible therapy with hyperbaric oxygen: (a) carboxyhemoglobin level higher than 25%; (b) carboxyhemoglobin level higher than 15% in a child or in a patient with cardiovascular disease; (c) carboxyhemoglobin level higher than 10% in a pregnant woman (and monitor fetus); (d) abnormal or ischemic chest pain or ECG abnormality; (e) abnormal chest x-ray; (f) presence of hypoxia, myoglobinuria, or abnormal renal function; (g) history of unconsciousness, syncope, or neuropsychiatric symptoms. Most important indication for hyperbaric chamber is history of unconsciousness. A list of hyperbaric oxygen chambers can be obtained by contacting a Regional Poison Control Center. (6) Treat seizures with intravenous diazepam. (7) Monitor ECG, chest radiograph, and serum CPK and lactate dehydrogenase levels. (8) Treat cerebral edema with elevation of the patient's head, minimizing intravenous fluid, hyperventilation, and, if needed, mannitol and intracranial pressure monitor. (9) Reevaluate after recovery for neuropsychiatric sequelae. *Laboratory aids:* Arterial blood gases show metabolic acidosis and normal oxygen tension but reduced oxygen saturation, as measured by a co-oximeter.

Carbon Tetrachloride. See Hydrocarbons.

Caustics and Corrosives. Common acid substances are hydrochloric acid, sulfuric acid (battery acid), carbolic acid (phenol), nitric acid, oxalic acid, hydrofluoric acid, and aqua regia (mixture of hydrochloric and nitric acids). These are used as cleaning agents. Common alkali substances are sodium or potassium hydroxide (lye), sodium hypochlorite (Clorox) (bleach), sodium carbonate (nonphosphate detergents), potassium permanganate, ammonia, electric dishwashing agents, cement, and flat disk batteries. *Toxicity:* Acids produce mucosal coagulation necrosis. They usually do not penetrate deeply (exception: hydrofluoric acid). The gastric mucosa is the primary site of injury. Alkalis produce liquefaction necrosis and saponification and penetrate deeply. Oropharyngeal and esophageal damage by solids is more frequent than by liquids. Liquids are more likely to produce gastric damage. *Toxic dose:* Adult potential fatal dose of concentrated acid/alkali is 5 mL. The absence of oral burns does not exclude the possibility of esophageal burns (10 to 15%). *Management:* (1) Dilute with milk or water immediately up to 30 mL in children or 250 mL in adults. Neutralization with acidic or alkalinic agents is contraindicated. Dilute only if patient can swallow. Contradictions to dilution are an inability to swallow, signs of respiratory distress, shock, or esophageal perforation. (2) Gastrointestinal decontamination is contraindicated. In acid ingestions, however, some authorities advocate nasogastric intubation and aspiration in the early postingestion phase. Patient should receive only intravenous fluids following dilution until surgical consultation is obtained. Dermal and ocular decontamination should be carried out. (3) Endoscopy at 12 to 48 hours may be indicated postingestion to assess severity of burn. (4) Steroids are controversial. (5) Antibiotics are not useful prophylactically. (6) Barium swallow may be necessary at 10 days to 3 weeks to assess severity of damage. (7) Esophageal dilation may need to be performed at 2- to 4-week intervals if evidence of stricture is found. (8) Intraposition of the colon may be necessary if dilation fails to provide an adequate-sized esophagus. (9) Inhalation management requires immediate removal from the environment, and clinical, x-ray, and arterial blood gas evaluation when appropriate. Oxygen and respiratory support may be required.

Chloral Hydrate. See Sedative Hypnotics.

Chlordane. See Organochlorine Insecticides.

Chlordiazepoxide (Librium) See Benzodiazepines.

Chlorine Gas. Chlorine gas is a yellow greenish gas with an irritating odor used in bleach, in manufacture of plastics, and for water purification. Exposure usually results from transportation mishaps, industrial accidents, chemistry experiments, the mixing of household cleaners with bleach containing hypochlorite; and accidental release around swimming pools. Its density is greater than that of air, and an odor is detected at concentrations of less than 0.04 to 0.2 PPM. Chlorine acts as an oxidizing agent and also acts with tissue water to form hypochlorous and hydrochloric acid and generate free oxygen radicals. *Toxic dose:* The threshold limit value is less than 1 PPM, but mild mucous irritation occurs in some patients; 30 PPM produces choking and chest pain; 60 PPM produces pulmonary edema; 400 PPM for 30 minutes is lethal; and 1000 PPM is fatal in a few minutes. *Management:* (1) Remove the patient from contaminated environment and stabilize vital functions. Decontamination procedures for dermal and ocular contamination as indicated. Protect rescue personnel with breathing apparatus. There are patients who have responded to nebulized 3.75% sodium bicarbonate (4 mL) (prepared by diluting 2 mL of 7.5% IV sodium bicarbonate with 2 mL saline). Classification—If symptomless or with a cough that clears up in less than 1 hour, rest for 12 hours and report if symptoms occur; no vigorous exercise for 24 hours. If symptoms persist beyond period of exposure, admit to hospital and treat with bronchodilators (use aerosol beta agonists and theophylline, not epinephrine) and humidified oxygen. Noncardiac pulmonary edema is treated with PEEP; corticosteroids are controversial; furosemide (Lasix) may be used. For conjunctival irritation, copious water irrigation and fluorescein stain for corneal damage. For dermal burns, copious water irrigation and conventional treatment of burns. *Laboratory aids:* Chest radiograph (may not reflect damage for 24 hours), arterial blood gases, cardiac monitor for dysrhythmias.

Chlorpromazine (Thorazine). See Phenothiazines and Other Major Neuroleptics.

Clinitest Tablets. See Caustics and Corrosives.

Cocaine (Benzoylmethylecgonine). *Toxic dose:* The potential fatal dose is 1200 mg, but death has occurred with 20 mg parenterally. *Toxicokinetics:* See Table 14. *Manifestations:* Hypertension, convulsions, hyperthermia, and cardiac dysrhythmias. *Management:* (1) Supportive care. Avoid induction of emesis or gastric lavage because of rapid onset of action of cocaine. Blood pressure and thermal monitoring. Phenytoin may be effective for ventricular dysrhythmias, whereas lidocaine may be ineffective and enhance toxicity. Nitroprusside infusion, 0.5 to 10 μg per kg per minute, may be used for severe hypertension. Avoid propranolol. Control anxiety and convulsions with diazepam. Labetalol intravenously (Antidote 27, Table 4) has been used to control life-threatening hypertension and tachycardia. A nonthreatening environment to reduce all sensory stimuli and protect patient from injury is required. Apply precautions against suicide attempts and monitor the fetus if patient is a pregnant woman. The management of the "body packer" and "body stuffer" is to administer repeated doses of activated charcoal (except plastic vials), secure venous access, and have drugs readily available for treating life-threatening manifestations until contraband is passed in the stool. Surgical removal may be indicated if material does not pass the pylorus. Endoscopy may be used to remove hard plastic vials, but not the bags, containing crack. Whole-body irrigation may be useful if plastic vials or bags were ingested.

Codeine. See Opioids.

Corrosives. See Caustics and Corrosives.

Cyanide. See Table 15. Hydrocyanic acid and sodium and potassium salts act rapidly and are extremely poisonous. The acid is extremely volatile, producing cyanide, which has a distinctive odor of bitter almonds and can produce death within minutes after inhalation. Cyanide interferes with the cytochrome oxidase system.

TABLE 14. **Pharmacotoxicokinetics of Cocaine**

Type	Route	Onset	Peak	Duration Half-life (min)	Possible Fatal Dose (Adult)
Hydrochloride	Insufflation	1–5 min	15–60 min	60–75	750–800 mg
	Ingested	Delayed	50–90 min	Sustained	1.4 gm
	IV	30–120 sec	5–11 min	60–90	20–800 mg
Coca paste	Smoked			Not known	
Crack and free base	Smoked	(Fastest) 5–10 sec	5–11 sec	Up to 20 min	Not known

Classes of cyanides and derivatives: (1) Hydrogen cyanide and simple salts in large doses act to produce death in 15 minutes. (2) Halogenated cyanides, such as cyanogen chloride, produce irritant and vesicant gases that may cause pulmonary edema. (3) Nitriles, such as acrylonitrile and acetonitrile (artificial nail removers). (4) Residential fires. Cyanides are used as fumigants (hydrogen cyanide), in synthetic rubber (acrylonitrile), in fertilizers (cyanamide), in metal refining (salts), and in the home in some silver and furniture polishes. Cyanide in the seeds of fruit stones is harmful only if the capsule is broken. *Manifestations:* Seizures, stupor, cardiac dysrhythmias, pulmonary edema, lactic acidemia, decreased arterial venous oxygen difference. Bright red venous blood. *Management:* Attendants should not administer mouth-to-mouth resuscitation. (1) Immediately, 100% oxygen. If inhaled, remove patient from contaminated atmosphere. (2) Cyanide antidote kit (Antidote 14, Table 4). Use antidote only if certain of diagnosis or residential fires involving plastics, urethane, or upholstery plus: (a) significant toxicity (impairment of consciousness); (b) manifestations not corrected by oxygen and out of proportion to carboxyhemoglobin level; and (c) lactic acidosis and bright red venous blood with high or normal PaO_2. (3) Gastrointestinal decontamination by gastric lavage. *No* syrup of ipecac. Activated charcoal is used but is not very effective (1 gram binds only 35 mg of cyanide). (4) Treat seizures with intravenous diazepam. (5) Correct acidosis. (6) Other antidotes: In Europe, dicobalt edetate, 600 mg, is used intravenously, followed by 300 mg if the response is not satisfactory. Hydroxycobalamin (vitamin B_{12}) is a useful antidote but must be given immediately after exposure in large doses. Dose: 1800 mg of vitamin B_{12} per dL of potassium cyanide (KCN) is usually required (forms cyanocobalamin).

DDT and Derivatives. See Organochlorine Insecticides.

Desipramine (Norpramin, Pertofrane). See Tricyclic Antidepressants.

Diazepam (Valium). See Benzodiazepines.

Digitalis Preparations. See Table 16. *Mani-* *festations:* Manifestations may be delayed 9 to 18 hours. Abdominal pain, nausea, vomiting, diarrhea, dysrhythmias, heart block, CNS depression, colored-halo vision. No dysrhythmia on ECG is characteristic of digitalis toxicity. *Management:* (1) Gastrointestinal decontamination. Avoid ipecac syrup; it may increase the vagal effect if patient is symptomatic. Repeated doses of activated charcoal may interrupt enterohepatic recirculation. (2) Treat ventricular premature contractions, including bigeminy, trigeminy, quadrigeminy, ventricular tachycardia, and atrial tachycardia, with phenytoin. Lidocaine also may be administered for ventricular dysrhythmias. Magnesium sulfate, 20 mL 20% IV slowly over 20 minutes, has been useful for malignant ventricular dysrhythmias, such as torsades de pointes. (3) Treat bradycardia and second-degree and third-degree atrioventricular block with atropine or low-dose phenytoin, 25 mg per dose IV in adults. Insertion of a pacemaker should be seriously considered. Avoid isoproterenol, which causes dysrhythmias. External pacing may be needed. (4) Treat hyperkalemia (above 5.5 mEq per liter) with Fab (antibody fragments) (Digibind) (Antidote 22, Table 4). Hemodialysis is treatment of choice for severe or refractory hyperkalemia. (5) Direct current countershock may cause life-threatening dysrhythmias. (6) Specific Fab antibody fragments (Digibind) (Antidote 22, Table 4) have been used if cardiac arrest or shock is imminent; 10 mg in an adult, 4 mg (or over 0.3 mg per kg) in a child, or lower doses (0.2 mg per kg) in an adolescent are ingested, for hyperkalemia (>5.5 mEq per liter), or serum digoxin toxicity (>10 ng per mL in adults or >5 ng per mL in children) at 6 to 8 hours postingestion, or life-threatening dysrhythmias. Contact Poison Control Center for calculation of Fab or use package insert. *Laboratory aids:* Monitor ECG and potassium and digitalis levels. Draw digoxin levels 6 to 8 hours postingestion, as well as when it is given by the IV route. An endogenous digoxin-like substance that cross-reacts with most common immunoassay antibodies, with values as high as 4.1 ng per mL, has been reported in new-

TABLE 15. **Sources of Cyanide and Their Toxicity**

Plants Containing Cyanide Glycosides

Common Name	Part of Plant	Botanical Name
Apple	Seeds	*Malus* spp
Apricot		*Prunus armeniaca*
Arrow grass		*Triglochin* spp
Bamboo	Sprouts, stems	Tribe Bambuseae
Bermuda grass		*Cynodon dactylon*
Bird's-foot trefoil		*Lotus corniculatus*
Bitter almond		*Prunus amygdalus amara*
Blackthorn, sloe		*Prunus spinosa*
Calabash tree		*Crescentia cujete*
Cassava	Beans and roots	*Manihot esculenta*
Catclaw		*Acacia greggi*
Cherry laurel		*Prunus laurocerasus*
Chokecherry		*Prunus virginiana*
Cotoneaster		*Cotoneaster* spp
Cycad nut		*Zamia pumila*
Elderberry	Leaves and shoots	*Sambucus* spp
Eucalyptus		*Eucalyptus cladocalyx*
False sago palm		*Cycas circinalis*
Flax		*Linum usitatissimum*
Hyacinth bean	Bean	*Dolichos lablab*
Hydrangea	Leaves and bulb	*Hydrangea* spp
Jetbead		*Rhodotypos tetrapetala*
Johnson grass		*Sorghum halepense*
Lima bean		*Phaseolus lunatus* (not in United States)
Mountain mahogany		*Cercocarpus montanus*
Passionflower (African)		*Adenia volkensii*
Peach		*Prunus persica*
Pear	Seeds	*Pyrus communis*
Plains bahia		*Bahia oppositifolia*
Plum		*Prunus domestica*
Poison suckleya		*Suckleya suckleyana*
Queen's delight		*Stillingia sylvatica*
Sudan grass		*Sorghum* spp.
Velvet grass		*Holcus lanatus*
Vetch	Seed	*Vicia sativa*

Hydrogen Cyanide Liberated from Samples of Carcinogenic Glycosides

Sample	HCN (mg/gm or mL)
Laetrile (amygdalin)	
Sigma	55.9
Tablet yellow	400
Kemdalin	14.1
Apricot seeds	2.92
Peach seeds	2.60
Apple seeds	0.61
Laetrile is 500-mg tablet for oral use, which is 6% cyanide by weight	

Forms of Cyanide and Their Toxicity

Product	Toxicity (Potential Lethal Dose)
Hydrocyanic acid	50 mg (1.0 mg/kg)
Potassium/sodium cyanide	150–300 mg (2 mg/kg)
Ferriferrocyanide (Prussian blue)	50 gm
Sodium nitroprusside	5 mg/kg causes toxicity
Bitter almonds	
Oil	2 oz
Almonds	50–60 (each contains 0.001 gm of cyanide)
Pulp	240 gm
Apricot	
Wild	100 gm of moist seed = 217 mg of cyanide
Cultivated	100 gm = 8.7 mg of cyanide

borns, patients with chronic renal failure, and patients with abnormal immunoglobulin levels. The bound digoxin blood concentrations rise after use of Fab, but the free (usually unmeasured) digoxin level falls.

Diphenhydramine (Benadryl). See Anticholinergic Agents.

Doxepin (Sinequan, Adapin). See Tricyclic Antidepressants.

Ethchlorvynol (Placidyl). See Sedative Hypnotics.

Ethyl Alcohol. See Alcohols.

Ethylene Glycol (solvent, antifreeze). *Toxic dose:* Death has occurred after a 60-ml ingestion; fatal dose = 1.4 mL per kg of 100% solution. The TLV is 50 PPM. *Toxicokinetics:* Time of onset, 30 minutes to 12 hours for CNS and metabolic abnormalities to occur (Phase I). Twelve to 36 hours postingestion, cardiopulmonary depression (Phase II). In Phase III (2 to 3 days postingestion), renal failure occurs. The $t\frac{1}{2}$ is 3 hours (during ethanol therapy this is prolonged to 17 hours). Urine oxalate or monohydrate crystals may be seen 4 to 8 hours postingestion but are not always present. *Management:* (1) Gastrointestinal decontamination up to 30 minutes postingestion. Activated charcoal and cathartics are not indicated. (2) Treat seizures with intravenous diazepam. Exclude hypocalcemia and treat if necessary. (3) Correct acidosis with intravenous sodium bicarbonate. (4) Initiate ethanol therapy to block metabolism (Antidote 21, Table 4) if the blood ethylene glycol level is higher than 20 mg per dL, or if the patient is symptomatic or acidotic with increased anion gap or osmolar gap. Ethanol should be administered intravenously or orally to produce a blood ethanol concentration of 100 to 150 mg per dL. (5) Early hemodialysis is indicated if the ingestion was large; if the blood ethylene glycol level is greater than 50 mg per dL; if severe acid-base or electrolyte abnormalities occur despite conventional therapy; or if renal failure occurs. (6) Thiamine (100 mg) and pyridoxine (50 mg four times daily) have been recommended for 48 hours but have not been extensively studied. (7) Continue therapy (ethanol and hemodialysis) until the plasma ethylene glycol level is below 10 mg per dL, the acidosis has cleared, the creatinine level is normal, and urinary output is adequate. *Laboratory aids:* Complete blood count, electrolytes, urinalysis (look for oxalate ["envelope"] and monohydrate ["hemp seed"] crystals), and arterial blood gases. The oral mucosa and urine fluoresce if ethylene glycol is present. Obtain ethylene glycol and ethanol levels, plasma osmolarity (use freezing point depression method). Calcium, creatinine, and blood urea nitrogen studies. An ethylene glycol level of 20 mg per dL is usually toxic (levels are very difficult

TABLE 16. **Toxicity and Kinetics of Common Digitalis Preparations**

Characteristic	Digoxin	Digitoxin
Trade name	Lanoxin	Crystodigin
Loading dose (LD) over 18–24 h	Varies with age	Varies with age
Premature	0.005 mg/kg	
Range <10 years	0.020–0.060 mg/kg	<2 years 0.025–0.04 mg/kg
Range >10 years	0.010–0.015 mg/kg	>2 years 0.020–0.02 mg/kg
Total adult	0.5–7.5 mg	0.8–1.4 mg
Maintenance dose (MD)	25–35% of LD	10% of LD
Total adult	0.125–0.50 mg	0.05–0.2 mg
Toxic dose		
Child	0.3 mg/kg	NA
Normal adult	2 mg	3–5 mg
Adult fatal dose	10–20 mg	3–10 mg
GI absorption	50–80%	90–100%
Tablet bioavailable	60–75%	
Capsule bioavailable	95%	
Elixir bioavailable	85%	
Onset oral	15–30 min	25–120 min
Peak IV	1.5–6 h	4–12 h
Peak oral	3–6 h	4–12 h
Duration of action	3–6 days	2–3 weeks
Protein bound	25%	>90%
Vd		
In neonate	7.5–10 L/kg	
In infants and children	16 L/kg	
In adults	5–8 L/kg	0.6 L/kg
Fetal plasma concentrations equal maternal concentrations		
Half-life		
In premature	37–170 h	
In neonates	35–69 h	
In infants	19–35 h	
In adults	26–45 h (1½ days)	6–8 days or longer
Shorter in overdose	6–22 h	
Elimination	Renal 75%	Liver 80%
Active metabolite	None	8% converted digoxin
Plasma concentration should be measured 6–8 h after last dose		
Therap plasma conc	0.5–2 ng/mL	15–30 ng/mL
Toxic plasma conc	>2.5 ng/mL varies	>35 ng/mµg/mL
There is considerable overlap between therapeutic and toxic ranges		
Normal blood concentrations do not exclude toxicity		
Serious toxic conc	>10 ng/mL	
Healthy children tolerate high concentrations better than adults		
Enterohepatic recirculation	Up to 14%	30%
Availability		
Capsules	0.05, 0.1, 0.2 mg	
Tablets	0.125, 0.25, 0.50 mg	0.05, 0.1, 0.15, 0.2 mg
Elixir	0.05 mg/mL	0.05 mg/mL

Sources: Clinical Data Handbook 1988, pp 472–474; AMA Drug Evaluations 1986, pp 425–427.
SI conversion factor ng/ml × 1.281 = mmol/L; NA = not available.

to obtain). The oral mucosa and urine will fluoresce under Wood's light if ethylene glycol is present.

Flurazepam (Dalmane). See Benzodiazepines.

Fluoxetine (Prozac). *Toxic dose:* >3.5 mg/kg in children. Adult fatal dose, 6 grams. Over 1800 mg has produced seizures. *Manifestations:* Minimal risk of cardiovascular or neurologic complica-

tions. *Toxicokinetics:* See Table 30. *Management:* See Tricyclic Antidepressants.

Glutethimide (Doriden). See Sedative Hypnotics.

Hallucinogens

1. LSD (lysergic acid diethylamide). *Toxic dose:* ≥35 µg. Street doses are typically 50 to 300 µg. *Toxicokinetics:* Peak effect, 1 to 2 hours. Dura-

tion, 12 to 24 hours. t½, 3 hours. Route of elimination, hepatic.

2. MORNING GLORY SEEDS (*Rivea corymbosa* or *Ipomoea*). These have one-tenth the potency of LSD.

3. MESCALINE/PEYOTE (trimethoxyphenylethylamine or *Lophophora williamsii*). *Toxic dose:* ≥5 mg per kg. Each button of mescaline contains 45 mg (4 to 12 produce symptoms). *Toxicokinetics:* Peak effect, 4 to 6 hours. Duration, 14 hours.

4. PSILOCYBIN. Similar in effect to LSD but short acting. Peak effect, 90 minutes. Duration, 5 to 6 hours.

5. NUTMEG (*Myristica*). *Toxic dose:* 5 to 15 grams (1 to 3 nutmegs). Peak effect, 3 to 6 hours. Duration, up to 60 hours.

6. MARIJUANA (*Cannabis sativa*) (Δ⁹-tetrahydrocannabinol, THC). One joint equals 500 mg of marijuana; when smoked, 50% is destroyed. *Toxicokinetics:* Time of onset, 2 to 3 minutes (smoked). Duration, 2 to 3 hours. t½, 28 to 47 hours (shorter for chronic user). *Note:* 1% of the metabolite can be detected in urine up to 2 weeks after use. *Manifestations:* Visual illusions, sensory perceptual distortions, depersonalization, and derealization. *Management:* "Talk-down" technique.

7. INHALANTS. Nitrites (amyl and isobutyl nitrite)—act immediately; aromatic hydrocarbon in airplane model glues, plastic cements (benzene, toluene, xylene)—see Hydrocarbons; *nitrous oxide* and *halogenated hydrocarbons.*

8. TRYPTAMINE DERIVATIVES (DMT, *N*-dimethyltryptamine; DET, diethyltryptamine; DPT, dipropyltryptamine). Rapid onset of action, but duration is only 1 to 2 hours.

9. STP OR DOM (2,5-dimethoxy-4-methylamphetamine). Acts like LSD but lasts 72 hours or longer.

10. MDA (3-methoxy-4,5-ethylenedioxyamphetamine). Related to amphetamine, produces a mild LSD-like reaction lasting 6 to 10 hours ("love pill").

See also Alcohols, Amphetamines, Anticholinergic Agents, Barbiturates, Cocaine, Opioids, Phencyclidine, Phenothiazines and Other Major Neuroleptics, and Tricyclic Antidepressants.

Haloperidol (Haldol). See Phenothiazines and Other Major Neuroleptics.

Heroin. See Opioids.

Hydrocarbons

1. PETROLEUM DISTILLATES. Gasoline (petroleum spirit), 2 to 5% benzene; kerosene (coal oil, kerosene, jet aviation fuel No. 1, charcoal lighter fluid); petroleum naphtha (cigarette lighter fluid, ligroin, racing fuel); petroleum ether (benzine); turpentine (pine oil, oil of turpentine); and mineral spirits (Stoddard solvent, white spirits, varsol, mineral turpentine, petroleum spirit). *Mani-*

festations: Materials aspirated during the process of ingestion may produce pneumonitis. Hypoxia associated with aspiration is the cause of CNS depression, not absorption. It is *unlikely* that a child accidentally or an adult during siphoning would ingest a sufficient quantity to warrant the induction of emesis.

2. AROMATIC HYDROCARBONS. *Benzene,* a solvent used in manufacturing dyes, phenol, and nitrobenzene, has a TLV of 10 PPM by inhalation according to the Occupational Safety and Health Administration (OSHA). The National Institute for Occupational Safety and Health (NIOSH) value is 1 PPM. The adult ingested toxic dose is 15 mL. Chronic exposure may cause leukemia. Two hundred PPM is fatal in 5 minutes. *Toluene,* used in manufacturing TNT, has an OSHA TLV of 200 PPM by inhalation; the NIOSH figure is 100. The adult ingested toxic dose is 50 mL. *Styrene* has an OSHA TLV of 100 PPM by inhalation. *Xylene,* used in the manufacture of perfumes, has an OSHA TLV of 100 PPM by inhalation. The adult ingested toxic dose is 50 mL. *Manifestations:* Asphyxiation, CNS depression, defatting dermatitis, and aspiration pneumonitis. A bite into a tube of household plastic cement by a young child does not warrant the induction of emesis. Ingestion of hydrocarbon with a benzene fraction over 5% may warrant induction of emesis.

3. ALIPHATIC HALOGENATED HYDROCARBONS. See Table 17 for common examples. *Manifestations:* Myocardial sensitization and irritability, hepatorenal toxicity, and CNS depression. Dichloromethane may be converted into carbon monoxide in the body. Trichloroethylene concentrates in the fetus (pregnant women should not be exposed) and causes a disulfiram (Antabuse) reaction ("degreaser's flush") when associated with ingestion of ethanol. The decision to induce emesis must be based on the toxicity of the agent.

4. DANGEROUS ADDITIVES. Dangerous additives to the hydrocarbons, such as heavy metals, nitrobenzene, aniline dyes, insecticides, and demothing agents, may warrant the induction of emesis.

5. HEAVY HYDROCARBONS. These have high viscosity, low volatility, and minimal absorption, so emesis is unwarranted. Examples are asphalt (tar), machine oil, motor oil (lubricating oil, engine oil), diesel oil (engine fuel, home heating oil), petrolatum liquid (mineral oil, suntan oils), petrolatum jelly (Vaseline), paraffin wax, transmission oil, cutting oil, and greases and glues.

6. PRODUCTS TREATED AS PETROLEUM DISTILLATES. Essential oils (e.g., turpentine, pine oil) are treated as petroleum distillates. Mineral seal oil (signal oil), found in some furniture polishes, is a heavy, viscous oil that *never* warrants emesis;

TABLE 17. **Common Examples of Aliphatic Halogenated Hydrocarbons**

Hydrocarbon	Estimated Fatal Dose (Ingested)	TLV-TWA (PPM)	Synonyms
1,1,1-Trichloroethane	15.7 gm/kg	50	Methyl chloroform, Triethane, chlorethane, Glamorene Spot Remover, Scotchgard
1,1,2-Trichloroethane	580 mg/kg	10	Vinyl trichloride
Trichloroethylene	Controversial, 3–5 mL/kg	50	—
Tetrachloroethanene	Not known	5	Acetylene tetrachloride
Dichloromethane	25 mL	100	Methylene chloride
Tetrachloroethylene	5 mL	50	Tetrachloroethene Perchloroethylene
Dichloroethane	0.5 mL/kg	200	—
Carbon tetrachloride	3–5 mL	5	—

it can produce severe pneumonia if aspirated. It has minimal absorption. *Management:* Dermal decontamination. Removal from the environment in inhalation.

FIRST AID TREATMENT. See Table 18. *The use of activated charcoal, oils, and cathartics is not advised in petroleum distillate ingestions. General management:* (1) In the asymptomatic patient: observe several hours for development of respiratory distress. (2) In the symptomatic patient: supportive respiratory care for respiratory distress. Bronchospasm may be treated with intravenous aminophylline. Avoid epinephrine. Monitor ECG; arterial blood gases; liver, pulmonary, and renal function; serum electrolytes; serial radiographs. Observe for intravascular hemolysis and disseminated intravascular coagulation. If cyanosis is present that does not respond to oxygen or the arterial PaO_2 is normal, suspect methemglobinemia that may require therapy with methylene blue. Steroids have not been shown to be beneficial. Antimicrobial agents are not useful in prophylaxis. (Fever or leukocytosis may be produced by the chemical pneumonitis itself.) It is not necessary to treat pneumatoceles. Most infiltrations resolve spontaneously in 1 week except for lipoid pneumonia, which may last up to 6 weeks.

Imipramine (Tofranil). See Tricyclic Antidepressants.

Iron. The iron content of some preparations appears in Table 19. *Toxic dose:* Range, 20 to 60 mg per kg or greater of elemental iron. Dose to induce emesis, ≥20 mg per kg. The potential fatal dose is 180 mg per kg (600 mg of elemental iron). *Toxicokinetics:* Absorption occurs chiefly in the small intestine. For excretion there is no normal route except blood loss or gastrointestinal desquamation. *Manifestations:* Phase I—mucosal injury possibly with hematemesis (1 to 6 hours postingestion). Phase II—patient appears improved (2 to 24 hours). Phase III—cardiovascular collapse and severe metabolic acidosis (12 to 48 hours). Phase IV—hepatic injury associated with jaundice (2 to 4 days). Phase V—sequelae of intestinal stricture and obstruction or anemia (2 to 6 weeks). Patients asymptomatic for 6 hours rarely develop serious intoxication manifestations. *Management:* (1) Gastrointestinal decontamination. Emesis should be induced in ingestions of elemental iron of over 20 mg per kg.

TABLE 18. **Initial Management of Hydrocarbon Ingestions**

Symptoms	Contents	Amount	Initial Management
None	Petroleum distillate only	<2 mL/kg	None
None	Heavy hydrocarbon	Any amount	None*
	Mineral seal oil		None
	Petroleum distillate	>2 mL/kg	? Emesis
None	Petroleum distillate with dangerous additive (heavy metals, pesticides)	Depends on toxicity of additives	Emesis
	Aromatic	>1 mL/kg	Emesis
	Halogenated hydrocarbons		
	Trichlor compound	>1 mL/kg	Emesis
	Tetrachlor compound	Any amount ingested	Emesis
Loss of protective airway reflex, seizures	Petroleum distillate with dangerous additive, aromatic or halogenated hydrocarbon	Depends on toxicity	Use endotracheal tube before gastric lavage

*Emesis may be necessary if machine oil contains triorthocresyl phosphate (TOCP), which causes weakness, sensory impairment, and "partially reversible damage to the spinal cord."

TABLE 19. **Iron Content of Some Preparations**

Iron Salt	Elemental Iron Content (%)	Average Tablet Strength (mg)	Elemental Iron/ Tablet (mg)	Average FeSO₄ Strength Other Forms (mg)
Ferrous sulfate (hydrous)	20	300	60	Drp 75/0.6 mL
	20	SR 160	32	Syp 90/5mL
	20	195	39	Solu 125/mL
	20	325	65	Elxr 220/5mL
Ferrous sulfate (dried)	30	200	60	
	30	SR 160	48	
Ferrous gluconate	12	320	36	Elxr 320/5 mL
Ferrous fumarate	33	200	67	
	33	SR 324	107	Drp 45/0.6 mL
	33	Chewable 100	33	Susp 100/5 mL

Abbreviations: Drp = dropper; Syp = syrup; Solu = solution; Elxr = elixir; Susp = suspension.

Emesis should be followed by gastric lavage in an adult or in a child who has ingested a chewable or liquid preparation. The solution to be used for lavage is saline 0.9% or 1 to 1.5% sodium bicarbonate to form ferrous carbonate salts, which are poorly absorbed. One hundred milliliters of this solution should be left in the stomach (prepared by dilution of a sodium bicarbonate ampule with saline). The use of deferoxamine (Desferal) in the gastrointestinal tract is not recommended. The use of diluted Fleet's enema solution risks severe hypertonic phosphate poisoning. Activated charcoal is not recommended. (2) Postlavage abdominal radiograph—if significant amounts of residual radiopaque material are present, consider whole-bowel irrigation with polyethylene glycol solution first. Removal by endoscopy or surgery because coalesced tablets have produced hemorrhagic infarction and perforation peritonitis may also be required. (3) Diagnostic chelation test—deferoxamine not reliable. (4) Indications for chelation therapy with deferoxamine are serum iron level over 500 mg per dL, or systemic signs of intoxication independent of serum iron level. Chelation should be performed within 12 to 18 hours to be effective (Antidote 15, Table 4). *Laboratory aids:* Serum iron levels correlate with the clinical course. Iron levels taken at 2 to 6 hours that are below 350 mg per dL predict an asymptomatic course; levels of 350 to 500 are associated with mild gastrointestinal symptoms (rarely serious); and levels greater than 500 suggest the possibility of serious Phase III manifestations. Draw serum iron (SI) before administering deferoxamine because it interferes with analysis. Total iron-binding capacity is not necessary. An SI at 8 to 12 hours is useful to exclude delayed absorption from a bezoar or sustained-release preparation. White blood cell counts greater than 15,000 per μL, blood glucose levels over 150 mg per dL, radiopaque material present on abdominal radiograph, vomiting, and diarrhea predict iron levels greater than 300 mg per dL. Monitor complete blood counts, blood glucose, serum iron, stools, and vomitus for occult blood; electrolytes; acid-base balance; urinalysis and urinary output; liver function tests; blood urea nitrogen; and creatinine. Obtain type and match of blood in severe cases. Abdominal radiographs. Follow-up is necessary for sequelae in significant intoxications—gastrointestinal series for intestinal strictures and anemia secondary to blood loss. Patients who develop fever or toxic symptoms following iron overdose should have blood and stool cultures checked for *Yersinia enterocolitica.*

Isoniazid (INH, Nydrazid). This is an antituberculosis drug frequently used in suicide attempts by Native Americans and Eskimos. *Mechanism of toxicity:* It produces pyridoxine deficiency (doubles excretion of pyridoxine). *Toxic dose:* 1.5 grams, 35 to 40 mg per kg, produces convulsions; severe toxicity is seen at 6 to 10 grams; 200 mg per kg is an obligatory convulsant. *Toxicokinetics:* Absorption is rapid, with a peak in 1 to 2 hours (clinical symptoms may start in 30 minutes). Volume distribution is 0.6 liter per kg. It passes the placenta and into breast milk at 50% of the maternal serum level. Not protein bound. Elimination is by the liver, which produces a hepatotoxic metabolite, acetylisoniazid. The t½: Slow acetylators (2 to 4 hours) may develop peripheral neuropathy (50% of blacks and whites). Fast acetylators (0.7 to 2 hours) may develop hepatitis (90% of Asians and a majority of patients with diabetes). Excreted unchanged, 10 to 40%. *Major toxic manifestations:* Visual disturbances, convulsions (≥90% with one or more seizures), coma, resistant severe acidosis (due to lactate secondary to hypoxia, convulsions, and metabolic blocks). *Management:* (1) Control seizures with large doses of pyridoxine, 1 gram for each gram of isoniazid ingested (Antidote 38, Table 4). If the dose ingested is unknown, give at least 5 grams of pyridoxine intravenously. Diazepam is given and works synergistically to control seizures. (2) Correct acidosis with fluids and sodium bicarbonate (pyridoxine may spontaneously correct the acidosis). (3) After patient is stabilized, or if asymptomatic, gastrointestinal decontamination procedures may be carried out, keeping in mind the rapid onset of convulsions. Asymptomatic patients should be observed for 4 hours. (4) Hemodialysis is rarely needed but may be used as an adjunct for uncontrollable acidosis and seizures. Hemoperfusion has not been adequately evaluated. Diuresis is ineffective. *Laboratory aids:* Isoniazid toxic levels are above 10 to 20 μg per mL. Monitor the blood glucose (often hyperglycemia), electrolytes (often hyperkalemia), bicarbonate, arterial blood gases, liver function tests, blood urea nitrogen (BUN), and creatinine. If convulsions persist obtain an electroencephalogram (EEG). Monitor the temperature closely (often hyperpyrexia).

Isopropyl Alcohol. See Alcohols.

Kerosene. See Hydrocarbons.

Lead. *Acute* lead poisoning is rare. *Acute toxic dose:* 0.5 gram. *Management:* (1) Gastrointestinal decontamination. (2) Supportive care, including measures to deal with the hepatic and renal failure and intravascular hemolysis. (3) Ethylenediaminetetra-acetic acid (EDTA) in all severe cases if lead levels confirm absorption. *Chronic* lead poisoning occurs most often in children 6 months to 6 years of age who are exposed in their environment and in adults in certain occupations. *Chronic toxic dose:* Determined by blood lead level and clinical findings. A level of 10 μg per dL or over is the threshold of concern in children; 40 μg per dL or over in adult workers; 30 μg per dL or over for those planning pregnancy. Medical removal from work at 60 μg per dL. *Toxicokinetics:* Absorption—10 to 15% of the ingested dose is absorbed in adults; in children up to 40% is absorbed with iron deficiency anemia. Inhalation absorption is rapid and complete. Vd—95% present in bone. In blood, 95% is in red blood cells. t½, 35 days; in bone, 10 years. The major elimination route for inorganic lead is renal. Organic lead is metabolized in the liver to inorganic lead; 9% is excreted in the urine per day. *Manifestations of acute symptoms of chronic lead poisoning.* (ABCDE): Anorexia, apathy, anemia; behavior disturbances; clumsiness; developmental deterioration; and emesis. Manifestations of encephalopathy are "PAINT": *P*, persistent forceful vomiting; *A*, ataxia; *I*, intermittent stupor and lucidity; *N*, neurologic coma and convulsions; *T*, tired and lethargic. In adults, one may see peripheral neuropathies and "lead gum lines." *Management:* (1) Gastrointestinal decontamination with enemas if radiopaque foreign bodies are noted. Do not delay therapy until clear. (2) Remove from exposure. For children, see Table 20. Dimercaptosuccinic acid, a derivative of BAL, is an oral agent approved by the FDA for chelation of children only with venous blood lead >45 μg per dL. The recommended dose is 10 mg per kg every 8 hours for 5 days, then every 12 hours for 14 days (Antidote 42, Table 4). *Laboratory aids:* (1) Provocation mobilization test—500 mg per M² of EDTA for one dose given deeply intramuscularly with 0.5% procaine diluted 1:1 and collect the urine for 8 hours. A ratio of micrograms excreted in the urine to milligrams of Ca-EDTA administered greater than 0.6 represents an increased lead body burden, and chelation should be carried out. (2) Evaluate complete blood count, levels of serum iron, or ferritin; repeat blood lead levels and erythrocyte protoporphyrin. (3) Flat plate of the abdomen and long bone radiographs (knees usually). (4) Renal function tests. (5) Monitor electrolytes, serum calcium, phosphorus, blood glucose.

Lindane. See Organochlorine Insecticides.

Lithium (Eskalith, Lithane). Most cases of intoxication have occurred as therapeutic overdoses. The toxic dose is determined by serum levels, although intoxication has occurred with levels in the therapeutic range. *Toxicokinetics:* Absorption is rapid, with complete peaking in 1 to 4 hours. Vd is 0.5 to 0.9 liter per kg. It is not protein bound. The t½ therapeutically is 18 to 24 hours. Eighty-nine to 98% is excreted by the kidney unchanged, one-third to two-thirds in 6 to 12 hours. Excretion is decreased in the presence of hyponatremia and dehydration. The cerebrospinal fluid concentration is one-half the plasma concentration. The breast milk level is 50% of the maternal serum level—toxic to the nursling. *Manifestations:* The first sign of toxicity may be diarrhea. Fine tremor of hands, lethargy, weakness, polyuria and polydipsia, goiter and hypothyroidism, and fasciculations are side effects. Severe toxicity is manifested by ataxia, impaired mental state, coma, and seizures (limbs held in hyperextension with eyes open in "coma vigil"). Cardiovascular manifestations are dysrhythmias, hypotension, flat T waves, and increased QT interval. *Management:* (1) Gastrointestinal decontamination may not be useful after 2 hours because of rapid absorption. In slow-release preparations, decontamination may be useful up to 24 hours postingestion. Activated charcoal is not indicated. Sodium polystyrene sulfonate (Kayexalate), 60 mL orally four times a day, is useful in preventing absorption. (2) Hospitalize if intoxication is suspected, because seizures may occur unexpectedly. (3) Restore normothermia and fluid and electrolyte balance, particularly sodium. If diabetes insipidus is present, an infusion of sodium may cause hypernatremia. Current evidence supports saline infusion as enhancing excretion of lithium. (4) Hemodialysis is the treatment of choice for severe intoxication. Lithium is

TABLE 20. **Choice of Chelation Therapy Based on Symptoms and Blood Lead Concentration**

Clinical Presentation	Treatment	Comments
Symptomatic Children		

Acute encephalopathy	BAL, 450 mg/M²/24 h
	 CaNa₂-EDTA, 1500 mg/M²/24 h
		BAL, 75/M² q 4 h
		 After 4 h, start infusion of EDTA
		   or use IM* q 4 h†
		 Duration, 5 days
		 Interrupt therapy for 2 days
		 If blood Pb >70 µg/dL, BAL and EDTA for 5
		   more days; EDTA alone if blood Pb = 45–69
		   µg/dl
		 Other cycles depend on blood Pb rebound

Blood Pb >70 µg/dl	BAL, 300 mg/M²/24 h
	 CaNa₂-EDTA, 1000 mg/M²/24 h
	 Do not use CaNa₂-EDTA alone
	   if symptomatic
		BAL, 50 mg/M² q 4 h
		 After 4 h, start infusion of EDTA
		   or use IM q 4 h†
		 Duration, 5 days
		 Interrupt therapy for 2 days
		 Discontinue BAL in 3 days if blood Pb <50 µg/dl;
		   BAL and EDTA for 5 more days if blood Pb
		   >50 µg/dl
		 Other cycles depend on blood Pb rebound

Asymptomatic Children		
Before Treatment, Measure Venous Blood Lead		
Blood Pb > 70 µg/dl	BAL, 300 mg/M²/24 CaNa₂-EDTA, 100 mg/M²/24	BAL, 50 mg/M² IM q 4 h After 4 h, start infusion of EDTA or use IM q 4 h Duration, 5 days Discontinue BAL in 3 days if blood PB <50 µg/dl Give second course of EDTA if blood PB >45 µg/dl within 5 days Other cycles depend on blood Pb rebound

Blood Pb = 45–69 µg/dl‡	CaNa₂-EDTA, 1000 mg/M²/24 h	EDTA, IM q 4 h or IV
		 Duration, 5 days
		 Give second course of EDTA if blood Pb
		   >45 µg/dl within 7–14 days; wait 5–7 days
		   before giving second course
		 If lead exposure controlled, give single IV/IM
		   dose on outpatient basis
		 Other cycles depend on blood Pb rebound

Blood Pb = 25–44 µg/dl
   Ratio >0.6
   Ratio <0.6
	CaNa₂-EDTA, 1000 mg/M²/24 h	Provocation, EDTA test
		 Duration, 5 days IM or IV
		 Provocation test periodically

Guidelines for Chelation of Excess Lead in Adults		
Inorganic Lead§		
Symptomatic Cases		
Acute encepalopathy	BAL-EDTA	Same as for children

Abdominal pain, weakness,
   and colic
	BAL-EDTA	Course for 3–5 days followed by oral
		   penicillamine until urine lead is <500 µg/24 h
		   or 2 months, whichever less

Painless peripheral neuropathy	D-Penicillamine	For 1–2 months If blood lead >100 µg/dL, BAL-EDTA first Course 3–5 days, followed by oral penicillamine
Asymptomatic Cases		
Blood Lead Concentrations		
100 µg/dL	BAL-EDTA	
80–100 µg/dL	Penicillamine alone	
40–79 and EP >60 µg/dL	Provocative test	
Organic Lead	No chelation therapy	

Note: OSHA requires that workers be removed from the work environment when lead levels exceed 50 µg/dL and until they are below 40 µg/dL.

*Dimercaprol.

†Some physicians prefer to give EDTA IM to avoid large fluid volumes in high intracranial pressure.

‡DSMA may be used.

§Data from Rempel D: The lead exposed worker: JAMA 262:532–534, 1989. Copyright 1989, American Medical Association.

Abbreviations: Blood Pb = venous blood lead concentration; IM = intramuscularly; IV = intravenously.

Modified from Piomelli S, et al: Management of childhood lead poisoning. J Pediatr 103:527, 1984, and CDC Prevention of Childhood Lead Poisoning 1991.

the most dialyzable toxin known. Long runs should be used until the lithium level is less than 1 mEq per liter because of extensive re-equilibration rebound. Monitor levels every 4 hours after dialysis. Dialysis may have to be repeated. Expect a time lag in neurologic recovery. If hemodialysis is not available or delayed, peritoneal dialysis can be used but is less effective. (5) Monitor ECG. Refractory dysrhythmias may be treated with magnesium sulfate and sodium bicarbonate. (6) Avoid thiazides and spironolactone diuretics, which increase lithium levels. *Laboratory aids:* Lithium level determinations should be performed every 4 hours. Although they do not always correlate with the manifestations at low levels, they are predictive in severe intoxications. Levels of 0.6 to 1.2 mEq per liter are usually therapeutic. Levels over 4.0 mEq per liter are usually severely toxic. Other tests to be monitored are complete blood count (lithium causes leukocytosis), renal function, thyroid, ECG, and electrolytes. Factors that predispose to lithium toxicity are febrile illness, sodium depletion, concomitant drugs (thiazide and spironolactone diuretics), impaired renal function, advanced age, and fluid loss in vomiting and diarrheal illness.

Lomotil (Diphenoxylate and Atropine). See Opioids and Anticholinergic Agents.

LSD (Lysergic Acid Diethylamide). See Hallucinogens.

Marijuana. See Hallucinogens.

Meperidine (Demerol). See Opioids.

Meprobamate (Equanil, Miltown). See Sedative Hypnotics.

Mercury. *Management:* (1) Inhalation of elemental mercury—remove from exposure. (2) Ingestion of mercuric salt—gastrointestinal decontamination. Do not induce emesis. A protein solution such as egg white or 5% salt-poor albumin can be given to reduce salt to mercurous ion (less toxic). (3) Chelating agents (do not use Ca-EDTA because of nephrotoxicity): Dimercaprol (BAL) enhances mercury excretion through the bile as well as the urine and would be the choice if there were renal impairment from the mercury (Antidote 17, Table 4). Penicillamine (Antidote 34, Table 4) or *N*-acetyl-DL-penicillamine (investigational use). Use of BAL in methyl mercury intoxication increases the brain mercury and appears to be contraindicated; penicillamine and its analogue should be used (decreases mercury in brain). Another chelator, 2,3-dimercaptosuccinic acid, holds promise of less toxicity and more specific therapy.* (4) Monitor fluid and electrolyte levels, renal function, hemoglobin levels. Obtain blood and urine mercury levels (consult the labo-

---

*Not approved by the FDA for this purpose.

ratory for proper collection technique and containers). (5) Hemodialysis early in the symptomatic patient is useful. (6) Newer but not established approaches are Polythiol resin to bind the methyl mercury excreted in the bile; heat and sauna treatment to increase mercury excretion through perspiration; and a regional dialyzer system using L-cysteine. (7) Surgical excision of *local injection sites. Laboratory aids:* (1) Blood levels are below 2 to 4 µg per dL and urine levels below 10 to 20 µg per liter in 90% of the adult population. Levels above 4 µg per dL in blood and 20 µg per liter in urine probably should be considered abnormal. Blood levels are not always reliable. Exposed industrial workers' urine levels are 150 to 200 µg per liter. (2) In asymptomatic patients with urine levels under 300 µg per liter, a chelating challenge with BAL or penicillamine may bring a significant increase that may aid in establishing the diagnosis. (3) Approximately 150 µg per liter of mercury in urine is equivalent to 3.5 µg per dL in blood. (4) Methyl mercury is excreted mainly through the feces, so urine mercury would not be a reliable measurement. (5) Mercury is also excreted in the sweat and saliva. The parotid fluid level is approximately two-thirds that of the blood. Because the hair is porous, it may absorb mercury from the atmosphere; however, hair concentrations of 400 to 500 µg per gram are likely to be associated with neurologic symptoms.

Methadone. See Opioids.

Methanol. See Alcohols.

Methaqualone. See Sedative Hypnotics.

Methyprylon (Noludar). See Sedative Hypnotics.

Narcotic Analgesics. See Opioids.

Neuroleptics. See Phenothiazines and Other Major Neuroleptics.

Nitrites (NO$_2$) and Nitrates (NO$_3$). These are readily available in both inorganic and organic forms. Organic nitrates used for angina pectoris are listed in Table 21. Inorganic nitrates have more toxicologic importance in natural foods and contaminated well water. *Potential fatal doses:* Nitrite, 1 gram; nitrate, 10 grams; nitrobenzene, 2 mL; nitroglycerin, 0.2 gram; and aniline dye (pure), 5 to 30 grams. *Toxicokinetics:* Onset of action of nitroglycerin sublingually is 1 to 3 minutes, with a peak action of 3 to 15 minutes and a duration of 20 to 30 minutes. Other routes have a slower onset (2 to 5 minutes) and longer duration of action (1.5 to 6 hours). Nitrites are potent oxidizing agents converting ferrous to ferric iron, which cannot carry oxygen. Normally humans have 0.7% of methemoglobin, which is converted by methemoglobin reductase into oxygen-carrying hemoglobin. Liver detoxification by dinitration is the route of elimination. *Toxic manifesta-*

TABLE 21. Organic Nitrates for Angina Pectoris

Drug and Route	Trade Name	Onset (min)	Duration (h)
Nitroglycerin			
Oral	Many	Varies	4–6
Sublingual	Many	1–3	¼–½
2% ointment	Nitro-Bid Nitrol	Varies	3–6
Isosorbide dinitrate	Isordil		
Sublingual		1–3	1.3–3
Oral		2–5	4–6
Chewable		2–5	2–3
Timed release		Varies	—
Pentaerythritol tetranitrate, oral	Peritrate	2–5	3–5
Erythrityl tetranitrate, oral	Cardilate	2–5	4–6

tions depend on the level of methemoglobinemia. At 10%, "chocolate cyanosis" occurs; at 10 to 20%, headache, dizziness, and tachypnea occur; and at 50%, mental alterations are present and coma and convulsions may occur. Headache, flushing, and sweating are due to the vasodilatory effect; hypotension, tachycardia, and syncope may also occur. Severe hypoxia may produce pulmonary edema and encephalopathy. Levels above 50% produce metabolic acidosis and ECG changes; cardiovascular collapse occurs at levels of 70%. *Management:* (1) Dermal decontamination, if indicated. Aniline dyes may be removed with 5% acetic acid (vinegar). (2) Gastrointestinal decontamination if ingested. (3) Hypotension can be treated by the Trendelenburg position and fluid challenge. Vasoconstrictors (dopamine or norepinephrine) are rarely needed. (4) Methylene blue (Antidote 29, Table 4) is indicated for methemoglobin levels above 30%, dyspnea, metabolic acidosis (lactic acidosis), or an altered mental state. (5) Oxygen, 100%, or a hyperbaric chamber should be used in symptomatic patients if methylene blue fails or is not effective, e.g., as in chlorate intoxication or glucose-6-phosphate dehydrogenase deficiency. *Laboratory aids:* Methemoglobin levels, arterial blood gases. Blood has a chocolate-brown appearance and fails to turn red on exposure to oxygen. Methemoglobulin levels and oxygen saturation should be measured by cooximeter, not by pulse oximetry.

Nortriptyline (Aventyl, Pamelor). See Tricyclic Antidepressants.

Opioids (Narcotic Opiates). See Table 22. The major metabolic pathway differs for each opioid but they are 90% metabolized in the liver. Patients should be observed for CNS and respiratory depression and hypotension. Pulmonary edema is a potentially lethal complication of mainlining (intravenous use). *Manifestations:* All opiate agonists produce miotic pupils (except meperidine and Lomotil early), respiratory and CNS depression, physical dependence, and withdrawal. *Management:* (1) Supportive care, particularly an endotracheal tube and assisted ventilation. (2) Gastrointestinal decontamination up to 12 hours postingestion, because opiates delay gastric emptying time, but this is of no benefit if overdose is by injection. Convulsions occur rapidly with propoxyphene (Darvon) and codeine

TABLE 22. Opioids (Narcotic Opiates)*

Drugs		Equivalent IM Dose† (mg)	Oral† (mg)	Peak Action (h)	Half-life (h)	Duration of Action (h)	Potential Toxic Dose (mg)
Generic	*Trade*						
Alphaprodine	Nisentil	40–60	—	—	2	1–2	—
Butorphanol	Stadol	2	—	0.5–1.0	3	2.5–3.5	—
Camphorated tincture of opium	Paregoric	—	25 mL	—	—	4–5	—
Codeine	Various	120	200	—	3	4–6	800
Diacetylmorphine	Heroin	5	60	—	0.5	3–4	100
Hydrocodone	Hycodan	5–10	—	—	—	3–4	100
Diphenoxylate	Lomotil	—	10	Delayed by atropine	2.5	14	300
Fentanyl	Sublimaze	0.1–0.2	—	0.5	4–6	0.5–2	—
Hydromorphone	Dilaudid	1.5	6.0	0.5–1.5	2–3	2–4	100
Meperidine	Demerol	50–100	75–100	0.5–1	2–5	3–4	1000
Methadone	Dolophine	10.0	20	2–4	22–97	4–12	120
Morphine	Various	10.0	60	0.3–1.5	2–3	3–4	200
Nalbuphine	Nubain	10.0	—	0.5–1.0	3–4	3–4	—
Oxycodone	Percodan	—	15	—	—	3–4	—
Oxymorphone	Numorphan	1.0	—	1	2–3	4–5	—
Pentazocine	Talwin	—	30–60	1	2–6	3–4	—
Propoxyphene	Darvon	—	65–100	2–4	8–24	2–4	500

*"Ts and blues" are a combination of pentazocine (Talwin) and tripelennamine (Pyribenzamine) used intravenously. Pentazocine now has naloxone added to it to counter this abuse. Innovar is fentanyl plus droperidol, used as an IV anesthetic.

†Dose equivalent to 10 mg of morphine.

overdose, and this may be an indication not to use an emetic for gastrointestinal decontamination in this drug overdose. (3) Naloxone (Narcan) (Antidote 30, Table 4) may be given in bolus intravenous doses and by continuous drip. Naloxone must be titrated against the clinical response and precipitation of withdrawal in narcotic addicts. It should be repeated as often as necessary, because many opioids in overdose can last 24 hours to 48 hours, whereas the action of naloxone lasts only 2 to 3 hours. *Larger doses are needed for buprenorphine, codeine, designer drugs, dextromethorphan, diphenoxylate, methadone, pentazocine, and propoxyphene.* (4) Pulmonary edema does not respond to naloxone and needs respiratory supportive care. Fluids should be given cautiously in opioid overdose because these agents stimulate antidiuretic hormone effect and pulmonary edema is frequent. (5) *If the patient is comatose, give 50% glucose* (3 to 4% of comatose narcotic overdose patients have hypoglycemia). (6) *If the patient is agitated,* consider hypoxia rather than withdrawal and treat as such. (7) *Observe for withdrawal* (nausea, vomiting, cramps, diarrhea, dilated pupils, rhinorrhea, piloerection). If these occur, stop naloxone.

OPIOID ADDICT WITHDRAWAL SCORE. Symptoms of withdrawal are diarrhea, dilated pupils, gooseflesh, hyperactive bowel sounds, hypertension, insomnia, lacrimation, muscle cramps, restlessness, tachycardia, and yawning. Each sign or symptom is given 0, 1, or 2 points, depending on the severity. A score of 1 to 5 is mild; 6 to 10, moderate; and 11 to 15, severe. Seizures are unusual with withdrawal. They indicate severity regardless of the rest of the score. *Management:* Mild withdrawal is treated with diazepam orally, 10 mg every 6 hours; moderate withdrawal, with intramuscular diazepam; and severe withdrawal, with diazepam and diphenoxylate (Lomotil) for the diarrhea. Methadone orally may be used, 20 to 40 mg every 12 hours, decreased by 5 mg every 12 hours. When 10 mg is reached, add Lomotil. Clonidine (Catapres), 6 μg per kg every 6 hours, can be used with informed consent. (This is an unlisted use of clonidine; the manufacturer states that relief from withdrawal symptoms has been reported with 0.8 mg per day.) *Laboratory aids:* For acute overdose obtain levels of blood gases, blood glucose, and electrolytes; chest x-ray; and ECG. Blood opioid levels confirm diagnosis but are not useful for making a therapeutic decision. For drug abusers, consider testing for hepatitis B, syphilis, and human immunodeficiency virus (HIV) antibody (HIV testing usually requires consent).

PROPOXYPHENE (Darvon). *Manifestations:* Onset may be as early as 30 minutes after ingestion. Convulsions occur early. Patients may develop diabetes insipidus, pulmonary edema, and hypoglycemia. *Elimination:* Metabolism is 90% by demethylation in the liver. Peak plasma level of 1 to 2 hours after oral dose. Half-life is 1 to 5 hours. As little as 10 mg per kg has caused symptoms, and 35 mg per kg has caused cardiopulmonary arrest. Therapeutic blood level is less than 200 μg per mL. *Treatment* (in addition to the general management): (1) Emesis can be dangerous because of the rapid onset of seizures. (2) Indications for naloxone are respiratory depression, seizure activity, coma, and miotic pupils. Signs of naloxone effect are dilation of pupils, increased rate and depth of respirations, reversal of hypotension, and improvement of obtunded or comatose state. Larger doses of naloxone are often required and can be continued as an infusion of the initial response dose every hour. (3) Naloxone and intravenous glucose should be tried first to control seizures. If these fail, diazepam may be tried.

Organochlorine Insecticides (DDT Derivatives). See Table 23 for a listing of these agents. The *toxic dose* varies greatly. Chlorophenothane (DDT), 200 to 250 mg per kg, is fatal; 16 mg per kg causes seizures. Methoxychlor, 500 to 600 mg per kg, is fatal. Chlordane, 200 mg per kg, is fatal (chlordane house air guidelines are below 5 μg per M^3; the occupational TLV is 500 μg per M^3). These insecticides interfere with axon transmission of nerve impulses. Metabolism varies; they resist degradation in human tissue and the environment. They accumulate in adipose tissue; the elimination route is via the liver. *Manifestations:* CNS stimulation, convulsions, late respiratory depression, increased myocardial irritability usually develop within 1 to 2 hours and may last for 1 week or more. Endrin produces liver toxicity with guarded prognosis. Chronic exposure causes liver and kidney damage. *Management:* (1) Dermal decontamination, discard contaminated leather goods. Protect personnel. Gastrointestinal decontamination, no oils. Emesis can be dangerous, owing to rapid seizures. Many of these agents are dissolved in petroleum distillates, presenting an aspiration hazard. (2) No adrenergic stimulants (epinephrine) should be used because of myocardial irritability. (3) Cholestyramine, 4 grams every 8 hours, has been reported to increase the fecal excretion. (4) Anticonvulsants, if needed.

Organophosphate and Carbamate Insecticides (OPI). These may cause (1) irreversible inhibition of cholinesterase, either direct (TEPP) or delayed (parathion or malathion), or (2) reversible inhibition of cholinesterase (carbamates). Examples of OPI are listed in Table 24. Absorption is by all routes. The onset of acute toxicity is usually before 12 hours and always before 24 hours, unless they are absorbed by the dermal

TABLE 23. **Organochlorine Pesticides (DDT Derivatives)**

Chemical Name	Trade Name	Toxicity Rating	Fatal Dose (Adult)	Elimination Time	Comment
Endrin	Hexadrin	Highest	NA	Hours–days	Banned
Lindane	1% in Kwell; Benesan; Isotox; Gamene	Moderate to high	10 gm	Hours–days	Scabicide; general garden insecticide
Endosulfan	Thiodan	Moderate	NA	Hours–days	
Benzene hexachloride	BHC, HCH	Moderate	NA	Weeks–months	Banned, produces porphyria (cutanea tarda)
Dieldrin	Dieldrite	High	3 gm	Weeks–months	Banned in 1974
Aldrin	Aldrite	High	3 gm	Weeks–months	Banned in 1974
Chlordane (10% is heptachlor)	Chlordan	High	3 gm	Weeks–months	Restricted in 1979; termiticide
Toxophene	Toxakil Strobane-T	High	2 gm	Hours–days	
Heptachlor	—	Moderate	NA	Weeks–months	Malignancy in rats; banned in 1976
Chlorophenothane	DDT	Moderate	NA	Months–years	Banned in 1972
Mirex	—	Moderate	NA	Months–years	Banned; red anticide
Chlordecone	Kepone	Moderate	NA	Months–years	Tidewater, Virginia, contamination
Methoxychlor	Marlate	Low	600 mg/kg	Hours–days	
Ethylan	Perthane	Low	NA	Hours–days	
Dicofol	Kelthane	Low	NA	Hours–days	
Chlorobenzilate	Acaraben	Low	NA	Hours–days	Banned

Abbreviation: NA = not available.

route or are liquid soluble (fenthion), which may delay onset for 24 hours. Inhalation produces intoxication within minutes. *Toxic manifestations:* Garlic odor of the breath, gastric contents, or container; miosis and muscle twitching are helpful clues to acute OPI poisoning. Early, cholinergic crisis—cramps, diarrhea, excess secretion, bronchospasms, bradycardia. Later, sympathetic and nicotine effects occur—twitching, fasciculations, weakness, tachycardia and hypertension, and convulsions. CNS effects are anxiety, confusion, emotional lability, and coma. Delayed respiratory paralysis and neurologic disorders have been described. *Management:* (1) Basic life support and decontamination with careful protection of personnel. (2) Atropine (Antidote 7, Table 4), if symptomatic, every 10 to 30 minutes until drying of secretions and clearing of lungs occur. Maintain for 12 to 24 hours, then taper the dose and observe for relapse. (3) Intravenous pralidoxime (2-PAM) is required after atropinization (Antidote 36, Table 4). It should be given early. Its use may require reduction in the dose of atropine. (4) Careful dermal and gastrointestinal decontamination when stable. (5) Suction secretions until atropinization drying is achieved. Intubation and assisted ventilation may be needed. (6) *Do not* use morphine, aminophylline, phenothiazine, or reserpine-like drugs or succinylcholine. *Laboratory aids:* Draw blood for red blood cell cholinesterase determination before giving pralidoxime.

Levels are usually more than 90% depressed for severe symptoms. A postexposure rise of 10 to 15% determined at least 10 to 14 days without exposure is important in the diagnosis. Monitor chest radiograph, blood glucose, arterial blood gases, ECG, blood coagulation status, liver function, and the urine for the metabolite alkyl phosphate *p*-nitrophenol. *Note:* If the diagnosis is probable, do not delay therapy until it is confirmed by laboratory tests. Atropine is both a diagnostic and a therapeutic agent. A test dose of 1 mg in adults and 0.01 mg per kg in children may be administered parenterally. In the presence of severe cholinesterase inhibition, the patient fails to develop signs of atropinization.

PROPHYLAXIS. It is not medically advisable to administer atropine or pralidoxime prophylactically to workers exposed to organophosphate pesticides.

CARBAMATES (esters of carbonic acid). Carbamates cause reversible carbamylation of acetylcholinesterase. Pralidoxime is usually not indicated in the management but atropine may be required. The major differences from OPI are (1) toxicity is less and of shorter duration, (2) they rarely produce overt CNS effects because of poor penetration, and (3) cholinesterase returns to normal rapidly so blood values are not useful in confirming the diagnosis. Some common examples of carbamates are Ziram, Temik (alkicarb) (taken up by plants and fruit), Matacil (amino-

TABLE 24. **Examples of Common Organophosphate Insecticides (OPI)**

Common Name	Synonym	EFD (gm/70 kg)	LD$_{50}$ mg/kg
Agricultural Products (25–50% Formulations, Highly Toxic; LD$_{50}$ is 1–40 mg/kg)			
Azinphosmethyl	Guthion	0.2	10.0
Chlortriphos	Calathion		
Demeton[1]	Systox		1.5
Disulfoton[1]	Di-Syston	0.2	12.0
Ethyl-nitrophenyl thiobenzene PO$_4$	EPN		
Fonofon	Dyfonate		
Mevinphos	Phosdrin	0.15	
Methamidophos[2]	Monitor		
Monocrotophos	Azodrin		21.0
Octamethyldiphosphoramide	OMPA, Schradan		
Parathion	Thiophos	0.10	2.5
Ethyl parathion	Parathion		
Methyl	Dalf		
Phorate	Thimet		
Terbufos	Counter		
Tetraethyl pyrophosphate	TEPP, Tetron	0.05	1.5
Animal Insecticides (Moderately Toxic; LD$_{50}$ is 40–200 mg/kg)			
Chlorfenvinophos (tick dip)	Supona, Dermaton		
Coumaphos	Co-ral		
DEF	DeGreen		
Dichlorvos[3]	DDVP, Vapona		46
Dimethoate[4]	Cygon, De-fend		>500
Fenthione[5]	Baytex		40
Leptophos	Phosvel		
Phosmet	Imidon		
Ronnel	Korlan	10.0	
Trichlorfon	Dylox		
Household and Garden Pest Control (1–2% Formulations, Low Toxicity; LD$_{50}$ is 200–1400 mg/kg)			
Acephate[6]	Oerthene		>1000
Bromophos			>1000
Chlorpyrifos[7] toxic dose is 300 mg/kg	Lorsban, Dursban, Pyrinex		>500
Diazinon[1,8]	Spectracide, Dimpylate	25.0	>400
Dichlorvos[9]	DDVP, Vapona (plastic strip)		
Malathion (>92%, <24 h)	Cythion	60.0	1375
Merphos	Folex		>1000
Temephos	Abate		<2000

[1]Most OPI degrade in the environment in a few days to nontoxic radicals. These may be taken up by the plants and fruits.
[2]Delayed neuropathy.
[3]Found in flea collars and No-Pest Strips.
[4]Half-life is <24 h.
[5]Long-acting.
[6]Half-life is 1–6 days.
[7]Some authors classify this as moderately toxic; half-life is 27 h.
[8]In rats, half-life is 12 h.
[9]Some authors classify this as moderately toxic.
Abbreviations: EFD = estimated fatal dose, common lawn chemical as 14.3%; LD$_{50}$ = dose that is fatal in 50% of animals.

carb, carazol), Vydate (oxamyl), Isolan, furadan (Carbofuran), Lannate (methomyl, Nudrin), Zectran (mexacarbate), and Mesural (methiocarb). These agents are all highly toxic. Moderately toxic are Baygon (propoxur) and Sevin (carbaryl). Some of these agents may be formulated in wood alcohol and have the added toxicity of methyl alcohol.

Paradichlorobenzene. See Hydrocarbons.

Paraquat and Diquat. Paraquat is a quaternary ammonia herbicide rapidly inactivated in the soil by clay particles. Nonindustrial preparations of 0.2% are unlikely to cause serious intoxications. *Toxic dose:* Commercial preparations such as Gramoxone 20% are very toxic; one mouthful has produced death. Systemic absorption in the course of occupational use is apparently minimal. Paraquat on marijuana leaves is pyrolyzed to nontoxic dipyridyl. *Toxicokinetics:* "Hit and run" toxin. Less than 20% is absorbed. The peak is 1 hour postingestion. The route of elimination is the kidney. Most of the dose is eliminated in the first 40 hours; it is detected in urine for 15 days. Volume distribution is over 500 liters per kg. *Manifestations:* Local corrosive effect on skin and mucous membranes. Acute renal failure in 48 hours (often reversible). Pulmonary effects in 72 hours are progressive, and oxygen aggravates the pulmonary fibrosis. Diquat does not produce effects on the lungs but produces convulsions and gastrointestinal distention. Long-term exposure may cause cataracts. Chlormequat's target organ is the kidney. *Management:* (1) Gastrointestinal decontamination despite corrosive effects should be done cautiously with a nasogastric tube. Repeated doses of activated charcoal are recommended. Dermal and ocular decontamination as needed. (2) Hemodialysis and hemoperfusion may be carried out in tandem. Hemoperfusion with charcoal alone, if started within 2 hours after ingestion, may be effective; if started after 2 hours, however, the results are poor. Continue hemoperfusion until blood paraquat levels cannot be detected. (3) Diuresis may be of value but consider the risk of fluid overload. (4) Niacin and vitamin E have not been effective. (5) Avoid oxygen unless absolutely necessary (PaO_2 below 60 mmHg) because this aggravates fibrosis. Some use hypoxic air, F_IO_2 10 to 20%. (6) Corticosteroids may help prevent adrenocortical necrosis. (7) Sepsis often develops within 7 to 10 days and should be treated appropriately. *Laboratory aids:* Blood levels above 2 μg per mL at 4 hours or above 0.10 μg per mL at 24 hours are usually fatal. Blood level testing and advice may be obtained from ICI American, 800–327–8633. Monitor renal, liver, and pulmonary functions and chest radiographs. Urine test for paraquat exposure—alkalinization and sodium dithionite give an intense blue-green color in exposure.

Parathion. See Organophosphate Insecticides.

Pentazocine (Talwin). See Opioids.

Perphenazine. See Phenothiazines and Other Major Neuroleptics.

Petroleum Products. See Hydrocarbons.

Phencyclidine (Angel Dust, PCP, Peace Pill, Hog). This is the "drug of deceit" because it is substituted for many other drugs, such as THC and mescaline. There are now at least 38 analogues. Smoking may give cyanide poisoning. Improper mixing has caused explosions. *Toxic dose:* Two to 5 mg smoked or "snorted" produces drunken behavior, agitation, and excitement. Five to 10 mg produces stupor, coma, and myoclonus convulsions. Ten to 25 mg smoked, snorted, or taken orally results in prolonged coma and respiratory failure. It is usually fatal over 25 mg (250 ng per mL blood concentration). *Toxicokinetics:* Weak base. Rapidly absorbed when smoked, snorted, or ingested and secreted into stomach gastric juice. Absorbed in alkaline intestine, but ion trapping takes place in acid gastric media. Half-life is 30 to 60 minutes. Lipophilic drug with extensive Vd. The onset of action if smoked is 2 to 5 minutes (peak in 15 to 30 minutes); orally, 30 to 60 minutes. The duration at low doses is 4 to 6 hours and normality returns in 24 hours. At large over-

doses, coma may last 6 to 10 days (waxes and wanes). An adverse reaction in overdose occurs in 1 to 2 hours. *Route of elimination:* By liver metabolism (50%). Urinary excretion of conjugates and free PCP. *Manifestations:* Sympathomimetic, cholinergic, cerebellar. Observe for violent behavior, paranoid schizophrenia, self-destructive behavior. Clues to diagnosis are bursts of horizontal, vertical, and rotary nystagmus, coma with eyes open. *Management* (avoid overtreatment of mild intoxications): (1) Gastrointestinal decontamination up to 4 hours postingestion, but this may not be effective because PCP is rapidly absorbed. Insert nasogastric tube into stomach for administration of activated charcoal every 6 hours because PCP is secreted into the stomach even if it is smoked or snorted. (2) Protect patient and others from harm. "Talk down" is usually ineffective. Low sensory environment. Diazepam (Valium) may be used orally or intramuscularly in the uncooperative patient. (3) For behavioral disorders and toxic psychosis—diazepam. (4) Seizures and muscle spasm—control with diazepam, 2.5 mg, up to 10 mg (Antidote 16, Table 4). (5) Dystonia reaction—diphenhydramine (Benadryl) intravenously (Antidote 19, Table 4). (6) Hyperthermia—external cooling. (7) Hypertensive crisis (dopaminergic)—use nitroprusside, 0.3 to 2 μg per kg per minute. Maximum infusion rate—10 μg per kg per minute; should never last more than 10 minutes. (8) Acid diuresis ion trapping (controversial). Ammonium chloride use is not recommended because of rhabdomyolysis and the danger of myoglobin precipitation in the renal tubules (Antidote 2, Table 4). (9) Avoid phenothiazines in the acute phase of intoxication because they lower the convulsive threshold. May be needed later for psychosis. *Laboratory aids:* (1) Elevation of CPK level is a clue to the amount of rhabdomyolysis occurring and the chance of myoglobinuria developing. Values up to 20,000 units have been reported. (2) Test urine for myoglobin and pigmented casts. Test urine with orthotoluidine; a positive test without red blood cells on microscopic examination suggests myoglobinuria. (3) Monitor urine and blood pH and urinary output if acidifying patient. (4) Measure PCP level. (5) Evaluate blood urea nitrogen, ammonia, electrolytes, blood glucose levels (20% of patients have hypoglycemia). (6) Test for PCP in gastric juice; levels are 40 to 50 times higher than in blood. *Complications:* Rhabdomyolysis, myoglobinuria, and renal failure. Dopaminogenic hypertensive crisis, cerebrovascular accident, encephalopathy, and malignant hyperthermia. Schizophrenic paranoid psychosis (induced in chronic users or precipitated in acute users). Loss of memory for months. Delayed toxicity and "flashbacks" occur. Teratogenic cases have been reported. Children have been intoxicated from inhalation in a room where adults were smoking PCP. PCP-induced depression and suicide.

Phenobarbital. See Barbiturates.

Phenothiazines and Other Major Neuroleptics. Phenothiazines are represented by aliphatic compounds: chlorpromazine (Thorazine), promethazine (Phenergan), promazine (Sparine), triflupromazine (Vesprin), methoxypromazine (Tentone); piperazine compounds (dimethylamine series); acetophenazine (Tindal), fluphenazine (Prolixin), prochlorperazine (Compazine), perphenazine (Trilafon), trifluoperazine (Stelazine); and piperidine compounds: mesoridazine (Serentil), thioridazine (Mellaril), pipamazine (Mornidine). Nonphenothiazines are the thioxanthines: chlorprothixene (Taractan), thiothixene (Navane); butyrophenones: haloperidol (Haldol), droperidol (Inapsine); dibenzoxazepines: loxapine (Loxitane, Daxolin); and dihydroindolones: molindone (Moban, Lidone). These have pharmacologic properties similar to those of the phenothiazines. See Table 25. *Manifestations:* If patient is asymptomatic, monitor vital signs and ECG for at least 6 to 12 hours. Clues to phenothiazine overdose are miosis, tremor, hypotension, hypothermia, respiratory depression, radiopaque pills on radiograph of abdomen, and increased QT waves in the ECG. Anticholinergic actions are also present. Major problems are respiratory depression, myocardial toxicity (quinidine-like), neurogenic hypotension (antidopaminergic), and idiosyncratic reaction, which may occur at therapeutic levels. Idiosyncratic reaction consists of opisthotonos, torticollis, orolingual dyskinesis, and oculogyric crisis (painful upward gaze) and can be mistaken for a psychotic episode. Extrapyramidal crisis is frequent in children and women. Malignant neuroleptic syndrome may occur. It is characterized by hyperthermia, muscle rigidity, and autonomic dysfunction. Death is usually due to cardiac effects. Phenothiazines are metabolized by the liver into many metabolites. Some remain in the body longer than 6 months. *Management:* (1) Gastrointestinal decontamination. Emesis induction may be useful if symptoms have not occurred. If symptoms are already present, many of these agents have antiemetic action, so lavage may be required. Always provide gastric lavage to comatose patients after the airway is protected regardless of the time of ingestion because of inhibition of gastric motility. (2) Extrapyramidal signs (idiosyncratic reaction) can be treated with diphenhydramine (Benadryl) (Antidote 19, Table 4), or benztropine (Cogentin), 1 to 2 mg intravenously slowly. Symptoms recur, and these drugs should be continued orally for 2 to 3 days. *This is not the treatment of overdose,* only of the idiosyncratic reaction. (3) Monitor ECG for dysrhythmias and treat with antidysrhythmic agents. (4) Hypotension is treated with the Trendelenburg position or fluid challenge or both. Vasopressors are used only if these fail. Dopamine (Intropin) should not be used to treat the hypotension because these drugs are antidopaminogenic. If a pressor agent is needed, use norepinephrine (Levarterenol, Levophed). (5) Treat neuroleptic malignant syndrome by discontinuing the offending agent, reducing temperature with external cooling, and correcting any metabolic imbalance. Dantrolene, bromocriptine, and amantadine are agents that have been shown to be useful pharmacologic adjuncts for the management of this syndrome. (6) Treat hypothermia or hyperthermia with external physical measures (not drugs). (7) Physostygmine should be avoided because it can produce seizures and cardiac toxicity. *Laboratory aids:* A ferric chloride test of urine can confirm exposure to phenothiazines if there is a sufficient blood level. Blood levels are *not* useful in management. A radiograph of the abdomen is useful to detect undissolved tablets, which may be radiopaque. Monitor arterial blood gases, renal and hepatic function, and levels of electrolytes and blood glucose for creatinine kinase and myoglobinemia in neuroleptic malignant syndrome.

Phenylpropanolamine (PPA). See Amphetamines.

Primidone. See Anticonvulsants.

Propoxyphene. See Opioids.

Propranolol and Beta Blockers. Some of these agents available in the United States at this time are listed in Table 25. Beta blockers generally act as negative cardiac ionotropes and chronotropes, although some have partial agonist activity with the opposite effect. *Toxic dose:* Varies considerably. *Toxicokinetics:* Peak action is 1 to 2 hours orally and lasts 24 to 48 hours. In drugs with long half-lives, e.g., nadolol, it may take many days to recover from overdose toxicity (Table 26). *Manifestations:* Observe for bradycardia and hypotension. Fat-soluble drugs have more CNS effects. Partial agonists may initially produce tachycardia and hypertension (oxprenolol, pindolol). ECG changes include varying degrees of atrioventricular conduction delay or frank asystole. May cause hypoglycemia. *Management:* (1) Gastrointestinal decontamination with gastric lavage and activated charcoal/cathartic. Before gastric lavage, treatment with atropine, 0.01 mg per kg for a child and 0.5 mg for an adult, has been suggested to decrease the vagal effect in patients with bradycardia or significant intoxications. Avoid induced emesis because of early onset of seizures and vagal stimulation. Asymptomatic patients may be discharged after 12 to 24 hours of observation. (2) Treat hy-

TABLE 25. **Pharmacokinetics of Phenothiazines and Related Compounds**

Medication	Metabolism	Dose Equivalent	Absorption	Vd (L/kg)	Half-life (h)	Therapy
Aliphatic						
Moderate cardiotoxic and hypotensive effects; low sedation; moderate extrapyramidal effects; moderate anticholinergic effects						
Chlorpromazine (Thorazine) (high sedation)	Hepatic	100 mg	Rapid	10–20	16–30	PO: child, 2 mg/kg/24 h; max <12 years old, 75 mg/24 h; adult, 200–2000 mg/24 h
Fluphenazine HCl (Prolixin) (injectible deconate salt)	Hepatic	2 mg	Rapid	—	2–12 (6.8–9.6 days)	PO: adult, 2.5–10 mg/24h
Promethazine (Phenergan)	Hepatic	25 mg	Rapid	—	12	PO: child, 0.1–0.5 mg/kg/dose; adult; 12.5–25 mg/dose (25–200 mg/24 h)
Piperazine						
Least cardiotoxicity and hypotensive effects; very high extrapyramidal effects; moderate anticholinergic effects						
Prochlorperazine (Compazine)	Hepatic	15 mg	Slow	10–35	8–12	PO: child, 0.1 mg/kg/dose (not <2 years old); adult, 10 mg/dose
Piperidine						
Highest cardiotoxic and hypotensive effects: low extrapyramidal effects; high anticholinergic effects						
Theoridazine (Mellaril) (high sedation)	Hepatic	100 mg	Slow	3.5	26–36	PO: child, 1 mg/kg/24 h (not <3 years old); adult, 150–300 mg/24 h
Butyrophenone						
Low cardiotoxicity and hypotensive effects; low sedation; very high extrapyramidal effects; very low anticholinergic effects						
Haloperidol (Haldol) (sedation)	Hepatic	2–15 mg	Rapid	20–30	12–22	PO: child, 0.1 mg/kg/24 h; adult, 20–100 mg/24 h
Droperidol (Inapsine)	Hepatic	2.5–10 mg	N/A	Large	2.2	IM/IV: child, 0.1–1.5 mg/kg/dose; adult, 2.5–10 mg/dose
Thioxanthene						
Low cardiotoxic and hypotensive effects: low sedation; high extrapyramidal effects; low anticholinergic effects						
Thiothixene (Navane)	Hepatic	2 mg	N/A	Large	34	PO: child, 0.25 mg/kg/24 h; adult, 16–60 mg/24 h (max, 60 mg)
Dibenzorazepine						
Low cardiotoxic and hypotensive effects; low sedation; high extrapyramidal effects; low anticholinergic effects						
Loxapine (Loxitane)	Hepatic	15 mg	N/A	Large	3–4	PO: adult, initially 10 mg bid to max of 50 mg
Dihydroindolones						
Molindone (Moban)	Hepatic	10 mg	Rapid	Large	1.5	PO: adult, initially 50–75 mg/24 h increased up to 225 mg.

*Peak levels occur mainly 1–4 h postingenstion, and they have enterohepatic recirculation. The pharmacokinetics of most phenothiazines resemble those of chlorpromazine. See kinetics for details.

Abbreviations: PO = per os (orally); IM = intramuscularly; IV = intravenously; N/A = not available.

poglycemia (frequent in children) and hyperkalemia. (3) Control convulsions. (4) Cardiovascular manifestations: Bradycardia—if hemodynamically stable and asymptomatic, no therapy. If unstable (hypotension or atriovenous block), use atropine, isoproterenol, glucagon, and pacemaker. Ventricular tachycardia or premature beats—use lidocaine, phenytoin, or overdrive pacing. Myocardial depression and hypotension—correct dysrhythmias, institute Trendelenburg positioning, and fluids. Monitor with PAWP catheter. If low cardiac output with low PAWP, give more fluids. If low cardiac output with normal PAWP, use glu-

cagon (Antidote 26, Table 4). Avoid quinidine, procainamide, and disopyramide (Norpace). Glucagon is probably the drug of choice because it works through an adenyl cyclase mechanism not affected by the beta blockers. It is given as a bolus and may be continued as an infusion (Antidote 26, Table 4). If bronchospasm, give aminophylline. Hemodialysis or hemoperfusion for low volume distribution drugs that are low protein binding and water soluble (nadolol and atenolol), particularly with evidence of renal failure. If hypoglycemia, give intravenous glucose. *Laboratory aids:* Monitor blood glucose, potassium, ECG,

TABLE 26. **Pharmacokinetic Properties of Beta Blockers**

Drug Name	Solubility and Absorption (%)	Plasma Half-life (h)	Elimination Route	Peak Concentration (h)	Protein Bound (%)	Vd (L/kg)	Beta$_1$ Cardiac Selective
Acebutolol* (Sectral) Dose: 400–800 mg MDD: 800 mg TPC: 200–2000 ng/mL	Moderate, lipid (90)	3–4, metabolite diacetolol	Hepatic, active metabolite	—	26	1.2	+
Alprenolol* (Aptin, Betapin; Betacard) Dose: 200–800 mg MDD: 800 mg TPC: 50–200 ng/mL	Lipid (10)	3.1	Hepatic	1–3	85	3.4	−
Atenolol (Tenormin) Dose: 50–100 mg MDD: 100 mg TPC: 200–500 ng/mL	Water (46–62)	6–9	Renal, 95%	2–4	3–10	0.7	+
Betaxolol (Betoptic) Dose: 1 drop in eye twice daily MDD: Not available	Water (70–90)	12–22	Hepatic, 3–12%	—	50–60	4.9–13	+
Esmolol (Brevibloc) Dose: IV 50–500 μg/kg/min (loading dose) MDD: 300 μg/kg/min	Water	9 min	Hepatic, plasma esterases	—	55	3.4	+
Labetalol (Normodyne, Trandate) Dose: 400–800 mg MDD: 1–2 gm	Water (50)	6–8	Hepatic, 95% Blocks alpha (weakly) and beta activity	—	50	11	−
Levobunolol (Betagan) Dose: Ophthalmologic: 1 drop twice daily, 0.5%, 1%	Water (100)	6.1	Hepatic	—	—	—	−
Metoprolol (Lopressor) Dose: 50–100 mg MDD: 450 mg TPC: 50–100 ng/mL	Lipid (>95)	3–4	Hepatic	1–2	10	5.6	+
Nadolol (Corgard) Dose: 40–320 mg MDD: 320 mg TPC: 20–400 ng/mL	Water (15–25)	14–23	Renal, 70%	3–4	25	2.1	−
Oxprenolol (Trasicor) Dose: 80–320 mg MDD: 480 mg TPC: 80–100 ng/mL	Lipid (70–95)	1.5–3	Hepatic	1–2	80	1.5	−
Pindolol* (Visken) Dose: 20–60 mg MDD: 60 mg TPC: 50–150 ng/mL	Lipid (>90)	3–4	Hepatic, 60%; renal, 40%	1.25	57	2.0	−
Practolol* (Eraldin)			No longer available in United States because of adverse reactions				
Dose: 25–600 mg MDD: 800 mg TPC: 1500–5000 ng/mL	Water (100)	6–8	Renal	3	40	—	+
Propranolol (Inderal) Dose: 40–160 mg MDD: 480 mg TPC: 50–100 ng/mL	Lipid (100) (70% first pass)	2–3	Hepatic; renal (<1%), active hydroxy metabolite	1.5	90–95	3.6	−
Sotalol (Beta-cardone, Sotacor)			Prolongs QT and may produce torsade de pointes				
Dose: 80–320 mg MDD: 480 mg TPC: 500–4000 ng/mL	Water (70)	5–13	Renal	2–3	54	0.7	−

TABLE 26. **Pharmacokinetic Properties of Beta Blockers** *Continued*

Drug Name	Solubility and Absorption (%)	Plasma Half-life (h)	Elimination Route	Peak Concentration (h)	Protein Bound (%)	Vd (L/kg)	Beta₁ Cardiac Selective
Timolol†‡ (Blocadren) Dose: 20 mg; ophthalmologic (Timoptic, 0.25%, 0.5%), 1 drop twice daily MDD: 60 mg TPC: 5–10 ng/mL	Lipid (>90)	3–5	Hepatic, 80%; renal, 20%	4–5	<10	5.5	–

Abbreviations: MDD = maximum daily dose; TPC = therapeutic plasma concentration.
*Partial agonists.
†Substantial first pass.
‡Mitochondrial calcium protection during ischemia.

PAWP. Fatal blood level of propranolol is 0.8 to 1.2 mg per dL (8 to 12 μg per mL).

Quinidine and Quinine (Antidysrhythmic and Antimalarial Agents). *Toxic dose:* Quinidine in child is 60 mg per kg; in adult, 2 to 8 grams. Quinine is 15 mg per kg, child; 1 gram, adult. *Toxicokinetics:* There is 95 to 100% absorption, with peak action in 2 to 6 hours. Half-life is 3 to 4 hours (quinidine gluconate, 8 to 12 hours). Large Vd. Metabolized predominantly by the liver. *Manifestations:* Cinchonism (headache, nausea, vomiting, tinnitus, deafness, diplopia, dilated pupils). Myocardial depression, dysrhythmias, ECG changes—prolongation of PR, QRS, and QT intervals. Rashes and flushing. Hemolysis in glucose-6-phosphate dehydrogenase deficiency. Dementia reported. Quinidine produces more cardiovascular damage and quinine produces more ocular damage. *Management:* (1) Obtain an immediate cardiac consultation. Electrophysiologic support of the heart should be readily available. (2) Gastrointestinal decontamination. Avoid emesis because of rapid onset of seizures and coma. (3) Monitor ECG and liver function. (4) May need antidysrhythmic drugs (but avoid Class IA antidysrhythmics), and pacemaker and alkalinization. Treat torsades de pointes with magnesium sulfate, 2 grams IV over 2 to 3 min-

utes, in adults. *Laboratory aids:* Quinidine: Therapeutic level 2 to 6 μg per mL. Toxic greater than 8 μg per mL. Fatal greater than 16 μg per mL. Quinine: Therapeutic level 7 μg per mL. Toxic greater than 10 μg per mL.

Salicylates. *Toxic dose:* See Table 27. Methyl salicylate (oil of wintergreen): 1 ml equals 1.4 grams of salicylate. One teaspoonful equals 21 adult aspirins. *Toxicokinetics:* Plasma concentration is significant in 30 minutes and peaks in 1 to 2 hours but may be delayed 6 hours or more in overdose with enteric-coated, sustained-release preparations or concretions. Half-life is 3 to 6 hours (therapeutic) to 12 to 36 hours (toxic). Urine pH influences urine salicylate elimination. *Manifestations of acute ingestion* (see Table 27): The metabolic disturbance in adults and older children is usually respiratory alkalosis; in children younger than 5 years of age, the initial respiratory alkalosis usually changes to metabolic or mixed metabolic acidosis and respiratory alkalosis, with acidosis predominating within a few hours. *Management:* (1) Gastrointestinal decontamination is useful up to 12 hours postingestion because some factors delay absorption (food, enteric-coated tablets, other drugs); pylorospasm may delay emptying; and concretions may form. Activated charcoal should be administered every

TABLE 27. **Quantities of Aspirin Ingested: Deposition and Manifestations***

Category	Amount Ingested (mg/kg)	Toxicity Expected	Gastrointestinal Decontamination	Manifestations Anticipated
Nontoxic	<150	No	No	None
Mild intoxication	150–200	Yes	Yes (ECF)	Vomiting, tinnitus, mild hyperventilation
Moderate intoxication	200–300	Yes	Yes (ECF)	Hyperpnea, lethargy or excitability
Severe intoxication	300–500	Yes	Yes (ECF)	Coma, convulsions, severe hyperpnea
Very severe intoxication	>500	Yes	Yes (ECF)	Potentially fatal

Abbreviation: ECF = emergency care facility.
*See toxic dose indications for gastrointestinal decontamination.

TABLE 28. **Recommendations for Fluid Management for Moderate or Severe Salicylism***

Purpose	Rate (mL/kg/h)	Duration (h)	Na	K	Cl	HCO$_3$	Glucose
			mEq/L				
Volume expansion	20	0.5–1.0	100	0	77	23	5–10
Administered as 0.45% saline with 23 mEq/L NaHCO$_3$							
Hydration Ongoing losses Alkalinization	4–8	Until therapeutic blood serum concentration 30 mg/dL	56	40	56	1–2 mEq/kg child; 50–100 mEq adult	5–10
Administered as 0.33% saline and NaHCO$_3$ to obtain urine pH 7.5–8.0, blood pH 7.5							
			mEq/kg/day				
Maintenance	2–6	—	3	2	4		

*For severe acidosis pH <7.15, may require 1–2 mEq/kg of sodium bicarbonate every 1–2 h. Usual fluid loss is 200–300 mL/kg, but carefully monitor for fluid overload. Potassium may be needed in excess of 40 mEq/L when alkalinizing.

4 hours until stools are black. Concretions may be removed by lavage, whole-body irrigation, endoscopy, or gastrostomy. (2) Intravenous fluid should be given as recommended in Table 28. Alkalinization enhances salicylate excretion. Potassium is essential to produce adequate alkalinization. Monitor both the urine and blood pH. Do not use the urine pH alone to assess the need for alkalinization (Antidote 39, Table 4). (3) Fluid retention can be treated with mannitol (20%), 0.5 gram per kg over 30 minutes, or furosemide, 1 mg per kg intravenously. (4) Hyperpyrexia should be treated with external cooling. (5) Abnormal bleeding or hypoprothrombinemia will need vitamin K, 10 to 50 mg intravenously, and, if bleeding continues, fresh blood or platelet transfusion (Antidote 43, Table 4). (6) Dialysis (hemodialysis) or hemoperfusion is indicated if there is persistent acidosis (pH <7.1) and lack of response to fluid or alkali in 6 hours; if serum salicylate levels are initially greater than 160 mg per dL or greater than 130 mg per dL at 6 hours postingestion (do *not* use the salicylate level as the sole criterion for dialysis); or if there are coma and uncontrollable seizures, congestive heart failure, acute renal failure, and progressive deterioration despite good management. (7) Chronic toxicity is usually a more severe intoxication because of the cumulative pharmacokinetics of salicylates. Management needs are outlined in Table 29. *Laboratory aids:* The metabolic acidosis of salicylism has a moderately elevated anion gap. Hyperglycemia or hypoglycemia may exist. Serum salicylate levels used in conjunction with the Done nomogram (Fig. 3) are useful predictors of expected severity following *acute single ingestions.* The Done nomogram is *not* useful in chronic intoxications, methyl salicylate, phenyl salicylate, or homomethyl salicylate ingestions. The salicylate level for use in the Done nomogram should be obtained 6 hours postingestion. Before 6 hours, levels in the toxic range should be treated, and patients with levels below the toxic range should be retested if a potentially toxic dose is ingested. Monitor urine output, urine pH, electrolytes, arterial blood gases, blood glucose, prothrombin time, renal function, serum salicylate level, and urine salicylate with the ferric chloride test. Arterial blood pH should be kept at 7.5. *Prognosis:* Persistent vigorous treatment of salicylate ingestion is essential because recovery has occurred despite decerebrate rigidity.

Sedative Hypnotics, Nonbarbiturate. See Table 30. *Management:* Primarily supportive (especially intubation and ventilator therapy with continuous positive airway pressure for adult

TABLE 29. **Management of Chronic Salicylate Intoxication**

Classification	Urine pH	Blood pH	Hydration	NaHCO$_3$ (mEq/L)	Potassium (mEq/L)
Mild	Alkaline	Alkaline	Yes	Yes†	20
Moderate	Acid*	Alkaline	Yes	pH 7.5†	40
Severe	Acid	Acid	Yes	pH 7.5	40‡ 80§

*Paradoxical acid urine and alkaline blood indicate potassium depletion.
†Bicarbonate administered to keep blood pH 7.5 and urine pH 7.5–8.0.
‡Normal serum potassium and electrocardiogram (ECG).
§Low serum potassium and/or abnormal ECG indicating potassium deficiency.

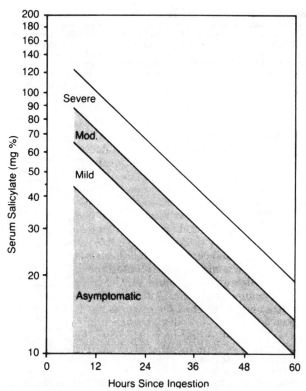

Figure 3. The Done nomogram for salicylate intoxication. For limitations of use, see *Laboratory aids.* (Redrawn from Done A: Salicylate intoxication: Significance of measurements of salicylate in blood in cases of acute ingestion. Pediatrics *26:*800, 1960. Reproduced by permission of Pediatrics.)

respiratory distress syndrome) and with the use of hemoperfusion or hemodialysis in patients who are severely intoxicated and fail to respond to good supportive care and whose intoxication is life-threatening. Avoid emesis because of rapid onset of convulsions, apnea, and coma. (1) *Chloral hydrate* management includes cautious gastrointestinal decontamination. Avoid the use of epinephrine and catecholamines that may produce dysrhythmias. Propranolol, 0.1 mg per kg in 1-mg increments, appears to be more effective than lidocaine for ventricular dysrhythmias. Charcoal hemoperfusion may effectively remove chloral hydrate and its metabolite in patients who fail to respond and have potentially fatal plasma levels (20 μg per mL or higher). Hemodialysis may be ineffective because of lipid solubility. (2) *Ethchlorvynol* management includes gastrointestinal decontamination up to several hours postingestion. Charcoal hemoperfusion is the best method of extracorporeal removal when other measures fail in a life-threatening situation (ingestion of over 10 grams or 100 mg per kg, with serum levels of over 100 μg per mL in the first 12 hours or 70 μg per mL after 12 hours in patients with prolonged life-threatening coma).

External rewarming if temperature is below 32° C. (3) *Glutethimide* management includes gastrointestinal decontamination up to several hours postingestion. Concretions may form. Charcoal hemoperfusion appears to be the best method of extracorporeal removal in life-threatening protracted coma when the patient has ingested over 10 grams and has a serum level of over 30 μg per mL. Treat hyperthermia with external cooling. (4) *Meprobamate* management includes gastrointestinal decontamination up to several hours postingestion, with charcoal hemoperfusion in prolonged coma with life-threatening complications. Concretions may form in the stomach and may require whole-bowel irrigation, endoscopy, or surgical removal. (5) *Methaqualone* management includes gastrointestinal decontamination up to 12 hours postingestion. Forced diuresis, dialysis, and hemoperfusion are not indicated. Fatalities are rare. (6) *Methyprylon* management includes gastrointestinal decontamination and may require treatment of the hypotension with vasopressors of the alpha-adrenergic variety—levarterenol (Levophed). The hypotension usually does not respond to position or fluids alone. This is a dialyzable drug, but dialysis usually is not necessary. Fatalities are rare.

Strychnine. Primarily available as a rodenticide and component of cathartics and "tonics." Adulterant of "street drugs," particularly marijuana and cocaine. *Toxic dose:* 5 to 10 mg; fatal in doses of 15 to 30 mg. *Toxicokinetics:* Rapid absorption. Manifestations may occur within 15 to 30 minutes. Low protein binding. Hepatic metabolism, which appears to be saturable. Twenty percent is excreted in urine. Has been found in the urine up to 48 hours after a 700-mg dose. *Manifestations:* Interferes with postsynaptic neurotransmitter inhibition by glycine. Hyperacusis is often the first sign. Mild cases—face stiffness (trismus and risus sardonicus). Moderate cases—extensor muscle thrusts. Severe cases—tetanic convulsions with opisthotonos. Death occurs within 1 to 3 hours after ingestion. The prognosis for survival improves if the patient survives beyond 5 hours. The complications of intoxication are lactic acidosis, hyperthermia, rhabdomyolysis and renal damage from precipitation of myoglobin in the renal tubules, and death from hypoxia. *Management:* (1) Emesis is contraindicated because of rapid absorption and the early onset of seizures. Gastric aspiration and lavage may be used after the seizures are controlled. Activated charcoal should be given and repeated. (2) Control convulsions with diazepam or phenobarbital. (3) Supportive care for respiratory depression. (4) Acid diuresis and dialysis do not appear to be justified on the basis of available studies. (5) Paralysis with assisted ventilation is useful.

TABLE 30. **Nonbarbiturate Sedative Hypnotic Drugs**

Drug	Absorption and Toxic Dose	Peak (h)	Vd (L/kg)	Protein Bound (%)	Elimination Route	Serum Half-life (h)	Toxic Level (μg/mL)	Manifestations and Comment*
Chloral hydrate (Noctec)	Rapid TD, 2 gm FD, 4–10 gm	1–2	0.75–0.9	40	Hepatic 90% to active metabolite trichloro-ethanol (TCE)	4–8 Min TCE: 8–12 h	100 (80 TCE— very toxic)	Pear-like odor; dysrhythmias (especially ventricular), hepatotoxicity, irritant to mucosa of GI tract; ARDS; radiopaque capsules
Ethchlorvynol (Placidyl)	Rapid TD, 2.5 gm FD, 10–25 gm	1–2	3–4	35–50	Hepatic 90%	10–25 in OD over 100	20–80	Prolonged coma up to 200 h, apnea, hypothermia, pulmonary edema, pink gastric aspirate, pungent odor
Glutethimide (Doriden) (highest mortality of all sedative-hypnotics, 14%)	Slow, erratic TD, 5 gm FD, 10 gm	6	Large, 2–2.7	50	Hepatic 98% to toxic metabolite 4-hydroxyglutarimide	10–40 in OD over 100	20–80	Prolonged, cyclic comas up to 120 h, anticholinergic signs, convulsions, recurrent apnea, hyperthermia
Meprobamate (Equanil, Miltown)	Rapid TD, 10–20 gm FD, 10–20 gm	4–8	10	20	Hepatic 90%	6–16	30–100	Coma, convulsions, pulmonary edema, apnea, concretions in stomach
Methaqualone (Quaaludes, "love drugs")	Rapid TD, 800 mg FD 3–8 gm	1–3	2–6	80	Hepatic 90%	10–40	8–10	Hypertonia, hyper-reflexia, convulsions, apnea, acts "drunk," bleeding tendencies
Methyprylon (Noludar)	Rapid TD, 3 gm FD, 8–20 gm	2–4	1–2	—	Hepatic 97%	3–6 in OD over 50	30	Hyperactive, coma lasts 30 h, miosis, persistent hypotension, pulmonary edema; mortality rare

Abbreviations: TD = toxic dose; FD = fatal dose; OD = overdose; ARDS = adult respiratory distress syndrome; GI = gastrointestinal.

*Comment includes other features besides the typical manifestations of all these agents—coma, respiratory depression, psychological and physiologic withdrawal, hypotension, hypothermia (except glutethimide hyperthermia).

Tear Gas (Lacrimators). CS (chlorobenzylidine), "riot control"; CN powder (chloroacetophenone, 1%); Mace (chloroacetophenone). *Management:* Dermal and ocular decontamination. Protect attendants from contamination. Ophthalmologic evaluation. Oxygen therapy may be needed for dyspnea and respiratory distress.

Theophylline. *Toxic dose:* Acute, single dose greater than 10 mg per kg yields mild toxicity. Greater than 20 mg per kg, moderate manifestations. *Toxicokinetics:* Absorption is complete. Peak levels occur within 60 minutes after ingestion of liquid preparations; 1 to 3 hours after regular tablets; and 3 to 10 hours after slow-release preparations. Vd, 0.3 to 0.7 liter per kg. Protein binding, 15 to 40%. Half-life varies: 3.5 hours average in a child and 4.5 hours in an adult (range from 3 to 9 hours). In neonates and young infants the drug's half-life is much longer. Overdose increases the half-life. *Elimination:* Hepatic metabolism, 90% (demethylation and oxidation); 8 to 10% is excreted unchanged in the urine. *Manifestations:* Acute toxicity generally correlates with blood levels; chronic toxicity does not. Ten to 20 μg per mL is the therapeutic range, but some

mild gastrointestinal toxicity may occur. Twenty to 40 μg per mL is moderate toxicity, with gastrointestinal and CNS stimulation. Over 50 μg per mL—seizures and dysrhythmias may occur, but they may also occur at lower levels and without gastrointestinal symptoms. Children tolerate higher serum levels. Chronic intoxication is more serious and difficult to treat. Many factors increase theophylline concentration. *Management:* (1) Gastrointestinal decontamination in acute overdose, up to 4 hours with regular preparations and up to 8 to 12 hours with slow-release preparations. Test aspirate or vomitus for blood. Give activated charcoal every 4 hours until serum theophylline levels are less than 20 μg per mL. Do not induce emesis if hematemesis exists. If there is intractable vomiting, administer the antiemetic metoclopramide, 0.4 mg per kg per dose intravenously (maximum, 0.5 mg per kg per 24 hours) in infants and children, and 10 mg slowly over 15 minutes every 6 to 8 hours in adults. Alternative: droperidol, 2.5 mg intravenously or 0.05 to 0.1 mg per kg per dose every 6 to 8 hours if needed. Both drugs may cause extrapyramidal symptoms. (2) Monitor ECG, obtain theophylline levels every 4 hours until in the therapeutic range of 10 to 20 μg per mL. (3) Control seizures with diazepam. If coma, convulsions, or vomiting exists, intubate immediately. (4) Hypotension is treated with fluid challenge and if this fails, vasopressors. (5) Hematemesis is managed with saline lavage and blood replacement if needed. (6) Charcoal hemoperfusion is the management of choice in life-threatening convulsions, dysrhythmias, hematemesis, or intractable vomiting refractory to conventional measures. It is recommended for acute intoxications with serum theophylline concentrations 70 to 100 μg per mL or with chronic overdoses of 40 to 60 μg per mL especially if the patient has risk factors that increase serum levels, i.e., younger than 6 months, older than 60 years, liver disease, heart failure, viral infections, pneumonia, fever greater than 102° F; medications: macrolid antibiotics, oral contraceptives, cimetidine, beta blockers, carbamazepine, and caffeine. Differences in slow-release preparations from regular preparations: few or no gastrointestinal symptoms with high levels; peak concentration times may be 10 to 24 hours postingestion; and onset of seizures may occur 10 to 12 hours postingestion. *Laboratory aids:* Monitor theophylline levels, check for occult blood in vomitus and stools, monitor vital signs and hemoglobin and hematocrit (for hemorrhage). Monitor cardiac, renal, and hepatic function, electrolytes, blood glucose, arterial blood gases, and acid-base balance.

Toluene. See Hydrocarbons.

Tranquilizers. See Sedative Hypnotics.

Trichloroethylene. See Hydrocarbons.

Tricyclic Antidepressants (TCAD). See Table 31. These agents are generally rapidly absorbed from the gastrointestinal tract, but absorption may be prolonged in overdose owing to anticholinergic action. Their bioavailability has considerable variation among patients, and they are highly bound to plasma and tissue proteins. Protein binding decreases with decreasing pH. The Vd is large, usually 10 to 20 liters per kg. The TCAD are metabolized primarily in the liver. *N*-Demethylation of the tertiary amines yields the active secondary amine metabolites; hydroxylation gives rise to inactive metabolites. Forty percent is excreted in the feces and only 3% in the urine unchanged. The t½ varies from 9 to 198 hours. In an overdose, the half-life may be much longer. Tricyclic tertiary amines (metabolized to active metabolites) are amitriptyline (Elavil), imipramine (Tofranil), and doxepin (Sinequan). Tricyclic secondary amines (metabolized to nonactive metabolites) are desipramine (Norpramin, Pertofrane), protriptyline (Vivactil), and nortriptyline (Pamelor). Tricyclic dibenzoxazepine (metabolized to a major metabolite) is amoxapine

(Asendin). *Manifestations:* The onset of action varies from less than 1 hour to 12 hours after ingestion. The phases of intoxication are (1) consciousness with dry mouth, mydriasis, ataxia, increased deep tendon reflexes, and changes in the ST segment; (2) Stages I and II coma with hypertension, tachycardia above 160, mydriasis, and supraventricular tachycardia; and (3) Stages III and IV coma with hypotension, heart rate under 120, respiratory depression, tonic-clonic seizures, and ventricular dysrhythmias. The CNS effects occur early, and seizures are common. *Cardiovascular toxicity* is frequent in the serious poisonings and results from anticholinergic effects, sympathomimetic activity (by blocking reuptake of catecholamines), quinidine activity, catecholamine depletion, and alpha-adrenergic blockage. Cardiotoxic effects include cardiac dysrhythmias, hypertension, hypotension, and pulmonary edema.

Toxic dose: The TCAD have a narrow margin of safety. In a child, a 375-mg dose and in adults, as little as 500 to 750 mg has been fatal. The following dosages may serve as a guide to the degree of imipramine toxicity: Less than 10 mg per kg produces light coma, mydriasis, and tachycardia and has a good prognosis. At 20 mg per kg, Stage III manifestations are produced. At 30 mg per kg, fatalities may result. At 50 mg per kg, the mortality rate is increased. Over 70 mg per kg is rarely survived. Relative adult dosage equivalents may serve as a guide: amitryptyline, 100 mg; amoxapine, 125 mg; desipramine, 75 mg; doxepin, 100 mg; imipramine, 75 mg; maprotiline, 75 mg; nortriptyline, 50 mg; and trazodone, 200 mg (see Table 30). Therapeutic blood levels are in the range of 50 to 170 ng per mL. If the QRS interval is less than 0.10 second for 6 hours, the prognosis is good. If it is greater than 0.10 second, seizures may occur, and if it is over 0.16 second, serious dysrhythmia may occur. In general, most antidepressants possess anticholinergic activity. The tricyclics produce dysrhythmias, hypotension, and seizures. The tetracyclics (amoxaprine, maprotiline) produce convulsions that may result in rhabdomyolysis and renal dysfunction. The new agents trazodone and fluoxetine appear to have mild sedative effects and cardiotoxicity, although orthostatic hypotension, vertigo, and priapism have been reported. Bupropion (Wellbutrin) is a phenylaminoketone antidepressant that produces dose-related seizures. Nomifensine (Merital) was withdrawn in 1986 because of reports of hemolytic anemia associated with it. *Management:* (1) Maintenance of vital functions. If the patient is asymptomatic, there should be less vascular access, and cardiac monitoring should continue for at least 6 hours from admission or 8 to 12 hours postingestion. All children should be observed closely for 24 hours in

TABLE 31. **Kinetics of Cyclic Antidepressants**

Antidepressant (Trade Name)	Absorption	Peak (h)	Vd (L/kg)	Half-life (h)	Protein Binding (%)	Elimination	Toxic Level (ng/mL)	Availability	Therapeutic Plasma Level (Range)	Usual Dose Adult (mg)	Usual Dose Child (mg/kg/24 h)
Tricyclic Tertiary Amines (metabolized to active metabolites)											
Amitriptyline (Elavil)	Slow	2–12	8–10	15–19	82–96	Hepatic	>500	Tab 10, 25, 75, 100, 150, mg	50–250	75–300	1.5–2.0
Imipramine (Tofranil)	Rapid (29–77%)	1–2	5–20	8–16	76–96	Hepatic	>500	Tab 10, 25, 50, mg; Cap 75, 100, 125, 150 mg	150–250	75–300	3–7
Doxepin (Sinequan, Adapin)	Rapid complete	2–4	20	15–19	95	Hepatic	>150	Cap 25, 50, 75, 100, 150 mg	150–250	75–300	
Tricyclic Secondary Amines (metabolized to nonactive metabolites)											
Desipramine (Norpramin, Pertofrane)	Rapid incomplete	4–6	28–60	18–28	73–92	Hepatic	>500	Tab 10, 25, 50, 100, 150 mg; Cap 10, 50 mg	125–300	75–300	
Protriptyline (Vivactil)						Hepatic	NA	Tab 5, 10 mg	70–260	20–60	
Nortriptyline (Aventyl)	Slow (46–77%)	7–8	21–57	50–150	93–65	Hepatic	>500	Cap 10, 25, 75 mg	50–150	75–200	1.5–2.0
Trimipramine (Surmontil)	Rapid	2	NA	NA	Large	Renal		Cap 25, 50, 100 mg	100–200	75–300	
Tetracyclic Dibenzoxapines (metabolized to major metabolites)											
Amoxapine (Asendin)	Rapid	1.5	Large	8–30	90	Renal and hepatic	NA	Tab 25, 50, 100, 150 mg	200–600	150–600	
Maprotiline (Ludiomil)		8–24	22.6	27–58	88	Hepatic	Over 300	Tab 25, 50, 75 mg	200–600	75–300	
Triazolopyridines											
Trazodone (Desyrel)	Rapid	0.5–2	NA	4–13	89–95	Hepatic	NA	Tab 50, 100, 150 mg	800–1600	50–600	
Unclassified or Bicyclics (metabolized to active metabolite)											
Fluoxetine (Prozac)	Rapid	4–6	14–102	24–96	94	Hepatic	>400	Cap 20 mg; Syrup 20 mg/5 mL 4-oz bottles	NA	20–80	
Norfluoxetine (active metabolite) peak 76 h, half-life 5–7 days											
Dibenzazepines											
Clomipramine* (Anafranil)	Rapid	3–5	12	21	98	Hepatic	500	Cap 25, 50, 75 mg		25 increasing up to 100, max 200	
Dimethylclomipramine (DM) (primary active metabolite) half-life 54–77 h											
Aminoketones											
Bupropion (Wellbutrin)	Rapid 5–20% bioavailability	2	NA	8–24	80%	Hepatic	NA	Tab 75, 100 mg		100 bid increasing up to 150 tid	
Several active metabolites relate to toxicity											

Abbreviations: Toxic Level = toxic serum concentration; NA = not available; Tab = tablets; Cap = capsules.
*Available to psychiatrists free of charge to treat patients 1–800–842–2422 (Med Lett 30:102–104, 1988).

an intensive care unit. If symptomatic, obtain cardiac consultation and monitor in an intensive care unit until the patient is asymptomatic and shows no ECG abnormalities for at least 72 hours. (2) Gastrointestinal decontamination (omit emesis) if the patient is alert. Intact pills have been recovered by lavage up to 18 hours after ingestion. Suspected cases should have ECG monitoring. (3) Activated charcoal initially with a cathartic and repeated every 4 to 6 hours without a cathartic, and continuous nasogastric suction for the first 48 hours, may interrupt enterohe-patic recycling of tricyclic antidepressants. (4) Control seizures with intravenous diazepam. Intravenous phenytoin (Dilantin) may be added for seizures not responding to diazepam alone. (5) All cardiovascular complications of TCAD should *first* be treated by alkalinization of blood with sodium bicarbonate to a pH of 7.5 to 7.55 (Antidote 39, Table 4). Alkalinization increases the protein binding of the TCAD. Serum potassium levels should be monitored because a sudden increase in blood pH can aggravate or precipitate hypokalemia. Specific cardiovascular complications should be treated as follows: *Hypotension*—norepinephrine (Levophed), a predominantly alpha-adrenergic drug, is preferred over dopamine. (Hypertension that occurs early rarely requires treatment.) *Serious conduction defects* are best managed with phenytoin, and patients may need a temporary transvenous pace maker. *Sinus tachycardia* usually does not require treatment except for alkalinization. *Supraventricular tachycardia* with hemodynamic instability requires synchronized cardioversion, 0.25 to 1.0 watt-seconds per kg after sedation. *Ventricular tachycardia*—after alkalinization and phenytoin, intravenous lidocaine (for one dose only) may be required for persistent ventricular tachycardia. Synchronized cardioversion may be needed if lidocaine fails. *Ventricular fibrillation* should be treated with direct current countershock. *Torsades de pointes* is treated with magnesium sulfate IV 20%, 2 grams over 2 to 3 minutes, followed by a continuous infusion of 5 to 10 mg per minute, of isoproterenol, lidocaine, phenytoin, and bretylium and atrial or ventricular overdrive pacing to shorten the QT interval. *Laboratory aids:* Arterial blood gases with blood pH, ECG, serum electrolytes, blood urea nitrogen and creatinine, serum phenytoin level, urine output, and, in severe cases, central venous pressure, PAWP, or both should be monitored.

Turpentine. See Hydrocarbons.

Xylene. See Hydrocarbons.

Appendices and Index

REFERENCE VALUES FOR THE INTERPRETATION OF LABORATORY TESTS

method of
WILLIAM Z. BORER, M.D.
Thomas Jefferson University Hospital
Philadelphia, Pennsylvania

Most of the tests performed in a clinical laboratory are quantitative in nature; that is, the amount of a substance present in blood or serum is measured and reported in terms of concentration, activity (e.g., enzyme activity), or counts (e.g., blood cell counts). The laboratory must provide reference values to assist the clinician in the interpretation of laboratory results. These reference ranges constitute the physiologic quantities of substance (concentrations, activities, or counts) to be expected in healthy persons. Deviation above or below the reference range may indicate the presence of a disease process, and the severity of the disease process may be indicated by the magnitude of the deviation. Unfortunately, there is rarely a sharp demarcation between physiologic and pathologic values, and the transition between these two is often gradual as the disease process progresses.

The terms "normal" and "abnormal" have been used to describe the laboratory values that fall inside and outside the reference range, respectively. Use of these terms is now discouraged because it is virtually impossible to define normality and because "normal" may be confused with the statistical term "Gaussian." Reference ranges are established from statistical studies in groups of healthy volunteers. Although these study subjects must be free of disease, their lifestyles or habits may result in subtle variations in their laboratory values. Examples of these variables include diet, body mass, exercise, and geographic location. Age and gender may also affect reference values. When the data from a large cohort of healthy subjects fit a Gaussian distribution, the usual statistical approach is to define the reference limits as two standard deviations above and below the mean. By definition, the reference range excludes the highest and the lowest 2.5% of the population.

Non-Gaussian distributions are handled by different statistical methods, but the results are similar in that the reference range is defined by the central 95% of the population. In other words, the odds are 1 in 20 that a healthy person's laboratory result will fall outside the reference range. If 12 laboratory tests are performed, the odds increase to about 1 in 2 that at least one of the results will be outside the reference range. This means that all healthy persons are likely to have a few unexpected laboratory results. The clinician must then integrate these data with other clinical information such as the history and physical examination results to arrive at the appropriate clinical decision. The reference ranges for many tests (especially enzyme and immunochemical measurements) vary with the method used. It is important that each laboratory establish reference ranges appropriate for the methods that it employs.

SI UNITS

During the past decade a concerted effort has been made to introduce SI units (le Système International d'Unités). The rationale for conversion to SI units is sound: laboratory data are scientifically more informative when the units are based on molar concentration rather than on mass concentration. For example, the conversion of glucose to lactate and pyruvate or the binding of a drug to albumin is more easily understood in units of molar concentration. Another example is illustrated as follows:

TABLE 1. **Base SI Units**

Property	Base Unit	Symbol
Length	Meter	m
Mass	Kilogram	kg
Amount of substance	Mole	mol
Time	Second	s
Thermodynamic temperature	Kelvin	K
Electric current	Ampere	A
Luminous intensity	Candela	cd

TABLE 2. **Derived SI Units**

Derived Property	Derived Unit	Symbol
Area	Square meter	m²
Volume	Cubic meter	m³
	Litre	L
Mass concentration	Kilogram/cubic meter	kg/m³
	Gram/liter	gL
Substance concentration	Mole/cubic meter	mol/m³
	Mole/liter	mol/L
Temperature	Degree Celsius	$C = K - 273.15$

Conventional Units

1.0 gram of hemoglobin
Combines with 1.37 mL of oxygen
Contains 3.4 mg of iron
Forms 34.9 mg of bilirubin

SI Units

4.0 mmol of hemoglobin
Combines with 4.0 mmol of oxygen
Contains 4.0 mmol of iron
Forms 4.0 mmol of bilirubin

Another advantage of SI units involves the standardization of nomenclature to facilitate global communication of medical and scientific information. The units, symbols, and prefixes employed in the SI are shown in Tables 1, 2, and 3.

Unfortunately, problems have arisen with the implementation of SI units in the United States. Their introduction in 1987 prompted many medical journals to report laboratory values in both SI and conventional units in anticipation of complete conversion to SI units in the early 1990s. The lack of a coordinated effort toward this goal has forced a retrenchment on the issue. Physicians continue to think and practice with laboratory results expressed in conventional units, and few if any American hospitals or clinical laboratories use SI units exclusively. It is not likely that complete conversion to SI units will occur in the foreseeable future, but most medical journals will probably continue to publish both set of units. For this reason, the tables of reference ranges in this appendix are given in both conventional units and SI units.

REFERENCES

AMA Drug Evaluations, 6th ed. Chicago, American Medical Association, 1992.

Bick RL (ed): Hematology—Clinical and Laboratory Practice. St. Louis, Mosby–Year Book, 1993.

Borer WZ: Selection and use of laboratory tests. *In* Tietz NW, Conn RB, and Pruden EL (eds): Applied Laboratory Medicine. Philadelphia, WB Saunders Co, 1992, pp 1–5.

Campion EW: A retreat from SI units. N Engl J Med *327:*49, 1992.

Friedman RB, and Young DS: Effects of Disease on Clinical Laboratory Tests, 2nd ed. Washington, DC, AACC Press, 1989.

Henry JB: Clinical Diagnosis and Management by Laboratory Methods, 18th ed. Philadelphia, WB Saunders Co, 1991.

Hicks JM, and Young DS: DORA '92–93: Directory of Rare Analyses. Washington, DC, AACC Press, 1992.

Jacobs DS, Kasten BL, Demott WR, and Wolfson WL: Laboratory Test Handbook, 2nd ed. Baltimore, Williams & Wilkins Co, 1990.

Kaplan LA, and Pesce AJ: Clinical Chemistry—Theory, Analysis, and Correlation, 2nd ed. St. Louis, CV Mosby, 1989.

Kjeldsberg CR, and Knight JA: Body Fluids—Laboratory Examination of Amniotic, Cerebrospinal, Seminal, Serous and Synovial fluids, 3rd ed. Chicago, ASCP Press, 1993.

Laposata M: SI Unit Conversion Guide. Boston, New England Journal of Medicine Books, 1992.

Scully RE, McNeely WF, Mark EJ, and McNeely BU: Normal reference laboratory values. N Engl J Med *327:*718–24, 1992.

Speicher CE: The Right Test—A Physician's Guide to Laboratory Medicine, 2nd ed. Philadelphia, WB Saunders Co, 1993.

Tietz NW (ed): Clinical Guide to Laboratory Tests, 2nd ed. Philadelphia, WB Saunders Co, 1990.

Wallach J: Interpretation of Diagnostic Tests—A Synopsis of Laboratory Medicine, 5th ed. Boston, Little, Brown and Co, 1992.

Young DS: Implementation of SI units for clinical laboratory data, Ann Intern Med *106:*114–29, 1987.

Young DS: Determination and validation of reference intervals. Arch Pathol Lab Med *116:*704–9, 1992.

Young DS: Effects of Drugs on Clinical Laboratory Tests, 3rd ed. Washington, DC, AACC Press, 1990.

TABLE 3. **Standard Prefixes**

Prefix	Multiplication Factor	Symbol
atto	10^{-18}	a
femto	10^{-15}	f
pico	10^{-12}	p
nano	10^{-9}	n
micro	10^{-6}	μ
milli	10^{-3}	m
centi	10^{-2}	c
deci	10^{-1}	d
deca	10^{1}	da
hecto	10^{2}	h
kilo	10^{3}	k
mega	10^{6}	M
giga	10^{9}	G
tera	10^{12}	T

TABLES OF REFERENCE VALUES

Some of the values included in the tables have been established by the Clinical Laboratories at Thomas Jefferson University Hospital, Philadelphia, Pennsylvania, and have not been published elsewhere. Other values have been compiled from the sources just cited. These tables are provided for information and educational purposes only. They are intended to complement data derived from other sources, including the medical history and physical examination. Users must exercise individual judgment in using the information provided in this appendix.

Reference Values for Hematology

	Conventional Units	SI Units
Acid hemolysis (Ham test)	No hemolysis	No hemolysis
Alkaline phosphatase, leukocyte	Total score, 14–100	Total score, 14–100
Cell counts		
Erythrocytes		
Males	4.6–6.2 million/mm^3	4.6–6.2 × 10^{12}/L
Females	4.2–5.4 million/mm^3	4.2–5.4 × 10^{12}/L
Children (varies with age)	4.5–5.1 million/mm^3	4.5–5.1 × 10^{12}/L
Leukocytes, total	4500–11,000/mm^3	4.5–11.0 × 10^9/L
Leukocytes, differential*		
Myelocytes	0%	0/L
Band neutrophils	3–5%	150–400 × 10^6/L
Segmented neutrophils	54–62%	3000–5800 × 10^6/L
Lymphocytes	25–33%	1500–3000 × 10^6/L
Monocytes	3–7%	300–500 × 10^6/L
Eosinophils	1–3%	50–250 × 10^6/L
Basophils	0–1%	15–50 × 10^6/L
Platelets	150,000–350,000/mm^3	150–350 × 10^9/L
Reticulocytes	25,000–75,000/mm^3	25–75 × 10^9/L
	(0.5–1.5% of erythrocytes)	
Coagulation tests		
Bleeding time (template)	2.75–8.0 min	2.75–8.0 min
Coagulation time (glass tube)	5–15 min	5–15 min
Factor VIII and other coagulation factors	50–150% of normal	0.5–1.5 of normal
Fibrin split products (Thrombo-Wellco test)	<10 μg/mL	<10 mg/L
Fibrinogen	200–400 mg/dL	2.0–4.0 gm/L
Partial thromboplastin time (PTT)	20–35 s	20–35 s
Prothrombin time (PT)	12.0–14.0 s	12.0–14.0 s
Coombs' test		
Direct	Negative	Negative
Indirect	Negative	Negative
Corpuscular values of erythrocytes		
Mean corpuscular hemoglobin (MCH)	26–34 pg/cell	26–34 pg/cell
Mean corpuscular volume (MCV)	80–96 μm^3	80–96 fL
Mean corpuscular hemoglobin concentration (MCHC)	32–36 gm/dL	320–360 gm/L
Haptoglobin	20–165 mg/dL	0.20–1.65 gm/L
Hematocrit		
Males	40–54 mL/dL	0.40–0.54
Females	37–47 mL/dL	0.37–0.47
Newborns	49–54 mL/dL	0.49–0.54
Children (varies with age)	35–49 mL/dL	0.35–0.49
Hemoglobin		
Males	13.0–18.0 gm/dL	8.1–11.2 mmol/L
Females	12.0–16.0 gm/dL	7.4–9.9 mmol/L
Newborns	16.5–19.5 gm/dL	10.2–12.1 mmol/L
Children (varies with age)	11.2–16.5 gm/dL	7.0–10.2 mmol/L
Hemoglobin, fetal	<1.0% of total	<0.01 of total
Hemoglobin A$_{1c}$	3–5% of total	0.03–0.05 of total
Hemoglobin A$_2$	1.5–3.0% of total	0.015–0.03 of total
Hemoglobin, plasma	0.0–5.0 mg/dL	0–3.2 μmol/L
Methemoglobin	30–130 mg/dL	19–80 μmol/L
Sedimentation rate (ESR)		
Wintrobe		
Males	0–5 mm/h	0–5 mm/h
Females	0–15 mm/h	0–15 mm/h
Westergren		
Males	0–15 mm/h	0–15 mm/h
Females	0–20 mm/h	0–20 mm/h

*Conventional units are percentages; SI units are absolute counts.

Reference Values* for Clinical Chemistry (Blood, Serum and Plasma)

	Conventional Units	SI Units
Acetoacetate plus acetone		
Qualitative	Negative	Negative
Quantitative	0.3–2.0 mg/dL	30–200 μmol/L
Acid phosphatase		
(Thymolphthalein monophosphate substrate), serum	0.1–0.6 U/L	0.1–0.6 U/L
ACTH (see corticotropin)		
Alanine aminotransferase (ALT, SGPT), serum	1–45 U/L	1–45 U/L
Albumin, serum	3.3–5.2 gm/dL	33–52 gm/L
Aldolase, serum	0.0–7.0 U/L	0.0–7.0 U/L
Aldosterone, plasma		
Standing	5–30 ng/dL	140–830 pmol/L
Recumbent	3–10 ng/dL	80–275 pmol/L
Alkaline phosphatase (ALP), serum		
Adult	35–150 U/L	35–150 U/L
Adolescent	100–500 U/L	100–500 U/L
Child	100–350 U/L	100–350 U/L
Ammonia nitrogen, plasma	10–50 μmol/L	10–50 μmol/L
Amylase, serum	25–125 U/L	25–125 U/L
Anion gap, serum, calculated	8–16 mEq/L	8–16 mmol/L
Ascorbic acid, blood	0.4–1.5 mg/dL	23–85 μmol/L
Aspartate, aminotransferase (AST, SGOT), serum	1–36 U/L	1–36 U/L
Base excess, arterial blood, calculated	0 ± 2 mEq/L	0 ± 2 mmol/L
Bicarbonate		
Venous plasma	23–29 mEq/L	23–29 mmol/L
Arterial blood	21–27 mEq/L	21–27 mmol/L
Bile acids, serum	0.3–3.0 mg/dL	0.8–7.6 μmol/L
Bilirubin, serum		
Conjugated	0.1–0.4 mg/dL	1.7–6.8 μmol/L
Total	0.3–1.1 mg/dL	5.1–19 μmol/L
Calcium, serum	8.4–10.6 mg/dL	2.10–2.65 mmol/L
Calcium, ionized, serum	4.25–5.25 mg/dL	1.05–1.30 mmol/L
Carbon dioxide, total, serum or plasma	24–31 mEq/L	24–31 mmol/L
Carbon dioxide tension (PCO_2), blood	35–45 mmHg	35–45 mmHg
Beta-carotene, serum	60–260 μg/dL	1.1–8.6 μmol/L
Ceruloplasmin, serum	23–44 mg/dL	230–440 mg/L
Chloride, serum or plasma	96–106 mEq/L	96–106 mmol/L
Cholesterol, serum or EDTA plasma		
Desirable range	<200 mg/dL	<5.20 mmol/L
Low-density lipoprotein cholesterol	60–180 mg/dL	1.55–4.65 mmol/L
High-density lipoprotein cholesterol	30–80 mg/dL	0.80–2.05 mmol/L
Copper	70–140 μg/dL	11–22 μmol/L
Corticotropin, plasma (ACTH), 8 A.M.	10–80 pg/mL	2–18 pmol/L
Cortisol, plasma		
8:00 A.M.	6–23 μg/dL	170–630 nmol/L
4:00 P.M.	3–15 μg/dL	80–410 nmol/L
10:00 P.M.	<50% of 8:00 A.M. value	<50% of 8:00 A.M. value
Creatine, serum		
Males	0.2–0.5 mg/dL	15–40 μmol/L
Females	0.3–0.9 mg/dL	25–70 μmol/L
Creatine kinase (CK, CPK), serum		
Males	55–170 U/L	55–170 U/L
Females	30–135 U/L	30–135 U/L
Creatine kinase MB isoenzyme, serum	<5% of total CK activity <5.0 ng/mL by immunoassay	
Creatinine, serum	0.6–1.2 mg/dL	50–110 μmol/L
Ferritin, serum	20–200 ng/mL	20–200 μg/L
Fibrinogen, plasma	200–400 mg/dL	2.0–4.0 gm/L
Folate		
Serum	2.0–9.0 ng/mL	4.5–20.4 nmol/L
Erythrocytes	170–700 ng/mL	385–1590 nmol/L

Table continued on following page

Reference Values* for Clinical Chemistry (Blood, Serum and Plasma) *Continued*

	Conventional Units	SI Units
Follicle-stimulating hormone (FSH), plasma		
Males	4–25 mU/mL	4–25 U/L
Females, premenopausal	4–30 mU/mL	4–30 U/L
Females, postmenopausal	40–250 mU/mL	40–250 U/L
Gamma-glutamyltransferase (GGT), serum	5–40 U/L	5–40 U/L
Gastrin, fasting, serum	0–110 pg/mL	0–110 mg/L
Glucose, fasting, plasma or serum	70–115 mg/dL	3.9–6.4 nmol/L
Growth hormone (hGH), plasma, adult, fasting	0–6 ng/mL	0–6 µg/L
Haptoglobin, serum	20–165 mg/dL	0.20–1.65 gm/L
Immunoglobulins, serum (see Immunologic Procedures)		
Insulin, fasting, plasma	5–25 µU/mL	36–179 pmol/L
Iron, serum	75–175 µg/dL	13–31 µmol/L
Iron-binding capacity, serum		
Total	250–410 µg/dL	45–73 µmol/L
Saturation	20–55%	0.20–0.55
Lactate		
Venous blood	5.0–20.0 mg/dL	0.6–2.2 mmol/L
Arterial blood	5.0–15.0 mg/dL	0.6–1.7 mmol/L
Lactate dehydrogenase (LD, LDH), serum	110–220 U/L	110–220 U/L
Lipase, serum	10–140 U/L	10–140 U/L
Lutropin, serum (LH)		
Males	1–9 IU/L	1–9 U/L
Females		
Follicular	2–10 IU/L	2–10 U/L
Midcycle	15–65 U/L	15–65 U/L
Luteal	1–12 U/L	1–12 U/L
Postmenopausal	12–65 U/L	12–65 U/L
Magnesium, serum	1.3–2.1 mg/dL	0.65–1.05 mmol/L
Osmolality	275–295 mOsm/kg H_2O	275–295 mOsm/kg H_2O
Oxygen, blood, arterial, room air		
Partial pressure (PaO$_2$)	80–100 mmHg	80–100 mmHg
Saturation (SaO$_2$)	95–98%	95–98%
pH, arterial blood	7.35–7.45	7.35–7.45
Phosphate, inorganic, serum		
Adult	3.0–4.5 mg/dL	1.0–1.5 mmol/L
Child	4.0–7.0 mg/dL	1.3–2.3 mmol/L
Potassium		
Serum	3.5–5.0 mEq/L	3.5–5.0 mmol/L
Plasma	3.5–4.5 mEq/L	3.5–4.5 mmol/L
Progesterone, serum, adult		
Males	0.0–0.4 ng/mL	0.0–1.3 mmol/L
Females		
Follicular phase	0.1–1.5 ng/mL	0.3–4.8 mmol/L
Luteal phase	2.5–28.0 ng/mL	8.0–89.0 mmol/L
Prolactin, serum		
Males	1.0–15.0 ng/mL	1.0–15.0 µg/L
Females	1.0–20.0 ng/mL	1.0–20.0 µg/L
Protein, serum, electrophoresis		
Total	6.0–8.0 gm/dL	60–80 gm/L
Albumin	3.5–5.5 gm/dL	35–55 gm/L
Globulins		
Alpha$_1$	0.2–0.4 gm/dL	2–4 gm/L
Alpha$_2$	0.5–0.9 gm/dL	5–9 gm/L
Beta	0.6–1.1 gm/dL	6–11 gm/L
Gamma	0.7–1.7 gm/dL	7–17 gm/L
Pyruvate, blood	0.3–0.9 gm/dL	0.03–0.10 mmol/L
Rheumatoid factor	0.0–30 IU/mL	0.0–30.0 kIU/L
Sodium, serum or plasma	135–145 mEq/L	135–145 mmol/L
Testosterone, plasma		
Males, adult	300–1200 ng/dL	10.4–41.6 nmol/L
Females, adult	20–75 ng/dL	0.7–2.6 nmol/L
Pregnant females	40–200 ng/dL	1.4–6.9 nmol/L

Reference Values* for Clinical Chemistry (Blood, Serum and Plasma) *Continued*

	Conventional Units	SI Units
Thyroglobulin	3–42 ng/mL	3–42 μg/L
Thyrotropin (hTSH), serum	0.4–4.8 μIU/mL	0.4–4.8 mIU/L
Thyrotropin releasing hormone (TRH)	5–60 pg/mL	5–60 ng/L
Thyroxine, free (FT$_4$), serum	0.9–2.1 ng/dL	12–27 pmol/L
Thyroxine (T$_4$), serum	4.5–12.0 μg/dL	58–154 nmol/L
Thyroxine-binding globulin (TBG)	15.0–34.0 μg/mL	15.0–34.0 mg/L
Transferrin	250–430 mg/dL	2.5–4.3 gm/L
Triglycerides, serum, 12-h fast	40–150 mg/dL	0.4–15.0 gm/L
Triiodothyronine (T$_3$), serum	70–190 ng/dL	1.1–2.9 nmol/L
Triiodothyronine uptake, resin (T$_3$RU)	25–38%	0.25–0.38
Urate		
Males	2.5–8.0 mg/dL	150–480 μmol/L
Females	2.2–7.0 mg/dL	130–420 μmol/L
Urea, serum or plasma	24–49 mg/dL	4.0–8.2 nmol/L
Urea nitrogen, serum or plasma	11–23 mg/dL	8.0–16.4 nmol/L
Viscosity, serum	1.4–1.8 × water	1.4–1.8 × water
Vitamin A, serum	20–80 μg/dL	0.70–2.80 μmol/L
Vitamin B$_{12}$, serum	180–900 pg/mL	133–664 pmol/L

*May vary, depending on the method and sample source used.

Reference Values for Therapeutic Drug Monitoring (Serum)

	Therapeutic Range	Toxic Concentrations	Proprietary Names
Analgesics			
Acetaminophen	10–20 µg/mL	>250 µg/mL	Tylenol
			Datril
Salicylate	100–250 µg/mL	>300 µg/mL	Aspirin
			Ascriptin
			Bufferin
Antibiotics			
Amikacin	25–30 µg/mL	Peak >35 µg/mL	Amikin
		Trough >10 µg/mL	
Chloramphenicol	10–20 µg/mL	>25 µg/mL	Chloromycetin
Gentamicin	5–10 µg/mL	Peak >10 µg/mL	Garamycin
		Trough >2 µg/mL	
Tobramycin	5–10 µg/mL	Peak >10 µg/mL	Nebcin
		Trough >2 µg/mL	
Vancomycin	5–10 µg/mL	Peak >40 µg/mL	Vancocin
		Trough >10 µg/mL	
Anticonvulsants			
Carbamazepine	5–12 µg/mL	>15 µg/mL	Tegretol
Ethosuximide	40–100 µg/mL	>150 µg/mL	Zarontin
Phenobarbital	15–40 µg/mL	40–100 ng/mL (varies widely)	
Phenytoin	10–20 µg/mmL	>20 µg/mL	Dilantin
Primidone	5–12 µg/mL	>15 µg/mL	Mysoline
Valproic acid	50–100 µg/mL	>100 µg/mL	Depakene
Antineoplastics and Immunosuppressives			
Cyclosporin-A	50–400 ng/mL	>400 ng/mL	Sandimmune
Methotrexate (high dose, 48 h)	Variable	>1 µmol/L 48 h after dose	Mexate
			Folex
Bronchodilators and Respiratory Stimulants			
Caffeine	3–15 ng/mL	>30 ng/mL	
Theophylline (Aminophylline)	10–20 µg/mL	>20 µg/mL	Accurbron
			Elixophyllin
			Quibron
			Theobid
Cardiovascular Drugs			
Amiodarone*	1.0–2.0 µg/mL	>2.0 µg/mL	Cordarone
Digitoxin†	15–25 ng/mL	>35 ng/mL	Crystodigin
Digoxin‡	0.8–2.0 ng/mL	>2.4 ng/mL	Lanoxin
Disopyramide	2–5 µg/mL	>7 µg/mL	Norpace
Flecainide	0.2–1.0 ng/mL	>1 ng/mL	Tambocor
Lidocaine	1.5–5.0 µg/mL	>6 µg/mL	Xylocaine
Mexiletine	0.7–2.0 ng/mL	>2 ng/mL	Mexitil
Procainamide	4–10 µg/mL	>12 µg/mL	Pronestyl
Procainamide plus NAPA	8–30 µg/mL	>30 µg/mL	
Propranolol	50–100 ng/mL	Variable	Inderal
Quinidine	2–5 µg/mL	>6 µg/mL	Cardioquin
			Quinaglute
Tocainide	4–10 ng/mL	>10 ng/mL	Tonocard
Psychopharmacologic Drugs			
Amitriptyline	120–150 ng/mL	>500 ng/mL	Amitril
			Elavil
			Triavil
Bupropion	25–100 ng/mL	Not applicable	Wellbutrin
Desiprimine	150–300 ng/mL	>500 ng/mL	Norpramin
			Pertofrane
Imipramine	125–250 ng/mL	>400 ng/mL	Tofranil
Lithium§	0.6–1.5 mEq/L	>1.5 mEq/L	Lithobid
Nortriptyline	50–150 ng/mL	>500 ng/mL	Aventyl
			Pamelor

*Specimen must be obtained >8 h after last dose.
†Specimen must be obtained 12–24 h after last dose.
‡Specimen must be obtained >6 h after last dose.
§Specimen must be obtained 12 h after last dose.

Reference Values* for Clinical Chemistry (Urine)

	Conventional Units	SI Units
Acetone and acetoacetate, qualitative	Negative	Negative
Albumin		
Qualitative	Negative	Negative
Quantitative	10–100 mg/24 h	0.15–1.5 μmol/day
Aldosterone	3–20 μg/24 h	8.3–55 nmol/day
δ-aminolevulinic acid (δ-ALA)	1.3–7.0 mg/24 h	10–53 μmol/day
Amylase	<17 U/h	<17 U/h
Amylase/creatinine clearance ratio	0.01–0.04	0.01–0.04
Bilirubin, qualitative	Negative	Negative
Calcium (regular diet)	<250 mg/24 h	<6.3 nmol/day
Catecholamines		
Epinephrine	<10 μg/24 h	<55 nmol/day
Norepinephrine	<100 μg/24 h	<590 nmol/day
Total free catecholamines	4–126 μg/24 h	24–745 nmol/day
Total metanephrines	0.1–1.6 mg/24 h	0.5–8.1 μmol/day
Chloride (varies with intake)	110–250 mEq/24 h	110–250 mmol/day
Copper	0–50 μg/24 h	0–0.80 μmol/day
Cortisol, free	10–100 μg/24 h	27.6–276 nmol/day
Creatine		
Males	0–40 mg/24 h	0–0.30 mmol/day
Females	0–80 mg/24 h	0–0.60 mmol/day
Creatinine	15–25 mg/kg/24 h	0.13–0.22 mmol/kg/day
Creatinine clearance (endogenous)		
Males	110–150 mL/min/1.73 m^2	110–150 mL/min/1.73 m^2
Females	105–132 mL/min/1.73 m^2	105–132 mL/min/1.73 m^2
Cystine or cysteine	Negative	Negative
Dehydroepiandrosterone		
Males	0.2–2.0 mg/24 h	0.7–6.9 μmol/day
Females	0.2–1.8 mg/24 h	0.7–6.2 μmol/day
Estrogens, total		
Males	4–25 μg/24 h	14–90 nmol/day
Females	5–100 μg/24 h	18–360 nmol/day
Glucose (as reducing substance)	<250 mg/24 h	<250 mg/day
Hemoglobin and myoglobin, qualitative	Negative	Negative
Homogentisic acid, qualitative	Negative	Negative
17-Ketogenic steroids		
Males	5–23 mg/24 h	17–80 μmol/day
Females	3–15 mg/24 h	10–52 μmol/day
17-Hydroxycorticosteroids		
Males	3–9 mg/24 h	8.3–25 μmol/day
Females	2–8 mg/24 h	5.5–22 μmol/day
5-Hydroxyindoleacetic acid		
Qualitative	Negative	Negative
Quantitative	2–6 mg/24 h	10–31 μmol/day
17-Ketosteroids		
Males	8–22 mg/24 h	28–76 μmol/day
Females	6–15 mg/24 h	21–52 μmol/day
Magnesium	6–10 mEq/24 h	3–5 mmol/day
Metaneprhines	0.05–1.2 ng/mg creatinine	0.03–0.70 mmol/mmol creatinine
Osmolality	38–1400 mOsm/kg H$_2$O	38–1400 mOsm/kg H$_2$)
pH	4.6–8.0	4.6–8.0
Phenylpyruvic acid, qualitative	Negative	Negative
Phosphate	0.4–1.3 g/24 h	13–42 mmol/day
Porphobilinogen		
Qualitative	Negative	Negative
Quantitative	<2 mg/24 h	<9 μmol/day
Porphyrins		
Coproporphyrin	50–250 μg/24 h	77–380 nmol/day
Uroporphyrin	10–30 μg/24 h	12–36 nmol/day
Potassium	25–125 mEq/24 h	25–125 mmol/day
Pregnanediol		
Males	0–1.9 mg/24 h	0–6.0 μmol/day
Females		
Proliferative phase	0–2.6 mg/24 h	0–8.0 μmol/day
Luteal phase	2.6–10.6 mg/24 h	8–33 μmol/day
Postmenopausal	0.2–1.0 mg/24 h	0.6–3.1 μmol/day

Reference Values* for Clinical Chemistry (Urine) *Continued*

	Conventional Units	SI Units
Pregnanetriol	0–2.5 mg/24 h	0–7.4 μmol/day
Protein, Total		
Qualitative	Negative	Negative
Quantitative	10–150 mg/24 h	10–150 mg/day
Protein/creatinine ratio	<0.2	<0.2
Sodium (regular diet)	60–260 mEq/24 h	60–260 mmol/day
Specific gravity		
Random specimen	1.003–1.030	1.003–1.030
24-Hour collection	1.015–1.025	1.015–1.025
Urate (regular diet)	250–750 mg/24 h	1.5–4.4 mmol/day
Urobilinogen	0.5–4.0 mg/24 h	0.6–6.8 μmol/day
Vanillylmandelic acid (VMA)	1–8 mg/24 h	5–40 μmol/day

*May vary, depending on the method used.

Reference Values for Toxic Substances

	Conventional Units	SI Units
Arsenic, urine	<130 μg/24 h	<1.7 μmol/d
Bromides, serum, inorganic	<100 mg/dL	<10 mmol/L
Toxic symptoms	140–1000 mg/dL	14–100 mmol/L
Carboxyhemoglobin, blood		
Urban environment	<5% (% saturation)	<0.05 (saturation)
Smokers	<12% (% saturation)	<0.12 (saturation)
Symptoms		
Headache	>15%	>0.15
Nausea and vomiting	>25%	>0.25
Potentially lethal	>50%	>0.50
Ethanol, blood	<0.05 mg/dL (<0.005%)	<1.0 mmol/L
Intoxication	>100 mg/dL (>0.1%)	>22 mmol/L
Marked intoxication	300–400 mg/dL (0.3–0.4%)	65–87 mmol/L
Alcoholic stupor	400–500 mg/dL (0.4–0.5%)	87–109 mmol/L
Coma	>500 mg/dL (>0.5%)	>109 mmol/L
Lead, blood		
Adults	<25 μg/d	<1.2 μmol/L
Children	<15 μg/dL	<0.7 μmol/L
Lead, urine	<80 μg/24 h	<0.4 μmol/d
Mercury, urine	<30 μg/24 h	<150 nmol/d

Reference Values for Cerebrospinal Fluid

	Conventional Units	SI Units
Cells	<5/mm³; all mononuclear	<5 × 10⁶/L, all mononuclear
Electrophoresis	Predominantly albumin	Predominantly albumin
Glucose	50–75 mg/dL (20 mg/dL less than in serum)	2.8–4.2 mmol/L (1.1 mmol less than in serum)
IgG		
Children under 14	<8% of total protein	<0.08 of total protein
Adults	<14% of total protein	<0.14 of total protein
IgG index $\left(\dfrac{\text{CSF/serum IgG ratio}}{\text{CSF/serum albumin ratio}}\right)$	0.3–0.6	0.3–0.6
Oligoclonal banding on electrophoresis	Absent	Absent
Pressure	70–180 mmH₂O	70–180 mmH₂O
Protein, total	15–45 mg/dL	150–450 mg/L

Reference Values for Tests of Gastrointestinal Function

	Conventional Units
Bentiromide test	6-h urinary arylamine excretion greater than 57% rules out pancreatic insufficiency
Beta-carotene, serum	60–260 µg/dL
Fecal fat estimation	
Qualitative	No fat globules seen on high-power microscopy
Quantitative	<6 gm/24 h (>95% coefficient of fat absorption)
Gastric acid output	
Basal	
Males	0–10.5 mmol/h
Females	0–5.6 mmol/h
Maximum (after histamine or pentagastrin)	
Males	9–48 mmol/h
Females	6–31 mmol/h
Ratio: basal:maximum	
Males	0–0.31
Females	0–0.29
Secretin test, pancreatic fluid	
Volume	>1.8 mL/kg/h
Bicarbonate	>80 mEq/L
D-Xylose absorption test, urine	More than 20% of ingested dose excreted in 5 h

Reference Values for Immunologic Procedures

	Conventional Units	SI Units
Complement, Serum		
C3	85–175 mg/dL	0.85—1.75 gm/L
C4	15–45 mg/dL	150–450 mg/L
Total hemolytic (CH$_{50}$)	150–250 U/mL	150–250 U/mL
Immunoglobulins, Serum, Adult		
IgG	640–1350 mg/dL	6.4–13.5 gm/L
IgA	70–310 mg/dL	0.70–3.1 gm/L
IgM	90–350 mg/dL	0.90–3.5 gm/L
IgD	0–6.0 mg/dL	0–60 mg/L
IgE	0–430 ng/dL	0–430 µg/L

Antigen	Cell Type	Percentage	Absolute
Lymphocyte Subsets, Whole Blood, Heparinized			
CD3	Total T cells	56–77%	860–1880
CD19	Total B cells	7–17%	140–370
CD3 and CD4	Helper-inducer cells	32–54%	550–1190
CD3 and CD8	Suppressor-cytotoxic cells	24–37%	430–1060
CD3 and DR	Activated T cells	5–14%	70–310
CD2	E rosette T cells	73–87%	1040–2160
CD16 and CD56	Natural killer (NK) cells	8–22%	130–500

Helper:suppressor ratio: 0.8–1.8.

Reference Values for Semen Analysis

	Conventional Units	SI Units
Volume	2–5 mL	2–5 mL
Liquefaction	Complete in 15 min	Complete in 15 min
pH	7.2–8.0	7.2–8.0
Leukocytes	Occasional or absent	Occasional or absent
Spermatozoa		
Count	60–150 × 10^6/mL	60–150 × 10^6/mL
Motility	>80% motile	>0.80 motile
Morphology	80–90% normal forms	0.80–0.90 normal forms
Fructose	>150 mg/dL	>8.33 mmol/L

NOMOGRAM FOR THE DETERMINATION OF BODY SURFACE AREA OF CHILDREN AND ADULTS

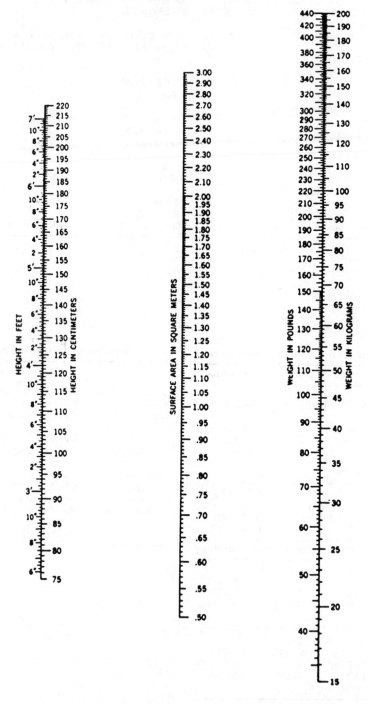

From Boothby WM, Sandiford RB: Boston Med Surg J *185*:337, 1921.

Index

Note: Page numbers followed by (t) refer to tables; page numbers in *italics* refer to illustrations.